*Oxford Textbook of* **Palliative Nursing**

# Oxford Textbook of
# Palliative Nursing

## THIRD EDITION

EDITED BY

### Betty R. Ferrell, RN, PhD, MA, FAAN, FPCN
*Research Scientist*
*Department of Nursing Research and Education*
*City of Hope National Medical Center*
*Duarte, California*

### Nessa Coyle, PhD, APRN, FAAN
*Pain and Palliative Care Service*
*Department of Medicine*
*Memorial Sloan-Kettering Cancer Center*
*New York, New York*

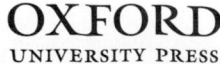
OXFORD
UNIVERSITY PRESS

2010

# OXFORD
## UNIVERSITY PRESS

Oxford University Press, Inc., publishes works that further
Oxford University's objective of excellence
in research, scholarship, and education.

Oxford  New York
Auckland  Cape Town  Dar es Salaam  Hong Kong  Karachi
Kuala Lumpur  Madrid  Melbourne  Mexico City  Nairobi
New Delhi  Shanghai  Taipei  Toronto

With offices in
Argentina  Austria  Brazil  Chile  Czech Republic  France  Greece
Guatemala  Hungary  Italy  Japan  Poland  Portugal  Singapore
South Korea  Switzerland  Thailand  Turkey  Ukraine  Vietnam

Published by Oxford University Press, Inc.
198 Madison Avenue, New York, New York 10016
www.oup.com

**Library of Congress Cataloging-in-Publication Data**
Oxford textbook of palliative nursing / edited by
Betty R. Ferrell, Nessa Coyle. —3rd ed.
    p. ; cm.
Rev. ed. of: Textbook of palliative nursing. 2nd ed. 2006.
Includes bibliographical references and index.
ISBN 978-0-19-539134-3
1. Palliative treatment.   2. Nursing.   3. Terminal care.
I. Ferrell, Betty.   II. Coyle, Nessa.   III. Textbook of palliative nursing.
IV. Title: Textbook of palliative nursing.
[DNLM: 1. Nursing Care.   2. Palliative Care.   3. Terminal Care. WY 152 O98 2010]
RT87.T45T49 2010
616′.029—dc22        2009029410

9  8  7
Printed in the United States of America
on acid-free paper

# FOREWORDS TO THE FIRST EDITION

Dame Cicely Saunders, OM, DBE, FRCP
*Chair*
*St. Christopher's Hospice*
*Syndenham, London*
*United Kingdom*

Palliative care stems from the recognition of the potential at the end of life for discovering and for giving, a recognition that an important dimension of being human is the lasting dignity and growth that can continue through weakness and loss. No member of the interdisciplinary team is more central to making these discoveries possible than the nurse. Realizing how little had been written and even less studied in this field, Peggy Nuttall, a former nursing colleague and then editor of the *Nursing Times* in London, invited me to contribute a series of six articles on the care of the dying in the summer of 1959.[1] A registered nurse and qualified medical social worker, I had trained in medicine because of a compulsion to do something about the pain I had seen in patients and their families at the end of life. During 3 years as a volunteer nurse in an early home for such patients, I had persuaded the thoracic surgeon, Norman Barrett, for whom I was working, to follow up a few of his mortally ill patients both there and in their homes. "Go and read medicine," he said. "It's the doctors who desert the dying, and there's so much more to be learned about pain. You'll only be frustrated if you don't do it properly, and they won't listen to you." He was right and I obeyed. After 7 years' work, the first descriptive study of 1,100 patients in St. Joseph's Hospice, London, from 1958 to 1965[2] was coupled with visits to clinical pain researchers such as Harry Beecher in Boston and many U.S. homes, social workers, and nurses in 1963. This visit included an all-important meeting with Florence Wald at Yale. A prodigious program of fundraising letters, professional articles, and meetings led to the opening of St. Christopher's Hospice in 1967, the first inpatient, home care, research, and teaching hospice. All of those early contacts and countless other interested people led to the hospice movement and the palliative care that developed within and from it.

Nurses were the first to respond to this challenge and remain the core of the personal and professional drive to enable people to find relief, support, and meaning at the end of their lives. All of the expertise described in this important collection is to this end. The window to suffering can be a window to peace and opportunity. The nurse, in her or his skilled competence and compassion, has a unique place to give each person the essential message: "You matter because you are you, and you matter to the last moment of your life. We will do all we can to help you, not only to die peacefully but to live until you die."[3]

*Dame Cicely Saunders died in July 2005. The editors and all nurses in hospice and palliative care are grateful for her life contributions.*

## REFERENCES

1. Saunders CM. Care of the dying. Nursing Times reprint. London: Macmillan, 1976.
2. Clark D. "Total pain," disciplinary power and the body in the work of Cicely Saunders, 1958–67. Soc Sci Med 1999; 49:727–736.
3. Saunders C. Care of the dying. 1. The problem of euthanasia. Nurs Times 1976;72:1003–1005.

## Florence Wald, RN, FAAN
*Branford, Connecticut*

Nurses of my generation in the second half of the twentieth century were fortunate to be part of the hospice movement and to respond to an eager public with an alternative way of care for the dying. Medical sociologists' studies of hospital culture showed what many nurses already knew, that when technological intervention failed to stop the course of disease, physicians could not see that the treatment was futile or join the patient in a willingness to cease.

By 1950, nurses began to carry out studies as principal investigators and were on their way to being respected by other disciplines. Two outstanding leaders were Hilde Peplau and Virginia Henderson, both educated nurses in clinical practice who established a foundation for the advanced nurse practitioner to be a valued member of an interdisciplinary team.

This surfaced first in psychiatric nursing, but as hospice care came into being, the nurse became a pivotal part of the interdisciplinary team. "Hospice nursing," Virginia Henderson said, "was the essence of nursing"; volunteers came quickly into hospice care, proving Henderson's precept and giving the lay individual "the necessary strength, will, and knowledge to contribute to a peaceful death."[1]

Physicians in the forefront of medical ethics, such as Edmund Pellegrino and Raymond Duff, encouraged physicians to recast their roles as decision makers and communicators so that the whole team could keep the patients' values and the families' wants the prime concern.

The works of those who have brought alternative therapies into use, for example, Martha Rogers and Barbara Dossey, have added to the spiritual dimensions of care. The growth of the religious ministry movement and the creative addition of the arts and environment round out the cast of contributors.

Reviewing the progress we nurses have made allows us to proceed more effectively.

*Florence Wald died in November 2008 at her home in Bradford, Connecticut at the age of 91. The editors and all nurses in hospice and palliative care are grateful for her life contributions.*

### REFERENCE

1. Henderson V. Basic Principles of Nursing Care. London: International Council of Nurses, 1961:42.

## Jeanne Quint Benoliel, DNSc, FAAN

*Professor Emeritus*
*Psychosocial and Community Health School of Nursing*
*University of Washington*
*Seattle, Washington*

At the end of the Second World War in 1945, people in Western societies were tired of death, pain, and suffering. Cultural goals shifted away from war-centered activities to a focus on progress, use of technology for better living, and improvements in the health and well-being of the public. Guided by new scientific knowledge and new technologies, health care services became diversified and specialized and lifesaving at all costs became a powerful driving force. End-of-life care was limited to postmortem rituals, and the actual caregiving of dying patients was left to nursing staff. Palliative nursing in those days depended on the good will and personal skills of individual nurses, yet what they offered was invisible, unrecognized, and unrewarded.

Thanks to the efforts of many people across the years, end-of-life care is acknowledged today as an important component of integrated health care services. Much knowledge has accrued about what makes for good palliative care, and nurses have been in the forefront of efforts to improve quality of life for patients and families throughout the experience of illness. This book is an acknowledgment of the important part played by nurses in helping patients to complete their lives in a context of care and human concern.

# PREFACE

## Compassion and Competence

Betty R. Ferrell, RN, PhD, MA, FAAN, FPCN
*Research Scientist*
*Department of Nursing Research and Education*
*City of Hope National Medical Center*

Nessa Coyle, PhD, APRN, FAAN
*Pain and Palliative Care Service*
*Department of Medicine*
*Memorial Sloan-Kettering Cancer Center*

This third edition of the Textbook comes at a time when palliative nursing has truly come of age. The lessons of hospice nursing paved the way to the broad field of palliative care nursing and, in doing so, care of the seriously ill has expanded across diagnosis and settings of care. We dedicated our second edition, released in 2006, "For Every Nurse—A Palliative Care Nurse," in recognition that nurses across settings and specialties were providing care that exemplifies palliative care principles.

This edition bears a new name *Oxford Textbook of Palliative Nursing.* This official designation by Oxford University Press recognizes that this book is a leading resource for the field. We are greatly indebted to our contributing authors, whose quality chapters have made this textbook a success. As this textbook has matured, so has our profession, and raising the bar has meant better care for patients and families.

Many years ago, Dame Cicely Saunders said that our patients need both our compassion and our competence. Patients and their families need compassionate care to address their suffering, grief, despair, and loneliness. Compassionate care, as described in these pages, includes spiritual care and attention to depression: it recognizes hope in the face of illness and leads patients and families to moments of joy amidst sorrow. Competent care insures optimum relief of pain, wound care, relief of terrifying dyspnea, and artful skill in approaching ethical issues, complex cultural considerations, and intense family dynamics. Palliative care nursing, which is both compassionate and competent, is as Florence Nightingale described, "an art and a science."

It is our hope that this third edition continues to strengthen nurses, individually and collectively, and that as a profession we continue to grow into the fullness of what Cicely Saunders and Florence Nightingale envisioned: compassionate and competent nurses practicing the art and science of palliative nursing.

## About the Forewords

On the previous pages, readers will find three Forewords, written for the first edition by three pioneers in the field of palliative nursing: Dame Cicely Saunders (deceased), founder of the modern hospice movement; Florence Wald (deceased), founder of the first hospice in America; and Jeanne Quint Benoliel, pioneer in psychosocial nursing and the role of nursing in caring for the terminally ill. We have reprinted the forewords from these pioneers in this edition because we believe that their legacy is an enduring contribution to all that has come to be known as palliative nursing care. We are indebted to these women and to the many other nurses who have brought the field of palliative care to the forefront, and whose dedication will provide a foundation for us in the future.

## Acknowledgments

The editors acknowledge the assistance of Licet Garcia and Andrea Hayward, who served as our research assistants throughout the process of this third edition.

# CONTENTS

# CONTRIBUTORS

**Paula R. Anderson, RN, MN, OCN**
Oncology Research Initiatives
University of Texas Southwestern Medical Center
Moncrief Cancer Center
Fort Worth, Texas

**Abby Baguma, BA**
Partnerships Manager
African Palliative Care Association
Kampala, Uganda, Africa

**Rev. Pamela Baird, AS**
End-of-Life Practitioner
Seasons of Life
Arcadia, California

**Marie Bakitas, APRN, DNSc, ACHPN, AOCN, FAAN**
Assistant Professor, Clinical Researcher
Dartmouth Medical School
Nurse Practitioner
Department of Anesthesiology, Section of Palliative
  Medicine
Dartmouth Hitchcock Medical Center
Lebanon, New Hampshire

**Barbara M. Bates-Jensen, PhD, RN, CWOCN**
Associate Professor
UCLA School of Nursing & David Geffen School
  of Medicine, Geriatrics
Los Angeles, California

**Susan Berenson, RN, MSN, OCN**
Clinical Nurse Specialist
Department of Integrative Medicine
Memorial Sloan-Kettering Cancer Center
New York, New York

**Patricia Berry, PhD, APRN, ACHPN, FAAN**
Associate Professor
University of Utah Hartford Center of Geriatric Nursing
    Excellence
College of Nursing
Salt Lake City, Utah

**Margaret Firer Bishop, MS, ARNP**
Adult Nurse Practitioner
Department of Anesthesiology, Section of Palliative
    Medicine
Dartmouth Hitchcock Medical Center
Lebanon, New Hampshire

**Barton T. Bobb, MSN, FNP-BC, ACHPN**
Palliative Care & Pain Consult Team NP
Virginia Commonwealth University Massey Cancer Center
Thomas Palliative Care Program
Richmond, Virginia

**Marilyn Bookbinder, RN, PhD**
Director of Nursing and Quality
Department of Pain Medicine and Palliative Care
Beth Israel Medical Center
New York, New York

**Tami Borneman, MSN, RN, PHN, CNS, FPCN**
Senior Research Specialist
Division of Nursing Research and Education
City of Hope National Medical Center
Duarte, California

**Laura Bourdeanu, MS, PhD**
Nurse Practitioner
Nursing Support, Medical Oncology
City of Hope National Medical Center
Duarte, California

**Marina Boykova, MSc, RN**
Doctoral Student
University of Oklahoma
Oklahoma City, Oklahoma

**Katherine Brown-Saltzman, RN, MA**
Executive Director
University of California, Los Angeles, Ethics Center
Assistant Clinical Professor
University of California, Los Angeles, Medical Center
University of California, Los Angeles, School of Nursing
Los Angeles, California

**Margaret L. Campbell, RN, PhD, FAAN**
Director, Nursing Research
Detroit Receiving Hospital
Assistant Professor—Research
Wayne State University, College of Nursing
Detroit, Michigan

**Paula A. Caron, MS, ARNP, AOCNP, ACHPN**
Adult Nurse Practioner
Department of Anesthesiology, Section of Palliative
    Medicine
Dartmouth Hithcock Medical Center
Lebanon, New Hampshire

**Garrett K. Chan, APRN, PhD, ACHPN, CEN, FAEN**
Lead Advanced Practice Nurse and Associate Medical
    Director
Emergency Department Observation Unit
Stanford Hospital & Clinics
Stanford, California
Assistant Clinical Professor
University of California San Francisco
Department of Physiological Nursing
San Francisco, California

**Nathan I. Cherny, MBBS, FRACP, FRCP**
Director
Cancer Pain and Palliative Medicine
Shaare Zedek Medical Center
Jerusalem, Israel

**Douglas Cluxton, MA, LPC**
Vice President, Education
Ohio Hospice and Palliative Care Organization
Columbus, Ohio

**Audrey Kurash Cohen, MS, CCC-SLP**
Clinical Specialist
Department of Speech, Language and Swallowing Disorders
Massachusetts General Hospital
Boston, Massachusetts

**Peggy Compton, RN, PhD**
Associate Professor
University of California, Los Angeles, School of Nursing
Los Angeles, California

**Inge B. Corless, RN, PhD, FAAN**
Professor
MGH Institute of Health Professions School of Nursing
Boston, Massachusetts

**Valerie T. Cotter, DrNP(c), CRNP, FAANP**
Advanced Senior Lecturer
Director, Adult Health Nurse Practitioner Program
University of Pennsylvania School of Nursing
Philadephia, Pennsylvania

**Nessa Coyle, PhD, APRN, FAAN (Editor)**
Pain and Palliative Care Service
Memorial Sloan-Kettering Cancer Center
New York, New York

**Patrick J. Coyne, MSN, APRN, ACHPN, FAAN, FPCN**
Clinical Director
Thomas Palliative Care Services
Virginia Commonwealth University /Massey Cancer Center
Richmond, Virginia

**Constance M. Dahlin, ANP, BC, ACHPN, FPCN**
Clinical Director
Palliative Care Service
Massachusetts General Hospital
Boston, Massachusetts

**Barbara J. Daly, PhD, RN, FAAN**
Professor
Case Western Reserve University
Director
Clinical Ethics
University Hospitals Case Medical Center
Cleveland, Ohio

**Betty Davies, RN, PhD, FAAN**
Professor Emerita
Department of Family Health Care Nursing
School of Nursing
University of California, San Francisco
San Francisco, California
Professor and Senior Scholar
School of Nursing
University of Victoria
Victoria, British Columbia, Canada

**Henry Ddungu, MBChB, MMed**
Advocacy Manager
African Palliative Care Association
Kampala, Uganda, Africa

**Grace E. Dean, PhD, RN**
Assistant Professor of Nursing
University at Buffalo
Adjunct Assistant Professor of Oncology
Roswell Park Cancer Institute
Buffalo, New York

**Susan Derby, RN, MA, GNP-BC**
Nurse Practitioner
Pain and Palliative Care Service
Memorial Sloan-Kettering Cancer Center
New York, New York

**Julia Downing, MMedSci, BN(Hons) Dip CN RGN, PhD**
Deputy Executive Director
African Palliative Care Association
Kampala, Uganda, Africa

**Deborah Dudgeon, MD, FRCPC**
W. Ford Connell Professor of Palliative
    Care Medicine
Queen's University
Kingston, Ontario, Canada

**Anna R. Du Pen, RN, MN, ARNP**
Adult Nurse Practitioner
Kitsap Medical Group
Bremerton, Washington

**Denice Caraccia Economou, RN, MN, AOCN**
Senior Research Specialist
City of Hope
Division of Nursing Research and
    Education
Duarte, California

**Kathleen A. Egan City, MA, BSN, CHPN**
Executive Director
Suncoast Hospice
Clearwater, Florida
Executive Committee
The Center for Hospice, Palliative Care and End-of-Life
    Studies
University of South Florida
Tampa, Florida

**Nancy English, PhD, APRN**
Assitant Professor
University of Colorado
College of Nursing
Aurora, Colorado

**Elizabeth Ercolano, DNSc, RN, AOCNS**
Associate Research Scientist
Yale University School of Public Health
New Haven, Connecticut

**Mary Ersek, PhD, RN, FAAN**
Associate Professor
University of Pennsylvania
School of Nursing
Philadelphia, Pennsylvania

**Laura A. Espinosa, RN, MS, CS**
Administrative Director of Heart and
    Vascular Services
Memorial Hermann Hospital
Houston, Texas

**Betty R. Ferrell, RN, PhD, MA, FAAN, FPCN (Editor)**
Research Scientist
Division of Nursing Research and Education
City of Hope National Medical Center
Duarte, California

**Iris Cohen Fineberg, PhD, MSW**
Lecturer
International Observatory on End of Life Care
Division of Health Research
School of Health and Medicine
Lancaster University
Lancaster, United Kingdom

**Regina M. Fink, RN, PhD, FAAN, AOCN**
Research Nurse Scientist
University of Colorado Hospital
Aurora, Colorado

**Mei R. Fu, PhD, RN, APRN-BC**
Assistant Professor
Course Coordinator
Fundamentals of Nursing
College of Nursing
New York University
New York, New York

**Wayne L. Furman, MD**
Member
Department of Hematology-Oncology
St. Jude's Children's Research Hospital
Memphis, Tennessee

**Michelle Schaffner Gabriel, RN, MS, ACHPN**
Palliative Care Coordinator
Department of Veterans Affairs
VA Sierra Pacific Network
Palo Alto, California

**Rose A. Gates, RN, PhD, NP, AOCN**
Oncology Nurse Practitioner
Rocky Mountain Cancer Center
Colorado Springs, Colorado

**Elaine Glass, RN, MS, ACHPN**
Clinical Nurse Specialist
Palliative Care at Grant Medical Center
Columbus, Ohio

**Tessa Goldsmith, MA, CCC/SLP, BRS-S**
Assistant Director
Department of Speech, Language and Swallowing
    Disorders
Massachusetts General Hospital
Boston, Massachusetts

**Mary Layman Goldstein, RN, MS, APRN, BC**
Nurse Practitioner
Pain and Palliative Service
Memorial Sloan-Kettering Cancer Center
New York, New York

**Linda M. Gorman, RN, MN, CNS-BC, CHPN, OCN**
Clinical Nurse Specialist
Palliative Care
Cedars-Sinai
Los Angeles, California

**Marcia Grant, DNSc, RN, FAAN**
Research Scientist and Director
Division of Nursing Research and Education
City of Hope National Medical Center
Duarte, California

**Mikel Gray, PhD, FNP, PNP, CUNP, CCCN, FAAN**
Professor and Nurse Practitioner
Department of Urology and School of Nursing
University of Virginia
Charlottesville, Virginia

**Julie Griffie, RN, MSN, ACNS-BC, AOCN**
Clinical Nurse Specialist
Froedtert Hospital
Milwaukee, Wisconsin

**Penny Hansford, RN, RM, HV, MSc**
Director of Nursing
St. Christophers's Hospice
London, England

**Debra E. Heidrich, MSN, RN, CHPN, AOCN**
Palliative Care Clinical Nurse Specialist
Bethesda North Hospital, TriHealth, Inc.
Cincinnati, Ohio

**Marjorie J. Hein, MS**
Nurse Practitioner
Nursing Support, Medical Oncology
City of Hope National Medical Center
Duarte, California

**Melody Brown Hellsten, RN, MS, PNP-BC**
Pediatric Nurse Practitioner
University of Texas Health Science Center,
    San Antonio
Program Coordinator
Pediatric Palliative and Supportive Care
CHRISTUS Santa Rosa Children's Hospital
San Antonio, Texas

**Pamela S. Hinds, PhD, RN, FAAN**
Director of Nursing Research
Children's National Medical Center
Professor of Pediatrics
George Washington University
Washington, DC

**Jay R. Horton, ACHPN, FNP-BC, MPH**
Clinical Program Coordinator
The Lilian and Benjamin Hertzberg Palliative
    Care Institute
The Brookdale Department of Geriatrics and Palliative
    Medicine
Mount Sinai School of Medicine
New York, New York

**Nancy G. Houlihan, RN, MA, AOCN**
Clinical Program Manager, Survivorship Program
Memorial Sloan-Kettering Cancer Center
New York, New York

**Peter L. Hudson, RN, PhD**
Director and Associate Professor
Centre for Palliative Care Education & Research
St. Vincent's Hospital and The University of
    Melbourne
Fitzroy, Victoria, Australia

Jayne Huggard, NZRN, Dip Couns., Dip AdTertEd,
  MHSc (Hons) MNZAC
Staff and Family Support, Mercy Hospice Auckland
Senior Tutor, School of Nursing
Faculty of Medical and Health Sciences
University of Auckland
Auckland, New Zealand

Anne Hughes, RN, PhD, ACHPN, FAAN
Advance Practice Nurse, Palliative Care
Laguna Honda Hospital & Rehabilitation Center/SFDPH
San Francisco, California

Dennie Hycha, RN, MN
Program Director
Regional Palliative Care Program
Alberta Health Services, Capital Health
Grey Nuns Community Hospital
Edmonton, Alberta, Canada

Rose Anne Indelicato, RN, MSN, ANP-BC, ACHPN, OCN
Nurse Practitioner, Palliative Care
Sound Shore Medical Center of Westchester
New Rochelle, New York
Instructor of Medicine
New York Medical College
Valhalla, New York

Marianne Jensen Hjermstad, RN, MPH, PhD
Associate Professor
Pain and Palliation Research Group
Department of Cancer Research and Molecular Medicine
Faculty of Medicine
Norwegian University of Science and Technology (NTNU)
Trondheim, Norway
Senior Researcher
The Cancer Center
Oslo University Hospital HF, Ulleval
Oslo, Norway

Juhye Jin, RN, MS, PhD
PhD Graduate
Department of Family Health Care Nursing
School of Nursing
University of California, San Francisco
San Francisco, California

Barbara Jones, MSW, PhD
Assistant Professor
Co-Director, The Institute for Grief, Loss, and
  Family Survival
The University of Texas at Austin
Austin, Texas

Gloria Juarez, RN, PhD
Assistant Professor
Division of Nursing Research and Education
City of Hope National Medical Center
Duarte, California

Marta H. Junin, RN
Palliative Care Service
Bonorino Udaondo Hospital
Palliative Care Nurse Educator
University of Buenos Aires
Buenos Aires, Argentina

Stein Kaasa, MD, PhD
Professor
Pain and Palliation Research Group
Department of Cancer Research and Molecular Medicine
Faculty of Medicine
The Norwegian University of Science and Technology
  and The Palliative Medicine Unit
St. Olavs Hospital
Trondheim, Norway

Peggy Kalowes, RN, PhD, CNS
Director, Center for Women's Cardiac Health
  and Research
Memorial Heart and Vascular Institute
Long Beach Memorial Medical Center
Long Beach, California

Pamela Kedziera, RN, MSN, AOCN
Clinical Nurse Specialist
Pain Management Center
Fox Chase Cancer Center
Philadelphia, Pennsylvania

Charles Kemp, FNP, FAAN
Senior Lecturer
Baylor University
Dallas, Texas

Carole Kenner, DNS, RNC-NIC, FAAN
Dean/Professor
School of Nursing
Northeastern University
Boston, Massachusetts

Boon Han Kim, RN, PhD
Professor
Department of Nursing, Hanyang University
President
Korean Hospice Palliative Nurses Association
Seoul, South Korea

Hyun Sook Kim, PhD, RN
Associate Professor
Department of Elderly Health & Welfare, Chungju National
  University
Director
Research Institute of Health, Welfare & Education, Chungju
  National University
Chungju, South Korea

**Cynthia King, PhD, NP, MSN, CNL, FAAN**
Professor and Nurse Scientist
Presbyterian School of Nursing
Queens University of Charlotte
Owner and Consultant
Special Care Consultants
Charlotte, North Carolina

**Kenneth L. Kirsh, PhD**
Assistant Professor
Assistant Director for Research
Symptom Management and Palliative Care Program
Division of Hematology/Oncology
Department of Internal Medicine
Markey Cancer Center
University of Kentucky
Lexington, Kentucky

**Carl A. Kirton, DNP, RN, ANP-BC, ACRN**
Nurse Practitioner and Clinical Manager
The AIDS Center
Mount Sinai Hospital and Medical Center
New York, New York

**Fatia Kiyange, BA, MA**
Education and Standards Manager
African Palliative Care Association
Kampala, Uganda, Africa

**Patti Knight, RN, MSN, CS, CHPN**
Palliative Care Unit Patient Manager
Department of Palliative Care and
   Rehabilitation Medicine
University of Texas MD Anderson Cancer Center
Houston, Texas

**Kate Kravits, RN, MA, LPC, ATR-BC, HNB-BC**
Senior Research Specialist
Division of Nursing Research
Department of Population Sciences
City of Hope National Medical Center
Duarte, California

**Mary J. Labyak, MSW, LCSW**
President and Chief Executive Officer
Suncoast Hospice
Clearwater, Florida

**Philip J. Larkin, RN, RSCN, RHV, RNT, BSc(Hons),**
   **MSc, PhD**
Associate Professor
Clinical Nursing [Palliative Care]
School of Nursing, Midwifery & Health Systems
University College Dublin
Belfield, Dublin, Ireland

**Marcia Levetown, MD, FAAP**
HealthCare Communication Associates
Houston, Texas

**Rana Limbo, PhD, RN, PMHCNS-BC**
Director of Bereavement and Advance Care Planning
   Services
Faculty Associate, University of Wisconsin—Madison
   School of Nursing
Gundersen Lutheran Medical Foundation, Inc.
La Crosse, Wisconsin

**Laurel J. Lyckholm, MD**
Professor and Fellowship Program Director
Hematology/Oncology and Palliative Care Medicine
The Massey Cancer Center
Virginia Commonwealth University School of Medicine
Richmond, Virginia

**Pam Malloy, MN, RN, OCN, FPCN**
Project Director
ELNEC Project
American Association of Colleges of Nursing
Washington, DC

**Marianne Matzo, PhD, GNP-BC, FPCN, FAAN**
Professor and Frances E. and A. Earl Ziegler Chair
   in Palliative Care Nursing
Sooner Palliative Care Institute
University of Oklahoma
College of Nursing
Adjunct Professor, Department of Geriatric Medicine
Oklahoma City, Oklahoma

**Terri L. Maxwell, PhD, APRN, ACHPN**
Vice President of Clinical Initiatives
Hospice Pharmacia, A Division of excelleRx, Inc.,
Philadelphia, Pennsylvania

**Polly Mazanec, PhD, ACNP-BC, AOCN**
Assistant Professor
Frances Payne Bolton School of Nursing
Case Western Reserve University
& CNS, Ireland Cancer Center, University
   Hospitals Case Medical Center
Cleveland, Ohio

**Jennifer McAdam, PhD, RN**
Assistant Professor
Dominican University of California
Department of Nursing
San Rafael, California

**Mary S. McCabe, RN, BA, MA**
Director
Survivorship Program
Memorial Sloan-Kettering Cancer Center
New York, New York

**Ruth McCorkle, PhD, FAAN**
Florence S. Wald Professor of Nursing and Director
Center for Excellence in Chronic Illness Care
Yale University School of Nursing
New Haven, Connecticut

**Glen Medellin, MD, FAAP**
Assistant Professor, Division of General Pediatrics
Interim Greehey Distinguished Chair in Palliative Care for
    Children
Clerkship Director, Department of Pediatrics
University of Texas Health Science Center, San Antonio
San Antonio, Texas

**Kathleen Michael, PhD, RN, CRRN**
Assistant Professor
University of Maryland
Baltimore, Maryland

**Paula Milone-Nuzzo, PhD, RN, FAAN, FHHC**
Dean and Professor
School of Nursing
The Pennsylvania State University
University Park, Pennsylvania

**Pamela A. Minarik, MS, APRN, BC, FAAN**
Professor of Nursing
Professor, Office of International Affairs
Yale University School of Nursing
Psychiatric Consultation Liaison Clinical Nurse
    Specialist
Yale-New Haven Hospital
New Haven, Connecticut

**Betty D. Morgan, PhD, PMHCNS, BC**
Associate Professor, Department of Nursing
School of Health and Environment
University of Massachusetts Lowell
Lowell, Massachusetts

**Faith N. Mwangi-Powell, Msc(Econ), PhD**
Executive Director
African Palliative Care Association
Kampala, Uganda, Africa

**Leslie Nield-Anderson, APRN, BC, PhD**
Private Practice
Geropsychiatric Consultant
Sunhill Medical Center
Sun City Center, Florida

**Linda L. Oakes, MSN, RN, CCNS**
Pain Clinical Nurse Specialist
St. Jude's Children's Research Hospital
Memphis, Tennessee

**Margaret O'Connor, RN, DN, MN, B.Theol**
President, Palliative Care Australia
Vivian Bullwinkel Chair in Palliative Care
    Nursing
Palliative Care Research Team, Monash
    University
Frankston, Victoria, Australia

**Sean O'Mahony, MBBCh, BAO**
Medical Director
Palliative Care Service
Montefiore Medical Center
Assistant Professor
Albert Einstein College of Medicine
Bronx, New York

**Shirley Otis-Green, MSW, LCSW, ACSW, OSW-C**
Senior Research Specialist
Division of Nursing Research and Education
City of Hope National Medical Center
Duarte, California

**Judith A. Paice, PhD, RN, FAAN**
Director, Cancer Pain Program
Division of Hematology-Oncology
Northwestern University
Feinberg School of Medicine
Chicago, Illinois

**Joan T. Panke, APRN, ACHPN**
Palliative Care Nurse Practioner
Nurse Educator
Capital Hospice
Washington, DC

**Jeannie V. Pasacreta, PhD, APRN**
Director
Integrated Mental Health Services LLC
Newtown, Connecticut

**Steven D. Passik, PhD**
Associate Attending Psychologist
Memorial Sloan-Kettering Cancer Center
New York, New York

**Melany A. Piech**
Research Assistant
State University of New York at Buffalo
Holland, New York

**Richard A. Powell, BA, MA, MSc**
Monitoring, Evaluation and Research Manager
African Palliative Care Association
Kampala, Uganda, Africa

**Maryjo Prince-Paul, PhD, APRN, ACHPN**
Assistant Professor
Frances Payne Bolton School of Nursing
Case Western Reserve University
Research Associate
Hospice of the Western Reserve
Cleveland, Ohio

**Kathleen Puntillo, RN, CNS, DNSc, FAAN**
Professor of Nursing and Research Scientist
Department of Physiological Nursing
University of California, San Francisco
San Francisco, California

Patrice Rancour, MS, RN, PMHCNS-BC
Prospective Health Care Program Manager
The Ohio State University Faculty/Staff Wellness Program
Columbus, Ohio

Jeanne Robison, RN, MN, ARNP
Oncology Nurse Practitioner
Rockwood Cancer Treatment Center
Spokane, Washington

Ora Rosengarten, MD
Oncologist, Palliative Care Physician
Department of Medical Oncology
Shaare Zedek Medical Center
Jerusalem, Israel

Mayuko Sakae, MD
Pediatrician
University of Florida Pediatric Residency Programs
Jacksonville, Florida

Colleen Scanlon, RN, JD
Senior Vice President, Advocacy
Catholic Health Initiatives
Denver, Colorado

Susie Seaman, MSN, NP, CWOCN
Nurse Practitioner
Sharp Rees-Stealy Medical Group Wound Clinic
San Diego, California

Denice K. Sheehan, PhD, RN
Assistant Professor
College of Nursing
Kent State University
Kent, Ohio

Deborah Witt Sherman, PhD, APRN, ANP, BC, ACHPN, FAAN
Professor and Assistant Dean for Research
Co-Director of the Center for Excellence in Palliative
    Care Research
Senior Faculty for Palliative Care and Center for  Excellence
Baltimore, Maryland

Terran Sims, RN, MSN, ACNP
Nurse Practitioner
Department of Urology
Univeristy of Virginia
Charlottesville, Virginia

Jean K. Smith, RN, MS, OCN
Lymphedema Clinical Nurse Specialist
Centura Health Penrose Cancer Center
Colorado Springs, Colorado

Thomas J. Smith, MD, FACP
Massey Endowed Professor for Palliative Care
    Research
Medical Director, Thomas Palliative Care Unit
Richmond, Virginia

Rose Steele, RN, PhD
Professor
School of Nursing
Faculty of Health, York University
Toronto, Ontario, Canada

Lizabeth H. Sumner, RN, BSN
Director
The Center for Compassionate Care
The Elizabeth Hospice
Escondido, California

Virginia Sun, PhD(c), RN
Senior Research Specialist
Division of Nursing Research and Education
City of Hope National Medical Center
Duarte, California

Sayaka Takenouchi, RN, BSN, MPH
PhD Student
Kyoto University Graduate School of Medicine
Department of Biomedical Ethics
Osaka, Japan

Keiko Tamura, RN, PhD, OCNS
Nurse Manager/Certified Nurse Specialist in Cancer Nursing
Yodogawa Christian Hospital
Osaka, Japan

Dana Tarcatu, MD
Temporary Physician
Pain and Palliative Care Service
City of Hope National Medical Center
Duarte, California

Elizabeth Johnston Taylor, PhD, RN
Associate Professor
School of Nursing
Loma Linda University
Loma Linda, California
Mary Potter Hospice
Wellington, Aotearoa New Zealand

Roma Tickoo, MD, MPH
Pain and Palliative Care Physician
Pain & Palliative Care Service
Memorial Sloan-Kettering Cancer Center
New York, New York

Pamela R. Tryon, MS
Nurse Practitioner
Nursing Support, Medical Oncology
City of Hope National Medical Center
Duarte, California

Mary L. S. Vachon, RN, PhD
Psychotherapist and Consultant in Private Practice
Professor
Department of Psychiatry and Dalla Lana
    School of Public Health
University of Toronto
Toronto, Ontario, Canada

**Rose Virani, RNC, MHA, OCN, FPCN**
Senior Research Specialist
Nursing Research and Education
City of Hope National Medical Center
Duarte, California

**Deborah L. Volker, PhD, RN, AOCN**
Associate Professor
The University of Texas at Austin
School of Nursing
Austin, Texas

**Lynn Whitten, BN, MSA, CHPCN(c)**
Manager
Palliative and Hospice Care Service
Alberta Health Services, Calgary Health Region
Calgary, Alberta, Canada

**Dorothy Wholihan, MSN, ANP-BC, AHPCN**
Program Coordinator
Adult Primary Care/Palliative Care Nurse Practitioner
    Program
New York University College of Nursing
New York, New York

**Donna J. Wilson, RN, CNS**
Clinical Nurse Specialist/Fitness Coordinator
Department of Integrative Medicine
Memorial Sloan-Kettering Cancer Center
New York, New York

**Sarah A. Wilson, PhD, RN**
Associate Professor
Director, Institute for End-of-Life Education
Marquette University College of Nursing
Milwaukee, Wisconsin

**Robert Zalenski, MD, MA**
Professor of Emergency Medicine
Wayne State University School of Medicine
Director of Research
Maggie Allesee Center for Quality of Life
Hospice of Michigan
Detroit, Michigan

# I
# General Principles

# 1

*Nessa Coyle*

# Introduction to Palliative Nursing Care

*My life's work is done but I am not able to die. How can the day-to-day time I have left be given a sense of meaning? The hardest thing is living without a goal, a new way of being—just being. That's the hardest thing. I know that I'm going to die at some point but I don't want it to be a painful and undignified death. This is the most important time in my life and yet I feel disconnected from it. It's hard to talk to my family about how I feel—they don't understand.*
*—Palliative care patient*

♦ **Key Points**
♦ *Palliative nursing reflects "whole person" care.*
♦ *Palliative nursing combines a scientific approach with a humanistic approach to care.*
♦ *The caring process is facilitated through a combination of science, presence, openness, compassion, mindful attention to detail, and teamwork.*
♦ *The patient and family are the unit of care.*

The goal of palliative nursing is to promote quality of life across the illness trajectory through the relief of suffering, including care of the dying and bereavement follow-up. As reflected by the words of the patient quoted, illness both affects and is affected by all aspects of the individual's being. The potential for healing in the face of progressive disease is a potential rooted in the special relationship between the healer and sufferer.[1] The genuine, warm and compassionate relationship of a palliative care or hospice nurse with his or her patient is frequently a healing relationship. The nurse gives attention to the physical, psychological, social, spiritual, and existential aspects of the patient and family—whole person care. Palliative nursing care is a combination of state-of-the-art clinical competence with fidelity to the patient, the ability to listen and to remain present in the face of much suffering and distress, and communication at a deeply personal level with the patient and family. Palliative care nursing involves having a genuine interest in the person as an individual, and the ability to convey hope even in the face of death.

What appears in the abstract to be a daunting task is practiced every day throughout the world by skilled and compassionate palliative care nurses. Specialized education and training, as well as mentoring by seasoned palliative care nurses, is recognized as a needed foundation for palliative care and hospice nursing. Without such training, nurses will inevitably find themselves in situations where they are unable to provide the necessary symptom control and amelioration of suffering for those living with advanced progressive disease and those near death.

"I failed to care for him properly because I was ignorant"—these are haunting thoughts, sometimes expressed in words, other times borne silently, by the nurse. This experience is as true today as it was several decades earlier. Nurses cannot practice what they do not know, so patient and family needs are not met. However, when under the care of a skilled palliative care nurse, patients and their families struggling to live in the face of progressive, symptomatic, and debilitating disease can be well cared for and supported throughout this process—and find meaning and peace even in the face of death. This is the essence of skilled palliative nursing care—to facilitate the "caring" process through a combination of science, presence, openness, compassion, mindful attention to detail, and teamwork. It remains true, however, that although we have both the knowledge and the art to control the majority of symptoms that occur during the last months, weeks, and days of life, we still have much to learn about how to alleviate the psychological and spiritual distress that comes with life-threatening illness.[2] Listening to the experts—our patients and their families—will help us obtain this necessary knowledge.

Advanced-practice palliative care nurses have pioneered models of palliative nursing care in many different settings in the United States, as well as elsewhere around the world. For example, a former critical care nurse may now provide palliative care at an urban/trauma emergency center. Her focus is on patients who are not expected to survive their hospital stay, many of whom are respirator dependent. She may not work as part of a standing palliative care team, but has access to the multiple disciplines within the institution whom she can call on as needed. Another nurse practices at an urban acute care teaching hospital as part of a palliative care team. The patients he works with may not be actively dying, but are in need of symptom management, psychosocial support, grief and bereavement counseling, discharge planning, and/or long-term care planning. Continuity of care is emphasized, as well as education of nursing and medical staff. A third nurse practices at a large inner-city hospital serving a disadvantaged urban population. She heads the interdisciplinary End-of-Life Consultation Service and sees patients and their families concerning pain, grief and ethical questions.

In contrast, a nurse with expertise in both geriatrics and palliative care works at a university-affiliated geriatric practice. Generally, the patients she serves have advanced chronic illness such as end-stage heart and lung disease, dementia or cancer. Many of these patients are at risk for "falling through the cracks," as their prognosis and trajectory of dying may be uncertain and they do not fit into established categories for provision of home care. A fifth example is a nurse practitioner who works in a rural primary care practice with an emphasis on palliative care. He focuses on integrating palliative care into traditional health services for an underserved, sparsely populated rural community. As in the case of many senior palliative care nurses, this nurse practitioner mentors graduate and undergraduate students. A last example of this diversity in practice settings is a clinical specialist who practices at a long-term care facility—a setting where palliative care needs of patients have only recently begun to receive due attention. This nurse's focus is to integrate palliative care into the normal flow of clinical care at the nursing home.

The role of the Advanced-Practice Palliative Care Nurse is addressed in detail in Chapter 60. Other examples of advanced-practice palliative care nursing are illustrated throughout the text, including Part IX—International Models of Palliative Care reflecting various stages of development.

## Shifting the Paradigm of End-of-Life Care to Palliative Care

Advances in health care have changed the trajectory of dying. Improved nutrition and sanitation, preventive medicine, widespread vaccination use, the development of broad-spectrum antibiotics, and an emphasis on early detection and treatment of disease have resulted in fewer deaths in infancy and childhood, and fewer deaths from acute illness. The combination of a healthier population in many developed countries and effective treatments for disease has resulted in the ability to prolong life. This has led to both benefits and challenges for society. For example, in the United States, more than 70% of those who die each year are 65 years of age or older. The majority of these deaths, however, occur after a long, progressively debilitating chronic illness, such as cancer, cardiac disease, renal disease, lung disease, or acquired immunodeficiency syndrome (AIDS).[3,4]

It is also now recognized that the palliative-care needs and end-of-life needs of children have long been ignored.[5] The field of palliative care nursing has expanded in response to these challenges. It has built on the long tradition of hospice care and the models of excellent nursing care within hospice.

## The Relationship of Hospice Care to Palliative Care in the United States of America

The hospice model of care was developed to address the specific needs of the dying and of their families, so long neglected by the medical system of care. The modern hospice movement started in England in 1967, through the work of Dame Cicely Saunders (who was trained as a nurse, a social worker and a physician) and colleagues at St. Christopher Hospice in London. The hospice movement came to the United States in the mid-1970s, when Dr. Florence Wald, a nursing pioneer, led an interdisciplinary team to create the first American hospice.[6]

Hospice care became a Medicare benefit in the 1980s. Patients traditionally followed in hospice programs could no longer receive life-prolonging therapy, and it was required that they be certified by a physician as having a life expectancy of 6 months or less. This presented a problem for patients living with a chronic debilitating disease, whose life expectancy was unclear or was greater than 6 months, or who, for a variety of reasons, did not want to be "identified" as a hospice patient. The palliative care and family-centered care provided through hospice programs was needed, but the rationing of hospice programs (based on prognosis) and the requirement of denying life-prolonging therapies were barriers that deprived many individuals of the benefit of such care.

The palliative care model evolved from the traditional hospice perspective to address quality-of-life concerns for those patients living for prolonged periods with a progressive, debilitating disease. It recognized the change in the trajectory of dying in many industrial countries, from that of a relatively short illness leading to death, to one involving a progressive and prolonged debilitating illness frequently associated with multiple factors affecting the quality of life. It recognized that such factors required skilled and compassionate palliative care interventions, regardless of prognosis, life-prolonging therapy, or closeness to death.

In looking at the relationship between hospice and palliative care, perhaps hospice can best be described as a program through which palliative care is intensified as an individual moves closer to death. Ideally, patients and families living with a chronic, debilitating and progressive disease receive palliative care throughout the course of their disease and its treatment. As they come closer to death, they are able to transition seamlessly and without added distress into a hospice program of care.

The "Open Access" hospice approach—a blended model between curative and palliative care—is a recent development with the goal of mainstreaming hospice care into the current system of care. The goal of open access is to deliver hospice care concurrently with the patient's other treatments, allowing state-of-the-art end-of-life care for a much longer period. The hope was that patients would access hospice earlier and would have the space and support to come to terms with their ambivalence about dying.[7] Eligibility for hospice services would be determined solely by the regulatory requirements. However, open access programs remain the exception because of cost. According to the Centers for Medicare and Medicaid Services (CMS), only 2.5% of the country's over 4,000 hospices have an average daily census above 400—the commonly considered minimum requirement for open access programs.[7] With a large average daily census of patients, the hospice program is able to balance the cost of patients opting to continue with expensive palliative therapies, with those who prefer to have comfort measures alone.

### World Health Organization Definition of Palliative Care

In recognition of the changing trajectory of dying and the implications for palliative care, the World Health Organization (WHO) modified its 1982 definition of palliative care to the following: "Palliative care is an approach to care which improves quality of life of patients and their families facing life-threatening illness, through the prevention, assessment and treatment of pain and other physical, psychological and spiritual problems."[8]

The new WHO definition broadens the scope of palliative care beyond end-of-life care and suggests that such an approach can be integrated with life-prolonging therapy and should be enhanced as death draws near. In a similar vein, the National Comprehensive Cancer Network (NCCN) developed guidelines to facilitate the "appropriate integration of palliative care into anticancer therapy."[9] The focus of all these efforts is to change the standard practice of palliative care (identified as "too little, too late")—in which there is a distinct separation between diagnosis, treatment, and end-of-life care—to a vision of the future in which there is "front-loading" of palliative care.[10] This means, for example, that at the time of the cancer diagnosis and initiation of treatment, the patient would also have access to psychological counseling, nutrition services, pain management, fatigue management, and cancer rehabilitation.[10] Such a model is appropriate for other chronic diseases as well. MediCaring, a national demonstration project spearheaded by the Center to Improve Care of the Dying, is an example of an attempt to integrate palliative care into medical and disease management for seriously ill cardiac and pulmonary-disease patients who have a life expectancy between 2 to 3 years. The intent is to make this program a Medicare benefit, as is the case with hospice care.[11]

### The Distinctive Features of Palliative Care Nursing

With this as a background, it is important to define the field of palliative care nursing and to recognize how it differs in essence from other areas of nursing care. In this way, nurses can be educated and trained appropriately, and the special nature of such education and training can be recognized. Palliative care nursing reflects a "whole-person" philosophy of care implemented across the lifespan and across diverse health care settings. The patient and family are the unit of care. The goal of palliative nursing is to promote quality of life along the illness trajectory through the relief of suffering, and this includes care of the dying and bereavement follow-up for the family and significant others in the patient's life. Relieving suffering and enhancing quality of life include the following: providing effective pain and symptom management; addressing psychosocial and spiritual needs of the patient and family; incorporating cultural values and attitudes into the plan of care; supporting those who are experiencing loss, grief, and bereavement; promoting ethical and legal decision-making; advocating for personal wishes and preferences; using therapeutic communication skills; and facilitating collaborative practice.

In addition, in palliative nursing, the "individual" is recognized as a very important part of the healing relationship. The nurse's individual relationship with the patient and family is seen as crucial. This relationship, together with knowledge and skills, is the essence of palliative care nursing and sets it apart from other areas of nursing practice. However, palliative care as a therapeutic approach is appropriate for all nurses to practice. It is an integral part of many nurses' daily practice, as is clearly demonstrated in work with the elderly, the neurologically impaired, and infants in the neonatal intensive care unit.

The palliative care nurse frequently cares for patients experiencing major stressors, whether physical, psychological, social, spiritual, or existential.[12,13] Many of these patients recognize themselves as dying and struggle with this role. To be dying and to care for someone who is dying are two sides of a complex social phenomenon. There are roles and obligations for each person.[12,14] To be labeled as "dying" affects how others behave toward an individual and how the individual behaves toward self and others.[12,14] The person is dying, is "becoming dead" (personal communication, Eric Cassell, January 1, 2000), with all that implies at both an individual and a social level. A feeling of failure and futility may pervade the relationship between the patient and a nurse or physician not educated or trained in hospice or palliative care. They may become disengaged, and the potential for growth on the part of both patient and clinician may be lost—"I failed to care for him properly because I was ignorant…the memory haunts me."

## The Palliative Care Nurse and the Interdisciplinary Palliative Care Team: Collaborative Practice

The composition of teams providing palliative care varies tremendously, depending on the needs of the patients and the resources available. The one common denominator is the presence of a nurse and a physician on the team. Regardless of the specific type of palliative care team, it is the nurse who serves as a primary liaison between the team, patient, and family, and who brings the team plan to the bedside, whether that is in the home, the clinic, or the inpatient setting. Because of the close proximity of the nurse to the patient and family through day-to-day observation and care, there is often a shift in the balance of decision-making at the end of life from physician to nurse. However, continued involvement of the physician in palliative care should still be fostered and encouraged; it is a myth that the physician need be less involved as the goal of care shifts from cure to comfort. Not uncommonly, a physician oriented toward life-prolonging therapies, who has provided care for a given patient over a number of years, may feel lost, helpless, overwhelmed, and uncertain of his or her role in the care of the dying. Yet, the patient and family may feel very close to that physician and have a great need for him or her at this time. Fear of abandonment by the patient, and the physician's desire to "do everything" rather than abandon the patient, may result in inappropriate and harmful treatments being offered and accepted. A nurse who is educated and trained in palliative care and end-of-life care can do much to guide and support the physician during this transition, and to redirect or reframe the interventions from "doing everything" toward "doing everything to provide comfort and healing."

There may be other reasons why patients want to continue aggressive, life-prolonging interventions in the face of impending death. Understanding why patients sometimes seek aggressive medical care and life-prolonging measures is an integral part of the role of the nurse on the palliative care team. This is illustrated in the following case example:

CASE STUDY
*Mr. Stevens, a Patient with Lung Cancer*

Mr. Stevens, a 30-year-old man with far-advanced, non-small cell lung cancer and rapidly failing pulmonary status, wanted every measure to be taken to maintain his life, including experimental chemotherapy and ventilator support if needed. He had a 9-month-old daughter and a wonderful and caring wife and extended family. Whatever he wanted was what they wanted. As Mr. Stevens' respiratory status continued to deteriorate, the nurses who were involved in his care felt that by respecting his wishes in providing what they considered "futile care,"they were doing harm. After discussion with the patient's attending physician, a palliative care consult was initiated with the purpose of addressing goals of care and the benefits and burdens of ongoing experimental chemotherapy. Code status also needed to be addressed.

An experienced palliative care nurse met with the patient and his wife and the following story unfolded. Mr. Stevens had emigrated from Russia to the United States as a child. He had overcome a difficult childhood, and had finally achieved what he wanted: a family of his own and a job that allowed him to care for them. He had overcome seemingly insurmountable odds in the past, and found it impossible to accept that his life was coming to an end—a life that was only just beginning. It was too painful for him. After many sessions in which the palliative care nurse bore witness to his grief at losing all that he loved, as well as the grief of his wife, Mr. Stevens gradually came to terms with the powerful legacy that he was leaving behind. He recognized that his life, however short, had made a difference, that he would not be forgotten, and that he had a loving wife, a child, and a legacy of courage, love and achievement. When the "silence" of his pending death was broken, friends and family were able to share with him how he had influenced their lives and what he meant to them. Although Mr. Stevens decided to continue in chemotherapy for several more weeks, when the burden became too great for him he was able to say "enough is enough," that he had fought the disease as long as he could and now was the time to rest and be at peace. He had done what he could. Mr. Stevens died at home, and though never quite accepting hospice support, received excellent palliative and supportive care in a manner that was acceptable to him.

Although other members of the interdisciplinary team, including the chaplain and social worker, were involved with this patient and family's care, and in family and staff "debriefing" and bereavement follow-up sessions, the palliative care nurse played a central coordinating and mentoring role in meeting the needs of the patient, family, physician, and nursing staff. However, clearly no single discipline can meet all the needs of most patients and their families; an interdisciplinary team greatly enhances such care.[15]

How little is known about patients, their families, and their aspirations, is illustrated in this case.[16] What seems to be an irrational choice to health care providers may be eminently sensible to the patient and family. The frequent struggle and suffering of nurses and physicians as they grapple with their own mortality and with being asked to provide care they think is inappropriate or harmful for dying patients is also demonstrated.[17] Assessment and communication skills, as well as a firm foundation in the ethical principles of palliative care and end-of-life care when treating such patients, are clearly important.

## End-of-Life Care in the United States Today: Improving But Still a Long Way To Go

The inadequacy of care for the dying, who are among the most voiceless and vulnerable in our society, came into national focus during the debates over the past two decades surrounding physician-assisted suicide and euthanasia. The national dialogue was fueled by: the actions of Dr. Jack Kevorkian and his suicide machine; the rulings of two United States Appeals Courts on the right to die[18,19]; findings from the Study to Understand Prognoses and Preferences for Outcomes and Risks of Treatments (SUPPORT)[20]; interviews with family caretakers[21]; a review of end-of-life content in nursing and medical texts[22,23]—which reflected minimal to no such content—and the Institute of Medicine's reports on end-of-life care, with its series of recommendations to address deficiencies in care of the chronically ill and dying, both children and adults.[3,5]

*Means to a Better End*, a report card generated by Last Acts (a Robert Wood Johnson-funded coalition created with almost 1,000 national partner organizations dedicated to end-of-life reform), was the first attempt at a comprehensive report on the state of end-of-life care in the United States.[24] Between August 30 and September 1, 2002, slightly more than 1,000 Americans were surveyed by telephone and asked their opinions regarding the quality of health care at the end of life. Three quarters of those surveyed had suffered the loss of a family member or close friend in the last 5 years. Each of the 50 states and the District of Columbia were represented in the survey and were rated on eight criteria: state advance directive policies, location of death, hospice use, hospital end-of-life care services, care in intensive care units at the end of life, pain among nursing home residents, state pain policies, and the presence of palliative care-certified nurses and doctors.

The findings suggested that, "despite many recent improvements in end-of-life care and greater public awareness about it, Americans had no better than a fair chance of finding good care for their loved ones or for themselves when facing a life-threatening illness." For example, nationally only 25% of deaths occur at home, although 70% of Americans say that they would prefer to die at home; about half of all deaths occur in hospitals, but fewer than 60% of the hospitals

in any given state offer specialized end-of-life services; and most states have only "fair" hospice use.[24] In 2007, there were approximately 4,700 hospice programs in the United States, caring for over 1.4 million patients and their families, indicating that about 38.8% of all deaths in America are under hospice care. Of these patients, approximately 50% had a cancer diagnosis, 12% had end-stage cardiac disease, 10% had dementia, 3% had end-stage kidney disease, and 2% had end-stage liver disease.[25]

Although the 2002 state report card measures were very disturbing, activities at the federal, state, and community levels continue to work toward improving access to skilled palliative care and end-of-life care.[25] Some broad examples of these initiatives by professional organizations supported through philanthropic funding include the following:

- Promoting Excellence in End-of-Life Care, a program of the Robert Wood Johnson Foundation that provides grants and technical support to innovative programs throughout the United States to improve care of the dying.[26]
- The End-of-Life Nursing Education Consortium (ELNEC), a national and international education program to improve end-of-life care.[27]
- The Education on Palliative and End-of-Life Care (EPEC) project, a national program for physicians to improve end-of-life care.[28]
- The pain standards supported by the Joint Commission on Accreditation of Healthcare Organizations (JCAHO), which hold institutions accountable for assessment and management of pain among the patients in their care.[29]

In addition, philanthropically supported programs to improve care of the dying have been developed at a community level to meet the needs of specific populations (e.g., the Missoula Demonstration Project[30]) or underserved communities (e.g., the Harlem Palliative Care Network[31]). Unfortunately, many such philanthropically supported programs are unable to self sustain once the financial support comes to an end. There are also a growing number of palliative care programs being developed within institutions and long-term care facilities, as well as end-of-life pathways and critical care pathways for the dying.[32] Home hospice programs that offer palliative care consultation services to the broader patient population are a recent innovation that may improve access to palliative care in non-hospice patients. Board certification in palliative nursing and palliative medicine are also important milestones in recognizing the specific body of knowledge and expertise necessary to practice with competence in this specialty.

Many professional, state, and community initiatives address the barriers identified by the National Cancer Policy Board that keep individuals with progressive cancer from receiving excellent palliative care.[33] These barriers include

- The separation of palliative and hospice care from potentially life-prolonging treatment within the health care system, which is both influenced by and affects reimbursement policy.

- Inadequate training of health care personnel in symptom management and other end-of-life skills.
- Inadequate standards of care and lack of accountability in caring for dying patients.
- Disparities in care, when available, for African Americans and other ethnic and socioeconomic segments of the population.
- Lack of information and resources for the public dealing with end-of-life care.
- Lack of reliable data on the quality of life for patients dying of cancer (as well as other chronic diseases).
- Low public sector investment in palliative care and end-of-life care research and training.

The National Institute of Medicine Report on improving care at the end of life[3] suggested that people should be able to achieve a "decent" or "good" death—"one that is free from avoidable distress and suffering for patients, families, and caregivers; in general accord with patients' and families' wishes; and reasonably consistent with clinical, cultural and ethical standards" (p. 24). The report and recommendations focused on the interdisciplinary nature of palliative care, of which nursing is the core discipline. Traditionally, nursing has been at the forefront in the care of patients with chronic and advanced disease, and recent advances in symptom management, combined with the growing awareness of palliative care as a public health issue, have provided the impetus for bringing together this compendium of nursing knowledge.

The general public and the health care community, of which nurses are the largest group, have been confronted with facts about care for the dying and with the task of determining how to achieve quality of life even at the end of life.[34,35] In December 2001, a consortium of five national palliative care organizations came together in New York because of the identified need to: expand access to palliative care for patients and families; to increase the number of reliable, high-quality programs; and to ensure quality.[34] Participants from these organizations were nominated by their peers, with palliative care nursing leadership well represented by Connie Dahlin, Betty Ferrell, Judy Lentz, and Deborah Sherman.

## The National Consensus Project for Quality Palliative Care

The National Consensus Project consisted of four key national palliative care organizations: American Academy of Hospice and Palliative Medicine; Center to Advance Palliative Care; Hospice and Palliative Nurses Association; and the National Hospice and Palliative Care Organization. The consensus project had five goals: (1) to build national consensus concerning the definition, philosophy, and principles of palliative care through an open and inclusive process that includes the array of professionals, providers, and consumers involved in and affected by palliative care; (2) to create voluntary clinical practice guidelines for palliative care that describe the highest quality services to patients and families; (3) to broadly disseminate the clinical practice guidelines to enable existing and future programs to define better their program organization, resource requirements, and performance measures; (4) to help clinicians provide the key elements of palliative care in the absence of palliative care programs; and (5) to promote recognition, stable reimbursement structure, and accreditation initiatives.[34]

The clinical practice guidelines cover in detail eight domains identified as being crucial to the delivery of comprehensive palliative care: the structure and process of care; the physical domain; the psychological and psychiatric domain; the social domain; the spiritual, religious, and existential domain; the cultural domain; the imminently dying patient; and ethics and the law. The guidelines were released in April 2004, and a revised version released in March 2009. These guidelines are outlined in Appendix 1–1.

Progress is being made and palliative care nurses have been involved each step of the way. There are a growing number of palliative care programs being developed within institutions and long-term care facilities. Some hospice programs offer palliative care consultation services to the broader patient population—a fairly recent innovation that may improve access to palliative care for non-hospice patients. Board certification in palliative nursing at both the generalist and advanced-practice levels are also important milestones in recognition of the specific body of knowledge and expertise necessary to practice with competence in this area. In addition, as mentioned earlier, there has been a steady growth in hospice programs over the past decade. In 2007, there were over 4,700 hospice providers in the United States, with hospice reaching 38.8% of all deaths. Hospice nurses would have been intimately involved in the care of each of these patients and their families. The number of patients served has increased to over 1.4 million and more patients followed by hospice are dying in the place they call "home." This includes a private residence, nursing home or residential facility.[25] The number of palliative care programs in hospitals has also increased significantly over the past 5 years. In 2006, 30% of hospitals had a palliative care program, up from 15% in the year 2,000. In addition, 64.4% of hospices report provision of palliative care outside of their hospice program.[25]

## The Scope and Aims of the Third Edition of the Textbook of Palliative Nursing Reflect State-of-the-Art Palliative Nursing Care

Palliative nursing is a world of many connections. To see the world of the individual, a multidimensional, multi-lens perspective is needed. Often, this complexity is best conveyed through simple stories.[36,37] This duality of complexity and simplicity is incorporated into the structure of the current and expanded third edition of the *Oxford Textbook of Palliative Nursing*. Each chapter is introduced by a quotation from a patient or family member to illustrate the content of the chapter. Key Points are included as a quick reference and also as an overview of the chapter content. In addition, brief case examples are used to anchor the theoretical and practical content of the chapter in real-life situations.

The textbook, which includes an international perspective, is intended as a comprehensive resource for nurses in the emerging field of palliative care. The approach has been to incorporate the principles of palliative care nursing throughout the course of a chronic, progressive, incurable disease rather than only at the end of life. The scope is broad. The content, contributed by more than 100 national and international nursing experts and divided into 78 chapters in ten parts, covers the world of palliative care nursing.

Part I provides a general introduction to palliative nursing care and includes an in-depth discussion of hospice care as a model for quality end-of-life care, the principles of family assessment, and the principles of communication in palliative care. Part II moves into the critical area of symptom assessment and management. Each of the 28 chapters in this section addresses the assessment and pathophysiology of the symptoms, pharmacologic interventions, non-drug treatments, and patient/family teaching within the goals of palliative care. Based on suggestions from readers of the previous edition of the textbook, two additional chapters have been added to this section: Insomnia and Withdrawal of Life Sustaining Treatment. Part III addresses psychosocial support in palliative care and at the end of life. Here the focus is on the meaning of hope at the end of life, bereavement, family support, and planning for the death and death rituals. Spiritual care and meaning in illness are addressed in Part IV. The impact of spiritual distress on quality of life at the end of life has become increasingly clear, and the ability of the nurse to recognize such distress in patients and their families, and to make appropriate interventions and referrals, is an essential component of palliative care. Much remains to be learned in this area.

In Part V, the needs of special populations and cultural considerations in palliative care are addressed. Included here are the elderly, the poor and underserved, individuals with AIDS, and care for the drug-addicted patient at the end of life. Additional chapters have been added to this section, including Caring for those with Chronic Illness, Palliative Care in Psychiatric Illness, and Cancer Survivorship. Part VI focuses on improving the quality of end-of-life care across settings. After a practical overview on monitoring quality and development of pathways and standards in end-of-life care, subsequent chapters discuss long-term care, home care, hospital care, intensive care, rehabilitation, and care in the outpatient or office setting.

Part VII remains entirely devoted to pediatric palliative care across care settings. Part VIII moves into special issues for nurses in end-of-life care that include ethics, public policy, requests for assistance in dying, nursing education, and

nursing research. Two additional chapters have been added to this section: The Advanced Practice Nurse, and Teamwork in Palliative Care. Part IX explores international models of palliative care reflecting various stages of national development. Four new chapters have been added representing palliative care in Canada, Africa, Japan, and Korea. Part X gives voice to the patient and family, exploring the concept of "a good death" through a detailed case discussion. The appendix provides a very comprehensive and useful list of community and professional resources.

The purpose of the *Oxford Textbook of Palliative Nursing* is to organize and disseminate the existing knowledge of experts in palliative care nursing and to provide a scientific underpinning for practice. The focus is on assessment and management of the wide range of physical, psychosocial, and spiritual needs of patients, their families, and staff in palliative care across clinical settings. Topics frequently cited as challenges in nursing care at the end of life—including palliative sedation, communication, ethics, research, and providing care for the underserved and homeless—are specifically addressed. As illustrated throughout, the world of palliative care nursing is complex, scientifically based, and immensely rewarding.

REFERENCES

1. Kearney M. Mount B. Spiritual care of the dying patient. In: Chochinov HM, Breitbart W, eds. Handbook of Psychiatry in Palliative Medicine. Oxford: Oxford University Press, 2000:357–373.
2. Kuhl D. What Dying People Want: Practical Wisdom for the End of Life. New York: Public Affairs, 2002.
3. Field M, Cassel C. Approaching Death: Improving Care at the End of Life. Committee on Care at the End of Life, Institute of Medicine. Washington, DC: National Academy Press, 1997.
4. Corr C. Death in modern society. In: Doyle D, Hanks WC, MacDonald N, eds. Oxford Textbook of Palliative Medicine, 2nd ed. Oxford: Oxford University Press, 1998:31–40.
5. Institute of Medicine. When Children Die: Improving Palliative and End-of-life Care for Children and their Families. Washington, DC: National Academy Press, 2003.
6. Wald FS. Hospice care in the United States: A conversation with Florence S. Wald. JAMA 1999;281:1683–1685.
7. Wright AA, Katz IT. Letting go of the ropes—aggressive treatment, hospice care, and open access. N Eng J Med 2007; 357:324–327.
8. World Health Organization. Palliative care. Available at: http://www.who.int/cancer/palliative/definition/en (accessed November 16, 2008).
9. National Comprehensive Cancer Network (NCCN). Practice guidelines in oncology: Palliative care, version 1.2004. Available at: http://www.nccn.org (accessed October 12, 2008).
10. Oncology Roundtable. Culture of Compassion: Best Practices in Supportive Oncology. Washington, DC: The Advisory Board Company, 2001:98–99.
11. Washington Home Center for Palliative Care Studies (CPCS). MediCaring. Available at: http://www.medicaring.org (accessed December 1, 2008).

12. Cassell EJ. Diagnosing suffering: A perspective. Ann Intern Med 1999;131:531–534.

13. Aries P. Western attitudes towards death: From the Middle Ages to the present. Baltimore, Md.: Johns Hopkins University Press, 1974.

14. Cherny N, Coyle N, Foley KM. Suffering in the advanced cancer patient. Part I: A definition and taxonomy. J Palliat Care 1994; 10:57–70.

15. Ingham J, Coyle N. Teamwork in end-of-life care: A nurse–physician perspective on introducing physicians to palliative care concepts. In: Clark D, Hockley J, Ahmedzai S. New Themes in Palliative Care. Buckingham: Open University Press, 1997:255–274.

16. Coyle N. Suffering in the first person. In: Ferrell BF, ed. Suffering. Boston: Jones and Bartlett, 1996:29–64.

17. Ferrell BF, Coyle N. The Nature of Suffering and the Goals of Nursing. Oxford: Oxford University Press, 2008

18. United States Court of Appeals for the Ninth Circuit. Compassion in Dying v. State of Washington. Fed Report. 1996 Mar 6 (date of decision);79:790–859.

19. United States Court of Appeals for the Second Circuit. Quill v. Vacco. Fed Report. 1996 Apr 2 (date of decision);80:716–743.

20. SUPPORT Principal Investigators. A controlled trial to improve care for seriously ill hospitalized patients: The Study to Understand Prognoses and Preferences for Outcomes and Risks of Treatments (SUPPORT). JAMA 1995;274:1591–1598.

21. Lynn J, Teno JM, Phillips RS, Wu AW, Desbiens N, Harrold J, Claessens MT, Wenger N, Kreling B, Connors AF Jr. for SUPPORT investigators. Perceptions by family members of the dying experience of older and seriously ill patients. Study to Understand Prognoses and Preferences for Outcomes and Risks of Treatments. Ann Intern Med 1997;126:97–106.

22. Ferrell BR, Virani R, Grant M, Juarez G. Analysis of palliative care content in nursing textbooks. J Palliat Care 2000;16:39–47.

23. Rabow MW, Hardie GE, Fair JM, McPhee SJ. End-of-life care content in 50 textbooks from multiple specialties. JAMA 2000; 283:771–778.

24. Last Acts. Means to a better end: A report card on dying in America today. November 2002. Available at: http://www.rwjf.org/files/publications/other/meansbetterend.pdf (accessed November 16, 2009).

25. National Hospice and Palliative Care Organization. NHPCO facts and figures. Available at: http://www.nhpco.org/files/public/statistics_Research/NHPCO_facts_and_figures.pdf (accessed November 16, 2009).

26. Promoting Excellence in End-of-Life Care website. Available at: http://www.promotingexcellence.org (accessed December 12, 2008).

27. American Association of Colleges of Nurses. End-of-Life Nursing Education Consortium (ELNEC) website. Available at: http://www.aacn.nche.edu/ELNEC/ (accessed December 11, 2008).

28. The Education on Palliative and End-of-Life Care (EPEC) project website. Available at: http://www.epec.net (accessed December 8, 2008).

29. Joint Commission on Accreditation of Healthcare Organizations and National Pharmaceutical Council, Inc. Improving the quality of pain management through measurement and action. Available at: http://www.reliefinsite.com/downloads/Improving_the_Quality_of_Pain_Mgmt_Thru_Measurement_and_Action_JCAHO.pdf (accessed November 16, 2009).

30. Life's End Institute. Missoula demonstration project. Available at: http://www.missoulademonstration.org (accessed December 8, 2008).

31. Payne R, Payne TR. The Harlem Palliative Care Network. J Palliat Med 2002;5:781–792.

32. Coyle N, Schacter S, Carver AC. Terminal care and bereavement. Neurol Clin 2001;19:1005–1025.

33. Institute of Medicine and National Research Council. Improving Palliative Care for Cancer: Summary and Recommendations. Washington, DC: National Academy Press, 2001:5.

34. National Consensus Project for Quality Palliative Care. Clinical practice guidelines for quality palliative care. 2004. Available at: http://www.nationalconsensusproject.org (accessed December 8, 2008).

35. National Quality Forum. National framework and preferred practices for palliative and hospice care. 2006. Available at: http://www.qualityforum.org/Projects/n-r/Palliative_and_Hospice_Care_Framework/Palliative_Hospice_Care_Framework_and_Practices.aspx (accessed November 16, 2009).

36. Steeves RH. Loss, grief and the search for meaning. Oncol Nurs Forum 1996;23:897–903.

37. Ferrell BR. The quality of lives: 1525 voices of cancer. Oncol Nurs Forum 1996;23:907–915.

APPENDIX 1–1
# Summary of the National Consensus Project Clinical Practice Guidelines

## Domain 1: Structure and Practice of Care
- Care starts with a comprehensive interdisciplinary assessment of the patient and family.
- Addresses both identified and expressed needs of the patient and family.
- Education and training available.
- Team is commitment to quality improvement.
- Emotional impact of work on team members is addressed.
- Team has a relationship with hospice.

## Domain 2: Physical
- Pain, other symptoms, and treatment side effects are managed using best practice.
- Team documents and communicates treatment alternatives, permitting patient/family to make informed choices.
- Family is educated and supported to provide safe/appropriate comfort measures to the patient.

## Domain 3: Psychological and Psychiatric
- Psychological and psychiatric issues are assessed and managed based on best available evidence.
- Team employs pharmacologic, non pharmacologic and Complementary and Alternative Medicine (CAM) as appropriate.
- Grief and bereavement program is available to patients and families.

*Domain 4: Social*
- Assessment includes family structure, relationships, medical decision-making, finances, sexuality, caregiver availability, access to medications and equipment.
- Individualized comprehensive care plans lessens caregiver burden and promotes well-being.

*Domain 5: Spiritual, Religious, and Existential*
- Assesses and addresses spiritual concerns.
- Recognizes and respects religious beliefs—provides religious support.
- Makes connections with community and spiritual religious groups or individuals as desired by patient/family.

*Domain 6: Cultural*
- Assesses and aims to meet cultural-specific needs of patients and families.
- Respects and accommodates range of language, dietary, habitual, and religious practices of patients and families.

- Team has access to/uses translation resources.
- Recruitment and hiring practices reflect cultural diversity and community.

*Domain 7: The Imminently Dying Patient*
- Team recognizes imminence of death and provides appropriate care to the patient and family.
- As patient declines, team introduces hospice referral option.
- Team educates the family on signs/symptoms of approaching death in a developmentally, age, and culturally appropriate manner.

*Domain 8: Ethics and Law*
- Patient's goals, preferences, and choices are respected and form basis for plan of care.
- Team is knowledgeable about relevant federal and state statutes and regulations.

*(Source: National Consensus Project, reference 34.)*

# 2

## Hospice Palliative Care for the 21ˢᵗ Century: A Model for Quality End-of-Life Care

*Kathleen A. Egan City and Mary J. Labyak*

*My dad and I would like to thank hospice for the support, help, information, guidance, love and compassion they provided during the entire time my mom was in hospice care. They were so knowledgeable and everyone worked so quickly and efficiently that they became instant and trusted friends. Somehow they knew just when to explain what was going on and what to expect with each phase of her illness. We would have been heartbroken if we weren't able to keep her at home. With the support of hospice, we learned how to keep her comfortable, how to decrease her anxiety, and even how to find moments of laughter and joy as we grew closer remembering our lives together. Ultimately, hospice gave us confidence and peace of mind that our mother and wife was finally receiving the type of care she needed to peacefully and comfortably find the path to the next stage of her existence. A heartfelt thanks to everyone at hospice.—Adult daughter of a hospice patient.*

- ◆ **Key Points**
- ◆ *Nurses must understand and honor each patient's and family's unique experiences near life's end, addressing the physical, emotional, and spiritual dimensions of the experience through holistic care guided by what is most important to the patient and family at this time in their lives.*
- ◆ *Hospice blends compassion and strategic skilled services to support patients and families through life-limiting illnessess so they may find meaning and purpose, optimizes dignity and comfort at life's completion, enhance meaningful closure of relationships for the patient and family.*
- ◆ *Hospice care models are expanding to serve people across the lifespan and across care settings with a variety of services that are helpful from the time of diagnosis of a life-limiting condition through bereavement. including preventive approaches found in public health models.*
- ◆ *By understanding the impact of illness on people's lives and their hopes, dreams, and relationships, nurses gain more insights into the value of hospice and how to introduce it to patients and families in a supportive way.*
- ◆ *Nurses working with the dying and bereaved can experience cumulative loss, and can balance that with experiences of great meaning and purpose in their work.*

To provide care and services that optimally support patients and families in the last years of life, one must first understand the experiences of illness and their impact on the patient and family. The experiences of illness, caregiving, dying and bereavement are more than physical events focused on disease and symptom management. The specialty of hospice palliative care nursing provides this broader perspective, with an understanding that illness and dying include suffering beyond the physical aspects for both the person who is ill and his or her family. People who are dying experience all the emotions people feel through the course of a lifetime. As much as they might know fear, loneliness, guilt, shame, and despair, they can also experience hope, joy, love, compassion and intimacy. Dying is not void of the painful emotions we experience in living. At the same time dying, like living, presents opportunities for personal growth and development, renewal or repair of relationships, and review of the meaning of life's experiences.[1] It is within the framework of this realization that nurses can learn the skills to be present with, communicate with, and compassionately foster patient and family resolution and a dignified closure that honors their lives and relationships.

Instead of asking the patient and family members to fit into a caregiving system, hospice extends services according to their unique situation and personal values, and focuses through holistic, compassionate care. Compassionate care by its very nature is shaped to fit the individual needs and values of the people involved. Rather than having professionals direct the patient and family experiences, hospice establishes a relationship of care and support that is directed by the patient and family, focusing on the individual's and family's world, encouraging personal choices and meaningful experiences around the process of illness, dying, death, and bereavement.

The "Hospice Experience Model" and "experience approach" blends compassion and skill to assist patients and their families in creating their own experiences around their life-limiting illnesses and caregiving. Ultimately, patients and families can experience optimal comfort and dignity, gain or retain control over their lives, reflect on what is most important to them at this time in their lives, and unwind their lives or relationships in a way that is meaningful.

Hospice is a program of care provided across all care and home settings that involves a variety of services. Based on the understanding that dying is part of the life cycle, hospice manages disease symptoms but does not stop there. It offers excellent disease and symptom management so the patient and family can have the energy and ability to focus on what is most important to them at this time. Dr. David Kuhl spent years researching the end of life experiences of patients. He stresses the importance of people simply wanting to tell their stories, to relate to someone about living with dying. He summarizes their stories by outlining nine concerns or themes that capture their experiences, and that include:

1. Their changing perceptions of time, what it means, and how to spend it.
2. The suffering that resulted from the experience of hearing their terminal diagnosis for the first time and the need to communicate effectively with health care professionals.
3. Physical pain, its reality, and its effect on who they were.
4. The importance of being touched and being "in touch."
5. The natural process of reviewing one's life (looking back) once one understands that dying is a reality.
6. Speaking and hearing truth.
7. Longing to belong, that is, to understand who they were in the past with regard to their original families, as well as in the present with regard to their chosen (adult) family.
8. Asking the question, "Who am I?" in the search to know who they are in the present, free of the expectations of others.
9. Experiencing transcendence–meaning, value, God, spirituality, a higher being greater than oneself.

As people experience this last phase of life, hospice provides comprehensive palliative medical and supportive services, compassion, and care with the goals of comfort and meaningful life completion for the patient and relationship closure for the family. A hospice supports the patient through the dying process and the family through the experience of caregiving, the patient's illness, dying, and their own bereavement. Understanding that the last phase of life is as individual as each person who experiences it, hospice advocates so that people may live the remainder of their lives with dignity and in a manner that is meaningful to them.

Hospice focuses on caring, not curing, and in most cases, care is provided in the patient's home. Hospice care also is provided in freestanding hospice centers, hospitals, and nursing homes and other long-term care facilities. Hospice services are available to patients of any age, religion, race, or illness.

Typically, a family member serves as the primary caregiver and, when appropriate, helps make decisions for the terminally ill individual. Members of the hospice staff make regular visits to assess the patient and provide additional care or other services. Hospice staff is available through 24 hours a day, seven days a week to assist patients and families through this journey.[2]

## Hospice in the United States

Hospice began in the United States as a grassroots effort to improve the quality of the dying experience for patients and their families in communities where the traditional medical systems fell short. Historically, health care delivery systems have been disease driven, with the focus on cure and rehabilitation. Approaches have focused on scientific knowledge of diseases, which drives the care processes. However, approaches to care are different when cure is the goal and when cure is no longer possible. End-stage disease progression and resulting symptoms produce different physiological responses, as well as different emotional responses. Hospice care began to fill the gap where systems fell short of addressing those differences.

The beginning of the contemporary hospice movement is credited to Dame Cicely Saunders. Beresford[3] described her pioneering work as follows: "Her concept of hospice was to combine the most modern medical techniques in terminal care with the spiritual commitment of the medieval religious orders that had once created hospices as way stations for people on pilgrimages." Learning from Dame Saunders, Florence Wald became one of the first pioneers promoting the growth of hospice in the United States.

When Wald was dean of the nursing school in the 1960s, the medical establishment was focused entirely on cures, with little attention given to palliative care and the patients' wishes about their care. In particular, most physicians were loath to prescribe narcotics to ease terminal patients' pain for fear that the patients would become addicted.

Her transformation of the situation had its germ in a 1963 lecture at Yale by Dr. Cicely Saunders, founder of St. Christopher's Hospice in London. Saunders' lecture emphasized minimizing pain in terminal cancer patients so that they could focus on their relationships and prepare for death. Wald immediately began reshaping the nursing school curriculum to put more focus on patients and their families and to emphasize care of the dying. But feeling that further effort was required, Wald resigned as dean and went to London to study at St. Christopher's. Upon her return, she organized the first U.S. hospice in Branford in 1971, Connecticut Hospice, which began by offering in-home care but eventually built its own inpatient facility and became a model for hospice care here and abroad.

"Hospice care for the terminally ill is the end piece of how to care for patients from birth on," she wrote. "As more and more people—families of hospice patients and hospice volunteers—are exposed to this new model of how to approach end-of-life care, we are taking what was essentially a hidden scene—death, an unknown—and making it a reality. We are showing people that there are meaningful ways to cope with this very difficult situation." In the process, she made nurses an integral part of the care of patients and forged a new coalition between doctors, nurses and patients—replacing the long-held tradition that the doctor reigns supreme. The core idea of this new coalition was that, when hope for a cure is gone, attention should shift to a dying patient's physical, emotional and spiritual comfort. "In some ways, we have to reform our end goals," she said in a recent interview before her death in 2008. "We need to cure sometimes but care always."[4]

No specific therapy is excluded from consideration. The test of palliative care lies in the agreement between the individual, his or her physicians, the primary caregiver, and the hospice team that the expected outcome is relief from distressing symptoms, the easing of pain, and/or enhancement of the quality of life. The decision to intervene with active palliative care is based on an ability to meet stated goals rather than affect the underlying disease. An individual's needs must continue to be assessed, and all treatment options must be explored and evaluated in the context of the individual's values and symptoms. The individual's choices and decisions regarding care are paramount and must be followed.

Hospice palliative care is considered to be the model for quality, compassionate care at the end of life. Hospice care involves a team-oriented approach to expert medical care, pain management, and emotional and spiritual support expressly tailored to the patient's needs and wishes. Support is extended to the patient's family as well. At the center of hospice is the belief that each of us should be able to live and die free of pain, with dignity, and that our families should receive the necessary support to allow us to do so.[4]

The *Standards of Practice for Hospice Programs* of the National Hospice and Palliative Care Organization (NHPCO) describes palliative care as follows:

> *Patient and family-centered care that optimizes quality of life by anticipating, preventing, and treating suffering. Palliative care throughout the continuum of illness involves addressing physical, intellectual, emotional, social, and spiritual needs and to facilitate patient autonomy, access to information, and choice. (Definition recommended by CMS in the Medicare Hospice Conditions of Participation and adopted by the National Quality Forum (NQF), with agreement by NHPCO and CAPC.)[5]*

Statewide surveys completed by the American Association of Retired People (AARP) show similar results that were seen in Massachusetts. More than 90 percent surveyed said they have heard of hospice, although fewer than four in ten know that Medicare pays for it. Three quarters of those who know about hospice would want hospice care if they were dying. Members surveyed are willing to think and talk about these important end-of-life decisions, but they need help to start these conversations and understand end-of-life care issues. This provides an opportunity for the medical, legal, and spiritual professionals to be well-versed in end-of-life issues so they can help their clients have these important conversations and make well-informed decisions for their end-of-life care.[6]

Comparing the AARP statistics with the national statistics on hospice utilization, there continues to be a large gap between what people want and how they are cared for at life's end. In 2007, an estimated 1.4 million patients received services from hospice compared to 950,000 in 2003. For 2007, NHPCO estimates that approximately 38.8% of all deaths in the United States were under the care of a hospice program. Half of hospice patients received care for less than three weeks and half received care for more than three weeks.[7] These statistics reflect how important it is for nurses and other health professionals to be more aware of when to think about hospice and how to communicate the value of hospice to patients and families sooner.

※

## Hospice Palliative Care: A Holistic Approach Focusing on the Experiences of the Patient and Family

Understanding the need for a better way to care for the dying, the hospice movement began to provide alternatives to the traditional curative model. Hospice expanded the traditional model, not only to address end-stage disease and symptom management but also to provide for the emotional, social, and spiritual dimensions of the patient's and family's experiences around their illness, dying, caregiving, and bereavement.

The experience of the last phase of life is an individual journey involving one's mind, body, and spirit. Cassell[8] described a theory of personhood reflecting that each person is a holistic being with dynamic, interrelated dimensions that are affected by the changes and adaptations experienced with progressive illness and dying. These dimensions involve the physical experience of end-stage disease, the emotional experience of one's relationships, and the way in which one defines spiritual existence.[9] As the disease progresses and the physical dimensions decline, the other dimensions (i.e., interpersonal and spiritual) take on added meaning and purpose. What one defines as quality of life changes substantially for people with life-limiting illnesses. Life perspectives, goals, and needs change. It is a time of reflection on a broader sense of meaning, purpose, and relationships, based on each individual's values.

Hospice grew from this understanding of full personhood; it is designed to offer expert end-of-life care to patients and families that addresses all of these dimensions through a holistic approach. Each patient and family is supported by an interdisciplinary group (IDG) consisting of physicians, nurses, social workers, counselors, chaplains, therapists, home health aides, and volunteers. These disciplines reflect the expertise needed to address the varied dimensions that are affected through the course of illness, caregiving, dying, and bereavement.

## The Medicare Hospice Benefit Service

The initial design of the Medicare Hospice Benefit program is still consistent in its overall structure including the following hospice services: nursing care, medical and social services, physician services, counseling/pastoral services, short-term inpatient and respite care, medical appliances and supplies including drugs and biologicals, home health aide and homemaker services, therapies (physical, occupational, speech), dietary/nutrition counseling, bereavement counseling, and drugs for symptom management and pain control.[10]

The levels of care outlined in the Medicare Hospice Benefit reflect the variations in care intensity that are required to meet patient and family needs in the last phase of life. Medicare provides coverage for hospice care to Medicare beneficiaries who have elected the hospice benefit and who have been certified as terminally ill with a prognosis for a life expectancy of 6 months or less. Once elected, Medicare pays one of four prospective, per diem rates for hospice care: routine home care, continuous home care, respite care, general inpatient care. Each of these payment categories is defined later. Changing the level of care is determined through a collaborative effort by the hospice IDG, patient, family, and primary physician.

The four levels of care include:

1. **Routine Home Care:** Routine home care is provided in the patient's home, nursing home, or residential care setting or wherever the patient and family reside.
2. **Continuous Home Care:** A continuous home care day is a day on which a patient receives hospice care consisting predominantly of nursing care on a continuous basis at home. Home health aide or homemaker services, or both, may also be provided on a continuous basis. Continuous home care is only furnished during brief periods of crisis and only as necessary to maintain the terminally ill patient at home.
3. **General Inpatient Care:** Patient receives general inpatient care in an inpatient facility for pain control or acute or chronic symptom management which cannot be managed in other settings.
4. **Inpatient Respite Care:** Patient receives care in an approved facility on a short-term basis in order to provide respite for the family caregiver.[7]

Continuity across all care settings with hospice professional management of care was and continues to be a strong underpinning of the benefit.

## Aging in the United States and End-of-Life Care

The aging of America has changed the nature and needs of people who are in their last years of life. The Medicare Hospice

Benefit was designed to provide substantial professional and material support (e.g., medications, equipment) to families caring for dying individuals at home during their last 6 months of life. The benefit was designed for, and lends itself well to, the predictable trajectory of end-stage cancers but not as well to unpredictable chronic illnesses such as congestive heart failure, chronic lung disease, stroke, and dementing illnesses.[11] An examination of hospice care and the delivery of quality end-of-life services must reflect the societal change in aging demographics and the resulting varied needs in end-of-life care models.

In our society, the overwhelming majority of dying people are elderly, and they typically die of a slowly progressing, chronic disease or of multiple coexisting problems that result in multisystem failure. Their final phase of life, which often lasts several years before death, is marked by a progressive functional dependence and associated family and caregiver burden. Hospice programs in demographic areas that represent the future of our aging society, such as Florida, have expanded their care and service options well beyond the original definition of the MHB to more fully respond to the frail elderly in their communities who are dying of chronic, progressive illnesses. These expanded hospice delivery models (Table 2–1) are: applying hospice approaches through a variety of services throughout the lifespan, long before the last 6 months of life, recognizing the variable dying process; and providing an array of services so that individuals may age in their own homes, or wherever they choose, until death.

The expanded services models are reflected in the 69.8% percent of hospices operating service delivery programs outside of the Medicare Hospice Benefit model and include:

- From 15.9% operating formal pediatric palliative care programs with specialized staff.
- 79.6% offering palliative consult services in any setting.
- 73.4% offering palliative care services at home or in an inpatient facility.
- 62.5% offering post-hospice support programs for patients discharged alive.[12]

## Expanded Hospice Palliative Care Models

Although hospice appears to add value to end-of-life care, and although it does not cost government payers significantly more, the Medicare Hospice Benefit alone is not meeting all the needs of communities for comprehensive, high-quality hospice and palliative end-of-life care.[13] The most prevalent model of U.S. hospice care, the "Medicare hospice model," is not viewed as the answer to the challenge of just or equitable access to hospice care nationwide.[14] Hospices compatible with this model provide all or almost all of their care within the eligibility requirements and funding parameters of the Medicare (and Medicaid) hospice benefit; this creates numerous access barriers. These hospice models are much less likely

**Table 2-1**
**Suncoast Hospice Coordinated Continuum of Hospice Services Across the Lifespan**

| | | Center for Caring | | |
|---|---|---|---|---|
| Center for Community | Center for Living & Wellness | Palliative Care | Hospice | Center for Loss & Healing |
| • Public Engagement<br>• Community Mobilization<br>• Advocacy<br>• Web Access/& Virtual Communities<br>• Advance Directive Campaigns<br>• Community Ethics Center<br>• Advisory Counsels<br>• Community Education/End of Life Issues<br>• Speakers Bureau<br>• Workplace Awareness<br>• Community Library<br>• Faith In Action<br>• Hospice Teen Volunteers<br>• Hospice Youth Promoting Excellence<br>• Veterans Partnership<br>• Child and Family Support –Children's Education<br>• AIDS Service of Pinellas –Preventive Education<br>• Diversity Initiatives<br><br><u>PERSONS SERVED</u><br>• Everyone in Our Community<br>• Worried Well<br>• Friends, Neighbors, Caregivers | • Welcome/Comfort<br>• Service Inquiries<br>• Information & Referral Resources<br>• Care Planning<br>• Decision Making Consults<br>• PATH<br>• Advance Directives<br>• Patient/Caregiver/Client Counseling<br>• Wellness and Spiritual Direction<br>• Workplace Initiatives Regarding Illness & Caregiving<br>• Family & Children's Counseling (CFSP)<br>• AIDS Testing and Counseling<br><br><u>PERSONS SERVED</u><br>• All Who Come to The Center Seeking Our Services<br>• Clients Needing Assistance—Not Physical Care | • Palliative Care—Decisions—Consults<br>• Hospitals/NH—Palliative Care Partnerships<br>• Suncoast Supportive Care >1yr Life Expectancy<br>• Palliative Home Care<br>• Partners in Caring: Together for Kids (CFSP)<br>• Home Health Care<br>• AIDS Medicaid Waiver (ASAP)<br>• HIV Specialty Home Care<br>• Clinical Education in the Community<br><br><u>EMERGING/INNOVATION</u><br>• EOL as Disease State Mgmt.<br>• Disease Specific Care Programs<br>• Pain Programs<br>• Case Management<br>• Long Distance Case Mgmt.<br>• Waiver Programs<br>• Chronic Care Program<br>• Private Pay Home Care<br>• Senior Companion Service<br><br><u>PERSONS SERVED</u><br>• Patient with >1 yr. Life Expectancy & Their Care Givers | • Hospice at Home<br>• Continuous Care/Respite<br>• Hospice in Long Term Care<br>• Hospice in ALFs<br>• Inpatient Hospice in Hospitals & Nursing Homes<br>• Woodside Hospice House Inpatient<br>• Residential<br>• Caregiver Program<br>• Caregiver Support<br>• Education/Inspiration<br>• Caregiving Network Incl. Families Out of Area<br>• Jewish Hospice<br>• Children's Hospice<br>• HIV Hospice<br>• Team IMPACT<br>• IV Team<br>• Pharmacy<br>• DME<br>• Bereavement Care<br>• Quality of Life Funds<br>• Palliative Arts<br>• Suncoast Supportive Care <1 yr Life Expectancy<br><br><u>PERSONS SERVED</u><br>• Persons with <1yr Life Expectancy<br>• Medicare Hospice Benefit Patients/Families | • Bereavement Care for Community Survivors<br>  –Individual Counseling<br>  –Family Counseling<br>  –Groups<br>  –Support Programs<br>  –Social Events<br>  –Camps/Retreats/Education<br>• EAP Grief in the Workplace<br>• Resources/Literature/Library<br>• Emergency Response<br>• Sudden Death Interventions<br>  –Mass Losses<br>  –CISD for Responders<br>  –Traumatology Specialists<br>• Specialized Bereavement Care<br>  –Suicide Survivors<br>  –Homicide Survivors<br>  –Accidents/Sudden loss<br>• CFSP<br>  –Children's Bereavement Care<br>  –Pediatric Loss Programs<br>  –Perinatal Loss<br>  –Bereavement camps/retreats<br>• ASAP<br>  –Loss from HIV/AIDS<br>• High Risk Hospice Survivors<br><br><u>PERSONS SERVED</u><br>• All in the Community Who Have Experienced/Been Touched by Loss |

*Source:* Copyright © 2009 Suncoast Hospice. Reprinted with permission.

to admit individuals who do not meet Medicare hospice eligibility requirements (i.e., those without a 6-month terminal prognosis and those who do not choose to relinquish all curative care options). They are also less able to admit individuals whose palliative care treatments and medications are costly, although the receipt of costly beneficial palliative care treatment has increased.[14]

With the understanding that the Medicare hospice model needs to expand to meet the growing needs for palliative care, hospice programs nationally are developing expanded models. Jennings and colleagues[15] described two models of hospice care that provide care beyond the Medicare hospice model (Table 2–2). The first of these is the *Community Hospice*; hospices compatible with this model rely on Medicare hospice revenue but also provide services that reach beyond the Medicare hospice patient to individuals who may not meet the eligibility requirements of the MHB or who do not wish to choose Medicare hospice. However, although the community hospice model is considered superior to the Medicare hospice model, a third form—the *Comprehensive Hospice Center*

model—was believed by Jennings and colleagues to be better for addressing the hospice and palliative care needs of communities. Comprehensive hospices provide all the care and services provided by community hospices but, in addition, they also have a dedicated academic mission.[15] Considering this, comprehensive hospices are "centers of excellence" for hospice and palliative care.

Since the Jennings study an expanded model of the "Comprehensive Hospice" has evolved and includes all the features of the previous models but adds a focused structure and processes to integrate and collaborate with care and service partners in the community it serves. This model focuses on building communities of caring through social responsibility and change. Examples of types of programs added would be *Faith in Action*—a partnership program between faith communities and hospices that train and support volunteers to care for others in their community. Another may be a partnership *day care program* with a senior center, or a partnership *teen volunteer program* with school systems.[16]

**Table 2–2**
**Services Provided by the Medicare Hospice Model and Extended Hospice Models**

| Medicare Hospice Model | Community Hospice Model (in Addition to All Medicare Hospice Model Services) | Comprehensive Hospice Model (in Addition to All Medicare Hospice Model and Community Hospice Model Services) |
|---|---|---|
| Core services, required by law: Florida Statutes Section 400.609(1) <br>   Physician <br>   Nursing <br>   Social work <br>   Pastoral or counseling <br>   Dietary counseling <br>   Bereavement counseling <br><br> As needed services, provided or arranged for patient <br>   Physical therapy <br>   Occupational therapy <br>   Speech therapy <br>   Massage therapy <br>   Home Health Aide services <br>   Infusion therapy <br>   Medical supplies <br>   Durable medical equipment <br>   Day care <br>   Homemaker/Chore services <br>   Funeral services | Services and care for patients and families <br>   Community support groups/programs <br>   Palliative care treatments <br>   General palliative care <br>   Caregiver programs <br>   Specialized staff in hospitals for supportive palliative care and pain and symptom control <br>   Special hospice therapy programs <br>   Veteran's initiative <br>   Telephone installation in patient's home <br>   Assistance with home renovation or modification <br>   Caregiver/Companion funded program <br>   Durable medical equipment <br>   Pharmacy <br>   Specialized HIV/AIDS care teams <br><br> Services and programs for communities at large <br>   Community education programs <br>   Workplace initiatives and support <br>   Community support groups and programs <br>   Community programs to youth <br>   Community programs for crisis/emergency <br>   Professional education <br>   Faith-based initiatives <br>   Cultural/Diversity initiatives <br>   Community programs for the needy | Research/Academic endeavors <br>   Structured sharing of knowledge through presentations and publications <br>   Best practice protocols and services—designing, assessing, and educating staff <br>   Academic-based research affiliations <br>   Research on end-of-life care <br><br> Community advocacy <br>   Partner in a community coalition on end-of-life issues |

*Source:* Jennings et al., reference 15.

## Hospice Palliative Care Approach

Hospice approach supports the long-term objective of creating a personalized experience with each patient and family at the end of life, with a particular focus on opportunities to find meaning, growth, and quality end-of-life and relationship experiences in the midst of a very difficult time. Promoting quality of life and relationships, as well as death with dignity, hospice assists the patient and family to live each day as fully as possible for their remaining time together.

## Honoring the Patient's and Family's Experience

The experiences of advanced illness, dying, and caregiving have significant and profound effects on both the patient and the family. Therefore, hospice supports both patient and family as the unit of care. Family is defined as not only the biological relatives, but also those people who are identified by the patient as significant.

Patients and families face many changes and losses during the last years of life. Patients often become concerned about the burden they may cause their family and how their family will survive after they are gone. Families become concerned about how to care for the patient, how to adapt to role changes, their reactions to their losses, and how their lives will change after the death. Families provide varying degrees and types of support, love, and compassion during times of change and crisis. As the patient becomes more dependent on others for care, families become even more significant in this process. Yet, many families have never experienced caring for a loved one who is dying or actually losing someone so close to them.

By understanding the importance of these relationships and family dynamics, hospice can minimize patient and family suffering and enhance experiences through education, support, and services. Hospice honors the intimate and important role of the family in caregiving and offers resources, education, and support, so that family members can be involved in a meaningful way with the care of their loved one.

The death of an individual is an unwanted but also an inevitable and unavoidable event within the life of every family. In addition to responding to family members' suffering, when a patient is not expected to survive, supportive counseling of families extends to offering suggestions for interacting, touching, or spending time with the patient and, when appropriate, encouraging culturally consonant ways of completing relationships, celebrating shared lives, and saying goodbye.[7]

Care does not stop after the death of the patient. Just as the patient's death experience involves the physical, emotional, spiritual, and social dimensions, survivors' reactions to caregiving and loss are experienced through the same dimensions. There is continued commitment to bereavement services for both family members of hospice patients and for the community at large. For a minimum of one year following their loved one's death, grieving families can receive hospice bereavement education and support. In 2007, for each patient death, an average of two family members received bereavement support from their hospice. This support included follow-up phone calls, support groups, specialty bereavement groups for traumatic deaths, educational sessions, visits and mailings throughout the post-death year. Most hospice agencies (94.7%) also offer some level of bereavement services to the community members whose loved one was not served by hospice.[7]

## Care Is Directed by Patient and Family Choices and Values

The hospice approach supports the understanding that dying is the patient's and family's experience. Nurses are challenged to approach the hospice care process differently from other situations. Hospice care begins and continues with ongoing facilitated discussions with the patient and family, to discern what is most important to them—their values, choices, wishes, and needs for the remaining life and death. This information becomes the foundation that directs the team in the provision of care and services. Goals become patient–and-family goals rather than nurse-directed goals. It is not about what nurses feel is best, but about what the patient and family choose and decide for themselves. The care plan becomes the "patient/family care plan," and the care process is defined by what the patient and family decide is important for this time. A care process directed by patient and family values begins to differentiate the specialty of hospice nursing. This goal is achieved when the nurses and other team members continuously offer opportunities for the patient and family to identify what is most important in completing their relationships, finding meaning in life closure, and reaching personal goals before and after the death.

## Hospice Care, Palliative Care, and Curative Care

Hospice is a defined, integrated model of palliative care, which can be as aggressive as curative care, focusing on comfort, dignity, quality of life/relationship closure, directed by patient/family goals and choices. Palliative care extends the approaches and principles of hospice care to a broader population that could benefit from receiving this type of care earlier in their illness or disease process. Palliative care, ideally, would segue into hospice care as the illness progresses and p care is most supportive when it is experienced throughout the care continuum, even concurrently with curative approaches. A patient receiving curative chemotherapy or radiation therapy could certainly benefit from palliative symptom management. From a psychological and spiritual perspective, patients and their families begin to think about the aspects of life and relationship closure from the time they recognize that the patient has an incurable disease. This is when they begin to think about both their own future course and about their loved ones—during as well as after death. Worries, fears and hopes are paramount, and it is vital to open the dialogue as soon as possible so patients' questions can be answered, and options and choices for dealing with their concerns can be offered. Questions that go unanswered or issues that are not discussed only create additional suffering. Questions answered and concerns brought to some resolution allow for a more peaceful life and death. Emotional and spiritual support from the time of diagnosis, including preparation for remaining life, advancing illness, caregiving, preparation for family left behind, death, and bereavement, creates optimal experiences.

Aggressive treatments in the last week of life increase difficult symptoms during dying, while longer time in hospice care appears to reduce distress at the time of death for people with advanced cancer. As part of the Coping with Cancer study, researchers found the more time patients spent under hospice care, the greater their quality of death. For example, patients who received at least five weeks of hospice care were in less physical distress in their last week of life than those who lived less than a week with hospice, and those who received no hospice at all were in the most physical distress at the end of their lives. These results suggest that when patients are actively dying, the use of aggressive treatments should be considered with caution and only pursued with the full understanding of patients or their surrogate decision makers. Researcher Silverman pointed out that discussions about prognosis, goals of care, and treatment preferences, including the option of hospice care, should occur with more patients and earlier in the course of the disease.[18]

When a patient's disease process is no longer curable or reversible, aggressive curative treatment becomes increasingly inappropriate. An aggressive curative approach to care may actually cause more suffering if cure is no longer possible, or it may needlessly extend the period of suffering. As a patient advocate, the hospice nurse and other team members must understand the differences between curative and palliative interventions to avoid futile care, to prevent unnecessary suffering, and to be able to have conversations with the patient and family about the benefits and burdens of different care options.

The curative model of care has an inherent problem orientation. Practitioners are often trained to assess and identify "problems" and then determine how to reverse the problem and its effects. Palliative care moves beyond problem identification. The specialty of hospice nursing involves the expert management of end-stage disease symptomatology as a prerequisite to providing the opportunity for patients and families to experience life completion and relationship closure in ways that are personally meaningful. Hospice expands the traditional *disease, problem-oriented model* to a proactive, preventive, *quality of life experiences approach* that reflects the full scope of the patient's and family's illness, dying, and caregiving experiences.

Through anticipation and prevention of the negative effects of physical symptoms, suffering can be decreased; this allows the patient and family the time and personal resource energy to attend to their living while dying. Moving beyond a simple problem orientation, the focus has become one of prevention of suffering and opportunity for growth rather than simply the physical reaction to disease.

A search for meaning and purpose in life is a common experience for people in their last years of life and for their families. From the individual experience of suffering, death can be a time for personal growth, deepening or reconnecting interpersonal and spiritual relationships, and preparing for death and afterlife with enrichment of meaning.

## Autonomy and Choice

The hospice approach promotes patient and family autonomy in which illness, caregiving, and dying are directed by the patient's and family's desires. Hospice strongly believes in patient choice regarding all aspects of living, caregiving, dying, and grieving, including where they will die, how they will die, and with whom they will die. Respecting the patient's and family's choices is paramount to quality hospice palliative care.

One of the greatest concerns of the dying patient and the family is the fear of loss of control. Many losses are anticipated and experienced by terminally ill patients and their families, including loss of bodily functions, loss of independence and self-care, loss of income with resulting financial burdens, loss of the ability to provide for loved ones, loss or lack of time to complete tasks and mend relationships, and loss of decision-making capacity. Dying patients have a right to remain in control of their lives and their deaths. They are often concerned that their wishes will not be honored, that their requests will not be answered, and that, when they are too ill to prevent it, control of their lives will be taken from them. It is critical to provide continued opportunities for choice, input, informed decision making, and the ability to change decisions as situations change.

The National Hospice Foundation outlines what patients and families want at this time in their lives, which includes:

1. The best of medical treatment, to improve function where possible and ensure comfort always.
2. Never having to endure overwhelming pain, shortness of breath, or other symptoms.
3. Care that is continuous, comprehensive, and coordinated.
4. Being prepared for everything that is likely to happen in the course of the illness.
5. Having their wishes sought and respected, and followed whenever possible.
6. Having the opportunity to make the best of every day.[17]

## Informed Decisions and Autonomy

The hospice approach has been built on the ethical principle of veracity, or truth-telling. Patients' wishes for information about their condition are respected. Patients and families have the right to be informed about their conditions, treatment options, and outcomes so that they can make autonomous, informed choices and spend the rest of their lives the way they choose.

Truth-telling is the essence of open, trusting relationships. A sense of knowing often relieves the burden of the unknown. Knowing and talking about diagnosis and prognosis aids in making informed decisions. Patients who have not been told about their illness naturally suspect that something is wrong or being hidden from them, which can result in frustrating, unanswered questions. When patients and families are not told the truth, or when information is withheld, they can no longer make informed choices about the end of life.

Autonomy results in empowerment of the patient and family to make their own informed decisions regarding life and death. Hospice encourages the discussion of advance directives but does not influence those decisions. Hospice nurses and other interdisciplinary team members educate on these issues and offer support while the patient and family discuss and choose what is best for them. Their choices may change over time as the disease progresses, the patient becomes more dependent, or they accomplish their life and relationship closure goals.

When advance directives such as living wills, health care surrogacy, durable power of attorney, and do-not-resuscitate orders are honored, the patient's wishes can be carried out even if he or she is no longer able to communicate or to make health care decisions. With advance preparation, these directives can act in place of the patient's verbal requests to ensure that her or his wishes are honored. When patient and family members discuss advance directives together, there is often less conflict over decisions and family members are more comfortable supporting the patient's choices. When advance directives are combined with hospice approach, they can serve as preventive measures to ensure that patient's choices will be communicated, supported, and carried out, avoiding ethical dilemmas. It is critical to provide continued opportunities for discussions, choice, input, informed decision-making, and ability to change decisions as situations change. Hospice team members are trained to facilitate personal and family decision-making regarding care, service, and life closure issues. Often, simply having professionals comfortable enough to approach these issues allows patients and families to express their inner feelings, desires, and wishes.

Hospice care supports sensitivity in truth-telling to the degree that the patient and family choose, encouraging open communication among the patient, the family, physicians, and the hospice team. Preparation for death becomes difficult if communication is not open and truthful. With a truthful understanding and freedom of informed choice, patients are more able to control their own living and dying instead of being controlled by the disease or by the treatment plans of others. They can put their affairs in order, say their goodbyes, and prepare spiritually in a way that promotes quality and dignity.

## Dignity and Respect for Patients and Families

Quality end-of-life care is most effective from the patient and family perspective when the patient's lifestyle choices are maintained and his or her philosophy of life is respected. Individual patient's and family's needs vary depending on values, cultural orientation, personal characteristics, and environment. Dignity is provided when individual lifestyles are supported and respected. This requires respect for ethnicity, cultural orientation, social and sexual preferences, and varied family structures. Hospice nursing requires the provision of nonjudgmental, unconditional, positive regard when caring for patients and families, honoring each person's experience as unique and valuable.

Each person and family has individual coping skills, varied dynamics, strengths and weaknesses. It is our responsibility to accept patients and families "where they are," approaching living and dying in their own way. Patients and families should be encouraged to express any emotion, including anger, denial, or depression. By listening without being judgmental, the hospice nurse accepts the patient's and family's coping mechanisms as real and effective.

Dying patients have their own needs and wants, and hospice nurses must be open to accept direction from the patient. A patient's focus may include saving all of one's energy for visits from loved ones, loving and being loved, sharing with others one's own philosophy of life and death, reviewing one's life and family history, and sharing thoughts and prayers with one's family or caregivers. Patients' goals may include such things as looking physically attractive or intrinsically exploring the purpose and meaning of their lives. Hospice workers' openness and ability to accept and support the patient's and family's direction on any given visit helps facilitate achievement of their goals. The patient's and family's own frame of reference for values, preferences, and outlook on life and death is considered and respected without judgment.

Respecting patients requires hospice nurses to approach their communications and care in a way that ensures patients and families can express their values and opinions, participate in care planning, make decisions regarding how they choose to spend their time, and participate in their own care. Fostering an environment that allows the patient and family to retain a sense of respect, control, and dignity is the foundation of hospice care and services.

## The Hospice Nurse as Advocate

Enhancing quality of life and relationships is the primary goal of hospice and palliative care. Patients who, in the later stages of their life, have chosen to receive palliative care have a right to have their wishes honored and respected at all points of entry into and across the health care continuum. Optimizing quality of life and respecting patient's and family's wishes involves a great deal of commitment, collaboration, and communication. In promoting patient autonomy, hospice nurses participate as patient advocates across all care settings, supporting the choices and goals that the patient and family have selected for the remainder of their lives.

By integrating the hospice approach and values, the hospice nurse acts as advocate for the patient and family to preserve their rights and protect the goals of their palliative care plan. The hospice nurse's role of professional advocacy involves collaboration with patients, families, physicians, health care institutions, health care systems and faith communities. She or he may be involved in advocating for appropriate symptom management, identifying valuable resources, and coordinating the utilization of community resources and services. Clinicians have a responsibility to provide accurate information to patients and families, conveyed in words they can understand, about the patient's condition and treatment options and to guide them in a decision-making process that respects the individual's and family's ethnic and cultural values. Ultimately, clinicians must respect the autonomy rights of individual patients to choose between available options for care and to refuse any indicated treatment that is offered.[19]

The patient, family, hospice IDG, physician, hospice organization, other health and human service providers, and legal institutions are all affected by patient choices. It is the responsibility of every care provider to respect and ensure the rights of dying patients and their families.

## Hospice Palliative Care Delivery Systems

Hospice care is not defined by a distinct physical setting or individual organizational structure. It is provided in a variety of settings. In 2007, 70.3% of hospice patients received care in their residence; 19.2% received care in an inpatient facility; and 10.5% of patients died in an acute care hospital setting. Although a majority of hospice patient time is spent in a personal residence, some patients live in long-term care facilities, assisted-living facilities, continuous care retirement communities, hospice care centers, or other group settings. In addition, some hospices provide day care programs. In 2007, approximately 3,500 hospice programs were in existence in the United States, for a total of 4,700 sites, including satellite offices, and 450 dedicated inpatient units and facilities. As identified by the NHPCO, the following organizational structures of hospice programs exist, with ever-expanding care and service designs to meet the needs of varied communities:[12]

Free-standing entities represent approximately 58.3% of hospice programs, and are defined as being independent of affiliation to a hospital, home health care agency, or other care agency.

Hospices affiliated with hospitals, home health agencies, or nursing homes are managed as departments or divisions of those systems and represent 41.7% of hospice programs.

Hospice dedicated inpatient unit or facilities were operated by 19.7% of hospice agencies.[12]

## Hospice Palliative Care and Service Sites

Private Homes. Encompassing the philosophical principle of autonomy, hospice supports patients and families wherever they choose to live and die. Therefore, hospice services are offered to patients' staying at home until death, if that is their choice. With so many people choosing to stay at home with family, hospice emphasizes the need to empower families so they may participate in meaningful ways in the care of their loved one. Hospice's ability to involve the family in caregiving often improves the family's perspectives and experiences.

Long-Term Care Settings. As the population ages, health care professionals are challenged to provide care and services in different ways. Hospices are increasingly serving elderly people, many older than 75 years of age, who live alone or with a frail family caregiver. As evidenced by the ongoing expansion of elder-care communities to meet the growing demand of the aging boomers, the definition of "home" has also changed for many elderly persons and can include a variety of residential settings with various levels of assistance. Some hospice patients are referred while residing in long-term care, whereas others are transferred into long-term care after being served by a hospice program at home. As patient and family needs change at the end of life, hospice home care patients may find long-term care placement a chosen, necessary alternative care setting.

There are many potential benefits to a partnership approach between hospices and nursing homes; their coordinated resources and efforts can result in optimal experiences for the resident and family. The potential benefits of a partnership to residents and their families or significant others are detailed in Table 2–3.

Research on the benefits of hospice care in nursing homes has focused on medical dimensions of support. This research has shown that hospice residents, compared to nonhospice residents, experience fewer hospitalizations near the end of life, have fewer invasive treatments (e.g., enteral tubes, intravenous fluids, intramuscular medications), and receive analgesic management for daily pain that is more in agreement with guidelines for management of chronic pain in long-term care settings.[13,20,21] Family members of persons who died in nursing homes perceived improvements in care after hospice admission; they cited fewer hospitalizations and lower levels of pain and other symptoms after hospice admission.[22] Nonhospice residents in nursing homes also appeared to benefit from hospice presence in the nursing home. Nonhospice residents residing in nursing homes with a greater hospice presence (i.e., a greater proportion of residents enrolled in hospice), compared with those in homes with limited or no hospice presence, were less frequently hospitalized at the end of life and more frequently had a pain assessment performed.[22,23] Considering the cited potential and actual benefits, collaboration seems to be a care alternative worthy of pursuit.

**Table 2–3**
**Benefits of Hospice and Long-Term Care Collaboration**

| Benefits to Patient/Family | Benefits to Long-Term Care Facility and Staff | Benefits to Hospice Provider |
|---|---|---|
| Access to care expertise in both long-term care and hospice care | Additional professionals to help with care planning and provision | Professionals expert in chronic residential care |
| Additional attention from the increased number of people involved in care | Interdisciplinary team expertise in the specialty of palliative care | Nursing home staff who know and support the resident as their extended family |
| Access to counseling and spiritual care disciplines to meet the intense and varied needs that surround the end-of-life experience | Shared expertise in pain and symptom management | Extended team to help in care of resident 24 hr/day, 7 days/wk |
| Access to hospice volunteers who spend time with residents and provide diversional and quality-of-life activities that nursing home staff do not have time to provide | Ethical decision-making consulting services | Clinical expertise in chronic care |
| Access to hospice volunteers who assist and support families and significant others so they can spend more quality time with residents | Family decision-making counseling | More people to provide services near life's end |
| Continuity of care team providers | Hospice nursing assistant visits to supplement the increasing intensity of hands-on care | |
| Coverage of medications, medical supplies, and equipment related to terminal illness | Validation of residents' palliative care (and care outcomes) needs to an outside reviewer (such as federal government quality indicator outcomes that, if observed for nonpalliative care patients, would be considered negative outcomes) | |
| Access to professionals who specialize in supporting residents and families to a more meaningful life closure | Expertise in documenting palliative care assessment, interventions, and expected outcomes that differ from restorative/rehabilitative outcomes | |
| Additional support for family members providing care and anticipating life without their loved one | Volunteers to sit with residents so they are not alone | |
| Bereavement support for family members for up to 12 months after the resident has died | Grief support for other residents | |
| | Grief support for nursing home staff who experience cumulative loss with the deaths of many residents | |
| | Education for staff on palliative care | |

*Source:* Miller SC, Egan KA, reference 26.

Many hospice programs also have arrangements to admit hospice home patients into long-term care facilities for respite care. *Respite care* is care for a limited period of time that provides a break for the family while the patient is cared for in another setting. Wherever the patient resides, hospice philosophy can be incorporated and care provided by the full IDG in collaboration with the long-term care staff.

The hospice IDG again advocates and supports autonomy in decision-making by providing information on many alternative care options to the patient and family when home care is no longer appropriate. The hospice nurse and team have the responsibility to educate the family about patient care needs and to respect and support the family's ability to set limits and acknowledge their own needs in placing their loved ones in other care settings.

*Assisted-Living and Comprehensive Care Retirement Community (CCRC) Settings.* With the aging of the population, there are a variety of elder-care living settings in which people may be dying. Recent expansion of adult living facilities (ALFs)

and CCRCs has presented the challenge to care for people while allowing them to "age in place" and to "die in place." In the past, facilities licensed as ALFs were required to transfer a resident out of their facility if they could not independently provide care. For many people, this removed them from their home environment as they came closer to death, often resulting in loss of all sense of control over their lives. These residents were prevented from "aging in place" and "dying in place."

Recognizing the detrimental effects of moving people at this time in their lives, residents in ALFs in many parts of the country are now able to stay in the ALF until death, as long as hospice is involved in their care. The end result supports patient autonomy related to where and how the patient chooses to live until life's end. Just as in other care settings, the hospice team remains the care manager in collaboration with the family and ALF staff to advocate for the patient's and family's palliative care goals.

*Hospice Inpatient and Residential Facilities.* Expanding as another alternative setting for people who can no longer stay in their own home is hospice inpatient and residential care. Inpatient or residential hospice care refers to the care provided in a facility that is staffed and owned by hospice programs. Patients and their families are given the choice of admission to a hospice facility setting if they are no longer able to care for themselves at home and do not have a caregiver, or if the caregiver is either frail or working and unable to provide care at home. Patients may also be admitted to a hospice facility when needs for care (especially highly skilled technical care) are more than the family can manage at home. The same hospice services are available at the hospice facility as in private homes. Family of patients at hospice facilities are encouraged to participate in the care to their level of comfort, but hospice staff and volunteers are available 24 hours a day to provide needed care, support, and assistance. The number of hospice facilities is growing as communities are realizing their value in filling a care need not provided in the same way in other settings.

Nearly one in five hospice agencies operate a dedicated inpatient unit or facility. Most of these facilities are either free standing or located on a hospital campus and provide a mix of general inpatient and residential care. Short-term inpatient care can be made available when pain or symptoms become too difficult to manage at home, or the caregiver needs respite time. NHPCO estimates that more than 450 inpatient facilities were operating in the U.S. in 2007.[7]

Children, adolescents, young adults, and the elderly can be cared for in hospice residential settings. Consistent with hospice philosophy, admittance to residential care should not depend on race, color, creed, or ability to pay. Admission to hospice residences is based on the needs and preferences of the patient and family. Some hospice programs have admission guidelines that restrict their residential care option to those who are closer to death (e.g., within 2 months). However, other programs have found this option of care to be beneficial for many different reasons and have not limited its use or length of stay to a specific time frame.

Hospice seeks to create a community of caring within its residences and facilities, striving to be flexible and home-like. Patients may follow their own personal schedule, and their visitors have unlimited access. Patients are usually free to come and go as they please and are encouraged to bring some of their belongings to create an environment that is most comforting to them. The residential setting promotes community and affirms life by offering group activities, group meals, events, and celebrations that promote socialization. Patient choice in participation is respected.

*Palliative Care Units.* One approach to meeting the expanding needs of patients and families is evident in the growing number of partnerships between hospital systems and hospice programs. A study conducted by the NHPCO and the Center to Improve Palliative Care identified various structures currently in place to meet the palliative care needs of patients in acute care. Their report, *Hospice–Hospital Collaborations: Providing Palliative Care Across the Continuum of Services,* offers glimpses of how some models of collaboration are contributing to the expansion

of palliative care in the hospital setting. Hospital–hospice collaboration is generally proceeding on two tracks. The first overall direction lies in enhanced use of the MHB for appropriate patients by promoting closer relationships between hospice programs and hospitals, offering education, developing specialized units, and encouraging the direct admission of hospitalized patients to hospice. The second track involves development of new, nonhospice benefit services, such as hospice palliative care management and consultation services.[24] It is now recognized that palliative care should not be an alternative to curative or life-prolonging treatment but should be offered in conjunction with such medical treatment. It is also recognized that this type of care is increasingly important as the health care system faces the need to find ways to treat the growing number of older adults with complex chronic illness.[24]

The Center to Advance Palliative Care report states that in 2007, there were over 2,000 hospitals in the United States with existing or developing palliative care programs. Many of these programs are in partnership with hospice programs to offer services across the continuum of care settings.[25]

These units offer a range of services within those facilities, including palliative care consultation, palliative case management, caregiver support and counseling services, and full MHB services. The expertise of acute care professionals coupled with that of hospice professionals allows for the combined benefits of both systems in care of patients at the end of life. Generally, there are patients in palliative care units who are placed there as hospice patients needing acute care interventions or as transfers from the acute care hospital settings. This usually occurs when a transition to hospice may be beneficial or the palliative care expertise of hospice will be beneficial earlier in the disease progression before Medicare model hospice services are instituted.

Palliative care units provide an option that allows attention to acute symptomatology by expert end-of-life clinicians, while encouraging comfort and dignity for patients and families. These units also provide the opportunity for a smooth transition from the curative to the palliative model of care.

*Hospital Settings and Hospice.* In addition to inpatient palliative care consultation and case management services, inpatient hospital care is an option for hospice patients and families, usually to meet their acute care needs. Most hospice patients admitted to the hospital setting are considered to be inpatients, as defined by the Medicare levels of care, receiving skilled care. Although most patients prefer to live out the remainder of their lives in their homes, there are times when inpatient hospitalization is requested or necessary to meet the changing needs of patients and families.

The reasons for hospitalization can vary. For some patients, the physician may request hospitalization for acute problems, including exacerbation of symptoms that are difficult to control in a home care setting. The patient may also require hospitalization for palliative surgical intervention. At times, hospice patients are admitted to the hospital for a condition that is not related to their terminal diagnosis. Physical needs resulting in hospitalization vary from patient to patient and should be an option in response to patient need and choice.

Some patients may request hospitalization for a fracture repair, whereas others may request to stay at home with medication for pain control. In situations involving possible hospitalization, it is important for the hospice nurse and the IDG to be available to explore with the patient the available choices in care and care setting before hospitalization. The patient and family should also remain involved in the plan of care, to determine how to best meet their changing needs. It is vital that the team provide the patient and family with other available services and care options, to prevent hospitalization if that is their wish.

While assessing the changing needs of patients and families, it is also important that the hospice nurse and IDG support patient and family choice regarding care setting and that they continue to honor the patient's and family's requests.

Other population groups receiving hospice care are the homeless and those in prison. These groups have posed challenges for hospice programs to expand service delivery options and provide care in all of these "homes."

### The Hospice Nurse's Responsibilities in Facility-Based Care Settings

Regardless of the type of setting, the hospice nurse and IDG are responsible for continuity of the patient's and family's palliative plan of care. When a patient is admitted to a facility, the hospice IDG remains the patient's care manager. Regulations also require collaborative care planning as well as documentation of mutually developed goals and interventions across care settings. (e.g., between long-term care facilities and hospice).[10]

To ensure the highest level of patient and family autonomy, hospice nurses have a responsibility to educate the facility staff about the philosophy, principles, and practices of hospice care. The staff should be able to integrate into their practice a dying patient's rights and their responsibility in allowing the patient to make his or her own decisions. The specialty of end-of-life symptom management and support of the emotional and spiritual aspects of life closure are still elusive to many nurses; therefore, hospice nurses are often involved in nonhospice settings, educating staff about protocols for pain and symptom management, as well as ways to assist patients and families with the emotional and spiritual aspects of closure of their life and relationships. Education of the staff improves the delivery of palliative care and makes the staff feel more confident and comfortable in caring for dying patients and their families—in contrast to the avoidance that sometimes comes from feelings of inadequacy.

Fundamentally, hospices and NHs do have common goals for residents and their families. If you were to ask the question, "What do you want for your resident?," the common response would be "comfort, compassion and dignity." Too often, these areas of common goals are misunderstood or overlooked, creating a barrier to collaborative care

approaches or openness to mutually respectful partner relationships. Optimal NH/hospice partnerships grow from understanding the value of common goals and collegial relationships. The misperception of differing goals prevents each partner from joining together toward common goals and instead creates a false belief that each partner's objectives are in opposition to the other. This misperception causes a failure to see or understand the value each brings to the partnership. What does differ between NHs and hospices is their usual care approaches. The NH is focused on restorative and rehabilitative approaches; the hospice concentrates on palliative care. An essential fact is that most nurses and nursing assistants do not receive training in palliative care in their core academic programs and therefore lack skill sets necessary for quality palliative care. Hospice is also responsible to provide this education to NH staff, helping to assure staff's competency in palliative care collaboration.

The following key factors were identified in successful NH/hospice partnerships and demonstrate principles of respectful collaboration:[26]

- Communicate commonalities—the resident's needs as primary drivers of collaboration.
- Be open to learn from each other, respecting the different areas of expertise each brings.
- Approach your partnership as if you wanted to provide the best possible service—not only to the resident and family, but to each other.
- Demonstrate knowledge, understanding and support of each other's schedules, systems, regulations, and challenges.
- Be proactive in anticipating and meeting each others' needs.

To provide continuity of care, the hospice nurse should be in contact with the facility staff to ensure the patient's and family's optimum physical, psychosocial, and spiritual status; that their goals and wishes are addressed; and that their decisions regarding advance directives are communicated. While respecting the policies and procedures of each setting, the hospice IDG must communicate and collaborate with the patient, family, physician, and facility staff to ensure continuity of the hospice plan of care.

### Hospice Care Provided Through an Interdisciplinary Group

#### The Hospice Experience Model: A Patient/Family Value-Directed Care Model

Nurses caring for patients and their families at the end of life need to first comprehend the basic differences between curative approaches and palliative end-of-life approaches that honor the unique experiences of patients and families.

Within the foundation of hospice philosophy, one of the significant differences in hospice nursing is the concept that the patient and family direct care, based on their personal values, culture, wishes, and needs. Such issues as dignity and quality can be defined only subjectively by those who are experiencing life changes associated with illness, caregiving, dying, and bereavement.

The *Hospice Experience Model,*[21] an end-of-life model based on patient/family choice and values, is founded on the following principles that apply to both the patient and family caregivers:

1. Illness, caregiving, dying & bereavement are unique, personal experiences.
2. People experience the last phase of life & relationships through many related dimensions (physical/symptom, function, interpersonal, well-being, transcendent).
3. The last phase of life and relationships provides continued opportunity for meaningful, positive experiences in the midst of suffering.

### Principle 1: Illness, caregiving, dying, and bereavement are unique personal experiences.

Respecting patients' individuality is the foundation of humane care. It requires confronting the fullness of the human context in which illness and aging occur. Individual patients must be the focus of attention, and their particular values, concerns, and goals must be recognized and addressed.[27]

Just as earlier stages of life for each individual are different, so is dying and end-of-life caregiving. How one adapts to changes brought on as a result of an end-stage disease process or by the normal slowing of systems associated with aging is a very personal response. This response reflects the diversity of an individual's life experiences. Looking to the future in end-of-life care and understanding the vast differences among individuals who are in the final phase of life, nurses must provide care that results in individualized, customized relationships that respect the values, culture, preferences, and expressed needs of the patient and family in the final phase of life and relationships.

What one person defines as quality of life in the final phase may differ drastically from the next person's definition, or differ at points in the life continuum. For one patient, self-determined life closure may mean not being dependent on life-sustaining machines, or having a living will. For another patient, it may mean being able to die at home, with family at the bedside. For the patient who has spent the last 3 years confined to a wheelchair, it may involve dying on the screened porch of a mobile home.

The hospice approach to care respects and honors the individual experiences of caregiving for the family and of illness and dying for the patient. To best meet the goal of supporting individualized dying experiences, nurses providing quality end-of-life care must use the guiding principles of autonomy or choice, advocacy, and acceptance.

### Principle 2: People experience the last phase of life and relationships through many related dimensions (physical/symptom, function, interpersonal, well-being, transcendent).

The caregiving and dying experience is one that affects all dimensions of a person. To comprehend the nature of suffering among the dying, it is essential to know and understand all dimensions of the person's experiences. Each dimension has a significant and dynamic impact on, and relationship with, the other dimensions. Understanding this dynamic relationship between dimensions guides the nurse in providing optimal end-of-life experiences for the patient and family.

Ira Byock and Melanie Merriman,[28] authors of the Missoula-VITAS Quality of Life Index (the only assessment tool designed to evaluate quality of life closure as an interdimensional, subjective experience of the patient), have developed an end-of-life construct based on Cassell's[29] topology of personhood. The basis for this construct is that people experience the last phase of life as multidimensional beings. In end-of-life care, as a person's physical and functional dimensions (experiences) decline, quality of life closure can be enhanced by additional attention to their interpersonal, well-being, and transcendent dimensions (experiences). Each dimension is briefly described as follows:

*Physical/Symptom Dimension:* a patient's experience of the physical discomfort associated with progressive illness, perceived level of physical distress; also, caregivers' experience of their physical response to caregiving, which may include fatigue or altered health as a result of the effects of caregiving or the lack of attention to their own health status.

*Function Dimension:* a patient's and family's perceived ability to perform accustomed functions and activities of daily living (ADLs), experienced in relation to expectations and adaptations to declining functionality; may include functional ADLs such as bathing, transfer, and feeding, but also includes the expanded aspects of those things that one does to "function" each day and within the social context, such as childcare, paying bills, maintaining a household, and employment or providing for family.

*Interpersonal Dimension:* degree of investment in personal relationships and perceived quality of one's relations with family, friends, and others; quality of relationships between the patient and others as well as the caregiver and others; from the caregivers experience, this specifically refers to the changes in their relationship with the patient as a result of the illness as well as the anticipated changes in the caregiver's life after the patient's death.

*Well-being Dimension:* self-assessment of internal condition, subjective sense of "wellness" or "dis-ease," contentment or lack of contentment, personal sense of well-being, how individuals feel within themselves; may include anxiety, sadness, restlessness, depression, fears, sense of peace, readiness, mindfulness, acceptance.

*Transcendent Dimension:* one's experienced degree of connection with an enduring construct; one's relationship on a transpersonal level, which may involve, but does not have to involve, spiritual or religious values; may involve one's perception of the meaning of life, caregiving, suffering, death, and afterlife.

Nurses must approach end-of-life care and caregiving with the understanding that a change in one of these dimensions affects the other dimensions. Assessing pain as a physical dimension without being prompted to assess how this has affected all of the other dimensions of that person's experience would neglect the full dying experience. Assessing fatigue of a family caregiver as a physical experience alone would not allow us to understand the full experience of the caregiver. In both of these cases, by not assessing the experiences from an interdimensional perspective, we miss the opportunity to affect the quality of the living experience that is resulting from illness or caregiving.

An example of a hospice nurse's assessment of a patient's shortness of breath and fatigue from an interdimensional perspective is illustrated in the following case study.

CASE STUDY

### Mrs. Palm, a Patient with End-stage Heart Failure

Mrs. Palm has increasing levels of fatigue and shortness of breath *(physical/symptom dimension)*. She can no longer walk from her bedroom to the bathroom or kitchen and is becoming more isolated and dependent on others *(functional dimension)*, *(interpersonal dimension)*. Mrs. Palm is showing signs of depression and withdrawal *(well-being dimension)*. She prays for God to take her, yet in the same prayers, asks for his forgiveness so she is worthy of heaven *(spiritual dimension)*.

Continuing with the understanding that the experiences of illness also impact the family, the nurse's interdimensional assessment of the family (Mrs. Palm's husband Charlie, who is frail himself and her primary caregiver) may be illustrated in the following.

Charlie is awakened many times during the night to assist Mrs. Palm and is becoming exhausted and often falls asleep in the chair during the daytime *(physical dimension)*. Charlie is no longer able to keep up with Mrs. Palm's care, the laundry, housecleaning, and cooking *(functional dimension)*. Afraid to leave Mrs. Palm alone *(well-being dimension)*, he no longer vists with his buddies in the mobile home clubhouse *(interpersonal dimension)*. He prays with Mrs. Palm, asking for strength, and praying that she will live as he does not know what he will do without her *(transcendent dimension)*.

Referred to as *interdimensional care*, this approach respects the full experiences of dying and caregiving and guides the nurse in affecting quality of life completion and relationship closure. If this patient's and family's situation were approached and assessed from a singular physical/symptom dimension perspective, opportunities to improve the quality of life completion and relationship closure for the patient and family in all of the other dimensions would be neglected.

When all dimensions are assessed and the patient or family member is able to direct her or his own care and support, an extraordinary possibility for growth, healing, dignity, and positive life and relationship closure can occur. There is opportunity for review, restitution, amends, exploration, development, and insight affecting all dimensions, thereby creating opportunities for positive experiences in the face of suffering.

Family caregivers also experience this phase of their lives through these related dimensions. With so many people choosing to stay at home with family, hospice emphasizes the importance of empowering families so that they can participate to the level they are able in providing care to the patient. In order to understand and honor the family's experience, it is important not to "take over" the care, but instead to provide resources, assistance and support so family members may find the potential for deep meaning and purpose in caregiving and the last phase of their relationship with the care-receiver. Hospice's ability to involve the family in caregiving often improves family members' perspectives and experiences. Research has shown significant differences in favor of hospice in three measures used to evaluate the quality of life of the primary caregiver (family). Primary caregivers for hospice patients were found to be find more gain in the caregiving experience, have a higher sense of confidence, and were better able to experience positive closure.[30]

**Principle 3: The last phase of life and relationship provides continued opportunity for meaningful, positive experiences in the midst of suffering.**

In his book, *Dying Well: The Prospect for Growth at the End of Life*, Ira Byock[31] first wrote about the opportunities for growth and development at the end of life. Sharing his observations of patients and families, he explained how people, in the midst of suffering, develop a sense of completion, find meaning in their lives, experience love of self and others, say their good-byes, and surrender to the unknown. Byock[32] conceptualized dying as a stage of the human life cycle that inherently holds opportunities to broaden the personal experience, determine "what matters most," influence the outcome for improved quality of life closure and, in so doing, reveal new sources of hope. He believes that individuality extends through the very end of life, characteristic challenges and meaningful developmental landmarks can be discerned, and representative tasks toward the achievement of goals for life completion and life closure can be identified. Byock elucidated the opportunity, during this last phase of life, for uncovering new or deeper sources of meaning in people's lives and in their dying.

It is important that a developmental approach to the end of life not be misconstrued as a set of prescribed requirements. Rather, these landmarks and tasks can become part of a conceptual framework in which to approach care processes, systems, and relationships. They can provide common language for clinicians to use with patients and families, helping them create meaningful experiences. How each patient and family chooses to attend to or accomplish these tasks will be specific to what is most important to them at this time in their lives, as reflected by their values, goals, and needs.

Byock's work was expanded and researched resulting in the *Aspects of Completion and Closure* (Table 2–4), which simplifies the language for clinicians, patients and families. *The Hospice Experience Model* incorporates the *Aspects of Completion and Closure* to address the interpersonal, well-being and transcendent dimensions of care.

They reflect the gradual process of life transition from worldly and social affairs, to individual relationships, and to intrapersonal and transcendent dimensions. In a landmark research project, *Caregiving at Life's End*, a national needs assessment of hospice family caregivers confirmed the hypothesis that family caregivers also experience these *Aspects of Completion and Closure* (Table 2–4), and the more they experience these aspects, the more comfort and gain they find in their caregiving experiences.[33]

In addition, the more family caregivers feel they have a positive impact on the life closure aspects for the care-receiver, the more meaning they find in the experience of caregiving. The aspects of completion and closure are closely interrelated for the patient and family caregiver, as illustrated in case examples shown in Table 2–5.

These *Aspects of Completion and Closure* offer a guide for professionals caring for patients and families in the last years of life. By first opening dialogue about the possibility of meaningful experiences related to the *Aspects of Completion and Closure*, we acknowledge and validate the patient's and family's experience. Then as each patient and family identify what is important, the hospice team helps to assess what is happening that is helping or hindering them from reaching their related goals while providing choices of interventions and support to reach their goals.

## Application of the Hospice Experience Model

Within our current culture, there seems to be an assumption that, once a terminal diagnosis has been given, meaningful life has ended. This limited perspective devalues and separates this last stage of life from the continuum of a person's existence, while minimizing hopes and possibilities for growth, comfort and peace. Hospice professionals have learned that dying and end-of-life caregiving are specific stages with unique experiences and accomplishments, and the *Hospice Experience Model* includes those lessons by integrating a framework for life completion and relationship closure.

Hospice nursing involves incorporating the three principles of the *Hospice Experience Model*: (1) Illness, caregiving, dying, and bereavement are unique, individual, and (2) interdimensional experiences of the patient and caregiver, with a (3) focus on finding meaningful, positive experiences utilizing the *Aspects of Completion and Closure*.

The ultimate goal is to guide patients and families as they identify what is important to them at this time in their lives, and focus their energies to realize their goals before the patient dies, and through the bereavement experience.

Quality of life closure is enhanced as the *Aspects of Completion and Closure* are realized by the patient and family.

Nurses along with their IDG members have the responsibility to attend to the physical and functional dimensions of care while supporting issues of life completion and relationship closure through the other dimensions (interpersonal, well-being, transcendent) so that patients and families can accomplish their goals to the extent that they choose. Accordingly, the hospice nurse's initial role is to work with the patient and family to prevent or minimize the suffering that results from the physical and functional decline of advancing age or from end-stage disease progression. It is after these dimensions are addressed and managed that the patient and family can attend to the life completion and relationship closure concerns that they feel are important. Nurses should be incorporating the spiritual and psychosocial team members in addressing the Aspects of Closure. When patients and families are able to attend to these aspects, their experiences become less burdensome, more positive, more peaceful and with less suffering.

Although each patient approaches the *Aspects of Completion and Closure* in his or her own way, there are some common characteristics. Generally, patients first address the aspects that relate to separating from and settling worldly affairs and community relationships, before those that involve moving away or separating from friends and family. Finally, they begin to move toward the tasks marked by introspection. As people get closer to death, it is common to observe a gradual withdrawal from worldly relationships, friends, and family as they begin the transition on their individual journey from life to death. The nurse's goal is to explain and normalize this experience, recruiting the IDG members to help preserve the patient's and family's opportunities to experience peace and comfort within themselves during their personal encounters with illness, caregiving, death, and bereavement.

Salmon and colleagues[33] confirmed the positive aspects of caregiver relationship closure through their research with hospice family caregivers. They found that hospice family caregivers:

- Indicated that they want practical information about caregiving, such as information that helps them to understand the illness, know how to

**Table 2–4**
**Aspects of Completion and Closure**
**The *Hospice Experience Model* of Care—Suncoast Hospice**

| Aspect | Core Content | Experiences and Activities |
|---|---|---|
| *The experience of caregiving at the end of life* | • The experience of caregiving<br>• Choice, advocacy, respect, dignity<br>• How caring affects caregivers | • Life as a caregiver<br>• Stories of caregiving<br>• Fears, wishes, concerns of caregivers<br>• Helping care receiver with physical, emotional & spiritual life transitions<br>• Focus on "How caregiving has affected you" & spending time on what is most important |
| *Aspects of completion and closure for the caregiver and the care-receiver* | • Self care redefined<br>• What is most important to caregiver & care-receiver<br>• Meaning & purpose<br>• Completion & closure<br>• Creating positive experiences | • Finding meaning and purpose in the experience<br>• "What is important to me and my loved one?"<br>• Creating positive experiences by focusing on what is important<br>• The experiences of relationship & life completion & closure<br>• Reframing the experiences of caregiving<br>• Conversation starters for difficult conversations |
| *Life affairs* | • Financial affairs<br>• Legal affairs<br>• Social affairs<br>• Family discussions & decisions<br>• Future care needs issues and plans | • Transfer of knowledge and/or responsibility from care receiver to caregiver (or others such as family members, legal guardian, etc.) for financial matters, legal matters, and/or health care decision-making<br>• Respect for and advocacy of care-receiver's wishes at the end of life<br>• Family discussions and planning for future care needs, wishes, concerns |
| *Relationships with community* | • Employment<br>• Social<br>• Congregational<br>• Organizational | • Changes and/or closure in multiple formal social relationships including employment, business, organizational, congregational, educational<br>• Expressing feelings regarding these changes such as regret, gratitude, appreciation, loss<br>• Maintain connections for care-receiver and self |
| *Personal relationships* | • Communication & acceptance<br>• Reconciliation in relationships<br>• Saying goodbye<br>• Family and personal legacies | • Life review—facilitating the telling of "one's story;" the telling of "our story" including the expression of meaning in care-receiver's life and relationships with caregiver, family, friends<br>• Acceptance of transmission of knowledge and wisdom from care-receiver<br>• Reconciliation of conflicts with care-receiver and other personal relationships<br>• Open, honest communication in important relationships<br>• Expression of regret, forgiveness and acceptance, gratitude and appreciation, affection and love, with family, friends<br>• Ways to "be present" with those who are important |
| *Experience of love of self and love of others* | • Acknowledging limitations/ expectations<br>• Forgiveness, worthiness, acceptance<br>• Unconditional love<br>• Validation, recognition | • Acknowledgement—affirmation and appreciation of self as a caregiver and as an individual<br>• Forgiveness—self-forgiveness, forgiveness to care receiver, others, a higher power/spiritual entity and acceptance of forgiveness from care receiver, others, spiritual entity/higher power<br>• Worthiness—worthy of giving and receiving love, of assistance with caregiving, of self-care<br>• Acceptance of strengths, limitations, realistic expectations, new role as caregiver and value of that role, of self beyond caregiving, of self as individual |

*(Continued)*

Table 2–4
Aspects of Completion and Closure
The *Hospice Experience Model* of Care—Suncoast Hospice *(Continued)*

| Aspect | Core Content | Experiences and Activities |
|---|---|---|
| *Acceptance of the finality of life* | • Feelings, attitudes and beliefs about death<br>• Physical, spiritual and psychosocial aspects of dying<br>• Anticipatory grief<br>• Finality of relationship and role | • Acknowledgment of the personal loss and personal tragedy represented by care-receiver's dying<br>• Anticipatory grief—Experience pain of loss (all losses, loss of care-receiver)<br>• Acknowledgement and/or acceptance of care-receiver's impending death<br>• Letting go—giving permission to die, assurance of your well-being, saying goodbye<br>• Understanding and/or acceptance of care-receivers withdrawal from worldly affairs, family, friends, caregivers and transition to the unknown<br>• Closure of relationship with care-receiver |
| *Meaning of life* | • Meaning & purpose as a caregiver<br>• Spiritual experience<br>• Sense of connectedness<br>• Acknowledgement of burdens and rewards | • Achieving a sense of awe about the journey, death and life<br>• Attending to the spiritual elements including recognition of life after death, recognition of a higher power, a connectedness with something greater than oneself, and/or spiritual growth, spiritual peace<br>• Acceptance of constant changes in life, growth in experiences<br>• Sense of meaning and purpose as a caregiver and in life |
| *Bereavement, renewal & resocialization* | • Readiness for death<br>• Acceptance of death<br>• Loss, mourning, grief<br>• The experience of renewal<br>• New life without loved one | • Loss of role as a caregiver<br>• The experiences and phases of grief<br>• New self beyond caregiver role<br>• Acknowledge, value and accept the new self<br>• Readiness for new life<br>• New self in personal relationships and community without your loved one |

*Sources:* Adapted from: Byock I. (1996), reference 32; The Hospice of the Florida Suncoast. Copyright © 2009 Suncoast Hospice.

give medications, make end-of-life decisions, communicate with health care professionals, and give hands-on care.
• Valued and felt comfortable with tasks such as understanding the illness and giving medications.
• Wanted to know what to expect at the time of death.
• Experienced greater caregiver gain when comfortable with what are known as the transformative tasks of caregiving—finding meaning and purpose, feeling closure, and self-acceptance.

These results support the principle of opportunity for gain and positive experiences in the face of suffering and clearly indicate the unique value of hospice services for family caregivers.

## The Experience of Illness and Dying: Nursing Process from a Hospice Perspective

Hospice nursing involves three broad areas: (1) approaching care from a patient- and family experience, interdimensional

care focus, as described earlier; (2) expertise in end-stage disease and symptom management; and (3) applying the nursing process as a member of the hospice IDG through a critical thinking approach that supports the Hospice Experience Model (Figure 2–1).

End-stage disease and symptom management present a unique challenge for many nurses when they begin hospice nursing. This challenge involves incorporating norms for disease progression and symptom management different from those applied in a curative model. Symptoms that are considered abnormal in a curative approach may become the expected norm for a person who is dying.

Pharmacological interventions for pain and symptom management are emerging as a body of knowledge that has not yet been integrated well into the core nursing curriculum. Nonpharmacological interventions that are considered appropriate for a patient on a curative path may actually increase suffering for a patient who is dying. An example may be encouraging intake of food and fluids. For a curative approach, this is appropriate to increase strength and healing. When a patient approaches death, however, the body's systems are

**Table 2-5**

Interrelatedness of Care-receiver and Caregiver Experiences & Aspects of Closure

| Care-receiver and Caregiver Tasks | Example of Interrelatedness (see Table 2–4) |
| --- | --- |
| *Care-receiver*: Sense of completion with worldly affairs<br>• Transfer of social responsibilities<br>*Caregiver*: Life affairs<br>• Transfer of knowledge and/or responsibility<br>• Advocacy of care-receiver's wishes | *Care-receiver*: Mr. Kent, the patient, wants his son (caregiver) to have power of attorney to manage his wife's financial accounts. Mrs. Kent has dementia, and he is concerned about having money available for her continued care after he dies.<br>*Caregiver*: Mr. Kent, an only child, does not want his dad to worry. He is willing to be the primary caregiver for his mother after his dad dies. He knows he will need to be able to manage the family money so that it is available for her care at home if he must hire additional help or if he needs to place her in a long-term care facility. |
| *Care-receiver*: Sense of completion in relationships with community<br>• Closure of multiple social relationships<br>• Expression of feelings<br>• Leave-taking<br>*Caregiver*: Relationships with community<br>• Changes and/or closure in multiple social relationships<br>• Expressing feelings<br>• Maintaining connections | *Care-receiver*: Mr. Jay wants to sell his business to his partner, because he can no longer attend to the clients.<br>*Caregiver*: Mrs. Jay does not want the business to be sold, especially because her husband worked so hard to make it successful. She was employed in the business until her spouse got very sick and could no longer care for himself. She feels she lacks some of the skills to be a partner but could team. She is hesitant to ask her husband about it, because he is so ill. She very much wants to spend time with her husband right now and has no time to attend to work. She feels she is losing both her husband and the family business. |
| *Care-receiver*: Sense of meaning about one's individual life<br>• Life review<br>• Telling "one's story"<br>• Transmission of knowledge and wisdom<br>*Care-receiver*: Sense of completion in relationships with family and friends<br>• Reconciliation, fullness of communication, and closure<br>• Expression of feelings<br>• Leave-taking<br>*Caregiver*: Personal relationships<br>• Facilitating the life review<br>• Acceptance of transmission of knowledge and wisdom<br>• Reconciliation of conflicts<br>• Open, honest communication<br>• Expression of feelings | *Care-receiver*: Mrs. Thomas is widowed and lives alone on the family farm. She has two daughters, both living in distant cities, having left the state for college, started careers, and seldom returned to the family home. When Mrs. Thomas became bed bound, her daughter, Judy, came to care for her and intends to share the caregiving with her sister. Mrs. Thomas tells stories about the girls' childhoods, trying to understand what she did to make her children want to leave the farm. She also tells stories about her own childhood and growing up on the family farm, her fame as the best cook in the county, and her willingness to take in stray animals. Judy is a successful corporate lawyer. Mrs. Thomas feels the need to relay to her daughter that success is not measured by money but by being "good to all creatures great and small."<br>*Caregiver*: Judy has taken a leave of absence from work to care for her mother for a month. She is very concerned about her job and corporate clients while she is away. When Judy returned home, she noticed the peace and quiet of her family home. As her mother told stories about her life and raising her and her sister, Judy realized how little she knew about the family tree and family history. She began to ask other questions about the family. As her mother provided advice about success and felt such accomplishment in what Judy considered "little things," Judy began questioning her own accomplishments and whether they really made a difference in anyone else's life. She began to examine her role as a caregiver and the difference it was making in her mother's life. |

*(Continued)*

**Table 2–5**
**Interrelatedness of Care-receiver and Caregiver Experiences & Aspects of Closure** (*Continued*)

| Care-receiver and Caregiver Tasks | Example of Interrelatedness (see Table 2–4) |
|---|---|
| *Care-receiver:* Experience of love of self<br>• Self-acknowledgment<br>• Self-forgiveness<br><br>*Care-receiver:* Experience of love of others<br>• Acceptance of worthiness<br>• Acceptance of forgiveness | *Care-receiver:* Mrs. Snider is dying from breast cancer, and her husband is her caregiver. Their son died when he was 4 years old; he drowned in the backyard pool while in her care. She was never able to forgive herself for the death of her son, and she believes her husband never really forgave her in the 50 years they have been together since that awful time. He grieved hard, and he punished her for her son's death by never really letting go of the grief. She feels she missed life because of her guilt and her husband's grief. With the help of the chaplain, Mrs. Snider has been able to forgive herself for her son's death, and she is glad that after death she will be reunited with him. She also realizes that her love of her husband allowed him to stay a shut-in, because she did not want to hurt him any more by leaving him. She only wishes he could forgive her. She did the best she could, and that is worth something. |
| *Care-receiver:* Sense of a new self beyond personal loss<br>• Acceptance of new definition of self<br>• Acknowledgment of the value of that new self<br><br>*Caregiver:* Experience of love of self and love of others<br>• Acknowledgment<br>• Forgiveness | *Caregiver:* After the death of his son, Mr. Snider felt he had no other reason to live. His legacy was gone, and he and his wife could not have any other children. They were so grief-stricken that he felt the need to protect both of them from the outside world, which became a lifelong pattern. They depended on each other for everything, never asking for help and never socializing with anyone. Since he lost his son, he has had difficulty loving anyone for fear he would lose them. Now he is losing his wife. Even though he tried not to love her for not being there when his son fell into the pool, he finds he still loves her. For the past 50 years, however, he has not shown his love to her. He also did not know he could care for anyone the way he has been able to care for his wife throughout this illness. The chaplain who visits is helping him feel better. He realizes that his grief filtered down to his relationships, and that it was okay to miss his son. He feels he had no right to punish his wife for this long; holding onto her so tightly to keep from losing someone else was not intentional and was a sign of love. Could she ever forgive him? He needs to show her his love and ask her forgiveness for his past actions. He is worried about life without her—he will have no one if he doesn't act now. Perhaps he will call his sister to help. |
| *Care-receiver:* Acceptance of the finality of life<br>• Acknowledgment of personal loss<br>• Expression of the depth of personal tragedy that dying represents<br>• Decthexis and cathexis<br>• Acceptance of dependency<br><br>*Care-receiver:* Surrender—"letting go"<br>• Will to die<br>• Acceptance of death<br>• Saying good-bye<br>• Withdrawal from family, friends, and professional caregivers | *Care-receiver:* Here she was, dying. She was so saddened to be leaving her kids, her husband, and her mother and father behind. There had been so much she wanted to do, such as seeing her children grow up and become mothers and fathers. She wanted to hold her grandchildren. She wanted to take care of her husband forever and her parents in their old age, not have her husband and parents take care of her. She wanted to learn how to play the piano. She would never be able to do any of these things. She could not even bathe or dress herself. The pain had become unbearable, and watching herself deteriorate was even more difficult. Flo counted on her faith and put all her troubles, the care of her children, and the care of her parents into God's hands. There was no turning back, and she began to welcome death. She said her good-byes and wrote letters to her children to be opened on special occasions after her death. She even wrote her memoirs so they would know the kind of person she was. She hired a nanny for the kids so that her husband could focus on his work and grief, and she gave him permission to remarry. As she became more ill, she withdrew and focused more on God and on the possibility of heaven and life after death. She was ready to die and wished God would take her now. |
| *Caregiver:* Acceptance of the finality of life<br>• Acknowledgment of personal loss/tragedy<br>• Anticipatory grief<br>• Acknowledgment and/or acceptance of the care-receiver's impending death<br>• Letting go—acceptance of care-receiver's withdrawal<br>• Closure of relationship with care-receiver | *Caregiver:* Michael was grieving the loss of his wife, his high school sweetheart. He had loved her forever. He had no idea how to raise the kids without her, how to go on without her. He had lost his future. He knew there was nothing more that could be done, and he was trying to support her as she prepared for her death. She was quickly withdrawing from everyone, including him, as she moved closer to death. She had asked him if he would be okay without her, and he had always said not to say that, because he would love her forever. He knew he had to say good-bye and tell her that he and the kids would be okay. But would he be okay? He did not think so, but perhaps she would help him from wherever she was. He said good-bye, and she died 3 hours later. |

*Care-receiver:* Sense of meaning about life in general
- Achieving a sense of awe
- Recognition of transcendent realm
- Developing/achieving a sense of comfort with chaos

*Caregiver:* Meaning of life
- Achieving a sense of awe
- Attending to the spiritual elements
- Acceptance of constant changes in life, growth in experiences
- Sense of meaning and purpose as a caregiver and in life

*Note:* The care-receiver and the caregiver usually do not go through this stage at the same time. The care-receiver usually finds meaning in life before he or she dies, whereas the caregiver may not find meaning in life until after the death, sometimes as a result of paralleling the care-receiver's journey and observing him or her make sense of death and look to the unknown with comfort. The care-receiver finds comfort with the chaos that surrounds dying, whereas the caregiver realizes that change is constant, that it is still affecting him or her, and that growth can result from change. In addition, while the care-receiver's focus becomes death, the caregiver's focus becomes one of life—a sense of awe about life, a new-found appreciation for life, a purpose in life (possibly a feeling of connectedness between this world and the next or between the self and a higher power or the universe). The caregiver may also find spiritual peace as he or she begins to feel that everything is connected, that there is meaning and purpose in caregiving and in life.

*Care-receiver:* Fred's health was declining rapidly. He became weaker and slept more. He was not eating and was taking only sips of fluids. He felt as though there was nothing more to do, nothing more to say, and he had somehow accepted death. He was comfortable with who he was and what he had accomplished. He felt in awe about life and what a wonderful gift it was to be able to live, but he also sensed that there was something greater, something beyond this place. While his daughter was running around and fretting about her job, her income, how much she had to do, and managing all his care and the community services he received, he found himself relaxing and actually trying to comfort her. He thought she was dumbfounded by how calm he was about dying. He was not sure he even knew why he was so calm, except that he knew there was nothing more he could do or had to do, and he instinctually felt that there was something beyond this world, something waiting for him, someone waiting for him. He hoped it was his wife and his favorite dog.

*Caregiver:* Katie missed her dad terribly, but she was glad her dad had died comfortably and peacefully. She felt as though he had somehow resigned himself to death a few weeks before he actually died. He tried to explain to her that he was not afraid and that she should take life less seriously, but she did not quite understand what he was saying, or perhaps she was too busy to think about it. She now felt privileged to have been a part of his life, his care, and his death. She never thought she could do it, but she had, and she very much wanted to tell other caregivers about how special it could be. Death was not as bad as she had thought it would be, either. It seemed so natural, and she felt such a sense of relief when her dad began talking to her mother, who had been deceased for 5 years. She felt a sense of hope about life after death, and a sense that life had a purpose even if she was not sure what that meant for her in the future. It would come to her; she just needed some time to grieve first. She also felt a renewed appreciation for life and hoped to enjoy it more fully when she felt more physically and emotionally able.

*Caregiver:* Bereavement—loss, mourning, and grief, renewal, resocialization
- Loss of role as caregiver
- Tasks of grief
- New self beyond caregiver role
- New definition of self
- Acknowledge, value, and accept the new self
- Readiness for new life
- New self in personal relationships and community
- Moving on

*Note:* Although the care-receiver is not physically present, the caregiver still honors and respects the memory of the deceased.

*Caregiver:* After the death of her partner, Joanne went through the stages of grief. It took her almost a year before she realized she was no longer a caregiver or the same person she had been before Susan died. She was partly her old self and partly someone stronger, more self-sufficient, and more appreciative of life. She now volunteers with the local branch of the Red Cross. She would never have given volunteering a thought before Susan died, but now she wants to make a difference in the lives of others. She still thinks about Susan frequently, especially during holidays and their anniversary, and when she is on the beach. The beach was where she and Susan met and where they shared their favorite activity of windsurfing. Just a few weeks ago, Joanne began windsurfing again. She hadn't done that since Susan became ill and she began caregiving. She also changed jobs to one she enjoyed. She likes her "new self." She still visits the gravesite every month to change the flowers and to honor the memory of her loved one. Lately, she has been thinking about dating again. She feels as though she will never find anyone like Susan and isn't sure she could love that deeply again, but she would enjoy some companionship.

*Source:* Adapted from Hospice Institute of the Florida Suncoast (2003), reference 33.

1. Have the primary team member (which is any discipline—the one most involved) begin by telling the story of who this patient/family are and were before the disease.

    IE: Mr. & Mrs. Johnson who have been married for 55 years and never without each other for more than a day. They lived in this town, were very active in community events as volunteers, and have raised three children who live out of state.

    IE: Mr. Smith has been a bachelor all his life. He was an elementary school teacher for the past 25 years, being awarded the "Teacher of the Year" three times. His mother lives in the next town and they have been very close, with Mr. Smith being her primary support. She can live alone but needs help with shopping, travel, and transportation to doctor, etc.

> **Critical Thinking Questions:**
>
> *Who are they as people?*
>
> *(Who are they aside from their disease/caregiving)*
>
> *What was their life like before the illness, changes as a result of the illness?*
>
> *How has their illness/caregiving changed the way they live?*

**Patient and Family Goals Directing IDG Care Planning**

2. Invite all of the disciplines who have been involved to share "How does that patient and family communicate their goals, wishes, needs at this time?"

> **Critical Thinking Questions:**
>
> *What is important to each of them?*
>
> *What experiences do they want now and/or for their future?*
>
> *What is meaningful with the current situation?*
>
> *What is not helpful or meaningful with their current situation?*
>
> *What would they still like to accomplish?*
>
> *How can that experience be addressed or reframed?*
>
> *What are the possibilities they may otherwise not consider?*

**Choices & Options:**
**Focusing on Patient & Family Strengths & Challenges**

**Choices & Options:**

3. Each discipline should then have the opportunity to share what they feel is happening with the team focusing on the patient/family strengths and challenges. All disciplines involved should have an opportunity to participate.
4. No issue, problem or opportunity is owned by any discipline because they belong to the patient/family. All disciplines can address and work on all dimensions (physical, functional, interpersonal, well-being, and spiritual).
5. Collaborate on how the team can help support their strengths, and provide options for them to choose to deal with their challenges.

> **Critical Thinking Questions:**
>
> *What is happening in this situation that is helping or hindering this patient and family from reaching their goals, wishes, needs?*
>
> *What choices and options can we offer this patient/family to support their strengths and minimize/reduce their challenges?*

**Figure 2–1.** The Hospice Experience Model of care: critical thinking approach to care planning and team discussion.

Outcome of Patient and Family Experiences:
Does Their Care Plan Help Them Meet Their Goals?

6.  IDG discussion on how the care plan choices and options have or have not changed the patient/family experience.
7.  Evaluation of effectiveness of care plan is based on whether or not the patient and family have been able to accomplish, meet, finish their end-of-life goals, wishes, and needs.
8.  Decisions to continue with current choices and options, add, change, delete.

*Critical Thinking Questions:*

*Have the patient goals been met?*

*Have the family goals been met?*

*How has the care plan interventions improved the quality of their experiences?*

*Now that they have met that goal, is there more they would like to happen?*

*What have they not even considered?*

**Figure 2–1.** Continued.

slowing. This slowing results in a decreased caloric requirement as well as a slowing of fluid perfusion. Forcing food and fluids could increase the demands on the gastrointestinal and circulatory systems, thereby creating increased discomfort. It becomes the responsibility of any nurse caring for patients at the end of life to gain specific knowledge and competence in end-stage disease and symptom management.

### Critically Thinking Through the End-of-Life Nursing Process

Illness, caregiving, suffering, dying, and bereavement evoke many interdimensional changes and reactions for both the patient and the family. By looking at the patient and family from this perspective, we begin to move away from a traditional, problem-oriented approach to a quality-of-life and relationship closure-oriented approach. All of the care processes and tools must therefore prompt a different critical thought process.[34]

Each step of the hospice interdimensional care process (assessment, care planning, goal setting, interventions, and evaluation) must involve three critical questions:

Question 1:  How do we honor the unique values, wishes, choices, hopes and experiences of those we serve?

Question 2:  How does an "experience" (issue/problem/opportunity) in one dimension affect other "experiences" (dimensions) of the patient and family?

Question 3:  Where are the opportunities for meaningful, positive experiences & quality of life completion and relationship closure?

The main steps of the hospice interdimensional care process are similar to the nursing process but with a focus on preventing and managing suffering and on quality of life completion and relationship closure rather than rehabilitation or cure. Nurses must also look beyond problem identification as they apply the interdimensional care process and anticipate changes to prevent suffering while preserving opportunity for growth. At each step of the care process (assessment, planning, intervention, and evaluation), the three critical thinking questions must be applied.

### Integrating the Hospice Experience Model with the IDG Care Process

Incorporating the nursing process into an interdimensional care process further defines the specialty of hospice nursing with the nurse working as a collaborative member of the IDG and expands the picture of the nursing process to an interdisciplinary, interdimensional care process. All disciplines on the hospice team are valued, and their expertise is combined. The steps of the hospice interdimensional care process are visualized with the *The Hospice Experience Model* and the IDG Care Process (Figure 2–2).

Each of the steps are outlined in the following paragraphs.

### Step 1: Assessing Interdimensional Experiences

Assessment begins with discussion soliciting information about the patient's and family's situation, including the values, wishes, and dreams that they identify as important. Data collection assesses all dimensions of a person and family as well as how changes in those dimensions affect the quality of life completion and relationship closure. Traditional nursing physical assessment is accomplished during this step, using norms for end-stage disease and symptom management.

Subjective and objective data are collected from a palliative, comfort care perspective and based on what patients and families define as important to them at this time. Their identified goals become the focus and driving force for the hospice team.

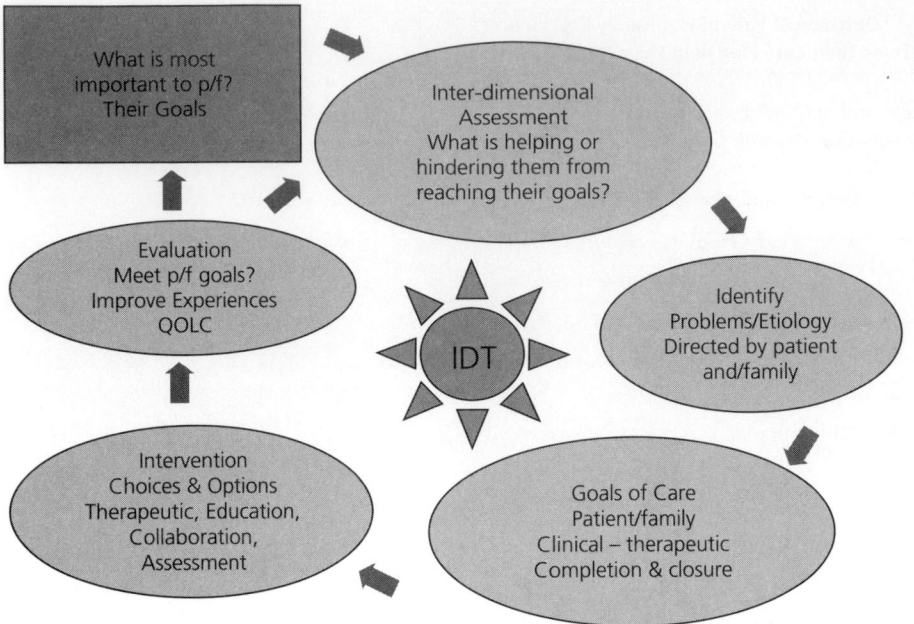

**Figure 2–2.** The *Hospice Experience Model* and the IDG Care Process. *Source:* Copyright © 2009 Suncoast Hospice. Reprinted with permission.

The focus of a palliative care assessment is to ask the question, "What is happening that is helping or hindering this patient and family from reaching their end-of-life goals?" From that perspective, the IDG supports integrated family systems theory, supporting the strengths of the patient and family while providing options for resources in areas of challenge.

### Step 2: Identifying Specific Issues, Problems, and Opportunities and Their Causes

The next step involves identifying specific issues, which is comparable to developing the nursing diagnosis. A specific issue, problem, or opportunity is defined from a palliative perspective, and the cause is identified. In this step, hospice differentiates between definitions of problems that are expected norms for the dying process and those that are unexpected or may cause secondary suffering for the patient or family.

For example, a patient may become incontinent as her or his systems fail and death is imminent. This is an expected physical change during the dying process. Assessment of this using an interdimensional approach might determine that the problem is the potential for skin breakdown (with the cause being incontinence), rather than incontinence as the primary problem secondary to advanced disease. Another problem or issue may be that the "spouse is exhausted from being awake all day and night changing the patient's linens" secondary to incontinence of the patient. What a nurse may instinctively identify as a problem in a curative model often becomes the *cause* of a problem in end-of-life care.

Another important difference in hospice nursing is that problems, issues, or opportunities are assessed and identified beyond the physical and functional dimensions, including the following for both patient and family:

- Physical symptoms and prevention of related suffering.
- Psychosocial symptoms and prevention of related suffering.
- Spiritual symptoms and prevention of related suffering.
- Attention to *Aspects of Completion and Closure* to the extent that the patient and family choose to participate.
- Issues and opportunities in the family dynamics and relationships.
- Issues of loss, grief, bereavement and healing.
- Functional status, safety and environmental status.

This step also involves determining the cause of the problem, issue, or opportunity. The cause of a physical problem can often be identified through physiological changes, but nurses must also take into consideration other causes related to all of the dimensions. For example, a patient with end-stage chronic obstructive pulmonary disease (COPD) may complain of shortness of breath. Initial reactions would be to identify the problem as shortness of breath "secondary to ineffective air exchange in the lung." Again, in end-stage COPD, this is an expected norm. With further interdimensional assessment, the patient identifies episodes of shortness of breath secondary to "anticipated fear of being alone at night." Obviously, the interventions are different if the full dimensions are assessed and the patient's and family's experiences direct the process.

The cause of a problem that is not physiologically based can often be attributed to the patient's or family's adaptation to the current situation, unfinished personal conflict related to the *Aspects of Completion and Closure* (see examples in

Table 2–4). In this step, opportunities can also be identified for prevention of problems or issues, or situations can be presented that would enhance personal growth, life completion and relationship closure.

For example, a patient with COPD who was imminently dying was becoming progressively anxious, with increased episodes of shortness of breath despite all medical interventions. On assessment of this problem, the patient shared that he had a son to whom he had not spoken in more than 20 years. The patient was afraid of dying before mending that relationship, apologizing to his son, and letting him know he loved him. The hospice team assisted in locating his son and arranging for a visit. The patient and son were able to spend time together, give and receive forgiveness, and, in so doing, mend their relationship. The patient's unfinished relationship issues and resulting anxieties were the cause of his physical episodes of shortness of breath. Hospice nursing involves a holistic approach that realizes the potential effect of one dimension (e.g., interpersonal) on all other dimensions and ensures that the nursing assessment gathers and uses all dimensional changes for optimal care.

### Step 3: Interdisciplinary Team Care Planning

Interdisciplinary care planning is a process that occurs from the time the patient is referred through the family's bereavement period. It occurs both in formal IDG care planning meetings or conferences and between meetings, as patient and family needs change and members of the IDG collaborate on care. Patients and families are assessed by the nurse and by a psychosocial professional on admission. As the care plan is developed, each discipline blends its own area of expertise with those of other team members to formulate shared interventions that support the patient's and family's goals.

Similar to the nursing process, this step involves planning the care, directed by patient and family goals with the appropriate staff and facilities; determining the best interventions to offer as choices; and devising a team plan for providing services.

*Collaboration.* Collaboration builds an interdisciplinary awareness of interdependence with a common mission, values, and patient/family goals for optimal care. Collaboration is essential for all hospice professionals as they develop innovative ideas and interventions are formulated. One of the key reasons for IDG collaboration is to share assessment data and feedback that each member was able to solicit from the patient and family based on their unique expertise, so that a comprehensive interdimensional care plan can be established and mutually understood by all team members caring for that patient and family. The hospice nurse therefore collaborates with the patient and family to determine their goals, and with other IDG members on a 24 hour, 7-day-a-week basis to ensure a holistic approach and continuity of care. If the patient is residing in a facility, the nurse must also include the staff of that facility in care planning. Collaboration ensures continuity of care.[10]

*Patient/Family-Directed Goal Setting.* A comprehensive plan is developed according to three types of goals: (1) patient/family goals, (2) aspects of life completion and relationship closure goals, and (3) clinical obligation goals.

*Patient/Family Goals.* Primarily the care plan should be directed by what the patient and family have defined as their goals. The hospice plan of care belongs to the patient and family; therefore, goals should be articulated from their perspective, not the nurse's perspective of how things "should happen." Eliminating goals that begin with "The patient will…", or "The family will…" keeps the focus on the experiences of the patient and family vs. the clinicians. Examples of goals articulated in words used by hospice patients and families may include: "Mr. Karst stated he wants to be able to care for a his wife at home while she is bedridden." Another may be: "Mrs. Arthur said she wants her pain at a 2 or less out of 10 at meal times so she can join the family at the table." Articulating goals from the perspective of the patient and family makes it apparent what direction each member of the IDG should take to collaboratively help them meet their goals. It also becomes apparent that the IDG as a group, not one discipline alone, is equipped to deal with complex issues associated with dying and bereavement.

*Aspects of Life Completion and Relationship Closure Goals.* Hospice nurses, as part of the IDG, add their expertise to support the patient and family in accomplishing aspects of completion and closure that are important to them through disease and symptom management as well as emotional and spiritual support. An example of a life completion goal as defined by the patient may be to take one last trip to visit and say good-bye to family and friends. The nurse may be involved by teaching energy conservation, the use of portable oxygen, transfer techniques for car transportation, or titration of medications to ensure comfort. Completion and closure goals may also include "creating a memory book for my grandchildren to have when I'm gone," or being forgiven by a spouse for a life transgression. Again, the focus becomes the patient's and family's goals and experiences; the nurse collaborates with other team members, such as the psychosocial counselor or chaplain, to help the patient and family accomplish these goals.

*Clinical Obligation Goals.* These are identified by the IDG only in those situations in which the patient or family is unable to identify the problem or issue. These goals are strictly related to clinical obligation situations such as neglect or suicide, in which the team must establish goals to ensure the patient's or family's safety.

*Interdisciplinary Team Planning of Intervention Choices.* Interventions are based on interdimensional assessment, with the overall goals of reducing or preventing suffering and accomplishing life and relationship closure in a way that is important and meaningful to the patient and family. Directed by the goals of the patient and family, with their input and approval, the hospice nurse and the other IDG members collaborate to determine the optimal choices of interventions that would move the patient and family closer to their goals.

The interdisciplinary planning process involves determining which discipline, or combination of disciplines, is most appropriate to assist patients and families in accomplishing their goals. Some patients and families may allow only one or two disciplines to be involved in their care. Some individuals expect nurses to provide care and are not always open to visits from social workers or chaplains. The nurse's role may then include communicating the value of other team members and facilitating their involvement to the degree that the patient and family are comfortable. In situations where the nurse may be the sole team representative, incorporating the expertise of all disciplines is paramount. If this happens, it becomes crucial that members of the IDG collaborate and share expertise so that interdisciplinary care can still be delivered and the patient's and family's goals can still be addressed.

### Step 4: Providing Intervention Choices to Meet Patient and Family Goals

The hospice care plan involves interventions in four areas: palliative therapeutic interventions, educational interventions, collaboration interventions, and assessment interventions.

*Palliative Therapeutic Interventions.* Palliative therapeutic interventions include those that have been identified to be conducive to meeting the patient's and family's care plan goals. These include both pharmacological and nonpharmacological interventions to best address the interdimensional adaptation and goals of the patient and family.

Hospice nurses must always be aware of not only the traditional medical interventions but also those interventions specific to the specialty of end-of-life care. An example is a patient who had a stroke that left him aphasic of both spoken and written word. During his lifetime, he had kept a scrapbook of articles from national newspapers and current events journals. In the scrapbook, he had written his perceptions of how an event may have been significant to his daughter's life. To assist this patient in finding meaning and purpose in his life, the nurse requested a volunteer to help the patient engage in life review. The volunteer visited the patient, reading the articles and the patient's philosophical messages to his daughter related to each event in the history of their lives together. Through the reading of these scrapbooks, the patient was able to sense his contribution and value as a parent, while is physical suffering exhibited by extreme restlessness was drastically reduced.

Again, hospice nursing is based on a holistic approach and the understanding that life completion and relationship closure is an interdimensional experience for both the patient and the family.

*Educational Interventions.* As with all nursing practice, patient and family education is a cornerstone of hospice nursing. Because most patients followed by hospice do stay in their homes until death, the primary role of the hospice team is to empower the patient and family caregivers so that they can develop the skills to comfortably provide care and find meaning and purpose in the experience.

The nurse becomes involved in education of the patient and family as it relates to personal care, prevention of problems such as skin breakdown, administration and management of medications, nonpharmacological interventions such as therapeutic touch, application of heat, breathing exercises, and functional assistance with ADLs. As the patient's disease progresses, the hospice nurse is also involved in educating the family about expected changes. Common responses to each stage of the disease and related interventions to decrease suffering are taught so that the patient and family are optimally prepared before the changes occur. When patients and families know what to expect, hospice can help to prevent or reduce anxiety related to the unknown. Critical to the specialty of hospice nursing is the ability to be comfortable having conversations with patients and families about the aspects of closure, offering opportunities for them to identify what is most important and finding ways to support their goals in these aspects.

Helping both patients and their family think about and plan for how they would like their time of death experienced allows for planning and fewer surprises. Educating them about the possibilities of a clam environment, favorite music playing, favorite pets in bed with the patient providing comfort, integration of religious or spiritual ritual, family presence or a choice to die alone are all examples of providing an individualized experience. Another crucial goal of education is to provide information and support so that patients and families can advocate for themselves in all care settings, with other providers, and with other family members.

*Collaboration Interventions.* Crucial to ensuring unified delivery of care to patients and families is the practice of collaboration. In planning interventions, it is crucial to ensure that the patient, the family, and the professional caregivers are all involved. Caregivers include IDG members, facility staff, attending and consulting physicians, therapists, and the family. For example, the hospice nurse collaborates with the attending physician about the need for medication for symptom management or with facility nurses to educate and ensure around-the-clock administration of pain medications. If a hospice patient is residing in a nursing facility, the hospice nurse must collaborate with the nursing facility staff, communicating and documenting the outcome of that collaboration. Communication of these interventions is paramount to ensure continuity of care among team members, caregivers, and care settings.

*Assessment Interventions.* The final type of hospice nursing intervention is ongoing assessment necessary to determine whether continuation of the care plan is effective or optimal. For hospice nursing, this may include closely monitored titration of opioids for pain control or respiratory status to determine effective doses as symptoms change or the patient's needs change throughout the trajectory of illness.

## Step 5: Evaluating Interventions, Continuation, or Revision of the Care Plan: Are the Patient and Family Goals Being Met?

With the patient and family at the core of the hospice team, evaluation begins with their perspective on their experiences impacted by the care plan interventions. Do the interventions help them to reach their goals? What has been most beneficial from their perspective? What do they want to continue or discontinue? It is crucial for the hospice nurse to involve the patient and family in evaluating the effectiveness of the care plan interventions on an ongoing basis.

By evaluating and documenting the effects of interventions, the hospice nurse shares his or her expertise as a valued member of the IDG. If the current care plan is effective at meeting the patient's and family's palliative care goals, then interventions continue. If interventions do not meet the patient's and family's goals, then the hospice nurse collaborates with the patient, family, and IDG for additional assessment and identification of meaningful choices and changes.

A significant difference between traditional nursing and hospice care is the involvement of the patient and the family as they guide the hospice IDG in providing palliative care and services that are most meaningful to them.

As hospice and palliative care continue to grow, the need to incorporate both qualitative and quantitative outcomes in care plan documentation is critical. The incorporation of outcome measures using standardized tools such as Palliative Performance Scale, Missoula-VITAS Quality of Life Index, Edmonton Sypmtom Assessment Score, bereavement risk assessments, spiritual assessments, along with quotes from the patient or family expressing the value of hospice care and services are critical.

## Key Elements of a Hospice Palliative Care Program

### Purpose and Process of Interdisciplinary Team Care Management

In *The Hospice Handbook*, Larry Beresford stated, "The glue that holds together this hospice approach to care is the interdisciplinary team."[3] The primary purpose of the IDG model of care management is to build a caring community between the patient, the family, and the hospice team. This integrated community is responsible for responding to the patient's and family's dynamic needs 24 hours a day, 7 days a week. The entire IDG is accountable for the physical, psychosocial, spiritual, and bereavement needs of both the patient and the family, ensuring that the palliative care plan is carried out across all care settings.

Because the physical, psychosocial, spiritual, and bereavement needs of patients and families are inseparable, the interdisciplinary approach is also the hospice approach to care. The team, not just the hospice nurse, becomes the care manager. The patient, family, and IDG are equally important in problem solving and goal formulation, collaborating with each other for expertise and input into care planning. The hospice approach is a holistic care process that is directed by the patient and family to best meet their interdimensional needs.

Under the 2008 Hospice Conditions of Participation, bringing the team together and working as a team is essential to meet the requirements of CoP §418.54 (Initial and Comprehensive Assessment of the Patient). The hospice IDG must now complete both an initial and a comprehensive assessment that identify the patient's need for medical, nursing, psychosocial, emotional and spiritual care. The initial assessment will determine the patient's and family's immediate needs and the comprehensive assessment forms the basis for the plan of care. Perhaps more importantly, the IDG is required to directly involve the patient, family and caregivers in their plan of care.[35]

Care management by the IDG is a process, not an event. This process begins at the time the patient is admitted to the hospice program and continues until well after the death of the patient, through bereavement services for the survivors. Effective IDG care management promotes daily, ongoing collaborative practice that incorporates shared goals, care planning, role blending, and shared leadership.

### Interdimensional Care Delivered by an Interdisciplinary Team

Chronic illness, aging, and terminal illness affect patients and families not only physically but psychologically, emotionally, spiritually, and financially. To provide effective, quality hospice care, all of these dimensions of the dying experience should be addressed. An IDG, incorporating the expertise of members from several disciplines who are trained to meet these varied needs of patients and families, provides the most effective holistic approach to end-of-life care.

In a traditional multidisciplinary approach to patient care, a member representing each discipline visits the patient and formulates goals depending on his or her own area of expertise. The patient and family may not always be considered together as a unit of care, and the specific goals of one discipline are not always shared by the other disciplines caring for the patient. Often, one discipline is the "case manager," having more direction and input than the others in the care-planning process. This lack of collaborative care planning and goal setting can create an inconsistent approach that lacks cohesion and continuity and often frustrates those receiving care. The focus is on the "discipline" (e.g., nurse, social worker) rather than the patient and family. The hospice IDG model improves on the multidisciplinary approach with a process that allows for the following:

- Patient and family direction of care and services and involvement in decision-making in all aspects of care.

- Determination of patient/family value-directed care plan goals.
- Collaboration of expertise from varied disciplines to meet patient/family goals.
- Identification of intervention choices that support patient/family goals.
- Role blending of expertise among disciplines toward common patient/family goals and outcomes.

The IDG model provides optimal interdimensional care by jointly assessing and determining goals and sharing ideas for interventions with the patient, the family, and all team members working toward patient/family goals and intervention choices. The success of the hospice IDG model lies in the partnership between patient/family and care professionals that best reflects the full scope and experience of illness, caregiving, dying, and bereavement—focusing on the choices, goals, wishes, and experiences of the patient and family.

### The Hospice Interdisciplinary Team Structure and Role Blending

The structure of the hospice IDG is designed to meet the interdimensional needs of patients and families. To be most effective, care teams must be designed to honor the experience of the patients and families they serve. End-of-life care teams, the disciplines that comprise the IDG, and how they function as a collaborative team mirror the patient's and family's complex experience of life-limiting illness, caregiving, dying, death, and bereavement. Collaboration as an IDG focuses on transforming the patient's and family's end-of-life experience. The critical components of this interdisciplinary model can and should be offered in all settings of care for patients and families near the end of life.[34]

As previously discussed, a number of dimensions define the full experience of patients and families. The related dimensions and the corresponding staff that form an effective hospice/palliative care team include the patient and their family and the following:

- *Physical/symptom dimension*: physicians, nurses, pharmacist, therapists, nutritionist, and volunteers.
- *Functional dimension*: nurses, nursing assistants/hospice aides, therapists, homemakers, and volunteers.
- *Interpersonal dimension*: counselors, social workers, psychologists, chaplains, and volunteers.
- *Well-being dimension*: counselors, social workers, psychologists, chaplains, and volunteers.
- *Transcendent dimension*: chaplain, counselors, social worker, psychologist, and volunteers.

Interdimensional care provided by an IDG focuses on the experiences of those served and the core disciplines that can best support that experience. By changing from a singular discipline to an interdimensional approach, all disciplines attend to all dimensions of the patient's and family's experience.[34]

Whereas each discipline of the IDG involves special areas of expertise, responsibilities, and duties, the IDG approach to care management requires that each team member expand and blend the traditional roles with those of other disciplines to provide a holistic approach to patient and family care.

One must be an expert in her or his own discipline and have the basic competence to provide physical, psychosocial, spiritual, and bereavement care. Assessment, planning, intervention, and evaluation are ongoing responsibilities of all team members, implying that each is attentive to all dimensions of patient and family care. Role blending is essential for providing coordinated, comprehensive hospice services. As such, roles need to be dynamic, changing, growing, and overlapping.

### Direct Responsibilities of Patient/Family Care Team Members

*Nurses, Including Advanced Registered Nurse Practitioners and Registered Nurses.* In the MHB model, the registered nurse is primarily responsible for the initial assessment, including the patient's physical condition and comfort, yet must also include assessment of the psychosocial and spiritual dimenstions of care, to address the patient and family from a holistic perspective. The initial and comprehensive assessment that establishes hospice services is completed in collaboration with other IDG members, and the primary physician.[10] She or he must be highly skilled in end-stage physical assessment, disease progression, and pain and symptom management. The nurse is also responsible for educating the patient and family regarding physical care, which includes such things as medication administration, equipment use, skin care, nutrition, catheter care, and transfers.

For those hospice programs that are MHB certified, regulations require the coordination of care by a registered nurse and primary physician in collaboration with the IDG. As a member of the IDG, the nurse's expertise related to disease and symptom management is one of the critical aspects of providing competent end-of-life care. The nurse's primary role involves managing and preventing the physical and functional decline, to reduce suffering so that the patient and family can attend to activities that promote quality of life completion and relationship closure.

The hospice nurse is also responsible for supervising related nursing personnel, including licensed practical nurses, certified nursing assistants, and home health aides. Communicating care plan goals and interventions and monitoring and evaluating the care provided by these other IDG members are the responsibilities of the hospice registered nurse.

Advanced registered nurse practitioners are most often used as collaborative primary care practitioners, providing palliative care consultation and care management for the expanded hospice palliative care programs (e.g., pain consultation in hospital and long-term care settings). Advanced registered nurse practitioners and clinical nurse specialists are also involved as consultants to the primary hospice team.

*Psychosocial Professionals.* Psychosocial professionals may include social workers and counselors who are competent in psychosocial assessment, family dynamics, social/emotional therapeutic interventions, grief and bereavement, and group work. They provide support to patients and families, assisting with psychological issues, emotional responses, and the overall adaptation of the patient, family, and significant others through counseling and utilization of community resources. They may also be involved with financial issues, legal issues, advance directives, and funeral arrangements. Overall, the psychosocial professional helps the patient and family as they adapt to, and cope with, a terminal illness, experience the Aspects of Completion and Closure, and the survivors as they adjust to life during the bereavement process. It is also crucial for nurses to possess expertise in end-of-life psychosocial issues because they, too, will be involved in addressing and supporting the patient's and family's psychosocial needs as members of the IDG. Both the psychosocial and the spiritual care team members are experts in addressing the Aspects of Completion and Closure.

*Spiritual Care Professionals.* Dying is only one part of life, but it is the one in which spiritual dimensions of the human condition are most clearly revealed. Spirituality is not confined to religion or belief in deity. The confrontation with death often evokes the need to make meaning of circumstances and to seek connection to something larger and more enduring than oneself. Evaluation of these aspects of a patient's and family's experience must be incorporated in routine procedures and supported by education, resources, and documentation tools.[19]

Spiritual care is a significant component in end-of-life care. The spiritual caregiver, also known as the chaplain, clergy person, or pastoral care worker, can be a paid hospice professional or a resource volunteer from the community. Hospice spiritual care is nonsectarian, nondenominational, and all-inclusive, with the goal of supporting the patient's and family's spiritual and/or religious practices. The hospice philosophy in terms of spiritual care is nonjudgmental and focuses on healing, forgiveness, and acceptance. Spiritual care is provided through direct spiritual counseling and support in collaboration with the patient's and family's own clergy or by working with patients who do not have a clergy person . Spiritual interventions can include helping patients and families experience the Aspects of Completion and Closure in ways that are most meaningful to them and can include interventions such as prayer, rites, rituals, life review, assistance in planning and performing funerals and memorial services, and assistance with ethical dilemmas and decision-making. Again, the nurse must have some level of expertise in the spiritual aspects of care to address the patient's and family's spiritual needs.

*Patient's Primary Physician.* The patient's primary physician is also part of the IDG. The primary physician is responsible for overseeing patient care. The physician often refers the patient to hospice; certifies the patient's terminal condition; and collaborates throughout the care process, providing the admitting diagnosis and prognosis, current medical findings, and orders for medications, treatments, and symptom management.

*Hospice Medical Director.* The hospice medical director is a member of the IDG. She or he is responsible for the overall medical management of patients in collaboration with the IDG. Depending on the structure of the hospice program, the medical director may also become a patient's primary physician. The role of the hospice medical director is to participate in the team care planning process as a collaborative member of the IDG. The director may also be responsible for the oversight of medical services provided by the hospice.

*Hospice Aide, Certified Nursing Assistant or Home Health Aide.* Certified nursing assistants provide basic physical and functional care if there is a need, as well as patient and family support. Often becoming the closest to the patient and family, they provide and educate caregivers on personal care assistance with ADLs, which may include bathing, grooming, mouth care, skin care, transfers, and repositioning, and sometimes with light housekeeping, shopping, cooking, and laundry. Visits vary depending on patient and family needs and what is most important to the patient at each visit. At times, a walk in the garden is more therapeutic than a bath. As with all disciplines, activities that improve the quality of life experiences are provided by hospice aide.

*Homemaker/Companion.* The homemaker/companion assists the patient and family by doing light housekeeping, meal planning and preparation, laundry, and shopping and by acting as a companion to the patient. The homemaker/companion does not provide direct, hands-on care. For elderly patients living alone, it is often the addition of a homemaker/companion that allows them to remain independent in their homes until they die.

*Patient and Family Care Volunteer.* Volunteers play an integral role in providing hospice care and are fundamental to the hospice philosophy. Hospice patient care volunteers are trained to work in a variety of roles. The most common role is working with a single patient and family in providing support through companionship, listening, diversion, delivering medications, running errands, taking patients to appointments or on outings, shopping, or preparing a special meal. They may provide companionship to patients in extended care facilities or respite time for the home patient's caregiver. Specialized volunteer roles may include bereavement volunteers, who work exclusively with grieving families and friends, or vigil volunteers who sit at the bedside during the dying process so no one dies alone. Specialty volunteers may also include both lay and professional pet, art, music, massage, touch, and drama therapies.

Hospice programs with higher use of volunteers per patient day are associated with bereaved family member reports that the hospice program quality of care was excellent . Those hospice programs in the lowest quartile of volunteer usage had lower overall satisfaction compared to those hospice programs in the highest quartile of volunteer use

(67.8% reported excellent overall quality of care in the lowest quartile compared to 75.8% in the highest quartile, $P < .001$). After adjustment for hospice program characteristics, hospice programs in the highest quartile had highest satisfaction (coefficient =.054; 95% CI, .02-.09). Their study concluded that bereaved family members who receive their care in hospice programs with higher use of volunteers report higher rates of satisfaction with hospice services.[36] The scope of volunteers' duties is all-inclusive, depending on the needs of the patient and family and their quality-of-life goals.

## Roles and Responsibilities of Consultative Team Members

Consultative team members participate in direct patient care as needed to meet the palliative care goals of the care plan. Consultative team members may include the hospice team medical director; consulting physician; psychologist or psychiatrist; nutritional counselor; community clergy; clinical pharmacist; occupational, physical, respiratory, speech, and language therapists; intravenous infusion nurse; and members of pharmacy, radiology, laboratory, and durable medical equipment services.[37] In addition, the palliative arts therapists such as music, art, aromatherapy, massage, etc. are often incorporated into the hospice plan of care.

## When Nurses Should Consider Hospice for Their Patients

All nurses must be familiar with the benefits and expanded scope of services of their local hospice programs, so that they can effectively educate and advocate for palliative care when their patients and families could benefit from this approach and scope of supportive services. Considering the expanding hospice models, there are many myths and misperceptions that must be eliminated—such as the need to be within 6 months of death to receive hospice services—so that patients and families can be optimally supported. The most common comment nationally on hospice family satisfaction surveys is, "I wish we had hospice sooner." The voices of these families support the need for earlier referral to hospice. It is important for nurses providing end-of-life care to consider when to think about hospice. Table 2–6 lists practical scenarios to guide nurses in offering hospice as a supportive service to patients and families throughout the lifespan. Hospice teams are expert at assessing palliative care needs and are available to assist nurses in determining which services may benefit a given patient. A call to collaborate with the local hospice provider can initiate this assessment.

~~~

## Coping with Cumulative Loss: Finding a Healthy Balance as a Caring Professional

The hospice approach to care emphasizes intense interpersonal care and active involvement with the patient and family, and creates more intense and more intimate relationships among the nurse, patient, and family than exist in traditional health care settings. Like families who grieve the loss of their loved ones, the hospice nurse also grieves the loss and, in fact, may need to grieve on a continuous basis due to the number of deaths that occur. As the hospice nurse adjusts to caring for dying patients and their families, the stress of coping with death on a daily basis can trigger many emotional feelings, reactions, and behaviors. It is critical to be aware of these reactions and develop a system to process emotions for a healthy personal balance.

Other factors may also influence a nurse's successful adaptation to caring for dying patients and their families. If the nurse has experienced death on a personal level or has experienced life changes that signify loss (e.g., children leaving home, divorce), caring for dying patients and families may trigger issues of unresolved grief. The nurse's ability to verbalize or process his or her feelings regarding death and loss with other members of the IDG is important for support and for normalizing these feelings.

Hospice nurses who are unable to process these losses through appropriate grief and personal death awareness may begin to distance themselves from emotional involvement with patients and families. This withdrawal may negatively affect not only the coping ability of the professional but also the quality of compassionate delivery of care and the ability to meet the needs of dying patients and their families during the terminal phases of an illness.

## Stages of Adaptation for the Hospice Nurse

Hospice nurses go through many stages when they begin caring for dying patients and their families. Successful progression through these stages and the support systems in place to facilitate successful progression are vitally important in determining whether the nurse will be comfortable and effective in caring for the dying.

As proposed by Bernice Harper,[38] an expert in anxiety issues in the professional caregiver, there are six stages of adaptation that characterize the hospice nurse's normal progression, adaptation, and coping in caring for the dying: intellectualization, emotional survival, depression, emotional arrival, deep compassion, and The Doer. Five of these stages, the emotions, behaviors, and reactions of each stage are shown in Figure 2–3 and Table 2–7.

*Intellectualization.* Intellectualization usually occurs during the first 1 to 3 months of caring for the dying. During this time, professional caregivers are usually confronted with their first experience of a hospice death. Nurses in this initial stage spend much of their energy learning the facts, tasks, policies, and procedures of the job. Emotional involvement in the dying and death of the patient may be inadvertently avoided, and the hospice nurse seldom reacts on an emotional level to the death.

**Table 2–6**
**When to Call Hospice**

| Call for a Consultation When | How Hospice May Help |
|---|---|
| Your patients and family members are calling more and more to ask questions about care | Hospice can provide support for the patient and family to help lessen their anxieties, normalize their feelings, connect them to community caregiver resources, and teach caregiving skills. |
| You would not be surprised by this patient's death within the next year | The number one comment made by hospice families after the death of a loved one is, "I wish we had hospice services earlier. We needed the help." Hospice can outline ways to support your patient and family earlier. |
| You see a sudden decline in the patient's condition | Hospice admissions staff and medical directors are experts at assessing for needed care and services. If the patient is not eligible for the Medicare Hospice Benefit, the patient and family may be offered other services, such as palliative care or counseling. |
| There is progressive loss of function | Loss of function is a key prognostic indicator for a life-limiting condition. Hospice can provide durable medical equipment, personal care, and other assistance. |
| Your patient has been hospitalized twice in the past year due to symptom exacerbation from a chronic illness | Two hospitalizations for the same chronic disease within 12 months is often an indicator of less than 1 year to live. Hospice interdisciplinary teams can assess the progression of the disease and help determine whether it a good time for hospice support. |
| There is an onset of multiple comorbidities and/or an increase in symptoms associated with comorbidities | Especially for the elder population, a rapid change in condition or progressive decline of functional abilities indicate it may be time for hospice. Call for an assessment and identification of support services. |
| Your patient would benefit from help with advance directive/care planning | Hospice staff are experienced in clarifying the various options for advance directives. They can assist patients and family members in having discussions to clarify end-of-life goals and make informed choices. |
| Your patient could benefit from palliative symptom management while still pursuing curative therapy | Through an array of programs, hospice may be able to provide palliative care coordination to patients along the care continuum. Physicians, nurse practitioners, and the hospice interdisciplinary team can help control side effects and other symptoms. |
| A patient is making decisions about transitioning to palliative care | Hospice counselors and peer volunteers can help your patients/families address options and fears and advocate for their wishes. Hospice staff assist patients and families in identifying and defining quality of life, so that decisions can be made with peace of mind. |
| Someone needs information about any end-of-life or related health care issues | Hospice has an extensive resource center with a broad range of topics including end of life, wellness, complementary therapies, and advance directives. |
| Your patient is in the intensive care unit and is considering comfort measures only | Hospice can provide family support in decision-making, resources on alternative placement options if the patient cannot be cared for at home, and the option for hospice residence placement. |
| The family or other caregivers are unable to care for the patient at home | Hospice can help patients and families to determine caregiving resources available through personal support systems, community groups/agencies and hospice. The hospice residence expands the available options. |
| At the time of diagnosis of a life-limiting illness | Someone to talk to may be the best support you can offer. Hospice reassurance volunteers are trained to help in these difficult situations. |
| It is time to have a difficult discussion | Hospice counselors can be present during these conversations or can meet with families afterward and provide resources to patients and families to guide conversations. |

*Source*: Copyright © 2009 Suncoast Hospice. Reprinted with permission.

*Emotional Survival.* Emotional survival generally occurs within 3 to 6 months of employment. Emotional involvement and a deeper connection with the patient and family occur. The nurse begins to confront the reality of the patient's death, to face her or his own mortality, and to feel sadness about the patient's situation and/or the loss of the patient. Often during this stage, the nurses begin to fully understand the magnitude of their roles and responsibilities and to question their abilities and desire to continue caring for dying patients and their families. This is a crucial time, and the nurse needs to be reassured and given support and resources to feel competent and confident so that he or she can progress successfully in the field.

*Depression.* Depression occurring at 6 to 9 months is often a time when hospice nurses process the losses rather than avoid them or remain emotionally detached. They begin to explore

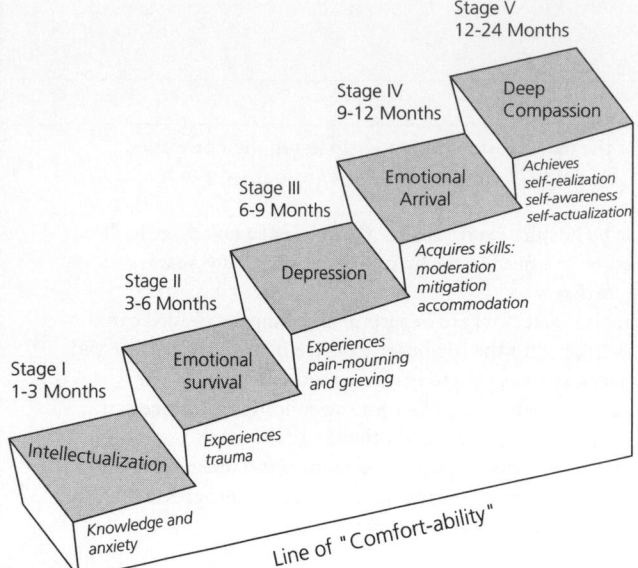

Stage V
12-24 Months

Stage IV
9-12 Months

Deep
Compassion

Stage III
6-9 Months

Emotional
Arrival

*Achieves
self-realization
self-awareness
self-actualization*

Stage II
3-6 Months

Depression

*Acquires skills:
moderation
mitigation
accommodation*

Stage I
1-3 Months

Emotional
survival

*Experiences
pain-mourning
and grieving*

Intellectualization

*Experiences
trauma*

*Knowledge and
anxiety*

Line of "Comfort-ability"

**Figure 2–3.** Cumulative loss and the caregiver: Five stages experienced by the hospice nurse while caring for the dying. *Source*: Harper (1994), reference 38.

their own feelings about death, accept their own mortality, and accept death as a natural part of life.

It is in this stage that hospice professionals positively move toward resolution of death and loss and accept the reality of death and dying, or negatively resolve death and loss by choosing to avoid the emotional pain. In positive resolution, hospice professionals emotionally arrive at a comfortable place in caring for dying patients and their families.

*Emotional Arrival.* Emotional arrival occurs within 9 to 12 months of caring for the dying. With positive resolution of the last stage, hospice professionals become sensitive to the emotional needs and issues associated with dying and death. They can now cope with and accept loss, participate in healthy grieving, experience and conceptually work within the principles of hospice philosophy by advocating for the patient and family, and become involved with patients and families on a deeper level.

*Deep Compassion.* Deep compassion occurs after the first year as a hospice nurse. In this stage, hospice professionals begin to refine their knowledge and skills and are comfortable in providing compassionate, physical, psychosocial, and spiritual care to dying patients and their families. This stage is characterized by personal and professional growth and development.

*The Doer.* This final stage is the culmination of nurses' experiencing the first five stages in a healthy and balanced manner; this outcome is characterized by hospice professionals who are efficient, vigorous, knowledgeable, and able to understand and comprehend humankind. Death has an inner meaning embedded in caring. Doers have grown and developed personally and professionally through the experiences of caring for the terminally ill.

## Support Systems

In caring for dying patients and their families, the hospice nurse is vulnerable to emotions, reactions, and behaviors that can ultimately affect his or her personal well-being and the delivery of quality palliative care. To effectively care for patients and families, the nurse must also be responsible for attending to her or his own emotional, physical, and spiritual needs. Successfully coping with and adapting to dying, death, and cumulative loss is possible only if a system is in place that provides support to the nurse. Support systems may include personal death awareness exercises, time to verbalize in one-on-one counseling or with the IDG or both, supervisor support, preceptors or mentors, spiritual support, funeral or memorial services for closure, joint visits with members of other disciplines, and educational opportunities. The nurse should also explore individually facilitated support systems through journal writing, exercise, relaxation, meditation, and socialization with family and friends. This individual support can even be found by reflecting on each patient/family relationship and asking, "What can I learn from this experience to either improve the care of other patients and families or grow myself professionally and personally?" By exploring and accessing support systems, hospice nurses can find satisfaction, fulfillment, and growth and development in their personal and professional lives as they provide compassionate end-of-life care to patients and their families.

## Access to Hospice Care

In the national dialogue about improving care at the end of life, access to hospice services has been raised as a public policy and public health concern. There is acknowledgment of the value of hospice care for patients who need palliative care, with the recognition that there are barriers to its full utilization. Often patients are referred for hospice care just a few days or even hours before their deaths. Innovative hospice demonstration projects continue testing how to care for patients who have an extended life expectancy or are receiving experimental or disease-modifying treatments. Many factors contribute to late referrals and access barriers, and communities are collaborating to ensure that palliative care is available across settings throughout the disease trajectory.[15]

The Access and Values project offered a wide array of hospice and nonhospice stakeholders in end-of-life care an opportunity to examine the cultural and regulatory barriers

**Table 2–7**
**Cumulative Loss and the Professional Caregiver**

| Stage I (0–3 mo) Intellectualization | Stage II (3–6 mo) Emotional Survival | Stage III (6–9 mo) Depression | Stage IV (9–12 mo) Emotional Arrival | Stage V (12–24 mo) Deep Compassion |
|---|---|---|---|---|
| Professional knowledge | Increasing professional knowledge | Deepening professional knowledge | Acceptance of professional knowledge | Refining professional knowledge |
| Intellectualization | Less intellectualization | Decreasing intellectualization | Normal intellectualization | Refining intellectual base |
| Anxiety | Emotional survival | Depression | Emotional arrival | Deep compassion |
| Some uncomfortableness | Increasing uncomfortableness | Decreasing uncomfortableness | Increasing comfortableness | Increased comfortableness |
| Agreeableness | Guilt | Pain | Moderation | Self-realization |
| Withdrawal | Frustration | Mourning | Mitigation | Self-awareness |
| Superficial acceptance | Sadness | Grieving | Accommodation | Self-actualization |
| Providing tangible services | Initial emotional involvement | More emotional involvement | Ego mastery | Professional satisfaction |
| Use of emotional energy in understanding the setting | Increasing emotional involvement | Overidentification with the patient | Coping with loss of relationship | Acceptance of death and loss |
| Familiarizing self with policies and procedures | Initial understanding of the magnitude of the area of practice | Exploration of own feelings about death | Freedom from concern about own death | Rewarding professional growth and development |
| Working with families rather than patients | Overidentification with the patient's situation | Facing own death | Developing strong ties with dying patients and families | Development of ability to give of one's self |
| | | Coming to grips with feelings about death | Development of ability to work with, on behalf of, and for the dying patient | Human and professional assessment |
| | | | Development of professional competence | Constructive and appropriate activities |
| | | | Productivity and accomplishments | Development of feelings of dignity and self-respect |
| | | | Healthy interaction | Ability to give dignity and self-respect to dying patient |
| | | | | Feeling of comfortableness in relation to self, patient, family, and the job |

*Source*: Harper (1994), reference 38.

to hospice access for dying Americans. The Access and Values project focused on external barriers to care. Importantly, the perspectives of that project's consumer and non-hospice representatives were largely responsible for seeding a movement within the hospice movement, now known as Open Access. Simply stated, the goal of Open Access is to optimize the response of hospice programs to community members in need of palliative services and specifically to those who are eligible for the Medicare Hospice Benefit. [15]

A fundamental tenet of Open Access is that everyone who wants hospice care and meets hospice's eligibility requirements should be admitted to hospice. As a service philosophy, Open Access further requires that every person requesting assistance by hospice be offered information, coaching and referral to community resources if they are not eligible for direct care by hospice, palliative care or bereavement teams.

The Open Access approach attempts to prevent the denial or delays of admissions to hospice caused by admission criteria, caregiver status, diagnosis, type and nature of palliative treatments, preferences for resuscitation, complexity of care, site of care, reimbursement source or cost of care. When hospice managers or staff limit admissions based solely on unreliable "predictive" prognostic guidelines, living conditions or type of palliative treatment, they contribute to a perspective that hospice is only for a narrow subset of terminally ill patients. These practices are "unfriendly" to a wide range of potential customers and do not position the hospice to serve the whole community of patients and families that need care.[39]

## A Death-Defying Society

The prevailing attitude of society toward death continues to be "death-defying." Unquestionable acceptance of innovation, efficiency, science, technological advances, and the ability to prolong life reflects the current perspective on health care. Therefore, acceptance of death as a natural process is difficult and offensive. As experts in the care of patients and families at the end of life, hospice workers will continue to shape the way in which people view dying and death.

## Access Barriers

At the request of the NHPCO, the Committee on the Medicare Hospice Benefit and End-of-Life Care spent almost a year addressing issues related to hospice and end-of-life care. As part of the committee's review and recommendations, barriers to achieving the characteristics of the ideal future hospice and extending hospice to more Americans were identified. The specific recommendations of the report were wide-ranging, from improving the MHB to changing the education of health and human service professionals to raising the expectations for performance by hospice programs. All are important, but the following steps were identified as having the highest priority:

- Eliminating the 6-month prognosis under the MHB and identifying alternative eligibility specifications.
- Collecting and analyzing comprehensive data on the cost of meeting patient and family needs through hospice, with the intent to address inadequacies in Medicare payments.
- Developing outcome measures for assessing the quality of end-of-life care.
- Engaging the public in a campaign to create wider understanding and utilization of hospice care.[40]

## Prognostic Limitations

One of the significant factors limiting access to hospice care is the determination of when hospice care should begin. There is mounting clinical evidence of the appropriateness of palliative care but few documented, valid, and reliable prognostic indicators of when palliative care should begin,

especially for patients with diagnoses of chronic noncancer disease or aging and multisystem failure. This ambiguity can cause delay in referral to hospice or toward any palliative care focus. Terminally ill persons, given physician-certified prognosis of 6 months or less to live, represent patients who are potentially eligible for the MHB model. From historical,[41] contemporary,[42] and scientific perspectives,[43] however, determination of terminal status is notoriously elusive.

In an effort to implement criteria to identify when hospice should begin, the Centers for Medicare and Medicaid (formerly the Health Care Financing Administration) implemented Medicare prognostic criteria called Local Medical Review Policies (LMRPs) through the national Fiscal Intermediaries in the mid-1990s. The appropriateness of the Medicare prognostic criteria (LMRPs) has been contested on several points including: the criteria appear to have limited scientific merit,[44] the criteria exclude nonphysical markers of disease progression and the LMRPs appear to disadvantage those who are less obviously and imminently terminally ill. The findings of the largest project testing the validity of the LMRPs as prognostic criteria strongly indicate that application of the LMRP criteria can yield considerable misclassification. Moore observed a consistent pattern of relatively low rates of false-positive error, representing those patients who will survive longer than 6 months as MHB-eligible. What seemed to be significantly more important was the much higher corresponding rates of false-negative error, representing those patients who would have been denied hospice based on the LMRP yet died within six months… Relative to the costs and benefits of regulatory innovation, false-negative errors most disadvantage patients, families, and providers, whereas false-positive errors most disadvantage payers of public services.[44] If admission criteria were solely based on the LMRPs, more people would be denied hospice care who would otherwise qualify and benefit.

Since then, Medicare and the Fiscal Intermediaries for hospice have updated and changed the LMRPs to LCDs—Local Coverage Determination criteria—to aid in determining and documenting terminal prognosis for some non-cancer diagnosis.

The MHB was initially implemented with the understanding that the IDG in collaborative assessment would be the ideal way to identify when someone is eligible for the core MHB. After years of practical use of the LMRPs/LCDs, the fiscal intermediaries reinforced the use of the LCDs as "guidelines" for admission and recertification assessment in collaboration with the IDG assessment and primary physician. Fiscal intermediaries outline four possible ways admission and recertification decisions can be made including:

1. Patient meets requirements of the general and disease specific LCD.
2. Patient meets some of the LCD requirements and had comorbid conditions that would impact their survival.
3. Patient meets some of the LCD and documented rapid decline.
4. Physician's clinical assessment in collaboration with IDG.[45]

Interestingly, a 2007 study of hospice outcomes has indicated a longer life expectancy with people enrolled in hospice compared to those with similar situations who were not enrolled in hospice care. Among the patient populations studied, the mean survival was 29 days longer for hospice patients than for non-hospice patients. In other words, patients who chose hospice care lived an average of one month longer than similar patients who did not choose hospice care. Researchers studied 4,493 terminally ill patients with either congestive heart failure or cancer of the breast, colon, lung, pancreas, or prostate. Longer lengths of survival were found in four of the six disease categories studied.

Researchers cited several factors that may have contributed to longer life among patients who chose hospice. First, patients who are already in a weakened condition avoid the risks of over-treatment when they make the decision to receive hospice care. Second, hospice care may improve the monitoring and treatment patients receive. Additionally, hospice provides in-home care from an interdisciplinary team focused on the emotional needs, spiritual well-being, and physical health of the patient. Support and training for family caregivers is provided as well. This may increase the patient's desire to continue living and may make them feel less of a burden to family members.[46]

### Eliminating Barriers and Improving Access

Hospice programs have begun to respond to these barriers and are now providing a broader range of services by using more liberal internal eligibility criteria, flexible state hospice licensing provisions, home health agency licensure, volunteer support programs, counseling centers, and other approaches. Many hospice programs have extended their services to incorporate new palliative treatments, eliminated access barriers by admitting patients who live alone or lack a family caregiver or stable home setting, and cared for more patients with diagnoses other than cancer, including children with life-threatening illnesses. Other hospice agencies have pursued a somewhat different path to the same goal of expanded access by labeling their broader service offerings as "palliative care."

According to the NHWG, Open Access programs vary across communities, but commonly have internal policy and practice in place in order to:

- Provide flexible intake processes designed to receive referrals/inquiries 24 hours a day, 7 days a week and provide same-day admissions.
- Admit physician-referred patients who are ambivalent about their treatment options and find it difficult to acknowledge the reality of their imminent death.
- Provide review of atypical and high-cost therapies on a daily/weekly basis to determine whether they are achieving the intended outcomes.
- Rigorously monitor the consequences of treatments. Open Access does not mean "anything goes."

- Fully use existing insurance benefits for those who will likely die within the next 6–12 months and want hospice care. These programs further position themselves as "community trusts." They do not define their mission or service availability solely by insurance regulations or reimbursement practices, but rather as a resource for all in the community. However, when the needs of patients do not completely conform to the regulations, these programs engage in discussion with insurers in order to address their needs.
- Establish very effective working relationships with other health care providers in hospitals, nursing homes, assisted living residences and other residential facilities.
- Actively involve local physicians in the hospice program.
- Maximize volunteers' involvement to meet challenging caregiver/staffing needs.
- Develop caregiver partnerships with other human service providers (Alzheimer's Association, American Cancer Society, Area Agency on Aging, etc.) and with families already in the chronic care continuum.
- Develop philanthropically funded programs that broaden access to the hospice's palliative programs and services.[39]

The Comprehensive Hospice Center model, described earlier, aligns care and services with the needs of an aging population; these centers are compatible with a public health paradigm reflecting the preventive and care needs of youth, middle-aged, and older persons—a birth-to-death public health paradigm (Figure 2–4). Comprehensive hospices provide primary prevention services to the community by offering education on terminal disease trajectories and end-of-life care and caregiving and by providing bereavement support to communities. Through such activities, these hospices have the potential to contribute to the occurrence of lower survivor morbidity and mortality—to contribute to the public's health.[15]

Comprehensive hospices provide educational programs and services in schools and universities, in workplaces, and in other public places within communities (e.g., churches); they sponsor culturally diverse initiatives and help in the creation and dissemination of new knowledge.

### The Funding of Hospice Programs

The original hospices were funded almost exclusively by charitable support, grants, and volunteer efforts. Some components of care were supported by Medicare or insurance, such as skilled nursing visits, medications, or durable medical equipment on a per-unit fee-for-service basis allowed under an acute care model.

The Medicare Hospice Benefit (MHB) enacted by Congress in 1982 is the dominant source of payment for hospice care.

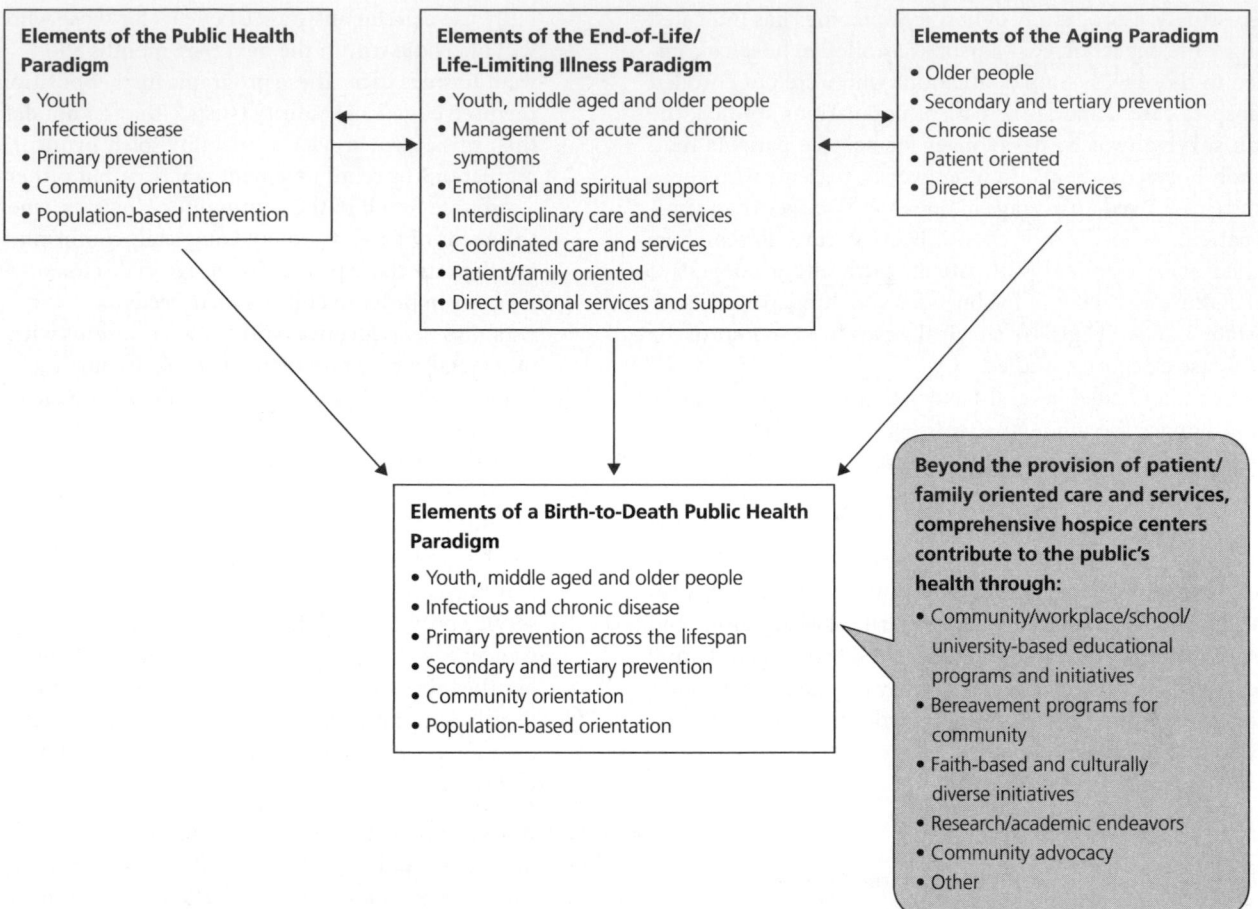

**Figure 2–4.** Elements of a birth-to-death public health paradigm: an extension of an integrated public health and aging model by Anderson and Pourat. *Sources*: Andersen R, Pourat N. Toward a synthesis of a public health agenda for an aging society. In: Hickey T, Speers MA, Prohaska TR, eds. Public Health and Aging. Baltimore: Johns Hopkins University Press, 1997, pp 311–324; Reprinted with permission.

Medicare pays for hospice care when qualifying criteria are met and documented. It is essential for hospice agencies to have a complete understanding of these criteria, as they have the right and responsibility, in collaboration with the physician, to decide if the beneficiary qualifies for services. The agency then must understand what services are covered, and how to document the outcomes, value and ongoing need for hospice services. To be eligible to elect the hospice benefit under Medicare, the beneficiary must be entitled to Part A of the Medicare benefit and be certified by a physician as terminally ill. A beneficiary is considered to be terminally ill if the medical prognosis for life expectancy is six months or less if the illness runs its normal course.[47]

Following the MHB benefit development, Medicaid and private insurance hospice benefits began to emerge. Ultimately, most states developed Medicaid benefits, which are mandated to be no less than the Medicare benefit. Private insurers frequently model their benefit on the MHB, although they are under no mandate to do so.

Most hospices are committed to providing care regardless of ability to pay, and they continue to be dependent on charitable dollars to provide such care. Additional supportive services, beyond the benefit, such as children's programs, in-home caregiver programs, hospice residences, and community bereavement and education programs, are provided in many hospice communities.

Although a small portion of all people receiving health care are at the end of life and receiving terminal care, the terminally ill consume a disproportionate percentage of all health care expenditures. There are several studies on the cost savings in hospice versus traditional health care at the end of life.

Findings of a 2007 major study of hospice care in America demonstrate that hospice services save money and meet the needs of patients and families. Given that hospice has been widely demonstrated to improve quality of life of patients and families, the Medicare program appears to have a rare situation whereby something that improves quality of life also appears to reduce costs. One often asked question about hospice care is: "What length of hospice use maximizes reduction in medical expenditures near death in the US Medicare program?" While previous studies have reported conflicting data regarding the costs savings of the Hospice Medicare Benefit, this study used improved methods that build on previous research on hospice costs to Medicare. Each hospice patient in the study was compared with 2 non-hospice patients with the same sex, diagnosis, age, and time period of care to achieve a more apples to apples comparison.

Researchers suggest that there should be a focus on lengthening the time patients received hospice care services. Not only does this allow people more opportunity to take advantage of care, but additional cost savings would be seen. They specifically demonstrated that increasing length of hospice use by just three days would increase savings due to hospice by nearly 10 percent, from around $2,300 to $2,500 per hospice user. In summary, the study used improved research methods to demonstrate that:

- Hospice saves Medicare money.
- Hospice is more cost effective for cancer patients for more than 7 months of care provided.
- Hospice is also more cost effective for non-cancer patients for more than 5 months of care.
- Hospice would further reduce Medicare costs if seven out of 10 people had hospice care longer.[48]

Hospice has remained a positive example of integrating a managed care model with proven cost savings while meeting patients' and families' needs and receiving high quality scores.

### The Medicaid Hospice Benefit

Medicaid coverage for hospice is patterned after the Medicare benefit, including both patient eligibility requirements and coverage for specific services. States do have some flexibility in developing their hospice benefit.

### Private Insurance Reimbursement and Managed Care

Private insurance companies have begun to realize the benefits of hospice care and are including a hospice benefit in their services. As with Medicaid, many private insurers pattern their benefit after Medicare. Some insurers have negotiated services with hospices, including those palliative care consultation and care management services of the Community Hospice Model, before the MHB services begin. Many managed care companies have also reflected the Medicare benefit in services provided to their members either through their own hospice programs or under contract with programs serving the patient's community.

### Hospice Conditions of Participation

When a hospice agency becomes certified by Medicare to provide services it agrees to abide by the *Hospice Conditions of Participation* (CoPs). For the first time since the Medicare

Hospice Conditions of Participations were created in 1983, the regulations for Medicare certified hospice providers issued by the Centers for Medicare and Medicaid Services were significantly revised and enacted in December 2008. The new CoPs are a welcome recognition of the value of hospice and the importance of quality practice. CMS worked with many stakeholders including NHPCO to provide a framework that will help improve—and standardize—the quality of care among the nation's providers. Hospice has always been centered around the patient and family and the new CoPs require that providers demonstrate this through data collection during the initial and comprehensive assessments and in the documentation processes–and then be sure this information is used to address the provision of care, as mandated by the Quality Assessment and Performance Improvement (QAPI) component (CoP §418.58). They focus on providing patient-centered care and putting the needs of the patient and family first.[10] The Quality Assessment and Performance Improvement component of the CoPs is new to the regulations. It requires hospices to: (1) conduct a 360-degree surveillance of their operation and assess the impact of the medical, psychosocial, and spiritual care provided to the patient/family; (2) initiate performance-improvement projects, where needed, to demonstrate measurable improvements; and (3) evaluate performance and continue to make improvements as needed.

Hospice nurses with other IDG members can play a vital role in assuring quality and supporting agency activities related to outcome and quality measures.

### Future Trends

*Innovative Expansion of Services.* Hospice Programs will continue to expand innovative services such as those already in place in the Comprehensive Hospice Model. "Be There" services, mostly provided through volunteers, are another innovative approach being developed to augment services so people can remain in their homes until death. "Be There" services for patients may include errands, transportation, home maintenance, gardening, sitting with patients at the doctor, evening "tuck-in" calls, and creating celebrations. "Be There" services for the family may include packing of a relative's home, communication with neighbors and distant family, food preparation for working caregivers, child care, errands, and sitting respite.

*Integrating Caring Technologies.* The most significant opportunity in technology lies with the use of the electronic health record (EHR) at the point-of-care. This contribution is not about documentation, but rather *Communication.* The laptop or other point-of-care device with an EHR places information about the patients and families we serve at the fingertips of care staff. Communication ensures that patients and families do not serve as conduits of information between multiple care providers that enter their home. All staff, regardless of when they work, have the information they need to assist the patient and family immediately and effectively. Quality outcomes and continuity of care are more manageable when communication is in "real time." The real time EHR can strengthen relationships with community partners such as nursing homes and hospitals. The ability to communicate during visits inside our partners' facilities can provide relevant data to place on their charts or share with physicians.

Distance family caregivers and working family caregivers are already utilizing email communications with care teams. Direct links with webcams to patients and between patients and families improve the quality of communications and have created a new form of "presence" when face-to-face may be delayed or not possible.

The third significant contribution of technology voice communication—cell phones, combination phone/personal data assistants, text pages, and instant messaging. These tools are essential to communication and responsiveness to our patients and families. As the baby boomers become part of the population we care for, we find that their children don't communicate by phone, but rather through e-mails sent at midnight, instant messaging in times of crisis, and cell phone voicemail as primary access tools. Once again these tools are operationally efficient for care staff providing real time access to patients and families, replacing the messaging systems of old, creating immediate emergency access to field staff.

## Outcome Measurement and Research

With the increased regulatory requirements for hospice reporting and the mandate through the new CoPs for an agency-wide QAPI program, integrating data is even more crucial to hospices. Hospices must have the ability to collect electronic data for the purpose of analysis, benchmarking, and quality measurement. When we use laptops at the point of care and collect structured data, we create the opportunity for business intelligence. We can mine the data to understand the basics such as census, and length of stay to guide our strategic planning and competitive awareness. In addition, we can begin to identify the interventions that best manage pain in 50-year-old male pancreatic cancer patients, how suffering relates to pain management, and what 90-year-old female patients living alone are most worried about. Within this data lies the knowledge needed to teach and train staff and volunteers best practice, improve outcomes, and decrease the trial and error methods of care planning. Data can make us more focused, more efficient in meeting the basic needs of our patients, and more available for providing our most important intervention "Presence."

Hospice and palliative care continues to be seen as a fairly new science and industry. Although hospice research has increased in the past 5 years, there continues to be a need for ongoing research in all areas that impact care, systems of care, workforce practices, and policy.

## Future Funding

Funding will continue to be a challenge for all of healthcare. Yet the responsibility to assure quality cost-effective care still resides with hospice providers. The hospice industry has grown tremendously with hospice Medicare expenditures in 2007 exceeding $10 billion annually. The Medicare Hospice Benefit (MHB) was initially designed, in part, to provide an alternative to traditional end-of-life care in a hospital setting by enabling patients to receive care in a less intensive, home-based setting at a lower cost to Medicare. Hospice must continue to be able to demonstrate this cost benefit to CMS. With the future of healthcare and the economic challenges of this country, hospices will be challenged to balance the caring sanctuary with a sound business.[35]

## Conclusion

Hospice is more than a program of health services. It is an approach and philosophy of care and services that strives to encompass and support the full experience of illness, aging, caregiving, dying, and bereavement for both the patient and the family. Although the last phase of life and relationship is a difficult time, with sensitive support it can be a time of tremendous growth and opportunity for the person who is dying and for loved ones—such as in the finding of meaning and purpose in one's suffering, the value of one's life accomplishments, the deepening of relationships, and the personal spiritual significance of the experience.

Nurses, along with their IDG team members, can positively affect this experience for others by allowing the patient's and family's personal values and goals to direct the support and care they offer as they are invited to share in this intimate time of life. Regardless of the site of care or type of program or services, nurses providing end-of-life care must be proficient in end-stage disease and symptom management. They also have a responsibility to be knowledgeable about the services a hospice program can offer their patients and families and to know when to consider offering hospice care. Nurses must be guided by dignity, compassion, love, and individual acceptance of patient and family values and choices to ensure quality end-of-life care.

REFERENCES

1. Kuhl D. What Dying People Want—Practical Wisdom for the End of Life. Public Affairs Percus Books Group, 2002.
2. Panke J, Coyne P. Conversations in Palliative Care. Pensacola, Fla.: Pohl Publishing Company, 2004.
3. Beresford L. The Hospice Handbook: A Complete Guide. Boston: Little, Brown, 1993.
4. Maugh TH. Florence S. Wald dies at 91; former dean of Yale's nursing program pioneered U.S. hospice care. AARP Bulletin Today. American Association of Retired People, November

2008. Available at http://www.bulletin.aarp.org (accessed December 10, 2008).

5. Standards and Accreditation Committee. Standards of Practice for Hospice Programs. Arlington, Va.: National Hospice and Palliative Care Organization, 2005.

6. (AARP) American Association of Retired Persons. AARP Massachusetts End of Life Survey. Knowledge Management. Washington, DC, 2005. Available at http://www.aarp.org/research/surveys/life/legal/eol/articles/ma_eol.html (accessed November 18, 2009).

7. National Hospice & Palliative Care Organization. NHPCO Facts & Figures: Hospice Care in America. Arlington, Va. October 2008. Available at http://www.nhpco.org/files/public/Statistics_Research/NHPCO_facts-and-figures_2008.pdf (accessed November 18, 2009).

8. Cassell EJ. The nature of suffering and the goals of medicine. N Engl J Med 1982;306:639–642.

9. Cassell EJ. The Nature of Suffering and the Goals of Medicine. Oxford: Oxford University Press, 1991.

10. Federal Register. Department of Health and Human Services Centers for Medicare & Medicaid Services 42 CFR Part 418 Medicare and Medicaid Programs: Hospice Conditions of Participation; Final Rule. Available at www.edocket.access.gpo.gov/2008/pdf/08-1305. (accessed December 16, 2008).

11. Meier DE, Morrison RS. Old age and care near the end of life. J Am Soc Aging 1999;23:7.

12. NHPCO FY2007 National Summary of Hospice Care. National Hospice and Palliative Care Organization. Alexandria, Va: Available at www.nhpco.org (accessed December 22, 2008).

13. Miller SC, Lima J. The Florida Model of Hospice Care: A Report for Florida Hospices and Palliative Care, Inc, pp 8–9. Tallahasee, Fla.: Florida Hospices & Palliative Care, Inc., 2004.

14. Huskamp HA, Buntin MB, Wang V, Newhouse JP. Providing care at the end of life: Do Medicare rules impede good care? Health Affairs 2001;20:204–211.

15. Jennings B, Ryndes R, D'Onofrio C, Baily MA. Access to Hospice Care: Expanding Boundaries, Overcoming Barriers. Hastings Center Report, March 1, 2003.

16. Labyak, M. Conversation About the Comprehensive Hospice. The Hospice of the Florida Suncoast, October 2008.

17. National Hospice Foundation. Quality End of Life Care. Arlington, Va. Available at www.nationalhospicefoundation.org (accessed December 27, 2008).

18. Barclay, L. Medscape Medical News, May 3, 2007 reporting on AGS 2007 Annual Scientific Meeting: Abstract P4 Silverman.

19. Byock I. Where Do We Go From Here? Crit Care Med 2006;34, 11 (Suppl.):416–420.

20. Miller SC, Mor V. The emergence of Medicare hospice in U.S. nursing homes. Palliat Med 201;15:471–480.

21. Miller SC, Mor V, Wu N, et al. Does receipt of hospice care in nursing homes improve the management of pain at the end-of-life? J Am Geriatr Soc 2002;50:507–515.

22. Wu N, Miller SC, Lapane K, Gozalo P. The problem of assessment bias when measuring the hospice effect on nursing home residents' pain. J Pain Symptom Manage 2003;26: 998–1009.

23. Miller SC, Gozalo P, Mor V. Hospice enrollment and hospitalization of dying nursing home patients. Am J Med 2001;111:38–44.

24. Hospital–Hospice Partnerships in Palliative Care: Creating a Continuum of Service. National Hospice and Palliative Care Organization and The Center to Advance Palliative Care in Hospitals and Health Systems. Arlington, Va.: NHPCO, 2002.

25. Center to Advance Palliative Care. Available at www.capc.org. (accessed January 10, 2007).

26. Miller SC, Egan KA. How can clinicians with diverse backgrounds and training collaborate with one another to care for patients at the end of life? Nursing Home/Hospice Partnerships. Brown University. January 2006.

27. Gerteis M, Edgman-Levitan S, Daley J, Delbanco TL, eds. Through the Patient's Eyes: Understanding and Promoting Patient-Centered Care. San Francisco: Jossey-Bass, 1993:20.

28. Byock I, Merriman MP. Measuring quality of life for patients with terminal illness: The Missoula-VITAS® Quality of Life Index. Palliat Med 1998;12:231–244.

29. Cassell EJ. The Nature of Suffering and the Goals of Medicine, 2nd ed. Oxford: Oxford University Press, 2004.

30. Salmon JR, Kwak J, Acquaviva K, Brandt K, Egan K. Transformative aspects of caregiving at life's end. J Pain Symptom Manage 2005;29(2):121–129,

31. Byock I. Dying Well: The Prospect for Growth at the End of Life. New York: G. P. Putnam's Sons, 1997.

32. Byock I. The nature of suffering and the nature of opportunity at the end-of-life. Clin Geriatr Med 1996;2:237–251.

33. Salmon JR, Deming AM, Kwak J, Acquaviva K, Brandt K, Egan K. Caregiving at Life's End: The National Needs Assessment and Implications for Hospice Practice. Executive Summary to The Hospice Institute of the Florida Suncoast. Tampa, Fla.: Florida Policy Exchange Center on Aging, University of South Florida, 2003:2–7.

34. Egan-City KA. The Hospice Experience Model: Discussion on the Specialty of Hospice and Palliative Care. Presentation to National Hospice & Palliative Care Clinical Team Conference. Dallas, Tx. October 2008.

35. Newsline Quarterly Insights Edition, The Hospice Team on the New CoPs. National Hospice & Palliative Care Organization. Arlington, Va. December 2008. Available at http://www.nhpco.org/files/public/newsline/NewsLine_Dec_08.pdf (accessed November 18, 2009).

36. Block EM, Cassarett DJ, Spence C, Gozalo P, Connor SR, Teno JM. Got Volunteers? Association of Hospice Use of Volunteers with Bereaved Family members Overall Rating of the Quality of Life Care. Abstract presented at AAHPM/HPNA 2009 Annual Assembly. p 62.

37. Connor SR, Egan KA, Wilosz DK, Larson DG, Reese DJ. Interdisciplinary approaches to assisting with end-of-life care and decision making. Am Behav Sci 2002;46:340–356.

38. Harper BC. Death: The Coping Mechanism of the Health Professional. Greenville, S.C.: Southeastern University Press, 1994.

39. National Hospice Work Group. The Access and Innovations Project: Enhancing Access to Quality Outcomes at the End of Life. May 2007.

40. Committee on the Medicare Hospice Benefit and End-of-Life Care. Final Report to the Board of Directors. Arlington, Va.: National Hospice Organization, 1998:23–25.

41. Christakis NA, Lamont EB. Extent and determinants of error in doctors' prognoses in terminally ill patients: Prospective cohort study. BMJ 2000;320:469–473.

42. Lynn J, Harrell FE, Cohn F, Wagner D, Conners AF Jr. Prognoses of seriously ill hospitalized patients on the days before death: Implications for patient care and public policy. New Horizons 1997;5:56–61.

43. Pearlman RA. Variability in physician estimates of survival for acute respiratory failure in chronic obstructive pulmonary disease. Chest 1987;91:515–521.

44. Moore HD. Evaluation of the Prognostic Criteria for Medicare Hospice Eligibility. A dissertation submitted in partial fulfillment of the requirements for the degree of Doctor of Philosophy, School of Aging Studies, College of Arts and Sciences, University of South Florida. March 2004.

45. Cahaba Government Benefit Administrators, LLC. Hospice Coverage Guidelines: Medicare Benefit Policy Manual (CMS Pub, 100-02, Ch. 9). Available at http://www.cms.hhs.gov/manuals/Downloads/bp102c09.pdf (accessed December 18, 2008).

46. Ferrell B, Connor S, Cordes A, etal. The National Agenda for Quality Palliative Care: The National Consensus Project and the National Quality Forum. J Pain Symptom Manage 2007;737–744.

47. Centers for Medicare and Medicaid Services. MS Medicare Coverage Database: LCD for Hospice: Determining Terminal Status (L13653). Available at www.cms.hhs.gov/mcd (accessed December 2, 2008).

48. Taylor DH, Ostermann J, Van Houtven, CJ, Tulsky, JA, Steinhauser, K. What length of hospice use maximizes reduction in medical expenditures near death in the US Medicare program? Social Sci & Med 2007;65:1466–1478.

# 3

*Marie Bakitas, Margaret Firer Bishop, and Paula A. Caron*

# Hospital-Based Palliative Care

*Palliative care is doing 500% more than it was five years ago, and our perceived need is about 800% more. The more we've used Palliative Care Services, the more we are coming to rely on them. The main difference now is that it's sort of like breathing—it's happening automatically. There are countless patients with pain management needs, or patients with bowel obstructions who had really terrible, hard-to-manage symptoms and needed G-tubes (for drainage) and complex medication management…and the Palliative Care Team was able to come up with a variety of interventions to help the patient stay home. Otherwise, they would have been in the hospital and really suffering. That is the difference!—An oncologist commenting on the growth of Palliative Care Services in the medical center.*

*People who say it cannot be done should not interrupt those who are doing it.—Chinese Proverb*

♦ ***Key Points***
♦ *The structure, clinical processes, and measurement of outcomes of specialized palliative and hospice services, organized as hospital-based palliative care (HBPC) programs, have grown in sophistication in response to documented, poor end-of-life care, growth of the elderly and chronic illness populations, and documented successes of pilot and maturing clinical palliative care programs.*
♦ *Standards, guidelines and other resources are now available to assist health systems to develop, sustain, or expand palliative care services for persons of all ages and stages of illness, along the entire care continuum. All hospitals and health care systems should develop palliative care services that are consistent with these standards and the mission, size, and scope of the health system.*
♦ *Processes of "best-practice" palliative care should address the right person, at the right time, and to the appropriate degree. Fundamental processes of HBPC include: introduction of palliative care services to patients and their families at the time of diagnosis with life-limiting illness; triggers for palliative care referral; standardized assessment; proactive advance care planning; treatment decision-making; crisis prevention; expert symptom management; attention to psychosocial, spiritual and physical needs; family care; and bereavement.*
♦ *Processes and infrastructures of care should exist "upstream" from palliative care services so that advance care plans documenting patients' values and preferences for care (including proxy decision-maker, site of care, symptom management, artificial nutrition and hydration, and resuscitation) can be honored.*
♦ *Establishing standardized assessment, measurement, and reporting of patient, family, and institutional outcomes is an essential component of every HBPC program both for program evaluation and research.*
♦ *Internal (e.g., quality improvement and ethics committees) and external (e.g., The Joint Commission, Center to Advance Palliative Care) resources can assist with the development or improvement of a high quality, cost effective HBPC program.*

After a battle victory in 1942, Winston Churchill, said: "Now this is not the end. It is not even the beginning of the end. But it is, perhaps, the end of the beginning." These same words could apply to the current status of hospital-based palliative care (HBPC). One hundred years ago, the cause, age, and place of death were very different compared to the beginning of the 21st century.[1] Table 3–1 compares some characteristics of dying in 1900 and in 2000. Chronic illness and longer life were the legacy of the 20th century. However, the health care system did not keep pace with medical advances. The hospital became a common location for a good portion of end-of-life (EOL) care despite Americans' stated preference for death at home.[1,2] An analysis of the experience of dying among chronically ill Medicare recipients (based on claims data for 2001–2005) demonstrated that the incidence of dying in hospitals varied, but in some regions of the United States it was greater than 40% (Figure 3–1).[3] An additional 25% to 35% of the nation's elderly die in nursing homes.[4,5] Although a percentage of seriously ill patients experienced their final admission in a critical care unit, by and large hospital deaths occurred in non-critical care units and could have been anticipated for hours or days before death actually occurred.[6] Despite this opportunity to provide comfort measures during the dying process, patients dying in the acute care hospital experienced pain, dyspnea, anxiety, and other distressing symptoms.[7–9]

As Berwick described the nature of system improvement: "Every system is perfectly designed to get the results it gets."[10] Hospitals were designed primarily to provide acute, episodic care to persons with acute illness, rather than comfort and continuity to persons who were not expected to survive a particular disease or episode of illness. Therefore, fundamental system reform and redesign was needed to improve (and possibly prevent) hospital care of persons with life-limiting illness. Such data served as a call to action, particularly for nurses. Since nursing care is the primary service provided during hospital admission, much of the care and the system that patients experience could be influenced by nurses at all organizational levels. Most other types of care, such as physician consultation, diagnostic tests, and pharmaceutical treatments, don't generally require inpatient admission.

HBPC programs have begun to change the quality and quantity of hospitalized deaths.[11–13] Nurses have served as leaders and active team members to define, direct, and lead multidisciplinary and interdisciplinary teams and modify efforts at multiple levels of the hospital care system to improve the complex care process for persons with life-limiting illness.[14,15] Improved palliative care structure, standards for care processes and the measurement of outcomes have begun to come about as a result of the development of HBPC programs. The new millennium marked the "end of the beginning" of the discipline of palliative care.

This chapter provides nursing leaders and others with historical and foundational information on HBPC for the purpose of improving access to high quality palliative and hospice services for the right person, at the right time, and in the right amount. The chapter begins with two cases. The first case describes how many patients experience life-limiting illness in many of our current health systems. The second case illustrates how serious illness can be experienced differently in a health system with a comprehensive HBPC program. The cases are followed by discussion of a variety of HBPC structures or models, palliative care delivery processes, quality improvement and outcomes measurement, and future directions in the evolution of HBPC programs. The information contained in this chapter is important for all nurses who care for persons with life-limiting illness, including senior nursing leaders, clinical nurse specialists, nurse practitioners,

**Table 3–1**
**Comparison of Death and Dying in 1900 and in 2000**

|  | 1900 | 2000 |
|---|---|---|
| Life expectancy | 47 y | 75 y |
| Usual place of death | Home | Hospital |
| Most medical expenses | Paid by family | Paid by Medicare |
| Disability before death | Usually not much | 2 y, on average |

*Source*: Data from Lynn and Adamson (2003), reference 1.

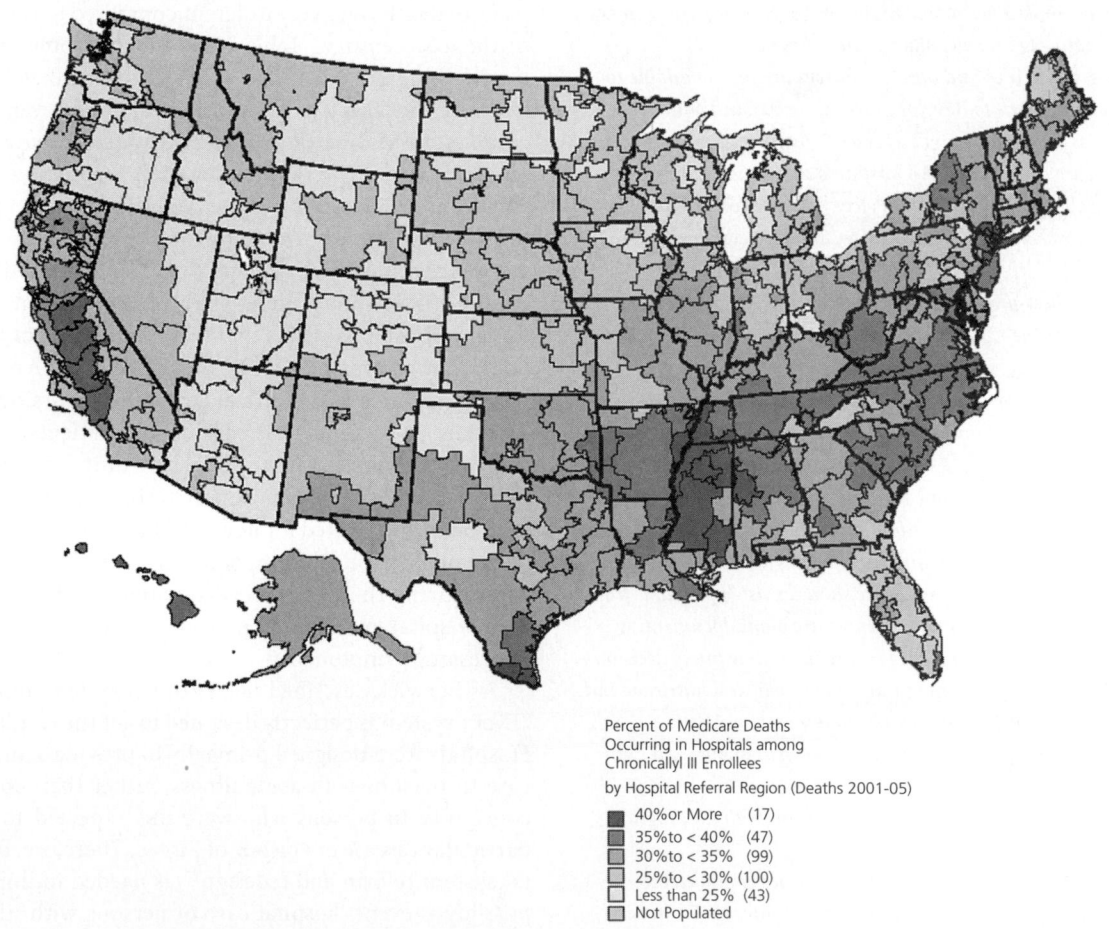

Percent of Medicare Deaths
Occurring in Hospitals among
Chronicallyl Ill Enrollees

by Hospital Referral Region (Deaths 2001-05)

- 40%or More    (17)
- 35%to < 40%  (47)
- 30%to < 35%  (99)
- 25%to < 30% (100)
- Less than 25%  (43)
- Not Populated

**Figure 3–1.** Percent of Medicare deaths occurring in hospitals among chronically ill enrollees. *Source*: Data from the Dartmouth Atlas Project and Wennberg, Fisher, et al., 2008. Reprinted with permission.

nurse managers, educators, quality improvement nurses, nurse researchers, and especially nurses on the front lines at the bedsides of patients with serious illness.

CASE STUDY

### Mr. F, a 75-Year-Old Man with Lung Cancer and Bilateral Hip Fractures

Mr. F, a 75-year-old man, was admitted to the medical/surgical unit with bilateral hip fractures after a fall at home. He underwent open reduction with internal fixation of his hips bilaterally. His past medical history was significant for metastatic lung cancer with bony involvement and chronic obstructive pulmonary disease. Postoperatively, he developed intermittent confusion, cough, and dyspnea. A chest radiograph revealed a right upper lobe infiltrate, and intravenous antibiotics, supportive oxygen therapy, nebulizer treatments, and close observation were instituted.

Mr. F's respiratory status worsened, and he required increasing oxygen via nasal cannula and then via face mask. As his condition declined, he was asked by the intern if he would "like everything done for him." He continuously nodded his head "Yes" to the question. Shortly after this "discussion," Mr. F suffered a respiratory arrest, for which he received CPR including intubation, and mechanical ventilation. He was transferred to the intensive care unit (ICU) in critical condition. No family members could be identified to assist the medical team with decision-making.

While he was in the ICU, a Swan-Ganz catheter and central line were inserted, multiple daily blood draws were taken, and Mr. F was heavily sedated to prevent him from dislodging his tubes. His medical condition progressively deteriorated, and the medical and nursing staff became increasingly frustrated, feeling helpless and not knowing Mr. F's goals of care. After multiple attempts, a neighbor was finally contacted who said he didn't really know the patient well enough to understand what he may have wanted done at this point. After a 2-week ICU stay, Mr. F developed sepsis. Eventually, he died in the ICU.

### Quality of Care Issues Identified in this Case

- Discussion of advance directives should take place with patients when they have capacity and are not in crisis.
- Early introduction of palliative care specialists may help to clarify and document patients' goals of care and pain/symptom management preferences.
- Lack of advance planning can result in health care provider frustration, fatigue, and moral distress.
- Medical and nursing staff education about advance directives, palliative care, and EOL issues can establish baseline competence levels.

- Unnecessary patient and staff suffering can be minimized if palliative care education, protocols, and policies are in place to support patient identification of goals of care.

CASE STUDY

### Mr. RL, a 71-Year-Old Man with Painless Jaundice

Mr. RL, a 71-year-old gentleman, presented to his family doctor in March with indigestion, bloating, and painless jaundice. He was diagnosed by endoscopic ultrasound and biopsy with adenocarcinoma of the head of the pancreas. Placement of a biliary stent relieved his jaundice and he was scheduled for further evaluation. On laparoscopic exam, he was found to have metastatic disease with multiple lesions on the surface of the liver. His family doctor referred Mr. RL to medical oncology and because of his stage of disease, the cancer center routine protocol called for referral to the palliative care team (PCT) for an initial assessment and consultation. Palliative care assessment revealed that he was relatively asymptomatic since relief of the jaundice and he was in the process of deciding whether or not to begin chemotherapy.

Mr. and Mrs. RL had been married for 44 years and they had 3 grown children who were involved and supportive. His wife was having particular problems coping with and adjusting to his illness. Before his recent retirement, Mr. RL worked in sales as a businessman and enjoyed traveling extensively. Although he lived in Hawaii, he had family near an NCI cancer center on the mainland and he chose to go there for his treatment. He often stayed in local hotels near the cancer center during treatments but returned frequently between treatments to his home in Hawaii. Mr. RL described himself as more spiritual than religious and routinely meditated twice daily. He understood this illness was incurable; however, he preferred not to openly discuss this much with his family. He often commented that he "wanted to fight and stay positive" and hoped he'd "be the one person to beat this."

Following the initial consultation, regular clinic visits with the palliative care nurse practitioner (NP), concurrent with his gemcitabine chemotherapy were arranged. The palliative care team also arranged visits with the spiritual care provider, who at the patient's request offered prayer and assisted Mr. and Mrs. RL to explore their religious beliefs and their wishes to re-engage in their relationship with God. The team social worker offered regular counseling to both Mr. and Mrs. RL regarding adjustment to illness and anticipatory grief. The healing arts practitioner offered Reiki and massage when the patient was receiving infusions and through occasional "home" visits at the nearby hotel where they were staying. Over this period of relative stability, the palliative care clinicians built trust and rapport and they were able to assist him and his wife with treatment decision-making and advance care planning. They also did much teaching regarding symptom management and "crisis prevention" and served as an initial contact (in conjunction with the oncology team) so that any uncomfortable symptoms could be evaluated by phone or in the clinic rather than in the emergency department. Their regular contact and knowledge of his symptoms averted two inpatient admissions for symptoms when a blocked stent was identified by the palliative care NP and MD and was replaced as an outpatient procedure, and when potential small bowel obstruction was managed conservatively at home through a constipation protocol.

Mr. RL did very well on gemcitabine from April to October, when he had evidence of disease progression. He was offered a "standard" second-line treatment or a Phase I trial. While making this difficult decision, he required much counseling with his oncologist and the palliative care team NP. He finally decided to take standard treatment as he felt that the Phase I study would interfere with too many of his valued activities. He progressed after 2 cycles of docetaxel. He began to experience significant weight loss and had a duodenal blockage which was relieved by stenting in November. As the disease progressed, Mr. RL struggled with decisions about DNR and whether to continue further therapy. With the support and trust of the palliative care NP, he was now able to have open discussions with his wife and family about end-of-life preferences, especially the place of death. He continued to wish to "fight" his disease and his oncologist suggested that there might be other treatments; however, with the support of the PCT, the patient and oncologist were able to see that his poor performance status and desire to spend quality time with family made pursuing additional treatment not consistent with Mr. RL's goals. A major wish of the patient was to be able to return to Hawaii. With the help and coordination between the PCT and local home hospice program in Hawaii, he was able to fly home immediately. The PCT continued contact with Mr. RL and his family after his return home. In early January, he died comfortably in his home surrounded by family. A bereavement contact was made by the PCT as well as the home hospice team. Over the course of his illness, Mr. RL received 17 outpatient PC visits and 5 inpatient PC visits to help with symptom management, healing arts, psychosocial and spiritual support, continuity and coordination of care, and advance care planning and treatment decision-making.

### Quality of Care Issues Identified in this Case

- The patient was identified early in the trajectory of illness.
- Patient and family's values and preferences for care were identified early and integrated into the plan of care.
- A team approach allowed for various members to assist with the patient's diverse needs across the entire episode of illness.

- Palliative care involvement occurred in and out of the hospital setting. Continuity occurred across all settings.
- The patient's preference for location of death was met.

### Brief History and Definitions of HBPC

In 1974, the Royal Victoria Hospital in Montreal, Canada, developed one of the first initiatives in North America to improve hospital-based palliative care. They developed a palliative care service to meet the needs of hospitalized patients who were terminally ill within the general hospital setting.[16] The palliative care service was an integral part of the Royal Victoria Hospital; a 1,000 bed teaching hospital affiliated with McGill University consisting of five complementary clinical components: (1) the Palliative Care Unit, (2) the home care service, (3) the consultation team, (4) the palliative care clinic, and (5) the bereavement follow-up program. Members of an interdisciplinary team were involved with the care of these patients, and the focus was on holistic care with pain control and symptom management.

Three decades later, these basic palliative care concepts are becoming more prevalent in many U.S. hospitals. In the U.S., a number of milestones over the past 4 decades have shaped the evolution of care of the seriously ill (see Table 3–2). In the 1970s, the concept of home-based hospice programs (often volunteer only) migrated to the U.S. from Europe and Canada. Since that time, a number of professional, medical, societal, and academic endeavors have coalesced in the form of hospital-based palliative care (HBPC) programs. HBPC adapts and "upstreams" many of the principles of hospice care into mainstream medicine. Although there is no requirement for all health care systems to have such a program, palliative care is gradually being recognized as a "standard of care." For organizations that still need convincing, Meier[17,18] makes the case by using at least 5 evidence-based arguments: (1) to improve clinical quality of care for seriously ill patients; (2) to increase patient and family satisfaction with care; (3) to meet the demand of a growing, chronically-ill, elderly demographic; (4) to serve as "classrooms" for the next generation of clinicians who need to provide better care to the seriously ill; and (5) to provide value-added, cost-effective care in the face of a national health care and economic crisis. A recent review of palliative care studies presents a compelling argument that, based on the amount of available evidence, HBPC is state-of-the-art care.[19]

Although much of the data to support the evolution of HBPC have come from care deficits identified in hospitalized patients at the very end of life (EOL)[2,6,8,9]; the goal of HBPC is to improve the quality of life of persons with life-limiting illness much earlier in the course of illness across all settings of health care.[20]

A number of definitions of HBPC exist, but contain similar elements. In 1990, the World Health Organization defined

**Table 3–2**
**Milestones in the Evolution from Home Hospice to Hospital-Based Palliative Care**

1970s Awareness of hospice philosophy transfers from Great Britain to United States

- 1976 Karen Ann Quinlan Case

1980s Recognition of aging population, chronic disease demographics, growth of National Institute on Aging and American Association of Retired Persons

- Passage of Medicare Hospice Benefit
- Recognition of AIDS

1990s National recognition in United States of the problem of end-of-life care

- 1990 Nancy Cruzan Case
- 1990–1997 Kevorkian assisted deaths
- 1991 Patient Self-Determination Act
- 1995– SUPPORT Study findings of poor EOL care
- 1997 Legalization of Assisted Suicide in Oregon
- 1997 Institute of Medicine Report (IOM) "Approaching Death: Improving Care at the End of Life"
- 1997 Institute for Health Care Improvement (IHI) EOL Breakthrough Collaborative
- 1998 First Palliative Care APN Programs (Ursuline College, New York University)
- 1999 Kevorkian convicted of first degree murder and imprisoned

2000 Baby boomers with aging parents achieve positions of leadership & authority (Project on Death In America [PDIA] scholars/leaders) entering and legitimizing Palliative Medicine as a specialty field

- 2001 Institute of Medicine Report: "Improving Palliative Care for Cancer"
- Public Broadcasting System (PBS) Bill Moyers Special "On our own terms"
- 1995–2003 Robert Wood Johnson Foundation EOL funded activities
  - Last Acts
  - Promoting Excellence in EOL Care
  - Partnership for Caring
  - Educating Physicians in End-of-Life Care (EPEC)
  - End-of-Life Nursing Education Consortium (ELNEC)
- Open Society/Project on Death In America (PDIA)
  - Faculty Scholars Program
- 2001 Disseminating End-of-Life Education to Cancer Centers (DELEtCC)
- 2002 Department of Veterans Affairs Initiates multiple Palliative/EOL programs
- Mayday, Kornfeld sponsored mini-fellowships (Northwestern, Memorial Sloan Kettering, etc.)
- Growth and development of specialty education and organizations
  - Shift of professional membership organizations from homes of the isolated to active change agents in policy, education, and clinical change: HPNA, AAHPM
  - Center to Advance Palliative Care & Palliative Care Leadership Centers
  - NHPCO, AAHPM, HPNA—membership organizations
    - Palliative Medicine achieves ABMS specialty status
    - Advanced and NA specialty nursing certification
    - Expansion of Harvard course, EPEC, ELNEC, JPM
- Development of (MD) fellowship programs
- 2004 National Consensus Project + 2008 NQF-Quality Guidelines
- 2005 Terry Schiavo case
- Research Evidence to support Palliative Care emerging and developing new funding sources
- NPCRC/ACS Junior Faculty & Pilot Project Awards
- 2008 The Joint Commission considers Palliative Care Certification Process

palliative care as care that "seeks to address not only physical pain, but also emotional, social, and spiritual pain to achieve the best possible quality of life for patients and their families. Palliative care extends the principles of hospice care to a broader population that could benefit from receiving this type of care earlier in their illness or disease process."[21] A HBPC program has been defined by the American Hospital Association (AHA) as: "an organized program providing specialized medical care, drugs, or therapies for the management of acute or chronic pain and/or the control of symptoms administered by specially trained physicians and other clinicians; and supportive care services, such as counseling on advance directives, spiritual care, and social services, to patients with advanced disease and their families."[22] The

Center to Advance Palliative Care defines HBPC as: "an interdisciplinary medical team focused on symptom management, intensive patient–physician–family communication, clarifying goals of treatment and coordination of care across health care settings" (p. 34).[23] In each of these definitions, a clear goal of the development of HBPC was to bring fundamental concepts of hospice care to persons with life-limiting illness—but to do so earlier in the trajectory of care and across all health care settings.

The good news is that since the AHA survey began to measure the availability of HBPC programs in 2000, there has been a steady growth (see Figure 3–2).[24] This positive movement is tempered by two issues. First, there is wide variability in patients' access to palliative care programs across the U.S. (see Figure 3–3). In particular, the southern region of the U.S. at 41% has the lowest availability of programs.[23,24] And second, despite definitions of HBPC, mandatory standards of care as yet do not exist; therefore, programs can vary in their quality, components, and their emphasis on the missions of service, research, and education.

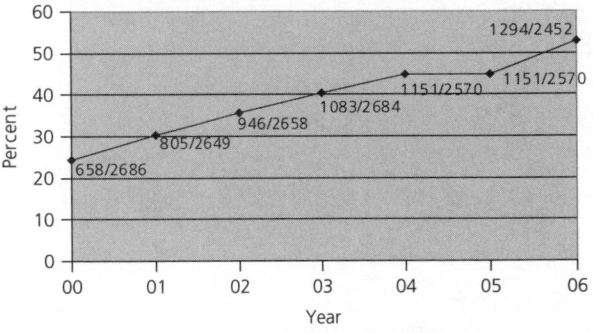

**Figure 3–2.** Percent of hospitals reporting an HBPC program. *Source*: Data from Goldsmith B, Dietrich, J. et al. (2008), reference 24.

## Primary, Secondary, Tertiary Models of Hospital-Based Palliative Care

Promoting HBPC requires a myriad of resources. Depending on the model of palliative care being introduced, the required resources can vary greatly. For example, some changes may require financial support via construction or addition of staff, whereas other changes are less resource intensive. Regardless of the health care system and the availability of resources, all health care practitioners have the ability to introduce palliative care concepts and use already established resources to develop or improve their palliative care services. According to von Gunten,[25] "One way that patients and their families will get better care is to ensure that clinical services focusing on the relief of suffering are available in every hospital" (p. 876). He suggests that hospitals (and health care systems) consider their mission and level of palliative care delivery (e.g., primary, secondary, tertiary)—as they do for other medical specialties and incorporate a model of palliative care resources in accordance with that level. Institutions with limited resources may choose a primary model which focuses on enhancing existing services and clinician education, while secondary and tertiary palliative care programs may provide multiple services, including inpatient and/or outpatient consult teams, an inpatient palliative care/hospice unit, and a home care program, all under the jurisdiction of a single hospital system. A full-service approach can ease transitions among different levels of care and has the potential to provide the optimum in seamless palliative care. Table 3–3 lists a variety of different models that have been described by the Center to Advance Palliative Care (CAPC). In addition to an extensive manual on developing a program,[18] CAPC offers a variety of other resources including individual consultation to developing programs via on-site visits and follow up consultations (see CAPC Leadership Centers below).

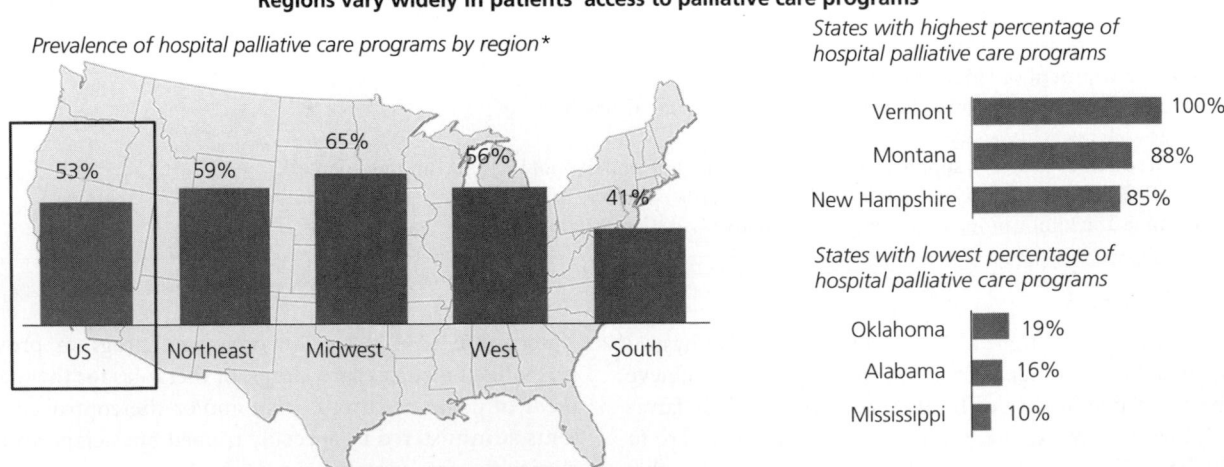

**Figure 3–3.** Variability in access to palliative care. *Source*: Nurse Executive Watch, 2008. Reprinted with permission.

**Table 3-3**
**Program Model Options**

The following chart is designed to help the planning team assess various options and their potential to provide this care in a manner that best meets hospital and patient needs.

| Characteristics | Solo Practitioner Model | Full Team Model | Geographic Model |
|---|---|---|---|
| **Philosophy/Approach** | • Consultative service<br>• Doctor (MD) or advanced nurse practitioner (ANP) provides initial assessment and communication with attending physician, nursing, and social work staff<br>• May or may not write patient orders<br>• MD or ANP refers patients to needed services (such as social work), discusses needs in conference, and communicates clinicians<br>• Assists patient and family with advance directives and plans for future | • Consultative service with full team of doctor, ANP or nurse, and social worker assesses and follows patients referred by attending physician<br>• Provides advice to primary physician, or may assume all or part of care of patient and/or write patient orders<br>• Doctor bills fee-for-service as a consultant physician<br>• Team refers patient to needed services and discharges to appropriate setting(s), discusses needs in conference, and communicates with all team members | • Inpatient program with all patients on designated unit<br>• Inpatient staff team (doctor, ANP, social worker, chaplain, therapists specially trained to provide palliative care) manages patients<br>• Staff is trained in palliative care and focuses on creating an inpatient environment supportive of patients and families<br>• Approach is milieu intensive as well as individual patient-focused<br>• Care reimbursed under licensure and guidelines (e.g., acute care) |
| **Service Model** | • MD or ANP receives referrals from attending physician, hospital staff, patient, or family<br>• All units in hospital deliver palliative care as part of their mission<br>• MD or ANP develops protocols for patient care in conjunction with treatment team, educates staff about palliative care and protocols | • Team works in unison to coordinate care plan and provide services<br>• Social worker on team may assume role of case manager<br>• Team develops and uses standing orders to manage patient<br>• All hospital units deliver palliative care as part of their mission | • Patients referred to palliative care program are screened by team for appropriateness<br>• Appropriate patients are transferred to service when they meet admission criteria<br>• Palliative care team assumes responsibility for patient management and discharge planning<br>• Patient may be followed on an outpatient basis after discharge |
| **Staffing and Budget Implications** | • One FTE MD or ANP<br>• 0.2 FTE clerical support<br>• Access to and time allotted for social worker, nursing, physical and occupational therapists (PT and OT), and pharmacy to respond to referrals (should be monitored for time requirements)<br>• 0.2 FTE finance person<br>• 0.2 FTE medical director (if ANP-led) | • 0.5 to one FTE medical director<br>• One FTE ANP<br>• 0.5 medical social worker<br>• One FTE clerical support<br>• Access to and time allotted for social work, nursing, PT, OT, and pharmacy to respond to referrals (should be monitored for time requirements)<br>• 0.2 FTE finance person | • 0.5 to one FTE medical director<br>• One FTE ANP<br>• 0.5–1.0 FTE medical social worker<br>• 0.5–1.0 FTE chaplain<br>• 0.2 FTE finance person<br>• Nurse manager<br>• Inpatient unit staffing<br>• Preferably, unit is situated where staff are likely to have training in fundamentals of palliative care<br>• An allocation of DRG revenues may be required when a patient transfers from another unit to palliative care. |

*(Continued)*

**Table 3-3**
**Program Model Options** (*Continued*)

| Characteristics | Solo Practitioner Model | Full Team Model | Geographic Model |
|---|---|---|---|
| **Patient Volume Thresholds** | • Patient coordination is intensive and ANP spends time with patient providing psychosocial support as well as symptom management and family teaching. Staff teaching as well.<br>• Literature does not define volume but anecdotal reports suggest maximum comfortable caseload of 4 new cases per day and average census of 10 patients/week | • Number varies, depending on whether patient is transferred to the team for all management<br>• Can reach the largest number of patients and does not restrict the number of beds occupied by patients requiring palliative care services | • Geographic unit approach allows the institution to designate beds, yet allow the number of beds to flex with patient volume<br>• Most efficient staffing with 12 or more beds, preferably in rooms with space for family members to stay and room for staff and family members to meet<br>• Because reimbursement is still acute care-oriented, the unit can flex to a capacity deemed appropriate to staffing levels and clinical expertise |
| **Benefits/Advantages** | • Lower start-up costs and financial risk<br>• Opportunity to develop a program based on existing patient population<br>• Less threatening to medical staff<br>• Builds on existing programs and services and uses them whenever possible | • More medical expertise available<br>• Provides alternative to medical staff that struggle with implementing new skills and knowledge<br>• Consultative service reaches largest number of nurses and physicians through bedside and nursing station teaching and role modeling<br>• Builds on existing programs and services and uses them whenever possible | • The program has a clinical milieu and staff to support it<br>• Greater control over patient care<br>• Higher visibility and influence within the hospital<br>• Inpatient unit can be made patient-and family-friendly<br>• May be easier to manage overuse of resources, length of stay<br>• Opportunity for philanthropic support more easily developed<br>• Can convert all or part of an existing unit to minimize additional staffing |
| **Disadvantages/Threats** | • Program rests on one individual's shoulders<br>• Patient volume quickly limited by workload<br>• Service effectiveness is dependent on staff knowledge and cooperation<br>• All units referring patients need to be educated | • Added costs for team with limited, or no, additional revenue<br>• Physician must establish rapport with many medical staff members; consultant serves as an advisor to the primary physician and recommendations may or may not be followed<br>• Service effectiveness is dependent on staff knowledge and cooperation<br>• All units referring patients need to be educated | • Geographic patient concentration deprives staff in other parts of the hospital from exposure to the service and learning opportunities<br>• May be viewed as the "death ward," making physicians reluctant to refer patients<br>• Unless beds can be shared efficiently with an adjacent unit, under-use of continuous nursing coverage beds due to low referral volume will translate into losses for the unit. |

*Source:* Copyright 2009: Center to Advance Palliative Care (CAPC). Reprinted from CAPC website with permission: http://www.capc.org/building-a-hospital-based-palliative-care-program/designing/characteristics/program-model-chart/document_view.

## Primary Palliative Care

Primary palliative care should be available at all hospitals. This level of care requires, at a minimum, clinician education in the basics of pain and symptom management. Primary palliative care refers to a level of care whereby basic skills and competencies are required of all physicians, nurses, and other health care practitioners who come in contact with persons with life-limiting illness. The National Consensus Project (NCP), the National Quality Forum (NQF), and the Joint Commission (TJC) have each identified standards that should be addressed in all hospitals and other settings (see later discussion). All practitioners should be competent at this level.

Clinicians can gain the knowledge, attitudes, and skills needed to provide palliative care to their patients through basic palliative care training and clinical practice. There is a growing availability of continuing education, including established formal programs for all disciplines to improve their knowledge of basic palliative care principles. The End-of-Life Nursing Education Consortium (ELNEC) and Education for Physicians on End-of-Life Care (EPEC) are two comprehensive educational programs that can provide such information. Both educational programs are further described later in this chapter and in Chapter 65.

## Secondary Palliative Care

Secondary palliative care refers to a model in which all providers have a minimum level of competence and, in addition, have specialists who provide palliative care through an interdisciplinary consultation team (IDT), specialized unit or both. The development and success of these specialized services will come about as a result of strong leadership, marketing and accessibility.[18] It is not necessary for an IDT or unit to evaluate every patient with palliative care needs who is admitted to the hospital, but these specially trained clinicians are available as a resource and guide for their colleagues.

## Tertiary Palliative Care

Teaching hospitals and academic centers with teams of experts in palliative care are classified as tertiary organizations. A tertiary-level program may serve as a consultant to primary and secondary level practices in difficult clinical situations or as model programs to assist developing centers. Practitioners and institutions involved at the tertiary level of palliative care are also involved in educational and research activities.[25] Multidisciplinary training programs for nurses and physicians are an important function of a tertiary center (see below). Tertiary centers also have an obligation to perform research to enhance the evidence base for palliative care.

It is the responsibility of all hospitals and health care organizations to be competent, at a minimum, at the primary level of palliative care. Organizations at different levels may choose among different components of care to incorporate into their model. Some components are less resource intense (e.g., staff education, care pathways), while others may require additional allocations of budget and personnel. The latter resources include Interdisciplinary Consult Team (IDTs), specialized palliative care units (PCUs), outpatient/ambulatory palliative care clinics, and structured outreach or strong relationships with skilled nursing facilities (SNF) and home-based hospice programs.

## The Inpatient Interdisciplinary Consult Team

A growing literature summarizes the development of palliative care consultation teams within hospitals to offer specialized consultation and expertise to patients, families, and other health care providers.[26-31] Dunlop and Hockley published a manual in 1990 and a second edition in 1998 describing the experience in England.[32,33] They described the movement as one that tries to take the hospice philosophy of care and bring it into the hospital using a consultancy team. A number of U.S. and Canadian hospital-based teams have described their experiences.[34-36] Among the components of successful teams are an interdisciplinary approach, physician and non-physician referral, rapid response to requested consultations, around-the-clock availability, and ability to follow patients through all care settings.

IDTs can be effective in modeling behaviors that are supportive of appropriate HBPC, but they should also recommend infrastructure and organizational changes as part of their approach to consultation. Gathering data about demographic statistics about the location and nature of regular consultations may help to identify the need for particular institutional policies and procedures. For example, if a particular unit or care provider has difficulty managing patients with dyspnea on a regular basis, targeted educational approaches and treatment algorithms or standardized orders may help achieve consistent and long-lasting change. Theoretically, an IDT could "put itself out of business" with such an approach. However, teams to date have not reported the need to dissolve as an outcome of implementing system changes.

Studies have begun to examine the impact of IDTs on the overall care of hospitalized, seriously ill patients.[26-31,35,37] However, this is challenging research and, as in any multi-component intervention, it is difficult to identify exactly which components or processes of the team are responsible for the outcomes. Valid, reliable measures and multi-method research are likely to be needed to capture this information.[38] Maintaining an IDT can be costly; therefore, it is imperative to continue to evaluate programs and strengthen the evidence base to provide economic justification for many hospitals. A consensus panel has recommended minimum data that should be collected by all consultation services[39] (see *Measurement* later in this chapter).

## Inpatient Hospice and Palliative Care Units (PCUs)

Some hospitals, faced with the problem of providing high-quality palliative care, have found the development of a specialized unit to be the solution. In the United Kingdom, these units have been developed from preexisting oncology units, as part of another unit, or sometimes in a separate building that is distinct but near the hospital it serves.[33] U.S. hospitals have varying amounts of experience with opening specialized units for the care of patients with hospice, or palliative care needs.[40-42] An inpatient unit has some advantages and disadvantages. Advantages include:

- Patients requiring palliative care have a familiar place to go during the exacerbations and remissions that come with progressive disease.
- Unit staff and policies are under the control and financing of experts trained as a team who are skillful at difficult care and communications.
- Patients may get palliative care earlier if other care teams see the advantages of this approach and trust that patients will receive good care.

Providers who monitor their patients on these units (if allowed) can learn valuable lessons about palliative care that can be carried forward to future patients. These future patients may not require admission to the PCU for some types of care. Some disadvantages of creating a PCU include:

- It can prevent others from learning valuable palliative care techniques if the PCU staff are seen as "specialized" and are secluded in one area.
- Care providers may come to rely on this expertise instead of learning palliative care techniques themselves.
- If PCU transfer includes a transfer of doctors to a palliative care specialist, patients and families may feel abandoned by their primary team in the final hours.
- Hospice providers fear loss of the hospice philosophy when a PCU exists in the context of the general hospital.

### Outpatient/Ambulatory Palliative Care Clinics

In an ideal world, patients with life-limiting illness spend the majority of their time outside of the hospital with only occasional need for attention by a palliative care specialist. Transitions of care are a common area of difficulty for patients with palliative care needs. An outpatient service can serve as an initial point of referral for patients early in their disease process[43] or it may allow a discharged patient to continue to have specialized management of their symptoms and other needs. A number of models of delivering outpatient care exist[44-50] including a consultative model in which palliative care clinicians participate in other disease-focused outpatient visits (e.g., in clinics serving patients with congestive heart failure, cancer, amyotrophic lateral sclerosis (ALS), dialysis unit, etc.) to geographic space allotted only to palliative care clinicians and patients. Outpatient services are still considered a novel, less frequent service component of HBPC in most organizations.

### Liaisons with Skilled Nursing Facilities and Home Hospice

Perhaps one of the most important ways to improve HBPC is to develop strong relationships with other health care agencies outside of the hospital, so that alternatives to inpatient admission for palliative care exist. Alternatives such as home hospice care or skilled hospice care within assisted-living centers, free-standing hospices, or specially-designated areas in nursing homes or rehabilitation facilities can provide expert palliative and hospice care. However, some areas of the United States lack these options. For example, in some rural areas, health care services such as visiting nurses agencies, home care, hospice, and skilled nursing facilities are sparse, or staff may feel unprepared to care for people who require intensive palliative care. Some visiting nurse and home care agencies may see so few symptomatic, seriously ill patients that it is difficult for staff to maintain adequate palliative care and hospice expertise in these agencies. There continues to be a need to develop models and strengthen relationships between HBPC programs and community agencies that will provide palliative care services prior to or following hospital palliative care services.[45,51-56]

### Bereavement Services

Improving HBPC does not end with the development of mechanisms to ensure peaceful, pain-free patient death. Although accomplishing this goal is surely a comfort to family and friends, bereavement care for survivors is an important final step in the process of HBPC. Which families are most in need of specific services? Identifying families at the greatest risk has been the topic of palliative care research, particularly in evaluating the quality of palliative care services.[57-62]

Bereavement services for survivors are an important part of the total care plan after the patient's death (see Chapters 30 and 58). NQF preferred practices standard for bereavement care indicates organizations should: "Facilitate effective grieving by implementing in a timely manner a bereavement care plan after the patient's death, when the family remains the focus of care."[63] Adverse physical and psychological outcomes of unsupported grief are known to occur during the bereavement period.[64] Because of this, bereavement services are a typical component of the services offered to families when patients die as part of a hospice program. Because not all deaths in the United States have hospice involvement, a large portion of families must rely on bereavement follow-up offered by other care providers. Although historically, few hospitals routinely offered bereavement services to families after patients died in the hospital,[58] a growing interest in implementing such programs has come about as a result of implementing HBPC programs.

Bereavement services can address currently unmet needs of survivors, who can benefit from resources that offer information and support on coping with the loss.[60-62,65] Having follow up contact with decedents' family members can also provide HBPC programs with information about the effectiveness of EOL care. Families' perspectives should be sought about what went well and what could be improved. For example, results of a focus group of bereaved family members indicated that, although the family was quite satisfied with pain management, breathing changes and dyspnea were not anticipated and were very distressing.[66] Hence, this became a target for improving EOL care in one hospital.

Use of family proxy perspectives is an emerging area of research and quality improvement.[52,67–72] (Measurement issues are described later in this chapter). Press-Ganey, a healthcare measurement and improvement company that is well-known for collecting patient satisfaction data after hospital discharge, now also has a survey to collect family perspectives on the end-of-life experience in the hospital.[73] This survey asks about topics such as care at the time of death, care provided by nurses, physicians, chaplains, social workers and others, environment, family care, symptoms, and overall satisfaction with care.

Standardized bereavement care can take many forms and can result in improved family satisfaction with care.[65] These actions might include sending a note of sympathy or establishing some other contact from a staff member, mailing a list of local bereavement resources or a pamphlet, and delaying the time before a hospital bill is mailed out to prevent its coinciding with funeral or memorial services. A variety of bereavement services have been developed for parents that specifically address their needs after the death of an infant or child. [65,74]

## Interdisciplinary Education: A Key Component of Palliative Care

It is imperative that staff that care for patients with life-limiting illness have sufficient and appropriate palliative care knowledge and skills. Organizations with or without HBPC programs should encourage staff members to participate in conferences on EOL and palliative care and also should support them through the continuing education process (e.g., becoming certified in a specialty). The value of improved education is not only in direct patient care, but in the role modeling that takes place. The majority of students in medical, nursing, and other health care disciplines receive clinical training for practice in hospitals. However, few hospitals provided role models for teaching palliative care practices. The following is one of several comments made by family members about the insensitive way the act of "pronouncing" the death of their loved one was handled by an inexperienced new medical intern[66]:

*I was holding his hand when he stopped breathing.*
*I called the nurse, who called the doctor. He went*
*over and looked at him lying in the bed, listened for a*
*heartbeat with his stethoscope and said, "He's dead,"*

*and walked out of the room. That's it —not "I'm sorry."*
*No, "Is there anything we can do?" Just, "He's dead."*
*It was painful, and made us think that the staff didn't*
*care.*

A study by Ferris and colleagues[75] documented that medical schools devote little time to care of dying patients. A survey of medical interns revealed significant concern and fear about providing these services with no or little supervision. The traditional "See one, do one, teach one" supervisory principle of medical education was ineffective. One resident explained that the pronouncing experience was not one that was perceived as causing harm when performed by the inexperienced. Another stated, "I felt really inadequate, I had absolutely no idea what to do when the nurse called me to pronounce this patient whom I had never met—my first night on call. I was never taught the steps—how long should I listen to the chest to be sure there was no heartbeat; what, if anything else, I should do; what should I say to the family. Thankfully, the death coordinator was there to help me fill out the paperwork." Conversely, in states where nurses are allowed to pronounce deaths, some course work exists to teach a process that gives attention to the family. For resident education, there is a comprehensive, multimedia program called "The Art of Compassionate Death Notification."[76] The program includes a facilitator's guide, manuals for learners, a pocket card of the process, and videos demonstrating communication skills.

The lack of role models for students in the clinical setting is further compounded by the lack of palliative care content in student curricula[77] and major textbooks.[78,79] When major medical and nursing texts were analyzed, they were found to be sorely lacking in the content that would inform students about the basics of palliative symptom management, decision-making, and critical communication skills. On a positive note, however, there is evidence that this situation is changing; medical and nursing school curricula and textbooks have begun to incorporate some palliative care-focused content.[80] Other creative ways to actively engage learners in palliative care education include:

- Arrange for clinician role models to provide lectures to students and faculty.
- Assist with curriculum review of current EOL care training.
- Change elective coursework and clinical work in hospice and palliative care to required status, and include these subjects in other mandatory clinical assignments.
- Use texts that contain clinically relevant palliative care content.
- Include content on ambulatory-based symptom management and decision-making that defines patient preferences for care.
- Encourage students to describe evidence-based approaches to palliative care and to challenge their mentors about approaches and interventions that

increase the burden of care without clear patient benefit.

- Encourage students to learn from staff role models appropriate ways of communicating bad news and of presenting options that respect patient preferences and values.
- Identify opportunities for undergraduate or graduate fellowships in palliative care.
- Encourage quality improvement teams to offer students opportunities to participate in, and to collect data from, patients, charts, and staff.

Experienced health care providers also have needs for specialty palliative care educational experiences. (See Chapter 65 for a detailed discussion on the topic.) Both the nursing and medical professions have embraced the concept of palliative care continuing education, advanced academic training, and certification.

In the area of continuing education, The End-of-Life Nursing Education Consortium (ELNEC) and Education for Physicians on End-of-Life Care (EPEC) are exemplary programs. The ELNEC program is a collaboration of the City of Hope Medical Center and the American Association of Colleges of Nursing, and the program has a variety of curricula for different audiences (undergraduate and graduate nursing faculty, nurses working in critical care, pediatrics, or geriatric settings, etc.). The American Medical Association (AMA) and EPEC programs address similar issues for physicians. Both curricula are widely available as a means to educate practicing nursing and medical staff.

## The Harvard Medical School Program in Palliative Care Education and Practice

Another example of palliative care continuing education is sponsored by The Harvard Medical School Center for Palliative Care. In response to the need for leaders in palliative care education in nursing and medicine, the Harvard program offers intensive learning experiences for physician and nurse educators who wish to become expert in the clinical practice and teaching of comprehensive, interdisciplinary palliative care, as well as to gain expertise in leading and managing improvements in palliative care education and practice at their own institutions. The program includes a special pediatric track. The course is delivered in two sections: Part 1 consists of 7 days of intensive learning, followed by a 6-month interim where participants work on an individual project and contribute to weekly e-mail discussions of problematic clinical, educational, and program development cases presented by other participants through e-mail exchanges. Part 2 is a second 7-day block that includes continued experiential learning and training focused on communication, teaching methods, teamwork and leadership.

The curriculum features content on how to: (1) teach the fundamentals of palliative care (assessment of physical causes of distress, psychosocial and spiritual assessment, ethical and cultural issues, palliative care in geriatric and pediatric populations, depression, and bereavement); (2) communicate at the end of life (understanding the experience of life-threatening illness, breaking bad news, communicating across cultural barriers, family meetings, providing feedback to learners); (3) manage challenges in palliative care education (principles of adult learning, understanding, learning styles, new teaching methodologies); and (4) develop and promote clinical and educational programs in palliative care (assessing institutional structure and culture, evaluating readiness to change, dealing with resistance, developing and financing palliative care programs, and fund-raising strategies).

The course faculty includes physicians, nurses, social workers, and educators from within the Harvard teaching hospitals, as well as outside experts. Complete information can be accessed at: http://www.hms.harvard.edu/cdi/pallcare/pcep.htm.

## Advanced Education and Certification in Palliative Care

As standards of care are increasingly applied to HBPC programs, advanced specialty training in palliative care will likely become a requirement. Academic opportunities for education and preparation as an advanced palliative care practitioner currently exist in a number of programs (see Chapter 65 for additional details).

Following these programs and other specialized training, nurses may take advanced certification in palliative care through the National Board for Certification of Hospice and Palliative Nurses (NBCHPN). Eligible nurse practitioners and clinical nurse specialists can acquire the credential of ACHPN® (Advanced Certified Hospice and Palliative Nurse). Certification exams are also available for registered nurses, licensed vocational nurses, nursing assistants, and nurse administrators. Hundreds have become nationally board certified as palliative care specialists since the examinations' inception.

A major advance in the field came about in 2007 when the American Board of Medical Specialties voted to approve hospice and palliative medicine as a recognized medical subspecialty. The application to recognize the subspecialty had broad support and was co-sponsored by 10 medical specialty boards. As a result, physicians in a number of specialties—including internal medicine, family medicine, pediatrics, psychiatry, neurology, surgery, emergency medicine, and obstetrics and gynecology—are able to seek this certification. Prior to that time, this certification exam was offered by the American Board of Hospice and Palliative Medicine (ABHPM). In the first decade of certification, over 2,100 physicians obtained certification from ABHPM. The ABHPM was not recognized by the American Board of Medical Specialties (ABMS), but worked successfully over the course of the decade to persuade the ABMS to recognize Hospice and Palliative Medicine as a medical subspecialty. Although voluntary, this recognition is used by the government, health care systems, and insurers as evidence of high standards. There are currently 24 member boards of the ABMS (see www.abms.org). These 24 member boards constitute the officially recognized allopathic specialties of medicine in the United States.

⚘

## Developing Standards for HBPC

A number of organizations have worked together to develop standardized palliative care practices.

### National Consensus Project

In April 2004, The National Consensus Project (NCP) for Palliative Care released Clinical Practice Guidelines for Quality Palliative Care. An updated second edition of the guidelines was published in 2009. The guidelines, which can be downloaded free of charge from their website (http://www.nationalconsensusproject.org), represent a consensus of four major United States palliative care organizations: the American Academy of Hospice and Palliative Medicine, the Center to Advance Palliative Care (CAPC), the Hospice and Palliative Nurses Association (HPNA), and the National Hospice and Palliative Care Organization (NHPCO). The guidelines identify core precepts and structures of clinical palliative care programs. Domains of palliative care from the guidelines are listed in Table 3–4. The domains were intended as a framework for HBPC programs to develop and evaluate their approaches to delivering comprehensive palliative care services. Although voluntary, one potential outcome for these guidelines is to provide a framework for certification or mandatory accreditation.[81]

### National Quality Forum

In 2007, in response to a need for national quality standards, the National Quality Forum (NQF) released a document listing "preferred practices."[63] The NQF collaborated with NCP in developing these 38 "best practices" or performance measures which are organized under the NCP 8 domains of care (Table 3–4). The practices are evidence-based or endorsed by expert consensus and apply to hospice and palliative care services across all care settings.

The NQF is a nonprofit, public-private partnership organization whose mission is to develop ways to improve the quality of U.S. health care. The NQF has representation from national, state, regional, and local organizations representing consumers, public and private insurers, employers, professionals, health plans, accrediting bodies, labor unions, and other organizations representing health care research and quality improvement. They rely on or use consensus-building processes to develop national standards for measurement and public reporting of health care performance that is safe, timely, beneficial, patient-centered, equitable, and efficient. These standards have served in other areas of care as a method to link performance with reimbursement.

The NQF used the following definition of palliative care to develop the practices: "Palliative care is both a philosophy of care and an organized, highly structured system for delivering care. The goal of palliative care is to prevent and relieve suffering and to support the best possible quality of life for patients and their families, regardless of the stage of the disease or the need for other therapies. Palliative care expands traditional disease-model medical treatments to include the goals of enhancing quality of life for patients and family, , optimizing function, helping with decision making, and providing opportunities for personal growth."[63]

### Center to Advance Palliative Care (CAPC)

One of the major efforts to improve hospital-based palliative care programs in the United States is led by the CAPC. Originally formed and funded by a 4-year grant from the RWJ Foundation in 2000, the national center was established at Mount Sinai School of Medicine in New York City. The Aetna Foundation, the Brookdale Foundation, the JEHT Foundation, and The John A. Hartford Foundation also provide support. The Center, directed by Diane Meier, MD, has a mission to make information on how to establish high-quality palliative care services available to hospitals and health systems nationwide.

CAPC assists hospitals with the planning, development, and implementation of HBPC programs. In addition to assisting hospitals and other health systems in program development, CAPC facilitates collaboration among hospitals, hospices, and nursing homes; promotes educational initiatives in palliative care; and encourages growth and development of new and innovative mechanisms for financing palliative care programs.[82] More recently, they have collaborated on the development of a strong evidence base and palliative care research with the National Palliative Care Research Center (described later in this chapter).

CAPC has developed six Palliative Care Leadership Centers (PCLCs) to assist organizations that wish to learn the practical aspects of developing a palliative care program. The six organizations are Fairview Health Services, Minneapolis, MN; Massey Cancer Center of Virginia Commonwealth University Medical Center, Richmond, VA; Medical College of Wisconsin, Milwaukee, WI; Mount Carmel Health System, Columbus, OH; Palliative Care Center of the Bluegrass, Lexington, KY; and University of California, San Francisco, CA. Each represents a different type of health care system and palliative care delivery model. They serve as exemplary organizations offering site visits, hands-on training, and technical assistance to support development of palliative care programs nationwide. Further information regarding the PCLC can be found on the CAPC website (http://www.capc.org).

Building on the work of the NCP and NQF, in 2008 a consensus panel of CAPC staff, consultants, and PCLC faculty convened to determine which operational details were essential for program sustainability and growth for HBPC. They identified "must have" and "should have" elements that are arranged under 12 domains (see Table 3–5).[83] Each of these activities is described further in Table 3–5.

**Table 3–4**
**National Quality Forum Preferred Practices Organized by National Consensus Project: Domains of Quality Palliative Care**

| NCP Domains of Quality Palliative Care | NQF Preferred Practices |
|---|---|
| 1. Structure and processes of care | 1. Provide palliative and hospice care by an interdisciplinary team of skilled palliative care professionals, including, for example, physicians, nurses, social workers, pharmacists, spiritual care counselors, and others who collaborate with primary healthcare professional(s). [**4. STAFFING**] |
| | 2. Provide access to palliative and hospice care that is responsive to the patient and family 24 hours a day, 7 days a week. [**3.AVAILABILITY**] |
| | 3. Provide continuing education to all healthcare professionals on the domains of palliative care and hospice care. [**8. EDUCATION**] |
| | 4. Provide adequate training and clinical support to assure that professional staff are confident in their ability to provide palliative care for patients. [**12. STAFF WELLNESS**] |
| | 5. Hospice care and specialized palliative care professionals should be appropriately trained, credentialed, and/or certified in their area of expertise. [**4. STAFFING**] |
| | 6. Formulate, utilize, and regularly review a timely care plan based on a comprehensive interdisciplinary assessment of the values, preferences, goals, and needs of the patient and family and, to the extent that existing privacy laws permit, ensure that the plan is broadly disseminated, both internally and externally, to all professionals involved in the patient's care. |
| | 7. Ensure that upon transfer between healthcare settings, there is timely and thorough communication of the patient's goals, preferences, values, and clinical information so that continuity of care and seamless follow-up are assured.[**11. CONTINUITY OF CARE**] |
| | 8. Healthcare professionals should present hospice as an option to all patients and families when death within a year would not be surprising and should reintroduce the hospice option as the patient declines. [**11. CONTINUITY OF CARE**] |
| | 9. Patients and caregivers should be asked by palliative and hospice care programs to assess physicians'/healthcare professionals' ability to discuss hospice as an option. |
| | 10. Enable patients to make informed decisions about their care by educating them on the process of their disease, prognosis, and the benefits and burdens of potential interventions. |
| | 11. Provide education and support to families and unlicensed caregivers based on the patient's individualized care plan to assure safe and appropriate care for the patient. |
| 2. Physical aspects of care | 12. Measure and document pain, dyspnea, constipation, and other symptoms using available standardized scales. [**5. MEASUREMENT & 6. QI**] |
| | 13. Assess and manage symptoms and side effects in a timely, safe, and effective manner to a level that is acceptable to the patient and family. [**5. MEASUREMENT & 6. QI**] |
| 3. Psychological and psychiatric aspects of care | 14. Measure and document anxiety, depression, delirium, behavioral disturbances, and other common psychological symptoms using available standardized scales. [**5. MEASUREMENT & 6. QI**] |
| | 15. Manage anxiety, depression, delirium, behavioral disturbances, and other common psychological symptoms in a timely, safe, and effective manner to a level that is acceptable to the patient and family. [**5. MEASUREMENT & 6. QI**] |
| | 16. Assess and manage the psychological reactions of patients and families (including stress, anticipatory grief, and coping) in a regular, ongoing fashion in order to address emotional and functional impairment and loss. [**5. MEASUREMENT & 6. QI**] |
| | 17. Develop and offer a grief and bereavement care plan to provide services to patients and families prior to and for at least 13 months after the death of the patient. [**9. BEREAVEMENT**] |
| 4. Social aspects of care | 18. Conduct regular patient and family care conferences with physicians and other appropriate members of the interdisciplinary team to provide information, to discuss goals of care, disease prognosis, and advance care planning, and to offer support. |
| | 19. Develop and implement a comprehensive social care plan that addresses the social, practical, and legal needs of the patient and caregivers, including but not limited to relationships, communication, existing social and cultural networks, decision-making, work and school settings, finances, sexuality/intimacy, caregiver availability/stress, and access to medicines and equipment. [**4. STAFFING**] |

*(Continued)*

**Table 3-4**
**National Quality Forum Preferred Practices Organized by National Consensus Project: Domains of Quality Palliative Care**
*(Continued)*

| NCP Domains of Quality Palliative Care | NQF Preferred Practices |
|---|---|
| 5. Spiritual, religious, and existential aspects of care | 20. Develop and document a plan based on an assessment of religious, spiritual, and existential concerns using a structured instrument, and integrate the information obtained from the assessment into the palliative care plan. **[4. STAFFING]**<br>21. Provide information about the availability of spiritual care services, and make spiritual care available either through organizational spiritual care counseling or through the patient's own clergy relationships. **[4. STAFFING]**<br>22. Specialized palliative and hospice care teams should include spiritual care professionals appropriately trained and certified in palliative care. **[4. STAFFING]**<br>23. Specialized palliative and hospice spiritual care professionals should build partnerships with community clergy and provide education and counseling related to end-of-life care. **[4. STAFFING]** |
| 6. Cultural aspects of care | 24. Incorporate cultural assessment as a component of comprehensive palliative and hospice care assessment, including but not limited to locus of decision-making, preferences regarding disclosure of information, truth telling and decision-making, dietary preferences, language, family communication, desire for support measures such as palliative therapies and complementary and alternative medicine, perspectives on death, suffering, and grieving, and funeral/burial rituals.<br>25. Provide professional interpreter services and culturally sensitive materials in the patient's and family's preferred language. |
| 7. Care of the imminently dying patient | 26. Recognize and document the transition to the active dying phase, and communicate to the patient, family, and staff the expectation of imminent death.<br>27. Educate the family on a timely basis regarding the signs and symptoms of imminent death in an age-appropriate, developmentally appropriate, and culturally appropriate manner.<br>28. As part of the ongoing care planning process, routinely ascertain and document patient and family wishes about the care setting for the site of death, and fulfill patient and family preferences when possible. **[11. CONTINUITY OF CARE]**<br>29. Provide adequate dosage of analgesics and sedatives as appropriate to achieve patient comfort during the active dying phase, and address concerns and fears about using narcotics and of analgesics hastening death.<br>30. Treat the body after death with respect according to the cultural and religious practices of the family and in accordance with local law. **[9. BEREAVEMENT]**<br>31. Facilitate effective grieving by implementing in a timely manner a bereavement care plan after the patient's death, when the family remains the focus of care. **[9. BEREAVEMENT]** |
| 8. Ethical and legal aspects of care | 32. Document the designated surrogate/decisionmaker in accordance with state law for every patient in primary, acute, and long-term care and in palliative and hospice care.<br>33. Document the patient/surrogate preferences for goals of care, treatment options, and setting of care at first assessment and at frequent intervals as conditions change.<br>34. Convert the patient treatment goals into medical orders, and ensure that the information is transferable and applicable across care settings, including long-term care, emergency medical services, and hospital care, through a program such as the Physician Orders for Life-Sustaining Treatment (POLST) program.<br>35. Make advance directives and surrogacy designations available across care settings, while protecting patient privacy and adherence to HIPAA regulations, for example, by using Internet-based registries or electronic personal health records.<br>36. Develop healthcare and community collaborations to promote advance care planning and the completion of advance directives for all individuals, for example, the Respecting Choices and Community Conversations on Compassionate Care programs.<br>37. Establish or have access to ethics committees or ethics consultation across care settings to address ethical conflicts at the end of life.<br>38. For minors with decision-making capacity, document the child's views and preferences for medical care, including assent for treatment, and give them appropriate weight in decision-making. Make appropriate professional staff members available to both the child and the adult decision-maker for consultation and intervention when the child's wishes differ from those of the adult decision-maker. |

*[BOLDED] entries refer to corresponding domain from "Operational Features for Hospital Palliative Care Programs: Consensus Recommendations" (Weissman and Meier 2008).

*Source*: http://www.nationalconsensusproject.org/guidelines.pdf and www.qualityforum.org.

**Table 3–5**
**Consensus Recommendations: Operational Features for Hospital Palliative Care Programs**

| Domain | NQF* | RECOMMENDATIONS | |
|---|---|---|---|
| | | **Must have** | **Should have** |
| **1. Program Administration** <br> To effectively integrate palliative care services into hospital culture and practice, so that the program's mission is aligned with that of the hospital, the program must have both visibility and voice within the hospital management structure. This can best be accomplished by (1) ensuring that a program has a designated program director, with dedicated funding for program director duties and (2) a routine mechanism for program reporting and planning that is integrated into the hospital management committee structure. | | Palliative care program staff integrated into the management structure of the hospital to ensure that program consideration of hospital mission/goals. Processes, outcomes, and strategic planning are developed in consideration of hospital mission/goals. | Systems that integrate palliative care practices into the care of all seriously ill patients, not just those seen by the program. |
| **2. Types of Services** <br> The three components of a fully integrated palliative care program are an inpatient consultation service, outpatient practice, and geographic inpatient unit. All three serve different but complementary functions to support patients/families through the illness experience. Because a consultation practice has the ability to serve patients throughout the entire hospital, this is typically recommended as the first point of program development. | | A consultation service that is available to all hospital inpatients. | Resources for outpatient palliative care services, especially in hospitals with more than 300 beds. An inpatient palliative care geographic unit, especially in hospitals with more than 300 beds. |
| **3. Availability** <br> Patients, families and hospital staff need palliative care services that are available for both routine and emergency services. | 2 | Monday–Friday inpatient consultation availability and 24/7 telephone support. | 24/7 inpatient consultation availability, especially in hospitals with more than 300 beds. |
| **4. Staffing** <br> The following disciplines are essential to provide palliative care services: physician, nursing, social work and chaplaincy. In addition, mental health services must be available. Depending on the institution and staff, basic mental health screening services can be provided by an appropriately trained social worker, chaplain, or nurse with psychiatric training. Ideally a psychologist or psychiatrist are also available for complex mental health needs. Social work, chaplaincy, and mental health services can be provided by dedicated palliative care fulltime equivalent positions or by existing hospital staff, although their work in support of the palliative care program will still need to be accounted and paid for, and not just "added on" to their existing job responsibilities. | 1, 5, 19, 20, 21, 22, 23 | Specific funding for a designated palliative care physician(s). All certified in hospice and palliative medicine (HPM) or committed to working toward board certification. Specific funding for a designated palliative care nurse(s), with advance practice nursing preferred. All program nurses must be certified by the National Board for Certification of Hospice and Palliative Nursing (NBCHPN) or committed to working toward board certification. Appropriately trained staff to provide mental health services. Social worker(s) and chaplain(s) available to provide clinical care as part of an interdisciplinary team. Administrative support (secretary/administrative assistant position) in hospitals with either more than 150 beds or a consult service with volume >15 consults per month. | |
| **5. Measurement** <br> Providing evidence of the value of palliative care programs to patients, families, referring physicians and hospital administrators is critical for program sustainability and growth. Key outcome measures can be divided into four domains (examples provided): | 12, 13, 14, 15, 16 | Operational metrics for all consultations. Customer, clinical and financial metrics that are tracked either continuously or intermittently. | |

- Operational Metrics: (number of consults, referring physician, disposition)
- Clinical Metrics: (improvement in pain, dyspnea, distress)
- Customer Metrics: (patient/family/referring physician satisfaction)
- Financial Metrics: (cost avoidance, billing revenue, length of stay).

| Domain | NQF* | Description |
|---|---|---|
| **6. Quality Improvement**<br>Palliative care programs must be held accountable to the same quality-improvement standards as other hospital clinical programs. | 12, 13, 14, 15, 16 | Quality improvement activities, continuous or intermittent, for (a) pain, (b) non-pain symptoms, (c) psychosocial/spiritual distress and (d) communication between health care providers and patients/surrogates. |
| **7. Marketing**<br>As a new specialty, the palliative care program is responsible for making its presence and range of services known to the key stakeholders for quality care. | | Marketing materials and strategies appropriate for hospital staff, patients, and families. |
| **8. Education**<br>As a new specialty, the palliative care program is responsible for helping develop and coordinate educational opportunities and resources to improve the attitudes, knowledge, skills, and behavior of all health professionals. | 3 | Palliative care educational resources for hospital physicians, nurses, social workers, chaplains, health professional trainees, and any other staff the program feels are essential to fulfill its mission and goals. |
| **9. Bereavement Services**<br>There are no currently accepted *best practice* features of bereavement services to recommend. Common elements present in many programs include telephone or letter follow-up, sympathy cards, registry of community resources for support groups and counseling services, an remembrance services. All programs are encouraged to develop a bereavement policy and make changes as needed through quality-improvement initiatives. | 17, 30, 31 | A bereavement policy and procedure that describes bereavement services provided to families of patients impacted by the palliative care program. |
| **10. Patient Identification**<br>In most hospitals, palliative care consultations originate from a physician order. To facilitate referrals for "at-risk" patients, many hospitals have begun adopting screening. | | A working relationship with the appropriate departments to adopt palliative care screening criteria for patients in the emergency department, general med/surgical wards and intensive care units. |
| **11. Continuity of Care**<br>Coordination of care as patients move from one care site to another is especially critical for patients with serious, often life-limiting diseases, and is a cornerstone of palliative care clinical work. | 7, 8, 28 | Policies and procedures that specify the manner in which transitions across care sites (e.g., hospital to home hospice) will be handled to ensure excellent communication between facilities.<br>A working relationship with one or more community hospice providers. |
| **12. Staff Wellness**<br>The psychological demands on palliative care staff are often overwhelming, placing practitioners at risk for burnout and a range of other mental health problems. Common examples of team wellness activities are team retreats, regularly scheduled patient debriefing exercises, relaxation-exercise training and individual referral for staff counseling. | 4 | Policies and procedures that promote palliative care team wellness. |

*The numbers in the NQF column represent the specific National Quality Forum Hospice and Palliative Medicine Preferred Practice. A National Framework and Preferred Practices for Palliative and Hospice Care Quality: A Consensus Report ©2006 National Quality Forum, www.qualityforum.org, Washington, DC (See Table 3–4)

Sources: Adapted from National Quality Forum (2006), reference 63 & Weissman DE, Meier DE (2008), reference 83.

## The National Palliative Care Research Center

The mission of the National Palliative Care Research Center (NPCRC) is to improve care for patients with serious illness and the needs of their families by promoting palliative care research. In partnership with the Center to Advance Palliative Care, the NPCRC aims to rapidly translate these findings into clinical practice. The NPCRC uses three mechanisms to accomplish their aims:

- Establish priorities for palliative care research;
- Develop a new generation of researchers in palliative care;
- Coordinate and support studies focused on improving care for patients and families living with serious illness.

The NPCRC, located in New York City, is headed by Dr. Sean Morrison and receives direction and technical assistance from the Mount Sinai School of Medicine. Prior to the establishment of the NPCRC, there was no organizing force promoting and facilitating the conduct of palliative care research. Because departments or divisions of palliative medicine do not yet exist in most medical schools, palliative care research is conducted by a small number of highly successful investigators working in isolation at a limited number of universities and clinical settings in the United States.

The NPCRC provides an administrative home to promote intellectual exchange, sharing of resources (e.g., biostatisticians) and access to data from ongoing studies to plan and support new research. Furthermore, the Center takes a collaborative approach to establishing its funding priorities. As such, it is a key force in the development of an evidence base from which standards of HBPC can be developed and measured. (For more information about activities, see http://www.npcrc.org.)

## The Joint Commission

The Joint Commission (TJC) is one of the paramount accreditation organizations for hospitals and other health care organizations. The purpose of TJC is to continuously improve the safety and quality of care provided to the public. TJC is an independent, not-for-profit organization, and perhaps its most important benefit is that TJC accredited organizations make a commitment to continuous improvement in patient care. During an accreditation survey, TJC evaluates a group's performance by using a set of standards that cross eight functional areas: (1) rights, responsibilities, and ethics; (2) continuum of care; (3) education and communication; (4) health promotion and disease prevention; (5) leadership; (6) management of human resources; (7) management of information; (8) improving network performance.[84]

In 2004, a specific palliative care focus was introduced within two standards: (1) rights, responsibilities, and ethics and (2) the provision of care, treatment, and services. The goal of the ethics, rights, and responsibilities standard is to improve outcomes by recognizing and respecting the rights of each patient and working in an ethical manner. Care, treatment, and services are to be provided in a way that respects the person and fosters dignity. The performance standard states that a patient's family should be involved in the care, treatment, and services if the patient desires. Care, treatment, and services are provided through ongoing assessments of care; meeting the patient's needs; and either successfully discharging the patient or providing referral or transfer of the patient for continuing care.[84] More detailed information is available by contacting TJC or visiting their website at http://www.jcrinc.com.

These standards incorporated a stronger emphasis on palliative care practices within organizations. Hence, organizations are being held accountable for the manner in which they provide appropriate palliative care. It is in the public's best interest that TJC requires organizations to adhere to these provisions for a successful accreditation. In 2008, a process to develop specific "Certification for Palliative Care Programs" was begun. This process would create an evaluation mechanism of palliative care services across settings. Proposed eligibility for organizations included: having a clearly-defined palliative care program; providing services following clinical care guidelines or evidence-based practice; and the use of data to inform its performance improvement projects. Updates on TJC progress on standard development can be obtained from TJC website under "certification programs."[85,86]

## Veterans Health Administration Initiatives

The U.S. Department of Veterans Affairs (VA) health care system has shown leadership in improving palliative and EOL care in their hospitals through multiple initiatives that have been designed or implemented since the early 1990s. In 1992, Secretary Jesse Brown mandated that VA medical centers (VAMCs) establish hospice consultation teams to respond to the complex palliative care needs of patients with advanced disease. The VA provided training for team members during 1992 and 1993. One team reported success in pain and cost reduction while also undertaking significant institution-wide improvements through education of nurses and house staff and making pain management resources available.[87]

In 1997, the Veterans Health Administration began an intensive, system-wide, continuous quality improvement (CQI) initiative to improve pain management. This endeavor resulted from a 1997 survey that found both acute and chronic pain management services to be inconsistent, inaccessible, and non-uniform throughout the system. Two major thrusts formed the basis of the initiative: issuing a system-wide mandate and forming a permanent National Pain Advisory Committee to provide direction and encouragement to the development of the program. Thus, this initiative incorporated two essential elements found in all successful system-wide improvement strategies: an influential champion at the highest level of the organization and a mandate for organizational commitment to this activity. The charge document offered a variety of suggestions for system improvement: making pain more visible by enhancing current measurement and reporting methods (using the "Fifth Vital Sign" approach in all patient contacts in the system); increasing access to pain therapy and increasing professional education about pain; adopting the Agency for Health Care Policy and Research and American Pain Society guidelines for pain management; pursuing research on pain therapies for veterans; distributing and sharing pain management protocols via a central clearinghouse; and exploring methods to maintain cost-effective pain therapy.

Also in 1997, the VA incorporated a palliative care measure in the performance criteria of its regional directors. In this program, performance of the directors is evaluated based on the number of charts that contain information about veterans' preferences regarding various palliative care indicators.[88]

In 1998, the Robert Wood Johnson Foundation Last Acts program created a Clinical Palliative Care Faculty leadership program and awarded a 2-year grant to promote development of 30 faculty fellows from VA-affiliated internal medicine training programs. Their goal was to develop curricula to train residents in the care of dying patients, to integrate relevant content into the curricula of residency training programs, and to add internal medicine faculty leaders and innovators to the field of palliative medicine.

In 2001, the VA Hospice and Palliative Care initiative began. This was a two-phase initiative to improve EOL care for veterans. Phase 1 of the project was funded in part by the National Hospice and Palliative Care Organization (NHPCO) and the Center for Advanced Illness Coordinated Care. This phase of the initiative was designed to accelerate access to hospice and palliative care for veterans. A major product of the program was the Hospice-Veteran Partnership Toolkit. It also created 2.5 full-time equivalent employee positions in Geriatrics and Extended Care, to be used for hospice and palliative care presence in the VA system.

In 2004, phase 2 of the project was launched. It was funded in part by Rallying Points and the NHPCO. It built on the success of phase 1 and developed a Hospice-Veterans Administration Partnership in every state to build an enduring infrastructure for the Accelerated Administrative and Clinical Training Program. In a statement made in 2002 regarding the VA national initiatives, the VA made a clear commitment to improving hospice and palliative care for their patients. The Geriatrics and Long Term Care strategic plan states[88]: "All VAMCs will be required to have designated inpatient beds for hospice and palliative care, or access to these services in the community, and an active hospice and palliative care team for consult, care and placement." Funding continues to be designated to build palliative care consult teams at every facility, to fund new Palliative Care Units, and to enhance existing Palliative Care Units. For example, in 2009, the New England Network of VAs received awards for 3 new Palliative Care Units and enhancement funding for 2 existing units. Additional national efforts include partnerships with CAPC, HPNA, NHPCO and EPEC to provide veterans-specific palliative and EOL education.

As the services continue to grow, the VA has also taken a leadership role in evaluating these services through the use of the Family Assessment of Treatment at End-of-life (FATE) tool.[70,89] This 32-item tool assesses family members' impressions of care received by the deceased veteran in the last month of life. It includes topics such as well-being and dignity, information and communication, respect for treatment preferences, emotional and spiritual support, management of symptoms, care around the time of death, access to outpatient services and access to benefits and services after the patient's death.[89] To date this tool has demonstrated improved outcomes at end-of-life (as judged by the family member) in those veterans who received specialized palliative care consultations.[89] As a result of their initiatives, nearly 50% of veterans dying in VA facilities received the services of a palliative care team.[90] Together, these initiatives address the need for improvement on multiple fronts and create a momentum in the VA system that can set an example for other large hospital-based systems of care.

## Professional Societies Contribute to Palliative Care Development

Multiple professional societies have made contributions to the development of HBPC generalized or specialty population-specific palliative care standards, guidelines, or consensus statements by raising professional and public awareness of the unique issues of palliative care. A few selected organizations and their initiatives are described below.

### National Hospice and Palliative Care Organization

The National Hospice and Palliative Care Organization (NHPCO) was founded in 1978 as the National Hospice Organization. The organization changed its name in February 2000 to include palliative care. Many hospice care programs added palliative care to their names to reflect the range of care and services they provide, as hospice care and palliative care share the same core values and philosophies.

According to their website, the NHPCO is the largest nonprofit membership organization representing hospice and palliative care programs and professionals in the United States. NHPCO is committed to improving end-of-life care and expanding access to hospice care with the goal of profoundly enhancing quality of life for people dying in America and their loved ones. The NHPCO advocates for the terminally ill and their families. It also develops public and professional educational programs and materials to enhance understanding and availability of hospice and palliative care; convenes frequent meetings and symposia on emerging issues; provides technical informational resources to its membership; conducts research; monitors Congressional and regulatory activities; and works closely with other organizations that share an interest in end-of-life care.

## Hospice and Palliative Nurses Association (HPNA)

Incorporated in 1987 as the Hospice Nurses Association, the organization was created to establish a network and support for nurses in this specialty. In 1998, HPNA formally added palliative care to the organization to recognize the needs of nurses working in palliative care settings separate from hospice. HPNA has become the nationally recognized organization providing resources and support for advanced practice nurses, registered nurses, licensed practical nurses, and nursing assistants who care for people with life-limiting and terminal illness. As such they have developed a number of position statements and standards to guide best practices that are available to members and non-members on a variety of topics.

## Processes for Providing HBPC

HBPC programs are increasing in number; however, many organizations are contemplating enhancing palliative resources or developing a program. Such an endeavor requires careful planning, as these programs are not "one-size-fits all." Patience, persistence, and consensus building are key to successful program development.[18] As described earlier, CAPC has taken a leadership role in assisting organizations of all types to build a successful program that is suited to their unique patient population, resources, and organizational culture.

Particular to integrating palliative care principles into cancer centers through a multi-year grant, the City of Hope developed the Disseminating End of Life Education to Cancer Centers (DELETec).[91] In this multi-year project, they invited 2 person teams to attend a 3-day workshop conducted by nationally recognized expert faculty to focus on best practices in palliative oncology care. The teams had additional follow up support and assistance to help ensure successful program implementation. In all 400, participants from 199 different cancer programs/institutions from 42 states attended one of their 4 programs.

A complete primer on developing a HBPC program is beyond the scope of this chapter; however, some of the most important care processes are described below. Those wishing more complete information are referred to the excellent resources mentioned earlier in the chapter.[18]

### Process of Program Development

Regardless of organizational type, the first step in developing a HBPC program is to perform a system assessment or "organizational scan" to identify existing organizational strengths, resources, potential partnerships, and collaborators.[18] A task force or team of interested clinicians, administrators, and possibly consumers might be a first good start. Examples of possible existing resources include clinicians from all disciplines

with interest and training in palliative care, existing relationships with hospice, case management, discharge planners, and hospital chaplaincy programs. The needs assessment should determine the hospital focus on length of stay, ventilator days and pharmacy/ancillary costs per day, palliative care leadership based on personal experience or professional interest, pre-existing pain programs, and trustee/philanthropic interest in, and support for, palliative care.

Second, after the system assessment is performed, identifying areas of need within the organization can highlight where palliative care programs can make the greatest contribution. Many institutions have easy access to data that can help to "build the case" for palliative care. Selling the idea of palliative care to an institution or gaining institutional support is more likely when benefits (such as economical, efficiency, improved clinical care) can be shown. Common areas of need that have shown improvement as a result of HBPC programs include pain and symptom management, patient and family satisfaction, nurse retention and satisfaction, bed and ICU capacity, and length of stay. Other outcomes may include pharmacy costs, establishment and strengthening of hospice partnerships, and improving fragmented subspecialty care.

CAPC provides a Systems Assessment Tool and a Needs Assessment Checklist that can be found at http://www.capc.org/building-a-hospital-based-palliative-care-program/designing/system-assessment to assist organizations with the complexities of the planning process.

## The Process of Providing Palliative Care: Developing an Interdisciplinary Team

The holistic process of providing palliative care to patients and their families is rarely accomplished by one individual or discipline. The interdisciplinary team (IDT) is the foundation of the HBPC service and in many ways is unique in contrast to how medical care is traditionally provided. The core IDT typically consists of specially-trained palliative care professionals including: physicians; nurses at all levels of training (registered nurses, nursing assistants, and advanced practice nurses [APNs]); social workers; pharmacists; spiritual care counselors; healing arts/complementary practitioners; hospice representatives; and volunteers.

Identifying which team member(s) can best serve a patient's needs is a key part of the initial assessment.[92,93] One clinician may be designated to receive initial consults and organize distribution of work for the day. A team may decide that all new consults are seen first by a medical provider: either the physician or APN. The physician also serves as the medical resource person for other team members, and supervises physician learners. APNs may work independently or collaboratively with the attending physician to conduct initial consultations. If resources allow, this may be done together; however, workload and resources may dictate that new consults are divided among the medical providers.

In organizations that support learners, after a period of supervision and observation, it may be that the learner (e.g., fellow, resident, medical or nursing student) conducts an initial chart review, patient and/or family interview and then presents the patient to the physician or APN—after which the pair will revisit the patient. At all times the team should be aware of the patient's energy level and the learner's level of expertise in deciding if this format is appropriate. During the initial consult, the medical provider assesses psycho/social/spiritual needs are identified and other team members are integrated into the plan of care.[94]

A palliative care certified physician and/or APN may be responsible for the initial assessment and day-to-day medical care of most patients. However, depending on the patient's needs, another member of the team might take the lead in care. For example, if the patient's primary concern is physical, then a medical provider may direct the plan of care. If the patient's primary concern is existential in nature, the spiritual care provider may take the lead. Alternatively, if the patient's primary need is for family support, the social worker may be the most active care provider. Healing arts and complementary medicine practitioners and volunteers are also integral members of the IDT.

Healing arts/complementary medicine practitioners are providers from a variety of backgrounds who can provide massage, energy work or instruction in guided imagery or meditation. Palliative care volunteers are specifically trained to see palliative care patients and are overseen by a volunteer coordinator. They provide presence, active listening, and company for patients and families. Although some tasks are seemingly small, such as reading, playing cards, or running small errands, these are often essential aspects of care from the patient/family perspective.

Pharmacists, healing arts/complementary therapy clinicians, hospice liaisons and volunteers may or may not be part of the core team in some organizations. For example, even though medication needs may be complex, few teams have the ability to have a dedicated pharmacist who could round daily with the team. Hence, it may be more realistic to have a pharmacist present during regularly scheduled IDT meetings. Similarly, local hospice liaisons, healing arts/complementary therapy practitioners, etc. may only be available to meet with a team weekly.

Non-clinical members of the team including administrative, financial or practice managers and secretarial support are responsible for holding the IDT together by providing the supportive infrastructure within which the team can operate. These key team members may serve as representatives or liaisons on important institutional committees. Another important function of program administrators is the collection of data for clinical and fiscal evaluation for quality improvement, program justification to the institution or research. The receptionist/secretarial support may be the first contact for patients and referring clinicians and can become the "face or voice of the program." Individuals selected for these positions should be skilled, patient, and caring to enable

them to deal with the stress of people in crisis and urgency of consultations.

After an initial consultation, depending on the patients' needs, they may continue to be seen in follow up throughout their hospitalization. Some patients may have acute needs (such as uncontrolled pain) that may require them to be seen more than once daily. Other patients may be seen several times a week or weekly or until the goal of the initial consultation is achieved. Some patients may be visited by the medical provider, the spiritual care provider, the healing arts provider, and a volunteer—all on the same day. In the earlier case of Mr. RL, visits from the APN medical provider, the spiritual care provider, the healing arts practitioner and a volunteer were frequent, and some occurred on the same visit.

## Processes to Support IDT Communication

Communication may be the most challenging and crucial aspect of providing palliative care.[95,96] Intra-team communications that are regular and efficient will allow for seamless care to be delivered. Teams will likely explore a variety of mechanisms to achieve optimal communication about not only issues of patient care but also about team function. The purpose of regular patient care-related team meetings is to allow all disciplines to contribute to the development and implementation of comprehensive care plans that reflect the values, preferences, goals and needs of each individual patient.

Practicing as a true interdisciplinary team requires significant and ongoing intention and effort. Traditionally the medical model has driven health care delivery and, to a large extent, still does. However, in a holistic care model of palliative care, the psycho/social/spiritual care providers should have equal authority and input; for many clinicians, this represents a change in practice. Teams should be mindful of tendencies to become "efficient" that can sometimes lead to a focus only on the medical or physical aspects of care.

Minimally, a weekly face-to-face meeting, in which all IDT members gather, is considered an essential element of team function in order to provide high-quality, coordinated care. During the IDT meeting, active patients are presented and all team members have an opportunity to contribute their expertise in the development of the plan of care. In some cases, weekly meetings may not be enough and a team may choose to meet more frequently. These meetings are also a place to role model, for the learners, healthy and respectful team interactions that recognize the value and expertise of each team member.

## Performing the Palliative Care Consult

A palliative care consult can be initiated in a variety of different ways. Some services (or reimbursement mechanisms) require that a physician initiate the consult, rather than a nurse or other care provider. If someone other than the attending physician requests a consult on a hospitalized patient, it would still be important to include the attending (or primary care) physician in the consult. Most services choose to do this before seeing the patient.

## When is a Consult Made?

Consultations should be initiated any time a person with life-limiting illness has physical, psychological, social, or spiritual needs.[97] Palliative care programs began for many reasons, but one of them was to meet the end-of-life care planning and symptomatic needs of patients who are not yet hospice eligible, either because of life expectancy (greater than 6 months) or because they are receiving active disease-modifying treatment. Palliative care referrals do not hinge on the "less than 6 months" life expectancy as is often the case for hospice referrals. Referring patients with life-limiting illness early is one of the benefits of having a palliative care service.

Some organizations have built-in consult triggers, protocols, or algorithms for specific life-limiting illnesses in which, consults are recommended at diagnosis.[43,98,99] "Automatic referrals" would be generated for all patients who are newly-diagnosed with certain types of life-limiting cancers (e.g. pancreatic, brain, stage IIIB and greater lung, liver, etc.).[43] Table 3–6 provides some examples of patient types that might "trigger" an automatic referral. Non-cancer patient populations that may be considered for automatic referrals are those with amyotrophic sclerosis (ALS), heart failure, dialysis-dependent renal failure, and those who, regardless of diagnosis, experience frequent hospitalizations. These patient populations are typically highly in need of palliative care services. Careful planning and close collaboration with colleagues is necessary to establish a process for automatic referrals that ensures that the patients that are most in need of palliative care services have them "early and often." Some automatically scheduled palliative care consultations may occur in the outpatient setting or clinic, while some organizations have hospital "triggers" that may alert that primary team that a patient may benefit from these specialized services. Over time, in HBPC programs with high community visibility and/or marketing efforts, it may be common to have patients or family members self-refer.

## What is Included in the Initial Palliative Care Consultation?

The initial consult will lay the foundation for all further interactions with the patient and family. In addition to specialty expertise, the palliative care team may offer the unique resources of presence and time. Much has been written about the importance of setting during the initial consult.[100] Making sure there is adequate time to see the patient and family is crucial. If time restrictions are unavoidable—state these constraints at the outset of the consultation. Sitting down during the consultation and making sure everyone who is participating in the consult has a seat is important (see Chapter 5, communication). Depending on the resources available and the composition of the team, an initial consult can occur almost anywhere. For inpatient consults, it is often in the patient's room; for outpatient consults, it may be in the clinic exam room. If resources permit, consults can also be done at patient's homes or in local care facilities. The main concern is an environment that allows for privacy and quiet—often difficult to find in most acute care hospitals.

---

**Table 3–6**
**Possible Triggers for "Automatic" Palliative Care Assessment or Referral**

| Population | Possible Triggers |
|---|---|
| Cancer Outpatients | • Any newly diagnosed (advanced stage e.g. stage IIIb or IV diagnosis of selected cancers)<br>• Uncontrolled pain or other symptoms (with frequent hospitalizations)<br>• Decreased functional status (e.g. KPS 50 or less)<br>• Complex psychosocial situations |
| Hospital Inpatients | • Prolonged hospital stay (greater than hospital ALOS)<br>• Age 80 or greater with multiple comorbidities (or admitted from nursing home)<br>• Survived cardiac arrest<br>• Multiple admissions in past 3 months for same chronic condition (e.g. COPD, pneumonia, heart failure, complications of stroke)<br>• Advanced cancer<br>• Intensive Care Unit (e.g., prolonged ventilator dependent, Ethics Committee Consultation, tracheotomy or feeding tube decisions, ventilator withdrawal decision, etc.)<br>• Neurological conditions (feeding tube, ALS, Parkinson's disease with dementia, recurrent brain cancer)<br>• Cardiac (e.g. multiple admissions for heart failure, decision for placement of implantable cardioverter defibrillator (AICD))<br>• Pediatric/neonatal intensive care unit (e.g. prolonged or multiple admissions for chronic condition, prolonged ventilator-dependency) |

Many patients may be unfamiliar with the term "palliative" care or may associate it with hospice care and/or death. Patients who are early in their disease process may wonder why a consult to this service has been initiated. Establishing the patients' level of understanding and explaining the role and focus of the palliative care team is an important starting point to the consultation. Some patients and families may need reassurance that they are not being "abandoned" by their primary team. Explaining that the palliative care team consults and provides expert guidance to the primary team but does not replace them is important. Providing a clear and confident explanation of services will help everyone know what to expect. Providing a brochure or some written information about what palliative care is and who the team members are can be helpful. Assessing the patient/family knowledge and understanding their current situation is the next step. Health care providers often believe that they have done a complete and thorough job in explanations; however, patients are under stress and may need multiple explanations in very simple language before they fully understand their situation.

Next, a complete and thorough assessment is begun. This should include a review of symptoms and physical complaints, as well as an assessment of psychological, emotional, social and spiritual concerns. Understanding the patient's social support structure and family relationships is essential. Exploring what gives meaning to patients' lives and who they are as individuals will help direct care. Assessing and attending to cultural preferences will enhance communication and increase the effectiveness of interventions.

Other areas that are important to assess are goals of care, advance care planning wishes and treatment decision-making style. Due to time constraints and sometimes lack of skill, these complex issues are often overlooked or only superficially explored by the primary team. They are some of the most important pieces of the puzzle when constructing a plan of care. It is important to find out what the patient/family is hoping for from treatment interventions. What are their personal preferences and goals? Exploring, on the first visit, if they have ever considered and/or completed advance directives may elucidate this. Completing advance directives is a structured way of beginning to look at goals of care and what is meaningful when making treatment decisions. Some programs have developed standardized templates that remind the team (and the referring provider) of the important and comprehensive domains of care and intervention that are included in the consultation.

## Who Should be Present at an Initial Consultation?

While there are times that it is appropriate to conduct a consult without the patient present (e.g., the patient is in coma)—in most cases every effort is made to include the patient. The patient should decide which support members and/or family they want to include. There may be one or more members of the palliative care team present. A member from the referring team may want to attend—but this is less common on initial consult. If a focused family meeting is arranged—it is imperative for the referring team to be present so all decision makers are in the room together. Family meetings are a large part of palliative care interventions. During the initial consult, it may be clear that a family meeting is needed to proceed with discussion about care planning. Sometimes, this is organized as a part of the initial consult. Conducting a family meeting takes skill and planning. Resources are available to assist inexperienced team members with the important process of organizing and conducting a family meeting.[101]

## Continuing the Care: Day to Day Operations

Patients with serious illness may follow many different paths. Table 3–7 illustrates paths that may be typical in the current "care as usual" for a seriously ill patient, compared with an "ideal" or expected pathway in a health care system with a HBPC program. Numerous institutions have studied their processes of care and have created clinical pathways that can help standardize procedures and reduce the variation of care experienced by terminally ill or symptomatic palliative care patients as they traverse the complex health care system.[102] Usual components include attention to patient symptoms, as well as family needs at system entry and throughout the course of stay until discharge. Assigning time frames to address needs helps in monitoring progress and tracking outcomes that have been met, as well as those that continue to need attention.

Although published guidelines and standards may offer similar suggestions, the road map format of clinical pathways identifies practical and accountable mechanisms to keep patient care moving in the direction of specific identified outcomes. Some pathway forms allow for documentation of variation from the designated path. Analysis of several instances of variation might alert a care team about a potential system "defect" in need of improvement.

Many institutions have implemented standard orders or evidence-based algorithms to guide various aspects of care pertinent to EOL situations. Some of these include limitations of certain types of therapies such as CPR and blood pressure medications. In addition, preprinted order sheets that outline management of symptoms and side effects such as nausea, constipation, and pain are making it easier for physicians and trainees to reproduce comprehensive plans that do not vary because of individual opinion. These order forms can be valuable teaching tools in a setting of regularly changing care providers. Figure 3–4 shows a sample order sheet and the companion guidelines printed on the reverse for patients who are hospitalized and have a palliative focus of care. Certainly, important considerations in the development of such "recipes" for care include having broad, multidisciplinary, evidence-based input. The process of producing such documents is also potentially a care consensus and learning environment for many teams.

Care pathways and order also demonstrate what care is provided when a patient is no longer receiving curative care. In cases where curative care ceases, clinicians and patients may believe "there is nothing more to do." Order sheets,

**Table 3–7**
**How HBPC Programs Might Influence "Care as Usual" for Persons with Life-limiting Illness**

| Current Process of Care | Care Process with an Integrated HBPC |
|---|---|
| Patient with known life-limiting, chronic illness arrives in emergency department for relief of uncontrolled disease-related symptoms. | Patient with known life-limiting, chronic illness meets criteria and is referred for initial outpatient Palliative Care Team (PCT) Consultation and standardized holistic assessment<br><br>• PCT documents and communicates consultation to patient/ family & referring team<br>• Advance directives documents completed including patient's preference for resuscitation status<br>• Prospective symptom management plan identified<br>• Community-based resources in place<br>• Regular PCT follow up planned in conjunction with other medical appointments when possible (including MSW, chaplain, healing arts providers as appropriate). |
| ED workup and hospital admission to medical unit. | Patient develops disease-related symptoms which are managed by PCT staff by phone. |
| Inpatient/hospitalist medical team continues diagnostic workup. | Patient requires brief, planned hospital admit for symptom relief procedure; continuity of care ensured by preplanned inpatient PCT follow up over hospitalization. |
| Patient undergoes tests and procedures. Symptom management per medical team. | Symptoms are assessed using standardized tool & documented. Evidence-based symptom treatment is implemented and symptoms rapidly managed with standardized symptom assessment/management algorithm or pathway. (If patient is approaching end-of-life and cannot or does not wish to die outside of hospital then Comfort Measures standardized orders are implemented). |
| Patient's disease process is not able to be reversed. Patient develops acute deterioration and is transferred to the intensive care unit on ventilator. | Discharge plan coordinated by inpatient PCT for patient to have home care (or hospice care) as needed. |
| After prolonged stay, patient dies in hospital. | Patient dies in preferred site of death. Bereavement care offered to family after the death. |

algorithms and care pathways are common in complex acute care situations. Using these same tools palliative care can demonstrate the complex, aggressive care that can be directed at comfort. The patient and family can have confidence that everything will be done to provide pain management and relief of suffering. Nurses in particular can advocate through development of hospital policy, education, and individual practice for aggressive comfort care. The health care team must ensure that a positive approach—focusing on what can be done for patients with life-limiting illness and their families—is implemented. Pathways may go a long way towards reducing variation in care so that delays or unpredictable outcomes are avoided.[103] At a macro level of cancer care, the National Comprehensive Cancer Network[92] has published a care algorithm and extensively detailed "care standards" in the Palliative Care Clinical Guideline. This booklet is produced as a professional and patient guide and is available from http://nccn.org.

## Documenting Palliative Care Consultations

As in all aspects of health care delivery, documentation is the foundation for communicating with other providers, particularly across care settings. As a consultative service, including the primary care providers in the plan of care promotes collegiality and helps assure follow through. Recommendations for symptom management, identification of goals of care, advance planning and resuscitation wishes, or emotional counseling and support—are at the heart of the palliative care assessment and interventions.

An electronic medical record (EMR) may provide an immediate way to share information with all members of the care team. Pertinent members with whom the consult should be shared include the primary referral service (if the patient is inpatient), the primary care provider, and other specialties consulting on the patient. Providing a copy of the consultation note, electronically in real time, can assist with the timely communication and implementation of recommendations.

Documentation can also be a vehicle for education that should not be overlooked. Including specifics in the plan of care can help other providers learn aspects of palliative care. For example, breakthrough dosing for pain medications is often under-dosed by the primary team. When addressing pain management in the palliative plan of care, noting the total daily opioid use and writing the details of the calculation (10–20% of total daily need) in print can teach other providers how to prescribe adequate breakthrough medication in the future.

Finally, documenting goals of care, resuscitation wishes and advance care planning in a way that is visible to everyone is a challenge. Patients often complain that they have provided documents or information, such as an advance directive, but at the point of care the information is not easily located. As a quality improvement initiative, our institution created a visible tab embedded in the electronic medical record for advance directives. In this system, important documents (advance directives and Do Not Resuscitate orders) are scanned into the record and are readily available. For patients that have stated verbal wishes, but have not completed the official document, a clinician can complete a templated advance care planning note that carries the same force as an official form. This can be completed by any team member and can indicate the durable power of attorney as well as care wishes (e.g., resuscitation wishes, medically administered nutrition/hydration wishes, etc). The templated notes and actual documents are all located in the same section of the electronic medical record and are accessible to all providers (including in the Emergency Department and physician offices that are part of the medical center system).

## Completing the Process-Transitions of Care and Continuity

The palliative care team must remember that they are the consultants and ultimately most patients will remain under the guidance of the primary provider. While some referring providers welcome aggressive assistance in care, others may prefer to accept or decline palliative care team recommendations. Talking a case over with the primary team is always preferable to leaving a note in the record.

Continuity is improved dramatically when there is an outpatient, as well as an inpatient portion of HBPC. Our outpatient service is managed by the advance practice nurses and all inpatients can be followed in the outpatient setting (when indicated). This provides an opportunity to reinforce or adjust recommendations made while the patient was hospitalized. It also provides an opportunity to explore complex emotional topics or decision-making.

For patients who do not return to the center, providing continuity is difficult. Sending the initial palliative care consult and pertinent notes to the receiving team (including the patient's PCP) is useful. Being open to phone calls or proactively placing a personal call to the receiving provider will help to build bridges to the community and encourage community providers to see the palliative care team as a resource.

## Extending the Reach of HBPC: Advance Care Planning

The Patient Self-Determination Act (PSDA) of 1991 required that hospitals and other organizations receiving Medicare or Medicaid funding provide written information to patients about their rights to make decisions to accept or refuse medical care.[104] Further, it stipulated that advance directives, including living wills and appointment of a health care proxy, may be used to provide substituted judgment in the event of patients' inability to speak for themselves regarding health care decisions. Although this legislation was designed to allow patients to have a durable mechanism to outline their preferences for certain types of treatments, for many years it had little impact on yielding improvements in EOL care.[105] There are several reasons that this occurred. First, not all patients actually choose to complete advance directives. Often, inexperienced personnel distribute the information without providing appropriate explanation of the documents, leading to lack of completion by patients. Even for patients who complete them, they may not be specific enough to address the situation in which patients later find themselves. Second, even when a patient has taken the time to thoughtfully complete a document, the health care provider may not be aware of it[6,106] or the health care proxy may not interpret them as the patient intended.[107]

Staff of HBPC programs can play an important role in patient decision-making with each individual patient and within the larger health care system. At an individual patient level, consensus guidelines recommend that patients/families' preferences for surrogate decision makers and treatment goals be documented at the initial assessment and whenever there is a change in the patients' situation.[20] However this task is not complete until the information is both documented in the medical record and shared with the primary team. In addition to documenting the presence of advance directives, for hospitalized patients these wishes must be translated into medical orders (e.g., completion of Do Not Resuscitate forms if the patient prefers not to have this life-sustaining treatment applied). Furthermore, documentation of these preferences should accompany patients when transitioning to other health care settings. Different states have laws about how these orders are documented and transferred among settings. Many states' laws have provisions for patients at home who are dying and do not want to be resuscitated to use home labeling systems such as a "DNR bracelet," sticker, or forms. Some states may have "Physician Orders for Life-Sustaining Treatment (POLST)" programs to identify ambulatory/outpatient wishes outside of the hospital. (More information on individual state efforts regarding POLST-type programs is available at http://www.ohsu.edu/ethics/polst/about/index.htm.)

Health care providers who are not focused on palliative care needs may not gather information about advance directives and patient treatment preferences as an automatic component of their health history (such as occurs when identifying and documenting allergies and medications). Therefore, it is not uncommon for providers to be unaware of the presence of the patient's advance directive until the patient is in crisis. Such late awareness can result in patient's making choices under duress that they might not otherwise have made. For example, if the patient is experiencing respiratory distress

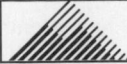 # DARTMOUTH-HITCHCOCK MEDICAL CENTER

One Medical Center Drive
Lebanon, New Hampshire 03756

Physician/ARNP Order Sheet
Comfort Measures
Any order preceded by a check box must have the box checked to enable the order. All other orders will be automatically implemented

☐ **DISCONTINUE ALL PREVIOUS ORDERS**

| | | | |
|---|---|---|---|
| **Activity:** | ☐ OOB as tolerated | ☐ OOB with assistance | ☐ Bedrest |
| **Hunger:** | ☐ Diet as tolerated | ☐ NPO | ☐ Other_____ |
| **Thirst:** | ☐ PO Fluids as tol. **IV Fluids:** | ☐ No IVF | ☐ Yes_____ |
| **Dyspnea:** | ☐ O₂ prn for patient comfort | ☐ No Oxygen | ☐ Fan at bedside |
| **Elimination:** | ☐ Insert Foley Catheter prn | | |
| **Oral Care:** | ☐ **per guideline (see reverse)** | ☐ **Other**_____ | |
| **Skin Care:** | ☐ **per guideline (see reverse)** | ☐ **Other**_____ | |

**Monitoring:**

Vital Signs:      ☐ No            ☐ Yes - specify_____

Weight:           ☐ No weights    ☐ Yes - specify_____

Labs:             ☐ No lab draws  ☐ Yes labs - specify_____

**Consider Other Consults (if not already involved):** ☐ Palliative Care  ☐ Pastoral Care

**Medication for Symptom Management**
Pain – Scheduled (If PCA use special sheet) :
Pain - Breakthrough:
Dyspnea:
Anxiety/Agitation:
Myoclonus:
Depression:
Sleep Disturbance:
Pruritus:
Fever:
Nausea/Vomiting:
Constipation:
Diarrhea:
Other Orders:

A generic equivalent may be administered when a drug has been prescribed by brand name unless the order states to the contrary.

_____          _____

Physician/ARNP  Signature              Date/Time

_____          _____

Print Physician/ARNP Name              Pager or Phone

_____

Secretary Transcribing

Original to the medical record       Yellow copy to Pharmacy      See Other Side
P&T Committee: 7/15/2004 (P-225)     Medical Records: 08/03/2004  Form #1826

**Figures 3–4 A&B.** Comfort Measures Orders sheet with guidelines for care as reference for staff education on the back (*see next page*).
*Source:* ©Dartmouth-Hitchcock Medical Center, June 2004. Used with permission.

*Guidelines for Comfort Measures Orders*

**D/C ALL PREVIOUS ORDERS** – Assess & reorder existing orders effective for comfort.

**Activity**: Goal is patient comfort.  Activity level and hygiene routine should be based on patient's preference.

**Hunger**: Goal is to respond to patient's hunger, not to maintain a "normal nutritional intake."

**Thirst**: Goal is to respond to patient's thirst, which is best accomplished by oral fluids, sips, ice chips, and mouthcare per patient desires, not IV hydration.

**IV Fluids**: Goal is to avoid over-hydration which can lead to discomfort from edema, pulmonary and gastric secretions, and urinary incontinence. A small volume of IV fluid may assist with medication metabolism and delirium.

**Dyspnea:** Respond to the patient's perception of breathlessness rather than "numerical abnormalities"; i.e. oxygen saturation via pulse oximetry. Interventions include medications (e.g. opioids, antianxiety agents, steroids), scopolamine patch and minimizing IV fluids to decrease secretions; oxygen therapy per nasal cannula prn for patient comfort—avoid face mask.
Fans at Bedside – Fans are available for patient comfort and are often more effective for perception of breathlessness than other interventions.

**Elimination**: Focus on managing distress from bowel or bladder incontinence. Insert Foley Catheter prn – per patient comfort and desire.

**Oral Care**: Studies show dry mouth is the most common & distressing symptom in conscious patients at end of life.
Ice chips and sips of fluid prn; humidify oxygen to minimize oral/nasal drying.
Mouth care q 2 hours and prn – sponge oral mucosa and apply lubricant to lips and oral mucosa.

**Skin Care**: Air mattress, Pressure Sore Prevention Measures per DHMC skin care guidelines.
Incontinent care every 2 hours and prn.

**Monitoring**: Focus monitoring on the patient's symptoms (e.g. pain) & responses to comfort measures.

**Psychosocial Consults**: Goal is to provide resources and support through the dying process.

**Medication for Symptom Management (Scheduled & PRN):**
Pain Management, scheduled and breakthrough: consider PCA/ IV/SQ/rectal analgesics.
Dyspnea Management: consider opioids, scopolamine patch, atropine for secretions.
Anxiety /Agitation Management: consider combination of lorazepam (Ativan) & haloperidol (Haldol).
Myoclonus: consider benzodiazepines &/or opioid rotation for myoclonus.
Depression Management: evaluate for antidepressants or methylphenidate.
Sleep Disturbance Management: consider diphenhydramine (Benadryl).
Pruritus Management: consider diphenhydramine (Benadryl) PO/IV.
Fever Management: consider acetaminophen (Tylenol) PO/ rectal
Nausea/Vomiting Management: consider prochlorperazine (Compazine), metoclopramide; 5-HT3 antagonist PO/IV.
Constipation Management: consider Narcotic Bowel Orders.
Diarrhea Management: consider diphenoxylate/atropine (Lomotil) or loperamide (Imodium).

**Figures 3–4 A&B.**  Continued.

and is asked if he "would like everything done" to help him to breathe better—the answer is understandably 'yes'. If the topic had been discussed earlier in his admission, he would have been provided with comprehensive information regarding his prognosis and probable course of illness, and multiple options for treating dyspnea at end-of-life (e.g. opioids and oxygen rather than intubation and ventilation). Meeting the patient and family's preferences for EOL care requires advance care planning that occurs early in the course of illness, or preferably in the primary health care setting while people are well and healthy. Intensive health care provider education on communicating with patients about advance care planning, before a health crisis occurs, is an area where a HBPC program can have influence beyond the bedside of the individual patient.

The case study of Mr. RL demonstrates the importance of early palliative care intervention so that advance directives and patient- and family-centered care can be planned.

The introduction of palliative care at the time of diagnosis allowed for appropriate and effective utilization of the palliative care services. When the patient is identified early in the course of illness, the palliative care team can act as a resource for advance care planning in addition to providing information about symptom and pain management and help with psychosocial issues. As the patient nears death, and the goal of care becomes focused more on comfort, the palliative care team will be a familiar member of the care team during a potentially stressful time.

## Outcomes and Their Measurement: The Role of QI and Research in HBPC

Measurement of outcomes is vital to demonstrate quality and to maintain viability and growth of HBPC programs.

Although the field is still developing, tools are beginning to emerge to measure care, assist with developing standards of care and, most importantly, to bring individual and organizational transparency and accountability to the care that is being delivered. Documentation of less than excellent outcomes may result in the organizational tension needed for change to occur. Such motivation can stimulate improvement and motivation for both administrators and clinicians.

As described earlier in this chapter, a number of organizations such as CAPC, NQF, and NCP have urged all programs to collect standardized measures across settings. In particular, CAPC has taken the lead in providing technical assistance in this regard. Examples of available CAPC resources for business, clinical, quality management, and strategic and financial planning are available on their website. Each category noted on the webpage is a link to the actual tools and instruments for measurement and planning of clinical care.

A number of efforts have been initiated to move the measurement of palliative care outcomes forward. The Institute of Medicine issued a report in 2007, "Cancer Care for the Whole Patient: Meeting Psychosocial Health Needs."[104] This report requested development of mechanisms to measure quality of care by organizations that are involved in developing and measuring standards of quality. In response, the American Society of Clinical Oncologists (ASCO), recognizing that oncologists had few reliable resources to assess and measure the quality of supportive care delivered in their practices, launched a Health Plan Program developed by its Quality Oncology Practice Initiative (QOPI).[46] Data is collected on a quarterly basis and, if desired, reported by ASCO to insurers. Measurement of data in this fashion has an impact on the quality of care delivered within an individual program, but also serves to promote evidence based practices as well as standardization across settings.

Another national effort was led by the University HealthSystem Consortium (UHC) recommending collection of data for the purpose of academic benchmarking nationally.[109] The UHC, comprised of over 100 academic medical centers and nearly 200 of their affiliates, is an alliance of US Academic Medical Centers (AMCs), whose goal is to provide resources to support transformational change leading to clinical and operational excellence. Through the consensus of an expert panel and based on other published guidelines, they developed 11 Key Performance Measures and collected data from the 35 centers that agreed to participate—some had palliative care consultation services, while others did not. The 11 measures included pain assessment, use of a pain rating scale, pain reduction, bowel regimen, dyspnea assessment and relief, comprehensive assessment, psychosocial assessment, patient/family meeting, documentation of discharge plan and arrangement for discharge services. They found significant variability across these centers, but identified 5 organizations that were found to be "better performers" overall. However, no organization reached the predetermined 90% benchmark on all parameters, while some hospitals achieved low or 0% achievement of some.[109] Despite its limitations, this

project demonstrated the importance of measurement of palliative care indicators.

As previously described, the NCP 8 domains and NQF 38 preferred practices are key resources for the development of measures to determine HBPC quality. Although voluntary, the preferred practices were intended to provide a standard of care for which measures could be developed for quality assessment. Other NQF guidelines have become the foundation for accreditation and reimbursement. It is the hope that this same outcome will occur in the palliative care preferred practices.

The CAPC website and a printed technical manual[18] contain tools for measuring HBPC outcomes. When assisting an organization to establish a program, CAPC encourages the incorporation of clinical, financial, operational and customer metrics.[39] In 2008, CAPC convened a consensus panel to discuss which operational metrics should be measured as programs "strive for quality, sustainability and growth" and which metrics can be used to "compare service utilization across settings." Twelve domains of operational data were agreed upon which may be used to compare service characteristics and impact within a program or between programs. The four categories of measurement to assure effectiveness and efficiency recommended by CAPC are: (1) Clinical (pain and symptom control) metrics; (2) Program Operational measures; (3) Customer metrics (satisfaction surveys of patients, families and providers); and (4) Financial metrics. Table 3–8 lists some examples of these measurement variables. Examples of actual tools to measure these characteristics are available on the CAPC website mentioned earlier.

Every program should have a plan to measure and monitor its effect on the quality of patient care, ideally from program inception. Some measures will be useful for internal

| Table 3–8 Metric Categories | |
|---|---|
| Metric Domain | Examples |
| Operational | Patient demographics (diagnosis, age, gender, ethnicity) referring clinician, disposition, hospital length of stay |
| Clinical | Symptom scores, psychosocial symptom assessment |
| Customer (patient, family, referring clinicians) | Patient, family, referring clinician satisfaction surveys |
| Financial | Costs (pre- and post-HBPC consultation), inpatient palliative unit, net loss/gain for inpatient deaths |

*Source*: Data from Weissman DE, Meier DE, Spragens LH. Center to Advance Palliative Care. Palliative Care Consultation Service Metrics: Consensus Recommendations. J Palliat Med 2008;11(10):1294–1298.

planning for staffing, need for program growth, and productivity goals. These same measures could then be compared to other programs as external benchmarks, especially for newer programs under development. Ultimately, the data collected can be used to assure that high quality palliative care is provided across organizations.[39]

## Economic Issues

Despite higher spending per individual on health care than any other country, over 50% of caregivers of hospitalized Americans with a life-threatening illness surveyed report suboptimal care.[71] Over 1.5 million Americans die of chronic illness each year, and more than 70% are admitted to a hospital during the last six months of life.[107,110] The number of people over age 85 will double to 10 million by the year 2030. Currently, 23% of Medicare patients with more than four chronic conditions account for 68% of all Medicare spending.[111] As the population ages and technology advances, the potential for prolonged care with minimal improvement in quality of life and associated human suffering looms large. The cost to an overburdened health care system could be disastrous over the long term. Just because the technology exists does not mean it should be used for everyone. The Dartmouth Atlas of Health Care reported that 98% of Medicare decedents spent at least some time in a hospital in the year before death. And of this group, 15–55% had at least one stay in a critical care unit in the 6 months before death.[108,112]

Palliative care has been demonstrated to lower costs for both hospitals and payers by reducing hospital lengths of stay as well as pharmacy and procedural costs. Morrison et al conducted a retrospective study reviewing hospital costs for eight hospitals with established palliative care programs over a two-year period.[113] Considerable cost savings (cost avoidance) were demonstrated when matching patients who had palliative care team involvement were compared to those patients who did not.

Although it is not the goal of palliative care to reduce costs, several studies have demonstrated this to be the case.[42,113–116] Reduction in costs by palliative care intervention may occur in multiple ways. Patients and their families are often stressed and burdened by a serious illness. Many times they are not clear about what to expect and may be experiencing the fragmentation of multiple specialty providers giving seemingly conflicting messages. Compounding this is the erroneous societal expectation that medicine is able to fix nearly any health challenge. It is no wonder that patients and families sometimes have unreasonable expectations and are unable to discern the larger picture when functional status is declining and treatment options offer fewer benefits to quality or quantity of life.

HBPC clinicians may be able to provide the family with "the big picture" of the illness situation. As an "objective" coordinator, the palliative care provider is particularly skilled at summarizing all relevant information and assisting the patient to match treatments with their own personal values and preferences. In so doing, patients and families are better able to apply their personal wishes and goals to the care that is being offered. They may elect to decline certain diagnostics or invasive treatments in favor of those that will provide comfort. Some may choose to not escalate care or perhaps discontinue treatments that were previously initiated. In the setting of a prolonged critical care stay where treatments are no longer resulting in positive progress, a Palliative Care consult may result in de-escalation of disease-modifying care in favor of increasing "low-tech" comfort care. Such changes in treatment can result in reducing suffering of the patient and family and, at times, has also resulted in significant cost avoidance. Consistent with criteria from the CAPC report card, the Palliative Care consult may "reduce unwanted, unnecessary and painful interventions."[23]

In the less costly hospital care that occurs in the critical care unit, the Palliative Care team can assist patients and families to select medical treatments and care that are consistent with their values and preferences. When patients and families have a clear understanding of their prognosis, and realistic information about proposed procedures or treatments, they may wish to decline further hospital care and return to home. In some situations when symptom relief procedures or family respite is indicated, palliative care involvement can facilitate timely occurrence of the needed procedures so that time in the hospital is minimized. Not only does this potentially reduce costs, but quality of care is also enhanced.[113]

In settings of seemingly futile care or conflict among healthcare providers, patients and families or among healthcare providers, involvement of palliative care in conjunction with an ethics committee consultation may help in a more rapid conflict resolution.[63] Cost savings can be accomplished in indirect ways as well. When the palliative care team is involved, they can spend the time at the bedside necessary to manage pain and other symptoms. This is invaluable to an already overburdened primary treating team who may be working with other patients who also have intensive care needs. Thus, quality of life and satisfaction for the patient and family as well as professional colleagues is enhanced. The palliative care team may also be invaluable in assisting with complex plans for discharge, coordinating care across settings, and enhancing communication between the treating team and the patient and their family.

## Influencing Institutional, State, and National Policy

It is not enough to provide excellent, comprehensive care to just the patients that are referred for consultation. The truly effective HBPC program must seek out ways to influence care for all patients with life-limiting illness by developing an awareness and ability to influence health care policy within their institutions, and at a state or national level. The influence should begin within the larger organization in two main ways: (1) by developing policies, procedures, and practices that will guide care of all persons' with life-limiting illness within the agency and any affiliates; and (2) by integrating palliative care education and competency standards into basic orientation and continuing (preferably mandatory) staff education. Examples of the former include development of consultation triggers, policies for advance care planning, limitations of life-sustaining treatments, "comfort measures," withdrawal of mechanical ventilation, and standardized pain and symptom assessment and management. This type of influence will likely necessitate regular or ad hoc participation or leadership on institutional practice or ethics committees. Staff orientation has grown in sophistication such that "simulated" patients and learning labs are becoming standard mechanisms for learning basic care skills. Practicing skills of communicating bad news, holding family meetings, and discussing advance care planning, are some possible activities that lend themselves to such environments. Similarly, most organizations hold staff accountable for mandatory cardiopulmonary resuscitation (CPR) certification. It would seem reasonable to require mandatory "do not resuscitate" classes in which staff learns effective care to provide when patients are near death but will not be resuscitated. Other educational endeavors include annual presentations at other department or affiliated agencies grand rounds on palliative care topics. Also holding annual regional palliative care conferences for professionals or the general public can bring attention to the program.

Acting locally at the state level in legislative or health policy forums can make a big difference in care of patients. Examples of vital work performed at the state level include crafting of advance directive documents and laws, expanding hospice coverage to Medicaid, opioid prescribing laws, and other practice issues. The National Quality Forum Preferred Practices include a recommendation to "develop health care and community collaborations to promote advance care planning and completion of advance directives for all individuals—for example, the Respecting Choices and Community Conversations on Compassionate Care programs."[20] Some states have palliative care or EOL task forces that make policy and legislative recommendations that will enhance care of the seriously ill. For example, in New Hampshire, an EOL task force was created by legislation in which palliative care clinicians participated to assist in revising advance care planning legislation (see http://www.healthynh.com/fhc/initiatives/performance/eol/endoflifecare.php). Expert input assisted to improve advance directives forms and incorporate APNs as providers who could write DNR orders among other improvements. Palliative care and survivorship were added as major initiatives to the State Cancer Plan, which mandates some palliative practices for organizations to strive for as well as potential designate grant funds for palliative care focused projects (see http://www.nhcancerplan.org).

In addition to supporting legislative initiatives to improve care, it is just as vital to be involved to monitor policy that could have a harmful effect on patient care. For example, overly restrictive prescribing policies can interfere with patients in pain obtaining adequate amounts of opioids. Activism around restrictive policies may have direct improvement in patients' outcomes. Legislators respect the input from healthcare professionals who are able to provide expert input and "real life" patient examples to assist in crafting legislation. Meier and Beresford offer a practical summary and multiple examples of ways in which palliative care professionals can contribute to state and national legislation and policy.

Collaborating with local organizations also lends power to individual efforts. For example, the National Hospice and Palliative Care Organization, the American Cancer Society, nursing and medical associations and professional organizations at local, state, or national levels often have lobbyists and resources to assist with legislative efforts. Chapter 63 contains a broader discussion on the nursing role in policy development. However, it is important for HBPC program staff and leaders to keep these initiatives in mind as they develop within a health care setting.

## Future Directions

This chapter began by suggesting that HBPC is at the "end of the beginning." Despite a strong foothold within mainstream medicine, there is much growth, improvement, and education to be done to sustain and expand palliative care. Calvin Coolidge is quoted as saying, "We cannot do everything at once, but we can do something at once." Table 3–9 lists some future professional and societal issues that need attention. Great strides have been made in providing a solid infrastructure for growth in the form of increasing research evidence,[19] consensus guidelines for practice,[20,39,63,81,83,85,92] reliable and valid outcome measures,[39] and specialty educational/certification standards. These standards need to be widely disseminated and adopted. As more HBPC programs develop, there is likely to be a shortage of specialty-trained personnel and the faculty to educate them. Additional sources of funding and support are needed to continue the current momentum of change.

However, palliative care programs must not remain insular. Good work and rigorous studies need to be disseminated outside of the specialty via "mainstream" health care journals and conferences. External agencies (e.g., TJC) must begin to require mandatory adherence to standards and those agencies that meet established standards should be properly reimbursed for their performance. Funding for palliative care research, adequate reimbursement, and support for faculty development must become national priorities. Perhaps consumer demand for patient and family-centered care will be the "tipping point" that will make palliative care services an

**Table 3–9**
**Future Growth of HBPC**

Within Specialty

- Full/mandatory implementation of NCP + NQF Guidelines
- Evaluate/expand requirement of palliative care programs to have specialty-certified clinicians
- Increase educational funding/support for palliative care specialty education
- Increase number of specialty-trained faculty and students
- Increase availability of technical support for new programs

External/Societal/Policy

- Publish palliative care studies in top tier journals
- Increase NIH funding for palliative care research
- Accreditation requirements for HBPC
- Improve fiscal policy for reimbursement for hospice and palliative care services
- Develop medical and nursing school departments of palliative care
- Faculty career development support
- Legislative initiatives that support/promote palliative care and patient/family-centered care

integral part of every organization that touches the lives of persons with life-limiting illness and their families.

## Acknowledgments

The authors would like to acknowledge the following colleagues who provided important information for the development of this chapter: Jay Horton, ARNP, Sean Morrison, MD, Lisa Morgan (Center for the Advancement of Palliative Care), Lisa Stephens, ARNP (Dartmouth-Hitchcock Palliative Care Team), and Melissa Thompson, RN, CHPN (VAMC: VISN 1 Palliative Care Coordinator).

REFERENCES

1. Lynn J, Adamson D. Living Well at the End of Life: Adapting Health Care to Serious Chronic Illness in Old Age. Santa Monica, CA: RAND Health Communications, 2003.
2. Field MJ, Cassel CK. Approaching Death: Improving Care at the End of Life. Washington, D.C.: National Academy Press, 1997.
3. Wennberg JE, Fisher ES, Goodman DC, Skinner JS. Tracking the Care of Patients with Severe Chronic Illness: The Dartmouth Atlas of Health Care 2008. Lebanon, NH: Dartmouth Institute for Health Policy and Clinical Practice, 2008.
4. Bercovitz A, Decker FH, Jones A, Remsburg RE. End-of-life care in nursing homes: 2004 National Nursing Home Survey. Natl Health Stat Report 2008;9:1–24.
5. Flory J, Young-Xu Y, Gurol I, Levinsky N, Ash A, Emanuel E. Place of Death: U.S. Trends Since 1980. Health Aff 2004;23:194–200.
6. SUPPORT Principal Investigators. A controlled trial to improve care for seriously ill hospitalized patients. JAMA 1995;274:1591–1598.
7. Elshamy M, Whedon MB. Symptoms and care during the last 48 hours of life. Quality of life: A nursing challenge. Quality Assessment 1997;5(2):21–29.
8. Goodlin S, Winzelberg G, Teno J, Whedon M, Lynn J. Death in the hospital. Arch Intern Med 1998;158:1570–1572.
9. Lynn J, Teno JM, Phillips R, et al., for the SUPPORT Investigators. Perceptions of family members of the dying experience of older and seriously ill patients. Ann Intern Med 1997; 126:97–106.
10. Berwick D. A primer on leading the improvement of systems. BMJ 1996;312:619–622.
11. Lynn J, Schuster JL. Improving Care for the End of Life: A Sourcebook for Health Care Managers and Clinicians. New York: Oxford University Press, 2000.
12. Miller FG, Fins JJ. A proposal to restructure hospital care for dying patients. N Engl J Med 1996;334:1740–1742.
13. Solomon M. The enormity of the task: SUPPORT and changing practice Hastings Cent Rep 1995;25:S28–S32.
14. Krammer LM, Muir JC, Gooding-Kellar N, Williams MB, von Guten CF. Palliative care and oncology: Opportunities for oncology nursing. Oncology Nursing Updates 1999;6:1–12.
15. Emnett J, Byock I, Twohig JS. Advanced Practice Nursing: Pioneering Practices in Palliative Care. Missoula, Montana: The Robert Wood Johnson Foundation: Promoting Excellence in End-of-Life Care, July 2002.
16. Ajemian I, Mount B. The Royal Victoria Hospital Manual on Palliative/Hospice Care: A Resource Book. Montreal: Palliative Care Service, Royal Victoria Hospital; 1980.
17. Palliative Care in Hospitals. Center to Advance Palliative Care, 2006. Available at www.capc.org (accessed December 1, 2008).
18. Meier DE, Spragens LH, Sutton S. A Guide to Building a Hospital-Based Palliative Care Program. New York: Center to Advance Palliative Care, 2004.
19. Tieman J, Sladek R, Currow D. Changes in the quality and level of evidence of palliative and hospice care literature: The last century. Am J Clin Oncol 2008;26:5679–5683.
20. National Consensus Project. Clinical Practice Guidelines for Quality Palliative Care. Brooklyn, NY: National Consensus Project for Quality Palliative Care, 2004.
21. World Health Organization. Cancer Pain Relief and Palliative Care. Geneva: World Health Organization; 1990.
22. American Hospital Association. Hospital Statistics. Chicago: Health Forum, 2002, 2003, 2004.
23. Center to Advance Palliative Care, National Palliative Care Research Center. America's Care of Serious Illness: A State-by-State Report Card on Access to Palliative Care in Our Nation's Hospitals. New York: Center to Advance Palliative Care, 2008: p 34.
24. Goldsmith B, Dietrich J, Qingling D, Morrison RS. Variability in access to hospital palliative care in the United States. J Palliat Med 2008;11:1094–1102.
25. von Gunten C. Secondary and tertiary palliative care in US hospitals. JAMA 2002;287:875–881.
26. Lorenz KA, Lynn J, Dy SM, et al. Evidence for improving palliative care at the end of life: A systematic review. Ann Intern Med 2008;148:147–159.

27. Teno JM. Palliative care teams: Self-reflection—past, present, and future. J Pain Symptom Manage 2002;23:94–95.

28. Hanks GW, Robbins M, Sharp D, et al. The imPaCT study: A randomised controlled trial to evaluate a hospital palliative care team. Br J Cancer 2002;87:733–739.

29. Higginson I, Finlay I, Goodwin D, et al. Do hospital-based palliative teams improve care for patients or families at the end of life? J Pain Symptom Manage 2001;23:96–106.

30. Francke AL. Evaluative research on palliative support teams: A literature review. Patient Educ Couns 2000;41:83–91.

31. Bascom PB. A hospital-based comfort care team: Consultation for seriously ill and dying patients. J Hosp Palliat Care 1997;14(2):57–60.

32. Dunlop RJ, Hockley JM. Terminal Care Support Teams. New York: Oxford University Press, 1990.

33. Dunlop RJ, Hockley JM. Hospital-Based Palliative Care Teams: The Hospital–Hospice Interface (Vol. 2) (2nd ed). New York: Oxford University Press, 1998.

34. O'Neill WM, O'Connor P, Latimer EJ. Hospital palliative care services: Three models in three countries. J Pain Symptom Manage 1992;7:406–413.

35. Manfredi P, Morrison S, Morris J, Goldhirsch S, Carter J, Meier D. Palliative care consultations: How do they impact the care of hospitalized patients? J Pain Symptom Manage 2002;20:166–173.

36. Weissman DE. Consultation in palliative medicine. Arch Intern Med 1997;157:733–737.

37. Pan CX, Morrison RS, Meier DE, et al. How prevalent are hospital-based palliative care programs? Status report and future directions. J Palliat Med 2001;4:315–324.

38. Zimmermann C, Riechelmann R, Krzyzanowska M, Rodin GC, Tannock I. Effectiveness of specialized palliative care: A systematic review. JAMA 2008;299:1698–1709.

39. Weissman DE, Meier DE, Spragens LH. Center to advance palliative care. Palliative care consultation service metrics: Consensus recommendations. J Palliat Med 2008;11:1294–1298.

40. Kellar N, Martinez J, Finis N, Bolger A, von Guten C. Characterization of an acute inpatient hospice palliative care unit in a US teaching hospital. JONA 1996;26:16–20.

41. Billings A, Pantilat S. Survey of palliative care programs in United States teaching hospitals. J Palliat Med 2004;4:309–314.

42. Smith TJ, Coyne P, Cassel B, Penberthy L, Hopson A, Hager MA. A high-volume specialist palliative care unit and team may reduce in-hospital end-of-life care costs. J Palliat Med 2003;6:699–705.

43. Bakitas M, Stevens M, Ahles T, et al. Project ENABLE: A palliative care demonstration project for advanced cancer patients in three settings. J Palliat Med 2004;7:363–372.

44. Rabow M, Dibble S, Pantilat S, McPhee S. The Comprehensive Care Team: A controlled trial of outpatient palliative medicine consultation. Arch Intern Med 2004;164:83–91.

45. Byock I, Twohig JS, Merriman M, Collins K. Promoting excellence in end-of-life care: A report on innovative models of palliative care. J Palliat Med 2006;9:137–151.

46. McNiff KK, Neuss MN, Jacobson JO, Eisenberg PD, Kadlubek P, Simone JV. Measuring supportive care in medical oncology practice: Lessons learned from the quality oncology practice initiative. J Clin Oncol 2008;26:3832–3837.

47. Follwell M, Burman D, Le LW, et al. Phase II Study of an outpatient palliative care intervention in patients with metastatic cancer. J Clin Oncol 2009;27:206–213.

48. Rabow MW, Dibble SL, Pantilat SZ, McPhee SJ. The comprehensive care team: A controlled trial of outpatient palliative medicine consultation. Arch Intern Med 2004;164:83–91.

49. Moore S, Corner J, Haviland J, et al. Nurse led follow up and conventional medical follow up in management of patients with lung cancer: Randomised trial. BMJ 2002;325:1145.

50. Bakitas M, Lyons K, Hegel M, et al. The project ENABLE II randomized controlled trial to improve palliative care for rural patients with advanced cancer: Baseline findings, methodological challenges, and solutions. Palliat Support Care 2009;7:75–86.

51. Wetle T, Shield R, Teno J, Miller SC, Welch L. Family perspectives on end-of-life care experiences in nursing homes. Gerontologist 2005;45:642–650.

52. Shield RR, Wetle T, Teno J, Miller SC, Welch L. Physicians "missing in action": Family perspectives on physician and staffing problems in end-of-life care in the nursing home. J Am Geriatr Soc 2005;53:1651–1657.

53. Casarett D, Karlawish J, Morales K, Crowley R, Mirsch T, Asch DA. Improving the use of hospice services in nursing homes: A randomized controlled trial. JAMA 2005;294(2):211–217.

54. Wetle T, Teno J, Shield R, Welch L, Miller SC. End of Life in Nursing Homes: Experiences and Policy Recommendations. Washington, DC: AARP Public Policy Institute, 2004.

55. Zerzan J, Stearns S, Hanson L. Access to palliative care and hospice care in nursing homes. JAMA 2000;284:2489–2494.

56. Castle NG, Mor V, Banaszak-Holl J. Special care hospice units in nursing homes. Hosp J 1997;12:59–69.

57. Kelly B, Edwards P, Synott R, Neil C, Baillie R, Battistutta D. Predictors of bereavement outcomes for family carers of cancer patients. Psychooncology 1999;8:237–249.

58. Billings JA, Kolton E. Family satisfaction and bereavement care following death in the hospital. J Palliat Med 1999;2:33–49.

59. Wright A, Zhang B, Ray A, et al. Associations between end-of-life discussions, patient mental health, medical care near death, and caregiver bereavement adjustment. JAMA 2008;300:1665–1673.

60. Valks K, Mitchell ML, Inglis-Simons C, Limpus A. Dealing with death: An audit of family bereavement programs in Australian intensive care units. Aust Crit Care 2005;18:146, 8–51.

61. Walsh T, Foreman M, Curry P, O'Driscoll S, McCormack M. Bereavement support in an acute hospital: An Irish model. Death Stud 2008;32:768–786.

62. Schachter SR. Developing and analyzing a hospital wide bereavement program in a comprehensive cancer center. Psychooncology 2003;12:19.

63. National Quality Forum. A National Framework and Preferred Practices for Palliative and Hospice Care Quality: A Consensus Report. Washington, DC: National Quality Forum, 2006.

64. Elwert F, Christakis NA. The effect of widowhood on mortality by the causes of death of both spouses. Am J Public Health 2008;98:2092–2099.

65. Harvey S, Snowdon C, Elbourne D. Effectiveness of bereavement interventions in neonatal intensive care: A review of the evidence. Semin Fetal Neonatal Med 2008;13:341–356.

66. Mulrooney T, Whedon M, Bedell A. Focus group of family members after death of a loved one in the hospital. DHMC—unpublished data, 1999.

67. Bakitas M, Ahles T, Skalla K, et al. Proxy perspectives regarding end-of-life care for persons with cancer. Cancer 2008;112:1854–1861.

68. Miyashita M, Morita T, Hirai K. Evaluation of end-of-life cancer care from the perspective of bereaved family members: The Japanese experience. J Clin Oncol 2008;26:3845–3852.

69. Grunfeld E, Folkes A, Urquhart R. Do available questionnaires measure the communication factors that patients and families consider important at end of life? J Clin Oncol 2008;26:3874–3878.

70. Finlay E, Shreve S, Cassarett D. Nationwide veterans affairs quality measure for cancer: The family assessment of treatment at end of life. Am J Clin Oncol 2008;26:3838–3844.

71. Teno J, Clarridge BR, Casey VA, et al. Family perspectives on end-of-life care at the last place of care. JAMA 2004;291:88–93.

72. Tang ST, McCorkle R. Use of family proxies in quality of life research for cancer patients at the end of life: A literature review. Cancer Invest 2002;20:1086–1104.

73. Press Ganey Associates. Patient/Family satisfaction with end-of-life care survey. Available at: http://www.pressganey.com/ (accessed January 1, 2009).

74. Macdonald M, Liben S, Carnevale F, et al. Parental perspectives on hospital staff-members' acts of kindness and commemoration after a child's death. Pediatrics 2005;116:884–890.

75. Ferris TGG, Hallward JA, Ronan L, Billings JA. When the patient dies: A survey of medical housestaff about care after death. J Palliat Med 1998;1:231–239.

76. Shively P, Midland D, eds. The Art of Compassionate Death Notification. La Crosse, WI: Gundersen Lutheran Medical Foundation, 1999.

77. Ferrell BR, Grant M, Virani R. Strengthening nursing education to improve end-of-life care. Nurs Outlook 1999;47:252–256.

78. Carron AT, Lynn J, Keaney P. End-of-life care in medical textbooks. Ann Intern Med 1999;130:82–86.

79. Ferrell BR, Virani R, Grant M. Analysis of end-of-life content in nursing textbooks. Oncol Nurs Forum 1999;26:869–876.

80. Bakitas M, Dahlin C, Bishop M. Palliative and end-of-life care. In: Buttaro TM, Trybulski J, Bailey PP, Sandberg-Cook J, eds. Primary Care: A Collaborative Approach (3rd ed). St. Louis: Mosby, 2007:70–79.

81. Ferrell B, Paice J, Koczywas M. New standards and implications for improving the quality of supportive oncology practice. J Clin Oncol 2008;26:3824–3831.

82. Center to Advance Palliative Care. Palliative Care Leadership Centers. Available at: www.capc.org (accessed December 1, 2008).

83. Weissman DE, Meier DE. Operational features for hospital palliative care programs: Consensus recommendations. J Palliat Med 2008;11:1189–1194.

84. Comprehensive Accreditation Manual for Hospitals: The Official Handbook (CAMH). The Joint Commission, 2008. Available at: http://www.jointcommission.org (accessed March 17, 2008).

85. The Joint Commission. Certification for Palliative Care Programs. 2008. Available at: www.jointcommission.org/CertificationPrograms/Pallative_Care/ (accessed March 17, 2008).

86. Hume M. Improving care at the end-of-life. Qual Lett Healthc Lead 1998;10(10):2–10.

87. Abrahm JL, Callahan J, Rossetti K, Pierre L. The impact of a hospice consultation team on the care of veterans with advanced cancer. J Pain Symptom Manage 1996;12:23–31.

88. Creating and expanding hospice and palliative care programs in VA, 2002. Available at: www.va.gov/oaa/flp/ (accessed November 24, 2009).

89. Casarett D, Pickard A, Bailey FA, et al. Do palliative consultations improve patient outcomes? J Am Soc Geriatr Dent 2008;56:593–599.

90. Edes T, Shreve S, Cassarett D. Increasing access and quality in Department of Veterans Affairs Care at the end of life: A lesson in change. J Am Soc Geriatr Dent 2007;55:1645–1649.

91. Grant M, Hanson J, Mullan P, Spolum M, Ferrell B. Disseminating end-of-life education to cancer centers: Overview of program and of evaluation. J Cancer Educ 2007;22:140–148.

92. Epstein R, Street R, Jr. Patient-Centered Communication in Cancer Care: Promoting Healing and Reducing Suffering. Bethesda, MD: National Cancer Institute. 2007. NIH Publication No. 07-6225.

93. Palliative Care: What is it? 2003. Available at: www.who.org (accessed November 24, 2009).

94. Byock I. Completing the continuum of cancer care: Integrating life-prolongation and palliation. CA Cancer J Clin 2000;50:123–132.

95. Schwartz CE, Wheeler HB, Hammes B, et al. Early intervention in planning end-of-life care with ambulatory geriatric patients: Results of a pilot trial. Arch Intern Med 2002;162:1611–1618.

96. Von Gunten C, Ferris F, Emanuel L. Ensuring competency in end-of-life care: Communication and relational skills. JAMA 2000;284:3051–3057.

97. End of Life/Palliative Education Resource Center. Fast Fact and Concept #016: Conducting a Family Conference 2nd Edition EPERC, 2008. Available at: http://www.eperc.mcw.edu/fastFact/ff_016.htm (accessed December 1, 2008).

98. Du Pen S, Du Pen AR, Polissar N, et al. Implementing guidelines for cancer pain management: Results of a randomized controlled clinical trial. Am J Clin Oncol 1999;17:361–370.

99. Stair J. Oncology critical pathways: Palliative care: A model example from the Moses Cone Health system. Oncology 1998;14(2):26–30.

100. Berwick DM. Controlling variation in health care: A consultation from Walter Shewhart. Med Care 1991;29:1212–1225.

101. Meisel A. The Right to Die. New York: John Wiley and Sons, 1995, 1998.

102. Teno J, Lynn J, Wenger N, et al. Advance directives for seriously ill hospitalized patients: Effectiveness with the patient self-determination act and the SUPPORT intervention. J Am Geriatr Soc 1997;45:500–507.

103. Sulmasy DP, Terry PB, Weisman CS, et al. The accuracy of substituted judgments in patients with terminal diagnosis. Ann Intern Med 1998;128:621–629.

104. Institute of Medicine. Cancer Care for the Whole Patient: Meeting Psychosocial Health Needs. Washington, DC: The National Academies Press, 2007.

105. Twaddle M, Maxwell T, Cassel J, et al. Palliative care benchmarks from academic medical centers. J Palliat Med 2007;10:86–98.

106. The Dartmouth Institute for Health Policy and Clinical Practice. Tracking the Care of Patients with Severe Chronic Illness: The Dartmouth Atlas of Health Care 2008. Lebanon, NH: Dartmouth Institute for Health Policy and Clinical Practice, 2008.

107. Anderson GF. Medicare and chronic conditions. N Engl J Med 2005;353:305–309.

108. The care of patients with severe chronic illness: An online report on the Medicare program by the Dartmouth Atlas Project: The Dartmouth Atlas of Health Care 2006. Center for the Evaluative Clinical Sciences, 2006. Available at: http://www.dartmouthatlas.org/atlases/2006_Chronic_Care_Atlas.pdf (accessed November 24, 2009).

109. Morrison RS, Penrod JD, Cassel JB, et al. Cost savings associated with US hospital palliative care consultation programs. Arch Intern Med 2008;168:1783–1790.

110. The Robert Wood Johnson Foundation. Accounting for the costs of caring through the end of life: Cost accounting peer workgroup recommendations to the field. The Robert Wood Johnson Foundation, 2004.

111. Solomon M, Romer A, Sellers D. Meeting the Challenge: Improving End-of-Life Care in Managed Care: Access, Accountability, and Cost. Newton, MA: Robert Wood Johnson, 1999.

112. Engelhardt J, McClive-Reed K, Toseland R, Smith TL, Larson DG, Tobin D. Effects of a program for coordinated care of advanced illness on patients, surrogates, and healthcare costs: A randomized trial. Am J Manag Care 2006;12:93–100.

113. Brumley R, Enguidanos S, Jamison P, et al. Increased satisfaction with care and lower costs: results of a randomized trial of in-home palliative care. J Am Geriatr Soc 2007;55:993–1000.

114. Sweeney L, Halpert A, Waranoff J. Patient-centered management of complex patients can reduce costs without shortening life. Am J Manag Care 2007;13:84–92.

115. Hughes SL, Cummings J, Weaver F, Manheim L, Braun B, Conrad K. A randomized trial of the cost effectiveness of VA hospital-based home care for the terminally ill. Health Serv Res 1992;26:801–817.

116. Meier DE, Beresford L. Palliative care professionals contribute to state legislative and policy initiatives. J Palliat Med 2008;11:1070–1073.

# 4

*Elaine Glass, Douglas Cluxton, and Patrice Rancour*

# Principles of Patient and Family Assessment

*To get to my body, my doctor has to get to my character. He has to go through my soul...I'd like my doctor to scan me, to grope for my spirit as well as my prostate. Without such recognition, I am nothing but my illness.*—Anatole Broyard

- ◆ **Key Points**
- ◆ *Comprehensive assessment of the patient and family is essential to planning palliative care.*
- ◆ *Assessment involves input from the interdisciplinary team with information shared verbally as well as in the patient record.*
- ◆ *Ongoing, detailed and comprehensive assessment is needed to identify the complex and changing needs of patients and families facing chronic or life-threatening illness.*

An effective assessment is key to establishing an appropriate nursing care plan for the patient and family. The initial palliative care nursing assessment may vary little from a standard nursing assessment.[1,2] In order to assess effectively, members of the health care team need to maximize their listening skills and minimize quick judgments. Groopman indicated that as many as 15% of all diagnoses are inaccurate due to physicians falling into cognitive traps.[3]

The goals of the palliative care plan that evolve from the initial and ongoing nursing assessments focus on enhancing quality of life. Ferrell's quality-of-life framework[4] is used to organize the assessment. The four quality-of-life domains in this framework are physical, psychological, social, and spiritual well-being. For the purpose of this chapter, the psychological and social domains are combined into one: the psychosocial domain.

Because the needs of patients and families change throughout the course of a chronic illness, these quality-of-life assessments are examined at four critical stages along the illness trajectory: at the time of diagnosis, during treatments, after treatments (long-term survival or terminal phase), and during active dying.

CASE STUDY
*Initial Description of Ladona and Her Family*

Ladona is a single, 26-year-old African-American female who lives with her parents while she gets established in her first teaching position at the local high school. Her parents are Jehovah's Witnesses and Ladona recently returned to her faith following a time of questioning during her college years. Ladona has a fiancé, Michael, whom she met in college. He is Roman Catholic. They are considering marriage in the near future. Ladona's parents are very involved in her life as a result of her life long struggle with sickle cell anemia.

## Malignant and Nonmalignant Chronic Illnesses

The experiences of chronically ill patients are dynamic in terms of the continuous or episodic declines they face throughout the illness trajectory. The focus of medical care for these patients is palliative rather than curative, including reduction of symptoms, improvement of quality of life, and optimization of the highest level of wellness. Examples of these kinds of illnesses today include acquired immune deficiency syndrome (AIDS); refractory cardiovascular, hepatic and renal diseases; diabetes; and neurological disorders such as multiple sclerosis, cerebral palsy, amyotrophic lateral sclerosis, Parkinson's disease, Alzheimer's disease, multiple types of cancer, and sickle cell disease. For some of these diseases, the focus of medical care may include attempting to extend life through research with the hope of finding a cure.

Non-malignant illness admissions to hospice reported by the National Hospice & Palliative Care Organization from 2007[5] include:

- Cardiac = 11.8%
- Debility unspecified = 11.2%
- Dementia, includes Alzheimer's = 10.1%
- Lung Disease = 7.9%

The person with cancer may repeatedly alter his or her expectations about the future. Words describing the status of the disease during a cancer illness include "no evidence of disease," "remission," "partial remission," "stable disease," "recurrence," "relapse," and "metastasis." Patients report experiencing a "roller-coaster ride," in which the hopeful points in remission are often followed by crises with relapse or disease progression. Patients may be told, more than once, that they are likely to die within a short period of time, only to recover and do well for awhile. As a result, the finality of death may be more difficult when it does occur.

## Introduction to Physical Assessment

Before beginning the assessment interview and physical examination, it is important for the nurse to establish a relationship with the patient by doing the following:

- Introducing himself or herself to the patient and others in the room.
- Verifying that this is the correct patient.
- Determining how the patient would like to be addressed: first name? last name? a nickname?
- Explaining the purpose of the interaction and the approximate length of time that the nurse intends to spend with the patient.
- Asking the patient's permission to proceed with the assessment, giving the patient an opportunity to use the restroom, and excusing others whom the patient does not wish to be present during the interview and examination. (Some patients may want significant others to be present during the interview, to assist with recall, but not during the examination. The nurse needs to modify the assessment routine to accommodate the patient's preferences.)
- Taking a seat near the patient, being respectful of the patient's cultural norms for physical closeness and eye contact.
- Inviting the patient to tell about how he or she learned of the illness.
- Taking care not to interrupt the patient too often; using communication techniques such as probing, reflecting, clarifying, responding empathetically, and asking open-ended questions to encourage greater detail if the patient's account is brief or sketchy.

Palliative care patients are often very ill and do not have the energy, patience, or interest in answering a myriad of questions—especially if the questions do not relate to their immediate needs. Therefore, individualized assessments, based on prioritized symptoms for each patient, are conducted using the following process:

- Print off a demographic sheet. During the assessment, ask the patient what name he or she would like to be called. Note the patient's next of kin and ask the patient and/or family who is the legal health care power of attorney (HCPOA). If no one has been legally designated and the default person is not who the patient wants to make his health care decisions, contact the appropriate resource persons (social worker or chaplain) to assist the patient in completing these legal documents. Also, record other close family members or friends (not listed on the demographic sheet) and include their names and phone numbers. Finally, note the patient's insurance coverage. For example, Medicaid may have a restricted medication formulary. If the patient does not have adequate insurance coverage, consider a social worker consult to help the patient access the necessary resources to obtain financial assistance.
- Print off the most recent history and physical (H&P) or consultation report to serve as the primary reference for the patient's current health care status. Read all the consultation reports available to see if any additional information is provided that is not on the printed H&P. Make note of this information on the printed H&P.
- Review labs and transcribe pertinent ones to the printed sheets. Particularly make note of the creatinine to assess kidney function, which will determine the use of morphine in the patient's care. Morphine typically is not used if the creatinine is higher than 2 (or over 1.5 in older adults), because metabolites that are not excreted may cause confusion. Review liver function tests, since some medications' efficacy may be altered with liver failure. Check the albumin (reflects the patient's nutritional intake for the past few months) and prealbumin (reflects the patient's nutritional intake for the past few days) to determine the patient's nutritional status. Note

the ejection fraction to determine if heart failure is contributing to the patient's symptoms. Finally, read recent radiology and pathology reports to collect further information on the severity of the patient's illness.

- Print out a list of the patient's current medications in the hospital. Check to make sure it includes pertinent home medications, including any over-the-counter and/or herbal preparations that contribute to the patient's comfort. Note if any newly ordered medications relate to the patient's comfort. During the initial assessment interview, confirm with the patient and/or the family that these medications are effective. Negotiate revisions as needed. Make note of medications that are not present for the following key symptoms: pain, bowel function, anxiety, and sleep, and for any symptoms mentioned in the H&P or indicated by the lab values or radiology reports. For example, patients with liver or kidney failure may have pruritus or nausea. During the interview, ask about any other symptoms that may be present from observing the patient, such as dyspnea, anorexia, somnolence/sedation or agitation. Inquire if any past medications have been effective in managing these symptoms. If the patient has no preferred medications, offer options and obtain the patient's or the family's agreement to the medication regimen recommended. When able, the patient and/or family should always be an active participant in the plan of care.
- Ask the patient and family about their interest in any complementary therapies that may be available to them, such as music therapy, guided imagery, massage therapy, healing touch, and aromatherapy.
- Many times, palliative care is requested to assist with the discussion and decision making about code status. One way to introduce the topic to the patient and/or family is, "We hope for the best, but try to prepare for the worst. If, despite our best efforts, your heart or breathing would stop, would you want us to allow you to die naturally or would you want us to try to revive you and put you on life support machines?" Depending on the patient's or family member's knowledge level, further conversation may be required regarding details about cardio-pulmonary resuscitation (CPR), defibrillation, intubation and ventilators.
- Finally, ask the patient and family if they can think of anything else that you might do for them that would contribute to their comfort.

## Introduction to Psychosocial Assessment

Tables 4–1 through 4–3 provide a framework for three key elements of assessment: conducting a psychosocial assessment, distinguishing normal grief from depression, and doing a general mental status assessment. Throughout the illness trajectory, the nurse can use these tools to monitor the patient's response to illness and treatment.

Anyone diagnosed with a serious or life-threatening illness experiences many losses. However, responses to illness vary tremendously among individuals. In addition, the same person may respond differently at various times during an illness. How a particular patient copes depends on the severity of the illness, the patient's history of coping with stressful life events, and available supports. Some individuals develop coping styles that are more helpful than others when facing a life-threatening illness.

The nurse needs to assess two very important parameters in order to assist the patient in coping in the most functional way possible. These parameters are the patient's need for information and her or his need for control in making decisions. Observers of "exceptional" patients, such as Bernie Siegel[6] have noted that patients who are proactive, assertive information-seekers often appear to experience better outcomes than patients who are passive in making decisions. Indicators of a person's expressed need for control may include the following:

- Expressed need for information.
- Comfort in asking questions.
- Willingness to assert own needs and wishes relative to the plan of care.
- Initiative taken to research print and Internet resources on the illness and treatment.

Table 4–1 provides details for doing a psychosocial assessment. More detailed information on the psychosocial aspects of oncology can be found in Holland's *Psychooncology.*[7]

Grief is a normal reaction to loss, especially a major loss such as one's health. In chronic illness, grief is likely to be recurrent as losses accumulate. This does not make it pathological, but it does form the basis of the "roller-coaster" phenomenon that many patients describe. Some patients with advanced disease have been able to integrate their losses in a meaningful way, managing to reconcile and transcend them. An example of such a person is Morrie Schwartz, who wrote about his illness in *Letting Go: Morrie's Reflections on Living While Dying.*[8] And, of course, while all this is going on with the patient, family members are also going through a myriad of their own reponses, which are often not in synch with one another. Refer to Chapter 31 of this text to learn about "Supporting Families in Palliative Care."

Table 4–2 contrasts and compares normal grief with depression, to assist the nurse in determining when a patient needs to be referred for counseling. For further information, consult John Schneider's classic work, "Clinically Significant Differences between Grief, Pathological Grief and Depression."[9] Information on the use of the Distress Thermometer as an assessment tool for emotional distress can be found in Chapter 48, "The Outpatient Setting." In addition, the Distress Thermometer has been validated as a screening tool for psychological distress.[10]

In some cases, patients may appear to be having difficulties in coping but the nurse cannot easily identify the specific

**Table 4–1**
**Framework for Psychosocial Assessment**

Determining the types of losses

**Physical losses**
Energy
Mobility
Body parts
Body function
Freedom from pain and other forms of physical dysfunction
Sexuality

**Observing emotional responses**
Anxiety
Anger
Denial
Withdrawal
Shock
Sadness
Bargaining
Depression
Acceptance

**Assessing the need for information**
Wants to know details
Wants the overall picture
Wants minimal information
Wants no information, but wants the family to know

**Psychosocial losses**
Autonomy
Sense of mastery
Body image alterations
Sexuality
Relationship changes
Lifestyle
Work changes
Role function
Money
Time

**Identifying coping styles**
*Functional:*
   Normal grief work
   Problem-solving
   Humor
   Practicing spiritual rituals, e.g. prayer, attending worship services
*Dysfunctional:*
   Aggression
   Fantasy
   Minimization
   Addictive behaviors
   Guilt
   Psychosis

**Assessing the need for control**
Very high
High
Moderate/average
Low
Absent—wants others to decide

**Spiritual losses**
Illusion of predictability/certainty
Illusion of immortality
Illusion of control
Hope for the future
Time

**Table 4–2**
**Differentiating Normal Grief from Depression**

| Normal Grief/Response to Loss of Health | Depression |
|---|---|
| Self-limiting but recurrent with each additional loss | Frequently not self-limited, lasting longer than 2 months |
| Preoccupied with loss | Self-preoccupied, rumination |
| Emotional states variable | Consistent dysphoria or anhedonia (absence of pleasure) |
| Episodic difficulties sleeping | Insomnia or hypersomnia |
| Lack of energy, slight weight loss | Extreme lethargy, weight loss |
| Identifies loss | May not identify loss or may deny it |
| Crying is evident and provides some relief | Crying absent or persists uncontrollably |
| Socially responsive to others | Socially unresponsive, isolated |
| Dreams may be vivid | No memory of dreaming |
| Open expression of anger | No expression of anger |
| Adaptation does not require professional intervention | Adaptation requires professional treatment |

problem. The nurse may need to make a more thorough mental health assessment to determine the most appropriate referral. Key elements in such an assessment are found in Table 4–3. For more detailed psychosocial information, consult Holland's *Psycho-oncology*.[7] In such instances, a referral to a behavioral health professional may be warranted.

## Introduction to Spiritual Assessment

Although Chapter 33, entitled "Spiritual Assessment," provides additional information on spiritual assessment, the following discussion illustrates the importance of assessing the spiritual domain as a component of a comprehensive evaluation.

**Table 4–3**
**General Mental Health Assessment**

| | |
|---|---|
| **Appearance** | **Psychomotor behavior** |
| Hygiene | Gait |
| Grooming | Movement |
| Posture | Coordination |
| Body language | Compulsions |
| **Mood and affect** | Energy |
| Interview behavior | Observable symptoms (tics, perseveration) |
| Specfic feelings expressed | **Speech** |
| Facial expressions | Pressured, slow, rapid |
| **Intellectual ability** | Goal-oriented, rambling, incoherent, fragmented, coherent |
| Attention | Relevant, irrelevant |
| Concentration | Poverty of speech |
| Concrete/abstract thinking | Presence of latencies (delayed ability to respond when conversing) |
| Comprehension | **Thought patterns** |
| Insight | Loose, perseverating |
| Judgment | Logical, illogical, confused |
| Educational level | Oriented, disoriented |
| **Sensorium/level of consciousness** | Tangential, poorly organized, well-organized |
| Alert | Preoccupied |
| Somnolent | Obsession |
| Unresponsive | Paranoid ideas of reference |
| | Delusions |
| | Hallucination, illusions |
| | Blocking, flight of ideas |
| | Neologisms (made-up words) |
| | Word salad (meaningless word order) |
| | Presence of suicidal or homicidal ideation |

Attempts to define spirituality can often result in feelings of dismay and inadequacy. It is like trying to capture the wind or grasp water. Therefore, assessing and addressing the spiritual needs of patients can be a formidable challenge. Spirituality may include one's religious identity, beliefs, and practices, but it involves much more. The person without an identified religious affiliation is no less spiritual. Indeed, the desire to speak one's truth, explore the meaning of one's life and illness, and maintain hope are fundamental human quests that reflect the depth of the spirit. Haase and colleagues[11] concluded that the spiritual perspective is "an integrating and creative energy based on belief in, and feeling of interconnectedness with, a power greater than self." Amenta[12] viewed spirituality as "the life-force springing from within that pervades our entire being." Hay[13] defined it as "the capacity for transcending in order to love or be loved, to give meaning, and to cope." Doyle[14] wrote, "Spiritual beliefs may be expressed in religion and its hallowed practices, but a person can and often does have a spiritual dimension to his or her life that is totally unrelated to religion and not expressed or explored in religious practice." He further noted that "a prerequisite to discussion of spiritual issues with a patient is to create a situation which permits speaking of spiritual problems, i.e. environment, ambiance, and attitude."[14]

The spiritual issues that arise after the diagnosis of a serious or life-threatening illness are abundant and varied.

As a person progresses through the phases of an illness (diagnosis, treatment, post-treatment, and active dying), he or she is confronted with mortality, limitations, and loss. This frequently leads to questions such as, "What is my life's purpose?," "What does all this mean?," "What is the point of my suffering?," "Why me?," and "Is there life after death?" Indeed, Victor Frankl,[15] in his classic work, *Man's Search for Meaning*, affirmed that the quest to find meaning is one of the most characteristically human endeavors. To find meaning in suffering enhances the human spirit and fosters survival.

According to Abraham Maslow's[16] theory, human needs can be placed on a hierarchy that prioritizes them from the most basic physical and survival needs to the more transcendent needs. Thus, a patient's ability and willingness to engage in dialogue about issues of meaning, to discuss successes and regrets, and to express his or her core values may occur only after more fundamental needs are addressed. This reality in no way diminishes the spiritual compared with the physical; rather, it supports the need for an interdisciplinary approach that provides holistic care of the entire person. For example, if a physician relieves a young woman's cancer pain and a social worker secures transportation for her to treatments, she and her family may be more able to address the vital concerns of her soul. Religious or spiritual advisor consultation may be indicated.

The sensitivity of the nurse to a patient's spiritual concerns improves the quality of palliative care throughout the illness

---

**Table 4–4**
**Categories of Spiritual Assessment**

**Substantive information: The "what" of spiritual life**
Present religious affiliation or past religious background
Beliefs about God, the transcendent, an afterlife
Present devotional practice and spiritual disciplines, like
    praying, attending worship services, significant religious
    rituals meditation, yoga, etc.
Identification of membership in a faith community and the
    degree of involvement and level of support

**Functional information: The "how" of spiritual life**
Making meaning
Retaining hope
Securing a source of inner strength and peace
Exploring the relationship between beliefs, practices, and
    health
Surviving losses and other crises

---

trajectory. When members of the health care team serve as "companions" to a patient and family during their journey with an illness, they offer vital and life-affirming care.

Responding to the spiritual needs of patients and families is not solely the domain of the chaplain, clergy, or other officially designated professionals. All members of the health care team share the responsibility of identifying and being sensitive to spiritual concerns.

It is vital that a patient be viewed not in isolation but in the context of those who are affected by the illness. Thus, the focus of spiritual assessment includes both the patient and the family or significant others. This perspective affirms the power of a systems view, which sees the patient and family as interdependent and connected. Providing support to family members not only assists them directly but may also contribute to the patient's comfort secondarily, as she or he sees loved ones being cared for as well.

The purpose of a spiritual assessment is to increase the health care team's knowledge of the patient's and family's sources of strength and areas of concern, in order to enhance their quality of life and the quality of care provided. The methods of assessment include direct questioning, acquiring inferred information, and observing. This is most effectively accomplished when a basis of trust has been established. Fitchett[17] noted that spiritual assessments consist of both "substantive" and "functional" information. Table 4–4 examines these categories of spiritual assessment.

One of the fundamental principles underlying spiritual assessment and care is the commitment to the value of telling one's story. Alcoholics' Anonymous, a very successful program with spiritual tenets, acknowledges the power of story. This might be paraphrased as follows: in the hearing is the learning, but in the telling is the healing. Similarly, Thompson and Janigan[18] developed the concept of "life schemes," which provide a sense of order and purpose for one's life and promotes a perspective on the world, oneself, events, and goals. Simple, open-ended questions, such as, "How is this illness affecting you?" and "How is the illness affecting the way you relate to the world?" provide the opportunity for validation and exploration of the patient's life scheme.

## Cultural Competence

It is unrealistic to expect that health care professionals will know all of the customs, beliefs, and practices of patients from every culture. There are useful reference sources to assist in gaining cultural competence.[19] However, all providers should strive for some degree of cultural competence, which has been defined as "an educational process, which includes the ability to develop working relationships across lines of difference. This encompasses self-awareness, cultural knowledge about illness and healing practices, intercultural communication skills and behavioral flexibility."[20] The *Inclusion and Access Toolbox,* by the National Hospice & Palliative Care Organization, is a collection of suggestions and successes based on the thoughts and experiences of hospice providers in many settings throughout the United States, highlighting populations with diverse economic, education, sexual preferences, and disabilities.[21]

The members of the health care team can increase their cultural competence by concentrating on the following:

- Being aware of one's own ethnocentrism, the unconscious tendency to assume that one's own worldview is superior to that of others.
- Assessing the patient's and family's beliefs about illness and treatments.
- Conveying respect, such as saying, "I am unfamiliar with your culture. Please help me understand why you think you got sick and what you think will make you better."
- Soliciting the patient and family as teachers and guides regarding cultural practices.
- Asking about the patient's personal preferences and avoiding expectations for any individual to represent his or her whole culture.
- Respecting cultural differences regarding personal space and touch, such as requesting, "Whom do I ask for permission to examine you?" and "May I touch you here?"
- Determining needs and desires regarding health-related information, such as asking, "When I have information to tell you, how much detail do you want to know and to whom do I give it?"
- Noting and affirming the use of complementary and integrative health care practices.
- Incorporating the patient's cultural healing practices into the plan of care.
- Responding to resistance from the patient and family about the recommended treatment plan with understanding, negotiation, and compromise.
- Being sensitive to the need for interpreter services (Table 4–5).

**Table 4-5**
**Meeting the Need for Interpreter Services**

A child or family member should not be used as an interpreter for major explanations or decision-making about health care. Even adult children may feel uncomfortable speaking with their parents or grandparents about intimate topics. Furthermore, many lay people do not know or understand medical terms in their own language. Informed consent requires that the patient receive accurate information that he or she can understand, before making a health care decision.

It is recommended that the health care team obtain the services of a certified medical interpreter, if possible.

In the absence of an on-site certified translator, use AT&T interpreters. In the United States or Canada, call 1-800-752-6096 to set up an account and obtain a password.

A new technology service is available in the USA via computer called Language Access Network or Marti (My Accessible Real-Time Trusted Interpreter). It is HIPPA compliant and available 24/7, 365 days a year. Contact customer service at 866-449-4428 or visit their Website at www.languageaccessnetwork.com.

## The Time of Diagnosis

### Assessment at the Time of Diagnosis

The goals of a palliative care nursing assessment at the time of diagnosis are as follows:

1. Determine the baseline health of the patient and family.
2. Document problems and plan interventions with the patient and family to improve their quality of life.
3. Identify learning needs to guide teaching that promotes optimal self-care.
4. Recognize patient and family strengths to reinforce healthy habits and behaviors for maximizing well-being.
5. Discern when the expertise of other health care professionals is needed (e.g., social worker, registered dietitian).

### Physical Assessment at Diagnosis

When the patient has finished telling his or her story about the illness, the nurse needs to do an individualized, focused physical assessment, based on data previously collected from the medical record. This assessment might use the general categories of head and neck, shoulders and arms, chest and spine, abdomen, pelvis, legs and feet. The nurse obtains data by observing, interviewing, and examining the patient. The format, policies, procedures, and expectations of the health care agency in which the assessment occurs guide the specific

details that are collected and documented. Figure 4-1 shows cues to guide a head-to-toe physical assessment.

Because the family is so important to the palliative care focus on quality of life, the overall health of other family members needs to be documented. Identification of the major health problems, physical limitations, and physical strengths of family members serves as a basis for planning. The physical capabilities and constraints of the caregivers available to assist and support the patient may affect the plan of care, especially in relation to the most appropriate setting for care. This information also provides direction for the types of referrals that may be needed to provide care.

### Psychosocial Assessment at Diagnosis

The primary psychosocial feature of a new diagnosis is anticipatory grief. Patients' responses to receiving bad news range from shock, disbelief, and denial to anger and fatalism. As further losses occur along the illness continuum, this grief mechanism is retriggered, and losses become cumulative. Statements such as, "I can't believe this is happening to me" or "Why is this happening to us?" are signals to the health care professional that the patient and family are grappling heavily with this threat to their equilibrium. There is already a sense that life will be forever changed. A longing emerges to return to the way things were.

In response to these emotional states, the health care team is most helpful when they do the following:

- Normalize the patient's and family's experiences: "Many people share similar reactions to this kind of news."
- Use active listening skills to facilitate grief work: "Of all that is happening to you right now, what is the hardest part to deal with?"
- Create a safe space for self-disclosure, and build a trust relationship: "No matter what lies ahead, you will not face it alone."
- Develop a collaborative partnership to establish a mutual plan of care: "What would help you the most right now?"
- Respect the patient's or family's use of denial in the service of coping with harsh realities: "It must be hard to believe this is happening."
- Assess the patient's and family's coping styles: "When you have experienced difficult times in the past, how did you get through them?"
- Reinforce strengths. "It sounds like this has helped you before."
- Maximize a sense of control, autonomy, and choice. "It seems you really have a handle on this."
- Assess the patient's need for information: "What do you know about your illness?," "Are you the kind of person who likes to know as much as possible, or do you function on a need-to-know basis only?," "What would you like to know about your illness now?"
- Check the need for clarification: "What did you hear?" or "Summarize in your own words how you understand your situation now."

**Head & Neck:**

| | | |
|---|---|---|
| Hair | – | Texture, fullness, shine, dandruff, well-kept, bald? Complexion-Skin condition? Scars? Make-up? |
| Mind | – | Alert & Oriented x3? MMSE needed? Capacity for decision-making? Speech, language, vocabulary? Education? Ability to read? Memory & attention span? General mood? Stress level? Hx of anxiety, depression, phobias? Hx headaches? Seizures? Knowledge & experience with illness? Perception of illness? Meds? |
| Senses | – | Sight – PERRLA? Visual acuity? Glasses/contacts? Redness, itching, puffiness, icterus? Eye drops needed? Hearing – Deficits? Use of aids? Tinnitus? Dizziness? Pain? Inspect for excess wax, signs of infection. Smell – Ability? Sensitivities? Interest in aromatherapy? Taste – Flavor likes and dislikes? |
| Nose | – | Hx of sinusitis or other sinus problems? Nose bleeds? Frequency of URIs? Pain? Meds? |
| Mouth | – | Inspect condition of teeth, gums, & mucous membranes? Dryness? Sores? Infection? Brushing & flossing habits? Semi-annual cleanings & dental exams? Dentures, bridges? Hx of sore throats? Pain? |
| Lips | – | Dry or cracked? Hx of fever blisters? |
| Neck | – | Quality & clarity of voice? Full ROM? Hx of problems swallowing, laryngitis, esophagitis, reflux? Swollen lymph nodes? Venous distension? Carotid pulses? Pain? |

**Shoulders & Arms:**

Full ROM? Strength? Dexterity? Coordination? Crepitus?
Deformities? Swelling? Joint/muscle pain or stiffness?
Neuropathies? Changes in sensation? Reflexes?
Venous access? Access devices? Condition of nails?

**Chest & Spine:**

| | | |
|---|---|---|
| Lungs | – | Respiratory rate; SOB? DOE? Orthopnea? Lung sounds? Cough? Sputum? CXR? Shape of chest? Smoking hx? Hx of infections,asthma, or night sweats? Pain? Meds? |
| Heart | – | Heart rate & rhythm? Murmurs? BP? EKG? Hx of palpitations, CP, MI? CAD/CHF? Pedal edema? Meds? |
| Breasts | – | Appearance, lumps, discharge? BSE? Mammogram? Regular HCP Exam? Pain/tenderness? |
| Spine | – | Hx of back pain, problems, or injuries? Flexibility? Deformities? |

**Legs & Feet:**

Full ROM? Strength? Crepitus? Ability to walk &/or
run? How far? Gait? Coordination? Balance?
Weakness? Paralysis? Deformities? Use of DME?
Hx of problems? Muscle/joint pain or stiffness?
Reflexes? Change in sensation? Temperature?
Edema? Pedal pulses? Dryness? Cellulitis? Venous
stasis? Skin discoloration? Condition of toenails?
Neuropathies?

**Abdomen:**

| | | |
|---|---|---|
| General | – | Appearance? Ascites? Masses? Tenderness? Surgery scars? |
| Stomach | – | Usual diet? Appetite? Caffeine intake? Vitamin use? Hx of problems? -PUD? Belching? Pain? Motion sickness? N & V with pregnancy? |
| Liver | – | Alcohol intake? Hx hepatitis? LFTs? |
| GB | – | Hx of indigestion? Pain? |
| Pancreas | – | Hx of diabetes? Pancreatitis? |
| Bowels | – | Normal habits? Recent changes? Color, form? Diarrhea? Incontinence? Constipation? Laxative use? Gas? Pain? Fat & fiber in diet? Hemorrhoids? Rectal bleeding? Hemoccult tests? Regular HCP rectal exams? Colonoscopy? |

**Pelvis:**

| | | |
|---|---|---|
| Kidneys /Urine | – | Color, frequency? Nocturia? Pain? Hx of UTIs? Incontinence? Other problems? |
| Male | = | TSE? DRE? PSA? Hx BPH? Meds? Hernia? Sexually active? Hx of STDs? Contraception? Circumcised? Sexual function concerns? Impotence? Erectile Dysfunction? Importance to self concept, relationships, & quality of life? |
| Female | = | Gx Px? Contraception? LMP? Menarche age? Usual menses cycle? Break through bleeding? Menses pain or problems? Menopause – age? ERT? Pelvic exam & PAP smear? Vaginal discharge, dryness, odor, infection? Sexually active? Sexual function concerns? Importance to self concept, relationships, & quality of life? |

**General:**

Allergies? Temperature? Height? Weight? -loss, gain, ideal?
Functional Status?Exercise tolerance? Needs related to ADLs?

| | | |
|---|---|---|
| Appearance | – | Personal hygiene, dress, posture, body language, sweating? Intolerance to heat or cold? |
| Skin | – | Color, turgor, bruising, rashes, itching? Moles? -ABCD? Wounds? Previous surgical sites healed? |
| General | – | Aches, pains? Muscle twitching, tingling, cramps? Hx broken bones? Hx of major illness, injuries, surgeries? Family hx of illnesses? Past health & well-being? Sleep patterns/problems? Prevention habits? Rest, relaxation, recreation? Immunizations? Use of alternative therapies? |

**Figure 4–1.** Assessment at the time of diagnosis: obtaining a baseline of the patient's health status. *Source:* Courtesy of Elaine Glass, ACHPN.

- Avoid "medspeak," which is medical terminology unfamiliar to the average person, such as the use of abbreviations, acronyms, etc. (for example, UTI, CHF, PEG).
- Mentor patients and families who have had little experience with the health care system, including coaching them in conversations with their physicians and teaching them ways to navigate the complexities of the health care system.

The nurse must remember that, while the patient is feeling strong emotions, the family is also experiencing intense feelings. Similar assessments of family members will help to mobilize resources at critical times. Family members experience their grief reactions at their own individual rates throughout the course of the illness. Each family member has his or her own particular coping style and need for information. (See Chapter 31: "Supporting Families in Palliative Care.")

The nurse and other members of the health care team assist the patient and family when they do the following:

- Observe changes in family members' roles and responsibilities (e.g., the breadwinner becomes a caregiver, the homemaker begins working outside the home).
- Identify external community support systems.
- Assist the patient and family in identifying coping strategies to use while awaiting test results, which is one of the most stressful times and which recurs throughout the illness.
- Help the patient and family explore the benefits and burdens of various treatment options when changes are needed in the plan of care.
- Assess parental readiness to assist children with their adaptation needs: "How do you plan to tell your children?"
- Identify family communication ground rules and seek to improve communication among family members: "Is it OK if we discuss this subject with you and your family?"
- Assess the coping of children within the family by being aware of their fears and concerns.

Table 4–6 describes some common responses of children to having an adult loved one who is ill.

Assisting in the process of making initial treatment decisions can be an opportunity to begin a relationship that will continue to grow. Members of the health care team may ask questions such as, "What is most important to you in life?" and "Is quality of life or quantity of life most meaningful?" Assisting the patient and family in identifying and expressing their values will guide them in subsequent decision-making.

**Spiritual Assessment at Diagnosis**

The diagnosis of a serious illness generally brings with it a sense of shock to the patient and family. It may threaten many of their assumptions about life, disrupt their sense of control,

---

**Table 4–6**
**Common Responses of Children to Serious Illness in the Family**

Magical thinking that results in feelings of guilt (e.g., "I once told Mommy I wished she were dead.")
Fears of abandonment, especially in younger children
Fears of contracting the disease
Anger, withdrawal, being uncooperative, especially in adolescents
Acting-out behavior with lack of usual attention
Frustrations with an altered lifestyle because of decreased financial resources, less family fun activities because of the ill person's inability to participate, etc.
Inability to concentrate and focus, especially regarding schoolwork

---

and cause them to ask "Why?" The health care team can be most helpful at this time if they do the following:

- Determine the patient's and family's level of hopefulness about the future: "What are you hoping for?" or "How do you see the future at this time?"
- Inquire about how the patient and family have dealt with past crises of faith, meaning, or loss: "What helped you get through that?"
- Determine the patient's and family's comfort level in talking about the spiritual life: "Some people need or want to talk about these things; others don't. How is it for you?"
- Inquire about spiritual support persons available to the patient and family (e.g., pastor, rabbi, counselor, spiritual advisor).
- Determine the patient's or family's need or desire to speak with a spiritual support person.
- Ask about spiritual self-care practices to promote healthy coping: "How are you taking care of yourself at this time?"
- Listen for comments from the patient and family regarding the importance of their religious traditions and practices.

Spiritual goals at this phase are to normalize initial concerns, to provide information that fosters positive coping, and to encourage the patient and family to seek supportive spiritual resources.

CASE STUDY
*Ladona at the Time of Diagnosis of Sickle Cell Disease*

Ladona was diagnosed with sickle cell anemia at birth when the mandatory state test came back positive. Her parents read extensively about the illness and followed the hematologist's orders to the letter. They did everything they could to prevent Ladona from having crises. They took her to yoga and stress management classes. They were diligent in taking her for physical checkups every six months, including seeing a retinal ophthalmologist and getting periodic ultrasound scans of her brain to look for early signs of stroke. Ladona was a compliant child and followed her parents' example of eating a healthy diet and drinking plenty of fluids. She was also conscientious in taking the medications prescribed for her by the hematologist. Until she was five, she took penicillin and folic acid daily. As she grew older, her medications included butyric acid, nitric oxide and hydroxyurea—and more recently, decitadine. Fortunately, Ladona only had minor pain episodes during her childhood and teenage years and she never had to be hospitalized. Her parents encouraged her to pursue a career that would avoid exposure to extremes in heat and cold and that would not require strenuous physical labor. Ladona has always been an avid reader and she chose a career in teaching literature and history to high school students.

The goals of care during the time of diagnosis were to:

- Encourage adherence to the medical plan of care.
- Provide resources to her parents and to Ladona so they can learn about how to live and cope effectively with this lifelong, incurable illness.
- Assist Ladona in assuming responsibility for her own health as she grows into a young adult.
- Offer supportive encouragement to both Ladona and her parents and screen for depression and challenging behaviors, offering counseling and antidepressants if needed.
- Introduce the subject of advance directives and provide the necessary forms when Ladona reaches adulthood.

## During Treatments

### Assessment During Treatments

The goals of a palliative care assessment during active treatment are as follows:

1. Assess the patient's systems in all domains that are at risk for problems, considering both the patient's baseline problems and any side effects of the treatments.
2. Record the current and potential problems and plan early interventions with the patient and family.
3. Ascertain the need for teaching to prevent, minimize, and manage problems with the goal of maximizing quality of life.
4. Reinforce patient and family strengths, healthy habits, and behaviors to maximize well-being.
5. Recognize when other health care professionals' expertise is needed and make appropriate referrals (e.g., physical therapist, pharmacist).

### Physical Assessment During Treatments

Reassessments during treatment determine the changes that have occurred since the initial assessment. Knowledge of the usual disease process and the side effects of treatment assists the nurse in focusing reassessments on those body systems most likely to be affected.

In addition to the patient's physical assessment, the nurse should make periodic observations and inquiries about the health of other family members. It is important to document any changes in their health problems or physical limitations and physical strengths that might have an impact on the patient's care and the family's overall quality of life.

### Psychosocial Assessment During Treatments

Once a treatment plan has been initiated, patients often express relief that "something is finally being done." Taking action frequently reduces anxiety. The most important psychosocial intervention at this stage is the amelioration of as many treatment side effects as possible. After basic needs for physical well-being are assessed and symptoms are controlled, the patient is able to explore and meet higher needs, including the needs for belonging, self-esteem, and self-actualization.[16] Patients who are preoccupied with pain and nausea or vomiting have no energy or ability to explore the significance of their illness or their feelings about it. Effective management of physical symptoms is mandatory before the patient can begin to work on integrating the illness experience into the tapestry of his or her life.

After several months or years of treatment, the effects of having a chronic illness may exhaust even the hardiest person. Patients may begin to weigh the benefits versus the burdens of continuing aggressive therapies. Initially, patients will endure almost anything if they believe a cure is possible. As time unfolds, their attitudes may change as they watch their quality of life erode with little prospect of a more positive outcome. Patients may also reprioritize what is most important to them. For example, the workaholic may find less satisfaction at the office, or the homemaker may experience less fulfillment from daily routines around the house. Change, transition, and existential questioning characterize this phase.[22]

The nurse and other members of the health care team will assist the patient and family when they do the following:

- Inquire about the patient's newly emerging identity as a result of the illness: "What activities and which relationships bring you the most joy and meaning?" or "Have you been able to define a new purpose for yourself?"
- Assess for signs of anxiety and depression, which remain the two most common psychosocial problems associated with severe illness (Table 4–7); for more information contrasting anxiety and depression, consult Holland's *Psycho-oncology*.[23,24]

**Table 4–7**
**Assessment of Anxiety and Depression**

| Signs and Symptoms of Anxiety | Signs and Symptoms of Depression |
|---|---|
| Excessive worry | Sad mood |
| Trouble falling or staying asleep | Insomnia and hypersomnia |
| Irritability, muscle tension | Anhedonia (absence of pleasure) |
| Restlessness, agitation | Psychomotor retardation |
| Unrealistic fears (phobias) | Feelings of worthlessness or inappropriate guilt |
| Obsessions (persistent painful ideas) | Diminished ability to concentrate, make decisions or remember |
| Compulsions (repetitive ritualistic acts) | Recurrent thoughts of death, suicidal ideation (lethality assessed by |
| Frequent crying spells, headaches, gastrointestinal upsets, palpitations, shortness of breath | expressed intent, presence of a plan and the means to carry it out, previous attempts, and provision for rescue) |
| Self-medication | Marked weight loss or weight gain |
| Anorexia or overeating | Fatigue |
| Thoughts interfere with normal activities of daily living | |

- Screen for suicidal ideation in cases of depression: "Have you been feeling so bad that you've been thinking of a way to hurt yourself?" and "Do you have a plan for how to do it?"
- Refer for counseling and possible psychotropic medication to enhance positive coping and comfort.

## Spiritual Assessment During Treatments

With the treatment of a serious illness comes the introduction of an additional stressor to the patient and family. It is important to assess how they incorporate the demands of treatment into their daily routine and how these changes have affected the meaning of their lives.

The nurse and other members of the care team will be helpful to the patient and family if they normalize the stress of treatment and do the following:

- Inquire about the patient's and family's hopes for the future.
- Assess the level and quality of support they are receiving—for instance, from other family members, faith community, and neighbors.
- Explore expressions of anxiety and fear by asking, "What is concerning you the most at this time?"
- Assess how the patient and family are coping with the rigors of treatment: "What is the most challenging part of this for you?" and "What is helping you day by day?" Consider referrals to a chaplain or faith community as needed.
- Inquire about the patient's and family's definitions of quality of life and the impact of treatment on these aspects of their lives: "What is most important to you in life now?"
- Determine their use of spiritual practices and offer assistance in developing these (e.g., meditation, relaxation, prayer).

- Ask how the patient or family members feel about their current practices: "Are these helpful or not?"
- Discuss the completion of advance directives: "Who would you want to make your health care decisions for you if you were not able to make them yourself?" Also, revisit the subject of code status. If patients say they would want to be revived and put on life support, explain to them what usually happens if life support cannot be removed in about two weeks: that is, the placement of a tracheostomy and feeding tube (PEG). Encourage patients to discuss all these matters and options with their loved ones, especially their surrogate decision makers (health care power of attorneys).

The health care team's goals are to reinforce positive coping, mobilize existing spiritual resources, invite the patient and family to develop new skills for self-care, and continue disclosures in an atmosphere of trust.

CASE STUDY
*Ladona During Sickle Cell Crisis Treatment*

Ladona arrives at the emergency department with shortness of breath and extreme pain in her long bones, joints, and abdomen. The staff recognizes the emergent signs as those of a sickle cell crisis. In addition to her pain, she is found to have marked anemia (hemoglobin is 6.5 and hematocrit is 20) and is severely dehydrated. It is determined that the current crisis might be precipitated by Ladona's newly-discovered pregnancy. She is given IV fluids to counter the dehydration and analgesics to stabilize her pain. The hematologist consults the palliative care team to assist in titrating her pain medications and in providing additional support. The staff decides to admit her due to the pregnancy (eight weeks), to control her pain and the need to monitor her during this crisis.

The goals of care during crisis treatments are to:

- Stabilize the sickle cell crisis with rehydration, intensive pain management and relief of nausea which is a common cause of dehydration in the first trimester.
- Address anemia by assessing iron, B-12 and folate stores and providing iron and folic acid supplementation if needed. A nutrition referral for reinforcement of sickle crisis prevention and prenatal nutritional needs is also recommended.
- Refer for pre-natal care and for family counseling due to repercussions from pregnancy before marriage, which conflicts with her recent acceptance of her parents' faith beliefs and her membership in the Jehovah's Witness church.
- Respect Ladona's insistence that no blood products be used to address her health problems.
- Revisit a discussion about advance directives and provide information about the Jehovah's Witness blood directive form, since Ladona and her parents are Jehovah's Witnesses but her fiancé, Michael, is not.

## After Treatments

### Assessment After Treatments (Long-Term Survival or Terminal Phase)

The goals of a palliative care assessment after treatments are as follows:

1. Examine the benefits and burdens of all interventions to manage the residual symptoms remaining from the treatments and/or the disease process.
2. Determine the current physical problems that are most distressing to the patient and family, and plan rehabilitative interventions.
3. Assess learning needs and provide teaching to aggressively manage problems with the goal of maximizing quality of life.
4. Continue to reinforce patient and family strengths, healthy habits, and behaviors to enhance well-being and to prevent problems.

Survivors are defined as those patients whose diseases are cured, who go into long remissions, or who become chronically ill. These individuals may require some degree of palliative care for the rest of their lives. Examples of survivors likely to require ongoing palliative care include those with graft-versus-host disease (GVHD), irreversible peripheral neuropathies, or structural alterations of the integumentary, gastrointestinal, and genitourinary systems (e.g., mastectomies, amputations, colostomies, ileostomies, laryngectomies).

Psychosocial issues for survivors include fear of recurrence as well as practical considerations such as insurance and job discrimination. Many patients make major life changes regarding work and relationships as a result of their illness experiences. These patients, even if cured, live with the ramifications of the disease and its treatment for the rest of their lives.

Some patients begin to explore, in new ways, the spiritual foundations and assumptions of their lives. Often, patients relate that in spite of the crisis of an illness and its treatment, the experience resulted in a deepened sense of meaning and gratitude for life. Examples of such growth experiences as a result of surviving cancer can be found in *Cancer as a Turning Point: A Handbook for People with Cancer, Their Families and Health Professionals.*[25]

### Physical Assessment After Treatments

The patient is reassessed after treatments are finished to determine the changes that have occurred since previous assessments; the focus is on the systems that have been affected and altered by the disease and treatments. Thorough assessment of the residual problems and changes in the patient's body are critical to successful symptom management. Effective management of symptoms with rehabilitative interventions achieves the goal of maximizing the patient's and family's quality of life, whether in long-term survival or during the terminal phase. Two examples of functional assessment tools used in physical rehabilitation are the Functional Assessment of Cancer Therapy (FACT) Scale[26] and the Rotterdam Symptom Checklist.[27]

In addition to the patient's physical assessment, the nurse should continue to make periodic observations and inquiries about the health of other family members. Noting changes in family members' health, physical limitations, and physical strengths is important to ascertain any impact on the patient's care and the family's lifestyle. Research suggests that a strong correlation exists between caregiver stress and morbidity.[28] This is especially true of caregiver stress that effects blood pressure and mental health stress responses such as chronic depression. For additional information, refer to Chapter 31: "Supporting Families in Palliative Care."

An emerging issue that relates to family members' health is genetic testing for familial diseases. The health care team needs to ask patients with diseases that could have a genetic origin whether they would be interested in receiving more information. Patients or family members who desire more facts will benefit from written materials and referral to an experienced genetic counselor. Table 4–8 provides resource information on genetic counseling.

### Psychosocial Assessment After Treatments

For those patients who are free of disease, palliative care focuses on post-treatment-related symptoms and fears of recurrence. For others, recurrence is most often signaled by

| Table 4–8<br>Genetic Counseling Information |
| --- |
| To locate a genetic counselor in a particular region of the United States, contact<br>**National Society of Genetic Counselors**<br>610–872–7608<br>www.nsgc.org |

| Table 4–9<br>Assessment of Family Members' Risk Factors<br>for Complicated Bereavement |
| --- |
| Concurrent life crises<br>History of other recent or difficult past losses<br>Unresolved grief from prior losses<br>History of mental illness or substance abuse<br>Extreme anger or anxiety<br>Marked dependence on the patient<br>Age of the patient and the surviving loved ones, developmental phases of the patient and family members<br>Limited support within the family's circle or community<br>Anticipated situational stressors, such as loss of income, financial strain, lack of confidence in assuming some of the patient's usual responsibilities<br>Illnesses among other family members<br>Special bereavement needs of children in the family<br>The patient's dying process is difficult (e.g., poorly controlled symptoms such as pain, shortness of breath, agitation, delirium, anxiety)<br>Absence of helpful cultural and/or religious beliefs |

the appearance of advancing physical symptoms. When this happens, the patient's worst nightmare has been realized. A recurrence is experienced differently from an initial diagnosis, because the patient is now a "veteran" of the patient role and may understand all too well what the recurrence means.

Attention to concerns at this phase of illness include the following:

- Revisit the quality versus quantity of life preferences as the patient and family weigh the benefits and burdens of further treatment. Beginning these conversations earlier rather than later in the illness helps make them discussible and creates an ongoing dialogue that will help patient, family and health care providers alike when further treatment becomes, in essence, futile.
- Be sensitive to the patient's readiness to discuss a transition in emphasis from curative to comfort care only. The patient often signals his or her readiness by statements such as, "I'm getting tired of spending so much time at the hospital" or "I've had it with all of this." Ask: "What has your physician told you that you can expect now?" or "How do you see your future?"
- Explore readiness to set new goals of treatment: "I know you understand that your illness has not responded to the treatments as we had hoped. I'd like to talk with you about changing your health care goals."
- Revisit the need for advance directives.
- Consider a discussion about hospice if the patient begins to question the efficacy of treatments. Present hospice as the gold standard for end-of-life care. A hospice referral should never be made as a gesture indicating that "There is nothing more that we can do for you." The benefits of increased availability of services, such as symptom management and bereavement care for the family, should be emphasized.
- Determine the patient's and family's interest or need for education about death and dying.
- Discern the risk factors for complicated bereavement in family members, as described in Table 4–9.

### Spiritual Assessment After Treatments

After treatment, the patient embarks on a journey leading to long-term survival, chronic illness, or recurrence and the terminal phases of the illness. The nurse and other caregivers can provide valuable spiritual support at these junctures when they do the following:

- Determine the quality and focus of the patient's and family's hopes for the future. Listen for a transition from hoping for a cure to another kind of hope (e.g., hope for a remission, hope to live until a special family event occurs). For an in-depth, practical, and inspiring discourse on hope, refer to *Finding HOPE: Ways to See Life in a Brighter Light*.[29]
- Listen for comments that suggest a crisis of belief and meaning. For example, at recurrence, a patient may feel abandoned or experience an assault on his or her faith. Questions such as "Why?" and "Where is God?" and "Why are my prayers not being answered?" are very common. The nurse can best respond to these questions by normalizing them and emphasizing that to question God or one's faith can indicate a vitality of faith, not its absence.
- Assess the patient's and family's use of spiritual practices: "What are you doing to feel calmer and more peaceful?" Consider a chaplain referral if the patient or family are interested and open to such an intervention.
- Inquire regarding the desire for meaningful rituals, such as communion or anointing. Consult with local clergy or a hospital chaplain to meet these needs.
- Assess the level and quality of community supports: "Who is involved in supporting you and your family at this time?"
- Listen for indicators of spiritual suffering (e.g., unfinished business, regrets, relationship discord, diminished faith, fears of abandonment): "What do

**Table 4-10**
**Assessment of Funeral Plans and Preferences**

Has the patient and/or family selected a funeral home?

Has the patient and/or family decided about the disposition of the body: organ, eye, and/or tissue donation; autopsy; earth burial (above ground or below ground); cremation; and/or total body donation to a medical school?

Has the decision been made regarding a final resting place?

Does the patient want to make his or her wishes known regarding the type of service, or will the family decide these details? For example: clothes to be buried in, favorite songs to be sung or played, poems to be read, open or closed casket.

you find yourself thinking about at this time?" and "What are your chief concerns or worries?"

- Assess the need and desire of the patient and family to talk about the meaning of the illness, the patient's declining physical condition, and possible death.
- Ask questions to foster a review of critical life incidents, to allow grieving, and to explore beliefs regarding the afterlife: "What do you believe happens to a person at the time of death?"
- Determine the need and desire for reconciliation: "Are there people with whom you want or need to speak with about anything?" and "Do you find yourself having any regrets?"
- Invite a discussion of the most meaningful, celebratory occurrences in life to foster integrity, life review, and a sense of meaning.
- Assess the patient's and/or the family's readiness to discuss funeral preferences and plans and desired disposition of the body, as noted in Table 4-10. Encourage referral to hospice for end-of-life care if the death of the patient might be anticipated within the year. Ask the physician: "Would it surprise you if this person would die within the year?"

The main spiritual goal of this phase of illness is to provide the patient and family a "place to stand" in order to review the past and look toward the future. This encourages grieving past losses, creating a sense of meaning, and consolidating strengths for the days ahead.

CASE STUDY
*Ladona After Completion of Sickle Cell Crisis Treatment*

After discharge from the hospital, Ladona is followed closely for her sickle cell disease as well as for her pregnancy. She tries to reduce her stress levels by using counseling to build support for her relationship with her fiancé, whom she still plans to marry. Her parents, after dealing with the shock of the pregnancy, feel they can only support Ladona's decision to marry if her fiancé, Michael, agrees to either convert to their faith or he provides reassurance that he accepts

Ladona's naming her parents as her surrogate health care decision makers. The goals of care after crisis treatments are to:

- Try to reestablish a higher hemoglobin and hematocrit.
- Take measures to prevent further sickle cell crises and infections.
- Continue prenatal care and prepare for eventual delivery.
- Continue to work on relationship building within the family system to reduce everyone's stress levels.
- Establish Ladona's wishes regarding advance directives and the Jehovah's Witness blood directive, and complete the forms.

## Actively Dying

### Assessment During Active Dying

The goals of a palliative care assessment when the patient is actively dying are as follows:

1. Observe for signs and symptoms of impending death, aggressively managing symptoms and promoting comfort (Table 4-11).
2. Determine the primary source of the patient's and family's suffering and plan interventions to provide relief.
3. Identify the primary sources of strength for the patient and family members so that they can be used to provide support.
4. Ascertain the patient's and family's readiness and need for teaching about the dying process.
5. Look for ways to support the patient and family to enhance meaning during this intense experience.

**Table 4-11**
**Common Physical Symptoms Experienced by People Who Are Actively Dying**

Pain or discomfort from the illness and/or immobility

Dyspnea

Sleepiness

Confusion

No interest in eating or drinking

Gurgling sounds in the back of the throat from not being able to swallow saliva

Agitation/restlessness/delirium

Coolness in extremities that progresses from distal to proximal during the last 2–3 hours of life

Incontinence

Skin breakdown from immobility

6. Determine whether the family members and friends who are important to the patient have had the opportunity to visit in person or on the telephone, as desired by the patient and family.

## Physical Assessment During Active Dying

Physical assessment during the active dying process is very focused and is limited to determining the cause of suffering and identifying sources of comfort. Figure 4–2 shows common areas to assess in the last few days of a person's life.

In addition to the patient's physical assessment, the nurse should monitor the health of other family members to prevent and minimize problems that could compromise their health during this very stressful time.

Hospice team members have excellent skills in making palliative care assessments at the end of life. The goal of hospice is to support the terminally ill patient and family at home, if that is their wish. Many hospice teams also provide palliative care in acute care settings, nursing homes, and specially designed inpatient hospice facilities. Unfortunately, many patients die without the support of hospice services in any of these settings.

## Psychosocial Assessment During Active Dying

Many people believe that the transition from life to death is as sacred as the transition experienced at birth. Keeping this in mind, the nurse can help to create a safe environment in which patients and families are supported in their relationships and the creation of meaningful moments together. The patient may also still be reviewing his or her life. Common psychosocial characteristics of the person who is actively dying include social withdrawal, decreased attention span, and decreasing ability to concentrate, resulting in gradual loss of consciousness. Experiences normally considered to be psychotic in Western culture, such as visions and visitations from deceased relatives or spiritual/religious figures, are often viewed as transcendent—and normal—at this stage of life by those with strong spiritual beliefs. In Western medicine, there is a tendency to medicalize transcendent experiences.

Members of the health care team can assist the patient and family in the following vital ways:

- Avoid the assumption that the patient's reports of seeing deceased loved ones or visions are evidence of confusion or other mental health problems. Consultation with a behavioral health professional may be indicated to distinguish such experiences from delirium.
- Encourage continued touching and talking to the patient, even if he or she is unconscious.
- Assist communication among the patient, family members, and close friends, by suggesting reminiscing, story-telling, and other familiar ways of relating to each other—for example, joking, laughing and singing.[30,31]

- Invite family members to "give permission" to the patient "to let go," providing reassurance that the family will remain intact and learn to deal effectively with the person's absence.
- Assess the patient's and family's need for continued education about death and dying.
- Observe family members for evidence of poor coping and consider making referrals for additional support.
- Encourage family members to consider "shift rotation" in the face of lengthy, exhausting vigils at the bedside.
- Revisit any complementary and alternative medical (CAM) therapies that the family might find effective.[32]

## Spiritual Assessment During Active Dying

When the patient enters the phase of active dying, spiritual realities often increase in significance. The nurse and other members of the care team will facilitate adaptation during the process of dying and provide much valuable support when they do the following:

- Determine the need for different or more frequent visits by the patient's or family's spiritual support person: "Is there anyone I can call to be with you at this time?" and "Are there any meaningful activities or rituals you want to do?"
- Inquire about dreams, visions, or unusual experiences (e.g., seeing angels or persons who have died). Normalize these if they are disclosed. Ask if these experiences are sources of comfort or fear. Encourage further discussion if the patient is interested.
- Foster maintenance of hope by asking, "What are you hoping for at this time?" Reassure the patient and family that they can be hopeful and still acknowledge that death is imminent. Moving toward a transcendent hope is vital. Observe that earlier, the focus of hope may have been on cure, remission, or an extension of time; now, hope may be focused on an afterlife, the relief of suffering, or the idea of living on in loved ones' memories.
- Listen for and solicit comments regarding the efficacy of spiritual practices. For instance, if the patient is a person who prays, ask, "Are your prayers bringing you comfort and peace?"
- Realize that expressions of fear, panic attacks, or an increase in physical symptoms such as restlessness, agitation, pain, or shortness of breath may indicate intense spiritual distress. A chaplain's intervention may provide spiritual comfort and assist the patient in reaching peace. This may reduce the need for medications.
- Determine the need and desire of the patient and family to engage in forgiveness, to express feelings to one another, and to say their good-byes.
- Recognize that a prolonged dying process may indicate that the patient is having difficulty "letting

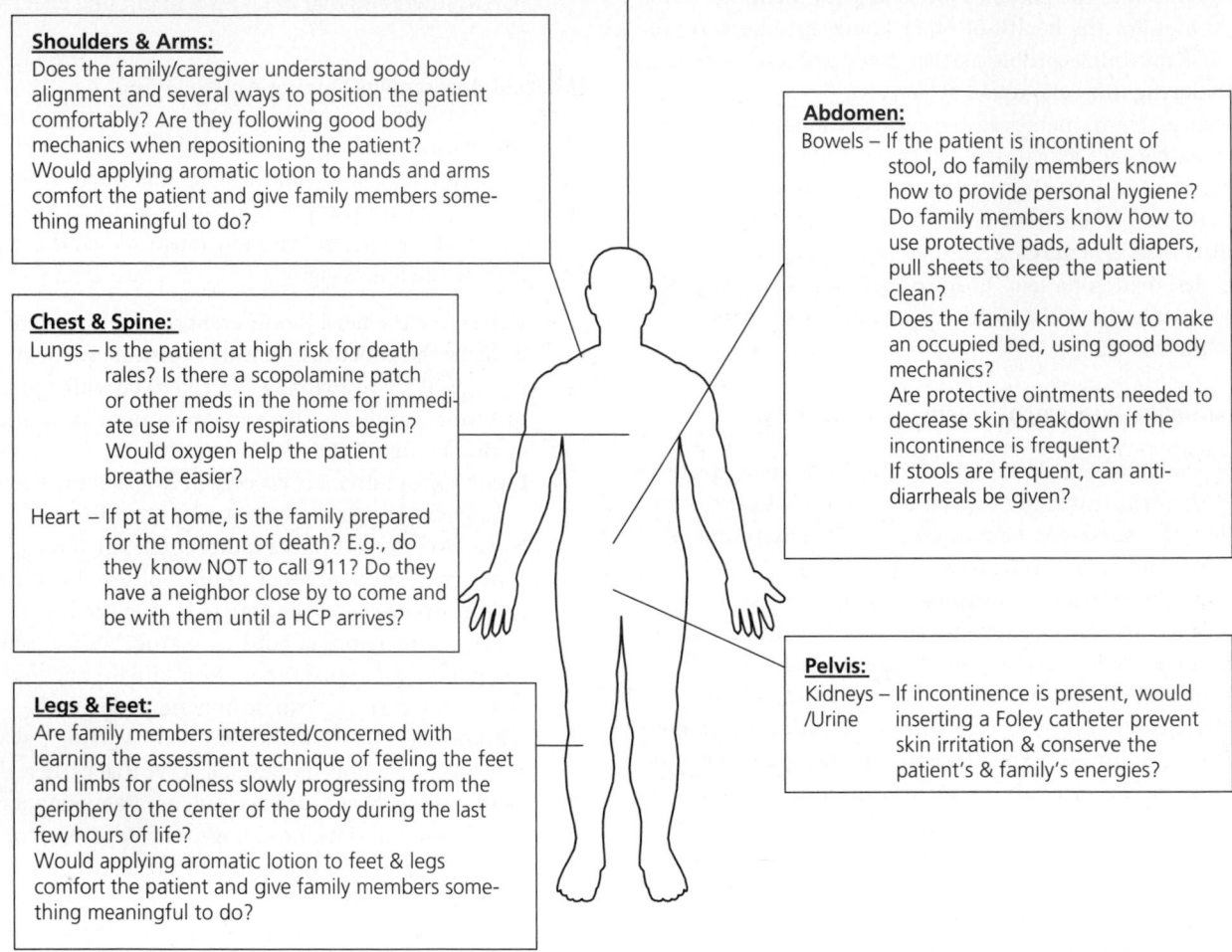

**Head & Neck:**
Mind – How important is level of alertness versus control of pain and anxiety which may cause sedation?
Senses: Sight – What objects at the bedside provide comfort when seen by the patient? Family photos? Children's drawings?
　　　　Special objects? Pets? Loved ones sitting nearby? What degree of lighting does the patient prefer? Does
　　　　darkness increase anxiety? Would scented candles provide solace?
　　　Hearing – What sounds most comfort the patient? Music? Family chatting nearby? The TV or radio on in the back-
　　　　ground? Someone reading to him or her? Silence?
　　　Smell – What scents does the patient enjoy? Would aromatic lotions be soothing?
　　　Taste – What are the patient's favorite flavors? Would mouth care to relieve dryness be more acceptable with fruit
　　　　punch, apple juice, beer, or coffee?
Mouth /Lips – Does the family/caregiver understand how to provide good, frequent mouth and lip care, especially if the patient
　　　　is a mouth -breather?

**Shoulders & Arms:**
Does the family/caregiver understand good body alignment and several ways to position the patient comfortably? Are they following good body mechanics when repositioning the patient? Would applying aromatic lotion to hands and arms comfort the patient and give family members something meaningful to do?

**Abdomen:**
Bowels – If the patient is incontinent of
　　　　stool, do family members know
　　　　how to provide personal hygiene?
　　　　Do family members know how to
　　　　use protective pads, adult diapers,
　　　　pull sheets to keep the patient
　　　　clean?
　　　　Does the family know how to make
　　　　an occupied bed, using good body
　　　　mechanics?
　　　　Are protective ointments needed to
　　　　decrease skin breakdown if the
　　　　incontinence is frequent?
　　　　If stools are frequent, can anti-
　　　　diarrheals be given?

**Chest & Spine:**
Lungs – Is the patient at high risk for death
　　　　rales? Is there a scopolamine patch
　　　　or other meds in the home for immedi-
　　　　ate use if noisy respirations begin?
　　　　Would oxygen help the patient
　　　　breathe easier?

Heart – If pt at home, is the family prepared
　　　　for the moment of death? E.g., do
　　　　they know NOT to call 911? Do they
　　　　have a neighbor close by to come and
　　　　be with them until a HCP arrives?

**Pelvis:**
Kidneys – If incontinence is present, would
/Urine　　inserting a Foley catheter prevent
　　　　skin irritation & conserve the
　　　　patient's & family's energies?

**Legs & Feet:**
Are family members interested/concerned with learning the assessment technique of feeling the feet and limbs for coolness slowly progressing from the periphery to the center of the body during the last few hours of life?
Would applying aromatic lotion to feet & legs comfort the patient and give family members something meaningful to do?

**General:**
• Are the patient's pain & other symptoms well controlled? Would massage, healing touch or other integrative therapies add
　to patient's comfort?
• Are family members capable & comfortable with continuing to provide physical care for the patient? Are family members
　getting enough sleep and rest to maintain their own health? Are additional resources needed to support the family?
• Is the home the best place for the patient to die? Has the family thought about their comfort in living in the house if their
　loved one dies there?
• Does the family know whom to call on a 24-hour basis for advice and support?

**Figure 4–2.** Assessment when the patient is actively dying: determining causes of pain and discomfort and identifying sources of comfort. HCP = health care professional; pt = patient. *Source*: Courtesy of Elaine Glass, ACHPN.

go," perhaps due to some unfinished business or fears related to dying. Assist the patient and family in exploring what these issues might be. A referral to a chaplain may be very helpful.

- Encourage celebration of the life of the loved one by acknowledging his or her contributions to family members, close friends, and the community.
- Explore the need and desire for additional comfort measures in the environment, such as soothing music, devotional readings, gazing out a window at nature, or increased quiet.
- Ask the family about their anticipated needs and preferences at the time of death: "Is there anyone you will want us to call for you?" "What can the health care team do to be most supportive?" "Are there specific practices regarding the care of the body that you want the team to carry out?"

The goals of spiritual care at this phase of illness are as follows:

- Facilitate any unfinished business among the patient and significant others (e.g., expressions of love, regret, forgiveness, gratitude).
- Promote the integrity of the dying person by honoring his or her life. One way to do this is by encouraging reminiscence at the bedside of the patient, recalling the "gifts" the patient bestowed on the family—that is, his or her legacy of values and qualities passed on to survivors.
- Assist the patient and family in extracting meaning from the dying experience.
- Provide sensitive comfort by being present and listening, or determine the patient's and family's need for privacy.
- Provide information regarding bereavement support groups and/or counseling if indicated.

CASE STUDY
*Ladona's Death*

At about seven-and-a-half month's gestation, Ladona wakes up in the middle of the night in sickle cell crisis and discovers that she is having severe vaginal bleeding. She is experiencing intense abdominal pain, nausea and vomiting, and is running a fever of 101.8. She is rushed to the emergency room where efforts to staunch the bleeding are initially unsuccessful. She is rushed to intensive care where she is put on life support with non-blood volume expanders. No fetal heartbeat can be ascertained and it is presumed that the fetus is dead. Her temperature continues to spike and her hemoglobin and hematocrit continue to drop precipitously. Ladona loses consciousness. She never did complete her advance directives.

Ladona's fiancé insists that she be given blood transfusions as the transfusion alternatives are not working. Ladona's parents forbid such blood products as a transgression against their daughter's expressed religious beliefs. The surgeons are afraid of removing the fetus without access to transfusion due to her severe blood loss already. They try to pressure Ladona's parents into consenting to blood products, especially after talking to Ladona's fiancé.

The healthcare team is unsuccessful in convincing Ladona's parents to allow her to have transfusions. The parents express their faith beliefs that when a Christian abstains from blood, he or she is, in effect, expressing faith that only the shed blood of Jesus Christ can truly redeem him or her and save his or her life.[33,34]

Michael is furious with Ladona's parents and becomes verbally abusive. In addition to calling Security, the social worker on the Palliative Care Team is paged. He has had a good relationship with Michael and he takes Michael aside to allow him to vent and express his grief. Michael knows Ladona will die without transfusions and he cannot bear the thought of losing her. With the help of the social worker, Michael is able to go to Ladona's side and hold her hand while she dies. Ladona's parents are on the other side of the bed. Everyone is weeping, including members of the staff. Some staff walk away because they cannot tolerate seeing Ladona die a death that seems so unnecessary and unfortunate to them.

The goals of care during the actively dying phase are to:

- Respect the patient's religious and cultural preferences despite absence of written advance directives. (In some states, her parents are the default primary decision-makers, as Michael has no legal authority since he and Ladona are not yet legally married.)
- Negotiate end-of-life care preferences with an eye toward successful conflict resolution in order to improve patient and family outcomes.
- Encourage Ladona's parents and Michael to participate in the local hospice's community grief program.
- Invite staff to a "debriefing" session to help them express their frustrations with caring for someone with a faith that appeared to contribute to her death in ways that seemed confusing or unreasonable to them.

## Summary of a Comprehensive Palliative Care Assessment

A comprehensive assessment of the patient and family provides the foundation for mutual goal setting, devising a plan of care, implementing interventions, and evaluating the effectiveness of care. Reassessments are done throughout the patient's illness, to ensure that quality of life is maximized (Table 4–12). Further sources of information are listed in the bibliography.

**Table 4-12**
**Best Practice Tip**

Clinicians who are in ambulatory settings may find the use of an abbreviated symptom assessment form helpful to track the efficacy of palliative care interventions. Whereas pain is usually plotted along the familiar 0–10 scale, other symptoms such as nausea, vomiting, diarrhea, constipation, fatigue, anxiety, and depression can be quickly evaluated on a flow sheet as, mild, moderate, or severe. These kinds of tools assist in interdisciplinary evaluation of symptoms without requiring paging through lengthy progress notes. In this way, treatment can be highly individualized and more evidence based.

Finally, as Colleen Scanlon[35] reminds us, two of the most important assessment questions that nurses and other health care team members can ask the patient and family, regardless of the phase or focus of the assessment, are, "What is your greatest concern?" and "How can I help?"

REFERENCES

1. Craven RF, Hirnle CJ. Fundamentals of Nursing: Human Health and Function, 4th ed. Philadelphia: Lipincott, Williams and Wilkins, 2003.
2. Jarvis C. Physical Examination and Health Assessment, 4th ed. St. Louis: Saunders, 2004.
3. Groopman J. How Doctors Think. New York: Houghton Mifflin, 2007.
4. Ferrell BR. The impact of pain on quality of life: A decade of research. Nurs Clin North Am 1995;30:609–624.
5. NHPCO's Facts and Figures. Available at http://www.nhpco.org/i4a/pages/index.cfm?pageid=5763 (accessed November 29, 2008).
6. Siegel BS. Love, Medicine and Miracles. New York: Harper and Row, 1986.
7. Holland J, ed. Psycho-oncology. New York: Oxford University Press, 2001.
8. Schwartz M. Letting Go: Morrie's Reflections on Living While Dying. New York: Delta, 1997.
9. Schneider JM. Clinically significant differences between grief, pathological grief and depression. Patient Counsel Health Educ 1980;4:267–275.
10. Bultz B, Holland J. Emotional Distress in Patients with Cancer: the Sixth Vital Sign. Community Oncology 2006;3:311–314.
11. Haase J, Britt T, Coward D, Leidy N, Penn P. Simultaneous concept analysis of spiritual perspective, hope, acceptance, and self-transcendence. Image J Nurs Sch 1992;24:141–147.
12. Amenta M. Nurses as primary spiritual care workers. Hospice J 1988;4:47–55.
13. Hay MW. Principles in building spiritual assessment tools. Am J Hospice Care 1989;6:25–31.
14. Doyle D. Have you looked beyond the physical and psychosocial? J Pain Symptom Manage 1992;7:303.
15. Frankl V. Man's Search for Meaning. Boston: Beacon Press, 1959.
16. Maslow AH. Motivation and Personality, 3rd ed. Hummelstown, PA: Scott Foresman-Addison Wesley, 1987.
17. Fitchett G. Assessing Spiritual Needs. Minneapolis: Augsburg, 1993.
18. Thompson S, Janigan A. Life schemes: A framework for understanding the search for meaning. J Soc Clin Psychol 1988;7:260–280.
19. Purnell L, Paulanka B. Guide to Culturally Competent Health Care. Philadelphia: F.A. Davis & Co., 2006.
20. Andrews M, Boyle J. Competence in transcultural nursing care. Am J Nurs 1997;8:16AAA–16DDD.
21. Inclusion and Access Toolbox, 2007. NHPCO. Available at www.nhpco.org/i4a/pages/Index.cfm?pageid=5162 (accessed December 2, 2008).
22. Rancour P. Using archetypes and transitions theory to assist patients to move from active treatment to survivorship. Clin J Oncol Nurs 2008;12:935–941.
23. Noyes R, Holt CS, Massie MJ. Anxiety disorders. in: Holland J, ed. Psycho-oncology. New York: Oxford University Press, 1998: 548–563.
24. Massie MJ. Depressive disorders. In: Holland J, ed. Psycho-oncology. New York: Oxford University Press, 1998:518–540.
25. Shehan L. Cancer as a Turning Point: A Handbook for People with Cancer, Their Families and Health Professionals. Revised Edition. Long Beach, CA: Plume, 1994.
26. Cella DF, Tulsky DS, Gray G, et al. The Functional Assessment of Cancer Therapy Scale: Development and Validation of the General Measure. J Clin Oncol 1984;11:570–579.
27. de Haes JCJM, van Knippenberg FCE, Neijt JP. Measuring psychological and physical distress in cancer patients: Structure and application of the Rotterdam Symptom Checklist. Br J Cancer 1990;62:1034–1038.
28. Fisher Center for Alzheimer's Research Foundation. Available at www.alzinfo.org/alzheimers-caregiving.asp (accessed December 13, 2008).
29. Jevene RF, Miller JE. Finding Hope: Ways to See Life in a Brighter Light. Fort Wayne, Ind.: Willowgreen, 1999.
30. Threshold Choir. Available at http://www.thresholdchoir.org/music.htm (accessed December 13, 2008).
31. The Chalice of Repose Project, Inc. Available at http://www.thresholdchoir.org/music.htm (accessed December 13, 2008).
32. Rancour P. Integrating Complementary and Alternative Therapies into End-of-Life Care. InTouch: A Hospice and Palliative Care Resource of the Ohio Hospice & Palliative Care Organization 2008;12:8–10.
33. Watchtower Publications. How Can Blood Save Your Life. Watchtower, 1990;24.
34. Watchtower Publications. Awake! August 2006;11.
35. Scanlon C. Creating a vision of hope: The challenge of palliative care. Oncol Nurs Forum 1989;16:491–496.

BIBLIOGRAPHY

Back AL, Arnold RM, Quill TE. Hope for the Best, and Prepare for the Worst. Ann Intern Med 2003;138:439–443.
Bolen JS. Close to the Bone: Life Threatening Illness and the Search for Meaning. New York: Scribner, 1996.
Byock I. Dying Well: Peace and Possibilities at the End of Life. New York: Riverhead Books, 1998.

Carroll-Johnson R. Psychosocial Nursing Care Along the Cancer Continuum. Pittsburgh, Pa.: Oncology Nursing Press, 1998.

Center for Blood Conservation at Grant Medical Center, Columbus Ohio. (To obtain a copy of a blood directive form.) Available at, http://www.ohiohealth.com/bodygrant.cfm?id=3640 (accessed December 3, 2008).

Davis L, Keller A. At the Close of Day: A Person Centered Guide Book on End-of-Life Care. Charleston, NC: Streamline Press, 2004.

Emanuel L, Ferris FD, von Gunten CF, Von Roenn JH. The Last Hours of Living: Practical Advice for Clinicians. CME/CE. Available at: http://www.medscape.com/viewprogram/5808 (accessed December 13, 2008).

Foos-Graber A. Deathing. York Beach, Maine: Nicolas-Hays, 1989.

Glass E, Cluxton D. Truth-telling: ethical issues in clinical practice. J Hosp Palliat Care 2004;6:232–242.

Grauer P, Shuster J, Protus BM. Palliative Care Consultant: A reference guide for palliative care—Guidelines for Effective Management of Symptoms, 3rd ed. Dubuque, IA: Kendallhunt Professional, 2007.

Greenspan M. Healing Through the Dark Emotions: The Wisdom of Grief, Fear and Despair. Shambhala, 2003.

Hutchinson J, Rupp J. May I Walk You Home? Courage and Comfort for Caregivers of the Very Ill. Notre Dame, Ind.: Ave Maria Press, 1999.

Jehovah's Witnesses Official Web Site. Available at http://www.watchtower.org (accessed December 19, 2008).

Kramp E, Kramp D. Living with the End in Mind: A Practical Checklist for Living Life to the Fullest by Embracing Your Mortality. New York: Three Rivers Press, 1998.

Lo B, Quill T, Tulsky J. Discussing palliative care with patients. American College of Physicians–American Society of Internal Medicine End-of-Life Care Consensus Panel. Ann Intern Med 1999;130:744–749.

Lynn J, Harrold J. Handbook for Mortals: Guidance for People Facing Serious Illness. New York: Oxford University Press, 1999.

Meraviglia M, Sutter R, Gaskamp CD, Adams S, Titler MG. Evidence-Based Guideline: Providing Spiritual Care to Terminally Ill Older Adults. J Gerontol Nurs 2008;34:8–14.

Miller JE. One You Love Is Dying: 12 Thoughts to Guide You On the Journey. Fort Wayne, Ind.: Willowgreen Publishing, 1997.

Miller JE. When You Know You're Dying: 12 Thoughts to Guide You Through the Days Ahead. Fort Wayne, Ind.: Willowgreen Publishing, 1997.

Miller JE. Willowgreen. Available at http://www.willowgreen.com (accessed December 13, 2008).

National Family Caregivers Association website. Available at: http://www.nfcacares.org (accessed December 13, 2008).

National Selected Morticians. Arranging a funeral; A friend's guide to funeral services; Funeral services by religion. Available at http://www.selectedfuneralhomes.org (accessed December 13, 2008).

Ohio State University Medical Center, Columbus, Ohio. Patient education materials are available at: http://medicalcenter.osu.edu/patientcare/patient_education/ (accessed December 13, 2008).

Rancour P. Those tough conversations. Am J Nurs: Crit Care Suppl 2000;100:24HH–24LL.

Rancour P. Catapulting through life stages: When young adults are diagnosed with life-threatening illness. Psychosocial Nursing and Mental Health Services 2002;40(2):32–37.

Robertson C. Let the Choice Be Mine: A Personal Guide to Planning Your Own Funeral. Standpoint, Idaho: MCR, 1995. (Available from MCR, P.O. Box 1922, Sandpoint, ID 83864; telephone 208-263-8960.)

Sickle Cell Anemia, National Institutes of Health. Available at: http://www.nlm.nih.gov/medlineplus/sicklecellanemia.html (accessed December 13, 2008).

Steel K, Ljunggren G, Topinkova E, Morris JN, Vitale C, Parzuchowski J, Nonemaker S, Frijters DH, Rabinowitz T, Murphy KM, Ribbe MW, Fries BE. The RAI-PC: An assessment instrument for palliative care in all settings. Am J Hospice Palliat Med 2003;20:211–219.

Stoll R. Guidelines for spiritual assessment. Am J Nurs 1979;79:1574–1577.

Tanyi RA. Spirituality and family nursing: Spiritual assessment and interventions for families. Issues and Innovations in Nursing Practice 2006;287–294.

Taylor R. Check your cultural competence. Nurs Manage 1998;3:30–32.

Timmons F, Kelly J. Spiritual assessment in intensive and cardiac nursing. Br Assoc Crit Care Nurses, Nurs Crit Care 2008;13:124–131.

Warm E, Weissman D. Fast fact and concept #21: Hope and truth telling. EPERC: Educational Materials Fast Facts. Available at: http://www.eperc.mcw.edu/ff_index.htm (accessed December 13, 2008).

# 5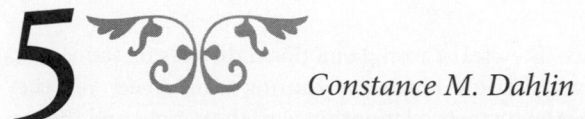

*Constance M. Dahlin*

# Communication in Palliative Care: An Essential Competency for Nurses

*The best thing about palliative care was the constant presence and discussion of the important issues. We knew what was happening and what was going to happen. We knew the team understood Roni's wishes and her definition of quality of life. When it came time that there was no quality of life, all the prior conversations made the process bearable. And the palliative care nurse was with us throughout the process.—Surviving husband of 65 year old with ALS*

♦ **Key Points**

♦ *In order to provide optimal palliative care, effective communication is the fundamental intervention to ensure qaulity care.*

♦ *Communication is a learned skill that includes 80% non-verbal communication and 20% verbal communication, both of which are important.*

♦ *The art of nursing presence includes listening and silence.*

Communication is a complex, continual transactional process that occurs between persons by which information, feelings, and meaning are conveyed through verbal and nonverbal messages.[1] It is the essential aspect to good nursing practice and some studies would suggest that communication training is mandatory for any nurse working in palliative care.[2] In 1998, the American Association of Colleges of Nursing (AACN) developed a document, "A Peaceful Death," which entailed 15 competencies for nursing in providing care at the end of life.[3] This document serves as the basis for formal educational preparation for nurses, particularly in communication.

The third AACN Peaceful Death competency states that the nurse should "Communicate effectively and compassionately with the patient, family, and health care team members about end-of-life issues."[3] With good communication skills, the nurse is able to assess various domains related to the patient's illness. These domains relate to many areas such as health belief systems, information needs, physical symptoms, as well as psychological, cultural, and spiritual issues. Therefore, it is essential that nurses develop effective communication skills. Only then can the nurse optimize skill in his or her nursing practice and provide both the art and science of palliative care.

However, long before this document was created, the rich origin of palliative care was founded within the principles of nursing care. Nursing has been prominent in the provision of the care of the dying throughout history: from the early nurses of Greek and Roman times; through the nuns who provided care in the middle ages; to Florence Nightingale and Clara Barton who created the role of the modern nurse to care for dying soldiers; to modern times when Cecily Saunders, beginning her health career as a nurse, realized care of the dying needed to be improved; and finally to Florence Wald, who created the hospice curriculum at the Yale University School of Nursing.[4] The reason for this is that the essence of nursing is being present and providing palliative caring at the bedside. The close proximity of nurses allows for communication at all levels, often in a less formal and less threatening discussion. Patients quickly develop trust in the nurse and realize the nurse is their advocate.

Unlike other conditions that may only affect a subset of the population, such as diabetes or infection, heart or lung conditions, death is inevitable. It is not a matter of *if* patients will die; it is a matter of how and when. Palliative care is one aspect of nursing that cuts across all specialties of practice. It is important to remember that palliative care is an inherent tenet of nursing, upon which modern nursing was developed. Thus nurses in all areas of practice will always be exposed to dying patients and will always need solid communication skills.

Because death is universal, various teams will be involved in the care of patients. Teams may be divided by specialty or discipline. Often, specialty teams have cared for particular patients over long periods of time, such as in heart failure, amyotrophic sclerosis, or HIV. Communication and collaboration are vital to optimal care, as no one health care provider can attend to all aspects of the needs of the patient and family. With needs changing as the disease progresses, various disciplines will be needed to assure holistic care. Teams that communicate effectively provide better care, even when they disagree. Nurses, as primary members of the team, do well to learn negotiation skills and strategies for conflict resolution to assist in advocating for the patient.

This Chapter examines many important aspects of communication as a competency for nursing. It begins with a discussion of the fundamental role of the nurse in the communication process. It reviews the phases of communication in the nurse patient relationship. The essential elements of communication are described. Consideration of the communication process for palliative care patients, across the spectrum of care from diagnosis to death, is explored. Strategies for successful family meetings are reviewed along with the exploration of the focus of difficult communication such as advanced care planning, breaking bad news and code status. Finally, there is discussion of the elements of collaboration, which includes negotiation and conflict resolution.

## Overview

During the course of their studies and training, few nurses receive formal death education. Twenty years ago, Degner and Gow (1988) wrote about this lack of education and how nurses in training were protected from death education until they graduated.[5] Then, as new nurses, they were exposed to the reality of care. This phenomenon continues today in many nursing programs. The result is that new graduate nurses must care for patients with life threatening illnesses without any experience, mentoring, or coaching to do so. Many of their senior colleagues have had little training and are unable to serve as guides in this process. In this author's experience, when nurses are asked about their fears concerning caring for patients, most fear saying the wrong thing to patients. They fear causing emotional distress or sadness, as well as saying too much and causing team strife. Yet, they underestimate their relationship with the patient and the significance of their presence.

CASE STUDY
*Mrs. R: An Example of the Importance of Presence*

GRADUATE NURSE JASON: Mrs. R, I am your nurse, Jason. How are you today?

MRS. R: I am not feeling so well and the doctors said they wanted to talk to me. I am worried.

JASON: What are you worried about?

MRS. R: What if they have bad news? Will you be here if they do?

JASON: I am not sure what the doctors have to say. However, I will ask them if they are planning a meeting and let you know if that is the case. In the meantime, I will be here all day to support you. We can plan a schedule and I will let you know when I leave for a break. Is that helpful?

MRS. R: Yes, I just don't want to be alone and would appreciate you checking in on me.

JASON: Of course, Mrs. R, you will not be alone.

With skilled interactions, trusting relationships are established and the nurse can promote a respectful dying process for the patient and family. Effectively communicating with patients provides accurate assessment of physical, psychological, spiritual, and social dimensions of care. Patients with an uncertain future require open and honest discussion to facilitate expression of feelings and concerns. Often this discussion provides patients time and space to reflect upon their priorities, to consider their values, and to articulate their needs in the remaining time. Preferences and beliefs are ascertained, and goals of care can be developed. Simultaneously, since both the patient and the family are the unit of care, good communication facilitates the inclusion of family members, allowing expression of their feelings, concerns, and needs in caring for their loved one.[6] Without effective communication, the patient's experience of suffering is unknown, and effective symptom control is impossible.[7,8]

There are several levels of communication for the nurse to address. One is day-to-day interactions surrounding the tasks in caring for the patient. On a simple level, this may involve small talk, or discussion of basic treatment issues, such as pain medication schedules, activities of daily living, or personal care. Another level is assessment of treatments. The nurse approaches the patient in an open manner to allow the patient to honestly evaluate the effectiveness of treatments, hoping to gain more specific information concerning distress or pain. The third and most complex level of communication is the existential level. This occurs at the level of the patient's deepest sense of self. Communication at this level is sensitive and often nuanced because the existential aspects of end-of-life include disclosure, searching for meaning, and suffering.[9,10] Exploration at this level can help a patient with a life-threatening illness to live while dying, lessen fear, achieve quality of life, and have psychological healing during this process.[11]

## The Role of the Nurse in Palliative Care

Many researchers have written on the role of the nurse in patients who are dying. Indeed, there seems to be agreement that communication is a core aspect of nursing care of patients with life-threatening illness. The essential skills require effective listening, appropriate non-verbal communication, counseling skills with the elements of reflection, clarification, and empathy, and supportiveness.[2] The development of these skills requires self-awareness, which is best fostered in formal and supportive educational venues.

Good communication allows for optimal palliative care, as it is the basis of the relationship.[12] It is grounded in the establishment of a strong nurse-patient relationship that provides a therapeutic basis for the care.[2] Various researches have described the roles of the nurse interactions within the following categories support, caring, collaboration, continuous presence, fostering of hope, and advocacy for the patient.[13-16] Research speaks to the various aspects of communication: active listening, presence, eliciting preferences and facilitating communication choices.[17] There seems to be agreement that the establishment of trust, continuity, and understanding foster good relationships.[12] Moreover, it is also important that the nurse has a healthy coping style and understanding of timing in communication.

In the National Consensus Project for Quality Palliative Care *Clinical Guidelines for Quality Palliative Care*, communication is emphasized throughout the document. Communication is the basis of *Domain 1: Structure and Processes of Care*, which describes how care is delivered. Guideline 1.2 states: "The care plan is based on the identified and expressed preferences, values, and needs of the patient and family and is developed with professional guidance and support for decision making."[18] Criteria to support this guideline include ongoing assessment and the creation of an evolving care plan created by the whole team, including the patient and family. The interdisciplinary team is responsible for communication with all involved, including the patient and family. This is articulated through documentation. Nurses have an important role in the team process and need to promote optimal communication among the team, patient, and family.

According to the American Nurses Association, nurses have several responsibilities in the care of dying patients. They have a duty to educate patients and families about end-of-life issues, to encourage the discussion of life preferences, to communicate relevant information for any decision, and to advocate for the patient.[19] However, many nurses—feel uncomfortable communicating with dying patients. This

discomfort stems from lack of training and education, lack of confidence to integrate this into their practice, and lack of mentoring in this skill.

Various studies have identified a lack of communication in addressing care wishes and inadequate knowledge and skill in end-of-life-care communication.[20,21] Indeed, in American culture, the importance of designating a health care proxy has been emphasized—but without stressing the importance of accompanying conversation about values and preferences regarding limits of health care in futile situations. The nurse has the opportunity to facilitate a process that allows the patients to state their care wishes and the family to hear those wishes.

Nonetheless, nurses are often one of the first health care providers to identify issues in patients with life threatening illness. These may be related to advanced care planning, goals of care, conflict between patient and family wishes, and use of life-sustaining measures for patients with life threatening illnesses. They glean this information from their direct care provision and constant presence at the bedside. This information gathering is encouraged by the team, as it is useful to direct care. Fallowfield[22] suggested that some physicians believe nurses are more capable than physicians in talking with distressed patients and families.

Across the palliative care spectrum, communication occurs at critical junctures. Depending on the diagnosis of the patient, these communications may occur over a long or a short period of time. Since it has been estimated that 80–90% of all patients who die have a chronic illness,[23] there is much potential for communication to take place over the long course of that illness. Within the relationship between a nurse and a patient, Perrin[24] speaks about three stages. The introductory phase is where the nurse and the patient learn about each other's styles. The middle phase involves establishing a working relationship in which the work is done, such as pain and symptom management, discussions about the meaning of life, along with legacy work and family work. Finally, final and third phase is termination, in which the nurse and the patient say goodbye to each other either because the patient is leaving the system or is dying.[24]

The initial communication or introductory phase consists of the introduction of the nurse as a member of the care team. During this time, the nurse assesses the patient and the patient determines the style of the nurse. The tasks of the nurse include exploring the patient's understanding of his or her illness, eliciting personality and coping styles and identifying any existing advanced care planning. Another task is assessing the patient's learning styles and discerning the patient's ability to understand the seriousness of the illness. The process itself varies according to the age and cognitive development of the patient. For children and some older adults, the family or support unit is primarily involved in the information process. The introductory phase leads into the working phase.

The working phase may extend over a long period of time. It can include pain and symptom management interventions initiated by the nurse and critical conversations related to disease progression. Disease progression usually causes anxiety and distress for the patient and family. At this point, the patient and family seek trust and reassurance from the nurse, based on continued presence. The nurse is able to have insight into patient and family coping and articulate their concerns, or perceptions of care. Later, there may be a discussion of bad news. Best practice mandates that the nurse be present during these conversations. This allows for later reinforcement of the information and the usage of similar language. At this time, the nurse, according to Pierce,[25] fulfills three critical communication tasks in end-of-life care: (1) creates an environment conducive to communication; (2) eases interaction between physician and patient; and (3) facilitates interaction between family and patient.

As the patient begins to die, the termination phase commences. The nurse offers continued presence and reassurance. Communication with the patient and family often focuses on support of decision-making, the assurance of comfort in the presence of pain and symptoms, information about the dying process, and solace in anticipatory grieving. Most importantly, the nurse monitors the patient while they are dying and provides intensive caring to both the patient and family in this process. The nurse and the patient are able to come to some closure as the patient dies. Immediately following the death, the nurse can play a critical role in providing family support to promote a more healthy grief and bereavement process.

Within the spectrum of health care, nurses are trusted members of the health care team at the time of diagnosis, during treatment, and in the final stages of life. Through effective communication, the nurse has a pivotal role in accompanying the patient through this journey. Indeed, the nurse may have the best opportunity to learn the patient's hopes, fears, dreams, and regrets. Using this information, the nurse can create a healing environment within a poignant situation.

CASE STUDY
*Information Gathering: Ms. Bee, a 63-Year-Old with ALS*

Ms. Bee, a 63-year-old woman with amyotrophic lateral sclerosis, has progressed with the disease since her diagnosis 5 years ago. She wants to consolidate her care at the hospital and meets a new primary care team consisting of a nurse, physical therapist, and physician. The nurse wants to get to know Ms. Bee.

> NURSE: Hi, Ms. Bee. I am the nurse with the primary care team. I know you are here to meet us and we would like to get to know you. Can you tell us how you have been doing?
>
> MS. BEE: I am okay, but I am in pain. So many people have been poking at me.
>
> NURSE: Can you tell me a little about your pain?
>
> MS. BEE: My chest hurts like they said it would. But there is nothing more they can do. I guess I should just forget about it and try to make the best of it.
>
> NURSE: What did the doctors tell you?

> MS. BEE: They said I would have a hard time moving and breathing. I knew it was coming but it is worse now that it is here.
>
> NURSE: In what way?
>
> MS. BEE: I have tried to be strong. But I now have a breathing machine at night. I can't move myself. This tube in my stomach hurts. I just feel overwhelmed.
>
> NURSE: That must be hard.
>
> MS.BEE: I get tired and sometimes I just cry. But it could be worse.
>
> NURSE: What happens when you cry?
>
> MS.BEE: It makes it hard to breathe and my family just says I am feeling sorry for myself.
>
> NURSE: What gives you strength?
>
> MS.BEE: My faith.
>
> NURSE: Do you belong to a church?
>
> MS. BEE: I do and they call in.
>
> NURSE: Is that enough support?
>
> MS.BEE: Not really.
>
> NURSE: Is there anyone else?
>
> MS. BEE: Well I live with my ex-husband and his mother. They just let me stay in the back room.
>
> NURSE: That must be isolating.
>
> MS. BEE: It is and I can't do anything about it.
>
> NURSE: Have you spoken to our social worker or the ALS society?
>
> MS.BEE: Not really.
>
> NURSE: Do you want to try that and see?
>
> MS. BEE: Okay

Here the nurse promotes an open environment for the patient to express feelings. She explores the patient's support system and offers some problem solving.

## Historical Perspective of Communication at the End of Life

Communication about the end of life has changed dramatically since the 1960s, when death and dying were closed, unacknowledged topics. The patient lay in a hospital bed, clearly declining, with no one interacting or communicating to them any information about what was occurring. There was no effort by health care professionals to elicit any feelings or concerns from the patient. Many people died alone and in silence without being allowed the opportunity to say goodbye. Field and Copp[26] discuss an interesting observations in communication with dying patients. Initially, the topic of death was avoided with patients and was discussed only among health care providers. This may have been in part because communication skills were considered to be intuitive or inherited traits. Practitioners either had empathetic and effective communication skills, or not.[7] For patients being cared for by an uncommunicative or ineffective clinician, dying could be an isolating, anxious, fearful, mistrustful experience that translated into a sense of abandonment. In such a situation, families experience complex grief and bereavement and increased stress. For nurses, this indirect communication and lack of truth-telling in the dying process resulted in greater stress, anxiety, and inauthentic communication, which translated to guilt, internal conflict, and a sense of failure.

From the 1960s to the 1980s, the principles of informed consent and autonomy became valued aspects of health care. In the 1990s, truth telling became a central focus of terminal care, allowing death to become a more open topic of discussion for patients. The pendulum swung the other way. Instead of holding back information, patients and families were informed of all aspects of death and dying. This was irrespective of their wishes to know such information, be involved in decision-making, or any consideration of the uniqueness of patient/family systems. Active participation of patients in their care became the underlying value that led to a greater sense of control and diminished anxiety. Simultaneously, a shift in communication theory occurred. The research demonstrated that communication skills, like any other skills, could be acquired by health care providers.[7]

The current communication trend is a conditional process that supports the patient's individual coping style. There has been a movement of health care systems toward the practice of patient and family centered care, whereby the needs of the patient and family dictate care, not the providers. This allows for care to follow the patient's individual personality, particularly in terms of the patient's level of acceptance or denial of the dying process. It also promotes the importance of family in decision-making. And since communication is an acquired skill, nurses at all levels of practice, need to learn basic skills in communication with palliative care patients.

## Nursing Communication Skills

In the health care environment, communication, whether intentional or not, occurs all the time between nurses and patients in every aspect of care. Patients consider communication skills to be very important. Bailey and Wilkerson[27] performed a qualitative study that evaluated patients' perceptions of nurses' communication skills and the attributes of a good nurse. Twenty-nine patients were surveyed about communication. Patients specified the following: nurses must have good verbal and nonverbal skills, be approachable, sympathetic, and nonjudgmental, as well as caring. Patients also felt that a good nurse has the personal characteristic of being a good listener and the professional quality of being a good communicator. Though the patients interviewed in this study were not palliative care patients, their feelings reflect how essential communication is to expert nursing care.

Communication skills affect the success of the nurse in his/her various therapeutic roles, including advocacy, support, information-sharing, empowerment, validation, and

psychological ventilation.[23] In order to participate fully in these areas, the nurse has focused areas of skill acquisition: the basics of initiating conversations, asking questions, developing a comfortable vocabulary, and listening and attending to behaviors. In addition, the nurse needs current state-of-the-art knowledge in end-of-life care, factual information about the progression of various diseases, realistic dying trajectories, and the care entailed for families and professional care givers. Finally, the nurse needs education about the process of patient and family centered care, as well as the institutional and collegial empowerment to participate and communicate in death and dying discussions.[27,28]

There are two levels of necessary communication skills for nurses. These are based on education and expertise. At the registered nurse or generalist level, critical communication skills include, but are not limited to: presence; listening and supporting patients in coping with their disease; providing appropriate information necessary for decision-making; participation at bad news discussions and family meetings; reinforcing information provided by the health care team; supporting decision-making; advocating for the patient and family; information sharing about signs and symptoms of dying; facilitating communication between the patient and family; and providing support in grief and bereavement. Some generalist nurses consider the role of information sharing and any discussion of diagnosis and treatment to be outside their scope of practice. However, from the perspective of the advocacy role in nursing, information sharing empowers the patient to make informed decisions. Moreover, the very proximity of the nurse in the direct bedside caregiving function affords the nurse a trusted role, providing many opportunities to create positive communication encounters. The plethora of opportunities to begin dialogue about death and dying include—in addition to planned meetings—moments of privacy between nurse and patient during bathing, feeding, and self-care activities.

At the master's or advanced practice (APN) level, critical nursing communication skills include discussions of diagnosis, treatment options, and prognosis; delivery of bad news with disease progression and transition into palliative care; discussions of life-sustaining treatment; facilitation of family meetings; discussion of post-death options such as autopsy or organ donation; and grief and bereavement support. The APN may serve in a dual consultative role. In the medical model, the focus of consultation is on the APN to provide expert palliative care. In the nursing model, the focus of consultation is the APN's role in coaching or mentoring other nurses or providers to administer palliative care.

CASE STUDY
### Mrs. L and Nurse Rose: An Example of Nurse Patient Relationship

Mrs. L is a 73-year-old woman with lung cancer. She is a former hospice nurse and is now on 3rd line treatment. Rose, her nurse, is helping her with a.m. care. Mrs. L has been dismissing people who talk to her. She sent out the social worker and the palliative care team. As she is getting things ready, Rose decides to talk to Mrs. L in a non-threatening way.

ROSE: Mrs. L, I have noticed the past few days, you have not wanted to talk to many people.

MRS. L: I am tired of talking. I know what is going on and I don't want to think about it.

ROSE: Is there some way we can support you? You seem so sad.

MRS. L: Things are just bad. How do you feel you can help?

ROSE: Well, we have known each other a long time. I wonder if you are more down these days.

MRS. L: Things are bad at home. I can't get out much. And this treatment wipes me out.

ROSE: Do you think you are depressed?

MRS. L: I am not sure.

ROSE: Is there anything that brings you joy?

MRS. L: My grandson, but he takes too much energy.

ROSE: Perhaps we should think about if we can treat your fatigue and lack of joy. What do you think?

MRS. L: Well, maybe. Let's talk to my oncologist.

Here, Rose uses her long standing relationship with Mrs. L to explore the patient's depressive mood.

## Barriers to Communication

The barriers to such communication can be seen from the perspective of patient, family, and nurse. Patients often avoid talking about their pain, anger, sense of loss, sense of guilt, and fears due to embarrassment, shyness, confusion, or cultural prohibitions. They may also fear that talking about something may make it happen, or that it will cause too much distress for themselves and/or their families. Families may find it too painful to talk about the advanced state of their loved one's illness. Moreover, it is not uncommon that family members have little knowledge of the patient's preferences for types of care. In order to maintain hope, families tend to overestimate the possibility of cure. They also fear future regrets if they do not pursue or demand further curative treatment.

Nursing barriers to communication include fear, perceived scope-of-practice issues, and legal concerns. There may also be difficulty or discomfort with communication due to personal cultural norms, struggles of unresolved grief, fear of their own mortality, or fear of being emotional in front of a patient.[29,30] Lack of education or training, or lack of personal and professional experience with death and dying means they have little exposure to end-of-life communication.[31,32] One myth is that bringing up issues related to death and dying will cause too much emotional distress to the patient and family. Additionally, nurses fear conflict between patient and family. Consequently, with patients facing difficult issues at end of life, nurses may employ several mechanisms to avoid discussion. A nurse may focus more on the biomedical aspects, particularly using technical medical jargon, and thereby avoid eliciting, allowing for, and responding to a patient's thoughts and feelings.[33,34] A nurse may focus only on the present time, thereby preventing the patient from expressing concerns about a previous time. For example, rather than listening to the patient relate concerns from an earlier time, the nurse may stop the conversation by saying, "But how are you now?" Another way of avoiding discussion is to change the focus or the subject. For example, if the patient says, "I am nauseated," the nurse may divert the conversation by saying, "So, how is your family?" Sometimes the nurse may interrupt the conversation by offering advice: "Of course, you will get over this in time. It won't last for too long." Another avoidance technique is responding to a patient's expressed difficulties by stating, "Clearly you need to talk to the social worker about your issues."[35] Finally, nurses and physicians may collude with patients in avoiding discussions of death and dying.[36,37] In this way, the nurse prevents opportunities to offer any information on the patients' condition.[34]

## Information Needs

To best provide supportive care to patients and families, it is necessary to understand their information and communication needs. Patients require information around treatment, management of symptoms, support from family and friends, fulfillment of family or cultural expectations, attaining meaning, and maintaining dignity and control.[38] Correspondingly, the communication needs for the patient include disease specifics, rationale for care, being listened to, and the opportunity to participate in important discussions.[39] The role of the nurse is to assess the patient's knowledge and concerns in these areas, offer reinforcement of information, and to facilitate information to the rest of the care team.

The communication needs of the family and other supportive people depend on their role in the family system, age, decision-making ability, and other rules within and specific to the family. To participate in the patient's care, families need communication regarding several issues: reassurance of the patient's comfort; support in coping with the patient's condition; understanding the evolving care plan; and what care currently includes.[38] Families may be very involved in care, but may have multiple home and work obligations. Therefore, it may be a challenge for family members to be participating directly in meetings at the bedside. Families may experience a high level of stress from their need for constant updates of information.

One factor that may affect communication is anxiety. As Pasareta and colleagues[40] described, a person who is mildly anxious may be able to process information and, in fact, may be quite creative. Indeed, mild anxiety helps most people do their work by being alert to issues, identifying problems, and facilitating creative solutions. Some patients experience mild anxiety simply by participating in a preventive health encounter. In this situation, the nurse may provide basic health information. However, as anxiety increases toward a moderate level, as often occurs with receiving news about disease progression, information processing becomes selective. In terms of patients, this means that when something scary or threatening is communicated, the patient may not be able to take in much information. For instance, a patient may be told that an x-ray film looks abnormal. At that point, the patient has a heightened awareness and may be thinking of possible issues. In this case, the nurse supports the patient by allowing him or her to voice fears and concerns and by reiterating information that the team has provided.

In cases of severe anxiety and panic, such as when hearing bad news in the form of a short prognosis or lack of options, a patient's information processing may be totally impaired.[40] This occurs when a patient is given a terminal diagnosis. As soon as the physician or the advanced practice nurse gives bad news, the patient may not hear anything else. He or she may have gone into shock or panic about the news and cannot take in any other information. Understanding this point is important for the nurse's communication timing—he or she will refrain from sharing further information until the patient has had time to process the bad news. Nurses have an important role in validating the patient's reactions and offering support in determining what further information the patient may need.

Similarly, a nurse may have anxiety in caring for a dying patient. In some cases, the nurse may be quite able to understand and respond to patient and family cues. However, if there are factors that make care more difficult, such as the patient being close in age to the nurse or resembling members of the nurse's family, the nurse may become more anxious and unable to attend and be present to the patient and family. Moreover, as the patient's needs escalate or there are more complex family dynamics to attend to, the nurse may not be able to communicate as well. Finally, if a patient has a sudden emergency or decline, causing the nurse to become more emotional and/or overwhelmed by care need. Thus, communication skills may become compromised just when they are needed most. Thus, it is important for the nurse to monitor his or her own anxiety in caring for the patient.

## Communication Framework

Communication comprises both verbal expression, through the use of language, and nonverbal expression, using the body to convey messages. Verbal communication must be considered in terms of the educational level of content, the emotional content, and the nature of the relationship between the health care provider and the patient.[21] Communication can be affected by myriad factors including, but not limited to, education of the patient and family; literacy of the patient and family; cultural issues of the patient and family; English not as first language; stress, coping, and anxiety of patient and family; use of medical jargon, particularly three-letter acronyms; and assumed common understanding of particular vocabulary.[41,42]

Nurses often act as translators between the various health disciplines and providers and the patient/family. By the virtue of their constant bedside presence, nurses must create the optimal method of interaction with a patient. In setting the tone for future communication, the nurse can ask several open-ended questions to begin a conversation. These include:

- Tell me about your condition?
- How much information do you want to know?
- How do you make decisions?
- Is there anyone else you want to know or whom we should talk to about your condition, treatment or process?
- Are there any cultural considerations to your health care that I should know?[43]

It is also important to emphasize the use of interpreters for patients for whom English is a second language. It has become clear that the use of medical interpreters can bridge communication in a sensitive and appropriate way. In fact, federal law mandates the use of interpreters for any facilities receiving federal funds.[44] In this author's experience, it is always alarming when critical discussions such as disease progression or code status have occurred with families who do not have command of the English language. This may damage trust and sets up an awkward relationship. Often, family members had been used as interpreters. This practice should be discouraged, in particular the use of children as translators. Children lack the medical vocabulary and health literacy to interpret with any accuracy.[45] Furthermore, the use of trained interpreters can guide difficult conversations by helping the clinician use culturally appropriate language and avoid making cultural faux-pas.[46]

## Elements of Communication

Working within the phases of the nurse patient relationship, there are four basic elements to communication: imparting information, listening, information gathering, and presence and sensitivity. Realistically, these elements do not occur in a linear fashion but may occur concurrently. However, for the sake of simplicity, they are discussed separately.

### Imparting Information

A primary role of the nurse is to impart information. This may include education about the illness, medications, or general information about treatments. APNs may offer other information, including diagnosis and treatment options. The task of imparting information is complex, because information alone is not enough. Rather, information must be provided within the appropriate context of educational level, the appropriate developmental level, consideration to the stress level, and within the various time constraints of a healthcare setting. The patient's educational level and understanding of medical language affects his or her information processing. If a patient hasn't completed high school, he may not understand complex words. If English is a second language, attention must be paid to medical terminology. Developmentally appropriate language refers to the age of the patient and his or her ability to reason. Younger children do not have complex reasoning abilities, whereas adolescents do. Information for pediatric patients and families must meet their particular needs, and with modifications to make the language simpler and more concrete. The same is true for those patients with developmental delays or cognitive deficits. The stress of being in a health care setting impairs a person's ability to process information. The more anxious a person is, the less able she or he is to process information. Therefore, imparting information usually means providing information incrementally, at a fifth or sixth grade education level to allow patients and families to best hear and process what is being said.

CASE STUDY
*JQ, A 35-Year-Old with Gastric Cancer: Imparting Information*

JQ: I can't believe this. I want to go out with my friends. I can't be sick now. I have too much going on. They did the tests too quickly and didn't read them properly. They will just have to redo everything as I don't believe it.

NURSE: It must be hard to go through this.

JQ: Go through what? They just didn't do the tests right. I plan on leaving here and I will come back when they can focus on me. There have been too many people. Besides, my parents told me not to worry.

NURSE: Can you tell me what your doctor told you?

JQ: My cancer doctor told me I was cured of cancer. But I just have a little spot on my stomach. They just need to work on it. It is no big deal.

NURSE: What is your understanding of your type of cancer?

JQ: I have melanoma, which they can cut out and give me chemotherapy. They just need to figure out what to cut.

NURSE: This must be hard to take in. Would it be helpful to set a time to talk with your doctor again?

Here the nurse listens to the patient to hear what she understands and to assess her ability to process new information. Because the young woman is having difficulty processing the news, the nurse allows her to vent and validates her feelings.

**Listening**

Listening is an active process that requires full presence and attention. Specifically, one both listens to the words and interprets nonverbal gestures. Often it is very helpful to hear the patient's story in his or her own words. One helpful technique is to ask an open-ended question such as, "What brought you to the hospital?" or "Tell me about what has been going on?" This allows better understanding of the patient's journey within the disease trajectory and of how the patient is processing information. The nurse observes both the spoken verbal content in the patient's responses as well as the words left unsaid. Concurrently, the nurse observes the nonverbal expressions of emotion and any psychological or spiritual distress.[47]

During this process, the nurse listens to the patient's words and concerns without interrupting. The use of silence by the nurse is paramount. It is best to be present in the moment and not be mentally preparing answers or replies. In this way, the nurse uses self-reflection and conveys empathy. The nurse clarifies what has been heard by such comments as, "Hmm" or "Tell me more." By acknowledging the patient's comments and emotions and exploring their meaning in a compassionate and supportive way, the nurse encourages the patient to explain difficult issues and concerns.[48] There may be times when the patient is silent. In this circumstance, it may appropriate for the nurse to just sit quietly, letting the patient reflect on the moment and the current situation. It is at these moments of silence that a patient may relate an important concern at a deeper level because he or she has been given the opportunity and permission to do so.

CASE STUDY
*AS, A 54-Year-Old with Stage IV Lung Cancer: An Example of Listening*

AS is 54-year-old male with stage IV lung cancer

AS: I know I only have 6 months left. It is just so hard to talk about.

NURSE: Are there things in particular that are bothering you?

AS: Well, I am trying to plan things out. I used to like to go to the office just to get out. But now, everyone there, well they just ask me about my cancer. It is too hard emotionally. I hate having them feel sorry for me.

NURSE: What is it that happens?

AS: Well, once I get to the office, everyone tiptoes in and gives me the sad look. I can't stand it.

NURSE: Hmm.

AS: And then everyone is careful with me and won't disagree. We used to have such good debates.

NURSE: What would you like them to do?

AS: Fight with me as we did before. But I can see it in their eyes—"he is dying." I don't want to be reminded all the time.

NURSE: Do you think that is all they are thinking—that you are dying?

AS: I am not sure. They just don't know what to say. Sometimes, I think I should be home more. But then, my wife can't stand it. She won't talk about it. Do you notice she never comes in here when I have chemo?

NURSE: I did notice that. How does that make you feel?

AS: Sad. That is why I talk to you. I worry about her though. I wish she would come and talk with you too because it helps.

Here the nurse listens to the patient and his language. She shows that she is really listening by asking more questions so as not to assume meaning. The nurse also provides support by not trying to have all the answers and by letting the patient guide the conversation.

**Information Gathering**

To gather information from patients, the use of open-ended questions is most effective. This allows the patient to tell his or her story in narrative. During this process, the nurse therapeutically uses open-ended questions rather than "yes-or-no" questions or closed-ended questions. Open-ended questions allow the patient to tell his or her story, whereas closed-ended questions limit the patient's answers and thereby inhibit elaboration, explanations, and clarifications from the patient. Open-ended questions promote a richness in hearing the patient's words and nonverbal cues, which express issues of importance and priorities of care.[23] Open-ended questions may take many directions in terms of coping, life priorities, and spiritual concerns. Closed-ended questions include leading questions, questions that focus on physical symptoms, questions that do not address affect or coping, and questions that evoke advice giving rather that discussion.[35]

A nurse may not be able to ask many questions. However, a few key questions can set a tone of a caring relationship with the nurse. Table 5–1 offers a list of questions. Once such a question is asked, it is essential to listen to the answer. Often important questions are asked but, as the patient starts to answer, the conversation moves on, with no time or attention being given to hearing what the patient is expressing, no

---

Table 5–1
**Sample of Open-Ended Questions to Begin Discussions about Life-Threatening Illness**

What concerns you about your illness?
How are you doing with your illness?
How is treatment going for you?
What are your worries?
What are your hopes?
Who is important to you?
Who provides support to you?
What gives you meaning in your life?
What gives you joy in your life?
What provides you with the strength to live each day ?
Do you consider yourself spiritual or religious?
What rituals are important to you?
Is there any unfinished business you need to attend to?
What relationships are the most important to you?

*Sources:* Adapted from references 7, 23, 43.

---

further elaboration, and no response to the patient's verbal and nonverbal messages. This can cause resentment in the patient if he or she has shared something intimate without receiving acknowledgment of its significance.

CASE STUDY
*HR, A Patient with ESRD: An Example of Information Gathering*

HR is a 60-year-old female with ESRD and colon cancer. She is on hemodialysis. She has already undergone chemotherapy and surgery and is found to have another lesion in her colon.

HR: So what is going on here? I come in for a routine test for my kidneys and now I have colon cancer. I don't understand what the cancer is. Can you explain this to me?
NURSE: What do you need explained?
HR: I thought they had treated the cancer and it has come back. How could that be?
NURSE: Do you remember the principles of cancer?
HR: No not really.
NURSE: Well, once you have cancer, it can return. So yours has returned and you need more treatment for the cancer.
HR: But that is all a problem. I was trying to get on the list for a kidney transplant. Now, with the cancer I cannot. I had one year already and I needed two more years of cancer-free scans. Now I have to start over. How will they treat me?
NURSE: What did the oncologist tell you?
HR: She said 1 round of chemo and then surgery. Is that true?
NURSE: Yes that is true. You will be seeing the surgeon tomorrow who will confirm this.
HR: What type of chemo?
NURSE: It looks like the same as last time. How did you tolerate it?
HR: Okay. But I cannot think any more. I just have to take it one step at a time.
NURSE: That is okay. I can give you more information when you are ready.

Here the nurse evaluates the patient's knowledge of her disease and how much information she can handle. She is able to see that the patient cannot take in any more information.

**Sensitivity**

Sensitivity, another term for cultural competence, includes issues pertaining to religious, spiritual, cultural, ethnic, racial, gender, and language issues and is a very important element of communication. Not only is it important to appreciate verbal cues, but also it is critical to interpret nonverbal cues. Communication varies in different cultures. In many

Table 5–2
**Useful Cultural Assessment Questions**

Where were you born and raised?

What do you want to know about your medical condition/
illness?

How do you describe your medical condition/illness?

How have you treated your medical condition/illness?

Who else, if anyone, do you want to know about your
medical condition/illness?

Who else, if anyone, should we talk to about your
medical condition/illness, treatment options, and the
disease process?

Who is responsible for your health care decisions?

Who are important people in your community?

What do you fear most about your condition and its
treatment?

Are there any important rituals that are important to your
health care?

Are you spiritual or religious? How should we address that?

*Sources:* Adapted from references 7, 23, 25, 43.

situations, beneficence takes precedence over autonomy. Disclosure and nondisclosure must be viewed within the context of the patient and the family, with understanding of, and respect for, their values and beliefs.

In these situations, nurses must first examine their own cultural backgrounds and reflect upon their own ethical values and beliefs. Then, they can assess the communication patterns of the patient and the family, using questions from Table 5–2. For example, the nurse may ask the patient how she wants to receive medical information. The patient may state she wants to hear it directly, or she may defer to family members. Next, the nurse helps the patient identify others whom she wishes to be told about her medical issues. The nurse then may help the patient state who she wants to make health care and treatment decisions.

If the patient and family do not speak English as a first language, it is incumbent to use an interpreter for any discussions. Too often, family members are asked to interpret from English to another language, which puts them in a double bind. Culturally, although they may be translators, they must also act within their family roles and consequently they may need to protect the patient from information. This may result in the withholding of information if they are uncomfortable with what is being discussed. Therefore, it may be very unclear what the patient has actually been told.[49] For this reason, a professional interpreter should be used.

CASE STUDY
*LB, A Female from Ghana: An Example of Sensitivity*

LB is a woman from Ghana who is newly diagnosed with metastatic pancreatic cancer. Her family is her son and

daughter. She has been shy about questions. The family has told the nurse not to give LB any information.

LB: What is wrong with me? I am so nauseous? I cannot walk?
NURSE: What has the doctor told you?
LB: He says my liver is sick. I am not so sure. I went to a medicine man lately and he said I needed to use these herbs and pray more often.
NURSE: What has your family told you?
LB: They said I would get well soon. I just needed to try hard, and pray. I need to offer myself to God.
NURSE: Is that helpful?
LB: Sometimes, but other times I hurt so much. That is why I have my Bible here and my special crucifix.
NURSE: Would it be helpful to pray now?
LB: No, I will wait for my daughter.
NURSE: Well if you have any questions or you want any other support let me know.

Here the nurse clarifies and validates the patient's information preferences while respecting the patient's religious and cultural beliefs.

## Methods of Communications

The context in which communications occur influences the process and outcomes of interactions. Important information is best conveyed face-to-face, allowing observation of verbal as well as nonverbal communication by various team members. Scheduled meetings are good for both patients and health care providers. For the interdisciplinary health care team, scheduled meetings allow for preparation of the important information to be shared, including medical facts, prognosis, treatment options, and sources of support and guidance. They promote collaborative care by allowing the team (nurse, physician, social worker, and other clinicians) to review the information in order to provide a unified and consistent message to the patient and family. They also allow the bedside nurse to organize his or her day so as to be part of these important discussions.

The timing of communication is important. Quill and colleagues[50] defined the following "urgent" situations that necessitate immediate communication: (1) the patient is facing imminent death; (2) the patient is talking about wanting to die;[51] (3) the patient or family is inquiring about hospice; (4) the patient has recently been hospitalized for severe, progressive illness; and (5) the patient is experiencing severe suffering and poor prognosis.

Less urgent situations that require more routine planned meetings include (1) the discussion of prognosis, particularly if life expectancy is thought to be between 6 and 12 months; (2) the discussion of treatment options with low probability of success; and (3) the discussion of hopes and fears. End-of-life communication in more "routine" circumstances, when stability or recovery is predicted, normalizes the discussion of advanced care planning. These discussions assist the determination of the patient's values, goals, fears, and concerns while also developing the core issues for patient education, including the right to high-quality pain control and symptom management.[36]

## Scheduled Meetings

Scheduled meeting times are critical in allowing the patient to prepare emotionally and psychologically for any potential news. This includes allowing for the presence of the patient's support network to hear and validate information conveyed. Nurses play a vital role in these meetings because they are often responsible for arranging the meeting and securing a comfortable space. Before the meeting, the nurse may assess the patient's physical, emotional, and psychological concerns. This information can assist the team in planning discussion points at the scheduled meetings. After the meeting, the nurse can follow up and reinforce information conveyed.

Because of their perceived formality, scheduled meetings tend to take on more importance than informal meetings. Several steps are important to their success. After introductions have been done, the goals of the meeting can be stated. Then the patient can be asked about his or her understanding of the medical condition and situation. This is followed up by ascertaining the patient's worries and fears, how much information the patient wishes to know,[52] and which other people the patient wishes to be informed or involved in his or her care. A patient who is hesitant to express emotional concerns may need prompting or an invitation to speak. With overbearing families, it may be important to reinforce the goals of the meeting and to restate that the focus of care is on the patient.[53] The nurse may facilitate the initial conversation by serving as a reference point for the patient and family in conveying important concerns or worries from previous interactions. Often this occurs at the beginning of the meeting and personalizes the discussions to the specific needs of the patient and family. In addition, the nurse may act as a translator between the medical team and the patient, facilitating information sharing, interpreting information and medical jargon in language the patient understands, and also ensuring that the members of the care team understand the patient's words and language.

## Effective Communication

Effective communication, as viewed by terminally ill patients, their families, and health care professionals, primarily consists of providing accurate information in a sensitive, simple, and straightforward manner and in understandable language. Studies indicate that patients want their healthcare providers to be honest and straightforward, as well as hopeful. Therefore, the nurse should encourage questions from the patient and be responsive to his or her readiness to talk about death.[54] This can best be achieved by discussing outcomes other than cure, such as improved functional status or independence in care needs.

Focusing on quality of life offers hope and meaning to the patient, helping the patient prepare for losses and leaving open the possibility of "miracles."[55] The significance of nursing presence at any discussions between physician and patient—particularly when important information is conveyed—cannot be over-emphasized. Sometimes the nurse may be reticent and wait to be invited, rather than being proactive and offering to participate. Sometimes, the team needs to be reminded of the nurse's important role in advocating for the patient and being able to follow up in subsequent discussions. If the primary nurse is not able to participate in the delivery of difficult information, a nursing colleague may participate. If this is not possible, it is essential that the team review the specifics about the conversation with the nurse—in particular the news delivered, the wording used and the patient's response. This allows the nurse to provide collaborative follow-up support.

The context in which communications occur influences the process and outcomes of interactions. Because of the rapidly changing complexity of health care, important information is best conveyed in face-to-face meetings between health care providers and patients and families. This allows the patient and family to plan their schedules and formulate questions and concerns. Moreover, having all providers in the room at the same time promotes unity and consistency in the messages being delivered. Planned meetings also allow the bedside nurse to organize his or her day so as to be part of these important discussions. For the interdisciplinary health care team, meetings allow for optimal preparation and delivery of important information, including medical facts, prognosis, treatment options, and sources of support and guidance.

## Patient and Family Meetings

Patient and family meetings are a wonderful but greatly underutilized tool. Moreover, with even simple technology, family meetings can include members not actually present by means of cell phones, teleconferencing, or videoconferencing. Most clinicians, with the exception of social workers, have not been taught how to effectively run a family meeting. Family meetings help the family understand the involvement of various health care providers, the disease process, and options of care. They also reassure families that a plan is in place and everyone is working toward a consistent goal. The family meeting also provides clinicians an opportunity to collaboratively formulate a plan of care that is consistent with the goals and wishes of the patient and family.

These meetings promote the respectful and sensitive conveyance of information. Nurses play a vital role in these meetings because they are often responsible for arranging the meeting and securing a comfortable space. Before the meeting, the nurse may assess the patient's physical, emotional, and psychological concerns. This information can assist the team in planning discussion points at the meeting. After the meeting, the nurse can follow up and reinforce information conveyed.

Before calling a family meeting, it is important to clarify the goal for the meeting, to maximize the effective use of time. This can range simply from an update of care to discussing withdrawal of technological interventions. Consideration should be given to the attendance of key and central health care providers, who should meet at least a few minutes before the meeting to clarify the messages to be conveyed. For more complex or contentious families, having a meeting specifically to plan strategies to deal with a difficult family is time well spent.

The actual steps for a family meeting are fairly straightforward and based on common sense. There are eight steps.[28] (1) finding an appropriately private space for the meeting, (2) introductions of all the participants at the meeting, (3) using open-ended questions to establish what the patient (and family) knows, (4) determining how the patient wishes the information to be presented, (5) presenting information in a straightforward manner, using understandable language, in small quantities and with pauses for processing and questions to assess understanding, (6) responding to emotions, (7) clarifying goals of care and treatment priorities, and (8) establishing a plan.

The patient may or may not attend depending on his or her condition, decision-making capacity, and preference for involvement. Sometimes the family may not have met various members of the team and not all health care providers know each other. One clinician should take the lead, ensuring that everyone in the room is introduced, and reviewing the goal of the meeting. The nurse may facilitate the initial conversation by serving as a focal point for continuity of care. The meeting may proceed as suggested under the section of Scheduled Meetings. This includes determining the both the patient and family understanding of illness, their values, preferences, and beliefs along with their informational needs for decision-making (see Table 5–3).

At this point, the family's understanding and perception of the patient's current condition should be sought. Sometimes overbearing families may shift the conversation to their own needs and concerns. It is important to reinforce the goals of the meeting and to restate that the focus of care is on the patient.[53] The speaker may offer a summary of the care. The next part of the meeting addresses questions and issues that require clarification. After this discussion, the lead person can summarize the issues and collaboratively develop a plan of care. If the patient/family agrees to the plan, the meeting can end with a synopsis of the meeting and the decisions made. If the family disagrees, another meeting can be suggested. One of the most important tasks after the meeting is documentation. The names and titles of the people who attended, the issues discussed, and the decisions made should be documented in the medical record, as outlined in Table 5–4.

---

**Table 5–3**
**Questions to Address Patients' and Families' Coping**

Have you/your family been through something like this before? How did you/your family react/cope?

Do you have a belief in a higher power that supports you?

Is there anyone you'd like us to call?

Can you anticipate any potential areas of concern for you and your family?

Who could you call if you started to feel really sad?

Did the patient ever tell you what they wanted for themselves?

Is there anyone you think the patient would like to see?

Who is supporting you now?

Who can you call when things get more difficult?

---

**Table 5–4**
**The Family Meeting**

**Calling a family meeting**

1. Clarify goals of meeting with patient and family and staff.
2. Providers should meet beforehand to assure consistency of message and process.
3. Decide the appropriate people to attend—patient, family, and health care providers.

**The actual meeting**

4. Arrange appropriate setting.
5. Introductions of everyone in room and relationship to patient.
6. Review goal of meeting.
7. Elicit patient/family understanding of care to date.
8. Review of current medical condition.
9. Questions.
10. Options for care.
11. Elicit response from patient if decisional.
12. Elicit response from family in terms of what patient would choose for him or her if he/she could.

**Summary**

13. Review plan. If agreement—then decision.
    If no agreement—what follow-up is planned?
14. Document meeting—who attended, what was discussed, and plan.

*Sources:* Adapted from references 7, 36, 99.

---

## Types of Patient and Family Meetings

There are several types of meetings that occur within the context of palliative care: information meetings, advanced care planning meetings, bad news discussions and code status discussions. The first is straightforward information meetings. These can occur to start the relationship between the patient and family and the care team. These may have no particular agenda other than to convey information about the patient's current status. There may be no decisions to be made and no future planning. Advanced care planning is a process that ideally begins when a patient enters a health care system. However, it should always be revisited upon diagnosis of a life limiting illness. Bad news discussions occur when disease progression occurs. Finally, code status discussions take place when a crisis occurs, the patient's status is unstable, and a decision must be made as to whether to transfer to a critical care setting or initiate life sustaining therapies. These discussions should ideally take place before a crisis occurs.

## Advance Care Planning

The National Consensus Project for Quality Palliative Care *Clinical Practice Guidelines for Quality Palliative Care* has several guidelines that refer to communication. Under *Domain 1: Structure and Processes of Care*, Guideline 1.2 states "the care plan is based on the identified and expressed preferences, values, goals, and needs of the patient and the family and is developed with professional guidance and support for decision making."[18] Under *Domain 8: Ethical and Legal Aspects of Care*, Guideline 8.1 states "the patients' goals, preferences, and choices are respected within the limits of applicable state and federal law, within current accepted standards of medical care, and form the basis for the plan of care.[18] Thus, the importance of advanced care planning, as much as possible, is paramount to palliative care.

The nurse's role in this has been delineated by The American Nurses Association (ANA). The ANA stated that nurses "have a responsibility to facilitate informed decision-making, including but not limited to advance directives."[56] Nurses play a critical role in advocating for and implementing the patient's wishes and preferences and communicating these to family members and other health care providers. As such, the nurse has a role in advocating the implementation of the patient's wishes.[56] Nurses at all levels provide important assistance in helping patients define their goals and wishes and express their cultural and religious practices and preferences.

Advanced care planning is a social process based on the ethical principle of autonomy of the patient. It focuses on completing written advance directive forms, to promote the relief of the burden of decision-making on other people. For the patient, advanced care planning may be regarded as a mechanism to prepare for death. For the health care provider, advanced care planning prepares for the possibility that the patient may become incapable of making decisions. These discussions are best completed over time, allowing the patient opportunity for reflection and discussion with family and friends about possible scenarios, which in itself may prepare the patient for the course of disease.

It is widely agreed that discussions about advanced care planning and completion of advance directives should occur before acute, disabling events and hopefully before the end stage of a terminal illness. However, these conversations do not occur earlier, for a number of reasons: reluctance to initiate such discussions due to time constraints, lack of comfort with such discussions, lack of skills in such communications, and fear of upsetting the patient even though she or he may wish to have the conversation. A study of patients 50 years of age and older who had at least one chronic, morbid medical condition (ischemic heart disease, chronic heart failure, chronic obstructive pulmonary disease, cerebrovascular disease, cancer, chronic renal disease, or chronic liver disease) found that greater satisfaction with the primary care physician was expressed if advance directives were discussed during outpatient visits.[57]

Although patients may differ in the extent to which they wish to participate in treatment decisions, a number of studies have indicated preference to participate in a collaborative process. Being provided with adequate information is critical. However, simply being offered choices, particularly without any direction, can cause a patient to feel excessively burdened and responsible. The weight of these decisions can cause patients and families to feel a sense of self blame or to lose confidence in the physician, particularly if the outcome is poor. Therefore, it is critically important to identify how much the patient wishes to be involved in decision-making at all stages of disease.[58]

The process of advanced care planning involves setting goals of therapy, developing care directives, and making decisions about specific forms of medical therapy. It is more effective if the patient has previous experience with poor health and death of family members.[26,59] For chronically ill, debilitated, and terminally ill patients, advanced care planning includes making decisions about life-sustaining therapies (code status), artificial feeding and hydration, and palliative and hospice care. Performing advanced care planning prepares for both incapacity and death, relieves burdens on others, solidifies relationships,[59] and identifies appropriate surrogates and delineates their authority.[60,61] For the terminally ill patient, the health care provider may begin the discussion about planning for the future by asking any of a number of questions, as described in Table 5–5.

Because survival estimates affect the decisions patients make, patients need accurate prognostic information. The disparity of estimated survival times may confuse patients, particularly with other references such as the Internet readily available. Interviews of 56 terminally ill patients concluded that all patients wanted their physicians to be honest about the prognoses conveyed.[62] However, physicians often do poorly at estimating and reporting accurate survival times to patients.[63,64] Therefore, it is very helpful for nurses to be in attendance when such information is delivered. The patient's wish to hear optimistic information and the physician's reluctance to present information on disease progression may impair accurate portrayal of the patient's condition.[37] Given their knowledge and working with professional colleagues, nurses may also temper the overly optimistic survival times.

Discussions between patients and providers about complementary treatments are essential to promote realistic outcomes.[65] Some of this information, including complementary and alternative treatments, may be inaccurate, harmful, or

Table 5–5
Questions for Advance Directive Conversations

**Normalizing comments/questions:**
I'd like to talk with you about possible health care decisions in the future.
I'd like to discuss something I discuss with all patients admitted to the hospital.
We often like to make sure we understand patients' preferences and wishes for aggressive care when there is serious change in condition. I would like to discuss your feelings about going to the emergency room, the intensive care unit, and being on life support.

**Inquiries of patient's understanding of illness:**
What do you understand about your current health situation?
What do you understand from what the doctors have told you?

**Inquiries to elicit hopes and expectations:**
What do you expect in the future?
Have you ever thought about if things don't go the way you hoped?
How can we help you live in the best way possible for you?
How do you wish to spend whatever time you have left?
What activities or experiences are most important for you to do to maximize the quality of your life?

**Inquiries to elicit thoughts regarding cardiopulmonary resuscitation:**
If you should stop breathing or your heart stops breathing, would you want us to use 'heroic measures' to bring you back?
Have you ever thought about if something were to happen to you and you could not breathe or your heart won't work on your own?
Have you ever thought about life support?
Have you given any thought to what kinds of treatment you would want or not want if you become unable to speak for yourself in the future?

**For the family**
Did the patient ever tell you what he or she wanted for him or herself?
Did he or she ever talk about life prolonging therapies?
Did he or she ever talk about the care of another family member and state whether they would have wanted the same type of treatment?

A change in focus from future cure-oriented treatments to goals of current living may facilitate discussions of 1meaning and purpose.[66] Having the patient consider such questions as, "What if we are not sure whether we will be able to get you off the breathing machine?" can help facilitate thought and decision about how much chance of success a patient needs to have to make certain decisions.[67] After patients understand their condition, options for therapy, and potential circumstances of death, they may share their values and express their preferences for care. The result may be a sense of control, a sense of trust with health care providers, and a sense of resolution in aspects of one's life.

Studies have been conducted on patients', families', physicians', and other caregivers' preferences regarding preparing for the end of life. All agree on the importance of (1) naming someone to make decisions, (2) knowing what to expect about one's physical condition, (3) having financial affairs in order, (4) having treatment preferences in writing, and (5) knowing that one's physician is comfortable talking about death and dying. Not surprisingly, patients were less inclined to talk about personal fears than were families, physicians, and other caregivers.[68] Patients, more than others, want to know the timing of death and make funeral plans. Identified as the most important factors in achieving quality at the end of life were the relief of pain and other distressing symptoms, communication with one's physician, preparation for death, and the opportunity to achieve a sense of completion. In spite of widespread agreement about the importance of preparation, such discussions often are not included in clinical encounters.[68]

Quill[36] emphasized the importance of these end-of-life conversations in their early, systematic occurrence. He described how the early introduction of such conversations in the disease process promotes better outcomes. These outcomes include more informed choices, better palliation of symptoms, and more opportunity for resolution of important issues. Such questions as, "Are there things that would be left undone if you were to die sooner rather than later?" stimulate thought and discussion about dying and important life closure issues such as healing relationships and completing financial transactions. However, a nurse may ask this in a different way, such as, "Are there things you need to do in case things do not go as well as we hope?"[69] Encouraging patients to hope for the best outcome while preparing for the possibility that treatment may not work is helpful in guiding the patient.[70] Again, the nurse advocate role facilitates the provision of all essential information the patient needs to make choices.

Nurses may be particularly helpful in advocating for patients when they are unable to speak for themselves. The nurse may assist the surrogate to convey the patient's wishes. If the surrogate is not certain about the patient's wishes or if no advance directive is available, the nurse, by posing questions such as those recommended by Harlow in "Family Letter Writing,"[71] can be very helpful. Such questions include, "What type of person was the patient?," "Did she/he ever comment on another person's situation when they were

inapplicable when put in context of the patient's situation. Promoting open dialogue of complementary and alternative therapies allows for a more honest discussion as to the utilization of such therapies. Just as a nurse discusses the benefits and burdens of traditional treatment, patients need to also be informed of the benefits and burdens of complementary and alternative therapies. Moreover, it establishes a more collaborative relationship between patient and nurse, as well as nurse and complementary provider.

incapacitated or on life support?," "Did she/he relate those experiences to her/his own personal views of her/himself?," and "What vignettes can you recall from his/her life that illustrates his/her values?"[71] In addition to helping to clarify a patient's wishes, addressing these questions may also serve as a healing review of the person's life and help identify what has brought them meaning. The nurse is often the best person to engage the family in such reflections and discussions, as they have had ample opportunity to talk during patient care.[72]

## Bad News Discussions

Bad or unfavorable medical news may be defined as "any news that drastically and negatively alters the patient's view of her or his future."[73] In palliative care, bad news includes, but is not limited to, disease diagnosis, recurrence, disease progression, lack of further curative treatments, transition to comfort care, and a terminal prognosis for a patient's condition. Nurses, particularly APNs, along with their physician colleagues, generally have the responsibility of communicating such information to a patient. The decision as to who delivers the news may depend on the relationship of the patient with the team, the clinician the patient most trusts and, sometimes, institutional culture or practice guidelines.

Two survey studies of oncology physicians conducted by Baile and colleagues provide insight. One study reported that 22% of oncology physicians had no consistent manner of communicating bad news, and 51.9% used several techniques or tactics without having an overall plan.[74] The second study revealed considerable variability in disclosing diagnoses and prognoses, reporting the absence of further curative treatments, discussing resuscitation, and making recommendations for hospice services.[75] There have been no such surveys among nurses but, given the lack of education in this area, there is a high probability that the findings would be similar.

Coyle and Sculco beautifully describe the emotional setting of giving bad news for the clinician and the patient (p. 212).[76]

> Is it possible for any news, transmitted by a doctor [or nurse] to a patient, to be "good news" in the face of advancing disease that is not responsive to chemotherapy? The doctor [or nurse] is in a position of having to give information that the patient does not want to hear, and yet the patient needs to have the information in order to make necessary life decisions. Does it matter how the information is given when medical information itself can remove hope for continued existence? In a way, both parties—the doctor and the patient—are engaged in a communication dance of vulnerability. The physician is vulnerable because he/she must deliver the facts, whatever they may be, and the patient is vulnerable because he/she doesn't want to hear any more bad news.

Moreover, both physicians and nurses can be part of this communication dance. From this author's experience and the literature, patients with advanced disease generally do want to have the information. Nurses may feel in the middle of a rock and a hard place, wanting to tell patients more but feeling it is not within their scope of practice, while physicians may want to tell less because they don't want to feel they have failed the patient. In addition, families may try to prevent any difficult communication. In a report by Yun and colleagues,[77] 96% of 380 cancer patients and 76.9% of 280 family members stated that patients should be informed of a terminal illness. Not surprisingly, some discrepancy was apparent between the opinions of patients and those of family members regarding disclosure. Another study of cancer patients' perspectives concluded that the most important factors when receiving bad news were the expertise of the physician and being given pertinent information about their condition and treatment options. Other lesser, but still important, aspects of bad news delivery related to content, setting, and supportive aspects of the meetings.[55]

It should be noted that, although patients may want to have the information, they may be reluctant to initiate such a discussion.[78] Moreover, patients may not be actively invited to express their feelings and concerns. One study showed that patients not provided with an opportunity to disclose concerns before the information is provided tended to remain silently preoccupied with the information and were more likely to develop a pessimistic sense of their situation, compared with patients who were invited to share and discuss their concerns.[79]

Behaviors used in presenting unfavorable information may be grouped into four domains: (1) preparation, (2) delivering the content of the message, (3) dealing with the responses of the patient (and family), and (4) closing the encounter.[80] Essential within the preparation of giving bad news is attention to the health care provider's own emotional stress. There may be a range of possible feelings: guilt, lack of control, failure, loss, fear, or resentment.[81] Awareness of these feelings allows for clarity in ownership of issues and a more objective encounter. Nurses, in particular, may also need to deal with their own sense of anxiety that results from closely empathizing with the patient.[82]

Recommended guidelines that have been developed for delivering unfavorable or bad news are similar to those of scheduled meetings. Based on a review of the literature and a consensus panel of patients and physicians, Girgis and Sanson-Fisher[83] recommended the following: (1) ensuring privacy and adequate time, (2) assessing patients' understanding, (3) providing information about diagnosis and prognosis simply and honestly, (4) avoiding the use of euphemisms, (5) encouraging patients to express their feelings, (6) being empathetic, (7) giving a broad but realistic time frame regarding prognosis, and (8) arranging review or follow-up. Other points are summarized in Table 5–6.

In response to presenting bad news, patients may ask difficult questions, such as, "Why me?" One approach to

**Table 5–6**
**Delivering Bad News**

1. Create a physical setting consisting of a quiet, comfortable room with all participants sitting and free of interruptions. Obtain interpreter as needed. Prepare for the meeting.
2. Determine who should be present.
3. Clarify and clearly state your and the patient's goals for the meeting.
4. Determine what the patient and family know about the patient's condition and what they have been told.
5. Provide the foundation of a brief overview of the patient's course and condition for understanding of the entire group.
6. Give a warning—"Unfortunately, I have some bad news to share with you." Others have suggested stating, "I wish things were different,"[33] then pause.
7. Sit quietly and allow the patient and family to absorb the information. Wait for the patient to respond. After being silent, check in with the patient such as by saying, "I have just told you some pretty serious news. Do you feel comfortable sharing your thoughts about this?" This may help the patient verbalize concerns.[52]
8. Listen carefully and acknowledge the patient's and family's emotions such as by reflecting on both the meaning and the affect of their responses. Give an opportunity for questions and comments.

answering the question is to maintain a sense of openness and curiosity,[84] and not to assume that it is a direct question that necessitates and answer. An acknowledgment, such as "That is a tough question," allows the nurse to comment and explore further without feeling the need to solve or "fix" the assumed source of the patient's question or comment. This can be followed up by, "Please tell me what you are concerned about." The nurse, by acknowledging and normalizing the patient's feelings, invites the patient to voice his or her thoughts, feelings, and concerns. By sharing the patient's distress, the nurse may reduce the patient's sense of isolation and suffering.

Another common and difficult question is the patient's response to such news with the questions, "How long do I have to live?" Responding to and acknowledging such a question normalizes the discussion around death and dying. The nurse may choose to answer in several ways, depending on his or her comfort in these discussions. One response is, "Are you asking something specific?" Here the nurse is trying to ascertain whether the patient is asking about dying or is thinking of a certain event that he or she wishes to live to experience. Another response is, "How long do you think you have to live?" This allows the patient to voice his or her concern about time. The patient may say, "Not long, but I wanted to see how long you thought," as if to compare input from different members of the team. A third response is, "Why do you ask?" This invites the patient to share his or her fears and concerns about dying. The nurse may also reflect on difficult information with, "I imagine it is very frightening not

knowing what will happen and when. Do you have particular fears and concerns?" Finally, if the anticipated survival time is short or the nurse is uncomfortable, the reply, "What has the team told you?" may be used. In this case, the patient may state that the team has given a certain estimate of time, or the patient may be seeking validation of the prediction.

After listening to the patient's and family members' fears and concerns, it is essential to provide accurate, hopeful information while deliberately addressing the issue of abandonment. This can be done with such words as, "I wish things were different. But no matter what, I will be there to support you in your decisions and focus on your quality of life." This allays fear that because the patient can no longer tolerate treatment, the providers will no longer have contact with them.

## Discussions of the Use of Life-Sustaining Therapies or Code Status

Often when patients are critically ill and have advanced disease, the health care team seeks clarification on how aggressively to initiate life-sustaining measures. "Code status" is commonly defined as the use, or limitation of use, of life-sustaining therapy in the event of clinical deterioration of respiratory function and/or cardiac arrest. Life-sustaining measures include nasotracheal intubation and mechanically assisted ventilation and cardiac resuscitation, the combination of which is called Cardiopulmonary Resuscitation or CPR. Other measures may include pressers to help the heart pump more efficiently and effectively, dialysis for kidney failure, and antibiotics for infections. If a patient in any setting experiences a cardiac arrest and/or respiratory failure, usually emergency personnel are called upon to respond to keep the patient alive. CPR is performed unless the patient, or the patient's surrogate, has indicated the patient's desire not to be resuscitated (DNR) and/or not to be intubated and supported with mechanical ventilation (DNI). When patient's wishes for or against application of these medical interventions or treatments are being discussed and documented in the medical record, the process is often referred to as "getting the code status" or discussing "Do-Not-Resuscitate" orders.[85]

There are several important concepts around code status discussions. Just discussing code status alone is worthless as it offers little insight into the patient's preferences, values or beliefs. Alone, a code status tells the health care team whether or not to perform a procedure. Use of medical vernacular, such as "full code" or "no code" and "Do you want everything done?" is ambiguous at best, and offers little guidance. Rather, it is helpful to promote a discussion on quality of life for the patient which guides care in avoiding unacceptable conditions. Particular to this discussion, it is essential to place the conversation in the context of the patient's wishes for goals of therapy. It is imperative to convey to the patient or health care agent the very low likelihood of survival after CPR in the presence of terminal illness.[86]

**Table 5-7**
**Further Questions to Consider End-of-Life Discussions**

How can we help you live in the best way possible for you?

How do you wish to spend the time you have left?

What activities or experiences are most important for you to do to maximize the quality of your life?

What fears or worries do you have about your illness, about or medical care?

Do you have other worries or fears?

What do you hope for your family?

What needs or services would you like to talk about?

What do you now find particularly challenging in your life?

Do you have religious or spiritual beliefs that are important to you?

What would make this time especially meaningful for you?

How would you describe quality of life?

What would not be quality of life?

What makes life worth living for you?

What would be an unacceptable life?

Patients are less likely to opt for CPR knowing that almost no patients with severe, multiple, chronic illnesses who receive CPR in a hospital survive to discharge.[67,87] Table 5-7 lists questions that may be helpful in facilitating communications about advance directives.

The goal of these discussions is to review the anticipated benefits and burdens of interventions without placing any responsibility on the patient and family. Important elements of this discussion include sensitivity to, acknowledgment of, and response to emotions of the patient, family, and surrogate. To dispel concerns of abandonment, it is particularly important to reassure the patient, family, and surrogate that even though CPR will not be performed, all beneficial care will be actively provided. The final task is to develop and document a plan and share this information with other health care professionals caring for the patient.[88] This may be done through documenting the conversation and completing state-recognized comfort care/DNR order forms.

As stated before, the process is similar to other patient and family meetings. The recommended steps include: (1) establishing an appropriate setting, (2) inquiring of patient and family what they understand of the patient's condition, (3) finding out what the patient expects for the future, (4) discussing the DNR order with the patient in the context of the patient's understanding of present condition and thoughts of the future, including the context in which resuscitation would be considered, (5) responding to the patient's emotions, and (6) developing a plan.[89]

Nurses are heavily invested in clarification of code status. They are often the ones who find the patient with a life threatening illness in respiratory or cardiac arrest and must initiate a code. Most nurses want to quickly establish the code status with providers familiar with the patient's medical condition. Nurses fear situations in which the primary physician is unavailable, and they must deal with a covering physician unfamiliar with the patient and goals of care. It is not uncommon that the wish for code status clarification arises from concerned nurses who do not want to call a code unless the patient and family want to undergo that procedure.

Because of the 24-hour presence with the patient, the nurse may be the one to whom the patient and family turn for explanations, recommendations, reassurance, validation, and support. Questions to the nurse may focus on the meaning of medical jargon such as "CPR/DNR/DNI", presser support, ventilators, etc. This may include queries from the patient and family such as, "What do you think?" or "What should I do?" The nurse can offer the facts and reflect back the patient's values and preferences such as, "Mr. X, you told me you want to be comfortable and not return to the hospital. We can get support at home to keep you comfortable and aggressively treat any symptoms." Reassurance and support for the appropriateness of preferences and decisions develops from questions such as, "Do you feel I made the right decision?" or "What would you do?" They may need reassurance that the nurses will continue to provide care. By educating the patient about the actual intervention and likely outcome, a nurse may be able to reassure the patient.[72]

There are often circumstances when the patient and family convey their overwhelming sense of pressure or responsibility about the decisions they are being asked to make. When this occurs, it may be that the responsibility of making such a decision is too great for patients and families. They may feel that by making a choice to refuse resuscitation, they are "pulling the plug." In these situations, the nurse can offer a plan and then ask for agreement from the patient and family. Thus, they are reaching decision-making by assent to a procedure rather than informed consent. Assent means the families if told of an option and they agree to it. Consent means the families is offered a range of options and they chose which option. By assenting, the burden of the decision is removed from the family and placed on the care team. The patient and family don't have to decide from a range of options but rather just agree to the plan. For many families, this feels like less of a burden as the team makes the difficult decision. It may still be the same plan, but the team has allowed the patient and family to "un-shoulder" the burden or weight of the decision.

## Conversations About Artificial Hydration and Nutrition

Numerous cultures place great social and cultural importance on drinking and eating. When patients are not able to take food or fluid by mouth, artificial hydration and nutrition may be provided through the gastrointestinal tract using a nasogastric or gastric tube or administering intravenously. Many people believe that not eating and drinking causes great physical suffering. Therefore, it is necessary to discuss the potential benefits and burdens of both instituting and withholding artificial hydration and nutrition. The rationale for and against these procedures is discussed in Chapter 62,

"Ethical Considerations." Nonetheless, there are several important communication points regarding artificial hydration and nutrition. Thus discussion with the patient and/or the patient's surrogate should include: (1) perception of the benefits and burdens of artificial hydration and the suffering with or without these interventions; (2) any values, beliefs, and culture of the patient and family that affect the decision or need for such interventions; (3) the available data regarding the benefits and burdens of the interventions; and (4) collaborative decision-making about these interventions to meet the patient's goals.

The risks and burdens of artificial hydration and nutrition include lung congestion and increased respiratory tract secretions, increased edema with its attendant pain at sites of tumors and inflammation, more urine production, more peripheral swelling (particularly in the setting of liver or kidney disease), and skin breakdown. Feeding tubes and intravenous lines may be painful, carry risks of infections, and may be fraught with complications. These may include restraint of the patient to prevent removal, which can cause secondary agitation and may also result in accelerated skin breakdown from less turning in bed.

The benefits of artificial hydration and nutrition may be comfort, particularly for patients who have nausea and vomiting related to dehydration or electrolyte imbalances. Patients with hypercalcemia may be more alert. Extra fluids may prolong a dying process, which may be necessary for life closure. Finally, for some cultures, intravenous fluids and nutrition may be necessary for any prohibitions on hastening death. Artificial hydration and nutrition may alleviate any guilt for patients and family arising out of the feeling that they had not tried everything.

There are myriad nursing interventions to replace artificial nutrition and hydration. Maximal safe and appropriate intake can be evaluated by a speech and language pathologist or a swallowing therapist if appropriate. Families can be taught to provide relief with sips of water, ice chips, and conscientious mouth and lip care.[85]

## Conversations About the Transition to Palliative Care or Hospice

The transition from curative to palliative care is often an emotional time for patients, families, and clinicians alike. Patients may feel a sense of sadness, anger, denial, and loss of control to the disease. Families may suddenly understand the serious nature of the illness in its real sense. Physicians may feel a sense of failure for not curing the disease, a lack of confidence in not knowing what else they can do for the patient, and perhaps worry about their own personal reactions as well as patients' emotions.[80] Nurses may feel frustration and disappointment if a patient is not well informed on how to accomplish life closure.

A number of specific questions may address feelings of powerlessness, uncertainty, isolation, and helplessness that otherwise could lead to a sense of hopelessness in the patient.

| Table 5–8<br>Questions for Changing Goals of Care |
| --- |
| Tell me about the history of your illness. |
| What do you understand as your treatment options? |
| What are some of the concerns you have at this time? |
| What, if anything, are you worried about or afraid of? |
| Have you had other family members or other loved ones die? How was their death? What was that like for you? |
| What practical problems is your illness creating for you? |
| Are there any family members of loved-ones who need to know what's going on? |
| Given the severity of your illness, what is most important for you to achieve? |
| What are your most important hopes? |
| What are your biggest fears? |
| What makes life most worth living for you? |
| Would there be any circumstances under which you would find life not worth living? |
| What do you consider your quality of life to be like now? |
| Have you seen or been with someone who had a particularly good death or particularly difficult death? |
| Have you given any thought to what kinds of treatment you would want (and not want) if you become unable to speak for yourself in the future? |
| Are there important things you need to do for closure? |
| How is your family handling your illness? What are their reactions? |
| Are there any spiritual issues you are concerned about at this point? |
| Has religion been an important part of your life? |
| We want to focus on maximal comfort and optimal functioning with as much support as possible. Is that okay? |

These queries focus on expectations regarding the patient's decline and the patient's involvement in decision-making, as well as encouraging relationships and connections with important people.[90] Such discussions lend themselves to strategies for life closure in identifying patient goals and purposes, preparation for death, leaving a legacy for loved ones, and often legal and financial issues. Completing these tasks frees the patient to concentrate on emotional and spiritual matters and to enjoy the company of loved ones.[91]

Guidelines for initiating end-of-life conversations during the last phase of life include (1) focusing on the patients' unique experiences of illness, (2) helping patients confront their fears, (3) helping patients address practical issues, (4) facilitating the shift to palliative care, and (5) helping the patient achieve a peaceful and dignified death.[92] This means that each situation is individual and cannot be determined by an algorithm or recipe approach (Table 5–8).

This conversation is vital to help the patient and family prepare for death in as comfortable and meaningful a way as possible. The focus shifts to the psychological and spiritual aspects of care.[85,93,94] A direct approach is helpful such as, "We do not have any more therapies to cure your disease. We would like to focus on comfort and maximal pain and

**Table 5–9**
**Questions to Facilitate Quality-of-Life Discussions**

How is your quality of life?

Is this how you thought it would be?

How do you spend your days?

If you were not ill, how would you spend your time or how would you like to spend your time?

Which symptoms bother you the most?

How has your disease interfered with your daily activities?

How are things with family and friends?

Have you been feeling worried, sad or frightened about your illness?

How have your religious or spiritual beliefs been affected by your illness?

Do you have a preference for where you spend your time, at home, in the hospital, or at appointments?

symptom management. We also have specially trained nurses who care for patients with life threatening illness and help them stay at home. We will work with them to focus on maximal functioning and quality of life." This allows patient and families to know that they will continue to be cared for and not abandoned. Both patients and physicians display reluctance to discuss psychosocial issues unless the other party initiates the discussion.[53] It behooves nurses, along with social work colleagues, to initiate such conversations, because the evidence suggests that little time is devoted to quality-of-life issues during outpatient palliative care visits.[95] Table 5–9 lists open-ended questions that help facilitate quality-of-life discussions with patients.[87,95]

Nursing has a central role in helping patients and their families at times of transition. The nurse in the hospital helps the transition to a home care or hospice team and reinforces for patient and family the skills of the new specialized health care providers. The APN may also assist the patient in this transition and develop orders for the treatment plan. Once the patient is at home, the hospice nurses begin to empower family and friends to care for the patient through the implementation of the plan of care.

CASE STUDY

*Mack, A 73-Year-Old with Esophageal Cancer: Example of APN Discussing Changing Disease*

Mack is a 73 year old with recently diagnosed esophageal cancer. He has been in the hospital three times for confusion and weakness. His pain is worse. Mary, the APN, talks with him about his worries.

MARY: Mack, you have been in the hospital three times in the last 8 weeks. I am worried about how you are doing with treatment.

MACK: I am fine. I just am weak, that's all. If I get a bit stronger and if I could eat more, I could take the treatment just fine.

MARY: Well, we haven't been able to give you treatment because you have been so weak.

MACK: Well, that is okay, we can keep trying.

MARY: Mack, if you continue to be this weak, we won't be able to give you treatment. Then that will mean we have nothing to contain the cancer.

MACK: Are you saying that if I can't get stronger, there is no treatment?

MARY: Yes.

MACK: If I don't have treatment, then I will die.

MARY: Yes.

MACK: How can that be possible?

MARY: Well, remember when you came in, we discussed your cancer. Remember that you had been experiencing symptoms for awhile. Remember that when we discussed treatment, we stated it was no longer for cure, but for palliation.

MACK: Yes.

MARY: So we said we would try to get you strong enough to take chemotherapy. However, if you remained weak, that the chemotherapy would do more harm than good.

MACK: Yes, I remember that.

MARY: Mack, we are at that point. We think that chemotherapy would cause more burden than benefit. At this point, we need to focus on treating your symptoms and optimizing your quality of life rather than trying to give you treatment that will continue to cause more distress and symptoms.

MACK: I worried that we might be at that point, but I hadn't wanted to think about it. Does my wife know this yet?

MARY: No, would you like help in talking to her?

MACK: Yes, she will be back in a bit and she will know something is wrong. We can talk to her then.

Here the APN helps the patient review his own symptoms to realize how ill he is. She then helps Mack focus on quality of life.

## Transition to Death

When curing is no longer viable and this message is communicated to or intuited by the patient, a pregnant moment for healing arises for both physician and patient. The focus and fight for life can give way to a new alliance based on sharing the inevitability of the human contract. This sharing, in and of itself, can have an exponential benefit on the patient's subjective sense of well-being.[96]

As death draws near, the nurse's communications with the patient and family may facilitate comfort and healing in a number of ways. The nurse should review the actual physiological and biological process of dying in language that also addresses the benefits and burdens of various interventions. Pain and symptom management is based upon a patient's previously stated preferences regarding alleviation versus desired level of alertness, as well as preferences around artificial hydration and nutrition. Often this includes discussion about the withdrawal of ineffective and/or burdensome medical treatments. Simple presence, listening, and attending to the basic humanity of the dying patient may be one of the nurse's most powerful contributions.

The simple act of visitation, of presence, of taking the trouble to witness the patient's process can in itself be a potent healing affirmation—a sacramental gesture received by the dying person who may be feeling helpless, diminished, and fearful that he or she has little to offer others. The patient may also fear that he or she has failed....I and many dying persons would agree that beyond pain control, the three elements we most need are feeling cared about, being respected, and enjoying a sense of continuity—be it in relationships or in terms of spiritual awareness.[96]

The communication skills required include: being present with the patient in his or her state of vulnerability and decline; consciously and non-judgmentally listening and bearing witness to the patient; and encouraging the patient to express all feelings while resisting defensiveness if the patient voices anger or disappointment about dying.

The willingness to extend freshness, innocence, and sincere concern to the patient far outweighs any technique or expertise in the art of listening. Practice and exposure hone these skills and deepen one's personal awareness, which in itself is the fertile soil for end-of-life completion work for both parties.[96]

Nurses, by virtue of explaining the dying process, may reduce anxiety and help prepare patients and families. In response to patients' desires to articulate the meaning and purpose of their lives as they face death, nurses may use interventions to help relieve spiritual suffering. Performing a life review serves many purposes. It facilitates healing in helping patients resolve past conflicts, gain forgiveness and reconciliation, recognize purpose and meaning, and achieve a sense of personal integration and inner peace. Meditation, guided imagery, music, reading, and art that focuses on healing may be comforting.[48]

Role modeling for families the art of being present to the dying person is important. Encouraging the family to engage in loving, physical contact, such as holding hands, embracing, or lying next to the patient, may help the patient in his or her transition and may help the survivors in their anticipatory grieving. For families who want to be present at the time of death, explaining that patients often wait until they are alone to die may prevent the family from feeling a sense of guilt if they are away from the patient at the time of death. Allowing the family to be with the patient after death may help the surviving family members grieve the loss of their loved one.

Nurses' awareness of anticipatory grief and bereavement and communications with family members and other loved ones may help them through these painful times. Bereaved families are often in most need of having someone to listen to them. One of the nurses' most important roles in working with grieving patients and bereaved families is active, compassionate listening. Encouraging the bereaved to tell stories of their loss, including details of the days and weeks around the death of their loved one; encouraging the sharing of memories of the person; asking about how things are different now; and helping to identify sources of support, of coping, and of accomplishing practical daily activities may be of great assistance.[97]

## Family Communication

Zerwekh[98] suggests a family hospice caregiving model whereby communication—in particular the nurse's communication—sets the tone for all care. In this model, the role of the nurse is to help guide the care. Speaking the truth enables the nurse to connect with family members and empower them to make choices, but also to be collaborative, to comfort, to guide the dying process, and to provide spiritual support.

Nurses, by the nature of their practice, understand that the focus of care is on patients and their families. Because the essence of nursing is to care for actual and potential health problems of the patient and family, the scope of care is broad. Challenges arise when the patient and the family are in conflict. In these times of nursing shortages, interference from family members at the bedside may overwhelm the nurse in her best efforts to provide care for the patient.

Communication with family members is as important as communication with the patient. One challenge is a mismatch of patient and family needs for information and communication and differences in coping styles. A patient may need little communication, whereas certain family members may need constant updates, partially because they are unable to attend appointments with the patient. The family may not understand as much as the patient does, or the family may understand more than the patient. The family's questions and comments may focus on their coping and coming to terms with the patient's potential death. Being at different places in coping may also create tension between a patient and his or her family. A patient may be coping well and adjusting to the physical changes, whereas a family member may just be beginning to deal with the diagnosis of a life-threatening illness and not be able to even conceptualize a prognosis. On the other hand, a patient may be too overwhelmed by symptoms to deal with psychological aspects of care, whereas a family member may be more objective. It should be remembered that because of their knowledge of the patient, families may serve as the best advocates for their ill family member.[19] This is well illustrated in pediatrics, where parents are considered to be the experts on their children.

The nurse often interacts with many family members. The nurse has a daunting task to determine the patient's important relationships and who should get what information. This work is very labor intensive, because different family members have varying needs for information and reassurance. Often this ultimately requires that one family member serve as the spokesperson. The communication needs of the family are varied. Families often need education in various aspects of physical caregiving, including transfers and personal care.[99] They may also need assistance in rallying support to care for loved ones and identifying and accessing community services. To successfully ascertain the situation, the nurse needs to know about the communication style of the family. Duhamel and Dupuis[100] offered the following questions:

- What is helping you the most?
- Where are you getting support?
- What information do you need right now?

To best work with families, the nurse can use several strategies. First, frequent interaction with family members can help the family feel included and not avoided. Second, understanding of the family's communication styles can help in these interactions. As part of the nursing assessment, a determination of the family's understanding of the patient's condition helps facilitate communication. Third is to acknowledge the family's roles and responsibilities and support their efforts and sacrifices as caregivers. This is critically important when working in partnership with patients and their families.[101] Finally, the nurse is invaluable to the family in their anticipatory grieving and bereavement. Eliciting the coping mechanisms of the patient and family is an important part of patient assessment, as the patient transitions in care and later progresses to dying, and also of family assessment during these times and during bereavement.

Sometimes, there are family structures with unhealthy functioning. This includes families with histories of physical, emotional, sexual, and substance abuse, to name but a few. Patient care can be affected because these issues take on more importance than issues around the diagnosis. Teamwork is essential in these situations, particularly in maintaining objectivity and realizing these circumstances cannot be changed or fixed. Focused interventions by social worker and chaplains can be extremely helpful.

## Team Communication and Teamwork

It is well known that palliative care is best delivered in a team fashion.[18] The underlying reasoning is that well-functioning interdisciplinary teams can share responsibility for care, are able to balance multiple perspectives in care, can support each other in the provision of care, and can provide more comprehensive care, compared with a sole individual clinician.[99] More simply put, a team is more capable of achieving better results than are individuals working in isolation.[100] To create a good team necessitates the following

- Consensus of Goals/Objectives/Strategies.
- Recognition of individual contribution of team members.[102]

- Competence of team member in discipline and respect for the competence of other team members.[103]
- Clear definition of tasks and responsibilities and means for communication within the team.
- Competent leadership—with shared accountability.
- Process for evaluating quality and effectiveness of team.[104]
- Bereavement support for team.
- Respect of patient.[105]

Good teams promote collaboration with effective communication, coordination, cooperation, and competence.[38,106,107] Witnessing interactions that highlight good communication skills among health care professionals is reassuring to patients and their families.[108]

Nurses must work closely with physicians at various levels, depending on their role and practice.[109] Different environmental and organizational cultures dictate the nature of the work together as collaborative, deferential, or hierarchical. Collaborative practice is the outcome of good teamwork and communication.

Nurses and physicians differ in their communication styles. Whereas physicians often want facts and numbers, nurses often emphasize process and reflection. Because of these different styles, the nurse should be clear on the goal of the communication interaction. If the contact is about information sharing, the nurse may need to be brief. If a treatment change is warranted, the nurse should have the supporting evidence. For example, if calling about pain and symptoms, the nurse should know the medications the patient is taking, when they were last taken and the patient's pain scores, and should offer a suggested plan. Part of working as a team is to develop a working relationship and understand team members' communication styles.[110]

A struggle often occurs because much of palliative care is care that nurses have historically provided. Indeed, the central caregiver in hospice is the nurse. In palliative care, the more academic aspect of end-of-life care, physicians now are taking on many aspects of the nursing role. Because of the interdependence of the members of the team, interdisciplinary roles may become blurred. This can result in a favorable collaboration, but it may also result in friction and competition among members of the inter-professional team. Tension may exist due to the fact that much of palliative care is still the 24-hour care provided by the bedside nurse.[111] Therefore, it is important to work out the conflicts and to recognize the role of each team member in the care of the patient.

There can be some darker sides of team interactions. According to Kane,[112] stress and tension can arise from ethical conflicts among team members and conflicting goals regarding patient care. Eight problems may occur within a team: (1) overwhelming the patient, (2) making the patient part of the team, (3) squelching of individual team members, (4) lack of accountability, (5) team process trumping client outcome, (6) orthodoxy and groupthink, (7) overemphasis on health and safety goals, and (8) squandering of resources. All of these issues can occur at various times within the palliative care team and necessitate good communication and conflict resolution. Examples of these problems include the following:

1. Overwhelming the patient—This occurs often at a family meeting, where there may be the patient, one family member, and many health care professionals. The patient or family may feel outnumbered and hesitant to talk about the goals of care.

2. Making the patient part of the team—Patients are told that they are part of the decision-making team and are asked for input. However, the fact is that patients who are dying may not have the energy to advocate for themselves. Rather, they want other people to advocate for them.

3. Squelching of individual team members—The team may explicitly say that everyone's input is equal when implicitly that is not the case. Non-physician voices may be dismissed. The nurse must often work hard to be heard.

4. Lack of accountability—This is often a challenge when there is a primary team working with other consultants such as palliative care teams. The team is consulted to do a certain thing. There can be tension if they see other things that should be done but they have not been asked to address these issues.

5. Team process trumping client outcome—Often, in providing end-of-life care, health care providers have certain ideas or feelings about what is right or wrong. The challenge is to allow an open process to occur and not to limit it to one particular pathway simply because that is the way it is always done.

6. Orthodoxy and groupthink—A group can become insular and not incorporate new ideas. The team becomes unable to assess itself, and obvious problems are overlooked. In end-of-life situations, this often happens in relation to the dying process. Nurses may see that the patient is dying, but other health professionals look for a specific symptom and treat it. The fact that the patient is dying is overlooked.

7. Overemphasis on health and safety goals—The care plan takes over, in preference to the patient's needs.

8. Squandering of resources—Needs of patients are missed, and high-cost interventions are implemented.

In summary, interdisciplinary teams have much to offer patients and families. Together, the various disciplines can meet the needs of the whole person. However, teams have their own dynamics, just as a family does, because they are, in effect, social systems. With good leadership, role delineation, and flexibility, interdisciplinary teams work well, creating a synergy that promotes positive outcomes.[113] There are inherent issues that may make teams less helpful if they do not take the time to reflect on their process. To look at its effectiveness, a team needs to assess its process. First, the participation of all members is essential; the degree of involvement may depend on the issues of the patient and family. Second,

each team member should have a voice in the process. Third, the mission and goals should be periodically reviewed so that all members are working on the same premise. Finally, each team member should understand his or her role in patient care and maintain the process of the group. With a periodic review of these issues, the group will work more effectively and efficiently as a team. Reflection helps a team mature, avoiding some of the pitfalls of teamwork.

## Collaboration

Collaboration is a vital force for teams working with dying patients. In fact, there are some important reasons for it. These include an imperative for good care, a financial imperative to appropriate resource allocation, and a healthcare imperative in which clinicians have different knowledge about the patient and various expertise to promote good care.[114] Collaboration enables the sustainability of the team to care for a population of patients that is demanding in all the domains of care: physically, psychologically, spiritually, and emotionally.

Most literature on collaboration is in nursing journals. Thus there is a tension within collaboration, which stems from the nature of nursing practice which focuses on—caring rather than curing. Hanson and Spross[115] describe collaboration as "dynamic interpersonal process in which two or more individuals make a commitment to each other to interact authentically and constructively to solve problems and to learn from one another to accomplish identified goals, purposes, or outcomes. The individuals recognize and articulate the shared values that make this commitment possible."

To promote collaboration, each team member should have a clear role and that role must be respected. If done well, the team identity as a palliative care team member supersedes the individual member's discipline such as nurse, social worker, physician, etc. Members share information and work both independently and together to develop goals. This necessitates good communication and negotiation. Leadership is shared among team members depending on the task at hand. This means there must be respect for different styles, trust in clinical competence, and compassion for each other.[116–118]

Barriers to effective teamwork include lack of training, hierarchical team structures, organizational rules, and reimbursement. Often team members' roles are not clearly defined and there may be ineffective communication. This results in ineffective leadership without the ability to share mission and vision. Poor communication results in conflicts and ultimately team demoralization.[119]

## Conflict Resolution

Conflict is a situation in which the concerns of two or more people or parties appear to clash.[120] This may occur between a patient and a nurse, between a nurse and a doctor, or between two health care teams. Conflict is inevitable and healthy. If managed well, it helps people look at different perspectives and can allow for creativity and positive movement. If dismissed or ignored, it can breed demoralization and negativity. Nurses on the front line deal with conflict all the time. The challenge is to recognize the conflict and the nature of the conflict.

There are several methods to resolve conflict between team members, or between a colleague and a patient. The two extremes are conflict avoidance and continued conflict. Between the extremes on this spectrum are negotiation, accommodation, and collaboration. What differentiates these processes is the perceived power differences. Nurses, depending on their level of practice, practice site, and experience, may deal with conflict differently. Even within nursing, there may be tension between generalists and APNs. Historically, an imbalance of power has existed between attending physicians and nurses. However, with social work colleagues, nurses have felt equal, with a balanced or similar power. Often, nurses avoid conflict if they constantly have difficulty dealing with a team member who will not talk about disagreements. However, in palliative care, the goal should be collaboration in which all problems are discussed and mutual solutions are reached. In order to best solve conflict, there are several strategies. Common issues of team conflict include information, goals, role expectations, and differences in underlying values.[106]

Conflict resolution occurs through a process (Table 5–10). This involves looking at the facts of a conflict, the feelings of a conflict and the identity in the conflict.[119]

First, the nurse identifies the source of the conflict in terms of reviewing the facts of what happened, and what the impact was. Second, the nurse reflects on the emotional aspect of the conflict—these are the feelings. Then the nurse addresses goal of conflict resolution in terms of what she or he hopes to accomplish as it relates to the patient and or family. Sometimes, this may be looking at the role each provider has at stake and then thinking what is best for the patient.

There are several steps in meeting with a team member about a conflict. Be curious about your colleague's perspective by learning his or her story. In doing so, the two parties share their common purposes and differing interests. Express your views, including statements of feelings, and take the time to LISTEN. This leads to exploration of the conflict and letting each party tell his or her perspective while acknowledging feelings and each party's version of the events. Among the hardest things to learn to say are "I am sorry," "I was wrong," and "You could be right." Don't feel pressured to agree instantly, as it is important to discuss the range of the issue to process it more fully rather than submerging the conflict. Problem-solve together with the common goal of the patient's well-being and decide on a tack of resolution.[109, 110,115]

### Achieving Expertise in Communication

Achieving expertise in communication requires a long-term commitment. First, a nurse must assess his or her own

---

| Table 5–10 |
| --- |
| **Approaches to Effective Conflict Negotiation** |

**I. Reflection of the conflict**
A. Identify source of conflict—the facts
   What happened?
   What emotions contributed to conflict?
   What impact has the situation has on you?
   What did you contribute to the problem?
B. Identify the goal of conflict resolution
   What do you hope to accomplish?
   What is best way to raise issue?
   What's at stake for you?

**II. Negotiation of the conflict**
A. Address the conflict
   When and how is the best way to raise the issue and achieve the purpose?
B. Identify each individual's purpose to conflict resolution—the feelings
   Where do the individuals share purposes?
   Where do the individual's interests differ?
C. Explore the conflict—problem-solve with patient's best interest as goal
   Listen to other individual and explore the story.
   Acknowledge feelings behind story and paraphrase them.
   Ask other individual to "listen to you as you share your version of events and your intentions."
D. Problem solving
   Invent options to meet each side's most important concerns and interests.
   Decide tack of resolution—avoidance, collaborate, compromise.
   Use objective criteria or gold standard of palliative care for what should happen.
   Include approach for future communication.

*Sources:* Adapted from references 119 and 120.

---

strengths and weaknesses in communication. Then, the nurse must evaluate his or her skills specifically in the area of death and dying. Completing a death awareness questionnaire helps identify areas of comfort and discomfort regarding discussions of death and dying. Often, it is helpful for the nurse to ask colleagues to observe how he or she talks with patients and to give honest feedback. Working within palliative care necessitates self-awareness; therefore, nurses must examine their own feelings about death and dying, receive support for their personal grief, and seek mentoring to improve communication skills. This skill should include education in cancer patients as well as non-cancer patients, as the conversations are different.[120] It may also be helpful to spend some time with hospice and palliative nurses who can discuss more about the communication process. Reflection of a nurse's own areas of strength and style of communication is helpful. Language and words are individual to one's experience and practice.

Recently, there has also been more research into the use of simulation communication training, particularly for nurses at the advanced practice level. Usually this involves role plays, in which other clinicians or actors play the part of patients with advanced illnesses. The simulations can be focused on real end-of-life scenarios to encourage nursing language and allow the nurse to focus on the communication aspect of the nurse/patient/family relationship rather the treatment aspects of care.[121] As a follow up to the training, it is helpful to have a place for the nurse to develop and acquire skills. This may occur through a formal preceptorship, formal education, or mentoring with expert nurse colleagues. Sometimes, this can be augmented through writing a narrative about a difficult case, doing a case review, or participating in peer supervision of cases of patients with life-threatening illnesses. Structured formats include coursework in death and dying, continuing education forums, and psychotherapy. Informal structures include support groups, committee work on quality improvement processes, participation in ethics committees or forums, and informal work with spiritual caregivers.

## Conclusion

Because death is universal, palliative care is one aspect of nursing practice that cuts across all specialties of practice. Communication is a complex, continual transactional process that occurs between persons. Information, feelings, and meaning are conveyed through verbal and nonverbal messages.[1] Because communication is the cornerstone of end-of-life care, communication skills are an essential competency for nurses. Communication serves as the foundation of the nurse–patient relationship in every aspect of care. This includes from assessment to intervention, from diagnosis to death, and all aspects of care: physical, psychological, spiritual and social. Communication facilitates the expression of feelings by the patient and family members. It allows patients to articulate their hopes, dreams, priorities, values, and needs in the last stages of life.[122] And it allows the team to work collaboratively to provide comprehensive care to the patient and family.

REFERENCES

1. Dunne K. Effective communication in palliative care. Nursing Standard 2005;20:57–64.
2. Johnston B, Smith L. Nurses' and patients' perceptions of expert palliative nursing care. J Adv Nurs 2006;54:700–709.
3. American Association of Colleges of Nursing. Peaceful Death Competencies: Recommended Competencies and Curricular Guidelines for End-of-Life Nursing Care. Washington, DC: AACN, 2002.
4. Campbell L. History of the hospice movement. Cancer Nursing 1986;9:333–338.
5. Degner L, Gow C. Evaluations of death education in nursing—A critical review. Cancer Nursing 1988;11:151–159.
6. Steinhauser KE, Christakis NA, Clipp EC, et al. Factors considered important at the end of life by patients, family, physicians, and other care providers. JAMA 2000;284:2476–2482.
7. Buckman R. Communication skills in palliative care. Neurol Clin 2001;19:989–1004.
8. Ferrell BR, Coyle N. The nature of suffering and the goals of nursing. Oncology Nursing Forum 2007;35(2):241–247.
9. Vachon MLS. Caring for the caregiver in oncology and palliative care. Semin Oncol Nurs 1998;14:152–157.
10. Greisinger A, Lorimor R, Aday, Winn R, Baile W. Terminally ill cancer patients: their most important concerns. Cancer Pract 1997;5:147–154.
11. McSkimming S, Hodges M, Super A, Driever M, Schoessler FS, Lee M. The experience of life-threatening illness: Patients' and their loved ones' perspectives. J Palliat Med 1999; 2:173–184.
12. Lowey S. Communication between the nurse and family caregiver in end-of-life care—A review of the literature. J Hospice Palliat Nurs 2008;10:35–48.
13. Dobratz M. Hospice nursing: Present perspectives and future directives. Cancer Nursing. 1990;13:112–122.
14. Herth K. Fostering hope in terminally ill people. J Adv Nurs 1990;15:1250–1259.
15. Degner L, Gow C. Critical nursing behaviors in care for the dying. Cancer Nursing 1991;14:246–253.
16. Steeves R, Cohen M, Wise C. An analysis of critical incidents describing the essence of oncology nursing. Oncology Nurs Forum Suppl 1994;218:19–25.
17. Wilson S, Coenen A, Doorenbos A. Dignified dying as a nursing phenomenon in the United States. J Hospice Palliat Nursing 2006;8:34–41.
18. National Consensus Project for Quality Palliative Care. Clinical Practice Guidelines for Palliative Care, 2009. Available at www.nationalconsensusproject.org (accessed March 1, 2009).
19. American Nurses Association. Position Statement on Nursing Care and Do-Not-Resuscitate (DNR) Decisions. Revised 2003. Washington, DC. Available at http://www.nursingworld.org/EthicsHumanRights (accessed January 21, 2009).
20. SUPPORT Principal Investigators. A controlled trial to improve care for seriously ill patients. JAMA 1995;274:1591–1598.
21. Marvel MK, Epstein RM, Flowers K, Beckman HB. Soliciting the patient's agenda: Have we improved? JAMA 1999;281:283–287.
22. Fallowfield L. Communication and palliative medicine: Communication with the patient and family in palliative medicine. In: Doyle D, Hanks G, Cherny N, Calman K, eds. The Oxford Textbook of Palliative Medicine, 3rd ed. Oxford, England: Oxford University Press, 2004:101–115.
23. City of Hope National Medical Center and the American Association of Nursing. End-of-Life Nursing Education Consortium (ELNEC) Core Curriculum. Duarte, CA: Authors, 2008.
24. Perrin K. Communicating with seriously ill and dying patients, their families and their health care providers. Palliative Care Nursing—Quality Care to the End-of-Life. In: Matzo M, Sherman D, eds. 2nd ed. New York: Springer Publishing, 2006: 221–246.
25. Pierce SF. Improving end-of-life care: Gathering questions from family members. Nurs Forum 1999;34:5–14.
26. Field D, Copp G. Communication and awareness about dying in the 1990s. Palliat Med 1999;13:459–468.

27. Bailey E, Wilkerson S. Patients' views on nurses' communication skills: A pilot study. Int J Palliat Nurs 1998;4:300–305.

28. von Gunten CF, Ferris FD, Emanuel LL. Ensuring competency in end-of-life care: Communication and relational skills. JAMA 2000;284:3051–3057.

29. Kruijver IP, Kerkstra A, Bensing JM, van de Wiel HB. Nurse-patient communication in cancer care: A review of the literature. Cancer Nurs 2000;23:20–31.

30. Andershed B, Ternestedt BM. Being a close relative of a dying person: Development of concepts, "involvement in the light and the dark." Cancer Nurs 2000;23:151–159.

31. White K, Coyne P, Patel DW. Are nurses adequately prepared for end-of-life care? J Nurs Scholarship 2001;33:147–151.

32. Ferrell B, Virani R, Grant M. Review of communication and family caregivers content in nursing texts. J Hospice Palliat Nurs 1999;1:97–100.

33. Maguire P. Breaking bad news. Eur J Surg Oncol 1998; 24:188–191.

34. Zanchetta M, Moura S. Self-determination and information seeking in end-stage cancer. Clin J Oncol Nurs 2006;10:803–807.

35. Heaven C, Magure P. Communication issues. In: Lloyd-Williams M, ed. Psychosocial Issues in Palliative Care. Oxford: Oxford University Press, 2003:13–34.

36. Quill TE. Initiating end-of-life discussions with seriously ill patients: Addressing the "elephant in the room." JAMA 2000;284:2502–2507.

37. The A-M, Hak T, Koeter G, van der Wal G. Collusion in doctor–patient communication about imminent death: An ethnographic study. BMJ 2000;321:1376–1381.

38. Cist A, Truog R, Brackett S, Hurford W. Practical guidelines on the withdrawal of life-sustaining therapies. Int Anesth Clin 2001;39(3):87–102.

39. Wilkerson S, Mula C. Communication in care of the dying. In: Ellershaw J, Wilkerson S, eds. Care of the Dying: A Pathway to Excellence. New York: Oxford University Press, 2003.

40. Pasareta JV, Minarik PA, Nield-Anderson L. Anxiety and depression. In: Ferrell B, Coyle N, eds. Textbook of Palliative Nursing. New York: Oxford University Press, 2001:269–289.

41. Kristjanson L. Establishing goals of care: Communication traps and treatment lane changes. In: Ferrell BR, Coyle N, eds. Textbook of Palliative Nursing. New York: Oxford University Press, 2001:331–338.

42. Fischberg D. Talking to Families. In Session: Do Everything! Responding to Request for Non-Beneficial Treatment. Annual Assembly. AAHPM and HPNA. Phoenix, AZ, January 22, 2004.

43. Bartel J, Dahlin C, Fordham P, Griffie J, Hedges L, Montana B, Muchka S. Advanced Skills for the Advanced Hospice and Palliative Care Nurse. Core Curriculum for the Advanced Practice Hospice and Palliative Nurse. In: Perley M, Dahlin C, eds. Pittsburgh: Hospice and Palliative Nurses Association, 2007.

44. Karliner L, Perez-Stable E, Gildenforin G. The language divide—the importance of training in the use of interpreters for outpatient practice. J Gen Intern Med 2004;19:175–183.

45. Levine C. Use of children as interpreters. JAMA; 2006. 296(23):2802.

46. Hudelson P. Improving patient–provider communication: Insights from interpreters. Fam Prac 2005;22:311–316.

47. Rousseau P. Spirituality and the dying patient. J Clin Oncol 2003;21(Suppl.):54s–56s.

48. Fogarty LA, Curbow BA, Wingard JR, McDonnell K, Somerfield MR. Can 40 seconds of compassion reduce patient anxiety? J Clin Oncol 1999;17:371–379.

49. Lapine A, Wang-Cheng R, Goldstein M, Nooney A, Lamb G, Derse A. When cultures clash: Physicians, patient, and family wishes in truth disclosure for dying patients. J Palliat Med 2001;4:475–480.

50. Quill TE, Arnold RM, Platt F. "I wish things were different": Expressing wishes in response to loss, futility, and unrealistic hopes. Ann Intern Med 2001;135:551–555.

51. Block SD, Billings JA. Patient requests to hasten death: Evaluation and management in terminal care. Arch Intern Med 1994;154:2039–2047.

52. Neff P, Lyckholm L, Smith T. Truth or consequences: What to do when the patient doesn't want to know. J Clin Oncol 2002;20:3035–3037.

53. Detmar SB, Aaronson NK, Wever LD, Muller M, Schornagel JH. How are you feeling? Who wants to know? Patients' and oncologists' preferences for discussing health-related quality-of-life issues. J Clin Oncol 2000;18:3295–3301.

54. Wenrich MD, Curtis JR, Shannon SE, et al. Communicating with dying patients within the spectrum of medical care from terminal diagnosis to death. Arch Intern Med 2001;161:868–874.

55. Parker PA, Baile WF, de Moor C, et al. Breaking bad news about cancer: Patient preferences for communication. J Clin Oncol 2001;19:2049–2056.

56. American Nurses Association. Position Statement on Nursing and the Patient Self-Determination Acts. Revised 1991. Washington, DC. Available at: http://www.nursingworld.org/EthicsHumanRights (accessed January 21, 2009).

57. Tierney WM, Dexter PR, Gramelspacher GP, Perkins AJ, Zhou X-H, Wolinsky FD. The effect of discussions about advance directives on patients' satisfaction with primary care. J Gen Intern Med 2001;16:32–40.

58. Maguire P. Improving communications with cancer patients. Eur J Cancer 1999;35:1415–1422.

59. Singer PA, Martin DK, Lavery JV, Thiel EC, Kelner M, Mendelssohn DC. Reconceptualizing advance care planning from the patient's perspective. Arch Intern Med 1998;158:879–884.

60. Hammes B. What does it take to help adults successfully plan for future medical decisions? J Palliat Med 2001;4:453–456.

61. Barnard D. Advanced care planning is not about "getting it right." J Palliat Med 2002;5:475–481.

62. Kutner JS, Steiner JF, Corbett KK, Jahnigen DW, Barton PL. Information needs in terminal illness. Soc Sci Med 1999; 48:1341–1352.

63. Christakis NA, Lamont EB. Extent and determinants of error in doctors' prognoses in terminally ill patients: Prospective cohort study. BMJ 2000;320:469–472.

64. Lamont EB, Christakis NA. Prognostic disclosure to patients with cancer near the end of life. Ann Intern Med 2001;134:1096–1105.

65. Cassileth BR. Enhancing doctor–patient communications. J Clin Oncol (Suppl) 2001;19(18s):61s–63s.

66. Fischer GS, Arnold RM, Tulsky JA. Talking to the older adult about advanced directives. Clin Geriatr Med 2000;16:239–254.

67. Weeks SC, Cook EF, O'Day SJ, et al. Relationship between cancer patients' predictions of prognosis and their treatment preferences. JAMA 1998;279:1709–1714.

68. Steinhauser KE, Christakis NA, Clipp EC, McNeilly M, Grambow S, Parker J, Tulsky JA. Preparing for the end of life: Preferences of patients, families, physicians, and other care providers. J Pain Symptom Manage 2001;22:727–737.

69. Lo B, Quill T, Tulsky J, for the ACP-ASIM End-of-Life Care Consensus Panel. Discussing palliative care with patients. Ann Intern Med 1999;130:744–749.

70. Back AL, Arnold RM, Quill TE. Hope for the best, and prepare for the worst. Ann Intern Med 2003;138:439–443.

71. Family letter writing: An interview with Nathan Harlow. Innovations in end of life care: An international on-line forum for leaders in end of life care 1999.

72. Matzo ML, Sherman DW, eds. Palliative Care Nursing: Quality Care to the End of Life, 2nd ed. New York: Springer Publishing Company, 2006.

73. Buckman R. How to Break Bad News: A Guide for Health Care Professionals. Baltimore, Md.: The Johns Hopkins University Press, 1992.

74. Baile WF, Buckman R, Lenzi R, et al. SPIKES: A six-step protocol for delivering bad news—Application to the patient with cancer. Oncologist 2000;5:302–311.

75. Baile WF, Lenzi R, Parker PA, Buckman R, Cohen L. Oncologists' attitudes toward and practices in giving bad news: An exploratory study. J Clin Oncol 2002;20:2189–2196.

76. Coyle N, Sculco L. Communication and patient/physician relationship: Phenomenological inquiry. J Support Oncol 2003;1:206–215.

77. Yun YH, Lee CG, Kim S-Y, Heo DS, Kim JS, Lee KS, Hong YS, Lee JS, You CH. The attitudes of cancer patients and their families toward disclosure of terminal illness. J Clin Oncol 2004;22:307–314.

78. Hancok K, Clayton J, Parker S, Wal der S, Butow P, Carrick S, Currow D, Chersi D, Glare PR, Tattersall M. Truth telling in discussing prognosis in advanced life-limiting illnesses: a systematic review. Palliative Medicine 2007; 21:506–517.

79. Buchanan J, Borland R, Cosolo W, Millership R, Haines I, Zimet A, Zalcberg J. Patient's beliefs about cancer management. Supportive Care Cancer 1996;4:110–117.

80. Fischer GS, Tulsky JA, Arnold RM. Communicating a poor prognosis. In: Portenoy RK, Bruera E, eds. Topics in Palliative Care, Vol. 4. New York: Oxford University Press, 2000.

81. Quill TE, Townsend P. Bad news: Delivery, dialogue, and dilemmas. Arch Intern Med 1991;151:463–468.

82. Friedrichsen MJ, Strong PM, Carlsson ME. Breaking news in the transition from curative to palliative cancer care: Patients' view of doctors giving the information. Supportive Care Cancer 2000;8:472–478.

83. Girgis A, Sanson-Fisher RW. Breaking bad news: Consensus guidelines for medical practitioners. J Clin Oncol 1995;13:2449–2456.

84. Faulkner A. ABC of palliative care: Communication with patients, families, and other professionals. BMJ 1998;316:130–132.

85. Dunn H. Hard Choices for Loving People: CPR, Artificial Feeding, Comfort Care, and the Patient with a Life-Threatening Illness, 4th ed. Herndon, Va.: A&A Publishers, 2001.

86. Saklayen M, Liss H, Markert R. In-hospital cardiopulmonary resuscitation. Survival in 1 hospital and literature review. Medicine (Baltimore) 1995;74:163–175.

87. Waisel DB, Truog RD. The cardiopulmonary resuscitation-not-indicated order: Futility revisited. Ann Intern Med 1995;122:304–308.

88. von Gunten CF. Discussing do-not-resuscitate status. J Clin Oncol (Suppl) 2003;21(9):20s–25s.

89. von Gunten CF. Discussing hospice care. J Clin Oncol (Suppl) 2003;21(9):31s–36s.

90. van Servellen G. Communicating with patients with chronic and/or life-threatening illness. In: Communication for the Health Care Professional: Concepts and Techniques. Gaithersburg. MD: Aspen, 1997: Chapter 13.

91. Schapira L, Eisenberg PD, MacDonald N, Mumber MP, Loprinzi C. A revisitation of "Doc, how much time do I have?" J Clin Oncol 2003 (Suppl);21:8s–11s.

92. von Gunten CF. Discussing hospice care. J Clin Oncol 2002;20:1419–1424.

93. Finucane T, Christmas C, Travis K. Tube feedings in patients with advanced dementia: A review of the evidence. JAMA 1999;282:1365–1370.

94. Weissman DE. Consultation in palliative medicine. Arch Int Med 1997;157:733–737.

95. Detmar SB, Muller MJ, Wever LD, et al. The patient–physician relationship. Patient–physician communication during outpatient palliative treatment visits: An observational study. JAMA 2001;285:1351–1357.

96. Fahnestock DT. Partnership for good dying. JAMA 1999;282:615–616.

97. Cassett D, Kutner JS, Abrahm J, for the End-of-Life Care Consensus Panel. Life after death: A practical approach to grief and bereavement. Ann Intern Med 2001;134:208–215.

98. Zerwekh J. Nursing Care at the End of Life—Palliative Care for Patients and Families. New York: FA Davis, 2006.

99. Rabow M, Hauser J, Adams J. Supporting family caregivers at the end of life. JAMA 2004;291:483–489.

100. Duhamel F, Dupuis F. Families on palliative care: Exploring family and healthcare professionals' beliefs. Int J Palliat Nurs 2003;9:113–119.

101. Levine C, Zuckerman C. The trouble with families: Toward an ethic of accommodation. Ann Intern Med 1999;130:148–152.

102. Hudson P, Sanchia A, Kristjianson L. Meeting the supportive needs of family caregivers in palliative care: Challenges for health professionals. J Palliat Med 2004;7:19–25.

103. Billings J, Dahlin C, Dungan S, Greenberg D, Krakauer E, Lawless N, Montgomery P, Reid C. Psychosocial training in a palliative care fellowship. J Palliat Med 2003;6:355–363.

104. Long DM, Wilson NL, eds. American Congress on Rehabilitation Medicine. Houston Geriatric Interdisciplinary Team Training Curriculum. Houston: Baylor College of Medicine, Huffington Center on Aging, 2001.

105. Norelle Lickiss J, Turner K, Pollack M. The interdisciplinary team. The Oxford Textbook of Palliative Medicine, 3rd ed. In: Doyle D, Hanks G, Cherney N, Calman K, eds. New York: Oxford University Press, 2005:42–45.

106. Hyer K, Flaherty S, Fairchild S, Bottrell M, Mezey M, Fulmer T. Geriatric Interdisciplinary Team Training Program (GITT) Curriculum Guide. New York: New York University, 2001.

107. Mystakidou K. Interdisciplinary working: A Greek perspective. Palliat Med 2001;15:67–68.

108. Hill A. Multiprofessional teamwork in hospital palliative care teams. Int J Palliat Nurs 1998;4:214–221.

109. Lockhart-Wood, K. Nurse–doctor collaboration in cancer pain management. Int J Palliat Nurs 2001;7:6–16.

110. Berry P, Miller G. Leading the way in Provider Communications. Pittsburgh, PA: Hospice and Palliative Nurses Association, 2006.

111. Coyle N. Interdisciplinary collaboration in hospital palliative care: Chimera or goal? Palliat Med 1997;11:265–266.

112. Kane R. Avoiding the dark side of geriatric teamwork. In: Mezey MD, Cassel CK, Bottrell MM, Hyer K, Howe JL, Fuher TT, eds. Ethical Patient Care: A Casebook for Geriatric Health Care Teams. Baltimore: John Hopkins Press, 2002:187–207.

113. Crawford G, Price S. Team working: Palliative care as a model of interdisciplinary practice. Med J Aust 2003(Suppl);6(179): s32–s34.

114. Hanson C, Spross J. In: Hamric A, Spross J, Hanson C, eds. Advanced Practice Nursing—An Integrative Approach, 3rd ed. St. Louis: Elsevier Saunders, 2004.

115. Hanson C, Spross J. In: Hamric A, Spross J, Hanson C, eds. Advanced Practice Nursing—An Integrative Approach, 4th ed. St. Louis: Elsevier Saunders, 2009:283–314.

116. Feudtner C. Collaborative Communication in Pediatric Palliative Care: A foundation for problem-solving and decision-making. Pediatric Clinics of North America 2007:54, 583–607.

117. Lindeke L, Sieckert A. Nurse–Physician Workplace Collaboration. *Online Journal of Issues in Nursing.* 2005; 10(1): Manuscript 4. Available at http://www.nursingworld.org/MainMenuCategories/ANAMarketplace/ANAPeriodicals/OJIN/TableofContents/Volume102005/No1Jan05/tpc26_416011.aspx (accessed January 12, 2008).

118. Gianakos D. Physicians, nurses and collegiality. Nursing Outlook 1997;45:57–58.

119. Stone D, Patton B, Heen S. Difficult Conversations: How to Discuss What Matters Most. New York: Penguin Books, 1999.

120. Skilbeck J, Payne S. End of life care: A discursive analysis of specialist palliative care nursing. J Adv Nurs 2005; 51:325–334.

121. Hanna M, Fins J. Power and communcation; why simulation training ought to be complemented by experiential and humanist learning. Acad Med 2006;81:265–270.

122. Fisher R, Shapiro D. Beyond Reason—Using Emotions as You Negotiate. New York: Viking, 2005.

# II
# Symptom Assessment and Management

# 6

*Regina M. Fink and Rose A. Gates*

# Pain Assessment

*Indeed, the most intense feeling we know of, intense to the point of blotting out all other experiences, namely, the experience of great bodily pain, is at the same time the most private and least communicable of all.—Hannah Arendt, 1958 [1]*

♦ **Key Points**
♦ *Pain is multifactorial and affects the whole person.*
♦ *There are multiple barriers to pain assessment.*
♦ *Patients or residents should be screened for pain on admission to a hospital, clinic, nursing home, hospice, or home care agency.*
♦ *If pain or discomfort is reported, a comprehensive pain assessment should be performed at regular intervals, whenever there is a change in the pain, and after any modifications in the pain management plan.*
♦ *Reassessment of pain intensity should occur within one hour of analgesic administration or other nonpharmacologic intervention.*
♦ *The patient's self report of pain is the gold standard, even for those patients who are nonverbal or cognitively impaired.*
♦ *Standard pain scales should be used in combination with clinical observation and information from health care professionals and family caregivers.*

Pain is a common companion of birth, growth, death, and illness; it is intertwined intimately with the very nature of human existence. Most pain can be palliated, and patients can be relatively pain free. To successfully relieve pain and suffering, accurate, continuous pain assessment and reassessment is mandatory. However, evidence demonstrates that pain is undertreated in the palliative care setting, contributing significantly to patient discomfort and suffering at the end of life. Studies suggest that as many as 25% of newly diagnosed cancer patients, 60% of those undergoing treatment, and 75% of those in the terminal phase of disease, have unrelieved pain.[2-6] Results from a recent systematic review of pain prevalence in cancer patients report that greater than one third of those experiencing pain report moderate to severe pain.[6] Kutner and colleagues[7] report that, even in the care-oriented culture of hospice, 82% of their patients in the Population-based Palliative Care Research Network listed pain as the most bothersome symptom and required more intensive pain management during the last weeks of life, at times requiring sedation. Unrelieved pain is one of the most frequent reasons for palliative care consultation.[8] Although nursing homes are increasingly becoming the most common site of death for the elderly,[9,10] pain relief in long-term care facilities varies widely, with 45% to 80% of residents having substantial pain with suboptimal pain management.[11-17] Pain continues to be poorly assessed with over one third of long-term care residents having no formal pain assessment.[18]

This chapter considers various types of pain, describes barriers to optimal pain assessment, and reviews current clinical practice guidelines for the assessment of pain in the palliative care setting. A multifactorial model for pain assessment is proposed, and a variety of instruments and methods that can be used to assess pain in patients at the end of life are discussed.

## Types of Pain

According to the International Association for the Study of Pain (IASP), pain is defined as "an unpleasant sensory or emotional experience associated with tissue damage. The inability to communicate verbally does not negate the possibility that an individual is experiencing pain and is in need of appropriate pain-relieving treatment."[19] Pain has also been clinically defined as "whatever the experiencing person says it is, existing whenever the experiencing person says it does."[20]

Pain is commonly described in terms of categorization along a continuum of duration. Acute pain may be associated with tissue damage, inflammation, a disease process that is relatively brief, or a surgical procedure. Regardless of its intensity, acute pain is of relatively brief duration: hours, days, weeks, or a few months.[21] Acute pain serves as a warning that something is wrong and is generally viewed as a time-limited experience. In contrast, chronic or persistent pain worsens and intensifies with the passage of time, lasts for an extended period (months, years, or a lifetime), and adversely affects the patient's function or well-being.[22] Chronic pain has been further subclassified into chronic malignant and chronic non-malignant pain. Cancer pain may be nociceptive, neuropathic, or sympathetically maintained;[23] it may be related to primary or metastatic disease in two thirds of patients, may be the result of treatment (surgery, chemotherapy, biotherapy, radiation therapy, or procedures), or other causes (side effects, infection).[5,24] Chronic pain may accompany a disease process such as human immunodeficiency virus (HIV) infection and acquired immune deficiency syndrome (AIDS), arthritis or degenerative joint disease, osteoporosis, chronic obstructive pulmonary disease, heart failure, neurological disorders (e.g., multiple sclerosis, cerebrovascular disease), fibromyalgia, sickle cell disease, cystic fibrosis, and diabetes. It may also be associated with an injury that has not resolved within an expected period of time, such as low back pain, trauma, spinal cord injury, reflex sympathetic dystrophy, or phantom limb pain.

The American Geriatric Society (AGS) Panel on Persistent Pain in Older Persons[13] has classified persistent pain in pathophysiological terms that assist the health care professional to determine the cause of pain and select the appropriate pain management interventions. The four pain subcategories that have been delineated are nociceptive pain (visceral or somatic pain resulting from stimulation of pain receptors), neuropathic pain (pain caused by peripheral or central nervous system stimulation), mixed or unspecified pain (having mixed or unknown pain mechanisms), and pain due to psychological disorders.

## Barriers to Optimal Pain Assessment

Inadequate pain control is not the result of a lack of scientific information. Over the last three decades, a plethora of research has generated knowledge about pain and its management. Reports that document the inability or unwillingness of health care professionals to use knowledge from research and advances in technology continue to be published. The armamentarium of knowledge is available to assist professionals in the successful assessment and management of pain; the problems lie in its misuse or lack of use. Undertreatment of pain often results from clinicians' failure or inability to evaluate or appreciate the severity of the patient's problem. Although accurate and timely pain assessment is the cornerstone of optimal pain management, studies of nurses and other health care professionals continue to demonstrate the contribution of suboptimal assessment and documentation to the problem of inadequate pain management.[2,22,25-27]

Multiple barriers to the achievement of optimal pain assessment and management have been identified (Table 6–1).[25,28-36] The knowledge and attitudes of health care professionals toward pain assessment are extremely important, because these factors influence the priority placed on pain treatment.[37]

## Pain Assessment Guidelines and Standards

Recognition of the widespread inadequacy of pain assessment and management has prompted corrective efforts within many health care disciplines, including nursing, medicine, pharmacy, and pain management organizations. Representatives from various health care professional groups have convened to develop clinical practice guidelines and quality assurance standards and recommendations for the assessment and management of acute, cancer, and end-of-life pain.[5,13,14,36,38-45] The establishment of a formal monitoring program to evaluate the efficacy of pain assessment and interventions has been encouraged. The American Pain Society (APS) Guidelines for the Management of Cancer Pain in Adults and Children, APS Recommendations for Improving Quality of Acute and Cancer Pain Management, the APS Position Statement on Treatment of Pain at the End of Life, the Oncology Nursing Society (ONS) Position Paper on Cancer Pain Management, the National Comprehensive Cancer Network Guidelines, the American Society of Pain Management Nurses Position Statements on Pain Management at the End of Life and Pain Assessment in the Nonverbal Patient, the American Geriatrics Society Panel on Persistent Pain in Older Persons, the American Geriatrics Society Panel on the Pharmacological Management of Persistent Pain in Older Person, the American Medical Directors Association Pain Guidelines, and an Interdisciplinary Expert Consensus Statement on Assessment of Pain in Older Persons are reflective of the national trend to assess quality of care in high-incidence patients by monitoring outcomes as well as assessing and managing pain.

Joint Commission surveyors routinely inquire about pain assessment and management practices and quality improvement activities designed to monitor pain assessment and

---

**Table 6–1**
**Barriers to Optimal Pain Assessment**

**Health care professional barriers**

Lack of identification of pain assessment and relief as a
    priority in patient care

Inadequate knowledge about the performance of a pain
    assessment

Perceived lack of time to conduct and document a pain
    assessment and reassessment

Failure to use validated pain measurement tools

Inability of clinician to empathize or establish rapport with
    patient

Lack of continuity of care

Lack of communication among the health care
    professional team

Prejudice and bias in dealing with patients

**Health care system barriers**

A system that fails to hold health care professionals
    accountable for pain assessment

Lack of criteria or availability of culturally sensitive
    instruments for pain assessment in health care settings

Lack of institutional policies for performance and
    documentation of pain assessment

**Patient/family/societal barriers**

The highly subjective and personal nature of the pain
    experience

Lack of patient and family awareness about the importance
    of speaking out about pain

Lack of patient communication with health care professionals
    about pain

- Patient reluctance to report pain
- Patient not wanting to bother staff
- Patient fears of not being believed
- Patient age-related stoicism
- Patient doesn't report pain because "nothing helps"
- Patient concern that curative therapy might be
    curtailed with pain and palliative care
- Lack of a common language to describe pain
- Presence of unfounded beliefs and myths about pain
    and its treatment

*Sources:* Adapted from references 25, 28–36.

---

reassessment practices, patient satisfaction, and outcomes within healthcare institutions. The Joint Commission provides standards for assessing and managing pain in hospital, ambulatory, home care, and long-term care settings, recommending that culturally sensitive, age-appropriate pain rating scales be available to assist with assessment activities. The Joint Commission recently launched a national campaign, the Speak Up™ program, to help persons with pain become better informed and more involved with their pain management plan of care.[45] Patient-centered care requires that health care professionals seek opportunities to empower patients and families in decision-making about their care, taking into account their personal preferences and values. Involving patients and families in the pain assessment process is key to improving pain management with the desired outcome of decreased pain for patients.

Health care reform processes require that patients be discharged sooner, without adequate time to assess pain or to evaluate newly prescribed pain management regimens. Therefore, the prevalence of inadequate pain assessment and management may be even greater than reported, because more persons may be suffering silently in their homes. Health care professionals may not be aware of the patient's pain; have the time to communicate, or understand the meaning of the pain experience for the patient; or be available due to less than adequate resources. With the influences and increasing demands of managed care and changes in the delivery of health care, pain assessment and management may not be a priority.

## Process of Pain Assessment

Accurate pain assessment is the basis of pain treatment; it is a continuous process that encompasses multidimensional factors. In formulating a pain management plan of care, an assessment is crucial to identify the pain syndrome or the cause of pain. A comprehensive assessment addresses each type of pain and includes the following: a detailed history, including an assessment of the pain intensity, its characteristics, and its effects on function, and history of previous substance abuse; a physical examination with pertinent neurological examination, particularly if neuropathic pain is suspected; a psychosocial and cultural assessment; and an appropriate diagnostic workup to determine the cause of pain.[5,36] Attention should be paid to any discrepancies between patients' verbal descriptions of pain and their behavior and appearance. The physical examination should focus on an examination of the painful areas, as well as common referred pain locations. In frail or terminally ill patients, physical examination maneuvers and diagnostic tests should be performed only if the findings will potentially change or facilitate the treatment plan. The burden and potential discomfort of any diagnostic test must be weighed against the potential benefit of the information obtained. Ongoing and subsequent evaluations are necessary to determine the effectiveness of pain relief measures and to identify any new pain. Patients or residents should be asked whether they have pain (screened for pain) on admission to a hospital, clinic, nursing home, hospice, or home care agency. If pain or discomfort is reported, a comprehensive pain assessment should be performed at regular intervals, whenever there is a change in the pain, and after any modifications in the pain management plan. Reassessment of pain intensity should occur within one hour of analgesic administration or other nonpharmacologic intervention.[5,46] Pain reassessment is crucial since subsequent actions of the pain algorithm depend on the patient's response. The frequency of a pain assessment and reassessment is determined by the patient's or resident's clinical situation. Pain assessment and reassessment should be individualized and documented so that all multidisciplinary team members involved will have an understanding of the pain problem. Information about the patient's pain can be obtained from multiple sources: verbal self-report, observations, interviews with the patient and significant others, review of medical data, and feedback from other health care providers.

Pain is uniquely personal and subjective. The first opportunity to understand the pain experience is at the perceptual level. Perception incorporates the patient's self-report and the results of a pain assessment accomplished by the health care provider. *Perception* is "the act of perceiving, to become aware directly in one's mind, through any of the senses; especially to see or hear, involving the process of achieving understanding or seeing all the way through; using insight, intuition, or knowledge gained"; *assessment* is defined as "the act of assessing, evaluating, appraising, or estimating by sitting beside another."[47] Perception is an abstract process in which the person doing the perceiving is not just a bystander but is immersed in understanding of the other's situation and has the capacity for such insight. Perception is influenced by "higher-order" processes that characterize the cognitive and emotional appraisal of pain—what people feel and think about their pain and their future with the pain. Perception also includes the interpersonal framework in which the pain is experienced (with family or friends or alone), the meaning or reason for the pain, the person's coping pattern or locus of control, the presence of additional symptoms, and others' concerns (e.g., significant others' distress). Alternatively, assessment is a value judgment that occurs by observing the other's experience.

Assessment and perception of the patient's pain experience at the end of life is essential before planning interventions. However, the quality and usefulness of any assessment is only as good as the ability of the assessor to be thoroughly patient-focused. This means listening empathetically, maintaining open communication, and validating and legitimizing the concerns of the patient and significant others. A clinician's understanding of the patient's pain and accompanying symptoms confirms that there is genuine personal interest in facilitating a positive pain management outcome.

Pain does not occur in isolation. Other symptoms and concerns experienced by the patient compound the suffering associated with pain. Total pain has been described as the sum of all of the following interactions: physical, psychological, social, and spiritual.[48] At times, patients describe their whole life as painful. The provision of palliative care to relieve pain and suffering is based on the conceptual model of the whole person experiencing "total pain."

It is not always necessary or relevant to assess all dimensions of pain in all patients or in every setting. At the very least, both the sensation and intensity of pain and the patient's response to pain management must be considered during an assessment. The extent of the assessment should be dictated by its purpose, the patient's condition or stage of illness, the clinical setting, feasibility, and the relevance of a particular dimension to the patient or health care provider. For example, a comprehensive assessment may be appropriate for a patient in the early stage of palliative care, whereas only a pain intensity score is needed when evaluating a patient's response to an increased dose of analgesic. Incorporation of the multidimensional factors described in the following section into the pain assessment will ensure a comprehensive approach to understanding the patient's pain experience.

## Multifactorial Model for Pain Assessment

Pain is a complex phenomenon involving many interrelated factors. The multifactorial pain assessment model is based on the work of a number of researchers over the last three decades.[49–53] An individual's pain is unique; it is actualized by the multidimensionality of the experience and the interaction among factors both within the individual and in interaction with others.

Melzack and Casey[50] suggested that pain is determined by the interaction of three components: the sensory/discriminative (selection and modulation of pain sensations), the motivational/affective (affective reactions to pain via the brain's reticular formation and limbic system), and the cognitive (past or present experiences of pain). Evidence presented by Ahles[51] supported the usefulness of a multidimensional model for cancer-related pain by describing the following theoretical components of the pain experience: physiologic, sensory, affective, cognitive, and behavioral. McGuire[49,54] expanded the work of Ahles and colleagues by proposing the integration of a sociocultural dimension to the pain model. This sociocultural dimension, comprising a broad range of ethnocultural, demographic, spiritual, and social factors, influences an individual's perception of, and responses to, pain. Bates[52] proposed a biocultural model, combining social learning theory and the gate control theory, as a useful framework for studying and understanding cultural influences on human pain perception, assessment, and response. She believed that different social communities (ethnic groups) have different cultural experiences, attitudes, and meanings for pain that may influence pain perception, assessment, tolerance, and neurophysiological, psychological, and behavioral responses to pain sensation. Hester[53] proposed an environmental component, referring to the setting, environmental conditions, or stimuli that affect pain assessment and management. Excessive noise, lighting, or adverse temperatures may be sources of stress for individuals in pain and may negatively affect the pain experience.

Given the complexity of the interactions among the factors, if a positive impact on the quality of life of patients is the goal of palliative care, then the multifactorial perspective provides the foundation for assessing and managing pain. Some questions that can guide a multifactorial pain assessment are reviewed in Table 6–2.

**Table 6–2**
**Multifactorial Pain Assessment**

| Factors | Question |
|---|---|
| Physiologic/ sensory | What is causing the patient's pain? |
| | How does the patient describe his/her pain? |
| Affective | How does the patient's emotional state affect his/her report of pain? |
| | How does pain influence the patient's affect or mood? |
| Cognitive | How do the patient's knowledge, attitudes, and beliefs affect their pain experience? |
| | What is the meaning of the pain to the patient? |
| | How does the patient's past experience with pain influence the pain? |
| Behavioral | How do you know the patient is in pain? |
| | What patient pain behaviors or nonverbal cues inform you that pain is being experienced? |
| | What is the patient doing to decrease his or her pain? |
| Sociocultural | How does the patient's sociocultural background affect the pain experience, expression, and coping? |
| Environmental | How does the patient's environment affect the pain experience or expression? |

## Physiological and Sensory Factors

The physiological and sensory factors of the pain experience explain the cause and characterize the person's pain. Over 80% of cancer patients with advanced metastatic disease suffer pain due to direct tumor involvement.[55] Patients should be asked to describe their pain, including its quality, intensity, location, temporal pattern, and aggravating and alleviating factors. The five key factors included in a basic pain assessment are outlined in Figure 6–1. [56] (Note: this pain assessment guide is available in seven other languages: Spanish, French, Bosnian, Croatian, Arabic, Chinese, and Vietnamese.) In the palliative care setting, the patient's cause of pain may have already been determined. However, changes in pain location or character should not always be attributed to these preexisting causes, but should instigate a reassessment. Treatable causes, such as infections or fractures, may be the cause of new or persistent pain.

*Words.* Patients are asked to describe their pain or discomfort using words or qualifiers. Table 6–3 summarizes various pain types, word qualifiers, etiological factors, and choice of analgesia based on pain type. Identifying the qualifiers enhances understanding of the patient's pain etiology and should optimize pain treatment. Not doing so may result in an incomplete pain profile. Screening tools are available to enhance and refine neuropathic pain assessment.[57]

*Intensity.* Although an assessment of intensity captures only one aspect of the pain experience, it is the most frequently used parameter in clinical practice. Obtaining a pain intensity score will quantify how much pain a person is experiencing. Pain intensity should be evaluated not only at the present level, but also at its least, worst, and at rest or with movement. Patients should be asked how their pain compares with yesterday or with their worst day. They should be asked for a personal comfort goal describing the level of pain that will allow functional and psychosocial comfort. A review of the amount of pain experienced after analgesic or adjuvant drug administration, and/or use of nonpharmacologic approaches can also add information about the patient's level of pain. Pain intensity can be measured quantitatively with the use of a visual analog scale, numeric rating scale, verbal descriptor scale, faces scale, or pain thermometer. In using these tools, patients typically are asked to rate their pain on a scale of 0 to 10: no pain = 0; mild pain is indicated by a score of 1 to 3; moderate pain, 4 to 6; and severe pain, 7 to 10.[5] No single scale is appropriate for all patients. During instrument selection, the nurse must consider the practicality, ease, and acceptability of the instrument's use by terminally ill patients. (For a description of these instruments, see later discussion.) To ensure consistency, staff should carefully document which scale worked best for the patient, so that all members of the health care team will be aware of the appropriate scale to use.

*Location.* The majority of persons with cancer have pain in two or more sites;[58] therefore, it is crucial to ask questions about pain location. Encourage the patient to point or place a finger on the area involved. This will provide more specific data than verbal self-report. Separate pain histories should be acquired for each major pain complaint, since their causes may differ and the treatment plan may need to be tailored to the particular pain type. For example, neuropathic pain may radiate and follow a dermatomal path; pain that is deep in the abdomen may be visceral; and when a patient points to an area that is well-localized and nonradiating, the pain may be somatic, possibly indicating bone metastasis. Metastatic bone pain is the most common pain syndrome in cancer patients, with up to 79% of patients experiencing severe pain.[59]

*Duration.* Learning whether the pain is persistent, intermittent, or both will guide the selection of interventions. Patients may experience "breakthrough" pain (BTP)—an intermittent, transitory flare of pain.[60] Several subtypes of BTP have been delineated—incidental, spontaneous, or end-of-dose pain.[61] BTP pain requires a fast-acting opioid, whereas persistent pain is usually treated with long-acting, continuous-release opioids. Patients with progressive diseases such as cancer and AIDS may experience chronic pain that has an ill-defined onset and unknown duration.

## PAIN ASSESSMENT GUIDE
### TELL ME ABOUT YOUR PAIN

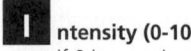 **W** ords to describe pain

| | | |
|---|---|---|
| aching | throbbing | shooting |
| stabbing | gnawing | sharp |
| tender | burning | exhausting |
| tiring | penetrating | nagging |
| numb | miserable | unbearable |
| dull | radiating | squeezing |
| crampy | deep | pressure |

#### Pain in other languages

| | | | |
|---|---|---|---|
| itami | Japanese | dolor | Spanish |
| tong | Chinese | douleur | French |
| dau | Vietnamese | bolno | Russian |

**I** ntensity (0-10)
if 0 is no pain and 10 is the worst pain imaginable, what is your pain now?... in the last 24 hours?

**L** ocation
Where is your pain?

**D** uration
Is the pain always there?
Does the pain come and go? (Breakthrough Pian)
Do you have both types of pain?

**A** ggravating and Alleviating Factors
What makes the pain better?
What makes the pain worse?

#### How does pain affect

| | | |
|---|---|---|
| sleep | energy | relationship |
| appetite | activity | mood |

#### Are you experiencing any other symptoms?

| | | |
|---|---|---|
| nausea/vomiting | itching | urinary retention |
| constipation | sleepiness/confusion | weakness |

#### Things to check
vital signs, past medication history, knowledge of pain, and use of noninvasive techniques

REFERENCES: Jacox A, Carr DB, Payne R, et al. Management of Cancer Pain. Clinical Practice Guidence No. 9. AHCPR Publication No. 94-0592. Rockville, MD. Agency for Health Care Policy and Research, U.S. Department of Health and Human Services, Public Health Service, March 1994. —Wong, D, and Whaley, L: Clinical Handbook of Pediatric Nursing, ed.2, The C.V. Mosby Company, St. Louis, 1986, p. 373.

**FIGURE 6–1.** A pocket pain assessment guide for use at the bedside. The health professional can use this guide to help the patient identify the level and intensity of pain and to determine the best approach to pain management in the context of overall care. *Source:* © 1996 Regina Fink, University of Colorado Denver, used with permission.

*Aggravating and Alleviating Factors.* If the patient is not receiving satisfactory pain relief, inquiring about what makes the pain better or worse—the alleviating and aggravating factors—will assist in determining which diagnostic tests need to be ordered or which nonpharmacologic approaches can be incorporated into the plan of care. Pain interference with functional status can be measured by determining the pain's effects on activities such as walking, sleeping, eating, energy, activity, relationships, sexuality, and mood. Researchers have found that pain interference with functional status is highly correlated with pain intensity scores; for example, a pain intensity score greater than 4 has been shown to significantly interfere with daily functioning.[2]

### Affective Factor

The affective factor includes the emotional responses associated with the pain experience and, possibly, such reactions as depression, anger, distress, anxiety, decreased ability to concentrate, mood disturbance, and loss of control. A person's feelings of distress, loss of control, or lack of involvement in the plan of care may affect outcomes of pain intensity and patient satisfaction with pain management.

### Cognitive Factor

The cognitive factor refers to the way pain influences the person's thought processes; the way the person views himself or herself in relation to the pain; the knowledge, attitudes, and beliefs the person has about the pain; and the meaning of the pain to the individual. Past experiences with pain may influence one's beliefs about pain. Whether the patient feels that another person believes in his or her pain also contributes to the cognitive dimension. Bostrom and colleagues[62] interviewed 30 palliative care patients with cancer-related pain to examine their perceptions of the management of their pain. Patients expressed a need for open communication with health care professionals about their pain problem and a need for being involved in the planning of their pain treatment. Those who felt a trust in their health care organization, their nurse, and their doctor described an improved ability to participate in their pain management plan.

Patients' knowledge and beliefs about pain play an obvious role in pain assessment, perception, function, and response to treatment. Patients may be reluctant to tell the nurse when they have pain; they may attempt to minimize its severity, may not know they can expect pain relief, and may be concerned about taking pain medications for fear of deleterious effects. A comprehensive approach to pain assessment includes evaluation of the patient's knowledge and beliefs about pain (Table 6–4) and its management and common misconceptions about analgesia.[33,56,63]

### Behavioral Factor

Pain behaviors may be a means of expressing pain or a coping response.[64] The behavioral factor describes actions the person exhibits related to the pain, such as verbal complaints, moaning, groaning, crying, facial expressions, posturing, splinting, lying down, pacing, rocking, or suppression of the expression of pain. Other cues can include anxious behaviors, insomnia, boredom, inability to concentrate, restlessness, and fatigue.[65] Unfortunately, some of these behaviors or cues may relate to causes or symptoms other than pain. For example, insomnia caused by depression may complicate the pain assessment.

Nonverbal expression of pain can complement, contradict, or replace the verbal complaint of pain[66] (see later discussion). Observing a patient's behavior or nonverbal cues, understanding the meaning of the pain experience to the patient, and collaborating with family members and other

**Table 6–3**
**Pain Descriptors**

| Pain Type | Qualifiers | Possible Etiological Factors | Intervention |
|---|---|---|---|
| Neuropathic (deafferentation) | Burning, numb, tingling, radiating, pricking, lancinating, "fire-like", "pins and needles", short-lasting shooting, electric or shock-like pains | Nerve involvement by tumor (cervical, brachial, lumbosacral plexi), postherpetic or trigeminal neuralgia, diabetic neuropathies, HIV associated neuropathy (viral or antiretrovirals), chemotherapy-induced neuropathy, post stroke pain, post radiation plexopathies, phantom pain | Anticonvulsants, local anesthetics, antidepressants, benzodiazepines, Tramadol hydrochloride, opioids, steroids, nerve blocks |
| Visceral (poorly localized) | Squeezing, cramping, gnawing, pressure, distention, deep, stretching, bloated feeling, diffuse | Bowel obstruction, venous occlusion, ischemia, liver metastases, ascites, thrombosis, post-abdominal or thoracic surgery, pancreatitis | Opioids (caution must be used in the administration of opioids to patients with bowel obstruction), nonsteroidal anti-inflammatory drugs (NSAIDs) |
| Somatic (well localized) | Dull, achy, throbbing, sore | Bone or spine metastases, fractures, arthritis, osteoporosis, injury to deep musculoskeletal structures or superficial cutaneous tissues, immobility | NSAIDs, steroids, muscle relaxants, bisphosphonates, opioids and/or radiation therapy (bone metastasis) |
| Psychologic | All-encompassing, everywhere | Psychologic disorders | Psychiatric treatments, support, nonpharmacologic approaches |

**Table 6–4**
**Common Patient Concerns and Misconceptions about Pain and Analgesia**

Pain is inevitable. I just need to bear it.
If the pain is worse, it must mean my disease (cancer) is spreading.
I had better wait to take my pain medication until I really need it or else it won't work later.
My family thinks I am getting too "spacey" on pain medication; I'd better hold back.
If it's morphine, I must be getting close to the end.
If I take pain medicine (such as opioids) regularly, I will get "hooked" or addicted.
If I take my pain medication before I hurt, I will end up taking too much. It's better to "hang in there and tough it out."
I'd rather have a good bowel movement than take pain medication and get constipated.
I don't want to bother the nurse or doctor; they're busy with other patients.
If I take too much pain medication, it will hasten my death.
Good patients avoid talking about pain.

*Sources*: Jones et al. (2005), reference 33; Fink (1997), reference 56; Gordon and Ward (1995), reference 63.

health care professionals to determine their thoughts about the patient's pain, are all part of the pain assessment process.

The behavioral dimension also encompasses the unconscious or deliberate actions taken by the person to decrease the pain. Pain behaviors include, but are not limited to, using both prescribed and over-the-counter analgesics; seeking medical assistance; using nonpharmacological approaches and other coping strategies such as removing aggravating factors (e.g., noise and light). Behaviors used to control pain in patients with advanced-stage disease include assuming special positions, immobilizing or guarding a body part, rubbing, and adjusting pressure to a body part.

### Sociocultural Factor

The sociocultural factor encompasses all of the demographic variables of the patient experiencing pain. The impact of these factors (e.g., age, gender, ethnicity, spirituality, marital status, social support) on pain assessment, treatment, and outcomes have been examined in the literature. Although many studies have promoted each individual dimension, few have concentrated on their highly interactive nature. Ultimately, all of these factors can influence pain assessment.

*Age.* Much of the pain literature has called attention to the problem of inadequate pain assessment and management in the elderly in a palliative care setting. Elderly patients suffer disproportionately from chronic painful conditions and have multiple diagnoses with complex problems and accompanying pain. Elders have physical, social, and psychological needs distinct from those of younger and middle-aged adults, and they present particular challenges for pain assessment and management. Pain assessment may be more problematic in elderly patients because their reporting of pain may differ from that of younger patients due to their increased stoicism.[33] Elderly people often present with failures in memory, depression, and sensory impairments that may hinder history taking; they may also underreport pain because they expect pain to occur as a part of the aging process.[67,68] Moreover, dependent elderly people may not report pain because they do not want to bother the nurse or doctor and are concerned that they will cause more distress in their family caregivers.[69]

Studies have documented the problem of inadequate pain assessment in the eldery.[70] Cleeland and colleagues[2] studied 1308 outpatients with metastatic cancer and found that those 70 years of age or older were more likely to have inadequate pain assessment and analgesia. Approximately 40% of elderly nursing home patients with cancer experience daily pain according to Bernabei, who reviewed Medicare records of more than 13,625 cancer patients aged 65 years or older discharged from hospitals to almost 1500 nursing homes in five states.[71] Pain assessment was based on patient self-report and determined by a team of nursing home personnel involved with the patients. Of the more than 4000 patients who complained of daily pain, 16% were given a nonopioid drug, 32% were given a weak opioid, 26% received morphine, and 26% received no analgesic. As age increased, a greater proportion of patients in pain received no analgesia (21% of patients aged 65 to 74 years, 26% of those aged 75 to 84 years, and 30% of those 85 years of age and older; $P = 0.001$). Fewer than half of over 2000 elderly residents with predictably recurrent pain were prescribed scheduled pain medication.[17] Therefore, it is imperative to pay particular attention to pain assessment in the elderly patient, so that the chance of inadequate analgesia is decreased. Dementia, cognitive and sensory impairments, and disabilities can make pain assessment and management more difficult (see later discussion). Also, residents in long-term care facilities are likely to have multiple medical problems that can cause pain.

*Gender.* Gender differences affect sensitivity to pain, pain tolerance, pain distress, willingness to report pain, exaggeration of pain, and nonverbal expression of pain .[72–75] Multiple studies have demonstrated that men show more stoicism than women, women exhibit lower pain thresholds and less tolerance to noxious stimuli than men, women become more upset when pain prevents them from doing things they enjoy, and women seek care of pain sooner.[75–79] Responses to analgesics and the prevalence of pain in various disease conditions may also vary according to sex and gender.[80,81] For example, in a study of pain in advanced cancer,[82] women experienced more visceral pain, whereas men had more somatic pain (bone metastases). Interestingly, differences in pain threshold between the sexes diminish with increasing age, particularly after the age of 40.[83] One study found that there were no sex differences in pain scores or postoperative morphine requirements among elderly patients over the age of 70.[81] Although a large amount of data support the finding that men respond better to mu opioid agonists and women respond better to kappa opioid analgesics, a research study challenged the previous findings.[84]

Although coping with pain and the experience of pain may be influenced by an individual's gender,[85,86] the reasons for these differences remain unclear or unidentified. It is important to note that gender or sex differences in pain response are not universal and do not exert a large effect.[80] Explanations that require further investigation include molecular and genetic mechanisms, hormonal influences, as well as social, cultural, psychological, and experimental bias.[87] Nurses and other health care professionals need to be mindful of possible gender differences when assessing pain and planning individualized care for persons in pain. However, until there is more definitive data, men and women should receive similar pain care based upon individual assessments.

*Ethnicity.* The term ethnicity refers to one or more of the following[88]: (1) a common language or tradition, (2) shared origins or social background, and (3) shared culture and traditions that are distinctive, passed through generations, and create a sense of identity. Ethnicity may be a predictor of pain expression and response. While assessing pain, it is important to remember that certain ethnic groups and cultures have strong beliefs about expressing pain and may hesitate to complain of unrelieved pain.[89] The biocultural model of Bates and associates[90] proposed that culturally accepted patterns of ethnic meanings of pain may influence the neurophysiological processing of nociceptive information that is responsible for pain threshold, pain tolerance, pain behavior, and expression. Thus, the manner in which a person reacts to the pain experience may be strongly related to cultural background. The biocultural model also hypothesizes that social learning from family and group membership can influence psychological and physiological processes, which in turn can affect the perception and modulation of pain. Bates stressed that all individuals, regardless of ethnicity, have basically similar neurophysiological systems of pain perception. Early clinical studies of pain expression and culture concluded that the preferred values and traditions of culture affected an individual's handling and communication of pain.[91–93]

Studies reveal that racial and ethnic minorities are not adequately assessed for pain and are at risk for undertreatment of pain.[2,94–96] Differences in cultural backgrounds between health care providers and patients can result in misunderstandings, mistrust, and lack of communication about pain.[97]

It is important to realize that racial and ethnic disparities exist in pain care and that too little is known about how culture and ethnicity affect pain responses, pain interventions, and pain measurement. Although pain assessment or pain tools may be available in languages spoken by the patients, the translations may be inadequate or may not capture cultural nuances or meanings.[98] When caring for any patient who is experiencing pain, the nurse must avoid cultural stereotyping and provide culturally sensitive assessment and educational materials, enlisting the support of an interpreter when appropriate.

*Marital Status and Social Support.* The degree of family or social support in a patient's life should be assessed, because these factors may influence the expression, meaning, and perception of pain and the ability to comply with therapeutic recommendations. Few studies have examined the influence of marital status on pain experience and expression. Dar and coworkers[99] studied 40 patients (45% women, 55% men) with metastatic cancer pain and found that patients minimized their pain when their spouses were present. When asked if and how their pain changed in the presence of spouses, 40% of the patients said the pain was better and 60% reported no change; none reported that the pain was worse. The majority (64%) of patients agreed that they conceal their pain so that their spouses will not be upset, even though spouses were generally accurate in their estimates of the patients' pain levels. Almost all patients reported a very high degree of satisfaction with the way their spouses helped them cope with pain.

*Spirituality.* Spross and Wolff Burke[100] believed that the spiritual dimension mediates the person's pain response and expression and influences how the other aspects of pain are experienced. Whereas pain refers to a physical sensation, suffering refers to the quest for meaning, purpose, and fulfillment. Although pain is often a source of suffering, suffering may occur in the absence of pain. Many patients believe that pain and suffering are meaningful signs of the presence of a higher being and must be endured; others are outraged by the pain and suffering they must endure and demand alleviation. The nurse must verify the patients' beliefs and give them permission to verbalize their personal points of view. Assessing a patient's existential view of pain and suffering is important because it can affect the processes of healing and dying. Wachholtz and colleagues explored the relationship between spirituality, coping, and pain and offer suggestions for future research.[101] Understanding patients' use of spiritual comfort strategies is also an area to explore. Dunn and Horgas[102] found that elderly women and older patients of minority background reported using religious coping strategies (prayer or spiritual comfort) to manage their pain more often than did older Caucasian men. Spiritual assessment is covered in greater detail in Chapter 33.

### Environmental Factor

The environmental factor refers to the the environment in which the person receives pain management. Creating a peaceful environment free from bright lights, extreme noise, and excessive heat or cold may assist in alleviating the patient's pain.

Context of care, setting, or where the patient receives care may also refer to the environmental aspect. Health care providers may perceive an individual's pain differently. Nurses and other health care professionals are inconsistent in their reliance on patient self-report as a major component in the assessment process. Agreement between patients' perceptions and health care professionals' perceptions was relatively low and was generally an inadequate substitute for patients' reports of pain.[103-106] Health care providers' ratings corresponded more with patients' ratings when pain was severe.[104,106] Additionally, when nurses' pain assessments were documented over time, early assessments were more accurate than later ones.[107]

A multifactorial framework describing the influences of all of these factors on the assessment of pain and the pain experience is desirable to attain positive pain outcomes. The factors comprising the framework are assumed to be interactive and interrelated. Use of this framework for pain assessment has clear implications for clinical practice and research.

## Quantitative Assessment of Pain

Although pain is a subjective, self-reported experience of the patient, the ability to quantify the intensity of pain is essential to monitoring a patient's responsiveness to analgesia.

### Pain Intensity Assessment Scales

The most commonly used pain intensity scales—the visual analog scale (VAS), the numeric rating scale (NRS), the verbal descriptor scale (VDS), the Wong–Baker FACES pain scale, the Faces Pain Scale (FPS), the Faces Pain Scale-Revised (FPS-R), and the pain thermometer—are illustrated and reviewed in Table 6–5 with advantages and disadvantages delineated. These scales have proved to be very effective, reproducible means of measuring pain and other symptoms, and they can be universally implemented and regularly applied in many care settings. How useful these tools are in the assessment of pain in the palliative care patient is a question that still needs to be answered.

Although no one scale is appropriate or suitable for all patients, universal adoption of a 0-to-10 scale, rather than a 0-to-5 or a 0-to-100 scale, for clinical assessment of pain intensity in adult patients is recommended.[129] Jensen and colleagues examined the maximum number of levels needed to measure pain intensity in patients with chronic pain and concluded that an 11-point scale (0 to 10) provided sufficient levels of discrimination when compared with a 0-to-100 scale.[130] Standardization may promote collaboration and consistency in evaluation among caregivers across multiple settings (i.e., inpatient, ambulatory, home care/hospice or long-term care environments) and would facilitate pain research across sites. Collection of comparative data would be enabled, allowing for simplification of the analytical process. Detailed explanation of how to use the pain scales is necessary before use by patients in any clinical care area.

Another concern is health care professionals' inconsistent use of word anchors on pain intensity scales. The intention behind the use of a word anchor to discriminate pain intensity is to provide a common endpoint; although that point may have not been reached by a patient, it would provide a place for any pain experienced to date or pain that may be experienced in the future. Some of the common endpoint word anchors that have been used are "worst possible pain," "pain as bad as it can be," "worst pain imaginable," "worst pain you have ever had," "most severe pain imaginable," and "most intense pain imaginable." Inconsistent or different

**Table 6–5**
**Pain Intensity Assessment Scales**

| Scale | Description | Advantages | Disadvantages |
|---|---|---|---|
| Visual Analogue Scale (VAS) | A vertical line of 10 cm (or 100 mm) in length anchored at each end by verbal descriptors (e.g., no pain and worst possible pain). Patients are asked to make a slash mark or X on the line at the place that represents the amount of pain experienced. | Positive correlation with other self-reported measures of pain intensity and observed pain behaviors.[108,109] Sensitive to treatment effects and distinct from subjective components of pain.[110,111] Qualities of ratio data with high number of response categories make it more sensitive to changes in pain intensity.[109,112]. | Scoring may be more time-consuming and involve more steps.[113] Patients may have difficulty using and understanding a VAS measure.[113] Too abstract for many adults, and may be difficult to use with elderly, non-English-speaking, and patients with physical disability, immobility, or reduced visual acuity, which may limit their ability to place a mark on the line.[113–115] |
| Numeric Rating Scale (NRS) | The number that the patient gives represents his/her pain intensity from 0 to 10 with the understanding that 0= no pain and 10 = worst pain possible. | Validity and demonstrated sensitivity to VAS.[116] Verbal administration to patients allows those by phone or who are physically and visually disabled to quantify pain intensity.[117] Ease in scoring, high compliance, high number of response categories.[117] Scores may be treated as interval data and are correlated with VAS.[118] | Lack of research comparing sensitivity to treatments impacting pain intensity. |
| Verbal Descriptor Scale (VDS) | Adjectives reflecting extremes of pain are ranked in order of severity. Each adjective is given a number which constitutes the patient's pain intensity. | Short, ease of administration to patients, easily comprehended, high compliance.[108] Easy to score and analyze data on an ordinal level.[63] Validity is established.[110] Sensitivity to treatments that are known to impact pain intensity.[109] | Less reliable among illiterate patients and persons with limited English vocabulary.[118] Patients must choose one word to describe their pain intensity even if no word accurately describes it.[108] Variability in use of verbal descriptors is associated with affective distress.[113] Scores on VDS are considered ordinal data; however, the distances between its descriptors are not equal but categorical.[117] |
| FACES Scale (Wong-Baker)[119] | The scale consists of six cartoon-type faces. The no pain (0) face shows a widely smiling face and the most pain (10) face shows a face with tears. The scale is treated as a Likert scale and was originally developed to measure children's pain intensity or amount of hurt. It has been used in adults. | Validity is supported by research reporting that persons from many cultures recognize facial expressions and identify them in similar ways.[120] Simplicity, ease of use, and correlation with VAS makes it a valuable option in clinical settings.[121,122] Short, requires little mental energy and little explanation for use.[123] | Presence of tears on the "most pain" face may introduce cultural bias when the scale is used by adults from cultures not sanctioning crying in response to pain.[124] |
| Faces Pain Scale—Revised (FPS-R)[125] | The Faces Pain Scale Revised (FPS-R) was adapted from the FPS[126] in order to make it compatible with a 0-10 metric scale.[120] The FPS-R measures pain intensity consists of six oval faces ranging from a neutral face (no pain) to a grimacing, sad face without tears (worst pain). | Easy to administer. Oval-shaped faces without tears or wide smiles are more adult-like in appearance, possibly making the scale more acceptable to adults. | Facial expressions may be difficult to discern by patients who have visual difficulties. The FPS-R may measure other constructs (anger, distress, and impact of pain on functional status) than just pain intensity. |
| Pain Thermometer[127] | Modified vertical verbal descriptor scale which is administered by asking the patient to point to the words that best describe his/her pain.[122] | Increased sensitivity. Preferred for patients with moderate to severe cognitive deficits or those with difficulty with abstract thinking and verbal communication.[128] | Allow for practice time to use this tool. |

word anchors may yield different pain reports. Therefore, it is important to come to some consensus about consistent use of word anchors.

## Comparison of Pain Scales

Several studies have been systematically reviewed,[43,108,131] and although many are limited in sample size and population, a positive correlation has been demonstrated among the VAS, VDS, NRS, Wong–Baker FACES scale, FPS, and FPS-R. Each of the commonly used rating scales appear to be adequately valid and reliable as a measure of pain intensity in both cancer patients and elders.

Herr and Mobily[115] studied 49 senior citizens 65 years of age with reported leg pain to determine the relationships among various pain intensity measures, to examine the ability of patients to use the tools correctly, and to determine elderly people's preferences. The VAS consisted of 10-cm horizontal and vertical lines; the VDS had six numerically ranked choices of word descriptors, including "no pain," "mild pain," "discomforting," "distressing," "horrible," and "excruciating"; the NRS had numbers from 1 to 20; and the pain thermometer had seven choices, ranging from "no pain" to "pain as bad as it could be." The scale preferred by most respondents was the VDS. Of the two VAS scales, the vertical scale was chosen most often because the elderly subjects had a tendency to conceptualize the vertical presentation more accurately. Elderly patients may have deficits in abstract ability that make the VAS difficult to use.[133] Increased age is associated with an increased incidence of incorrect response to the VAS.[108]

Paice and Cohen[117] used a convenience sample of 50 hospitalized adult cancer patients with pain to study their preference in using the VAS, the VDS, and the NRS. Fifty percent of the patients preferred using the NRS. Fewer patients preferred the VDS (38%), and the VAS was chosen infrequently (12%). Twenty percent of the patients were unable to complete the VAS or had difficulty in doing so. Problems included needing assistance with holding a pencil, making slash marks that were too wide or not on the line, marking the wrong end of the line, and asking to have instructions read repeatedly during the survey.

Additional problems exist with use of the VAS. When multiple horizontal scales are used to measure different aspects or dimensions (e.g., pain intensity, distress, depression), subjects tend to mark all of the scales down the middle. Pain intensity has been noted to be consistently higher on each scale for depressed and anxious patients compared with nondepressed, nonanxious patients.[132] Photocopying of VAS forms may result in distortion so that the scales may not be exactly 10 cm long and the reliability of measurement may be in question. Physical disability or decreased visual acuity may limit the ability of the palliative care patient to mark the appropriate spot on the line. The VAS also requires pencil and paper and requires the patient to be knowledgeable about various English pain adjectives. In conclusion, a VAS may be more difficult to use with elderly patients and has a higher failure rate, compared with an NRS or a VDS; in addition, the failure rate is slightly greater with an NRS compared with a VDS.

The use of a faces pain scale to measure pain intensity avoids language and may cross cultural differences.[133] Several faces pain scales have been used[119,125,126] to assess pain in both pediatric and adult populations. Jones and colleagues[134] asked elderly nursing home residents to choose which of three pain intensity scales (NRS, VDS, and FPS) they preferred to use to rate their pain. Of those able to choose, the VDS was the most commonly selected (52%); 29% chose the NRS; 19% preferred the FPS. More men than women and those residents with moderate to severe pain preferred the NRS; a higher percentage of minority (Hispanic) residents preferred the FPS.

Findings from various studies indicated that patients used the FPS to measure pain appropriately and that the FPS should be considered an alternative to the NRS or VAS in various populations. However, the literature regarding choice of scale among ethnic groups is equivocal. Carey and colleagues[135] asked hospitalized patients which of several scales they preferred to use: a modified Wong–Baker FACES scale (tears were removed), a NRS, or a vertical VAS. They found that less educated adults, both African American and Caucasian American, preferred the Wong–Baker FACES scale; more educated patients preferred the NRS. Stuppy[123] also found that patients preferred the FPS to the NRS, VAS, or VDS, with no significant differences noted between African American and Caucasian American participants. Taylor and Herr[127,133] discovered that both cognitively impaired and intact African American elders preferred the FPS to the NRS or the VDS, and they found support for the ordinal nature of the FPS. Participants clearly agreed that the FPS represented pain but also agreed that the FPS may represent other constructs, such as sadness or anger, depending how they were cued; this may suggest that the FPS may be measuring pain affect, not just intensity. Other researchers[136,137] found that Hispanic patients preferred the FPS-R over the Iowa Pain Thermometer (IPT) and other instruments used to measure pain intensity.

In summary, a variety of scales have been used to assess pain in varied patient populations. Each has been widely used in clinical research and practice. Little research has been done on the appropriateness of pain scales in the palliative care setting. Intellectual understanding and language skills are prerequisites for such pain assessment scales as the VAS and VDS. These scales may be too abstract or too difficult for palliative care patients. Because most dying patients are elderly, simple pain scales, such as the NRS or a faces scale, may be more advantageous.

## Multifactorial Pain Instruments

There are several pain measurement instruments that can be used to standardize pain assessment, incorporating patient demographic factors, pain severity scales, pain descriptors, and other questions related to pain. Four instruments have been considered short enough for routine clinical use with cancer patients. All of these instruments provide a quick way of measuring pain subjectively; however, their use in seriously ill, actively dying patients needs further study.

*The Short Form McGill Pain Questionnaire* (SF-MPQ)[138] has been developed and includes 15 words to describe pain. Each word or phrase is rated on a four-point intensity scale (0 = none, 1 = mild, 2 = moderate, and 3 = severe). Three pain scores are derived from the sum of the intensity rank values of the words chosen for sensory, affective, and total descriptors. Two pain measures are also included in the SF-MPQ: the Present Pain Intensity Index (PPI) and a 10-cm VAS. The SF-MPQ has demonstrated reliability and validity and is available in multiple languages.

*The Brief Pain Inventory* (BPI)[139] is a multifactorial instrument that address pain etiology, history, intensity, quality, location, and interference with activities. Patients are asked to rate the severity of their pain at its worst, least, average, and at present. Using an NRS (0 to 10), patients are also asked for ratings of how much their pain interferes with walking ability, mood, general activity, work, enjoyment of life, sleep, and relationships with others. The BPI also asks patients to represent the location of their pain on a drawing and asks about the cause of pain and the duration of pain relief.

*The Memorial Pain Assessment Card* (MPAC)[140] is a simple, valid tool consisting of three VAS, for pain intensity, pain relief, and mood, and one VDS to describe the pain. The MPAC can be completed by patients in 20 seconds or less and can distinguish between pain intensity, relief, and psychological distress.

*The City of Hope Patient and Family Pain Questionnaires*[141] were designed to measure the knowledge and experience of patients with chronic cancer pain and their family caregivers. The 16-item surveys use an ordinal scale format and can be administered in inpatient or outpatient settings.

Because terminally ill patients have multiple symptoms, it is impossible to limit an assessment to only the report of pain. Complications or symptoms related to the disease process may exacerbate pain, or interventions to alleviate pain may cause side effects that result in new or worsening symptoms, such as constipation or nausea. Symptoms such as fatigue and anxiety are distressful and may affect quality of life in seriously ill cancer and noncancer patients.[142] Therefore, pain assessment must be accompanied by assessment of other symptoms. Various surveys or questionnaires not only assess pain but also incorporate other symptoms into the assessment process. Many of these instruments are discussed in other chapters.

❧❧

## Pain Assessment in Nonverbal or Cognitively Impaired Patients

The patient's self-report, the gold standard for pain assessment, is not always feasible in patients who cannot verbalize their pain and for patients with severe cognitive impairment (e.g., dementia and delirium). Cognitive impairment and the inability to communicate by speaking, writing, or signing represent major barriers to adequate pain assessment and treatment. As noted by the International Association for the Study of Pain (IASP), "the inability to communicate verbally does not negate the possibility that an individual is experiencing pain and is in need of appropriate pain-relieving treatment."[19]

The potential for unrelieved and unrecognized pain is greater in patients who cannot verbally express their discomfort. Older, nonverbal, and cognitively impaired patients are at increased risk for pain, as well as underassessment and undertreatment of pain.[11–18,43,143–146] Patients who are nonverbal or cognitively impaired are usually excluded from pain studies; thus, pain assessment and treatment in these groups are poorly understood.[147]

The inability to communicate effectively due to impaired cognition and sensory losses is a serious problem for many patients with severe critical and terminal illnesses. Cognitive failure develops in the majority of cancer patients before death, and agitated delirium is frequently observed in patients with advanced cancer.[148,149] Loss of consciousness occurs in almost half of dying patients during the final three days of life.[150] These complications have been shown in part to be significantly correlated with a higher dose requirement of opioids and the presence of icterus.[151] Clearly, pain assessment techniques and tools are needed that apply to patients, whether mentally incompetent or nonverbal, who communicate only through their unique behavioral responses (Figure 6–2).

In addition to verbal self-reports, other ways to assess pain, such as observation of behaviors or surrogate reporting, must be utilized in persons who cannot verbally communicate their pain. It is important to remember that "No single objective assessment strategy, such as interpretation of behaviors, pathology, or estimates of pain by others, is sufficient by itself"[42]. *ASPMN Position Statement on Pain Assessment in the Nonverbal Patient*[42] provides recommendations for assessing pain in special populations including nonverbal older adults with dementia and those who are intubated and/or unconsious. Pain assessment can be guided by the following principles and framework:

1. Use the hierarchy of pain assessment techniques[152]
   a. Obtain self-report, if possible.
   b. Search for potential causes of pain or other pathologies that could cause pain.
   c. Observe patient behaviors that are indicative of pain.
   d. Obtain surrrogate reporting (family members, parents, caregivers) of pain and behavior/activity changes.
   e. Attempt an analgesic trial to assess a reduction in possible pain behaviors.

**A. Visual Analog Scale**

Worst possible
pain

No pain

**B. Numeric Rating Scale**

0–10 Numeric Rating Scale

| 0 | 1 | 2 | 3 | 4 | 5 | 6 | 7 | 8 | 9 | 10 |

No
pain

Moderate
pain

Worst
possible
pain

**D. Wong-Baker FACES Scale**

Wong-Baker FACES Pain Rating Scale

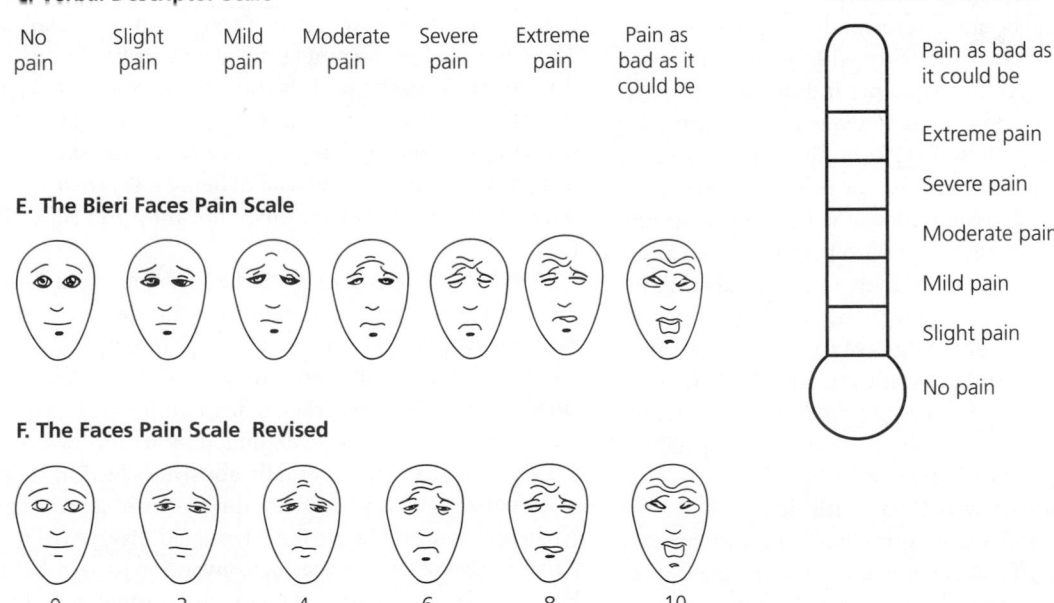

| 0 | 2 | 4 | 6 | 8 | 10 |

No
hurt

Hurts
little
bit

Hurts
little
more

Hurts
even
more

Hurts
whole
lot

Hurts
worst

Explain to the resident that each face is for a person who feels happy because he has no pain (hurt) or sad because he has some or a lot of pain. On the 0–5 scale, Face 0 is very happy because he doesn't hurt at all. Face 2 hurts just a little bit. Face 4 hurts a little more. Face 6 hurts even more. Face 8 hurts a whole lot. Face 10 hurts as much as you can imagine, although you don't have to be crying to feel this bad. Ask the person to choose the face that best descibes how he is feeling.

*Source:* Adapted from Wong & Baker (1988), reference 111.

**C. Verbal Descriptor Scale**

No
pain   Slight
pain   Mild
pain   Moderate
pain   Severe
pain   Extreme
pain   Pain as
bad as it
could be

**E. The Bieri Faces Pain Scale**

**F. The Faces Pain Scale Revised**

| 0 | 2 | 4 | 6 | 8 | 10 |

**G. Pain Thermometer**

Pain as bad as
it could be

Extreme pain

Severe pain

Moderate pain

Mild pain

Slight pain

No pain

**Figure 6–2.** Commonly used pain intensity scales. Refer to Table 6–5 for descriptions, advantages, and disadvantages. *Source*: Adapted with permission from Wong DL, Baker CM. Pain in children: comparison of assessment scales. Pediatr Nurs 1988;14:9–17.

Table 6–6
**Possible Pain Behaviors in Nonverbal and Cognitively Impaired Patients or Residents**

| Behavior Category | Possible Pain Behaviors |
| --- | --- |
| Facial expressions | Grimace, frown, wince, sad or frightened look, wrinkled forehead, furrowed brow, closed or tightened eye-lids, rapid blinking, clenched teeth or jaw |
| Body movements | Restless, agitated, jittery, "can't seem to sit still", fidgeting, pacing, rocking, constant or intermittent shifting of position, withdrawing |
| Protective mechanisms | Bracing; guarding; rubbing or massaging a body part; splinting; clutching or holding onto side rails, bed, tray table, or affected area during movement |
| Verbalizations | Saying common phrases such as "help me", "leave me alone" , "get away from me", "don't touch me", "ouch", cursing, verbally abusive, praying out loud |
| Vocalizations | Sighing, moaning, groaning, crying, whining, oohing, aahing, calling out, screaming, chanting, breathing heavily |
| Mental status changes | Confusion, disorientation, irritability, distress, depression |
| Changes in activity patterns, routines, or interpersonal interactions | Decreased appetite, sleep alterations, decreased social activity participation, change in ambulation, immobilization, aggressive, combative, resisting care |

*Sources*: Adapted from references 13, 14, 145, 155–157.

2. Establish a procedure for pain assessment.
3. Use behavioral pain assessment tools, as appropriate.
4. Minimize emphasis on physiologic indicators.
5. Reassess and document.

## Pain Behaviors

It may be more complicated to assess nonverbal cues in the palliative care setting because terminally ill patients with chronic pain, in contrast to patients with acute pain, may not demonstrate any specific behaviors indicative of pain. It is also not satisfactory and even erroneous to assess pain by reliance on involuntary physiological bodily reactions, such as increases in blood pressure, pulse, or respiratory rate and depth.. Elevated vital signs may occur with sudden, severe pain; but they usually do not occur with persistent pain after the body reaches physiological equilibrium.[153] The absence of behavioral or involuntary cues does not negate the presence of pain. Assessment of behavior for signs of pain during rest and movement provides a potentially valid and reliable alternative to verbal and physiological indices of pain.[154,155] Examples of pain behaviors in cognitively impaired or nonverbal patients or residents are displayed in Table 6–6.[113,14,155–157]

Pain indicators in elderly patients with dementia identified by nursing home staff members included specific physical repetitive movements, facial expressions, vocal repetitions, physical signs of pain, and changes in behavior from the norm for that person.[158,159] It should be noted that observations of facial expressions may not be valid in those patients with some types of dementia in which facial expressions are muted[145] or in conditions that result in distorted facial expressions, such as Parkinson's disease or stroke. Cultural influences on behavioral expressions and interpretation of behavior must also be considered.

## The Pain Experience in Patients with Cognitive Failure

Pain behaviors in individuals with cognitive failure or dementia may be different from those of patients or residents who are cognitively intact. There is a tendency for patients with increased levels of cognitive impairment to report less severe pain[133,160–163] and for patients with progressive dementia to have fewer pain complaints.[164,165] The decreased pain complaints are most likely related to a diminished capacity or difficulty in communicating pain.[145] As reflected in several studies,[166–168] "there is no consistent evidence to indicate that persons with dementia experience less pain sensation."[145] Instead of being less sensitive to pain, older adults with dementia may not interpret sensations as painful.[169]

Behavior or responses caused by noxious stimuli in individuals with cognitive impairment or dementia may not necessarily reflect classic or typical pain behaviors. There is considerable variability and uniqueness in behavior expressions of pain in nonverbal older adults with dementia.[145] For example, pain may be exhibited by withdrawn behavior, aggressive behavior, or verbally abusive behavior. In a study of 26 patients with painful conditions from a nursing home Alzheimer's unit, Marzinski[170] reported diverse responses to pain that were not typical of conventional pain behaviors. For example, with pain, a patient who normally moaned and rocked became quiet and withdrawn. Pain in another nonverbal patient caused rapid blinking. Other patients who normally exhibited disjointed verbalizations could, when experiencing pain, give accurate descriptions of their pain. Parmelee[161] and Huffman[164] and their colleagues also found that verbal pain reports by patients with dementia are accurate and valid.

**Table 6–7**
**Assessment and Treatment of Pain in the Nonverbal or Cognitively Impaired Patient or Resident**

Is there a reason for the patient to be experiencing pain? Review the patient's diagnoses.

Was the patient previously treated for pain? If so, what regimen was effective (include pharmacologic and nonpharmacologic interventions)?

How does the patient usually act when he/she is in pain? (Note: the nurse may need to ask family/significant others or other health care professionals.)

What is the family/significant others' interpretation of the patient's behavior? Do they think the patient is in pain? Why do they feel this way?

Try to obtain feedback from the patient, e.g., ask patient to nod head, squeeze hand, move eyes up or down, raise legs, or hold up fingers to signal presence of pain.

If appropriate, offer writing materials or pain intensity charts that patient can use or point to.

If there is a possible reason for or sign of acute pain, treat with analgesics or other pain-relief measures.

If a pharmacologic or nonpharmacologic intervention results in modifying pain behavior, continue with treatment.

If pain behavior persists, rule out potential causes of the behavior (delirium, side effect of treatment, symptom of disease process); try appropriate intervention for behavior cause.

Explain interventions to patient and family/significant other.

Questions and suggestions in Table 6–7 can be used as a template for assessment and treatment of pain in the nonverbal or cognitively impaired patient or resident.

## Instruments Used to Assess Pain in Nonverbal or Cognitively Impaired Patients

### Pain Behavioral Scales

Assessing pain in patients/residents who are nonverbal or cognitively impaired and are unable to verbally self-report pain presents a particular challenge to clinicians. An instrument that could detect the presence of or a reduction in pain behaviors could facilitate effective pain management plans. However, because pain is not just a set of pain behaviors, the absence of certain behaviors does not necessarily mean that the patient is pain free.[171] As evident from several excellent reviews of pain tools[43,145,169,172], many health care providers and researchers have attempted to develop an easy-to-use, yet valid and reliable instrument for the assessment of pain in this vulnerable population. There is no one current tool based on nonverbal pain behaviors that can be recommended for general applicability in clinical practice and palliative care settings. A basic summary of instruments used to assess

pain in nonverbal or cognitively impaired patients is found in Table 6–8. Herr and colleagues[145] have performed an extensive and critical evaluation of many of these existing tools (conceptualization, subject/setting, reliability and validity data based on research, administration/scoring methods, strengths/weaknesses) with the intent of providing up-to-date information to clinicians and researchers as it becomes available. This detailed review can be accessed at http://prc.coh.org/PAIN-NOA.htm.

Additionally, the Edmonton Symptom Assessment System (ESAS) is a validated tool for use in the palliative care setting.) Originally tested in palliative care inpatients, 83% of symptom assessments were completed by nurses or patients' relatives.[192] The ESAS is a brief and reproducible scale consisting of separate visual analog or numeric scales that evaluate pain and eight additional symptoms (activity, nausea, depression, anxiety, drowsiness, appetite, sensation of well-being, and shortness of breath). If patients are unable to complete the form, a space is provided for the person completing the assessment. If patients or residents are unresponsive and incapable of reporting their own pain (e.g., during the final days of life), observer judgments of pain become necessary. In this situation, the main caregiver completes the Edmonton Comfort Assessment Form (ECAF). Although the ESAS has been considered useful to display the symptom prevalence, some investigators have found it to be impractical in patients with a poor performance status.[193] To evaluate pain and other symptoms, an individualized approach may be a more appropriate practice than completing health-related checklists.

### Pain Intensity Scales

Research[43,133,136,161,194–196] indicates that the verbal descriptor scale (VDS), the numeric rating scale (NRS), the faces pain scales (FPS and FPS-R), and the Iowa pain thermometer (IPT), are reliable and valid in older adults with mild to moderate degrees of cognitive impairment. Cognitively impaired older adults are able to accurately complete one or more pain intensity scales;[133,136,144,195–198] however, there is concern about the reliability of their short-term pain reports.[199] Ware et al. recommend consideration of the FPS when repeat assessments are indicated, in older cognitively impaired minority adults.[136] While the FPS-R is generally favored for *both* cognitively intact and cognitively impaired older adults, it should be noted that the FPS-R may not clearly represent pain intensity only but may also represent a broader construct "pain affect."[136] Because the FPS-R is easy to use and easily understood, it can be offered to minority older adults as an alternative if other validated tools, such as the VDS and NRS, are not usable by this population because of language barriers.

### Proxy Pain Assessment in the Nonverbal or Cognitively Impaired Patient or Resident

Just as the experience of pain is subjective, observing and interpreting a patient's or resident's pain is a subjective

**Table 6–8**
**Pain Assessment Tools for the Cognitively Impaired or Nonverbal Patient or Resident**

| Tool | Goal | Dimensions/Parameters | Comments |
|---|---|---|---|
| Abbey Pain Scale[173] | Assess pain in late stage demented patients in nursing homes. | Vocalization<br>Facial expression<br>Change in body language<br>Behavioral change<br>Physiological change<br>Physical change | Based on previous research[174,175] this scale was developed for use with end/late stage dementia residents unable to express needs. Six behavioral indicators are scored with three grades of severity (0 = absent through 3 = severe) for a total possible score of 18. |
| Assessment of Discomfort in Dementia Protocol (ADD)[176–178] | Improve the recognition and treatment of pain and discomfort in patients with dementia who cannot report their internal states, with the added goal of decreasing inappropriate use of psychotropic medication administration. | Facial expression<br>Mood<br>Body language<br>Voice<br>Behavior | Based on DS–DAT items, the ADD protocol includes more overt symptoms (physical aggression, crying, calling out, resisting care, and existing behaviors). Protocol implementation when basic care interventions failed to ameliorate behavioral symptoms resulted in significant decreases in discomfort, significant increases in the use of pharmacologic and nonpharmacologic comfort interventions and improved behavioral symptoms.[176–178] |
| Checklist of Nonverbal Pain Indicators (CNPI)[155,160] | Measure pain behaviors in cognitively impaired elders. | Nonverbal Vocalizations<br>Facial Grimaces/winces<br>Bracing<br>Rubbing<br>Restlessness<br>Verbalizations | Modified from the University of Alabama-Birmingham Pain Behavior Scale for chronic pain patients.[179] Rates the absence or presence of six behaviors, at rest and on movement. A summed score of the number of nonverbal pain indicators observed at rest and on movement is calculated (total possible score = 0–12). |
| Discomfort Scale for Dementia of the Alzheimer Type (DS–DAT)[174] | Measure discomfort, defined as a negative state, in elders with advanced dementia who have decreased cognition and verbalization. | Noisy breathing<br>Negative vocalizations<br>Contented facial expression<br>Sad facial expression<br>Frightened facial expression<br>Frown<br>Relaxed body language<br>Tense body language<br>Fidgeting | The negative state could be pain, anguish, or suffering. Scoring is based on evaluation of frequency, intensity, and duration of the behaviors and may be cumbersome, requiring more training and education than is feasible or realistic for clinicians in hospital or long term care settings. Although the DS–DAT has been criticized for being too complex for routine nursing care,[180] it has been revised.[181] |
| Doloplus-2[182,183] | Assess pain in nonverbal elders experiencing chronic pain. | Somatic<br><br>• Somatic complaints<br>• Protective body<br>• postures at rest<br>• Protection of sore areas<br>• Expression<br>• Sleep pattern<br>• Psychomotor<br>• Washing and/ordressing<br>• Mobility<br>• Psychosocial<br>• Communication<br>• Social life<br>• Behavioral problems | Each of the ten items is given a score (0–3) representing increased severity and summed for a total score ranging from 0–30. A total score of 6 or above indicates pain. |
| FLACC[184] | Measure pain severity in postoperative children. Has also been tested in cognitively impaired older adults. | Face<br>Legs<br>Activity<br>Cry<br>Consolability | Each of the five items is given a score (0–2) representing increased severity and summed for a total score ranging from 0–10. |

*(continued)*

**Table 6–8**

**Pain Assessment Tools for the Cognitively Impaired or Nonverbal Patient or Resident** (*continued*)

| Tool | Goal | Dimensions/Parameters | Comments |
|---|---|---|---|
| Non-communicative Patient's Pain Assessment Instrument (NOPPAIN)[185] | Assess pain behaviors in patients with dementia by nursing assistants. | Activity<br>Behaviors and intensity<br><br>• Pain words<br>• Pain noises<br>• Pain faces<br>• Bracing<br>• Rubbing<br>• Restlessness<br><br>Pain thermometer | Developed as a nursing assistant-administered instrument. Pain is observed at rest and on movement while nursing assistants perform resident care (bathing, dressing, and transferring). Pain behaviors are observed and pain intensity is scored using a pain thermometer. |
| Pain Assessment for the Dementing Elderly (PADE)[186,187] | Assess pain behaviors in patients with advanced dementia. | Physical<br>• Facial expression<br>• Breathing pattern<br>• Posture<br><br>Global<br>• Proxy pain intensity<br><br>Functional<br>• Dressing<br>• Feeding oneself<br>• Wheelchair to bed transfers | Twenty-four items (three domains) were developed after a literature review, interviews with nursing staff, and observations of residents in a dementia unit. |
| Pain Assessment Tool in Confused Older Adults (PATCOA)[188] | Observe nonverbal cues to assess pain in acutely confused older adults. | Quivering<br>Guarding<br>Frowning<br>Grimacing<br>Clenching jaws<br>Points to where it hurts<br>Reluctance to move<br>Vocalizations of moaning<br>Sighing | An ordinal scale includes nine items of nonverbal pain cues rated as absent or present while the patient is at rest; higher scores indicate higher pain intensity. |
| Pain Assessment in Advanced Dementia (PAINAD)[181] | Assess pain in patients with advanced dementia. | Breathing (independent of vocalization)<br>Negative vocalization<br>Facial expression<br>Body language<br>Consolability | Derived from the behaviors and categories of the FLACC,[184] DS-DAT,[174] and clinicians' pain descriptors of dementia. The intent is to simply measure pain using a 0–10 score (each item is scored as 0-2 and summed) in noncommunicative individuals. |
| Pain Assessment Behavioral Scale (PABS)[189] | Assess pain in nonverbal hospital critically ill inpatients. | Face<br>Restlessness<br>Muscle tone<br>Vocalization<br>Consolability | Each of the five items is given a score (0–2) representing increased severity and summed for a total score ranging from 0–10. The patient is observed at rest and with movement. Two scores are generated; the higher score is documented. |
| Pain Assessment Checklist for Seniors with Limited Ability to Communicate (PACSLAC)[43, 190] | Assess common and subtle behaviors in seniors with advanced dementia. | Facial expressions<br>Activity and body movements<br>Social/personality/mood indicators<br>Physiological indicators/eating and sleeping/vocal behaviors | Can differentiate between pain and distress; scores were positively correlated with cognitive impairment level. |
| PAINE[191] | Assess pain in non-communicative elders. | Facial expressions<br>Verbalizations<br>Body movements<br>Changes in activity/patterns<br>Nurse-identified physical and vocal behaviors<br>Visible pain cues | 22 item scale with a 6-point rating scale (1=never to 7 =several times an hour) to measure frequency of occurrence of pain behaviors. |

experience. Without verbal validation from the patient, the clinician must rely not only on behavioral observations but on intuition and personal judgment. It is also particularly important to elicit the opinions of the individuals closest to the patient, which are also subjective.

Nurses and other health care providers reflect the difficulty of accurately assessing pain in nonverbal or cognitively impaired patients in studies that show low concurrence between patients' self-ratings of pain and clinicians' ratings.[200-202] Other findings are equivocal, with some studies suggesting that family caregivers or significant others accurately estimate the amount of pain cancer patients experience[89] and others proposing that family caregivers overestimate patients' pain.[203-205] Bruera and colleagues[206] studied relatives and the nurses who cared for 60 unresponsive, dying patients. Both were asked to rate a patient's discomfort level—six observed behaviors (grimacing, groaning, shouting, touching or rubbing an area, purposeless movement, labored breathing), and the suspected reason for the discomfort. Although the mean levels of perceived discomfort were similar, relatives reported significantly more observed behaviors and more often indicated pain as a reason for discomfort than did the nurse caregivers. According to Cohen-Mansfield,[207] relatives of cognitively impaired nursing home residents are better able to interpret facial expressions and other pain behaviors if they visit their loved ones at least once a week and have a close relationship. To detect pain in cognitively impaired nursing home residents, it is essential for family members and certified nursing assistants (CNAs) to know the resident's usual behavior and patterns to be able to detect pain.[208]

**Implications for Treatment**

Although pain assessment in the nonverbal or cognitively impaired patient or resident presents a challenge to clinicians, it should not pose a barrier to optimal pain management. If patients are no longer able to verbally communicate whether they are in pain or not, the best approach is to assume that their underlying disease is still painful and to continue pain interventions based on analgesic history.[42] Nonverbal patients should be empirically treated for pain if there is preexisting pain or evidence that any individual in a similar condition would experience pain. Likewise, palliative measures should be considered in nonverbal patients with behavior changes potentially related to pain.

**Summary**

In summary, multiple factors should be incorporated into the assessment of the pain experience. The following case examples include some of the pain assessment techniques discussed in this chapter and may prove beneficial in applying this content for nurse clinicians.

CASE STUDY
*Judy, A Hospice Patient with Pain*

Judy is a 68-year-old African-American woman with breast cancer metastatic to bones, lung, and liver. Her treatments have included surgery, hormonal therapy, chemotherapy, samarium, and palliative radiotherapy. A year after her presentation with metastatic disease, she suffered an acute stroke resulting in left-sided weakness and difficulty with speech. Her bone pain, particularly in her sternum, left ribs, and left hip, is usually well controlled with long acting oxycodone 40 mg every 12 hours with immediate-release oxycodone for breakthrough pain. She generally rates her pain intensity as a 4 or 5 out of 10. She and her supportive husband have a strong belief in God and believe that God will not let her suffer. After CT scans revealed progressive disease in the liver and lungs, Judy elected to stop chemotherapy and receive hospice care at home. Two weeks after admission into home hospice, Judy's condition rapidly declined and she became verbally non-communicative. She is only awake for an hour or two during the day. Most of the time, she seems peaceful. Intermittently, she is restless and clutches at her chest.

1. What type of pain is Judy experiencing?
2. What are ways to assess that Judy is having pain?
3. What pharmacological approaches are recommended when Judy can no longer take oral analgesics?
4. Identify possible barriers to optimal assessment and treatment of pain in Judy.

CASE STUDY
*Lyle, A Cognitively Impaired Resident with Pain*

Lyle is an 91-year-old man with a history of pneumonia, degenerative joint disease, mild osteoporosis, diabetes, Alzheimer's dementia, and myelodysplastic disorder who has been admitted to your facility. Lyle is extremely depressed. The certified nursing assistants caring for Lyle report that he moans and groans when they bathe and change him (he is incontinent of bowel and bladder) and screams, "You're so mean to me!" He often is combative, tearful, has a sad facial expression, and is very restless.

1. What kind of pains might Lyle be having? What is the etiology?
2. What can be done for his pain?
3. Did he take any pain medication previously? How would you know?
4. What does his family think?
5. How can his caregivers tell if the pain has been controlled?

REFERENCES

1. Arendt H. The Human Condition: Introduction by Margaret Canovan, 2nd ed. Chicago: The University of Chicago Press, 1998:50–51.
2. Cleeland CS, Gonin R, Hatfield AK, Edmonson JH, Blum RH, Stewart JA, Pandya KJ. Pain and its treatment in outpatients with metastatic cancer. N Engl J Med 1994;330: 592–596.
3. Desbiens NA, Wu AW, Broste SK, Wenger NS, Connors AF Jr, Lynn J, Yasui Y, Phillips RS, Fulkerson W. Pain and satisfaction with pain control in seriously ill hospitalized adults: Findings from the SUPPORT research investigations. Crit Care Med 1996;24:1953–1961.
4. Hearn J, Higginson IJ. Cancer pain epidemiology: A systematic review. In Bruera ED, Portenoy RK, eds. Cancer Pain, Assessment and Management. Cambridge, UK: Cambridge University Press, 2003:19–37.
5. National Comprehensive Cancer Network (NCCN). Adult Cancer Pain. Clinical Practice Guidelines in Oncology, version 1.2008. Available at http://www.nccn.org/professionals/physician_gls/PDF/pain.pdf (accessed January 14, 2009).
6. van den Beuken-van Everdingen MH, de Rijke JM, Kessels AG, Schouten HC, van Kleef M, Patijn J. Prevalence of pain in patients with cancer: A systematic review of the past 40 years. Ann Oncol 2007;18:1437–1449.
7. Kutner JS, Bryant LL, Beaty BL, Fairclough DL. Time course and characteristics of symptom distress and quality of life at the end of life. J Pain Symptom Manage 2007;34:227–236.
8. Weissman DE, Griffie J. The palliative care consultation service of the Medical College of Wisconsin. J Pain Symptom Manage 1994;9:474–479.
9. Miller SC, Mor V, Teno J. Hospice enrollment and pain assessment and management in nursing homes. J Pain Symptom Manage 2003;26:791–799.
10. Sloane PD, Zimmerman S, Hanson L, Mitchell CM, Riedel-Leo C, Custis-Buie V. End-of-life care in assisted living and related residential care settings: Comparison with nursing homes. J Am Geriatr Soc 2003;51:1587–1594.
11. Bernabei R, Gambassi G, Lapane K, Landi F, Gatsonis C, Dunlop R, Lipsitz L, Steel KL, Mor V. Management of pain in elderly cancer patients. JAMA 1998;279:1877–1882
12. Teno JM, Weitzen S, Wetle T, Mor V. Persistent pain in nursing homes: Validating a pain scale for the Minimum Data Set. Gerontologist 2001;41:173–179.
13. American Geriatrics Society (AGS) Panel on Persistent Pain in Older Persons. Clinical practice guideline: The management of persistent pain in older persons. J Am Geriatr Soc 2002;50(6 Suppl):S205–S224.
14. American Medical Directors Association. Pain Management in the Long-Term Care Setting: Clinical Practice Guideline. Columbia, MD: AMDA, 2009:1–45.
15. Teno JM, Kabumoto G, Wetle T, Roy J, Mor V. Daily pain that was excruciating at some time in the previous week: prevalence, characteristics, and outcomes in nursing home residents. J Am Geriatr Soc 2004; 52:762–767.
16. Won A, Lapane K, Vallow S, Schein J, Morris J, Lipsitz L. Persistent nonmalignant pain and analgesic prescribing patterns in elderly nursing home residents. J Am Geriatr Soc 2004;52:867–874.

17. Hutt E, Pepper GA, Vojir C, Fink R, Jones KR. Assessing the appropriateness of pain medication prescribing practices in nursing homes. J Am Geriatr Soc 2006;54:231–239
18. Williams C, Zimmerman S, Sloane P, Reed P. Characteristics associated with pain in long-term care residents with dementia. The Gerontologist 2005;45:68–73.
19. Merskey H, Bogduk N eds. Classification of Chronic Pain, 2nd ed. International Association for the Study of Pain, Task Force on Taxonomy. Seattle, WA: IASP Press, 1994: 209–214.
20. McCaffery M. Nursing Practice Theories Related to Cognition, Bodily Pain, and Man–Environment Interactions. Los Angeles, CA: UCLA Press, 1968:95.
21. Turk DC, Melzack R. The measurement of pain and the assessment of people experiencing pain. In: Turk DC, Melzack R, eds. Handbook of Pain Assessment. New York, NY: Guilford Press, 1992:3–14.
22. Chodosh J, Solomon D, Roth C, Chang JT, MacLean CH, Ferrell BA, Shekelle PG, Wenger NS. The quality of medical care provided to vulnerable older patients with chronic pain. J Am Geriatr Soc 2004;52:756–767.
23. Fine PG, Miaskowski C, Paice JA. Meeting the challenges of cancer pain management. Supp Oncol 2004;2:5–22.
24. Bruera E, Kim HN. Cancer pain. JAMA 2003;290:2476–2479.
25. Ferrell BR, Dean GE, Grant M, Coluzzi P. An institutional commitment to pain management. J Clin Oncol 1995;13:2158–2165.
26. Jones K, Fink R, Hutt E, Pepper G, Hutt E, Vojir CP, Scott J, Clark L, Mellis K. Improving nursing home staff knowledge and attitudes about pain. The Gerontologist 2004;44:469–478.
27. Goldberg GR, Morrison RS. Pain management in hospitalized cancer patients: A systematic review. J Clin Oncol 2007;25: 1792–1801.
28. Gunnarsdottir S, Donovan HS, Serlin RC, Voge C, Ward S. Patient-related barriers to pain management. The Barriers Questionnaire II (BQ-II). Pain 2002;99:385–396.
29. Weiner DK, Rudy TE. Attitudinal barriers to effective treatment of persistent pain in nursing home residents. J Am Geriatr Soc 2002;50:2035–2040.
30. Coyle N. In their own words: Seven advanced cancer patients describe their experience with pain and the use of opioid drugs. J Pain Symptom Manage 2004;27:300–309.
31. Tarzian A, Hoffmann D. Barriers to managing pain in the nursing home: Findings from a statewide survey. J Am Med Dir Assoc 2004;5: 82–88.
32. Anderson KO, Mendoza TR, Payne R, Valero V, Palos GR, Nazario A, Richman SP, et al. Pain education for underserved minority cancer patients: A randomized controlled trial. J Clin Oncol 2004;22:4918–4925.
33. Jones K, Fink R, Clark L, Hutt E, Vojir CP, Mellis BK. Nursing home resident barriers to effective pain management: Why nursing home residents may not seek pain medication. J Am Med Dir Assoc 2005;6:10–17.
34. Vallerand, AH, Collins-Bohler D, Templin T, Hasenau S. Knowledge of and barriers to pain management in caregivers of cancer patients receiving homecare. Cancer Nurs 2007;30:31–37.
35. Chih-Yi Sun V, Borneman T, Ferrell B, Piper B, Koczywas M, Choi K. Overcoming Barriers to Cancer Pain Management: An Institutional Change Model. J Pain Symptom Manage 2007;34:359–369.

36. Miakowski C, Cleary J, Burney R, et al. Guideline for the Management of Cancer Pain in Adults and Children. APS Clinical Practice Guidelines, Series No. 3. Glenview, IL: APS, 2005.

37. Cleeland CS. The impact of pain on the patient with cancer. Cancer 1984;58:2635–2641.

38. Gordon DB, Dahl JL, Miaskowski C, et al. American pain society recommendations for improving the quality of acute and cancer pain management. Arch Intern Med 2005;165: 1574–1580.

39. Oncology Nursing Society position paper on cancer pain management (revised) October 2006. Available at: http://www.ons.org/publications/positions/CancerPainManagement.shtml (accessed January 14, 2009).

40. Max M, Cleary J, Ferrell BR, Foley K, Payne R, Shapiro B. Treatment of pain at the end of life: A position statement from the American Pain Society. American Pain Society Bulletin 1997;7:1–3.

41. American Society of Pain Management Nurses Position Statement on Pain Management at the End of Life. Available at: http://www.aspmn.org/Organization/documents/EndofLifeCare.pdf (accessed Janurary 14, 2009).

42. Herr K, Coyne PJ, Key T, Manworren R, McCaffery M, Merkel S, Pelosi-Kelly J, Wild L. Pain assessment in the nonverbal patient: Position statement with clinical practice recommendations. Pain Manage Nurs 2006;7:44–52.

43. Hadijistavropoulos T, Herr K, Turk DC, Fine PG, Dworkin RH, Helme R, Jackson K, Parmelee PA, Rudy TE, Beattie BL, Chibnall JT, et al. An interdisciplinary expert consensus statement on assessment of pain in older persons. Clin J Pain 2007; 23: S1–S43.

44. American Geriatrics Society (AGS) Panel on the Pharmacological Management of Persistent Pain in Older Persons. Pharmacological management of persistent pain in older persons. J Am Geriatr Soc 2009;57:1331–1346.

45. The Joint Commission. Speak Up: What You Should Know About Pain Management. Available at: http://www.jointcommission.org/PatientSafety/SpeakUp/Speak_up_pain_managment.htm (accessed January 14, 2009).

46. Idell CS, Grant M, Kirk C. Alignment of pain reassessment practices and national comprehensive cancer network guidelines. Oncol Nurs Forum 2007;34:661–671.

47. American Heritage Dictionary of the English Language. Boston, MA: Houghton Mifflin, 2000.

48. Twycross RG, Wilcock A. Symptom Management in Advanced Cancer. Oxford, UK: Radcliffe Publishers, 2001:18.

49. McGuire D. The multiple dimensions of cancer pain: A framework for assessment and management. In: McGuire D, Yarbro CH, Ferrell BR, eds. Cancer Pain Management, 2nd ed. Boston: Jones and Bartlett, 1995:1–17.

50. Melzack R, Casey KL. Sensory, motivational, and central control determinants of pain: A new conceptual model. In: Kenshalo D, ed. The Skin Senses. Springfield, IL: Charles C Thomas, 1968:423–439.

51. Ahles TA, Blanchard EB, Ruckdeschel JC. The multidimensional nature of cancer-related pain. Pain 1983;17:277–288.

52. Bates MS. Ethnicity and pain: A biocultural model. Soc Sci Med 1987;24:47–50.

53. Hester NO. Assessment of acute pain. Baillieres Clin Paediatr 1995;3:561–577.

54. McGuire DB. Comprehensive and multidimensional assessment and measurement of pain. J Pain Symptom Manage 1992;7:312–319.

55. Jost L, Roila F. Management of cancer pain: ESMO Clinical Recommendations. Ann Oncol 2008;19:119–121.

56. Fink RM. Pain assessment: The cornerstone to optimal pain management. Analgesia 1997;8:16–21.

57. Bennett MI, Attal N, Backonja, et al. Using screening tools to identify neuropathic pain. Pain 2007;127:199–203.

58. Goudas L, Carr DB, Bloch R, et al. Management of cancer pain, Volume 1 #35. Agency for Healthcare Research and Quality, 2001.

59. Janjan N. Bone metastases: approaches to management. Semin Oncol 2001;28(4 Suppl 11):28–34.

60. Portenoy RK, Hagen NA. Breakthrough pain: Definition, prevalence, and characteristics. Pain 1990;41:273–281.

61. Zeppetella G. Breakthrough pain in cancer patients. Adv Pain Manage 2001;1:5–11.

62. Bostrom B, Sandh M, Lundberg D, Fridlund B. Cancer-related pain in palliative care: Patients' perceptions of pain management. J Adv Nurs 2004;45:410–419.

63. Gordon DB, Ward SE. Correcting patient misconceptions about pain. Am J Nurs 1995;95:43–45.

64. McGuire D, Kim HJ, Lang X. Measuring pain. In: Frank Stromberg M, Olsen SJ, eds. Instruments for Clinical Health Care Research, 3rd ed. Boston, MA: Jones and Bartlett, 2004:603–644.

65. Turk DC, Matyas TA. Pain-related behaviors: Communication of pain. Am Pain Soc J 1992;1:109–111.

66. Craig KD. The facial expression of pain: Better than a thousand words? Am Pain Soc J 1992;1:153–162.

67. Ferrell BA. Overview of aging and pain. In: Ferrell BR, Ferrell BA, eds. Pain in the Elderly. Seattle, WA: IASP Press, 1996:1–10.

68. Miaskowski C. The impact of age on a patient's perception of pain and ways it can be managed. Pain Manage Nurs 2000; 1(Suppl 1):2–7.

69. Ferrell BR. Patient education and nondrug interventions. In: Ferrell BR, Ferrell BA, eds. Pain in the Elderly. Seattle, WA: IASP Press, 1996:35–44.

70. Cleeland CS. Undertreatment of cancer pain in elderly patients. JAMA 1998;279:1914–1915.

71. Bernabei R, Gambassi G, Lapane K, Landi F, Gatsonia C, Dunlop R, Lipsitz L, Steel K, Mor V. Management of pain in elderly patients with cancer. SAGE Study Group. JAMA 1998;279:1877–1882.

72. Vallerand AH. Gender differences in pain. Image J Nurs Sch 1995;27:235–237.

73. Miaskowski C. Women and pain. Crit Care Nurs Clin North Am 1997;9:453–458.

74. Berkley KJ. Sex, drugs and.... Nat Med 1996;2:1184–1185.

75. Unruh AM. Gender variations in clinical pain experience. Pain 1996;65:123–167.

76. Miaskowski C, Levine JD. Does opioid analgesia show a gender preference for females? Pain Forum 1999;8:34–44.

77. Vallerand AH, Polomano RC. The relationship of gender to pain. Pain Manage Nurs 2000;1(Suppl 1):8–15.

78. Dubreuil D, Kohn P. Reactivity and response to pain. Person Indiv Diff 1986;7:907–909.

79. Robin O, Vinard H, Varnet-Maury E, Saumet JL. Influence of sex and anxiety of pain threshold and tolerance. Func Neurol 1987; 2:73–179.

80. Hurley RW, Adams MCB. Sex, gender, and pain: An overview of a complex field. Anesthesia & Analgesia 2009;107:309–317.

81. Aubrun F, Salvi N, Coriat P, Riou B. Sex- and age-related differences in morphine requirements for postoperative pain relief. Anesthesiology 2005;103:156–60.

82. Mercadante S, Casuccio A, Pumo S, Fulfaro F. Factors influencing opioid response in advanced cancer patients with pain followed at home: The effects of age and gender. Support Care Cancer 2000;8:123–130.

83. Pickering G, Jourdan D, Eshalier A, Dubray C. Impact of age, gender and cognitive functioning on pain perception. Gerontology 2002;48:112–118.

84. Kroin JS, Buvanendran A, Nagalla SK, Truman KJ. Postoperative pain and analgesic responses are similar in male and female Sprague-Dawledy rats. Can J Anaesth 2003;50:904–908.

85. LaResche L. Sex, gender, and clinical pain. Proceedings of the 11th World Congress on Pain. In: Flor H, Kalso E, eds. IASP Press, 2006:543–554.

86. Keogh E, Herdenfeldt M. Gender, coping and the perception of pain. Pain 2002;97:195–201.

87. Chin ML, Rosequist R. Sex, gender, and pain: "Men are from Mars, women are from Venus." Anesthesia & Analgesia 2008;107:4–5.

88. Senior PA, Bhopal R. Ethnicity as a variable in epidemiological research. BMJ 1994;309:327–330.

89. Fink RS, Gates R. Cultural diversity and cancer pain. In: McGuire DB, Yarbro CH, Ferrell BR, eds. Cancer Pain Management, 2nd ed. Boston, MA: Jones and Bartlett, 1995:19–39.

90. Bates MS, Edwards WT, Anderson KO. Ethnocultural influences on variation in chronic pain perception. Pain 1993;52:101–112.

91. Lipton JA, Marbach JJ. Ethnicity and the pain experience. Soc Sci Med 1984;19:1279–1298.

92. Zborowski M. People in Pain. San Francisco, CA: Jossey-Bass, 1969.

93. Zola IK. Culture and symptoms: An analysis of patients' presenting complaints. Am Soc Rev 1996;31:615–630.

94. Martin ML. Ethnicity and analgesic practices [editorial]. Ann Emerg Med 2000;35:77–79.

95. Anderson KO, Richman SP, Hurley J, Palos G, Valero V, Mendoza TR, Gning I, Cleeland CS. Cancer pain management among underserved minority outpatients: Perceived needs and barriers to optimal control. Cancer 2002;94:2295–2304.

96. Green GR, Anderson KO, Baker TA, Campbell LC, Decker S, Fillingim RB Kalaoukalani DA, Lasch KE, Myers C, Tait RC, Todd KH, Vallerand AH. The unequal burden of pain: Confronting racial and ethnic disparities in pain. Pain Med 2003;4:277–294.

97. Beck, SL. An ethnographic study of factors influencing cancer pain management in South Africa. Cancer Nurs 2000;23:91–99.

98. Gélinas C, Loiselle CG, LeMay S, Ranger M, Bouchard E, McCormack D. Theoretical, psychometric, and pragmatic issues in pain measurement. Pain Manage Nurs 2008;9:120–130.

99. Dar R, Beach CM, Barden PL, Cleeland CS. Cancer pain in the marital system: A study of patients and their spouses. J Pain Symptom Manage 1992;7:87–93.

100. Spross J, Wolff Burke M. Nonpharmacological management of cancer pain. In: McGuire DB, Yarbro CH, Ferrell BR, eds. Cancer Pain Management, 2nd ed. Boston, MA: Jones and Bartlett, 1995:159–205.

101. Wachholtz AB, Pearce MJ, Koenig H. Exploring the relationship between spirituality, coping, and pain. J Behav Med 2007;30:311–318.

102. Dunn KS, Horgas AL. Religious and nonreligious coping in older adults experiencing chronic pain. Pain Manage Nurs 2004;5:19–28.

103. Brunelli C, Costantini M, Di Giulio P, Gallucci M, Fusco F, Miccinesi G, Paci E, Peruselli C, Morino P, Piazza M, Tamburini M. Quality of life evaluation: When do terminally ill cancer patients and health-care providers agree? J Pain Symptom Manage 1998;15:151–158.

104. Grossman SA, Sheidler VR, Swedeen K, Mucenski J, Piantadosi S. Correlation of patient and caregiver ratings of cancer pain. J Pain Symptom Manage 1991;6:53–57.

105. Ferrell BR, Eberts M, McCaffery M, Grant M. Clinical decision making and pain. Cancer Nurs 1991;14:289–297.

106. Carpenter JS, Brockopp D. Comparison of patients' ratings and examination of nurses' responses to pain intensity rating scales. Cancer Nurs 1995;18:292–298.

107. Puntillo KA, Miaskowski C, Kehrle K, Stannard D, Gleeson S, Nye P. Relationship between behavioral and physiological indicators of pain, critical care patients, self-reports of pain, and opioid administration. Crit Care Med 1997;25:1159–1166.

108. Jensen M. The validity and reliability of pain measures in adults with cancer. J Pain 2003;4;2–21.

109. Ohnhaus EE, Adler R. Methodological problems in the measurement of pain: A comparison between the verbal rating scale and the visual analogue scale. Pain 1975;1:379–384.

110. Ahles TA, Ruckdeschel JC, Blanchard EB. Cancer-related pain: II. Assessment with visual analogue scales. J Psychosom Res 1984; 28:121–124.

111. Scott J, Huskisson EC. Graphic representation of pain. Pain 1976;2:175–184.

112. Revill SI, Robinson JO, Rosen M, Hogg MIJ. The reliability of a linear analogue for evaluating pain. Anaesthesia 1976;31:1191–1998.

113. Kremer E, Atkinson J. Pain language: Affect. J Psychosom Res 1984;28:125–132.

114. Shannon MM, Ryan MA, D'Agostino N, Brescia FJ. Assessment of pain in advanced cancer patients. J Pain Symptom Manage 1995;10:274–278.

115. Herr KA, Mobily PR. Comparison of selected pain assessment tools for use with the elderly. Appl Nurs Res 1993;6:39–49.

116. Wallenstein SL, Heidrich G, Kaiko R, Houde RW. Clinical evaluation of mild analgesics: The measurement of clinical pain. Br J Clin Pharmacol 1980;10:319S–327S.

117. Paice JA, Cohen FL. Validity of a verbally administered numeric rating scale to measure cancer pain intensity. Cancer Nurs 1997;20:88–93.

118. Ferraz MB, Quaresma MR, Aquino LRL, Atra E, Tugwell P, Goldsmith CH. Reliability of pain scales in the assessment of literate and illiterate patients with rheumatoid arthritis. J Rheumatol 1990;17:1022–1024.

119. Hockenberry MJ, Wilson D. Wong's Essential of Pediatric Nursing, 8th ed. St. Louis: Mosby, 2009.

120. Matsumoto D. Ethnic differences in affect intensity, emotion judgments, display rule attitudes, and self-reported emotional expression in an American sample. Motiv Emot 1993;17:107–123.

121. Frank AJM, Moll JMH, Hort JF. A comparison of three ways of measuring pain. Rheumatol Rehabil 1982;21:211–217.

122. Wilson JS, Cason CL, Grissom NL. Distraction: An effective intervention for alleviating pain during venipuncture. J Emerg Nurs 1995;21:87–94.

123. Stuppy DJ. The Faces Pain Scale: Reliability and validity with mature adults. Appl Nurs Res 1998;11:84–89.

124. Casas JM, Wagenheim BR, Banchero R, Mendoza-Romero J. Hispanic masculinity: Myth or psychological schema meriting clinical consideration. Hisp J Behav Sci 1994;16:315–331.

125. Hicks CL, von Baeyer CL, Spafford P, van Korlaar I, Goodenough B. The Faces Scale—Revised: Toward a common metric in pediatric pain measurement. Pain 2001;93:173–183.

126. Bieri D, Reeve R, Champion GD, Addicoat L, Ziegler JB. The Faces Pain Scale for the self assessment of the severity of pain experienced by children: Development, initial validation, and preliminary investigation for ratio scale properties. Pain 1990;41:139–150.

127. Herr K. Assessment of pain intensity in older adults: Is there a better way? Paper presented at the 19th Annual American Pain Society Scientific Meeting, Atlanta, GA, 2001.

128. Herr KA, Garand L. Assessment and measurement of pain in older adults. Clin Geriat Med 2001;17:457–478.

129. Dalton JA, McNaull F. A call for standardizing the clinical rating of pain intensity using a 0 to 10 rating scale. Cancer Nurs 1998; 21:46–49.

130. Jensen MP, Turner JA, Romano JM. What is the maximum number of levels needed in pain intensity measurement. Pain 1994;58:387–392.

131. Rodriguez CS. Pain measurement in the elderly: A review. Pain Manage Nurs 2001;2:38–46.

132. Kremer E, Hampton Atkinson J, Ignelzi RJ. Measurement of pain: Patient preference does not confound pain measurement. Pain 1981;10:241–248.

133. Taylor LJ, Herr K. Pain intensity assessment: A comparison of selected pain intensity scales for use in cognitively intact and cognitively impaired African American older adults. Pain Manage Nurs 2003;4:87–95.

134. Jones K, Fink R, Hutt E, Vojir C, Pepper G, Scott-Cawiezell J, Mellis BK. Measuring pain intensity in nursing home residents. J Pain Symtom Manage 2005;30:519–527.

135. Carey SJ, Turpin C, Smith J, Whatley J, Haddox D. Improving pain management in an acute care setting: The Crawford Long Hospital of Emory University experience. Orthopaedic Nurs 1997;16:29–36.

136. Ware LJ, Epps CD, Herr K, Packard A. Evaluation of the revised faces pain scale, verbal descriptor scale, numeric rating scale, and Iowa pain thermometer in older minority adults. Pain Manage Nurs 2006;7:117–125.

137. Miro J, Huguet A, Nieto R, Paredes S, Baos J. Evaluation of reliability, validity, and preference for a pain intensity scale for use with the elderly. J Pain 2005;6:727–735.

138. Melzak R. The short-form McGill Pain Questionnaire. Pain 1987;30:191–197.

139. Daut RL, Cleeland CS, Flanery R. Development of the Wisconsin Brief Pain Inventory to assess pain in cancer and other diseases. Pain 1983;17:197–210.

140. Fishman B, Pasternak S, Wallenstein SL, Houde RW, Holland JC, Foley KM. The Memorial Pain Assessment Card: A valid instrument for the evaluation of cancer pain. Cancer 1987;60:1151–1158.

141. Ferrell BR. Patient and family pain questionnaires. Available at: http://prc.coh.org/res_inst.asp (accessed January 14, 2009).

142. Tranmer J, Heyland D, Dudgeon D, Groll D, Squires-Graham M, Coulson K. Measuring the symptom experience of seriously ill cancer and noncancer hospitalized patients near the end of life with the Memorial Symptom Assessment Scale. J Pain Symptom Manage 2003;25:420–429.

143. Weiner D, Peterson BL, Ladd K, McConnell E, Keefe FJ. Pain in nursing home residents: An exploration of prevalence, staff perspectives, and practical aspects of measurement. Clin J Pain 1999;15:92–101.

144. Morrison RS, Siu AL. A comparison of pain and its treatment in advanced dementia and cognitively intact patients with hip fracture. J Pain Symptom Manage 2000;19:240–248.

145. Herr K, Bjoro K, Decker S. Tools for assessment of pain in non-verbal older adults with dementia: a state of the science review. J Pain Symptom Manage 2006; 31:170–192.

146. Reynolds KS, Hanson LC, De Vellis RF, . Disparities in pain management between cognitively intact and cognitively impaired nursing home residents. J Pain Symptom Manage 2008;35:388–396.

147. Bachino C, Snow AL, Kunik ME, Cody M, Wristers K. Principles of pain assessment in non-communicative demented patients. Clin Gerontol 2001;23:97–115.

148. Bruera E, Fainsinger RL, Miller MJ, Kuehn N. The assessment of pain intensity in patients with cognitive failure: A preliminary report. J Pain Symptom Manage 1992;7:267–270.

149. Stiefel F, Fainsinger R, Bruera E. Acute confusional states in patients with advanced cancer. J Pain Symptom Manage 1992;7:94–98.

150. Lynn J, Teno JM, Phillips RS, Wu AW, Desbiens N, Harrold J, Claessens MT, Wenger N, Kreling B, Connors AF Jr. Perceptions by family members of the dying experience of older and seriously ill patients. SUPPORT Investigators. Study to Understand Prognoses and Preferences for Outcomes and Risks of Treatment. Ann Intern Med 1997;126:97–106.

151. Morita T, Tei Y, Inoue S. Impaired communication capacity and agitated delirium in the final week of terminally ill cancer patients: Prevalence and identification of research focus. J Pain Symptom Manage 2003;26:827–834.

152. McCaffery M, Pasero C. Assessment. Underlying complexities, misconceptions, and practical tools. In: McCaffery M, Pasero C, eds. Pain: Clinical Manual, 2nd ed. St. Louis, MO: Mosby, 1999:35–102.

153. McCaffery M, Ferrell BR. How vital are vital signs? Nursing 1992;22:43–46.

154. Wilkie DJ, Keefe FJ, Dodd MJ, Copp LA. Behavior of patients with lung cancer: Description and associations with oncologic and pain variables. Pain 1992;51:231–240.

155. Feldt KS. The Checklist of Nonverbal Pain Indicators (CNPI). Pain Manage Nurs 2000;1:13–21.

156. Jones K, Fink R, Hutt E, Clark L, Pepper G, Scott J, et al. Improving Pain Management in Nursing Homes. Staff Training Workbook—Nursing Edition. OTR04054-0404. Aurora, CO: University of Colorado Denver, College of Nursing, 2003.

157. Herr K, Decker S. Assessment of pain in older adults with severe cognitive impairment. Ann Long-Term Care 2004;12:46–52.

158. Cohen-Mansfield J, Creedon M. Nursing staff members' perceptions of pain indicators in persons with severe dementia. Clin J Pain 2002;18:64–73.

159. Manfredi PL, Breuer B, Meier DE, Libow L. Pain assessment in elderly patients with severe dementia. J Pain Symtom Manage 2003;25:48–52.

160. Feldt KS, Ryden MB, Miles S. Treatment of pain in cognitively impaired compared with cognitively intact elder patients with hip fracture. J Am Geriatr Soc 1998;46:1079–1985.

161. Parmelee PA, Smith B, Katz IR. Pain complaints and cognitive status among elderly institution residents. J Am Geriatr Soc 1993;41:517–522.

162. Fisher-Morris M, Gellatly A. The experience and expression of pain in Alzheimer patients. Age Aging 1997;26:497–500.

163. Werner P, Cohen-Mansfield J, Watson V, Pasis S. Pain in participants of adult day care centers: Assessment by different raters. J Pain Symptom Manage 1998;15:8–17.

164. Huffman JC, Kunik ME. Assessment and understanding of pain in patients with dementia. Gerontologist 2000;40:574–581.

165. Nygaard HA, Jarland M. Are nursing home patients with dementia diagnosis at increased risk for inadequate pain treatment? Int J Geriatr Psychiatry 2005;20:730–737.

166. Gibson SJ, Voukelatos X, Ames D, Flicker L, Helme RD. An examination of pain perception and cerebral event-related potentials following carbon dioxide laser stimulation in patients with Alzheimer's disease and age-matched control volunteers. Pain Res Manag 2001;6:126–132.

167. Gibson SJ, Farrell M. A review of age-related differences in the neurophysiology of nociception ad the perceptual experience of pain. Clin J Pain 2004;20:227–239.

168. Helme RD, Meliala A, Gibson SJ. Methodologic factors which contribute to variations in experimental pain threshold for older people. Neurosci Lett 2004;361:144–146.

169. Bjoro K, Herr K. Assessment of pain in the nonverbal or cognitively impaired older adult. Clin Geriat Med 2008;24:237–262.

170. Marzinski LR. The tragedy of dementia: Clinically assessing pain in the confused nonverbal elderly. J Gerontol Nurs 1991;17:25–28.

171. Keefe FJ, Dunsmore J. Pain behavior: Concepts and controversies. Am Pain Soc J 1992;1:92–100.

172. Hjermstad MJ, Gibbins J, Haugen DF, Caraceni A, Loge JH, Kaasa S. Pain assessment tools in palliative care: An urgent neeed for consensus. Palliat Med 2008;22:895–903.

173. Abbey J, Piller N, De Bellis A, Esterman A, Parker D, Giles L, Lowcay B. The Abbey Pain Scale: A 1-minute numerical indicator for people with end-stage dementia. Int J Palliat Nurs 2004;10:6–13.

174. Hurley AC, Volicer BJ, Hanrahan PA, Houde S, Volicer L. Assessment of discomfort in advanced Alzheimer patients. Res Nurs Health 1992;15:369–377.

175. Simons W, Malabar R. Assessing pain in elderly patients who cannot respond verbally. J Adv Nurs 1995;22:663–669.

176. Kovach CR, Weissman D, Griffie J, Matson S, Muchka S. Assessment and treatment of discomfort for people with late-stage dementia. J Pain Symptom Manage 1999;18:412–419.

177. Kovach CR, Noonan PE, Griffie J, Muchka S, Weissman DE. Use of the Assessment of Discomfort in Dementia protocol. Appl Nurs Res 2001;14:193–200.

178. Kovach CR, Noonan PE, Griffie J, Muchka S, Weissman DE. The Assessment of Discomfort in Dementia protocol. Pain Manage Nurs 2002;3:16–27.

179. Richards JS, Neopomuceno C, Riles M, Suer Z. Assessing pain behavior: The UAB Pain Behavior Scale. Pain 1982;14:393–398.

180. Miller J, Neelson V, Dalton J, Ng'andu N, Bailey DJ, Layman E, Hosfeld A. The assessment of discomfort in elderly confused patients: A preliminary study. J Neurosci Nurs 1996;28:175–182.

181. Warden V, Hurley AC, Volicer L. Development and psychometric evaluation of the Pain Assessment in Advanced Dementia (PAINAD) scale. J Am Med Dir Assoc 2003;9–15.

182. Wary B. Doloplus-2: A scale for pain measurement. Soins Gerontol 1999;19:25–27.

183. Lefebvre-Chapiro S. The Doloplus-2 scale—evaluating pain in the elderly. Eur J Palliat Care 2001;8:191–194.

184. Merkel SI, Voepel-Lewis T, Shayevitz JR, Malviya S. The FLACC: A behavioral scale for scoring postoperative pain in young children. Pediatr Nurs 1997;23:293–297.

185. Snow AL, Weber JB, O'Malley KJ, Cody M, Beck C, Bruera E, Ashton C, Kunik ME. NOPPAIN: A nursing assistant-administered pain assessment instrument for use in dementia. Dement Geriatr Cogn Disord 2004;17:240–246.

186. Villanueva MR, Smith TL, Erickson JS, Lee AC, Singer C. Pain Assessment for the Dementing Elderly (PADE): Reliability and validity of a new measure. J Am Med Dir Assoc 2003;4:1–8.

187. Cohen-Manfield J, Lipson S. The utility of pain assessment for analgesic use in persons with dementia. Pain 2008;134:16–23.

188. Decker SA, Perry AG. The development and testing of the PATCOA to assess pain in confused older adults. Pain Manage Nurs 2003;4:77–86.

189. Campbell M. Psychometric Testing of a New Pain Assessment Behavior Scale (PABS). Abstract presented at the 29th Annual MNRS Research Conference, 2005.

190. Fuchs-Lacelle S, Hadjistavropoulos T. Development and preliminary validation of the Pain Assessment Checklist for Seniors with Limited Ability to Communicate (PACSLAC). Pain Manage Nurs 2004;5:37–49.

191. Cohen-Mansfield J. Pain assessment in noncommunicative elderly persons—PAINE. Clin J Pain 2006;22: 569–575.

192. Bruera E, Kuehn N, Miller MJ, Selmser P, MacMillan K. The Edmonton Symptom Assessment System (ESAS): A simple method for the assessment of palliative care patients. J Palliat Care 1991;7:6–9.

193. Rees E, Hardy J, Ling J, Broadley K, A'Hearn R. The use of the Edmonton Symptom Assessment Scale within a palliative care unit in the UK. Palliat Med 1998;12:75–82.

194. Herr KA, Mobily PC, Kohart FJ, Wagenaar D. Evaluation of the faces pain scale for use with the elderly. Clin J Pain 1998;14:29–38.

195. Manz BD, Mosier R, Nusser-Gerlach MA, Bergstrom N, Agrawal S. Pain assessment in the cognitively impaired and unimpaired elderly. Pain Manage Nurs 2000;1:106–115.

196. Chibnall JT, Tait RC. Pain assessment in cognitively impaired and unimpaired older adults: A comparison of four scales. Pain 2001;92:173–186.

197. Closs SJ, Barr B, Briggs M, Cash K, Seers K. A comparison of five pain assessment scales for nursing home residents with varying degrees of cognitive impairment. J Pain Symptom Manage 2004;27:196–205.

198. Kamel H, Phlavan M, Malekgoudarzi B, Gogel P, Morley JE. Utilizing pain assessment scales increases the frequency of diagnosing pain among elderly nursing home residents. J Pain Symptom Manage 2001;21:450–455.199.

199. Buffum M, Miaskowski C, Sands L, Brod M. A pilot study of the relationship between discomfort and agitation in patients with dementia. Geriatr Nurs 2001;22:80–85.

200. Weiner D, Peterson B, Keefe F. Chronic pain associated behaviors in the nursing home: Resident versus caregiver perceptions. Pain 1999;80:577–588.

201. Cohen-Mansfield J. Nursing staff members' assessment of pain in cognitively impaired nursing home residents. Pain Manage Nurs 2005;6:68–75.

202. Scherder E, van Manen F. Pain in Alzheimer's disease: Nursing assistants' and patients' evaluations. J Adv Nurs 2005;52:151–158.

203. Clipp EC, George LK. Patients with cancer and their spouse caregivers. Cancer 1992;69:1074–1079.

204. Madison JL, Wilkie DJ. Family members' perceptions of cancer pain: Comparisons with patient sensory report and by patient psychologic status. Nurs Clin North Am 1995;30:625–645.

205. Yeager KA, Miaskowski C, Dibble SL, Wallhagen M. Differences in pain knowledge and perceptions of the pain experience between outpatients with cancer and their family caregivers. Oncol Nurs Forum 1995;22:1235–1241.

206. Bruera E, Sweeney C, Willey J, Palmer JL, Strasses F, Strauch E. Perception of discomfort by relatives and nurses in unresponsive terminally ill patients with cancer: A prospective study. J Pain Symptom Manage 2003;26:818–826.

207. Cohen-Mansfield J. Relatives assessment of pain in cognitively impaired nursing home residents. J Pain Symptom Manage 2002;24:562–571.

208. Mentes JC, Teer J, Cadogan MP. The pain experience of cognitively impaired nursing home residents: Perceptions of family members and certified nursing assistants. Pain Manage Nurs 2004;5:118–125.

# 7

*Judith A. Paice*

# Pain at the End of Life

*The world is full of suffering, it is also full of overcoming it.—Hellen Keller*

♦ **Key Points**
♦ *Pain is highly prevalent in palliative care, yet the majority of individuals can obtain good relief with available treatment options.*
♦ *An awareness of barriers to adequate pain care allows palliative care nurses to assess for and to plan interventions to overcome these obstacles when caring for patients. Advocacy is a critical role of the palliative care nurse.*
♦ *Assessment of pain, including a thorough history and comprehensive physical exam, guides the development of the pharmacological and nonpharmacological treatment plan.*
♦ *Pharmacological therapies include nonopioids, opioids, coanalgesics, cancer therapies and, in some cases, interventional techniques.*
♦ *Intractable pain and symptoms, although not common, must be treated aggressively. In some cases, palliative sedation may be warranted.*

Of the many symptoms experienced by those at the end of life, pain is one of the most common and most feared.[1] However, this fear is largely unfounded because the majority of patients with terminal illness can obtain relief. Nurses are critical members of the palliative care team, particularly in providing pain management. The nurse's role begins with assessment and continues through the development of a plan of care and its implementation. During this process, the nurse provides education and counsel to the patient, family, and other team members. Nurses also are critical for developing institutional policies and monitoring outcomes that ensure good pain management for all patients within their palliative care program. To provide optimal pain control, all health care professionals must understand the frequency of pain at the end of life, the barriers that prevent good management, the assessment of this syndrome, and the treatments used to provide relief.

## Prevalence of Pain

The prevalence of pain in the terminally ill varies by diagnosis and other factors. Approximately one third of persons who are actively receiving treatment for cancer and two thirds of those with advanced malignant disease experience pain.[2-6] Individuals at particular risk for undertreatment include the elderly, minorities, and women.[7,8] Almost three quarters of patients with advanced cancer admitted to the hospital experience pain upon admission.[9] In a study of cancer patients very near the end of life, pain occurred in 54% at 4 weeks and 34% at 1 week before death.[10] In other studies of patients admitted to palliative care units, pain often is the dominant symptom, along with fatigue and dyspnea.[1a] Children dying of cancer also are at risk for pain and suffering.[11]

The prevalence of pain in those with human immunodeficiency virus (HIV) disease varies widely and can have a profound negative effect on quality of life.[12-14] Headache, abdominal pain, chest pain, and neuropathies are the most frequently reported types of pain. Lower CD4 cell counts and HIV-1 RNA levels are associated with higher rates of neuropathy.[15] Numerous studies have reported undertreatment of persons with HIV disease, including those patients with a history of addictive disease.[16,17]

Unfortunately, there has been little characterization of the pain prevalence and experience of patients with other life-threatening disorders. However, those working in palliative care are well aware that pain frequently accompanies many of the neuromuscular and cardiovascular disorders, such as multiple sclerosis and stroke, seen at the end of life.[18–22] Furthermore, many patients in hospice and palliative care are elderly and more likely to have existing chronic pain syndromes, such as osteoarthritis or low back pain.[23]

Additional research is needed to fully characterize the frequency of pain and the type of pain syndromes seen in patients at the end of life. This information will lead to improved detection, assessment and, ultimately, treatment. Unfortunately, pain continues to be undertreated, even when prevalence rates and syndromes are well understood. The undertreatment is largely due to barriers related to health care professionals, the system, and patients and their families.

---

**Table 7–1**
**Barriers to Cancer Pain Management**

**Problems related to health care professionals**
Inadequate knowledge of pain management
Poor assessment of pain
Concern about regulation of controlled substances
Fear of patient addiction
Concern about side effects of analgesics
Concern about patients' becoming tolerant to analgesics

**Problems related to the health care system**
Low priority given to cancer pain treatment
Inadequate reimbursement
Restrictive regulation of controlled substances
Problems of availability of treatment or access to it

**Problems related to patients**
Reluctance to report pain
Concern about distracting physicians from treatment of underlying disease
Fear that pain means disease is worse
Concern about not being a "good" patient

**Reluctance to take pain medications**
Fear of addiction or of being thought of as an addict
Worries about unmanageable side effects
Concern about becoming tolerant to pain medications

*Sources:* Adapted from references 38 and 39.

---

## Barriers to Pain Relief

Barriers to good pain relief are numerous and pervasive. Often, because of lack of education, misconceptions, or attitudinal issues, these barriers contribute to the large numbers of patients who do not get adequate pain relief.[24,25] Careful examination of these barriers provides a guide for changing individual practice, as well as building an institutional plan within the palliative care program to improve pain relief (Table 7–1). Most studies address the barriers associated with cancer pain. Therefore, barriers facing individuals with other disorders commonly seen in palliative care are not well characterized. One might suggest that these individuals are affected to an even greater extent, as biases may be more pronounced in those with noncancer diagnoses.

### Health Care Providers

Fears related to opioids held by professionals lead to underuse of these analgesics. Numerous surveys have revealed that physicians, nurses, and pharmacists express concerns about addiction, tolerance, and side effects of morphine and related compounds.[26] Inevitability of pain is also expressed, despite evidence to the contrary. Not surprisingly, lack of attention to pain and its treatment during basic education is frequently cited.[27–29] Those providing care at the end of life must evaluate their own knowledge and beliefs, including cultural biases, and strive to educate themselves and colleagues.[30]

### Health Care Settings

Lack of availability of opioids is pervasive, affecting not only sparsely populated rural settings but also inner-city pharmacies reluctant to carry these medications.[31–33] Pain management continues to be a low priority in some health care settings, reimbursement for these services is poor and, as a result, some settings lack qualified professionals with expertise in pain management. All of this is complicated by the cost of analgesic therapies and other treatments.[34]

### Patients and Families

Understanding these barriers will lead the professional to better educate and better counsel patients and their families.[35,36] Since these fears are insidious, patients and family members or support persons should be asked if they are concerned about addiction and tolerance (often described as becoming "immune" to the drug by laypersons).[37] Studies have suggested that these fears lead to undermedication and increased intensity of pain.[38] Concerns about being a "good" patient or belief in the inevitability of cancer pain lead patients to hesitate in reporting pain.[39] In these studies, less educated and older patients were more likely to express these beliefs.[40–42] Patients seeking active treatment may believe that admitting to pain or other symptoms may reduce their eligibility for clinical trials. Adherence to the medication regimen, complicated by a lack of understanding, can lead to unrelieved pain.[43] Some patients and family members delay taking opioids, believing they are only for the dying.[44]

At the end of life, patients may need to rely on family members or other support persons to dispense medications. Each person's concerns must be addressed or provision of medication may be inadequate. Studies suggest that little concordance exists between patients' and family members' beliefs regarding analgesics.[45,46] The interdisciplinary team is essential, with nurses, social workers, chaplains, physicians, volunteers, and others providing exploration of the meaning of pain and possible barriers to good relief. Education, counseling, reframing, and spiritual support are imperative. Nurses are particularly well trained to offer the education and "coaching" that has been shown to provide improved relief.[47] A recent randomized controlled clinical trial demonstrated that integrated video and print materials presented by oncology nurses could reduce patient barriers and improve pain control.[48] Ersek provided an excellent review of the assessment and interventional approaches indicated for specific patient barriers.

## Effects of Unrelieved Pain

Although many professionals and laypersons fear that opioid analgesics lead to shortened life, there is significant evidence to the contrary. Inadequate pain relief hastens death by increasing physiological stress, potentially diminishing immunocompetence, decreasing mobility, worsening proclivities toward pneumonia and thromboembolism, and increasing work of breathing and myocardial oxygen requirements.[49,50] For example, a large study of men with prostate cancer revealed a significant association between pain interference scores and risk of death.[51] Furthermore, pain may lead to spiritual death as the individual's quality of life is impaired.[52] Therefore, it is the professional and ethical responsibility of clinicians to focus on, and attend to, adequate pain relief for their patients and to properly educate patients and their caregivers about opioid analgesic therapies.

## Assessment and Common Pain Syndromes

Comprehensive assessment of pain is imperative. This must be conducted initially, regularly throughout the treatment, and during any changes in the patient's pain state.[53] A randomized controlled trial using algorithms found that the comprehensive pain assessment integral to these algorithms contributed to reduced pain intensity scores.[54] For a complete discussion of pain assessment, see Chapter 6.

## Pharmacological Management of Pain in Advanced and End-Stage Disease

A sound understanding of pharmacotherapy in the treatment of pain is of great importance in palliative care nursing. First, this knowledge allows the nurse to contribute to and fully understand the comprehensive plan of care. Thorough understanding also allows the nurse to recognize and assess medication-related adverse effects, to understand drug–drug and drug–disease interactions, and to educate patients and caregivers regarding appropriate medication usage. This will assure a comfortable process of dying for the well-being of the patient and for the sake of those in attendance.

This section provides an overview of the most commonly used agents and some of the newer pharmaceutical agents available in the United States for the treatment of unremitting and recurrent pain associated with advanced disease. The intent of this section is to arm the reader with a fundamental and practical understanding of the medications that are (or should be) available in most contemporary care settings, emphasizing those therapies for which there is clear and convincing evidence of efficacy. For an extensive review of mechanisms of pain and analgesia, pharmacological principles of analgesics, and more-detailed lists of all drugs used for pain control throughout the world, the reader is referred to recent comprehensive reviews.[55–59] Since patients or family members are not always aware of the names of their medications, or they may bring pills to the hospital or clinic that are not in their original bottles, several web-based resources provide pictures that can assist the nurse in identifying the current analgesic regimen. These can be found at http://www.webmd.com/pill-identification/default.htm or http://www.drugs.com.

### Nonopioid Analgesics

#### Acetaminophen

Acetaminophen has been determined to be one of the safest analgesics for long-term use in the management of mild pain or as a supplement in the management of more intense pain syndromes. It is especially useful in the management of nonspecific musculoskeletal pains or pain associated with osteoarthritis, but acetaminophen (also abbreviated as APAP) should be considered an adjunct to any chronic pain regimen. It is often forgotten or overlooked when severe pain is being treated, so a reminder of its value as a "coanalgesic" is warranted. However, acetaminophen's limited anti-inflammatory effect should be considered when selecting a nonopioid. Reduced doses or avoidance of acetaminophen is recommended in the face of renal insufficiency or liver failure, and particularly in individuals with significant alcohol use and possibly in those with muscular dystrophies.[60–62]

**Table 7-2**
**Acetaminophen and Selected Nonsteroidal Antiinflammatory Drugs**

| Drug | Dose If Patient > 50 kg | Dose If Patient < 50 kg |
|---|---|---|
| Acetaminophen*† | 4000 mg/24h q 4–6h | 10–15 mg/kg q 4h (oral) |
| | | 15–20 mg/kg q 4h (rectal) |
| Aspirin*† | 4000 mg/24h q 4–6h | 10–15 mg/kg q 4h (oral) |
| | | 15–20 mg/kg q 4h (rectal) |
| Ibuprofen*† | 2400 mg/24h q 6–8h | 10 mg/kg q 6–8h (oral) |
| Naproxen*† | 1000 mg/24h q 8–12h | 5 mg/kg q 8h (oral/rectal) |
| Choline magnesium trisalicylate*§ | 2000–3000 mg/24h q 8–12 h | 25 mg/kg q 8h (oral) |
| Indomethacin† | 75–150 mg/24h q 8–12h | 0.5–1 mg/kg q 8–12h (oral/rectal) |
| Ketorolac‡ | 30–60 mg IM/IV initially, then 15–30 mg q 6h bolus IV/IM or continuous IV/SQ infusion; short-term use only (3–5 days) | 0.25–1 mg/kg q 6h short-term use only (3–5 days) |
| Celecoxib§¶ | 100–200 mg PO up to b.i.d. | No data available |

*Commercially available in a liquid form.
†Commercially available in a suppository form.
‡Potent antiinflammatory (short-term use only due to gastrointestinal side effects).
§Minimal platelet dysfunction.
¶Cyclooxygenase-2-selective nonsteroidal antiinflammatory drug.

## Nonsteroidal Antiinflammatory Drugs

Nonsteroidal antiinflammatory drugs (NSAIDs) affect analgesia by reducing the biosynthesis of prostaglandins, thereby inhibiting the cascade of inflammatory events that cause, amplify, or maintain nociception. These agents also appear to reduce pain by influences on the peripheral or central nervous system independent of their antiinflammatory mechanism of action. This secondary mode of analgesic efficacy is poorly understood. The "classic" NSAIDs (e.g., aspirin or ibuprofen) are relatively nonselective in their inhibitory effects on the enzymes that convert arachidonic acid to prostaglandins.[63] As a result, gastrointestinal (GI) ulceration, renal dysfunction, and impaired platelet aggregation are common.[64,65] The cyclooxygenase-2 (COX-2) enzymatic pathway is induced by tissue injury or other inflammation-inducing conditions.[66] It is for this reason that there appears to be less risk of GI bleeding with short-term use of the COX-2 selective NSAIDs.[67] However, although several studies demonstrate prolonged GI-sparing effects,[68] others suggest that these benefits may not extend beyond 6 to 12 months, and there may be a risk of cardiovascular events with prolonged COX-2 selective NSAID use.[69-74] Additionally, because there is cross-sensitivity, patients allergic to sulfa-containing drugs should not be given celecoxib (Table 7–2).

The NSAIDs, as a class, are very useful in the treatment of many pain conditions mediated by inflammation, including those caused by cancer.[64,75] There are insufficient data to determine whether the COX-2 agents have any specific advantages over the nonselective NSAIDs in the management of pain due to conditions such as metastatic bone pain. The NSAIDs do offer the potential advantage of causing minimal nausea, constipation, sedation, or other effects on mental functioning, although there is evidence that short-term memory in older patients can be impaired by them.[76] Therefore, depending on the cause of pain, NSAIDs may be useful for moderate to severe pain control, either alone or as an adjunct to opioid analgesic therapy. The addition of NSAIDs to opioids has the benefit of potentially allowing the reduction of the opioid dose when sedation, obtundation, confusion, dizziness, or other central nervous system effects of opioid analgesic therapy alone become burdensome.[77] As with acetaminophen, decreased renal function and liver failure are relative contraindications for NSAID use. Similarly, platelet dysfunction or other potential bleeding disorders contraindicate use of the nonselective NSAIDs due to their inhibitory effects on platelet aggregation, with resultant prolonged bleeding time. Proton pump inhibitors can be given to prevent GI bleeding.[78]

## Opioid Analgesics

As a pharmacological class, the opioid analgesics represent the most useful agents for the treatment of pain associated with advanced disease. The opioids are nonspecific insofar as they decrease pain signal transmission and perception throughout the nervous system, regardless of the pathophysiology of the pain. Moderate to severe pain is the main clinical indication for the opioid analgesics. Despite past beliefs that opioids were ineffective for neuropathic pain, these agents have been found to be useful in the treatment of this complex pain syndrome.[79] Other indications for opioid use include the treatment of dyspnea, use as an anesthetic adjunct, and as a form of prophylactic therapy in the treatment of psychological dependence to opioids (e.g., methadone maintenance for those with a history of heroin abuse).[80-82]

The only absolute contraindication to the use of an opioid is a history of a hypersensitivity reaction (rash, wheezing,

**Table 7–3**
**Definitions**

**Addiction:**

Addiction is a primary, chronic, neurobiological disease, with genetic, psychosocial, and environmental factors influencing its development and manifestations. It is characterized by behaviors that include one or more of the following: impaired control over drug use, compulsive use, continued use despite harm, and craving.

**Physical dependence:**

Physical dependence is a state of adaptation that is manifested by a drug-class-specific withdrawal syndrome that can be produced by abrupt cessation, rapid dose reduction, decreasing blood level of the drug, and/or administration of an antagonist.

**Tolerance:**

Tolerance is a state of adaptation in which exposure to a drug induces changes that result in a diminution of one or more of the drug's effects over time.

**Pseudoaddiction:**

Pseudoaddiction is the mistaken assumption of addiction in a patient who is seeking relief from pain.

**Pseudotolerance:**

Pseudotolerance is the misconception that the need for increasing doses of drug is due to tolerance rather than disease progression or other factors.

*Sources:* Adapted from reference 53.

---

**Table 7–4**
**Guidelines for the Use of Opioids**

Clinical studies and experience suggest that adherence to some basic precepts will help optimize care of patients who require opioid analgesic therapy for pain control:

- Intramuscular administration is highly discouraged except in "pain emergency" states when nothing else is available. (Subcutaneous delivery is almost always an alternative.)
- Noninvasive drug delivery systems that "bypass" the enteral route (e.g., the transdermal and the oral transmucosal routes for delivery of fentanyl for treatment of continuous pain and breakthrough pain, respectively) may obviate the necessity to use parenteral routes for pain control in some patients who cannot take medications orally or rectally.
- Anticipation, prevention, and treatment of sedation, constipation, nausea, psychotomimetic effects, and myoclonus should be part of every care plan for patients being treated with opioid analgesics.
- Changing from one opioid to another or one route to another is often necessary, so facility with this process is an absolute necessity. Remember the following points:
  —Incomplete cross-tolerance occurs, leading to decreased requirements of a newly prescribed opioid.
  —Use morphine equivalents as a "common denominator" for all dose conversions in order to avoid errors.

*Sources:* Adapted from reference 53.

---

edema). Allergic reactions are almost exclusively limited to the morphine derivatives. In the rare event that a patient describes a true allergic reaction, one might begin therapy with a low dose of a short-acting synthetic opioid (e.g., IV fentanyl) or try an intradermal injection as a test dose. The rationale for using a synthetic opioid (preferably one without dyes or preservatives since these can cause allergic reactions) is that the prevalence of allergic reactions is much lower. If the patient does develop a reaction, using a low dose of a short-acting opioid will produce a reduced response for a shorter period of time when compared to long-acting preparations.

Because misunderstandings lead to undertreatment, it is incumbent upon all clinicians involved in the care of patients with chronic pain to clearly understand and differentiate the clinical conditions of tolerance, physical dependence, addiction, pseudoaddiction, and pseudotolerance (Table 7–3).

It is also critically important for clinicians who are involved in patient care to be aware that titration of opioid analgesics to affect pain relief is rarely associated with induced respiratory depression and iatrogenic death.[83,84] In fact, the most compelling evidence suggests that inadequate pain relief hastens death by increasing physiological stress, decreasing immunocompetence, diminishing mobility, increasing the potential for thromboembolism, worsening inspiration and thus placing the patient at risk for pneumonia, and increasing myocardial oxygen requirements.[49,50] Furthermore, in a recent survey

of high-dose opioid use (299-mg oral morphine equivalents) in a hospice setting, there was no relationship between opioid dose and survival.[85] And, finally, in a small study of opioid use for the treatment of dyspnea, there was no increased risk of respiratory depression in opioid naïve patients when compared to those patients who had been receiving opioids.[86]

In a study of patients with advanced cancer, no reliable predictors for opioid dose were identified.[9] There is significant inter- and intraindividual variation in clinical responses to the various opioids, so in most cases, a dose-titration approach should be viewed as the best means of optimizing care. This implies that close follow-up is required to determine when clinical end points have been reached. Furthermore, idiosyncratic responses may require trials of different agents to determine the most effective drug and route of delivery for any given patient. Table 7–4 lists more specific suggestions regarding optimal use of opioids.

Another factor that needs to be continually considered with opioid analgesics is the potential to accumulate toxic metabolites, especially in the face of decreasing drug clearance and elimination as disease progresses and organ function deteriorates.[87] Due to its neurotoxic metabolite, normeperidine, meperidine use is specifically discouraged for chronic pain management.[88] Propoxyphene (e.g., Darvocet N-100) also is discouraged for use in palliative care due to the active metabolite, norpropoxyphene, its weak analgesic efficacy, and the

**Table 7–5**
**Approximate Equianalgesic Doses of Most Commonly Used Opioid Analgesics**

| Drug | Parenteral Route | Enteral Route |
|---|---|---|
| Morphine[†] | 10 mg | 30 mg |
| Codeine | 130 mg | 200 mg (not recommended) |
| Fentanyl[‡‡‡] | 50–100 mcg | OTFC and buccal available[‡] |
| Hydrocodone | Not available | 30 mg |
| Hydromorphone[§] | 1.5 mg | 7.5 mg |
| Levorphanol[¶] | 2 mg acute, 1 chronic | 4 mg acute, 1 chronic |
| Methadone[¶] | See text & Table 7–7 | See text & Table 7–7 |
| Oxycodone[††] | Not available | 20–30 mg |

[*]Dose conversion should be closely monitored since incomplete cross-tolerance may occur.

[†]Available in continuous and sustained-release pills and capsules, formulated to last 12 or 24 hours. Interindividual variation in duration of analgesic effect is not uncommon, signaling the need to increase the dose or shorten the dose interval.

[‡]Also available in transdermal and oral transmucosal forms, see package insert materials for dose recommendations. OTFC=oral transmucosal fentanyl citrate.

[§]Available as a continuous-release formulation lasting 24 hours.

[¶]These drugs have long half-lives, so accumulation can occur; close monitoring during first few days of therapy is very important.

[**]Available in several continuous-release doses, formulated to last 12 hours. Interindividual variation in duration of analgesic effect is not uncommon, signaling the need to increase the dose or shorten the dose interval.

[††]Fentanyl 100 mcg patch ≈ 4 mg IV morphine/h.

*Sources:* Adapted from references 53, 56, 57, 59.

significant acetaminophen dose found in some formulations.[53] As well, the mixed agonist–antagonist agents, typified by butorphanol, nalbuphine, and pentazocine, are not recommended for the treatment of chronic pain. They have limited efficacy, and their use may cause an acute abstinence syndrome in patients who are otherwise using pure agonist opioid analgesics.

## Morphine

Morphine is most often considered the "gold standard" of opioid analgesics and is used as a measure for dose equivalence (Table 7–5).[53] Although some patients cannot tolerate morphine due to itching, headache, dysphoria, or other adverse effects, common initial dosing effects such as sedation and nausea often resolve within a few days. In fact, one should anticipate these adverse effects, especially constipation, nausea, and sedation, and prevent or treat appropriately (see below). One metabolite of morphine, morphine-3-glucuronide (M3G) is active and may contribute to myoclonus, seizures and hyperalgesia (increasing pain), particularly when patients cannot clear the metabolite due to renal impairment.[87,89] Side effects and metabolic effects can be differentiated by the time course. Side effects generally

occur soon after the drug has had time to absorb, whereas there usually is a delay in metabolite-induced effects by several days. If adverse effects exceed the analgesic benefit of the drug, convert to an equianalgesic dose of a different opioid. Because cross-tolerance is incomplete, reduce the calculated dose by one third to one half and titrate upward based on the patient's pain intensity scores (see Chapter 19 for more information on the neurotoxicity of opioids).[53]

Morphine's bitter taste may be prohibitive, especially if "immediate-release" tablets are left in the mouth to dissolve. When patients have dysphagia, several options are available. The 24-hour, long-acting morphine capsule can be broken open and the "sprinkles" placed in applesauce or other soft food.[90] Oral morphine solution can be swallowed, or small volumes (0.5–1 mL) of a concentrated solution (e.g., 20 mg/mL) can be placed in the mouth of patients whose voluntary swallowing capabilities are more significantly limited.[91,92] Transmucosal uptake of morphine is slow and unpredictable due to its hydrophilic chemical nature. In fact, most of the analgesic effect of a morphine tablet or liquid placed buccally or sublingually is due to drug trickling down the throat and the resultant absorption through the GI tract. Furthermore, again due to the hydrophilic nature of morphine, creams, gels and patches that contain morphine do not cross the skin and therefore do not provide systemic analgesia.[93] Another useful route of administration when oral delivery is unreasonable is the rectal route.[94] Commercially prepared suppositories, compounded suppositories, or microenemas can be used to deliver the drug into the rectum or stoma.[95] Sustained-release morphine tablets have been used rectally, with resultant delayed time to peak plasma level and approximately 90% of the bioavailability achieved by oral administration.

## Fentanyl

Fentanyl is a highly lipid soluble opioid that has been administered parenterally, spinally, transdermally, transmucosally, and by nebulizer for the management of dyspnea.[75,96] Because of its potency, dosing is usually conducted in micrograms.

*Transdermal Fentanyl.* Transdermal fentanyl, often called the fentanyl patch, is particularly useful when patients cannot swallow, do not remember to take medications, or have adverse effects to other opioids.[97] Opioid-naive patients should start with a 12.5-mcg/h patch (currently the lowest available dose) or a 25-mcg/h patch after evaluation of effects with immediate-release opioids (Table 7–6). Patients should be monitored by a responsible caregiver for the first 24 to 48 hours of therapy until steady-state blood levels are attained. Fever, diaphoresis, cachexia, morbid obesity, and ascites may have a significant impact on the absorption, predictability of blood levels, and clinical effects of transdermal fentanyl; thus, this form of administration may not be appropriate in those conditions.[98,99] The specific effects of body mass and temperature on absorption have not been studied. Some believe the changes in fat stores (seen with cachexia) alter the fat depot

---

**Table 7–6**
**Fentanyl Patch Instructions to Patients and Caregivers**

1. Place patch on the upper body in a clean, dry, hairless area (clip hair, do not shave). The patch does not need to be placed over the site of pain.
2. Choose a different site when placing a new patch, then remove the old patch.
3. If a skin reaction consistently occurs despite site rotation, spray inhaled steroid (intended for inhalational use in asthma) over the area, let dry and apply patch (steroid creams prevent adherence of the patch).
4. Remove the old patch or patches and fold sticky surfaces together, then flush down the toilet.
5. Wash hands after handling patches.
6. All unused patches (patient discontinued use or deceased) should be removed from wrappers, folded in half with sticky surfaces together, and flushed down the toilet.

*Sources:* Adapted from references 97–99.

---

needed for absorption of this lipid-soluble compound. There is some suggestion that transdermal fentanyl may produce less constipation when compared to long-acting morphine.[97] Further study is needed to confirm these findings.

Some patients experience decreased analgesic effects after only 48 hours of applying a new patch; this should be accommodated by determining if a higher dose is tolerated with increased duration of effect or a more frequent (q 48 h) patch change should be scheduled. As with all long-acting preparations, breakthrough pain medications should be made available to patients using continuous-release opioids such as the fentanyl patch. Several reports have documented the safe and effective use of subcutaneous fentanyl when the transdermal approach could no longer provide relief or side effects occurred with other opioids.[97] However, parenteral fentanyl is commercially available in a 50-mcg/mL concentration. Higher doses may preclude the subcutaneous route. When this occurs, the intravenous (IV) route is warranted.

*Oral Transmucosal Fentanyl Citrate.* Oral transmucosal fentanyl citrate (OTFC) is composed of fentanyl on an applicator that patients rub against the oral mucosa to provide rapid absorption of the drug.[100,101] This formulation of fentanyl is particularly useful for breakthrough pain, described later in this chapter. One example of OTFC use would be pain relief of rapid onset or during a brief but painful dressing change. Adults should start with the 200-mcg dose and monitor efficacy, advancing to higher dose units as needed.[102] Clinicians must be aware that, unlike other breakthrough pain drugs, the around-the-clock dose of opioid does not predict the effective dose of OTFC. Pain relief can usually be expected in about 5 minutes after beginning use.[103] Patients should use OTFC over a period of 15 minutes because too-rapid use will result in more of the agent being swallowed rather than being absorbed transmucosally. Any remaining partial units

should be disposed of by placing under hot water or inserting the unit in a child-resistant temporary storage bottle provided when the drug is first dispensed.

*Buccal.* The fentanyl buccal tablet has been shown to be effective and to provide more rapid onset of pain relief for breakthrough pain.[104] When compared with OTFC, fentanyl buccal tablets produce a more rapid onset and greater extent of absorption.[105] The adverse effects are similar to those seen with other opioids, although a small percentage of patients do not tolerate the sensation of the tablet effervescing in the buccal space.[106] There does not seem to be a significant difference in absorption of the drug when comparing individuals who have mucositis with those who do not have an altered oral mucosa.[107] For patients who cannot place the tablet buccally (between the gum and cheekpouch), sublingual (under the tongue) administration produced comparable bioequivalence.[108] Bioadhesive films impregnated with fentanyl are under investigation as an alternate to tablet formulations.[109]

## Oxycodone

Oxycodone is a synthetic opioid available in a long-acting formulation (OxyContin), as well as immediate-release tablets (alone or with acetaminophen) and liquid. It is approximately as lipid soluble as morphine, but has better oral absorption.[110] The equianalgesic ratio is approximately 20–30 mg:30 mg of oral morphine. Side effects appear to be similar to those experienced with morphine; however, one study comparing these two long-acting formulations in persons with advanced cancer found that oxycodone produced less nausea and vomiting.[111] Despite significant media attention to OxyContin and its role in opioid abuse, it does not appear to be inherently "more addicting" than other opioids used in palliative care. Because of this attention, however, several states have restricted the number of tablets that will be distributed to an individual per month.

## Methadone

Methadone has several characteristics that make it useful in the management of severe, chronic pain.[112–114] The half-life of 24 to 36 hours or longer allows prolonged dosing intervals, although for pain control, every-eight-hour dosing is recommended.[115] Methadone may also bind as an antagonist to the N-methyl-D-aspartate (NMDA) receptor, believed to be of particular benefit in neuropathic pain.[116] Additionally, methadone can be given orally and parenterally, and sublingual administration is under investigation.[117] Furthermore, methadone is much less costly than comparable doses of proprietary continuous-release formulations, making it potentially more available for patients without sufficient financial resources for more costly drugs.

Despite these advantages, much is unknown about the appropriate dosing ratio between methadone and morphine, as well as the safest and most effective time course for conversion from another opioid to methadone.[118] Early studies

**Table 7-7**
**Rotation to Methadone from Other Opioids in Oral Morphine Equivalents**

| Bruera, E. & Sweeney, C.[113] | |
| --- | --- |
| If oral morphine < 100 mg, change to methadone 5 mg every 8 hours.<br>If oral morphine > 100 mg, use 3-day rotation period:<br>Day 1—Reduce oral morphine dose by 30%–50% and replace opioid using a 10:1 ratio. Administer methadone every 8 hours.<br>Day 2—Reduce oral morphine by another 35%–50% of original dose and increase methadone if pain is moderate to severe.<br>Supplement with short-acting opioids.<br>Day 3—Discontinue oral morphine and titrate methadone dose daily. | Begin methadone at 10 mg or less per day given in divided doses (every 8 hours). Do not increase the dose by more than 25%–50% weekly |

*Source*: www.zerodeaths.org (accessed November 30, 2009).

suggested the ratio might be 1:1, and this appears to be true for individuals without recent prior exposure to opioids. Newer data suggest the dose ratio increases as the previous dose of oral opioid equivalents increases.[119-121] Systematic review of exisiting studies do not favor one approach over another[122] (Table 7-7). Furthermore, although the long half-life is an advantage, it also increases the potential for drug accumulation before achieving steady-state blood levels, putting patients at risk for oversedation and respiratory depression. This might occur after 2 to 5 days of treatment with methadone. Close monitoring of these potentially adverse or even life-threatening effects is required and most experts suggest that methadone only be prescribed by experienced clinicians.[123,124] Myoclonus has been reported with methadone use.[125] Finally, recent studies suggest high doses of methadone may lead to QT wave changes (also called torsade de pointes).[126-128]

Methadone is metabolized primarily by CYP3A4, but also by CYP2D6 and CYP1A2. As a result, drugs that induce CYP enzymes accelerate the metabolism of methadone, resulting in reduced serum levels of the drug. This may be demonstrated clinically by shortened analgesic periods or reduced overall pain relief. Examples of these drugs often used in palliative care include several antiretroviral agents, dexamethasone, carbamazepine, phenytoin, and barbiturates.[129] Drugs that inhibit CYP enzymes slow methadone metabolism, potentially leading to sedation and respiratory depression. These include ketoconazole, omeprazole, and SSRI antidepressants such as fluoxetine, paroxetine, and sertraline.[113,115]

Patients currently receiving methadone as part of a maintenance program for addictive disease will have developed cross tolerance to the opioids and, as a result, require higher doses than naive patients.[130] Prescribing methadone for addictive disease requires a special license in the United States. Therefore, prescriptions provided for methadone to manage pain in palliative care should include the statement "for pain."

### Hydromorphone

Hydromorphone (Dilaudid) is a useful alternative when synthetic opioids provide an advantage. It is available in oral tablets, liquids, suppositories, and parenteral formulations, and a long-acting formulation is under investigation in the United States (these are currently available in Canada and elsewhere).[131] As a synthetic opioid, hydromorphone provides an advantage when patients have true allergic responses to morphine, or when inadequate pain control or intolerable side effects occur. Recent experience suggests that the metabolite hydromorphone-3-glucuronide (H3G) may lead to the same opioid neurotoxicity seen with morphine metabolites: myoclonus, hyperalgesia, and seizures.[89,132,133] This is of particular risk in persons with renal dysfunction.[134-136]

### Oxymorphone

Oxymorphone is a semi-synthetic opioid that has been available in a parenteral formulation for almost 50 years and is now available in oral immediate-release and extended-release formulations. The safety and efficacy profile in people with cancer is similar to other opioids, such as morphine and oxycodone.[134,135] In a study of people with low back pain, the equianalgesic dosage of extended-release oxymorphone was approximately 50% of the oxycodone extended-release dose.[137]

### Other Opioids

Codeine, hydrocodone, levorphanol, oxymorphone and tramadol are other opioids available in the United States for treatment of pain. Their equianalgesic comparisons are included in Table 7-5. Buprenorphine, a partial agonist, is typically used as part of an opioid maintenance program instead of methadone. A buprenorphine patch has been used in Europe for relief of cancer pain; however, this is not yet available in the United States.[138] Furthermore, because of its partial agonist properties, an appropriate breakthrough medication (oral buprenorphine) is not currently available in the United States.

## Alternative Routes of Administration for Opioid Analgesics

Many routes of administration are available when patients can no longer swallow or when other dynamics preclude the oral route or favor other routes. These include transdermal, transmucosal, rectal, vaginal, topical, epidural, and intrathecal. In a study of cancer patients at 4 weeks, 1 week, and 24 hours before death, the oral route of opioid administration was continued in 62%, 43%, and 20% of patients, respectively. More than half of these patients required more than one route of opioid administration. As patients approached death and oral use diminished, the use of intermittent subcutaneous injections and IV or subcutaneous infusions increased.[10]

Thus, in the palliative care setting, nonoral routes of administration must be available. Enteral feeding tubes can be used to access the gut when patients can no longer swallow. The size of the tube should be considered when placing long-acting morphine "sprinkles" to avoid obstruction of the tube. The rectum, stoma, or vagina can be used to deliver medication. Thrombocytopenia or painful lesions preclude the use of these routes. Additionally, delivering medications via these routes can be difficult for family members, especially when the patient is obtunded or unable to assist. Because the vagina has no sphincter, a tampon covered with a condom or an inflated urinary catheter balloon may be used to prevent early discharge of the drug.[139] As previously discussed, transdermal, transmucosal or buccal fentanyl are useful alternatives to these techniques.

Parenteral administration includes subcutaneous and IV delivery (intramuscular opioid delivery is inappropriate in the palliative care setting).[140] The IV route provides rapid drug delivery but requires vascular access, placing the patient at risk for infection and potentially complicating the care provided by family or other loved ones. Subcutaneous boluses have a slower onset and lower peak effect when compared with IV boluses.[53] Subcutaneous infusions may include up to 10 mL/h (although most patients absorb 2 to 3 mL/h with least difficulty).[141,142] Volumes greater than these are poorly absorbed. Hyaluronidase has been reported to speed absorption of subcutaneously administered drugs.

Intraspinal routes, including epidural or intrathecal delivery, may allow administration of drugs, such as opioids, local anesthetics, and/or α-adrenergic agonists. One randomized controlled trial demonstrated benefit for cancer patients experiencing pain.[143] However, the equipment used to deliver these medications is complex, requiring specialized knowledge for health care professionals and potentially greater caregiver burden. Risk of infection is also of concern. Furthermore, cost is a significant concern related to high-technology procedures. See Chapter 24 for a review of high-technology procedures for pain relief.

## Preventing and Treating Adverse Effects of Opioid Analgesics

*Constipation.* Patients in palliative care frequently experience constipation, in part due to opioid therapy.[1a,144] Always begin a prophylactic bowel regimen when commencing opioid analgesic therapy. Most clinicians recommend a laxative/softener combination, although a recent study found that senna alone was more effective than senna and docusate.[145] Avoid bulking agents (e.g., psyllium) since these tend to cause a larger, bulkier stool, increasing desiccation time in the large bowel. Furthermore, debilitated patients can rarely take in sufficient fluid to facilitate the action of bulking agents. Fluid intake should be encouraged whenever feasible. Senna tea and fruits may be of use. A novel compound, methylnaltrexone, has been shown to be effective in relieving opioid-induced constipation when given subcutaneously at doses of 0.15 mg//kg.[146,147] For a more comprehensive review of bowel management, refer to Chapter 12.

*Sedation.* Excessive sedation may occur with the initial doses of opioids. If sedation persists after 24 to 48 hours and other correctable causes have been identified and treated if possible, the use of psychostimulants may be beneficial. These include dextroamphetamine 2.5 to 5 mg PO q morning and midday or methylphenidate 5 to 10 mg PO q morning and 2.5 to 5 mg midday (although higher doses are frequently used).[148,149] Adjust both the dose and timing to prevent nocturnal insomnia and monitor for undesirable psychotomimetic effects (such as agitation, hallucinations, and irritability). Interestingly, in one study, as-needed dosing of methylphenidate in cancer patients did not result in sleep disturbances or agitation, even though most subjects took doses in the afternoon and evening.Modafinil, a newer agent approved to manage narcolepsy, has been reported to relieve opioid-induced sedation with once-daily dosing.[150]

*Respiratory Depression.* Respiratory depression is rarely a clinically significant problem for opioid-tolerant patients in pain.[53] When respiratory depression occurs in a patient with advanced disease, the cause is usually multifactorial.[83,74] Therefore, other factors beyond opioids need to be assessed, although opioids are frequently blamed for the reduced repirations. When undesired depressed consciousness occurs along with a respiratory rate less than 8/min or hypoxemia ($O_2$ saturation <90%) associated with opioid use, cautious and slow titration of naloxone, which reverses the effects of the opioids" should be instituted. Excessive administration may cause abrupt opioid reversal with pain and autonomic crisis. Dilute 1 ampule of naloxone (0.4 mg/mL) in 10 mL of injectable saline (final concentration 40 mcg/mL) and inject 1 mL every 2 to 3 minutes while closely monitoring the level of consciousness and respiratory rate. Because the duration of effect of naloxone is approximately 30 minutes, the depressant effects of the opioid will recur at 30 minutes and persist until the plasma levels decline (often four or more hours) or until the next dose of naloxone is administered.[53] A relatively recently identified phenomenon is the onset, or exacerbation of, sleep apnea in patients taking opioids for pain.[151] Although this has been described in nonmalignant pain populations,[152] this may be of concern for some palliative care patients. Risk factors appear to be the use of methadone, concomitant use of benzodiazepines or other sedative agents, respiratory infections and obesity (which is a risk factor for sleep apnea).

*Nausea and Vomiting.* Nausea and vomiting are common with opioids due to activation of the chemoreceptor trigger zone in the medulla, vestibular sensitivity, and delayed gastric emptying, but habituation occurs in most cases within several days.[153] Assess for other treatable causes. In severe cases or when nausea and vomiting are not self-limited, pharmacotherapy is indicated. The doses of nausea-relieving medications and antiemetics listed below are to be used initially but can be increased as required. See Chapter 10 for a thorough discussion of the assessment and treatment of nausea and vomiting.

*Myoclonus.* Myoclonic jerking occurs more commonly with high-dose opioid therapy, although it has also been reported with lower dosing.[154–156] If this should develop, switch to an alternate opioid, since evidence suggests this symptom is associated with metabolite accumulation, particularly in the face of renal dysfunction.[89,125,132,157] A lower relative dose of the substituted drug may be possible, due to incomplete cross-tolerance, which might result in decreased myoclonus. Clonazepam 0.5 to 1 mg PO q 6 to 8 hours, to be increased as needed and tolerated, may be useful in treating myoclonus in patients who are still alert, able to communicate, and take oral preparations.[158] Lorazepam can be given sublingually if the patient is unable to swallow. Otherwise, parenteral administration of diazepam is indicated if symptoms are distressing. Grand mal seizures associated with high-dose parenteral opioid infusions have been reported and may be due to preservatives in the solution.[159] Preservative-free solutions should be used when administering high-dose infusions. (See Chapter 19 for more specific information.)

*Pruritus.* Pruritus appears to be most common with morphine, in part due to histamine release, but can occur with most opioids. Fentanyl and oxymorphone may be less likely to cause histamine release.[53] Most antipruritus therapies cause sedation, so this side effect must be viewed by the patient as an acceptable trade-off. Antihistamines (such as diphenydramine) are the most common first-line approach to this opioid-induced symptom when treatment is indicated. Ondansetron has been reported to be effective in relieving opioid-induced pruritus, but no randomized controlled studies exist.[160]

## Coanalgesics

A wide variety of nonopioid medications from several pharmacological classes have been demonstrated to reduce pain caused by various pathological conditions (Table 7–8). As a group, these drugs have been called analgesic "adjuvants," but this is something of a misnomer since they often reduce pain when used alone. However, under most circumstances, when these drugs are indicated for the treatment of severe neuropathic pain or bone pain, opioid analgesics are used concomitantly to provide adequate pain relief.

## Antidepressants

The mechanism of the analgesic effect of tricyclic antidepressants appears to be related to inhibition of norepinephrine and serotonin.[161] Despite the absence of positive controlled clinical trials in cancer pain or other palliative care pain conditions, the tricyclic antidepressants are generally believed to provide relief from neuropathic pain.[162] One consensus panel listed this category as one of five first-line therapies for neuropathic pain.[163] Side effects often limit the use of these agents in palliative care. Cardiac arrhythmias, conduction abnormalities, narrow-angle glaucoma, and clinically significant prostatic hyperplasia are relative contraindications to the tricyclic antidepressants. The delay in onset of pain relief, from days to weeks, may preclude the use of these agents for pain relief in end-of-life care. However, their sleep-enhancing and mood-elevating effects may be of benefit.[164]

Both older antidepressants and newer atypical agents have been shown to be effective in relieving neuropathic pain, although there remains little support for the analgesic effect of serotonin-selective uptake inhibitors (SSRIs).[165] Atypical antidepressants, venlafaxine and duloxetine, have been shown to reduce neuropathy associated with chemotherapy-induced neuropathy in experimental animal models and in humans,[166,167] as well as following treatment for breast cancer.[168]

## Anticonvulsants

The older anticonvulsants, such as carbamazepine and clonazepam, relieve pain by blocking sodium channels.[164] Often referred to as membrane stabilizers, these compounds are very useful in the treatment of neuropathic pain, especially those with episodic, lancinating qualities. Gabapentin and pregabalin act at the alpha-2delta subunit of the voltage-gated calcium channel.[169] Additional evidence supports the use of these agents in neuropathic pain syndromes seen in palliative care, such as thalamic pain, pain due to spinal cord injury, and cancer pain, along with restless leg syndrome.[172–174] Pregabalin has undergone extensive testing in pain due to diabetic neuropathy and has been found to be effective.[170,171] Withdrawal from either compound should be gradual.[175] Other anticonvulsants have been used with success in treating neuropathies, including lamotrigine, levetiracetam, tiagabine, topiramate, and zonisamide, yet no randomized controlled clinical trials are currently available.[163]

## Corticosteroids

Corticosteroids inhibit prostaglandin synthesis and reduce edema surrounding neural tissues.[176] This category of drug is

**Table 7–8**
**Adjuvant Analgesics**

| Drug Class | Daily Adult Starting Dose* (Range) | Routes of Administration | Adverse Effects | Indications |
|---|---|---|---|---|
| Antidepressants | Nortriptyline 10–25 mg | PO | Anticholinergic effects | Neuropathic pain |
| | Desipramine 10–25 mg | PO | | |
| | Venlafaxine 37.5 mg BID | PO | Nausea, dizziness | |
| | Duloxetine 30 mg | PO | Nausea | |
| Anticonvulsants | Clonazapam 0.5–1 mg hs, bid or tid | PO | Sedation | Neuropathic pain |
| | Carbamazapine 100 mg q day or tid | PO | | |
| | Gabapentin 100 mg tid Pregabalin 50 mg TID | PO | | |
| Corticosteroids | Dexamethasone 2–20 mg q day; may give up to 100 mg IV bolus for pain crises | PO/IV/SQ | "Steroid psychosis," dyspepsia | Cerebral edema, spinal cord compression, bone pain, neuropathic pain, visceral pain |
| | Prednisone 15–30 mg tid, qid | PO | | |
| Local anesthetics | Mexiletine 150 mg tid | PO | Lightheadedness, arrhthymias | Neuropathic pain |
| | Lidocaine 1–5 mg/kg hourly | IV or SQ infusion | | |
| N-Methyl-D-aspartate antagonists | Dextromethorphan, effective dose unknown | PO | Confusion | Neuropathic pain |
| | Ketamine (see Pain Crises) | IV | | |
| Bisphosphonates | Pamidronate 60–90 mg over 2h every 2–4 wk | IV infusion | Pain flare | Osteolytic bone pain |
| Calcitonin | 25 IU/day | SQ/nasal | Hypersensitivity reaction, nausea | Neuropathic pain, bone pain |
| Capsaicin | 0.025–0.075% | Topical | Burning | Neuropathic pain |
| Baclofen | 10 mg q day or qid | PO | Muscle weakness, cognitive changes | |
| Calcium channel blockers | Nifedipine 10 mg tid | PO | Bradycardia, hypotension | Ischemic pain, neuropathic pain, smooth muscle spasms with pain |

*Pediatric doses for pain control not well established.
*Sources:* Adapted from references 161–198.

particularly useful for neuropathic pain syndromes, including plexopathies, and pain associated with stretching of the liver capsule due to metastases.[176,177] Corticosteroids are also highly effective for treating bone pain due to their anti-inflammatory effects, as well as relieving malignant intestinal obstruction.[178] Dexamethasone produces the least amount of mineralocorticoid effect, leading to reduced potential for Cushing's syndrome. Dexamthasone is available in oral, IV, subcutaneous, and epidural formulations. The standard dose is 16 to 24 mg/day and can be administered once daily due to the long half-life of this drug.[53] Doses as high as 100 mg may be given with severe pain crises. IV bolus doses should be pushed slowly, to prevent uncomfortable perineal burning and itching.

## Local Anesthetics

Local anesthetics work in a manner similar to the older anticonvulsants—by inhibiting the movement of ions across the neural membrane.[179] They are useful for relieving neuropathic pain. Local anesthetics can be given orally, topically, intravenously, subcutaneously, or spinally.[179] Mexiletine has been reported to be useful when anticonvulsants and other adjuvant therapies have failed. Doses start at 150 mg/day and increase to levels as high as 900 mg/day in divided doses.[180,181] Local anesthetic gels and patches have been used to prevent the pain associated with needlestick and other minor procedures. Both gel and patch (Lidoderm) versions of lidocaine have been shown to reduce the pain of postherpetic neuropathy.[182]

IV lidocaine at 1 to 5 mg/kg (maximum 500 mg) administered over 1 hour, followed by a continuous infusion of 1 to 2 mg/kg/hour has been reported to reduce intractable neuropathic pain in patients in inpatient palliative care and home hospice settings.[183] Epidural or intrathecal lidocaine or bupivacaine delivered with an opioid can reduce neuropathic pain.[184]

### N-Methyl-D-Aspartate Antagonists

Antagonists to NMDA are believed to block the binding of excitatory amino acids, such as glutamate, in the spinal cord. Ketamine, a dissociative anesthetic, is believed to relieve severe neuropathic pain by blocking NMDA receptors (see the section "Pain Crisis," below). Case reports and small studies suggest that intravenous or oral ketamine can be used in adults and children for their relief of neuropathic pain or to reduce opioid doses.[185,186] A Cochrane review found insufficient trials conducted to determine safety and efficacy in cancer pain.[187] Routine use often is limited by cognitive changes and other adverse effects. Oral compounds containing dextromethorphan have been tested, but were found to be ineffective in relieving cancer pain.[188]

### Bisphosphonates

Bisphosphonates inhibit osteoclast-mediated bone resorption and alleviate pain related to metastatic bone disease and multiple myeloma.[189,190] Pamidronate disodium reduces pain, hypercalcemia, and skeletal morbidity associated with breast cancer and multiple myeloma.[191,192] Dosing is generally repeated every four weeks and the analgesic effects occur in two-to-four weeks. Interestingly, a recent randomized, controlled trial of pamidronate in men experiencing pain due to prostate cancer failed to demonstrate any benefit.[193] Zoledronic acid is a newer bisphosphonate that has been shown to relieve pain due to metastatic bone disease.[194] It is somewhat more convenient because it can be infused over a shorter duration of time. Ibandronate is a bisphosphonate that is taken either orally or intravenously and has been shown in a small trial to reduce pain in women with metastatic breast cancer.[195,196] Clodronate and sodium etidronate appear to provide little or no analgesia.[197]

### Calcitonin

Subcutaneous calcitonin may be effective in the relief of neuropathic or bone pain, although studies are inconclusive.[198] The nasal form of this drug may be more acceptable in end-of-life care when other therapies are ineffective. Usual doses are 100 to 200 IU/day subcutaneously or nasally.

### Radiation Therapy and Radiopharmaceuticals

Radiotherapy can be enormously beneficial in relieving pain due to bone metastases or other lesions.[199,200] In many cases, single-fraction external beam therapy can be used to facilitate treatment in debilitated patients.[200] Goals of treatment should be clearly articulated so that patients and family members understand the role of this therapy. Targeted therapies, also referred to as radiosurgery, can be effective in selected situations.[201] Radiolabeled agents such as strontium-89 and samarium-153 have been shown to be effective at reducing metastatic bone pain.[202–204] Thrombocytopenia and leukopenia are relative contraindications since strontium-89 causes thrombocytopenia in as many as 33% of those treated and leukopenia up to 10%.[202] Because of the delayed onset and timing of peak effect, only those patients with a projected life span of greater than 3 months should be considered for treatment. Patients should be advised that a transitory pain flare can occur after either external beam therapy or radiolabeled agents; additional analgesics should be provided in anticipation.[205]

### Chemotherapy

Palliative chemotherapy is the use of anti-tumor therapy to relieve symptoms associated with malignancy. Patient goals, performance status, sensitivity of the tumor, and potential toxicities must be considered.[206] Examples of symptoms that may improve with chemotherapy include hormonal therapy in breast cancer to relieve chest wall pain due to tumor ulceration, or chemotherapy in lung cancer to relieve dyspnea.[207]

### Other Adjunct Analgesics

Topical capsaicin is believed to relieve pain by inhibiting the release of substance P. This compound has been shown to be useful in relieving pain associated with post-mastectomy syndrome, post-herpetic neuralgia, and post-surgical neuropathic pain in cancer.[176] A burning sensation experienced by patients is a common reason for discontinuing therapy. A high concentration topical capsaicin patch is being studied in the relief of HIV associated painful neuropathy.[208]

Patients often ask about cannabinoids for the relief of pain or spasticity. Major advances, such as the characterization of the cannabinoid receptors (CB1 and CB2) have increased our understanding of the role of these receptors in pain and have allowed the development of more selective agents that might provide analgesia without the central nervous system depressant effects seen with tetrahydrocannabinol (THC). Evidence exists for the efficacy of some of these new selective compounds in animal models of noncancer and cancer pain.[209,210] However, review of existing literature evaluating the role of cannabinoids currently approved for human use suggests that these agents are moderately effective with comparable adverse effects.[211] Questions regarding the long-term safety and regulatory implications remain.[212]

Baclofen is useful in the relief of spasm-associated pain. Doses usually begin at 10 mg/day, increasing every few days. A generalized feeling of weakness and confusion or hallucinations often occurs with doses above 60 mg/day. Intrathecal baclofen has been used to treat spasticity and resulting pain, primarily due to multiple sclerosis and spinal cord injury, although a case report describes relief from pain due to spinal cord injury and ALS.[213–215]

Calcium channel blockers are believed to provide pain relief by preventing conduction. Nifedipine 10 mg, taken orally, may be useful to relieve ischemic or neuropathic pain syndromes.[216]

## Interventional Therapies

In addition to previously discussed spinal administration of analgesics, interventional therapies to relieve pain at end of life can be beneficial, including nerve blocks, vertebroplasty, kyphoplasty, radiofrequency ablation of painful metastases, procedures to drain painful effusions and other techniques.[53,217–219] Few of these procedures have undergone controlled clinical studies. One technique, the celiac plexus block, has been shown to be superior to morphine in patients with pain due to unresectable pancreatic cancer.[220,221] A relatively new approach to providing analgesia is the administration of botulinum toxin (sometimes referred to as botox). Injections of this substance into areas of muscle spasticity, tightness and pain can result in relief. This has been used extensively in migraine treatment and chronic pain conditions and, more recently, has been used to relieve pain in people with cancer who experience radiation fibrosis, such as cervical dystonia, trigeminal nerve pain and headache.[222] Botulinum toxin has also been used to reduce postoperative pain associated with tissue expander placement after mastectomy.[223]

A complete review of interventional procedures can be found in a variety of sources. Choosing one of these techniques is dependent upon the availability of experts in this area who understand the special needs of palliative care patients, the patient's ability to undergo the procedure, and the patient's and family's goals of care.

## Nonpharmacological Therapies

Non-drug therapies, including cognitive–behavioral techniques and physical measures, can serve as adjuncts to analgesics in the palliative care setting. This is not to suggest that when these therapies work, the pain is of psychological origin.[224] The patient's and caregivers' abilities to participate must be considered when selecting one of these therapies, including their fatigue level, interest, cognition, and other factors.[225]

Cognitive–behavioral therapy often includes strategies to improve coping and relaxation, such as relaxation, guided imagery, music, prayer, and reframing.[224,226–229] In a randomized clinical trial of patients undergoing bone marrow transplantation, pain was reduced in those patients who received relaxation and imagery training and in those who received cognitive-behavioral skill development with relaxation and imagery.[230] Patients who received treatment as usual or those randomized to receive support from a therapist did not experience pain relief. More recent trials have employed multiple measures,

such as education, exercise, coaching, coping and other support, to effectively relieve cancer-related pain.[231,232]

Physical measures, such as massage, reflexology, heat, chiropractic and other techniques, produce relaxation and relieve pain.[233–237] In a study of massage in hospice patients, relaxation resulted as measured by blood pressure, heart rate, and skin temperature.[238] A 10-minute back massage was found to relieve pain in male cancer patients.[239] Rhiner and colleagues[240] employed a comprehensive non-drug program for cancer patients that included education; physical measures such as heat, cold, and massage; and cognitive–behavioral strategies such as distraction and relaxation. All therapies were rated as useful, with distraction and heat scoring highest. More research is needed in the palliative care setting regarding non-drug therapies that might enhance pain relief.

## Difficult Pain Syndromes

The above therapies provide relief for the majority of patients (Table 7–9). Unfortunately, complex pain syndromes may

---

**Table 7–9**
**Guidelines for Pain Management in Palliative Care**

- Sustained-release formulations and around-the-clock dosing should be used for continuous pain syndromes.
- Immediate-release formulations should be made available for breakthrough pain.
- Cost and convenience (and other identified issues influencing compliance) are highly practical and important matters that should be taken into account with every prescription.
- Anticipate, prevent, and treat predictable side effects and adverse drug effects.
- Titrate analgesics based on patient goals, requirements for supplemental analgesics, pain intensity, severity of undesirable or adverse drug effects, measures of functionality, sleep, emotional state, and patients'/caregivers' reports of impact of pain on quality of life.
- Monitor patient status frequently during dose titration.
- Discourage use of mixed agonist–antagonist opioids.
- Be aware of potential drug–drug and drug–disease interactions.
- Recommend expert pain management consultation if pain is not adequately relieved within a reasonable amount of time after applying standard analgesic guidelines and interventions.
- Know the qualifications, experience, skills, and availability of pain management experts (consultants) within the patient's community before they may be needed.

These basic guidelines and considerations will optimize the pharmacologic management of all patients with pain, particularly those in the palliative care setting.

*Sources:* Adapted from references 55–59.

require additional measures. These syndromes include break-through pain, pain crises, and pain control in the patient with a past or current history of substance abuse.

## Breakthrough Pain

Intermittent episodes of moderate to severe pain that occur in spite of control of baseline continuous pain are common in patients with advanced disease.[241] Studies suggest that although breakthrough pain in cancer patients at home is common, short-acting analgesics are frequently not provided and patients do not take as much as is allowed.[241–243] Mostly described in cancer patients, there is evidence that patients with other pain-producing and life-limiting diseases commonly experience breakthrough pains a few times a day, lasting moments to many minutes.[244,245] Several studies of patients with cancer and non-cancer diagnoses at end of life demonstrate an average of 4–5 breakthrough episodes per day, with the majority of these episodes occuring without any warning.[246,247] The risk of increasing the around-the-clock or continuous-release analgesic dose to cover breakthrough pains is that of increasing undesirable side effects, especially sedation, once the more short-lived, episodic breakthrough pain has remitted. Guidelines for categorizing, assessing, and managing breakthrough pain are described below:

*Incident Pain.* Incident pain is predictably elicited by specific activities. Use a rapid-onset, short-duration analgesic formulation in anticipation of pain-eliciting activities or events. Use the same drug that the patient is taking for baseline pain relief for incident pain whenever possible. Educate patients and family members regarding the need to administer short acting opioids approximately 30–60 minutes prior to the activity to prevent pain.

*Spontaneous Pain.* Spontaneous pain is unpredictable and not temporally associated with any activity or event. These pains are more challenging to control. The use of adjuvants for neuropathic pains may help to diminish the frequency and severity of these types of pain (see Table 7–8). Otherwise, immediate treatment with a potent, rapid-onset opioid analgesic is indicated.

*End-of-Dose Failure.* End-of-dose failure describes pain that occurs toward the end of the usual dosing interval of a regularly scheduled analgesic. This results from declining blood levels of the around-the-clock analgesic before administration or uptake of the next scheduled dose. Appropriate questioning and use of pain diaries will assure rapid diagnosis of end-of-dose failure. Increasing the dose of around-the-clock medication or shortening the dose interval to match the onset of this type of breakthrough pain should remedy the problem. For instance, a patient who is taking continuous-release morphine every 12 hours and whose pain "breaks through" after about eight to 10 hours is experiencing end-of-dose failure. The dosing interval should be increased to every eight hours or, if this is not reasonable, the dose should be increased by 25% to 50%.

## Bone Pain

Pain due to bone metastatis or pathological fractures can include extremely painful breakthrough pain, often associated with movement, along with periods of somnolence when the patient is at rest.[216] In one study of cancer patients admitted to an inpatient hospice, 93% had breakthrough pain, with 72% of the episodes related to movement or weight bearing.[248] Treatment of bone pain includes the use of corticosteroids, bisphosphonates if indicated, radiotherapy or radionuclides if consistent with the goals of care, and long-acting opioids along with short-acting opioids for the periods of increasing pain.[199] Vertebroplasty or kyphoplasty may stabilize the vertebrae if tumor invasion leads to instability.[217]

## Pain Crisis

Most nociceptive (i.e., somatic and visceral) pain is controllable with appropriately titrated analgesic therapy.[249] Some neuropathic pains, such as invasive and compressive neuropathies, plexopathies, and myelopathies, may be poorly responsive to conventional analgesic therapies, short of inducing a nearly comatose state. Widespread bone metastases or end-stage pathological fractures may present similar challenges.[216,250] When confronted by a pain crisis, the following considerations will be helpful:

- Differentiate terminal agitation or anxiety from "physically" based pain, if possible. Terminal symptoms unresponsive to rapid upward titration of an opioid may respond to benzodiazepines (e.g., lorazepam, midazolam).
- Make sure that drugs are getting absorbed. The only route guaranteed to be absorbed is the IV route. Although invasive routes of drug delivery are to be avoided unless necessary, if there is any question about oral or transdermal absorption of analgesics or other necessary palliative drugs, parenteral access should be established.
- Preterminal pain crises that respond poorly to basic approaches to analgesic therapy merit consultation with a pain management consultant as quickly as possible. Radiotherapeutic, anesthetic, or neuroablative procedures may be indicated.[216]

## Management of Refractory Symptoms at the End of Life

Sedation at the end of life is an important option for patients with intractable pain or other symptoms. The most commonly employed agents include benzodiazepines, including midazolam or lorazepam, barbiturates, and in some cases, propofol.[251–254] Palliative sedation is best delivered under the guidance of experts in palliative care and is usually reserved for those patients who are expected to die within hours to days.[255] Light sedation may first be attempted to allow communication with loved ones, although in some circumstances this may be

**Table 7–10**
**Protocol for Using Ketamine to Treat a Pain Crisis**

1. Bolus: ketamine 0.1 mg/kg IV. Double the dose if no clinical improvement in 5 minutes. Repeat as often as indicated by the patient's response. Follow the bolus with an infusion. Decrease opioid dose by 50%.
2. Infusion: ketamine 0.015 mg/(kg/min) IV (about 1 mg/min for a 70 kg individual). Subcutaneous infusion is possible if IV access is not attainable. In this case, use an initial IM bolus dose of 0.3–0.5 mg/kg. Decrease opioid dose by 50%.
3. It is advisable to administer a benzodiazepine (e.g., diazepam, lorazepam) concurrently to mitigate against the possibility of hallucinations or frightful dreams because moribund patients under these circumstances may not be able to communicate such experiences.
4. Observe for problematic increases in secretions; treat with glycopyrrolate, scopolomine, or atropine as needed.

*Sources:* Adapted from reference 260.

insufficient to relieve the intractable symptoms. See Chapter 26 for additional discussion regarding palliative sedation.

Parenteral administration of ketamine is also useful for some patients with refractory pain at the end of life.[256] Ketamine is a potent analgesic at low doses and a dissociative anesthetic at higher doses.[257] In particular, ketamine can be used for the management of severe neuropathic pain and can be effective as an opioid-sparing agent, allowing in some cases increased interactive capability. Adverse effects are often dose-related and include psychotomimetic effects (hallucinations, dysphoria, nightmares) as well as excess salivation[258] (Table 7–10).[259,260] Haloperidol can be used to treat the hallucinations, and scopolamine may be needed to reduce the excess salivation seen with this drug. Ketamine is commercially available in the United States only in a parenteral formulation. If the oral route is indicated, a palatable solution can be compounded or the parenteral solution ingested, usually mixed with juice or other liquids to mask the bitter taste. Because the opioid sparing effect is so pronounced, the opioid dose should be reduced by 25 to 50% when initiating ketamine. More research is needed regarding the efficacy of and adverse effects associated with the use of ketamine for intractable pain in the palliative care population.

## Pain Control in People with Addictive Disease

The numbers of patients entering palliative care with a current or past history of addictive disease are unknown, yet thought to be significant.[14,261] As approximately one third of the U.S. population has used illicit drugs, it would logically follow that some of these individuals will require palliative care. In one uncontrolled survey of people with cancer or HIV, more than half of those with HIV considered themselves to be recovering addicts.[262] Therefore, all clinicians must be aware of the principles and practical considerations necessary to adequately care for these individuals (see Chapter 42 for a complete discussion of care for the addicted patient at the end of life).

The underlying mechanisms of addiction are complex, including the pharmacological properties of the drug, personality and psychiatric disorders, as well as underlying genetic factors.[263] Caring for these patients can be extremely challenging. Thorough assessment of the pain and their addictive disease is critical. Defensive behavior is to be expected; therefore, the interview should begin with general questions about the use of caffeine and nicotine and gradually become more specific about illicit drug use.[264] Patients should be informed that the information will be used to help prevent withdrawal from these drugs, as well as ensure adequate doses of medications used to relieve pain.

Patients can be categorized in the following manner: (1) individuals who used drugs or alcohol in the past but are not using them now; (2) patients in methadone maintenance programs who are not using recreational drugs or alcohol; (3) persons in methadone maintenance programs but who continue to actively use drugs or alcohol; (4) people using drugs or alcohol occasionally, usually socially; and (5) patients who are actively abusing drugs.[265,266] Treatment is different for each group.

A frequent fear expressed by professionals is that they will be "duped," or lied to, about the presence of pain. One of the limitations of pain management is that pain, and all its components, cannot be proven. Therefore, expressions of pain must be believed. As with all aspects of palliative care, an interdisciplinary team approach is indicated. This may include inviting addiction counselors to interdisciplinary team meetings. Realistic goals must be established. For example, recovery from addiction is impossible if the patient does not seek this rehabilitation. The goal in that case may be to provide a structured and safe environment for patients and their support persons. Comorbid psychiatric disorders are common, particularly depression, personality disorders, and anxiety disorders. Treatment of these underlying problems may reduce relapse or aberrant behaviors and may make pain control more effective.[267]

The pharmacological principles of pain management in the person with addictive disease are not unlike those in a person without this history. Nonopioids may be used, including antidepressants, anticonvulsants, and other adjuncts. However, psychoactive drugs with no analgesic effect should be avoided in the treatment of pain. Tolerance must be considered; thus, opioid doses may require more rapid titration and may be higher than for patients without previous exposure to opioids.[268] Requests for increasing doses may be due to psychological suffering, so this possibility must also be explored.

An additional complicating factor is that many people with addictive disease have limited psychological, social, and financial resources. Part of the reason for self-medication may be mental illness. The lack of resources makes provision of care difficult, as many of these patients may have lost their jobs and homes and have alienated friends and family members. Innovative programs offering palliative care of homeless patients living in shelters include attention to treatment of substance abuse. [269,270]

Consistency in the treatment plan is essential. Inconsistency can increase manipulation and lead to staff frustration. Setting limits is a critical component of the care plan, and medication contracts may be indicated.[271] In fact, one primary clinician may be designated to handle the pharmacological management of pain. Prescriptions may be written for 1-week intervals if patients cannot manage an entire month's supply.[270] The prescriptions may be delivered to one pharmacy to reduce the potential for altered prescriptions or prescriptions from multiple prescribers. Writing out the number for the dose and the total number of tablets will prevent alterations of the prescription (e.g., increasing the number of tablets from 10 to 100). Use long-acting opioids whenever possible, limiting the reliance upon short-acting drugs.[264] Require patients bring in pill bottles to all clinic visits to conduct pill counts.[272] Avoid bolus parenteral administration, although at the end of life, infusions can be effective and diversion limited by keeping no spare cassettes or bags in the home. Weekly team meetings provide a forum to establish the plan of care and discuss negative attitudes regarding the patient's behavior. Family meetings may be indicated, particularly if they are also experiencing addictive behaviors.

Withdrawal from drugs of abuse must be prevented or minimized. These may include cocaine, benzodiazepines, and even alcohol. Alcoholism in palliative care has been underdiagnosed.[273] Thus, a thorough assessment of recreational drug use, including alcohol, must be conducted. This provides evidence for adherence to the treatment plan.[274] Urine toxicology studies may be necessary. One resource is the Fast Fact Urine Drug Testing for Opioids and Marijuana available at http://www.eperc.mcw.edu.

Patients in recovery may be extremely reluctant to consider opioid therapy. Patients may need reassurance that opioids can be taken for medical indications, such as cancer or other illnesses. If patients currently are treated in a methadone maintenance program, continue the methadone but add another opioid to provide pain relief. Communicate with the program to ensure the correct methadone dose. Nondrug alternatives may also be suggested. An excellent resource for information about addiction treatment is http://www.opiateaddictionrx.info.

## Nursing Interventions: Outcomes and Documentation

Quality-improvement measures to relieve pain in the palliative care setting include setting outcomes, developing strategies to maintain or meet these outcomes, and then evaluating effectiveness.[275,276] Some suggested goals and outcome measures that can be used in each patient's care plan are listed in Table 7–11.

Documentation is also essential to ensure continuity of care. Recommendations for documentation in the medical record include the following:

---

**Table 7–11**
**Outcome Indicators for Pain Control in the Palliative Care Setting**

- *Initial Evaluation:* Pain that is not well controlled (patient self-report of 3 out of 10 or greater than the patient's acceptable comfort level) is brought under control within 48 hours of a patient's initial evaluation.
- *Ongoing Care:* Pain that is out of control is assessed and managed with effective intervention(s) within a predetermined time frame in all patients (set an appropriate time limit).
- *Terminal Care:* No patient dies with pain out of control.
- *Adverse Effects:* Analgesic adverse effects and side effects are prevented or effectively and quickly managed in all patients.

*Sources:* Adapted from references 275 and 276.

---

- Initial assessment, including findings from the comprehensive pain assessment; the current pain management regimen; prior experience with pain and pain control; patient and caregiver understanding of expectations and goals of pain management; elaboration of concerns regarding opioids; and a review of systems pertinent to analgesic use, including bowels, balance, memory, function, etc.[277]
- Interdisciplinary progress notes, including ongoing findings from recurrent pain assessment; baseline pain scores; breakthrough pain frequency and severity with associated causes and timing of episodes; effect of pain and pain treatment on function, sleep, activity, social interaction, mood, etc.; types and effects (outcomes) of intervention, including adverse effects (bowel function, sedation, nausea/vomiting assessments); documentation of specific instructions, patient/caregiver understanding, and compliance; and patient/caregiver coping.[277]

Comprehensive strategies to improve pain outcomes in the hospice setting have included improving professional education, developing policies and procedures, enhancing pain documentation, advancing the use of computer-based technologies, and instituting other performance-improvement measures.[275–280] These have resulted in reduction of pain-intensity scores and other changes. More research is needed in the development of quality-improvement strategies that most accurately reflect the needs of patients and families in palliative care settings.

CASE STUDY
*Ms. Jones, A Patient with Breast Cancer and Multiple Bone Metastases*

Mrs. Jones is a 32-year-old woman who was diagnosed with painful bone metastases (ribs, spine) due to advanced breast cancer. Her family, incuding her husband, two daughters, ages 5 and 7, her parents and two siblings, along with a large network of friends, was very supportive. During the course of her illness, the pain was fairly well-controlled with opioids and NSAIDs while receiving multiple courses of chemotherapy and hormonal therapy, as well as monthly bisposphonates. However, the cancer had spread to her liver and to additional boney sites of pain, causing the pain to escalate. This could not be effectively managed at home and she was admitted to the hospital. The Palliative Care Consult Service (including an advanced practice nurse, physician and social worker) was asked to see her on the inpatient oncology unit to assist in pain management . A thorough pain assessment revealed severe (9/10 intensity scale) pain in the right hip, which increased to 10+ when standing or weight bearing. She described the pain as aching, stabbing, and throbbing and denied radiation of the pain from the spine to legs or other locations. She also had pain in several ribs and her left shoulder, areas of documented metastases. Oral NSAIDs were discontinued and dexamethasone 8 mg every morning was started for pain control. Omeprazole was started for gastrointestinal protection. Her total daily oral opioid dose of 780 mg (long acting morphine 100 mg every 8 hours and approximately 8 doses of immediate release morphine 60 mg in the past 24 hours) was converted to 260 mg of intravenous morphine. To deliver this dose, patient controlled analgesia was initiated at 10 mg of morphine/hour with bolus doses of 10 mg every 15 minutes. After several hours, the pain was better controlled and radiotherapy to the new lesion in the hip was started. The team continued to titrate the dose upward with the goal to provide optimal control with limited adverse effects. Stimulant laxatives and softeners were escalated to provide more regular bowel movements. Anesthesia was consulted to determine if any interventional procedures might be useful.

As her physical symptoms were more effectively managed, the palliative care team could more meaningfully address Mrs. Jones' goals of care. Although the oncologist had suggested hospice several weeks ago, she had not been able to consider this option and wished to pursue more anticancer therapy. She wanted to stay in her own home with her family, although she was very worried about the effects of the illness on her children. She had tried desparately to spare them from knowing much about her illness or how much pain she was having. She expressed fear of the dying process and was reluctant to discuss advance directives. The APN and social worker spent more time exploring Ms. Jones' understanding of her illness, her fears, and her care needs. With Mrs. Jones' approval, child life therapists were consulted to meet with the children. A chaplain was also consulted to address existential concerns and to address advance care planning. Her husband, parents and other family members were included in these discussions. After these interventions, her goals of care became more focused on comfort rather than cure and she expressed interest in hospice.

In preparation for going home with hospice, the palliative care team considered returning her to oral morphine for ease of administration in the home. There was concern as she was becoming more lethargic that she might have difficulty swallowing the number of pills required to equal the current opioid dose. The intravenous morphine dose (now at 20 mg of morphine/hour with an average of 6 boluses of 20 mg/bolus) was 600 mg/24 hours. By multiplying by 3 to convert to oral equivalents, the daily oral intake would have been 1800 mg of oral morphine. Although the long-acting morphine comes in 200 mg tablets and would require 3 tablets every 8 hours, the breakthrough dose would have been 180 to 360 mg of short-acting morphine. Because these tablets come in 30 mg, she would have required 6–12 tablets for each dose. The team considered transdermal fentanyl patches, but this would have required 6 patches. As a result, the team, along with the patient, family and the hospice team, decided to continue PCA at home. Dexamethasone was continued.

Mrs. Jones was discharged home to hospice. She continued to obtain relief with PCA morphine until her death one month later.

## Conclusion

Pain control in the palliative care setting is feasible in the majority of patients. For patients whose pain cannot be controlled, sedation is always an option. Understanding the barriers that limit relief will lead to improved education and other strategies to address these obstacles. Developing comfort and skill with the use of pharmacological and nonpharmacological therapies will enhance pain relief. Quality improvement efforts within a palliative care setting can improve the level of pain management within that organization and ultimately the pain relief experienced by these patients. Together, these efforts will reduce suffering, relieve pain, and enhance the quality of life of those at the end of life.

REFERENCES

1. Ng K, von Gunten CF. Symptoms and attitudes of 100 consecutive patients admitted to an acute hospice/palliative care unit. J Pain Symptom Manage 1998;16:307–316.
2. Valeberg BT, Rustoen T, Bjordal K, Hanestad BR, Paul S, Miaskowski C. Self-reported prevalence, etiology, and characteristics of pain in oncology outpatients. Eur J Pain 2008: 12:582–590.
3. Salminen E, Clemens K, Syrjanen K, Salmenoja H. Needs of developing the skills of palliative care at the oncology ward: An audit of symptoms among 203 consecutive cancer patients in Finland. Supportive Care in Cancer 2008;16:3–8.
4. van den Beuken-van Everdingen MH, de Rijke JM, Kessels AG, Schouten HC, van Kleef M, Patijn J. High prevalence of pain in patients with cancer in a large population-based study in The Netherlands. Pain 2007;132:312–320.

5. van den Beuken-van Everdingen MH, de Rijke JM, Kessels AG, Schouten HC, van Kleef M, Patijn J. Prevalence of pain in patients with cancer: a systematic review of the past 40 years. Ann Oncol 2007;18:1437–1449.

6. Teunissen SC, Wesker W, Kruitwagen C, de Haes HC, Voest EE, de Graeff A. Symptom prevalence in patients with incurable cancer: a systematic review. J Pain & Symptom Manage 2007;34:94–104.

7. Cleeland CS, Gonin R, Baez L, Loehrer P, Pandya KJ. Pain and treatment of pain in minority patients with cancer. The Eastern Cooperative Oncology Group Minority Outpatient Pain Study. Ann Intern Med 1997;127:813–816.

8. Cleeland CS, Gonin R, Hatfield AK, Edmonson JH, Blum RH, Stewart JA, et al. Pain and its treatment in outpatients with metastatic cancer. N Engl J Med 1994;330:592–596.

9. Brescia FJ, Portenoy RK, Ryan M, Krasnoff L, Gray G. Pain, opioid use, and survival in hospitalized patients with advanced cancer. J Clin Oncol 1992;10:149–155.

10. Coyle N, Adelhardt J, Foley KM, Portenoy RK. Character of terminal illness in the advanced cancer patient: pain and other symptoms during the last four weeks of life. J Pain Symptom Manage 1990;5:83–93.

11. Wolfe J, Grier HE, Klar N, Levin SB, Ellenbogen JM, Salem-Schatz S, et al. Symptoms and suffering at the end of life in children with cancer. N Engl J Med 2000;342:326–333.

12. Vanhems P, Dassa C, Lambert J, Cooper DA, Perrin L, Vizzard J, et al. Comprehensive classification of symptoms and signs reported among 218 patients with acute HIV-1 infection. J Acquir Immune Defic Syndr 1999;21:99–106.

13. Breitbart W, Dibiase L. Current perspectives on pain in AIDS. Oncology (Huntingt) 2002;16:964–968, 972; discussion 972, 977, 980, 982.

14. Douaihy AB, Stowell KR, Kohnen S, Stoklosa JB, Breitbart WS. Psychiatric aspects of comorbid HIV/AIDS and pain, Part 1. AIDS Reader 2007;17:310–314.

15. Simpson DM, Haidich AB, Schifitto G, Yiannoutsos CT, Geraci AP, McArthur JC, et al. Severity of HIV-associated neuropathy is associated with plasma HIV-1 RNA levels. AIDS 2002;16: 407–412.

16. Vogl D, Rosenfeld B, Breitbart W, Thaler H, Passik S, McDonald M, et al. Symptom prevalence, characteristics, and distress in AIDS outpatients. J Pain Symptom Manage 1999;18:253–262.

17. Swica Y, Breitbart W. Treating pain in patients with AIDS and a history of substance use. West J Med 2002;176:33–39.

18. Ehde DM, Gibbons LE, Chwastiak L, Bombardier CH, Sullivan MD, Kraft GH. Chronic pain in a large community sample of persons with Mult Scler. Mult Scler 2003;9:605–611.

19. Svendsen KB, Jensen TS, Overvad K, Hansen HJ, Koch-Henriksen N, Bach FW. Pain in patients with Mult Scler: a population-based study. Arch Neurol 2003;60:1089–1094.

20. Kong KH, Woon VC, Yang SY. Prevalence of chronic pain and its impact on health-related quality of life in stroke survivors. Arch Phys Med Rehabil 2004;85:35–40.

21. Douglas C, Wollin JA, Windsor C. Illness and demographic correlates of chronic pain among a community-based sample of people with multiple sclerosis. Arch Phys Med Rehabil 2008;89:1923–32.

22. Naess H, Beiske AG, Myhr KM. Quality of life among young patients with ischaemic stroke compared with patients with multiple sclerosis. Acta Neurologica Scandinavica 2008;117:181–5.

23. Woolf AD, Pfleger B. Burden of major musculoskeletal conditions. Bull World Health Organ 2003;81:646–656.

24. Soares LG. Poor social conditions, criminality and urban violence: Unmentioned barriers for effective cancer pain control at the end of life. J Pain Symptom Manage 2003;26:693–695.

25. Sun VC, Borneman T, Ferrell B, Piper B, Koczywas M, Choi K. Overcoming barriers to cancer pain management: an institutional change model. J Pain & Symptom Manage 2007;34:359–369.

26. Lasch K, Greenhill A, Wilkes G, Carr D, Lee M, Blanchard R. Why study pain? A qualitative analysis of medical and nursing faculty and students' knowledge of and attitudes to cancer pain management. J Palliat Med 2002;5:57–71.

27. O'Brien S, Dalton JA, Konsler G, Carlson J. The knowledge and attitudes of experienced oncology nurses regarding the management of cancer-related pain. Oncol Nurs Forum 1996;23: 515–521.

28. Von Roenn JH, Cleeland CS, Gonin R, Hatfield AK, Pandya KJ. Physician attitudes and practice in cancer pain management. A survey from the Eastern Cooperative Oncology Group. Ann Intern Med 1993;119:121–126.

29. Singh RM, Wyant SL. Pain management content in curricula of U.S. schools of pharmacy. J Am Pharm Assoc 2003;43:34–40.

30. Cornelison AH. Cultural barriers to compassionate care—patients' and health professionals' perspectives. Bioethics Forum 2001;17:7–14.

31. Anderson KO, Richman SP, Hurley J, Palos G, Valero V, Mendoza TR, et al. Cancer pain management among underserved minority outpatients: perceived needs and barriers to optimal control. Cancer 2002;94:2295–2304.

32. Baltic TE, Whedon MB, Ahles TA, Fanciullo G. Improving pain relief in a rural cancer center. Cancer Pract 2002;10 (Suppl 1): S39–44.

33. Morrison RS, Wallenstein S, Natale DK, Senzel RS, Huang LL. "We don't carry that"—failure of pharmacies in predominantly nonwhite neighborhoods to stock opioid analgesics. N Engl J Med 2000;342:1023–1026.

34. Simone CB 2nd, Vapiwala N, Hampshire MK, Metz JM. Internet-based survey evaluating use of pain medications and attitudes of radiation oncology patients toward pain intervention. Int J Radiat Oncol, Biol Phys 2008;72:127–133.

35. Keefe FJ, Ahles TA, Porter LS, Sutton LM, McBride CM, Pope MS, et al. The self-efficacy of family caregivers for helping cancer patients manage pain at end-of-life. Pain 2003;103(1–2):157–162.

36. Vallerand AH, Collins-Bohler D, Templin T, Hasenau SM. Knowledge of and barriers to pain management in caregivers of cancer patients receiving homecare. Cancer Nurs 2007;30:31–37.

37. Paice JA, Toy C, Shott S. Barriers to cancer pain relief: fear of tolerance and addiction. J Pain Symptom Manage 1998; 16:1–9.

38. Potter VT, Wiseman CE, Dunn SM, Boyle FM. Patient barriers to optimal cancer pain control. Psychooncology 2003;12:153–160.

39. Gunnarsdottir S, Donovan HS, Serlin RC, Voge C, Ward S. Patient-related barriers to pain management: the Barriers Questionnaire II (BQ-II). Pain 2002;99:385–396.

40. Anderson KO, Mendoza TR, Valero V, Richman SP, Russell C, Hurley J, et al. Minority cancer patients and their

providers: pain management attitudes and practice. Cancer 2000;88:1929–1938.

41. Weiner DK, Rudy TE. Attitudinal barriers to effective treatment of persistent pain in nursing home residents. J Am Geriatr Soc 2002;50:2035–2040.

42. Davis GC, Hiemenz ML, White TL. Barriers to managing chronic pain of older adults with arthritis. J Nurs Scholarsh 2002;34:121–126.

43. Valeberg BT, Miaskowski C, Hanestad BR, Bjordal K, Moum T, Rustoen T. Prevalence rates for and predictors of self-reported adherence of oncology outpatients with analgesic medications. Clin J Pain 2008;24:627–36.

44. Reid CM, Gooberman-Hill R, Hanks GW. Opioid analgesics for cancer pain: symptom control for the living or comfort for the dying? A qualitative study to investigate the factors influencing the decision to accept morphine for pain caused by cancer. Ann Oncol 2008;19:44–8.

45. Ward SE, Berry PE, Misiewicz H. Concerns about analgesics among patients and family caregivers in a hospice setting. Res Nurs Health 1996;19:205–211.

46. Berry PE, Ward SE. Barriers to pain management in hospice: a study of family caregivers. Hosp J 1995;10:19–33.

47. Fahey KF, Rao SM, Douglas MK, Thomas ML, Elliott JE, Miaskowski C. Nurse coaching to explore and modify patient attitudinal barriers interfering with effective cancer pain management. Oncol Nurs Forum Online 2008;35:233–40.

48. Syrjala KL, Abrams JR, Polissar NL, Hansberry J, Robison J, DuPen S, Stillman M, Fredrickson M, Rivkin S, Feldman E, Gralow J, Rieke JW, Raish RJ, Lee DJ, Cleeland CS, DuPen A. Patient training in cancer pain management using integrated print and video materials: a multisite randomized controlled trial. Pain 2008;135(1–2):175–186.

49. Page GG. The immune-suppressive effects of pain. Adv Exp Med Biol 2003;521:117–125.

50. Page GG, Blakely WP, Ben-Eliyahu S. Evidence that postoperative pain is a mediator of the tumor-promoting effects of surgery in rats. Pain 2001;90(1–2):191–199.

51. Halabi S, Vogelzang NJ, Kornblith AB, Ou SS, Kantoff PW, Dawson NA, Small EJ. Pain predicts overall survival in men with metastatic castration-refractory prostate cancer. J Clin Oncol 2008;26:2544–2549.

52. Hwang SS, Chang VT, Kasimis B. Dynamic cancer pain management outcomes: the relationship between pain severity, pain relief, functional interference, satisfaction and global quality of life over time. J Pain Symptom Manage 2002;23:190–200.

53. American Pain Society. Principles of Analgesic Use in the Treatment of Acute Pain and Cancer Pain, 5th ed. Glenview, IL: American Pain Society, 2003.

54. Du Pen SL, Du Pen AR, Polissar N, Hansberry J, Kraybill BM, Stillman M, et al. Implementing guidelines for cancer pain management: results of a randomized controlled clinical trial. J Clin Oncol 1999;17:361–370.

55. Lorenz KA, Lynn J, Dy SM, Shugarman LR, Wilkinson A, Mularski RA, Morton SC, Hughes RG, Hilton LK, Maglione M, Rhodes SL, Rolon C, Sun VC, Shekelle PG. Evidence for improving palliative care at the end of life: a systematic review. Ann Inter Med 2008;148:147–159.

56. Bruera E, Kim HN. Cancer pain. JAMA 2003;290:2476–2479.

57. Fallon M, Hanks G, Cherny N. Principles of control of cancer pain. BMJ 2006;332(7548):1022–1024.

58. Foley KM, Gelband H. Improving Palliative Care for Cancer. Washington, D.C.: Institute of Medicine and National Research Council, 2001.

59. Cherny NI. The management of cancer pain. Ca 2000;50:70–116; quiz 117–120.

60. Schiodt FV, Rochling FA, Casey DL, Lee WM. Acetaminophen toxicity in an urban county hospital. N Engl J Med 1997;337:1112–1117.

61. Tanaka E, Yamazaki K, Misawa S. Update: the clinical importance of acetaminophen hepatotoxicity in non-alcoholic and alcoholic subjects. J Clin Pharm Thera 2000;25:325–332.

62. Pearce B, Grant IS. Acute liver failure following therapeutic paracetamol administration in patients with muscular dystrophies. Anaesthesia 2008;63:89–91.

63. Rainsford KD. Anti-inflammatory drugs in the 21st century. Sub-Cellular Biochemistry 2007;42:3–27.

64. Mercadante S. The use of anti-inflammatory drugs in cancer pain. Cancer Treat Rev 2001;27:51–61.

65. Perez Gutthann S, Garcia Rodriguez LA, Raiford DS, Duque Oliart A, Ris Romeu J. Nonsteroidal anti-inflammatory drugs and the risk of hospitalization for acute renal failure. Arch Intern Med 1996;156:2433–2439.

66. Dabu-Bondoc S, Franco S. Risk-benefit perspectives in COX-2 blockade. Current Drug Safety 2008;3:14–23.

67. Simon LS, Weaver AL, Graham DY, Kivitz AJ, Lipsky PE, Hubbard RC, et al. Anti-inflammatory and upper gastrointestinal effects of celecoxib in rheumatoid arthritis: a randomized controlled trial. JAMA 1999;282:1921–1928.

68. Silverstein FE, Faich G, Goldstein JL, Simon LS, Pincus T, Whelton A, et al. Gastrointestinal toxicity with celecoxib vs nonsteroidal anti-inflammatory drugs for osteoarthritis and rheumatoid arthritis: the CLASS study: a randomized controlled trial. Celecoxib Long-term Arthritis Safety Study. JAMA 2000;284:1247–1255.

69. Juni P, Rutjes AW, Dieppe PA. Are selective COX 2 inhibitors superior to traditional nonsteroidal anti-inflammatory drugs? BMJ 2002;324:1287–1288.

70. Juni P, Dieppe P, Egger M. Risk of myocardial infarction associated with selective COX-2 inhibitors: questions remain. Arch Intern Med 2002;162:2639–2640; author reply 2630–2632.

71. Wright JM. The double-edged sword of COX-2 selective NSAIDs. CMAJ 2002;167:1131–1137.

72. Shi S, Klotz U. Clinical use and pharmacological properties of selective COX-2 inhibitors. Eur J Clin Pharmacol 2008;64:233–52.

73. Scott PA, Kingsley GH, Smith CM, Choy EH, Scott DL. Nonsteroidal anti-inflammatory drugs and myocardial infarctions: comparative systematic review of evidence from observational studies and randomised controlled trials. Ann Rheum Dis 2007;66:1296–1304.

74. Kerr DJ, Dunn JA, Langman MJ, Smith JL, Midgley RS, Stanley A, Stokes JC, Julier P, Iveson C, Duvvuri R, McConkey CC. VICTOR Trial Group. Rofecoxib and cardiovascular adverse events in adjuvant treatment of colorectal cancer. NEJM 2007;357:360–369.

75. Lucas LK, Lipman AG. Recent advances in pharmacotherapy for cancer pain management. Cancer Pract 2002;10(Suppl 1):S14–S20.

76. Hoppmann RA, Peden JG, Ober SK. Central nervous system side effects of nonsteroidal anti-inflammatory drugs. Aseptic meningitis, psychosis, and cognitive dysfunction. Arch Intern Med 1991; 151:1309–1313.

77. Mercadante S, Fulfaro F, Casuccio A. A randomised controlled study on the use of anti-inflammatory drugs in patients with cancer pain on morphine therapy: effects on dose-escalation and a pharmacoeconomic analysis. Eur J Cancer 2002;38:1358–1363.

78. Wolfe MM, Lichtenstein DR, Singh G. Gastrointestinal toxicity of nonsteroidal antiinflammatory drugs. N Engl J Med 1999; 340:1888–1899.

79. Rowbotham MC, Twilling L, Davies PS, Reisner L, Taylor K, Mohr D. Oral opioid therapy for chronic peripheral and central neuropathic pain. N Engl J Med 2003;348:1223–1232.

80. Viola R, Kiteley C, Lloyd NS, Mackay JA, Wilson J, Wong RK. Supportive Care Guidelines Group of the Cancer Care Ontario Program in Evidence-Based Care. The management of dyspnea in cancer patients: a systematic review. Supp Care Cancer 2008;16:329–37.

81. Ben-Aharon I, Gafter-Gvili A, Paul M, Leibovici L, Stemmer SM. Interventions for alleviating cancer-related dyspnea: a systematic review. J Clin Oncol 2008;26:2396–2404.

82. Jennings AL, Davies AN, Higgins JP, Broadley K. Opioids for the palliation of breathlessness in terminal illness. Cochrane Database Syst Rev 2001:CD002066.

83. Sykes N, Thorns A. Sedative use in the last week of life and the implications for end-of-life decision making. Arch Intern Med 2003;163:341–344.

84. Sykes N, Thorns A. The use of opioids and sedatives at the end of life. Lancet Oncol 2003;4:312–318.

85. Bercovitch M, Waller A, Adunsky A. High dose morphine use in the hospice setting. A database survey of patient characteristics and effect on life expectancy. Cancer 1999;86:871–877.

86. Clemens KE, Quednau I, Klaschik E. Is there a higher risk of respiratory depression in opioid-naive palliative care patients during symptomatic therapy of dyspnea with strong opioids? J Palliat Med 2008;11:204–216.

87. Andersen G, Jensen NH, Christrup L, Hansen SH, Sjogren P. Pain, sedation and morphine metabolism in cancer patients during long-term treatment with sustained-release morphine. Palliat Med 2002;16:107–114.

88. Kaiko RF, Foley KM, Grabinski PY, Heidrich G, Rogers AG, Inturrisi CE, et al. Central nervous system excitatory effects of meperidine in cancer patients. Ann Neurol 1983;13: 180–185.

89. Smith MT. Neuroexcitatory effects of morphine and hydromorphone: evidence implicating the 3-glucuronide metabolites. Clin Exp Pharmacol Physiol 2000;27:524–528.

90. O'Brien T, Mortimer PG, McDonald CJ, Miller AJ. A randomized crossover study comparing the efficacy and tolerability of a novel once-daily morphine preparation (MXL capsules) with MST Continus tablets in cancer patients with severe pain. Palliat Med 1997;11:475–482.

91. Coluzzi PH. Sublingual morphine: efficacy reviewed. J Pain Symptom Manage 1998;16:184–192.

92. Zeppetella G. Sublingual fentanyl citrate for cancer-related breakthrough pain: a pilot study. Palliat Med 2001;15:323–328.

93. Paice JA, Von Roenn JH, Hudgins JC, Luong L, Krejcie TC, Avram MJ. Morphine bioavailability from a topical gel formulation in volunteers. J Pain Symptom Manage 2008; 35:314–320.

94. Walsh D, Tropiano PS. Long-term rectal administration of high-dose sustained-release morphine tablets. Supp Care Cancer 2002;10:653–655.

95. Du X, Skopp G, Aderjan R. The influence of the route of administration: a comparative study at steady state of oral sustained release morphine and morphine sulfate suppositories. Ther Drug Monit 1999;21:208–214.

96. Coyne PJ, Viswanathan R, Smith TJ. Nebulized fentanyl citrate improves patients' perception of breathing, respiratory rate, and oxygen saturation in dyspnea. J Pain Symptom Manage 2002;23:157–160.

97. Muijsers RB, Wagstaff AJ. Transdermal fentanyl: an updated review of its pharmacological properties and therapeutic efficacy in chronic cancer pain control. Drugs 2001;61:2289–2307.

98. Menten J, Desmedt M, Lossignol D, Mullie A. Longitudinal follow-up of TTS-fentanyl use in patients with cancer-related pain: results of a compassionate-use study with special focus on elderly patients. Curr Med Res Opin 2002;18:488–498.

99. Radbruch L, Sabatowski R, Petzke F, Brunsch-Radbruch A, Grond S, Lehmann KA. Transdermal fentanyl for the management of cancer pain: a survey of 1005 patients. Palliat Med 2001;15: 309–321.

100. Egan TD, Sharma A, Ashburn MA, Kievit J, Pace NL, Streisand JB. Multiple dose pharmacokinetics of oral transmucosal fentanyl citrate in healthy volunteers. Anesthesiology 2000;92:665–673.

101. Gordon, DB. Oral transmucosal fentanyl citrate for cancer breakthrough pain: a review. Oncol Nurs Forum Online 2006; 33:257–64.

102. Coluzzi PH, Schwartzberg L, Conroy JD, Charapata S, Gay M, Busch MA, et al. Breakthrough cancer pain: a randomized trial comparing oral transmucosal fentanyl citrate (OTFC) and morphine sulfate immediate release (MSIR). Pain 2001;91:123–130.

103. Payne R, Coluzzi P, Hart L, Simmonds M, Lyss A, Rauck R, et al. Long-term safety of oral transmucosal fentanyl citrate for breakthrough cancer pain. J Pain Symptom Manage 2001;22:575–583.

104. Blick SK, Wagstaff AJ. Fentanyl buccal tablet: in breakthrough pain in opioid-tolerant patients with cancer. Drugs 2006;66: 2387–2393; discussion 2394–2395.

105. Darwish M, Kirby M, Robertson P Jr, Tracewell W, Jiang JG. Absolute and relative bioavailability of fentanyl buccal tablet and oral transmucosal fentanyl citrate. J Clin Pharmacol 2007;47:343–350.

106. Portenoy RK, Taylor D, Messina J, Tremmel L. A randomized, placebo-controlled study of fentanyl buccal tablet for breakthrough pain in opioid-treated patients with cancer. Clin J Pain 2006;22:805–811.

107. Darwish M, Kirby M, Robertson P, Tracewell W, Jiang JG. Absorption of fentanyl from fentanyl buccal tablet in cancer patients with or without oral mucositis: a pilot study. Clin Drug Inves 2007;27:605–611.

108. Darwish M, Kirby M, Jiang JG, Tracewell W, Robertson P Jr. Bioequivalence following buccal and sublingual placement of fentanyl buccal tablet 400 microg in healthy subjects. Clin Drug Inves 2008;28:1–7.

109. Diaz del Consuelo I, Falson F, Guy RH, Jacques Y. Ex vivo evaluation of bioadhesive films for buccal delivery of fentanyl. J Contr Rel 2007;122:135–140.

110. Davis MP, Varga J, Dickerson D, Walsh D, LeGrand SB, Lagman R. Normal-release and controlled-release oxycodone: pharmacokinetics, pharmacodynamics, and controversy. Support Care Cancer 2003;11:84–92.

111. Lauretti GR, Oliveira GM, Pereira NL. Comparison of sustained-release morphine with sustained-release oxycodone in advanced cancer patients. Br J Cancer 2003;89:2027–2030.

112. Shaiova L, Sperber KT, Hord ED. Methadone for refractory cancer pain. J Pain Symptom Manage 2002;23:178–180.

113. Bruera E, Sweeney C. Methadone use in cancer patients with pain: a review. J Palliat Med 2002;5:127–138.

114. Bruera E, Palmer JL, Bosnjak S, Rico MA, Moyano J, Sweeney C, et al. Methadone versus morphine as a first-line strong opioid for cancer pain: a randomized, double-blind study. J Clin Oncol 2004;22:185–192.

115. Davis MP, Walsh D. Methadone for relief of cancer pain: a review of pharmacokinetics, pharmacodynamics, drug interactions and protocols of administration. Support Care Cancer 2001;9:73–83.

116. Morley JS, Bridson J, Nash TP, Miles JB, White S, Makin MK. Low-dose methadone has an analgesic effect in neuropathic pain: a double-blind randomized controlled crossover trial. Palliat Med 2003;17:576–587.

117. Hagen NA, Fisher K, Stiles C. Sublingual methadone for the management of cancer-related breakthrough pain: a pilot study. J Palliat Med 2007;10:331–337.

118. Mercadante S, Casuccio A, Fulfaro F, Groff L, Boffi R, Villari P, et al. Switching from morphine to methadone to improve analgesia and tolerability in cancer patients: a prospective study. J Clin Oncol 2001;19:2898–2904.

119. Watanabe S, Tarumi Y, Oneschuk D, Lawlor P. Opioid rotation to methadone: proceed with caution. J Clin Oncol 2002;20: 2409–2410.

120. Moryl N, Santiago-Palma J, Kornick C, Derby S, Fischberg D, Payne R, et al. Pitfalls of opioid rotation: substituting another opioid for methadone in patients with cancer pain. Pain 2002;96:325–328.

121. Santiago-Palma J, Khojainova N, Kornick C, Fischberg DJ, Primavera LH, Payne R, et al. Intravenous methadone in the management of chronic cancer pain: safe and effective starting doses when substituting methadone for fentanyl. Cancer 2001;92:1919–1925.

122. Weschules DJ, Bain KT. A systematic review of opioid conversion ratios used with methadone for the treatment of pain. Pain Med 2008;9:595–612.

123. Hanks GW, Conno F, Cherny N, Hanna M, Kalso E, McQuay HJ, et al. Morphine and alternative opioids in cancer pain: the EAPC recommendations. Br J Cancer 2001;84:587–593.

124. Nicholson, AB. Methadone for cancer pain. Cochrane Database Syst Rev 2007;(4):CD003971.

125. Sarhill N, Davis MP, Walsh D, Nouneh C. Methadone-induced myoclonus in advanced cancer. Am J Hosp Palliat Care 2001;18:51–53.

126. Kornick CA, Kilborn MJ, Santiago-Palma J, Schulman G, Thaler HT, Keefe DL, et al. QTC interval prolongation associated with intravenous methadone. Pain 2003;105:499–506.

127. Krantz MJ, Kutinsky IB, Robertson AD, Mehler PS. Dose-related effects of methadone on QT prolongation in a series of patients with torsade de pointes. Pharmacotherapy 2003;23:802–805.

128. Sekine R, Obbens EA, Coyle N, Inturrisi CE. The successful use of parenteral methadone in a patient with a prolonged QTc interval. J Pain Sympt Manage 2007;34:566–569

129. Bernard SA, Bruera E. Drug interactions in palliative care. J Clin Oncol 2000;18:1780–1799.

130. Doverty M, Somogyi AA, White JM, Bochner F, Beare CH, Menelaou A, et al. Methadone maintenance patients are cross-tolerant to the antinociceptive effects of morphine. Pain 2001;93:155–163.

131. Wallace M, Rauck RL, Moulin D, Thipphawong J, Khanna S, Tudor IC. Conversion from standard opioid therapy to once-daily oral extended-release hydromorphone in patients with chronic cancer pain. J Int Med Res 2008;36:343–352.

132. Wright AW, Mather LE, Smith MT. Hydromorphone-3-glucuronide: a more potent neuroexcitant than its structural analogue, morphine-3-glucuronide. Life Sci 2001;69: 409–420.

133. Patel S, Roshan VR, Lee KC, Cheung RJ. A myoclonic reaction with low-dose hydromorphone. Ann Pharmacotherapy 2006;40:2068–2070.

134. Chamberlin KW, Cottle M, Neville R, Tan J. Oral oxymorphone for pain management. Ann Pharmacotherapy 2007; 4:1144–1152.

135. Gabrail NY, Dvergsten C, Ahdieh H. Establishing the dosage equivalency of oxymorphone extended release and oxycodone controlled release in patients with cancer pain: a randomized controlled study. Curr Med Res Opinion 2004; 20:911–918.

136. Lee MA, Leng ME, Tiernan EJ. Retrospective study of the use of hydromorphone in palliative care patients with normal and abnormal urea and creatinine. Palliat Med 2001;15:26–34.

137. Hale ME, Dvergsten C, Gimbel J. Efficacy and safety of oxymorphone extended release in chronic low back pain: results of a randomized, double-blind, placebo- and active-controlled phase III study. J Pain 2005;6:21–28.

138. Sittl R. Transdermal buprenorphine in cancer pain and palliative care. Palliat Med 2006;20(Suppl 1):s25–30.

139. McCaffery M, Martin L, Ferrell BR. Analgesic administration via rectum or stoma. J ET Nurs 1992;19:114–121.

140. Walsh D, Perin ML, McIver B. Parenteral morphine prescribing among inpatients with pain from advanced cancer: a prospective survey of intravenous and subcutaneous use. Amer J Hospice Palliat Med 2006;23: 353–359.

141. Nelson KA, Glare PA, Walsh D, Groh ES. A prospective, within-in-patient, crossover study of continuous intravenous and subcutaneous morphine for chronic cancer pain. J Pain Symptom Manage 1997;13:262–267.

142. Watanabe S, Pereira J, Hanson J, Bruera E. Fentanyl by continuous subcutaneous infusion for the management of cancer pain: a retrospective study. J Pain Symptom Manage 1998;16:323–326.

143. Smith TJ, Staats PS, Deer T, Stearns LJ, Rauck RL, Boortz-Marx RL, et al. Randomized clinical trial of an implantable drug delivery system compared with comprehensive medical management for refractory cancer pain: impact on pain, drug-related toxicity, and survival. J Clin Oncol 2002;20: 4040–4049.

144. Potter J, Hami F, Bryan T, Quigley C. Symptoms in 400 patients referred to palliative care services: prevalence and patterns. Palliat Med 2003;17:310–314.

145. Hawley PH, Byeon JJ. A comparison of sennosides-based bowel protocols with and without docusate in hospitalized patients with cancer. J Palliat Med 2008;11:575–581.

146. Portenoy RK, Thomas J, Moehl Boatwright ML, Tran D, Galasso FL, Stambler N, Von Gunten CF, Israel RJ. Subcutaneous methylnaltrexone for the treatment of opioid-induced constipation in patients with advanced illness: a double-blind, randomized, parallel group, dose-ranging study. J Pain Symptom Manage 2008;35:458–468.

147. Thomas J, Karver S, Cooney GA, Chamberlain BH, Watt CK, Slatkin NE, Stambler N, Kremer AB, Israel RJ. Methylnaltrexone for opioid-induced constipation in advanced illness. N Engl J Med 2008;358:2332–2343.

148. Breitbart W, Rosenfeld B, Kaim M, Funesti-Esch J. A randomized, double-blind, placebo-controlled trial of psychostimulants for the treatment of fatigue in ambulatory patients with human immunodeficiency virus disease. Arch Intern Med 2001;161:411–420.

149. Bruera E, Driver L, Barnes EA, Willey J, Shen L, Palmer JL, et al. Patient-controlled methylphenidate for the management of fatigue in patients with advanced cancer: a preliminary report. J Clin Oncol 2003;21:4439–4443.

150. Webster L, Andrews M, Stoddard G. Modafinil treatment of opioid-induced sedation. Pain Med 2003;4:135–140.

151. Teichtahl H, Wang D. Sleep-disordered breathing with chronic opioid use. Expert Opinion on Drug Safety 2007;6:641–649.

152. Webster LR, Choi Y, Desai H, Webster L, Grant BJ. Sleep-disordered breathing and chronic opioid therapy. Pain Med 2008;9:425–432.

153. Wood GJ, Shega JW, Lynch B, Von Roenn JH. Management of intractable nausea and vomiting in patients at the end of life: "I was feeling nauseous all of the time…nothing was working." JAMA 2007;298:1196–1207.

154. Nunez-Olarte J. Opioid-induced myoclonus. Eur J Palliat Care 1995;2:146–150.

155. Ito S, Liao S. Myoclonus associated with high-dose parenteral methadone. J Palliat Med 2008;11:838–841.

156. Patel S, Roshan VR, Lee KC, Cheung RJ. A myoclonic reaction with low-dose hydromorphone. Ann Pharmacotherapy 2006;40:2068–2070.

157. Sjogren P, Thunedborg LP, Christrup L, Hansen SH, Franks J. Is development of hyperalgesia, allodynia and myoclonus related to morphine metabolism during long-term administration? Six case histories. Acta Anaesthesiol Scand 1998;42:1070–1075.

158. Eisele JH Jr., Grigsby EJ, Dea G. Clonazepam treatment of myoclonic contractions associated with high-dose opioids: case report. Pain 1992;49:231–232.

159. Hagen N, Swanson R. Strychnine-like multifocal myoclonus and seizures in extremely high-dose opioid administration: treatment strategies. J Pain Symptom Manage 1997;14:51–58.

160. Larijani GE, Goldberg ME, Rogers KH. Treatment of opioid-induced pruritus with ondansetron: report of four patients. Pharmacotherapy 1996;16:958–960.

161. Max MB, Lynch SA, Muir J, Shoaf SE, Smoller B, Dubner R. Effects of desipramine, amitriptyline, and fluoxetine on pain in diabetic neuropathy. N Engl J Med 1992;326:1250–1256.

162. Hammack JE, Michalak JC, Loprinzi CL, Sloan JA, Novotny PJ, Soori GS, et al. Phase III evaluation of nortriptyline for alleviation of symptoms of cis-platinum-induced peripheral neuropathy. Pain 2002;98:195–203.

163. Dworkin RH, Backonja M, Rowbotham MC, Allen RR, Argoff CR, Bennett GJ, et al. Advances in neuropathic pain: diagnosis, mechanisms, and treatment recommendations. Arch Neurol 2003;60:1524–1534.

164. Farrar JT, Portenoy RK. Neuropathic cancer pain: the role of adjuvant analgesics. Oncology (Huntingt) 2001;15:1435–1442.

165. Saarto T, Wiffen PJ. Antidepressants for neuropathic pain. Cochrane Database Syst Rev 2007;(4):CD005454.

166. Durand JP, Goldwasser F. Dramatic recovery of paclitaxel-disabling neurosensorytoxicity following treatment with venlafaxine. Anti-Cancer Drugs 2002;13:777–780.

167. Add Xiao W, Naso L, Bennett GJ. Experimental studies of potential analgesics for the treatment of chemotherapy-evoked painful peripheral neuropathies. Pain Med 2008; 9:505–517.

168. Tasmuth T, Hartel B, Kalso E. Venlafaxine in neuropathic pain following treatment of breast cancer. Eur J Pain 2002;6:17–24.

169. Johannessen Landmark, C. Antiepileptic drugs in non-epilepsy disorders: relations between mechanisms of action and clinical efficacy. CNS Drugs 2008;22:27–47.

170. Tassone DM, Boyce E, Guyer J, Nuzum D. Pregabalin: a novel gamma-aminobutyric acid analogue in the treatment of neuropathic pain, partial-onset seizures, and anxiety disorders. Clin Therapeutics 2007;29:26–48.

171. Baron R, Brunnmuller U, Brasser M, May M, Binder A. Efficacy and safety of pregabalin in patients with diabetic peripheral neuropathy or postherpetic neuralgia: Open-label, non-comparative, flexible-dose study. Eur J Pain 2008;12:850–858.

172. Garcia-Borreguero D, Larrosa O, de la Llave Y, Verger K, Masramon X, Hernandez G. Treatment of restless legs syndrome with gabapentin: a double-blind, cross-over study. Neurology 2002;59:1573–1579.

173. Pandey CK, Bose N, Garg G, Singh N, Baronia A, Agarwal A, et al. Gabapentin for the treatment of pain in guillain-barre syndrome: a double-blinded, placebo-controlled, crossover study. Anesth Analg 2002;95:1719–1723.

174. Ahn SH, Park HW, Lee BS, Moon HW, Jang SH, Sakong J, et al. Gabapentin effect on neuropathic pain compared among patients with spinal cord injury and different durations of symptoms. Spine 2003;28:341–346.

175. Barrueto F Jr., Green J, Howland MA, Hoffman RS, Nelson LS. Gabapentin withdrawal presenting as status epilepticus. J Toxicol Clin Toxicol 2002;40:925–928.

176. Mercadante S, Fulfaro F, Casuccio A. The use of corticosteroids in home palliative care. Support Care Cancer 2001;9:386–389.

177. Wooldridge JE, Anderson CM, Perry MC. Corticosteroids in advanced cancer. Oncology (Huntingt) 2001;15:225–234; discussion 234–236.

178. Feuer DJ, Broadley KE. Corticosteroids for the resolution of malignant bowel obstruction in advanced gynaecological and gastrointestinal cancer. Cochrane Database Syst Rev 2000:CD001219.

179. Mao J, Chen LL. Systemic lidocaine for neuropathic pain relief. Pain 2000;87:7–17.

180. Sloan P, Basta M, Storey P, von Gunten C. Mexiletine as an adjuvant analgesic for the management of neuropathic cancer pain. Anesth Analg 1999;89:760–761.

181. Wallace MS, Magnuson S, Ridgeway B. Efficacy of oral mexiletine for neuropathic pain with allodynia: a double-blind, placebo-controlled, crossover study. Reg Anesth Pain Med 2000;25:459–467.

182. Galer BS, Rowbotham MC, Perander J, Friedman E. Topical lidocaine patch relieves postherpetic neuralgia more effectively than a vehicle topical patch: results of an enriched enrollment study. Pain 1999;80:533–538.

183. Ferrini R, Paice JA. Infusional lidocaine for severe and/or neuropathic pain. J Support Oncol 2004;2:90–94.

184. Deer TR, Caraway DL, Kim CK, Dempsey CD, Stewart CD, McNeil KF. Clinical experience with intrathecal bupivacaine in combination with opioid for the treatment of chronic pain

related to failed back surgery syndrome and metastatic cancer pain of the spine. Spine J 2002;2:274–278.

185. Finkel JC, Pestieau SR, Quezado ZM. Ketamine as an adjuvant for treatment of cancer pain in children and adolescents. J Pain 2007;8:515–521.

186. Campbell-Fleming JM, Williams A. The use of ketamine as adjuvant therapy to control severe pain. Clin J Oncology Nurs 2008;12:102–107.

187. Bell R, Eccleston C, Kalso E. Ketamine as an adjuvant to opioids for cancer pain. Cochrane Database Syst Rev 2003:CD003351.

188. Mercadante S, Casuccio A, Genovese G. Ineffectiveness of dextromethorphan in cancer pain. J Pain Symptom Manage 1998;16:317–322.

189. Walker K, Medhurst SJ, Kidd BL, Glatt M, Bowes M, Patel S, et al. Disease modifying and anti-nociceptive effects of the bisphosphonate, zoledronic acid in a model of bone cancer pain. Pain 2002;100:219–229.

190. Wong R, Wiffen PJ. Bisphosphonates for the relief of pain secondary to bone metastases. Cochrane Database Syst Rev 2002: CD002068.

191. Groff L, Zecca E, De Conno F, Brunelli C, Boffi R, Panzeri C, et al. The role of disodium pamidronate in the management of bone pain due to malignancy. Palliat Med 2001;15:297–307.

192. Lipton A, Theriault RL, Hortobagyi GN, Simeone J, Knight RD, Mellars K, et al. Pamidronate prevents skeletal complications and is effective palliative treatment in women with breast carcinoma and osteolytic bone metastases: long term follow-up of two randomized, placebo-controlled trials. Cancer 2000; 88:1082–1090.

193. Small EJ, Smith MR, Seaman JJ, Petrone S, Kowalski MO. Combined analysis of two multicenter, randomized, placebo-controlled studies of pamidronate disodium for the palliation of bone pain in men with metastatic prostate cancer. J Clin Oncol 2003;21:4277–4284.

194. Lipton A, Small E, Saad F, Gleason D, Gordon D, Smith M, et al. The new bisphosphonate, Zometa (zoledronic acid), decreases skeletal complications in both osteolytic and osteoblastic lesions: a comparison to pamidronate. Cancer Invest 2002;20(Suppl 2):45–54.

195. Clemons M, Dranitsaris G, Ooi W, Cole DE. A Phase II trial evaluating the palliative benefit of second-line oral ibandronate in breast cancer patients with either a skeletal related event (SRE) or progressive bone metastases (BM) despite standard bisphosphonate (BP) therapy. Breast Cancer Res Treatment 2008;108:79–85.

196. Gralow J, Tripathy D. Managing metastatic bone pain: the role of bisphosphonates. J Pain Symptom Manage 2007; 33:462–472.

197. Jagdev SP, Purohit P, Heatley S, Herling C, Coleman RE. Comparison of the effects of intravenous pamidronate and oral clodronate on symptoms and bone resorption in patients with metastatic bone disease. Ann Oncol 2001;12: 1433–1438.

198. Martinez MJ, Roque M, Alonso-Coello P, Catala E, Garcia JL, Ferrandiz M. Calcitonin for metastatic bone pain. Cochrane Database Syst Rev 2003:CD003223.

199. Janjan N. Bone metastases: approaches to management. Semin Oncol 2001;28(4 Suppl 11):28–34.

200. Jeremic B. Single fraction external beam radiation therapy in the treatment of localized metastatic bone pain. A review. J Pain Symptom Manage 2001;22:1048–1058.

201. Ryu S, Jin R, Jin JY, Chen Q, Rock J, Anderson J, Movsas B. Pain control by image-guided radiosurgery for solitary spinal metastasis. J Pain Symptom Manage 2008;35:292–298.

202. Serafini AN. Therapy of metastatic bone pain. J Nucl Med 2001;42:895–906.

203. Kraeber-Bodere F, Campion L, Rousseau C, Bourdin S, Chatal JF, Resche I. Treatment of bone metastases of prostate cancer with strontium-89 chloride: efficacy in relation to the degree of bone involvement. Eur J Nucl Med 2000;27:1487–1493.

204. Sciuto R, Festa A, Pasqualoni R, Semprebene A, Rea S, Bergomi S, et al. Metastatic bone pain palliation with 89-Sr and 186-Re-HEDP in breast cancer patients. Breast Cancer Res Treat 2001;66:101–109.

205. Loblaw DA, Wu JS, Kirkbride P, Panzarella T, Smith K, Aslanidis J, Warde P. Pain flare in patients with bone metastases after palliative radiotherapy—a nested randomized control trial. Support Care in Cancer , 2007;15:451–455.

206. Prommer E. Guidelines for the use of palliative chemotherapy. AAHPM Bulletin 2004;5:1–4.

207. Geels P, Eisenhauer E, Bezjak A, Zee B, Day A. Palliative effect of chemotherapy: objective tumor response is associated with symptom improvement in patients with metastatic breast cancer. J Clin Oncol 2000;18:2395–2405.

208. Simpson DM, Brown S, Tobias J. NGX-4010 C107 Study Group. Controlled trial of high-concentration capsaicin patch for treatment of painful HIV neuropathy. Neurology 2008;70:2305–2313.

209. Khasabova IA, Khasabov SG, Harding-Rose C, Coicou LG, Seybold BA, Lindberg AE, Steevens CD, Simone DA, Seybold VS. A decrease in anandamide signaling contributes to the maintenance of cutaneous mechanical hyperalgesia in a model of bone cancer pain. J Neurosci 2008;28:11141–52.

210. Rahn EJ, Zvonok AM, Thakur GA, Khanolkar AD, Makriyannis A, Hohmann AG. Selective activation of cannabinoid CB2 receptors suppresses neuropathic nociception induced by treatment with the chemotherapeutic agent paclitaxel in rats. J Pharmacol Exper Therapeutics 2008; 327:584–591.

211. Ashton JC, Milligan ED. Cannabinoids for the treatment of neuropathic pain: clinical evidence. Current Opinion Invest Drugs, 2008;9:65–75.

212. Wang T, Collet JP, Shapiro S, Ware MA. Adverse effects of medical cannabinoids: a systematic review. CMAJ Canadian Med Assoc J 2008;178:1669–1678.

213. Thompson E, Hicks F. Intrathecal baclofen and homeopathy for the treatment of painful muscle spasms associated with malignant spinal cord compression. Palliat Med 1998; 12:119–121.

214. Schapiro RT. Management of spasticity, pain, and paroxysmal phenomena in Mult Scler. Curr Neurol Neurosci Rep 2001;1:299–302.

215. McClelland S 3rd, Bethoux FA, Boulis NM, Sutliff MH, Stough DK, Schwetz KM, Gogol DM, Harrison M, Pioro EP. Intrathecal baclofen for spasticity-related pain in amyotrophic lateral sclerosis: efficacy and factors associated with pain relief. Muscle & Nerve 2008; 37:396–398.

216. Fine PG. Analgesia issues in palliative care: bone pain, controlled release opioids, managing opioid-induced constipation and nifedipine as an analgesic. J Pain Palliat Care Pharmacother 2002;16:93–97.

217. Alvarez L, Perez-Higueras A, Quinones D, Calvo E, Rossi RE. Vertebroplasty in the treatment of vertebral tumors: post-procedural outcome and quality of life. Eur Spine J 2003;12:356–360.

218. Brubacher S, Gobel BH. Use of the Pleurx Pleural Catheter for the management of malignant pleural effusions. Clin J Oncol Nurs 2003;7:35–38.

219. Goetz MP, Callstrom MR, Charboneau JW, Farrell MA, Maus TP, Welch TJ, et al. Percutaneous image-guided radiofrequency ablation of painful metastases involving bone: a multicenter study. J Clin Oncol 2004;22:300–306.

220. Wong GY, Schroeder DR, Carns PE, Wilson JL, Martin DP, Kinney MO, et al. Effect of neurolytic celiac plexus block on pain relief, quality of life, and survival in patients with unresectable pancreatic cancer: a randomized controlled trial. JAMA 2004;291:1092–1099.

221. Add Zhang CL, Zhang TJ, Guo YN, Yang LQ, He MW, Shi JZ, Ni JX. Effect of neurolytic celiac plexus block guided by computerized tomography on pancreatic cancer pain. Digestive Dis Sci 2008;53:856–860.

222. Stubblefield MD, Levine A, Custodio CM, Fitzpatrick T. Botulinum toxin for radiation-induced facial pain and trismus. Arch Phys Med Rehabil 2008;89:417–421.

223. Layeeque R, Hochberg J, Siegel E, Kunkel K, Kepple J, Henry-Tillman RS, Dunlap M, Seibert J, Klimberg VS. Botulinum toxin infiltration for pain control after mastectomy and expander reconstruction. Ann Surg 2004;240:608–613.

224. Kwekkeboom KL, Hau H, Wanta B, Bumpus M. Patients' perceptions of the effectiveness of guided imagery and progressive muscle relaxation interventions used for cancer pain. Compl Ther Clin Pract 2008;14: 185–194.

225. Kwekkeboom KL, Kneip J, Pearson L. A pilot study to predict success with guided imagery for cancer pain. Pain Manage Nurs 2003;4:112–123.

226. Magill L. The use of music therapy to address the suffering in advanced cancer pain. J Palliat Care 2001;17:167–172.

227. Sahler OJ, Hunter BC, Liesveld JL. The effect of using music therapy with relaxation imagery in the management of patients undergoing bone marrow transplantation: a pilot feasibility study. Altern Ther Health Med 2003;9:70–74.

228. Anderson KO, Cohen MZ, Mendoza TR, Guo H, Harle MT, Cleeland CS. Brief cognitive-behavioral audiotape interventions for cancer-related pain: Immediate but not long-term effectiveness. Cancer , 2006;107:207–214.

229. Tatrow K, Montgomery GH. Cognitive behavioral therapy techniques for distress and pain in breast cancer patients: a meta-analysis. J Behav Med 2006;29:17–27.

230. Syrjala KL, Donaldson GW, Davis MW, Kippes ME, Carr JE. Relaxation and imagery and cognitive-behavioral training reduce pain during cancer treatment: a controlled clinical trial. Pain 1995;63:189–198.

231. Robb KA, Williams JE, Duvivier V, Newham DJ. A pain management program for chronic cancer-treatment-related pain: a preliminary study. J Pain 2006;7:82–90.

232. Sherwood P, Given BA, Given CW, Champion VL, Doorenbos AZ, Azzouz F, Kozachik S, Wagler-Ziner K, Monahan PO. A cognitive behavioral intervention for symptom management in patients with advanced cancer. Oncol Nurs Forum Online 2005;32:1190–1198.

233. Ernst E. Manual therapies for pain control: chiropractic and massage. Clin J Pain 2004;20:8–12.

234. Post-White J, Kinney ME, Savik K, Gau JB, Wilcox C, Lerner I. Therapeutic massage and healing touch improve symptoms in cancer. Integr Cancer Ther 2003;2:332–344.

235. Stephenson N, Dalton JA, Carlson J. The effect of foot reflexology on pain in patients with metastatic cancer. Appl Nurs Res 2003;16:284–286.

236. Zappa SB, Cassileth BR. Complementary approaches to palliative oncological care. J Nurs Care Qual 2003;18:22–26.

237. Stephenson NL, Weinrich SP, Tavakoli AS. The effects of foot reflexology on anxiety and pain in patients with breast and lung cancer. Oncol Nurs Forum 2000;27:67–72.

238. Meek SS. Effects of slow stroke back massage on relaxation in hospice clients. Image—the J Nurs Scholarsh 1993;25:17–21.

239. Weinrich SP, Weinrich MC. The effect of massage on pain in cancer patients. Appl Nurs Res 1990;3:140–145.

240. Rhiner M, Ferrell BR, Ferrell BA, Grant MM. A structured nondrug intervention program for cancer pain. Cancer Pract 1993; 1:137–143.

241. Mercadante S, Radbruch L, Caraceni A, Cherny N, Kaasa S, Nauck F, et al. Episodic (breakthrough) pain: consensus conference of an expert working group of the European Association for Palliative Care. Cancer 2002;94:832–839.

242. Ferrell BR, Juarez G, Borneman T. Use of routine and breakthrough analgesia in home care. Oncol Nurs Forum 1999;26: 1655–1661.

243. Miaskowski C, Dodd MJ, West C, Paul SM, Tripathy D, Koo P, et al. Lack of adherence with the analgesic regimen: a significant barrier to effective cancer pain management. J Clin Oncol 2001;19:4275–4279.

244. Caraceni A, Portenoy RK. An international survey of cancer pain characteristics and syndromes. IASP Task Force on Cancer Pain. International Association for the Study of Pain. Pain 1999;82:263–274.

245. Portenoy RK, Hagen NA. Breakthrough pain: definition, prevalence and characteristics. Pain 1990;41:273–281.

246. Zeppetella G, O'Doherty CA, Collins S. Prevalence and characteristics of breakthrough pain in patients with non-malignant terminal disease admitted to a hospice. Palliat Med 2001; 15:243–246.

247. Zeppetella, G. Opioids for cancer breakthrough pain: a pilot study reporting patient assessment of time to meaningful pain relief. J Pain Symptom Manage 2008;35(5):563–567.

248. Swanwick M, Haworth M, Lennard RF. The prevalence of episodic pain in cancer: a survey of hospice patients on admission. Palliat Med 2001;15:9–18.

249. Hagen NA, Elwood T, Ernst S. Cancer pain emergencies: a protocol for management. J Pain Symptom Manage 1997;14:45–50.

250. Clohisy DR, Mantyh PW. Bone cancer pain. Cancer 2003;97 (3 Suppl):866–873.

251. Braun TC, Hagen NA, Clark T. Development of a clinical practice guideline for palliative sedation. J Palliat Med 2003;6: 345–350.

252. Fainsinger RL, Waller A, Bercovici M, Bengtson K, Landman W, Hosking M, et al. A multicentre international study of sedation for uncontrolled symptoms in terminally ill patients. Palliat Med 2000;14:257–265.

253. Hanks-Bell M, Paice J, Krammer L. The use of midazolam hydrochloride continuous infusions in palliative care. Clin J Oncol Nurs 2002;6:367–369.

254. Golf M, Paice JA, Feulner E, O'Leary C, Marcotte S, Mulcahy M. Refractory status epilepticus. J Palliat Med 2004;7:85–88.

255. de Graeff A, Dean M. Palliative sedation therapy in the last weeks of life: a literature review and recommendations for standards. J Palliat Med 2007;10(1):67–85.

256. Legge J, Ball N, Elliott DP. The potential role of ketamine in hospice analgesia: a literature review. Consult Pharmacist 2006;21(1):51–57.

257. Hocking G, Cousins MJ. Ketamine in chronic pain management: an evidence-based review. Anesth Analg 2003;97:1730–1739.

258. Campbell-Fleming JM, Williams A. The use of ketamine as adjuvant therapy to control severe pain. Clin J Oncol Nurs 2008;12(1):102–107.

259. Bell RF, Eccleston C, Kalso E. Ketamine as adjuvant to opioids for cancer pain. A qualitative systematic review. J Pain Symptom Manage 2003;26:867–875.

260. Fine PG. Low-dose ketamine in the management of opioid nonresponsive terminal cancer pain. J Pain Symptom Manage 1999;17:296–300.

261. Katz N. Neuropathic pain in cancer and AIDS. Clin J Pain 2000;16(2 Suppl):S41–S48.

262. Passik SD, Kirsh KL, McDonald MV, Ahn S, Russak SM, Martin L, et al. A pilot survey of aberrant drug-taking attitudes and behaviors in samples of cancer and AIDS patients. J Pain Symptom Manage 2000;19:274–286.

263. Cami J, Farre M. Drug addiction. N Engl J Med 2003;349: 975–986.

264. Whitcomb LA, Kirsh KL, Passik SD. Substance abuse issues in cancer pain. Curr Pain Headache Rep 2002;6:183–190.

265. Newshan G. Pain management in the addicted patient: practical considerations. Nurs Outlook 2000;48:81–85.

266. Kirsh KL, Whitcomb LA, Donaghy K, Passik SD. Abuse and addiction issues in medically ill patients with pain: attempts at clarification of terms and empirical study. Clin J Pain 2002;18(4 Suppl):S52–S60.

267. Passik SD, Theobald DE. Managing addiction in advanced cancer patients: why bother? J Pain Symptom Manage 2000;19:229–234.

268. Kaplan R, Slywka J, Slagle S, Ries K. A titrated morphine analgesic regimen comparing substance users and non-users with AIDS-related pain. J Pain Symptom Manage 2000;19:265–273.

269. Podymow T, Turnbull J, Coyle D. Shelter-based palliative care for the homeless terminally ill. Palliative Medicine 2006;20:81–6.

270. Kushel MB, Miaskowski C. End-of-life care for homeless patients: "she says she is there to help me in any situation." JAMA 2006;296:2959–2966.

271. Fishman SM, Kreis PG. The opioid contract. Clin J Pain 2002;18(4 Suppl):S70–75.

272. Kirsh KL, Passik SD. Palliative care of the terminally ill drug addict. Cancer Investigation 2006 Jun-Jul;24:425–431.

273. Bruera E, Moyano J, Seifert L, Fainsinger RL, Hanson J, Suarez-Almazor M. The frequency of alcoholism among patients with pain due to terminal cancer. J Pain Symptom Manage 1995;10:599–603.

274. Fishman SM, Wilsey B, Yang J, Reisfield GM, Bandman TB, Borsook D. Adherence monitoring and drug surveillance in chronic opioid therapy. J Pain Symptom Manage 2000;20:293–307.

275. Braveman C, Rodrigues C. Performance improvement in pain management for home care and hospice programs. Am J Hosp Palliat Care 2001;18:257–263.

276. Higginson IJ. Clinical and organizational audit in palliative medicine. In: Doyle D, Hanks G, Cherny N, Calman K, eds. Oxford Textbook of Palliative Medicine, 3rd ed. Oxford: Oxford University Press, 2004:183–196.

277. Gordon DB, Pellino TA, Miaskowski C, McNeill JA, Paice JA, Laferriere D, et al. A 10-year review of quality improvement monitoring in pain management: recommendations for standardized outcome measures. Pain Manage Nurs 2002; 3:116–130.

278. Hall P, Schroder C, Weaver L. The last 48 hours of life in long-term care: a focused chart audit. J Am Geriatr Soc 2002;50:501–506.

279. Oderda GM. Outcomes research: what it is and what it isn't. J Pain Palliat Care Pharmacother 2002;16:83–89.

280. Elvidge K. Improving pain & symptom management for advanced cancer patients with a clinical decision support system. Stud Health Technol Informatics 2008;136:169–174.

# 8

*Paula R. Anderson, Grace E. Dean, and Melany A. Piech*

# Fatigue

*Everyone sees the difference in me. When I sit, I have to have my elbows support me. When I stand, I have to have something to lean on...and when I lie down, I am asleep. It's like I became old overnight.—A patient with COPD*

- ◆  **Key Points**
- ◆  *Fatigue is the most common chronic symptom associated with cancer and other chronic progressive diseases.*
- ◆  *Ongoing research has provided lines of evidence for improved patient outcomes through both pharmacologic and nonpharmacologic measures.*
- ◆  *Thorough assessment of all patient comorbidities and symptoms is critical to accurately diagnose and treat chronic progressive disease-related fatigue.*
- ◆  *Education interventions in fatigue directed at health care providers, patients and families provide an important opportunity for consistent integration of current guidelines into practice.*

Chronically ill patients often do not have the energy or forethought to communicate to health care professionals about what may be viewed as a non-urgent symptom. They find it difficult to convey just how exhausted they feel. Fatigue is a devastating, multidimensional symptom that involves the entire person, touching every facet of daily life. It can progressively interfere with a patient's physical and social activities resulting in increased withdrawal. Fatigue is a symptom that possibly has the greatest potential to interfere with quality of life at the end of life.[2]

## Definitions of Fatigue

*Please, please put me to bed. I don't have the strength to keep my arms on the pads of the wheelchair. I'm so tired that I'm just going to collaspe in a heap right here. I barely have the strength left... to take a deep breath. —An elderly cancer patient.*

Fatigue is an example of a complex phenomenon that has been studied by many disciplines but has no widely accepted definition.[3] The discipline of nursing is no exception. Even within different specialties of nursing, there has been little agreement on a definition of fatigue. In oncology, for example, patients perceive fatigue differently depending on where in the disease trajectory fatigue occurs. Fatigue is often the symptom that causes the patient with an undiagnosed cancer to seek medical treatment. Once diagnosed, the cancer patient experiences fatigue as a side effect of treatment. The patient who has finished treatment and is in recovery discovers a "new normal" level of energy. The patient who has experienced a recurrence of cancer considers fatigue to be as much an enemy as the diagnosis itself. Finally, the patient who is in the advanced stages of cancer interprets fatigue as the end of a very long struggle, as something to be endured.

The National Comprehensive Cancer Network (NCCN) Fatigue Practice Guidelines Panel, charged with synthesizing research on fatigue to develop recommendations for care, defines fatigue as "a distressing, persistent, subjective sense of physical, emotional and/or cognitive tiredness or exhaustion related to cancer or cancer treatment that is not proportional to recent activity and interferes with usual functioning."[4] The European Association for Palliative Care identified a working definition of fatigue as a subjective feeling of tiredness, weakness or lack of energy.[5] Cancer-related fatigue is defined by the American Cancer Society as "feeling tired—physically, mentally, and emotionally. It means having less energy to do the things you normally do or want to do"[6] This definition is similar to that of a multiple sclerosis panel that defined fatigue as a subjective lack of physical and/or mental energy perceived by individuals that interferes with usual and desired activities.[7] Sufferers of non-malignant diseases such as stroke and end-stage heart failure define fatigue as being "tired and physically and mentally exhausted" and perceive it as one of their worst symptoms, yet receiving little attention.[8] While other definitions have been proposed, the two key elements that are dominant in most definitions of fatigue are: (1) subjective perception with physical, emotional and cognitive features and (2) interference with the ability to function.[5–8]

As with adults, no universal definition has been agreed upon for fatigue in children. A description of fatigue derived from a group of 7- to -12-year-old pediatric oncology patients consisted of "a profound sense of being weak or tired, or of having difficulty with movement such as using arms or legs, or opening eyes." In the same study of 13- to -18-year-old pediatric oncology patients, fatigue was described as "a complex, changing state of exhaustion that at times seems to be a physical condition, at other times a mental state, and still other times to be a combination of physical and mental tiredness."[9] The children's definition emphasizes a physical sensation (weakness), whereas the adolescents' definition accentuated both physical and mental exhaustion. These researchers concluded that fatigue existed within the greater context of the child's developmental stage and that the developmental stage might have a greater impact when evaluating fatigue than has yet been appreciated.

More recently, researchers identified three different types of fatigue in a study of pediatric oncology patients, 5 to 15 years of age: typical tiredness (normal ebb and flow of energy), treatment fatigue (energy loss greater than replenishment), and shutdown fatigue (profound, sustained loss of energy).[10] Research is currently underway focusing on the confounding symptom clusters seen in children and adolescents with cancer. A triad of fatigue, sleep disturbance and pain and their interrelationship forms a framework for improving the quality of life of pediatric patients.[11] Additional exploratory research continues to be needed to expand these findings.

## Prevalence

*I can't "do" anything that I want to do. Just watching my family from my chair exhausts me. I am incapable of even watching life go on…it's going by me and not including me. Is that crazy? Every hour I seem incapable. This cannot be me. —A young cancer patient during treatment*

Fatigue has been reported to be the most common symptom that is linked to the clinical course of cancer and other chronic diseases. Estimates of prevalence are between 60% and 90%. This depends upon the diagnostic category, length of disease, course of treatment, complications, physical state and psychosocial factors.[12] Research in the palliative care arena has focused primarily on adults.[11–13] One prospective study of fatigue compared advanced cancer patients to age- and sex-matched controls. The control group had a moderate excess of women (57%), with 49% (48/98) who were overweight and 50% having at least one concomitant medical problem, such as arthritis, airflow limitation, or hypertension. Although both advanced cancer patients and controls complained of a degree of fatigue, the severity of symptoms in cancer patients was much worse. The prevalence of severe subjective fatigue (defined as a score on the fatigue scale of greater than the 95th percentile of controls) was 75% in the advanced cancer group. In this patient group, there were a variety of cancer diagnoses (breast, lung, and prostate) and many of the patients were also taking opioid medications.[12]

Another relevant study, conducted by the World Health Organization, included 1,840 palliative care patients.[14] The prevalence of nine symptoms (pain, nausea, dyspnea, constipation, anorexia, weakness, confusion, insomnia, and weight loss) was examined in seven palliative care centers from the United States, Europe, and Australia. With the exception of moderate to severe pain, weakness was the most common symptom, reported by 51% of patients.[14]

Cancer is only one of many diseases in which fatigue is a common symptom. Fatigue prevalence rates for a variety of common chronic illnesses are identified in Figure 8–1. Of note, 11% to 25% of patients present with chronic fatigue as their chief complaint in primary care settings.[15] Of these, 20% to 45% will have a primary organic cause and 40% to 45% will have a primary psychiatric disorder diagnosed. The remaining patients will either meet the diagnostic criteria for chronic fatigue syndrome or remain undiagnosed.[15] In a comparison review of symptom prevalence in a diverse population of patients with cancer, AIDS, heart disease, chronic obstructive pulmonary disease and renal disease, fatigue was reported in 32%–90% of patients for all five diseases.[16] Symptoms rarely occur in isolation, and there is enough evidence to support the occurrence of multiple clusters of symptoms and the concept of "symptom burden."[17] The increase in symptom cluster research, particularly in the context of cancer and comorbid conditions is expanding. Sixty percent of subjects reported fatigue when cancer was a comorbid condition with rheumatoid arthritis.[18] Other studies suggest a correlation between fatigue, physical function, and systemic inflammatory response and psychological distress in advanced cancer.[19]

The majority of fatigue research over the past two decades has been conducted on the adult population.[20] Fatigue

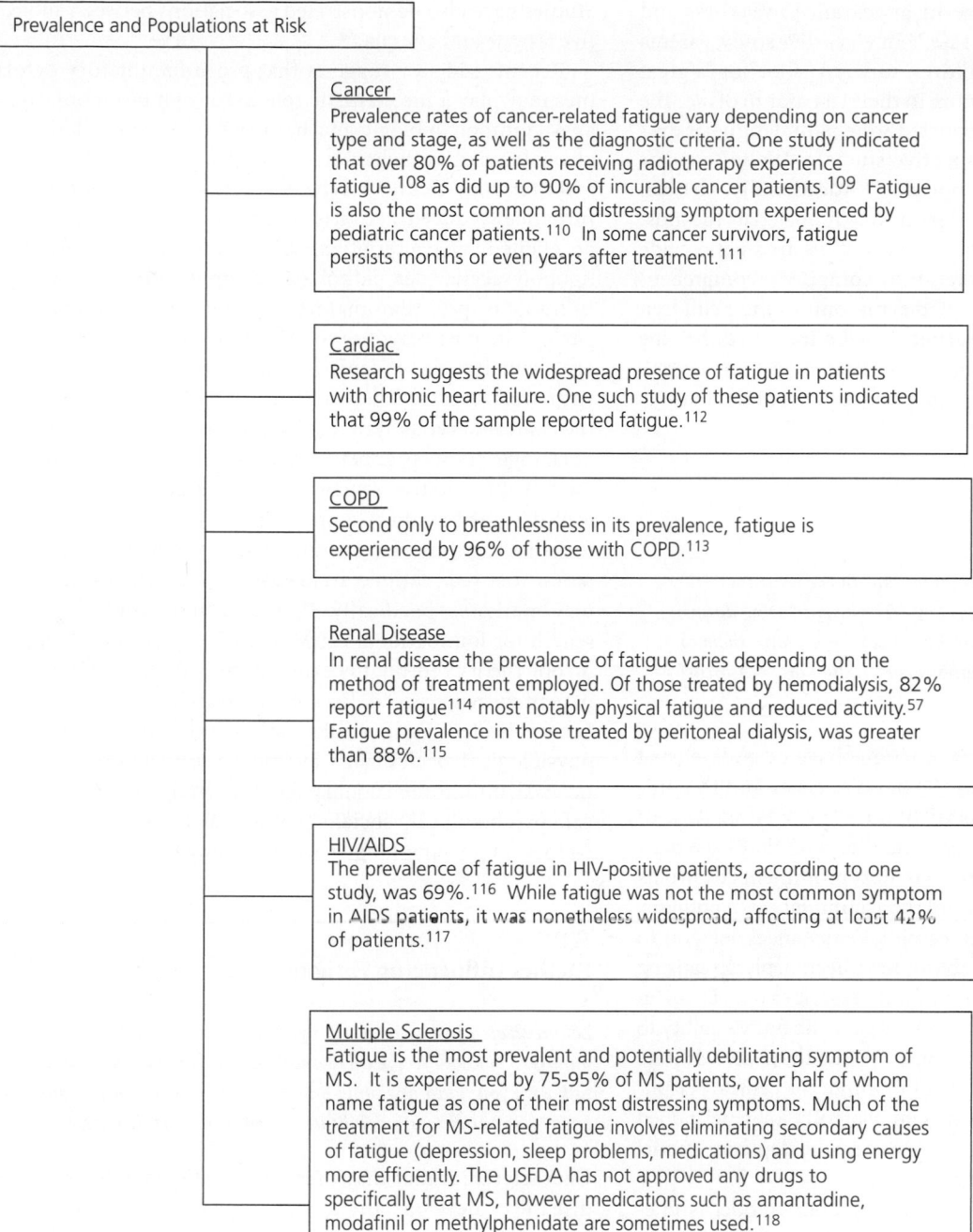

Prevalence and Populations at Risk

**Cancer**
Prevalence rates of cancer-related fatigue vary depending on cancer type and stage, as well as the diagnostic criteria. One study indicated that over 80% of patients receiving radiotherapy experience fatigue,[108] as did up to 90% of incurable cancer patients.[109] Fatigue is also the most common and distressing symptom experienced by pediatric cancer patients.[110] In some cancer survivors, fatigue persists months or even years after treatment.[111]

**Cardiac**
Research suggests the widespread presence of fatigue in patients with chronic heart failure. One such study of these patients indicated that 99% of the sample reported fatigue.[112]

**COPD**
Second only to breathlessness in its prevalence, fatigue is experienced by 96% of those with COPD.[113]

**Renal Disease**
In renal disease the prevalence of fatigue varies depending on the method of treatment employed. Of those treated by hemodialysis, 82% report fatigue[114] most notably physical fatigue and reduced activity.[57] Fatigue prevalence in those treated by peritoneal dialysis, was greater than 88%.[115]

**HIV/AIDS**
The prevalence of fatigue in HIV-positive patients, according to one study, was 69%.[116] While fatigue was not the most common symptom in AIDS patients, it was nonetheless widespread, affecting at least 42% of patients.[117]

**Multiple Sclerosis**
Fatigue is the most prevalent and potentially debilitating symptom of MS. It is experienced by 75-95% of MS patients, over half of whom name fatigue as one of their most distressing symptoms. Much of the treatment for MS-related fatigue involves eliminating secondary causes of fatigue (depression, sleep problems, medications) and using energy more efficiently. The USFDA has not approved any drugs to specifically treat MS, however medications such as amantadine, modafinil or methylphenidate are sometimes used.[118]

**Figure 8–1.** Prevalence and populations at risk.

research in children and adolescents has received little attention.[21] The prevalence of fatigue in children is difficult to gauge from the general lack of research, but one study in 75 school-aged children receiving cancer treatments reported a prevalence rate of 50%.[22] Fatigue was expressed by the children as being tired, not sleeping well, and not being able to do the things they wanted to do. More than half the children were not as active as before the illness and reported playing less. An exploratory study with cohorts of adolescents with cancer investigated fatigue and its impact on quality of life during and after treatment. The results suggest that fatigue may extend deep into the post-treament phase and prevent the child from engaging with their adolescent peers.[23] One review of fatigue in adolescents with cancer summarized the state of evidence and designed clinical strategies for the fatigue management in this population.[21]

In a recent study on fatigue in children with advanced cancer, 18 cancer-related symptoms of concern were identified by parents during the last days of their children's life. The most frequently cited symptoms included changes in behavior and breathing, pain, change in appearance, weakness and fatigue and change in heart rate.[24] In an earlier study, parents reported that 89% of the children suffered "a lot" or "a great deal" from at least one symptom in their last month of life. The most common symptoms reported were pain, fatigue or dyspnea.[25] A subsequent retrospective study by Wolfe supports the occurrence of these symptoms.[26] Additionally, physical fatigue, reduced mobility and pain were reported as the most frequent symptoms in the last month of life in a nationwide follow-up study.[27] Further, one study compiled a comprehensive inventory of parent-reported symptoms of their children who had died six months earlier. Results indicated that the most frequently parent-reported physical symptoms experienced by the children were pain, poor appetite and fatigue.[28]

## Pathophysiology

*No matter how determined I am to be "me" in the morning, I cannot even get through making my bed without sitting down. My legs and arms should work right…I can't even force them to do the things they used to do without even a thought. —A breast cancer patient*

Models to explain the causes of fatigue have been developed by a variety of disciplines in the basic sciences and by clinicians. Figure 8–2 represents distinctive theories, models, or frameworks to explain cancer-related fatigue that have been reported in the literature. The two most prominent constructs are the depletion hypothesis and the accumulation hypothesis. In the depletion hypothesis, essential substances integral to muscle activity are not available or have been depleted causing fatigue. The accumulation hypothesis describes a mechanism where waste products collect and outpace the body's ability to dispose of them resulting in fatigue. While these models were developed with the cancer patient in mind, the central peripheral model (central nervous system control)[151] may be applied to the patient with multiple sclerosis and the depletion model may be applied to end-stage renal disease.

A well known example of the depletion model is anemia. A deficiency of red blood cells or lack of hemoglobin that leads to a reduction in oxygen-carrying capacity of the blood, anemia has a profound impact on patients experiencing the associated complications of fatigue, dyspnea, palpitations, dizziness, and decreased cognitive function.[29] Anemia is a common occurrence in patients with advanced disease or those receiving aggressive therapy.[30] Multiple studies evaluating recombinant erythropoietin in patients with end-stage renal failure, orthopedic surgery, and those receiving chemotherapy for cancer have demonstrated a reduction in fatigue and an improvement in exercise capacity, muscle strength, and performance of daily activities.[31] Randomized trials have revealed a direct relationship between increases in hemoglobin and improvements in fatigue and quality of life in patients with chronic anemia and patients with cancer.[32–35]

Studies have also demonstrated associations between subjective fatigue and anemia.[24]

Recent evidence suggests that pro-inflammatory cytokines may play a mechanistic role in the symptom of fatigue as a common biologic mechanism.[36,37] A constellation of physiologic and behavioral responses observed in animals termed "sickness behavior" (hyperalgesia, sleep disturbance, reduced activity, reduction in food intake) can be elicited by bacterial infections and administration of lipopolysaccharides-pathologic components of bacteria.[38] In humans, proinflammatory cytokines may be released as part of the host response to infection, a tumor, tissue damage from injury or depletion of immune cells associated with treatments.[38] These inflammatory stimuli can signal the central nervous system (CNS) to generate fatigue, as well as changes in sleep, appetite, reproduction and social behavior.[39] A quantitative review of the strength of evidence (18 well-designed studies) supporting the relationship between inflammation and fatigue found significant positive correlations between fatigue and levels of circulating inflammatory markers, specifically, IL-6, IL-1 and neopterin.[40] The search for foundational causes of fatigue continues because no one theory thoroughly explains the basis for fatigue in the patient with advanced disease. The search for such a theory is complicated. Fatigue, like pain, is not only explained by physiological mechanisms, but must be understood as a multicausal, multidimensional phenomenon that includes physical, psychological, social, and spiritual aspects. As such, factors influencing fatigue are beginning to be addressed.

## Factors Influencing Fatigue

*Let me sleep, I just can't get up right now, maybe in a few minutes…I know you're there and I want to open my eyes and talk with you, but I just don't have the energy to keep my eyelids open. —A patient with debilitating cardiovascular disease*

Characteristics that may predispose patients with advanced disease to develop fatigue have not been comprehensively studied. Oncology research has placed importance on patient characteristics in treatment-related fatigue. Table 8–1 provides a list of factors that have been associated with cancer-related fatigue. Several of these factors have been studied and are presented in some detail below.

Age has been examined in several studies of treatment-related fatigue in oncology. The majority of research indicates that younger adult patients with cancer report more fatigue than older patients with cancer.[41,42] This suggests that fatigue may be influenced by the developmental level of the adult. For example, young adults may have heavy responsibilities of balancing career, marriage, and child-rearing, while older adults may be at the end of their careers or retired with empty nests. Additionally, the older adult often has more than one simultaneous medical condition and may attribute the fatigue to advancing age and

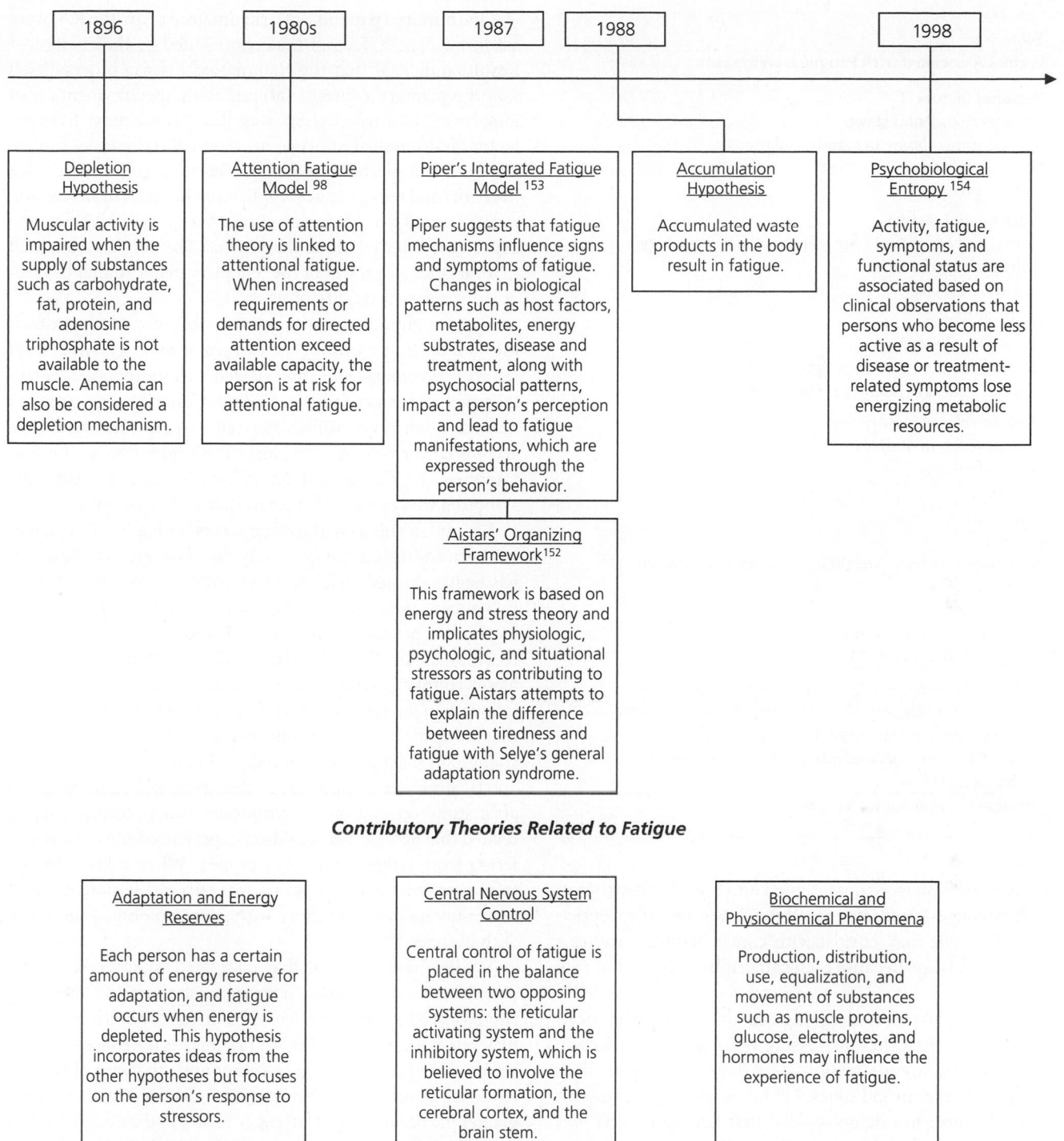

**Figure 8–2.** Chronology of fatigue theories, models, and frameworks.[151]

view the fatigue as normal. These may partially explain why studies report that younger adults have fatigue more frequently. However, in a study of older cancer patients aged 70–90, it was reported that fatigue occurrence in this elderly group was a long lasting complication of cancer and treatment and might actually cause as well as accelerate their functional decline.[43]

Depression has been linked to patients with cancer-related fatigue.[44-46] Depression and fatigue are two related concepts.

Fatigue is part of the diagnostic criteria for depression,[47] and depression may develop as a result of being fatigued.[48] While depression is less frequently reported than fatigue, feelings of depression are common in patients with cancer, with a prevalence rate in the range of 20% to 25%.[49,50] One study exploring correlates of fatigue found a fused relationship between depression and fatigue. This research indicated that fatigued women scored twice as high on the depression

**Table 8–1**
**Factors Associated with Fatigue Development**

**Personal factors**
Age (developmental stage)
Marital status (home demands, isolation)
Menopausal status
Income/insurance

**Psychosocial factors**
Mental and emotional state (depression, fear, anxiety, distress, conflicts)
Culture/ethnicity
Living situation

**Care-related factors**
Number/cohesiveness of caregivers
Responsiveness of health care providers

**Disease-related factors**
Stage and extent of disease
Co-morbidities
Anemia
Pain
Dyspnea
Nutritional changes (weight loss, cachexia, electrolyte imbalance)
Continency
Sleep patterns/interruptions

**Treatment-Related factors**
Any treatment-related effect from surgery, chemotherapy or radiation (skin reaction, temporary altered energy level, urinary/bowel changes, pain)
Medication issues (side effects, polypharmacy, taste changes, OTC's)
Permanent physiologic changes

scale as those who were not fatigued and also that depression was the strongest predictor of fatigue.[51] Additionally, depression and fatigue may coexist with cancer without having a causal relationship, because each can originate from the same pathology.[48,52]

Fatigue in patients undergoing cancer treatment has been closely linked with other distressing symptoms, such as pain, dyspnea, anorexia, constipation, sleep disruption, depression, anxiety, and other mood states.[53–55] Research on patients with advanced cancer has demonstrated that fatigue severity was significantly associated with similar symptoms.[56]

The value of assessing the "most troublesome" symptom when symptom clusters are identified, was examined. In 146 palliative care patients, 590 symptoms were reported by patients to be present. Among all of the symptoms reported, fatigue and pain were reported most frequently as the "most severe" and the "most troublesome."[56] Like patients with cancer, patients with end-stage renal disease on chronic dialysis complained of a high level of fatigue that was associated with other symptoms.[57] The other symptoms identified were headaches, cramps, itching, dyspnea, sleep disruption (highest mean score), nausea, chest pain, and abdominal pain.

One hundred patients with rheumatoid arthritis (RA) were asked to identify factors that contributed to their fatigue.[58] Results indicated that the rheumatoid disease process itself was the primary cause of fatigue, with specific mention of joint pain. Disturbed sleep was the second most frequent factor, and physical effort to accomplish daily tasks ranked third. Patients with RA indicated that they had to exert twice the effort and energy to accomplish the same amount of work. Another study of patients with RA reported that women experienced more fatigue than men.[59] The authors explained this variance as a result of the female patients' higher degrees of pain and poor quality of sleep.

Various physical symptoms were also identified as affecting fatigue in a study of 80 women with congestive heart failure.[60] Women were interviewed 12 months after hospitalization for heart failure. A second interview occurred 18 months later. Sleep difficulties, chest pain, and weakness accounted for a unique variance in fatigue during the first interview. By the second interview, dyspnea was the only symptom that explained the variance in fatigue level.[60]

Fatigue in children and adolescents with advanced cancer has been addressed, but is in early stages of research. Research has begun on pediatric oncology patients' reports of factors influencing their fatigue.[9,61] In one study, for example, 7- to 12-year-old patients with cancer viewed hospital noises, new routines, changing sleep patterns, getting treatment, and low blood counts as contributing factors to the development of fatigue.[61] In the same study, 13- to 18-year-old patients reported that going for treatment, noisy nurses and inpatient children, changes in sleep position, boredom, being fearful or worried, and treatment side effects led to their fatigue. In another pediatric study on end-of-life symptoms and suffering, parents related that 89% of their children experienced substantial suffering from fatigue, pain, or dyspnea. When asked whether treatment for these symptoms was successful, parents indicated success in 27% of those with pain and only 16% of those with dyspnea.[25]

Studies have reported that compared to controls, cancer patients are more fatigued, have worse sleep quality, more disrupted circadian rhythms, worse quality of life and lower activity levels.[62] The scientific literature supports the conclusion that the advanced stage of disease compounds the level of fatigue. Evidence demonstrates that the more advanced the cancer, the greater the occurrence of fatigue.[63] Fobair and colleagues interviewed 403 long-term survivors of Hodgkin's disease who had completed their initial therapy between one and 21 years prior. Patients were asked if their energy had changed and, if it had, how long it took to return to normal. Patients whose energy level had not returned to normal were more frequently found to be in the later stages of the disease.[63] Additional research by Wang and colleagues[64] examined fatigue severity and fatigue interference in hematological malignancies. They found that patients with acute leukemia reported more severe fatigue than those with chronic leukemia or non-Hodgkin's lymphoma. Their research also indicated that nausea was a clinical predictor of severe fatigue. Olson and colleagues suggest from their research that fatigue consists of three distinct, yet interrelated, concepts of tiredness, fatigue and exhaustion which are not merely degrees of one state.[65] Their work with varied cancer populations indicates clear delineation between the fatigue experienced by those receiving treatment and the palliative care patients.[156] However, a noted consensus group emphasized that cancer-related fatigue did not seem to be qualitatively different from the fatigue of the healthy, but simply represented one end of a "continuum of intensity."[5]

Little research on factors influencing fatigue in patients with advanced cancer has been conducted. Results from treatment-related fatigue research do, however, give direction for assessment and management of fatigue in the palliative care setting.

As illustrated by the following case report, patient perceptions may be influenced by other symptoms.

CASE STUDY
*Mr. Ives, A Patient with Stage IV Small-Cell Lung Cancer*

At 54 years old, Mr. Ives has had lymphoma, heart surgery, and now lung cancer. He has been receiving intensive concurrent chemotherapy with radiation therapy. Current laboratory values: hemoglobin 8.0 g/dl, hematocrit 28%, platelet count 155,000 mm$^3$, white blood cell count 3,400 mm$^3$, and absolute granulocyte count of 1,800 cells/mm$^2$. All of his blood chemistries were within normal limits.

Though he used to sleep 7–8 hours each night, since his treatment for lung cancer, Mr. Ives now rarely obtains four hours of rest each night even with the aid of a sleeping pill (Ambien). Mr. Ives often lays awake on the couch for hours before falling asleep, only to wake up a few hours later. He has trouble getting comfortable in bed and frequently tries to sleep on the couch. Mr. Ives explains that when he was first discharged from the hospital (for diagnostic purposes), he felt very tired (fatigue rated "7" out of 10). Although he was tired, he couldn't get his mind to rest. He reported, "I don't have deep sleep. I'm sleeping, but my brain is still going." His difficulty sleeping also seems interwoven with the emotional impact of his illness. Besides feeling afraid to fall asleep because he may not wake up, Mr. Ives speaks of "all kinds of feelings coming out. I can't control them."

Mr. Ives is used to working in the outdoors, doing physical work such as construction. His functional ability has been impacted by his illness and has greatly narrowed the time he spends outside. He is unable to work on projects that give him purpose and satisfaction, such as rebuilding a car or riding his motorcycle.

Mr. Ives acknowledges the severity of his condition and has in mind to prepare for the worst-case scenario. He frequently worries about what will happen to his family, yet has difficulty in carrying out his intention to make plans. He relates, "I can't bring myself to plan my death. I'm too tired" (fatigue rating "8" out of 10). Mr. Ives acknowledges that his family may be able to help him with these decisions.

His extended family has been supportive of him during his illness, taking him to the hospital and helping him pay for his prescriptions.

## Case Study Assessment

When considering patient assessment for treatment-related fatigue, this case study illustrates the importance of evaluating all physical, psychosocial, and emotional contributing factors that may respond to intervention. An analysis of the patient's condition is a continuous process. Because of the high prevalence of fatigue, patients should be screened for fatigue throughout the diagnosis and illness trajectory. A focused history and physical assessment to determine causative and contributing factors are warranted. Prior to his treatment, the patient, Mr. Ives, complained of a fatigue level at a "7," while during treatment his fatigue level peaked at "8." Both of these indicate a severe level of fatigue and require intervention. The patient has a variety of factors contributing to his cancer-related fatigue. (1) He has anemia, but may require further testing to determine the exact type of anemia (treatment-related versus iron deficiency anemia). After the anemia is treated, the fatigue level should be re-evauated. (2) He is experiencing emotional distress which may be causing or contributing to his sleep disruption. His emotional distress level was not assessed in this scenario. However, a distress level of $\geq 4$ on a scale of 0–10 would require referral to a psychologist, social worker and/or pastoral care, depending on the apparent cause and the patient response to the referral. A reduction in the distress level may result in improved sleep, but this too requires consistent re-evaluation. (3) His reduced activity level may be the result of his medical history, current diagnosis, current treatment regimen and/or other contributing factors along with deconditioning. A referral to physical therapy for evaluation will identify the specific level of muscle deconditioning and will assist with a plan of care. Remaining active, energy conservation, and energy restoration are all interventions that may be of benefit to Mr. Ives. A thorough history and physical/psychosocial assessment will lead to individualized interventions to help alleviate patients' symptoms and enhance quality of life.

## Assessment of Fatigue

*They told me that I might experience fatigue. But I thought, "Who cares about that, I have cancer." Now I know what they meant. It is a suffocating cloud that slowly overtakes my thinking and my responses. I cannot find words when I speak and I cannot make myself get going. I could have never anticipated how completely consuming the fatigue would be. —A breast cancer long-term survivor.*

Fatigue assessment of the whole person is essential—of the mind and spirit as well as the body. When assessing fatigue,

---

**Table 8–2**
**Proposed Criteria for Diagnosing Cancer-Related Fatigue**

These symptoms have been present almost every day
during the same 2-week period in the past month:
Significant fatigue, diminished energy or increased need of
rest, disproportionate to any recent change in activity as
well as five or more of the following:

1. Complaints of generalized weakness or limb heaviness
2. Diminished concentration or attention
3. Decreased motivation or interest in engaging in usual
   activities
4. Insomnia or hypersomnia
5. Sleep is unrefreshing or nonrestorative
6. Perceived need to struggle to overcome inactivity
7. Marked emotional reactivity to feeling fatigued (sadness,
   frustration, irritability)
8. Difficulty in completing daily tasks attributed to feeling
   fatigued
9. Perceived problems with short-term memory
10. Post-exertional malaise lasting several hours

The symptoms cause clinically significant distress or
impairment in social, occupational or other important
areas of functioning.
There is evidence from the history, physical examination
or laboratory findings that symptoms are a consequence of cancer or cancer-related therapy.
The symptoms are not primarily the consequence of
comorbid psychiatric disorders, such as major depression,
somatization disorder, somatoform disorder or delirium.

*Source*: Adapted from Cella (1998), reference 66

---

the literature on pain assessment is useful. In pain assess-ment, the patient is considered the expert on his or her pain. Pain is whatever the patient says it is; so, too, it should be with fatigue. Caregiver or staff perceptions may be quite different from those of the person experiencing fatigue. There is no agreement on one definition for fatigue—it is the patient's definition or description of fatigue that counts. This personal fatigue may include any reference to a decrease in energy, weakness, or a tired or 'wiped out' feeling.

There are numerous methods of assessing and diagnos-ing fatigue. Recognizing the importance of cancer-related fatigue, the diagnosis has been proposed for inclusion in the International Classification of Diseases[66] (Table 8–2). However, some researchers suggest that the diagnostic cri-teria are too stringent and the strict exclusion of those with possible "mood disorders" is of concern and may underesti-mate fatigue occurrence.[62]

Many scales have been developed to measure fatigue in the adult, with varying levels of validity and reliability. Examples of fatigue measurement tools include the Multidimensional Assessment of Fatigue, the Symptom Distress Scale, the Fatigue Scale, the Fatigue Observation Checklist, and a Visual Analogue Scale for Fatigue.[67] These scales are available for use in research and may be used in the clinical area. A comprehensive review by Piper and colleagues[68] describes the advantages and disadvantages of the single item as well as multi-item, multidimensional cancer-related fatigue mea-sures currently in use. The European Association for Palliative Care compiled a list of assessment instruments that have been used in research for fatigue in the palliative care group.[5] One scale that has been used extensively in the oncology popula-tion is the Piper Fatigue Scale. This questionnaire has 22 items that measure four dimensions of fatigue: affective meaning, behavioral/severity, cognitive/mood, and sensory. This scale measures perception, performance, motivation, and change in physical and mental activities.[68]

In clinical practice, however, a verbal rating scale may be the most efficient. Fatigue severity may be quickly assessed using a "0" (no fatigue) to "10" (extreme fatigue) scale. As with the use of any measure, consistency over time and a specific frame of ref-erence are needed. During each evaluation, the same instruc-tions must be given to the patient. For example, the patient may be asked to rate the level of fatigue for the past 24 hours.

Fatigue, as with any symptom, is not static. Changes take place daily and sometimes hourly in the patient with an advanced illness. As such, fatigue bears repeated evaluation on the part of the health care provider. One patient, noticing the dramatic change in his energy level, remarked "Have I always been this tired?" He seemed unable to discern whether there had ever been a time when he did not feel overwhelmed by the impact of fatigue. The imperative for palliative care nursing is to consistently take the initiative and ask the patient—and then continue to ask—about fatigue, keeping in mind that the ulti-mate goal is the patient's comfort. An example of a thorough assessment of the symptom of fatigue is found in Table 8–3, which utilizes both a subjective and objective framework to ascertain patient fatigue and possible underlying physiological events that may exacerbate the fatigue.

Fatigue assessment tools for use in the young pediatric population are in the developmental stages, but research has been progressing. Many fatigue questionnaires and guide-lines developed for the adult patient with cancer may provide a framework for use in pediatrics. Three instruments to assess fatigue in children with cancer between the ages of seven and 12 have been tested and demonstrated strong initial validity.[69] The tools consisted of a parallel parent, staff and child assess-ment of fatigue. Although larger patient samples are needed, results from the Childhood Fatigue Scale are encouraging. The PedsQL Multidimensional Fatigue Scale has also been used in the pediatric oncology population.[70] Until a valid and reliable tool is available , a simple assessment of fatigue sever-ity may be used.

In the adolescent patient population, the assessment of fatigue is equally challenging. One researcher used a Fatigue and Quality of Life Diary to elicit the depth of the problem for this age group across three phases of illness. Patients were evaluated while undergoing treatment, in early remis-sion and in the follow-up stage.[23] Other studies focusing on adolescents employ a variety of tools. A review by Erickson[21]

---

**Table 8–3**
**Primary Fatigue Assessment**

*Physical exam based on subjective symptom*: Review of systems. Significant co-morbidities? Is there anything on exam that could account for the fatigue (recurrence, progression of disease, nerve damage, dehydration, cachexia)?

*Medications*: Is the patient taking any medications that could contribute to the fatigue (pain or sleep medication, OTC medications, supplements, new medication changes)?

*Location*: Where on the body is the fatigue located: Upper/lower extremities? All muscles of the body? Is there mental/attentional fatigue? Is rising from a chair difficult?

*Intensity/severity*: Does the fatigue interfere with activities (work, role/responsibilities at home, social interaction), patient's usual enjoyable activities?

*Duration:* How long does the fatigue last (minutes, hours, days, time of day)? Has it become chronic (lasting more than 6 months duration)? What is the pattern (wake up from a night's sleep exhausted, evening fatigue, transient, unpredictable, unfading, are circadian rhythms affected)? Any changes over time?

*Aggravating factors*: What makes it worse (rest, activity, social interaction, other symptoms, environmental heat, cold, noise)?

*Alleviating factors*: What relieves it (a good night's rest, food, fluids, caffeine, listening to music, exercise)?

*Knowledge of fatigue*: Had the patient been prepared for fatigue occurrence? What meaning does the patient assign to the symptom of fatigue (getting worse, disease progression, dying)?

*Muscle strength*: Tests to elicit muscle strength are available if necessary (Jamar grip strength, nerve conduction studies).

*General appearance*: Assess general appearance and look for pallor, monotone voice, slowed speech, dull facial expression, stooped shoulders or weight loss.

*Vital signs*: Anything out of the ordinary to explain fatigue (fever, low blood pressure, irregular heart rate, shortness of breath, weight/caloric intake changes).

*Laboratory results*: Oxygenation status (pulse oximeter, hemoglobin, hematocrit), electrolytes, thyroid and adrenal status, increased white count, increased erythrocyte sedimentation rate).

*Level of activity*: Has the patient's usual activity changed? How many hours/day in bed or resting?

*Affect*: What is the mood of the patient (anxious, depressed, sad, apathetic, withdrawn, flat)?

*Source:* Adapted from NCCN v.1.2008, reference 4.

---

indicates that often a single-item fatigue assessment is utilized. Although a small number of adolescents have participated, results indicate that fatigue continues to be a problem lasting well into the post-treatment phase for adolescents.

## Management/Treatment of Fatigue

*I fall into bed exhausted. I can't wait one minute longer or speak one more sentence. But within a couple of hours, I'm wide awake. My eyes will not rest, my mind will not rest. I hear every sound in the neighborhood. It's horrible not being able to sleep when I know I'm completely spent. I try to numb myself with a sleeping pill and wine. It doesn't help. —A palliative care patient at home*

When considering palliative care, the management of fatigue is extremely challenging. By its very definition, palliative care may encompass a prolonged period before death, when a person is still active and physically and socially participating in life, to a few weeks before death, when participatory activity may be minimal. With fatigue interventions, the wishes of the patient and family are paramount. One must consider management in the context of the extent of disease, other symptoms (pain, nausea, diarrhea, etc.), whether palliative treatment is still in process, age and developmental stage, and the emotional "place" of the patient. Barriers to fatigue assessment as well as intervention exist and must be considered in the context of the patient, health care provider, and within the health care system itself. Patients may feel that their fatigue is not a paramount problem compared to other disease and treatment-related side effects unless their physician asks. Health care providers and their systems may not have the time/staff to routinely assess fatigue, and may believe that disease-related fatigue has no concrete solution potential. Current results in translational research on the implementation of a patient and staff fatigue education program using the NCCN fatigue guidelines indicate a significant decrease in barriers and fatigue in the intervention sample.[71]

Interventions for fatigue have been suggested to occur at two levels: the management of symptoms that contribute to fatigue, and the prevention of additional or secondary fatigue by maintaining a balance between restorative rest and restorative activity.[72] Fatigue interventions have been grouped into two broad categories: pharmacologic interventions and nonpharmacologic interventions.

## Pharmacologic Intervention

Pharmacological approaches to treat fatigue in patients with cancer and chronic progressive diseases have increased (Table 8–4). The categories outlined in the table include both FDA approved medications, as well as complementary alternative medications. The most promising randomized controlled trials of drug therapies as well as non-pharmaceutical interventions targeting adult cancer patients are outlined in an extensive review and meta-analysis.[73] Pharmacologic therapies include: antidepressants, psychostimulants, progestional steroids, tumor necrosis factor alpha, micronutrients such as L-carnitine and various other classes of drugs.[74,75] Methylphenidate, a psychostimulant, has been shown to improve quality of life when given to depressed, terminally ill patients. It has also been shown to counteract opioid somnolence, enhance the effects of pain medication, improve cognition, and increase patient activity level.[12,76] Appropriate initial dosing for this drug is between 5 mg–10 mg orally at breakfast and 5 mg at lunch daily. Some patients require higher doses. The elderly may require a downward dose adjustment. However, further research is needed to confirm methylphenidate use in cancer-related fatigue.[20]

Pemoline had been used in the past to treat fatigue. Reports of liver toxicities resulted in this drug being withdrawn from the market. Dextroamphetamines, a potent CNS stimulant, may also be used. They are quickly absorbed from the gastrointestinal tract with high concentrations in the brain.

Antidepressants have shown some effectiveness when a patient experiences both fatigue and depression. Efficacy has been shown with both nortriptyline and amitriptyline.[74] The use of Sertraline in advanced cancer patients has shown no significant effect on fatigue,[77] whereas Bupropion, used with cancer patients with a concomitant psychiatric diagnosis, showed improvement in fatigue.[78] Corticosteroids have been used to increase energy levels at a dose of about 20 mg–40 mg/day. Prednisone has been shown to decrease the degree of fatigue experienced in some patients. Results from one study indicated an increase in activity level when palliative care patients were treated with methylprednisolone.[79] The side effects that may occur with these drugs are always a concern. Both progestational steroids and paroxetine showed no superiority over placebo in treating cancer related fatigue.[20]

Anemia as a result of chemotherapeutic regimens has been very responsive to interventions. Erythropoietin alpha has been important in increasing hemoglobin levels for some cancer patients to improve quality of life. Doses varying from 10,000U subcutaneously given three times per week, to 40,000U given once a week, have resulted in a similar increase in hemoglobin level.[58] In one study of 4382 anemic cancer patients, the highest quality of life was experienced when hemoglobin was maintained between 11 g–13 g/L with the use of epoetin alfa.[80] Although results suggest that erythropoietin has a positive effect on fatigue, two studies terminated their drug trials early due to safety concerns over possible thromboembolic events.[81,82]

Other drugs have been used to combat chronic disease-related fatigue. Clinical trials of Tumor Necrosis Factor Alpha (etanercept) for fatigue have had varied results. In cancer patients receiving docetaxel, there was a significant decrease in fatigue and improved tolerability of the chemotherapy.[141] In rheumatoid arthritis, human immunodeficiency virus and acquired immunodeficiency disease, this drug may reduce fatigue and shows promise for improvement of cachexia.[83,84] Modafanil has been useful predominately in patients with multiple sclerosis, where some studies report clear improvement in fatigue.[85,86] Levo-Carnitine, a micronutrient, was used in a small group of advance cancer patients with carnitine deficiency and appeared to provide fatigue improvement.[87] A trial using Bisphosphonate Ibandronate in over 400 breast cancer patients showed significant improvement in fatigue and possibly in overall quality of life.[88] Initial research of Co-enzyme Q10[89] and American Ginseng[90] for fatigue is underway. Exploration and positive findings with multi-use drugs and alternative medicines are very encouraging for patients with chronic progressive disease and associated fatigue.

## Non-pharmacological Interventions

Interventions for cancer-related fatigue encompass several disciplines. Historically, nurse clinicians and researchers have been the trailblazers in assessing and managing fatigue in the clinical setting. Research has been conducted on all of the fatigue management strategies listed in Table 8–5. Included are: patient and staff educational interventions; studies on disrupted sleep patterns; nutritional deficits and their effect on patient quality of life; symptom management; and physical and attentional fatigue. Sample sizes have often been small and groups homogeneous, but the studies highlight the contribution of nurse researchers.

A recent review on the effect of exercise on fatigue has been undertaken with the evaluation of twenty-eight studies representing 2083 participants. The outcome measures were diverse and included, but were not limited to, the Functional Assessment of Cancer Therapy-Fatigue (FACT-F), Profile of Mood States (POMS), Piper Fatigue Scale, the Brief Fatigue Inventory and the SF-35 vitality scale. The authors concluded that the use of exercise can be beneficial for cancer-related fatigue during and after cancer treatment.[91] An additional meta-analysis of 14 studies concentrating on breast cancer patients and survivors by McNeely et al.[92] concluded that exercise has an effect on improving quality of life, fitness, physical functioning and decreasing fatigue. Several other investigators have reported the benefits of a consistent exercise regimen in breast cancer patients.[93–96] Their research confirmed that exercise decreased perceptions of fatigue and increased quality of life, and indicated that those patients who exercised reported half the fatigue level of those who did not exercise.

In palliative care, a group exercise program was piloted for those with incurable cancer and a short life expectancy. Outcomes indicated that physical fatigue was reduced.[97]

**Table 8-4**
**Selected Pharmacologic Studies for Fatigue in Cancer and Chronic Progressive Diseases**

| Drug Category | Medication/Action | Description of Trial | Subjects/N | Measurement Tool | Findings |
|---|---|---|---|---|---|
| **Antidepressants** | Paroxetine Hydrochloride (Paxil) Serotonin reuptake inhibitor | Roscoe 2005[119] (DBPC) | **Breast cancer** patients on treatment N = 94 | Fatigue Symptom Checklist plus single item fatigue measure | No difference between paroxetine and placebo for CRF. |
| | | Morrow 2003[120] Double Blind Placebo Controlled (DBPC) | **Ambulatory cancer patients** on chemotherapy Breast Cancer more than 50% of patients N = 479 | Fatigue Symptom Checklist, plus one item fatigue measure | Increase in mood, no fatigue difference between paroxetine and placebo. |
| | Sertraline (Zoloft) Selective serotonin reuptake inhibitor | Stockler 2007[77] (DBPC) | **Palliative care/Advanced cancer patients** N = 189 | FACT-F and FACT-G | No significant effect on fatigue. Measured effects on symptoms and survival. |
| | Bupropion (Wellbutrin-SR) Non serotonergic antidepressant with psychostimulant properties | Moss 2006[121] Convenience sample referred for depression | **Various cancer diagnoses** (Brain, breast, hematological, head and neck, others ) N = 21 | Brief Fatigue Inventory, Hamilton Depression Scale, City of Hope QOL scale. | Improvement in depression & fatigue in small sample of depressed and non depressed group. |
| | | Cullum 2004[78] Prospective open label trial | **Various cancer diagnoses** N = 15 | Global Clinical Improvement Scale | Improvement in fatigue. 13/15 pts. psychiatric diagnosis. |
| **Psychostimulants** | Methylphenidate (Ritalin) Stimulates the CNS by blocking presynaptic dopamine reuptake | Bruera 2006[122] Randomized (DBPC) | **Cancer patients** off active treatment. Patient controlled dosing. N = 112 | FACIT-F (13 item fatigue subscore) | Significant fatigue improvement day 8 both drug and placebo. No improvement in FACIT-F score. |
| | | Hanna 2006[123] Convenience sample. Drug with dose escalation @ week 2 if needed | **Stage I-III breast cancer** patients w/o disease or treatment for 6 months. N = 32 | FACT-F and Brief Fatigue Inventory | Suggests that women with moderate to severe fatigue will have benefit. |
| | | Roth 2006[124] Randomized (DBPC) | **Ambulatory Prostate Cancer Patients** N = 24 | Self Report of Fatigue | Preliminary report indicates fatigue reduction, 6/17 withdrew due to cardio effects. |
| | | Breitbart 2001[125] Randomized (DBPC) Methylphenidate vs. Pemoline vs. placebo | **Ambulatory Human Immunodeficiency Virus (HIV)** patients N = 144 | Piper Fatigue Scale and Visual Analog Scale | Ritalin & Pemoline, significant fatigue improvement vs. placebo. No difference between drugs. |

*(Continued)*

**Table 8–4**
**Selected Pharmacologic Studies for Fatigue in Cancer and Chronic Progressive Diseases** (*continued*)

| Drug Category | Medication/Action | Description of Trial | Subjects/N | Measurement Tool | Findings |
|---|---|---|---|---|---|
| | | Sarhill 2001[149] Open label pilot | **Advanced cancer patients,** various tumor types N = 11 | | 9/11 patients had improvement. No valid fatigue measure used. Findings suggest drug may be effective. |
| | | Sugawara 2002[126] Preliminary study | **Advanced cancer patients** referred to psychiatrist for fatigue N = 16 | Visual Analogue Scale | |
| | | Schwartz 2002[150] Methylphenidate plus exercise comparison to historical control | **Melanoma** patients pilot study of interferon induced fatigue N = 12 | Schwartz Cancer Fatigue Scale, Medical Outcomes Study Short Form 36 (SF36) | Fatigue lower for exercise and drug group. Randomized trial is needed. |
| | Dexmethylphenidate d-MPH (Focalin) | Fleishman 2005[127] Randomized (DBPC) Patients on single blind placebo without improvement, randomized to double blind with dosing adjustment | **All cancer patients** treated with chemo, breast cancer patients = 110/152 N = 152 | FACIT-F | Significantly effective treating fatigue over placebo. |
| | Modafanil (Provigil) CNS stimulant, adrenergic agonist. | Morrow 2007[128] Modafanil vs. placebo | **Cancer patients** receiving chemotherapy | Brief Fatigue Inventory, POMS, Fatigue Severity Scale | No published results. |
| | | Kaleita 2006[29] Double blind dose-controlled randomized | **Primary Brain cancer** or non malignant brain tumor patients N = 21 | Fatigue Severity Scale and Visual Analogue Fatigue Scale (VAFS) | Improved fatigue outcome measures. Side effects included headache, insomnia, dizziness. |
| | | Morrow 2005[130] Modafanil vs. placebo Prospective open label | **Breast cancer** patients completed treatment 2 years prior N = 51 | Visual Analog Scale? | Improvement in fatigue that had persisted for 2 years. |
| | | Stankoff 2005[31] Randomized (DBPC) | **Multiple Sclerosis** patients N = 115 | Modified Fatigue Impact Scale | No significant improvement in fatigue compared to placebo. |
| | | Rabkin 2004[132] Open-label | **HIV patients** on antiretroviral medication N = 30 | Fatigue Severity Scale | Significant improvement in all measures of fatigue. |

| | | | | |
|---|---|---|---|---|
| | Rammohan 2002[86] Single blind pilot study at 2 centers. Modafinil vs. placebo | **Multiple Sclerosis** patients N = 72 | Modified Fatigue Impact Scale, VAS-F | Significant fatigue improvement vs placebo. Six patients stopped due to adverse events. |
| | Zifko 2002[85] Open label 2 center, dose escalating trial | **Multiple Sclerosis** patients N = 50 | Fatigue Severity Scale | Reported clear improvement in fatigue in 43 patients. |
| **Progestational Steroids** Megestrol Acetate or Medroxyprogesterone Acetate (Megace) | Bruera 1998[133] DBPC cross-over study | **Advanced solid tumor cancer patients** off active treatment. N = 84 | Piper Fatigue Scale | Significant difference in progestational steriods and placebo for CRF. |
| | DeConno 1998[134] (DBPC) | **Advanced cancer** all tumor types N = 42 | POMS fatigue subscale | No significant change in fatigue. |
| | Simons 1996[135] Randomized (DEPC) | **Advanced stage** any cancer type N = 206 | EORTC QLQ 30 fatigue subscale | General QOL indicated no measurable effect. |
| | Westman 1999[136] Randomized (DBPC) | **Advanced stage** any tumor type not receiving treatment N = 244 | EORTC QLQ 30 fatigue subscale | Did not show improved QOL. |
| **Hemopoetic Growth Factors** Epoetin Alpha (Procrit) 13 trials Mimicks erythropoietin stimulates RBC production | Selected Studies Minton 2008[20] | 11/13 trials of cancer **patients on chemotherapy** 13 trials N = 3735 | | All showed evidence of effect of erythropoietin over placebo for CRF. |
| | O'Shaughnessy 2005[137] Randomized (DBPC) | **Breast cancer patients** on Anthracycline therapy N = 94 | FACT-AN | Results suggest epoetin attenuated cognitive impairment and fatigue. |
| | Leyland Jones 2005[81] (DBPC) | **Breast cancer patients** N = 939 | FACT-AN VAS | Epoetin group had increased 4 month mortality. Trial ended early possibly due to thromboembolis. |

*(Continued)*

**Table 8–4**
**Selected Pharmacologic Studies for Fatigue in Cancer and Chronic Progressive Diseases** (*continued*)

| Drug Category | Medication/Action | Description of Trial | Subjects/N | Measurement Tool | Findings |
|---|---|---|---|---|---|
| | | Wright 2007[82] Randomized multicenter (DBPC) | **Non Small cell lung cancer.** N = 300 | FACT-AN | Decreased survival in Epoetin group compared to placebo. Terminated trial early due to safety concerns. |
| | Darbopoetin (Aranesp) Synthetic of erythropoietin, longer duration. 4 trials combined[20] | Hedenus 2003[138] Kotasek 2003[139] Smith 2003[140] Vansteenkiste 2002[35] (All trials placebo controlled) | **Hematologic malignancies, lung cancer, various tumors types** N = 1650 | FACT-F Used by all investigators | Small but statistically significant difference between darbopoetin and placebo for CRF. |
| **Tumor Necrosis Factor Alpha Blockade (TNF-alpha)** | Etanercept (Enbrel) TNF decoy receptor | Monk 2006[141] Open label | **Any cancer patients** on Docetaxel for 18 weeks. N = 12 | Fatigue Symptom Inventory | Statistically significant decrease in fatigue QOL tool. |
| | | Moreland 2006[83] Multicenter Randomized DBPC 12 months then open label for 12 months. Methotrexate vs. study drug | **Rheumatoid Arthritis** (RA) | Health Assessment Questionnaire Vitality Domain | Etanercept reduced fatigue in recent onset RA and established RA. |
| | | Ting 2006[84] | **HIV and AIDS** patients to examine safety | | TNF may improve ulcers, cachexia, dementia and fatigue. Shows promise in this patient group. |
| | Under current study with Etanercept | Thomas 2007[142] Etanercept vs. placebo | **Lung & Prostate patients** receiving radiation | Quality of Life | |
| **Ongoing Medication/ CAM Studies** | Donepezil (Aricept) Reversible inhibitor of acetyl-cholinesterase (AChE) appears to enhance cholinergic function | Bruera 2007[143] Randomized (DBPC) | **Any cancer patient** receiving strong opioids experiencing sedation. N = 142 | FACIT-F | No significant fatigue improvement between groups. |

| Treatment | Study | Population | Measurement | Results |
| --- | --- | --- | --- | --- |
| Levo Carnitine (L-carnitine) Micronutrient important for acids and energy production. | Cruciani 2008[144] L. Carnitine vs. placebo double blind phase followed by open label phase | **Advanced cancer patients** both on or off chemo with carnitine deficiency N = 29 | FACT-AN fatigue subscale | Showed significant fatigue improvement when treatment phases combined. Suggests a larger study justified. |
| | Gramignano 2006[145] L. Carnitine open label non-randomized | **Advanced solid tumor cancer patients** with concurrent anti-cancer treatment. N = 12 | Multidimensional Fatigue Symptom Inventory-SF and QOL | Fatigue decreased significantly. Limited sample size. No adverse events. |
| Bisphosphonate Ibandronate Binds on bone, Delays skeletal events, improves bone pain. | Diel 2004[88] Randomized (DBPC) | **Breast cancer patients** only. Dose open label due to infusion volume. N = 466 | EORTC QLQ 30 fatigue subscale | Significant improvement in fatigue in patients receiving 6 mg. May improve overall QOL. |
| Co-Enzyme Q10 Dietary supplement that boosts the immune system | Lesser 2008[89] Drug vs. placebo | **Breast cancer** patient on chemo | FACIT-F | Results unpublished. |
| American Ginseng May lessen sense of fatigue that cancer patients experience. | Barton 2008[90] American Ginseng vs. placebo | **Any tumor type.** Stratified by stage of disease | Brief Fatigue Inventory, POMS | Results unpublished. |
| Adenosine 5'- Triphosphate (ATP) Intracellular energy-transferring role . Extracellular ATP is involved in neurotransmission, muscle contraction | Beijer 2007[146] RCT Open label infusion vs. usual care | **Palliative home care cancer patients** all tumor types. N = 100 | Short Fatigue Questionnaire 4 Items and QLQ-C30 | Changes in QOL including fatigue final results in analysis. |
| Dexamphedamine Causes stimulation of cerebral cortex, respiratory, vasomotor centers. | Auret 2008[247] Randomized (DBPC) | **Advanced Cancer** all tumor types. N = 50 | Brief Fatigue Inventory | Transient fatigue improvement but no statistical difference in fatigue. |
| Amantadine Releases endogenous dopamine from basal ganglia and acts as a central stimulator | Zifko 2004[148] Review article summarizing 4 studies | **Multiple Sclerosis** Total N = 213 over 4 studies | Various measurements utilized. | Found to be superior to placebo in some not all endpoints. Not all studies used blinding or randomization. |

**Table 8–5**
**Non-Pharmacologic Symptom Management Strategies for Fatigue**

| Problem | Intervention | Rationale |
|---|---|---|
| Lack of information or lack of preparation | Explain complex nature of fatigue and importance of communication of fatigue level with health care providers. Explain causes of fatigue in advanced cancer and chronic progressive diseases and evaluate fatigue level with each visit.<br>• Fatigue can increase in advanced disease.<br>• Cancer cells can compete with body for essential nutrients.<br>• Palliative treatments, infection and fever increase the body's need for energy.<br>• Anxiety, depression and tension can contribute to fatigue.<br>• Changes in daily schedules, or interrupted sleep schedules contributes to fatigue development.<br>Prepare patient for planned ADL and daily events (eating, moving, visitors, healthcare provider appointments). | Preparatory sensory information reduces anxiety and fatigue.<br>Realistic expectations decrease distress and fatigue. |
| Disrupted rest/sleep patterns | Evaluate/establish sleep routine:<br>• Usual sleep pattern, length of uninterrupted sleep, temperature in room, activity prior to sleep.<br>• Eating habits prior to sleep, medications, exercise.<br>• Establish/continue regular, routine bedtime and awakening.<br>• Obtain as long sleep sequences as possible, plan uninterrupted time.<br>• Take short rest periods/naps that do not interfere with night sleep.<br>• Use light sources to cue the body into a consistent sleep rhythm.<br>• Pharmacologic management of insomnia should be used when behavioral and cognitive approaches have been exhausted. | Minimizing time in bed helps patients feel refreshed, avoids fragmented sleep, and strengths circadian rhythm. |
| Deficient nutritional status | Recommend to patient:<br>• High protein, nutrient dense food to "make every mouthful count."<br>• Use protein supplements to augment diet.<br>• Suggest small, frequent meals.<br>• Coordinate time up in chair with meal arrival time.<br>• Socialization may increase oral intake.<br>• Encourage adequate intake of fluids, 8 glasses/day or whatever is tolerated, unless contraindicated.<br>• Consider requesting an appetite stimulant like Medroxyprogesterone Acetate (Megace). | Increased nutrition will raise energy level. Less energy is needed for digestion with small, frequent meals. |

**Table 8–5**
**Non-Pharmacologic Symptom Management Strategies for Fatigue** (*Continued*)

| Problem | Intervention | Rationale |
|---|---|---|
| Multi-symptom occurrence | Assess and control symptoms contributing to or coexisting with fatigue such as: Pain, sleeplessness, depression, nausea, diarrhea, constipation, electrolyte imbalances, dyspnea, dehydration, infection.<br>Assess for symptoms of anemia and evaluate for the possibility of pharmacologic intervention or transfusion. | Multiple distressing symptoms drain energy and will contribute to marked physical/ mental fatigue. |
| Decreased energy reserves | Plan/Schedule Activities:<br>• Identify a person to be in charge (fielding questions, answering the phone, organizing meals).<br>• Adjust method/pace of care and move slowly when providing care.<br>• Prioritize and save energy for the most important events.<br>• Eliminate or postpone noncritical activities.<br>• Learn to listen to body; if fatigued, rest.<br>Obtain Physical Therapy Consult:<br>• Mild physical therapy may help joint flexibility & prevent pain.<br>• Engage in individually tailored, team approved exercise/yoga program.<br>Use Distraction/Restoration<br>• Encourage activities to restore energy: spending time in natural environment, gardening, listening to music, praying, meditating, engaging in hobbies (art, reading, journaling).<br>• Spend time with family/friends, joining in passive activities (riding in car, watching meal preparation). | Energy conservation helps to reduce fatigue burden and efficiently use energy available.<br>Pleasant activities may reduce/relieve mental (attentional) fatigue. |

Toward the end of life, the NCCN guidelines recommend general strategies for fatigue management that begin with energy conservation techniques, prioritizing activities, delegating, taking rest periods and using labor-saving devices. They also recommend optimizing patient activity levels with the consideration of a referral to both physical and occupational therapy. Increased caution was emphasized for those with bone metastases and immunosupression.[4]

Attentional fatigue has been noted to be disturbing to many patients. It is defined by one author as a decreased capacity to concentrate or direct attention during stressful situations. When attention-restoring interventions were used with cancer patients, it was found that attention capacity was enhanced and fatigue was reduced.[98,99] Restorative activities are based on a program that required patients to select and engage in a favorite activity for 30 minutes three times a week. The use of this technique provided restorative distraction and replaced boredom and understimulation. Included in the activities were spending time in a natural environment, participating in favorite hobbies, writing, fishing, music, and gardening. Regardless of the limitations of the patients with advanced disease, incorporation of some of these activities may prove helpful.

Nutritional consultation for patients has been shown to be key to managing the physiological deficiencies from cachexia, nausea and anorexia.[100] Adequate hydration and the replacement of lost electrolytes enable the fatigue-sufferer to have the best opportunity to control fatigue symptoms that are physiologically based.

The National Institutes of Health identified a major barrier to effective fatigue management as a lack of knowledge and awareness among physicians and patients.[101] Educational intervention at all levels opens a broad category for fatigue intervention including taking advantage of every educational opportunity during the advanced disease course. With education of both the patient and the family as a constant theme, every attempt should be made to forewarn of changes in disease progression, procedures, treatment, medication side effects, or scheduling. Even a personnel change can be enough to impact the physical and emotional energy reserves. Nurse-initiated and planned educational sessions with both the patient and family give a forum in which to field forgotten questions, reinforce nutritional information, and together manage symptoms.

Sleep disruption is a common problem encountered by the patient with advanced chronic progressive disease as identified in the case study. Sleep cycles may be negatively affected by innumerable internal and external factors.[155] The disturbances may be actual or perceived but result in daytime impairment. Common sleep disturbances include insomnia, breathing disorders, and movement disorders. Complete measurement of sleep–wake disturbances are described extensively by Page et al and include an evaluation of: total sleep time, sleep latency, awakenings and wakefulness after sleep onset. Additional measurements include an evaluation of time spent napping, excessive daytime sleepiness, perceived quality of sleep, sleep efficiency and circadian rhythm.[102] Simple changes in environment and habits may improve sleep distress tremendously. One study evaluated the feasibility of sleep interventions while patients underwent adjuvant chemotherapy. Components of the intervention included sleep hygiene (maintaining regular sleep schedule, low lighting, cool room), relaxation therapy (warm bath, reading, massage), stimulus control and sleep-restriction techniques (use bed for sleeping and sex only—avoid day napping).[103] For those situations where pharmacological intervention is necessary, a thorough assessment of past and current sleep habits is essential. The temporary use of sleep medications such as Ambien (zolpidem tartrate) may be used to minimize sleep deprivation enough to energize the patient into trying non-pharmacological measures.

Psychosocial techniques are the last broad category of fatigue intervention. A recent meta-analysis of cancer related fatigue research aimed to evaluate both physical and psychosocial interventions (cognitive behavioral therapy and counseling), as well as behavioral and alternative treatments (massage, yoga) and their effect on fatigue. The findings provide evidence that psychosocial interventions, restorative approaches, and counseling therapies have a moderate to strong effect in not only reducing fatigue, but in increasing vigor and vitality as well.[104] Additionally, a review of 22 studies of psychosocial treatment with cancer patients reported findings that indicate psychosocial support and individualized counseling have a fatigue-reducing effect.[105] If deemed appropriate, the patients and/or family should be encouraged to participate in disease-specific support groups. If unable to travel, there are support groups offered by telephone and/or internet. Individual counseling by nurses, social workers, or psychologists may also help.

Fatigue-management interventions need to be considered within the cultural context of the patient and family. For some cultures, this may include only the "nuclear" family, whereas in other cultures, there are ritual or extended relatives. When information is shared and decisions are made regarding an intervention, the "family" is acknowledged formally, and care should be made inclusive of these cultural variations.[106]

Management of, and interventions for, fatigue in pediatric oncology have mirrored intervention techniques used in adults. Taking into account the developmental stage of the pediatric patient will provide the structure needed to be effective.[9] Children up to 13 years old with cancer consider taking a nap or sleeping, having visitors, and participating in fun activities to be fatigue alleviating behaviors. Adolescent patients with cancer add their own perceptions of what helps their fatigue by including interventions such as going outdoors, having protracted rest time, keeping busy, taking medication for sleep, receiving physical therapy as well as blood transfusions.[9] Pediatric interdisciplinary palliative care teams are becoming more common and can provide a comprehensive range of non-pharmacologic interventions for fatigue including exercise, psychosocial interventions, and complementary and alternative therapy.[107]

As the practice guidelines and standards for fatigue management in palliative care continue to evolve,[152–154] the NCCN fatigue guidelines provide a framework for adults, children and adolescents suffering from cancer-related fatigue. Consolidation of the standards provides recommendations that: fatigue commonly occurs with other symptoms and all patients—regardless of age or extent of disease—should be screened, assessed and managed according to clinical practice guidelines, by a multidisciplinary team, at regular intervals throughout the disease course. They also recommend patient, family and health care provider education programs be ongoing and that quality of fatigue management be implemented as continuous quality improvement projects. Finally, guidance is given that suggests that medical care contracts include reimbursement for fatigue and that disability insurance address coverage for long-lasting fatigue.[4]

## Summary

This chapter has provided an overview of fatigue as it spans the illness trajectory and end-of-life experience for patients with chronic progressive disease. While fatigue is a complex phenomenon that has been widely studied, there is no universally accepted definition. Fatigue is experienced by individuals with cancer and many other chronic, progressive diseases. It is influenced by many factors such as age, psychological state, social support, stage of disease, polypharmacy issues, cognitive impairment and other comorbid conditions. Fatigue has a myriad of causes. The authors have provided a fatigue-assessment checklist that can be used to identify potential sources and/or antecedents for the patient's fatigue. As there is no instant fix for fatigue, the patient may become frustrated, and feel too fatigued to introduce life changes that require the habitual practice of non-pharmacologic interventions. Nurses are challenged to provide ongoing fatigue management education and to support and encourage the patient to actively participate in fatigue-management strategies. Patient referral to appropriate members of the treatment team and utilization of their services is always warranted.

In the last stages of life, many patients experience fatigue in the context of multiple symptoms and comorbidities. Assessment of all treatable factors known to contribute to fatigue will impact on fatigue amelioration. As patients decline toward end of life, fatigue may provide a comforting form of protection and an insulation from suffering. It is essential to identify the point at which active fatigue intervention is no longer appropriate.

## REFERENCES

1. Yennurajalingam S, Bruera E. Palliative management of fatigue at the close of life "It feels like my body is just worn out". JAMA 2007; 297:295–304.

2. Mustian KM, Morrow GR, Carroll JK, Figueroa-Moseley CD, Jean-Pierre P, Williams GC. Integrative nonpharmacologic behavioral interventions for the management of cancer-related fatigue. The Oncologist 2007;12(Suppl 1):52–67.

3. Nail LM. Fatigue in patients with cancer. Oncol Nurs Forum 2002;537–546.

4. National Comprehensive Cancer Network. Practice Guidelines in Oncology Cancer Related Fatigue. Rockledge, Pa: National Comprehensive Cancer Network; January 2008. Available at www.nccn.org/index.asp (accessed December 2008).

5. Radbrunch L, Strasser F, Elsner F, Goncalves JF, Loge J, Kaasa S, Nauck F, Stone P. Fatigue in palliative care patients—an EAPC approach. Pall Med 2008;22:13–32.

6. American Cancer Society. Fatigue. Available at www.cancer. org, (accessed December 31, 2008).

7. National Multiple Sclerosis Society. Fatigue: what you should know. A guide for people with muliple sclerosis. Available at http://www.nationalmssociety.org/living-with-multiple-sclerosis/you-can/manage-fatigue/index.aspx (accessed January 2, 2008).

8. Smith ORF, van den Brock KC, Renkens M, Denollet J. Comparison of fatigue levels in patients with stroke and patients with end-stage heart failure: Application of the fatigue assessment scale. J Am Geriat Soc 2008;56:1915–1919.

9. Hinds PS, Hockenberry-Eaton M, Gilger E, et al. Comparing patient, parent, and staff descriptions of fatigue in pediatric oncology patients. Cancer Nurs 1999;22:277–289.

10. Davies B, Whitsett SF, Bruce A, McCarthy P. A typology of fatigue in children with cancer. J Ped Oncol 2002;19:12–21.

11. Hockenberry M, Hooke MC. Symptom clusters in children with cancer. Seminars Oncol Nurs 2007;23:152–157.

12. Barnes EA, Bruera E. Fatigue in patients with advanced cancer: a review. Int J Gynecol Cancer 2002;12:424–428.

13. Priovano M, Maltoni M, Nanni O, et al. A new palliative prognostic score: a first step for the staging of terminally ill cancer patients. J Pain Symptom Manage 1999;17:231–239.

14. Vainio A, Auvinen A. Prevalence of symptoms among patients with advanced cancer: an international study. J Pain Symptom Manage 1996;12:3–10.

15. Epstein KR. The chronically fatigued patient. Med Clin North Am 1995;79:315–327.

16. Solano JP, Gomes B, Higginson IJ. A comparison of symptom prevalence in far advanced cancer, AIDS, heart disease, chronic obstructive pulmonary disease and renal disease. J Pain Sympt Manage 2006;31:58–69.

17. Cleeland CS. Symptom burden: Multiple symptoms and their impact as patient-reported outcomes. J Nat Cancer Instit Mono 2007;37:16–21.

18. Bender CM, Engberg SJ, Donovan HS, Cohen SM, Houze MP, Rosenzweig MO, Mallory GA, Dunbar-Jacob U, Sereika SM. Symptom clusters in adults with chronic health problems and cancer as a comorbidity. Oncol Nurs Forum 2008;35:E1–E11.

19. Brown DJF, McMillan DC, Milroy R. The correlation between fatigue, physical function, the systemic inflammatory response, and psychological distress in patients with advanced lung cancer. Cancer 2005;103:377–382.

20. Minton O, Stone P, Richardson A, Sharpe M, Hotopf MM. Drug therapy for the management of cancer related fatigue. Cochrane Database Syst Rev 2008, Issue 1.Art.No.:CD006704. DOI:10.1002/14651858.CD006704.pub2.

21. Erickson JM. Fatigue in adolescents with cancer: a review of the literature. Clin J Oncol Nurs 2004;8:139–145.

22. Bottomly S, Teegarden C, Hockenberry-Eaton M. Fatigue in children with cancer: clinical considerations for nursing. J Pediatr Oncol Nurs 1996;13:178.

23. Ream E, Gibson F, Edwards J, Sjeption B, Mulhass A, Richardson A. Experience of fatigue in adolescents living with cancer. Cancer Nurs 2006;29:317–326.

24. Pritchard M, Brughen E, Srivastava DK, Okuma J, Anderson L, Powell B, Furman WL, Hinds PS. Cancer-related symptoms most concering to parents during the last week and last day of their child's life. Pediatrics 2008;121:e1301–e1309.

25. Wolfe J, Holcombe GE, Klar N, Levin SB, Ellenbogen JM, Salem-Schatz S, Emanuel EJ, Wees JC. Symptoms and suffering at the end of life in children with cancer. N Engl J Med 2000;342:326–333.

26. Wolfe J, Hammel JF, Edwards KE, Duncan J, Comeau M, Breyer J, Aldridge SA, Grier HE, Berde C, Dussel V, Weeks JC. Easing of suffering in children with cancer at the endo of life: Is caring changing? J Clin Oncol 2008;26:1717–1723.

27. Jalmsell L, Kreicbergs U, Onelov E, Steineck G, Henter JI. Symptoms affecting children wit malignancies during the last month of life: A nationwide follow-up. Pediatrics 2006;117:1314–1320.

28. Theunissen JMJ, Hoogerbrugge PM, vanAchterberg T, Prins JB, Vernooij-Dassen MJFJ, vandenEnde CHM. Symptoms in the palliative phase of children with cancer. Pediat Blood Cancer 2007;49:160–165.

29. Hurter B, Bush MK. Cancer-related anemia: a clinical review and management update. Clin J Oncol Nurs 2007;11:349–359.

30. Bosanquet N, Tolley K. Treatment of anaemia in cancer patients: implications for supportive care in the National Health Service Cancer Plan. Curr Med Res Opin 2003;19:643–650.

31. Carson JL, Terrin ML, Jay M. Anemia and postoperative rehabilitation. Can J Anaesth 2003;50(6 suppl):S60–S64.

32. Agnihotri P, Teifer M, Butt Z, Jella A, Cella D, Kozma CM, Ahuja M, Riaz S, Akamah J. Chronic anemia and fatigue in elderly patients: results of a randomized, double-blind, placebo-controlled, cross-over exploratory study with epoetin alfa. J Am Geriatr Soc 2007;55:1557–1565.

33. Cella D, Kallich J, McDermott A, Xu X. The longitudinal relationship of hemoglobin, fatigue and quality of life in anemic cancer patients: Results from five randomized clinical trials. Ann Oncol 2004;15:979–986.

34. Gabrilove JL, Cleeland CS, Liningston RB, Sarokhan B, Winer E, Einhorn LH. Clinical evaluation of once-weekly dosing of epoetin alfa in chemotherapy patients: Improvements in hemoglobin and quality of life are similar to three-times-weekly dosing. J Clin Oncol 2001;19:2875–2882.

35. Vansteenkiste J, Pirker R, Massuti B, Barata F, Font A, Fiegl M and Aranesp 980297 Study Group. Double-blind, placebo-controlled, randomized phase III trial of darbopoetin alfa in lung cancer patients receiving chemotherapy. J Nat Cancer Instit 2002; 94:1211–1220.

36. Barsevick AM, Whitmer K, Nail LM, Beck SL, Dudley WN. Symptom cluster research: Conceptual design, measurement, and analysis issues. J Pain Symptom Manage 2006;31:85–95.

37. Wang XS, Fairclough DL, Liao Z, Komaki R, Chang JY, Mobley GM, et al. Longitudinal study of the relationship between chemoradiation therapy for non-small cell lung cancer and patient symptoms. J Clin Oncol 2006;24:4485–4491.

38. Cleeland CS, Bennett GJ, Dantzer R, Dougherty PM, Dunn AJ, Meyers CA, Miller AH, et al. Are the symptoms of cancer and cancer treatment due to a shared biologic mechanism? A cytokine-immunologic model of cancer symptoms. Cancer 2003;97:2919–2925.

39. Kent S, Bluthe RM, Kelley KW, Dantzer R. Sickness behavior as a new target for drug development. Trends Pharmacol Sci 1992;13:24–28.

40. Schubert C, Hong S, Natarajan L, Mills PJ, Dimsdale JE. The association between fatigue and inflammatory marker levels in cancer patients: A quantitative review. Brain, Behavior and Immunity 2007;21:413–427.

41. Ashbury FD, Findlay H, Reynolds B, McKerracher K. A Canadian survey of cancer patients' experiences: Are their needs being met? J Pain Symptom Manage 1998;16:298–306.

42. Woo B, Dibble SL, Piper BF, Keating SB, Weiss MC. Differences in fatigue by treatment methods in women with breast cancer. Oncol Nurs Forum 1998;25:915–920.

43. Luciani A, Jacobsen PB, Extermann M, Foa P, Marussi D, Overcash JA, Balducci L. Fatigue and functional dependence in older cancer patients. American J Clin Oncol 2008;31:424–430.

44. Hardman A, Maguire P, Crowther D. The recognition of psychiatric morbidity on a medical oncology ward. J Psychosom Res 1989;33:235–239.

45. Kathol RG, Noyes R, Williams J. Diagnosing depression in patients with medical illness. Psychosomatics 1990;31:436–449.

46. Valente SM, Saunders JM, Cohen MZ. Evaluating depression among patients with cancer. Cancer Pract 1994;2:65–71.

47. American Psychiatric Association. Diagnostic and Statistical Manual of Mental Disorders, 4th ed. Washington DC: American Psychiatric Association, 1994:317–391.

48. Visser MRM, Smets EMA. Fatigue, depression and quality of life in cancer patients: How are they related? Support Care Cancer 1998;6:101–108.

49. Hayes JR. Depression and chronic fatigue in cancer patients. Prim Care 1991;18:327–339.

50. Ibbotson T, Maguire P, Selby P, Priestman T, Wallace L. Screening for anxiety and depression in cancer patients: the effects of disease and treatment. Eur J Cancer 1993;30:37–40.

51. Bower JE, Ganz PA, Desmond KA, Rowland JH, Meyerowitz BE, Belin TR. Fatigue in breast cancer survivors: occurrence, correlates, and impact on quality of life. J Clin Oncol 2000;18:743–753.

52. Redd WH, Jacobson PB. Emotions and cancer. Cancer 1988; 62:1871–1879.

53. Aaronson LS, Teel CS, Cassmeyer V, et al. Defining and measuring fatigue. Image—J Nurs Sch 1999;31:45–50.

54. Blesch K, Paice J, Wickman R, et al. Correlates of fatigue in people with breast or lung cancer. Oncol Nurs Forum 1991;18:81–87.

55. Gift A, Pugh G. Dyspnea and fatigue. Nurs Clin North Am 1993;28:373–384.

56. Hoekstra J, Vernooij-Dassen MJFJ, de Vos R, Bindels PJE. The added value of assessing the "most troublesome" symptom among patient with cancer in the palliative phase. Patient Educ Counsel 2007; 65:223–229.

57. O'Sullivan D, McCarthy G. An exploration of the relationship between fatigue and physical functioning in patients with end-stage renal disease receiving haemodialysis. J Clin Nurs 2007;16:276–284.

58. Crosby L. Factors which contribute to fatigue associated with rheumatoid arthritis. J Adv Nurs 1991;16:974–981.

59. Belza B, Henke C, Yelin E, Epstein W, Gilliss C. Correlates of fatigue in older adults with rheumatoid arthritis. Nurs Res 1993;42:93–109.

60. Friedman M, King K. Correlates of fatigue in older women with heart failure. Heart Lung 1995;24:512–518.

61. Hinds PS, Hockenberry-Eaton M, Quargnenti A, et al. Fatigue in 7- to 12-year-old patients with cancer from the staff perspective: an exploratory study. Oncol Nurs Forum 1999;26: 37–45.

62. Fernandes R, Stone P, Andrews P, Morgan R, Sharma S. Comparison between fatigue, sleep disturbance, and circadian rhythm in cancer impatients and healthy volunteers: Evaluation of diagnostic criteria for cancer-related fatigue. J Pain and Sympt Manage 2006;32:245–254.

63. Fobair P, Hoppe RT, Bloom J, Cox R, Varghese A, Spiegel D. Psychosocial problems among survivors of Hodgkin's disease. J Clin Oncol 1986;4:805–814.

64. Wang XS, Giralt SA, Mendoza TR, Engstrom MC, Johnson BA, Peterson N, Broemeling LD, Cleeland CS. Clinical factors associated with cancer-related fatigue in patients being treated for leukemia and non-Hodgkin's lymphoma. J Clin Oncol 2002;20:1319–1328.

65. Olson K. A new way of thinking about fatigue: A reconceptualization. Oncol Nurs Forum 2007;34:93–99.

66. Cella D, Peterman A, Pasik S, et al. Progress toward guidelines for the management of fatigue. Oncology 1998;12:369–377.

67. Aaronson LS, Teel CS, Cassmeyer V, Neuberger GB, Pallikkathayil L, Pierce J, Press AN, Williams PD, Wingate A. Defining and measuring fatigue. Image—J Nurs Sch 1999; 31:45–50.

68. Piper BF, Borneman T, Chih-Yi Sun V, Koczywas M, Uman G, Ferrell B, James RL. Cancer-related fatigue: role of oncology nurses in translating National Comprehensive Cancer Network assessment guidelines into practice. Clin J Oncol Nurs 2008;12:37–47.

69. Hockenberry MJ, Hinds PS, Barrera P, et al. Three instruments to assess fatigue in children with cancer: The child, parent and staff perspectives. J Pain Symptom Manage 2003;25:319–328.

70. Varni JW, Bruwinkle TM, Katz ER, et al. The PedsQL in pediatric cancer: Reliability and validity of the Pediatric Quality of Life Inventory Generic Core Scales, Multidimensional Fatigue Scale and Cancer Module. Cancer 2002;94:2090–2106.

71. Ferrell BR, Koczywas M, Borneman T, Sun V, Piper BF. Barriers to pain and fatigue management in medical oncology. J Clin Oncol 2008; 26:(May 20 supplement; abstract 9546).

72. Winningham ML. Strategies for managing cancer-related fatigue syndrome: A rehabilitation approach. Cancer 2001;92 (4 Suppl):988–997.

73. Minton O, Richardson A, Sharpe M, Hotopf M, Stone P. A systematic review and meta-analysis of the pharmacological treatment of cancer-related fatigue. J Natl Cancer Inst 2008;100:1155–1166.

74. Escalante CP. Treatment of cancer-related fatigue: An update. Supp Care Cancer 2003;11:79–83.

75. Carroll JK, Kohli S, Mustian K, Roscoe JA, Morrow GR. Pharmacologic treatment of cancer related fatigue. The Oncol 2007;12(Suppl 1):43–51.

76. Rozans M, Dreisbach A, Lertora JJ, Kahn MJ. Palliative uses of methylphenidate in patients with cancer: a review. J Clin Oncol 2002;20:335–339.

77. Stockler MR, O'Connell R, Nowak AK, Goldstein D, Turner J, Wilcken NR, Wyld D, et al. Effect of sertraline on symptoms and survival in patients with advanced cancer, but without major depression: A placebo-controlled double-blind randomised trial. Lancet Oncol 2007;8:603–612.

78. Cullum JL, Wojciechowski AE, Pelletier G, Simpson JS. Bupropion sustained release treatment reduces fatigue in cancer patients. Canad J Psych 2004;49:139–144.

79. Bruera E, Roca E, Cedaro L, Carraro S, Chacon R. Action of oral methylprednisolone in terminal cancer patients: A prospective randomized double-blind study. Cancer Treat Rep 1985;69:751–754.

80. Crawford J, Cella D, Cleeland CS, Cremieux PY, Demetri GD, Sarokhan BJ, Slavin MB, Glaspy JA. Relationship between changes in hemoglobin level and quality of life during chemotherapy in anemic cancer patients receiving epoetin alfa therapy. Cancer 2002;95:888–895.

81. Leyland-Jones B, Semiglazov V, Pawlicki M, Peinkowski T, Tjulandin S, Manikhas G, et al. Maintaining normal heloglobin levels with epoetin alfa in mainly nonanemic patients with metastatic breast cancer receiving first-line chemotherapy: a survival study. J Clin Oncol 2005;23:5960–5972.

82. Wright JR, Ung YC, Julian JA, Pritchard KI, Whelan TJ, Smith C, et al. Randomized, double-blind, placebo-controlled trial of erythropoietin in non-small cell lung cance with disease-related anemia. J Clin Oncol 2007;25:1–6.

83. Moreland LW, Genovese MC, Sato R, Singh A. Effect of etanercept on fatigue in patients with recent or established rheumatoid arthritis. Arthritis Rheum 2006;55:287–293.

84. Ting PT, Koo JY. Use of etanercept in human immunodeficiency virus (HIV) and acquired immunodeficiency syndrome (AIDS) patients. Internat J Dermat 2006;45:689–692.

85. Zifko UA, Rupp M, Schwarz S, Zipko HT, Maida Em. Modafinil in treatment of fatigue in multiple sclerosis: result of an open-label study. J Neurol 2002;249:983–987.

86. Rammohan KE, Rosenberg JH, Lynn DJ, Blumenfled AM, Pollak CP, Nagaraja HN. Efficacy and safety of modafinil (Provigil) for the treatment of fatigue in multiple sclerosis: a two centre phase 2 study. J Neurol Neurosurg Psychiatry 2002;72:179–183.

87. Cruciani RA Dvorkin E, Homel P, Culliney B, Malamud S, Lapin J, Protneoy RK, Esteban-Cruciani N. Safety, tolerability and symptom outcomes associated with L-carnitine supplementation in patients with cancer, fatigue, and carnitine deficiency: a phase I/II study. J Pain Symptom Manage 2007;32:551–559.

88. Diel IJ, Body JJ, Lilchinitser MR, Kreuser ED, Dornoff W, Gorbunova VA, Budde M, Bergstron B, et al. Improved quality of life after long-term treatment with the bisphosphonate ibandronate in patients with metastatic bone disease due to breast cancer. Eur J Cancer 2004;40:1704–1712.

89. Lesser GJ. Coenzyme Q 10 in relieving treatment-related fatigue in women with breast cancer. 2008. [NCT00096356]. Available at www.clinicaltrials.gov (accessed December 31, 2008).

90. Barton D. American ginseng in treating patients with fatigue caused by cancer. 2008. [NCT00719563]. Available at www.clinicaltrials.gov (accessed December 31, 2008).

91. Cramp F, Daniel J. Exercise for the management of cancer-related fatigue in adults (review). Cochrane Database Syst Rev 2008; 2: CD006145. DOI: 10.1002/14651858.CD006145.pub.2.

92. McNeely ML, Campbell KL, Rowe BH, Klassen TP, Mackey JR, Courneya KS. Effects of exercise on breast cancer patients and survivors: a systematic review and meta-analysis. Canad Med Assoc J 2006;175:34–41.

93. Mock V, Dow KH, Meares CJ, et al. Effects of exercise on fatigue, physical functioning, and emotional distress during radiation therapy for breast cancer. Oncol Nurs Forum 1997;24:991–1000.

94. Winningham M, MacVicar M, Burke C. Exercise for cancer patients: guidelines and precautions. Physician Sportsmed 1986;14:125.

95. Courneya KS, Segal RJ, Gelmon K, Reid RD, Mackey JR, Friedenreich CM, Prouix C, Lane K, Ladha AB, Vallance JK, Liu Q, Yasui Y, McKenzie DC. Six-month follow up of patient rated outcomes in a randomized controlled trial of exercise training during breast cancer chemotherapy. Cancer Epidemiol Biomarkers Prev 2007;16:2572–2578.

96. Mock V, Frangakis C, Davidson NE, Ropka ME, Poniatowski B, Stewart KJ, Cameron L, Zawacki K, Podewils LJ, Cohen G, McCorkle R. Exercise manages fatigue during breast cancer treatment: a randomized controlled trial. Psycho-oncology 2005;14:464–477.

97. Oldervoll LM, Loge JH, Paltiel H, Asp MB, Vidvei U, Wiken AN, Hjermstad MJ, Kaasa S. The effect of a physical exercise program in palliative care: A phase II study. J Pain and Symptom Manage 2006;32:421–430.

98. Cimprich B. Attentional fatigue following breast cancer surgery. Res Nurs Health 1992;15:199–207.

99. Cimprich B, Ronis DL. An environmental intervention to restore attention in women with newly diagnosed breast cancer. Cancer Nurs 2003;26:284–292.

100. Brown JK. A systematic review of the evidence on symptom management of cancer-related anorexia and cachexia. Oncol Nurs Forum 2002;29:517–532.

101. National Institutes of Health state of the science conference statement Symptom management in cancer: Pain, depression, and fatigue. July 15–17, 2002. Natl Cancer Inst Monogr 2004;32:9–16.

102. Page MS, Berger AM, Johnson LB. Putting evidence into practice: evidence-based interventions for sleep-wake disturbances. Clin J Oncol Nurs 2006;10:753–767.

103. Berger AM, VonEssen S, Kuhn BR, Piper BF, Farr L, Agrawal A, Lynch JC, Higginbotham P. Feasibility of a sleep intervention during adjuvant breast cancer chemotherapy. Oncol Nurs Forum 2002;29:1431–1441.

104. Kangas M, Bovbjerg DH, Montgomery GH. Cancer-related fatigue: A systematic and meta-analytic review of non-pharmacological therapies for cancer patients. Psycholog Bull 2008;134:700–741.

105. Trijsburg R, van Knippengerg F, Rijpma S. Effects of psychological treatment on cancer patients: A comparison of strategies. Psychosom Med 1992;54:489–517.

106. Kagawa-Singer M. A multicultural perspective on death and dying. Oncol Nurs Forum 1998;25:1752–1756.

107. Ullrich CK, Mayer OH. Assessment and management of fatigue and dyspnea in pediatric palliative care. Pediatrc Clin N Am 2007;54:735–756.

108. Hickok JT, Morrow G, Roscoe JA, et al. Occurrence, severity, and longitudinal course of twelve common symptoms in 1129 consecutive patients during radiotherapy for cancer. J Pain Symptom Manage 2005;30:433–442.

109. Collins S, de Vogel-Voogt E, Visser A, van der Heide A. Presence, communication and treatment of fatigue and pain complaints in incurable cancer patients. Pat Educ Counsl 2008;72:102–108.

110. Goldman A, Hewitt M, Collins GS, et al. Symptoms in children/young people with progressive malignant disease: United Kingdom Children's Cancer Study Group/Paediatric Oncology Nurses Forum survey. Pediatr 2006;117:1179–1186.

111. Bower JE. Cancer-related fatigue: Links with inflammation in cancer patients and survivors. Brain, Behavior and Immunity 2007;21:863–871.

112. Falk K, Swedberg K, Gaston-Johansson F, Ekman I . Fatigue is a prevalent and severe symptom associated with uncertainty and sense of coherence in patients with chronic heart failure. Eur J Cardio Nurs 2007;6:99–104.

113. Elkington H, White P, Addington-Hall J, Higgs R, Edmonds P. The healthcare needs of chronic obstructive pulmonary disease patients in the last year of life. Pall Med 2005;19:485–491.

114. Merkus MP, Jager KJ, Dekker FW, de Haan RJ, Boeschoten EW, Krediet RT. Physical symptoms and quality of life in patients on chronic dialysis: results of The Netherlands Cooperative Study on Adequacy of Dialysis (NECOSAD). Neph Dialysis Transpl 1999;14:1163–1170.

115. Uhlin PY, Edéll-Gustafsson U. Self-reported subjective sleep quality and fatigue in patients with peritoneal dialysis treatment at home. Internat J Nurs Pract 2006;12:143–152.

116. Grierson J, Mission S, MacDonald K, Pitts M, O'Brien M. HIV Futures 3: Positive Australians on Services, Health and Well-Being. Psychoso Med 2002;60:759–764.

117. Norval, D. Symptoms and sites of pain experienced by AIDS patients. South African Med J 2004;94:450–454.

118. National Multiple Sclerosis Society. Management of MS-related fatigue. Available at http://www.nationalmssociety.org (accessed January 12, 2009).

119. Roscoe JA, Morrow GR, Hickok JT, Mustian KM, Griggs JJ, Matteson SE, Bushunow P, Qasi R, Smith B. Effect of paroxitine hydrochloride (Paxil) on fatigue and depression in breast cancer patients receiving chemotherapy. Breast Cancer Res Treatment 2005;89:243–249.

120. Morrow GR, Hickock JT, Roscoe JA, Raubertas RF, Andrews PL, Flynn PJ, et al. Differential effects of paroxetine on fatigue and depression: A randomized, double-blind trial from the University of Rochester Cancer Center Community Clinical Oncology Program. J Clin Oncol 2003;21:4635–4641.

121. Moss E, Simpson SA, Pelletier G, Forsyth P. An open-label study of the effects of Bupropion SR on fatigue, depression and quality of life of mixed-site cancer patients and their partners. Psycho-Oncol 2006;15:259–267.

122. Bruera E, Valero V, Driver L, Shen L, Willey J, Zhang T, Palmer JL. Patient-controlled Methylphenidate for cancer fatigue: A double-blind, randomized, placebo-controlled trial. J Clin Oncol 2006;24:2073–2078.

123. Hanna A, Sledge G, Mayer ML, Hanna N, Einhorn L, Monahan P, Daggy J, Bhatia S. A phase II study of methylphenidate for the treatment of fatigue. Supportive Care Cancer 2006;14:210–215.

124. Roth AJ, Nelson CJ, Rosenfelf B, O'Shea N, Slovin S, Scher HI, Breitbart W. Randomized controlled trial testing Methylphenidate as treatment for fatigue in men with prostate cancer. ASCO Prostate Cancer Symposium 2006. Available at www.asco.org (accessed December 31, 2008).

125. Breitbart W, Rosenfeld B, Kaim M, Funesti-esch J. A randomized, double-blind, placebo-controlled trial of psychostimulants for the treatment of fatigue in ambulatory patients with human immunodeficiency virus disease. Arch Intern Med 2001;161:411–420.

126. Sugawara Y, Skechi T, Shima Y, Okuyama T, Akizuki B, Nakano T, Uchitomi Y. Efficacy of methylphenidate for fatigue in advanced cancer patients: a preliminary study. Pall Med 2002;16:261–263.

127. Fleishman S, Lower E, Zeldis J, Faleck H, Manning D. A phase II, randomized, placebo-controlled trial of the safety and efficacy of dexmethylphenidate (d-MPH) as a treatment for fatigue and "chemobrain" in adult cancer patients. Breast Cancer Res Treatment 2005;94:S214.

128. Morrow GR. Modafinil in treating fatigue in patients receiving chemotherapy for cancer. [NCT00042848]. Available at www.clinicaltrials.gov (accessed December 31, 2008).

129. Kaleita TA, Wellisch DK, Graham CA, Steh B, Nghiemphu P, Fort JM, Lai A, Peak S, Cloughesy TF. Pilot study of modafinil for treatment of neurobehavioral dysfunction and fatigue in adult patients with brain tumors. J Clin Oncol 2006; ASCO Meeting Proceedings Part 1;24:18S:1503.

130. Morrow GR, Gillies LJ, Hickok JT, Roscoe JA, Padmanaban D, Griggs JJ. The positive effect of the psychostimulant Modafinil on fatigue from cancer that persisits after treatment is completed. J Clin Oncol 2005; ASCO Meeting Proceedings Part 1;23:16S:8012.

131. Stankoff B, Waubant E, Confavreux C, Edan G, Debouverie M, Rumbach L, Moreau T, Pelletier J, Lubetzki C, Clanet M; French Modafinil Study Group. Neurology 2005;64:1139–1143.

132. Rabkin JG, McElhiney MC, Rabkin R, Ferrando SJ. Modafinil treatment for fatigue in HIV+ patients: A pilot study. J Clin Psych 2004;65:1688–1695.

133. Bruera E, Ernst S, Hagen N, Spachynski K, Belzile M, Hanson J, Summers N, Brown B, Dulude H, Gallant G. Effectiveness of megestrol acetate in patients with advanced cancer: A randomized, double-blind, crossover study. Cancer Prevent Contr 1998;2:74–78.

134. DeConno F, Martini C, Zecca E, Balzarini A, Venturino P, Groff L, Caraceni A. Megestrol acetate for anorexia in patients with far-advanced cancer: A double-blind controlled clinical trial. Eur J Cancer 1998;34:1705–1709.

135. Simons JP, Aaronson NK, Vansteenkiste JF, Ten Velde GP, Muller MJ, Drenth BM, et al. Effects of medroxyprogesterone acetate on appetite, weight and quality of life in advanced stage non-hormone sensitive cance: A placebo controlled multicenter study. J Clin Oncol 1996;14:1077–1084.

136. Westman G, Bergman B, Albertsson M, Kadar L, Gustavsson G, Thaning L, Andersson M, et al. Megestrol acetate in advanced, progressive, hormone-insensitive cancer. Effects on quality of life: A placebo-controlled, randomised, multicentre trial. Eur J Cancer 1999;35:586–595.

137. O'Shaughnessy JA, Vukelja SJ, Holmes FA, Savin M, Jones M, Royall D, George M, Von Hoff D. Feasibiliity of quantifying the effects of epoetin alfa therapy on cognitive function in women with breast cancer undergoing adjuvant or neoadjuvant chemotherapy. Clin Breast Cancer 2005;5:439–446.

138. Hedenus M, Adriansson M, San Miguel J, Kramer MHH, Schipperus MR, Juvonen E, et al. Efficacy and safety of darbopoetin alfa in anemic patients with lymphoproliferative malignancies: A randomized, double-blind, placebo-controlled study. Brit J Haemat 2003;122:394–403.

139. Kotasek D, Steger G, Faught W, Underhill C, Poulson E, Colowick AB, et al. Darbopoetin alfa administered every 3 weeks alleviates anemia in patients with solid tumors receiving chemotherapy; results of a double-blind, placebo controlled randomized study. Eur J Cancer 2003;39:2026–2034.

140. Smith RE Jr, Tchekmedyian NS, Chan D, Meza LA, Northfelt Dw, Patel R, et al. A dose-and schedule-finding study of darbopoetin apfa for the treatment of chronic anemia of cancer. Brit J of Cancer 2003;88:1851–1858.

141. Monk JP, Phillips G, Waite R, Kuhn J, Schaaf LJ, Otterson GA, Guttridge, D, Rhoades C, Shah M, Criswell T, Caligiuri MA, Villalona-Calero MA. Assessment of tumor necrosis factor alpha blockade as an intervention to improve tolerability of dose-intensive chemotherapy in cancer patients. J Clin Oncol 2006;24:1852–1859.

142. Thomas CR. Enbrel versus placebo with radiation therapy to combat fatigue and cachexia. [NCT00127387]. Available at www.clinicaltrials.gov (accessed December 31, 2008).

143. Bruera E, El Osta B, Valero V, Driver LC, Pei BL, Shen L, Poulter VA, Palmer JL. Donepezil for cancer fatigue: A double-blind, randomized, placebo-controlled trial. J Clin Oncol 2007; 25: 3475–3481.

144. Cruciani RA, Dvorkin E, Homel P, Culliney B, Malamud S, Lapin J, Protneoy RK, Esteban-Cruciani N. L-Carnitine supplementation in patients with advanced cancer and carnitine deficiency: A double-blind, placebo-controlled study. J Pain Symptom Manage 2009;37:622–631.

145. Gramignano G, Lusso MR, Madeddu C, Massa E, Serpe R, Deiana L, LaMonica G, Dessi M, Spiga C, et al. Efficacy of L-carnitine administration of fatigue, nutritional status, oxidative stress, and related quality of life in 12 advanced cancer patients undergoing anticancer therapy. Nutrition 2006;22:136–145.

146. Beijer S, van Rossum E, Hupperets PS, Spreeuwenberg C, van den Beuken M, Winkens RA, Ars L, van den Borne BE, de Graeff A, Dagnelie PC. Application of adenosine 5'-triphosphate (ATP) infusions in palliative home care: design of a randomized clinical trial. BioMed Centr Pub Health 2007;7:4–11.

147. Auret KA, Schug SA, Bremner AP, Bulsara M. A randomized, double-blind, placebo-controlled trial assessing the impact of dexamphetamine on fatigue in patients with advanced cancer. J Pain Symptom Manage 2009;37:613–621.

148. Zifko UA. Management of fatigue in patients with multiple sclerosis. Drugs 2004;64:1295–1304.

149. Sarhill N, Walsh D, Nelson KA, Homsi J, Lerand S, Davis MD. Methylphenidate for fatigue in advanced cancer: A prospective open-label pilot study. Am J Hospice Palliat Care 2001;8:187–192.

150. Schwartz AL, Thompson JA, Masood N. Interferon-induced fatigue in patients with melanoma: A pilot study of exercise and Methylphenidate. Oncol Nurs Forum Online Exclusive 2002;29:E85–E90.

151. Barnett ML. Fatigue. In: Otto SE, ed. Oncology Nursing 3rd ed. St. Louis: Mosby, 1997:670.

152. Aistars J. Fatigue in the cancer patient: A conceptual approach to a clinical problem. Oncol Nurs Forum 1987;15:199–207.

153. Piper BF, Lindsey AM, Dodd MJ. Fatigue mechanisms in cancer patients: Developing nursing theory. Oncol Nurs Forum 1987;21:17–23.

154. Winningham ML, Nail LM, Burke MB, Brophy L, Cimprich B, Jones LS, Pickard-Holley S, Rhodes V, St. Pierre B, Beck S, et al. Fatigue and the cancer experience: The state of the knowledge. Oncol Nurs Forum 1994;21:23–36.

155. Berger AM, Mitchell SA. Modifying cancer-related fatigue by optimizing sleep quality. J National Compre Cancer Network 2008;6:3–13.

156. Olson K, Krawchuk A, Quddusi T. Fatigue in individuals with advanced cancer in active treatment and palliative settings. Cancer Nurs 2007;30:E1–E10.

# 9

*Dorothy Wholihan and Charles Kemp*

# Anorexia and Cachexia

*When my husband stopped wanting to eat, I knew it was the beginning of the end. He made an effort sometimes because he knew how much I worried when he didn't eat. I brought him food from home but he only took a few bites to please me. I felt so helpless. I watched him just start to waste away, and I knew he would be going sooner than I was ready for. It was heartwrenching.—Wife of a man with metastatic colon cancer*

◆ **Key Points**
◆ *Anorexia and cachexia are a distressing part of advanced illness.*
◆ *They are distinct syndromes but clinically difficult to differentiate.*
◆ *Metabolic alterations are the primary cause of anorexia/cachexia syndrome.*
◆ *Assessment and treatment of anorexia and cachexia include determining whether exogenous etiologies such as nausea and pain are involved and vigorous treatment of any such etiologies if present.*

Anorexia is defined as the loss of desire to eat[1] and is a symptom which accompanies many common illnesses. In acute events, anorexia usually resolves with resolution of the illness, and any weight lost may be replaced with nutritional supplements or increased intake.[2] Unchecked, anorexia leads to insufficient caloric intake and protein-calorie malnutrition. Weight loss from this starvation phenomenon usually involves loss of fat, rather than muscle tissue.[3] Anorexia is common among patients with advanced cancer and acquired immune deficiency syndrome (AIDS), but also characterizes the clinical course of patients with other chronic progressive disease, such as COPD, CHF, and end-stage renal disease.[4]

Anorexia and cachexia are two distinct clinical syndromes, but are often intertwined in chronic progressive disease. Cachexia is a complex syndrome that usually involves anorexia, along with significant weight loss, loss of muscle tissue as well as adipose tissue, and generalized weakness.[3] The word "cachexia" is derived from the Greek *kakos*, meaning bad, and *hexis*, meaning condition or appearance; throughout medical history, cachexia has been associated with the gravely ill.[5] The first clinical definition can be traced to Hippocrates earlier than 400 BC: "The flesh is consumed and becomes water...the abdomen fills with water, the feet and legs swell, the shoulders, clavicles, chest and thighs melt away...the illness is fatal."[6] It is important to differentiate the cachexia syndrome from simple anorexia or starvation. Anorexia resulting in decreased intake is usually a component of both phenomena, but cachexia can still be found in the absence of decreased appetite. Anorexia alone does not account for the magnitude of weight loss seen in diseases like cancer, and nutritional supplementation does not restore the lean body mass of cancer anorexia/cachexia syndrome.[1] Cachexia is defined as a state of "general ill health and malnutrition, marked by weakness and emaciation"; it occurs in more than 80% of patients with cancer before death and is the main cause of death in more than 20% of such patients.[7] In contrast to the starvation seen in anorexia, in cachexia there is approximately equal loss of fat and muscle, significant loss of bone mineral content, and no response to nutritional supplements or increased intake.

Weight loss, regardless of etiology, has a decidedly negative effect on survival, and loss of lean body mass has an especially deleterious effect.[2] Evidence-based reviews about prognosis reveal a significant correlation between anorexia/cachexia and survival in newly diagnosed cancer patients[8] and in patients with advanced disease.[9] Weight loss is also linked to decreased survival in congestive heart failure,[10] chronic obstructive lung disease,[5] end-stage renal disease, and AIDS.[11] The term anorexia/cachexia syndrome (ACS) has been used mostly in reference to patients with cancer, and is sometimes termed cancer-related anorexia/cachexia (C-ACS).[7] Varying terminology has been used to describe the syndrome in other disease states for instance, HIV wasting syndrome, cardiac cachexia, pulmonary cachexia syndrome, and, in patients with advanced renal disease, the ACS has been named "malnutrition-inflammation-cachexia syndrome" (MICS).[5] Table 9–1 lists the various terms used to describe anorexia–cachexia and estimated prevalence in different disease states. The pathophysiology and clinical presentation of ACS overlap in these various diseases, even though the underlying metabolic and neurohormonal imbalances may differ. The basic issue of underlying chronic inflammation can be seen in them all.[12] For the purposes of this chapter, the term ACS shall refer to all chronic, advanced disease-related anorexia/cachexia syndromes.

The anorexia/cachexia syndrome of all diseases is characterized by a variety of signs and symptoms that represent interference with energy intake (decreased appetite, early satiety, taste changes, etc.) and nutritional status, i.e. increased metabolic rate, weight loss, hormonal alterations, muscle and adipose tissue wasting, fatigue and decreased performance status.[4] Whatever the specific disease, the development of ACS poses a significant clinical problem. It is a grave prognostic sign, but also has a detrimental effect on quality of life, as documented by studies of all the above major diagnoses.[5] This syndrome leads to serious physical and functional deficits, and can be devastating to self-image, social and family relationships, and spiritual well being.

## Pathophysiology of ACS

The basic etiologies of anorexia/cachexia syndrome are: (1) decreased food intake, (2) metabolic abnormalities, (3) the actions of proinflammatory cytokines, (4) systemic inflammation, (5) neurohormonal dysregulation, (6) tumor by-products, and (7) the catabolic state.[7] These result in derangement of function with negative effects on survival and quality of life. There is within some of these mechanisms a mutually reinforcing aspect; for example, anorexia leads to fatigue, fatigue increases anorexia, anorexia increases fatigue, and so on. Table 9–2 summarizes the mechanisms and effects of ACS.

The anorexia/cachexia syndrome is categorized as primary or secondary, depending on its etiology. Primary ACS results from endogenous metabolic abnormalities such as cytokine production which stimulates chronic inflammation and resulting catabolism. The syndrome is called secondary if it results from exogenous etiologies, caused by symptoms which interfere with the intake or absorption of nutrients. Examples of such interfering symptoms are pain, nausea, intestinal obstruction, or psychosocial distress.[7]

---

**Table 9–1**
**Anorexia/Cachexia Syndrome in Various Disease States**

| Disease | Terminology | Estimated Prevalence: Highest In Advanced Disease |
|---------|-------------|---------------------------------------------------|
| Cancer | Cancer-related ACS | Up to 86% |
| CHF | Cardiac cachexia | 16–36% |
| COPD | Pulmonary cachexia syndrome | 30–70% |
| HIV disease | HIV wasting syndrome | 10–35% |
| Renal disease | MIC: Malnutrition-Inflammation Cachexia syndrome | 30–60% |

*Sources*: Adapted from Bennani-Baiti & Davis (2008), reference 1; Morley et al. (2006), reference 3; Tan & Fearon (2003), reference 5.

---

**Table 9–2**
**Mechanisms and Effects of ACS**

| Mechanisms | Effect |
|------------|--------|
| Loss of appetite | Generalized host tissue wasting, nausea or "sick feeling," loss of socialization and pleasure at meals |
| Reduced voluntary motor activity (fatigue) | Skeletal muscle wasting and inanition (fatigue) |
| Reduced rate of muscle protein synthesis | Skeletal muscle wasting and asthenia (weakness) |
| Decreased immune response | Increased susceptibility to infections |
| Decreased response to therapy | Earlier demise and increased complications of illness |

*Sources*: Adapted from Bennani-Baiti & Davis (2008), reference 1; Morley et al. (2006), reference 3; Strasser (2005), reference 13.

## Primary ACS

The pathogenesis of primary ACS is multifactorial, complex, and incompletely understood. Accumulating evidence suggests that chronic illness disrupts the homeostatic function of the central nervous system leading to profound metabolic changes. Peripheral input causes the awareness of threats such as a growing tumor, or cardiac or renal failure, and this promotes a catabolic effect which results in increased energy expenditure, reduced intake, increased muscle breakdown, and loss of adipose tissue.[4]

## Metabolic Alterations

Metabolic alterations are common in cancer and other diseases and are thought to be due in large part to the systemic inflammatory response and stimulation of cytokine production (principally tumor necrosis factor alpha [TNF-$\alpha$], prostaglandins [PG], interleukin-1 [IL-1], interleukin-6 [IL-6], interferon $\alpha$ [IFN-$\alpha$], and interferon $\beta$ [IFN-$\beta$]). Other catabolic tumor-derived factors thought to play a role in cachexia include proteolysis-inducing factor (PIF) and lipid mobilizing factor (LMF).[7] Major metabolic alterations include glucose intolerance, insulin resistance, increased lipolysis, increased skeletal muscle catabolism, negative nitrogen balance and, in some patients, increased basal energy expenditure.[7]

A number of different theories regarding the pathophysiology of ACS are under study. The maladaptive activation of oxidative processes which may be seen in chronic illness are also thought to be partially responsible for the cachexia syndrome.[12] Recent advances in genomics suggest that specific genetic polymorphisms contribute to the prominent inflammatory component of this problem.[12] The melanocortin system of the hypothalamus which coordinates appetite and feeding is influenced by peptide hormones such as leptin[7] and ghrelin.[13] Disturbances in these hormonally regulated feedback loops appear to play a role in ACS. Other potential mediators of ACS include testosterone, insulin-like growth factor-1, myostatin, and adrenal hormones.[3] In sum, the underlying pathophysiological processes of ACS are complex and not yet fully understood. Researchers postulate that the above mechanisms play different roles of varying importance in different diseases.[7] The relative importance of these factors and the interplay among them remains unclear. However, irrespective of the underlying mechanism or specific medical illness, patients experience progressive worsening of their clinical condition, and ultimately they perish soon after the development of cachexia.[11]

## Secondary ACS

Secondary causes of ACS include exogenous factors that can frequently lead to weight loss, anorexia, fatigue, or other symptoms associated with this wasting syndrome.

## Physical Symptoms

A number of physical symptoms of advanced disease may contribute to or cause anorexia, including pain, dysguesia (abnormalities in taste, especially aversion to meat), ageusia (loss of taste), hyperosmia (increased sensitivity to odor), hyposmia (decreased sensitivity to odor), anosmia (absence of sense of smell), stomatitis, dysphagia, odynophagia, dyspnea, hepatomegaly, splenomegaly, gastric compression, delayed emptying, malabsorption, intestinal obstruction, nausea, vomiting, diarrhea, constipation, inanition, asthenia, various infections (see below), and early satiety. Alcoholism or other substance dependence may also contribute to or cause anorexia. Primary or metastatic disease sites have an effect on appetite, with cancers, such as gastric and pancreatic, having direct effects on organs of alimentation.[15]

In general, people who are seriously ill and/or suffering distressing symptoms have poor appetites. In addition, in cancer, metabolic paraneoplastic syndromes such as hypercalcemia or hyponatremia (SIADH) may also cause anorexia or symptoms such as fatigue that contribute to anorexia. Patients with HIV disease may also develop primary muscle disease, leading to weight loss. Many cancer or human immunodeficiency virus (HIV) treatments have deleterious effects on appetite or result in side effects leading to anorexia and/or weight loss.[15,16] Each of these should be ruled out as a contributing cause of anorexia and, if present, treated as discussed elsewhere in this book.

## Treatment Side Effects

Many interventions used to treat advanced chronic disease have adverse effects on nutritional status. The many medications used to treat HIV/AIDS and its sequela are an excellent example. Despite the success of HAART in curbing ACS in many patients, the myriad of medications involved in the prevention and treatment of AIDS complications often lead to anorexia and malabsorption themselves.[17] Cytotoxic drugs can be emetogenic, cause taste changes, or cause other GI side effects such as oral stomatitis and diarrhea.[16] Radiotherapy can also lead to significant side effects, including nausea, vomiting, diarrhea, xerostomia, and severe fatigue.[16] Among patients with advanced renal disease on dialysis, there is a high prevalence of protein-energy malnutrition.[18]

## Psychological and/or Spiritual Distress

Psychological and spiritual distress are often overlooked causes of anorexia. The physical effects of the illness and/or treatment coupled with psychological responses (especially anxiety and depression) and spiritual distress, may result in little enthusiasm or energy for preparing or eating food. As weight is lost, and energy decreases, changes in self image occur. Appetite and the ability to eat are key determinants of physical and psychological quality of life. [15] Cultural influences must always be considered. For example, for Southeast and East Asians, some degree of obesity is perceived as a sign of good health and weight loss is seen as a clear sign of declining health.[19] For many patients, the net result of ACS and weight loss constitute a negative-feedback loop of ever-increasing magnitude and increased suffering in multiple dimensions. Clinicians evaluating patients with anorexia are encouraged to review basic principles for the assessment and management of depression, as covered in detail in Chapter 20. Treatment of underlying depression can improve appetite considerably.

## Oral Issues

Special attention should be directed toward the oral cavity of patients with advanced disease. The fit of dentures may change with illness, or already poorly fitting dentures may not be as well tolerated in advanced disease. Dental pain may be overlooked in the context of terminal illness. Oral and esophageal infections and complications increase with disease progression and immunocompromise. Xerostomia and worsening of tooth decay can occur with radiation therapy. Basic oral hygiene can often be neglected in the setting of advanced illness. Aphthous ulcers, mucositis, candidiasis, aspergillosis, herpes simplex, and bacterial infections cause oral or esophageal pain and, thus, anorexia.[15,16,20]

## Assessment

Anorexia and weight loss may begin insidiously with slightly decreased appetite and slight weight loss characteristic of virtually any illness. As the disease progresses and comorbid conditions increase in number and severity, anorexia and malnutrition increase, and a mutually reinforcing process may emerge. For example, poor appetite and intake leads to fatigue, which in turn leads to more pronounced anorexia and malnutrition, which then leads to increased fatigue and weakness that may accelerate the metabolic processes of ACS.

With ACS common, and in many cases inevitable, among patients with advanced or terminal illness, identifying specific causes is an extremely challenging task. There is of yet no clear and widely accepted definition or diagnostic criteria for ACS. There have been standardized tools for the general assessment of nutrition status, but none specific to ACS for palliative care.[21] Nevertheless, anorexia from some etiologies is treatable; hence, assessment of the possible presence of etiologies noted above is integral to quality palliative care. Assessment parameters are used according to the patient's ability to tolerate and benefit from the assessment.

Assessment parameters should include appetite, nutritional intake, and basic nutritional status.[21] Appetite is a component of several well validated tools of global symptom assessment, such as the Edmonton Symptom Assessment Scale[23] or the Memorial Symptom Assessment Scale.[24] In addition, simple assessment questions about change in appetite can be transformed into a numerical assessment scale. Intake can be measured retrospectively by recall or prospectively by calorie count. Detailed exploration with appropriate physical examination can identify associated factors (i.e., dysphagia, nausea, oral issues, or pain). Open ended questions can be helpful in eliciting specific characteristics of the eating problem.

A variety of methods can be used to assess nutritional status, from basic tools such as the Subjective Global Assessment for Nutrition (SGA) to sophisticated anthropometric and laboratory testing.[22] Common lab values may reveal decreased serum albumin, a prognostic indicator of increased morbidity and mortality, as well as changes in several electrolyte and mineral levels.[16]

Perhaps the most important component of assessment in ACS involves the patient's goals of care. Since palliative care encompasses the entire disease continuum, stage of illness and goals of care should be clearly determined before detailed assessment and intervention are planned or initiated. It is imperative to evaluate the degree of suffering or distress experienced as a result of the ACS. A cost/benefit analysis should be undertaken to determine if a diagnostic workup is valuable in light of the effort, cost, or discomfort it may incur. At some point in the illness, even basic assessments, such as weight, serve only to decrease the patient's quality of life. Assessment parameters are summarized in Table 9–3.

---

**Table 9–3**
**Assessment Parameters in Anorexia and Cachexia**

The patient is likely to report anorexia and/or early satiety.

Weakness (asthenia) and fatigue are present.

Mental status declines, with decreased attention span and ability to concentrate. Depression may increase concurrently.

Inspection/observation may show progressive muscle wasting, loss of strength, and decreased fat. There often is increased total body water, and edema may thus mask some wasting.

Weight may decrease. Weight may reflect nutritional status or fluid accumulation or loss.

Increased weight in the presence of heart disease suggests heart failure.

Triceps skinfold thickness decreases with protein calorie malnutrition (PCM, skinfold thickness and mid-arm circumference vary with hydration status).

Mid-arm muscle circumference decreases with PCM.

Serum albumin concentrations decrease as nutritional status declines. Albumin has a half-life of 20 days; hence, it is less affected by current intake than other measures.

Other lab values associated with anorexia/cachexia syndrome include anemia, increased triglycerides, decreased nitrogen balance, and glucose intolerance.[1,3,7,13]

*Sources:* Bennani-Baiti & Davis (2008), reference 1; Morley, et al. (2006), reference 3; Innui (2002), reference 7; Strasser (2005), reference 13.

Assessment also includes a psychosocial evaluation, particularly concerning food, determining usual intake patterns, food likes and dislikes, and the meaning of food or eating to the patient and family. Too often, a family member attaches huge significance to nutritional intake and exerts pressure on the patient to increase intake: "If he would just get enough to eat." Giving sustenance is a fundamental means of caring and nurturing, and it is no surprise that the presence of devastating illness often evokes an almost primitive urge to give food.

In some cases the patient is less troubled than the family by poor nutritional intake. Clinicians should explore the meaning of feeding in the context of the family's cultural and religious background, and help identify other ways in which the family can participate in caring for the patient.[25]

## Interventions

The palliative approach to care of the patient with ACS focuses on improving patient comfort and minimizing distress caused by the anorexia and weight loss. Assisting patients and families to adapt to progressive symptoms and alleviating symptoms which may be exacerbating the problem are two foci of interventions. Interventions may combine a variety of approaches, including exogenous symptom management, nutritional support, enteral and parenteral nutrition, pharmacological management, and psychosocial support.

### (Exogenous) Symptom Management

The presence of symptoms that may cause or exacerbate secondary anorexia and weight loss should be evaluated. For example, if anorexia is due to an identifiable problem, such as pain, nausea, fatigue, depression, or taste disorder, appropriate interventions as discussed elsewhere in this book should be instituted.

### Nutritional Support

Oral nutritional support, to increase intake or to maximize nutritional content, may be helpful to some extent, especially early in the disease process or in specific disease states. For example, there is strong evidence that nutritional supplementation can be effective in patients with COPD.[5] However, cancer related ACS studies have been disappointing. The current evidence reveals that improving the quantity and quality of nutrition does not improve lean body mass in patients with cancer.[27] A recent systematic review on non-pharmacologic interventions found that interventions which were able to increase protein and calorie intake showed no resulting improvement in nutritional status, tumor response, survival, or quality of life.[29]

Helping family members understand nutritional needs and limitations in terminal situations is essential. Consultation with a nutritionist is usually warranted for the purpose of education and recommendation of appropriate supplements. General guidelines for nutritional interventions include the following:[16,19, 22, 25–28]

- The nutritional quality of intake should be evaluated and, if possible and appropriate, modified to improve the quality. Patients who are not moribund may benefit from supplementary sources of protein and calories. Clinicians should determine the meaning to the patient and family of giving, taking, and refusing food. Strong and even unconscious beliefs about food are difficult to modify, and many families require education and frequent support in the face of helplessness and frustration related to ever-diminishing intake.

- Culturally appropriate or favored foods should be encouraged. Preserving cultural or social traditions around meals may also be helpful. Families should be encouraged to share mealtime with patients or continue habits such as a glass of wine with meals, if medically appropriate.
- Small meals, on the patient's schedule and according to the taste and whims of the patient, are helpful, at least emotionally, and should be instituted early in the illness so that eating does not become burdensome.
- Foods with different tastes, textures, temperatures, seasonings, degrees of spiciness, degrees of moisture, and colors, for example, should be tried, but the family should be cautioned against overwhelming the patient with a constant parade of foods to try. Room temperature and less spicy foods are preferred by many patients.
- Different liquids should also be tried. Cold, clear liquids are usually well tolerated and enjoyed, though cultural constraints may exist. For example, patients with illnesses that are classified as "cold" by some Southeast Asians and Latinos are thought to be harmed by taking drinks or foods that are either cold in temperature or thought to have "cold" properties.
- Measures as basic as timing intake may also be instituted. Patients who experience early satiety, for example, should take the most nutritious part of the meal first. Filling fluids without nutritional value (such as carbonated soda) should be avoided at mealtime Oral care must be considered an integral part of nutritional support. Hygiene and management of any oral pain are essential in nutritional support. Procedures, treatments, psychological upsets (negative or positive), or other stresses or activities should be limited prior to meals.

### Enteral and Parenteral Nutrition

Enteral feeding (via nasoenteral tube, gastrostomy, or jejunostomy) may be indicated in a small subset of terminally ill patients. Many clinicians postulate that there exist certain patients with a relevent starvational secondary component to their ACS, and that these patients may benefit from invasive nutritional interventions. Examples include patients with head and neck cancer with severe dysphagia who are undergoing radiation therapy, patients with slow growing tumors causing bowel obstruction, patients undergoing certain surgeries for UGI malignancies, or those undergoing bone marrow transplant.[12] However, the evidence remains insufficient to recommend specific guidelines, and the clinical indications in non-cancer diagnoses are less defined.[26]

The use of parenteral nutrition in ACS has been controversial within the palliative care field.[17,30] Some guidelines recommend the use of PPN or TPN for a subset of patients who meet the following criteria: total gastrointestinal failure, limited life expectancy were TPN not initiated, expected survival of more than a few months, and sufficient performance status, QOL, and home environment for the successful use of the intervention.[30] However, sytstematic reviews evaluating the use of TPN in cancer patients found very limited benefit.[22] The use of parenteral nutrition should be carefully assessed on an individual basis. Although it may have clinical implications in a few patients, it has greater potential for complications than does enteral nutrition, seldom improves outcomes, and thus is rarely indicated in terminally ill patients with advanced disease.[2,13] The choice of nutritional support depends on the cause of the malnutrition, the expected survival, goals of care and planned therapy, and patient preferences. General consensus within palliative care is that the indications for parenteral nutrition are limited and routine use should be discouraged.[13]

## Pharmacological Interventions

A plethora of pharmacologic studies have targeted cancer-related ACS,[1,7,26] and recent work includes other chronic advanced disease.[4,11,13,14] The most frequently prescribed and most studied drug is Megestrol Acetate (MA), a synthetic progestogen agent which acts to increase appetite and weight gain. Although the mechanisms by which MA operate are not well understood, most hypothesis suggest that the medication acts on cytokines, inhibiting the tumor necrosis factor.[30]

A recent Cochrane review[31] reviewed 34 trials which examined different aspects of the use of MA to stimulate appetite and weight gain. The review found that MA significantly increased both appetite and weight in cancer patients, but there was not enough evidence to make definitive conclusions about its effect on quality of life, the optimal medication dose, or the effects of MA on patients with other underlying diagnoses. Side effects of Megestrol Acetate include hypoadrenalism, hypogonadism, and most concerning, thrombosis and DVT. However, the recent systematic reviews[30,31] found the rate of adverse effects to be insignificant, and concluded that MA is an effective and safe medication for improving appetite and weight in cancer patients. The medication has also shown positive results in patients with COPD and AIDS.[32,36] The benefit of Megestrol in other non-cancer diagnoses remains unclear; more study is needed to make conclusive recommendations. However, it has not been studied in heart failure, and more study is needed to make conclusive recommendations in non-cancer diagnoses.

Glucocorticoids are widely used in the palliative care setting to address a number of symptoms, including pain, dyspnea, and nausea.[15] In cancer patients, steroids have been shown to have a limited positive effect (up to four weeks) on appetite, nutritional intake, and sense of well being, but no demonstrable effect on weight.[7] The wide range of side effects, including adrenal suppression, hyperglycemia, and peptic ulceration may preclude its use in some patients.

Cannabinoids have shown similar positive effects: improved appetite and mood, but without weight gain.[7] However, the CNS side effects also limit use of this medication. Commonly used pharmacological options with indications and notable side effects are presented in Table 9–4.

**Table 9–4**
**Medications Commonly Used in ACS**

| Medication Effects and Common Dosing | Indications | Side Effects and Considerations |
|---|---|---|
| **Progestational agents** esp: Megestrol acetate 160–800 mg/day | Improves appetite, weight gain, and sense of well being | Thromboembolic events, glucocorticoid effects, GI upset, heart failure, menstrual abnormalities, tumor flare |
| **Corticosteroids** e.g.: Decadron 4 mg/day | Improves appetite and sense of well being | Immunosuppression, masks infection, HTN, myopathy, GI disturbances, dermal atrophy, increased ICP, electrolyte imbalances, avoid abrupt cessation |
| **Cannabinoids** Dronabinol 5–20 mg/day | Increases appetite and decreases anxiety | Somnolence, confusion, dysphoria, especially in elderly |
| **Metoclopramide** 10 mg before meals | Improves gastric emptying, decreases early satiety, improves appetite | Diarrhea, restlessness, fatigue, drowsiness, extrapyrimidal S/E |

*Sources:* Innui (2002), reference 7; Rosenzweig (2006), reference 16; Berenstain & Ortiz (2008), reference 32; Bruera et al. (2005), reference 33.

## Table 9-5
### Components of a Multimodal Approach to ACS

1. Early and ongoing determination of goals of care.
2. Optimal treatment of underlying disease according to goals of care.
3. Prevention, recognition, and prompt treatment of exogenous causes.
4. Guidance from nutrition specialists.
5. Appropriate pharmacologic interventions.
6. Resistance exercise as appropriate.
7. Compassionate counseling to patient, family, and significant caregivers.

*Sources:* Rosenzweig (2006), reference 16; Fainsinger & Pereira (2005), reference 22; Institute for Clinical Systems Improvement (2008), reference 25; Andrew et al. (2007), reference 28; Zinna & Yarasheski (2003), reference 35.

Future directions in pharmacologic management target various pathways implicated in ACS. Neurohormonal manipulation, cytokine inhibition, and anti-inflammatory interventions all show some promise in clinical trials.

The peptide hormone ghrelin is a circulating mediator of appetite and has been implicated in ACS. Early trials which supplement ghrelin in various illnesses have shown short-term increases in caloric intake in patients with cancer and renal failure, and improved lean body mass and exercise capacity in those with COPD and CHF.[14]

Thalidomide is a controversial medication of interest to ACS researchers. Previously withdrawn from the market due to its teratogenic side effects, thalidomide is now under study in advanced disease due to its potent anti-emetic and TNF inhibitor activity. Although its safety profile remains a concern, this medication may be a useful option and is under study.[1,33,34] Other medications under study include melanocortin (thought to decrease circulating TNF), various anabolic steroids, such as growth factor, insulin-like growth factor, and testosterone derivatives, N-3 polyunsaturated fatty acids (as found in fish oils), B-adrenergic agonists, and anti-inflammatory medications.[7,11,12]

## Multimodal Approach

The devastating consequences, pathophysiologic complexities, and treatment resistance of ACS lead inevitably to consideration of a multimodal approach.[15,16,22,25,28] A summary of what should be included in this approach is summarized in Table 9-5.

CASE STUDY
### Some Issues Commonly Associated with ACS

Mr. WD was an 84-year-old man with hormone refractory prostate cancer treated with radiation therapy for bone metastasis in his thoracic spine. He was residing in a long-term care facility while undergoing rehabilitative therapy for deconditioning. A community hospice consulted on his care. Although Mr. D's previous symptom of bone pain was well controlled on opioids, the staff noted that he had become less energetic, more withdrawn, staying in his room, and eating less. His weight had dropped eight pounds in the past month. Six months previously he had developed a left DVT while on Megestrol Acetate, so this was not a therapeutic option.

Upon closer assessment, the nurse discovered that Mr. D had been experiencing opioid-induced constipation and fatigue (felt to be related to his past radiation and underlying anemia of chronic disease). He complained of anorexia and early satiety. He was started on Decadron 4 mgm QD, and his constipation resolved with an improved bowel regimen. The patient initially felt more energy and slight increase in appetite, but this was short lived, and within two weeks, he refused to get out of bed and barely interacted with staff and family. At this point, he only took about ½ can of supplement drink for each meal. His wife became despondent and frustrated that he was "giving up."

The staff performed a basic screen and felt that the patient was depressed. He was started on Methylphenidrate 2.5 mgm at 8 AM and 12 PM. with resulting increase in activity, mood, and appetite. He continued to lose weight, but with counseling, his wife understood that his anorexia and weight loss were mostly related to his underlying cancer. The patient's daughter arrived from out of state to assist with care, and he was able to return home where he died peacefully three weeks later.

## Summary

Increasingly, ACS is recognized as a serious aspect of advanced or terminal illness and as an area requiring further research, especially with respect to (1) the pathophysiology of cachexia and (2) increasing treatment options.

The management of ACS is complicated by numerous obstacles, including lack of clear definition and guidelines, inconsistency in assessment and management strategies, and knowledge deficits about this complex clinical syndrome in health professionals and caregiving families. The challenge is compounded by the interwoven emotional symbolism of food and nurturance. As palliative care providers, we should strive to support, understand, and translate the developing evidence which guides our care . The complex and potentially devastating impact of this problem demands a holistic response. Palliative care nurses are optimally situated to coordinate and drive the necessary multidisciplinary approach to address anorexia and cachexia in advanced, progressive disease.

Current understanding of ACS includes the following:

- Anorexia and cachexia are distinct syndromes but clinically difficult to differentiate.

- Anorexia is characterized by decreased appetite that may result from a variety of causes (including unmanaged symptoms such as nausea and pain) It results primarily in loss of fat tissue, and resultant weight loss is reversible.
- Cachexia is a complex metabolic syndrome thought to result from the production of proinflammatory cytokines such as TNF and IL-1. In cachexia, there is approximately equal loss of fat and muscle and significant loss of bone mineral content. Weight loss from cachexia does not respond to nutritional interventions.
- Assessment and treatment of ACS include determination of whether exogenous etiologies such as nausea or pain are involved, the vigorous treatment of any such etiologies, and nutritional support if indicated.
- Treatment of cachexia is unsatisfactory, but some temporary gains may occur with progestational agents, especially megestrol acetate and a multimodal approach such as discussed above.

## REFERENCES

1. Bennami-Baiti N, Davis MP. Cytokines and the cancer anorexia cachexia syndrome. Am J Hosp Palliat Care 2008;25:407–409.
2. Van Halteran HK, Bongaerts GPA, Wagener DJ. Cancer cachexia: what is known about its etiology and what should be the current treatment approach? Anticancer Res 2003;23:5111–5116.
3. Morley JE, Thomas DR, Wilson MG. Cachexia: pathophysiology and clinical relevance. J Clin Nutr 2006;83:735–743.
4. Laviano A, Innui A, Marks DL, Meguid MM, Pichard C, Fanelli Fr, Seelander M. Neural control of the anorexia-cachexia syndrome. Am J Physiol Endrocrinol Metab 2008;298:E1000–E1008.
5. Tan BH, Fearon KC. Cachexia: prevalence and impact in medicine. Curr Opin Clin Nutr Metab Care 2003;11:400–407.
6. Doehner W. Cardiac cachexia in early literature: a review of research. Int J Cardiol 2002;85:7–14.
7. Innui A. Cancer anorexia–cachexia syndrome: current issues in research and management. CA: Cancer J Clin 2002;52:72–91.
8. Hauser C, Stockler M, Tattersall M. Prognostic factors in patients with recently diagnosed incurable cancer: a systematic review. Support Care Cancer 2006;14:999–1011.
9. Maltoni M, Caraceni A, Brunelli C, Broeckaert B, Christakis N, Eychmueller S, Glare P, Nabal M, Vigano A, Larkin P, DeConno F, Hanks G, Kaasa S. Prognostic factors in advanced cancer patients: evidence-based clinical recommendations—a study by the steering committee of the European Association for Palliative Care. J Clin Oncol 2005;23:6240–6248.
10. Anker S, Negrassa A, Coat AJ, Afzal R, Poole-Wilson RA, Cohn JN, Yusuf S. Prognostic importance of weight loss in chronic heart failure and the affect of treatment with angiotensin-converting enzyme: an observational study. The Lancet 361:1077–1083.
11. Lainscak M, Podbregar M, Anker SD. How does cachexia influence survival in cancer, heart failure, and other chronic diseases? Curr Opin Supp Pall Care 2007;1:299–305.
12. Kalantar-Zadeh K, Anker SD, Horwich TB, Fonarow GC. Nutritional and anti-inflammatory interventions in chronic heart failure. Am J Card 2008;101:89E–103E.
13. Strasser F. Pathophysiology of the anorexia/cachexia syndrome. In: Doyle D, Hank G, Cherny NI, Calman K, eds. Oxford Textbook of Palliative Medicine, 3rd ed. Oxford: Oxford University Press, 2005:520–530.
14. Ashby D, Choi P, Bloom S. Gut hormones and the treatment of disease cachexia. Proc Nut Soc 2008;67:263–269.
15. Cunningham RS. The anorexia–cachexia syndrome. In: Yarbro CH, Frogge MH, Goodman M, eds. Cancer Symptom Management, 3rd ed. Boston: Jones and Bartlett, 2004: 137–167.
16. Rosenzweig MQ. Anorexia/cachexia. In: Camp-Sorrell D, Hawkins RA, eds. Clinical Manual for the Oncology Advanced Practice Nurse, 2nd ed. Pittsburgh: Oncology Nursing Society, 2006.
17. Woodruff R, Glare P. AIDS in adults. In: Doyle D, Hanks G, Cherny NI, Calman K, eds. Oxford Textbook of Palliative Medicine, 3rd ed. Oxford: Oxford University Press, 520–530.
18. Kalantar-Zadeh K, Ikizler TA, Block G. Malnutrition–inflammation–cachexia syndrome in dialysis patients: causes and consequences. Am J Kidney Dis 2003;42:864–881.
19. Kemp C, Rasbridge L. Refugee & Immigrant Health. Cambridge: Cambridge University Press, 2004.
20. Stroll RA, Camp-Sorrell D. Stomatitis/xerostomia. In: Camp-Sorrell D, Hawkins RA, eds. Clinical Manual for the Oncology Advanced Practice Nurse, 2nd ed. Pittsburgh: Oncology Nursing Society, 2006.
21. Churm D, Andrew IM, Holden K, Hildreth AJ, Hawkins C. A questionnaire study of the approach to the anorexia–cachexia syndrome in patients with cancer by staff in a district general hospital. Support Care Cancer, 2009;17:503–507.
22. Fainsinger RL, Pereira J. Clinical assessment and decision-making in cachexia and anorexia. In: Doyle D, Hanks G, Cherny NI, Calman K, eds. Oxford Textbook of Palliative Medicine, 3rd ed. Oxford: Oxford University Press, 200: 520–530.
23. Bruera E, The Edmonton Symptom Assessment Scale: A simple method for the assessment of palliative care patients. J Pall Care 1991;2:6–9.
24. Chang VT, Hwang SS, Kasimis B, Thaler B. Shorter symptom assessment instruments: The Condensed Memorial Symptom Assessment Scale (CMSAS). Cancer Invest 2004;22:526–536.
25. Institute for Clinical Systems Improvement. Clinical Practice Guideline: Palliative Care 2008. Retrieved November 15 from: http://www.guideline.gov/summary/summary.aspx?doc_id=12618&nr=0065268&string=cachexia.
26. Lennie TA, Nutritional self-care in heart failure: state of the science. J Cardiovasc Nurs 2008;23:197–204.
27. Brown JK. A systematic review of the evidence on symptom management of cancer-related anorexia and cachexia. Oncol Nurs Forum 2002;29:517–532.
28. Andrew I, Hawkins C, Waterfield K, Kirkpatrick G, Williams S. Anorexia–cachexia syndrome—improving the patient experience. Hosp Pharmacist 2007;14:265–266.
29. Yavuzsen T, Davis MP, Walsh D, LeGrand S, Lagman R. Systematic review of the treatment of cancer-associated anorexia and weight loss. J Clin Oncol 2005;23:8500–8511.

30. Mirhosseini MD, Fainsinger RL, Baracos V. Parenteral nutrition in advanced cancer: indications and clinical practice guidelines. J Pall Med 8:914–918.

31. Lopez AP, Figuls MR, Cuchi GU, Berenstain EG, Pasies BA, Alegre MB, Herdman M. Systematic review of megestrol acetate in the treatment of anorexi cachexia syndrome. J Pain & Symptom Mange 27:360–369.

32. Berenstain EG, Ortiz Z. Megestrol aceate for treatment of anorexia–cachexia syndrome. Cochrane Database Syst Rev 2008;4:1–8.

33. Bruera E, Sweeney C. Pharmacological interventions in cachexia and anorexia. In: Doyle D, Hanks G, Cherny NI, Calman K, eds. Oxford Textbook of Palliative Medicine, 3rd ed. Oxford: Oxford University Press, 2005:520–530.

34. Tassineri D, Santelmo C, Tombesi P, Sartori S. Thalidomide in the treatment of cancer cachexia. J Palliat Care 2008;24:187–189.

35. Zinna EM, Yarasheki KE. Exercise treatment to counteract protein wasting of chronic diseases. Curr Opin Clin Nutr Metab Care 2003;6:87–93.

36. Weisberg J, Wanger J, Olson J, Streit B, Fogaraty C, Martin T, Casaburi, R. Megestrol acetate stimulates weight gain and ventilation in underweight COPD patients. Chest 2002;121:1070–1078.

# 10 &#127803; Cynthia King and Dana Tarcatu

# Nausea and Vomiting

*I feel so nauseated all the time. I am miserable. Even the smell of food makes me retch. It is hard on my family. —Palliative care patient*

♦ **Key Points**

♦ *Nausea and vomiting are common and significant symptoms experienced by over 50% of patients with advanced diseases.*

♦ *There are multiple receptors in the central nervous system which are involved in the development of nausea.*

♦ *Blocking of these receptors forms the basis of antiemetic medications. These receptors are: dopaminergic, muscarinic, cholinergic, histaminic, and serotonergic.*

♦ *The choice of antiemetic therapy should be based on the presumed underlying cause of the nausea, i.e. a mechanism-based approach.*

♦ *Nurses in all settings can play an important role in advancing the knowledge and skills related to nausea and vomiting in palliative care.*

Nausea and vomiting are symptoms commonly experienced by patients with advanced disease. The majority of available research on nausea and vomiting deals with cancer patients.[1] Therefore, this chapter will use advanced cancer patients as a model for assessment and treatment of nausea and vomiting, but these principles can be extrapolated to other patients with advanced non-oncological diseases. For cancer patients, nausea and vomiting may be experienced secondary to the underlying malignancy, as well as to the frequent treatment toxicities. To date, most research has been focused on treatment-induced nausea and vomiting in patients receiving chemotherapy used either with curative or palliative intent. Unfortunately, there is a paucity of literature on the assessment and management of nausea and vomiting in cancer patients who are experiencing these symptoms from causes other than chemotherapy or terminal illness.[2]

Research has shown that over 50% of patients with advanced cancer experience nausea and/or vomiting. These symptoms are more common in patients under 65 years old, in women, and in patients with cancer of the gastro-intestinal tract or breast. For stomach cancer, the high frequency may be due to local causes such as gastric outlet obstruction. For breast cancer, the causes may be multifactorial and include metabolic abnormalities like hypercalcemia, increased intracranial pressure from brain metastases, medications, and gender.[3–5] Ross and Alexander[5] describe the "11 Ms" of nausea and vomiting in terminally ill patients. These include: (1) metastases (cerebral or liver), (2) meningeal irritation, (3) movement (causing vestibular stimulation), (4) mentation (e.g., cerebral cortex), (5) medications (e.g., opioids, chemotherapy), (6) mucosal irritation (e.g., hyperacidity, gastroesophageal reflux), (7) mechanical obstruction (e.g., constipation, obstipation, tumor), (8) motility (e.g., ileus), (9) metabolic imbalance (e.g., hypercalcemia, hyponatremia), (10) microbes (e.g., esophagitis), and (11) myocardial dysfunction (e.g., ischemia, congestive heart failure).

The level of distress associated with nausea and vomiting may be profound.[6,7] If these symptoms are left untreated, they can interfere with usual daily activities, increase anxiety and other symptoms, and impair quality of life (QOL).[7–13] It is essential that these symptoms be adequately treated throughout the trajectory of cancer care and across all settings. As more aggressive symptom control is provided in outpatient settings like patients' homes and hospices, it is important to involve the patients and their families in the management of nausea and vomiting. Nurses who provide palliative care to cancer patients of any age and in any setting need to have the skills to adequately assess for nausea and vomiting, and provide appropriate pharmacologic and nonpharmacologic interventions.[10]

Teaching of self-care to patients and families is essential, as is the evaluation of the outcomes of all interventions. The approach must be practical, with the goal being relief of symptoms as soon as possible. Management should be "mechanism based" and reflect the most likely underlying cause of the nausea and vomiting.

## Nausea and Vomiting and Quality of Life

The distress and disruption in daily activities caused by nausea and vomiting impairs QOL for patients with advanced disease. Although there is controversy over the number and exact dimensions of QOL, the City of Hope National Medical Center QOL model includes four dimensions: physical well-being, psychological well-being, social well-being, and spiritual well-being.[14] The impact of nausea and vomiting is reflected on one or all of the four dimensions of QOL (Figure 10–1).[15] Therefore adequate management of nausea and vomiting can positively affect all dimensions of a patient's QOL. The patient may regain a sense of control over his or her body and life, anxiety and fear as well as fatigue may decrease, some degree of appetite may be regained, and there may be an increase in the patient's physical, social, and cognitive functioning even at the end of life. Caregiver burden may also be markedly lessened.[13,15]

## Conceptual Concerns Related to Nausea and Vomiting

To thoroughly examine the problem of nausea and vomiting in palliative care, it is important to be clear about certain concepts. Symptoms such as nausea and vomiting are composed of subjective components and dimensions unique to each patient. Symptoms are different from signs, which are objective and can be observed by the health care professional.[16,17] Symptom occurrence is comprised of the frequency, duration, and severity with which the symptom presents.[13] Symptom distress involves the degree or amount of physical, mental or emotional upset and suffering experienced by an individual. This is different from symptom occurrence.[16,17] Lastly, symptom experience involves the individual's perception and response to the occurrence and distress of the symptom.[16,17]

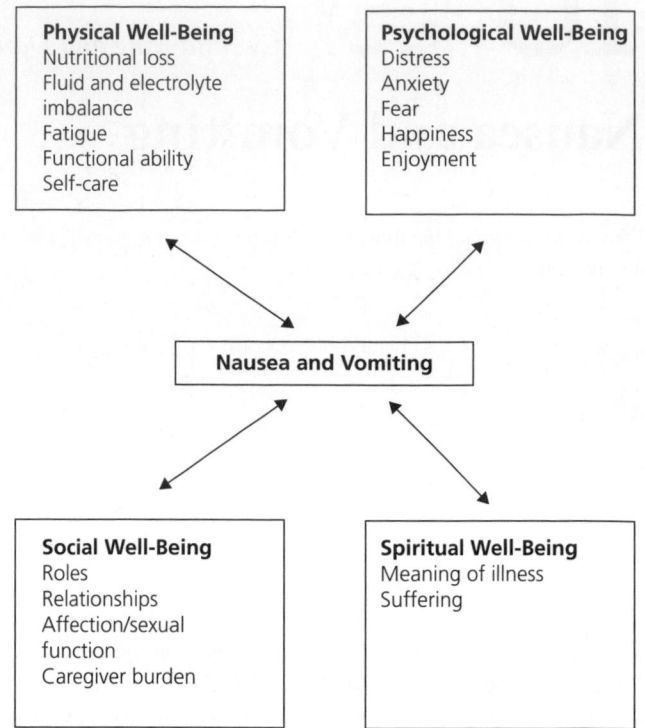

**Figure 10–1.** The effect of nausea and vomiting on the domains of quality of life (QOL). *Source*: Grant (1997), reference 15, used with permission.

The terms "nausea" and "vomiting" represent clearly distinct concepts. Unfortunately, terms used to describe them are frequently used interchangeably. This may result in confusion during assessment, measurement, treatment, or patient and family education. Nausea is a subjective symptom involving an unpleasant sensation experienced in the back of the throat and the epigastrium, which may or may not result in vomiting.[16–19] Other terms used by patients include "sick to my stomach," "butterflies," "queasiness" and "fish at sea." The symptoms of increased salivation, dizziness, light-headedness, difficulty swallowing, and tachycardia may accompany the feeling of nausea. Patterns of nausea include acute, delayed, and anticipatory. Acute nausea occurs within minutes or hours after events such as having chemotherapy. Delayed nausea generally occurs at least 24 hours after events like chemotherapy and may last for several days. Anticipatory nausea occurs before the actual stimulus and develops only after an individual has had a previous bad experience with an event such as chemotherapy that resulted in nausea or vomiting.[16,17,19–22]

Vomiting is often confused with nausea but is, in fact, a separate phenomenon and may or may not occur in conjunction with nausea. It is a self-protective mechanism by which the body attempts to expel toxic substances and involves the expulsion of gastric contents through the mouth, caused by forceful contraction of the abdominal muscles. Vomiting is frequently described as "throwing up," "pitching," "barfing," or "upchucking." Retching involves the spasmodic contractions of the diaphragm and abdominal muscles.[16–20]

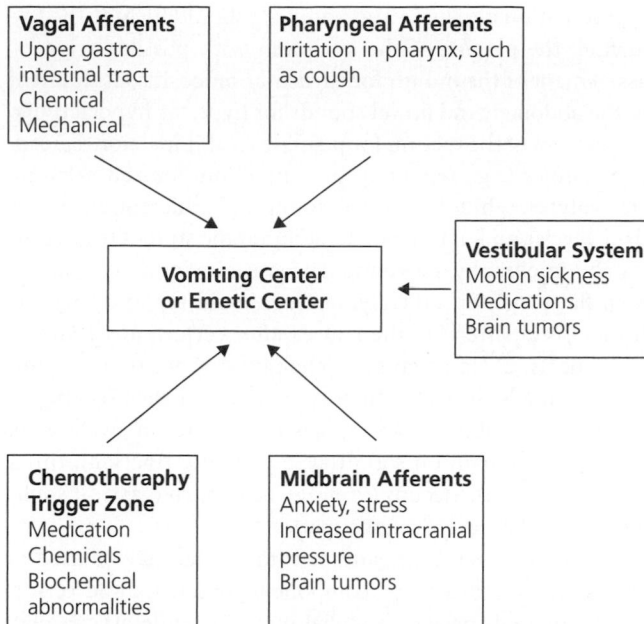

**Figure 10–2.** Physiological mechanisms of nausea and vomiting.

## Physiological Mechanisms of Nausea and Vomiting

After thoroughly understanding the concepts of nausea and vomiting, it is important to understand the physiological mechanisms and causes of this symptom complex.[19–21] Vomiting is controlled by stimulation of the vomiting center (VC) or emetic center, which is an area located in the medulla. There are multiple central and peripheral pathways that can stimulate the VC. It is important for nurses to understand these pathways to be able to determine a cause and to select appropriate treatments. The peripheral pathways include: the vagal afferents (from the gut and pharyngeal walls) and the vestibular system. The central pathways include afferents from the cerebral cortex, chemoreceptor trigger zone (CTZ) and vestibular nuclei (Figure 10–2).[18,20,23–25]

The vagal afferent pathway involves fibers located in the wall of the stomach and proximal small intestine, which sense mechanical or chemical changes in the upper gastrointestinal tract. The pharyngeal afferent pathway involves mechanical irritation of the glossopharyngeal nerve. Excessive coughing may cause nausea by irritating this pathway. The vestibular system involves stimulation starting in the inner ear. This mechanism is involved in nausea and vomiting resulting from vertigo, motion sickness and opioids. If a patient has a prior history of motion sickness, he or she may have an increased incidence of nausea and vomiting with treatments such as chemotherapy.[20,23,24]

The central pathways include the midbrain and the CTZ. Raised intracranial pressure, fear, anxiety, sights, sounds, or tastes may stimulate the midbrain afferent pathway. The CTZ is located at the area postrema of the fourth ventricle of the brain, is very vascular and lies outside the blood-brain-barrier. Cytotoxic chemotherapy, medications and metabolic derangements cause irrtiation of the CTZ through various neurotransmitters such as: serotonin, dopamine and histamine. The vagal afferents also enter the CTZ.[20–25]

In the past, it was hypothesized that chemotherapy-induced nausea and vomiting occurred as a result of stimulation of the CTZ by the chemotherapy or other drugs. Today there is more emphasis placed on understanding other mechanisms, such as the 5-hydroxytryptamine$_3$ ($5\text{-HT}_3$) receptors located in the wall of the small intestine. In newer theories, it appears that for patients receiving chemotherapy, abdominal radiotherapy, or who develop significant abdominal distention, the enterochromaffin cells of the mucosa of the small intestine release Serotonin. When $5\text{-HT}_3$ is released from these cells, it binds to specific receptors and these afferent impulses travel to the VC.[20,26]

More recently, a new ligand-receptor pair has been described as having an important role in nausea and vomiting. The three neurokinin receptors are called neurokinin-1, neurokinin-2, and neurokinin-3 receptors. Their preferred ligands are known as neurokinins(NK) or tachykinins. These are 11-amino-acid peptides including substance P, neurokinin A, and neurokinin B. The NK-1 receptor is stimulated by substance P and is thought to be involved in emesis.[17,27] Other neuroreceptors involved in emesis include acetylcholine, corticosteriod, histamine, and cannabinoid receptors which are located in the vomiting centers of the brain.

## Causes of Nausea and Vomiting

There are numerous potential causes of nausea and vomiting in cancer patients with advanced disease requiring palliative care. These are presented in Table 10–1 and are useful to remember when working with terminally ill patients. Often, the cause for nausea and vomiting is multifactorial.[4,5,20,22,25,28] For instance, there may be a metabolic derangement, such as a fluid and electrolyte imbalance (i.e. hypercalcemia, hyperglycemia, hyponatremia), occurring at the same time. In addition, the patient may be receiving opioids and/or nonsteroidal anti-inflammatory drugs (NSAIDs) to control pain. All of the factors can contribute to nausea and vomiting.[29] It has recently been hypothesized that patients' expectations may affect their experience of nausea and vomiting and the response to treatment. One study examined chemotherapy-related nausea and vomiting in treatment-naïve patients and found a statistically significant relationship (p = 0.015) between the patient's expectations of the symptom occurrence and their actual symptom distress.[17,30] Roscoe and colleagues[31] described two studies that found significant relationships between patients' expectations for nausea development measured before their first chemotherapy treatment and their mean post-chemotherapy nausea severity. Therefore, when considering nausea and vomiting from a QOL perspective (see Figure 10–1),[15] the nurse must keep in mind that psychological, social, and spiritual distress can cause or exacerbate nausea and vomiting.

**Table 10–1**
**Causes of Nausea and Vomiting**

| | |
|---|---|
| **Irritation/obstruction of gastrointestinal** | **Biochemical abnormalities** |
| Cancer | Hypercalcemia |
| Chronic cough | Hyponatremia |
| Esophagitis | Fluid and electrolyte imbalances |
| Peptic ulcer | Volume depletion |
| Gastric distention | Adrenocorticol insufficiency |
| Gastric compression | Liver failure |
| Delayed gastric | Renal failure |
|   emptying | |
| Bowel obstruction | **Drugs** |
| Constipation | Chemotherapy |
| Hepatitis | Opioids |
| Biliary obstruction | Digoxin |
| Chemotherapy | Antibiotics |
| Radiation | Anticonvulsants |
| | Aspirin and NSAIDs |
| **Sepsis** | |
| **metastases** | **Increased intracranial pressure** |
| CNS | Cerebral edema |
| Brain | Intracranial tumor |
| Meninges | Intracranial bleeding |
| Liver | Skull metastases |
| **Psychological** | |
| Fear | |
| Anxiety | |

CNS = central nervous system; NSAIDs = nonsteroidal antiinflammatory drugs.

## Assessment of Nausea and Vomiting

Assessment is an important process and the foundation of all treatment-related decisions. It should be an ongoing process that begins with the initial patient contact. Without a complete and ongoing assessment, nausea and vomiting may be mismanaged. This can result in unnecessary anxiety, suffering, and decrease in the QOL for the patient and family. Nurses working in all settings and with all age ranges of patients need to use skillful observation along with effective data collection techniques for a complete and comprehensive assessment. It is rare that patients present with nausea and vomiting as a first sign of advanced cancer. Generally, patients who complain of this symptom complex have a well-documented history of their disease, including diagnosis, prior treatment, and sites of metastases. If this information is not available, nurses should obtain a complete medical/surgical history, including previous episodes of nausea and vomiting, effectiveness of previous treatments, including the schedule of administration, and any current therapies that might be contributing to these symptoms. Information obtained by questionnaires or self-report tools such as diaries, journals, or logs is crucial for the identification and management of this symptom complex and for improving the patient's QOL.[16,23,25]

Evaluation of nausea and vomiting should include the following: the pattern of the symptom with possible triggers, assessment of the mouth for thrush or mucositis, assessment of the abdomen and bowel sounds for hyper or hypo activity, assessment of the rectum for possible fecal impaction, laboratory studies (e.g., renal and liver function, ionized calcium, electrolytes, white blood cell count and differential, serum drug levels), and, if indicated, radiographic studies (e.g., computed tomography, magnetic resonance imaging scan, abdomen flat plate). Specifically, nurses should try to determine if there is a pattern to the nausea after certain medications, after meals, on movement or changing in position, or with certain smells. It is also important to ask if there is epigastric pain (possibly indicating gastritis), pain on swallowing (oral thrush), pain on standing (mesenteric traction), thirst (hypercalcemia), hiccups (uremia), heartburn (gastro-esophageal reflux disease), or constipation.[32]

There are several measurement tools that may be used to assess one or more of the components of nausea and vomiting. Some tools provide a global measure while others measure a single component of the nausea/vomiting. Instruments may involve checklists, visual analogue scales, patient interviews, or Likert scales. Almost all involve self-report by the patient.[18,19,33-39] The most commonly used tools with reliability and validity reproducible in research studies are shown in Table 10–2.[17,19,33,40,41]

The tools used by nurses should be evaluated and chosen carefully. The words on the tools should have the same meaning to all participants. It is also important not to burden the patient or family with lengthy or intrusive questions.[17] Rhodes[16] recommends the following points when using an instrument to measure nausea and vomiting: (1) use self-report tools instead of observational assessments; (2) determine and describe the symptoms and components; (3) consider the

**Table 10–2**
**Tools to Measure Nausea and Vomiting**

| Instrument | Type | Reliability/Validity |
|---|---|---|
| Visual Analog Scale (VAS) | 100-mm line, with anchor descriptors at each end | Reliability is a strength. |
| Morrow Assessment of Nausea and Emesis (MANE) | 16 item, Likert scale (onset, severity–intensity) | Test/retest reliability 0.61–0.78 |
| Rhodes Index of Nausea and Vomiting Form 2 (INV-2) | 8 item, Likert scale | Split-half reliability 0.83–0.99 Cronbach's alpha 0.98 Construct validity 0.87 |
| Functional Living Index Emesis (FLIE) | 18 item, Likert scale | Content and criterion validity Internal consistency |

clarity, cultural sensitivity, and understandability of the tool; (4) check reliability and validity; (5) use an instrument with an easy-to-read format; (6) consider the purpose of the tool, the target population, and whether it is for acute, delayed, or anticipatory nausea and vomiting or for patients with advanced cancer; and (7) consider the type of score obtained (total versus subscale scores) and the ease of scoring.

Self-report tools such as journals, logs, or diaries can be especially helpful for assessing nausea and vomiting. They can be completed by the patient, a family member, caregiver. By using these tools, patients and families can develop experience with problem-solving and a sense of control. For health care providers, journals, logs, and diaries can offer useful information on patterns of symptom occurrence, self-care strategies, and situational events.[17] Goodman[42] provided examples of a chemotherapy treatment diary that could be adapted for use with terminally ill patients to record nausea and vomiting (Figure 10–3).

Name

**Medications to Take for Nausea & Vomiting**

| Medication | Time to take | How to take |
|---|---|---|
| | | |
| | | |
| | | |
| | | |

Special instructions:

________________________________

________________________________

________________________________

________________________________

If you have difficulty drinking fluids or your nausea and/or vomiting does not go away, you must call your doctor or hospice.

Doctor's phone____________________

Hospice phone____________________

**Nausea Log**

| Date | Drug | Time | Degree of Nausea* | Vomiting (#of times) | Effect of Drug** |
|---|---|---|---|---|---|
| | | | | | |
| | | | | | |
| | | | | | |

*0 = no nausea; 1 = slight nausea; 2 = moderately severe nausea, interferes with activities and eating; 3 = severe nausea, intolerable.
**Effect of drug: 1 = very effective, 2 = moderately effective, 3 = not effective.

**Figure 10–3.** Nausea diary. *Source*: Goodman (1997). Copyright 1997 by Oncology Nursing Society. Reproduced with permission.

CASE STUDY

***Gail, A Patient with Worsening Chronic Nausea Due to POD (Progression of Disease) and Escalation of Opioid Dosages***

Gail, a 40-year-old mother of a ten-year-old boy, has been referred to hospice with metastatic pancreatic cancer. She tells you she has had severe ongoing sharp pain in her right side that radiates to the back, associated with abdominal bloating. She reports intemittent nausea that keeps her from being able to eat. She feels like she will vomit but only has dry heaves. She currently has four 100 mcg/h transdermal fentanyl patches that are changed every 48 hours. She also uses oral hydromorphone 8 mg every 3 hrs as needed for breakthrough pain. She recently started using hydromorphone around the clock due to uncontrolled pain and thinks that her nausea has been more pronounced since then. Gail does not want to eat or drink fluids because of the nausea, dry heaves and the fear that her pain will worsen. You perform a thorough assessment of this chronic but worsening symptom by (1) asking the patient/family about the severity/intensity of the nausea, duration of nausea, frequency of nausea, pattern of nausea, triggers (e.g., with movement, after eating or drinking), and presence of vomiting; (2) asking the patient/family about epigastric pain, pain on swallowing, pain on standing, thirst, hiccups, heartburn, constipation, and any changes in medications; and (3) performing a thorough examination of the abdomen and bowel sounds, and of the rectum.

Through your assessment, you discover that her abdomen is distended, bowel sounds are present but diminished in all quadrants, and there is severe tenderness with palpation of the right upper quadrant in the area of the liver. She is uncomfortable lying flat. You think that if she didn't have to take so much hydromorphone, she wouldn't have such a bad nausea.

You decide to consult with the hospice physician and do opioid rotation, by changing the fentanyl patches and hydromorphone to methadone. You also anticipate that the nausea is likely to persist for few more days despite changing to a different opioid. In addition, 10 mg of metoclopramide every 6 hours is added to her regimen, with additional 10 mg doses as needed for severe nausea. A combination of Senokot and Colace is prescribed preemptively for constipation. Within 3 days, Gail's pain is under better control, and her nausea and dry heaves have improved significantly. She is having regular bowel movements, and she is able to take some fluids, food, and medications by mouth.

## Pharmacological Management of Nausea and Vomiting

Significant progress has been made through research in managing chemotherapy-induced nausea and vomiting.[37,38]

However, there have been few changes in clinical practice when treating nausea and vomiting in patients with far-advanced disease. The challenge is to provide appropriate antiemetic interventions for these patients in the setting in which they are receiving palliative care, while appreciating the demand for cost containment in health care delivery. Individuals with advanced cancer range from pediatric patients to elderly patients and receive end-of-life care in many health care settings (e.g., home, hospitals, inpatient hospice units, hospice houses, and outpatient and ambulatory units). The array of antiemetics available has increased (Table 10–3),[4,16,25,42–45] allowing for individualized protocols. Thus, it is important for nurses to continually reassess the effectiveness of the implemented treatments. Additionally, it is essential that nurses use and teach the patients and their families nonpharmacological methods to prevent and decrease nausea and vomiting.

In recent years, health care associations and groups of health care providers have developed recommendations or guidelines for the use of antiemetics in clinical practice. However, only a few of these mention the use of antiemetics for terminally ill patients.[27,43,46–48]

According to Kaye,[32] the overall plan of management for palliative care of nausea and vomiting should be as follows:

1. Make an assessment.
2. Identify the causes if possible.
3. Choose the antiemetic(s).
4. Choose the route.
5. Change the protocol if it is not working.
6. Consider steroids.
7. Consider antacids .
8. Decrease or change the opioid for pain (opioid rotation).
9. Remember that anxiety can cause nausea.

Woodruff[24] adds that pharmacological management should include adequate doses of antiemetics, combinations of antiemetics, and use of intravenous (IV), subcutaneous (SC) and rectal routes if necessary. If nausea and vomiting continue, consider psychological factors like untreated anxiety, and reassess for missed physical and or pharmacological causes. Different combinations of antiemetics should also be tried.

For intractable nausea and vomiting, a multimodal approach combining antiemetics targeting different rceptors is recommended. Similar to the setting of ongoing pain, ongoing nausea requires regular dosing of antiemetics rather than just on an as-needed basis.

### Classes of Antiemetics

There are currently 10 classes of drugs used as antiemetics in palliative care: butyrophenones, prokinetic agents, cannabinoids, phenothiazines, antihistamines, anticholinergics, steroids, benzodiazepines, 5-HT$_3$ receptor antagonists, and NK1 receptor antagonists.

Mannix[4] recommends seven steps to choosing an appropriate antiemetic protocol for palliative care. The first step involves identifying the likely cause(s) of the symptoms. In the second step, the clinician should try to identify the pathway by which each cause is triggering nausea and vomiting (see Figure 10–3). In step three, it is helpful to identify the neurotransmitter receptor that may be involved in the pathway, such as the 5-HT$_3$ receptor. Once the receptor is identified, step four requires selection of the most potent antagonist to that receptor. Step five involves selecting a route of administration that will ensure that the drug will reach the site of action. Once the route is chosen, step six is to titrate the dose carefully and give the antiemetic around the clock. Lastly, in step seven, if symptoms continue, review the likely cause(s) and consider additional treatment that may be required for an overlooked cause.

The clinical practice guidelines developed by the American Society of Clinical Oncologists (ASCO)[46] provides levels and grades of evidence for the guidelines. The five levels of evidence include:

Level I: Evidence is obtained from meta-analysis of multiple, well-designed, controlled studies.
Level II: Evidence is obtained from at least one well-designed experimental study.
Level III: Evidence is obtained from well-designed, quasi-experimental studies such as nonrandomized, controlled, single-group, pre-post, cohort, time, or matched case-control studies.
Level IV: Evidence is obtained from well-designed, non-experimental studies, such as comparative and correlational descriptive and case studies.
Level V: Evidence is obtained from case reports and clinical examples.

There are four grades in the ASCO guidelines. They are:

A: There is evidence of Level I or consistent findings from multiple studies of Levels II, III, and IV.
B: There is evidence of Level II, III, and IV, and findings are generally consistent.
C: There is evidence of Level II, III, and IV, but findings are inconsistent.
D: There is little or no systematic empirical evidence.

Butyrophenones are dopamine antagonists (D2 subtype) and are rated by the ASCO guidelines as Level I and grade A. Haloperidol and droperidol are the medications in this class, and they are most potent at the CTZ (see Figure 10–3). Butyrophenones are major tranquilizers whose mode of action, other than dopamine blockade, is not well understood. In general, they are less effective at controlling nausea and vomiting than other classes of drugs except for the phenothiazines. They are effective, however, when used in combination with other medications, especially with the 5-HT$_3$ receptor antagonists. Butyrophenones can be effective when anxiety and anticipatory symptoms aggravate the intensity

**Table 10-3**
**Antiemetic Drugs in Palliative Care**

| Drug | Indication | Dosage, Route, and Schedule | Side Effects | Comments |
|---|---|---|---|---|
| **Butyrophenones** | | | | |
| Haloperidol | Opioid-induced nausea, chemical and mechanical nausea | Oral; 0.5–5 mg every 4–6 h<br>IM: 5 mg/mL every 3–4 h<br>IV: 0.5–2 mg every 3–4 h | Dystonias, dyskinesia, akathisia | Side effects are less at low doses. Butyrephenones may be as effective as phenothiazines, may have additive effects with other CNS depressants. Use when anxiety and anticipatory symptoms aggravate intensity of nausea and vomiting. |
| Droperidol | | IV, IM: 1.25–2.5 mg every 2–4 h | | |
| **Prokinetic agents** | | | | |
| Metoclopramide | Gastric stasis, ileus | Oral: 5–10 mg every 2–4 h<br>IV: 1–3 mg/kg every 2–4 h | Dystonias, akathisia, esophageal spasm, colic if gastrointestinal obstruction, headache, fatigue, abdominal cramps, diarrhea | Infuse over 30 min to prevent agitation and dystonic reactions; use diphenhydramine to decrease extrapyramidal symptoms. |
| Domperidone | | Oral: 10–30 mg every 2–4 h<br>PR: 30–90 mg every 2–4 h | | |
| **Cannabinoids** | | | | |
| Dronabinol | Second-line anti-emetic | Oral: 2–10 mg every 4–6 h | CNS sedation, dizziness, disorientation, impaired concentration, dysphoria hypotension, dry mouth, tachycardia | More effective in younger adults. |
| **Phenothiazines** | | | | |
| Prochlorperazine | General nausea and vomiting. Not as highly recommended for routine use in palliative care | Oral: 5–25 mg every 3–4 h<br>PR: 25 mg every 6–8 h<br>IM: 5 mg/mL every 3–4 h<br>IV: 20–40 mg every 3–4 h | Drowsiness, irritation, dry mouth, anxiety hypotension, extrapyramidal side effects | May cause excessive drowsiness in elderly, IM route is painful. |
| Thiethylperazine | | Oral: 10 mg every 3–4 h<br>IM: 10 mg/2 mL every 3–4 h<br>PR: 10 mg every 6–8 h | | |
| Trimethobenzamide | | Oral: 100–250 mg every 3–4 h<br>PR: 200 mg every 3–4 h<br>IM: 200 mg/2 mL every 3–4 h | | |
| **Antihistamines** | | | | |
| Diphenhydramine | Intestinal obstruction, peritoneal irritation, vestibular causes, increased ICP | Oral: 25–50 mg every 6–8 h<br>IV: 25–50 mg every 6–8 h | Dry mouth, blurred vision, sedation | Cyclizine is the least sedative, so it is a better choice. |
| Cyclizine | | Oral: 25–50 mg every 8 h<br>PR: 25–50 mg every 8 h<br>SQ: 25–50 mg every 8 h | | |

*(Continued)*

**Table 10–3**
**Antiemetic Drugs in Palliative Care** *(Continued)*

| Drug | Indication | Dosage, Route, and Schedule | Side Effects | Comments |
|---|---|---|---|---|
| **Anticholinergics** | | | | |
| Scopolamine | Intestinal obstruction, peritoneal irritation, increased ICP, excess secretions | Sublingual: 200–400 mcg every 4–8 h SQ: 200–400 mcg every 8 h Transdermal: 500–1500 mcg every 72 h | Dry mouth, ileus, urinary retention, blurred vision, possible agitation | Useful if nausea and vomiting co-exist with colic. |
| **Steroids** | | | | |
| Dexamethasone | Given alone or with other agents for nausea and vomiting | Oral: 2–4 mg every 6 h IV: 2–4 mg every 6 h | Insomnia, anxiety, euphoria, perirectal burning | Compatible with 5-HT$_3$ receptor antagonists or metoclopramide. Taper dose to lowest effective dose to lessen adverse side effects. |
| **Benzodiazepine** | | | | |
| Lorazepam | Effective for nausea and vomiting as well as anxiety | Oral: 1–2 mg every 2–3 h IV: 2–4 mg every 4–8 h | Sedation, amnesia, pleasant hallucinations | Use with caution with hepatic or renal dysfunction or debilitated patients. |
| **5-HT$_3$ receptor antagonists** | | | | |
| Ondansetron | Chemotherapy, abdominal radiotherapy, postoperative nausea and vomiting | Oral, IV: 0.15–0.18 mg/kg every 12 h | Headache, constipation, diarrhea, minimal sedation | Indicated for moderate to highly emetogenic chemotherapy. Ideal for elderly and pediatric patients. |
| Granisetron | | Oral: 1 mg every 12 h IV: 10 mcg/kg every 12 h | | Effectiveness is increased if used with dexamethasone. |
| **Miscellaneous** | | | | |
| Octreotide acetate | Nausea and vomiting associated with intestinal obstruction | SQ (recommended), IV bolus (emergencies): 100–600 mcg SQ in 2–4 doses/day | Diarrhea, loose stools, anorexia, headache, dizziness, seizures, anaphylactic shock | May interfere as others with insulin and β-adrenergic blocking agents; watch liver enzymes. |
| Dimenhydrinate | Nausea, vomiting, dizziness, motion, sickness | Oral: 50–100 mg q 4 h, not > 400 mg/day IM, IV: 50 mg prn | Dry mouth, blurred vision, sedation | Geriatric clients may be more sensitive to dose. |

IM = intramuscular; SQ = subcutaneous; IV = intravenous; PR = per rectum; ICP = intracranial pressure; prn = as required; 5-HT = 5-hydroxytryptamine.
*Sources:* Baines (1997), reference 3; Mannix (2004), reference 4; Rhodes & McDaniel (2001), reference 17; Fallon (1998), reference 25; Enck (1994), reference 28; Goodman (1997), reference 42; Gralla et al. (1999), reference 46.

of a patient's nausea and vomiting. The side effects include: extrapyramidal dystonic reactions, akathisia, sedation, and postural hypotension.[4,17,24,27,42,46]

Prokinetic agents (see Table 10–3) include metoclopramide and domperidone. ASCO rates these agents as Level I and grade A for nausea and vomiting. They are also called "substituted benzamides." Metoclopramide is the most commonly used medication in this category. It has some antidopaminergic activity at the CTZ and stimulates 5-HT$_4$ receptors, which helps to bring normal peristalsis in the upper gastrointestinal tract and to block 5-HT$_3$ receptors in the CTZ and gut. Extrapyramidal side effects are common. Infusing the drug over 30 minutes and administering diphenhydramine 25 mg to 50 mg at the same time may lessen these side effects. Metoclopramide also enhances gastric emptying, decreases the sensation of fullness caused by gastric stasis, decreases the heartburn caused by chemotherapy, and slows the colonic transit time caused by the 5-HT$_3$ receptor antagonists. Although initially used as a single agent, metoclopramide is now the main component of several combination protocols.[17,27,46] In the setting of complete bowel obstruction, the use of prokinetic agents such as metoclopramide may result in increased pain and cramping and should be discontinued.

Cannabinoids (see Table 10–3), such as dronabinol, are options limited for patients who are refractory to other antiemetics. These substances presumably target higher CNS structures to prevent nausea and vomiting. According to the ASCO guidelines, there is Level I and grade A evidence that cannabinoids have antiemetic activity when used alone or in combination with other agents. Marijuana is the best known cannabinoid, but dronabinol is the plant extract preparation available for prescription use. The semisynthetic agents are nabilone and levonantradol. Marijuana, however, may be more effective when smoked. The actual site of action is not known, but it is thought to be at the cortical level. Cannabinoids are especially helpful in younger adults who do not have a history of cardiac or psychiatric illness. Younger patients may have a more positive experience, while older adults tend to have more neuroexcitatory side effects. These include hallucinations and feeling "high," although these side effects may be decreased by low-dose phenothiazines. Because the central sympathomimetic activity may increase with the use of cannabinoids, these drugs should be used with caution in patients with hypertension or heart disease or in those who are receiving psychomimetic medications.[4,17,24,27,42,46,49,50]

Phenothiazines (see Table 10–3) were once considered the mainstay of antiemetic therapy. ASCO rates them as level I, grade A. They act primarily as dopamine receptor antagonists at the CTZ, having both antiemetic and sedative effects. They can be used as single agents or in combination protocols. One major advantage of this class is that active substance is available in different formulations (oral, rectal suppository, parenteral, and sustained-release preparation), offering more flexibilty in the outpatient setting. The phenothiazines are especially effective for acute or delayed nausea, either used alone or in combination with $5-HT_3$ receptor antagonists and dexamethasone. The most common side effects are extrapyramidal (e.g., dystonia, akathisia, dyskinesia, akinesia). These symptoms appear with greater incidence in patients who are less than 30 years old. Frequently, 25 mg to 50 mg of diphenhydramine is given to prevent the extrapyramidal side effects.[4,17,24,27,42,46,49]

Antihistamines act on histamine receptors (H1) in the VC and vestibular nuclei. Diphenhydramine is often used in combination protocols to minimize the development of extrapyramidal side effects. Dimenhydrinate can be used for motion induced nausea. Cyclizine is less sedative than scopolamine (an anticholinergic) and can be given subcutaneously (SQ). These are rarely used as single agents for nausea and vomiting in palliative care, and the ASCO guidelines rate the level of evidence as II and grade as B.[4,17,24,46,49]

Anticholinergics act on the nicotinic receptors at the vomiting center or the muscarinic receptors found in the vestibular nuclei. They are not used frequently as antiemetic therapy due to the wide range of side effects: dry mouth, ileus, urinary retention, and blurred vision. They also come in different formulations (sublingual, SQ, and transdermal), offering the advantage of a better bioavailability. Their anticholonergic properties are very useful in the palliative care setting to treat excessive respiratory secretions and reduce gastrointestinal peristalsis associated with abdominal colic.[4,24]

Corticosteroids, especially dexamethasone, are frequently a component of aggressive antiemetic regimens and are used as a second-line therapy after other antiemetics have failed.[17,27,51–54] Their use remains controversial and has not been sufficiently studied in the palliative care setting. They appear to exert their antiemetic effects through the inhibition of antiprostaglandin activity. Dexamethasone is available in oral and parenteral formulations and is compatible to be mixed in solutions with $5-HT_3$ receptor antagonists and metoclopramide. In general, corticosteroids are most effective in combination with other agents due to synergistic actions. The efficacy of ondansetron, granisetron, and metoclopramide can be enhanced by adding dexamethasone.[55] The use of corticosteroids for four to five days can prevent delayed nausea and vomiting. However, the dose should be tapered after several days to decrease the likelihood of developing side effects including insomnia, anxiety and euphoria. A trial of high-dose steroids should be used as first-line therapy if there is increased intracranial pressure from cerebral metastases, hypercalcemia of malignancy, or malignant pyloric stenosis.[17,24,32,42,49,56] The ASCO guidelines suggest that the level of evidence is II and grade is B for the use of single doses of corticosteroids.[46]

Benzodiazepines act on the GABA receptors of the cerebral cortex (see Table 10–3). Lorazepam may be used alone when the intent is to treat anticipatory nausea (due to its temporary amnestic effect) or when anxiety is a contributing factor to nausea or vomiting.[5,17,24,27,42,49] Malik and Khan[57] found that lorazepam decreased the incidence of anticipatory nausea and vomiting, as well as acute emesis. Pediatric patients may experience sedation and pleasant hallucinations. Lorazepam should be used with caution in debilitated patients or those with hepatic or renal dysfunction. Benzodiazepines are used most commonly in combination protocols. The ASCO guidelines recommend that benzodiazepines be used in combination regimens (level of evidence II and grade B).[46]

The serotonin receptor anatgonists have been used to treat chemotherapy-induced nausea and vomiting since 1986. At that time, the selective blockade of 5-HT "m" receptors was shown to counteract the vomiting induced by cisplatin. Since then, there has been a rapid creation of new drugs and increased knowledge of the sites and roles of 5-HT receptors. The $5-HT_3$ receptors have been discovered in the CTZ, in the VC (centrally), and in the gut wall (peripherally). The mechanism of action of the $5-HT_3$ receptor antagonists (see Table 10–3)—ondansetron, granisetron, and dolasetron mesylate—appears to be limited to serotonin inhibition. Therefore, they lack the extrapyramidal side effects associated with dopamine antagonists. Ondansetron was the first agent to become available for clinical use in 1991, followed by granisetron in 1994, and dolasetron mesylate in 1997. Each of these medications can be given orally or intravenously. The oral route is as effective as the intravenous one and is preferred when feasible. Granisetron is the most specific $5-HT_3$ receptor antagonist and has a higher potency and a longer duration of action than ondansetron. All medications in this class can be used in the pediatric and geriatric populations because the side effects profile is very limited.[4,17,24,27,42,44,46] The ASCO grading of the level of evidence for these medications is I and grade is A.[46] Many clinicians feel that there are no major differences in the efficacy and toxicity of the three FDA approved medications in this category.[27] Palonosetron is a pharmacologically distinct 5-HT$_3$ antagonist that has also been approved by the FDA. It appears to have 100-fold higher affinity for the receptor compared to ondansetron, granisetron and dolasetron.[27] Olanzapine is a newer atypical neuroleptic which is both a dopamine and 5HT receptor antagonist. It is used to treat refractory nausea and vomiting and has pronounced sedative effects.[58,59]

As previously discussed, there is a ligand-receptor pair which has been described as having an important role in nausea and vomiting. This class of medications is called substance P antagonists or neurokinin-1 antagonists.[27] Aprepitant is an oral drug that acts as an NK-1 antagonist. It has been shown to be effective when combined with ondansetron and dexamethasone to prevent acute and delayed chemotherapy-induced nausea and vomiting.[27]

A variety of miscellaneous agents can be helpful in nausea and vomiting. Octreotide acetate is a long-acting somatostatin analogue which may be helpful for nausea and vomiting associated with intestinal obstruction. Specifically, it inhibits gastric, pancreatic, and intestinal secretions and reduces gastrointestinal motility, making it useful in cases where there is high volume emesis. Dimenhydrinate contains both diphenhydramine, an antihistaminic, and chlorotheophylline. It is helpful for nausea, vomiting, and dizziness associated with motion sickness.

### Combination Protocols

Combining antiemetic drugs appears to improve efficacy, decrease side effects, and increase QOL. This practice is based on the theory that blocking different types of receptors and their neurotransmitters offers a better management of symptoms through synergistic actions. In some instances, single agents, such as granisetron, ondansetron, and prochlorperazine, may be used independently. However, the combination of a 5-HT$_3$ receptor antagonist and a corticosteroid may be the most effective antiemetic regimen.[4,17,42,49,60,61] The various agents used in combination are adjusted according to the individual's tolerance.

### Routes of Administration

Nausea and vomiting may be treated with a combination of oral medications. If tolerated by the patient, this may be the most cost-effective treatment and provide the best prophylaxis.[27] Sometimes, other routes are needed if the patient has severe vomiting or is unable to swallow. If the patient has IV access, IV administration is appropriate. The intramuscular route should be avoided because of the unpredictable

absorption and the painful administration. Other routes used in home care are: subcutaneous (SQ), rectal, sublingual, and transdermal. A continuous SQ infusion is useful for severe nausea and vomiting when venous access is not available, to avoid repeated injections.

## Nonpharmacological Management of Nausea and Vomiting in the Palliative Care Setting

There is enough evidence in the literature to support the use of complementary and alternative techniques for the prevention and treatment of nausea and vomiting.[7,53,63,64] There is, however, very limited literature addressing the use of these interventions for patients receiving end-of-life care.

Nonpharmacological management of nausea and vomiting may involve simple self-care techniques (Table 10–4)[23,28] or mind-body therapies based on using psychological interventions to control physiological responses.[65] There are many different nonpharmacological techniques available today that can be used for the management of nausea and vomiting in the palliative care setting.

Behavioral interventions involve the acquisition of new adaptive behavioral skills. These techniques may include relaxation, biofeedback, self-hypnosis, cognitive distraction, guided imagery, and systematic desensitization. Other therapies very commonly used by the integrative medicine specialists are acupuncture, acupressure, and music therapy (Table 10–5).[17,63,64,66]

Behavioral interventions can be used alone or in combination with antiemetic medications to prevent and control nausea and vomiting. All of these techniques attempt to induce relaxation as a learned response. They differ only in the manner in which they induce relaxation.[63] Their effectiveness is based on the following principles: (1) they produce relaxation,

---

**Table 10–4**
**Nonpharmacological Self-Care Activities for Nausea and Vomiting**

Provide oral care after each episode of emesis.
Apply a cool damp cloth to the forehead, neck, and wrists.
Decrease noxious stimuli such as odors and pain.
Restrict fluids with meals.
Eat frequent small meals.
Eat bland, cold, or room-temperature food.
Lie flat for 2 hours after eating.
Wear loose-fitting clothes.
Have fresh air with a fan or open window.
Avoid sweet, salty, fatty, and spicy foods.
Limit sounds, sights, and smells that precipitate nausea and vomiting.

*Sources:* Ladd (1999), reference 23; Enck (1994), reference 28.

**Table 10–5**
**Nonpharmacological Interventions for Nausea and Vomiting**

| Techniques | Description | Comments |
|---|---|---|
| **Behavioral interventions** | | |
| Self-hypnosis | Evocation of physiological state of altered consciousness and total body relaxation. This technique involves a state of intensified attention receptiveness and increased receptiveness to an idea. | Used to control anticipatory nausea and vomiting<br>Limited studies, mostly children and adolescents<br>No side effects<br>Decreases intensity and duration of nausea<br>Decreases frequency, severity, amount, and duration of vomiting |
| Relaxation | Progressive contraction and relaxation of various muscle groups | Often used with imagery<br>Can use for other stressful situations<br>Easily learned<br>No side effects<br>Decreases nausea during and after chemotherapy<br>Decreases duration and severity of vomiting<br>Not as effective with anticipatory nausea and vomiting |
| Biofeedback | Control of specific physiological responses by receiving information about changes in response to induced state of relaxation | Two types: electromyographic and skin temperature<br>Used alone or with relaxation<br>Easily learned<br>No side effects<br>Decreases nausea during and after chemotherapy<br>More effective with progressive muscle relaxation |
| Imagery | Mentally takes self away by focusing mind on images of a relaxing place | Most effective when combined with another technique<br>Increases self-control<br>Decreases duration of nausea<br>Decreases perceptions of degree of vomiting<br>Feel more in control, relaxed, and powerful |
| Distraction | Learn to divert attention away from a threatening situation and toward relaxing sensations | Can use videos, games, and puzzles<br>No side effects<br>Decreases anticipatory nausea and vomiting<br>Decreases postchemotherapy distress |
| Desensitization | Three-step process involving relaxation and visualization to decrease sensitization to aversive situations | Inexpensive<br>Easily learned<br>No side effects<br>Decreases anticipatory nausea and vomiting |
| **Other interventions** | | |
| Acupressure | Form of massage using meridians to increase energy flow and affect emotions | Inconclusive literature support<br>Acupressure wrist bands may be helpful to decrease nausea and vomiting |
| Music therapy | Use of music to influence physiological, psychological, and emotional functioning during threatening situations | Often used with other techniques<br>No side effects<br>Decreases nausea during and after chemotherapy<br>Decreases perceptions of degree of vomiting |

which can decrease nausea and vomiting; (2) they serve as a distraction from the stimulus causing nausea and vomiting; (3) they enhance feelings of control and decrease feelings of helplessness as patients are actively involved in decreasing their symptoms; (4) they have no side effects; (5) they are easily self-administered; and (6) they can be cost effective because they require limited time by a health care professional to teach these interventions.[14,63,66,67]

There is currently no convincing evidence favoring one method over another; rather, the effectiveness of these techniques appears to depend on the individual preference.

## Self-Hypnosis

Self-hypnosis was the first behavioral technique tested to control the symptom complex of nausea and vomiting. This used to be considered part of a psychoanalytical approach used in psychotherapy but, more recently, has been categorized as a behavioral intervention. Self-hypnosis allows individuals to learn to invoke a physiological state of altered consciousness and total-body relaxation. This results from the individual's intensified attention receptiveness toward a specific idea or feeling.[63,64] Unfortunately, hypnotic methods are not standardized, but all include relaxation and imagery. As with many of the behavioral techniques, there have been few controlled studies published on self-hypnosis. Most of the research has been performed with children and adolescents receiving chemotherapy. They appear to be more easily hypnotized than adults.[68-73] The results have been mixed, with only some patients having a decrease in the frequency, severity, amount, and duration of vomiting, as well as duration of nausea. The advantages of this method include: absence of side effects, no need for equipment, minimal physical effort, and minimal training. Health care professionals, including nurses, have successfully taught patients self-hypnosis techniques.[68,69] In a study by Marchioro and associates,[73] all subjects showed a complete remission of anticipatory nausea and vomiting and major responses regarding postchemotherapy nausea and vomiting; however, these were not terminally-ill patients. There is a need for more research to evaluate which behavioral interventions are most effective in patients of all ages with advanced diseases who are receiving end-of-life care.

### Progressive Muscle Relaxation

Progressive muscle relaxation (PMR), also called active relaxation, involves individuals learning to relax by progressively tensing and then relaxing different muscle groups in the body. Passive relaxation is considered relaxation that does not involve active tensing of the muscles. Often, PMR is used in combination with guided imagery, and research has shown that it can decrease chemotherapy-induced nausea and vomiting as well as depression and anxiety.[63,66,74-77] However, research has not been conducted on patients with advanced illnesses receiving palliative care.[17] Research on chemotherapy-induced nausea and vomiting and PMR showed that PMR can decrease anxiety, the physiological indices of arousal (e.g., heart rate and blood pressure),depression and the occurrence of vomiting.[77] One study[78] was conducted with 60 Japanese cancer patients receiving chemotherapy protocols similar to those used in the United States. The subjects were randomly assigned to the PMR intervention or a control group. The findings verified the effectiveness of PMR in reducing the total scores used to measure nausea, vomiting and retching, and subjective feelings of anxiety. Another study[79] was performed with Chinese breast cancer patients receiving chemotherapy to evaluate the use of PMR as an adjuvant intervention to pharmacological antiemetic treatment. The use of PMR significantly decreased the duration of nausea and vomiting in the experimental group as compared to the control group.

Interestingly, as many as 65% of patients who learned PMR while undergoing chemotherapy continued to use this technique after they completed chemotherapy.[80] However, there is still much to study and research about the use of PMR in cancer patients with advanced disease suffering from nausea and vomiting.

### Biofeedback

Biofeedback is a behavioral technique through which patients learn to control a specific physiological response (e.g., muscle tension) by receiving information about moment-to-moment changes in that response. Two specific types of biofeedback include electromyography (EMG) and skin temperature (ST). The purpose of EMG biofeedback is to induce a state of deep muscle relaxation from tense muscles. The purpose of ST biofeedback is to prevent and control skin temperature changes that precede nausea and vomiting.[63,69,74]

Research has shown that biofeedback may help individuals achieve a state of generalized relaxation.[69,74,82,83] However, it has not been shown that EMG or ST biofeedback are as effective as PMR at decreasing chemotherapy-induced nausea and vomiting.[72] Little definitive data exists regarding biofeedback as a useful behavioral technique for chemotherapy-induced nausea and vomiting, and even fewer datum demonstrates that either EMG or ST is effective at decreasing this symptom complex in patients with advanced disease.

### Guided Imagery

Guided imagery allows individuals with nausea and vomiting to mentally take themselves away from their current site to a place that is relaxing. Individuals may choose a familiar vacation spot, a safe place, a specific place at home, or can imagine any pleasant place where they would like to transport themselves. Experiencing and inducing different pleasant sensation by using all senses can mentally block the negative conditioned stimuli from the cerebral cortex and prevent nausea and vomiting and other symptoms. It is thought that the body physiologically adapts and responds to the created positive and pleasant image rather than to the negative conditioned stimuli.[63-65,84]

Research has suggested that guided imagery, or visualization, can facilitate relaxation, decrease anxiety, decrease anticipatory nausea and vomiting, and increase self-control.[85-87] Guided imagery has also been assessed in combination with other techniques including music therapy. The results were better in the group of patients who received combined modalities than the controls who received either intervention alone. Interestingly, the subjects' perceptions of the occurrence of nausea remained unchanged. However, the degree of vomiting was reduced significantly, and there was a trend toward a decreased duration of vomiting observed with combined music therapy/guided imagery intervention. In another study,[88] patients who received guided imagery plus the standard antiemetic therapy exhibited a significantly more positive response in terms of alleviation of the chemotherapy induced nausea and vomiting than those who did not. Unfortunately, guided imagery did not have an effect on patients' perceptions of the frequency of nausea and vomiting or the distress associated with these symptoms. The subjects did, however, express that they felt more prepared, in control, powerful, and relaxed when using guided imagery.

From the limited research available, it appears that guided imagery may be most effective at decreasing nausea and vomiting associated with chemotherapy and mostly when it is combined with another nonpharmacological technique, such as PMR or music therapy. There is little research that has examined guided imagery alone or in combination with another behavioral technique for patients receiving symptom management in the palliative care setting. The palliative care nurse plays a key role in educating and teaching the patients and their families about guided imagery contributing to their overall quality of life.

## Cognitive Distraction

Cognitive distraction is also known as attentional diversion. This behavioral technique is thought to act by shifting an individual's attention away from nausea, vomiting, and the stimuli associated with these phenomena while focusing their attention on an engaging and pleasant activity.[63,64,66,69,74,89] Research has shown that simply distracting children and adolescents with video games can decrease anticipatory nausea and vomiting.[89,90] Research with adults has demonstrated that cognitive distraction can significantly decrease postchemotherapy nausea, regardless of the pre-chemotherapy anxiety levels.[91] Further research is needed to demostrate the utility of this techinque in preventing or treating nausea and vomiting associated with anti-cancer therapies.. It is important for nurses to educate themselves about nonpharmacolgical interventions so that they can discuss them with patients and families who might benefit from such interventions.

## Systematic Desensitization

Systematic desensitization is a standardized intervention that has been used to counteract anxiety-laden maladaptive responses such as phobias.[66] There are three key steps to the desensitization process. First, the individual is taught a response, such as PMR, that is incompatible with the current maladaptive response (e.g., chemotherapy-induced nausea and vomiting). After this first step, the individual and teacher create a hierarchy of anxiety-provoking stimuli related to the feared situation (events related to receiving chemotherapy, such as driving to the clinic, entering the treatment room, and seeing the chemotherapy nurse). This hierarchy of anxiety-provoking stimuli range from the least to the most frightening. In the last step, the individual uses the alternative response while systematically visualizing the increasingly aversive scenes related to chemotherapy and nausea and vomiting.[63,66,69,92–94]

Studies demonstrated that systematic desensitization can be effective against anticipatory nausea and vomiting associated with chemotherapy.[81,92,95,96] Specifically, systematic desensitization can decrease not only the frequency, severity, and duration of anticipatory nausea and vomiting, but also the duration and severity of post-treatment nausea.This particular behavioral technique can be effectively implemented by a variety of trained health care professionals (e.g., nurses, physicians, and clinical psychologists).[92] More research is needed to validate and standardize these techiques.

## Other Nonpharmacological Interventions

Acupuncture and acupressure are Eastern health care therapies that have gained awareness and have become part of the complementary interventions in the field of palliative care. Acupressure is a form of massage that uses specific energy channels known as meridians. *Tsubos* are acupuncture/acupressure points. Tsubos are points of decreased electrical resistance running along the body's energy pathways that form the meridian system. It is believed that stimulating the tsubo improves the energy flow, affects organs distant from the area being stimulated, and positively affects emotions.[63,97] Most studies have been performed with chemotherapy-induced nausea and vomiting.[98–102] Some studies have shown acupuncture on P6 (Neiguan point) to be effective at decreasing nausea and vomiting for 8 hours, and if acupressure is applied immediately after P6 acupuncture, there is a prolonged antiemetic effect.[99–101] Aglietti and colleagues[103] treated women receiving cisplatin with metoclopramide, dexamethasone, and diphenhydramine with and without acupuncture. Patients had a temporary acupuncture needle for 20 minutes during the infusion of chemotherapy and then a more permanent needle 24 hours after chemotherapy. Acupuncture did decrease the intensity and duration of nausea and vomiting, but the investigators commented that it was difficult to perform acupuncture in daily practice. Dibble and associates[104] conducted a pilot study with women undergoing chemotherapy for breast cancer and reported that finger acupressure decreased nausea. An NIH Consensus Conference has stated that acupuncture for adult post-operative and chemotherapy-related nausea and vomiting is efficacious.[105] Additionally, several reviews of acupuncture and acupressure have concluded that these are efficacious methods for relieving nausea and vomiting and other symptoms.[106,107] One study that was conducted on terminally ill patients found that acupressure wristbands were ineffective at decreasing the intensity or frequency of nausea and vomiting.[108] The investigators experienced difficulty in obtaining complete data and found subject recruitment a problem. Thus, studies on terminally ill patients need to be repeated and extended to confirm the usefulness of acupuncture or acupressure, even though research with terminally ill patients is difficult to conduct.

Music therapy has been used as a tool to prevent or control nausea or vomiting in cancer patients. This technique uses music to induce a state of well-being and counteract the side effects of treatment. The objective is to influence the patient's physiological, psychological, emotional, and behavioral well-being.[109] Music therapy has most often been used in combination with other nonpharmacological techniques. Few studies have looked at the ability of music therapy to decrease nausea and vomiting in cancer patients.[17] Most of the studies have not used music therapy as a single intervention and have assessed only nausea and vomiting related to chemotherapy. Frank[87] combined music therapy with guided imagery. The duration of nausea and the patients' perceptions of the degree of vomiting were decreased; however, the patients' perceptions of nausea did not change, and there was only a slight decrease in the duration of vomiting. Standley[110] used music therapy alone as an intervention and assessed the effects on the frequency and degree of anticipatory nausea and vomiting, as well as vomiting during and after chemotherapy. The individuals who received the music intervention reported a shorter duration of nausea and a longer time before the onset of nausea. Ezzone and colleagues[111] evaluated whether a music intervention would decrease bone marrow transplant patients' perceptions of nausea and number of episodes of vomiting while receiving high-dose chemotherapy. Significant differences were found, with the music therapy patients having less nausea and fewer episodes of vomiting. The music should be quiet and should create a calm background rather than being disruptive.[112] Music therapy is an intervention that can be initiated independently by nurses in all settings and individualized for each patient. Additionally, music as an intervention for patients with advanced cancer receiving end-of-life care requires less time and energy to implement than relaxation or guided imagery, and therefore may be less taxing for the seriously ill patient. Certainly, the combination of music therapy with antiemetic therapy warrants further study to assess their effects on alleviating the distressing symptoms of nausea and vomiting.

## Nursing Interventions

Palliative care is by definition active total care; thus, it is essential that nurses have a proactive attitude towards assessing and promptly relieving nausea and vomiting for patients under their care. The National Comprehensive Cancer Network (NCCN) palliative care guidelines recommend aggressive symptom management clarification of the intent of treatments, anticipation of the needs of patients and their families and involvement of the caregivers in the treatment process, when appropriate.[47] As discussed in this chapter, the NCCN guidelines emphasize the need for ongoing assessement of symptoms, therapeutic interventions and measurement of their outcomes. The palliative care nurse plays a crucial role in this aspect of care and is instrumental in promoting a collaborative approach among team members caring for their patients.

It is vital that nurses in all settings (e.g., administrators, clinicians, educators, and researchers) lead the way in learning how to manage these symptoms appropriately in the palliative care setting. From a clinical perspective, nurses need to provide initial and ongoing assessment of the patient's symptom experience, implement appropriate pharmacologic and nonpharmacologic interventions, evaluate the outcomes of all interventions, and educate the patient and family. Administrators play a key role in providing the resources necessary for clinical nurses to give quality, but cost-effective, palliative care in all settings (hospitals, inpatient hospice units, hospice houses, homes, and outpatient/ambulatory units).

Family caregivers are often expected to participate in and monitor the overall symptom management of their loved one, as well as to provide emotional support, and help with daily activities and general care. In addition, a family member is frequently the communication link between the patient and the nurse. Nurses depend heavily on family members for information about the patient, especially when the patient's clinical status deteriorates. It is therefore essential that family be involved early in the patient's plan of care and participate in the educational sessions provided by nurses and others involved.[113]

Specific to nausea and vomiting, patients and family need to be taught how to systematically assess the symptoms. They may use a log, such as the one developed by Goodman[42] (see Figure 10–3). It is helpful to teach the patient and family members to rate the distress caused by these symptoms on a scale of 0 to 10. This provides more accurate information regarding the intensity of the non-physical symptoms associated with nausea and vomiting. The patient and family also need to be taught problem-solving skills for specific situations (e.g., when they can give an extra dose of antiemetic) and self-care activities (see Table 10–4). The importance of dosing the antiemetics regularly rather then as needed should be reinforced when nausea and vomiting are ongoing symptoms. Information regarding medications and instructions for self-care should be provided in written form. Specific instruction should be given as to when to call the physician or nurse. Lastly, it is very helpful to teach nonpharmacological methods for decreasing nausea and vomiting (e.g., music therapy or relaxation).

Nurse educators can work collaboratively with clinicians to develop educational tools for patients and families (pamphlets, videos, and audiotapes) in managing these symptoms. Additional nursing research and multidisciplinary research is very much needed regarding appropriate antiemetic regimens, nonpharmacological interventions, appropriate self-care activities, and QOL issues for patients receiving palliative care. Nurse researchers are not only actively involved in this research, but also in the dissemination of the results to clinicians and educators.

CASE STUDY

### BT, A 39-Year-Old Man Who Has Intractable Nausea and Vomiting

BT, a 39-year-old man with metastatic non-small cell lung cancer, is admitted to a palliative care unit with intractable nausea and vomiting. He is unable to tolerate any food or water and can no longer take any medications by mouth. He also has severe headache, anxiety, and sometimes panic attacks. He has told his family and friends that he doesn't want to die in a hospital. He currently has three 100 mcg fentanyl patches placed every 3 days and used to take two hydrocodone (7.5 mg hydrocodone with 750 mg acetaminophen) tablets every 3 to 4 hours for breakthrough pain. BT is no longer able to use the prochorperazine previously prescribed for nausea, nor any other medication that is administered by mouth. He has nothing prescribed for anxiety. You do a thorough assessment of his pain, nausea, and anxiety and learn the following: (1) His persistent headache is a 6 to 9 out of 10 and his fentanyl patches used to treat his bone pain from metastases do not provide any relief for his headaches. The headaches occur mostly in the morning and are relieved after he vomits. His nausea is a 10 out of 10; (2) Many years ago he he had learned transcendental meditation but has not practiced in 20 years. He plays the violin as a hobby, but hasn't practiced since he was diagnosed with cancer; (3) His anxiety and panic attacks are precipitated by planning his funeral and Will; (4) He can not tolerate morphine due an exacerbation of his severe nausea.

After a thorough assessment is made, there is a high suspicion that brain metastases are causing increased intracranial pressure, resulting in headaches and severe nausea and vomiting. An antiemetic regimen is instituted promptly with Dexamethasone 10 mg Q.A.M. IV in combination with metoclopramide 10 mg every 6 hours around the clock. The patient refuses to have an evaluation by MRI to rule out cerebral metastases. Lorazepam is ordered at 1 mg IV every 6 hours as needed for anxiety. A referral is made to the music therapist because of his love of music. After 3 days, the patient's headaches have improved with a severity of 2 to 4 out of 10, and nausea has decreased to a severity of 3 to 4 out of 10 He is titrated to only one dose of lorazepam per day for anxiety. BT and his family express great relief that his nausea and vomiting are under control. He is discharged home with hospice support.

## Conclusion

A major goal of palliative care is to improve QOL by addressing suffering in all its dimensions. This can be achieved in part through aggressive and expert symptom management, including adequate treatment of nausea and vomiting in terminally ill patients. It can be difficult for nurses to meet the challenge of providing high quality palliative care when there is limited evidence base for interventions used routinely. However, vigilant assessment, appropriate use and evaluation of pharmacological and nonpharmacological interventions, appropriate patient and family education and support, as well as further research, will go a long way in approaching the problem. Nausea and vomiting profoundly affect all aspects of a person's' well being. Adequately managing these symptoms, especially at end of life, is essential.

REFERENCES

1. Molassiotis A, Saunders MP, Valle J, Wilson G, Lorigan P, Wardley A, et al. A prospective observational study of chemotherapy-related nausea and vomiting in routine practice in a UK cancer centre. Support Care Cancer 2008;16:201–208.

2. Ferrell B, Virani R, Grant M. Analysis of end-of-life-content in nursing textbooks. Oncol Nurs Forum 1999;26:869–876.

3. Baines M. ABC of palliative care: Nausea, vomiting and intestinal obstruction. BMJ 1997;315:1148–1150.

4. Mannix KA. Palliation of nausea and vomiting. In: Doyle D, Hanks G, Cherny N, Calman K, eds. Oxford Textbook of Palliative Medicine. New York: Oxford University Press, 2004:459–468.

5. Ross D, Alexander C. Management of common symptoms in terminally ill patients: Part I. Am Fam Physician 2001;64:807–814.

6. Maibach B, Thurlimann B, Sessa C, Aapro M. Patients' estimation of overall treatment burden: Why not ask the obvious? J Clin Oncol 2002;20:65–72.

7. Ballatori E, Rolia F, Ruggeri B, Betti M, Sarti S, Soru G, et al. The impact of chemotheray-induced nausea and vomiting on health-related quality of life. Support Cancer Care 2007;15:179–185

8. Cohen L, de Moor CA, Eisenberg P, Ming EE, Hu H. Chemotherapy-induced nausea and vomiting—incidence and impact onpatient quality of life at community oncology settings. Support Care Cancer 2007;15:497–503.

9. Bosnjack S, Radulovic S, Neskovic-Konstantinovic. Patient statement of satisfaction with antiemetic treatment is related to quality of life. Am J Clin Oncol 2000;23:575–578.

10. Tipson JM, Mc Daniel RW, Barbour L, Johnston MP, Kayne M, LeRoy P, et al. Putting evidence into practice: Evidence-based interventions to prevent, manage, and treat chemotherpay induced nuasea and vomiting. Clin J Oncol Nurs 2007;11:69–78.

11. Grunberg S, Boutin N, Ireland A, Miner S, Silveira J, Ashikaga T. Impact of nausea/vomiting on quality of life as a visual analogue scale-derived utility score. Support Care Cancer 1996;4: 435–439.

12. Morrow G, Roscoe J, Hickock J, et al. Initial control of chemotherapy-induced nausea and vomiting in patient quality of life. Oncology 1998;3(suppl 4):32–37.

13. Osoba D, Zee B, Warr D, Latreille J, Kaizer L, Pater J. Effect of postchemotherapy nausea and vomiting on health-related quality of life. Support Care Cancer 1997;5:307–313.

14. Ferrell B, Grant M, Padilla G, Vemuri S, Rhiner M. The experience of pain and perceptions of quality of life: validation of a conceptual model. Hospice J 1991;7:9–24.

15. Grant M. Nausea and vomiting, quality of life and the oncology nurse. Oncol Nurs Forum 1997;24:5–7.

16. Rhodes V. Criteria for assessment of nausea, vomiting and retching. Oncol Nurs Forum 1997;24:13–19.

17. Rhodes V, McDaniel R. Nausea, vomiting, and retching: complex problems in palliative care. CA Cancer J Clin 2001;51:232–248.

18. Rhodes V, Watson P, Johnson M, Madsen R, Beck N. Patterns of nausea and vomiting and distress in patients receiving antineoplastic drug protocols. Oncol Nurs Forum 1987;14:35–44.

19. Rhodes V, McDaniel R. The index of nausea, vomiting, and retching: a new format of the index for nausea and vomiting. Oncol Nurs Forum 1999;26:889–894.

20. Hogan C, Grant M. Physiologic mechanisms of nausea and vomiting in patients with cancer. Oncol Nurs Forum 1997; 24:8–12.

21. Hesketh PJ. Chemotherapy-induced nausea and vomiting – Review article. NEJM 2008;358:2482–2494.

22. Nausea, vomiting, constipation, and bowel obstruction in advanced cancer. National Cancer Institute. Available at: http://www.cancer.gov/cancerinfo/pdq/supportivecare/nausea/HealthProfessional (accessed Febuary 2, 2009).

23. Ladd L. Nausea in palliative care. J Hospice Palliat Nurs 1999;1:67–70.

24. Woodruff R. Symptom Control in Advanced Cancer. Melbourne: Asperula, 1997.

25. Fallon B. Nausea and vomiting unrelated to cancer treatment. In: Berger A, Portenoy R, Weissman D, eds. Principles and Practice of Supportive Oncology. Philadelphia: Lippincott Williams & Wilkins, 1998:179–189.

26. Andrews P, Davis CJ. The mechanism of induced anticancer therapies. In: Andrews P, Sanger G, eds. Emesis in Anticancer Therapy: Mechanisms and Treatment. New York: Chapman and Hall, 1993:113–161.

27. National Comprehensive Cancer Network. Practice guidelines in oncology: antiemesis. National Comprehensive Cancer Network. Available at: http://www.nccn.org (accessed January 28, 2009).

28. Enck R. The Medical Care of Terminally Ill Patients. Baltimore: Johns Hopkins University Press, 1994.

29. Ventrafridda, VM, Tamruini A, Caraceni F, DeConno F, Naldi F. A validation study of the WHO method for cancer pain relief. Cancer 1987;59:850–856.

30. Rhodes V, Watson P, McDaniel R, Hanson B, Johnson M. Expectation and occurrence of postchemotherapy side effects. Cancer Pract 1995;3:247–253.

31. Roscoe J, Hickock J, Morrow G. Patient expectations as predictor of chemotherapy-induced nausea. Ann Behav Med 2000;22:121–126.

32. Kaye P. Symptom Control in Hospice and Palliative Care. Essex, CT: Hospice Education Institute, 1997.

33. Zhou Q, O'Brien B, Soeken K. Rhodes index of nausea and vomiting—Form 2 in pregnant women. Nurs Res 2001;50:251–257.

34. McDaniel R, Rhodes V. Symptom experience. Semin Oncol Nurs 1995;11:232–234.

35. Del Favero A, Tonato M, Roila F. Issues in the measurement of nausea. Br J Cancer 1992;66(Suppl 19):S69–S71.

36. Rhodes V, McDaniel R, Homan S, Johnson M, Madsen R. An instrument to measure symptom experience. Cancer Nurs 2000; 23:49–54.

37. Naeim A, Dy SM, Lorenz KA, Sanati H, Walling A, Asch SM. Evidence-based recommendations for cancer nausea and vomiting. Review article. J Clin Oncol 2008;26:3903–3910.

38. Jordon K, Hinke A, Grothey A, Voigt W, Arnold D, Wolf HH, et al. A meta-analysis comparing the efficacy of four 5-HT3-receptor antagonists for acute chemotherapy-induced emesis. Review article. Support Care Cancer 2007;15:1023–1033.

39. Heedman P, Strang P. Symptom assessment in advanced palliative home care for cancer patients using the ESAS: clinical apsects. Anticancer Res 2001;21:4077–4082.

40. Morrow G. A patient report measure for the quantification of chemotherapy induced nausea and emesis: psychometric properties of the Morrow assessment of nausea and emesis (MANE). Br J Cancer 1992;19(Suppl):S72–S74.

41. Martin A, Pearson J, Cai B, Elmer M, Horgan K, Lindley C. Assessing the impact of chemotherapy-induced nausea and vomiting on patients' daily lives: a modified version of the Functional Living Index-Emesis (FLIE) with 5-day recall. Support Care Cancer 2003;11(8):522–527.

42. Goodman M. Risk factors and antiemetic management of chemotherapy-induced nausea and vomiting. Oncol Nurs Forum 1997;26:20–32.

43. Koeller J, Aapro M, Gralla R, et al. Antiemetic guidelines: Creating a more practical treatment approach. Support Care Cancer 2002;10:519–522.

44. Lucarelli C. Formulary management strategies for type 3 serotonin receptor antagonists. Am J Health Syst Pharm 2003;60(Suppl 1):S4–S11.

45. Engstrom C, Hernandez I, Haywood J, Lilenbaum R. The efficacy and cost effectiveness of new antiemetic guidelines. Oncol Nurs Forum 1999;26(9):1453–1458.

46. Gralla R, Osoba D, Kris M, et al. Recommendations for the use of antiemetics: evidence-based, clinical practice guidelines. J Clin Oncol 1999;17:2971–2994.

47. National Comprehensive Cancer Network. Practice Guidelines in Oncology: Palliative Care. National Comprehensive Cancer Network. Available at: http://www.nccn.org (accessed January 14, 2009).

48. Finnish Medical Society Duodecim. Palliative treatment of cancer. Duodecim Medical Publications Ltd. Available at: http://www.duodecim.fi/ (accessed December 30, 2004).

49. Hogan C. Advances in the management of nausea and vomiting. Nurs Clin North Am 1990;25:475–497.

50. Gonzalea-Rosales F, Walsh D. Intractable nausea and vomiting due to gastrointestinal mucosal metastases relieved by tetrahydrocannabinol (dronabinol). J Pain Symptom Manage 1997;14:311–314.

51. Kris M, Gralla R, Clark R. Antiemetic control and prevention of side effects of anticancer therapy with lorazepam or diphenydramine when used in combination with metoclopramide plus dexamethasone. Cancer 1987;60:2816–2822.

52. Fox S, Einhorn L, Cox E, Powell N, Abdy A. Ondansetron versus onansetron, dexamethasone and chlorpromazine in the prevention of nausea and vomiting associated with mutliple-day cisplatin chemotherapy. J Clin Oncol 1993; 11:2391–2395.

53. Lotfi-Jam K, Carey M, Jefford M, Schofield P, Charleson C, Aranda S. Nonpharmacologic strategies for managing common chemotherapy adverse effects: A systematic review. J Clin Oncol 2008;26:5618–5629.

54. Roila F, Tonato M, Cognetti F, et al. Prevention of cisplatin-induced emesis: A double-blind multicenter randomized crossover study comparing ondansetron and ondansetron plus dexamethasone. J Clin Oncol 1991;9:675–678.

55. Joss R, Bacchi M, Buser K. Ondansetron plus dexamethasone is superior to ondansetron alone in the prevention of emesis in chemotherapy naive and previously treated patients. Ann Oncol 1994;5:253–258.

56. Levy M, Catalano R. Control of common physical symptoms other than pain in patients with terminal disease. Semin Oncol 1985;12:411–430.

57. Malik I, Khan W. Clinical efficacy of lorazepam prophylaxis of anticipatory, acute and delayed nausea and vomiting induced by high doses of cisplatin. Am J Clin Oncol 1995;18:170–175.

58. Passik S, Kirsh K, Theobald D, et al. A retrospective chart review of the use of olanzapin for the prevention of delayed emesis in cancer patients. J Pain Symptom Manage 2003;25:485–489.

59. Passik S, Lundberg J, Kirsh K, et al. A pilot exploration of the antiemetic activity of olanzapine for the relief of nausea in patients with advanced cancer and pain. J Pain Symptom Manage 2002;23:526–532.

60. Clinical Guidelines for Palliative Care (INCTR). Nausea and vomiting, 2008:49–52.

61. Ettinger D. Preventing chemotherapy induced nausea and vomiting: an update and review of emesis. Semin Oncol 1995; 22:6–18.

62. Bartlett N, Koczwara B. Control of nausea and vomiting after chemotherapy: what is the evidence? Intern Med J 2002;32: 401–407.

63. King C. Nonpharmacologic management of chemotherapy-induced nausea and vomiting. Oncol Nurs Forum 1997; 24(Suppl):41–48.

64. Redd W, Montgomery G, DuHamel K. Behavioral intervention for cancer treatment side effects. J Nat Cancer Inst 2001;93:810–823.

65. Yasko J. Holistic management of nausea and vomiting caused by chemotherapy. Top Clin Nurs 1985;7:26–38.

66. Matteson S, Roscoe J, Hickock J, Morrow G. The role of behavioral conditioning in the development of nausea. Am J Obstet Gynecol 2002;186:S239–S243.

67. Fallowfield L. Behavioral interventions and psychological aspects of care during chemotherapy. Eur J Cancer 1992;28A (suppl 1):S39–S41.

68. Cotanch P, Hockenberry M, Herman. Self-hypnosis as an antiemetic therapy in children receiving chemotherapy. Oncol Nurs Forum 1985;12:41–46.

69. Morrow G, Hickok J. Behavioral treatment of chemotherapy-induced nausea and vomiting. Oncol Nurs Forum 1993;7:83–89.

70. Redd W, Andresen G, Minagawa R. Hypnotic control of anticipatory emesis in patients receiving chemotherapy. J Consult Clin Psychol 1982;50:14–19.

71. Zeltzer L, LeBaron S, Zeltzer P. The effectiveness of behavioral interventions for reducing nausea and vomiting in children receiving chemotherapy. J Clin Oncol 1984;2:683–690.

72. Jacknow D, Tschann J, Link M, Boyce T. Hypnosis in the prevention of chemotherapy-related nausea and vomiting in children: A prospective study. J Dev Behav Pediatr 1994;15:258–264.

73. Marchioro G, Azzarello G, Vivani F, et al. Hypnosis in the treatment of anticipatory nausea and vomiting in patients receiving cancer chemotherapy. Oncology 2000;59:100–104.

74. Burish T, Tope D. Psychological techniques for controlling the adverse side effects of cancer chemotherapy: findings from a decade of research. J Pain Symptom Manage 1992;7:287–301.

75. Burish T, Carey M, Krozely M, Greco A. Conditioned side effects induced by cancer chemotherapy. Prevention through behavioral treatment. J Consult Clin Psychol 1987;55:42–48.

76. Burish T, Snyder S, Jenkins R. Preparing patients for cancer chemotherapy. Prevention through behavioral treatment. J Consult Clin Psychol 1991;59:518–525.

77. Lyles J, Burish T, Krozely M, Oldham R. Efficacy of relaxation training and guided imagery in reducing the aversiveness of cancer chemotherapy. J Consult Clin Oncol 1982;50:509–526.

78. Arakawa S. Relaxation to reduce nausea, vomiting, and anxiety induced by chemotherapy in Japanese patients. Cancer Nurs 1997;20:342–349.

79. Molassiotis A, Yung H, Yan B, Chan F, Mok T. The effectiveness of progressive muscle relaxation training in managing chemotherapy-induced nausea and vomiting in Chinese breast cancer patients: A randomized controlled trial. Support Care Cancer 2002;10:237–246.

80. Burish T, Vasterling J, Carey M, Matt D, Krozely M. Posttreatment use of relaxation training by cancer patients. Hospice J 1988;4:1–8.

81. Morrow GC, Asbury R, Hamon S, Dobkin P, Caruso L, Pandya K, Rosenthal S. Comparing effectiveness of behavioral treatments for chemotherapy-induced nausea and vomiting when administered by oncologists, oncology nurses, and clinical psychologists. Health Psychol 1992;11(4):250–256.

82. Burish T, Jenkins R. Effectiveness of biofeedback and relaxation training in reducing the side effects of cancer chemotherapy. Health Psychol 1992;11:17–23.

83. Morrow G, Angel C, DuBeshter B. Autonomic changes during cancer chemotherapy induced nausea and emesis. Br J Cancer 1992;66(suppl 19):S42–S45.

84. Mundy E, DuHamel K, Montgomery G. The efficacy of behavioral interventions for cancer treatment-related side effects. Semin Clin Neuropsych 2003;8:253–275.

85. LaBaw W, Holton C, Tewell K, Eccle D. The use of self-hypnosis by children with cancer. Am J Clin Hypn 1975;17:233–238.

86. Achterberg J, Lawlis F. Imagery and health intervention. Top Clin Nurs 1982;3:55–60.

87. Frank J. The effects of music therapy and guided visual imagery on chemotherapy induced nausea and vomiting. Oncol Nurs Forum 1985;12:47–52.

88. Troesch L, Rodehaver C, Delaney E, Yanes B. The influence of guided imagery on chemotherapy-related nausea and vomiting. Oncol Nurs Forum 1993;20:1179–1185.

89. Redd W, Jacobsen, PB, Die-Trill M, Dermatis H, McEvoy M, Holland J. Cognitive-attentional distraction in the control of conditioned nausea in pediatric cancer patients receiving chemotherapy. J Consult Clin Psychol 1987;55:391–395.

90. Kolko D, Rickard-Figueroa J. Effects of video games in the adverse corollaries of chemotherapy in pediatric oncology patients: A single case analysis. J Consult Clin Psychol 1985;53:223–225.

91. Vasterling J, Jenkins R, Tope D. Cognitive distraction and relaxation training for the control of side effects due to cancer chemotherapy. J Behav Med 1993;16:65–80.

92. Morrow G, Asbury R, Hammon S, et al. Comparing the effectiveness of behavioral treatment for chemotherapy-induced nausea and vomiting when administered by oncologists, oncology nurses, and clinical psychologists. Health Psychol 1992;11: 250–256.

93. Morrow G, Dobkin P. Anticipatory nausea and vomiting in cancer patients undergoing chemotherapy treatment. Prevalence, etiology, and behavioral interventions. Clin Psychol Rev 1988;8:517–556.

94. Redd W. Behavioral intervention for cancer treatment side effects. Acta Oncol 1994;33:113–117.

95. Hailey B, White J. Systematic desensitization for anticipatory nausea associated with chemotherapy. Psychosomatics 1983;24: 287–291.

96. Hoffman M. Hypnotic desensitization for the management of anticipatory emesis in chemotherapy. Am J Clin Hypn 1983;25: 173–176.

97. Hare M. Shiatsu acupressure in nursing practice. Holistic Nurs Pract 1988;2:68–74.

98. Dundee J, Ghaly R, Fitzpatrick K. Randomized comparison of the antiemetic effects of metoclopramide and electroacupuncture in cancer chemotherapy. Br J Clin Pharmacol 1988;25:678P–679P.

99. Dundee J, Ghaly R, Fitzpatrick K, Abram W, Lynch G. Acupuncture prophylaxis of cancer chemotherapy-induced sickness. J R Soc Med 1989;82:268–271.

100. Dundee J, Yang J. Acupressure prolongs the antiemetic action of P6 acupuncture. Br J Clin Pharmacol 1990;29:644P–645P.

101. Dundee J, Yang J. Prolongation of the antiemetic action of P6 acupuncture by acupressure in patients having cancer chemotherapy. J R Soc Med 1990;83:360–362.

102. Dundee J, Yang J, Macmillan C. Non-invasive stimulation of the P(6) (Neiguan) antiemetic acupuncture point in cancer chemotherapy. J R Soc Med 1991;84:210–212.

103. Aglietti L, Roila F, Tonato M, et al. A pilot study of metoclopramide, dexamethasone, diphenhydramine and acupuncture in women treated with cisplatin. Cancer Chemother Pharmacol 1990;26:239–240.

104. Dibble S, Chapman J, Mack K, Shih A. Acupressure for nausea: results of a pilot study. Oncol Nurs Forum 2000;27:41–47.

105. Anonymous. NIH Consensus Conference. Acupunture. JAMA 1998;280:1518–1524.

106. Roscoe J, Matteson S. Acupressure and acustimulation bands for control of nausea: A brief review. Am J Obstet Gynecol 2002;188:S244–S247.

107. Vickers A. Can acupuncture have specific effects on health? A systematic review of acupuncture antiemesis trials. J Royal Soc Med 1996;89:303–311.

108. Brown S, North D, Marvel M, Fons R. Acupressure wrist bands to relieve nausea and vomiting in hospice patients. Do they work? Am J Hospice Palliat Care 1992;9:26–29.

109. Dossey B. Psychophysiologic self-regulation interventions. In: Dossey B, ed. Essentials of Critical Care Nursing: Body, Mind, Spirit. Philadelphia: J.B. Lippincott, 1990:42–54.

110. Standley J. Clinical applications of music and chemotherapy: the effects on nausea and emesis. Music Ther Perspect 1992;10: 27–35.

111. Ezzone S, Baker C, Rosselet R, Terepka E. Music as an adjunct to antiemetic therapy. Oncol Nurs Forum 1998;25:1551–1556.

112. Pervan V. Practical aspects of dealing with cancer therapy induced nausea and vomiting. Semin Oncol Nurs 1990;6 (Suppl):3–5.

113. Weitzner M, Moody L, McMillan S. Symptom management issues in hospice care. Am J Hospice Palliat Care 1997;14: 190–195.

# 11

*Constance M. Dahlin, Audrey Kurash Cohen, and Tessa Goldsmith*

# Dysphagia, Xerostomia, and Hiccups

*It seems ridiculous that with everything else going on, what bothers me the most is my difficulty swallowing and my dry mouth. Sometimes when I take lots of sips quickly to swallow, I get the hiccups. It exhausts me, making me no longer want to eat. It doesn't seem worth the effort.—Mark, 53-year-old ALS patient*

◆ ***Key Points***
◆ *Dysphagia, dry mouth, and hiccups affect quality of life and social interaction, and cause unnecessary suffering.*
◆ *Dysphagia has many etiologies and a multitude of management options.*
◆ *Xerostomia is a common complaint.*
◆ *Hiccups, though seemingly harmless, can be extremely frustrating for patients and can be difficult to treat.*
◆ *Comprehensive and regular mouth care relieves suffering and promotes comfort.*

Dysphagia and dry mouth are disturbing symptoms that occur frequently in progressive terminal illness. Hiccups, while less frequent, can be as distressing, adversely affecting quality of life. These problems impact the essence of pleasurable activities such as social interaction, communication, intimacy, and food consumption as well as impairing nutrition.

In a culture where food is both the core of life and a central focus of one's daily structure, disinterest in food and/or lack of the ability to eat can cause distress for both patients and families.

Patients at the end of life may lose interest and then withdraw from social interaction. Since the essence of nurturing is intertwined with the ability to provide and receive nourishment, the chronically ill patient, isolated from social interactions that take place around the consumption of food, becomes increasingly depressed. Family members may also refrain from eating around the dysphagic patient, further isolating him or her.[1] Families, with all good intentions, keep focusing on food. This creates a tension that may make the situation worse because the focus shifts from the patient to the importance of food. Thus, care for patients with terminal illnesses who are experiencing dysphagia, hiccups, or dry mouth, should focus on the following palliative care principles: (1) prevention and relief of suffering is the primary goal, (2) the patient and family are the unit of care, (3) dysphagia care is optimized by involvement of an interdisciplinary team whereby each specialist contributes his/her expert knowledge, and (4) care is best delivered with a plan that reflects the underlying aspect of the life-threatening disease, encompasses the goals of treatment, and determines where the plan of care can be adjusted as the situation demands.[2–4]

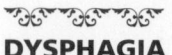

## DYSPHAGIA

### CASE STUDY
#### *AC, A Patient with Dementia and Recurrent Pneumonias*

AC, an 85-year-old man, was admitted to the acute care hospital with worsening shortness of breath and chest congestion and was diagnosed with a pneumonia and dehydration. Prior to this admission, he had been living in an assisted living facility due to his advancing dementia and other medical issues including diabetes, HTN and COPD. Although he was still able to ambulate independently, he required assistance for insulin administration, bathing, dressing and toileting, as he was becoming more forgetful and easily confused. Thus, the patient's daughter had hired a private caregiver to assist him.

Up until recently, he was able to go to family events, eat out at restaurants, and go shopping with her. Although no previous swallowing impairments were documented, upon investigation it was noted that over the past year he had lost 15 pounds, had been admitted to the hospital twice for pneumonia, and that his daughter had reported he would often hold food in his mouth for an extended period of time, benefiting from increasingly softer, moister items, and high calorie snacks.

Over the years, AC and his daughter had spoken about his wishes and he had always stated that he did not want to prolong his life with artificial hydration and nutrition if he could not enjoy being with his family and remain independent. His primary care physician had provided advance care planning to clarify his advance directives regarding life-sustaining treatment and to reflect his wishes for end-of-life care.

While in the hospital, AC had periods of agitation that required staff to periodically use soft wrist restraints and a sitter for risk of falls. A nasogastric tube was placed to temporarily provide him with his medications and an IV for hydration. During the swallowing evaluation done by the speech language pathologist, AC could participate for short periods but became easily fatigued and restless. His oral mechanism assesment did not reveal a vocal weakness although his voice was inconsistently wet sounding, thought to likely be due to spillage of saliva into his airway secondary to reduced swallowing frequency and efficiency. When stimulated, he produced a strong cough to clear these secretions. When observed with small amounts of oral intake, he required sensory cues to close his mouth around the spoon, had delayed oral manipulation of the bolus and a slow reflexive swallow. He could not coordinate drinking from the straw, so liquids were presented via a spoon. He did not show frank signs of aspiration with small, controlled amounts of puree and thickened liquids; however, for larger bolus sizes and for thin liquids, he displayed frank coughing and a gurgly voice that were clinically significant for aspiration.

It was decided that, although an instrumental evaluation such as a videofluoroscopic swallow study could provide more information as to why he was aspirating and clarify the safest consistencies and best swallowing strategies, they would not complete one, as it would likely not alter management nor impact the treatment plan. Given his advancing dementia, history of pneumonias, and declining swallowing ability, it was felt that his ability to safely and adequately maintain his nutrition was compromised and was likely to further decline. The palliative care team was consulted and a team meeting took place with AC's daughter in order to discuss best management and alternatives.

Given the patient's stated wishes and his notable discomfort and suffering with the nasogastric tube and restraints, everyone was in agreement that a gastrostomy tube for feeding was not what he would want. Based on his goals of care and the literature on feeding patients with dementia, it was determined that careful hand feeding would be most appropriate. A plan was devised for AC's daughter and private caregiver to feed him by mouth, acknowledging the inherent risks of pulmonary infection, dehydration and malnutrition. He was discharged to his daughter's house with hospice care and over the next two months, his oral intake diminished and his pulmonary status slowly deteriorated. AC passed away eight weeks after his discharge from the hospital surrounded by his daughter and her family.

## Definition

Dysphagia is defined as difficulty swallowing food or liquid. Typically, chronic difficulty swallowing affects the efficiency with which oral alimentation is maintained. In addition, airway protection or swallowing safety can be threatened. Patients may complain of food getting caught along the upper digestive tract anywhere from the throat to the esophagus. In addition, diversion of food or liquid into the trachea may occur, causing aspiration, choking or, in severe cases, asphyxiation. Chronic difficulty swallowing can be both frustrating and frightening for patients. Because nutrition is compromised, generalized weakness, appetite loss, and weight loss may ensue. In severe cases, malnutrition may occur. Aspiration pneumonia may also occur, causing fevers, malaise, shortness of breath and, rarely, death.

The psychological impact of dysphagia cannot be underestimated. The development of dysphagia may be a pivotal symptom that prompts the decision to consider end-of-life care.[5] Life is not compatible without water, and thus the moment when the patient cannot or does not drink is when death becomes imminent and certain.[6] The palliative care challenge in managing dysphagia is how to ensure comfort, even at the expense of optimal nutrition and hydration.

Understanding the physiology of normal and aberrant swallowing is critical to meeting this challenge.

## Physiology and Pathophysiology of Swallowing

### Normal Swallowing

Swallowing involves the passage of food or liquid from the oral cavity through the esophagus and into the stomach, where the process of digestion begins. Swallowing is an extremely complex physiological act, and demands exquisite timing and coordination of more than 30 pairs of muscles under both voluntary and involuntary nervous control. Because humans swallow hundreds of times per day and are largely unaware of the activity, it is remarkable that difficulties do not occur more frequently.

For purposes of discussion, the act of swallowing is divided into three stages (Figure 11–1). In reality, these stages occur simultaneously, with a blending and overlap of these stages. The act of swallowing takes less than 20 seconds from the moment of bolus propulsion into the pharynx until the bolus reaches the stomach. The longest phase comprises the transit of the bolus through the esophagus.

The first stage of swallowing (see Figure 11–1), the oral stage, is responsible for readying the bolus for swallowing. The duration of the oral stage is variable, depending on the viscosity or consistency of the food bolus and individual chewing styles. Bolus preparation is under voluntary control and can be halted or changed at any point. The primary activities of mastication include gathering and placement of semisoft and liquid boluses on the tongue. It is during this stage that one takes pleasure from the flavor and texture of food through the chemoreceptors of the tongue and palate. During mastication, the tongue moves the bolus to the dental arches to grind into smaller pieces.

The bolus must be partitioned into smaller portions and moistened by saliva. Sensory receptors within the oral cavity, including along the tongue, teeth, cheeks and jaw, as well as within the muscles and joints, assist in mediating saliva production, as well as determining the chewing force and the configuration of the oral cavity to accommodate the bolus type and size.[7] Opening the jaw as well as rotary and lateral movements achieves the masticatory process. Cohesive solid bolus formation is dependent on several factors: the presence of enzyme-rich saliva to bind the material together, the ability of the tongue to gather particles from the sulci of the cheek and the mouth floor, the prevention of food falling out

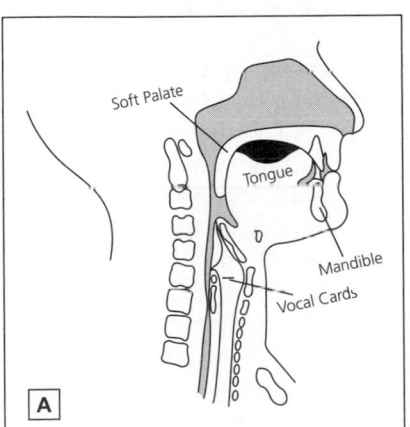
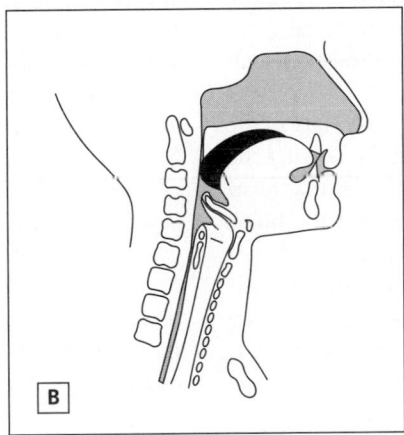
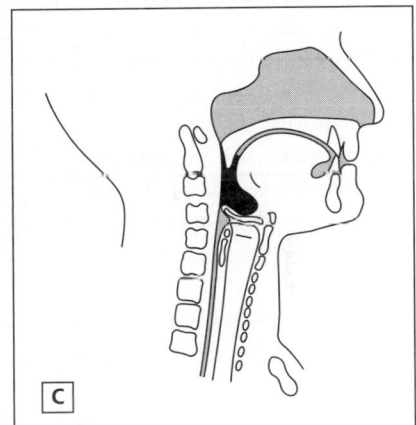
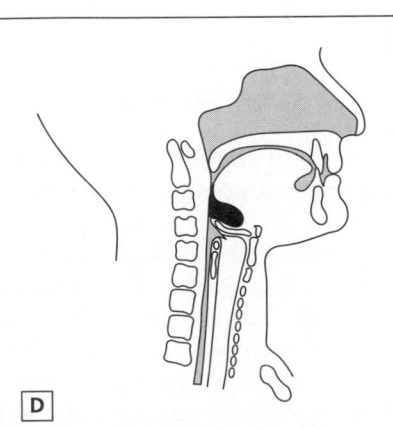
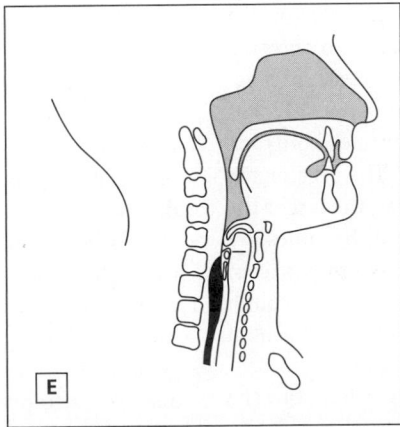

**Figure 11–1.** Stages of swallowing, beginning with voluntary initiation of the swallow by the tongue (A), oral transit (B), pharyngeal of swallowing with airway protection (C) and (D), and esophageal stage (E). *Source:* Logemann (1998), reference 8.

of the oral cavity anteriorly, and the premature spilling into the pharynx.[8] Once the bolus is formed, it is positioned on the tongue and is propelled posteriorly into the pharynx by contraction of the tongue and floor of mouth muscles. The soft palate elevates to prevent nasal regurgitation.

The second stage of swallowing, the pharyngeal stage (see Figure 11–1), is elicited as the posterior tongue retracts and descends, sending the bolus over the base of the tongue and past the faucial arches (the curved arches at the back of the mouth). The bolus passage stimulates the sensory impulses of the glossopharyngeal and vagus nerves to coordinate airway protection and opening of the esophagus. At this stage, the oral cavity and the pharynx become one continuous tube with the entrance to the larynx closed off.[8] The pharyngeal stage of swallowing is the most complex, requiring the most precise timing and coordination.

The process of airway protection—that is, closure of the larynx—is quite remarkable and intricate. Three levels of closure occur, including epiglottic inversion at the entrance to the larynx, closure of the true vocal folds, and closure of the false vocal folds. As the floor of the mouth/tongue muscles contract to propel the bolus from the oral cavity, the larynx moves upward and the epiglottis inverts, closing the laryngeal vestibule. Although the exact sequence and timing of these events is uncertain, it is known that these events occur in order to extrude any material that may have entered the laryngeal vestibule, as well as prevent further material from entering.[7] During the pharyngeal stage, respiration ceases on average of 1 second for a single sip of liquid.

Swallowing usually occurs during the expiratory stage of the respiratory cycle, with expiration preceding and following the swallow.[9] The three pharyngeal constrictor muscles that form semicircular bands progressively contract to send the bolus through the pharynx. As the bolus enters the pharynx, its tail is driven toward the hypopharynx and esophagus by the positive pressure generated from the base of the tongue contacting the pharyngeal walls. The pharyngeal constrictor muscles contract sequentially, and their topographic arrangement has the effect of stripping the bolus through the pharynx.

The upper esophageal sphincter (UES) separates the pharynx from the esophagus and prevents air from entering the esophagus and prevents esophageal contents from reentering into the pharynx.[10] Opening of the UES is the result of traction of the cricoid cartilage and larynx away from the posterior pharyngeal wall as the suprahyoid muscles contract, pulling the larynx upward and forwards.[11,12] The greater the excursion of the larynx and the larger the bolus, the larger the diameter of the opening of the upper esophagus becomes.[13,14]

This opening of the UES creates a negative pressure in the esophagus, further helping to propel the bolus through the pharynx and toward the esophagus.[15] The duration of the pharyngeal stage of swallowing is approximately 1 second. The order of contraction of muscles is invariant, but the timing and intensity of contraction depends on the viscosity and size of the bolus.[16,17] The biomechanical events involved in this stage of swallowing are under involuntary control and

carefully sequenced in a pattern by the central swallowing center in the lower medulla. In the medulla, sensory feedback continually modulates the motor response. For example, if the bolus is dense, the firing of a particular group of muscles of the tongue may be increased, or the opening of the upper esophagus may last longer with a large bolus volume. If the sensory feedback loop is disturbed, the onset of the pharyngeal stage of swallowing may be delayed or, in severe cases, absent.[8,16,18]

The esophageal stage or final stage of swallowing (see Figure 11–1) involves transport of the bolus from the upper esophageal segment, through the lower esophageal segment, and into the stomach, a distance of approximately 25 cm.[8,12] The esophageal stage is coordinated with the pharyngeal stage, with continued sequential contraction of muscles in the cervical esophagus. Like the pharyngeal phase of swallowing, the esophageal stage is under involuntary neuromuscular control. Unlike the pharyngeal stage, however, the speed of propagation of the bolus is much slower, with a rate of 3 to 4 cm/second compared to 12 cm/second in the pharynx.[14,19]

The upper portion or the cervical esophagus consists of approximately 8 cm of striated skeletal muscle, beginning at the upper esophageal segment. The outer fibers of the cervical esophagus are arranged longitudinally, while the inner fibers are arranged in a circular configuration. As the bolus reaches the esophagus, the longitudinal muscles contract, followed by contraction of the circular fibers, constituting the primary peristaltic wave. The lower portions of the esophagus are comprised of smooth muscle fibers. The primary peristaltic wave carries the bolus through the lower esophageal sphincter in a series of relaxation–contraction waves. The lower esophageal sphincter remains open until the peristaltic wave passes. A secondary peristaltic wave is generated where the striated muscle meets the smooth muscle and clears the esophagus of residue. This wave is reflexive in nature and initiated by distention of the esophagus during the primary peristaltic wave.[10,16] After passage of the bolus, the upper and lower esophageal sphincters contract to their resting, closed state. This position contains the gastric contents within the stomach and prevents regurgitation of material into the hypopharynx and airway.[13,14]

### Pathophysiology of Oropharyngeal Dysphagia

Difficulty swallowing can occur during, within, or across any of the above-described stages, depending on the underlying disease.

It is helpful to conceptualize the process of bolus transfer through the oral cavity according to a piston–chamber model proposed by McConnell and Cerenko in 1988,[11] while at the same time being aware that the pressure differential that is generated in the pharynx and throughout the esophagus also works to propel the bolus.[7] The oral cavity, or chamber, comprises the area extending from the lips anteriorly to the hard palate superiorly and the pharyngeal wall posteriorly, bounded by the floor of the mouth inferiorly.

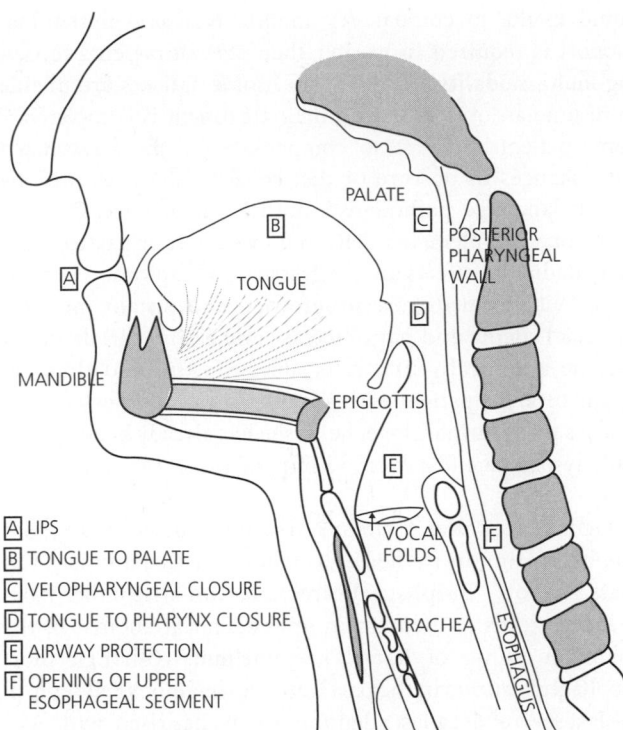

A LIPS
B TONGUE TO PALATE
C VELOPHARYNGEAL CLOSURE
D TONGUE TO PHARYNX CLOSURE
E AIRWAY PROTECTION
F OPENING OF UPPER
ESOPHAGEAL SEGMENT

**Figure 11–2.** Valves of the oral cavity illustrating twin function.

The tongue acts as the piston that creates pressure on the bolus to drive it into the esophagus. The ability of the oral cavity to fulfill its function as a closed chamber depends on the integrity of a number of muscular contractions, which form valves that open and close and are illustrated in Figure 11–2.

Bolus flow and, hence swallowing, is affected if there is dysfunction in the chamber or the piston. If the chamber leaks, residue, regurgitation, or aspiration may occur.

Inefficient bolus flow may result from weakness in the tongue-driving force on the bolus, reduced contraction of the pharynx, or reduced excursion of the hyolarynx. Patients with muscle weakness due to stroke, degenerative neuromuscular disease, or neoplastic lesions involving motor and sensory function of the lips and face may experience difficulty containing the bolus in the oral cavity, producing drooling. Patients with severe dementia who are not aware of food in their mouth may fail to close their lips. Patients with Parkinson's disease or ALS may experience lingual or facial weakness, resulting in oral pocketing of the bolus, making retrieval difficult, especially if buccal and lingual weakness coexist. In cases of reduced sensation, pocketed food may remain in the oral cavity for several hours, possibly increasing the risk of aspiration. Nasal regurgitation of liquids and particles of solids occurs when the velopharyngeal port is dysfunctional, such as in palate cancer where treatment involves resection, and in patients with progressive neuromuscular disease. Weak tongue-driving force during swallowing results in a significant amount of residue in the

pharyngeal recesses, loss of control over the bolus, or incomplete laryngeal closure, causing aspiration before, during, or after the swallow.

Valving of the larynx during the swallow is important for prevention of aspiration into the tracheobronchial tree. Failure of the larynx to close due to timing or muscular incompetence can result in aspiration of liquids or solid materials. Reduced sensory function and weakened laryngeal musculature impair expectoration of aspirated material. Functional and reliable laryngeal valving is crucial not only during oropharyngeal swallowing but also during periods of gastroesophageal reflux, regurgitation, or emesis. Failure of the upper esophagus to open completely results in residue in the pyriform sinuses superior to the pharyngoesophageal segment and, if abundant, may spill over into the unprotected larynx and trachea.[12]

### Etiology

A multitude of diseases can cause dysphagia, particularly in patients receiving palliative care. These include degenerative neuromuscular diseases, progressive cognitive decline disorders, recurrent or fatal neoplastic nervous system or gastrointestinal obstructive lesions, or pervasive debilitation from multisystem diseases. In some cases, side effects of treatment such as radiation therapy or chemotherapy are the precipitating causative factors of dysphagia, whereas in other cases, the progressive nature of the disease leads to unsafe and inefficient swallowing.

Understanding the physiological impact of the illness is critical in evaluation of the swallowing disorder and the method of management.

Generalized weakness of the oropharyngeal musculature may be evident in two patients—one with a diagnosis of ALS and another who has undergone chemoradiation therapy for a recurrent neck squamous cell carcinoma. Both patients may experience a weak pharyngeal swallow with difficulty clearing the bolus through the pharynx. In the patient with ALS, effortful swallows as a compensatory strategy or strengthening exercises would not be indicated due to fatigue. On the other hand, in the patient with neck cancer, encouraging effortful swallows to preserve motor flexibility may assist in protecting his airway to enable him to take some food by mouth in the short term. Some commonly encountered etiological categories in palliative care include cancer, and progressive neurodegenerative diseases which are dicussed below.

### Neoplasms

Tumors involving the nervous system, as well as the head and neck and upper aerodigestive tract can interfere with swallowing.

*Brain Tumors.* Brain tumors are classified into primary and secondary types. Primary brain tumors are a diverse group of neoplasms arising from different cells of the central nervous system. In contrast, secondary tumors originate elsewhere in the body and metastasize to the brain.

It has been estimated that 51,000 new cases of primary brain tumors, malignant or benign, are diagnosed each year.[20] Although dysphagia is rarely the presenting symptom, swallowing problems can develop directly or indirectly as the tumor increases in size and compresses surrounding structures and can be present in as many as 85% of brain tumor patients in the last stages of life.[21]

Extrinsic tumors located around the brain stem, such as acoustic neuromas and meningiomas, as well as those originating in the skull base, such as glomus jugulare, glomus vagale tumors, and chordomas, may compress or invade the lower medulla. Hence, the cranial nerves and their nuclei that are critical for swallowing will be affected, with the specific swallowing impairment dependent upon which cranial nerves are affected. In addition to direct tumor effects, swallowing and/or inability to maintain sufficient oral nutrition may be indirectly affected by depressed levels of consciousness, reduced awareness, fatigue, depression, seizures, sarcopenia, and need for opioids that is associated with tumor progression, mass effect and associated complications.[21–24]

*Head and Neck Cancer.* Oropharyngeal dysphagia is ubiquitous in patients with advanced-stage head and neck cancer. These tumors, most frequently squamous cell, occur in a variety of sites in the oral cavity, pharynx, larynx and upper esophagus and can affect nerve supply and muscle coordination and strength of movements involved in swallowing. Treatment approaches for advanced disease include surgery and chemoradiotherapy depending on the cell type, location, tumor size and presence of neck metastases. Radiation therapy forms the cornerstone of treatment even if other modalities are used. In extensive disease of the oral cavity or in cases of persistent or recurrent tumors, disfiguring surgical resection may be followed by reconstruction with a flap of tissue borrowed from another part of the body such as the fibula or radial forearm.

In the past two decades, "organ preservation" involving chemoradiation therapy has been the primary approach for treating cancers of the pharynx and larynx with the goal of sparing the organs involved in speech and swallowing. Survival at 5 years is about 60%.[25] Laryngectomy is seldom used as a first line treatment for cancer of the voice box but is used in cases of persistent or recurrent disease. Unfortunately, "organ preservation" is not synonymous with "functional preservation." In spite of advances in treatment methods, such as conformal intensity-modulated radiation therapy aimed at sparing normal tissue, and targeted chemotherapy agents, patients suffer from significant treatment toxicities including pulmonary aspiration, mucositis, edema, xerostomia, trismus (restricted jaw opening), and fibrosis affecting airway protection and opening of the upper esophagus.[26]

Swallowing becomes deliberate and effortful with coughing, food getting caught and the need for large volumes of liquid intake to combat dry mouth. Non-oral nutritional support is required in greater than 60% of patients receiving multi-modality treatment and some patients are unable to resume an oral diet once their treatment is completed.[27] Some patients manage to compensate for their dysphagia with changes in posture or diet consistencies suggested by speech language pathologists. Other patients rely on oral nutritional supplements delivered by mouth or gastrostomy tube. Radiation effects are progressive and aspiration is common. With local disease progression and distant metastasis, facial edema and pain increase and eating and drinking become chronically uncomfortable, effortful and difficult. By the time the patient with advanced head and neck cancer reaches the terminal stage, he or she has already been coping with dysphagia and its very visible consequences.

*Malignant Esophageal Tumors.* The incidence of malignant esophageal tumors in the U.S. is rising with as many as 15,500 cases in 2007.[28] Esophageal carcinoma can arise either from squamous cells of the mucosa or as adenocarcinomas of the columnar lining of Barrett's epithelium. Although most esophageal cancers in the past were the squamous cell type, in the last several decades, adenocarcinoma has risen, with adenocarcinoma now four to five times more prevalent in newly diagnosed cases.[29] Tumors of the squamous cell type are generally located in the upper or mid esophagus, while tumors of the adenocarcinoma type are located more distal.[19]

Treatment options and survival rate is much higher when the disease is detected early. Unfortunately, symptom presentation usually occurs late in the disease, resulting in diagnosis of advanced malignancy. Patients commonly complain of weight loss and progressive dysphagia with solid foods rather than liquids, throat pain and vomiting. In some cases, intractable cough may indicate extension of the tumor to the mediastinum or trachea. The presence of local extension to the aorta, trachea, or other mediastinal structures eliminates the possibility of surgical resection "Classic" symptom presentation for patients with adenocarcinoma is gastroesophageal reflux disease rather than dysphagia and weight loss.[30] Survival rates are reported to be between 10% and 20% at 5 years, and thus, palliative care is the foundation of management for this disease.[31]

If diagnosed early, esophagectomy or esophagogastrectomy may be the treatment of choice, although there is a 5% mortality rate and a 64% complication rate following this procedure.[32] However, in cases of unresectable advanced disease, symptomatic relief of dysphagia can be accomplished by radiation therapy, esophageal dilation, chemotherapy, placement of a plastic or wire mesh esophageal stent to open the lumen of the esophagus, tumor ablation via laser, or a newer procedure using photodynamic therapy. Concomitant radiation therapy and chemotherapy is more effective than radiation alone for localized esophageal cancer and is increasingly being used for palliative treatment.[33,34] Each of these treatments is associated with considerable side effects, including radiation-induced esophagitis and chemotherapy-induced mucositis, xerostomia, loss of taste, and lymphedema. Esophageal perforation during laser surgery or dilation and migration of the esophageal stents are potential complications from palliative procedures.[33] Frequently, jejunostomy tubes must be placed for nonoral feeding.

*Cancer, Non-head and Neck.* Oncology patients may develop transient or persistent oropharyngeal dysphagia due to a wide range of issues including presence of tumor, radiation, cytotoxic effects of chemotherapy, cancer-related weakness and fatigue and neurologic or respiratory compromise.[22,34] One study found that of 11 non-head and neck cancer patients receiving palliative care, nine of them reported either dysphagic symptoms, the need to modify their food texture to softer foods, and/or an impact on their quality of life due to swallowing difficulties at some point in the course of their disease.[22] Of particular note should be patients with intrathoracic malignancies, such as lung and mediastinal tumors that can invade the left recurrent laryngeal nerve and result in laryngeal nerve palsies, causing impaired airway protection and cough, as well as dysphagia. Alternatively, damage can occur during hilar lung tumor resection or mediastinal lymph node biopsy. Radiation therapy to the mediastinum may cause esophagitis, which can result in odynophagia, pain on swallowing. Chemotherapy can cause direct toxicity on the oral, pharyngeal or esophageal mucosa, or may result in infection during periods of myelosuppression. This can result in altered taste, pain, reduced appetite, nausea, mucosal bleeding and formation of lesions such as herpes simplex virus or varicella zoster.[35] Cancer patients suffering from dysphagia and/or odynophagia need extra support and nutritional interventions to ensure that their nutritional requirements are met.

## Progressive Neuromuscular Diseases

*Amyotrophic Lateral Sclerosis.* Amyotrophic lateral sclerosis, or ALS, is encountered with unfortunate regularity in patients on a palliative care service. A rapidly progressive degenerative disease of unknown etiology, ALS involves the motor neurons of the brain and spinal cord.[36,37] One quarter of ALS patients present with difficulty swallowing as their initial complaint, while other patients begin with distal weakness that travels proximally to involve the bulbar musculature. As the disease progresses, there is involvement with upper and lower motor neurons, affecting speaking, walking, writing, etc, and ultimately the respiratory system. Respiratory failure is the usual cause of death in patients with ALS because of weakness in diaphragmatic, laryngeal, and lingual function.[37]

Patients typically live between 3 and 5 years after diagnosis, making a multi-disciplinary team approach critical in caring for these patients.[38] Although there is no cure for ALS, numerous pharmacological agents are being researched to treat various symptoms of the disease. Riluzole, a glutamate antagonist, is currently the only pharmacologic treatment for ALS approved by the United States Food and Drug Administration and has been found to slow the progression of the disease and extend life expectancy by several months.[38–40] Non-invasive ventilation can help to manage respiratory failure due to neuromuscular weakness and may slow its rate of decline and prolong quality of life.[39]

Typically, patients with bulbar ALS experience a reduction in tongue mobility, oral and pharyngeal muscle weakness, and fatigue with eating. They experience progressive difficulty with the ability to chew and to control material in the mouth. They may experience nasal regurgitation of fluids and loss of control over liquids, resulting in aspiration and coughing before the swallow is triggered. With disease progression, heavier foods—even pureed—are difficult to manipulate, resulting in significant residue in the oral cavity. Reduced pharyngeal drive also results in residue in the pharynx. Diet modifications with calorie-dense foods and postural alterations are necessary if oral intake is to continue.

Many patients reach a point where the effort involved in eating is too great, significant weight loss and frequent choking may occur and the pleasure is lost. If the patient chooses, a gastrostomy tube is placed percutaneously (PEG) to provide nutrition, and sometimes supplemental oral intake for pleasure is possible. Early placement of a PEG tube may prolong survival, reduce complications and improve quality of life in some ALS patients when placed before body mass index has significantly dropped and before vital capacity drops below 50% anticipated. However, this has not been confirmed by large, randomized controlled trials.[8,37,39,41,42]

*Parkinson's Disease and Parkinsonian Syndromes.* Parkinson's disease is a relatively common, slowly progressive disease of the central nervous system, marked by an inability to execute learned motor skills automatically.[39] Classic motor symptoms include resting tremor, bradykinesia (slowness of movement) and rigidity, gait dysfunction and postural instability. Nonmotor features may include autonomic disturbances, sleep problems and cognitive dysfunction.[43] The largest etiological group is idiopathic; however, Parkinson-like symptoms may occur as a result of medications, toxins, head trauma, or degenerative conditions.[37]

Dysphagia in Parkinson's disease may be oral, pharyngeal and/or esophageal and is related to changes in striated muscles under dopaminergic control and in smooth muscles under autonomic control.[37] The oral stage is associated with rigidity of the lingual musculature rather than weakness.[44] Small-amplitude, ineffective tongue-rolling movements are observed as patients attempt to propel the boluses into the pharynx. As a result, pharyngeal swallow responses are delayed, with aspiration occurring before and during the swallow. Expectoration of cough-aspirated material is weak because of rigidity of the laryngeal musculature. Incomplete opening of the upper esophageal sphincter and esophageal dysmotility are also commonly observed in patients with Parkinson's disease.[34,37] Even mild swallowing impairments may cause changes in quality of life for patients with PD and their caregivers and often adds to their perceived burden and worries.[45]

In the early stages, antiparkinsonian medications such as levodopa or dopamine agonists improve flexibility and speed during swallowing. This medical therapy does not stop progression of the disease, however, and the majority of patients with PD continue to decline.[43] However, pharmacotherapy has only a limited amount to offer dysphagic patients with severe symptoms and sometimes non-oral feeding is necessary.[46] Dysphagia and resultant pneumonia is one of the most prevalent causes of death in patients with Parkinson's disease.[37,45]

Two other progressive neuromuscular diseases include progressive supranuclear palsy (PSP) and multiple system atrophy (MSA). PSP is often initially misdiagnosed as Parkinson's.[47] Early development of orthostasis, falls and vertical gaze palsy are cardinal features of PSP and distinguish it from Parkinson's disease.[48] Patients with PSP do not respond as well as patients with Parkinson's disease to pharmacological treatment, and thus their dysphagia may be more aggressive and more life threatening.[34] Multiple system atrophy is a progressive neurodegenerative disorder characterized by parkinsonism, ataxia, pyramidal signs such as spasticity, and autonomic failure such as orthostatic hypotension. Generally, most patients with MSA do not respond to L-dopa treament or respond only short-term.

*Myopathies.* Myopathy is a neuromuscular disorder that results in muscle weakness and can be either inherited or acquired. Some causes can be treated, such as infectious, toxic, endocrine, and alcohol related. The group of myopathies known as muscular dystrophies are chronic and progressive, resulting in progressive muscle weakness affecting oral, pharyngeal and esophageal muscles. Oculopharyngeal muscular dystrophy (OPMD) is an autosomal dominant muscle disorder with hallmark features of a slowly progressive ptosis and dysphagia, proximal limb and facial weakness and abnormal gait with onset generally occurring after age 40. The leading causes of death for patients with OPMD are recurrent aspiration pneumonia and malnutrition.[49]

Duchenne's muscular dystrophy is a childhood form that generally occurs in boys before the age of 6 and results in severe dysphagia by age 12.[34] The dysphagic symptoms include reduced palatal elevation, weak pharyngeal contraction, reduced hyolaryngeal excursion and reduced esophageal motility. Patients tend to have secretions that pool in their pharynx, aspiration, reflux and poor GI motility. Medical and drug treatments are not effective in treating the disease and thus treatment focuses on management of the symptoms. Surgically, there is some evidence that a myotomy of the UES/cricopharyngeus and/or upper esophageal dilation may be beneficial in cases of moderate/severe dysphagia where there has been no significant weight loss and with adequate pharyngeal contraction.[50]

*Multiple Sclerosis.* Multiple sclerosis (MS) is characterized by multifocal plaques of demyelination within the central nervous system that affects approximately 400,000 people in the US.[51] The scattered inflammatory white-matter lesions observed in the central nervous system result in varying combinations of motor, sensory, and cognitive deficits, which usually run a remitting–relapsing course that may then progress to the secondary progressive form within 10 years.[8,37] Symptoms that may affect quality of life include fatigue, spasticity, paroxysmal symptoms, pain, ataxia, bladder and bowel dysfunction, depression, cognitive problems and dysphagia.[52-54] Dysphagia has been found to occur in 34% of MS patients and was closely related to those patients with brainstem impairment and those who are non-ambulatory.[55] Dysphagia occurs primarily in the end stages, and is generally amenable to compensatory strategies in all but the most severe cases.[55] Difficulties arise with respect to the feeding process because of hand tremors and spasticity. Sclerosed plaques can be found in the cortex and the brain stem and can affect cranial nerves. Therefore, swallowing dysfunction will depend on the location of the lesions.

## Dementia

Dementia can result from many causes, including Alzheimer's disease, cumulative brain damage from multiple small cerebral infarcts (vascular dementia), advanced stages of other diseases such as Parkinson's or Huntington's disease, frontotemporal dementia, Lewy Body disease, and excessive and chronic alcohol use. In addition, patients can demonstrate cognitive decline from chronic metabolic derangement, sedating medications, and/or depression.[8] Dementia causes progressive memory loss, poor awareness, loss of language abilities, inactivity, agitation, and confusion.

Dysphagia in patients with dementia is extremely prevalent, and may be as high as 93%.[34] As a result, patients with dementia frequently encounter pneumonia, malnutrition and dehydration particularly in the advanced stages of the disease. Swallowing problems that arise in the late stages of dementia are generally not reversible, although treating concomitant infections, metabolic disarray and/or dehydration may result in improved functioning.[34,56]

No single dysphagia profile exists for demented patients because of the variety of causes of the disease. However, common observations include the inability to feed self independently and to remain focused for the duration of the meal. Some patients do not engage in the task of eating and swallowing. They may hold food in their mouth for prolonged periods without mastication or bolus formation, especially with uniformly textured foods such as pureed items or bland foods. Decreased consciousness predisposes patients to aspirate food and liquid. As a result of sensory impairments and lack of attention, the patient may fail to control the bolus in the mouth and lose it prematurely over the tongue base and into the larynx before the pharyngeal swallow has been elicited, resulting in aspiration. Moreover, their distractible or agitated behavior may prolong the feeding time and hence reduce the amount of nutrition and hydration received. As dementia progresses, patients develop a lack of desire in eating as a hallmark feature of late-stage dementia.[57] Malnutrition and dehydration can produce medical complications that in turn exacerbate the cognitive decline even further.[8,57]

There is growing consensus amongst medical care providers who work with the elderly and those with dementia that a palliative care approach should be taken, especially in late-stage dementia, including not using feeding tubes. The American Geriatrics Society (AGS) states, "The use of tube feedings, in patients with advanced dementia, is unlikely to provide medical benefit or improved comfort. In general, the benefits versus the burdens of TF do not support its use in these patients with advanced dementia."[56]

## Medical Etiologies

*Systemic Dysphagia.* The broadest category of causes of dysphagia includes inflammatory and infectious factors, which affect oral, pharyngeal, and esophageal stages of swallowing. Autoimmune inflammatory disorders can affect swallowing in either specific organs or the immune system as a whole. Pharyngeal and esophageal symptoms can be very common in this group of diseases. This category of diseases includes polymyositis, scleroderma, inflammatory myopathy and secondary autoimmune diseases. Sometimes, intrinsic obstruction is observed, such as in Wegener's granulomatosis. With other disorders, there is external compression, as in sarcoidosis, abnormal esophageal motility as in scleroderma, or inadequate lubrication as in Sjögren's syndrome.[34]

Poor esophageal motility restricts patients to small meals of pureed or liquid substances, and eating duration is long and drawn out. Patients report the sensation of solid foods getting caught in the esophagus. Weight loss is frequent. Gastroesophageal reflux results from poor esophageal peristalsis.[58] Candida esophagitis can occur in an immunocompromised host, such as in patients with AIDS or patients who have undergone chemotherapy. Dysphagia for solids is greater than for liquids, and patients frequently complain of food getting caught. Heartburn, nausea, and vomiting are other common complaints.[34]

*General Deconditioning.* Multisystem diseases, including the more frequently encountered progressive diseases such as end-stage chronic obstructive pulmonary disease, coronary artery disease, and chronic renal failure, cause insidious weakness. Weight loss in these patients is a common consequence because of reduced endurance for activities of daily living, including eating and swallowing. Patients with emphysema or COPD have difficulty coordinating swallowing and respiration, and may be unable to tolerate the obligatory cessation of breathing required for airway protection during the swallow. General immobility impairs spontaneous pulmonary clearance, resulting in an inability to expectorate material if it is aspirated. Patients are often discouraged and depressed by their loss of independence and declining health.

Dysphagia is often encountered in medical patients within the hospital setting who may have cachexia, loss of muscle mass, significantly compromised pulmonary systems that impede airway protection and/or general weakness and deconditioning from a multitude of illnesses and lengthy hospital stays. In these patients' fragile and immunocompromised condition, they are at much higher risk for suffering from pulmonary infections and negative outcomes should they aspirate, and fatigue may impede their ability to sustain their nutrition. Difficulty in completing oral care due to a low level of consciousness and/or presence of an endotracheal tube can promote colonization of oral bacteria in the hospitalized patient. Aspiration of colonized oropharyngeal contents (secretions, vomitus, food/liquid mixed with colonized secretions) has been found to be a major contributor to aspiration pneumonia.[59,60]

## Medications

Medications can create or worsen dysphagia. There are 160 known medications that list dysphagia as a potential adverse side effect.[61] The number of medications increases proportionally to the number of disorders to be treated, but their reactions may be exponential. Medications can affect all stages of swallowing including lubrication of the oral cavity and pharynx, taste and smell, reduced coordination or motor function, impaired consciousness, GI dysfunction and local mucosal toxicity.[34,61] Antipsychotic or neuroleptic medications can produce extrapyramidal motor disturbances, resulting in impaired function of the striated musculature of the oral cavity, pharynx, and esophagus. Long term use of antipsychotics may result in tardive dyskinesia, with choreiform tongue movements affecting the coordination of swallowing. Delayed swallow initiation is a reported side effect of some neuroleptic medications. Use of antipsychotic medications within the hospital setting has been found to result in impaired swallowing function with worsening of swallowing function as dosage increases.[62]

Anticonvulsants such as Phenobarbital, Tegretol and Dilantin may all have adverse effects and may impact CNS functioning, drowsiness and motor incoordination.[34] Antihistamines and anti-depressants may reduce taste and smell and decrease lubrication. Many of these medications can also alter GI motility, cause mucositis, or increase reflux including antipsychotics, antidepressants and antihistamines. Medications should always be reviewed to determine if they may be contributing to or causing a dysphagia.[61]

## Role of the Speech-Language Pathologist in End-of-Life Care

Speech-language pathologists (SLPs) are the expert specialists in assessment and management of communication and oropharyngeal swallowing disorders, although the traditional model of "rehabilitation" will likely need to be altered within the context of the goals of care of the palliative care patient. Their role as part of the multidisciplinary team in patients at the end of life can help to add comfort and maximize quality of life, as well as support the patient and family and help prepare them to deal with the progressive symptoms of dysphagia that may accompany their disease. The SLP can use his/her knowledge to carefully explain the swallowing process and disorder, use empirical data to determine swallowing potential and prognosticate in order to assist in decision making. The SLP may provide further assistance to the care team by determining ways to best communicate with a patient who has impaired communication abilities, including speaking valves for the tracheostomized or assistive and augmentative communication devices. This can improve the patient's ability to participate in decision making and in expressing their wishes—hallmark features of palliative care.[5,62]

A comprehensive swallow evaluation done by the SLP includes a thorough review of the patient's medical history and presenting complaint, evaluation of their alertness, hemodynamic stability and oromotor functioning, as well as observation of swallowing of various liquid and solid food consistencies, depending on the safety and appropriateness. An instrumental swallow evaluation may be indicated to further delineate swallowing physiology, determine effectiveness of various swallowing strategies and clarify or confirm aspiration risk (see below for more information). Treatment goals are individualized to the patient and may focus on improving swallow function, while for others they may focus on maximizing residual abilities, or maintaining some oral intake while ensuring safety and efficiency of nutrition. Speech-language pathologists who care for dying patients must carefully weigh what will benefit the patient and what will be burdensome. They need to be knowledgeable in the disease processes underlying the palliative care patient, cognizant of the spiritual and emotional issues, skilled in biomedical ethics and legal issues, and highly sensitive to the psychosocial ramifications of altering oral diets.[1,63–65]

## Assessment

Evaluation of dysphagia in patients receiving palliative care is best accomplished within a multidisciplinary framework where the patient's needs and wishes are held paramount. Approaching the evaluation of swallowing in the terminally ill patient demands a holistic view and reaches beyond the physiology of deglutition. While aspiration of food or liquid could realistically evolve into aspiration pneumonia, paradoxically, committing a patient to non-oral feeding or non per os (NPO) is also fraught with complications. It therefore behooves caregivers to carefully consider the multiple parameters in decision-making about oral nutrition in the terminally ill patient. The matter is not a simple decision of "if the patient is aspirating food, he or she should not receive nutrition orally."

For the patient with a life-threatening illness, the goals of the clinical swallowing evaluation are to: (1) identify the underlying physiological nature of the disorder; (2) determine whether any short-range interventions can alleviate the dysphagia; and (3) collaborate with the patient, family,

and caregivers on the safest and most efficacious method of nutrition and hydration. Balancing the safety and health of the patient with quality of life issues is integral to the assessment.[1]

## Clinical History

A comprehensive understanding of the difficulties involved in swallowing depends in large part on a detailed history from the patient and caregivers. Eliciting a description of the patient's complaints about swallowing is critical to painting a picture of the physiological basis of the problem and to integrating these hypotheses with attitudes and wishes about eating and not eating. Details of disease progression along with the accompanying emotional and psychological impact on the patient and the family should also be considered when determining the aggressiveness of a swallowing work-up and its treatment.

The swallowing history may indicate a mechanical obstruction etiology or an underlying neuromuscular cause. Asking the patient which foods are easier and which are avoided, with special focus on liquids versus solids, provides clues about the location of the disorder. For example, patients who complain of solid food dysphagia and localize the area of difficulty to the throat may present with bolus propulsion problems, whereas those who choke on liquids may have a sensory deficit with mistiming of airway protection. It is important to note low diagnostic specificity regarding the patient's localization of the problem with radiographic or endoscopic findings.[66]

Information about the patient's current eating habits and diet should be elicited. Does the patient choke on all consistencies of solid foods and fluids? Can the patient feed himself or herself? How have meal times changed since the illness? What is the total calorie intake the patient receives on a daily basis, and how far short does this fall from the patient's nutritional requirements? Length of meal times and effort required are indicators of eating efficiency. Additional areas of concern include appetite, factors that appear to alleviate or exacerbate the problem such as positioning, time of day, ability to swallow medication, and the presence of pain on swallowing. Table 11–1 lists frequently encountered complaints by patients regarding swallowing and their potential physiological counterparts.

The current complaints with respect to the physiology of swallowing are as important as the patient's previous attitudes toward eating. These attitudes form the foundation on which management strategies are implemented. The patient with a poor appetite, fatigue, and a sense of hopelessness will understandably be less compliant and less motivated to engage in a complex treatment program. Alternatively, the patient who derives much satisfaction from eating and drinking and wishes to continue with a regular diet, will not be satisfied with significant alterations in texture and consistency. Additionally, the patient and caregivers should understand and consider the competing benefits and risks regarding nutrition, with attention to the patient's preferences.

**Table 11–1**
**Patient Complaints of Swallowing Difficulty and Their Possible Physiological Correlates**

| Patient's Complaint | Physiological Impairment |
|---|---|
| Choking on fluids | Poor tongue control for oral manipulation |
| | Impaired laryngeal closure |
| | Delayed onset of pharyngeal swallow |
| Protracted meal times | Weak chewing |
| | Diminished endurance |
| Nasal regurgitation of fluids | Incompetent velopharyngeal mechanism |
| Difficulty getting swallow started | Reduced oral and hypopharyngeal sensation |
| Dry mouth | Reduced or impaired saliva production |
| Solids caught in throat | Weak tongue-driving force |
| | Impaired laryngeal excursion fails to open upper esophageal segment |
| Regurgitation or emesis after swallowing | Poor esophageal motility or esophageal obstruction |
| Sour taste in mouth after eating | Gastroesophageal reflux |
| Pain on swallowing | Esophagitis, mucositis, esophageal obstruction |
| Excessive drooling | Reduced frequency or efficiency of swallowing |
| Food sticking in thoracic or chest region | Poor esophageal motility or obstruction |

## Examination of Swallowing by Direct Observation

Direct observation by a perceptive clinician of the patient while eating, drinking, or taking medications can yield valuable information about the underlying disorder. As discussed previously, the speech-language pathologist is vigilant for indications of chewing inefficiencies, aspiration, or obstruction. Table 11–2 lists warning signs that can alert caregivers to possible swallowing problems.

Usually, the clinician assesses the patient's oral-motor and sensory function and cognitive communicative function, while observing the partaking of a variety of liquid and solid foods (e.g., semi-solid, soft solid, and, where appropriate, food requiring mastication). Speech and voice are analyzed to determine the underlying physiology of the swallowing disorder. Since aspiration may be silent in up to 40% of patients with dysphagia, close attention is paid to occult signs of aspiration, including wet vocal quality or gurgliness, frequent throat clearing, delayed coughing, and oral/pharyngeal residue.[8]

*Assessment of Airway Protection.* Functional airway protection is a critical predictor of safe swallowing and, thus, an important element of the clinical swallowing evaluation. Effective airway protection entails timely and complete laryngeal closure during swallowing and the efficient expectoration of material in response to aspiration. Audible strong cough at the glottis and pharyngeal contraction, which is necessary for bringing up a sputum sample, are required for functional airway protection. Patients who have weak voices and weak respiratory force for coughing and pulmonary clearance are at risk for pulmonary compromise. Airway protection cannot be definitively discerned from a clinical evaluation alone. Although the clinician may palpate moderate superior and anterior laryngeal elevation on swallowing, may

**Table 11–2**
**Indications of a Swallowing Disorder**

**Reduced alertness or cognitive impairment**
Coma, heavy sedation, dementia, delirium
Impulsivity with regard to eating, playing with food, inattention during eating

**Alterations in attitudes toward eating**
Refusal to eat in the presence of others
Avoidance of particular foods or fluids
Protracted meal times, incomplete meals, large amounts of fluids to flush solids
Changes in posture or head movements during eating
Laborious chewing, multiple swallows per small bites

**Signs of oral–pharyngeal dysfunction**
Dysarthria or slurred, imprecise speech
Dry mouth with thick secretions coating the tongue
And palate
Wet voice with "gurgly" quality
Drooling or leaking from the lips
Residual in the oral cavity after eating
Frequent throat clearing
Coughing or choking
Nasal regurgitation

**Specific patient complaints**
Sensation of food getting caught in the throat
Coughing and choking while eating
Regurgitation of solids after eating
Pain on swallowing
Food or fluid noted in tracheotomy tube
Inability to manage secretions
Drooling
Shortness of breath while chewing or after meals
Regurgitation of food or fluid through the nose
Difficulty initiating the swallow
Unexplained weight loss

perceive a normal vocal quality, and may not observe cough on swallowing, the patient may in fact be silently aspirating.[67] Silent aspiration can only be confirmed definitively with an instrumental examination. Previous radiation therapy, as well as cranial nerve IX (glossopharyngeal) and X (vagus) deficits, may all contribute to the picture of silent aspiration. Depending on the stage of progression of the patient's illness and overall management goals, it may be prudent to identify silent aspiration with the aim of limiting progression with behavioral strategies.

*Assessment of Oral Hygiene.* The status of the oral mucosa and general oral hygiene reflect a patient's ability to manage secretions and swallowing. As mentioned earlier, xerostomia may exacerbate, and in some cases even cause, difficulty swallowing. Patients who require supplemental oxygen delivered via a nasal cannula frequently experience dryness in the oral cavity. Severe illness and many medications may alter the normal oral environment, salivary production and the growth of oral bacteria.[68] It is not uncommon to find dry secretions crusted along the tongue, palate, and pharynx in patients who have not eaten orally in some time. Dental caries and dentures that are not well cared for can also contribute to a state of poor oral hygiene as well as poor quality of life. Before giving the patient food or liquids, even for assessment purposes, it is vital to clear the oral cavity of extraneous secretions, using mouth swabs, tongue scrapers, toothbrushes, and oral suction if necessary. If dried oral secretions are extensive, use of moist swabs alone is generally not effective and toothbrushes should be utilized. Use of a flashlight is recommended to assist in carefully inspecting the back of the mouth. Caution should be taken when completing oral care as dried oral secretions may loosen during trials of fluid and inadvertently obstruct the airway. Providing humidification via a shovel mask or face tent and consistent oral care for the hospitalized patient may help to loosen secretions, moisten the oropharyngeal mucosa, and maximize comfort.

*Screening of Swallowing Function.* In the last several years there has been increased awareness for the need to screen swallowing and assess risk for aspiration before giving patients anything to eat or drink, including oral medications.[69] This has been largely driven by the extensive research done on acute stroke patients and their high risk of aspiration (40–60%), the close relationship between aspiration and aspiration pneumonia, and the evidence that shows that mortality rates in acute stroke patients with pneumonia are three times higher than those without.[70] As a result, since 2005, several national regulatory and safety guidelines including JCAHO and American Heart Association state that all acute stroke patients should have their swallowing screened before being given anything orally. Although this currently relates to acute stroke patients, there is increasing awareness of the risk of aspiration and the need to determine swallowing safety in many hospitalized patient populations.[71,72] The swallow screening is typically done by the nurse and identifies potential aspiration risk, assists in determining if a patient is safe to start eating and drinking, and helps to determine if a patient requires a full evaluation by the SLP. It cannot, however, determine an etiology or underlying physiology of the swallowing disorder, and therefore cannot determine appropriate compensatory strategies, treatment or prognosis. Therefore, if a patient is felt to be at risk for aspiration, a comprehensive swallow evaluation should be completed.

*Evaluation of the Gag Reflex.* A word of caution is needed regarding the gag reflex and oropharyngeal swallowing. The gag reflex and the pattern of neuromuscular events comprising the swallow are very different, both in their innervation and in their execution. The gag reflex is a protective reflex that prevents noxious substances arising from the oral cavity or digestive tract from entering the airway. It involves simultaneous constriction of the pharyngeal and laryngeal muscles closing the airway and the pharyngeal lumen and results in anterior movement of the tongue.[73] A gag reflex is not elicited during the normal swallow and its assessment is not clinically relevant to ability to swallow.[74] In fact, 20% to 40% of normal, healthy adults do *not* have a gag reflex.[75] Unlike the pattern of events in the swallow, the gag reflex can be extinguished or reduced by a nasogastric feeding tube, endotracheal intubation, or repeated stimulation. Only evaluation of the biomechanical events of the swallow, not the gag reflex, can predict the safety of airway protection.

**Instrumental Evaluation**

The clinical examination of swallowing is not conclusive regarding location of the swallowing disorder or the underlying physiology. Radiographic or endoscopic evaluation of swallowing are functional examinations providing valuable information for management. Sometimes disease progression with its sequelae, including inability to travel, inability to sit upright, wakefulness, pain and/or somnolence, preclude instrumental examination. Management shifts from maintenance to comfort, with compensatory behaviors being inappropriate.

*Videofluoroscopic Evaluation of Swallowing.* Radiographic swallowing studies are helpful in understanding the underlying physiology of swallowing.[8] The videofluoroscopic swallowing study (commonly known as modified barium swallow study or MBS) examines oropharyngeal swallowing with the patient positioned upright while swallowing a variety of consistencies of barium-coated foods (liquids, semisolids, and solids) in controlled volumes. Speech-language pathologists and radiologists perform these studies together. The study is recorded digitally and reviewed following the study for closer inspection of the anatomy and physiology. The goal of this study is not only to determine the presence or absence of aspiration, but also to evaluate the effectiveness of compensatory swallowing strategies (described below) that may decrease the risk of aspiration and increase swallowing efficiency. The test is not invasive, takes a short time to administer, and provides valuable information that can be used in managing the dysphagia.[8,76]

In contrast to the videofluoroscopic swallowing study, which focuses on the oropharyngeal mechanism, a barium swallow study examines esophageal function and focuses on the anatomy of the esophagus, stomach and duodenum. The barium swallow identifies mucosal and anatomical abnormalities, esophageal strictures, and esophageal motility. It has less sensitivity for diagnosing gastroesophageal reflux, which is better assessed with pH monitoring and/or manonmetry.[10,77] This test is conducted with the patient positioned upright and in the supine position while swallowing liquid barium or, in some cases, a barium tablet. Since the esophagus is under involuntary neural control, compensatory swallowing strategies cannot be assessed with this procedure. However, recommendations can be made for changing to liquid consistencies in a patient with an esophageal stricture.

*Fiberoptic Endoscopic Evaluation of Swallowing (FEES).* Endoscopic examination of oropharyngeal swallowing can be performed at the bedside by a trained speech-language pathologist. The oropharynx and larynx can be visualized transnasally while the patient is swallowing food substances dyed with food coloring and the presence of laryngeal penetration, aspiration, and pharyngeal retention can be observed. As in the videofluoroscopic swallowing study, compensatory swallowing strategies such as postural modifications or swallowing maneuvers can be evaluated for their efficacy.[78] In contrast, endoscopic evaluation of the esophagus and stomach (Esophagogastroduodenoscopy or EGD) is completed by a Gastroenterologist and can confirm the presence of strictures and mucosal anomalies. The assistance of a gastroenterologist may be required in cases requiring palliative dilation of the esophagus.[34]

## Management

Effortless, efficient, and safe swallowing are important criteria for continued oral nutrition. Experience has shown that most patients prefer oral alimentation even if it means they do not receive sufficient nutrition. Patient autonomy in shared decision-making is a critical ethical principle to respect but should be accompanied by a clear understanding of the risks involved in eating by mouth. Specifically, families and patients should be informed about the risks and consequences of developing aspiration pneumonia and malnutrition. If the decision is to continue with oral intake, the safest diet should be suggested and aspiration precautions introduced, using assessment of the swallowing problem as a guide.

### Compensatory Swallowing Strategies

The physiologic information obtained from clinical and instrumental swallowing assessment facilitates on-line assessment of intervention strategies aimed at increasing swallowing safety and efficiency. These include alterations in head and neck posture, consistency of food, sensory awareness, and feeding behaviors. The chief advantage of these strategies is that they are simple for the patient to learn and to perform. In addition, once their effectiveness is determined, the patient can use the intervention during meals to improve swallowing function. In 2008, a large, multi-site, randomized clinical trial of patients with a diagnosis of dementia and/or Parkinson's disease was published examining the effects of three compensatory interventions to prevent aspiration of liquids, including chin-down posture, nectar-thickened liquids, and honey-thickened liquids. It demonstrated that determining which strategy or combination of strategies may be most effective is highly individualized, that there is no uniform effectiveness in any one of these strategies, and that effectiveness can only be determined by an objective swallowing evaluation.[79]

*Postural Modifications.* Postural changes during swallowing often have the effect of diverting the food or liquid to prevent aspiration or obstruction but do not change the swallowing physiology.[7,8] A commonly used strategy is the chin tuck posture. This posture has the advantage of increasing the pressure on the bolus and restricting the opening of the larynx during swallowing, thus potentially reducing the risk of laryngeal penetration and aspiration. However, in select cases, a chin tuck may exacerbate the aspiration, underscoring the need for radiographic evidence of its clinical value, if at all possible. Head rotation to the weak side in a patient with head and neck cancer is another postural change that may assist bolus flow down the intact side by obstructing the weak side and, hence, preventing residue or aspiration. These strategies may be used in isolation or in combination, depending on the nature of the underlying swallowing pathophysiology. Table 11–3 lists some of the postural strategies that the SLP may introduce, and their potential benefits on bolus flow.

*Changes in Texture and Consistency of Food.* Underlying physiological constraints, such as reduced tongue control or strength, may affect the safety of swallowing certain food consistencies. For example, a patient with profound tongue weakness, such as in advanced ALS, may exhibit signs of aspiration on thin liquids, but may have sufficient control to drink liquids thickened to nectar-like or honey-like consistency in small sips. Patients debilitated by chronic disease and who lack endurance to complete a meal may benefit from ground or pureed moist foods that require limited mastication. In certain circumstances, altered food consistency is the only way a patient can continue to eat orally—for example, in the patient with esophageal carcinoma or a severe esophageal motility disorder. Some nutritional supplement drinks are both thicker liquids and calorically fortified, providing a safer alternative to more solid consistencies.

Changes in the consistency of food and liquid are frequently difficult for patients because they often lack appeal.

Table 11–3
**Compensatory Postural Changes that Improve Bolus Flow and Reduce Aspiration and Residue During Swallowing**

| Postural Strategy | Effects on Bolus Flow |
| --- | --- |
| Chin tuck | Closes laryngeal vestibule, pushes tongue closer to posterior pharyngeal wall, and promotes epiglottic deflection |
| Head back | Promotes posterior bolus movement with assistance of gravity |
| Head tilt to stronger side | Directs bolus down stronger side with assistance of gravity |
| Head turned to weaker side | Diverts bolus away from weaker side by obstruction of weaker pharyngeal channel, promotes opening of upper esophagus |
| Head tilt plus chin tuck | Directs bolus down stronger side while increasing closure of laryngeal vestibule |
| Head rotation plus chin tuck | Diverts bolus away from weaker side while facilitating closure of laryngeal vestibule and vocal folds |

*Source*: Logemann (1998), reference 8.

Thus, this management strategy should be used as a last resort and reserved for patients who are unable to follow directions to use postural changes or for whom other compensatory strategies are not feasible.[8] See *Appendix 1* for a list of cookbooks that can assist patients and care providers in preparing foods and liquids that have altered textures and may be easier to swallow.

*Increased Sensory Awareness.* Sensory enhancement techniques include increasing downward pressure of a spoon against the tongue when presenting food in the mouth and presenting a sour bolus, a cold bolus, a bolus requiring chewing, or a large-volume bolus. These techniques may elicit a quicker pharyngeal swallow response while reducing the risk of aspiration. Some patients benefit from receiving food or liquid at a slower rate, while others are more efficient with larger boluses. Enhancing the bolus characteristics to include more texture can sometimes induce mastication and bolus formation more readily than a bolus that is both flavorless and homogenous in texture. This is particularly evident in patients with advanced dementia. Patient responses to these behaviors can be evaluated at the bedside, and the findings can be easily communicated to the caregivers.[8]

*Pharmacological Management.* There are no pharmacological agents that directly act on oropharyngeal swallowing function. However, there are agents for concurrent issues, which can exacerbate an underlying mucosal problem and medications that may effectively treat GI motility, reflux, and nausea and vomiting.[61] This includes yeast infections such as candidiasis, and sialorrhea or excess secretions.

Candida esophagitis requires oral antifungal agents such as nystatin topical. Other antifungal medications include ketoconazole, miconazole, fluconazole, and amphotericin B. Immunocompromised patients with candidiasis require potent systemic antifungal medications. Resistance can occur, however, in patients with long-term prophylaxis. Patients who fail the above regimen may be considered for antiviral agents.[80] A prokinetic agent may be prescribed for poor esophageal motility, and proton pump inhibitors or a histamine-2 blockers such as ranitidine have been found to be effective in patients with gastroesophageal reflux disease.[61] Botulinum toxin (Botox) injected into the lower esophageal sphincter can temporarily induce relaxation when LES spasm is present.[61]

*Sialorrhea and Secretion Management.* Sialorrhea, or excessive drooling due to the inability to control oral secretions, may often occur in patients with motor neuron disease and parkinsonian diseases due to impaired swallowing function, reduced frequency of swallowing, reduced oropharyngeal or laryngeal sensation, poor head posture, inability to close the oral cavity and a weak cough with poor clearance of secretions. Up to 80% of patients with Parkinson's Disease experience sialorrhea.[81,82] Excessive salivation can be embarrassing and socially disabling, as well as contribute to medical developments including skin irritation, poor oral health, dehydration and increased risk of aspiration pneumonia. In the early stages, behavioral, compensatory and strengthening exercises via speech-language therapy may be helpful.

In more severe disease, treatment options include anticholinergic medications (glycopyrrolate, scopolamine, benztropine); botulinum toxin; radiation therapy to the parotid and submandibular glands; and surgical resection of either the parasympathetic neural pathway or of the submandibular and salivary glands. However, each of these treatment options has significant side effects and may be contraindicated or poorly tolerated in various populations.[83–85] Patients with weakened cough and weakness of the respiratory muscles have an increased risk of mucus plugging, atelectasis and pneumonia. An insufflator-exsufflator or cough-assist device may help to improve air movement and strength of the cough and thus achieve greater pulmonary secretion clearance.[83]

**Table 11–4**
**Diet Modifications for Patients with Dysphagia**

| Diet | Definition | Example | Indication |
|---|---|---|---|
| Pureed diet | Blenderized food with added liquid to form smooth consistency; No chewing necessary | Applesauce, yogurt, moist mashed potatoes, puddings | Reduced tongue function for chewing, impaired pharyngeal contraction, esophageal stricture |
| Mechanically altered diet | Ground, finely chopped foods that form a cohesive bolus with minimal chewing | Pasta, soft scrambled eggs, cottage cheese, ground meats | Some limited chewing possible but protracted due to impaired tongue control |
| Soft, moist diet | Naturally soft foods requiring some chewing; food is cut in small pieces; serve with gravy to moisten | Soft meats, canned fruits, baked fish; avoid raw vegetables, bread, and tough meats | Reduced endurance for prolonged meal due to tongue weakness for chewing, reduced attention span |
| Liquids | Honey consistency | Similar in viscosity to honey; available in ready-to-serve packaging or use thickening agent | Reduced oral or lingual control, premature spillage, delayed swallow initiation and airway closure |
|  | Nectar consistency | Similar in viscosity to tomato juice; less thick than honey consistency | Reduced bolus control, premature spillage, delayed swallow and airway closure |

*Dietary Changes.* Evaluation results highlight the most appropriate nutritional method for the patient. If oral alimentation has been determined as safe, the guiding principle for diet is to ingest the maximum amount of calories for the least amount of effort. Examples of modified diets are listed in Table 11–4.

Nutritionists can provide individualized suggestions for calorie-dense foods or high calorie liquid supplements, depending on the patient's metabolic status. Patients with oropharyngeal dysphagia may require thickened liquids. Commercial thickening agents from modified food starch or gum-based (xanthan, guar, cellulose) can be used to thicken liquids. Gum-based thickeners have improved performance over starch-based in terms of stability over time and temperature.[86] Thickened liquids release the fluid in the gastrointestinal tract, do not alter the body's absorption rate of fluids, and provide water for hydration requirements.[87]

*Feeding the Patient.* While there is no cure for a swallowing disorder in the terminally ill patient, continued ability to eat by mouth may be facilitated by careful hand-feeding techniques and strategies employed by family and caregivers. These techniques will vary depending on the underlying swallowing/feeding difficulty. Compliance with feeding strategies is often related to understanding of the rationale. Family members are more likely to feed a patient a particular diet and in a particular manner if they understand the physiological and psychological reasons for the recommendation and if they have been included in the decision-making.[8] Although hand feeding is time consuming, it allows for continued intimate contact between patient and caregiver. Feeding the patient provides caregivers with a way to interact and connect and a way to demonstrate their care and compassion.[5]

Additional suggestions for feeding the patient include the following:

1. Remove distractions at mealtime. This is appropriate for patients who need to concentrate on swallowing to increase safety, such as patients with head and neck cancer who are using compensatory swallowing strategies, and for patients who easily lose their focus and need to be fed, such as patients with Alzheimer's dementia.[88]

2. Emphasize heightened awareness of sensory clues. Feeding patients larger boluses, increasing downward pressure of the spoon on the tongue to alert the patient that food is in the mouth, or feeding patients cold or sour boluses or foods requiring some mastication may improve oral sensation and awareness. Some patients with Alzheimer's disease demonstrate the most efficient swallow when offered finger foods that require chewing. These foods allow them to tap into the automatic motor rhythm of chewing and swallowing that is reminiscent of the patterns they have used all their lives.

3. Provide feeding utensils. Patients who have feeding difficulties associated with hand tremors or weakness may be aided with devices such as weighted cuffs or built-up utensils. Occupational therapists are often able to provide individualized assistive devices to patients.

4. Position the patient. Ensure optimal posture of the patient at meals. Sit the patient as upright as possible when eating, drinking or taking medications. Reduce the tendency to slump forward, which may cause loss of food from the oral cavity, or head extension, which

can promote an open airway and make the patient more vulnerable to aspiration.

5. Schedule meal times. Timing of meals to coincide with increased function, either due to effects from fatigue or medications, may enhance swallowing efficiency and safety. Increased frequency of small meals may help patients who do not have sufficient efficiency or endurance to complete an entire meal at one time.

*Non-oral Nutrition.* Some patients require primary non-oral feeding, and gastrostomy or jejunostomy tubes are placed endoscopically or in open surgical procedures. Some patients, such as those with esophageal cancer, head and neck cancer, or ALS, have had their feeding tubes in place for several months prior to the terminal period. For other patients, families and caregivers may have recently decided to pursue the non-oral feeding option. Irrespective of the scenario, the following should be considered:

1. Patients and their families need to be fully informed regarding benefits and risks of non-oral and oral feeding options in order to make fully informed decisions. Involving the patient and family in shared decision-making helps to ensure that the plan is consistent with their preferences.[3]

2. Knowing that progressive dysphagia and loss of appetite is typical for patients with many progressive diseases mentioned in this chapter, medical teams and families caring for these persons should begin to consider the patient's wishes early in the disease process in order to incorporate these wishes into the care plan.[56]

3. The presence of a feeding tube does not imply NPO, or nothing by mouth. Some patients are able to take small amounts of food for their pleasure. Restrictions to reduce the risk of aspiration may apply during these "trials" of oral intake, such as texture of the food, postural requirements, and length of the trial.

4. Patients who are fed non-orally remain at risk for aspiration and aspiration pneumonia from oral secretions and/or refluxed gastric contents, including tube feeding.[59] A long-term study by Langmore and associates[89] examined the predictors of aspiration pneumonia in 189 elderly patients, including such factors as oropharyngeal and esophageal dysphagia, medical and dental status, feeding status, and functional status. They found that the dominant risk factor for aspiration pneumonia was dependence for feeding—that is, inability to feed oneself. This variable included those patients who were tube-fed as well as those who were fed orally by a caretaker. This study found that patients who were tube-fed had a significantly increased risk of developing aspiration pneumonia. The authors posited that oral hygiene is frequently neglected in tube-fed patients, promoting colonization of bacteria, and aspiration of these secretions can result in pneumonia.

5. The decision to pursue the option of non-oral nutritional support has significant ramifications for both the patient and the family. The family may feel that they have neglected their obligation to nourish their loved one safely and may be overwhelmed by the demands of frequent nocturnal feedings, monitoring of gastric residuals, etc. However, in some disease processes and at early points in care, tube feeding may provide the patient with several more months of improved quality of life afforded by strength and endurance. Patients and families may also feel a sense of relief afforded to them because of the tube feeding.

6. Literature shows that feeding tubes have a limited role and are often overused in medical practice. Their placement should only be considered when the benefits (improving quality of life and/or mortality) clearly outweigh the burdens and are guided by the use of evidence-based placement guidelines.[90]

7. Seeking more creative solutions may help to ease the feeding decision. Hand feeding in small amounts and improving the care environment to maximize attention are two suggestions that have been made for patients with dementia. Interestingly, patients receiving hand feeding have in some cases had an equal duration of survival as those patients with gastrostomy tubes.[44] One prominent geriatrician has recently proposed creating new solutions, such as Ensure lollipops or sublingual high-calorie drops.[91,92]

*Gastroesophageal Reflux Precautions.* Poor esophageal motility or reduced tone of the lower esophageal sphincter can be managed either pharmacologically with the pro-motility agents described above or with nonpharmacological interventions. Ideally, a combination approach is most efficacious. Gastroesophageal reflux precautions include: elevation of the head of the bed to 45 degrees at night, inexpensively and effectively accomplished by placing blocks under the head of the bed; frequent small meals; upright posture for 45 to 60 minutes after eating; monitoring of gastric residuals in tube-fed patients; and avoidance of spicy foods, coffee, tea, chocolate, and alcohol.

*Administration of Medication.* Oral medications can present enormous challenges to patients with dysphagia. One study looking at pill swallowing in patients with chronic dysphagia found that more than 60% of subjects had difficulty swallowing tablets. Some of the physiologic difficulties they experienced included multiple swallows to clear the pill, residue in the pharynx after swallowing, increased time needed to swallow pills, use of liquid to assist in washing the pill down, and airway compromise.[93] Because difficulty swallowing may impact compliance with medications, finding alternative modes of presentation can be critical. Compounding, done by a pharmacist, creates a medication tailored to the specialized needs of an individual patient by producing an alternative form such as a powder, inhalor, liquid, lozenge, or suppository. Health care providers and patients should refer to the FDA statement on Regulation of Compounded Drugs found at: http://www.fda.gov/cder/pharmcomp/default.htm. Crushing medications or burying them whole in a semi-solid food such as applesauce or ice cream creates a uniform consistency and makes swallowing easier. Alternately, patients can be offered their medications in elixir form. Orally disintegrating medication technology has been used to formulate medications that rapidly disintegrate in the oral cavity. One study comparing this method of presentation to oral tablets found that dysphagic patients rated orally disintegrating medications easier to swallow.[93] Additionally, non-critical medications may be discontinued by the physician.

*Tracheostomy Tubes and Oral Intake.* The presence of a tracheostomy tube, with or without mechanical ventilation, does not preclude oral intake, although it may significantly alter swallowing function.[8] However, access to the upper respiratory tract via the trach improves pulmonary toilet in patients who have chosen to eat in spite of aspiration. Contrary to common thinking, an inflated trach tube cuff is not fully protective against aspiration.[2,47] The seal in the trachea is not complete, and secretions and/or liquid material may collect above the cuff and ultimately can be aspirated.[94] Ideally, the cuff should be deflated when the patient eats to reduce the tethering effect on hyolaryngeal excursion and improve oropharyngeal sensation and airflow in the upper airway.[95,96] In turn, this affords a more effective cough ability and airway clearance and increased swallowing efficiency. Tracheal suctioning should be performed after meals in patients with dysphagia who have chosen to eat.

## DRY MOUTH (XEROSTOMIA)

CASE STUDY
*Mr. M, A Patient with Cardiac Disease and Dry Mouth*

Mr. M was a 78-year-old man with a history of aortic stenosis, valve replacement and end-stage cardiac disease. One weekend, he developed shortness of breath and was admitted to the hospital. Work-up revealed infection of his valve and pneumonia. He was made NPO and placed on multiple antibiotics to prevent further infection. He became more agitated and more dyspnic, which necessitated intubation on a ventilator. It was difficult to wean him off the ventilator, but after several attempts, he was successful in breathing on his own. When he again became weak, he was placed back on intubation and is was difficult to wean him as before and took several attempts for him to breath on his own. His family decided that he would not want prolonged life support. The plan was that if anything happened, he would not undergo any further re-intubation. To protect

his airway, he was not allowed to eat or drink, because the team was afraid he would aspirate from his weakness and debility. However, because he was on high flow oxygen, he complained of thirst and dry mouth. After discussion with the family about his prognosis, the focus was changed to quality of life and allowing him to enjoy the food and drink he loved. The nurses gave him little spoonfuls of juice to relieve his dry mouth. They coated artificial saliva inside his mouth with an oral swab and applied lip balm. They brushed his teeth several times a day to stimulate saliva. His last wish was a martini. The family went across the street to a bar and ordered a drink to go. Mr. M was given the martini with mouth swabs, small bits of crushed ice, and by spoon. He enjoyed this with great pleasure.

## Definition

Xerostomia is the sensation of oral dryness, which sometimes may be accompanied by decreased salivary secretions. Although patients receiving palliative care commonly experience oral dryness,[97,98] it is often difficult to identify the exact underlying cause and contributing factors. Decreased salivary function and prolonged xerostomia cause myriad oral problems in the mouth, including dental caries, gum, tongue, and oral mucosal irritations and lesions, mouth infections, taste changes, and bad breath. In the esophageal region, problems include swallowing difficulties, along with alterations in speech formation and voice function.[97-99] Such conditions may cause physical discomfort and emotional suffering, resulting in the retreat from socializing. This means missing the essential daily encounters: communicating, laughing, smiling, and eating.[100,101] Treatment offers comfort to patients by focusing on both short and long term effects.

## Incidence

In a prevalence study of palliative care admissions, 55% experienced xerostomia.[102] Other authors estimate that xerostomia affects 30% of palliative care patients.[103,104] In palliative care, xerostomia is listed as a major source of discomfort in patients with cancer. Due to lack of studies outside of the cancer population, it is difficult to estimate the incidence of xerostomia. In noncancer, patients, there has not been much research except for Sjögren's disease. Nonetheless, it has been described more in the population of patients with end-stage renal failure and end-stage cardiac disease seondary to imposed fluid restrictions.[105,106] In the population at large, xerostomia increases with age and medical problems because medication therapy increases incidence.

## Pathophysiology

Although saliva is necessary for oral nutrition, it also facilitates chewing, swallowing, tasting, and talking. The properties of saliva allow oral lubrication, gum and tissue repair, as well as help in gustation with food-bolus formation, and food breakdown. Additionally, saliva breaks down bacterial substances, offering immunoprotection for oral mucosa and dental structures.[107,108] Saliva thereby inhibits dental caries and infections, while providing protection against extreme temperatures of food and drink.[100,107-109,111] In this way, it has antimicrobial properties, buffering properties, and liquid properties to help with gustation.

The function of saliva production is regulated by the nervous system. After experiencing smell, sight, or taste of food, the salivary glands are stimulated to produce saliva within 2 to 3 seconds.[111] There is a two-step process to saliva secretion: production at the acinar level of the cells, and secretion where saliva is actually secreted into the mouth via the ducts.[107] Saliva is comprised of several elements. Ninety-nine percent of saliva is fluid composed of water and mucus, providing a lubricative element. The remaining 1% of saliva is solid, containing salts, proteins, minerals such as calcium bicarbonate ions, and enzymes such as pytalin, antibodies, and other antimicrobial agents.[97,99,107-109]

Saliva is produced by numerous glands in the oropharynx[107,109]; the average healthy adult produces up to 1.5 liters of saliva a day. The parotid glands, the submandibular glands, and the sublingual glands produce 90% of saliva, with the other 10% produced in the oral pharynx. Parotid glands, located below and in front of each ear, produce a serous and watery saliva.[111] Therefore, damage to the parotid gland will produce a thicker saliva. Submandibular glands, located in the lower jaw, secrete mostly serous saliva with some mucinous elements.[111] Sublingual glands produce purely mucous saliva.[109,112] The overall viscosity of saliva is dependent on the functioning of the various glands.

There are four categories of the etiology of xerostomia: (1) reduced salivary secretions, (2) buccal erosion, (3) local or systemic dehydration, and (4) miscellaneous conditions. Reduced salivary secretion is commonly caused by both surgery and radiation to the head and neck regions, medication side effects, infections, hypothyroidism, autoimmune processes, and sarcoidosis. Oral dryness may result from oral diseases such as acute and chronic parotitis, or partial or complete salivary obstruction. Radiation to the head and neck can produce a 50% to 60% reduction of saliva within the first week of treatment because of inflammation.[112] Chemotherapy may also cause dry mouth, particularly in advanced disease.[112] Medications are notorious culprits of dry mouth, particularly several categories commonly used in palliative care.[107,112] These medications include sedatives, tranquilizers, antihistamines, anti-Parkinsonian medications, antiseizure medications, skeletal muscle relaxants, cytoxic agents, tricyclic antidepressants, and anticholinergics.

Buccal erosion can occur in cancer and cancer treatment, particularly chemotherapy and radiation, as well as in conditions that affect the immune system. Sjögren's syndrome, diabetes mellitus, HIV/AIDS, scleredema, sarcoidosis, lupus, Alzheimer's disease, and graft versus host disease, all may excerbate dry mouth.[107,112] Patients undergoing cancer therapy can have either tumor-induced salivary gland destruction or treatment-induced xerostomia from the destruction of salivary glands, debility and dehydration from surgery or radiation causes.[104] The duration of radiation and/or greater radiation doses affects the persistence and degree of salivary reduction.[104,113]

Local or systemic dehydration-induced xerostomia results from a wide spectrum of conditons, from anorexia, vomiting, diarrhea, fever, drying oxygen therapies, mouth breathing, polyuria, diabetes, hemorrhage, and swallowing difficulties. Mental health issues including depression, coping reactions, anxiety, and pain can produce xerostomia.[97,98,107,114] Dry mouth sensations are worse at night from their diurnal production, resulting in interrrupted sleep. Over longer periods of time, lack of sleep may cause anxiety, depression, and distress as part the stress response.[101]

There has been a long-standing myth that dry mouth occurs as part of the aging process. In fact, age is not the issue, but rather the potential for an increased number of comorbidities that may require medications.[107,108] Lack of saliva fosters plaque and gum disease, which can be difficult to manage. Patients undergoing cancer treatment or immunosuppressive therapies may either be too immunocompromised or weak to undergo oral surgery or treatment procedures. Thus, patients may experience both the underlying discomforts of their terminal disease and experience the distress from secondary oral problems.

## Assessment

Xerostomia may be accompanied by discomfort of both the oral mucosa and the tongue, such as burning, smarting, and soreness with or without the presence of ulcers. There may be difficulty with mastication, swallowing, and speech. Subsequently, there may be taste alterations, difficulty with dentures, and an increase in dental caries from the protection characteristics of saliva. Sleep, rest, and nutritional issues are common secondary concerns.[107,108] Therefore, a thorough history should review these problem areas, along with the subjective distress of xerostomia (Table 11–5).

A newer assessment tool is the Univeristy of Michigan Xerostomia. It is an 8-item interview in which the patient rates their xerostomia-related difficulties on a 1–10 scale.[115] The areas include talking, chewing, swallowing, sleeping, eating, resting, and the frequency of sipping liquids for eating and during the rest of the day. Although it was developed for patients undergoing radiation, it is very applicable to all palliative care patients.[112] Reviewing onset of oral dryness correlation with medication initiation may also be insightful in assessment.

| Table 11–5 |
| --- |
| **Assessment Questions for Xerostomia** |
| Do you frequently have a dry mouth? |
| Does it bother you? |
| Do you need to drink more fluids during the day and night? |
| Do you have difficulty speaking? |
| Do you have difficulty chewing? |
| Do you have difficulty swallowing? |
| Do you need extra fluids to swallow? |
| Is your sleeping interrupted by a dry mouth? |
| Have you experienced altered taste sensations? |
| Do you often do you use tobacco? |
| How often do you drink alcohol? |
| How much caffeine do you consume? |
| Are you taking any prescription medications, over the counter medications or preparations? |
| *Sources*: Sreebny and Valdini (1987), reference 98; Cooke et al. (1996), reference 109; Ship (2002), reference 107; Jensen et al., (2003), reference 108. |

| Table 11–6 |
| --- |
| **Dry Mouth Rating Scales** |
| **Oncology Nursing Society documentation for xerostomia** |
| 0 No dry mouth |
| 1 Mild dryness, slightly thickened saliva; little change in taste |
| 2 Moderate dryness, thick and sticky saliva, markedly altered taste |
| 3 Complete dryness of mouth |
| 4 Salivary necrosis |
| **Salivary gland changes:** **National Cancer Institute documentation of dry mouth** |
| 0 None |
| 1 Slightly thickened |
| 2 Thick, ropey, sticky saliva |
| 3 Acute salivary necrosis |
| 4 Disabling |
| *Sources*: National Cancer Institute (2003), reference 117; Oncology Nursing Society (2002), reference 116. |

| Table 11–7 |
| --- |
| **Stepwise Process for Managing Xerostomia** |
| Treat underlying infections |
| Review and alter current medications |
| Stimulate salivary flow |
| Replace lost secretions with saliva substitutes |
| Protect teeth |
| Rehydrate |
| Modify diet |

An intra-oral examination will reveal clear indications of dry mouth: pale and dry mucosal and buccal areas, the presence of a dry and fissured tongue, the absence of salivary pooling, and the presence of oral ulcerations, gingivitis, or candidiasis.[98,109] Salivary glands should be noted for swelling, indicating obstruction, and dentition should be examined for caries. Extra-oral examination reveals cracked lips, often with angular cheilitis or candida at the corners of the mouth.[107]

The standard bedside tests for xerostomia are the cracker biscuit test and the tongue blade test. The cracker biscuit test involves giving a patient a dry cracker or biscuit. If the patient cannot eat the cracker without extra fluids, xerostomia is present.[98] The tongue blade test is an extension of mouth inspection. After inspection is complete, the tongue blade is placed on the tongue. Since dry mouth makes a ropey, pasty saliva, the tongue blade will stick to the tongue of a patient with xerostomia.[109] Another, more aggressive test is unstimulated or stimulated sialometric measurement of saliva. This test measures the amount of saliva collected by spitting into a container, swabbing the mouth with a cotton-tipped applicator, or salivating into a test container at a set time.[98,109] However, for most palliative care patients, this may be a burdensome and unnecessary test.

To document the extent of xerostomia, it may be helpful to use rating scales specifically designed for this purpose. Two scales, contained in Table 11–6, rate xerostomia in a four-point system.[116,117]

## Management

There is little to offer patients to prevent oral dryness or treat it once it has occurred. Much of xerostomia management focuses on interventions to alleviate rather than interventions to eradicate or to prevent the symptom. The goal of management focuses on protecting patients from further complications, which may be more problematic.[118] The following stepwise approach should guide management and treatment: Table 11–7,

1. Treat underlying infection or disease such as candidiasis. Nystatin swish-and-swallow or fluconazole 150 mg PO can improve xerostomia.[97,104,107]

2. Review and alter current medications as appropriate. It is important to first evaluate the necessity of specific xerostomia-inducing drugs. There are some 500 medications that list oral dryness as a side effect.[107,112] Specifically, anticholinergics, antihistamines, phenothiazines, antidepressants, opioids, β-blockers, diuretics, anticonvulsants, sedatives, and tobacco all may cause oral dryness. Thus, patients with heart conditions, mental health issues, depression, anxiety, neurological disorders, and pain disorders may be at risk for dry mouth. If eliminating possible culprit medication is not

Table 11–8
Review of Interventions of Xerostomia

| Intervention | Role/Effect | Benefit | Side Effect |
|---|---|---|---|
| **Nonpharmacological** | | | |
| Peppermint water | Mucous saliva | Inexpensive | Interacts with metoclopromide |
| Vitamin C | Chemical reduction | Inexpensive Reduces viscosity | Can irritate mouth if sores present |
| Citric acid/#weets | Mucous saliva | Inexpensive | Can irritate like vitamin C. In sweets, can cause caries. |
| Chewing gum, mints | Watery saliva | Inexpensive More volume Only dentate | No side effects if sugarless, otherwise can promote caries |
| Acupuncture | Increase production | Noninvasive | Expensive |
| **Pharmacological** | | | |
| Pilocarpine | Nonselective muscarinic | Increases saliva production | Sweating, nausea, flushing, cramping |
| Bethanechol | M-3 muscarinic | Relieves side effect of TCA | |
| Methacholine | Parasympathetics | Increases salivation | Hypotension |
| Yohimbine | Blocks α-2 adrenoreceptors | Increases saliva | Drowsiness, confusion, atrial fibrillation |
| Cevimeline | M-1 & M-3 muscarinic agonist | Increases saliva | Less effects than pilocarpine |

*Sources*: Adapted from Amerongen (2003), reference 110; Ship (2002), reference 107.

possible, other possible strategies include decreasing the dosage to decrease dryness, or altering the schedule to assure that the peak effect of medication does not coincide with nighttime peak of decreased salivary production.[97,98,107,109]

3. Stimulate salivary flow. Salivary stimulation can occur with both nonpharmacological and pharmacological interventions.

4. Replace lost secretions with saliva substitutes. Saliva substitute are better tolerated than artificial saliva.[101] Oral spray preparations are best tolerated.[100] Saliva substitutes are based on aqueous solution and may contain carboxymethyl cellulose or mucin from animals. Attention must be paid to any philosophical, cultural or religious prohibitions concerning the animal ingredients of saliva substitutes.[105]

## Nonpharmacological Interventions

Nonpharmacological use of gustatory stimulation includes simple measures. Table 11–8 summarizes possible procedures. All of these interventions, except acupuncture, are inexpensive and are as efficacious as medications, without uncomfortable side effects. However, relief is not long lasting.[109]

- Peppermint water. Peppermint stimulates saliva and can be taken as needed. However, it should not be used with metoclopramide, as they have opposing actions.[97,98,107]

- Vitamin C. Use in lozenges or other forms as preferred. Disrupts salivary mucins to reduce viscosity of saliva.[110] Although inexpensive, vitamin C may be irritating to the mouth, particularly if the patient has mouth sores.[114] Also, there is a need to be careful, as continual vitamin C can erode dental enamel.[101,111]

- Citric acids. Present in malic acid or in sweets. Citric acids can act similarly to vitamin C in causing a burning sensation.[114]

- Chewing gum, mints. These are most preferred by patients, are inexpensive, and have no side effects. May create a buffer system to compensate for dietary acids.[110,114] Effective as salivary stimulants due to the effect on chemoreceptors and mechanical receptors, chewing gum is more effective than mints. In particular, a low tack gum is preferable for patients with dentures.[104] Preferably, gum is sugarless, to prevent caries and infections, because immunocompromised states promote cavities and infections. One study of dialysis patients revealed a preference for chewing gum. Attention must be paid to social acceptance of gum chewing, particularly in older populations.[105]

- Acupuncture. Effective with a variety of types of xerostomia, although mechanism not understood. Relief occurs as a single treatment with eight needles placed in three places: bilaterally in the ears and a single distal point in the radial aspect of the index finger.[111] One study showed that 6 weeks of twice-weekly treatment increased salivation for up to 1 year.[119] Another study used a 3-to-4 weekly regimen, with monthly maintenance visits to relieve xerostomia.[120]

- Humidity. Modulation of oxygen therapy and room environment.[121] This includes having oxygen modifications by changing humidified air and using vaporizors to add humidity to rooms, particularly since indoor heating and cooling systems are drying.
- Diet modifications. Soft texture foods are better tolerated than rough foods. Soups, pudding, mashed potatoes, and shakes rather than foods with rough edges such as crackers or toast.[122] Olive oil or another light oil to the gums and mucosa may help act as a lubricant.[123] Patients may sip such foods in milk, tea, or water to assist in swallowing. In addition, instruct patients to take fluids with all meals and snacks. The use of gravies and juices with foods can add moisture to swallowing. Education regarding the avoidance of sugars, spicy foods, sometimes salt, and dry or piquant foods is important, although preferred tastes may vary from one patient to the next. For dry mouth without oral ulcerations, provide carbonated drinks such as ginger ale, as well as cider, apple juice, or lemonade. Fresh fruits, papaya juice, or pineapple juice may help some patients refresh their mouths[14,101,124]; however, citrus products may be too acidic and irritating for other patients.[110]

## Pharmacological Interventions

- Pilocarpine. Pilocarpine is a parasympathetic agent that increases exocrine gland secretion and stimulates residual functioning tissue in damaged salivary glands. Saliva production is greatest after a dose and response lasts for about 4 hours.[110] Dose may be given at 5 mg TID or QID depending on how well patients tolerate the medication and its side effect.[111] Response varies with severity of xerostomia. Side effects include mild to moderate sweating, visual disturbances, nausea, rhinitis, chills, flushing, sweating, dizziness, increased urinary frequency, abdominal cramping, and asthenia,[109,110,114] but can be lessened if taken with milk.[110] New studies have shown that pilocarpine given before and during radiotherapy can reduce xerostomia.[114,124,125] However, due to the side effect profile, Pilocarpine should not be used in patients with chronic obstructive pulmonary disease, asthma, bradycardia, renal or hepatic impairment, glaucoma or bowel obstruction.[101,109,111,114]
- Bethanechol. Bethanechol relieves anticholinergic side effects of tricyclic antidepressants. Few studies have been done that focus specifically on xerostomia rather than the side effects of antidepressants.[109,114]

- Methacholine. Methacholine is a parasympathomimetic compound that increases salivation. Dose is 10 mg a day. One side effect is hypotension. It is short-acting.[109,114]
- Yohimbine. Yohimbine blocks $\alpha_2$-adrenoreceptors. Side effects include drowsiness, confusion, and atrial fibrillation, lasting up to 3 hours. Dose is 14 mg a day.[114,124]
- Cevimeline. Cevimeline is a muscarinic agonist that acts to increase saliva by inhibiting acetylcholinesterase. It works on salivary glands and lacrimal glands, promoting increased salivary flow and tears in the eyes. Used in a spray or mouthwash gargle, it lasts up to 6 hours.[110,111,126]
- Water. Water is simple and inexpensive. It is usually well tolerated and easily accessible. There is no research on whether optimal relief results from either warm or cold. Thus, temperature is a personal choice.[109,114]
- Artificial saliva. Artificial saliva contains carboxymethylcellulose or mucin; dose 2 mL every 3 to 4 hours.[109,114] Some examples include Glandosane, Xero-Lube, Orex, and Saliment.[107,110] It is important to consider patient preference of saliva stimulants over saliva substitutes.[114] If saliva substitutes are used, those with a mucin base appear to be better tolerated than those derived from carboxymethylcellulose.[127] However, both types of preparation bases are better tolerated as an oral spray than as a gel or rinse.[126,127]
- Protect teeth. Oral hygiene, such as frequent brushing with soft brushes, water jet, denture cleaning, fluoride rinses, mouthwash, and flossing, stimulate salivation. This can help prevent candidiasis, particularly since dentures can harbor infections.[107]
- Use of lip protectants such as balms, chapsticks, and other preparations prevents cracked lips, and use of saliva moistens lips. Care should be taken not to use products with alcohol, since these can be irritating.[111,114,116,117]
- Dentifrices. Several are manufactured for patients with dry mouth that contain antimicrobial enzymes to reduce oral infections and enhance mouth wetting. Examples are Biotene and Oral Balance.[107,110,111]
- Mouthwashes. Help rinse debris from mouth. Includes homemade mouthwashes made from saline, sodium bicarbonate, glycerin, and perhaps lemon.[107,111]
- Rehydration. Replenish oral hydration by sipping water, spraying water, and increasing humidity in the air.[67] To assist in sleep, instituting these measures at night may help rest.

## Nursing Interventions

Little research has focused on dry mouth prevention. Both the financial and physical burden of therapy may be of concern for patients. Many patients choose nonpharmacological therapy because it is inexpensive and has fewer side effects.[119] Other patients may consider nonpharmacological interventions depending on how many other symptoms they are experiencing or how many other medications they are currently taking. Therefore, to create an appropriate intervention, the nurse must assess the distress from xerostomia and facilitate a suitable therapy within financial constraints.

Nursing intervention will vary from one patient to the next based on the degree of xerostomia. Strong evidence supporting the efficacy of one treatment over another has not been demonstrated. The result is a lack of standardized oral care procedures, and protocols variation from one institution to another.[111] The nurse may help a family systematically go through a variety of therapies from nonpharmacological to pharmacological to achieve relief. If nonpharmacological interventions are unsuccessful, the pharmacological medications can be tried. However, medication interactions and side effects should be reviewed in the context of the patient's overall condition. Education about both the importance and comfort of good oral care is essential. As a patient declines, teaching the family how to provide mouth care offers a tangible and important role in the comfort of the patient.

# HICCUPS

CASE STUDY
*CJ, A Young Woman with Ovarian Cancer and Hiccups*

CJ is a 36-year-old woman with ovarian cancer. She has been undergoing treatment for 5 years. She has subseqeuntly anorexia, abdominal distention, and dyspnea. She is referred to hospice. Within the week, she is unable to sleep due to hiccups. She is assessed for constipation though this is ruled out as a source of the hiccups. She is assessed for ascites, which is a possible cause of the hiccups The nurse instructs her sleep on a wedge pillow. Various pharmacological regimens are discussed. Because she has small children and doesn't want to be sedated, a step wise approach to symptom relief is initiated. She is prescribed metaclopramide to decrease abdominal distention and lactulose to relieve constiption. Her shortness of breath and feelings of fullness are both diminished but she still has hiccups. She is then started on Baclofen 10 mg TID which results in the subsiding of the hiccups and allows

her to rest... A plan is made that if the hiccups persist, she will be placed on chlorpromazine 25 mg at night. Since this medication is very sedating, other measures will be considered for daytime to allow her to be alert as possible for her children.

## Definition

Hiccup, or singultus, is defined as sudden, involuntary contractions of one or both sides of the diaphragm and intercostal muscles, terminated by an abrupt closure of the glottis, producing a characteristic sound of "hic."[128–133] Hiccup frequency is commonly around 4 to 60 per minute.[134] Prolonged hiccups result in fatigue and exhaustion from both respiratory insufficiency and sleep interferences.[135] Anxiety, depression, and frustration may develop if eating and/or sleeping are routinely interrupted. Although seemingly insignificant, hiccups affect quality of life.[128,130,131,135]

## Prevalence and Impact

Hiccups, in the palliative care population, have not been well studied, resulting in a paucity of references devoted to the subject. Articles within the last 5 years pertain to case reports of a particular patient, but no research has been done about systematic studies on patient populations with specific diseases. Because of the perceived insignificance of hiccups, the incidence and prevalence are not well known. Estimates of prevalence of hiccups in cancer patients is about 10% to 20%.[136] Children appear more prone to hiccups than adults.[136]

## Pathophysiology

The precise pathophysiology and the physiological function of hiccups is unknown. What is known is that hiccups arise from a synchronous clonic spasm or spasmodic contraction of the diaphragm and the intercostal muscles, which results in sudden inspiration and prompt closure of the glottis, causing the hiccups sounds. Normally, the glottis pertains to the vocal cords and diaphragm, and the intercostal muscles pertain to respirations.[135] Nonetheless, hiccups are considered a primitive function, such as yawning or vomiting, that developed as an evolutionary process that now serves no discrete purpose.[128,131,137] The anatomical cause of hiccups is thought to be bimodal, with association either with the phrenic or vagus nerve,[135,138] or central nervous involvement, which causes misfiring.[131] It is hypothesized that a hiccup reflex arc is located in the phrenic nerves, the vagal nerves, and T6–T12 sympathetic fibers, as well as a possible hiccup center in either the respiratory center, the brain stem, or the cervical cord between C3 and C5.[139] However, there does not appear to be a discrete hiccup center, such as the chemoreceptor trigger zone for nausea.[134,137,140]

Evidence suggests an inverse relationship between partial pressure of carbon dioxide ($pCO_2$) and hiccups; that is, an increased $pCO_2$ decreases the frequency of hiccups and a decreased $pCO_2$ increases frequency of hiccups.[128] Interestingly, hiccups have a minimal effect on respiration. Hiccup strength or amplitude varies from patient to patient, as well as among separate episodes in an individual.[132] It is this characteristic that causes the distress, as continous strong hiccups are exhausting due to the energy used to hiccup.

There are three categories of hiccups: benign, persistent, and intractable hiccups. Benign, self-limiting hiccups, occur frequently. Such a bout of hiccups can last from several minutes to 2 days and is primarily associated with gastric distention.[140] Other causes are sudden changes in temperature, alcohol ingestion, excess smoking, and psychogenic alternations.[128,130-132] Persistent, or chronic, hiccups continue for more than 48 hours but less than 1 month. Third and last are intractable hiccups, which persist longer than 1 month.[128,130-132] For palliative care, the duration may not be as important as the amplitude or strength of the hiccup. For instance, a patient with ALS may have more distress than a cardiac patient, as they are already weak and breathing is compromised.[132]

Intractable hiccups have more than 100 different causes, varying from simple metabolic disturbances to complex structural lesions of the central nervous system or infections.[128,130,132] Particular causes can be consolidated into four categories: structural, metabolic, inflammatory, and infectious disorders.[128] Structural conditions specifically affect or irritate the peripheral branches of the phrenic and vagus nerves, such as in abdominal or mediastinal tumors, hepatomegaly, ascites, or gastric distention, and central nervous disorders. Persistant hiccups can indicate serious underlying disorders, such as thoracic aneurysm, brainstem tumors, metabolic and drug-related disorders, infectious diseases, and psychogenic disorders.[132,133,138] Common causes in terminal illness include neurological disorders such as stroke, brain tumors, and sepsis and metabolic imbalances; phrenic nerve irritations such as tumor compression or metastases; pericarditis, pneumonia, or pleuritis; and vagal nerve irritations such as esophagitis, gastric distention, gastritis, pancreatitis, hepatitis, and myocardial infarction.[130,131] Medications including steroids, chemotherapy, dopamine antagonists, megestrol, methyldopa, nicotine, opioids, and muscle relaxants may also cause hiccups.[136]

## Assessment

Extensive work-up for hiccups in palliative care is impractical, uncomfortable, and reveals little to assist in determining the etiology or delineating treatment. Indeed, a recent retrospective study revealed that laboratory studies neither assisted in treatment nor helped determine what treatment would be effective.[141] Nonetheless, assessment should include a subjective review of how much distress the hiccups cause the patient. For example, in a patient with an abdominal tumor, hiccups can cause excruciating pain, whereas in the obtunded patient in renal failure, hiccups may cause little distress at all.

In reviewing the distress of the hiccup, it is important to evaluate subsequent conditions. Patients may experience weight loss due to anorexia, fatigue, and inability to eat; shortness of breath from inability to take deep breaths; insomnia from hiccuping all night; heartburn from acid reflux; and depression resulting from all of the above, as well as the worry that hiccups are untreatable.[135] Subjective assessment includes the history and duration of the current episode of hiccups, previous episodes, and interference with rest, eating, or daily routines. Inquiry into possible triggers may be helpful, including patterns during the day, and activities preceding the hiccups such as eating, drinking, or positioning. A review of recent trauma, surgery, procedures, and acute illness, as well as a medication history, is important to help focus on potential causes.[128,137] There are case reports on oral and epidural steroid and bupivicaine induced hiccups.[142,143] Any wounds or infections should be examined, as well as the respiratory system.[135]

The presence of hiccups themselves is quite apparent. Further physical exam may not reveal much related to the hiccups themselves but, rather assists in ruling out other conditions. Oral examination may reveal signs of swelling or obstruction. Observation of the patient's general appearance includes inspection for signs of a toxic or septic process. More specifically, it includes evaluating for tenderness of the temporal artery, foreign bodies in the ear, infection of the throat, goiter in the neck, pneumonia or pericarditis of the chest, abdominal distention or ascites, and signs of stroke or delirium—all diagnoses that may have hiccups as part of the constellation of signs and symptoms.[128]

In very rare circumstances, specific testing may be warranted to eliminate other causes. Chest x-ray may rule out pulmonary or mediastinal processes, as well as phrenic/vagal irritation from peritumor edema in the abdominal area.[136] In addition, blood work including a complete blood count with differential electrolytes may rule out infection, as well as electrolyte imbalances and renal failure.[128,131,132] Sometimes a CT scan of the abdomen or head may be done to rule out abnormalities or a cerebral bleed.

## Management

The lack of research to increase understanding on the nature of hiccups has resulted in lack of consensus around treatment and anecdotal therapy. Consequentially, treatment is based

---

**Table 11–9**
**Nonpharmacological Interventions for Hiccups**

**Respiratory measures**
Breath holding
Rebreathing in a paper bag
Diaphragm compression
Ice application in mouth
Induction of sneeze or cough with spices or inhalants

**Nasal and pharyngeal stimulation**
Nose pressure
Stimulant inhalation
Tongue traction
Drinking from far side of glass
Swallowing sugar
Eating soft bread
Soft touch to palate with cotton-tipped applicator
Lemon wedge with bitters

**Miscellaneous vagal stimulation**
Ocular compression
Digital rectal massage
Carotid massage

**Psychiatric treatments**
Behavioral techniques
Distraction

**Gastric distention relief**
Fasting
Nasogastric tube to relieve abdominal distention
Lavage
Induction of vomiting

**Phrenic nerve disruption**
Anesthetic block

**Miscellaneous treatments**
Bilateral radial artery compression
Peppermint water to relax lower esophagus
Acupuncture

*Sources:* Lewis (1985), reference 128; Launois (1993), reference 137; Rousseau (2003), reference 132; Williams (2001), reference 131; Smith (2003), reference 130; and Kolodzik & Eilers (1991), reference 135.

---

on the bias of previous success rather than a systematic, evidence-based approach. Similar to treatment of dysphagia or xerostomia, treatment for hiccups should be focused on the underlying disease. If the etiology questionably includes simple causes such as gastric distention or temperature changes, "empiric" treatment should be initiated. Both non-pharmacological and pharmacological interventions may be used.[128,130–132] Therapies include physical maneuvers, medications, and various other procedures to interfere with the hiccup arc.[139] Otherwise, treatment for more complex episodes of hiccups without clear etiology will focus on various pharmacological interventions.

## Nonpharmacological Treatment

Nonpharmacological treatments can be divided into seven categories and are outlined in Table 11–9. The first category is simple respiratory maneuvers. These include breath holding, rebreathing in a bag, compression of the diaphragm, ice application in the mouth, and induction of sneeze or cough.[128,130–132] The second category is nasal and pharyngeal stimulation. These techniques use pressure on the nose, inhalation of a stimulant, traction of the tongue, drinking from the far side of a glass, swallowing sugar, eating a lemon wedge with bitters, eating soft bread, or soft touch to the palate with a cotton-tipped applicator.[131,132,134] The third category is miscellaneous vagal stimulation, including ocular compression, digital rectal massage, and carotid massage. The fourth category is psychiatric treatments, mainly behavioral therapy. The fifth category is relief of gastric distention, comprising of repositioning, fasting, a nasogastric tube to decrease distention, lavage, and induction of vomiting.[128,131] The sixth category is phrenic nerve disruption, such as an anesthetic injection or traditional acupuncture.[128,139] The seventh and final category is miscellaneous benign remedies, such as bilateral compression of radial arteries, peppermint water to relax the lower esophagus, use of distraction, or acupressure.[128,130–132]

## Pharmacological Treatment

Initial therapy should attempt to decrease gastric distention, the common cause in 95% of cases. Subsequent measures include hastening gastric emptying, and relaxing the diaphragm with simethicone and metoclopramide.[128,129,131,132,144] If ineffective, second-line therapy should focus on suppression of the hiccup reflex. Common pharmacological interventions, listed in Table 11–10, include the use of various classes of medications: muscle relaxants such as baclofen, midazolam, and chlordiazepoxide; anticonvulsants such as gabapentin, carbamazepine, and valproate[144–146]; corticosteroids such as dexamethasone and prednisone; dopamine antagonists such as haloperidol, droperidol, and chlorpromazine[149]; calcium channel blockers/antiarrhythmics such as nifedipine, nimodipine, nefopam, phenytoin, lidocaine, quinidine[139,144,147]; SSRI antidepressants, specifically sertraline; and various other medications such as ketamine, THC, and methylphenidate.[136,144,148–150] Third-line therapy is the use of other drugs to disrupt diaphragmatic irritation or other possible causes of hiccups, which may include anesthesia and phrenic and cervical blocks.[139,151–153]

## Nursing Interventions

Although hiccups appear to be a simple reflex, their specific mechanism of action is unclear due to myriad etiologies. Many patients are frustrated because their discomfort and disruption were not taken seriously. The nurse can help discuss with the patient their concerns about treatment and their desire for comfort. Nursing interventions should focus on information regarding the broad range of strategies to eliminate the hiccups. Thus, the nursing role is one of advocate to promote comfort, empathetic listener, and educator.

The extent of aggressive treatment will depend on the degree of distress of the hiccups and the interference with

**Table 11–10**
**Suggested Pharmacological Treatment for Hiccups**

| Agent | Site of Effect | Side Effect |
|---|---|---|
| **Agents to decrease gastric distention** | | |
| Simethicone 15–30 mL po q 4 h | Gas | Promotes emptying |
| Metochopromide 10–20 mg po/IV q 4–6 h (cannot use with peppermint water) | Blocks dopamine | Promotes gastric emptying |
| **Muscle relaxants** | | |
| Baclofen 5–10 mg PO q 6–14 h up to 15–25 mg/d | Sedation, nausea | Acts at synaptic level |
| Midazalem 5–10 mg q 4 h | Transient drowsiness | Reduces muscles spasm |
| **Anticonvulsants** | | |
| Gabapentin 300–600 mg PO TID | Drowsiness, HA, flu-like symptoms | Acts on cortex area |
| Carbamazepine 200 mg PO QID-TID | Drowsiness | |
| Valproic acid 15 mg/kg PO divided in one or three doses then may increase by 250 mg/wk until hiccups stop | | |
| Diphenylhydantoin 200 mg IV × 1, then 100 mg PO QID | | |
| **Corticosteroids** | | |
| Dexamethasone 40 mg PO QD | | |
| **Dopamine agonists** | | |
| Haloperidol 1–5 mg PO/IV/SQ q 4–12 h | Drowsiness | Reduces muscle spasm |
| Chlorpromazine 5–50 mg PO/IM/IV q 4–8 h | Sedation, extrapyramidal effects | Blocks dopamine and Alpha adrenergic receptors |
| **Calcium channel blockers** | | |
| Lidocaine 1 mg/kg w/ infusion fo 2 mg/min | Cardiac effects | Blocks sodium channels |
| Nifedipine 10–80 mg PO QD | Hypotension | |
| **Other medications** | | |
| Ketamine 0.4 mg/kg | Respiratory and cardiac suppression | Acts on cortex and limbic system |
| Amitriptyline 25–90 mg po QD | Dizziness, urinary retention | Inhibits serotonin and norepinephrine uptake |

*Source:* Sarhill and Mahmous (2007), reference 153.

quality of life—in particular, the extent of impact that hiccups have on the daily routine, specifically on sleep and nutrition. Information should include nonpharmacological maneuvers such as respiratory maneuvers, nasal and pharyngeal stimulation, distraction, and peppermint waters. If these measures fail to eradicate the hiccups, the nurse can discuss the range of pharmcologicaloptions, offer reassurance to continue various efforts because patients respond differently. Antacids may decrease gas, antiemetics may affect dopamine levels, and muscle relaxants may affect both gamma-aminobutyric acid channels and skeletal muscle.[130,132,136] Separately, they may be ineffective, but together they target several regions that trigger hiccups.

If all of these medications fail to induce hiccup reduction or cessation, the nurse should suggest a referral to a palliative care service, a pain service, or an anesthesia service to explore further treatment options. These services can consider possible invasive procedures such a nerve block, or infusion. However, as always, discussion with the patient should include prognosis and the benefit and burden of any procedure. If hiccups become extremely burdensome and all therapies have failed,

sedation may be a consideration. Again, the nurse may act as an advocate to provide the necessary information about the implications of sedation. For further discussion of palliative sedation, the reader is referred to Chapter 26.

## Summary

Dysphagia, xerostomia, and hiccups are common problems that have not garnered much interest in research. Many clinicians consider them minor symptoms; therefore, they appear to be underreported and underestimated.[55] Nurses at the bedside, whether in a facility or at home, may be the first to identify their presence and the negative impact on quality of life. The mere act of listening to a patient's distress offers affirmation of the existence of the symptoms and validation that the symptoms will be taken seriously. Given the lack of hard evidence to manage these symptoms, the nurse must be creative in the approach. Working with a team can offer relief to patients and their families.

APPENDIX 11-1
## Pureed Cookbooks

Eat Well Stay Nourished: A recipe and resources guide for coping with eating challenges. Compiled and edited by Nancy E. Leupold. Published by SPOHNC Support for People With Oral and Head and Neck Cancer, 2000.

Easy-to-Swallow, Easy-to-Chew Cookbook: Over 150 Tasty and Nutritious Recipes for People Who Have Difficulty Swallowing. Donna Weihoffen, JoAnne Robbins, Paula Sullivan. John Wiley & Sons, Inc., 2002.

The Dysphagia Cookbook. Elayne Achilles. Cumberland House Publishing, 2004

I-Can't-Chew Cookbook. J. Randy Wilson and Mark A. Piper. Hunter House, Inc Publishers, 2003.

Puree Gourmet. J William Richman. American Institutional Products, 1994.

REFERENCES

1. Davis LA. Quality of life issues related to dysphagia. Top Geriatr Rehabil Dysphagia in Older Adults, Part II 2007; 23(4):352–365.
2. von Gunten CF, Twaddle ML. Terminal care for noncancer patients. Clin Geriatr Med 1996;12(2):349–358.
3. Sharp HM, Wagner LB. Dysphagia in Older Adults, Part I. Ethics, informed consent, and decisions about non-oral feeding for patients with dysphagia. Top Geriatr Rehabil 2007; 23(3):240–248.
4. National Consensus Project: What is Palliative Care. Available at: www.nationalconsensusproject.org/WhatIsPC.asp (accessed December 31, 2008).
5. Pollens R. Role of the speech-language pathologist in palliative hospice care. J Palliat Med 2004;7(5):694–702.
6. Schmidlin E. Artificial hydration: The role of the nurse in addressing patient and family needs. Int J Palliat Nurs 2008;14(10):485.
7. Corbin-Lewis K, Liss JM, Sciortino KL. Clinical Anatomy and Physiology of the Swallow Mechanism. New York: Thomson Delmar Learning, 2004.
8. Logemann JA. Evaluation and Treatment of Swallowing Disorders. Austin, TX: Pro-Ed, 1998.
9. Martin-Harris B. Integration of breathing and oropharyngeal swallowing: A historical perspective and 13-year research experience. Perspect Swallow Swallow Disord (Dysphagia) 2003;12(3):6–11.
10. Easterling CS. Getting acquainted with the esophagus. Perspect Swallow Swallow Disord (Dysphagia) 2003;12(2):3–7.
11. McConnel FM, Cerenko D, Mendelsohn MS. Manofluorographic analysis of swallowing. Otolaryngol Clin North Am 1988;21:625–635.
12. Cook IJ, Dodds WJ, Dantas RO, et al. Opening mechanisms of the human upper esophageal sphincter. Am J Physiol 1989;257(5 Pt 1):G748–G759.
13. Benson TM. Physiology of oral cavity, pharynx, and upper esophageal sphincter. Available at: http://www.nature.com/gimo/contents/pt1/full/gimo2.html (updated 2006, accessed December 28, 2008).
14. Mashimo H, Goyal RK. Physiology of esophageal motility. Available at: http://www.nature.com/gimo/contents/pt1/full/gimo2.html (updated 2006, accessed December 28, 2008).
15. Kendall KA, Leonard RJ, McKenzie SW. Sequence variability during hypopharyngeal bolus transit. Dysphagia 2003; 18(2):85–91.
16. Shaker R, Hogan WJ. Normal physiology of the aerodigestive tract and its effect on the upper gut. Am J Med 2003;115 Suppl 3A:2S–9S.
17. Miller AJ. The Neuroscientific Principles of Swallowing and Dysphagia. San Diego: Singular Publishing, 1999.
18. Bieger D, Neuhuber W. Neural circuits and mediators regulating swallowing in the brainstem. Available at: http://www.nature.com/gimo/contents/pt1/full/gimo74.html (updated 2006, accessed December 28, 2008).
19. Rubenstein JH. Esophageal etiologies of dysphagia: A guide for SLP's. Perspect Swallow Swallow Disord (Dysphagia) 2007; 16(4):1–6.
20. 2007–2008 Statistical report: Primary brain tumors in the Unites States, 2000–2004. Available at: http://www.cbtrus.org/reports/reports.html (updated 2008, accessed December 28, 2008).
21. Pace A, Lorenzo CD, Guariglia L, Jandolo B, Carapella CM, Pompili A. End of life issues in brain tumor patients. J Neurooncol 2009;91(1):39–43.
22. Roe JW, Leslie P, Drinnan MJ. Oropharyngeal dysphagia: The experience of patients with non-head and neck cancers receiving specialist palliative care. Palliat Med 2007;21(7):567–574.
23. Oberndorfer S, Lindeck-Pozza E, Lahrmann H, Struhal W, Hitzenberger P, Grisold W. The end-of-life hospital setting in patients with glioblastoma. J Palliat Med 2008;11(1):26–30.
24. Drappatz J, Schiff D, Kesari S, Norden AD, Wen PY. Medical management of brain tumor patients. Neurol Clin 2007;25(4):1035–1071, ix.
25. Argiris A, Karamouzis MV, Raben D, Ferris RL. Head and neck cancer. Lancet 2008;371(9625):1695–1709.
26. Goldstein NE, Genden E, Morrison RS. Palliative care for patients with head and neck cancer: "I would like a quick return to a normal lifestyle." JAMA 2008;299(15):1818–1825.
27. Caudell JJ, Schaner PE, Meredith RF, et al. Factors associated with long-term dysphagia after definitive radiotherapy for locally advanced head-and-neck cancer. Int J Radiat Oncol Biol Phys 2008.
28. What is Esophageal Cancer? Available at: http://www.ecaware.org/EC_Information.htm (updated 2008, accessed December 28, 2008).
29. Classen M, Tytgat GNJ, Lightdale CJ. Gastroenterological Endoscopy. Thieme Publishing, 2002.
30. Gibbs JF, Rajput A, Chadha KS, et al. The changing profile of esophageal cancer presentation and its implication for diagnosis. J Natl Med Assoc 2007;99(6):620–626.
31. Detailed guide: Esophagus cancer. What are the key statistics about esophageal cancer? Available at: http://www.cancer.org/docroot/CRI/content/CRI_2_4_1X_What_are_the_key_statistics_for_esophagus_cancer_12.asp?sitearea= (updated 2006, accessed December 28, 2008).
32. Wilson JA. Management of esophageal dysphagia: The otolaryngolgist's perspective updated. Perspect Swallow Swallow Disord 2007;16(4):7–10.
33. McLoughlin MT, Byrne MF. Endoscopic stenting-where are we now and where can we go? World J Gastroenterol 2008; 14(24):3798–3803.

34. Murry T, Carrau RL. Clinical Management of Swallowing Disorders (2nd ed). San Diego, CA: Plural Publishing, 2006.

35. DeConti RC. Chemotherapy. In: Sullivan P, Guilford AM, eds. Swallowing Intervention in Oncology. Singular Publishing Group, Inc., 1999:27–46.

36. Ferguson TA, Elman LB. Clinical presentation and diagnosis of amyotrophic lateral sclerosis. NeuroRehabilitation 2007;22(6):409–416.

37. Yorkston KM, Miller RM, Strand EA, Levesque RJ. Management of Speech and Swallowing in Degenerative Diseases (2nd ed). Austin, TX: Pro-Ed, 2004.

38. Shoesmith CL, Strong MJ. Amyotrophic lateral sclerosis: Update for family physicians. Can Fam Physician 2006; 52(12):1563–1569.

39. Elman LB, Houghton DJ, Wu GF, Hurtig HI, Markowitz CE, McCluskey L. Palliative care in amyotrophic lateral sclerosis, Parkinson's disease, and multiple sclerosis. J Palliat Med 2007;10(2):433–457.

40. Miller RG, Mitchell JD, Lyon M, Moore DH. Riluzole for amyotrophic lateral sclerosis (ALS)/motor neuron disease (MND). Cochrane Database Syst Rev 2007;(1)(1):CD001447.

41. Mitsumoto H, Davidson M, Moore D, et al. Percutaneous endoscopic gastrostomy (PEG) in patients with ALS and bulbar dysfunction. Amyotroph Lateral Scler Other Motor Neuron Disord 2003;4(3):177–185.

42. Langmore SE, Kasarskis EJ, Manca ML, Olney RK. Enteral tube feeding for amyotrophic lateral sclerosis/motor neuron disease. Cochrane Database Syst Rev 2006;(4)(4):CD004030. 10.1002/14651858.CD004030.pub2.

43. Halbig TD, Tse W, Olanow CW. Neuroprotective agents in Parkinson's disease: Clinical evidence and caveats. Neurol Clin 2004;22(3 Suppl):S1–S17.

44. Micieli G, Tosi P, Marcheselli S, Cavallini A. Autonomic dysfunction in Parkinson's disease. Neurol Sci 2003;24 Suppl 1:S32–S34.

45. Miller N, Noble E, Jones D, Burn D. Hard to swallow: Dysphagia in Parkinson's disease. Age Ageing 2006;35(6):614–618.

46. Deane KH, Whurr R, Clarke CE, Playford ED, Ben-Shlomo Y. Non-pharmacological therapies for dysphagia in Parkinson's disease. Cochrane Database Syst Rev 2001;(1)(1):CD002816.

47. Warren NM, Burn DJ. Progressive Supranuclear Palsy. Pract Neurol 2007;(7):16–23.

48. Wenning GK, Seppi K, Scherfler C, Stefanova N, Puschban Z. Multiple system atrophy. Semin Neurol 2001;21(1):33–40.

49. Ruegg S, Lehky Hagen M, Hohl U, et al. Oculopharyngeal muscular dystrophy—an under-diagnosed disorder? Swiss Med Wkly 2005;135(39–40):574–586.

50. Hill M, Hughes T, Milford C. Treatment for swallowing difficulties (dysphagia) in chronic muscle disease. Cochrane Database Syst Rev 2004;(2)(2):CD004303.

51. Hauser SG, Goodin DS. Multiple sclerosis and other demyelinating diseases. In: Braunwalk E, Fauci AS, Kasper DL, Hauser SL, Longo DL, Jameson JL, eds. Harrison's Principles of Internal Medicine. New York: McGraw-Hill, 2005:2461–2471.

52. Schapiro RT. Managing symptoms of multiple sclerosis. Neurol Clin 2005;23(1):177–187, vii.

53. Bagert B, Camplair P, Bourdette D. Cognitive dysfunction in multiple sclerosis: Natural history, pathophysiology and management. CNS Drugs 2002;16(7):445–455.

54. Siegert RJ, Abernethy DA. Depression in multiple sclerosis: A review. J Neurol Neurosurg Psychiatr 2005;76(4):469–475.

55. Calcagno P, Ruoppolo G, Grasso MG, De Vincentiis M, Paolucci S. Dysphagia in multiple sclerosis—prevalence and prognostic factors. Acta Neurol Scand 2002;105(1):40–43.

56. American Geriatrics Society clinical recommendations. Feeding tube placement in elderly patients. Available at: http://www.americangeriatrics.org/education/cp_index.shtml (updated 2005, accessed December 28, 2008).

57. Chen JH, Chan DC, Kiely DK, Morris JN, Mitchell SL. Terminal trajectories of functional decline in the long-term care setting. J Gerontol A Biol Sci Med Sci 2007;62(5):531–536.

58. Schechter GL. Systemic causes of dysphagia in adults. Otolaryngol Clin North Am 1998;31(3):525–535.

59. Marik PE, Kaplan D. Aspiration pneumonia and dysphagia in the elderly. Chest 2003;124(1):328–336.

60. Leibovitz A, Plotnikov G, Habot B, Rosenberg M, Segal R. Pathogenic colonization of oral flora in frail elderly patients fed by nasogastric tube or percutaneous enterogastric tube. J Gerontol A Biol Sci Med Sci 2003;58(1):52–55.

61. Carl LC, Johnson PR. Drugs and Dysphagia: How Medications Can Affect Eating and Swallowing. Austin, TX: Pro-Ed, 2006.

62. Rudolph JL, Gardner KF, Gramigna GD, McGlinchey RE. Antipsychotics and oropharyngeal dysphagia in hospitalized older patients. J Clin Psychopharmacol 2008;28(5):532–535.

63. Brady Wagner LC. Dysphagia: Legal and ethical issues in caring for persons at the end of life. Perspect Swallow Swallow Disord (Dysphagia) 2008;17:27–32.

64. End of life issues in speech-language pathology. Available at: www.asha.org/members/slp/clinical/endoflife.htm (accessed January 4, 2009).

65. Levy A, Dominguez-Gasson, Brown E, Frederick C. Technology at end of life questioned. ASHA Leader 2004:1–14.

66. Cook IJ, Kahrilas PJ. AGA technical review on management of oropharyngeal dysphagia. Gastroenterology 1999;116(2):455–478.

67. Ramsey D, Smithard D, Kalra L. Silent aspiration: What do we know? Dysphagia 2005;20(3):218–225.

68. Ashford JR, Skelley M. Oral care and the elderly. Perspect Swallow Swallow Disord (Dysphagia) 2008;17:19–26.

69. Hinchey JA, Shephard T, Furie K, et al. Formal dysphagia screening protocols prevent pneumonia. Stroke 2005;36(9):1972–1976.

70. Sharma JC, Fletcher S, Vassallo M, Ross I. What influences outcome of stroke—pyrexia or dysphagia? Int J Clin Pract 2001;55(1):17–20.

71. Terre R, Mearin F. Prospective evaluation of oro-pharyngeal dysphagia after severe traumatic brain injury. Brain Inj 2007;21(13–14):1411–1417.

72. Wesling M, Brady S, Jensen M, Nickell M, Statkus D, Escobar N. Dysphagia outcomes in patients with brain tumors undergoing inpatient rehabilitation. Dysphagia 2003;18(3):203–210.

73. Leder SB. Gag reflex and dysphagia. Head Neck 1996; 18(2):138–141.

74. Leder SB. Videofluoroscopic evaluation of aspiration with visual examination of the gag reflex and velar movement. Dysphagia 1997;12(1):21–23.

75. Davies AE, Kidd D, Stone SP, MacMahon J. Pharyngeal sensation and gag reflex in healthy subjects. Lancet 1995; 345(8948):487–488.

76. Puntil Sheltman J. Fluoroscopic assessment of dysphagia: Which radiological procedure is best for your patient? Perspect Swallow Swallow Disord (Dysphagia) 2007; 16(4):11–14.

77. Kaul A, Miller C. Evaluation and management of esophageal disorders affecting feeding in pediatric patients. Perspect Swallow Swallow Disord (Dysphagia) 2003;1(2):12–16.

78. Langmore SE. Normal swallowing: The endoscopic perspective. In: Langmore SE, ed. Endoscopic Evaluation and Treatment of Swallowing Disorders. New York: Thieme, 2001.

79. Logemann JA, Gensler G, Robbins J, et al. A randomized study of three interventions for aspiration of thin liquids in patients with dementia or Parkinson's disease. J Speech Lang Hear Res 2008;51(1):173–183.

80. Sullivan DJ, Moran GP, Pinjon E, et al. Comparison of the epidemiology, drug resistance mechanisms, and virulence of *Candida dubliniensis* and *Candida albicans*. FEMS Yeast Res 2004;4(4–5):369–376.

81. Proulx M, de Courval FP, Wiseman MA, Panisset M. Salivary production in Parkinson's disease. Mov Disord 2005;20(2):204–207.

82. Volonte MA, Porta M, Comi G. Clinical assessment of dysphagia in early phases of Parkinson's disease. Neurol Sci 2002;23 Suppl 2:S121–S122.

83. Elman LB, Dubin RM, Kelley M, McCluskey L. Management of oropharyngeal and tracheobronchial secretions in patients with neurologic disease. J Palliat Med 2005;8(6):1150–1159.

84. Molloy L. Treatment of sialorrhoea in patients with Parkinson's disease: Best current evidence. Curr Opin Neurol 2007; 20(4):493–498.

85. Meningaud JP, Pitak-Arnnop P, Chikhani L, Bertrand JC. Drooling of saliva: A review of the etiology and management options. Oral Surg Oral Med Oral Pathol Oral Radiol Endod 2006;101(1):48–57.

86. Mills RH. Dysphagia management: Using thickened liquids. The ASHA Leader 2008;13(14):12–13.

87. Sharpe K, Ward L, Cichero J, Sopade P, Halley P. Thickened fluids and water absorption in rats and humans. Dysphagia 2007;22(3):193–203.

88. Mitchell SL, Buchanan JL, Littlehale S, Hamel MB. Tube-feeding versus hand-feeding nursing home residents with advanced dementia: A cost comparison. JAMDA 2004;5(2 suppl):s:22.

89. Langmore SE, Terpenning MS, Schork A, et al. Predictors of aspiration pneumonia: How important is dysphagia? Dysphagia 1998;13(2):69–81.

90. Plonk WM. To PEG or not to PEG. Pract Gastroenterol 2005;July:16–31.

91. Gillick MR, Volandes AE. The standard of caring: Why do we still use feeding tubes in patients with advanced dementia? J Am Med Dir Assoc 2008;9(5):364–367.

92. Mitchell SL, Kiely DK, Miller SC, Connor SR, Spence C, Teno JM. Hospice care for patients with dementia. J Pain Symptom Manage 2007;34(1):7–16.

93. Carnaby-Mann G, Crary M. Pill swallowing by adults with dysphagia. Arch Otolaryngol Head Neck Surg 2005; 131(11):970–975.

94. Donzelli J, Brady S, Wesling M, Theisen M. Secretions, occlusion status, and swallowing in patients with a tracheotomy tube: A descriptive study. Ear Nose Throat J 2006; 85(12):831–834.

95. Tippett DC. Swallowing, tracheostomy and ventilator dependency. In: Tippett DC, ed. Tracheostomy and Ventilator Dependency. Management of Breathing, Speaking and Swallowing. New York: Thieme, 2000.

96. Gross RD, Mahlmann J, Grayhack JP. Physiologic effects of open and closed tracheostomy tubes on the pharyngeal swallow. Ann Otol Rhinol Laryngol 2003;112(2):143–152.

97. Speilman A, Ben Aryad H, Gutman D, Szargel R, Duetsch E. Xerostomia—diagnosis and treatment. Oral Med 1981; 51:144–147.

98. Sreebny L, Valdini A. Xerostomia. Arch Intern Med 1987;147: 1333–1337.

99. Roh JL, Kim S, Kim AY. The effect of acute xerostomia on vocal function. Arch Otolaryngol Head Neck Surg 1006;132:543–546.

100. Mouly S, Orler JB, Tillet Y, Coudert AC, Oberli F, Presahw P, Bergmann F. Efficacy of a new oral psychotropic drug-induced xerostomia—a randomized controlled trial. J Clin Psychopharmacol 2007;27(5):437–443.

101. Hewett, J. Mouth Care. In Cooper J, ed. Stepping into Palliative Care: Care and Practice (2nd ed). Seattle: Radcliffe Press, 2006:89–102.

102. Ng K, von Gunton, CF. Symptoms and attitudes of 100 consecutive patients admitted to an acute hospice/palliative care unit. J Pain Symptom Manage 1998;16:307–316.

103. Mercandante S, Calderone L, Villari P, Serretta R, Sapio M, Casuccio A, Fulfaro F. The use of pilocarpine in opioid-induced xerostomia. Palliat Med 2000;14:529–531.

104. Davies A. The comparison of artificial saliva and chewing gum in the management of xerostomia in patients with advanced cancer. Palliat Med 2000;14:197–203.

105. Bots C, Brand H, Veerman E, Korevaar J, Valentijn-Benz M, Bezemer P, Valentijn R, Vos P, Bijlsma J, ter Wee P, Amerongen B, Amerongen A. Chewing gum and a saliva substitute alleviate thrist and xerostomia in patients on haemodialysis. Nephrol Dial Transplant 2005;20:578–584.

106. Cohen L, Moss A, Weisbord S, Germain M. Renal palliative care. J Palliat Med 2006;9(4):977–992.

107. Ship JA, Pillemer, SR, Baum BJ. Xerostomia and the geriatric patient. Geriatr Soc 2002; 50:535–543.

108. Jensen SB, Pedersen AM, Reibel, Nauntofte B. Xerostomia and hypofunction of the salivary glands in cancer therapy. Support Care Cancer 2003;11:207–225.

109. Cooke C, Admedzel S, Mayberry J. Xerostomia—a review. Palliat Med 1996;10:284–292.

110. Amerongen AV, Veerman EC. Current therapies for xerostomia and salivary gland hypofunction associated with cancer therapies. Support Care Cancer 2003;11:226–231.

111. Bruce S. Radiation-induced xerostomia: How dry is your patient. Clin J Oncol Nurs 2004;8:61–67.

112. Porter S, Scully C, Hegarty A. An update of the etiology and management of xerostomia. Oral Surg Oral Med Oral Pathol Oral Radiol Endod 2004;97:28–46.

113. Guchelaar H, Vermes A, Meerwaldt J. Radiation induced xerostomia: pathophysiology, clinical course, and supportive treatment. Support Care Cancer 1997;5:281–288.

114. Davies A. The management of xerostomia: A review. Eur J Cancer Care 1997;6:209–214.

115. Pacholke H, Amdure R, Morris C, Li J, Dempsey J, Hinerman R, Mendenhall W. Late xerostomia after intensity-modulated radiation therapy versus conventional radiotherapy. Am J Clin Oncol 2005;28:351–358.

116. Oncology Nursing Society. Radiation Therapy Patient Care Record. Pittsburgh: Oncology Nursing Society Press, 2002.

117. National Cancer Institute. Common terminology criteria for adverse events v3.0. Published December 12, 2003. Available

at: http://www.ctep.cancer.gov/forms/CTCAEv3.pdf (accessed December 28, 2008).

118. Guggenheimer J, Moore P. Xerostomia: Etiology, recognition and treatment. J Am Dent Assoc 2003;134:61–69.

119. Blom M, Dawidson I, Angmar-Mansson B. The effect of acupuncture on buccal blood flow assessed by laser doppler flowmetry: A pilot study. Caries Res 1992;24:428.

120. Johnstone, P, Niemtzow R, Riffenburgh RH. Acupuncture for xerostomia. Cancer 2002;94:1151–1156.

121. Dion D, Lapointe B. Mouth care. In: McDonaal N, Oneschuk D, Hagen N, Doyle D, eds. Palliative Medicine: A Case-based Manual (2nd ed). New York: Oxford Unitversity Press, 2005:317–331.

122. Miller E. Nutrition. In: Panke J, Coyne P, eds. Conversations in Palliative Care (2nd ed). Hospice and Palliative Nurses Association, 2006:107–115.

123. Diaz-Arnold A, Marak C. The impact of saliva on patient care: a literature review. J Prosthe Dent 2002;6:337–432.

124. Chatelut E, Rispail Y, Berlan M, Montastruc J. Yohimbine increases human salivary secretion. Br J Clin Pharmacol 1989;28:366–368.

125. Olasz L, Nyarady Z, Szentirmy M. Assessment of relieving symptoms of xerostomia with oral pilocarpine during irradiation in head-and-neck cancer patients. Cancer Detect Prev 2000;24(suppl 1):489.

126. Tagaki Y, Kimura Y, Nakamura T. Cevimeline gargle for the treatment of xerostomia in patients with Sjogren's syndrome. Ann Rheum Dis 2004;63:749.

127. Sweeney M, Bagg J, Baxter W, Aitchison T. Clinical trial of mucin-containing oral spray for treatment of xerostomia in hospice patients. Palliat Med 1997;11:225–232.

128. Lewis J. Hiccups: Causes and cures. J Clin Gastroenterol 1985;7:539–552.

129. Wilcock A, Twycross R. Midazolam for intractable hiccup. J Pain Symptom Manage 1996;12:59–61.

130. Smith H, Busracamwongs A. Management of hiccups in the palliative care population. Am J Palliat Care 2003;20:149–154.

131. Williams C. The unremitting hiccup. AAHPM Bull 2001; Summer:6–7.

132. Rousseau P. Hiccups in patients with advanced cancer: A brief review. Prog Palliat Care 2003;11:10–12.

133. Pollack M. Intractable hiccups: A serious sign of underlying systemic disease. J Clin Gastroenterol 2003;37:272–273.

134. Camp-Sorrell, D. Hiccups. In: Camp-Sorrell D, Hawkins R, eds. Clinical Manual for the Oncology Advanced Practice Nurse (2nd ed). Pittsburgh: Oncology Nursing Society, 2006:3–17.

135. Kolodzik P, Eilers M. Hiccups (singulatus): Review and approach to management. Ann Emerg Med 1991;20:565–573.

136. Regnaud C. Dysphagia, dyspepsia, and hiccup. In: Doyle D, Hanks G, Cherny N, Calman K, eds. Oxford Textbook of Palliative Medicine (3rd ed). New York: Oxford University Press, 2004:468–482.

137. Launois S, Bizec J, Whitelaw W, Cabane J, Derenne J. Hiccups in adults: An overview. Eur Respir J 1993;6:563–575.

138. Calvo E, Fernandez-Torre F, Brugarolas J. Cervical phrenic nerve block. J Nat Cancer Inst 2002;94:1175–1176.

139. Schiff E, River Y, Oliven A, Odeh M. Acupuncture therapy for persistent hiccups. Am J Med Sci 2002;323:166–168.

140. Pertel P, Till M. Intractable hiccups induced by the use of megestrol acetate. Arch Intern Med 1998;158:809–810.

141. Cymet TC. Retrospective analysis of hiccups in patients in a community hospital from 1995–2000. J Nat Med Assoc 2002;94:480–483.

142. McAllister R, Mcdonald A, Mayer T, Bittenbinder T. Recurrent persistent hiccups after epidural steroid injection and analgesia with bupivacaine. Anesth Analg 2005;100:1834–1836.

143. Dickerman R, Jaikumar S. The hiccup reflex arc and persistent hiccups with high-dose anabolic steroids: Is the brainstem the steroid-responsive locus? Clin Neurophamacol 2001;21(1):62–64.

144. Sanchek K. Hiccups—when the diaphragm attacks. J Palliat Med 2004;7(4);870–873.

145. Moretti R, Torre P, Antonello R, Ukmar M, Cazzato G, Bava A. Gabapention as a drug therapy of intractable hiccups because of vascular lesion: A three-year follow up. Neurologist 2004;10:102–106.

146. Petroianu P, Hein G, Stegmeier-Petroianu A, Bergler W, Rufer R. Gabapentin "Add-on Therapy" for idiopathic chronic hiccup (ICH). J Clin Gastroenterol 2000;30:321–324.

147. Bilotta F, Rosa G. Nefopam for severe hiccups. NEJM 2000;343:1973–1974.

148. Vaidya V. Sertraline in the treatment of hiccups. Psychosomatics 2000;41:353–355.

149. Cersosimo R, Brophy M. Hiccoughs with high dose dexametasone administration. Cancer 1998;82:412–414.

150. Marechal R, Berghmans T, Sculier JP. Succcessful treatment of intractable hiccup with methylphenidate in a lung cancer patient. Support Care Cancer 2003;11:126–128.

151. Lierz P, Felleiter P. Anesthesia as therapy for persistent hiccups. Anesth Analg 2002;95:494–495.

152. Cohen SP, Lubin E, Stojanovic M. Intravenous lidocaine in the treatment of hiccups. South Med J 2001;94:1124–1125.

153. Sarhill NB, Mahnind F. Hiccups and other GI symptoms. In: Berger A, Shuster J, Van Roem J, eds. Principles and Practice of Palliative Care and Supportive Oncology (3rd ed). Philadelphia, PA: Lippincott, Williams, & Wilkins, 2007:193–203.

# 12 ❦❦ *Denice Caraccia Economou*

# Bowel Management: Constipation, Diarrhea, Obstruction, and Ascites

*I am either constipated or have diarrhea. This bowel stuff is controlling my life—I don't know what to do. I am miserable—K.B., 60 year old with gastric cancer*

◆ *Key Points*

◆ *Multiple factors contribute to constipation. Proactive management is essential for successful outcomes.*

◆ *Treating diarrhea requires a thorough assessment and therapy directed at the specific cause.*

◆ *Palliative care should allow for a thoughtful and realistic approach to management of symptoms within the goals of care.*

## CONSTIPATION

Constipation affects 2% to 10% of the general population, but the incidence may be as high as 20% to 50% in older or ill persons.[1] Constipation is a major problem in cancer patients, with as many as 70% to 100% of cancer patients having this distressing symptom.[2] The use of opioids for pain is a contributory factor to constipation, and this side effect is the principal reason for their discontinuation.[3–5] Constipation is common and yet undertreated by both physicians and nurses.

### Definitions

Constipation is subjective to many patients, making assessment much more difficult. Constipation is defined as "a decrease in the frequency of passage of formed stools and characterized by stools that are hard and small and difficult to expel." Understanding the normal functioning of the bowel can provide insight into the contributing factors leading to constipation, diarrhea, and obstruction. Associated symptoms of constipation vary, but may include excessive straining, a feeling of fullness or pressure in the rectum, the sensation of incomplete emptying, abdominal distention, and cramps.[5,6] The subjective experience of constipation may vary for different individuals, underscoring the importance of individualized patient assessment and management.

### Prevalence and Impact

It is estimated that 50% of hospice patients are constipated; this may be an underestimate, as many of those patients are on opioids and stool softeners/laxatives at baseline.[1,6] Inpatient hospitalizaion and ambulatory clinic visits for constipation and related side effects cost the healthcare system $235 million annually.[7,10] Constipation is considered a symptom of

Bowel Dysfunction (BD) and Opioid Bowel Dysfunction (OBD) relating to opioid-induced constipation. The impact of constipation on quality of life is substantial. Constipation causes social, psychological, and physical distress for patients, which additionally impacts the caregiver and health care staff. Failure to anticipate and manage constipation in a proactive way significantly affects the difficulty a patient will experience in attempting to relieve this problem.

## Pathophysiology

Normal bowel function includes three areas of control: small intestinal motility, colon motility, and defecation. This includes the processes of secretion, absorption, transport, and storage.[6,8] Small-intestinal activity is primarily the mixing of contents by bursts of propagated motor activity that are associated with increased gastric, pancreatic, and biliary secretion. This motor activity occurs every 90 to 120 minutes, but is altered when food is ingested. Contents are mixed to allow for digestion and absorption of nutrients. When the stomach has emptied, the small intestine returns to regular propagated motor activity.[4]

The colon propels contents forward through peristaltic movements. The colon movement is much slower than that of the small intestine. Contents may remain in the colon for up to 2 to 3 days, whereas small-intestinal transit is 2–4 hours. Motor activity in the large intestine occurs approximately six times per day, usually grouped in two peak bursts. The first is triggered by awakening and breakfast, and a smaller burst is triggered by the afternoon meal. Contractions are stimulated by ingestion of food, psychogenic factors, and somatic activity. Sykes[6] found that 50% of the constipated patients in a hospice setting had a transit time between 4 and 12 days.

The physiology of defecation involves coordinated interaction between the involuntary internal anal sphincter and the voluntary external anal sphincter. The residual intestinal contents distend the rectum and initiate expulsion. The longitudinal muscle of the rectum contracts, and with the voluntary external anal sphincter relaxed, defecation can occur. Additional coordinated muscle activity also occurs and includes contraction of the diaphragm against a closed glottis, tensing of the abdominal wall, and relaxation of the pelvic floor.

The enteric nervous system plays an important role in the movement of bowel contents through the gastrointestinal (GI) tract as well. Smooth muscles in the GI tract have spontaneous electrical, rhythmic activity, resembling pacemakers in the stomach and small intestine, that communicate with the remainder of the bowel. There are both submucosal and myenteric plexuses of nerves. These nerves are connected to the central nervous system through sympathetic ganglia, splanchnic nerves, and parasympathetic fibers in the vagus nerve and the presacral plexus. Opioid medications affect the myenteric plexus, which coordinates peristalsis. Therefore, peristalsis is decreased and stool transit time is decreased, leading to harder, dryer, and less frequent stools, or constipation.[4,7]

Important factors that promote normal functioning of the bowel include the following:

1. *Fluid intake.* Nine liters of fluid (which includes 7 liters secreted from the salivary glands, stomach, pancreas, small bowel, and biliary system, and the average oral intake of 2 liters) are reduced to 1.5 liters by the time they reach the colon. At this point, water and electrolytes continue to be absorbed, and the end volume for waste is 150 mL.[8,9] Therefore, decreased fluid intake can make a significant difference in the development of constipation.[1]
2. *Adequate dietary fiber.* The presence of food in the stomach initiates the muscle contractions and secretions from the biliary, gastric, and pancreatic systems that lead to movement of the bowels.[7] The amount of dietary fiber consumed is related to stool size and consistency.[11]
3. *Physical activity.* Colonic propulsion is related to intraluminal pressures in the colon. Lack of physical activity and reduced intraluminal pressures can significantly reduce propulsive activity.[6]
4. *Adequate time or privacy to defecate.* Changes in normal bowel routines, such as morning coffee or reading the paper, can decrease peristalsis and lead to constipation. Emotional disturbances are also known to affect gut motility.[10,11]

## Primary, Secondary, and Iatrogenic Constipation

Causes of constipation in cancer patients are divided into three different categories.[4,6]

1. Primary constipation is caused by reduced fluid and fiber intake, decreased activity, lack of privacy and advanced age.
2. Secondary constipation is related to structural, metabolic or neurologic disorders. These changes may include tumor, partial intestinal obstruction, metabolic effects of hypercalcemia, hypothyroidism, hypokalemia, hyperglycemia, as well as spinal cord compression at the level of the cauda equina or sacral plexus, sacral nerve infiltration and cerebral tumors.
3. Iatrogenically induced constipation is related to pharmacological interventions. Opioids are the primary medications associated with constipation. In addition, Vinca alkaloid chemotherapies (vincristine, oxaliplatin, thalidomide), anticholinergic medications (belladonna, antihistamines), antiemetic therapy (5-HT$_3$ antagonists), tricyclic antidepressants (nortriptyline, amitriptyline), neuroleptics (haloperidol and chlorpromazine), antispasmodics, anticonvulsants (phenytoin and gabapentin), muscle relaxants, aluminum antacids, iron, diuretics (furosemide), and antiparkinsonian agents cause constipation.[4–6]

## Constipation Related to Cancer and Its Treatment

Multiple factors associated with cancer and its treatment cause constipation. When it primarily involves the GI system or is anatomically associated with the bowel, cancer itself causes constipation. Pelvic cancers, including ovarian, cervical, and uterine cancers, are highly associated with constipation and mechanical obstruction.[11] Malignant ascites, spinal cord compression, and paraneoplastic autonomic neuropathy also cause constipation. Cancer-related causes include surgical interruption of the GI tract, decreased activity, reduced intake of both fluids and food, changes in personal routines associated with bowel movements, bed rest, confusion, and depression.[4-7,12]

## Opioid-Related Constipation

Opioids affect bowel function primarily by inhibiting propulsive peristalsis through the small bowel and colon.[4,7,13] Chronic opioid use in non-cancer patients causes constipation in 40% of the patients; in advanced cancer patients, 50% to 90% will develop bowel dysfunction.[13,14] Opioids bind with the receptors on the smooth muscles of the bowel, affecting the contraction of the circular and longitudinal muscle fibers that cause peristalsis or the movement of contents through the bowel.[13,14] Colonic transit time is lengthened, contributing to increased fluid and electrolyte absorption and dryer, harder stools.[1,4,5] Peristaltic changes occur 5 to 25 minutes after administration of the opioid and are dose related. Patients do not develop tolerance to the constipation side effects even with long-term use of opioids.[15] There is evidence associated with transdermal fentanyl versus morphine and methadone compared to morphine or hydromorphone use that constipation severity may differ among opioids.[16,17] The use of laxatives and stool softeners with opioids represents a rational, proactive approach to opioid-induced constipation.

## Assessment of Constipation

### History

The measurement of constipation requires more than assessing the frequency of stools alone. Managing constipation requires a thorough history and physical examination.

The use of a quantifying tool can be helpful in understanding what the patient is experiencing and how different that may be from the usual or baseline bowel habit. A tool developed in 1989, the Constipation Assessment Scale (CAS), has been tested for validity and reliability and found to have a significant ability to measure constipation as well as its severity between moderate and severe constipation. It is a simple questionnaire that requires 2 minutes to complete (Figure 12–1).

*Direction: Circle the appropriate number to indicate whether, during the past three days, you have had NO PROBLEM, SOME PROBLEM or a SEVERE PROBLEM with each of the items listed.*

| Item | No Problem | Some Problem | Severe Problem |
|---|---|---|---|
| 1. Abdominal distension or bloating | 0 | 1 | 2 |
| 2. Change in amount of gas passed rectally | 0 | 1 | 2 |
| 3. Less frequent bowel movements | 0 | 1 | 2 |
| 4. Oozing liquid stool | 0 | 1 | 2 |
| 5. Rectal fullness or pressure | 0 | 1 | 2 |
| 6. Rectal pian with bowel movement | 0 | 1 | 2 |
| 7. Smaller stool size | 0 | 1 | 2 |
| 8. Urge but inability to pass stool | 0 | 1 | 2 |

Patient's Name                                    Date

**Figure 12–1.** Constipation Assessment Scale. *Source*: McMillan et al. (1989), reference 18. Reproduced with permission

The CAS includes eight symptoms associated with constipation: (1) abdominal distention or bloating, (2) change in amount of gas passed rectally, (3) less frequent bowel movements, (4) oozing liquid stool, (5) rectal fullness or pressure, (6) rectal pain with bowel movement, (7) small volume of stool, and (8) inability to pass stool.[18] These symptoms are rated as 0, not experienced; 1, some problem; or 2, severe problem. A score between 0 and 16 is calculated and can be used as an objective measurement of subjective symptoms for ongoing management.

The CAS gives a good sense of bowel function[6,18] and also outlines questions to use in taking a constipation history. It is important to start by asking patients when they moved their bowels last and to follow up by asking what their normal movement pattern is. Remember, what is considered constipated for one person is not for someone else. What are the characteristics of their stools and did they note any blood or mucus? Were their bowels physically difficult to move? This is especially important if they have cancer in or near the intestines or rectal area that may contribute to physical obstruction. Ovarian cancer patients usually complain of feeling severely bloated. They may say things like "If you stick a pin in me, I know I will pop!" Evaluating the abdomen or asking patients if they feel bloated or pressure in the abdomen is important. Does the patient feel pain when moving the bowels? Is the patient oozing liquid stool? Does the patient feel that the volume of stool passed is small? Many patients may experience unexplainable nausea.[4,5]

### Medication- or Disease-Related History

The patient's medical status and anticipated disease process are important in providing insight into areas where early intervention could prevent severe constipation or even obstruction. Constipation may be anticipated with primary and secondary bowel cancer, as well as with pelvic tumors, peritoneal mesothelioma or spinal cord compression, previous bowel surgery, or a history of Vinca alkaloid chemotherapy. Changes in dietary habits related to the above medications or the addition of new medications may contribute to constipation.[1,8,12] Anticholinergic medications, antihistamines, tricyclic antidepressants, aluminum antacids, and diuretics can cause constipation. Hypercalcemia, hyperglycemia and hypokalemia contribute to constipation by slowing down motility. Several factors aggravate and contribute to the experience of constipation including confusion, immobility and dehydration.[7] Ask patients if there are things they do to aid in defecation. Sometimes physical actions the patient may use can help causes related to rectocele, or rectal ulcer.[6] Table 12–1 outlines causes of constipation in cancer and other palliative care patients.

### Physical Examination

Begin the physical examination in the mouth, to ensure that the patient is able to chew foods and that there are no lesions or tumors in the mouth that could interfere with eating. Does the patient wear dentures? Patients who wear dentures and have lost a great deal of weight may have dentures that do not fit properly, which would make eating and drinking difficult. Patients may choose to eat only what they are able to chew as a result of their dentures or other dental problems. Therefore, they may not be eating enough fiber and, thus, contributing to primary constipation.

*Abdominal Examination.* Inspect the abdomen initially for bloating, distention, or bulges. Distention may be associated with obesity, fluid, tumor, or gas. Remember, the patient should have emptied the bladder. Auscultation is important to evaluate the presence or absence of bowel sounds. If no bowel sounds are heard initially, listen continuously for a minimum of 5 minutes. The absence of bowel sounds may indicate a paralytic ileus. If the bowel sounds are hyperactive, it could indicate diarrhea. Percussion of the bowel may result in tympany, which is related to gas in the bowel. A dull sound is heard over intestinal fluid and feces. Palpation of the abdomen should start lightly; look for muscular resistance and abdominal tenderness. This is usually associated with chronic constipation. If rebound tenderness is detected with coughing or light palpation, peritoneal inflammation should be considered. Deep palpation may reveal a "sausage-like" mass of stool in the left colon. Feeling stool in the colon indicates constipation. Although Sykes[6] points out that the distinction between tumor and stool is hard to make, recognizing the underlying anatomy is helpful in distinguishing the stool along the line of the descending colon or more proximal colon, including the cecum. A digital examination of the rectum may reveal stool or possible tumor or rectocele. If the patient is experiencing incontinence of liquid stool, obstruction must be considered. Examining for hemorrhoids, ulcerations, or rectal fissures is important, especially in the neutropenic patient. Patients with neutropenia can complain of rectal pain well before a rectal infection is obvious. Evaluating the patient for infection, ulceration, or rectal fissures is very important. Additionally, determine whether the patient has had previous intestinal surgery, alternating diarrhea and constipation, complaints of abdominal colic pain or nausea, and vomiting. Examining the stool for shape and consistency can also be useful. Stools that are hard and pellet-like suggest slow transit time, whereas stools that are ribbon-like suggest hemorrhoids. Blood or mucus in the stool suggests tumor, hemorrhoids, or possibly a preexisting colitis.[6] Elderly patients may experience urinary incontinence related to fecal impaction.[1,5,13] Abdominal pain may also be related to constipation. Patients will complain of colic pain related to the effort of colonic muscle to move hard stool. The history may be complicated by known abdominal tumors. Patients in pain should still be treated with opioids as needed.

### Management of Constipation

Preventing constipation whenever possible is the most important management strategy. Constipation can be extremely distressing to many patients and severely affects quality of life.[7,8] The complicating factor remains the individuality of a patient's response to constipation therapy. Therefore, there is no set rule for the most effective way to manage constipation. Patients with primary bowel cancers, pelvic tumors such as ovarian or uterine cancers, or metastatic tumors that press on colon structures will experience a difficult-to-manage constipation. It is not unusual for those patients to be admitted to the hospital to manage constipation and to rule out obstruction. To minimize those admissions whenever possible, as Dame Cicely Saunders, the founder of hospice recommends, "Do not forget the bowels." Nurses are at the bedside most often and are the ones who see the cumulated number and types of medication a patient may be taking. Understanding which medications and disease processes put a patient at high risk for constipation is essential for good bowel management.

Assessing the patient's constipation as discussed earlier is the best place to start. The patient's problem list should reflect the risk for constipation and the need for aggressive constipation management. For example, diabetic patients who are

**Table 12–1**
**Causes of Constipation in Cancer/Palliative Care Patients**

**Cancer-related**
Directly related to tumor site. Primary bowel cancers, secondary bowel cancers, pelvic cancers.
Hypercalcemia. Surgical interruption of bowel integrity.

**Etiology**
Intestinal obstruction related to tumor in the bowel wall or external compression by tumor. Damage to the lumbosacral spinal cord, cauda equina, or pelvic plexus. High spinal cord transection mainly stops the motility response to food. Low spinal cord or pelvic outflow lesions produce dilation of the colon and slow transit in the descending and distal transverse colon. Surgery in the abdomen can lead to adhesion development or direct changes in the bowel.

**Hypercalcemia**
Cholinergic control of secretions of the intestinal epithelium is mediated by changes in intracellular calcium concentrations. Hypercalcemia causes decreased absorption, leading to constipation, whereas hypercalcemia can lead to diarrhea.

**Secondary effects related to the disease**
Decreased appetite, decreased fluid intake, low-fiber diet, weakness, inactivity, confusion, depression, change in normal toileting habits.

**Etiology**
Decreased fluid and food intake leading to dehydration and weakness. Decreased intake, ineffective voluntary elimination actions, as well as decreased normal defecation reflexes. Decreased peristalsis; increased colonic transit time leads to increased absorption of fluid and electrolytes and small, hard, dry stools. Inactivity, weakness, changes in normal toileting habits, daily bowel function reflexes, and positioning affect ability to use abdominal wall musculature and relax pelvic floor for proper elimination. Psychological depression can increase constipation by slowing down motility.

**Concurrent disease**
Diabetes (hyperglycemia), hypothyroidism, hypokalemia, diverticular disease, hemorrhoids, colitis, chronic neurological diseases.

**Etiology**
Electrolytes and therefore water are transported via neuronal control. Like hypercalcemia, abnormal potassium can affect water absorption and contribute to constipation. Chronic neurological diseases affect the neurological stimulation of intestinal motility.

**Medication-related**
Opioid medications
Anticholinergic effects (hydroscine, phenothiazines)
Tricyclic antidepressants
Antiparkinsonian drugs
Iron
Antihypertensives, antihistamines
Antacids
Diuretics
Vinka alkaloid chemotherapy

**Etiology**
Opioids in particular suppress forward peristalsis and increase sphincter tone. Opioids increase electrolyte and water absorption in both the large and small intestine; this leads to dehydration and hard, dry stools. Morphine causes insensitivity of the rectum to distention, decreasing the sensation of the need to defecate. Vinca alkaloid chemotherapy has a neurotoxic effect that causes damage to the myenteric plexus of the colon. This increases nonpropulsive contractions. Colonic transit time is increased, leading to constipation. Antidepressants slow large bowel motility. Antacids (bismuth, aluminum salts) cause hard stools.

*Sources:* Levy (1991), reference 5; Sykes (1996), reference 21.

taking opioids for pain are at extremely high risk for constipation. Diabetes damages the sensory fibers that are most important for temperature and pain sensation, as well as the neuronal influence on intestinal motility.[3,6,13] In addition to assessing the extent of the patient's constipation, determining the methods the patient has used to manage the constipation in the past is essential. This can usually provide information regarding what medications the patient tolerates best and where to start with recommendations for management. According to Sykes,[1] using radiography to evaluate whether constipation has advanced to obstruction may be useful if there is indecision, but in palliative medicine, the use of x-ray procedures should be limited. He also suggests that blood work be limited to corrective studies; for example, if hypercalcemia or hyperkalemia can be reversed to improve constipation, such blood work may be useful.

Improving three important primary causes of constipation is essential. Encouraging fluid intake is a priority. Increasing or decreasing fluid intake by as little as 100 mL can effect constipation.[9] Increase dietary intake as much as possible. This is a difficult intervention for many patients. Focusing on food intake for some patients can increase their anxiety and discomfort. If a patient feels that bowel movements are less frequent, think about dietary intake. The Western diet is fiber-deficient.[5,6,12,19] Caution is needed for patients who use bulk laxatives such as psyllium, especially if they also are taking other bowel medications. Increasing the fiber intake for patients in general may be helpful, but in palliative care, high fiber in the diet can cause more discomfort and constipation. Fiber without fluid absorbs what little liquid the patient may have available in the bowel and makes the bowels more difficult to move.[5,13,14] For example, an elderly patient who experiences reduced appetite and decreased fluid intake related to chemotherapy or disease, and whose symptoms are nausea or vomiting with reduced activity, is at extreme risk for constipation. Encouraging activity whenever possible, even in end-of-life care, can be very helpful. Increased activity helps to stimulate peristalsis and to improve mood.[1,5] Physical therapy should be used as part of a multidisciplinary bowel-management approach. Providing basic range of motion, either active or passive, can improve bowel management and patient satisfaction.[12,13]

## Pharmacological Management

### Types of Laxatives

*Bulk Laxatives.* Laxatives can be classified by their actions. Bulk laxatives do just that—they provide bulk to the intestines to increase mass, stimulating the bowel to move. Increasing dietary fiber is considered a bulk laxative. The recommended dose of bran is 8 g daily. Other bulk laxatives include psyllium, carboxymethylcellulose, and methylcellulose.[6] Bulk laxatives are more helpful for mild constipation. Because bulk laxatives work best when patients are able to increase their fluid intake, they may be inappropriate for end-stage patients. In palliative care, patients may not ingest enough fluid. It is recommended that the patient increase fluids by 200 to 300 mL when using bulk laxatives. Patients may have difficulty with the consistency of bulk laxatives and find this approach unacceptable. Patients using bulk laxatives without the additional fluid intake are at risk of developing a partial bowel obstruction or, if an impending one exists, may risk complete bowel obstruction. The benefits of bulk laxatives in severe constipation are questionable.

Additional complications include allergic reactions, fluid retention, and hyperglycemia.[5] Bulk laxatives produce gas as the indigestible or nonsoluble fiber breaks down or ferments. The result can be uncomfortable bloating and gas.

The recommended dosage of bulk laxatives is to start with 8 g daily, then stabilize at 3 to 4 g for maintenance.

Psyllium is recommended at 2 to 4 teaspoons daily as a bulk laxative. Action may take 2 to 3 days.

*Lubricant Laxatives.* Mineral oil is probably the most common lubricant laxative used. It can help by both lubricating the stool surface and softening the stool by penetration, leading to an easier bowel movement. Overuse of mineral oil can cause seepage from the rectum and perineal irritation. With chronic use it can lead to malabsorption of fat-soluble vitamins (vitamins A, D, E, and K). Levy[5] recommends caution when giving mineral oil at bedtime or giving it to patients at risk for aspiration. Aspiration pneumonitis or lipoid pneumonia is common in the frail and elderly patient. A complication should be noted when mineral oil is given with docusate(Colace). If patients are on daily docusate and are given mineral oil in addition to assist with constipation, the absorption of mineral oil increases, leading to a risk of lipoid granuloma in the intestinal wall.[5]

The recommended dosage of mineral oil is 10 to 30 mL/day, and action may occur in 1 to 3 days.

*Surfactant/Detergent Laxatives.* Surfactant/detergent laxatives reduce surface tension, which increases absorption of water and fats into dry stools, leading to a softening effect. According to Levy[5] and others,[8,14] medications such as docusate exert a mucosal contact effect, which encourages secretion of water, sodium, and chloride in the jejunum and colon and decreases electrolyte and water reabsorption in the small and large intestines.[9,20] At higher doses, these laxatives may stimulate peristalsis. Docusate is used in a compounded or fixed combination with bowel stimulants like casanthranol (Peri-Colace) or senna (Senokot S). Castor oil also works like a detergent laxative by exerting a surface-wetting action on the stool and directly stimulates the colon, but Levy[5] discourages its use in cancer-related constipation because results are difficult to control.

The recommended dosage of surfactant/detergent laxatives includes docusate starting at 300 mg daily and calcium salt (Surfak) at 240 mg daily to twice a day. (This may take 1 to 3 days to be effective.)

*Combination Medications.* Peri-Colace is a combination of a mild stimulant laxative, casanthranol, and the stool softener docusate. Combination softener/laxative medications have been shown to be more effective than softeners alone at a lower total dose.[21]

The recommended dosage of Senokot S is two tablets daily to twice a day (see Senokot S flow chart in Table 12–2). Senokot is a combination of senna as a laxative and a stool softener for smoother and easier evacuation. Results occur in 6 to 12 hours. Flexibility of dosing allows individual needs to be met. Combination medications are especially recommended for opioid related constipation. Remember as the dose of opioid increases, the dose of anticonstipation medications must also be increased.

*Osmotic Laxatives.* Osmotic laxatives are nonabsorbable sugars that exert an osmotic effect in both the small and, to a lesser extent, large intestines. They increase fluid secretions in the small intestines by retaining fluid in the bowel lumen.[7,12] They have the additional effect of lowering ammonia levels. This is helpful in improving confusion, especially in hepatic failure patients. Laxatives in this category include: Lactulose, Magnesium citrate, Magnesium hydroxide (Milk of Magnesia®), Polyethylene glycol (PEG 3350, MiraLax®), and Sodium biphosphate (Phospho-Soda®). These laxatives can be effective for chronic constipation, especially when related to opioid use. Onset of action is between 2–48 hours.[7] Milk of Magnesia can cause severe cramping and discomfort. This medication is recommended for use only as a last resort in chronically ill patients. Opioid-related constipation requires the use of aggressive laxatives earlier rather than later to prevent severe constipation, referred to as obstipation, which leads to obstruction.

Drawbacks of agents like Lactulose or Sorbitol are that effectiveness is completely dose-related and, for some patients, the sweet taste is intolerable. The bloating and gas associated with higher doses may be too uncomfortable or distressing to tolerate. Lactulose or sorbitol can be put into juice or other liquid to lessen the taste. Patients may prefer hot tea or hot water to help reduce the sweet taste. Lactulose is more costly than sorbitol liquid. A study that compared the two medications found that there was no significant difference, except with regard to nausea, which increased with lactulose (P = 0.05).[22]

The recommended dosage of lactulose/sorbitol is 30 to 60 mL initially for severe constipation every 4 hours until a bowel movement occurs. Once that happens, calculate the amount of lactulose used to achieve that movement, and then divide in half for recommended daily maintenance dose.[5] An example would be: it took 60 mL to have a bowel movement; therefore, 30 mL daily should keep the bowels moving regularly. The recommended dosage of Milk of Magnesia is 30 mL to initiate a bowel movement. For opioid-related constipation, 15 mL of Milk of Magnesia may be added to the baseline bowel medications either daily or every other day. Magnesium citrate comes in a 10-ounce bottle. For severe constipation, it is used as a one-time initial therapy. It can be titrated up or down, depending on patient response. For patients with abdominal discomfort or pain, it is recommended that obstruction be ruled out before using this medication. If the patient were obstructed, even only partially, this would only increase the discomfort or lead to perforation.[3,23]

Polyethylene glycol (PEG 3350), (MiraLax®) is used frequently and can be sprinkled over food. Recommended dose is 1 tablespoon. Evacuation can take between 2 to 4 days. If bowel obstruction is suspected, do not use.[24] Osmotic rectal compounds include glycerin suppositories and sorbitol enemas. Glycerin suppositories soften stool by osmosis and act as a lubricant.

*Bowel Stimulants.* Bowel stimulants work directly on the colon to increase motility. These medications stimulate the myenteric plexus to induce peristalsis. They also reduce the amount of water and electrolytes in the colon. They are divided into two groups: the diphenylmethanes and the anthraquinones. The diphenylmethanes are commonly known as phenolphthalein (Ex-Lax, Fen-a-Mint, Correctol, and Doxidan) and bisacodyl (Dulcolax). Phenolphthalein must be metabolized in the liver rather than in the colon. Levy[5] points out that because the effect

---

**Table 12–2**
**Senokot S Laxative Recommendations for Cancer-Related Constipation**

Day 0
- Senokot S 2 tablets at bedtime

If no BM on day 1
- Senokot S 2 tablets Bid.

If no BM on day 2
- Senokot S 3 or 4 tablets Bid or Tid.

If no BM on day 3
- Dulcolax 2 or 3 tablets Tid and/or Hs.
- If no BM, rule out impaction
- If impacted:
  - Lubricate rectum with oil-retention enema
  - Medicate with opioid and/or benzodiazepine
  - Disimpact
  - Give enemas until clear.
  - Increase daily laxative therapy per above
- If not impacted:
  Give additional laxatives:
  - Lactulose (45–60 mL PO)
  - Magnesium citrate (8 oz)
  - Dulcolax suppository (1 PR)
  - Fleet enema (1 PR)

At any step, if medication is ineffective, continue at that dose. If < 1 BM per day, increase laxative therapy per steps. If > 2 BM per day, decrease laxative therapy by 24% to 50%.

*Source:* Adapted from Levy (1991), reference 5.

---

is difficult to control and hepatic circulation is significant, this class of stimulants may not be appropriate for cancer-related constipation. The anthraquinones are bowel stimulants that include senna and cascara. They are activated in the large intestine by bacterial degradation into the large bowel, stimulating glycosides. The negative side of bisacodyl is its cramping side effect. This action causes a 6- to 12-hour delay when taken orally. Rectal absorption is much faster, at 15 to 60 minutes. It is recommended that bisacodyl be taken with food, milk, or antacids to avoid gastric irritation. One Senokot S® can counter the constipation caused by 120 mg of codeine.[5] Senna is available in a liquid form called X-Prep Liquid. This is used for bowel cleansing before radiology procedures; 72 mL of X-Prep is equivalent to 10 Senokot tablets. Cascara, another anthraquinone, is commonly combined with milk of magnesia to make a mixture referred to as "Black and White." This is a mild combination that reduces colic pain. Casanthranol is derived from cascara and is used as the stimulant component in Peri-Colace.

Recommendations for use are senna 15-mg tablets used alone or as Senokot S. Starting dose is two tablets daily (see Table 12–2). These stimulating laxatives are the most effective management for opioid-related constipation. Bisacodyl comes in 10-mg tablets or suppositories and is used daily. The suppository medication has a faster onset that is much appreciated in the uncomfortable, constipated patient. Onset of action can be within 12 hours.[7]

---

**MILK and MOLASSES ENEMA RECIPE**

8 oz. warm water
3 oz. powdered milk
4.5 oz. molasses

- Put water and powdered milk in a plastic jar. Close the jar and shake until the water and milk appear to be fully mixed.
- Add molasses, and shake the jar again until the mixture appears to have an even color throughout.
- Pour mixture into enema bag. Administer enema high by gently introducing tube about 12 inches. Do not push beyond resistance. Repeat every 6 hours until good results are achieved.

---

**Figure 12–2.** Milk and molasses enema recipe. *Sources*: Bisanz (2005), reference 11; Lowell (2003), reference 38.

*Suppository Medications.* As discussed above, bisacodyl (Dulcolax) comes in a suppository. Although the thought of rectal medications is unpleasant for many patients, suppositories' quick onset of action makes them more acceptable. Bisacodyl comes in 10 mg for adults and 5 mg as a pediatric dose. Suppositories should never be used in patients with severely reduced white cell or platelet counts due to the risk of bleeding or infection.

Liquid rectal laxatives or lubricants should be used infrequently. In severely constipated patients, they may be necessary. Most commonly, saline enemas are used to loosen the stool and to stimulate rectal or distal colon peristalsis. Repeated use can cause hypocalcemia and hyperphosphatemia, so it is important to use enemas cautiously. Enemas should never be considered part of a standing bowel regimen. Onset of action can be within 30 minutes.

Oil retention enemas, however, are particularly helpful for severely constipated patients, for whom disimpaction may be necessary. They work best when used overnight, to allow softening. Overnight retention is effective only if the patient is able to retain it that long. The general rule is that the longer the enema is retained, the better the results. Bisanz[11] recommends a milk-and-molasses enema (Figure 12–2) for patients with low impaction to ease stool evacuation in a non-irritating way. It is a low-volume enema of 300 mL and therefore thought to cause less cramping.

Combining an enema with an oral saline-type cathartic (Lactulose, Cephylac) is helpful when a large amount of stool is present.[5,11] This may help to push the stool through the GI tract.

If disimpaction is necessary, remember that it can be extremely painful; therefore, premedicate the patient with either opioid and/or benzodiazepine anxiolytics to reduce physical and emotional pain.[4,6,14] There are few studies outlining the efficacy of one enema over another. The reported success rates for rectal enemas within 1 hour includes phosphate enemas (100%), mini-enemas (Micralax) (95%), bisacodyl suppositories (66%), and glycerine suppositories (38%).[25] If none of the above enemas is effective, Sykes[21] recommends rectal lavage with approximately 8 liters of warmed normal saline. It is important to remember that if a patient's constipation requires this invasive intervention, you must change the usual bowel regimen once this bowel crisis is resolved. For severe constipation associated with opioids, Levy[5] suggests four Senokot S and three Dulcolax tablets three times a day and 60 mL of lactulose every other night for a goal of a bowel movement every other day (see Table 12–2).

### New Approaches to Constipation Management

Oral naloxone has been studied for the treatment of opioid-related constipation resistant to other treatments. Culpepper-Morgan and colleagues[26] found that the majority of opioid effect on the human intestine is mediated peripherally rather than centrally at the level of the GI tract itself.[3,24,25] Naloxone, which is an opioid antagonist, has less than 1% availability systemically when given orally, due to the first-pass effect in the liver. Oral naloxone has shown some relief of constipation, but dosing varies among patients. Sykes used 20% of the daily morphine dose but found that patients did develop some decreased analgesia. Liu and Wittbrodt did a very small study and even with the some improvement in their bowel frequency some had a reversal in analgesia.[21,27] Using naloxone in the outpatient setting is not recommended because of the increased risk of withdrawal or dose-benefit behavior.[25] The starting dose should be no more than 5 mg.[21] It was suggested that oral naloxone doses of greater than 12 mg should be used with caution.

The newest opioid antagonist is Methylnaltrexone (Relistor®). It is administered subcutaneously and is indicated for the treatment of opioid-induced constipation in patients with advanced illness. Results occurred within 4 hours and, unlike oral naloxone, it crosses the blood-brain barrier less readily so therefore is less likely to reverse centrally-mediated analgesia.[27,28]

Oral erythromycin has been shown to cause diarrhea in 50% of patients who use it as an antibiotic.[6] Currently, researchers are investigating its use to promote diarrhea. There is also interest in identifying a medication that would increase colon transit time without being antibacterial.

Many herbal medicines have laxative properties, such as mulberry and constituents of rhubarb, which are similar to senna. These herbs are being evaluated for use as laxatives. Patients have been known to develop rashes; in one patient, changes were found in warfarin (Coumadin) levels that were related to natural warfarin found in a laxative tea. Many patients prefer these options instead of pharmaceutical laxatives, but they should be cautious about where they purchase any herbal product and be alert to any unexplained side effects, as their content is unregulated.

### Nursing Interventions for Constipation

Nurses should always be proactive in initiating laxative therapy. Bowel function requires continued evaluation to follow the trajectory of the disease and the changes that occur in normal activities that affect bowel function. Nurses should also be alert to medications that can increase the risk of constipation (see Table 12–1). Some patients, especially those on long-term opioid therapy, sometimes need at least two different regimens that can be interchanged when one or the other loses its effectiveness for a time. Like opioids, over time, a standing laxative regimen may be less effective if tolerance develops.[5,6] It is also important to be aware of medication dosing changes, as it is common to forget to increase anticonstipation therapy when there is an increase in opioid therapy. Patients generally have increased risk of constipation when opioids are increased. Positioning patients to allow gravity to assist with bowel movements is helpful. Assisting with oral fluid intake, as well as dietary interventions are both helpful. Discuss patients' management needs as well as personal cultural perspectives and factors that may contribute to good bowel hygiene. Exercise within each patient's tolerance is recommended to aid in elimination. Fatigue, advanced disease, and decreased endurance all play a role in obstructing good bowel maintenance. The importance of effective bowel management cannot be stressed enough. It remains one of the most distressing symptom in end-stage cancer patients.

## DIARRHEA

Diarrhea has been a major symptom and significant problem associated with newer chemotherapeutic and biological and radiation treatment regimens.[20,24,29] It is a main symptom of 7% to 10% of hospice admissions.[29,30] Overgrowth of GI infections such as Candida can cause diarrhea as well.[6] Treating diarrhea requires a thorough assessment and therapy directed at the specific cause. Diarrhea is usually acute and short-lived, lasting only a few days, as opposed to chronic diarrhea, which lasts 3 weeks or more.[29] Diarrhea can be especially severe in human immunodeficiency virus (HIV)-infected patients.[6,30,31] Diarrhea of 500 mL/day or greater occurs in 35%–50% of bone marrow transplant patients related to radiation or graft versus host disease (GVHD).[29] Similar to constipation, this symptom can be debilitating and can severely affect quality of life.[24,28] Diarrhea can prevent patients from leaving their homes, increase weakness and dehydration, and contribute to feelings of lack of control and depression. Nurses play a significant role in recognizing, educating, and managing diarrhea and its manifestations.

### Definitions

Diarrhea is described as an increase in stool volume and liquidity resulting in three or more bowel movements per day.[6,29] Secondary effects related to diarrhea include abdominal cramps, anxiety, lethargy, weakness, dehydration, dizziness, loss of electrolytes, skin breakdown and associated pain, dry mouth, and weight loss. Diarrhea varies among patients depending on their bowel history. Acute diarrhea occurs within 24 to 48 hours of exposure to the cause and resolves in 7 to 14 days. Chronic diarrhea usually has a late onset and lasts 2 to 3 weeks, with an unidentified cause.

### Prevalence and Impact

Cancer patients may have multiple causes of diarrhea. It may be due to infections or related to tumor type or its treatment. A common cause of diarrhea is overuse of laxative therapy or dietary fiber. Additional causes include malabsorption disorders, motility disturbances, stress, partial bowel obstruction, enterocolic fistula, villous adenoma, endocrine-induced hypersecretion of serotonin, gastrin calcitonin, and vasoactive intestinal protein prostaglandins.[5,29] Treatment-related causes include radiation and chemotherapy, which cause overgrowth of bacteria, with endotoxin production that has a direct effect on the intestinal mucosa. Local inflammation and increased fluid and electrolyte secretion occur, resulting in interference with amino acid and electrolyte transport and a shift toward secretion by crypt cells with shortened villi.[29]

Diarrhea associated with radiation can occur by the 2nd or 3rd week of treatment and can continue after radiation has been discontinued.[6,32] Radiation-induced diarrhea is related to focus of radiation and total of radiation dose. Pelvic radiation alone has been shown to cause diarrhea of any grade in up to 70% of the patients receiving it. A grade 3 or 4 diarrhea is associated with approximately 20% of those patients.[29] The risk is increased in acquired immunodeficiency syndrome (AIDS), GVHD, or HIV patients. The end result could be a change in the intestinal mucosa that results in a limited ability to regenerate epithelium, which can lead to bleeding and ileus. The damaged mucosa leads to increased release of prostaglandins and malabsorption of bile salts, increasing peristaltic activity.[30–32]

Surgical patients who have had bowel-shortening procedures or gastrectomy related to cancer experience a "dumping syndrome," which causes severe diarrhea. This type of diarrhea is related to both osmotic and hypermotile mechanisms.[5,6] Patients may experience weakness, epigastric distention, and diarrhea shortly after eating.[33] The shortened bowel can result in a decreased absorption capacity and an imbalance in absorptive and secretory function of the intestine.

### Pathophysiology

Diarrhea can be grouped into four types, each with a different mechanism: osmotic diarrhea, secretory diarrhea, hypermotile diarrhea, and exudative diarrhea. Cancer patients rarely exhibit only one type. Understanding the mechanism of diarrhea permits more rational treatment strategies.[6,29,30,33]

*Osmotic Diarrhea.* Osmotic diarrhea is produced by intake of hyperosmolar preparations or nonabsorbable solutions such as enteral feeding solutions.[6,29] Enterocolic fistula can lead to both osmotic diarrhea from undigested food entering the colon and hypermotile diarrhea. Hemorrhage into the intestine can

**Table 12–3**
**National Cancer Institute Scale of Severity of Diarrhea**

| | National Cancer Institute Grade | | | | |
|---|---|---|---|---|---|
| | 0 | 1 | 2 | 3 | 4 |
| Increased number of loose stools/day | Normal | 2–3 | 4–6 | 7–9 | >10 |
| Symptoms | | None | Nocturnal stools and/or moderate cramping | Incontinence and/or severe cramping | Grossly bloody diarrhea and/or need for parenteral support |

cause an osmotic-type diarrhea because intraluminal blood acts as an osmotic laxative. Osmotic diarrhea may result from insufficient lactase when dairy products are consumed.

*Secretory Diarrhea.* Secretory diarrhea is most associated with chemotherapy and radiation therapy. The cause is related to mechanical damage to the epithelial crypt cells in the GI tract.[32] The necrosis that results, along with the inflammation and ulceration of the intestinal mucosa, leads to further damage related to exposure to bile and susceptibility to opportunistic infections, atrophy of the mucosal lining, and fibrosis. This all contributes to loss of absorption due to damaged villi, causing an increase in water, electrolytes, mucus, blood, and serum to be pulled into the intestine from immature crypt cells, and increased fluid secretion, resulting in diarrhea.[20,33–35]

Secretory diarrhea is the most difficult to control. Malignant epithelial tumors producing hormones that can cause diarrhea include metastatic carcinoid tumors, gastrinoma, and medullary thyroid cancer. The primary effect of secretory diarrhea is related to the hypersecretion stimulated by endogenous mediators that affect the intestinal transport of water and electrolytes. This results in accumulation of intestinal fluids.[20,29,30,31] Diarrhea associated with GVHD results from mucosal damage and can produce up to 6 to 8 liters of diarrhea in 24 hours.[32] Surgical shortening of the bowel, which reduces intestinal mucosal contact and shortens colon transit time, causing decreased reabsorption, leads to diarrhea. Active treatment requires vigorous fluid and electrolyte repletion, antidiarrheal therapy, and specific anticancer therapy.[5,20] Preventing diarrhea associated with chemotherapy and radiation is not always realistic, but being proactive in anticipating diarrhea and prompt management may be effective.[5,30,33] Initiation of medication with the first episode is suggested. The recommendation starts with loperamide 4 mg, then 2 to 4 mg every 2 to 4 hours (max 16 mg/24 h). If there is no response at 24 to 48 hours, then, based on grade, either increase the loperamide dose, then reevaluate in 24 hours, or start octreotide 100 to 500 mcg subcutaneously, three times a day for grades 3 to 4 diarrhea.[20] The somatostatin analogue octreotide is used for grades 3 to 4 diarrhea with success. One study in patients experiencing chemotherapy-induced diarrhea unresponsive to loperamide had a 92% response to octreotide SC 500 mcg three times daily.[36] The use of sustained release octreotide (LAR) for the treatment of diarrheal

syndromes, as well as treatment of malignant bowel obstruction related nausea, vomiting and pain has shown benefit.[36] The goal is to prevent high-grade diarrhea that results in dose reduction or cessation of chemotherapy regimens.[37] Cost is a major issue with this medication; dosing for only 3–7 days at $50–$250.00/day could run close to $1800.00.[10,20,38] However, along with preventing dose reduction of chemotherapy, the potential to reduce the number of episodes of diarrhea and minimize the additional effects on psychosocial issues and quality of life may make this approach worthwhile.

*Hypermotile Diarrhea.* Partial bowel obstruction from abdominal malignancies can cause a reflex hypermotility that may require bowel-quieting medications such as loperamide.[33] Enterocolic fistula can lead to diarrhea from irritative hypermotility and osmotic influence of undigested food entering the colon. Biliary or pancreatic obstruction can cause incomplete digestion of fat in the small intestine, resulting in interference with fat and bile salt malabsorption, leading to hypermotile diarrhea, also called steatorrhea. Malabsorption is related to pancreatic cancer, gastrectomy, ileal resection or colectomy, rectal cancer, pancreatic islet cell tumors, or carcinoid tumors. Chemotherapy-induced diarrhea is frequently seen with 5-fluorouracil or N-phosphonoacetyl-L-aspartate. High-dose cisplatin and irinotecan (Camptosar) cause severe hypermotility. Other chemotherapy drugs that cause diarrhea include cytosine arabinoside, nitrosourea, methotrexate, cyclophosphamide, doxorubicin, daunorubicin, hydroxyurea and biotherapy-2, interferon and topoisomerase inhibitors (capecitabine [5-FU prodrug]), oxaliplatin.[20,29]

*Exudative Diarrhea.* Radiation therapy of the abdomen, pelvis, or lower thoracic or lumbar spine can cause acute exudative diarrhea.[29] The inflammation caused by radiation leads to the release of prostaglandins. Treatment using aspirin or ibuprofen was shown to reduce prostaglandin release and decrease diarrhea associated with radiation therapy.[29] Bismuth subsalicylate (Pepto-Bismol) is also helpful for diarrhea caused by radiotherapy.[11]

According to Sykes,[6] there are multiple causes of diarrhea in palliative medicine. Concurrent diseases such as diabetes mellitus, hyperthyroidism, inflammatory bowel disease, irritable bowel syndrome, and GI infection (C. difficile) can contribute to the development of diarrhea. Finally, the dietary influences of fruit, bran, hot spices, and alcohol, as well as over-the-counter medications, laxatives, and herbal supplements, need to be considered as sources of diarrhea.[6,29]

## Assessment of Diarrhea

Diarrhea assessment requires a careful history to detail the frequency and nature of the stools. The National Cancer Institute Scale of Severity of Diarrhea uses a grading system from 0 to 4. Stools are rated by (1) number of loose stools per day and (2) symptoms (Table 12–3). This scale permits an objective score to define the severity of diarrhea.

The initial goal of assessment is to identify and treat any reversible causes of diarrhea. If diarrhea occurs once or twice a day, it is probably related to anal incontinence. Large amounts of watery stools are characteristic of colonic diarrhea. Pale, fatty, malodorous stools, called steatorrhea, are indicative of malabsorption secondary to pancreatic or small-intestinal causes. If a patient who has been constipated complains of sudden diarrhea with little warning, fecal impaction with overflow is the probable cause.[6,29]

Evaluate medications that the patient may be taking now or in the recent past. Is the patient on laxatives? If the stools are associated with cramping and urgency, it may be the result of peristalsis-stimulating laxatives. If stools are associated with fecal leakage, it may be the result of overuse of stool-softening agents such as Colace.[6,29] Depending on the aggressiveness of the treatment plan, additional assessment could include stool smears for pus, blood, fat, ova, or parasites. Stool samples for culture and sensitivity testing may be necessary to rule out additional sources of diarrhea through C. difficile toxin, Giardia lamblia, or other types of GI infection.[5] If patients have diarrhea after 2 to 3 days of fasting, secretory diarrhea should be evaluated. Osmotic and secretory causes are considered first; if ruled out, then hypermotility is the suspected mechanism.

## Management of Diarrhea

A combination of supportive care and medication may be appropriate for palliative management of diarrhea. The goal of diarrhea management should focus on minimizing or eliminating the factors causing the diarrhea, providing dietary interventions, and maintaining fluid and electrolyte balance as appropriate. Quality-of-life issues include minimizing skin breakdown or infections, relieving pain associated with frequent diarrhea, and maintaining the patient's dignity.[20,29]

If the patient is dehydrated, oral fluids are recommended over the IV route.[9,20] Oral fluids should contain electrolytes and a source of glucose to facilitate active electrolyte transport (Figure 12–3). Foods to be avoided in patients experiencing acute diarrhea include: spicey food, high-fat and fried foods, gas causing foods, alcohol and caffeine foods or high-sorbitol

| ADULT HOMEMADE ELECTROLYTE REPLACEMENT SOLUTION | |
|---|---|
| 1 tsp salt | 6 oz. frozen orange juice concentrate |
| 1 tsp baking soda | 6 cups water |
| 1 tsp corn syrup | 47 kcal/cup, 515 mg Na$^+$, 164 mg K$^+$ |

Following diarrhea, the diet should start with clear liquids, flat lemonade, ginger ale, and toast or simple carbohydrates. It is recommended that the patient avoid milk if diarrhea is related to infection due to acute lactase deficiency. Protein and fats can be added to the diet slowly as diarrhea resolves. Dietary management may help minimize amount of diarrhea.

**Figure 12–3.** Homemade electrolyte replacement solution for adults. *Source*: Weihofen & Marino (1998), reference 34.

juices. Milk and dairy products for some patients should be avoided as well.[20]

## Medication Recommendations

There are many nonspecific diarrhea medications that should be used unless infections are suspected as the cause. If *Shigella* or *C. difficile* are responsible, nonspecific antidiarrheal medications can make the diarrhea worse.[6] Loperamide (Imodium) has become the drug of choice for the treatment of nonspecific diarrhea. It is a long acting opioid agonist.[20] The 2-mg dose has the same antidiarrheal action as 5 mg, two tablets of diphenoxylate, or 45 mg of codeine.[4] The usual management of diarrhea begins with 4 mg of loperamide, with one capsule following each loose bowel movement. Most diarrhea is managed by loperamide 2 to 4 mg once to twice a day.[5,20] Diphenoxylate (Lomotil 2.5 mg with atropine 0.025 mg) is given as one or two tablets orally as needed for loose stools, maximum of eight/day. Diphenoxylate is derived from meperidine and binds to opioid receptors to reduce diarrhea. Atropine was added to this antidiarrheal to prevent abuse.[5] Diphenoxylate is not recommended for patients with advanced liver disease because it may precipitate hepatic coma in patients with cirrhosis.[5,20] Neither diphenoxylate nor loperamide is recommended for use in children under 12 years old.[5] Codeine as an opioid for the reduction of diarrhea can be helpful. It is also less expensive than some opioid medications. Most cancer-related diarrheas respond well to this drug. For specific mechanisms, other medications might be more beneficial. Tincture of opium works to decrease peristalsis, given at 0.6 mL every 4 to 6 hours. This is a controlled substance but may also provide some pain relief.[20] Absorbent agents such as pectin and methylcellulose may help provide bulk to increase consistency of the stools.[20]

Anticholinergic drugs such as atropine and scopolamine are useful to reduce gastric secretions and decrease peristalsis. Somatostatin analogues such as octreotide (Sandostatin) are also effective for secretory diarrhea that may result from endocrine tumors, AIDS, GVHD, or post-GI resection.[5,6,20,33]

They may be helpful for patients who experience painful cramping.[5] Side effects of that class of drug can complicate their use: dry mouth, blurred vision, and urinary hesitancy.

Mucosal antiprostaglandin agents such as aspirin, indomethacin, and bismuth subsalicylate (Pepto-Bismol) are useful for diarrhea related to enterotoxic bacteria, radiotherapy, and prostaglandin-secreting tumors. Octreotide (Sandostatin) is effective for patients with AIDS, GVHD, diabetes, or GI resection.[6,30,39] Octreotide is administered subcutaneously at a dose of 50 to 200 mcg two or three times per day. Ranitidine is a useful adjuvant to octreotide for patients with Zollinger-Ellison syndrome with gastrin-induced gastric hypersecretion.[5] Side effects include nausea and pain at injection site. Patients may also experience abdominal or headache pain.[5] Clonidine is effective at controlling watery diarrhea in patients with bronchogenic cancer. Clonidine effects an $\alpha_2$-adrenergic stimulation of electrolyte absorption in the small intestine.[5] Streptozocin is used for watery diarrhea from pancreatic islet cell cancer because it decreases intestinal secretions. Hypermotile diarrhea involves problems with fat absorption. The recommended treatment is pancreatin before meals. Pancreatin is a combination of amylase, lipase, and protease that is available for pancreatic enzyme replacement. Lactaid may also be helpful for malabsorption-related diarrhea.

## Nursing Interventions for Diarrhea

Nursing interventions should include nonpharmacological interventions focused on diet and psychosocial support (Tables 12–4 and 12–5).

---

**Table 12–4**
**Nutritional Management of Cancer-Related Diarrhea: Foods and Medication to Avoid**

**Medications**
Antibiotics, bulk laxatives (Metamucil, methylcellulose), magnesium-containing medications (Maalox, Mylanta), promotility agents (propulsid, metoclopramide), stool softeners/laxatives (Peri-Colace, Dulcolax), herbal supplements (milk thistle, aloe, cayenne, saw palmetto, Siberian ginseng).

**Foods**
Milk and diary products (cheese, yogurt, ice cream), caffeine- containing products (coffee, tea, cola drinks, chocolate), carbonated and high-sugar or high-sorbitol juices (prune pear, sweet cherry, peach, apple, orange juice), high-fiber/gas-causing legumes (raw vegetables, whole grain products, dried legumes, popcorn), high-fat foods (fried foods, high-fat spreads, or dressings), heavily spiced foods that taste "hot".

High risk foods—sushi, street vendors, buffets.

*Sources:* Adapted from Stern & lppoliti (2003), reference 20; Engelking (2004), reference 30.

---

- Evaluate medications currently being used to identify polypharmacy, where multiple medication side effects may be contributing to the problem.
- Minimize or prevent diarrhea accidents in an effort to reduce patient anxiety. Anticipate obstacles between the patient and the bathroom. Assist with access plans and timing needs. Recommend commode chair at bedside to allow easiest access and prevent falls or additional problems.
- Protecting the bed with Chux can be better accepted than diapers. It may also be better for skin integrity but requires multiple layers of Chux and drawsheets for best results.
- Applying skin ointment protection after cleaning and drying the area is also important. Thick protectant creams that apply a barrier on the skin are most beneficial. Eucerin cream, zinc oxide, and bag balm are three that have been used anecdotally with success.
- The psychosocial impact of diapers can be devastating for some patients. Encourage a discussion with patient and family about patient needs, fears, and perceptions.
- Along with focus on diet/medications, skin integrity, and psychosocial needs, odor management must also be addressed. Perfumed air fresheners sometimes only make it worse. Concentrate on being sure the perineum or periostomy area is clean and the linens are not soiled. Also be sure that dirty linens or trash are removed from the room. Using aromatherapy such as lavender may be soothing.
- Remember that there may be times when adult diapers are essential and can help alleviate distress to the patient; for example, when traveling or on necessary outings. Remind families to check them frequently to prevent skin breakdown and, again, be sure there is skin barrier ointment applied before the diaper padding.

## Conclusion

Managing diarrhea in the cancer patient is challenging at best. The nurse's role in helping the patient and caregivers talk about this difficult symptom is essential. It is important to respect comfort levels about the topic among nurse, patient, and caregiver to allow information sharing. Goals of diarrhea therapy should be to restore an optimal pattern of elimination, maintain fluid and electrolyte balance as desired, preserve nutritional status, protect skin integrity, and ensure the patient's comfort and dignity.[11,20]

## MALIGNANT OBSTRUCTION

As primary tumors grow in the large intestine, they can lead to obstruction. Obstruction is related to the site and stage of

**Table 12–5**
**Nursing Role in the Management of Diarrhea**

**Environmental assessment**
- Assess the patient's and/or caregiver's ability to manage the level of care necessary.
- Evaluate home for medical equipment that may be helpful (bedpan or commode chair).

**History**
- Frequency of bowel movements in last 2 wks.
- Fluid intake (normal 2 quarts/day).
- Fiber intake (normal 30–40 g/day).
- Appetite and whether patient is nauseated or vomiting. Does diet include spicy foods?
- Assess for current medications the patient has taken that are associated with causing diarrhea (laxative use, chemotherapy, antibiotics, enteral nutritional supplements, nonsteroidal antiinflammatory drugs).
- Surgical history that may contribute to diarrhea (gastrectomy, pancreatectomy, bypass or ileal resection).
- Recent radiotherapy to abdomen, pelvis, lower spine.
- Cancer diagnosis associated with diarrhea includes abdominal malignancies, partial bowel obstruction; enterocolic fistulae; metastatic carcinoid tumors; gastrinomas; medullary thyroid cancer.
- Immunosuppressed, susceptible to bacterial, protozoan, and viral diseases associated with diarrhea.
- Concurrent diseases associated with diarrhea: gastroenteritis, inflammatory bowel disease, irritable bowel syndrome, diabetes mellitus, lactose deficiency, hyperthyroidism.

**Physical assessment**
- Examine perineum or ostomy site for skin breakdown, fissures, or external hemorrhoids.
- Gentle digital rectal examination for impaction.
- Abdominal examination for distention of palpable stool in large bowel.
- Examine stools for signs of bleeding.
- Evaluate for signs of dehydration.

**Interventions**
- Treatment should be related to cause (i.e., if obstruction is cause of diarrhea, giving antidiarrheal medications would be inappropriate).
- Assist with correcting any obvious factors related to assessment (e.g., decreasing nutritional supplements, changing fiber intake, holding or substituting medications associated with diarrhea).
- If bacterial causes are suspected, notify physician and culture stools as instructed. *Clostridium difficile* is most common.
- Educate patient and family on importance of cleansing the perineum gently after each stool, to prevent skin breakdown. If patient has a colostomy, stomal area must also be watched closely and surrounding skin protected. Use skin barrier such as Desitin ointment to protect the skin. Frequent sitz baths may be helpful.
- Instruct patient and family on signs and symptoms that should be reported to the nurse or physician: excessive thirst, dizziness, fever, palpitations, rectal spasms, excessive cramping, water or bloody stools.

**Dietary measures**
- Eat small, frequent, bland meals.
- Low-residue diet—potassium-rich (bananas, rice, peeled apples, dry toast).
- Avoid intake of hyperosmotic supplements (e.g., Ensure, Sustacal).
- Increase fluids in diet. Approximately 3 liters of fluid a day if possible. Drinking electrolyte fluids such as Pedialyte may be helpful.
- Homeopathic treatments for diarrhea include: ginger tea, glutamine, and peeled apples.

**Pharmacologic management**
- Opioids—codeine, paregoric, dihenoxylate, loperamide, tincture of opium.
- Absorbents—pectin, aluminum hydroxide.
- Adsorbents—charcoal, kaolin.
- Antisecretory—aspirin, bismuth subsalicylate, prednisone, Sandostatin, ranitidine hydrochloride, indomethacin.
- Anticholinergics—scopolamine, atropine sulfate, belladonna.
- $\alpha_2$-Adrenergic agonists—clonidine.
Report to nurse or physician if antidiarrheal medication seems ineffective.

**Psychosocial interventions**
Provide support to patient and family. Recognize negative effects of diarrhea on quality of life:
- Fatigue.
- Malnutrition.
- Alteration in skin integrity.
- Pain and discomfort.
- Sleep disturbances.
- Limited ability to travel.
- Compromised role within the family.
- Decreased sexual activity.
- Caregiver burden.

*Sources:* Levy (1991), reference 5; Bisanz (2005), reference 11; Viele (2003), reference 29.

disease.[35,40,41] Tumors in the splenic flexure obstruct 49% of the time, but those in the rectum or rectosigmoid junction only 6% of the time.[40,41] Obstruction can occur intraluminally related to primary tumors of the colon. Intramural obstruction is related to tumor in the muscular layers of the bowel wall. The bowel appears thickened, indurated, and contracted.[6,42] Extramural obstruction is related to mesenteric and omental masses and malignant adhesions. The common metastatic pattern, in relation to primary disease in the pancreas, ovaries or stomach, generally goes to the duodenum, from the colon to the jejunum and ileum, and from the prostate or bladder to the rectum.[6,41,42] Bowel obstruction in cancer patients is not always due to their tumors. Hernias, radiation induced strictures, or adhesions may be the cause, so it is important that patients with obstructive symptoms be thoroughly evaluated to rule out a correctable cause.[6,41,42]

## Definition

Experts agree there is no standard definition for Malignant Bowel Obstruction (MBO)—it means different things to different physicians.[43,44] A current definition uses the criteria that there is "clinical evidence of bowel obstruction, obstruction beyond the ligament of Treitz (in the setting of intra-abdominal cancer with incurable disease), or non-intra-abdominal primary cancer with clear intraperitoneal disease."[45] The significance of an agreed upon definition is the ability to evaluate treatment plans for evidence-based recommendations.[43]

Clinical evidence of intestinal obstruction is occlusion of the lumen or absence of the normal propulsion that affects elimination from the GI tract.[38,40] Motility disruption, either impaired or absent, leads to a mechanical obstruction but without occlusion of the intestinal lumen. Mechanical obstruction results in the accumulation of fluids and gas proximal to the obstruction. Distention occurs as a result of intestinal gas, ingested fluids, and digestive secretions. It becomes a self-perpetuating phenomenon as when distention increases, intestinal secretion of water and electrolytes increases. A small-bowel obstruction causes large amounts of diarrhea. The increased fluid in the bowel leads to increased peristalsis, with large quantities of bacteria growing in the intestinal fluid of the small bowel.[38,40]

Obstruction is related to the surrounding mesentery or bowel muscle, such as in ovarian cancer. Additional factors include multiple sites of obstruction along the intestine and constipating medications (Table 12–6), fecal impaction, fibrosis, or change in normal flora of the bowel. The goal of treatment is to prevent obstruction from happening whenever possible.

## Prevalance and Impact

The best treatment options for bowel obstruction in a patient with advanced cancer remain undetermined.[43] Managing MBO is dependant on level of obstruction, disease status related to prognosis, prior treatments, as well as the patient's current health status.[41,42] As obstruction increases, bacteria levels increase and can lead to sepsis and associated multi-system failure and death.[40] The difficulty is knowing which patients will truly benefit from surgical intervention. The impact of obstruction on the patient and family is overwhelming. The patient and caregivers have been aggressively trying to manage the patient's constipation in an effort to prevent this very problem. Obstruction for patients means failure to manage constipation or a sign of growing disease. New interventions have been developed in an effort to provide additional noninvasive approaches for the management of bowel obstruction.[36,43,46]

Bowel obstruction can occur in between 5%–43% of patients with advanced disease. Intestinal obstruction related to benign causes in patients with a previous malignancy can be significant: 3%-48%. No specific guidelines for the management of malignant bowel obstructions (MBO) are defined.[41,43,44] Each case must be evaluated individually with care decisions based on goal of treatment. Unfortunately, studies also differ in agreeing on a successful outcome. Defining success may be evaluated based on ability to resume oral intake, on relief of pain, nausea or vomiting, extended survival or improvement in quality of life.[41,43,44] Further research needs to be done[42,47] to evaluate the effects of surgical intervention on quality as well as quantity of life. The effect of unrelieved intestinal obstruction on quality of life for the patient and loved ones is devastating.

## Assessment and Management of Malignant Obstruction

Patients may experience severe nausea, vomiting, and abdominal pain associated with a partial or complete bowel obstruction. In the elderly patient, fecal impaction may also cause urinary incontinence.[6] General signs and symptoms associated with different sites of obstruction are listed in Table 12–6.

**Table 12–6**
**Sites of Intestinal Obstruction and Related Side Effects**

| Site | Side Effects |
|---|---|
| Duodenum | Severe vomiting with large amounts of undigested food. Bowel sounds: succussion splash may be present. No pain or distention noted. |
| Small intestine | Moderate to severe vomiting; usually hyperactive bowel sounds with borborygmi; pain in upper and central abdomen, colic in nature; moderate distention. |
| Large intestine | Vomiting is a late side effect. Borborygmi bowel sounds, severe distention. Pain central to lower abdomen, colic in nature. |

*Source:* Ripamonte & Mercadante (2004), reference 25.

Providing thoughtful and supportive interventions may be more appropriate than aggressive, invasive procedures. The signs and symptoms of obstruction may be acute, with nausea, vomiting, and abdominal pain. A majority of the time, however, obstruction is a slow and insidious phenomenon, which may progress from partial to complete obstruction. Palliative care should allow for a thoughtful and realistic approach to management of obstruction within the goals of care. Radiological examination should be limited unless surgery is being considered Treatment options start with a non-surgical approach and emergent surgical intervention is usually not necessary unless the risk of perforation is eminent. Patients who would benefit from surgical intervention for MBO are evaluated based on age, tumor status, presence of ascites, nutritional status, previous chemotherapy or radiation treatments.[40,41,43,47] A surgical intervention would most likely not benefit a patient if they have ascites, multiple bowel obstructions, carcinomatosis or poor overall clinical status.[41]

## Surgical Intervention

A percentage of cancer patients may experience nonmalignant obstruction.[42] Therefore, assuming the obstruction is related to worsening cancer may prevent the health care team from setting realistic treatment goals. A thorough assessment should be done, with attention to poor prognostic factors.[6,38,41] These factors historically include general medical condition or poor nutritional status, ascites, palpable abdominal masses or distant metastases, previous radiation to the abdomen or pelvis, combination chemotherapy, and multiple small-bowel obstructions.[41,42]

Helyer and Easson[42] organize criteria for surgical interventions as, firstly, patient factors including advanced age, nutritional status, performance status, comorbidities and anti-cancer treatment history, psychological health and social support. Secondly, factors including disease-related etiology, tumor grade and tumor extent. Finally, operative factors. Will the procedure relieve symptoms for an extended amount of time with reasonable operative morbidity? The bottom line becomes balancing the risks and benefits of the surgery in contrast to nonsurgical options and the patient's goals of care. The use of laparoscopic surgical techniques have brought about changes in the use of open surgical techniques in the palliative care patient.

Surgical intervention should be a decision made between patient and physician within the established goals of care. The patient's right to self-determination is essential. As patient advocates, the nurse's role is to educate the patient and family. Helping them to understand physician recommendations, as well as considering their personal desires and options in an effort to develop the treatment plan, is essential. Surgical resection for obstructing cancers of the GI tract, pancreas, or biliary tracts were found to have a 3- to 7-month survival.[33] This study pointed out the importance of nutritional status at baseline and assessment of performance status for its relationship to "reasonable quality of life."[33] The important

conclusion of these studies was to leave the decision to operate with an informed patient. Mortality is possible. The need for additional surgeries remains high due to recurrence of the obstruction, wound infections, sepsis and further obstruction.[25] Survival rates with each subsequent surgery lessen.

New options for management of MBO have developed as laporoscopy has become more frequent and experienced providers are more available. The improvements in X-ray technologies have also improved the diagnosis of the cause of the MBO to help choose more appropriate interventions4especially in light of the high morbidity and mortality associated with surgery in this population.[40–42,46,48–51]

## Radiological Examination

Bowel obstruction may be diagnosed on the basis of a plain abdominal x-ray, but contrast may help identify the site and extent of the obstruction. CT exams have shown an accuracy of 94% in determining the cause of a bowel obstruction. The use of either CT or MRI to help develop a treatment plan for MBO has improved decision-making between a surgical or medical management approach.[42] Barium is not recommended because it may interfere with additional studies.[43]

## Alternative Interventions

Nasogastric or nasointestinal tubes have been used to decompress the bowel and/or stomach. Use of these interventions, although uncomfortable for the patient, has been suggested for symptom relief while evaluating the possibility of surgery. Venting gastrostomy or jejunostomy can be a relatively easy alternative, which is especially effective for severe nausea and vomiting. It can be placed percutaneously with sedation and local anesthesia. Patients can then be fed a liquid diet, with the tube clamped for as long as tolerated without nausea or vomiting.[43]

## Endoscopic Palliation

Laparoscopic surgical techniques have brought about new options for inoperable cancers. Gastroenterologists or interventional radiologists now have an increased role in palliating obstructions.[46] The use of enteral self-expandable metal stents (SEMS) are a permanent intervention that is performed through endoscopy to improve luminal patency and allow oral intake without surgery. The use of self-expanding metallic stents has been highly effective for MBO and, in some cases, has prevented the need for colostomy.[42,46] It is done in interventional radiology and requires close clinical observation, since perforation is a potential complication. At the minimum, it has allowed emergent relief of obstruction for surgical intervention in the future. Putting a patient through an x-ray of the abdomen may be helpful to confirm the obstruction and identify where it is, but defining the goal of therapy is essential.[42] When patients exhibit signs of obstruction, a physical exam may be helpful to assess the extent of the problem. Asking the patient for a bowel history, last bowel movement, and a description of consistency can be helpful. Does the patient complain of constipation? Physical examination should include gentle palpation of the abdomen for masses or distention. A careful rectal exam can identify the presence of stool in the rectum or a distended empty rectum. An empty, or "ballooned," rectum may be a symptom of high obstruction. It is also difficult to distinguish stool from malignant mass.[11,43] The ability to assess whether an impaction is low or high in the intestinal tract is important to help guide the intervention planning. As discussed above, lack of stool noted in the rectum during a digital exam is usually indicative of a high impaction. Stool has not or cannot move down into the rectum. The goal then would be to use careful assessment to be sure the obstruction is not a tumor and to concentrate on softening the stool and moving it through the GI tract. Again, using a stimulant laxative for this type of patient would result in increasing discomfort and possible rupture of the intestinal wall.[11,40] Low impactions are uncomfortable, and patients may need more comforting measures. Patients may need to lie down to decrease pressure on the rectal area and avoid drinking hot liquids or eating big meals, which may increase peristalsis and discomfort until the impaction can be cleared.[11]

Multiple types of stents are available. After evaluating 600 patients who had stent placement for malignant gastric outlet obstruction (GOO), Dormann et al. found technical success with confirmaton that bowel patency occurred for 97% of patients.[51] Eighty-seven % of post procedural patients were able to tolerate a full or soft solid diet. Patients were able to tolerate oral diets within 24 hours of the stent placement.[33] Complications of stent placement is divided into early or late effects. Early is related to stent misdeployment or malpositioning or perforation. Late complications include: tumor growth extending through the stent into the lumen or stent migration, bleeding or perforation.[46] The use of stents has been shown to be effective in relieving malignant bowel obstruction and, compared to surgery, is less invasive with faster resumption of oral intake and shorter hospital stays, which saved money. One study found that the cost for patients who had stent placement versus surgical interventions was $7,215 to $10,190 in US dollars.[52] For complete obstructions, especially in an emergency situation, surgery has been necessary to decompress the bowel and frequently results in a colostomy. Laparoscopy is difficult in these patients due to the acutely dilated colon and the increased risk of complications when using laparoscopic instruments on that type of tissue.[46,53] Stenting versus surgery has been found to reduce morbidity and mortality of patients who would be poor candidates for surgery. It provides a way to prevent the need for a colostomy and results in shorter hospitalizations, which reduces healthcare costs.[53]

### Decompression Tubes

Colonic decompression tubes are used to reduce acutely distended bowel to prevent perforation and prevent more invasive surgical procedures. They can be placed by endoscopy or over a guidewire. They are inexpensive and widely available and prevent surgical intervention with colostomy. Disadvantages include success being dependent on the person placing them and the risk of dislodgment of the tubes. The size of these tubes allows for bowel cleansing or stool removal. These tubes are recommended as a temporizing measure to relieve distention and hopefully allow for bowel cleaning. More research needs to be done on the success of these larger decompression tubes.[46]

### Symptom Therapy

Providing aggressive pharmacological management of the distressing symptoms associated with MBO can prevent the need for surgical intervention.[6] The symptoms of intestinal colic, vomiting, and diarrhea can be effectively controlled with medications for most patients.

Depending on the location of the obstruction, either high or low, symptom severity can be affected. As accumulation of secretions increases, abdominal pain also increases. Distention, vomiting, and prolonged constipation occur. With high obstruction, onset of vomiting is sooner and amounts are larger. Intermittent borborygmi and visible peristalsis may occur.[40] Patients may experience colic pain on top of continuous pain from a growing mass. In chronic bowel obstruction, colic pain subsides. There are multiple options to attempt in an effort to relieve the symptoms and obstruction of an MBO (Table 12–7).

As stated above, the goal of treatment is to prevent obstruction whenever possible. The use of subcutaneous

---

**Table 12–7**
**Obstruction Management Options**

1. Prevent obstruction if at all possible.
2. Octreotide—may prevent complete obstruction if used early.
3. Opioids IV/SQ relieve pain.
4. Antiemetic medications—haloperidol 5–15 mg/day, Metoclopromide 10 mg Q 4 h. SQ—only if no colicky pain.
5. Corticosteroids.
6. Fluids and nutrients as tolerated.
7. Antispasmodic medications—hyoscine butylbromide 60 mg/day SQ may ↑ to 380 mg/day to relieve colicky pain.
8. Laxative Meds-stimulating laxatives. **contraindicated** due to ↑ peristalsis. Stool softener meds may be helpful if a single obstruction only.
9. Antidiarrheal medications—subacute obstruction or fecal fistula—codeine, loperamide, or octreotide.
10. Endoscopic therapeutic devices—Self Expandable Metal Stents (SEMS)
11. Colonic decompression tubes
12. Surgery

*Sources:* Adapted from Frech & Adler (2007), reference 46; Helyer (2008), reference 42.

(SQ) or intravenous (IV) analgesics, anticholinergic drugs, and antiemetic drugs can be effective for reducing the symptoms of inoperable and hard-to-manage obstruction.[6,38,39,45] Octreotide may be an option in early management to prevent partial obstructions from becoming complete.[6,38,39,45] Although octreotide is used for diarrhea because it decreases peristalsis, it also slows the irregular and ineffective peristaltic movements of obstruction, reducing the activity and balancing out the intestinal movement.[20,35] It reduces vomiting because it inhibits the secretion of gastrin, secretin, vasoactive intestinal peptide, pancreatic polypeptide, insulin, and glucagon. Octreotide directly blocks the secretion of gastric acid, pepsin, pancreatic enzyme, bicarbonate, intestinal epithelial electrolytes, and water.[20,35] It has been shown to be effective in 70% of patients for the control of vomiting.[6] Octreotide is administered by SQ infusion or SQ injection every 12 hours. A negative aspect of this drug is its cost. It is expensive and requires SQ injections or SQ or IV infusions over days to weeks. The recommended starting dose is 0.3 mg/day and may increase to 0.6 mg/day.[6] Hyoscine butylbromide is thought to be as effective as octreotide at reducing GI secretions and motility. Hyoscine butylbromide is less sedating, since it is thought to cross the blood–brain barrier less due to its low lipid solubility.[38] A recent study compared octreotide and scopolamine butylbromide for inoperable bowel obstruction with nasogastric tubes.[35,38] Both medications relieve colicky pain; both reduce the continuous abdominal pain and distention. Although this was a small study done over 3 days, they were able to remove the nasogastric tube in three of the seven patients on the first dose of octreotide 0.3 mg/day subcutaneously; three more patients were able to have the nasogastric tube removed when the dose was doubled to 0.6 mg/day. Scopolamine was similar in results, but the octreotide regimen was felt to be more effective overall. The negative effect is associated with the cost of the drug a definite consideration for overall quality of life. Scopolamine is less expensive.

### Analgesic Medications

Opioid medications have been used to relieve pain associated with obstruction.[6] Providing the opioid through SQ or IV infusion via a patient-controlled analgesic (PCA) pump is beneficial for two reasons: patients may receive improved pain relief over the oral route due to improved absorption, and by giving access to a PCA pump, patients are allowed some control over their pain management. Alternative routes of opioid administration, such as rectal or transdermal, may also be effective, but usually are inadequate if the pain is severe or unstable or there are frequent episodes of breakthrough pain.

### Antiemetic Medications

The goal of relief of symptoms for patients with MBO from a pharmacologic approach include the use of antiemetics,

antisecretory drugs, steroids and analgesics.[6] Recent additions of the selective serotonin antagonists, the 5-hydroxytryptamine blockers (5-HT$_3$) have made a significant difference in the treatment of nausea, especially when combined with corticosteroids for chemotherapy-induced nausea (see also Chapter 9).[40,54] Metoclopramide at 10 mg Q 4 hours SQ, has been the drug of choice for patients with incomplete bowel obstruction without colicky pain.[40] It stimulates the stomach to empty its contents into the reservoir of the bowel. Once complete obstruction is present, metoclopramide is discontinued and haloperidol or another antiemetic medication is started. Haloperidol is less sedating than other antiemetic or antihistamine medications.[40] The usual dose ranges from 5 to 15 mg/day, and at some institutions, it is combined with cyclizine.[6] Corticosteroids are particularly helpful antiemetics, especially when related to chemotherapy.[40]

In practice, it is recommended that morphine, haloperidol, and hyoscine butylbromide be given together by continuous SQ infusion. If pain or colic increases, the dose of morphine and hyoscine butylbromide should be increased; if emesis increases, increase the haloperidol dose.[6,40] Fluid and nutrient intake should be maintained as tolerated. Usually, patients whose vomiting has improved will tolerate fluids with small, low-residue meals. Dry mouth is managed with ice chips, although this has been suspected to wash out saliva that is present in the mouth. The use of artificial saliva may be more beneficial.[39]

*Corticosteroid Medications.* Corticosteroids have been helpful as antiemetic medications. The recommended dose of dexamethasone is between 6 and 16 mg/day; the prednisolone dose starts at 50 mg/day (injection or SQ infusion).[40] Steroids increase absorption of water and salt and reduce water and electrolytes in the intestine.

### Antispasmodic Medications

Colic pain results from increased peristalsis against the resistance of a mechanical obstruction. Analgesics alone may not be effective. Hyoscine butylbromide has been used to relieve spasm-like pain and to reduce emesis.[40] Dosing starts at 60 mg/day and increases up to 380 mg/day given by SQ infusion.[38] Side effects are related to the anticholinergic effects, including tachycardia, dry mouth, sedation, and hypotension.[40] Using methods to relieve dry mouth with sips of oral fluids, ice chips and good mouth care is important.[40]

### Laxative Medications

Stimulant laxatives are contraindicated due to increased peristalsis against an obstruction. Stool-softening medications may be helpful if there is only a single obstruction in the colon or rectum. If the obstruction is in the small bowel, laxatives will not be of benefit.[40]

**Antidiarrheal Medications**

Patients who experience a subacute obstruction or a fecal fistula may complain of diarrhea. Antidiarrheal medicine, such as codeine or loperamide, may be helpful. The benefit of these medications is that they may also help to relieve pain and colic. Octreotide may be helpful with bowel obstruction due to its mechanism of action. By inhibiting the release of certain secretions of the gastric, biliary, and intestine, intestinal motility decreases and absorption of water and electrolytes is increased.[35,40]

Helping families cope with symptoms associated with obstruction is important. Historically, the management of obstruction involved aggressive surgical intervention or symptom management alone. The initial assessment should include: (1) evaluating constipation, (2) evaluating for surgery, (3) providing pain management, and (4) managing nausea with metoclopramide. If incomplete obstruction, use dexamethasone, haloperidol, dimenhydrinate, chlorpromazine, or hyoscine butylbromide.[35,38,40] The introduction of new medications, such as octreotide, as well as newer antiemetics, has made a difference in the quality of life a patient with a malignant bowel obstruction may experience. The important thing to remember is that the treatment plan must always be in agreement with the patient's wishes. Discussing the patient's understanding of the situation and the options available are essential to effective and thoughtful care of bowel obstruction in the palliative care patient.

# ASCITES

Ascites associated with malignancy results from a combination of impaired fluid efflux and increased fluid influx.[38] The effect of the accumulation of fluids leads to symptoms of abdominal distention, pain, nausea, early satiety, dyspnea and reduced mobility.[55,56] Extreme ascites can lead to vomiting caused by external pressure on the stomach or intestines.[55] Ascites may be divided into three different types. *Central ascites* is the result of tumor-invading hepatic parenchyma, resulting in compression of the portal venous and/or the lymphatic system.[57] There is a decrease in oncotic pressure as a result of limited protein intake and the catabolic state associated with cancer.[57] *Peripheral ascites* is related to deposits of tumor cells found on the surface of the parietal or visceral peritoneum. The result is a mechanical interference with venous and/or lymphatic drainage.[57] There is blockage at the level of the peritoneal space rather than the liver parenchyma. Macrophages increase capillary permeability and contribute to greater ascites. *Mixed-type ascites* is a combination of central and peripheral ascites. Therefore, there is both compression of the portal venous and lymphatic systems, as well as tumor cells in the peritoneum. Chylous malignant ascites occurs when tumor infiltration of the retroperitoneal space causes obstruction of lymph flow through the lymph nodes and/or the pancreas.[55,57] Additional sources of ascites not related to malignancy include the following:

- Preexisting advanced liver disease with portal hypertension
- Portal venous thrombosis
- Congestive heart failure
- Nephrotic syndrome
- Pancreatitis
- Tuberculosis
- Hepatic venous obstruction
- Bowel perforation

Severe ascites is associated with poor prognosis (40% 1-year survival, less than 10% 3-year survival).[57] The pathological mechanisms of malignant ascites make the prevention or reduction of abdominal fluid accumulation difficult.[57] Invasive management of ascites is seen as appropriate whenever possible, in contrast to intestinal obstruction. Although survival is limited, the effects of ascites on the patient's quality of life warrant an aggressive approach.[57]

Tumor types most associated with ascites include ovarian, endometrial, breast, colon, gastric, and pancreatic cancers.[57] Less common sources of ascites include mesothelioma, non-Hodgkin's lymphoma, prostate cancer, multiple myeloma, and melanoma.[57]

## Assessment of Ascites

### Symptoms Associated with Ascites

Patients complain of abdominal bloating and pain. Initially, patients complain of feeling a need for larger-waisted clothing and notice an increase in belt size or weight. They may feel nauseated and have a decreased appetite. Many patients will complain of increased symptoms of reflux or heartburn. Pronounced ascites can cause dyspnea and orthopnea due to increased pressure on the diaphragm.[55–57]

### Physical Examination

The physical examination may reveal abdominal or inguinal hernia, scrotal edema, and abdominal venous engorgement. Radiological findings show a hazy picture, with distended and separate loops of the bowel. There is a poor definition of the abdominal organs and loss of the psoas muscle shadows. Ultrasound and computed tomographic scans may also be used to diagnose ascites.[57]

### Management of Ascites

Traditionally, treatment of ascites is palliative due to poor prognosis.[54] Ovarian cancer is one of the few types where the presence of ascites does not necessarily correlate with a poor prognosis. In this case, survival rate can be improved through surgical intervention and adjuvant therapy.[57,58]

## Medical Therapy

Advanced liver disease is associated with central ascites. There is an increase in renal sodium and water retention. Therefore, restricting sodium intake to 100 mmol/day or less along with fluid restriction for patients with moderate to severe hyponatremia (125 mmol/L) may be beneficial. Using potassium-sparing diuretics is also important. Spironolactone (100 to 400 mg/day) is the drug of choice.[57] Furosemide is also helpful at 40 to 80 mg/day to initiate diuresis. Over-diuresis must be avoided. Over-diuresis may precipitate electrolyte imbalance, hepatic encephalopathy, and pre-renal failure. The above regimen of fluid and sodium reduction and diuretics may work for mixed-type ascites, which results from compression of vessels related to tumor and peripheral tumor cells of the parietal or visceral peritoneum as well. Because mixed-type ascites is associated with chylous fluid, adding changes to the diet, such as decreased fat intake and increased medium-chain triglycerides, may be important. Chylous ascites results from tumor infiltration of the retroperitoneal space, causing obstruction of lymphatic flow.[57]

Medium-chain triglyceride oil (Lipisorb) can be used as a calorie source in these patients. Because the lymph system is bypassed, the shorter fatty acid chains are easier to digest. For patients with refractory ascites and a shortened life expectancy, paracentesis may be the most appropriate therapy.[50,52] Paracentesis is the most common and effective treatment to relieve ascites.[55,56] It is recommended that a maximum of 5 liters of ascites fluid be taken off.[56] Although this procedure gives temporary relief of symptoms like the treatment of MBO, palliative care decisions should be based on the goals of care and patients quality of life. New advances in paracentesis treatment options have improved long-term use to minimize the need for frequent trips to the hospital for the procedure and repeated painful needle sticks.[55,56]

## Paracentesis Catheters

Peritoneovenous shunts (PVS) (Denver or LeVeen shunt) are helpful for the removal of ascites in 75% to 85% of patients.[57] These shunts are used primarily for nonmalignant ascites. The shunt removes fluid from the site, and the fluid is shunted up into the internal jugular vein.[57]

This type of shunt has the advantage of avoiding an external drainage device and can be placed with minimal invasive techniques under conscious sedation. The disadvantages are that they have a high rate of failure related to occlusion and have been associated with pulmonary edema, thrombosis of major veins, seroma formation, leaks and disseminated intravascular coagulation (DIC).[55]

## Pigtail Catheter

Pigtail drainage catheters are used for percutaneous abscess drainage as well as pleural effusions and percutaneous biliary and renal drainage.[55] They are placed under ultrasound or fluoroscopic guidance and can be intermittently drained to gravity or vacuum bottles. This can be done as an outpatient procedure.[55]

## Dialysis Catheters

Silastic peritoneal dialysis catheters re providing effective management of malignant ascites.[55,59] They also can be managed at home easily and can be on gravity drainage or vacuum bottle drainage as needed.

## Pleurex Catheter (Denver Biomedical, Denver, Colorado)

This is a single-cuff tunneled Silastic catheter approved for the drainage of malignant plural effusions and malignant ascites. It offers a one-way valve instead of a clamp and can be managed in the home as well.[55]

The management of all of these types of catheters requires careful handling and techniques to prevent infections. Peritonitis, cellulitis and catheter occlusion are risks.[55]

## Nursing Management

Ascites management involves initially understanding the mechanism, then using interventions appropriately. The reality of recurring ascites requiring repeated paracentesis is present. Acknowledging the risk/benefit ratio of repeated paracentesis is essential, especially in palliative care. The placement of an indwelling catheter can reduce the need for multiple needle sticks and improve patient quality of life.[55] Nurses need to remember good supportive care in addition to other resources. These include skin care, to help prevent breakdown, and comfort interventions, such as pillow support, and loose clothing whenever possible. Educating the patient and caregivers on the rationale behind fluid and sodium restrictions when necessary can help their understanding and compliance. The cycle of a patient who feels thirsty, receives IV fluids, and has more discomfort is difficult for the patient to understand. Careful explanations about why an intervention is or is not recommended can go a long way toward improving the quality of life for these patients.

REFERENCES

1. Sykes NP. The pathogenesis of constipation. J Support Oncol 2006;4(5):213–224.
2. McMillan SC. Assessing and managing narcotic induced constipation in adults with cancer. Cancer Control 1999; 6:198–204.
3. Thomas J. Opioid-induced bowel dysfunction. J Pain Symptom Manage 2008;35(1):103–113.
4. Massey RL, Haylock PJ, Curtiss C. Constipation. In: Yarbro MHFCH, Goodman M, eds. Cancer Symptom Management. Boston: Jones and Bartlett, 2004:512–527.
5. Levy MH. Constipation and diarrhea in cancer patients. Cancer Bull 1991;43:412–422.

6. Sykes NP. Constipation and diarrhoea. In: Doyle GWCHD, Cherny N, Calman K, eds. Oxford Textbook of Palliative Medicine. Oxford University Press, 2004:483–496.

7. Thomas JR, Cooney G. Palliative care and pain: New strategies for managing opioid bowel dysfunction. J Palliat Med 2008;11(Suppl 1):S1–S19.

8. Woolery M, Bisanz A Lyons HF, Gaido L, Yenulevich M, Fulton S, McMillan SC. Putting evidence into practice: Evidence-based interventions for the prevention and management of constipation in patients with cancer. Clin J Oncol Nurs 2008;12:317–332.

9. Bruera E, Fadul N. Constipation and diarrhea. In: Bruera IJHE, Ripamonti C, Von Gunten C, eds. Textbook of Palliative Medicine. New York: Oxford University Press, Inc., 2006:554–570.

10. Martin BC, Barghout V, Cerulli A. Direct medical costs of constipation in the United States. Manag Care Interface 2006;19(12):43–49.

11. Bisanz A. Bowel management in patients with cancer. In: Ajani JA, ed. Gastrointestinal Cancer. New York: Springer, 2005:313–345.

12. Davison D. Constipation. Clin J Oncol Nurs 2006;10(1):112–113.

13. Sykes NP. The relationship between opioid use and laxative use in terminally ill cancer patients. Palliat Med 1998;12:375–382.

14. Panchal SJ, Muller–Schwefe P, Wurzelmann JI. Opioid-induced bowel dysfunction: Prevalence, pathophysiology and burden. Int J Clin Pract 2007;61:1181–1187.

15. National Comprehensive Cancer Network (NCCN). Clinical Practice Guidelines in Oncology–Palliative Care V.1.2008. Constipation management recommendations. NCCN.org (accessed October 23, 2009).

16. Radbruch L, Sabatowski R, Loick G, Kolbe C, Kasper M, Grond S, Lehmann KA. Constipation and the use of laxatives: A comparison between TDF & oral morphine. Palliat Med 2000;13:159–160.

17. Adler HF, Atkinson AJ, Ivy AC. Effect of morphine and Dilaudid on the ileum and of morphine, Dilaudid and atropine on the colon of man. Arch Intern Med 1942;69:974–985.

18. McMillan SC, Williams FA. Validity and reliability of the constipation assessment scale. Cancer Nurs 1989;12:183–188.

19. AHCPR, Management of Cancer Pain guidelines. Vol. Pub. # 94–0592. 1994, Washington DC: AHCPR.

20. Stern J, Ippoliti C. Management of acute cancer treatment-induced diarrhea. Semin Oncol Nurs 2003;19(4):11–16.

21. Sykes NP. An investigation of the ability of oral naloxone to correct opioid-related constipation in patients with advanced cancer. Palliat Med 1996;10:135–144.

22. Lederle FA, Busch DL, Mattox KM, West MJ, Aske DM. Cost-effective treatment of constipation in the elderly: A randomized double-blind comparison of sorbitol and lactulose. Am J Med 1990;89:597–601.

23. Larkin PJ, Sykes NP, Centeno C, Ellershaw JE, Elsner F, Eugene B, Gootjes JRG, Nabal M, Noguera A, Ripamonti C, Zucco F, Zuurmond WWA. The management of constipation in palliative care: Clinical practice recommendations. Palliat Med 2008;22:796–807.

24. Galligan JJ, Vanner S. Basic and clinical pharmacology of new motility promoting agents. Neurogastroenterol Motil 2005;17:643–653.

25. Ripamonti C, Mercadante S. Pathophysiology and management of malignant bowel obstruction. In: Doyle GWCHD, Cherny N, Calman K, eds. Oxford Textbook of Palliative Medicine. Oxford: Oxford University Press, 2004:496–507.

26. Culpepper-Morgan JA, Inturrisi CE, Portenoy RK. Treatment of opioid-induced constipation with oral naloxone: A pilot study. Clin Pharmacol Ther 1992;52:90–95.

27. Liu M, Wittbrodt E. Low-dose oral naloxone reverses opioid induced constipation and analgesia. J Pain Symptom Manage 2002;23:48–53.

28. Thomas J, Karver S, Cooney GA, Chamberlain BH, Watt CK, Slatkin NE, Stambler N, Kremer AB, Israel RJ. Methylnaltrexone for opioid-induced constipation in advanced illness. N Engl J Med 2008;358:2332–2343.

29. Viele CS. Overview of chemotherapy-induced diarrhea. Semin Oncol Nurs 2003;19(Suppl 3):2–5.

30. Engelking C. Diarrhea. In: Yarbro MHFCH, Goodman M, eds. Cancer Symptom Management. Boston: Jones and Bartlett, 2004:528–557.

31. Anastasi JK, Capili B. HIV-related diarrhea and outcome measures. J Assoc Nurses AIDS Care 2001;12(suppl):44–50.

32. Jacobsohn DA, Vogelsang GB. Acute graft versus host disease. Orphanet J Rare Diseases 2007;2(35).

33. Gwede CK. Overview of radiation and chemoradiation-induced diarrhea. Semin Oncol Nurs 2003;19(suppl3):11–16.

34. Weihofen DL, Marino C. Cancer Survival Cookbook. Los Angeles: John Wiley & Sons, 1998:28.

35. Holt AP, Patel M, Ahmed MM. Palliation of patients with malignant gastroduodenal obstruction with self-expanding metallic stents: The treatment of choice? Gastrointest Endosc 2004;60(6):1010–1017.

36. Prommer EE. Established and potential therapeutic applications of octreotide in palliative care. Support Care Cancer 2008;16:1117–1123.

37. Massacesi C, Galeazzi G. Sustained release octreotide may have a role in the treatment of malignant bowel obstruction. Palliat Med 2006;20:715–716.

38. Lowell A. New strategies for the prevention and reduction of cancer-treatment induced diarrhea. Semin Oncol Nurs 2003;19(Suppl 3):17–21.

39. Ripamonti C, Mercadante S, Groff L, Zecca E, DeConno F, Casuccio A. Role of octreotide, scopolamine butylbromide, and hydration in symptom control of patients with inoperable bowel obstruction and nasogastric tubes: A prospective randomization trial. J Pain Symptom Manage 2000;19:23–34.

40. Beckman R, Siden R, Yanik GA, Levine JE. Continuous Octreotide infusion for the treatment of secretory diarrhea caused by acute intestinal graft-versus-host disease in a child. J Pediatr Hematol 2000;22(4):344–350.

41. Krouse RS. Surgical palliation of bowel obstruction. Gastroenterol Clin North Am 2006;35(1):143–151.

42. Helyer L, Easson AM. Surgical approaches to malignant bowel obstruction. J Support Oncol 2008;6(3):105–113.

43. Ripamonti CI, Malignant bowel obstruction: Tailoring treatment to individual patients. J Support Oncol 2008;6(3):114–115.

44. Krouse RS. Surgical management of malignant bowel obstruction. Surg Oncol Clin N Am 2004;13:479–490.

45. Anthony T, Baron T, Mercadante S. Report of the clinical protocol committee: Development of randomized trials for malignant bowel obstruction. J Pain Symptom Manage 2007;34(1 Suppl):S49–S59.

46. Frech EJ, Adler DG. Endoscopic therapy for malignant bowel obstruction. J Support Oncol 2007;5(7):303–310,319.

47. Krouse RS. The value of a systematic approach to malignant bowel obstruction. J Support Oncol 2008;6:116–117.

48. Targownik LE, Spiegel BM, Sack J, Hines OJ, Dulai G, Grainek IM, Farrell JJ. Colonic stent vs. emergency surgery for management of acute left-sided malignant colonic obstruction: A decision analysis. Gastrointest Endosc 2004;60(6): 865–872.

49. Siddiqui A, Spechler SJ, Huerta S. Surgical bypass versus endoscopic stenting for malignant gastroduodenal obstruction: A decision analysis. Dig Dis Sci 2007;52:276–281.

50. Ozkan O, Akinci D, Gocmen R, Cil B, Ozmen M, Akhan O. Percutaneous placement of peritoneal port–catheter in patients with malignant ascites. Cardiovasc Intervent Radiol 2007;30:232–236.

51. Dormann A, Meisner S, Verin N, Wenk Lang A. Self-expanding metal stents for gastroduodenal malignancies: Systematic review of their clinical effectiveness. Endoscopy 2004;36:543–550.

52. Johnsson E, Thune A, Liedman B. Palliation of malignant gastroduodenal obstruction with open surgical bypass or endoscopic stenting: Clinical outcome and health economic evaluation. World J Surg 2004;28:812–817.

53. Osman HS, Rashid HI, Sathananthan N, Parker MC. The cost effectiveness of self-expanding metal stents in the management of malignant left-sided large bowel obstruction. Colorectal Dis 2000;2:233–237.

54. Mannix KA. Gastrointestinal symptoms—palliation of nausea and vomiting. In: Doyle GWCHD, Cherny N, Calman K, eds. Oxford Textbook of Palliative Medicine. New York: Oxford University Press, 2004:459–468.

55. Rosenberg SM. Palliation of malignant ascites. Gastroenterol Clin North Am 2006;35(1):189–199.

56. Becker G, Galandi D, Blum HE. Malignant ascites: Systematic review and guideline for treatment. Eur J Cancer 2006;42:589–597.

57. Kichian K, Bain VG, Jaundice, ascites, and hepatic encephalopathy. In: Doyle GWCHD, Cherny N, Calman K, eds. Oxford Textbook of Palliative Medicine. Oxford: Oxford University Press, 2004:507–520.

58. Numnum TM, Rocconi RP, Whitworth J, Barnes MN. The use of bevacizumab to palliate symptomatic ascites in patients with refractory ovarian carcinoma. Gynecol Oncol 2006;102:425–428.

59. Rosenberg S, Courtney A, Nemcek AA Jr, Omary RA. Comparison of percutaneous management techniques for recurrent malignant ascites. J Vasc Interv Radiol 2004;15: 1129–1131.

# 13  *Michelle Schaffner Gabriel, Pamela Kedziera, and Nessa Coyle*

# Hydration, Thirst, and Nutrition

*I just don't feel like eating anything. I have no appetite and nothing tastes good anymore.*
*—A dying patient*

- *Key Points*
- *The last year of life for someone with a progressive debilitating disease is frequently associated with multiple distressing symptoms, comorbidities, and loss of independent function.*
- *Difficulties with eating and drinking are common during this period.*
- *Decisions regarding hydration and nutrition are confronted by patients, families, and staff at this time.*
- *Discussions regarding artificial hydration and nutrition are frequently couched in terms of ethics, religious beliefs, and strongly held personal views.*
- *Nurses need to know their state laws concerning provision of artificial hydration and nutrition in the dying patient.*
- *Decisions regarding hydration and nutrition at end of life are guided by goals of care, benefit versus burden, and the wishes of the patient and family.*
- *Patients have the right to refuse hydration and nutrition, whether parenteral or oral.*

There is lack of consensus in society and among experts as to whether it is physically, psychologically, socially, or ethically appropriate to provide artificial hydration and nutrition to a terminally ill person. Do these therapies improve the way an individual feels physically and emotionally? Do they cause harm? Can an individual die comfortably without these interventions? Decisions on whether to provide artificial hydration and nutrition are made taking into consideration a person's wishes, which are often based on cultural, religious, and personal values, and on the basis of whether the intervention will make the patient more comfortable. These elements are illustrated in the following two case reports.

## CASE STUDY
### *Two Patients Receiving Artificial Hydration and Nutrition*

Mrs. M was a 79-year-old woman with metastatic breast cancer. She was a Chinese immigrant, who had moved to the United States to be with her children after her husband passed away. Her family had brought her to the hospital with mental status changes. She was diagnosed with aspiration pneumonia. Although she was cachectic and hadn't been able to tolerate much food according to her family, they insisted upon her receiving hydration and enteral feedings via a nasogastric (NG) tube. The translator who participated in the discussions shared with the team that many Chinese will insist upon artificial hydration and nutrition even if there are risks because of their belief in ensuring they or their loved one has enough food and fluid for their journey in the afterlife. Mrs. M died two days later, receiving both hydration and enteral feedings at 25 mL/h.

In a different situation, Mr. Y was a 45-year-old man who had suffered from complications following neurosurgery for the removal of a benign tumor. After months of being in the intermediate intensive care unit, on a ventilator and receiving enteral feedings, the neurologists had determined that Mr. Y was in a persistent vegetative state, and no longer able to have meaningful interactions. Mr. Y had completed an advance directive, which revealed his wishes not to be kept alive should he have no chance of a meaningful recovery. He defined this as being able to live independently outside of a skilled nursing facility. After much deliberation, his family decided to wean him off the ventilator, and he was transferred to an inpatient hospice unit. Discussions with the hospice team continued about whether to stop his enteral feedings. His family decided to discontinue the feedings, as they felt that this intervention was contrary to Mr. Y's expressed wishes. He died one week later with his family present.

The meaning of food and water, and the meaning of discontinuing food and water, need careful exploration and ongoing discussion of the benefits and burden for each individual, taking into consideration his or her cultural and religious beliefs. There are no absolutes. Nurses have reported that patients knowingly refuse food and fluids to hasten death.[1] The following pages provide basic information on hydration and nutrition as a framework for the nurse when guiding a patient and family who are considering the benefits and burdens of artificial hydration and nutrition in the setting of advanced, progressive disease. In addition, the following questions are explored: What are the current practices with regard to managing hydration at the end of life, and how are these clinical strategies justified? How is dehydration clinically recognized? Should dehydration at end of life be treated, and if so, how?

## HYDRATION

Water is an essential component of the human body. Complex cellular functions, such as protein synthesis and metabolism of nutrients, are affected by hydration status. The maintenance of hydration depends on a balance between intake and output, which is regulated by neuroendocrine influences. Homeostasis is maintained through parallel neuroendocrine activity on excretion of fluid via the kidneys[2] and on intake via thirst. Increased osmotic pressure is the prime stimulus for thirst, stimulating the release of vasopressin. Renal excretion is mainly dependent on the action of vasopressin, which is secreted by the posterior pituitary gland. This hormone, known as antidiuretic hormone (ADH), increases water reabsorption in the collecting ducts of the kidneys.[3] Thirst stimuli include hypertonicity; depletion of the extracellular fluid compartment arising from vomiting, diarrhea, or hemorrhage; and renal failure, in which plasma sodium is low but plasma renin levels are high.[4]

### Dehydration

*Dehydration* is a loss of normal body water. There are several types of dehydration.[3,5] *Isotonic* dehydration results from a balanced loss of water and sodium. This occurs during a complete fast and during episodes of vomiting and diarrhea

with the loss of water and electrolytes in the gastric contents. Billings[6] theorized that terminally ill individuals have this type of balanced decrease in food and fluid intake, causing eunatremic dehydration (sodium levels in normal range) because of the simultaneous loss of salt and water. *Hypertonic* dehydration occurs if water losses are greater than sodium losses. Fever can cause this problem, by loss of water through the lungs and skin and a limited ability to take in oral fluids. *Hypotonic* dehydration occurs when sodium loss exceeds water loss. This typically occurs when water is consumed but food is not. Overuse of diuretics is a major factor. Osmotic diuresis (e.g., from hyperglycemia), salt-wasting renal conditions, third spacing (ascites), and adrenal insufficiency are other common causes of sodium loss.[7]

The methodology for assessing dehydration has not been well studied and tends to vary among practitioners. The clinical sensitivity of each method has not been determined. Clinical assessment should include mental status changes, thirst, oral/parenteral intake, urine output, and fluid loss. Physical findings, such as weight loss, dry mouth, dry tongue, reduced skin turgor, and postural hypotension should be noted. Laboratory test findings, including increased hematocrit, elevated serum sodium concentration, azotemia with a disproportionate rise in blood urea nitrogen in relation to creatinine, concentrated urine, and hyperosmolarity, are indicative of dehydration.

Physical findings (Table 13–1) are complicated to evaluate.[7] Comorbid conditions can be the cause of many of these symptoms in the chronically or terminally ill individual. Skin turgor, for example, can be hard to evaluate in the cachexic individual and is unreliable. Obtaining weights may be impractical, but rapid weight loss of greater than 3% is indicative of dehydration.[5] Postural hypotension can be related to medications and cardiac pathology. Discomfort, especially problems with xerostomia and thirst, may result from dehydration,[8] although there can be other causes as well. Dry mouth can be associated with mouth breathing or anticholinergic medication. Thirst may be absent or mild in patients with hyponatremic dehydration, although marked volume loss may stimulate ADH and water craving.

There is evidence that elderly individuals do not perceive thirst in the same manner as healthy young adults.[4] In a study comparing the role of thirst sensation and drinking behavior in young versus older men, water was restricted for 24 hours. Only the young, healthy study group reported a dry, unpleasant mouth and a general sense of thirst; the healthy elders had a deficit in the awareness of thirst despite plasma osmolarity and sodium and vasopressin concentrations that were greater than those in the younger group. During the rehydration period, the younger group consumed enough fluid to correct their laboratory values. Elder subjects did not consume enough fluid to correct the laboratory values.[9] There is not, however, any evidence to support this observation in terminally ill patients. In hypernatremia, thirst is a powerful stimulus, and persons with access to water usually will take in sufficient amounts of fluid. Confused or somnolent individuals and those who are unable to drink are at risk because water losses may not be adequately replaced. Dehydrated,

**Table 13–1**
**Signs and Symptoms of Dehydration**

| Hyponatremic Dehydration | Hypernatremic Dehydration | Isotonic Dehydration |
|---|---|---|
| Volume depletion | Thirst | Morose |
| Anorexia, taste alteration, and weight loss | Fatigue | Aggression |
| Nausea and vomiting | Muscle weakness | Demoralized |
| Diminished skin turgor | Mental status changes | Apathetic |
| Dry mucous membranes | Fever | Uncoordinated |
| Reduced sweat | | |
| Orthostatic hypotension | | |
| Lethargy and restlessness | | |
| Delirium | | |
| Seizures (related to cerebral edema) | | |
| Confusion, stupor and coma | | |
| Psychosis (rare) | | |
| **Laboratory Results** | | |
| Azotemia | Increased sodium | Minor or no abnormalities |
| Disproportionate blood urea nitrogen compared to creatinine | | |
| Hyponatremia | | |
| Hemoconcentration | | |
| Urine osmolarity with sodium concentration | | |

**Table 13–2**
**The Hydration Debate**

**Arguments for hydration**
Provides a basic human need.
Provides comfort and prevents uncomfortable symptoms: confusion, agitation, and neuromuscular irritability.
Prevents complications (eg, neurotoxicity with high-dose narcotics).
Relieves thirst, recognized as a sign of fluid needs.
Does not prolong life to any meaningful degree.
Allows providers to continue their efforts to find ways to improve comfort and life quality, despite the perception of a poor quality of life.
Provides minimum standards of care; not doing so would break a bond with the patient.
May set a precedent to withhold therapies from other patients who are compromised.

**Arguments against hydration**
Interferes with acceptance of the terminal condition.
Intravenous therapy is painful and Intrusive.
Prolongs suffering and the dying process.
Unnecessary since unconscious patients do not experience uncomfortable symptoms, such as pain or thirst.
Less urine output means less need for bed pan, urinal, commode, or catheter.
Less fluid in the GI tract and less vomiting.
Less pulmonary secretions and less cough, choking, and congestion.
Minimizes edema and ascites.
Ketones and other metabolic by-products in dehydration act as natural anesthetics for the central nervous system, causing decreased levels of consciousness and decreased suffering.

*Source*: Dalal & Bruera, reference 19.

terminally ill patients usually present with mixed disorders of fluid and salt loss.

Some palliative care clinicians suggest that dehydration at the end of life causes suffering in some patients, which should be relieved. This suffering may include thirst, dry mouth, fatigue, nausea, vomiting, confusion, muscle cramps, and perhaps the hastening of death.[10,11] Dehydration has been associated with an increased risk of bedsores and constipation, particularly in the elderly. Dehydration causes confusion and restlessness in patients with non-terminal disease. These same symptoms are frequently reported in terminally ill persons and could be aggravated by dehydration.[12] Dehydration as a cause of renal failure has been well documented.[13,14] Opioid metabolite accumulation can result from renal failure and cause confusion and myoclonus.[15] A study of terminally ill cancer patients, however, showed that the group receiving intravenous fluids at a rate of 1 to 2 L/day consistently had more abnormal laboratory values of serum sodium, urea, and osmolarity than the group who were not hydrated.[16] In a separate study of terminally ill cancer patients, the group receiving intravenous fluids at a rate of 1 L/day had significantly lower albumin levels 1 week prior to death (p = 0.005), and no effects on blood urea nitrogen/creatinine, sodium or potassium levels.[17]

Dehydration may improve physical caregiving for some patients. For example, urinary catheters may be avoided if the frequency of urination decreases. With dehydration, there is less gastrointestinal fluid, with fewer bouts of vomiting, and a reduction in pulmonary secretions, with less coughing, choking, and need for suctioning.[18] Table 13–2 shows the arguments for and against hydration.[19]

## Additional Research on Hydration

Many researchers have looked at the effects of hydration on general symptom control as well as on specific symptoms such as thirst and dry mouth, cognitive symptoms and mental status. One study that looked at the differences between a group of patients who decided against artificial nutrition and hydration (ANH) versus a group in which other end-of-life decisions were made found that in the former group, patients as a whole received fewer drugs to relieve symptoms at end of life.[20] Although the study did not separate out artificial hydration from nutrition, patients at the end of life who received neither artificial hydration or nutrition died of dehydration, not starvation.[21]

A study of 82 patients in the last 2 days before death showed no statistically significant relationship between the level of hydration, respiratory tract secretions, dry mouth, and thirst.[22] The researchers concluded that artificial hydration to alleviate these symptoms may be futile. These results contrast with those of a study of 100 palliative care patients receiving *hypodermoclysis* (infusion of fluids into the subcutaneous space); researchers concluded that this therapy was useful for achieving better symptom control.[23] Another randomized, comparative and prospective trial looked at hydration and its effect on thirst in cancer patients and found no longstanding effect on this symptom.[24]

Some experts suggest that hydration may relieve symptoms other than thirst, such as confusion, restlessness, myoclonus, sedation, and nausea.[25] An anecdotal study of three patients being hydrated by hypodermoclysis reported that hydration may have contributed to improved cognitive function and allowed patients to deal with end-of-life issues.[26] Another study found that hydration with low volumes (1 L/day), along with frequent cognitive monitoring and opioid rotation, correlated with a reduction in prevalence of agitated delirium in cancer patients; however, a study that tried to replicate the results did not arrive at the same finding.[27,28] Yet another study[24] looked at the impact of hydration on delirium and did not find any preventive effects on this symptom by hydration. In a randomized, controlled, double-blind study evaluating the effects of hydration on several target symptoms, the researchers found that the group who received hydration had a significant improvement on myoclonus and sedation compared to the group who did not receive hydration.[29] In the previously mentioned study,[24] the researchers found that out of the three symptoms evaluated for an effect from hydration, chronic nausea was the only one that had significant improvement.

Other experts who have looked at dehydration-related suffering have stressed the role of inappropriate medical interventions that cause their own problems. They contend that hydrating a patient can be associated with repetitive needlesticks, decreased mobility, increased secretions, increased edema, and possibly congestive heart failure.[30,31] It is also suggested that improving the cognition of a dying patient with pain may make the patient more aware of the pain, with the possiblity of decreasing cognition once more through increased opioid requirements. Others state that comatose patients feel no symptoms; fluids may prolong dying, and dehydration may act as an anesthetic.[13]

In a descriptive study of symptoms of dehydration in the terminally ill, no association was found between fluid intake, serum sodium, osmolality, blood urea nitrogen, and symptom severity.[10] A study looking at the effects of hydration on laboratory findings found an association between hydration and hypoalbuminemia, with no beneficial effects on correcting abnormal values of blood urea nitrogen/creatinine, sodium, or potassium levels.[17] A survey of Swiss physicians found that there was no consensus with respect to the assessment of "suffering" from dehydration or thirst. The physicians who chose artificial hydration were more likely to perceive suffering and thirst as serious problems. Two thirds of the doctors did not believe that artificial hydration was the best way to respond to terminal dehydration.[32]

In addition to surveys of providers' beliefs about the benefits and burdens of hydration, researchers have looked at the beliefs of patients and family members as well. One study found that in the group receiving the placebo (100 mL of hydration/day versus 1000 mL/day), 50% of patients thought the treatment to be successful.[29] Another survey of 54 patients admitted to an acute pain relief and palliative care unit and their caregivers found that the majority felt parenteral hydration to be useful, provided some nutrition, improved their clinical condition, was useful psychologically, and carried an acceptable burden.[33] Specific to the method of administration, patients and their caregivers favored the intravenous route versus the subcutaneous route.

The decision to use artificial means of hydration comes more from tradition than from science. To avoid unnecessary interventions in the course of the dying process, some practitioners have avoided artificial fluid replacement secondary to its perceived negative effects. Their conclusion—that artificial hydration may cause harm to some dying patients—keeps them from offering this therapy. Palliative care clinicians have noted that some individuals are more comfortable without artificial fluids, which may prolong the dying process, whereas others are more comfortable when artificial hydration is used. Emotional issues are often the driving force in the decision to provide or withdraw artificial hydration. The need to provide fluids may be directed by very strong cultural, religious, and/or moral convictions on the part of patients, families, and some caregivers, even if there is no certainty that the therapy relieves discomfort.

## Screening for Dehydration, Management, and Assessing the Effects of Interventions

Screening for dehydration in the palliative care setting may include recording intake and output, examining skin turgor and mucous membranes, and monitoring mental status and blood pressure. Subjective reports of fatigue, muscle weakness, anorexia, and taste alteration are correlated with these signs and laboratory values (see Table 13–1). The benefits and possible adverse effects of hydration should be discussed within a broad framework of goals of care and the wishes of the patient and family explored within that framework. Each situation has unique aspects that affect choices and the possible outcomes of therapy. Finally, there is a need for regular reassessment to allow for changes in therapy and frequent discussions with patients and families to provide opportunities to reevaluate decisions.

The treatment of dehydration starts with a review of medications and elimination, if possible, of any agents (e.g. diuretics) that may be contributing to the dehydration. Mouth care should be provided regularly. Treating dehydration with fluids may include various routes of administration. A standard goal for fluid intake is 1500 to 3000 mL, or 8 to 10 glasses, of water daily.[7] The least invasive approach to replacing fluids is to offer liquid orally at regular intervals. For those able to swallow, this approach can help the patient as well as promote the emotional well-being of the caregivers. Those who are very weak, depressed, confused, agitated, or demented may need significant assistance in getting the fluids in on a regular basis.

The benefit/burden ratio for the patient in aggressively pursuing such a fluid intake approach must be carefully weighed. Care must be taken to avoid overhydration by a well-meaning but misdirected aggressive approach, and the patient should be monitored for new orthopnea, shortness of breath, increased emotional distress, or change in mental status. If the ability to swallow is diminished, there is a risk of aspiration that can cause more distress to the patient. Small, frequent sips of fluid or ice chips can be provided. Choice of fluids should be patient driven. Some individuals find sports replacement fluids a good choice because they are easily absorbed by the stomach and can correct hypertonic dehydration.[5] Use of a fine mist spray can also help to keep mucous membranes moist.[34] Hot, humid weather conditions can add to the risk of dehydration, so the use of air conditioning and fans should be considered.

## Alternative Routes of Hydration When the Oral Route Is No Longer Reliable

If there are days or weeks of life expected, and if it is appropriate to the goals of care and wishes of the patient and family, a more reliable route of fluid replacement than the oral route may be chosen. Rehydration by *proctoclysis* is relatively risk-free and less expensive than parenteral means of administration.[35] Through a NG tube placed rectally, tap water or saline is instilled, starting at about 100 mL/h. If there is no discomfort, leakage, or tenesmus (spasm of the anal sphincter), the rate can be increased to 400 mL/h. One liter of fluid can be instilled over 6 to 8 hours. Care must be taken, however, not to overhydrate. Side effects of this route of hydration can include pain, edema, rectal leakage of fluid, and pain during insertion of the tube. Researchers report that although proctoclysis is effective, safe, and economical, most patients prefer hypodermoclysis.[35] It is possible to foresee cultural and social reluctance to accept the rectal mode of fluid administration. In an inpatient setting, clinical staff would administer the fluids, but in a home setting, it may be impractical to use professional staff daily for this treatment. Family caregivers or patients may be uncomfortable with relatives or friends having to assume this type of care.

Standard methods for replacement of fluids can be achieved by the use of enteral feeding tubes and by parenteral methods, such as subcutaneous or intravenous infusion. A feeding tube placed through the nose is often uncomfortable

| Table 13–3 | | |
|---|---|---|
| **Potential Complications of Routes for Artificial Hydration** | | |
| IV Peripheral | IV Central | SC Hypodermuclysis |
| Pain | Sepsis | Pain |
| Short duration of access | Hemothorax | Infection |
| Infection | Pneumothorax | Third spacing |
| Phlebitis | Central vein thrombosis | Tissue sloughing |
| | Catheter fragment thrombosis | Local bleeding |
| | Air embolus | |
| | Brachial plexus injury | |
| | Arterial laceration | |
| IV, intravenous; SC, subcutaneous. | | |

and may agitate the confused individual. Patients often extubate themselves when agitated. Endoscopic gastrostomy tubes have become more popular but are usually placed for decompression or feeding rather than for fluid replacement. If the individual has a feeding tube or a permanent intravenous access device (port or peripherally inserted central catheter), these may be used safely without any added burden for the patient. Placement of these devices, however, needs to be considered in the context of the overall goals of therapy.

*Hypodermoclysis* (subcutaneous fluid administration) does not require special access devices. This method has the advantage over the intravenous route in people who have poor venous access. Use of this method may prevent transfer to an acute setting for line placement. Hypodermoclysis can also be initiated in the patient's home. It does not require monitoring for clotting in the line, and there is no fear of letting the line "run dry." There can be local irritation at the site of infusion, however, as well as minor bleeding. Sloughing of tissue is possible with overinfusion, and abscess formation may occur (Table 13–3). Hypotonic or isotonic solutions, with or without hyaluronidase or corticosteroids, are administered through needles inserted into the subcutaneous tissue of the abdomen or anterior or lateral thigh. Most individuals can tolerate 100 mL/h or more. Up to 1500 mL can be administered into a single site.[9,36] The following case report illustrates the use of hypodermoclysis.

### CASE STUDY
### *Mr. P, A 73-Year-Old Man with Prostate Cancer*

Mr. P was a 73-year-old man who was admitted for end-of-life care to an inpatient hospice unit. When he was first admitted, he was alert and oriented, although fatigued. He had been declining at home, and the level of care he required was more than his wife could provide. During his admission, he developed delirium. His family requested that hydration be attempted to see if it could improve his cognitive status. The nurse inserted a subcutaneous needle into his anterior thigh in order to administer fluids by hypodermoclysis. He received 1 L/day of fluid, and within 24 hours had improved in his cognitive status with no more indicators of delirium, although he continued to experience fatigue. He died peacefully two days later.

Replacement of fluids by the *intravenous* route is more technically complicated, and access to a competent vein must be available. Some patients have permanent-access devices, placed for therapy earlier in their treatment, that are more than adequate for this type of administration. Others may wish to have a device placed. Use of a regular intravenous line for ongoing hydration at home can be hard to maintain; if ongoing parenteral fluids are required, placement of a central catheter or peripherally inserted central catheter (PICC) line is the norm in these situations. Small, portable pumps to regulate fluid flow are available for hydration of a patient in the inpatient or home setting. Some individuals choose to run fluids via the permanent-access devices only at night. This allows for more mobility during the daylight hours. There needs to be a competent caregiver to monitor the therapy, and because caregivers have many duties and responsibilties, this can be overwhelming to some.

Consensus on the appropriate volume or type of fluid replacement does not exist. Clinicians make choices based on their previous experience and knowledge of the patient's condition and wishes. Some practitioners allow the individual to have 1 L/day despite the fact that it is inadequate replacement. Considerations also include safety and reality of the care burden on all caregivers. Providing 1 L of fluid per day may only partially correct the patient's deficits, but it may relieve the emotional burden of needing to provide fluids. Administration of 1 L/day can often be worked into the patient's and family's schedule better. If fluids are given only at night, the patient may be more mobile during the day. Fluid administration can be scheduled to accommodate the goals of living. More aggressive fluid replacement often requires monitoring of serum electrolytes and blood counts by regular laboratory testing. This type of approach requires monitoring of laboratory results and making adjustments every 24 to 48 hours.

Patients and family members can be taught to manage hydration techniques at home. An assessment of their concerns should precede the instruction about the actual procedures. Adequate time must be allowed for education and return demonstration. Backup support should be provided, and repetitive sessions may be required. If possible, direct instruction to more than one caregiver should be provided to allow them to help each other with the tasks required. Printed materials that are age and reading level appropriate should be given. In addition, video instructions can be helpful, if they are available. Follow-up visits or calls should be scheduled to assess level of functioning, to give support, and to reinforce teaching. These therapies may mean more home visits to accommodate those who learn more slowly or are not able to master all or part of the procedure. Specific protocols vary among institutions and agencies; however, written policies and procedures should guide practice.

### Dry Mouth and Thirst

Other symptoms related to dehydration can be assessed and treated. In one study that looked at the impact of interventions besides hydration on the symptoms of dry mouth and thirst, the researchers found that routine care, defined as offering food and fluids, administering ice chips, and providing mouth care, helped to alleviate these symptoms.[18] Dry mouth is treated with an intensive, every-2-hour schedule of mouth care, including hygiene, lip lubrication, and ice chips or popsicles. Elimination of medications that cause dry mouth, such as tricyclic antidepressants and antihistamines, should be considered. Usually, however, the drugs that contribute to these symptoms are being administered to palliate other symptoms. Mouth breathing can also cause dry mouth. *Candida* infection, a frequent cause of dry mouth in the debilitated individual, can be treated. Agents such as pilocarpine (Salagen) can be used to increase salivation.

## NUTRITION

To observe an anorexic, fatigued, wasted, and debilitated patient is disheartening for the family. Food is more than nutrition; it plays an important role in maintaining hope. For those who are able to enjoy eating, every opportunity to offer nourishment should be taken. However, attempts at aggressive nutritional intervention for someone who is unable to eat may end up being frustrating for the family and add to the patient's suffering.[37]

Malnutrition is a common problem in patients with chronic, advanced, debilitating illnesses such as acquired immunodeficiency syndrome (AIDS) or cancer. *Anorexia*, a loss of appetite, occurs in most patients during the last weeks of life. *Cancer cachexia* is a complex syndrome characterized by loss of appetite, generalized tissue wasting, skeletal muscle atrophy, immune dysfunction, and a variety of metabolic alterations.[38,39] It is likely that *asthenia*, mental and physical fatigue coupled with generalized weakness, is directly related to malnutrition.[40–42]

Administration of nutrition in the terminally ill is sometimes proposed as a medical intervention for nutrition-related symptoms or management of side effects such as weight loss, weakness, constipation, pressure sores, intestinal obstruction, and dehydration. Nutritional intervention is also recommended to prevent further morbidity and to maintain quality of life by controlling blood sugars or electrolyte

**Table 13–4**
**Potential Complications of Enteral Support**

| Complication | Symptom | Cause |
|---|---|---|
| Aspiration | Coughing | Excess residual |
| | Fever | Large-bore tube |
| Diarrhea | Watery stool | Hyperosmotic solution |
| | | Rapid infusion |
| | | Lactose intolerance |
| Constipation | Hard, infrequent stools | Inadequate fluid |
| | | Inadequate fiber |
| Dumping syndrome | Dizziness | High volume |
| | | Hyperosmotic fluids |

imbalance. Lastly, nutritional therapy is offered to provide enough dietary intake to maintain energy.

Enteral and parenteral feedings are, however, interventions with the potential for associated morbidity and increased suffering (Table 13–4). The American Medical Directors Association (AMDA), a group that represents nursing home physicians, has published a white paper including a section that cautions against tube feeding in patients with advanced dementia unless they have clearly indicated their desire for such treatment. This group believes that there is no advantage to tube feeding and that less time is spent and fewer complications are encountered with hand feeding.[43] Until the literature is conclusive, the clinician must stay current with the research in this area.[44]

In cancer patients, anorexia is influenced by alterations in taste, alterations in the gastrointestinal system, changes in metabolism, and effects of the tumor itself. In addition, psychological factors such as depression or anxiety can change eating habits. Pain, fatigue, and nausea may also decrease the desire for oral intake. Many aspects of the cancer experience decrease caloric intake. Taste changes may result from the tumor itself or from various treatments such as chemotherapy, surgery, radiation, or antibiotics.[45] These taste changes may in turn decrease digestive enzymes and delay digestion.[46] The gastrointestinal tract may be altered by tumor, opportunistic infections such as *Candida*, or ulcerations resulting from chemotherapy or radiation that cause diarrhea. These alterations can interfere with ingestion, digestion, and absorption. Nausea and vomiting may ensue. Abnormalities in glucose metabolism, increases in circulating amino acids or lactic acid, and increases in free fatty acids can cause early satiety.[47] Increased blood sugar and serotonin levels in the brain may also decrease appetite.[48] In addition, cytokines such as interleukin-1 and tumor necrosis factor, released from tumors, may mediate anorexia and decrease gastric emptying.[49]

In other chronic illnesses, such as dementia, end-stage heart disease, chronic obstructive pulmonary disease, and advanced chronic kidney disease, loss of appetite is a common symptom, ranging in prevalence from 21% to 88%.[50–59] In end-stage dementia, patients lose the interest and ability to eat. Although, at first, dementia patients can ingest an adequate amount of food with assistance in feeding, in later stages there are increased feeding problems such as difficulties in chewing and swallowing, leading to choking and increased frequency of aspirations.[60] The patient with advanced chronic illness may have increased caloric needs due to changes in metabolism. The basal metabolic rate can be increased by infection or malignancy. Age, nutritional status, temperature, hormones, and trauma can also change the metabolic rate. Unlike healthy persons, these patients have no adaptation to a decrease in food intake; metabolism does not slow down. Cytokines increase resting energy expenditure and skeletal muscle wasting.[49] Nutrients that help to maintain immune function are decreased, and the resulting immunosuppression increases the risk of infection. Tumors invading the esophagus, stomach, or bowel can cause compression or obstruction and may limit oral intake. Surgery to remove tumors can remove all or part of the organs that produce digestive enzymes. This results in incomplete digestion. A shortened intestine reduces the number of villi available for absorption of nutrients.[47]

## Additional Research on Nutrition

Research on the use of nutrition, mainly artificial nutrition (AN) by enteral and parenteral methods, has been conducted on patients with cancer, ALS and dementia. It is standard practice to administer nutrition via percutaneous endoscopic gastrostomy (PEG) tube to patients being actively treated for head and neck cancers and in patients post acute stroke with dysphagia, as research has shown decreased morbidity and improved survival.[60] However, in an article reviewing 17 trials of patients with advanced cancer receiving parenteral nutrition, no trial showed a survival benefit.[61] For patients with amyotrophic lateral sclerosis (ALS), research has not shown an increase in quantity of life with nutrition via PEG; however, such nutritional support has been shown to help palliate by decreasing the effort to eat, improving fatigue, reducing the amount of time spent eating and taking medications, and reducing the fear of choking.[60]

In end-stage dementia patients, much research has looked at the impact of tube feeding on prolongation of life and control of distressing symptoms. Several studies looking at placement of a feeding tube in patients with advanced dementia found that survival was not associated with the intervention.[62,63] A review of the literature found that tube feeding did not: prevent aspiration of oral secretions or reduce risk of aspiration pneumonia; improve pressure sore outcomes; improve functional status or slow down the decline for demented patients with dysphagia; or make dysphagic demented patients more comfortable.[61] The same review documented adverse outcomes from tube feedings that included aspiration pneumonia, tube occlusion, leaking and local infection.

One study looking at use of medications to relieve symptoms in end-stage dementia patients for whom ANH was not initiated found that those patients used fewer medications for symptoms at end-of-life compared to other patients who received ANH, suggesting no increased suffering from the decision to forgo ANH.[20] In another study looking at providers' perceptions of end-stage dementia patients' general level of discomfort, the researchers found that in patients who did not initiate ANH, their levels of discomfort decreased from baseline.[64] Research to date has not documented improved survival outcomes for end stage diseases.

**Nutritional Assessment**

Within the framework of goals of care, disease status, and closeness to death, nutritional assessment starts with a diet history. The history should include the individual's usual dietary habits, current eating habits, and disease symptoms. Food preferences and aversions should be explored, as well as family support and the ability to obtain and prepare foods. The educational needs of the patient and of caregivers should also be assessed. A food diary may be helpful in this situation, and dietitians recommend a 72-hour history followed by weekly documentation. A physical examination to screen for changes in oral mucosa and dentition should be performed.

Anthropometric measurements are part of nutritional assessment. These are often limited in scope at the end stages of disease. A history of weight loss of 20% or greater is indicative of increased morbidity and mortality.[65] In the patient with advanced disease, weight gain may indicate the presence of edema or ascites, and weight loss may indicate dehydration. Other anthropometric measurements, such as skinfold thickness and midarm circumference, assess muscle and fat stores and can be used to monitor progress. Laboratory values are also used to estimate protein stores. These biochemical measurements are the mainstay for determining TPN. The appropriateness of each of these assessment parameters is determined on a case-by-case basis in the terminally ill.

**Nutritional Therapy**

Nutritional therapy is aimed at improving intake and managing cachexia. Increasing appetite is sometimes possible with pharmacological therapy. Steroids have been known to increase appetite, but their long-term use can cause muscle weakness. High-dose megestrol acetate has been shown to increase appetite with subsequent weight gain.[66,67] Hydrazine sulfate did not improve appetite more than placebo.[68] Metoclopramide, tetrahydrocannabinol, and insulin have resulted in some improvement, but toxicities were problematic and the data were often insufficient. Exercise has been shown to stimulate appetite; however, few end-stage patients are able to participate in the type of exercise that is necessary to increase appetite.

Nursing measures to promote oral intake include managing other symptoms (e.g., constipation, pain, nausea) that negatively affect appetite. In addition, patients may require more seasoning than usual for food to taste good. Good oral care and unhurried meals should be encouraged. Suggesting that the patient allow others to cook may preserve energy for eating as well as decrease the negative effects of food odors. Wine or beer has been known to stimulate appetite but may be poorly tolerated by terminally ill patients or those receiving multiple medications with sedating properties.

Enteral feedings use the gastrointestinal tract for delivery of nutrients, and oral supplementation of nutrients can be tried in individuals who have the capacity to swallow. Care must be taken, however, to monitor the use of these supplements. Caregivers and patients sometimes feel a moral obligation to provide food and "push" the supplements at the risk of harm to the patient, such as aspiration pneumonia or increased distress and decreased quality of life. Feedings may also be given through a NG tube, an esophagostomy tube, a gastrostomy tube, or a jejunostomy tube. In addition to the possibility of aspiration with enteral feedings, dumping syndrome, diarrhea, constipation, skin irritation at tube site insertion, and clogging of feeding tubes are potential complications. Finally, it is possible to provide nutrition parenterally. This approach may be useful for a small and carefully selected group of patients. However, TPN can be complicated by venous thrombosis, air embolism, infection, sepsis, hyperglycemia, hypoglycemia, and increased pain.

**Whether or Not to Provide Artificial Hydration and Nutrition at End of Life**

Controversy about providing hydration for terminally ill individuals stems from trying to balance the medical tradition of doing everything possible to heal and prolong life with the idea of allowing patients to die comfortably without unnecessary interventions. Empirical studies of clinical practice suggest that the setting of end-of-life care influences the use of artifical hydration at the end of life. Patients are more likely to receieve hydration if they are cared for in an acute care setting and are less likely to receive hydration if they are cared for in a hospice program.[69-73]

What is the role of medical intervention at the final stage of illness? In conventional medical management, dehydration is routinely avoided or reversed with fluid and electrolyte replacement. Similarly, whenever a terminally ill patient seeks to prolong life, and if the goal of care is to prolong life, maintaining hydration is accepted medical management. Conversely, if a terminally ill patient does not wish to delay death or even seeks to hasten dying, fluid replacement is generally inappropriate. Table 13–5 outlines the principles of ethical decision-making in regard to artificial hydration and nutrition in the terminally ill. Table 13–6 illustrates four clinical scenarios or paradigm cases that the nurse may encounter while caring for the terminally ill and that influence clinical decision-making.

Dehydration may aggravate or alleviate the discomfort of terminal disease (Table 13–7).[6] Current research does not clearly guide practice. Dehydration causes unpleasant symptoms, such as confusion and restlessness, in nonterminally ill patients. These problems are common in the dying.

**Table 13–5**

**Hydration and Nutrition in the Terminally Ill: Guiding Principles of Ethical Decision-Making**

- Everything in the terminal phase of an irreversible illness should be decided on the basis of whether it will make the patient more comfortable and whether it will honor his or her wishes.
- Treatments are evaluated principally according to their consequences—benefits and burdens, physical, psychosocial, and spiritual—weighed within the patient's value framework.
- Dehydration per se does not require treatment, but symptoms associated with dehydration do require palliation.
- When a patient is unable to express his or her wishes, advance directives or input from the health care proxy is followed.
- Although the focus is the patient, attention to the concerns and distress of the family is essential.

**Table 13–6**

**Nutrition and Hydration at the End of Life: Four Paradigm Cases**

**Paradigm case 1**

The dying patient who becomes too weak or too obtunded to maintain normal fluid intake, who will die soon but may die less comfortably and perhaps more quickly without rehydration.

**Paradigm case 2**

The terminally ill cancer patient who has an inoperable intestinal obstruction, feels hungry, and wants to be fed.

**Paradigm case 3**

The terminally ill patient whose inability to take oral food or fluid is precipitated by, or partially the result of, palliative medical management: for example, the patient who is sedated in an attempt to manage a refractory symptom such as pain, dyspnea, or agitated delirium.

**Paradigm case 4**

The dying patient who voluntarily stops eating and drinking in order to hasten death.

**Table 13–7**

**Hydration and Rehydration at the End of Life: Potential Effects**

| Body System | Effects of Dehydration | Effects of Rehydration |
|---|---|---|
| General appearance | Sunken eyes | Improved appearance |
| Mouth | Decreased saliva | Oral comfort |
| | Thirst | Relief of thirst |
| | Bad lasted | Improved taste |
| | Dry, cracked lips | |
| Pulmonary | Dry airway, viscous secretions | Facilitates productive cough |
| | Reduced death rattle | Easer suctioning |
| | Reduced secretions, cough | |
| | Reduced congestion, wheezing, dyspnea, pleural effusions | |
| Gastrointestinal tract | Constipation | More normal bowel function |
| | Decreased secretions | |
| | Less vomiting, diarrhea | |
| | Anorexia | |
| | Reduced ascites | Ascites |
| Urinary tract | Reduced renal function | Improved renal drug clearance |
| | Edema | Reduced toxic metabolites |
| | Possible drug accumulation | May need more drug administration |

*Source:* Billings (1998), reference 7.

Dehydration can cause renal failure with an accompanying accumulation of opioid metabolites, which causes further symptoms, such as myoclonus and even seizures. Dehydration is also associated with constipation and increased risk of bedsores. Clinicians report that these symptoms are mild and easily treated without hydration and that some symptoms, such as increased secretions, are actually made worse by rehydration.[6,10,30] Hospice nurses have reported that the dehydrated patient is not uncomfortable.[74,75] There is concern that artificial hydration diminishes quality of life by adding tubes, which create a physical barrier that separates the terminally ill from their loved ones. There is often fear that hydration unnecessarily prolongs dying. Those clinicians who support the use of hydration point to the prevention or relief of some symptoms, such as delirium.[11,16,27] Patients and families may be making decisions based on inadequate knowledge or misconceptions about artificial hydration, such as the idea that it is helpful at any stage of disease or that it can increase strength.[76]

As with hydration, there is some controversy with regards to providing artificial nutrition at end of life. Most recent is the case of Terry Schiavo, who lived in a persistent vegetative state for 15 years because she was supported by ANH. In cases such as hers, it is clear that death results from the cessation of fluids and nutrition. It is not as clear that the provision of AN for most end-stage diseases actually prolongs life; however, AN may improve the quality of someone's life through palliating symptoms or psychological distress associated with a decreasing appetite.

Because food and fluids are viewed by many as a symbol of life, not to maintain fluids or to withdraw artificial hydration and nutrition at the end of life may cause spiritual or emotional conflict. These issues are complex and involve not only physical, psychological, and social concerns, but also individual ethical dilemmas. The decision to administer artificial hydration and nutrition should be discussed within the framework of a patient's goals of care and expectations of treatment, taking into consideration the person's culture, values and religious beliefs.

## Summary

We inherit beliefs that govern our behavior. Among them are numerous contradictory notions that associate support with sustenance. Attitudes, preferences, and decisions may be influenced by race, gender, and culture.[77] The rites of family meals and celebrations provide bonding and sharing as well as food—fundamental components of personal and social life. The issues of hydration and nutrition at the end of life are complex and require a thoughtful, individualized approach.[78] Nurses and physicians are guided to institute or withdraw artificial hydration or nutrition based on the ethical principles of autonomy, beneficence and nonmaleficence.[79,80] Provision of accurate and complete information by the nurse can influence a patient's and family's decisions about these matters.

REFERENCES

1. Ganzini L, Goy E, Miller LL, Harvarth TA, Jackson A, Delorit MA. Nurses' experiences with hospice patients who refuse food and fluids to hasten death. N Engl J Med 2003;349:359–365.
2. Rolls BJ, Phillips PA. Aging and disturbances of thirst and fluid balance. Nutr Rev 1990;48:137–144.
3. Smith SA. Patient-induced dehydration: Can it ever be therapeutic? Oncol Nurs Forum 1995;22:1487–1491.
4. Rolls BJ, Wood RJ, Rolls ET. Thirst following water deprivation in humans. Am J Physiol 1980;8:R476–R482.
5. Weinberg AD, Minaker KL. Council on Scientific Affairs, American Medical Association. Dehydration evaluation and management in older adults. JAMA 1995;274:1552–1556.
6. Billings JA. Comfort measures for the terminally ill: Is dehydration painful? J Am Geriatr Soc 1985;33:808–810.
7. Billings JA. Dehydration. In: Billings JA, Berger A, Portenoy R, Weissman D, eds. Principles and Practice of Supportive Oncology. Philadelphia: Lippincott-Raven, 1998:589–601.
8. Sweeney MP, Bragg J. The mouth and palliative care. Am J Hosp Palliat Care 2000;17:118–124.
9. Phillips PA, Rolls BJ, Ledingham JG, et al. Reduced thirst after water deprivation in healthy elderly men. N Engl J Med 1984;311:753–759.

10. Burge FI. Dehydration symptoms of palliative care cancer patients. J Pain Symptom Manage 1993;8:454–464.
11. del Rosario B, Martin AS. Hydration for control of syncope in palliative care. J Pain Symptom Manage 1997;14:5–6.
12. MacDonald N. Ethical issues in dehydration and nutrition. In: Bruera E, Portenoy RK, eds. Topics in Palliative Care (Vol 2). New York: Oxford University Press, 1998:153–169.
13. Fainsinger RL, Bruera E. Hypodermoclysis for symptom control versus the Edmonton Injector. J Palliat Care 1991;7:5–8.
14. Fainsinger R, Bruera E. The management of dehydration in terminally ill patients. J Palliat Care 1995;10:55–59.
15. Hanks G, Cherny N, Fallon M. Opioid analgesic therapy. In: Doyle D, Hanks G, Cherny N, Calman K, eds. Oxford Textbook of Palliative Medicine (3rd ed). Oxford, England: Oxford University Press, 2004:316–341.
16. Waller A, Hershkowitz M, Adunsky A. The effect of intravenous fluid infusion on blood and urine parameters of hydration and on state of consciousness in terminal cancer patients. Am J Hospice Palliat Care 1994;11:22–27.
17. Morita T, Hyodo I, Yoshimi T, et al. Artificial hydration therapy, laboratory findings, and fluid balance in terminally ill patients with abdominal malignancies. J Pain Symptom Manage 2006;31:130–139.
18. McCann RM, Hall WJ, Groth-Juncker A. Comfort care for terminally ill patients: The appropriate use of nutrition and hydration. JAMA 1994;272:1263–1266.
19. Dalal S, Bruera E. Dehydration in cancer patients: To treat or not to treat. J Support Oncol 2004;2:467–479.
20. Buiting HM, can Delden JM, Rietjens JAC, et al. Forgoing artificial nutrition or hydration in patients nearing death in six European countries. J Pain Symptom Manage 2007; 34:305–314.
21. Hoefler JM. Making decisions about tube feeding for severely demented patients at the end of life: Clinical, legal, and ethical considerations. Death Stud 2000;24:233–254.
22. Ellershaw JE, Sutcliffe JM, Saunders CM. Dehydration and the dying patient. J Pain Symptom Manage 1995;10:192–197.
23. Fainsinger R, MacEachern T, Miller MJ, et al. The use of hypodermoclysis for rehydration in terminally ill cancer patients. J Pain Symptom Manage 1994;9:298–302.
24. Cerchietti L, Navigante A, Sauri A, Pallazo F. Hypodermoclysis. Int J Palliat Nurs 2000;6:370–374.
25. Fainsinger RL, Bruera E. When to treat dehydration in a terminally ill patient. Support Care Cancer 1997;5:205–211.
26. Yan E, Bruera E. Parenteral hydration of the terminally ill. J Palliat Care 1991;7:40–43.
27. Bruera E, Franco JJ, Maltoni M, Watanabe S, Suarez-Almazor M. Changing pattern of agitated impaired mental status in patients with advanced cancer: Association with cognitive monitoring, hydration, and opioid rotation. J Pain Symptom Manage 1995;10:287–291.
28. Morita T, Tei Y, Inoue S. Agitated terminal delirium and association with partial opioid substitution and hydration. J Palliat Med 2003;6:557–563.
29. Bruera E, Sala R, Rico MA, Moyano J, Centeno C, Willey J, Palmer JL. Effects of parenteral hydration in terminally ill cancer patients: A preliminary study. J Clin Oncol 2005;23:2366–2371.
30. Zerwekh J. The dehydration question. Nursing 1983;13:47–51.
31. Printz LA. Is withholding hydration a valid comfort measure in the terminally ill? Geriatrics 1988;43:84–88.

32. Collard T, Rapin CH. Dehydration in dying patients: Study with physicians in French-speaking Switzerland. J Pain Symptom Manage 1991;6:230–240.

33. Mercadante S, Ferrera P, Girelli D, Casuccio A. Patients' and relatives' perceptions about intravenous and subcutaneous hydration. J Pain Symptom Manage 2005;30:354–358.

34. Kemp C. Dehydration, fatigue and sleep. In: Kemp C, ed. Terminal Illness: A Guide to Nursing Care (2nd ed). Philadelphia: Lippincott, 1999:205–210.

35. Bruera E, Pruvost M, Schoeller T, Montejo G, Watanabe S. Proctoclysis for hydration of terminally ill cancer patients. J Pain Symptom Manage 1998;8:454–464.

36. Berger EY. Nutrition by hypodermoclysis. J Am Geriatr Soc 1984; 32:199–203.

37. Cimino JE. The role of nutrition in hospice and palliative care of the cancer patient. Top Clin Nutr 2003;18:154–161.

38. Rivadeneira DE, Envoy D, Fahey TJ, Lieberman MD, Daly JM. Nutritional support of the cancer patient. CA Cancer Clin 1998; 48:69–80.

39. Costa G. Cachexia, the metabolic component of neoplastic diseases. Cancer Res 1977;37:2327–2335.

40. Neuenschwander H, Bruera E. Asthenia. In: Doyle D, Hanks GWC, MacDonald N, eds. Oxford Textbook of Palliative Medicine (2nd ed). New York: Oxford University Press, 1998:573–581.

41. Bruera E. Clinical management of cachexia and anorexia in patients with advanced cancer. Oncology 1992;49(Suppl 2):35–42.

42. Storey P. Symptom control in advanced cancer. Semin Oncol 1994;21:748–753.

43. American Medical Directors Association. White Paper on Surrogate Decision-Making and Advanced Care Planning In Long-Term Care, 2003. Available at: http://www.amda.com/governance/whitepapers/surrogate/surrogate.pdf (accessed December 29, 2008).

44. Meares C. Nutritional issues in palliative care. Semin Oncol Nurs 2000;16:135–145.

45. Bender CM. Taste alterations. In: Yasko JM, ed. Nursing Management of Symptoms Associated with Chemotherapy (3rd ed). Columbus, Ohio: Adria Laboratories, 1993:67–74.

46. Kesner DL, DeWys WD. Anorexia and cachexia in malignant disease. In: Newell GR, Ellison NM, eds. Nutrition and Cancer: Etiology and Treatment. New York: Raven Press, 1981:303–317.

47. Tait NS. Anorexia-cachexia syndrome. In: Groenwald SL, Frogge MH, Goodman M, Yarbro CH, eds. Cancer Symptom Management. Boston: Jones and Bartlett, 1997:171–185.

48. Grant M, Ropka ME. Alterations in nutrition. In: Baird S, McCorkle R, Grant M, eds. Cancer Nursing: A Comprehensive Textbook. Philadelphia: WB Saunders, 1991:717–741.

49. Moldawer LL, Rogy MA, Lowry SF. The role of cytokines in cancer cachexia. J Parenter Nutr 1992;16(Suppl):43s–49s.

50. Cartwright JC, Hickman S, Perrin N, Tilden V. Symptom experiences of residents dying in assisted living. J Am Med Dir Assoc 2006;7:219–223.

51. Cohen LM, Moss AH, Weisbord SD, Germain MJ. Renal palliative care. J Palliat Med 2006;9:977–992.

52. Kutner JS, Bryant LL, Beaty BL, Fairclough DL. Time course and characteristics of symptom distress and quality of life at the end of life. J Pain Symptom Manage 2007;34:227–236.

53. Kutner JS, Kassner CT, Nowels DE. Symptom burden at the end of life: Hospice providers' perceptions. J Pain Symtom Manage 2001;21:473–480.

54. Nordgren L, Sörensen S. Symptoms experienced in the last six months of life in patients with end-stage heart failure. Eur J Cardiovasc Nurs 2003;2:213–217.

55. O'Mahony S, Blank A, Simpson J, et al. Preliminary report of a palliative care and case management project in an emergency department for chronically ill elderly patients. J Urban Health 2008;85:443–451.

56. Solano JP, Gomes G, Higginson IJ. A comparison of symptom prevalence in far advanced cancer, AIDS, heart disease, chronic obstructive pulmonary disease and renal disease. J Pain Symptom Manage 2006;31:58–69.

57. Tilden VP, Tolle SW, Drach LL, Perrin NA. Out-of-hospital death: Advance care planning, decedent symptoms, and caregiver burden. J Am Geriatr Soc 2004;52:532–539.

58. Tranmer JE, Heyland D, Dudgeon D, Groll D, Squires-Graham M, Coulson K. Measuring the symptom experience of seriously ill cancer and noncancer hospitalized patients near the end of life with the Memorial Symptom Assessment Scale. J Pain Symptom Manage 2003;25:420–429.

59. Walke LM, Byers AL, Tinetti ME, Dubin JA, McCorkle R, Fried TR. Range and severity of symptoms over time among older adults with chronic obstructive pulmonary disease and heart failure. Arch Intern Med 2007;167:2503–2508.

60. Ganzini L. Artificial nutrition and hydration at the end of life: Ethics and evidence. Palliat Support Care 2006:4;135–143.

61. Finucane TE, Christmas C, Travis K. Tube feeding in patients with advanced dementia. JAMA 1999;282:1365–1370.

62. Meier, D, Ahronheim, JC, Morris J, Baskin-Lyons, S, Morrison, RS. High short-term mortality in hospitalized patients with advanced dementia: Lack of benefit of tube feeding. Arch Intern Med 2001;61:594–599.

63. Murphy LM, Lipman TO. Percutaneous endoscopic gastrostomy does not prolong survival in patients with dementia. Arch Intern Med 2003;163:1351–1353.

64. Pasman HRW, Onwuteaka-Philipsen BR, Kriegsman DMW, Ooms ME, Ribbe MW, van der Wal G. Discomfort in nursing home patients with severe dementia in whom artificial nutrition and hydration is forgone. Arch Intern Med 2005;165:1729–1735.

65. Bernard M, Jacobs D, Rombeau J. Nutrient requirements. In: Bernard M, Jacobs J, Romeau D, eds. Nutritional and Metabolic Support of Hospitalized Patients. Philadelphia: WB Saunders, 1986:11–45.

66. Tchekmedyian NS, Hickman M, Siau J, Greco FA, Keller J, Browder H, Aisner J. Megestrol acetate in cancer anorexia and weight loss. Cancer 1992;69:1268–1274.

67. Schmoll E, Wilke H, Thole R, Preusser P, Wildfang I, Schmoll HJ. Megestrol acetate in cancer cachexia. Semin Oncol 1991;18(Suppl 2):32–34.

68. Loprinzi CL, Goldberg RM, Su JQ, et al. Placebo-controlled trial of hydrazine sulfate in patients with newly diagnosed non small-cell lung cancer. J Clin Oncol 1994;11:1126–1129.

69. Asch DA, Faber-Langendoen K, Shea JA, Christakis NA. The sequence of withdrawing lifesustaining treatment from patients. Am J Med 1999;107:153–156.

70. Faber-Langendoen K. A multi-institutional study of care given to patients dying in hospitals: Ethical and practical implications. Arch Intern Med 1996;156:2130–2136.

71. Wilson D. A report of an investigation of end-of-life care practices in health care facilities and the influences on those practices. J Palliat Care 1997;13:34–40.

72. Zerzan J, Stearns S, Hanson L. Access to palliative care and hospice in nursing homes. JAMA 2000;284:2489–2494.

73. Lanuke K, Fainsinger RL, deMoissac D. Hydration management at the end of life. J Palliat Care 2004;7:257–263.

74. Andrews M, Bell ER, Smith SA, Tischler JF, Veglia JM. Dehydration in terminally ill patients: Is it appropriate palliative care? Postgrad Med 1993;93:201–208.

75. Andrews MR, Levine AM. Dehydration in the terminal patient: Perception of hospice nurses. Am J Hospice Care 1989;1:31–34.

76. Chiu TC, Hu WY, Chuang RB, Cheng YR, Chen CY, Wakai S. Terminal cancer patients' wishes and influencing factors toward the provision of artificial nutrition and hydration in Taiwan. J Pain Symptom Manage 2004;27:206–214.

77. Phipps E, True G, Harris D, Cong U, Tester W, Chavin SI, Braitman LE. Approaching the end of life: Attitudes, preferences, and behaviors of African-American and white patients and their family caregivers. J Clin Oncol 2003;21:549–554.

78. Daly B. Special challenges of withholding artificial nutrition and hydration. J Gerontol Nurs 2000;26:25–31.

79. Day L, Drought T, Davis AJ. Principle-based ethics and nurses' attitudes towards artificial feeding. J Adv Nurs 1995; 21:295–298.

80. Slomka J. Withholding nutrition at the end of life: Clinical and ethical issues. Cleve Clin J Med 2003;70:548–552.

# 14 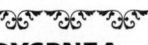 *Deborah Dudgeon*

# Dyspnea, Death Rattle, and Cough

*Have you ever choked on something and not been able to get your breath? That's what it feels like for me all of the time!—A patient*

*I can't go into the room. It sounds like she's drowning!!—A family member*

*At times I cough so much I vomit. I'm exhausted!—A patient*

---

◆ **Key Points**

◆ *Dyspnea is a subjective experience.*

◆ *Tachypnea is not dyspnea.*

◆ *Patients can be very frightened when breathless.*

◆ *Nursing and medical interventions are helpful for patients with dyspnea.*

◆ *Death rattle is common in dying patients.*

◆ *Death rattle is very distressing for people at the bedside.*

◆ *Family members need to receive good teaching and reassurance about death rattle.*

◆ *Anticholinergics are the drugs of choice for death rattle.*

◆ *Chronic cough can be very debilitating.*

◆ *Massive hemoptysis is very frightening and needs to be anticipated.*

◆ *Pharmacological and nonpharmacological interventions can help patients with chronic cough.*

## DYSPNEA

Dyspnea is a very common symptom in people with advanced disease and can severely impair their quality of life. The presence of dyspnea correlates with the probability of dying in the hospital.[1] In one international study, dyspnea prompted the use of terminal sedation in 25% to 53% of patients.[2] Management of breathlessness requires understanding and assessment of the multidimensional components of the symptom, knowledge of the pathophysiological mechanisms and clinical syndromes that are common in people with advanced disease, and knowledge of the indications and limitations of the available therapeutic approaches.

### Definition

The American Thoracic Society has defined *dyspnea* as the "term used to characterize a subjective experience of breathing discomfort that consists of qualitatively distinct sensations that vary in intensity."[3] Dyspnea, like pain, is multidimensional in nature, with not only physical elements but also affective components, which are shaped by previous experience.[4,5] In COPD, a neurophysiological model describes the variety of mechanisms that can lead to dyspnea: receptor → afferent impulse → integration/processing in the central nervous system (CNS) → efferent impulse → dyspnea.[5] Stimulation of a number of different receptors (Figure 14–1), and the conscious perception this stimulation invokes, can alter ventilation and result in a sensation of breathlessness.[4,5] It is proposed that dyspnea results from a "mismatch" between the afferent information to the CNS and the outgoing motor command to the respiratory muscles. This mismatch is called "neuroventilatory dissociation" or "afferent–efferent dissociation."[4]

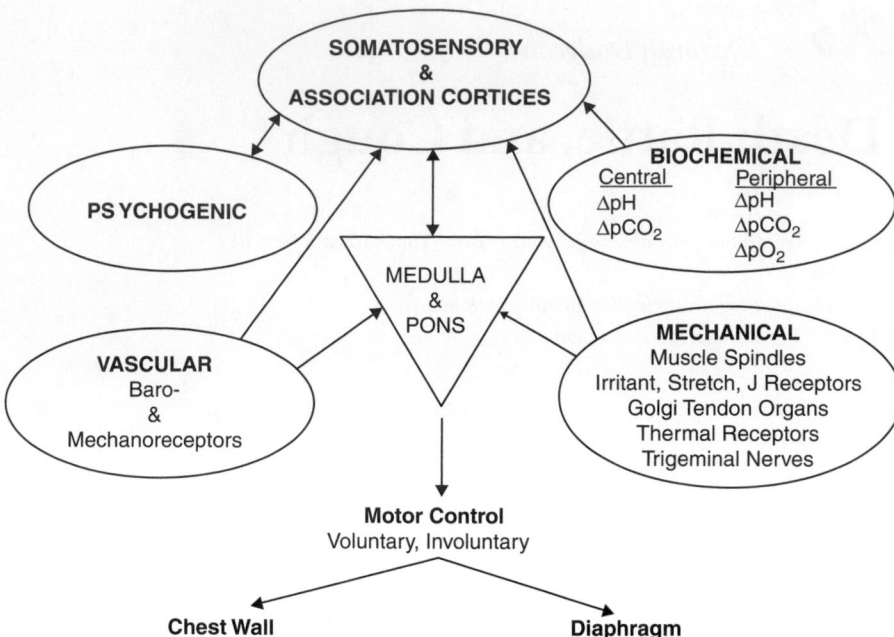

**FIGURE 14–1.** Schematic diagram of the neuroanatomical elements involved in the control of ventilation.

## Prevalence and Impact

The prevalence of the dyspnea varies according to the stage and type of underlying disease and the methodological design of the studies.[6] A systematic review of symptom prevalence in advanced cancer, AIDS, heart disease, chronic obstructive pulmonary disease (COPD) and renal disease found the prevalence of dyspnea was 10%–70% in patients with cancer, 11%–62% with AIDS, 60%–88% in heart disease, 90%–95% in COPD and 11%–62% in renal disease.[6] In a prospective study of 400 patients with inoperable lung cancer, the intensity of dyspnea was higher in patients closer to death and difficulties breathing was ranked as the most distressing among these patients.[7] Another study of patients with end-stage chronic obstructive pulmonary disease (COPD) found that 95% of the participants experienced extreme breathlessness and that it was the most distressing and debilitating symptom.[8] Dyspnea is also quite prevalent in people with advanced congestive heart failure (CHF): 56.3% experience dyspnea, 53.4% have it "frequently" or "almost constantly," 25.9% describe it as "severe" or "very severe," and 43.1% describe the distress associated with it as "quite a bit" or "very much."[9] Likewise, dyspnea occurs in 37% of patients with cerebrovascular accident (of whom 57% were breathless for >6 months)[10]; in 47% to 50% of patients with amyotrophic lateral sclerosis (ALS); and in 70% of those with dementia.[11]

In a study of late-stage cancer patients, Roberts and associates[12] used patient self-report surveys, chart audits of patients under the care of a hospice program, and interviews of patients and nurses in a home-care hospice program to examine the occurrence of dyspnea during the last weeks of

life. They found that 62% of the patients with dyspnea had been short of breath for >3 months. Various activities intensified dyspnea for these patients: climbing stairs, 95.6%; walking slowly, 47.8%; getting dressed, 52.2%; talking or eating, 56.5%; and resting, 26.1%. The patients universally responded by decreasing their activity to whatever degree would relieve their shortness of breath. Most of the patients had received no direct medical or nursing assistance with their dyspnea, leaving them to cope in isolation. Brown and colleagues[13] found that 97% of lung cancer patients studied had decreased their activities, and 80% believed they had socially isolated themselves from friends and outside contacts to cope with their dyspnea. Studies in patients with COPD, CVA, or end-stage heart or neurological diseases have also demonstrated the presence of significant dyspnea and other symptoms, functional disability, and impaired quality of life in the last year of their lives.[8,10,11,14,15]

Patients with advanced disease typically experience chronic shortness of breath with intermittent acute episodes.[13,16] Acute attacks of breathlessness are usually accompanied by feelings of anxiety, fear, panic, and, if severe enough, a sensation of impending death.[16] Patients and family members who were participants in a qualitative study using narrative analysis consistently expressed fear of dying during a future acute episode of breathlessness, or of watching helplessly as a loved one became increasingly breathless and died before receiving any help.[17] Many dying persons are terrified of waking in the middle of the night with intense air hunger.[18] They need providers who will anticipate their fears and provide symptomatic relief of their breathlessness and anxiety as they approach death.[17,18]

## Pathophysiology

Management of dyspnea of patients requires an understanding of its multidimensional nature and the pathophysiologic mechanisms that cause this distressing symptom. Exertional dyspnea in cardiopulmonary disease (Table 14–1) is caused by (1) increased ventilatory demand, (2) impaired mechanical responses, or (3) a combination of the two.[19] The effects of abnormalities of these mechanisms can also be additive.

## Increased Ventilatory Demand

Ventilatory demand is increased because of increased physiological dead space resulting from reduction in the vascular bed (from thromboemboli, tumor emboli, vascular obstruction, radiation, chemotherapy toxicity, or concomitant emphysema); hypoxemia and severe deconditioning with early metabolic acidosis (with excessive hydrogen ion stimulation); alterations in carbon dioxide output ($Vco_2$) or in the arterial partial pressure of carbon dioxide ($Pco_2$) set point; and

---

**Table 14–1**
**Pathophysiologic Mechanisms of Dyspnea**

**Increased ventilatory demand**
Increased physiological dead space

- Thromboemboli
- Tumor emboli
- Vascular obstruction
- Radiation therapy
- Chemotherapy
- Emphysema

Severe deconditioning
Hypoxemia
Change in $V_{CO_2}$ or arterial $P_{CO_2}$ set point
Psychological: anxiety, depression
Increased neural reflex activity

**Impaired mechanical response/ventilatory pump impairment**
Restrictive ventilatory deficit
  Respiratory muscle weakness

- Cachexia
- Electrolyte imbalances
- Peripheral muscle weakness
- Neuromuscular abnormalities
- Neurohumoral
- Steroids

  Pleural or parenchymal disease
  Reduced chest wall compliance
Obstructive ventilatory deficit

  Asthma
  Chronic obstructive pulmonary disease
  Tumor obstruction

Mixed obstructive/restrictive disorder (any combination of the above)

---

nonmetabolic sources, such as increased neural reflex activity, or psychological factors such as anxiety and depression.

### Impaired Mechanical Response/Ventilatory Pump Impairment

Impaired mechanical responses result in restrictive ventilatory deficits due to inspiratory muscle weakness,[20] pleural or parenchymal disease, or reduced chest wall compliance; airway obstruction from coexistent asthma or COPD, or tumor obstruction. Patients may also have a mixed obstructive and restrictive disorder.

### Multidimensional Assessment of Dyspnea

Dyspnea, like pain, is a subjective experience that may not be evident to an observer. *Tachypnea*, a rapid respiratory rate, is not dyspnea. Medical personnel must learn to ask for and accept the patient's assessments, often without measurable physical correlates. If patients say they are having discomfort with breathing, we must believe that they are dyspneic.

To determine whether dyspnea is present, it is important to ask more than the question, "Are you short of breath?" Patients often respond in the negative to this simple question because they have limited their activities so they won't become short of breath. It is therefore helpful to ask about shortness of breath in relationship to activities: "Do you get short of breath walking at the same speed as someone of your age?" "Do you have to stop to catch your breath when walking upstairs?" "Do you get short of breath when you are eating?"

### Qualitative Aspects of Dyspnea

Dyspnea is not a single sensation. Recent work suggests that the sensation of breathlessness encompasses several qualities.[21] Just as the descriptions "burning" or "numb" suggest neuropathic pain, phrases such as "chest tightness," "exhalation," and "deep" were among a cluster of words associated with asthma.[21] It is possible that dyspnea mediated by similar receptors evokes common word descriptors. From the research to date, it is not known whether qualitative assessments of dyspnea in breathless patients permit any discrimination among the various cardiopulmonary disorders. O'Donnell and coworkers[22–24] found that, although descriptor choices were clearly different between health and disease states, they provided no discrimination among various diseases (e.g., COPD, restrictive lung disease, and CHF). Others have suggested that changes in the quality of dyspnea may prompt patients with heart failure to go to the emergency department.[25]

### Clinical Assessment

Clinical assessments are usually directed at determining the underlying pathophysiology, deciding appropriate treatment, and evaluating the response to therapy.

The clinical assessment of dyspnea should include a complete history of the symptom, including its temporal onset (acute or chronic), whether it is affected by positioning, its qualities, associated symptoms, precipitation and relieving events or activities, and response to medications. A past history of smoking, underlying lung or cardiac disease, concurrent medical conditions, allergy history, and details of previous medications or treatments should be elicited.[26,27]

Careful physical examination focused on possible underlying causes of dyspnea should be performed. Particular attention should be directed at signs associated with certain clinical syndromes that are common causes of dyspnea. Examples are the dullness to percussion, decreased tactile fremitus, and absent breath sounds associated with a pleural effusion in a person with lung cancer; an elevated jugular venous pressure (JVP), audible third heart sound ($S_3$), and bilateral crackles audible on chest examination associated with CHF; and elevated JVP, distant heart sounds, and pulsus paradoxus in people with pericardial effusions.[26,27]

Gift and colleagues[28] studied the physiological factors related to dyspnea in subjects with COPD and high, medium, and low levels of breathlessness. There were no significant differences in respiratory rate, depth of respiration, or peak expiratory flow rates at the three levels of dyspnea. There was, however, a significant difference in the use of accessory muscles between patients with high and low levels of dyspnea, suggesting that this is a physical finding that reflects the intensity of dyspnea.

Diagnostic tests helpful in determining the cause of dyspnea include chest radiography; electrocardiography; pulmonary function tests; arterial blood gases; complete blood counts; serum potassium, magnesium, and phosphate levels; cardiopulmonary exercise testing; and tests specific for suspected underlying pathologies, such as an echocardiogram for suspected pericardial effusion.[26] The choice of appropriate diagnostic tests should be guided by the stage of disease, the prognosis, the risk/benefit ratios of any proposed tests or interventions, and the desires of the patient and family.

Nguyen and colleagues[29] found that the ratings of intensity of dyspnea during laboratory exercise, clinical measures of dyspnea such as the Oxygen Cost Diagram, and pulmonary function tests captured distinctly different information in patients with moderate to severe COPD. It is therefore not surprising that results of pulmonary function tests do not necessarily reflect the intensity of a person's dyspnea. Individuals with comparable degrees of functional lung impairment may also experience considerable differences in the intensity of dyspnea they perceive.[5] Factors such as adaptation, differing physical characteristics, and psychological conditions can modulate both the quality and the intensity of the person's perception of breathlessness.

The Visual Analog Scale (VAS) is one of the most popular techniques for measuring the perceived intensity of dyspnea. This scale is usually a 100-mm vertical or horizontal line, anchored at each end by words such as "Not at all breathless" and "Very breathless." Subjects are asked to mark the line at the point that best describes the intensity of their breathlessness. The scales can be used as an initial assessment, to monitor progress, and to evaluate effectiveness of treatment in an individual patient.[30] Numeric rating scales (NRS) are highly correlated with VAS ratings of breathlessness[31] and more repeatable measures that require a smaller sample size to detect a change in breathlessness.[31]

The modified Borg scale is a scale with nonlinear spacing of verbal descriptors of severity of breathlessness.[32] Patients are asked to pick the verbal descriptor that best describes their perceived exertion during exercise. It is usually used in conjunction with an exercise protocol with standardized power output or metabolic loads. When used in this manner, the slope of the Borg descriptors over time is very reproducible and reliable, permitting comparisons within individuals and across population groups.[33,34]

The Reading Numbers Aloud test was designed as an objective measure of the activity-limiting effect of breathlessness in people with cancer who were breathless at very low levels of exertion.[35,36] The test involves asking subjects to read a grid of numbers as quickly and clearly as possible for 60 seconds. The number of numbers read and the number read per breath are recorded.

In a systematic review of the usefulness of different assessment tools to measure breathlessness, Bausewein and colleagues[31] concluded that no one scale accurately reflected the effects of breathlessness on the patient with advanced disease and their family. They recommended that for general clinical questions, a VAS or modified Borg Scale were most useful; multidimensional tools if the focus was on quality of life; breathlessness-specific questionnaires if the focus was the sensation or functional impact of breathlessness; and a combination of instruments or methods (qualitative and quantitative) in a research setting.

## Dyspnea and Psychological Factors

The person's perception of the intensity of his or her breathlessness is also affected by psychological factors. Anxious, obsessive, depressed and dependent persons appear to experience dyspnea that is disproportionately severe relative to the extent of their pulmonary disease.[5] Gift and colleagues[28] found that anxiety was higher during episodes of high or medium levels of dyspnea, compared with low levels of dyspnea. Kellner and associates[37] found in multiple-regression analyses that depression was predictive of breathlessness. Studies in cancer patients by Dudgeon and Lertzman[20,38] and others[39–41] have also shown that anxiety is significantly correlated with the intensity of dyspnea ($r = 0.3$) but explains only 9% of the variance in the intensity of breathlessness. These studies were done in people with chronic dyspnea and when the person was at rest. Carrieri-Kohlman and colleagues[42] found higher correlations between dyspnea intensity and anxiety associated with dyspnea at the end of exercise ($r = 0.49$). It is also probable that anxiety is a more prominent factor during episodes of acute shortness of breath.

Table 14-2
**Management of Dyspnea**

Sit upright supported by pillows or leaning on overbed table
Fan +/- oxygen
Relaxation techniques and other appropriate
    nonpharmacological measures
Identify and treat underlying diagnosis (if appropriate)
Pharmacologic Management
Chronic
    Opioids
    Add phenothiazine (chlorpromazine, promethazine)
Acute
    Opioids
    Add anxiolytic

## Management

The optimal treatment of dyspnea is to treat reversible causes. If this is no longer possible, then both nonpharmacological and pharmacological methods are used (Table 14–2).

### Pharmacological Interventions

*Opioids.* Since the late 19th century, opioids have been used to relieve breathlessness of patients with asthma, pneumothorax, and emphysema.[43] Although most trials have demonstrated the benefit of opioids for the treatment of dyspnea,[43–53] some have been negative[54–57] or have produced undesirable side effects.[46,54]

In 2001, a systematic review examined the effectiveness of oral or injectable opioid drugs for the palliative treatment of breathlessness.[58] The authors identified 18 randomized, double-blind, controlled trials comparing the use of any opioid drug against placebo for the treatment of breathlessness in patients with any illness. In the studies involving non-nebulized routes of administration,[43,45,51,57,59–61] there was statistically strong evidence for a small effect of oral and parenteral opioids for the treatment of breathlessness.[58] Two recently published systematic reviews also support the use of oral or parenteral opioids for the management of dyspnea in cancer patients.[62,63]

In recent years, there has been tremendous interest in the use of nebulized opioids for the treatment of dyspnea. Opioid receptors are present on sensory nerve endings in the airways;[64] therefore, it is hypothesized that if the receptors were interrupted directly, lower doses, with less systemic side effects, would be required to control breathlessness. The 2001 systematic review[58] identified nine randomized, double-blind, controlled trials comparing the use of nebulized opioids or placebo for the control of breathlessness.[65–73] The authors concluded that there was no evidence that nebulized opioids were more effective than nebulized saline in relieving breathlessness.[58] In a recent double-blind, controlled, crossover study of the effects of nebulized hydromorphone, systemic hydromorphone and nebulized saline were compared for the relief of incident dyspnea in advanced cancer patients. Over time, breathlessness decreased significantly with all treatments and there weren't any significant differences between the treatments.[74] Although this study did not rule out the possibility that people's dyspnea improved because they stopped the activity that precipitated it, the results suggest that nebulized saline is an effective treatment for dyspnea. It is hard to justify the continued use of nebulized opioids.

Physicians have been reluctant to prescribe opioids for dyspnea since the potential for respiratory failure was recognized in the 1950s.[75] The 2001 systematic review of opioids for breathlessness identified 11 studies that contained information on blood gases or oxygen saturation after intervention with opioids.[58] Only one study reported a significant increase in the arterial partial pressure of carbon dioxide ($PaCO_2$), but it did not rise above 40 mm Hg.[59] In studies of cancer patients, morphine did not compromise respiratory function as measured by respiratory effort and oxygen saturation[44,45,76] or respiratory rate and $PaCO_2$.[44] In another study, authors found the patients' intensity of dyspnea and respiratory rates decreased significantly ($P = 0.003$) after the administration of an opioid, but there was no significant change in the transcutaneous arterial pressure of $CO_2$.[77] It is now known that the development of clinically significant hypoventilation and respiratory depression from opioids depends on the rate of change of the dose, the history of previous exposure to opioids, and possibly the route of administration.[78] Early use of opioids improves quality of life and allows the use of lower doses, while tolerance to the respiratory depressant effects develops.[79] Twycross[80] suggested that early use of morphine or another opioid, rather than hastening death in dyspneic patients, might actually prolong survival by reducing physical and psychological distress and exhaustion.

*Sedatives and Tranquilizers.* Chlorpromazine decreases breathlessness without affecting ventilation or producing sedation in healthy subjects.[81] Woodcock and colleagues[82] found that promethazine reduced dyspnea and improved exercise tolerance of patients with severe COPD. O'Neill and associates[81] did not find that promethazine improved breathlessness in healthy people, nor did Rice and coworkers[54] find that it benefited patients with stable COPD. McIver and colleagues[83] found that chlorpromazine was effective for relief of dyspnea in advanced cancer. The systematic review by Viola and colleagues concluded that promethazine could be used orally as an alternative when systemic opioids couldn't be employed.[62]

The results of clinical trials to determine the effectiveness of anxiolytics for the treatment of breathlessness have also been quite variable. Two studies showed that diazepam was effective in treating dyspnea,[82,84] and one showed a reduction in dyspnea.[85] Greene and colleagues[86] reported an improvement in dyspnea with alprazolam; however, a randomized, placebo-controlled, double-blind study did not find any relief of dyspnea with alprazolam.[87] Clorazepate was not found to be effective for breathlessness.[88] Buspirone, a nonbenzodiazepine anxiolytic, had no effect on pulmonary function tests or arterial blood gases in patients with COPD, but improved exercise tolerance and decreased dyspnea.[89] This drug warrants further study.

*Combinations.* In a double-blind, placebo controlled, randomized trial, Light and colleagues[60] studied the effectiveness of morphine alone, morphine and promethazine, and morphine and prochlorperazine for the treatment of breathlessness in patients with COPD. The combination of morphine and promethazine significantly improved exercise tolerance without worsening dyspnea, compared with placebo, morphine alone, or the combination of morphine and prochlorperazine.[60] Ventafridda and colleagues[90] also found the combination of morphine and chlorpromazine to be effective. In a randomized, single-blinded study, dyspneic cancer patients were given subcutaneous doses of: morphine routinely, every 4 hours, with breakthrough midazolam; routine midazolam with breakthrough morphine; or a routine dose of both midazolam and morphine.[91] After 24 hours, the patients who received the routine doses of morphine and midazolam had significantly less dyspnea with apparently no greater levels of sedation.

*Other Medications.* Indomethacin reduced exercise-induced breathlessness in a group of normal adults,[92] but no benefit was obtained in patients with diffuse parenchymal lung disease[93] or COPD.[94] Although inhaled bupivacaine reduced exercise-induced breathlessness in normal volunteers,[95] it failed to decrease breathlessness of patients with interstitial lung disease.[96] Inhaled lidocaine did not improve dyspnea in six cancer patients.[97] Dextromethorphan did not improve breathlessness of patients with COPD.[98] None of these medications can be recommended for the treatment of dyspnea at this time.

A recent review of nebulized furosemide for the management of dyspnea found encouraging results in patients with asthma, COPD and cancer with further study recommended.[99]

### Nonpharmacological Interventions

*Oxygen.* In hypoxic patients with COPD, oxygen supplementation improves survival, pulmonary hemodynamics, exercise capacity, and neuropsychological performance.[100] Guidelines for oxygen use in this setting are shown in Table 14–3. The usefulness of oxygen to relieve breathlessness in the person with refractory dyspnea is less clear.[101] In a Cochrane review (2008) to determine if oxygen therapy provided relief of dyspnea in chronic end-stage disease, Cranston and colleagues[102] identified 8 cross-over studies that met their inclusion criteria. There were 144 participants (97 cancer, 35 cardiac failure and 12 kyphoscoliosis). In the patients with cancer: the meta-analysis failed to demonstrate a signficant improvement of dyspnea at rest when oxygen was compared with air inhalation; improvement in dyspnea with oxygen inhalation was independent of resting hypoxia; and they perceived an improvement in dyspnea with inhalation of oxygen

---

| Table 14–3 |
| --- |
| **Guidelines for Oxygen Therapy** |

**Continuous oxygen**

$PaO_2 \leq 55$ mm Hg or oxygen saturation $\leq 88\%$ at rest

$PaO_2$ of 56 to 59 mm Hg or oxygen saturation of 89% in the presence of the following:

    Dependent edema suggesting congestive heart failure
    Cor pulmonale
    Polycythemia (hematocrit > 56%)
    Pulmonary hypertension

**Noncontinuous oxygen is recommended during exercise:**

$PaO_2 \leq 55$ mm Hg or oxygen saturation $\leq 88\%$ with a low level of exertion, or during sleep

$PaO_2$ of $\leq 55$ mm Hg or oxygen saturation $\leq 88\%$ associated with pulmonary hypertension, daytime somnolence and cardiac arrhythmias[100]

---

at rest and during exercise. In cardiac failure participants, high concentration oxygen provided relief of dyspnea at six minutes during exercise tests, but low-flow ambulatory oxygen during a submaximal exercise test did not provide relief. In a single study of oxygen inhalation during exercise in participants with kyphoscoliosis, oxygen improved dyspnea. The authors of this systematic review stated that their outcomes were inconclusive.[102] In a subsequent randomized, double-blind, crossover trial of the effect of oxygen versus air on the relief of dyspnea in 51 cancer patients, Philip and colleagues[103] found the mean sensation of dyspnea improved with both air and oxygen, with no significant differences in either VAS or patient preference between treatments. The 17 hypoxic patients also did not report a mean greater improvement with, or preference for, oxygen over air, despite improved oxygen saturations in all but 4 patients. The authors concluded that either air or oxygen via nasal prongs improved breathlessness.[103]

*Pleural Effusions.* Whether a malignant pleural effusion requires treatment is determined by the degree of symptomatic compromise, the stage of the disease, the patient's life expectancy, and the patient's estimated tolerance for more aggressive therapeutic approaches.[104,105] At the time of initial diagnostic or therapeutic tap of the pleural effusion, the removal of 1000 to 1500 mL of pleural fluid helps predict response to further therapies.[105] If symptoms are not relieved and the lung does not reexpand, then further thoracenteses or insertion of a chest tube is unlikely to be of any benefit, and treatment should include medications to relieve symptoms. In 97% of cases, fluid reaccumulates within 1 month after thoracentesis alone.[106] Repeated thoracenteses increase the risk for pneumothorax, empyema, and pleural fluid loculation and therefore should be limited to people with a short life span. Traditionally, tube thoracostomy was performed with large-bore chest tubes connected to wall suction; this treatment necessitated hospitalization and limited mobility, with substantial discomfort and expense.

Recent studies have shown the effectiveness of small-bore catheters and indwelling small pleural catheters in the outpatient setting.[107–109]

Instillation of any of several sclerosing agents into the pleural space after adequate drainage by tube thoracostomy creates a chemical pleuritis that obliterates the pleural space and prevents pleural fluid reaccumulation. Because pleurodesis is often painful, intrapleural lidocaine is administered before the instillation of the sclerosing agent to reduce local pain. Patients also should be premedicated and should have adequate analgesic available after the procedure.

*Pericardial Effusion.* As in all other situations, the approach to management of a pericardial effusion depends on the person's stage of disease, the prognosis, the potential benefits and complications, and the wishes of the patient and family. If pericardial tamponade with hemodynamic compromise is present and treatment is appropriate, an emergency pericardiocentesis is indicated, with aggressive intravenous fluid support and possible administration of a sympathomimetic agent to temporize.[110] Hemodynamic improvement usually occurs with removal of 50 to 100 mL of pericardial fluid. Continuous drainage can be achieved by placement of an indwelling pigtail catheter or creation of a pericardial window, or by percutaneous balloon pericardotomy.[111,112] Pericardial drainage can be followed by instillation of a sclerosing agent to obliterate the pericardial space.[113] Radiation or systemic chemotherapy could be considered if appropriate.[113]

### Nursing Interventions

Many patients obtain relief of dyspnea by leaning forward while sitting and supporting their upper arms on a table. This technique is effective in patients with emphysema,[114] probably because of an improved length-tension state of the diaphragm, which increases efficiency.[115]

Pursed-lip breathing slows the respiratory rate and increases intra-airway pressures, thus decreasing small airway collapse during periods of increased dyspnea.[116] Mueller and coworkers[48] found that pursed-lip breathing led to an increase in tidal volume and a decrease in respiratory rate at rest and during exercise in 7 of 12 COPD patients experiencing an improvement in dyspnea. Pursed-lip breathing reduces dyspnea in about 50% of patients with COPD.[117]

People who are short of breath often obtain relief by sitting near an open window or in front of a fan. Cold directed against the cheek[118] or through the nose[119,120] can alter ventilation patterns and reduce the perception of breathlessness, perhaps by affecting receptors in the distribution of the trigeminal nerve that are responsive to both thermal and mechanical stimuli.[118,119]

Randomized controlled trials support the use of acupuncture and acupressure to relieve dyspnea in patients with moderate to severe COPD.[121,122] Acupuncture provided marked symptomatic benefit in breathlessness and in respiratory rate in patients with cancer-related breathlessness.[123] Other randomized controlled trials support the use of muscle relaxation with breathing retraining to reduce breathlessness in COPD patients.[124,125]

Corner and colleagues[126] found that weekly sessions with a nurse research practitioner over 3 to 6 weeks, using counseling, breathing retraining, relaxation, and coping and adaptation strategies, significantly improved breathlessness and ability to perform activities of daily living compared with controls. Carrieri and Janson-Bjerklie[127] found that patients used self-taught relaxation to help control their breathlessness. Others have found that formal muscle relaxation techniques decrease anxiety and breathlessness.[128] Guided imagery[129] and therapeutic touch[130] resulted in significant improvements in quality of life and sense of well-being in patients with COPD and patients with terminal cancer, respectively, but without any significant improvement in breathlessness.

Nursing actions that intubated patients thought helpful included friendly attitude, empathy, providing physical support, staying at the bedside, reminding or allowing patients to concentrate on changing their breathing pattern, and providing information about the possible cause of the breathlessness and possible interventions.[131]

### Patient and Family Teaching

Carrieri and Janson-Bjerklie[127] identified strategies patients used to manage acute shortness of breath. These strategies could be taught to patients and their families. Patients benefited from keeping still with positioning techniques, such as leaning forward on the edge of a chair with arms and upper body supported, and using some type of breathing strategy, such as pursed-lip or diaphragmatic breathing. Some of the patients distanced themselves from aggravating factors, and others used self-adjustment of medications. Several subjects isolated themselves from others to gain control of their breathing and diminish the social impact. Others used structured relaxation techniques, conscious attempts to calm down, and prayer and meditation. The study of Carrieri and Janson-Bjerklie[127] and another by Brown and colleagues[13] demonstrated that most subjects reported some changes in activities of living, such as changes in dressing and grooming, avoidance of bending or stooping, advanced planning or reduction in activities, staying in a good frame of mind, avoidance of being alone, and acceptance of the situation.

Patients and families should be taught about the signs and symptoms of an impending exacerbation and how to manage the situation. They should learn problem-solving techniques to prevent panic, ways of conserving energy, how to prioritize activities, use of fans, and ways to maximize the effectiveness of their medications, such as using a spacer with inhaled drugs or taking an additional dose of an inhaled beta-agonist before exercise.[132] Patients should avoid activities in which their arms are unsupported, because these activities often increase breathlessness.[128]

Patients in distress should not be left alone. Social services, nursing, and family input need to be increased as the patient's ability to care for himself or herself decreases.[133]

CASE STUDY
*Mrs. P, A 58-Year-Old Woman with Dyspnea*

You are called to the room of Mrs. P and find her sitting at the bedside, gasping for breath. You know that Mrs. P is a 58-year-old woman with advanced non-small cell lung cancer. She has a large lung mass in the right hilar region which has received maximum radiation treatment. She says that she has been unable to lie flat for a number of months and describes a progressive onset of worsening breathlessness with less and less activity. She says that she had gone to the washroom to have a sponge bath and, while combing her hair, got quite breathless and struggled to make it back to her bed. While getting an overbed table and pillow for her to rest on, you calmly instruct her to take slow, deep breaths and to use the breathing technique that you had previously taught her. You note that she is cyanosed and institute oxygen and fan to help relieve her breathlessness. On further examination, you notice that her face is quite puffy. She has bilaterally elevated JVP's, distended vessels on her anterior chest and, when you raise her arm, her veins do not collapse until her hand is over her head. With institution of the oxygen, fan, and focused breathing, you note that she is slightly less distressed, but you ask her husband to stay with her while you prepare a dose of prn morphine. On your return 5 minutes later, Mrs. P's breathing has further improved but is still a little labored, so you administer the morphine. Her husband stays with her, and 15 minutes later, when you return, he has helped her back into bed, where she is resting comfortably.

## Summary

Dyspnea is a very common symptom in people with advanced disease. The symptom is often unrecognized and patients, therefore, receive little assistance in managing their breathlessness. Dyspnea can have profound effects on a person's quality of life, because even the slightest exertion may precipitate breathlessness.

# DEATH RATTLE

Noisy, rattling breathing in patients who are dying is commonly known as death rattle. This noisy, moist breathing can be very distressing for the family, other patients, visitors, and health care workers, because it may appear that the person is drowning in his or her own secretions.[134] Management of death rattle can present health care providers a tremendous challenge as they attempt to ensure a peaceful death for the patient.[135]

## Definition

*Death rattle* is a term applied to describe the noise produced by the turbulent movements of secretions in the upper airways that occur with the inspiratory and expiratory phases of respiration in patients who are dying.[136]

## Prevalence and Impact

Death rattle occurs in 23% to 92% of patients in their last hours before death.[136–142] Studies have shown that there is an increased incidence of respiratory congestion in patients with primary lung cancer,[138,141] cerebral metastases,[141,143] pneumonia, and dysphagia,[142] with the symptom more likely to persist in cases with pulmonary pathology.[141] The incidence of death rattle increases closer to death;[141] the median time from onset of death rattle to death is 8 to 23 hours.[139–141] Most commonly, this symptom occurs when the person's general condition is very poor, and most patients have a decreased level of consciousness.[141] If the person is alert, however, the respiratory secretions can cause him or her to feel very agitated and fearful of suffocating. Despite the identification of "noisy breathing" as a problem in 39% of patients dying in a long-term care setting, 49% of them received no treatment.[144] In one study of the attitudes of palliative care nurses about the impact of death rattle, 13% thought that death rattle distressed the dying patient; 100% thought it distressed the dying person's relatives, with 52% indicating that bereaved relatives had mentioned death rattle as a source of distress; and 79% thought that death rattle distressed nurses.[135] A qualitative study involving hospice staff and volunteers found that most participants had negative feelings about hearing the sound of death rattle and thought that relatives were distressed by it as well.[145] Studies of bereaved relatives, however, found that not all were distressed by the sound, and this was, in part, determined by whether the person appeared disturbed or if they saw fluid dribbling from the person's mouth.[146,147]

## Pathophysiology

The primary defense mechanism for the lower respiratory tract is the mucociliary transport system. This system is a protective device that prevents the entrance of viruses, bacteria, and other particulate matter into the body.[148–150] The surface of the respiratory tract is lined with a liquid sol phase near the epithelium and a superficial gel phase in contact with the air.[148] Ciliated epithelial cells, located at all levels of the respiratory tract except the alveoli and the nose and throat, are in constant movement to propel the mucus up the respiratory tract, to be either subconsciously swallowed or coughed out. The mucus is produced by submucosal glands, which are under neural and humoral control. The submucosal glands are under parasympathetic, sympathetic, and noncholinergic, nonadrenergic nervous control. Resting glands secrete approximately 9 mL/min., but mechanical, chemical, or pharmacological stimulation (via vagal pathways) of the airway epithelium can augment gland secretion. Surface goblet cells also produce mucus secretions, which can be increased with irritant stimuli (e.g., cigarette smoke). The secretory flow rate and amount, as well as the viscoelastic properties of the mucus, can be altered.[148]

The audible breathing of the so-called death rattle is produced when turbulent air passes over or through pooled secretions in the oropharynx or bronchi. The amount of turbulence depends on the ventilatory rate and airway resistance.[143] Mechanisms of death rattle include excessive secretion of respiratory mucus, abnormal mucus secretions inhibiting normal clearance, dysfunction of the cilia, inability to swallow, decreased cough reflex due to weakness and fatigue, and the supine, recumbent position. Factors that may contribute to respiratory congestion include infection or inflammation, pulmonary embolism producing infarction and fluid leakage from damaged cells, pulmonary edema or CHF,[150] dysphagia, and odynophagia. Although it has been suggested that a state of relative dehydration decreases the incidence of problematic bronchial secretions,[151] Ellershaw and colleagues[138] found no statistically significant difference in the incidence of death rattle in a biochemically dehydrated group of patients, compared with a group of hydrated patients.

Bennett[143] proposed two types of death rattle. Type 1 involves mainly salivary secretions, which accumulate in the last few hours of life when swallowing reflexes are inhibited. Type 2 is characterized by the accumulation of predominantly bronchial secretions over several days before death as the patient becomes too weak to cough effectively. This characterization has been empirically supported by Morita and colleagues[141] and therefore may prove useful to determine appropriate treatment.

## Assessment

Assessment of death rattle includes a focused history and physical examination to determine potentially treatable underlying causes. If the onset is sudden and is associated with acute shortness of breath and chest pain, it might suggest a pulmonary embolism or myocardial infarction. Physical findings consistent with CHF and fluid overload might support a trial of diuretic therapy; the presence of pneumonia indicates a trial of antibiotic therapy. The effectiveness of interventions should be included in the assessment. The patient's and family's understanding and emotional response to the situation should also be assessed so that appropriate interventions can be undertaken.

A recently developed and validated assessment tool, the Victoria Respiratory Congestion Scale (VRCS),[152] is clinically useful to determine the effectiveness of interventions. This instrument rates the congestion on a scale from 0 to 3, with 0 indicating no congestion heard at 12 inches from the chest; 1 indicating congestion audible only at 12 inches from the chest; 2 indicating congestion audible at foot of patient's bed; and 3 indicating congestion audible at door of patient's room. This scale has demonstrated interrater reliability

($\kappa = 0.53$, $P < 0.001$) and concurrent validity with a noise meter ($P < 0.001$). It was weakly correlated with a caregiver distress scale ($\kappa = 0.24$, $P < 0.001$).

## Management

### Pharmacological Interventions

Primary treatment should be focused on the underlying disorder, if appropriate to the prognosis and the wishes of the patient and family. If this is not possible, then anticholinergics are the primary mode of treatment. Hyoscine hydrobromide (scopolamine), atropine sulfate, hyoscine butylbromide (Buscopan), and glycopyrrolate (Robinul) are the anticholinergic agents that are used to treat death rattle. Anticholinergic drugs can prevent vagally induced increased bronchial secretions, but they reduce basal secretions by only 39%.[148] A recent evidence-based guideline stated that there is insufficient evidence to support the use of one drug over another, and that the decision should be based on the drug characteristics and the needs of the patient.[153]

*Hyoscine hydrobromide (scopolamine)* is the primary medication used for the treatment of death rattle. It inhibits the muscarinic receptors and causes anticholinergic actions such as decreased peristalsis, gastrointestinal secretions, sedation, urinary retention, and dilatation of the bronchial smooth muscle. It is administered subcutaneously, intermittently or by continuous infusion, or transdermally.[137,138,143,154] In one study,[155] hyoscine hydrobromide 0.4 mg subcutaneously was immediately effective and only 6% of the patients required repeated doses. In an open label study of the treatment of death rattle, 56% of patients who received hyoscine hydrobromide had a significantly reduced noise level after 30 minutes, compared with 27% of patients who had received glycopyrrolate ($P = 0.002$).[134] In other studies, between 22% and 65% of patients did not respond to hyoscine hydrobromide, and secretions recurred from 2 to 9 hours after the injection.[137] In a retrospective study of 100 consecutive deaths in a 22-bed hospice, 27% of patients received an infusion of hyoscine hydrobromide, with 5 of 17 requiring injections despite receiving an infusion.[143]

*Atropine sulfate* is another anticholinergic drug that is preferred by some centers for the treatment of respiratory congestion.[150] In a study of 995 doses of atropine, congestion was decreased in 30% of patients, remained the same in 69%, and increased in 1%.[150] Atropine is the drug of choice of this group, because it results in less CNS depression, delirium, and restlessness, with more bronchodilatory effect, than hyoscine hydrobromide. There is, however, the risk of increased tachycardia with atropine sulfate when doses >1.0 mg are given. Hyoscine hydrobromide is thought to have a more potent effect on bronchial secretions than atropine does,[136] but no comparative trials have been conducted in the palliative population.

*Glycopyrrolate (Robinul)* is also an anticholinergic agent. It has the advantages of producing less sedation and agitation and a longer duration of action than hyoscine hydrobromide.

In two studies in which its effectiveness was compared with that of hyoscine hydrobromide, glycopyrrolate was not as effective in controlling secretions.[134,137] However, others have disputed this finding and suggest it is also more cost-effective.[156] Glycopyrrolate is available in an oral form and can be useful for patients at an earlier stage of disease, when sedation is not desired.

*Hyoscine butylbromide* (Buscopan) is another anticholinergic drug, but it has not been evaluated for its effectiveness in this condition. It is available in injection, suppository, and tablet forms.

## Nonpharmacological Interventions

There are times when the simple repositioning of the patient may help him or her to clear the secretions (Table 14–4). Suctioning usually is not recommended, because it can be very uncomfortable for the patient and causes significant agitation and distress. Pharmacological measures are usually effective and prevent the need for suctioning. If the patient has copious secretions that can easily be reached in the oropharynx, then suctioning may be appropriate. In a study conducted at St. Christopher's Hospice, suctioning was required in only 3 of 82 patients to control the secretions.[138] In another study, 31% of the patients required only nursing interventions with reassurance, change in position, and occasional suctioning to manage respiratory congestion in the last 48 hours of life.[155]

## Patient and Family Teaching

The patient and the family can be very distressed by this symptom. It is important to explain the process, to help them understand why there is a buildup of secretions and that there is something that can be done to help. The Victoria Hospice group suggests using the term "respiratory congestion" as opposed to "death rattle," "suffocation," or "drowning in sputum," because these terms instill strong emotional reactions.[150] When explaining to families the changes that can occur before death, this is one of the symptoms that should be mentioned. If the person is being treated at home, the family should be instructed as to the measures available to relieve

---

| Table 14–4 |
| --- |
| **Management of "Death Rattle"** |
| Change position |
| Reevaluate if receiving IV hydration |
| Pharmacological management |
|   Chronic |
|     Glycopyrrolate or hyoscine hydrobromide patch |
|     *If treatment fails:* subcutaneous hyoscine hydrobromide or atropine sulfate |
|   Acute |
|     Subcutaneous hyoscine hydrobromide or subcutaneous atropine sulfate |

---

death rattle and to notify their hospice or palliative care team if it occurs, so that appropriate medications can be ordered.

CASE STUDY
### Mrs. S, A 60-Year-Old Woman with Metastatic Breast Cancer

When you start your shift and are walking down the hallway, you hear a loud gurgling noise as you pass Mrs. S's room. You enter and find her family surrounding the bed and looking extremely distressed. Mrs. S. has very advanced metastatic breast cancer to lung, bones, and brain. Her condition has deteriorated markedly over the past few days. She is very restless and is pulling at the intravenous line that is running at 125 mL/h. There are audible gurgling sounds as she breathes, with diffuse crackles throughout her chest, and 3+ pitting edema of all of her limbs. Her daughter, in tears, says, "It sounds like she is choking to death! Please do something!" While you help to reposition Mrs. S, you explain why this is happening and suction some of the mucus that has accumulated in her mouth. You go to the desk and get an order from the doctor for some furosemide, to change the intravenous line to a saline lock, and for an "as needed" dose of hyoscine hydrobromide subcutaneously. You administer the furosemide, but there is minimal improvement; therefore, you give Mrs. S an injection of hyoscine hydrobromide, and within 20 minutes she has settled.

## Summary

Although death rattle is a relatively common problem in people who are close to death, very few studies have evaluated the effectiveness of treatment. Anticholinergics are the drugs of choice at this time. Death rattle can be a very distressing for family members at the bedside, and they need to receive good teaching and reassurance.

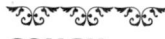

# COUGH

Cough is a natural defense of the body to prevent entry of foreign material into the respiratory tract. In people with advanced disease, it can be very debilitating, leading to sleepless nights, fatigue, pain and, at times, pathological fractures.

## Definition

*Cough* is an explosive expiration that can be a conscious act or a reflex response to an irritation of the tracheobronchial tree. Cough lasting 8 weeks is considered chronic.[154] A *dry cough* occurs when no sputum is produced; a *productive cough* is one in which sputum is raised. *Hemoptysis* occurs when the sputum contains blood. *Massive hemoptysis* is expectoration of at least 100 to 600 mL of blood in 24 hours.[155]

## Prevalence and Impact

Chronic cough is a common problem; recurrent cough is reported by 3% to 40% of the population.[157] In population surveys, men report cough more frequently than women do, but women appear to have an intrinsically heightened cough response.[157] Cough is often present in people with advanced diseases such as bronchitis, CHF, uncontrolled asthma, human immunodeficiency virus infection, and various cancers. In a study of 289 patients with non-small cell lung cancer, cough was the most common symptom (>60%) and the most severe symptom at presentation.[158] Eighty percent of the group had cough before death. Over time, cough and breathlessness were much less well controlled than the other symptoms in this group of patients.

In a study of 25 advanced cancer patients designed to evaluate treatment of cough, 88% of patients rated their cough as moderate or severe and 68% coughed >10 times per day.[159] Cough was found to interfere with breathing, sleep, and speech, and was associated with coughing spasms, pain, nausea, and vomiting.[159]

In patients with lung cancer, hemoptysis is the presenting symptom 7% to 10% of the time, 20% have it at some time during their clinical course, and 3% die of massive hemoptysis.[160] The mortality rate of massive hemoptysis in patients with lung cancer can be as high as 59% to 100%.[160]

## Pathophysiology

Cough is characterized by a violent expiration, with flow rates that are high enough to sheer mucus and foreign particles away from the larynx, trachea, and large bronchi. The cough reflex can be stimulated by irritant receptors in the larynx and pharynx or by pulmonary stretch receptor, irritant receptor, or C-fiber stimulation in the tracheobronchial tree.[161] Different mechanisms are involved in isolation or together in patients with cough of various causes.[162] The vagus nerve carries sensory information from the lung that initiates the cough reflex. Infection can physically or functionally strip away epithelium, exposing sensory nerves and increasing the sensitivity of these nerves to mechanical and chemical stimuli. It is also thought that inflammation produces prostaglandins, which further increase the sensitivity of these receptors, leading to bronchial hyperreactivity and cough. When cough is associated with increased sputum production, it probably results from stimulation of the irritant receptors by the excess secretion.[161] Cough is associated with respiratory infection, bronchitis, rhinitis, postnasal drip, esophageal reflux, medications including angiotensin-converting enzyme inhibitors,[161] asthma, COPD, pulmonary fibrosis, CHF, pneumothorax, bronchiectasis, and cystic fibrosis.[163] In the person with cancer, cough may be caused by any of these conditions; however, direct tumor effects (e.g.,

obstruction), indirect cancer effects (e.g., pulmonary emboli), and cancer treatment effects (e.g., radiation therapy) could also be the cause.[164]

Hemoptysis can result from bleeding in the respiratory tract anywhere from the nose to the lungs. It varies from blood streaking of sputum to coughing up of massive amounts of blood. There are multiple causes of hemoptysis, but some of the more common ones are a tracheobronchial source, secondary to inflammation or tumor invasion of the airways; a pulmonary parenchymal source, such as pneumonia or abscess; a primary vascular problem, such as pulmonary embolism; a miscellaneous cause, such as a systemic coagulopathy resulting from vitamin K deficiency, thrombocytopenia, or abnormal platelet function secondary to bone marrow invasion with tumor, sepsis, or disseminated intravascular coagulation; or an iatrogenic cause, such as use of anticoagulants, nonsteroidal antiinflammatory drugs, or acetylsalicylic acid.[165]

## Assessment

In assessing someone with cough, it is important to do a thorough history and physical examination. Because cough may arise from anywhere in the distribution of the vagus nerve, the full assessment of a patient with a chronic cough requires a multidisciplinary approach with cooperation between respiratory medicine, gastroenterology, and ear, nose, and throat (ENT) departments.[157] The assessment helps to determine the underlying cause and appropriate treatment of the cough. Depending on the diagnosis, the prognosis, and the patient's and family's wishes, it may be appropriate to perform diagnostic tests, including chest or sinus radiography, spirometry before and after bronchodilator and histamine challenge, and, in special circumstances in people with earlier-stage disease, upper gastrointestinal endoscopy and 24-hour esophageal pH monitoring. In patients with significant hemoptysis, bronchoscopy is usually needed to identify the source of bleeding.

In the history and physical examination, one should look for a link between cough and the associated factors listed in the previous section, whether the cough is productive, the nature of the sputum, the frequency and amount of blood, precipitating and relieving factors, and associated symptoms.

## Management

It is important to base management decisions on the cause and the appropriateness of treating the underlying diagnosis, compared with simply suppressing the symptom. This decision is based on the diagnosis, prognosis, side effects, and possible benefits of the intervention, and the wishes of the patient and family. Management strategies also depend on whether the cough is productive (Table 14–5). Theoretically, cough suppressants, by causing mucus retention, could be harmful in conditions with excess mucus production.[161]

> **Table 14-5**
> **Treatment of Non-Productive Cough**
>
> Nonopioid antitussive (dextromethorphan, benzonatate)
> Opioids
> Inhaled anesthetic (lidocaine, bupivacaine)

## Pharmacological Interventions

Antitussive drugs can be divided into two categories: centrally acting agents (opioids and nonopioids) and peripherally acting agents (which directly or indirectly act on cough receptors).[160]

## Centrally Acting Antitussives

*Opioids* suppress cough, but the dose is higher than that contained in the proprietary cough mixtures.[161] The exact mode of action is unclear, but it is thought that opioids inhibit the mu receptor peripherally in the lung; act centrally by suppressing the cough center in the medulla or the brainstem respiratory centers; or stimulate the mu receptor, thus decreasing mucus production or increasing mucus ciliary clearance.[161] Codeine is the most widely used opioid for cough; some authors claim that it has no advantages over other opioids and provides no additional benefit to patients already receiving high doses of opioids for analgesia,[166] whereas others state that the various opioids have different antitussive potencies.[160]

More than 200 synthetic *nonopioid antitussive agents* are available; most are less effective than codeine.[167] Dextromethorphan, a dextro isomer of levorphanol, is an exception; it is almost equiantitussive to codeine. Dextromethorphan acts centrally through nonopioid receptors to increase the cough threshold.[166] Benzonatate is a nonopioid antitussive with a sustained cough-depressing action[168] that provided excellent symptomatic relief for three cancer patients with opioid-resistant cough.[169] Opioid and nonopioid antitussives may act synergistically,[166] but further studies are needed to confirm this hypothesis.

## Peripherally Acting Antitussives

*Demulcents* are a group of compounds that form aqueous solutions and help to alleviate irritation of abraded surfaces. They are often found in over-the-counter cough syrups. Their mode of action for controlling cough is unclear, but it is thought that the sugar content encourages saliva production and swallowing, which leads to a decrease in the cough reflex; that they stimulate the sensory nerve endings in the epipharynx, and decrease the cough reflex by a "gating" process; or that demulcents may act as a protective barrier by coating the sensory receptors.[161]

*Benzonatate* is an antitussive that inhibits cough mainly by anesthetizing the vagal stretch receptors in the bronchi, alveoli, and pleura.[160] Other drugs that act directly on cough receptors include levodropropizine, oxalamine, and prenoxdiazine.[160]

Inhaled anticholinergic *bronchodilators*, either alone or in combination with $\beta_2$-adrenergic agonists, effectively decrease cough in people with asthma and in normal subjects.[170] It is thought that they decrease input from the stretch receptors, thereby decreasing the cough reflex, and change the mucociliary clearance.

The local anesthetic lidocaine is a potent suppressor of irritant-induced cough and has been used as a topical anesthetic for the airway during bronchoscopy. *Inhaled local anesthetics*, such as lidocaine and bupivacaine, delivered by nebulizer, suppress some cases of chronic cough for as long as 9 weeks.[161,171-173] Higher doses can cause bronchoconstriction, so it is wise to observe the first treatment. Patients must also be warned not to eat or drink anything for 1 hour after the treatment or until their cough reflex returns.

There are a number of treatments for cough which are under investigation including: newer opioids, neurokinin receptor antagonists, gamma-aminobutyric acid receptor agonists, cannabinoid $CB_2$ receptor agonists, compounds that block the transient receptor potential channels and other compounds that open potassium channels.[163]

## Productive Coughs

Interventions for productive coughs include chest physiotherapy, oxygen, humidity, and suctioning. In cases of increased sputum production, expectorants, mucolytics, and agents to decrease mucus production can be employed.[160] Opioids, antihistamines, and anticholinergics decrease mucus production and thereby decrease the stimulus for cough.

## Massive Hemoptysis

In patients with massive hemoptysis, survival is so poor that patients may not want any kind of intervention to stop the bleeding; in such cases, maintenance of comfort alone becomes the priority. For those patients who want intervention to stop the bleeding, the initial priority is to maintain a patent airway, which usually requires endotracheal intubation. Management options include endobronchial tamponade of the segment, vasoactive drugs, iced saline lavage, neodymium/yttrium-aluminum-garnet (Nd/YAG) laser photocoagulation, electrocautery, bronchial artery embolization, and external beam or endobronchial irradiation.[160]

## Nonpharmacological Interventions

If cough is induced by a sensitive cough reflex, then the person should attempt to avoid the stimuli that produce this. They should stop or cut down smoking and avoid smoky rooms, cold air, exercise, and pungent chemicals. If medication is causing the cough, it should be decreased or stopped if possible. If the cause is esophageal reflux, then elevation of the head of the bed may be tried. Adequate hydration, humidification of the air, and chest physiotherapy may help patients expectorate viscid sputum.[174] Radiation therapy to enlarged nodes, endoscopically placed esophageal stents for tracheoesophageal fistulas, or injection of Teflon into a paralyzed vocal cord may improve cough.[174]

## Patient and Family Education

Education should include practical matters such as proper use of medications, avoidance of irritants, use of humidification, and ways to improve the effectiveness of cough. One such way is called "huffing." The person lies on his or her side, supports the abdomen with a pillow, blows out sharply three times, holds the breath, and then coughs. This technique seems to improve the effectiveness of a cough and helps to expel sputum.

If the patient is having hemoptysis and massive bleeding is a possibility, it is important to educate the family about this possibility, to prepare them psychologically and develop a treatment plan. Dark towels or blankets can help to minimize the visual impact of this traumatic event. Adequate medications should be immediately available to control any anxiety or distress that might occur. Family and staff require emotional support after such an event.[175]

CASE STUDY
### JD, A 75-Year-Old Man with Metastatic Colon Cancer

JD is a 75-year-old man who presented to his family doctor 2 months ago with a 20-pound weight loss, a bowel obstruction, a cough, and shortness of breath. He was found to have metastatic colon cancer with lung and liver metastases. He was treated with surgery and chemotherapy. You are visiting him at home and find that he now has a dry, nonproductive cough that keeps him awake at night and is sometimes so forceful that he vomits. He is receiving hydromorphone 4 mg orally every 4 hours for pain. He has had a trial of demulcents, dextromethorphan, inhalers and opioids for his cough, with little effect. He is afebrile and has no evidence of pneumonia on physical examination, but does have some fine crackles. You suggest a trial of nebulized preservative-free lidocaine every 6 hours. When you next see him, he reports that his cough is much better and that he has been able to get some rest.

## Summary

Chronic cough can be a disabling symptom for patients. If the underlying cause is unresponsive to treatment, then suppression of the cough is the major therapeutic goal.

REFERENCES

1. Edmonds P, Higginson I, Altmann D, Sen-Gupta G, McDonnell M. Is the presence of dyspnea a risk factor for morbidity in cancer patients? J Pain Symptom Manage 2000;19:15–22.
2. Fainsinger R, Waller A, Bercovici M, Bengston K, Landman W, Hosking M, Nunez-Olarte JM, deMoissac D. A multicentre international study of sedation for uncontrolled symptoms in terminally ill patients. Palliat Med 2000;14:257–265.
3. American Thoracic Society. Dyspnea: Mechanisms, assessment, and management. A consensus statement. Am J Respir Crit Care Med 1999;159:321–340.
4. O'Donnell DE, Banzett RB, Carrieri-Kohlman V, et al. Pathophysiology of dyspnea in chronic obstructive pulmonary disease. A roundtable. Proc Am Thorac Soc 2007;4:145–168.
5. Mahler DA. Mechanisms and measurement of dyspnea in chronic obstructive pulmonary disease. Proc Am Thorac Soc 2006;3:234–238.
6. Solano JP, Gomes B, Higginson IJ. A comparison of symptom prevalence in far advanced cancer, AIDS, heart disease, chronic obstructive pulmonary disease and renal disease. J Pain Symptom Manage 2006;31(1):58–69.
7. Tishelman C, Petersson L-M, Degner LF, Sprangers MAG. Symptom prevalence, intensity, and distress in patients with inoperable lung cancer in relation to time of death. J Clin Oncol 2007;25(34):5381–5389.
8. Skilbeck J, Mott L, Page H, Smith D, Hjelmeland-Ahmedzai S, Clark D. Palliative care in chronic obstructive airways disease: A needs assessment. Palliat Med 1998;12:245–254.
9. Blinderman CD, Homel P, Billings JA, Portenoy RK, Tennstedt SL. Symptom distress and quality of life in patients with advanced congestive heart failure. J Pain Symptom Manage 2008;35(6):594–603.
10. Addington-Hall J, Lay M, Altmann D, McCarthy M. Symptom control, communication with health professionals, and hospital care of stroke patients in the last year of life as reported by surviving family, friends and officials. Stroke 1995;26:2242–2248.
11. Voltz R, Borasio GD. Palliative therapy in the terminal stage of neurological disease. J Neurol 1997;244(Suppl 4):S2–S10.
12. Roberts DK, Thorne SE, Pearson C. The experience of dyspnea in late-stage cancer: Patients' and nurses' perspectives. Cancer Nurs 1993;16:310–320.
13. Brown ML, Carrieri V, Janson-Bjerklie S, Dodd MJ. Lung cancer and dyspnea: The patient's perception. Oncol Nurs Forum 1986;13(5):19–24.
14. Barnes S, Gott M, Payne S, et al. Prevalence of symptoms in a community-based sample of heart failure patients. J Pain Symptom Manage 2006;32(3):208–216.
15. Gore JM, Brophy CJ, Greenstone MA. How well do we care for patients with end stage chronic obstructive pulmonary disease (COPD)? A comparison of palliative care and quality of life in COPD and lung cancer. Thorax 2000;55:1000–1006.
16. O'Driscoll M, Corner J, Bailey C. The experience of breathlessness in lung cancer. Eur J Cancer Care 1999;8:37–43.
17. Bailey PH. Death stories: Acute exacerbations of chronic obstructive pulmonary disease. Qual Health Res 2001;11:322–338.
18. Steinhauser KE, Clipp EC, McNeilly M, Christakis NA, McIntyre LM, Tulsky JA. In search of a good death: Observations of patients, families, and providers. Ann Intern Med 2000;132:825–832.

19. O'Donnell DE. Exertional breathlessness in chronic respiratory disease. In: Mahler D, ed. Dyspnea. New York: Marcel Dekker, 1998:97–147.

20. Dudgeon D, Lertzman M. Dyspnea in the advanced cancer patient. J Pain Symptom Manage 1998;16:212–219.

21. Simon PM, Schwartzstein RM, Weiss JW, Fencl V, Teghtsoonian M, Weinberger SE. Distinguishable types of dyspnea in patients with shortness of breath. Am Rev Respir Dis 1990;142:1009–1014.

22. O'Donnell DE, Chau LL, Bertley J, Webb KA. Qualitative aspects of exertional breathlessness in CAL: Pathophysiological mechanisms. Am J Respir Crit Care Med 1997;155:109–115.

23. O'Donnell DE, Chau LKL, Webb KA. Qualitative aspects of exertional dyspnea in interstitial lung disease. J Appl Physiol 1998;84:2000–2009.

24. D'Arsigny C, Raj S, Abdollah H, Webb KA, O'Donnell DE. Ventilatory assistance improves leg discomfort and exercise endurance in stable congestive heart failure (CHF). Am J Respir Crit Care Med 1998;157:A451.

25. Parshall MB, Welsh JD, Brockopp DY, Heiser RM, Schooler MP, Cassidy KB. Reliability and validity of dyspnea sensory quality descriptors in heart failure patients treated in an emergency department. Heart Lung 2001;30:57–65.

26. Silvestri GA, Mahler DA. Evaluation of dyspnea in the elderly patient. Clin Chest Med 1993;14:393–404.

27. Ferrin MS, Tino G. Acute dyspnea. Am Assoc Crit Care Nurs Clin Issues 1997;8:398–410.

28. Gift AG, Plaut SM, Jacox A. Psychologic and physiologic factors related to dyspnea in subjects with chronic obstructive pulmonary disease. Heart Lung 1986;15:595–601.

29. Nguyen HQ, Altinger J, Carrieri-Kohlman V, Gormley JM, Paul SM, Stulbarg MS. Factor analysis of laboratory and clinical measurement of dyspnea in patients with chronic obstructive pulmonary disease. J Pain Symptom Manage 2003;25:118–127.

30. Gift AG. Validation of a vertical visual analogue scale as a measure of clinical dyspnea. Am Rev Respir Dis 1986;133(4, Part 2):A163.

31. Bausewein C, Farquhar M, Booth S, Gysels M, Higginson IJ. Measurement of breathlessness in advanced disease: A systematic review. Respir Med 2006;101:399–410.

32. Burdon J, Juniper E, Killian K, Hargeave F, Campbell E. The perception of breathlessness. Am Rev Respir Dis 1982;126:825–828.

33. O'Donnell DE, Lam M, Webb KA. Measurement of symptoms, lung hyperinflation, and endurance during exercise in chronic obstructive pulmonary disease. Am J Respir Crit Care Med 1998;158:1557–1565.

34. Tattersall MHN, Boyer MJ. Management of malignant pleural effusions. Thorax 1990;45:81–82.

35. Wilcock A, Crosby V, Clarke D, Corcoran R, Tattersfield AE. Reading numbers aloud: A measure of the limiting effect of breathlessness in patients with cancer. Thorax 1999;54:1099–1103.

36. Neff TA, Petty TL. Tolerance and survival in severe chronic hypercapnia. Arch Intern Med 1972;129:591–596.

37. Kellner R, Samet J, Pathak D. Dyspnea, anxiety, and depression in chronic respiratory impairment. Gen Hosp Psychiatry 1992;14:20–28.

38. Dudgeon D, Lertzman M. Etiology of dyspnea in advanced cancer patients. Program Proc Am Soc Clin Oncol 1996;15:165.

39. Heyse-Moore LH. On Dyspnoea in Advanced Cancer. Southampton, UK: Southampton University, 1993.

40. Dudgeon DJ, Kristjanson L, Sloan JA, Lertzman M, Clement K. Dyspnea in cancer patients: Prevalence and associated factors. J Pain Symptom Manage 2001;21:95–102.

41. Bruera E, Schmitz B, Pither J, Neumann CM, Hanson J. The frequency and correlates of dyspnea in patients with advanced cancer. Personal communication, 1997.

42. Carrieri-Kohlman V, Gormley JM, Douglas MK, Paul SM, Stulbarg MS. Differentiation between dyspnea and its affective components. West J Nurs Res 1996;18:626–642.

43. Woodcock AA, Gross ER, Gellert A, Shah S, Johnson M, Geddes DM. Effects of dihydrocodeine, alcohol, and caffeine on breathlessness and exercise tolerance in patients with chronic obstructive lung disease and normal blood gases. N Engl J Med 1981;305:1611–1616.

44. Bruera E, Macmillan K, Pither J, MacDonald RN. Effects of morphine on the dyspnea of terminal cancer patients. J Pain Symptom Manage 1990;5(6):341–344.

45. Bruera E, MacEachern T, Ripamonti C, Hanson J. Subcutaneous morphine for dyspnea in cancer patients. Ann Intern Med 1993;119:906–907.

46. Cohen MH, Anderson AJ, Krasnow SH, Spagnolo SV, Citron ML, Payne M, Fossiek BE Jr. Continuous intravenous infusion of morphine for severe dyspnea. South Med J 1991;84(2):229–234.

47. Light RW, Muro JR, Sato RI, Stansbury DW, Fischer CE, Brown SE. Effects of oral morphine on breathlessness and exercise tolerance in patients with chronic obstructive pulmonary disease. Am Rev Respir Dis 1989;139:126–133.

48. Mueller RE, Petty TL, Filley GF. Ventilation and arterial blood gas changes induced by pursed lip breathing. J Appl Physiol 1970;28:784–789.

49. Masood AR, Subhan MMF, Reed JW, Thomas SHL. Effects of inhaled nebulized morphine on ventilation and breathlessness during exercise in healthy man. Clin Sci 1995;88:447–452.

50. Robin ED, Burke CM. Single-patient randomized clinical trial: Opiates for intractable dyspnea. Chest 1986;90:888–892.

51. Johnson MA, Woodcock AA, Geddes DM. Dihydrocodeine for breathlessness in "pink puffers." Br Med J 1983;286:675–677.

52. Sackner MA. Effects of hydrocodone bitartrate on breathing pattern of patients with chronic obstructive pulmonary disease and restrictive lung disease. Mt Sinai J Med 1984;51:222–226.

53. Timmis AD, Rothman MT, Henderson MA, Geal PW, Chamberlain DA. Haemodynamic effects of intravenous morphine in patients with acute myocardial infarction complicated by severe left ventricular failure. Br Med J 1980;280:980–982.

54. Rice KL, Kronenberg RS, Hedemark LL, Niewoehner DE. Effects of chronic administration of codeine and promethazine on breathlessness and exercise tolerance in patients with chronic airflow obstruction. Br J Dis Chest 1987;81:287–292.

55. Eiser N, Denman WT, West C, Luce P. Oral diamorphine: Lack of effect on dyspnoea and exercise tolerance in the "pink puffer" syndrome. Eur Respir J 1991;4:926–931.

56. Boyd KJ, Kelly M. Oral morphine as symptomatic treatment of dyspnea in patients with advanced cancer. Palliat Med 1997;11:277–281.

57. Poole PJ, Veale AG, Black PN. The effect of sustained-release morphine on breathlessness and quality of life in severe chronic obstructive pulmonary disease. Am J Respir Crit Care Med 1998;157(6 Pt 1):1877–1880.

58. Jennings AL, Davies A, Higgins JPT, Broadley K. Opioids for the palliation of breathlessness in terminal illness. Cochrane Datbase Syst Rev 2001;(4):CD002066.

59. Woodcock AA, Johnson MA, Geddes DM. Breathlessness, alcohol and opiates. N Engl J Med 1982;306:1363–1364.

60. Light RW, Stansbury DW, Webster JS. Effect of 30 mg of morphine alone or with promethazine or prochlorperazine on the exercise capacity of patients with COPD. Chest 1996;109:975–981.

61. Chua TP, Harrington D, Ponikowski P, Webb-Peploe K, Poole-Wilson PA, Coats AJ. Effects of dihydrocodeine on chemosensitivity and exercise tolerance in patients with chronic heart failure. J Am Coll Cardiol 1997;29:147–152.

62. Viola R, Kiteley C, Lloyd NS, Mackay JA, Wilson J, Wong RKS. The management of dyspnea in cancer patients: A systematic review. Support Care Cancer 2008;16:329–337.

63. Ben-Aharon I, Gafter-Gvili A, Leibovici L, Stemmer SM. Interventions for alleviating cancer-related dyspnea: A systematic review. J Clin Oncol 2008;26:2396–2404.

64. Belvisi MG, Chung KF, Jackson DM, Barnes PJ. Opioid modulation of non-cholinergic neural bronchoconstriction in guinea-pig in-vivo. Br J Pharmacol 1988;95:413–418.

65. Beauford W, Saylor TT, Stansbury DW, Avalos K, Light RW. Effects of nebulized morphine sulfate on the exercise tolerance of the ventilatory limited COPD patient. Chest 1993;104:175–178.

66. Davis CL, Hodder C, Love S, Shah R, Slevin M, Wedzicha J. Effect of nebulised morphine and morphine 6-glucuronide on exercise endurance in patients with chronic obstructive pulmonary disease. Thorax 1994;49:393P.

67. Davis CL, Penn K, A'Hern R, Daniels J, Slevin M. Single dose randomised controlled trial of nebulised morphine in patients with cancer related breathlessness. Palliat Med 1996;10:64–65.

68. Harris-Eze AO, Sridhar G, Clemens RE, Zintel TA, Gallagher CG, Marciniuk DD. Low-dose nebulized morphine does not improve exercise in interstitial lung disease. Am J Respir Crit Care Med 1995;152:1940–1945.

69. Jankelson D, Hosseini K, Mather LE, Seale JP, Young IH. Lack of effect of high doses of inhaled morphine on exercise endurance in chronic obstructive pulmonary disease. Eur Respir J 1997;10:2270–2274.

70. Leung R, Hill P, Burdon JGW. Effect of inhaled morphine on the development of breathlessness during exercise in patients with chronic lung disease. Thorax 1996;51:596–600.

71. Masood AR, Reed JW, Thomas SHL. Lack of effect of inhaled morphine on exercise-induced breathlessness in chronic obstructive pulmonary disease. Thorax 1995;50:629–634.

72. Noseda A, Carpiaux JP, Markstein C, Meyvaert A, de Maertelaer V. Disabling dyspnoea in patients with advanced disease: Lack of effect of nebulized morphine. Eur Respir J 1997;10:1079–1083.

73. Young IH, Daviskas E, Keena VA. Effect of low dose nebulised morphine on exercise endurance in patients with chronic lung disease. Thorax 1989;44:387–390.

74. Charles MA, Reymond L, Israel F. Relief of incident dyspnea in palliative cancer patients: A pilot, randomized, controlled trial comparing nebulized hydromorphone, systemic hydromorphone, and nebulized saline. J Pain Symptom Manage 2008;36(1):29–38.

75. Wilson RH, Hoseth W, Dempsey ME. Respiratory acidosis: I. Effects of decreasing respiratory minute volume in patients with severe chronic pulmonary emphysema, with specific reference to oxygen, morphine and barbiturates. Am J Med 1954;17:464–470.

76. Mazzocato C, Buclin T, Rapin CH. The effects of morphine on dyspnea and ventilatory function in elderly patients with advanced cancer: A randomized double-blind controlled trial. Ann Oncol 1999;10:1511–1514.

77. Clemens KE, Klaschik E. Symptomatic therapy of dyspnea with strong opioids and its effect on ventilation in palliative care patients. J Pain Symptom Manage 2007;33(4):473–481.

78. Dudgeon D. Dyspnea, death rattle, and cough. In: Ferrell BR, Coyle N, eds. Textbook of Palliative Nursing. New York: Oxford University Press, 2001:164–174.

79. Dudgeon D. Dyspnea: Ethical concerns. Ethics in Palliative Care: Part II. J Palliat Care 1994;10(3):48–51.

80. Twycross R. Morphine and dyspnoea. In: Twycross R, ed. Pain Relief in Advanced Cancer. New York: Churchill Livingstone, 1994:383–399.

81. O'Neill PA, Morton PB, Stark RD. Chlorpromazine: A specific effect on breathlessness? Br J Clin Pharmacol 1985;19:793–797.

82. Woodcock AA, Gross ER, Geddes DM. Drug treatment of breathlessness: Contrasting effects of diazepam and promethazine in pink puffers. Br Med J 1981;283:343–346.

83. McIver B, Walsh D, Nelson K. The use of chlorpromazine for symptom control in dying cancer patients. J Pain Symptom Manage 1994;9:341–345.

84. Sen D, Jones G, Leggat PO. The response of the breathless patient treated with diazepam. Br J Clin Pract 1983;37(June):232–233.

85. Mitchell-Heggs P, Murphy K, Minty K, Guz A, Patterson SC, Minty PS, Rosser RM. Diazepam in the treatment of dyspnoea in the "pink puffer" syndrome. Q J Med 1980;49:9–20.

86. Greene JG, Pucino F, Carlson JD, Storsved M, Strommen GL. Effects of alprazolam on respiratory drive, anxiety, and dyspnea in chronic airflow obstruction: A case study. Pharmacotherapy 1989;9:34–38.

87. Man GCW, Hsu K, Sproule BJ. Effect of alprazolam on exercise and dyspnea in patients with chronic obstructive pulmonary disease. Chest 1986;90:832–836.

88. Eimer M, Cable T, Gal P, Rothenberger LA, McCue JD. Effects of clorazepate on breathlessness and exercise tolerance in patients with chronic airflow obstruction. J Fam Pract 1985;21:359–362.

89. Argyropoulou P, Patakas D, Koukou A, Vasiliadis P, Georgopoulos D. Buspirone effect on breathlessness and exercise performance in patients with chronic obstructive pulmonary disease. Respiration 1993;60:216–220.

90. Ventafridda V, Spoldi E, De Conno F. Control of dyspnea in advanced cancer patients. Chest 1990;98:1544–1545.

91. Navigante AH, Cerchietti LCA, Castro MA, Lutteral MA, Cabalar ME. Midazolam as adjunct therapy to morphine in the alleviation of severe dyspnea perception in patients with advanced cancer. J Pain Symptom Manage 2006;31(1):38–47.

92. O'Neill PA, Stark RD, Morton PB. Do prostaglandins have a role in breathlessness? Am Rev Respir Dis 1985;132:22–24.

93. O'Neill PA, Stretton TB, Stark RD, Ellis SH. The effect of indomethacin on breathlessness in patients with diffuse parenchymal disease of the lung. Br J Dis Chest 1986;80:72–79.

94. Schiffman GL, Stansbury DW, Fischer CE, Sato RI, Light RW, Brown SE. Indomethacin and perception of dyspnea in chronic airflow limitation. Am Rev Respir Dis 1988;137:1094–1098.

95. Winning AJ, Hamilton RD, Shea SA, Knott C, Guz A. The effect of airway anaesthesia on the control of breathing and the sensation of breathlessness in man. Clin Sci 1985;68:215–225.

96. Winning AJ, Hamilton RD, Guz A. Ventilation and breathlessness on maximal exercise in patients with interstitial lung disease after local anaesthetic aerosol inhalation. Clin Sci 1988;74:275–281.

97. Wilcock A, Corcoran R, Tattersfield AE. Safety and efficacy of nebulized lignocaine in patients with cancer and breathlessness. Palliat Med 1994;8:35–38.

98. Giron AE, Stansbury DW, Fischer CE, Light RW. Lack of effect of dextromethorphan on breathlessness and exercise performance in patients with chronic obstructive pulmonary disease (COPD). Eur Respir J 1991;4:532–535.

99. Newton PJ, Davidson PM, Macdonald P, Ollerton R, Krum H. Nebulized furosemide for the management of dyspnea: Does the evidence support its use? J Pain Symptom Manage 2008;36(4):424–441.

100. Tarpy SP, Celli BR. Long-term oxygen therapy. N Engl J Med 1995;333:710–714.

101. Uronis H, McCrory DC, Samsa GP, Currow DC, Abernathy AP. Palliative oxygen for non-hypoxaemic chronic obstructive pulmonary disease (Protocol). Cochrane Library 2008; 3(4):1–7.

102. Cranston JM, Crockett A, Currow D. Oxygen therapy for dyspnea in adults (Review). Cochrane Library 2008;3(4):1–54.

103. Philip J, Gold M, Milner A, Di Iulio J, Miller B, Spruyt O. A randomized, double-blind, crossover trial of the effect of oxygen on dyspnea in patients with advanced cancer. J Pain Symptom Manage 2006;32(6):541–550.

104. Hausheer FH, Yarbro JW. Diagnosis and treatment of malignant pleural effusion. Semin Oncol 1985;1254–75.

105. Lynch TJ. Management of malignant pleural effusions. Chest 1993;4(Suppl):385S–389S.

106. Anderson CB, Philpott GW, Ferguson TB. The treatment of malignant pleural effusions. Cancer 1974;33:916–922.

107. Rauthe G, Sistermanns J. Recombinant tumour necrosis factor in the local therapy of malignant pleural effusion. Eur J Cancer 1997;33:226–231.

108. Grodzin CJ, Balk RA. Indwelling small pleural catheter needle thoracentesis in the management of large pleural effusions. Chest 1997;111:981–988.

109. Patz EF Jr. Malignant pleural effusions: Recent advances and ambulatory sclerotherapy. Chest 1998;113(1 Suppl):74S–77S.

110. Press OW, Livingston R. Management of malignant pericardial effusion and tamponade. JAMA 1987;257:1088–1092.

111. Vaitkus PT, Hermann HC, LeWinter MM. Treatment of malignant pericardial effusion. JAMA 1994;272:59–64.

112. Chong HH, Plotnick GD. Pericardial effusion and tamponade: Evaluation, imaging modalities, and management. Compr Ther 1995;21:378–385.

113. Mangan CM. Malignant pericardial effusions: Pathophysiology and clinical correlates. Oncol Nurs Forum 1992;19:1215–1223.

114. Barach AL. Chronic obstructive lung disease: Postural relief of dyspnea. Arch Phys Med Rehabil 1974;55:494–504.

115. Sharp JT, Drutz WS, Moisan T, Foster J, Machnach W. Postural relief of dyspnea in severe chronic obstructive pulmonary disease. Am Rev Respir Dis 1980;122:201–211.

116. Thoman RL, Stoker GL, Ross JC. The efficacy of pursed-lips breathing in patients with chronic obstructive pulmonary disease. Am Rev Respir Dis 1966;93:100–106.

117. Make B. COPD: Management and rehabilitation. Am Fam Physician 1991;43:1315–1324.

118. Schwartzstein RM, Lahive K, Pope A, Weinberger SE, Weiss JW. Cold facial stimulation reduces breathlessness induced in normal subjects. Am Rev Respir Dis 1987;136:58–61.

119. Burgess KR, Whitelaw WA. Effects of nasal cold receptors on pattern of breathing. J Appl Physiol 1988;64:371–376.

120. Burgess KR, Whitelaw WA. Reducing ventilatory response to carbon dioxide by breathing cold air. Am Rev Respir Dis 1984;129:687–690.

121. Jobst K, Chen JH, McPherson J. Controlled trial of acupuncture for disabling breathlessness. Lancet 1986;2:1416–1418.

122. Maa SH, Gauthier D, Turner M. Acupressure as an adjunct to a pulmonary rehabilitation program. J Cardiopulm Rehabil 1997;17:268–276.

123. Filshie J, Penn K, Ashley S, Davis CL. Acupuncture for the relief of cancer-related breathlessness. Palliat Med 1996;10:145–150.

124. Renfroe KL. Effect of progressive relaxation on dyspnea and state anxiety in patients with chronic obstructive pulmonary disease. Heart Lung 1988;17:408–413.

125. Rosser RM, Denford J, Heslop A. Breathlessness and psychiatric morbidity in chronic bronchitis and emphysema: A study of psychotherapeutic management. Psychol Med 1983;13:93–110.

126. Corner J, Plant H, A'Hern R, Bailey C. Non-pharmacological intervention for breathlessness in lung cancer. Palliat Med 1996;10:299–305.

127. Carrieri VK, Janson-Bjerklie S. Strategies patients use to manage the sensation of dyspnea. West J Nurs Res 1986;8:284–305.

128. van den Berg R. Dyspnea: Perception or reality. CACCN 1995;6:16–19.

129. Moody LE, Fraser M, Yarandi H. Effects of guided imagery in patients with chronic bronchitis and emphysema. Clin Nurs Res 1993;2:478–486.

130. Giasson M, Bouchard L. Effect of therapeutic touch on the well-being of persons with terminal cancer. J Holistic Nurs 1998;16:383–398.

131. Shih F, Chu S. Comparisons of American-Chinese and Taiwanese patients' perceptions of dyspnea and helpful nursing actions during the intensive care unit transition from cardiac surgery. Heart Lung 1999;28:41–54.

132. Tiep BL. Inpatient pulmonary rehabilitation: A team approach to the more fragile patient. Postgrad Med 1989;86:141–150.

133. Grey A. The nursing management of dyspnoea in palliative care. Nurs Times 1995;91:33–35.

134. Back IN, Jenkins K, Blower A, Beckhelling J. A study comparing hyoscine hydrobromide and glycopyrrolate in the treatment of death rattle. Palliat Med 2001;15:329–336.

135. Watts T, Jenkins K. Palliative care nurses' feelings about death rattle. J Clin Nurs 1999;8:615–616.

136. Wildiers H, Menten J. Death rattle: Prevalence, prevention and treatment. J Pain Symptom Manage 2002;23:310–317.

137. Hughes AC, Wilcock A, Corcoran R. Management of death rattle. J Pain Symptom Manage 1996;12:271–272.

138. Ellershaw JE, Sutcliffe JM, Saunders CM. Dehydration and the dying patient. J Pain Symptom Manage 1995;10:192–197.

139. Morita T, Ichiki T, Tsunoda J, Inoue S, Chihara S. A prospective study on the dying process in terminally ill cancer patients. Am J Hospice Palliat Care 1998;15:217–222.

140. Kass RM, Ellershaw JE. Respiratory tract secretions in the dying patient: A retrospective study. J Pain Symptom Manage 2003;26:897–902.

141. Morita T, Tsunoda J, Inoue S, Chihara S. Risk factors for death rattle in terminally ill cancer patients: A prospective exploratory study. Palliat Med 2000;14:19–23.

142. Morita T, Hyodo I, Yoshima T, et al. Incidence and underlying etiologies of bronchial secretion in terminally ill cancer patients: A multicenter, prospective, observational study. J Pain Symptom Manage 2004;27(6):533–539.

143. Bennett MI. Death rattle: An audit of hyoscine (scopolamine) use and review of management. J Pain Symptom Manage 1996;12:229–233.

144. Hall P, Schroder C, Weaver L. The last 48 hours of life in long-term care: A focused chart audit. J Am Geriatr Soc 2002;50:501–506.

145. Wee BL, Coleman PG, Hillier R, Holgate ST. Death rattle: Its impact on staff and volunteers in palliative care. Palliat Med 2008;22:173–176.

146. Wee BL, Coleman PG, Hillier R, Holgate SH. The sound of death rattle I: Are relatives distressed by hearing this sound? Palliat Med 2006;20:171–175.

147. Wee BL, Coleman PG, Hillier R, Holgate SH. The sound of death rattle II: How do relatives interpret the sound? Palliat Med 2006;20:177–181.

148. Nadel JA. Regulation of airway secretions. Chest 1985;87(1 Suppl):111S–113S.

149. Kaliner M, Shelhamer H, Borson B, Nadel JA, Patow C, Marom Z. Human respiratory mucus. Am Rev Respir Dis 1986;134:612–621.

150. Victoria Hospice Society. Medical Care of the Dying (3rd ed). Victoria, BC: Victoria Hospice Society, 1998.

151. Andrews MR, Levine AM. Dehydration in the terminal patient: Perception of hospice nurses. Am J Hosp Care 1989; 6:31–34.

152. Downing M. Victoria Respiratory Congestion Scale. 2004. Personal Communication.

153. Bennett M, Lucas V, Brennan M, Hughes A, O'Donnell V, Wee B. Using anti-muscarinic drugs in the management of death rattle: Evidence-based guidelines for palliative care. Palliat Med 2002;16:369–374.

154. Dawson HR. The use of transdermal scopolamine in the control of death rattle. J Palliat Care 1989;5:31–33.

155. Lichter I, Hunt E. The last 48 hours of life. J Palliat Care 1990;6:7–15.

156. Murtagh FEM, Thorns A, Oliver DJ. Correspondence: Hyoscine and glycopyrrolate for death rattle. Palliat Med 2002;16:449–450.

157. Morice AH, Kastelik JA. Cough 1: Chronic cough in adults. Thorax 2003;58:901–907.

158. Muers MF, Round CE. Palliation of symptoms in non-small cell lung cancer: A study by the Yorkshire Regional Cancer Organisation thoracic group. Thorax 1993;48:339–343.

159. Homsi J, Walsh D, Nelson KA. Important drugs for cough in advanced cancer. Support Care Cancer 2001;9:565–574.

160. Kvale PA, Simoff M, Prakash UBS. Palliative care. Chest 2003;123:284S–311S.

161. Fuller RW, Jackson DM. Physiology and treatment of cough. Thorax 1990;45:425–430.

162. Lalloo UG, Barnes PJ, Chung KF. Pathophysiology and clinical presentations of cough. J Allergy Clin Immunol 1996;98(5, Part 2):S91–S97.

163. Morice AH, McGarvey L, Pavord I. Recommendations for the management of cough in adults. Thorax 2006;61(Suppl 1):i1–i24; doi:10.1136/thx.2006.065144.

164. Dudgeon D, Rosenthal S. Pathophysiology and assessment of dyspnea in the patient with cancer. In: Portenoy RK, Bruera E, eds. Topics in Palliative Care. New York: Oxford University Press, 1999:237–254.

165. Ripamonti C, Fusco F. Respiratory problems in advanced cancer. Support Care Cancer 2002;10:204–216.

166. Hagen NA. An approach to cough in cancer patients. J Pain Symptom Manage 1991;6:257–262.

167. Eddy NB, Friebel H, Hahn KJ, Halbach H. Codeine and its alternatives for pain and cough relief. Potential alternatives for cough relief. Bull World Health Organ 1969;40:639–719.

168. Eddy NB, Friebel H, Hahn KJ, Halbach H. Codeine and its alternatives for pain and cough relief. Discussion and summary. Bull World Health Organ 1969;40:721–730.

169. Doona M, Walsh D. Benzonatate for opioid-resistant cough in advanced cancer. Palliat Med 1997;12:55–58.

170. Lowry R, Wood A, Johnson T, Higenbottam T. Antitussive properties of inhaled bronchodilators on induced cough. Chest 1988;93:1186–1189.

171. Louie K, Bertolino M, Fainsinger R. Management of intractable cough. J Palliat Care 1992;8:46–48.

172. Howard P, Cayton RM, Brennan SR, Anderson PB. Lignocaine aerosol and persistent cough. Br J Dis Chest 1977;71:19–24.

173. Sanders RV, Kirkpatrick MB. Prolonged suppression of cough after inhalation of Lidocaine in a patient with sarcoid. JAMA 1984;252:2456–2457.

174. Cowcher K, Hanks GW. Long-term management of respiratory symptoms in advanced cancer. J Pain Symptom Manage 1990;5:320–330.

175. Dudgeon D, Rosenthal S. Pathophysiology and treatment of cough. In: Portenoy R, Bruera E, eds. Topics in Palliative Care. New York: Oxford University Press, 2000:237–254.

# 15 ⟡ *Mikel Gray and Terran Sims*

# Urinary Tract Disorders

*As if being sick and dying isn't enough—it's all the indignity before you go. Losing control of my bladder and feeling like a baby in diapers has been the worst... when my daughter came and saw me like this (with the diaper), that's when she just lost it.—A patient*

◆ **Key Points**

◆ *The urinary system is frequently the cause of bothersome or deleterious symptoms that affect the patient receiving palliative care.*

◆ *A malignancy or systemic disease may affect urinary tract function and produce urinary incontinence, urinary retention, or upper urinary tract obstruction.*

◆ *Common lower urinary tract symptoms (LUTS) include urinary incontinence, daytime voiding frequency, nocturia, urgency, feelings of incomplete bladder emptying, and incomplete bladder emptying.*

◆ *Upper urinary tract symptoms include flank or abdominal pain and constitutional symptoms related to acute renal insufficiency or failure.*

◆ *Significant hematuria leading to clot formation and catheter blockage is an uncommon but significant complication of pelvic radiation therapy. Hematuria may occur months to years following radiotherapy.*

◆ *Initial treatment of hematuria includes continuous bladder irrigation to evacuate clots from the bladder vesicle until the fragile bladder wall heals. If hematuria recurs, more aggressive treatment options include intravesical alum or prostaglandins. Intravesical formalin treatments are reserved for very severe cases of blood loss.*

◆ *Bladder spasms (overactive detrusor contractions) may be associated with urinary tract infection or catheter blockage, or they may be idiopathic. Any apparent underlying cause of bladder spasms, such as a urinary tract infection, should be treated initially.*

◆ *An antimuscarinic medication should be used for long-term relief of bladder spasms. Extended-release or transdermal agents are usually preferred because of their favorable side effect profiles and avoidance of the need for frequent dosing. However, immediate release agents may be adminstered if bladder spasms prove refractory to extended release formulations.*

◆ *Indwelling catheterization is a viable option for managing urine elimination in the patient who is near death and has urinary retention, or when pain or immobility significantly impairs the ability to urinate. A suprapubic catheter may be used as an alternative to urethral catheterization after urethral trauma or in the presence of urethral obstruction in cases of urethral injury, strictures, prostate obstruction, after gynecologic surgery, or for long-term catheterization.*

In many ways, the techniques used for management of urinary symptoms are similar to those used for patients in any care setting. However, in contrast to traditional interventions, the evaluation and management of urinary tract symptoms in the palliative care setting are influenced by considerations of the goals of care and closeness to death.

Urinary system disorders may be directly attributable to a malignancy, systemic disease, or a specific treatment such as radiation or chemotherapy. This chapter provides an overview of the anatomy and physiology of the urinary system, which serves as a framework for understanding of the pathophysiology of bothersome symptoms and their management. This is followed by a review of commonly encountered urinary symptoms seen in the palliative care setting, including bothersome lower urinary tract symptoms (LUTS), lower urinary tract pain, urinary stasis or retention, and hematuria.

⟡

## Lower Urinary Tract Disorders

### Lower Urinary Tract Physiology

The lower urinary tract comprises the bladder, urethra, and supportive structures within the pelvic floor (Figures 15–1 and 15–2). Together, these structures maintain *urinary continence*, which can be simply defined as control over bladder filling and storage and the act of micturition. Continence is modulated by three interrelated factors: (1) anatomic integrity of the urinary tract, (2) control of the detrusor muscle, and (3) competence of the urethral sphincter mechanism.[1,2] Each may be compromised in the patient receiving palliative care, leading to bothersome LUTS, urinary retention, or a combination of these disorders.

### Anatomic Integrity

From a physiological perspective, the urinary system comprises a long tube originating in the glomerulus and

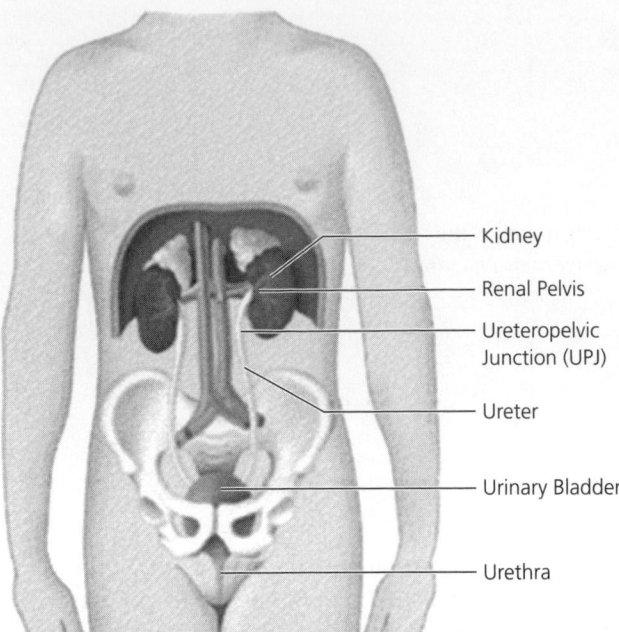

**Figure 15–1.** The female urinary tract.

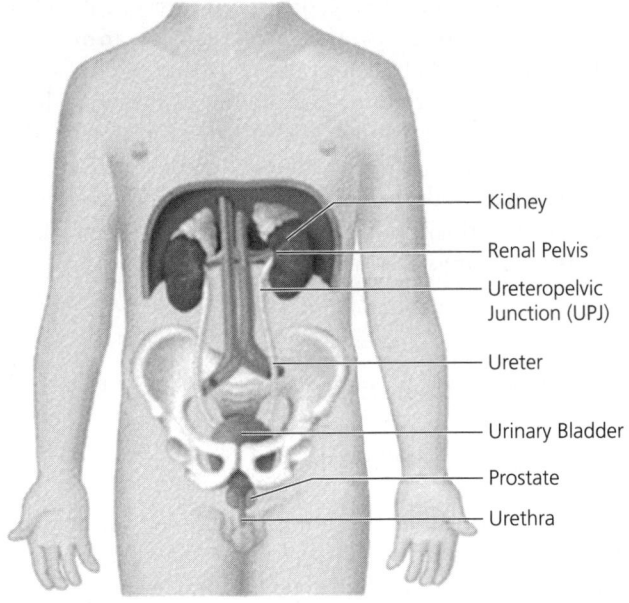

**Figure 15–2.** The male urinary tract.

terminating at the urethral meatus. When contemplating urinary continence, anatomic integrity of the urinary system is often assumed, particularly because extraurethral urinary incontinence (UI) is uncommon. However, anatomical integrity may be lost in the patient receiving palliative care when a fistula bypasses the urethral sphincter. This epithelialized tract allows continuous urinary leakage, which varies from an ongoing dribble in a patient with otherwise normal urine

elimination habits to total UI characterized by failure of bladder filling and micturition.

## Control of the Detrusor

In addition to a structurally intact urinary system, continence requires volitional control over detrusor contraction.[1,2] Control of this smooth muscle can be conceptualized on three levels. Multiple modulatory centers within the central nervous system modulate lower urinary tract function, ensuring low pressure bladder filling and micturition only when the person wishes to urinate. Detrusor control is also influenced by its histological characteristics, and on a molecular level by neurotransmitters released within the neuromuscular junction.

The nervous control of the detrusor arises from multiple modulatory areas within the brain and spinal cord.[3] Bilateral modulatory centers are found in the cerebral cortex; they are involved with bladder filling and storage, and more recent evidence suggests that they play a more active role in the decision to urinate than previously thought.[4] These modulatory centers interact with neurons in the thalamus,[5] hypothalamus,[6] basal ganglia,[7] and cerebellum[8] to modulate bladder filling and voiding. Data from functional MRI and PET scans reveal that each of these areas is involved with bladder filling and/or micturition, leading to new questions and new insights into the relationships between cognition, emotional state, mood and lower urinary tract symptoms.[3,4] Whereas modulatory centers within the brain are essential for continence, the primary integration centers for bladder filling and micturition are found within the brainstem.[9] Specific areas within the brainstem control bladder filling and storage under the influence of higher brain regions. These areas include the periaqueductal gray matter, which is responsible for coordinating multiple groups of neurons in the brainstem; the L and M regions, which modulate bladder filling and initiate the detrusor contraction; and the pontine micturition center, which coordinates the reflexive response of the urethral sphincter mechanism. Recognition of the significance of the brainstem micturition center is particularly important when providing palliative care, because a neurological lesion above the brainstem causes urge UI with a coordinated sphincter response, whereas lesions below this center affect bladder sensations and the coordination between the detrusor and the urethral sphincter, resulting in reflex UI.

The brainstem micturition center communicates with the bladder via spinal roots in the thoracolumbar and sacral segments.[3] Neurons in the thoracolumbar spine (T10–L2) transmit sympathetic nervous impulses that promote bladder filling and storage, whereas neurons in spinal segments S2–S4 transmit parasympathetic impulses to the bladder wall, promoting micturition under the influence of the brain and brain-stem. These impulses are carried through several peripheral nerve plexi, including the pelvic and inferior hypogastric plexi.

Histological characteristics of the detrusor also contribute to its voluntary control.[10] Unlike the visceral smooth muscle of the bowel, stomach, or ureter, the detrusor muscle bundles are innervated on an almost one-to-one basis, reflecting the critical importance of the neurological modulation described above. The smooth muscle bundles of the detrusor also lack gap junctions, observed in other visceral organs, which allow propagation of a contraction independent of nervous stimulation. These characteristics promote urinary continence because they discourage spontaneous contractions of the detrusor in response to bladder filling, as is characteristic of other visceral organs.

On a molecular level, specific chemical substances, commonly called neurotransmitters, exert local control over the detrusor muscle.[2] Several neurotransmitters are released from the axons of neurons within the bladder wall and act at specific receptors to produce smooth muscle contraction or relaxation. Norepinephrine acts through $\beta_3$-adrenergic receptors, promoting detrusor muscle relaxation, and acetylcholine acts through muscarinic receptors, leading to detrusor contraction and micturition. Although it has long been known that the cholinergic receptors within the detrusor are muscarinic, physiological studies have identified at least five muscarinic receptor subtypes (M1 through M5) in the human body.[11] Two receptor subtypes, M2 and M3, are believed to predominate within the bladder wall and are primarily responsible for the detrusor contraction that leads to micturition.[12] Identification of these receptor subtypes is clinically relevant because it has facilitated the development of drugs that act on the bladder but produce fewer central nervous system side effects than the older (nonselective) drugs traditionally used to manage urge UI or bladder spasms.

## Competence of the Urethral Sphincter Mechanism

The urethral sphincter is a combination of compressive and tension elements that form a watertight seal against urinary leakage, even when challenged by physical exertion or sudden increases in abdominal pressure caused by coughing, laughing, or sneezing.[1,2] The soft urethral mucosa interacts with mucosal secretions (glycosaminoglycans) and the submucosal vascular cushion to ensure a watertight seal that rapidly conforms to changes. Whereas the elements of compression provide a watertight seal for the urethra, striated and smooth muscle within the urethral wall and within the surrounding pelvic floor are necessary when sphincter closure is challenged by physical exertion. The muscular elements of the urethral sphincter include the smooth muscle of the bladder neck and proximal urethra (including the prostatic urethra in men), the rhabdosphincter, and the periurethral striated muscles. $\alpha_1$-Adrenergic receptors in the smooth muscle of the bladder neck and proximal urethra promote sphincter closure when exposed to the neurotransmitter norepinephrine.[13] Innervation of the rhabdosphincter is more complex. Acetylcholine acts on nicotinic receptors in the rhabdosphincter to stimulate muscle contraction. In addition, norepinephrine and serotonin (5HT) act on neurons within Onuf's nucleus (located at sacral spinal segments 2 through 4), modulating rhabdosphincter tone during bladder filling and storage.[14]

## Pathophysiology of Urinary Incontinence

*Urinary incontinence* is defined as the uncontrolled loss of urine of sufficient magnitude to create a problem.[15] It can be divided into two types: transient (acute) and chronic, based on onset and underlying etiology.[16] Factors resulting in transient UI clearly contribute to urinary leakage, but they often arise from outside the lower urinary tract. Therefore, treatment of transient UI is typically aimed at the contributing factor, rather than the urinary system itself. Several conditions associated with transient UI are commonly encountered when caring for patients in a palliative care setting; they include delirium, urinary tract infection, adverse side effects of various drugs, restricted mobility, and severe constipation or stool impaction (Table 15–1).

Chronic UI is subdivided into types according to its presenting symptoms or underlying pathophysiology.[16] Stress UI occurs when physical stress (exertion) causes urine loss in the absence of a detrusor contraction. Two conditions lead to stress UI—urethral hypermobility (descent of the bladder base during physical activity) and intrinsic sphincter deficiency (incompetence of the striated or smooth muscle within the urethral sphincter mechanism). Although urethral hypermobility is rarely the primary cause of significant stress UI in the patient receiving palliative care, intrinsic sphincter deficiency may compromise sphincter closure and lead to severe urinary leakage. Intrinsic sphincter deficiency occurs when the nerves or muscles necessary for sphincter closure are denervated or damaged.[17] Table 15–2 lists conditions that are likely to cause intrinsic sphincter deficiency in patients receiving palliative care.

Urge UI occurs when overactive detrusor contractions produce urinary leakage.[16] Urge UI is part of a larger symptom syndrome called *overactive bladder*. Overactive bladder is characterized by urgency (a sudden desire to urinate that is difficult to defer), and it is typically associated with daytime voiding frequency (more than every 2 hours) and nocturia ($\geq 3$ episodes per night). Reflex UI, in contrast, is caused by a neurological lesion below the brainstem micturition center.[18] It is characterized by diminished or absent sensations of bladder filling, neurogenic overactive detrusor contractions associated with urinary leakage, and a loss of coordination between the detrusor and sphincter muscles (detrusor-sphincter dyssynergia).

Functional UI occurs when long-standing deficits in mobility, dexterity, or cognition cause or contribute to urinary leakage. A variety of conditions may produce functional UI in the patient receiving palliative care. For example, neurological deficits or pain may reduce the patient's ability to reach the toilet in a timely fashion. Cognitive deficits caused by malignancies or diseases of the brain may predispose the patient to functional UI. In addition, sedative or analgesic

**Table 15–1**
**Causes of Acute Urinary Incontinence (DIAPERS Mnemonic)**

| Associated Factor | Effect on Continence |
| --- | --- |
| Delirium, confusion | Reduces patient's ability to recognize and respond to cues to urinate, resulting in daytime or nighttime UI episodes. |
| Urinary tract infection | May exacerbate or create transient UI, especially in patients with history of UI or overactive bladder dysfunction. |
| Various drugs | Multiple classes of drugs predispose vulnerable patients to UI; diuretics increase urine production, potentially increasing frequency and risk for overactive detrusor contractions; antidepressants, sedatives, sleeping medications, or opioid analgesics may reduce the individal's ability to detect or respond to cues to toilet. |
| Excessive urine output | Polyuria associated with diabetes mellitus, diabetes insipidus, chronic venous disease, chronic heart failure, renal insufficiency, or high volume fluid intake increases urine production, potentially increasing voiding frequency and risk for overactive detrusor contractions. |
| Restricted mobility | Immobility, secondary to pain to as a direct result of a disease process affecting neuromuscular function, impairs the individual's ability to respond to cues to toilet and to access toilet facilities. |
| Constipation or stool impaction | Exact mechanism is unknown; distension of the rectal valut may reduce bladder capacity and cause functional obstruction by reflex increase in pelvic floor muscle tone, as the valut fills with stool. |

**Table 15–2**
**Causes of Intrinsic Sphincter Deficiency in the Patient Receiving Palliative Care**

**Urethral surgery**
Radical prostatectomy
Transurethral prostatectomy
Cryosurgery
Multiple urethral suspensions in women

**Surgery indirectly affecting the urethra via local denervation**
Abdominoperineal resection
Pelvic exenteration
Radical hysterectomy

**Neurological lesions of the lower spine**
Primary or metastatic tumors of the sacral spine
Pathological fracture of the sacral spinal column
Multiple sclerosis
Tertiary syphilis

medications may reduce awareness of bladder fullness and the need to urinate, particularly in the patient who experiences nocturia. Recently, a Wound, Ostomy and Continence Nurse Practitioner worked with the US Centers for Medicare and Medicaid Services to define an ICD-9 code for Functional Incontinence, which will be particularly useful for palliative care nurses providing services for this common cause of urinary leakage.[19]

Extraurethral UI occurs when a fistula creates an opening between the bladder and the vagina or skin, allowing urine to bypass the urethral sphincter. Within the context of palliative care, fistulas are usually caused by invasive pelvic or gynecological malignancies, extensive pelvic surgery, or radiation treatment.

## Bladder Spasm

Bladder spasms may be defined as a painful contraction of the bladder. Their pathophysiology is not well understood, but they are probably caused by an overactive detrusor contraction against a closed or partially blocked bladder outlet. Patients with bladder outlet obstruction due to a urologic malignancy obstructing the bladder outlet, or secondary blockage from a tumor outside the urinary tract, are at risk for bladder spasm. Foreign objects within the urinary tract, such as indwelling urinary catheters or ureteral stents, are also associated with an increased risk for bladder spasm, presumably because of their irritative effect on the urinary mucosa.[20] Instillation of potentially caustic substances into the bladder to treat significant hematuria or a urothelial tumor, or recent urologic surgery also may result in bladder spasm owing to their irritative effects.[21,22]

## Assessment and Management of Bothersome LUTS

The results of a focused history, physical assessment, urinalysis, and bladder log are essential for the evaluation of UI in the patient receiving palliative care. Urine culture and sensitivity testing, blood tests, urodynamic evaluation, or imaging studies also may be completed in specific cases.

The history focuses on the duration of the problem and the probable cause of bothersome lower urinary tract symptoms. *Transient* UI is typically characterized by a sudden occurrence of urinary leakage or an acute exacerbation of preexisting symptoms. These symptoms are typically similar to those of urge or stress UI. In contrast, chronic or established UI usually evolves over a period of time, typically months or possibly years.

The history can also be used to provide clues about the type of chronic UI. Stress UI is characterized by urine loss occurring with physical exertion or a sudden increase in abdominal pressure caused by coughing or sneezing. It occurs in the absence of a precipitous and strong urge to urinate. Approximately 36% of patients with overactive bladder syndrome experience urge UI.[23] (The diagnosis of overactive bladder is based on a combination of symptoms: diurnal voiding frequency, nocturia, and urgency with or without the symptom of urge UI).[24] A diagnosis of overactive bladder cannot be inferred from a report of the symptom of urge UI alone.

Reflex UI is suspected in the patient who experiences a paralyzing neurological lesion that affects spinal segments below the brainstem and above S2.[18] The patient frequently reports periodic urination with little or no warning and little or no associated urgency. The urinary stream may be intermittent (stuttering), and the patient may perceive a sensation of incomplete bladder emptying or report additional urinary leakage soon after completion of micturition.

Bladder spasms are diagnosed when a patient reports painful episodes localized to the suprapubic or lower abdomen.[20,25] These pains are usually characterized by a sudden onset, and described as stabbing, cramping or colicky. They are often associated with urgency and may produce bypassing of urine around an indwelling urinary catheter or urethral leakage if a suprapubic catheter is in place.

Functional UI is suspected when a general evaluation of the patient reveals significant limitations in mobility, dexterity, or cognition.[26] Continuous urinary leakage that is not associated with physical exertion raises the suspicion of extraurethral UI associated with a fistula, but it is also associated with severe stress UI caused by intrinsic sphincter deficiency. A focused physical examination provides additional evidence concerning the UI type and its severity. A general examination is used to evaluate the presence of functional UI and to determine the influence of functional limitations on other types of UI. A pelvic examination is completed to assess perineal skin integrity, to identify the presence of obvious fistulas or severe sphincter incompetence, and to evaluate local neurological function. Altered skin integrity, particularly if accompanied by a monilial rash or irritant dermatitis, indicates high-volume (severe) urinary leakage. In certain cases, the source of severe leakage can be easily identified as a large fistula or massive intrinsic sphincter deficiency associated with a gaping (patulous) urethra. A local neurological examination, focusing on local sensations, pelvic floor muscle tone, and the presence of the bulbocavernosus reflex, provides clues to underlying neurological problems leading to voiding dysfunction.

A bladder log (a written record of the timing of urination, volume, timing of UI episodes, and fluid intake) is useful because it allows a semiquantitative analysis of the patterns of urinary elimination, UI, and associated symptoms. It can also be used to assess fluid intake or the patient's response to prompted voiding.[27] The patient is taught to record the time of voluntary urination, episodes of incontinence and associated factors (urgency, physical activity), and type and amount of fluids consumed. This record is used to determine voiding interval, frequency of UI episodes along with associated factors, and the total volume and types of fluids consumed. Recording fluid intake allows the nurse to calculate the cumulative volume of fluids consumed each day, as well as the proportion of fluids containing caffeine or alcohol—substances that exacerbate bothersome LUTS. A 3-day bladder log is strongly recommended, but valuable information can be obtained from a 1- or 2-day document if a 3-day record is not available.[28]

Urinalysis serves several useful purposes in the evaluation of the patient with UI. The presence of nitrites and leukocytes on dipstick analysis or bacteriuria and pyuria on microscopic analysis indicates a clinically relevant urinary tract infection. Blood in the urine may coexist with a urinary tract infection, or it may indicate significant hematuria demanding prompt management (see later discussion). In the patient receiving palliative care, glucosuria may indicate poorly controlled diabetes mellitus causing osmotic diuresis and subsequent UI. In contrast, a low specific gravity may indicate diabetes mellitus or excessive fluid intake from oral or parenteral sources.

Other diagnostic tests are completed when indicated. For example, a urine culture and sensitivity analysis is obtained if the urinalysis reveals bacteriuria and pyuria, and an endoscopy is indicated if significant hematuria is present without an obvious explanation. Urodynamic testing is indicated in selected patients after transient UI is excluded and when simpler examinations have failed to establish an accurate diagnosis leading to an effective plan for management.

The management of UI is based on its type, the desires of the patient and family, and the presence of complicating factors. Transient UI is managed by addressing its underlying cause.[29] Acute delirium is managed by treating the underlying infection of disease causing the delirium, if feasible. A urinary tract infection is treated with sensitivity-driven antibiotics. Similarly, medication regimens are altered as feasible if they produce or exacerbate UI. Fecal impaction must be relieved and constipation aggressively managed. After initial disimpaction, a scheduled elimination program is frequently indicated. This program usually combines a peristaltic stimulant, such as a warm cup of coffee or tea, a mini-enema, or a suppository, and a scheduled elimination program. In addition, stool softeners or laxatives may be used if simpler programs fail to alleviate constipation. These interventions are combined with increased fluid intake as indicated and addition of fiber to the diet whenever feasible. Refer to Chapter 12 for a detailed discussion of bowel elimination problems.

A number of techniques are used to manage chronic or established UI. Every patient should be counseled about lifestyle alterations that may alleviate or occasionally relieve UI and associated LUTS.[30,31] Patients are advised to avoid routinely restricting fluid intake to reduce UI, because this strategy only increases the risk of constipation and concentrates the urine, irritating the bladder wall. Instead, they should be counseled to obtain the recommended daily allowance for fluids (30 mL/kg or 0.5 oz/lb),[32] to sip fluids throughout the day, and to avoid intake of large volumes of fluids over a brief period. Patients may also be taught to reduce or avoid bladder irritants that increase urine production or stimulate detrusor muscle tone, including caffeine and alcohol, depending on the goals of care and the short-term prognosis.

Containment devices may be used to provide protection while treatments designed to address underlying UI are undertaken, or they may be used for added protection if these interventions improve but fail to eradicate urine loss.[33] Women and men should be counseled about the disadvantages of using home products and feminine hygiene pads when attempting to contain urine. Specifically, they should be counseled that home products, such as tissues or paper towels, are not designed to contain urine, and feminine hygiene products are designed to contain menstrual flow. As an alternative, patients should be advised about products specifically designed for UI, including disposable and reusable products, inserted pads, and containment undergarments.

If the patient experiences primarily stress UI, the initial management is with behavioral methods, often combined with use of absorptive products. Pelvic floor muscle training is strongly recommended for mild to moderate stress UI,[34] but its applicability in the palliative care setting is limited. Instead, the patient may be taught a maneuver called the "knack." The knack describes a pelvic floor muscle contraction completed in response to physical exertion.[35] The patient is taught to identify, contract and relax the pelvic floor muscles, typically using some form of biofeedback. Biofeedback provides sensory, audible or palpatory cues allowing the patient to identify the pelvic floor muscles, and to differentiate contraction of these muscles from the abdominals, gluteal or thigh muscles. Simple biofeedback maneuvers include assisting the patient to identify the pelvic floor muscles during a gentle vaginal or digital rectal examination, asking the patient to interrupt the urinary stream, or asking the patient to contract and relax while seated on a chair with a firm seat in order to maxzimize proprioception. After learning to identify, contract and relax the pelvic floor muscles, the patient is taught to maximally contract (squeeze) these muscles when performing a maneuver associated with urine loss such as coughing, sneezing, walking or bending over to don socks. This maneuver increases urethral closure and resistance to UI and relieves or prevents stress UI. It is generally preferred in the palliative care setting because it provides some relief from stress UI within a comparatively brief period of time (usually within days to a week) as compared to more formalized pelvic floor muscle training requiring 3–6 months.

Medications also may be used to treat stress UI in selected cases. Imipramine, a tricyclic antidepressant with both α-adrenergic effects that increase urethral resistance and anticholinergic actions, may be useful for patients who experience stress UI or mixed stress and urge UI symptoms.[36] Duloxetine, a norepinephrine and serotonin reuptake inhibitor, acts on neurons in Onuf's nucleus—nuclei located in spinal segments S2–4 that modulate rhabdosphincter tone in women and men—and has been found to relieve stress UI in women.[37] Duloxetine has been approved by the US Food and Drug Administration for treatment of depression, but not stress UI, and its use for this indication is classified as off-label. Although both imipramine and duloxetine have the potential to alleviate stress UI, their benefits must be weighed carefully against the potential for side effects. Common side effects of imipramine include anticholinergic effects such as dry mouth, blurred vision, flushing, and heat intolerance. Imipramine also may affect the central nervous system and may be associated with short-term memory impairment, hallucinations, and nightmares. These side effects may be particularly significant in aged patients and in those with preexisting cognitive defects related to a primary tumor or disease. Common side effects of duloxetine include nausea (occurring in up to 38%), drowsiness, dry mouth, and constipation. Among patients with clinical depression, it has been associated with anxiety, agitation, anger, panic attacks and temporary suicidal thoughts or actions.[38]

An indwelling catheter may be inserted if intrinsic sphincter deficiency and subsequent stress UI are severe. Although not usually indicated, a larger catheter size may be required to prevent urinary leakage (bypassing) around the catheter.[39] A detailed discussion of catheter management is provided later in this chapter.

Overactive bladder dysfunction, with or without urge UI, is also managed by behavioral or pharmacological modalities (or both) whenever possible.[40] Behavioral interventions include reduction or avoidance of bladder irritants such as caffeine and modification of fluid intake described previously. The patient can also be taught to identify, isolate, contract and relax the pelvic floor muscles using principles described above. These skills are applied to a technique called *urge suppression*, which is used to inhibit specific episodes of urgency before UI occurs. When a sudden urge to urinate occurs, the patient is taught to stop, tighten the pelvic muscles in rapid succession using several "quick flick" contractions until the urge has subsided, and proceed to the bathroom at a normal pace. The patient also may be taught relaxation or other distraction techniques to cope with specific urge episodes. Behavioral methods are particularly helpful for the patient who is at risk for falling and related injuries.

Antimuscarinic medications are often used to manage overactive bladder syndrome and urge UI. Multiple agents are available. Novel agents are usually preferred because they can be taken on daily basis promoting adherence,[41] and they tend to have less pronounced agents than the older classic drugs within this class.[40] Antimuscarinic medications block acetyl choline from binding to cholinergic receptors in the bladder wall. This increases functional bladder capacity, inhibits overactive detrusor contractions and associated incontinence episodes, and reduces voiding frequency. The principal side effect of all these agents is dry mouth, which can be severe

**Table 15-3**
**Pharmacologic Management for Overactive Bladder and Urge Urinary Incontinence**

| Antimuscarinic Drugs | Dosage | Nursing Considerations |
|---|---|---|
| Tolterodine ER (Detrol LA) | 2–4 mg daily | May be administered at night to reduce dry mouth; administration with antacid or proton pump inhibitor may reduce bioavailability of drug; does not cross blood–brain barrier as readily as oxybutynin IR; the lower (2 mg) dose is recommended for patients with imparied hepatic function. |
| Oxybutynin IR (Ditropan IR) | 5 mg twice daily to three times daily | Associated with higher incidence of moderate to severe dry mouth than extended release agents; readily crosses blood–brain barrier, potentially increasing the risk of central nervous side effects. |
| Oxybutinin ER (Ditropan XL) | 5–15 mg daily | Administered via osmotic releasing system; advise patient that skeleton of tablet will be pass in stool 24–48 hours after ingestion; incidence and severity of dry mouth less than IR formulation; may be administered at bedtime to reduce dry mouth. |
| Oxybutynin TDS (Oxytrol) | 3.9 mg patch twice weekly | Incidence of dry mouth not statistically different than placebo in pivotal trials; transdermal delivery systems avoids first-pass effects of oral drug formulations, increasing bioavailability of drug; local skin irritation associated with use of patch not seen with oral agents. |
| Solifenacin (Vesicare) | 5–10 mg daily | Half life of drug approximately 45–68 hours; may be administered at night to minimize dry mouth; use with caution in patients with impared hepatic function |
| Darifenacin (Enablex) | 7.5–15 mg daily | Drug has greater affinity for $M_3$ muscarinic receptors; this receptor type is common in the bladder wall, bowel and other periperal organs, but absent in the central nervous system, reducing the potential for adverse central nervous system side effects; constipation rates reported in pivotal trial for this drug are higher than other drugs, possibly associated with presence of $M_3$ receptors in bowel wall. |
| Trospium ER (Sactura XR) | 60 mg daily | Drug is primarily excreted in urine rather than metabolized in liver, should be administered on empty stomach to maximize bioavailability; comparatively large size of tropsium molecule (it is a quartenary amine) and lipophobic properties reduce likelihood drug will cross blood–brain barrier producing central nervous system side effects. |
| Fesoterodine ER (Toviaz) | 4–8 mg daily | Lower dosage not required for mild to moderate impairment of hepatic function; may be administered at bedtime to reduce dry mouth. |

and can interfere with appetite and mastication.[36] Other side effects include blurred vision, constipation, flushing, heat intolerance, and cognitive effects such as nightmares or altered short-term memory. Table 15-3 describes pharmacologic options for managing overactive bladder and urge UI and related nursing considerations.[41–45]

Although antimuscarinic medications are often viewed as an alternative to behavioral therapies, they are better viewed as complementary modalities.[46] Specifically, all patients who wish to use antimuscarinic medications for overactive bladder or urge UI should be advised to void according to a timed schedule (usually every 2 to 3 hours, depending on the urinary frequency documented on a bladder log obtained during assessment), and taught urge-suppression skills. Similarly, patients whose lower urinary tract symptoms are not managed adequately by behavioral methods should be counseled about antimuscarinic medications before placement of an indwelling catheter is considered. Nevertheless, use of a catheter is often necessary for patients managed in a palliative care setting. Traditionally, indwelling catheters have been preferred, but external collection devices often provide a viable alternative to indwelling devices in men.

CASE STUDY

*Mr. M, A Patient with Incontinence and Condom Catheter*

Mr. M is a 58-year-old male who was diagnosed with a high grade, small-cell carcinoma of the prostate. He initially responded to androgen deprivation therapy, but his tumor ultimately became hormone independent and he experienced local extension of the tumor and distant metastases. He began chemotherapy with cisplatin and etoposide but developed urinary incontinence. His oncology team stated that monitoring urinary output while on this chemotherapy regimen was important, and his urinary leakage rendered this especially challenging. In addition to the need to monitor urine output during chemotherapy, his urinary incontinence led to incontinence-associated dermatitis, characterized by inflamed and eroded skin. He wished to continue his work, which remained an essential part of his identity, as long as possible, but he was also bothered by the social stigma of urine loss and the need to wear an adult containment brief (an "adult diaper" as he described it). Mr. M was therefore referred for discussion of options to the urology clinic.

After discussing multiple options, he elected to have a #16 French, all silicone indwelling urinary catheter placed initially to control his urine loss and to enable monitoring of urinary output. However, he found the catheter uncomfortable, and reported experiencing bladder spasms. At this point, he wanted to explore other options for treating his urinary incontinence. Discussion with the oncology team also focused on the potential risk of infection using long-term catheters in a patient with chemotherapy immunosuppression. The urology nursing team was able to fit the patient with an external collecting device (condom catheter) for daily use and an adaptor for the collection bag connection. He was taught how to place the catheter securely and attach the collection bag. This option also enabled him to remove the catheter if he regained urinary continence following his chemotherapy. As the chemotherapy began to reduce the size of his prostatic tumor, Mr. M experienced increasing daytime continence and he was able to restrict use of the external collecting device to nights only. After three cycles of chemotherapy, he regained urinary control and no longer required the condom catheter until his tumor ultimately returned and death occurred. Nevertheless, Mr. M made a special trip to visit the urology nursing team and express how satisfied he was that he could remain "diaper free" and continue his work, which meant so much to his identity and self esteem.

Application of a condom catheter or hydrocolloid-based external collection device is indicated when urge UI is severe and refractory of other treatments.[47,48] Alternatively, an indwelling catheter may be inserted in women or men who are unable to wear an external device. Indwelling catheterization is also indicated if urge UI is complicated by clinically relevant urinary retention or if the patient is near death and immobile. Because reflex UI is typically associated with diminished sensations of bladder filling, it is not usually responsive to behavioral treatments.[18] A minority of patients with reflex UI retain the ability to urinate spontaneously, but most cases must be managed with an alternative program. For men, an external collection device may be used to contain urine. Several devices are available, including a hydrocolloid-based collection device.[47,48] This device attaches to the glans penis, without covering the penile shaft. Multiple condom catheters are also available. A latex-free device is typically selected, preferably with adhesive incorporated into the wall of the condom. In some patients, an α-adrenergic blocking agent such as terazosin, doxazosin, tamsulosin, or alfuzosin is administered, to minimize the obstruction caused by detrusor–sphincter dyssynergia.[49] Intermittent catheterization is encouraged whenever feasible. The patient and at least one significant other should be taught a clean intermittent catheterization technique. For the patient with reflex UI, an anticholinergic medication is usually required in addition to catheterization, to prevent UI. If intermittent catheterization is not feasible or if reflex UI develops near the end of life, an indwelling catheter may be inserted. Although the indwelling catheter is associated with serious long-term complications and is avoided in patients with spinal cord injury and a significant life expectancy, it remains a viable alternative for the patient receiving palliative care.

Functional UI is treated by minimizing barriers to toileting and the time required to prepare for urination.[50,51] Strategies designed to remove barriers to toileting are highly individualized and are best formulated with the use of a multidisciplinary team, combining nursing with medicine, as well as physical and occupational therapy as indicated. Strategies used to maximize mobility and access to the toilet include using assistive devices such as a walker or wheelchair, widening bathroom doors, adding support bars, and providing a bedside toilet or urinal. The time required for toileting may be reduced by selected alterations in the patient's clothing, such as substituting tennis shoes with good traction for slippers or other footwear with slick soles and substituting Velcro- or elastic-banded clothing for articles with multiple buttons, zippers, or snaps.

If the patient has significant contributing cognitive disorders, functional UI is usually managed by a prompted voiding program.[52,53] Baseline evaluation includes a specialized bladder log, which is completed over a 48- to 72-hour period. The caregiver is taught to assist the patient to void on a fixed schedule, usually every 2 to 3 hours. The caregiver is taught to help the patient move to the toilet and prepare for urination; the caregiver also uses this opportunity to determine whether the pad incontinence brief reveals evidence of UI since the previous scheduled toileting. Patients who are successful, dry, and able to urinate with prompting on more than 50% of attempts completed during this trial period are considered good candidates for an ongoing prompted voiding regimen; those who are unsuccessful are considered poor candidates and are managed by alternative methods, including indwelling catheterization in highly selected cases.

Because extraurethral UI is caused by a fistulous tract and produces continuous urinary leakage, it must be managed initially by containment devices and preventive skin care. The type of containment device depends on the severity of the UI; an incontinent brief is frequently required. In some cases, the fistula may be closed by conservative (nonsurgical) means. An indwelling catheter is inserted, and the fistula is allowed to heal spontaneously.[54] This intervention is most likely to work for a traumatic (postoperative) fistula. If the fistula is a result of an invasive tumor or radiation therapy, it is not as likely to heal spontaneously. In such cases, cauterization and fibrin glue may be used to promote closure.[55] Alternatively, a suspension containing tetracycline may be prepared and used as a sclerosing agent. The adjacent skin is prepared by applying a skin protectant (such as a petrolatum, dimethicone or zinc oxide-based ointment) to protect it from the sclerosing agent. Approximately 5 to 10 mL of the tetracycline solution is injected into the fistula by a physician, and the lesion is monitored for signs of scarring and closure. If UI persists for 15 days or longer, the procedure may be repeated under the physician's direction. For larger fistulas or those that fail to respond to conservative measures, surgical repair is undertaken if feasible.

All patients who experience UI are at risk for developing Incontinence Associated Dermatitis (IAD), particularly when they also experience fecal incontinence and when urinary leakage is managed by an absorptive containment brief.[56] Skin damage is characterized by inflammation, often accompanied by erosion. IAD is usually associated with burning and itching, and it increases the risk for pressure ulceration. Prevention focuses on a structured regimen of skin cleansing, moisturization, and application of a skin protectant.[57] An incontinence or perineal skin cleanser that contains a moisturizing agent such as an emollient or humectant may be selected, followed by application of an ointment-based skin protectant or alcohol-free liquid acrylate moisture barrier. Alternatively, these steps may be combined using a single use perineal cloth that combines a skin cleanser, moisturizer and dimethicone-based skin protectant. Treatment of IAD begins with establishment of a structured skin cleansing regimen unless one is already in place. IAD is often associated with cutaneous candidiasis, which may be treated by applying a thin layer of an antifungal powder covered by a skin protectant, or application of an ointment-based antifungal agent. An ointment containing as active ingredients Balsam Peru, castor oil and trypsin also may be applied for IAD; this ointment combines active ingredients that promote wound healing with a skin protectant, shielding the skin from additional exposure to urine or stool.

### Assessment and Management of Bothersome LUTS: Urinary Stasis or Retention

A precipitous drop or sudden cessation of urinary outflow is a serious urinary system complication that may indicate *oliguria* or *anuria* (failure of the kidneys to filter the blood and produce urine), *urinary stasis* (blockage of urine transport from the upper to lower urinary tracts), or *urinary retention* (failure of the bladder to evacuate itself of urine). The following sections review the pathophysiology and management of urinary stasis or acute postrenal failure caused by bilateral ureteral obstruction and urinary retention.

### Obstruction of the Upper Urinary Tract

Upper urinary tract stasis in the patient receiving palliative care is usually caused by obstruction of one or both ureters.[58] The obstruction is typically attributable to a primary or metastatic tumor, and most arise from the pelvic region. In men, prostatic cancer is the most common cause, whereas pelvic (cervical, uterine, and ovarian) malignancies produce most ureteral obstructions in women. In addition to malignancies, retroperitoneal fibrosis secondary to inflammation or radiation may obstruct one or both ureters. Unless promptly relieved, bilateral ureteral obstruction leads to acute renal failure with uremia and elevated serum potassium, which can cause life-threatening arrhythmias.

When a single ureter is obstructed, the bladder continues to fill with urine from the contralateral (unobstructed) kidney. In this case, urinary stasis produces symptoms of ureteral or renal colic. Left untreated, the affected kidney is prone to acute failure and infection, and it may produce systemic hypertension because of increased renin secretion.

### Urinary Retention

*Urinary retention* is the inability to empty the urinary bladder despite micturition.[59] Acute urinary retention is an abrupt and complete inability to void. Patients are almost always aware of acute urinary retention because of the increasing suprapubic discomfort produced by bladder filling and distention and the associated anxiety. Chronic urinary retention occurs when the patient is partly able to empty the bladder by voiding but a significant volume of urine remains behind. Although no absolute cutoff point for chronic urinary retention can be defined, most clinicians agree that a residual volume of 200 mL or more deserves further evaluation.

Urinary retention is caused by two disorders: bladder outlet obstruction or deficient detrusor contraction strength. Bladder outlet obstruction occurs when intrinsic or extrinsic factors compress the urethral outflow tract. For the patient receiving palliative care, malignant tumors of the prostate, urethra, or bladder may produce anatomic obstruction of the urethra, whereas lesions affecting spinal segments below the brainstem micturition center but above the sacral spine cause functional obstruction associated with detrusor–sphincter dyssynergia.[60] In addition, brachytherapy may cause inflammation and congestion of the prostate, producing a combination of urinary retention and overactive bladder dysfunction.[61] In the patient receiving palliative care, deficient detrusor contraction strength usually occurs as a result of denervation or medication. Alternatively, it may result from histological damage to the detrusor muscle itself, usually caused by radiation therapy or by detrusor decompensation after prolonged obstruction. Neurological lesions commonly associated with deficient detrusor contraction strength include primary or metastatic tumors affecting the sacral spine or spinal column, multiple sclerosis lesions, tertiary syphilis, and diseases associated with peripheral polyneuropathies, such as advanced-stage diabetes mellitus or alcoholism. Poor detrusor contraction strength also may occur as a result of unavoidable denervation from large abdominopelvic surgeries, such as abdominoperineal resection or pelvic exenteration.

### Assessment and Management of Upper Tract Obstruction and Urinary Retention

Accurate identification of the cause of a precipitous drop in urine output is essential, because the management of upper urinary tract obstruction and of urinary retention are different. Because both conditions cause a precipitous drop in urinary output, the LUTS reported by the patient may be similar. Patients usually report difficulty initiating urination and a dribbling, intermittent flow. In contrast, these conditions produce few or no bothersome symptoms in some instances. However, upper urinary tract obstruction is more likely to produce flank pain, whereas acute urinary retention is more likely to produce discomfort localized to the suprapubic area. The pain associated with upper urinary tract obstruction is usually localized to one or both flanks, although it may radiate to the abdomen and even to the labia or testes if the lower ureter is obstructed. Its intensity varies from moderate to intense. It typically is not relieved by changes in position, and the patient is often restless. The discomfort associated with acute urinary retention is typically localized to the suprapubic area or the lower back. The patient with acute urinary retention also may feel restless, although this perception is usually attributable to the growing and unfulfilled desire to urinate.

A focused physical examination assists the nurse to differentiate urinary retention from upper urinary tract obstruction. The patient with bilateral ureteral obstruction and acute renal failure may have systemic evidence of uremia, including nausea, vomiting, and hypertension. In some cases, obstruction may by complicated by pyelonephritis, causing a fever and chills. An abdominal assessment also should be performed. Physical assessment of the patient with upper urinary tract obstruction reveals a nondistended bladder, whereas the bladder is grossly distended and may extend above the umbilicus in the patient with acute urinary retention. Blood analysis reveals an elevated serum creatinine, blood urea nitrogen, and potassium in the patient with bilateral ureteral obstruction, but these values are typically normal in the patient with urinary retention or unilateral ureteral obstruction.[58] Ultrasonography of the kidneys and bladder reveals ureterohydronephrosis above the level of the obstruction or bladder distention in the patient with acute urinary retention.

In contrast to the patient with ureteral obstruction or acute urinary retention, many patients with chronic retention remain unaware of any problem, despite large residual volumes of 500 mL or more.[59] When present, LUTS vary and may include feelings of incomplete bladder emptying, a poor force of stream, or an intermittent urinary stream. Patients are most likely to complain of diurnal voiding frequency and excessive nocturia (often arising four times or more each night), but these symptoms are not unique to incomplete bladder emptying. Although acute renal failure is uncommon in the patient with chronic urinary retention, the serum creatinine concentration may be elevated, indicating renal insufficiency attributable to lower urinary tract pathology.

Obstruction of the upper urinary tract is initially managed by reversal of fluid and electrolyte imbalances and prompt drainage.[58] Urinary outflow can be reestablished by insertion of a ureteral stent (drainage tube extending from the renal pelvis to the bladder) via cystoscopy. A ureteral stent is preferred because it avoids the need for a percutaneous puncture and drainage bag. In the case of bilateral obstruction, a stent is placed in each ureter under endoscopic guidance; a single stent is placed if unilateral obstruction is diagnosed. The patient is advised that the stents will drain urine into the bladder. However, because the stents often produce bothersome LUTS, the patient is counseled to ensure adequate fluid intake while avoiding bladder irritants, including caffeine and alcohol. In certain cases, an antimuscarinic medication may be administered to reduce the irritative LUTS or bladder spasms that sometimes are associated with a ureteral stent. Alternatively, belladonna and opium (B&O) suppositories may be administered if painful ureteral spasms occur that are not responsive to antimuscarinic agents. B&O suppositories contain 16.2 mg of belladonna (an anticholinergic agent) and 30–60 mg of opium (an opoid analgesic). One to 2 suppositories are administered once or twice daily. The suppository should be moistened prior to insertion and care taken to place it immediately beside the rectal wall rather than in a bolus of stool. Potential side effects include anticholnergic effects such as dry mouth and constipation, as well as sensitivity to light, drowsiness and central nervous depression owing to their opium content.

If the ureter is significantly scarred because of radiation therapy or distorted because of a bulky tumor, placement of a ureteral stent may not be feasible and a percutaneous nephrostomy tube may be required. The procedure may be done in an endoscopy suite or an interventional radiographic suite under local and systemic sedation or anesthesia. Unlike the ureteral stent that drains into the bladder, the nephrostomy tube is drained via a collection bag. The patient and family are taught to monitor urinary output from the bag and to secure the bag to the lower abdomen or leg in a manner that avoids kinking. The success of placement of a ureteral stent or nephrostomy tube is measured by the reduction in pain and in serum creatinine and potassium concentrations, indicating reversal of acute renal insufficiency.

Acute urinary retention is managed by prompt placement of an indwelling urinary catheter.[59,62] The patient is closely monitored as the bladder is initially drained, because of the very small risk of brisk diuresis associated with transient hyperkalemia, hematuria, hypotension, and pallor.[63] This risk may be further reduced by draining 500 mL, interrupted by a brief period during which the catheter is clamped (approximately 5 minutes), and followed by further drainage until the retained urine is evacuated. The catheter is left in place for up to 1 month, allowing the bladder to rest and recover from the overdistension typical of acute urinary retention. After this period, the bladder may be slowly filled with saline, preferably heated to body temperature, and the catheter removed.[64] The patient is allowed to urinate, and the voided volume is measured. This volume is compared with the volume infused, to estimate the residual volume; or a bladder ultrasound study can be completed to assess the residual volume. If the patient is able to evacuate the bladder successfully, the catheter is left out and the patient is taught to recognize and promptly manage acute urinary retention. If the patient is unable to urinate effectively, the catheter may be replaced or an intermittent catheterization program may be initiated, depending on the cause of the retention and the patient's ability to perform self-catheterization.

The patient with chronic urinary retention may be managed by behavioral techniques, intermittent catheterization, or an indwelling catheter.[59,62] Behavioral methods are preferred because they are noninvasive and not associated with any risk of adverse side effects. Scheduled toileting with double voiding may be used in the patient with low urinary residual volumes (approximately 200 to 400 mL). The patient is taught to attempt voiding every 3 hours while awake and to double void (urinate, wait for 3 to 5 minutes, and urinate again before leaving the bathroom). Higher urinary residual volumes and clinically relevant complications caused by urinary retention, including urinary tract infection or renal insufficiency, are usually managed by intermittent catheterization or an indwelling catheter.

Many factors enter into the choice between intermittent and indwelling catheterization, including the desires of the patient and family, the presence of an obstruction or low bladder wall compliance (e.g., a small or contracted bladder), and the prognosis. From a purely urological perspective, intermittent catheterization is preferable because it avoids long-term complications associated with an indwelling catheter, including chronic bacteriuria, calculi, urethral erosion, and catheter bypassing. However, an indwelling catheter may be preferable in a palliative care setting when: the urethra is technically difficult to catheterize; the patient has a small capacity with low bladder wall compliance; the patient is experiencing significant pain or limited upper extremity dexterity that interferes with the ability to effectively evacuate the bladder via micturition; or UI is complicated by retention.

## Managing the Indwelling Catheter

Although the decision to insert a catheter may be directed by a physician or nurse practitioner, decisions concerning catheter size, material of construction, and drainage bag are usually made by the nurse.[39,65,66] A relatively small catheter is typically sufficient to drain urine from the bladder. A 14- to 16-French catheter is adequate for men and a 12- to 14-French catheter is usually adequate for women. Larger catheters (18 to 20 French) are reserved for patients with significant intrinsic sphincter deficiency, hematuria, or sediment in the urine. Silastic, Teflon-coated tubes are avoided if the catheter is expected to remain in place more than 2 to 3 days. Instead, a silicone-coated, all silicone or hydrogel-coated latex catheter is selected because of its increased comfort.[67] A hydrogel catheter coated with a silver alloy, or a silicone catheter impregnated with nitrofurazone, may be inserted when catheterization is anticipated to last for 2 weeks or less in order to reduce the risk of catheter-associated urinary tract infection.[62] However, these have not been found to provide protection when left indwelling more than 2 weeks and they are not recommended for patients managed by long-term catheters.

In men, water-soluble lubricating jelly should be injected into the urethra before catheterization and, in women, the gel is liberally applied to the catheter. A lubricant containing 2% Xylocaine may be used to reduce the discomfort associated with catheter insertion. The catheter is inserted to the bifurcation of the drainage port. The retention balloon is filled with 10 mL to fill the dead space in the port while ensuring proper inflation, and the inflated balloon is gently withdrawn to near the bladder neck.

A drainage bag that provides adequate storage volume and reasonable concealment under clothing should be chosen. A bedside bag is preferred for bed-bound patients and for overnight use in ambulatory persons. The bedside bag should hold at least 2000 mL, should contain an antireflux valve to prevent retrograde movement of urine from bag to bladder, and should include a drainage port that is easily manipulated by the patient or care provider. In contrast, a leg bag or belly bag is preferred for ambulatory patients. It should hold at least 500 mL, should be easily concealed under clothing, and should attach to the leg or waist by elastic straps or a cloth pocket rather than latex straps, which are likely to irritate the underlying skin.

The patient is taught to keep the drainage bag level with or below the symphysis pubis. All indwelling catheters should be secured using a manufactured leg strap or adhesive backed device to reduce unintentional traction against the bladder neck or inadvertent urethral trauma.[68] Typically, the patient is encouraged to drink at least the recommended daily allowance of fluids, and to drink additional fluids if hematuria or sediment is present. However, these recommendations may be altered depending on the clinical setting and the patient's short-term prognosis. The catheter is routinely monitored for blockage caused by blood clots, sediment, or kinking of the drainage bag above the urinary bladder. The patient and family are also advised to monitor for signs and symptoms of clinically relevant infection, including fever, new hematuria, or urinary leakage around the catheter. They are also advised that bacteriuria is inevitable, even with the use of catheters containing a bacteriostatic coating, and that only clinically relevant (symptomatic) urinary tract infections should be treated.

CASE STUDY

*DY, A Patient with an Indwelling Catheter, Hematuria, and Clot Retention*

DY is a 69-year-old white woman with type 2 diabetes mellitus, hypertension, and idiopathic cirrhosis with a mild coagulopathy. She was diagnosed with endometrial cancer at age 65 and treated with external beam radiation therapy and interstitial radium seed implants. She began noting

LUTS, including frequency, urgency, and dysuria, and she developed gross hematuria with clots approximately 3 years after completing radiation therapy. She was initially treated with continuous bladder irrigation, intravesical alum, and prostaglandin instillations with minimal response. She underwent a cystoscopy for evacuation of blood clots. At that time, random bladder biopsies were obtained, which revealed chronic inflammation, hemorrhage, hemosiderin-laden macrophages, and vascular telangiectasia. There was no evidence of malignancy. Several areas of bleeding were cauterized. Hyperbaric oxygen therapy was attempted, but the patient did not tolerate the procedure well and refused further treatments. Over the next 3 months, she continued to have intermittent episodes of gross hematuria and progressive weakness.

DY again sought assistance when she experienced a particularly severe episode of hematuria with clot retention and a hematocrit of 12%. She was admitted to the hospital for transfusions and management of recurring hemorrhagic cystitis. A voiding cystourethrogram (VCUG) was obtained on admission, and she was treated with transfusions and continuous bladder irrigations until her sixth hospital day, when she was taken to the operating room for a cystoscopy, performed under anesthesia. Before the cystoscopy, Vaseline gauze was placed on the perineal skin. Because left vesicoureteral reflux was noted on the VCUG, a Fogarty balloon was passed into the distal left ureter and inflated to occlude the ureter. The bladder was filled, and her capacity was determined to be 300 mL. A total of 150 mL of a 1% formalin solution was slowly infused into the bladder and retained for 20 minutes. The bladder was then drained and irrigated with saline. A three-way indwelling catheter was placed, and continuous bladder irrigation was restarted. Her hematuria partially resolved, and she returned to the operating room 3 days later for instillation of 150 mL of a 3% formalin solution. The hematuria resolved after this second instillation, and the continuous bladder irrigation was discontinued within 24 hours. At the time of discharge the next day, she was voiding well and her urine remained free of hematuria. Postprocedure pain was managed by a combination of urinary analgesics, such as phenazopyridine (Pyridium), and an oral narcotic analgesic (oxycodone). Both medications were discontinued 1 week after the final instillation.

Four months later, DY presented with recurrent dysuria, hematuria, and clots requiring transfusion and repeated cystoscopy with instillation of a 1% formalin solution. She responded to this treatment and was discharged 2 days after treatment.

This case demonstrates the risk of recurrent hemorrhagic cystitis after treatment with a combination of external beam and interstitial radiotherapy. This patient's coagulopathy may have exacerbated the risk for significant hematuria. In this case, the initial episode of hematuria occurred 3 years after therapy, and it recurred over a period of 22 months despite treatment with continuous bladder irrigation, cystoscopy with electrocauterization, hyperbaric oxygen, intravesical alum, and prostaglandin. Ultimately, the condition failed to respond to intravesical instillation of a 1% formalin solution, but it did respond to a 3% solution. Nonetheless, the patient experienced a single recurrence within a period of 4 months, which responded to a single instillation of a 1% formalin solution. She remained symptom-free at 1 year.

Fortunately, life-threatening blood loss is a rare complication of hemorrhagic cystitis and bladder tumors. Treatment usually begins with bladder irrigation, evacuation of clots, and intravesical instillations such as alum or silver nitrate and progresses to therapy with intravesical prostaglandin and formalin. Because of the significant risk of toxicity if formalin is absorbed, a Fogarty catheter must be introduced to prevent reflux of formalin into the upper urinary tract and renal capillaries. Alternatives include cystoscopy with electrical cauterization or laser coagulation of individual bleeding sites. Selective embolization or ligation of the hypogastric artery, palliative cystectomy, or radical nephrectomy may be required as a last resort. Table 15–4 summarizes the treatment options for hemorrhagic cystitis.

## Assessment and Management of Bothersome LUTS: Bladder Spasm

Irritative LUTS, including a heightened sense of urgency and urethral discomfort, are common in patients with a long-term indwelling catheter or ureteral stent. In certain cases, these irritative symptoms are accompanied by painful bladder spasms. Bladder spasms are characterized by intermittent episodes of excruciating, painful cramping localized to the suprapubic region. They are caused by high-pressure, overactive detrusor contractions in response to a specific irritation.[58] Urine may bypass (leak around) the catheter or cause urge UI in the patient with a stent. Painful bladder spasms may be the direct result of catheter occlusion by blood clots, sediment, or kinking; or they may be associated with a needlessly large catheter, an improperly inflated retention balloon, or hypersensitivity to the presence of the catheter or stent or to principal constituents. Other risk factors include pelvic radiation therapy, chemotherapeutic agents (particularly cyclophosphamide), intravesical tumors, urinary tract infections, and bladder or lower ureteral calculus.

Bladder spasms are managed by altering modifiable factors or by administering anticholinergic medications if indicated (Table 15–5). Changing the urethral catheter may relieve bladder spasms. An indwelling catheter is usually changed every 4 weeks or more often because of the risk of blockage and encrustation with precipitated salts, hardened urethral secretions, and bacteria.

In addition to changing the catheter, the nurse should consider altering the type of catheter. For example, a catheter with

**Table 15-4**
**Treatment Options for Hemorrhagic Cystitis**

| Agent | Action | Route of Administration/Dosage | Problems/Contraindications |
|---|---|---|---|
| ε-Aminocaproic acid | Acts as an inhibitor of fibrinolysis by inhibiting plasminogen activation substances | 5 g loading dose orally or parenterally, followed by 1–1.25 g hourly to max of 30 g in 24 h; Maximum response in 8–12 h | Potential thromboembolic complications<br>Increased risk of clot retention<br>Contraindicated in patients with upper urinary tract bleeding or vesicoureteral reflux<br>Decreased blood pressure |
| Silver nitrate | Chemical cautery | Intravesical instillation: 0.5% to 1.0% solution in sterile water instilled for 10–20 min followed by no irrigation; multiple instillations may be required | Reported as 68% effective<br>Case report of renal failure in patient who precipitated silver salts in renal collecting system, causing functional obstruction. |
| Alum (may use ammonium or potassium salt of aluminum) | Chemical cautery | Continuous bladder irrigation: 1% solution in sterile water, pH = 4.5 (salt precipitates at pH of 7) | Requires average of 21 h of treatment<br>Thought to not be absorbed by bladder mucosa; however, case reports of aluminum toxicity in renal failure patients |
| Formalin (aqueous solution of formaldehyde) | Cross-links proteins; exists as monohydrate methylene glycol and as a mixture of polymeric hydrates and polyoxyethylene glycols; rapidly "fixes" the bladder mucosa | Available as 37–40%, aqueous formaldehyde (= 100% formalin) diluted in sterile water to desired concentration (1% formalin = 0.37% formaldehyde); instillation: 50 mL for 4–10 min or endoscopic placement of 5% formalin-soaked pledgets placed onto bleeding site for 15 min and then removed | Painful, requires anesthesia<br>Vesicoureteral reflux (relative contraindication): patients placed in Trendelenburg position with low-grade reflux or ureteral occlusive balloons used with high-grade reflux<br>Extravasation causes fibrosis, papillary necrosis, fistula, peritonitis |

*Sources:* References 69,70.

**Table 15-5**
**Conditions Associated with Detrusor Overactivity in the Patient Receiving Palliative Care**

| Condition | Disorder |
|---|---|
| Neurological lesions above the brainstem micturition center | (Overactive bladder, with or without urge UI) Posterior fossa tumors causing intracranial pressure increased |
| Primary or metastatic tumors of the spinal segments | Cerebrovascular accident (stroke) |
| | Diseases affecting the brain, including multiple sclerosis, AIDS |
| Neurological lesions below the brainstem neicturition center but above sacral spinal segments | Reflex UI with vesicosphincter dyssynergia |
| | Primary or metastatic tumors of the spinal cord |
| | Tumors causing spinal cord compression because of their effects on the spinal column |
| | Systemic diseases directly affecting the spinal cord, including advanced-stage AIDS, transverse myelitis, Guillain-Barré syndrome |
| Inflammation of the bladder | (Overactive bladder, with or without urge UI) |
| | Primary bladder tumors, including papillary tumors or carcinoma in situ |
| | Bladder calculi (stones) |
| | Radiation cystitis, including brachytherapy |
| | Chemotherapy-induced cystitis |
| Bladder outlet obstruction | (Overactive bladder usually without urge UI) |
| | Prostatic carcinoma |
| | Urethral cancers |
| | Pelvic tumors causing urethral compression |

AIDS, acquired immunodeficiency syndrome; UI, urinary incontinence.

a smaller French size may be inserted if the catheter is larger than 16 French, unless the patient is experiencing a buildup of sediment causing catheter blockage. Similarly, a catheter with a smaller retention balloon (5 mL) may be substituted for a catheter with a larger balloon (30 mL), to reduce irritation of the trigone and bladder neck. Use of a catheter that is constructed of hydrophilic polymers or latex-free silicone may relieve bladder spasms and diminish irritative LUTS because of their greater biocompatibility when compared with Teflon-coated catheters.

Instruction about the position of the catheter, drainage tubes, and bags is reinforced; and the drainage tubes and urine are assessed for the presence of sediment or clots likely to obstruct urinary drainage. In certain cases, such as when the urethral catheter produces significant urethritis with purulent discharge from the urethra, a suprapubic indwelling catheter may be substituted for the urethral catheter. A suprapubic catheter also may be placed in patients who have a urethra that is technically difficult to catheterize, or who tend to encrust the catheter despite adequate fluid intake. Once established, these catheters are changed monthly, usually in the outpatient, home care, or hospice setting.

Patients with indwelling catheters who are prone to rapid encrustation and blockage present a particular challenge for the palliative care nurse. Options for management include frequent catheter changes (sometimes as often as one or two times per week) and irrigation of the catheter with a mildly acidic solution such as Renacidin. Irrigation may be completed once or several times weekly, and a small volume of solution is used (approximately 15 mL) to provide adequate irrigation of the catheter while avoiding irritation of the bladder epithelium.[71]

Bladder spasms also may indicate a clinically relevant urinary tract infection. The catheter change provides the best opportunity to obtain a urine specimen. This specimen should be obtained from the catheter and never from the drainage bag. Although bacteriuria is inevitable with a long-term indwelling catheter, cystitis associated with painful bladder spasms should be managed with sensitivity-guided antibiotic therapy.

The patient is taught to drink sufficient fluids to meet or exceed the recommended daily allowance of 30 mL/kg (0.5 oz/lb) whenever feasible. Reduced consumption of beverages or foods containing bladder irritants, such as caffeine or alcohol, also may alleviate bladder spasms in some cases.

If conservative measures or catheter modification fail to relieve bladder spasms, an anticholinergic medication may be administered. These medications work by inhibiting the overactive contractions that lead to painful bladder spasms.

### CASE STUDY
#### Mr. W, A Patient with Bladder Spasms in Hospice Care

Mr. W is an 81-year-old gentleman with progressive, metastatic lung cancer with significant pain and limited mobility. He developed urinary incontinence and a silastic,

18 French indwelling urethral catheter with a 30 mL retention balloon was placed based on hospice protocol. After a week spent with the indwelling catheter, the urology team was consulted for bladder spasms and leakage of urine around the Foley catheter (catheter bypassing). During this period, he also developed incontinence-associated dermatitis affecting his penis and the skin folds underneath the scrotum and on the inner thighs. The hospice nurse reported that the discomfort from his bladder spasm and skin irritation was not addressed by the opioid analgesics he was receiving for his metastatic lung cancer.

His indwelling catheter was replaced with a 16 French hydrogel-coated catheter, with a 5 mL retention balloon. A Velcro leg strap catheter securing device was placed to prevent traction of the retention balloon on the bladder neck. In addition, a skin care regimen comprising twice daily cleansing with a disposable washcloth containing a perineal cleanser, moisturizer, and 3% dimethicone cleanser was instituted. Mr. W initially experienced relief from bladder spasm, and his incontinence-associated dermatitis resolved within 7 days of beginning his skin care regimen. Unfortunately, his bladder spasms returned 2 days later, resulting in intermittent episodes of pain and catheter bypassing. In an effort to control leakage, the hospice nurses inflated the balloon to 10 and then 15 mL. However, the bladder spasms did not improve and appeared to increase, although the leakage diminished. Urology nursing was again consulted and suggested reduction in balloon inflation size, as this may have been contributing to spasms. The balloon was deflated to 5 mL and the patient started 2 mg extended release tolterodine capsules (Detrol™ LA) daily. This resulted in relief from his bladder spasms, but he reported a very dry mouth. The Detrol was discontinued and a 3.9 mg transdermal oxybutynin patch (Oxytrol) was prescribed. This transdermal medication reduced the need for one more oral agent on a daily basis, and it did not cause the dry mouth associated with the oral antimuscarinic. After 3 days of this medication, along with adjusted and reduced balloon size, the patient's bladder spasms and leakage stopped altogether.

This case illustrates several important aspects of indwelling catheter care, management of bladder spasms, and perineal skin care in the palliative care setting. Because of his metastatic lung cancer, Mr. W was experiencing significant pain and limited ability to ambulate. A decision to insert an indwelling catheter was made when he developed urinary incontinence in order to reduce the need for him to move to a toilet, to protect his skin from the potentially damaging effect of repeated exposure to urine, and to preserve him from the indignity of repeated episodes of urinary incontinence. However, the original indwelling catheter resulted in bladder spasms and catheter bypassing. Rather than increasing the catheter and balloon size, the urology team appropriately chose to reduce the catheter size to 16 French, and to reduce the retention balloon size to 5 mL. They also elected to insert a catheter with a hydrogel coating, and to employ a leg strap securing device, in an attempt to reduce irritation and traction at the bladder neck and within the urethra. These actions resulted in relief from bladder spasm for approximately 48 hours. When the spasms recurred, the hospice nurses increased the balloon size to 15 mL, which reduced urinary leakage around the catheter. However, increasing the balloon size probably increased the irritation at the level of the bladder neck, and failed to relieve the underlying bladder spasms. Instead, the patient was managed by reducing the balloon size to a standard 5 mL and an antimuscarinic medication was begun. This combination of interventions relieved the bladder spasms and catheter bypassing, but he experienced bothersome dry mouth. He was then switched to a transdermal oxybutynin patch, which avoids the first pass metabolic effect associated with oral agents, and is associated with a low occurrence of dry mouth. It relieved his painful bladder spasm and associated leakage without causing recurrence of his bothersome dry mouth.

## Hematuria

*Hematuria* is defined as the presence of blood in the urine. It results from a variety of renal, urological, and systemic processes. When gross hematuria presented as an initial complaint or finding in an adult, further evaluation in one study revealed that 23% of patients had an underlying malignancy.[66,72] In the palliative care setting, hematuria occurs more commonly after pelvic irradiation or chemotherapy, or as the result of a major coagulation disorder or a newly diagnosed or recurring malignancy.

Hematuria is divided into two subtypes according to its clinical manifestations. Microscopic hematuria is characterized by hemoglobin or myoglobin on dipstick analysis and more than 3 to 5 red blood cells (RBCs) per high-power field (hpf) under microscopic urinalysis, but the presence of blood remains invisible to the unaided eye. Macroscopic (gross) hematuria is also characterized by dipstick and microscopic evidence of RBCs in the urine, as well as a bright red or brownish discoloration that is apparent to the unaided eye.

In the context of palliative care, hematuria can also be subdivided into three categories depending on its severity.[69] Mild hematuria is microscopic or gross blood in the urine that does not produce obstructing clots or cause a clinically relevant decline in hematocrit or hemoglobin. Moderate and severe hematuria are associated with more prolonged and high-volume blood losses; hematuria is classified as moderate if < 6 units of blood are required to replace blood lost within the urine and as severe if ≥ 6 units are required. Both moderate and severe hematuria may produce obstructing clots that lead to acute urinary retention or obstruction of the upper urinary tract.

### Pathophysiology

Hematuria originates as a disruption of the endothelial–epithelial barrier somewhere within the urinary tract.[73] Inflammation of this barrier may lead to the production of cytokines, with subsequent damage to the basement membrane and passage of RBCs into the urinary tract. Laceration of this barrier may be caused by an invasive tumor, iatrogenic or other trauma, vascular accident, or arteriovenous malformation. Hematuria that originates within the upper urinary tract is often associated with tubulointerstitial disease or an invasive tumor, whereas hematuria originating from the lower urinary tract is typically associated with trauma, an invasive tumor, or radiation- or chemotherapy-induced cystitis.

In the patient receiving palliative care, significant hematuria most commonly occurs as the result of a hemorrhagic cystitis related to cancer, infection (viral, bacterial, fungal, or parasitic), chemical toxins (primarily from oxazaphosphorine alkylating agents), radiation, anticoagulation therapy, or an idiopathic response to anabolic steroids or another agent.[69] Radiation and chemotherapeutic agents account for most cases of moderate to severe hematuria.

Radiation cystitis is typically associated with pelvic radiotherapy for cancer of the uterus, cervix, prostate, rectum, or lower urinary tract. Most of these patients (80% to 90%) experience bothersome LUTS (diurnal voiding frequency, urgency, and dysuria) that reach their maximum intensity near the end of treatment and subside within 6 to 12 weeks after cessation therapy. However, about 10% to 20% of patients experience clinically relevant cystitis that persists well beyond the end of treatment or occurs months or even years after radiotherapy.[74,75] In addition to bothersome LUTS, these patients experience pain and hematuria caused by mucosal edema, vascular telangiectasia, and submucosal hemorrhage. They also may experience interstitial and smooth muscle fibrosis with low bladder compliance and markedly reduced bladder capacity.[69] Severe fibrosis associated with radiotherapy can lead to moderate to severe hematuria, as well as upper urinary tract distress (ureterohydronephrosis, vesicoureteral reflux, pyelonephritis, and renal insufficiency) caused by chronically elevated intravesical pressures.

Chemotherapy-induced cystitis usually occurs after treatment with an oxazaphosphorine alkylating agent, such as cyclophosphamide or isophosphamide.[69] A urinary metabolite produced by these drugs, acrolein, is believed to be responsible. Hemorrhage usually occurs during or immediately after treatment, but delayed hemorrhage may occur in patients undergoing long-term therapy. The effects on the bladder mucosa are similar to those described for radiation cystitis.

### Assessment

Because bleeding can occur at any level in the urinary tract from the glomerulus to the meatus, a careful, detailed history is needed to identify the source of the bleeding and to initiate an appropriate treatment plan. The patient should be asked whether the hematuria represents a new, persistent, or recurrent problem. This distinction is often helpful, because recurrent or persistent hematuria may represent a benign predisposing condition, whereas hematuria of new or recent onset is more likely to result from conditions related to the need for palliative care. A review of prior urinalyses also may provide clues to the onset and history of microscopic hematuria in particular. The patient is queried about the relation of grossly visible hematuria to the urinary stream. Bleeding limited to initiation of the stream is often associated with a urethral source, bleeding during the entire act of voiding usually indicates a source in the bladder or upper urinary tract, and bleeding near the termination of the stream often indicates a source within the prostate or male reproductive system.

The patient with gross hematuria should also be asked about the color of the urine: a bright red hue indicates fresh blood, whereas a darker hue (often described as brownish, rust, or "Coke" colored) indicates older blood. Some patients with severe hematuria report the passage of blood clots. Clots that are particularly long and thin, resembling a shoestring or fishhook, suggest an upper urinary tract source; larger and bulkier clots suggest a lower urinary tract source.

The patient is asked about any pain related to the hematuria; this questioning should include the site and character of the pain and any radiation of pain to the flank, lower abdomen, or groin. Flank pain usually indicates upper urinary tract problems, abdominal pain radiating to the groin usually indicates lower ureteral obstruction and bleeding, and suprapubic pain suggests obstruction or infection causing hematuria.

In addition to questions about the hematuria, the nurse should ask about specific risk factors, including a history of urinary tract infections; systemic symptoms suggesting infection or renal insufficiency including fever, weight loss, rash, and recent systemic infection; any history of primary or metastatic tumors of the genitourinary system; and chemotherapy or radiation therapy of the pelvic or lower abdominal region. A focused review of medications includes all chemotherapeutic agents used currently or in the past and any current or recent administration of anticoagulant medications, including warfarin, heparin, aspirin, nonsteroidal anti-inflammatory drugs, and other anti-coagulant agents.

### Physical Examination

Physical examination also provides valuable clues to the source of hematuria. When completing this assessment, the nurse should particularly note any abdominal masses or tenderness, skin rashes, bruising, purpura (suggesting vasculitis, bleeding, or coagulation disorders), or telangiectasia (suggesting von Hippel-Lindau disease). Blood pressure should be assessed, because a new onset or rapid exacerbation of hypertension may suggest a renal source for hematuria. The lower abdomen is examined for signs of bladder distention, and a rectal assessment is completed to evaluate apparent prostatic or rectal masses or induration.

### Laboratory Testing

A dipstick and microscopic urinalysis is usually combined with microscopic examination when evaluating hematuria. This provides a semiquantitative assessment of the severity of hematuria (RBCs/hpf), and it excludes pseudohematuria (reddish urine caused by something other than RBCs, such as ingestion of certain drugs, vegetable dyes, or pigments).

Urinalysis provides further clues to the likely source of the bleeding.[76] Dysmorphic RBCs, cellular casts, renal tubular cells, and proteinuria indicate upper urinary tract bleeding. In contrast, hematuria from the lower urinary tract is usually associated with normal RBC morphology.

Additional evaluation is guided by clues from the history, physical examination, and urinalysis. For example, the presence of pyuria and bacteriuria suggests cystitis as the cause of hematuria and indicates the need for culture and sensitivity testing. The calcium/creatinine ratio should be assessed in a random urine sample for patients with painful macroscopic hematuria, to evaluate the risk for stone formation, particularly for individuals with hyperparathyroidism or prolonged immobility. A random urine protein/creatinine ratio and measurement of the $C_3$ component of complement may be indicated in patients with proteinuria or casts, to evaluate for glomerulopathy or interstitial renal disease. Further studies also may be completed, to evaluate the specific cause of hematuria and implement a treatment plan.

### Imaging Studies

Ultrasonography is almost always indicated in the evaluation of hematuria in the patient receiving palliative care.[69] It is used to identify the size and location of cystic or solid masses that may act as the source of hematuria and to assess for obstruction, most stones, larger blood clots, and bladder-filling defects. An intravenous pyelogram also may be used to image the upper and lower urinary tracts, but its clinical use is limited by the risk of contrast allergy or nephropathy. Cystoscopy is performed if a bladder lesion is suspected, and ureteroscopy with retrograde pyelography may be completed if an upper urinary tract source of bleeding is suspected.

### Management

The management of hematuria is guided by its severity and its source or cause. Preventive management for chemotherapy-induced hematuria begins with administration of sodium 2-mercaptoethanesulfonate (mesna) to patients receiving an alkylating agent for cancer.[70] This is given parenterally, and it oxidizes to a stable, inactive form within minutes after administration. It becomes active when it is excreted into the urine, where it neutralizes acrolein (the metabolite postulated to cause chemotherapy-induced cystitis and hematuria) and slows degradation of the 4-hydroxy metabolites produced by administration of alkylating drugs. It is given with cyclophosphamide (20 mg/kg at time 0 and every 4 hours for 2 or 3 doses). When combined with vigorous hydration, it has been shown to protect the bladder from subsequent damage and hematuria.

Mild urinary retention is managed by identifying and treating its underlying cause. For example, sensitivity-guided antibiotics are used to treat a bacterial hemorrhagic cystitis, and extracorporeal lithotripsy may be used to treat hematuria associated with a urinary stone. While the hematuria persists, the patient is encouraged to drink more than the recommended daily allowance for fluids, to prevent clot formation and urinary retention. In addition, the patient is assisted in obtaining adequate nutritional intake to replace lost blood, and iron supplementation is provided if indicated.

In contrast to mild hematuria, moderate to severe cases often lead to the formation of blood clots, causing acute urinary retention and bladder pain. In these cases, complete evacuation of clots from the bladder is required before a definitive assessment and treatment strategy are implemented.[58] A large-bore urethral catheter (24 or 26 French in the adult) is placed, and manual irrigation is performed with a Toomey syringe. The bladder is irrigated with saline until no further clots are obtained and the backflow is relatively clear.[50] A 22- or 24-French three-way indwelling catheter is then placed, to allow continuous bladder irrigation using cold or iced saline. Percutaneous insertion of a suprapubic catheter is not recommended because of limitations of size and the potential to "seed" the tract if a bladder malignancy is present.

Unsuccessful attempts to place a urethral catheter or recurrent obstruction of the irrigation catheter provides a strong indication for endoscopic evaluation. Rigid cystoscopy is preferred because it allows optimal evacuation of bladder clots and further evaluation of sites of bleeding; retrograde pyelography or ureteroscopy may also be completed if upper urinary tract clots are suspected. Based on the findings of endoscopic evaluation, sites of particularly severe bleeding are cauterized or resected.

After the initial evacuation of obstructing clots, bladder irrigations or instillations may be completed if multiple sites of bleeding are observed or if the risk of recurrence is high, as in the case of radiation- or chemotherapy-induced hematuria. Table 15–4 summarizes treatment options for moderate to severe hematuria and their route, administration, and principal nursing considerations.

### CASE STUDY
#### Mr. J, A Patient with Urinary Obstruction and Percutaneous Nephrostomy

Mr. J is a 57-year-old African American male with prostate cancer. He was undergoing palliative chemotherapy for metastatic prostate cancer to the bone and pelvis lymph nodes when he developed persistent nausea, and his creatinine was found to be 2.8 mg/dL, up from his baseline 1.5 mg/dL. He was found to have incomplete bladder emptying and bladder outlet obstruction identified by ultrasound and non-contrast CT scan. Initially an indwelling urethral catheter was inserted that temporarily relieved his urinary retention and his creatinine dropped from 2.8 mg/dL to 1.6 mg/dL. His chemotherapy reduced the prostatic tumor volume and the severity of his bladder outlet obstruction. He underwent a trial of voiding and his indwelling urethral catheter was removed.

Four weeks later he again experienced a rising creatinine of 2.6 mg/dL accompanied by nausea and lower abdominal discomfort. Ultrasound at this point revealed bilateral hydronephrosis (enlargement of the renal pelvicaliceal systems). He was admitted to hospital after a difficult indwelling catheterization failed to relieve the hydronephrosis. His urologist performed a cystoscopy that revealed that growth of his prostate malignancy had led to obstruction of both the bladder outlet and both ureteral orifices. He was discharged from hospital with bilateral percutaneous tubes to drain bags. He was taken to the angiographic interventional radiology suite and bilateral percutaneous nephrostomy tubes were placed. This procedure relieved his hydronephrosis and his creatinine returned to baseline values (1.7 mg/dL).

Mr. J initially found his bilateral percutaneous nephrostomy tubes cumbersome. However, he also reported that they relieved his abdominal discomfort, improved his appetite, and enabled improved urinary drainage and a return of his serum creatinine to baseline values. His home health nurses worked to improve dressing comfort and the family was taught dressing care and tube management. By preserving maximal renal function, the patient was able to undergo further cycles of chemotherapy and remain out of the hospital. He also remained free of complaints of nausea and lower abdominal pain for many weeks while on palliative chemotherapy. Home health and, eventually, hospice nurses provided support in terms of nursing care of the nephrostomy tubes and drains. A waterproof covering was fashioned so the patient could shower on the days of the nurse visit. Then the dressings were changed and remained dry and free of complications.

Although Mr. J ultimately experienced progression of his prostatic malignancy and eventually was unable to undergo further chemotherapy, he expressed pleasure that the nephrostomy tubes allowed him an opportunity to try additional chemotherapeutic options in an attempt to slow progression of his disease. In addition, placement of nephrostomy tubes enabled him to spend valuable time with his family and to remain in his home with them on a special holiday. His family supported him at home with the help of hospice care.

This case illustrates the importance of evaluating the source of urinary tract obstruction, and the potentially beneficial effects of insertion of an indwelling urinary catheter or nephrostomy tubes in order to relieve obstruction and improve renal function. Initially, Mr. J experienced obstruction of the bladder outlet with incomplete bladder emptying transiently relieved by catheterization. Because chemotherapy initially reduced his tumor size, he was able to resume spontaneous voiding for a period of time. Ultimately, his tumor recurred, resulting in obstruction of both lower urinary tract and the ureteral outlets, leading to a rising creatinine and bilateral hydronephrosis. In this situation, insertion of an indwelling catheter was insufficient to relieve ureteral obstruction, and bilateral nephrostomy tube placement was required. Although the patient initially found the nephrostomy tubes cumbersome, he ultimately reported that their presence was worthwhile because they relieved his lower abdominal pain and nausea, and allowed him to pursue further chemotherapy—slowing progression of his cancer and allowing him to spend additional time with his family while remaining in a home care setting.

## Summary

Patients receiving palliative care frequently experience urinary system disorders. A malignancy or systemic disease may affect voiding function and produce UI, urinary retention, or upper urinary tract obstruction. In addition, upper acute renal insufficiency or renal failure may occur if the upper urinary tract becomes obstructed. These disorders may be directly attributable to a malignancy or systemic disease, or they may be caused by a specific treatment such as radiation, chemotherapy, or a related medication. Nursing management of patients with urinary system disorders is affected by the nature of the urological condition, the patient's general condition, and the nearness to death.

REFERENCES

1. Gray M, Brown KC. Genitourinary system. In: Thompson JM, McFarland GK, Hirsh JE, Tucker SM, eds. Clinical Nursing (5th ed). St. Louis: Mosby, 2002:917–999.

2. Gray ML. Physiology of voiding. In: Doughty DB, ed. Urinary and Fecal Incontinence: Current Management Concepts (3rd ed). St. Louis: Mosby-Elsevier, 2006:21–54.

3. Griffiths D, Tadic SD. Bladder control, urgency, and urge incontinence: Evidence from functional brain imaging. Neurourol Urodyn 2008;27:466–474.

4. Hruz P, Lovblad KO, Nirkko AC, Thoeny H, El-Koussy M, Danuser H. Identification of brain structures involved in micturition with functional magnetic resonance imaging (fMRI). J Neuroradiol 2008;35:144–149.

5. Kitta T, Kakizaki H, Furuno T, Moriya K, Tanaka H, Shiga T, Tamaki N, Yabe I, Sasaki H, Nonomura K. Brain activation during detrusor overactivity in patients with Parkinson's disease: A positron emission tomography study. J Urol 2006;175:994–998.

6. Sakakibara R, Hattori T, Yasuda K, Yamanishi T. Micturitional disturbance after hemispheric stroke: Analysis of the lesion site by CT and MRI. J Neurol Sci 1996;137:47–56.

7. Yamamoto T, Sakakibara R, Hashimoto K, Nakazawa K, Uchiyama T, Liu Z, Ito T, Hattori T. Striatal dopamine level increases in the urinary storage phase in cats: An in vivo microdialysis study. Neuroscience 2005;135:299–303.

8. Morrison JF. The discovery of the pontine micturition centre by F. J. F. Barrington. Exp Physiol 2008;93:742–745.

9. Kavia RB, Dasgupta R, Fowler CJ. Functional imaging and the central control of the bladder. J Comp Neurol 2005;493:27–32.

10. Andersson KE, Arner A. Urinary bladder contraction and relaxation: Physiology and pathophysiology. Physiol Rev 2004;84:935–986.

11. Eglen RM. Muscarinic receptor subtypes in neuronal and non-neuronal cholinergic function. Auton Autacoid Pharmacol 2006;26:219–233.

12. Anisuzzaman AS, Morishima S, Suzuki F, Tanaka T, Yoshiki H, Sathi ZS, Akino H, Yokoyama O, Muramatsu I. Assessment of muscarinic receptor subtypes in human and rat lower urinary tract by tissue segment binding assay. J Pharmacol Sci 2008;106:271–279.

13. de Groat WC, Fraser MO, Yoshiyama M, Smerin S, Tai C, Chancellor MB, Yoshimura N, Roppolo JR. Neural control of the urethra. Scand J Urol Nephrol Suppl 2001;207:35–43; discussion 106–125.

14. Thor KB. Serotonin and norepinephrine involvement in efferent pathways to the urethral rhabdosphincter: Implications for treating stress urinary incontinence. Urology 2003;62(4 Suppl):3–9.

15. Abrams P, Cardozo L, Fall M, Griffiths D, Rosier P, Ulmsten U, van Kerrebroeck P, Wein A. The standardization of terminology of lower urinary tract function: Report for the standardization sub-committee of the International Continence Society. Neurourol Urodyn 2002;21:167–178.

16. Gray M, Moore KN. Urologic disorders. Adult and Pediatric Care. St. Louis: Mosby-Elsevier, 2009:119–159.

17. McGuire EJ, English SF. Periurethral collagen injection and female sphincteric incontinence: Indications, techniques and result. World J Urol 1997;15:306–309.

18. Gray M. Pathology and management of reflex urinary incontinence/neurogenic bladder. In: Doughty DB, ed. Urinary and Fecal Incontinence: Nursing Management (3rd ed). St. Louis: Mosby-Elsevier, 2006:105–143.

19. Hurlow J. View from here: Functional urinary incontinence ICD-9. J Wound Ostomy Continence Nurs 2009;36:79–81.

20. Wilson M. Causes and management of indwelling urinary catheter-related pain. Br J Nurs 2008;17:232–239.

21. Chang D, Ben-Meir D, Pout K, Dewan PA. Management of postoperative bladder spasm. J Pediatr Child Health 2005;41(1–2):56–58.

22. Hendirckson K, Gleason D, Young JM, Saltsstein D, Gershman A, Lerner A, Witjes JA. Safety and side effects of immediate instillation of apaziquone following transurethral resection in patients with non-muscle invasive bladder cancer. J Urol 2008;180:116–120.

23. Stewart W, Herzog R, Wein A, et al. The prevalence and impact of overactive bladder in the U.S.: Results from the NOBLE program. Neurourol Urodyn 2001;20:406–408.

24. Gray M, Marx RM, Peruggio M, Patrie J, Steers WD. A model for predicting motor urge urinary incontinence. Nurs Res 2001;50:116–122.

25. Zhang B, Gao X, Wen XQ. Abderxit. [Analysis of the causes of postoperative chest or/and abdomen colic in benign

prostatic hyperplasia]. Zhong Hua Nan Ke Xue 2005;11:288–289, 295.

26. Jirovec MM, Wells TJ. Urinary incontinence in nursing home residents with dementia: The mobility–cognition paradigm. Appl Nurs Res 1990;3:112–117.

27. Robinson D, McClish DK, Wyman JF, Bump RC, Fantl JA. Comparison between urinary diaries with and without intensive patient instructions. Neurourol Urodyn 1996;15:143–148.

28. Sampselle CM. Teaching women to use a voiding diary. Am J Nurs 2003;103:62–64.

29. Ermer-Seltun J. Assessment and management of acute or transient urinary incontinence. In: Doughty DB, ed. Urinary and Fecal Incontinence: Current Management Concepts (3rd ed). St. Louis: Mosby-Elsevier, 2006:55–76.

30. Tomlinson BU, Doughery MC, Pendergrast JF, Boyington AR, Coffman PA, Pickens SM. Dietary caffeine, fluid intake and urinary incontinence in older rural women. Int J Urogynecol Pelvic Floor Dysfunct 1999;10:22–28.

31. Gray ML. Altered patterns of urinary elimination. In: Ackley BJ, Ladwig GB, eds. Nursing Diagnosis Handbook. St. Louis: Mosby, 1999:643–646.

32. National Academy of Sciences, Food and Nutrition Board. Recommended Daily Allowances (9th ed). Washington, DC: National Academy of Sciences, 1980.

33. Cottenden A, Fader M, Getliffe K, Paterson J, Szonyi G, Wilde M. Management with continence products. In: Abrams P, Cardozo L, Khoury A, Wein A, eds. Incontinence: Basics & Evaluation. Paris, France: Health Publications Ltd., 2005:149–254.

34. Gray M, Marx R. Results of behavioral treatment for urinary incontinence in women. Curr Opin Urol 1998;8:279–282.

35. Miller JM, Ashton-Miller JA, Delancey JO. A pelvic muscle precontraction can reduce cough-related urine loss in selected women with mild SUI. J Am Geriatr Soc 1998;46:870–874.

36. Ghoneim GM, Hassouna M. Alternative for the pharmacologic management of stress urinary incontinence in the elderly. J Wound Ostomy Cont Nurs 1997;24:311–318.

37. Hunsballe JM, Djurhuus JC. Clinical options for imipramine in the management of urinary incontinence. Urol Res 2001;29:118–125.

38. Duloxetine side effects. Available at: http://anxiety.emedtv.com/duloxetine/duloxetine-side-effects.html (accessed December 26, 2008).

39. Newman DK. The indwelling urinary catheter: Principles for best practice. J Wound Ostomy Continence Nurs 2007;34:655–661.

40. Burgio KL, Locher JL, Goode PS, Hardin JM, McDowell BJ, Dombrowski M, Candib D. Behavioral vs. drug treatment for urge urinary incontinence in older women: A randomized controlled trial. JAMA 1998;280:1995–2000.

41. D'Souza AO, Smith MJ, Miller LA, Doyle J, Ariely R. Persistence, adherence, and switch rates among extended-release and immediate-release overactive bladder medications in a regional managed care plan. J Manag Care Pharm 2008;14:291–301.

42. Michel MC. Fesoterodine: A novel muscarinic receptor antagonist for the treatment of overactive bladder syndrome. Expert Opin Pharmacother 2008;9:1787–1796.

43. Dmochowski RR, Sand PK, Zinner NR, Staskin DR. Trospium 60 mg once daily (QD) for overactive bladder syndrome: Results from a placebo-controlled interventional study. Urology 2008;71:449–454.

44. MacDiarmid SA. How to choose the initial drug treatment for overactive bladder. [Review] Curr Urol Rep 2007;8:364–369.

45. Andersson KE, Olshansky B. Treating patients with overactive bladder syndrome with antimuscarinics: Heart rate considerations. BJU Int 2007;100:1007–1014.

46. Burgio KL, Locher JL, Goode PS. Combined behavioral and drug therapy for urge incontinence in older women. J Am Geriatr Soc 2000;48:370–374.

47. Smith DA. Devices for continence. Nurse Pract Forum 1994;5:186–189.

48. Wells M. Managing urinary incontinence with BioDerm external continence device. Br J Nurs 2008;17:s24–s29.

49. Nickel JC. The use of alpha1-adrenoceptor antagonists in lower urinary tract symptoms: Beyond benign prostatic hyperplasia. Urology 2003;62(Suppl 1):34–41.

50. Anson C, Gray M. Secondary urologic complications of spinal injury. Urol Nurs 1993;13:107–112.

51. Van Gool JD, Vijverberg MA, Messer AP, Elzinga-Plomp A, De Jong TP. Functional daytime incontinence: Non-pharmacologic treatment. Scand J Urol Nephrol 1992;141:93–105.

52. Colling J, Ouslander J, Hadley BJ, Eisch J, Campbell E. The effects of patterned urge response toileting (PURT) on urinary incontinence among nursing home residents. J Am Geriatr Soc 1992;40:135–141.

53. Schnelle JF, Keeler E, Hays RD, Simmons S, Ouslander JG, Siu AL. A cost and value analysis of two interventions with incontinent nursing home residents. J Am Geriatr Soc 1995;43:1112–1117.

54. Golomb J, Ben-Chaim J, Goldwasser B, Korach J, Mashiach S. Conservative treatment of a vesicocervical fistula resulting from Shirodkar cervical cerclage. J Urol 1993;149:833–834.

55. Tostain J. Conservative treatment of urogenital fistula following gynecological surgery: The value of fibrin glue. Acta Urol Belg 1992;60:27–33.

56. Gray M, Bliss DZ, Doughty DB, Ermer-Seltun J, Kennedy-Evans KL, Palmer MH. Incontinence-associated dermatitis: A review. J Wound Ostomy Continence Nurs 2007;34:45–56.

57. Gray M. Perineal skin care for the continence professional. Continence UK J 2008;2:29–39.

58. Norman RW. Genitourinary disorders. In: Oxford Textbook of Palliative Medicine. Oxford: Oxford University Press, 1998:667–676.

59. Gray M. Urinary retention: Management in the acute care setting. Am J Nurs 2000;15:42–60.

60. Gray M. Functional alterations: Bladder. In: Gross J, Johnson BL, eds. Handbook of Oncology Nursing. Boston: Jones and Bartlett, 1998:557–583.

61. 61.Blaivas JG, Weiss JP, Jones M. The pathophysiology of lower urinary tract symptoms after brachytherapy for prostate cancer. BJU Int 2006;98:1233–1237.

62. Parker D, Callan L, Harwood J, Thompson DL, Wilde M, Gray M. Nursing interventions to reduce the risk of catheter-associated urinary tract infection. Part 1: Catheter selection. J Wound Ostomy Continence Nurs 2009;36:23–34.

63. Perry A, Maharaj D, Ramdass MJ, Naraynsingh V. Slow decompression of the bladder using an intravenous giving set. Int J Clin Pract 2002;56:619.

64. Thees K, Dreblow L. Trial of voiding: What's the verdict? Urol Nurs 1999;19:20–24.

65. Fiers S. Management of the long-term indwelling catheter in the home setting. J Wound Ostomy Cont Nurs 1995;22:140–144.

66. Copley JB. Asymptomatic hematuria in the adult. Am J Med Sci 1986;29:101–111.

67. Gray M. Does the construction material affect outcomes in long-term catheterization? J Wound Ostomy Cont Nurs 2006;33:116–120.

68. Gray M. Securing the indwelling catheter. Am J Nurs 2008;108:44–50.

69. DeVries CB, Fuad SF. Hemorrhagic cystitis: A review. J Urol 1990;143:1–7.

70. Droller MJ, Saral R, Santos G. Prevention of cyclophosphamide-induced hemorrhagic cystitis. Urology 1982;20:256.

71. Getliffe K. Managing recurrent urinary catheter blockage: Problems, promises, and practicalities. J Wound Ostomy Cont Nurs 2003;30:146–151.

72. Openbrier D. Asymptomatic hematuria. Adv Nurse Pract 2003;11:81–88.

73. Herrin JT. General urology: Workup of hematuria and tubular disorders. In: Gonzales ET, Bauer SB, eds. Pediatric Urology Practice. Philadelphia: Lippincott Williams & Wilkins, 1999:69–79.

74. Levenbach C, Eifel PJ, Burke TW, Morris M, Gershenson DM. Hemorrhagic cystitis following radio therapy for stage Ib cancer of the cervix. Gynecol Oncol 1994;55:206–210.

75. Dean RJ, Lytton B. Urologic complications of pelvic irradiation. J Urol 1978;119:64–67.

76. Stapleton FB. Morphology of urinary red blood cells: A simple guide in localizing the site of hematuria. Pediatr Clin North Am 1987;34:561–563.

# 16 ❧❧ Mei R. Fu and Jean K. Smith

# Lymphedema Management

*Until you get lymphedema, you cannot really know what it is. And, you are the only one who notices that the swelling is keeping growing.—A breast cancer survivor with lymphedema*

♦ **Key Points**

♦ *Lymphedema, or abnormal swelling is frequently neglected by healthcare providers.*

♦ *Lymphedema is a syndrome of abnormal accumulation of lymph fluid and multiple symptoms that is caused by irreversible damage to, or congenital malformation of, the lymphatic system.*

♦ *There is no cure for lymphedema, and management of lymphedema requires daily self-care and changes in lifestyle.*

♦ *Promotion of lymph fluid flow and prevention of infection is fundamental to achieve long-term effective lymphedema management.*

Lymphedema or abnormal swelling is seen regularly in palliative and acute care settings. Lymphedema is often neglected despite its capacity to cause pain, immobility, infection, skin problems, and significant patient distress. Because nurses have access to large, diverse patient populations, they constitute an ideal resource for improving patient care. This text prepares nurses to understand, assess, and manage lymphedema. Information is applicable to various clinical settings, including acute, outpatient, community, and palliative care.[1,2]

## ❧❧ Definitions

Lymphedema, a syndrome of abnormal swelling and multiple symptoms is a chronic condition, resulting from abnormal accumulation of fluid and other elements (e.g. protein) in the tissue spaces due to an imbalance between interstitial fluid production and transport.[3] *Edema,* a symptom, refers to excessive accumulation of fluid within interstitial tissues and is one of the manifestations of lymphedema. Long-term, neglected edema, such as lower extremity venous insufficiency, can develop into chronic lymphedema. Discerning the difference between edema and lymphedema allows appropriate treatment.

One or several factors precipitate an imbalance in extracellular fluid volume. Excess fluids, proteins, immunological cells, and debris in affected tissues can produce chronic inflammation and connective tissue proliferation, including hypertrophy of adipose tissue. Some degree of progression usually occurs and can produce subcutaneous and dermal thickening and hardening. Lymphedema and edema are contrasted in Table 16–1, which provides definitions, signs and symptoms, and basic pathophysiology.[2–5]

**Table 16–1**
**Comparison of Edema and Lymphedema**

|  | Edema | Lymphedema |
|---|---|---|
| Disorder | A symptom of various disorders | A chronic, currently incurable edema |
| Definition | Swelling caused by the excessive fluid in tissues (interstitially) due to imbalance between capillary filtration and lymph drainage over time | Swelling (edema) caused by accumulation of fluid within tissues as a result of lymphatic drainage failure, increased production of lymph over time, or both |
| Signs and symptoms | Swelling, decreased skin mobility<br>Tightness, tingling, or bursting<br>Decreased strength and mobility<br>Discomfort (aching to severe pain)<br>Possible skin color change<br>*Pitting scale is often used:*<br>   1+ Edema barely detectable<br>   2+ Slight indentation with depression<br>   3+ Deep indentation for 5–30 sec with pressure<br>   4+ Area 1.5–2 times greater than normal | Swelling, decreased skin mobility<br>Tightness, tingling or bursting sensations<br>Decreased strength and mobility<br>Discomfort (none to severe pain)<br>Progressive skin changes (color, texture, tone, temperature), integrity such as blisters, weeping (lymphorrhea), hyperkeratosis, warts, papillomatosis, and elephantiasis |
| Pathophysiology | Capillary filtration rate exceeds lymph transport capacity<br>*Example*: Heart failure, fluid overload, and/or venous thrombosis are common causes of increased capillary pressure, leading to an increased capillary filtration rate that causes edema<br>*Note*:<br>Timely treatment of the underlying cause or causes usually reduces edema<br>Prolonged, untreated edema can transition to lymphedema | Inadequate Lymph transport capacity<br>  *Primary*—Inadequately developed lymphatic pathways<br>  *Secondary*—Damage outside lymphatic pathways (obstruction/obliteration)<br>*Initial sequelae of transport failure:*<br>  Lymphatic stasis →<br>  Increased tissue fluid →<br>  Accumulated protein and cellular metabolites →<br>  Further increased tissue water and pressure<br>*Potential long-term sequelae:*<br>  Macrophages seek to decrease inflammation<br>  Increased fibroblasts and keratinocytes cause chronic inflammation<br>  Gradual increase in adipose tissue<br>  Lymphorrhea (leakage of lymph through skin)<br>  Gradual skin and tissue thickening and hardening progressing to hyperkeratosis, papillomatosis and other problems<br>  Ever-increasing risk of infection and other complications |

*Sources*: References 2, 4.

## Prevalence

The world prevalence of edema is unknown,[2] and that of lymphedema is poorly documented. According to the World Health Organization, lymphedema affects 250 million people worldwide and the global burden of lymphedema is estimated at 5.78 million disability-adjusted life years lost annually.[6] Primary lymphedema, a genetic disorder, is attributed to embryonic developmental abnormalities, which may be sporadic or part of a syndrome caused by either chromosomal abnormalities (e.g., Turner's syndrome) or inherited single-gene defects.[7,8] Primary lymphedema occurs in about one person in 6,000 individuals and is more common in women than men, with a 3:1 ratio.[9] The overall prevalence of lymphedema has been estimated as about 2%.[10] Secondary (acquired) lymphedema results from obstruction or obliteration of lymph nodes or lymphatic vessels.[3,10,11] Cancer, trauma, surgery, severe infections, cardiac disease, poor venous function, immobility or paralyzing diseases are major causes of secondary lymphedema.[10] In developed countries, cancer treatment is the main cause of lymphedema. Prevalences of 10–60% have been reported in breast cancer patients[11–13] and of 28–40% in patients treated for gynecological cancer.[14,15] Other cancers associated with lymphedema risk include prostate cancer; head and neck cancer; sarcoma; melanoma; and lymphoma. Infection, inflammation, and obesity are risk factors for the development of lymphedema in patients treated for cancers.[16,17]

Lymphatic filariasis, a parasitic infection transmitted by mosquitoes, is the predominant worldwide cause of secondary lymphedema in underdeveloped countries. Mosquitoes transmit filariasis nematodes, which embed in human lymphatics to cause progressive lymphatic damage. It is estimated that the worldwide incidence of filariasis is 750 million.[18,19]

## Impact

Often, the most visible manifestation of lymphedema is persistent swelling.[11,13,20] Yet, lymphedema is more than swelling alone. Undiagnosed and unmanaged, lymphedema exerts extensive impact on individual's quality of life, including physical discomfort, functional disabilities, impaired occupational roles, poor self-image, decreased self-esteem, interrupted interpersonal relationships, financial burden, and life-style changes.[21,22,24] Physically, lymphedema leads to the suffering of distressing symptoms such as swelling, firmness, tightness, heaviness, pain, fatigue, numbness, and impaired limb mobility.[11,24] Lymphedema also predisposes individuals to fibrosis, cellulitis, infections, lymphadenitis, or septicemia.[23] Prolonged fluid stasis can lead to severe skin and tissue symptoms, sometimes referred to as elephantiasis. Symptoms include hyperkeratosis (hard, reptile-like skin), warts, and papillomas (engorged and raised lymph vessels on the skin surface).[1] Chronic lymphedema, over a number of years, has also been associated with the development of the rare, usually fatal cancer, lymphangiosarcoma.[1,23] Functionally, lymphedema makes it difficult for individuals to accomplish house chores and impairs their abilities to fulfill work that involves heavy lifting, gripping, holding, fine motor dexterity, and repetitive movement of the affected limb.[20,21] Some individuals have to give up hobbies that aggravate lymphedema.[20] Psychologically, individuals feel stigmatized and a loss of sexual attractiveness because of obvious disfigurement, which often elicits social anxiety, depression, and disruption of interpersonal relationships.[21,23,25]

## Anatomy, Physiology, and Pathophysiology

### Edema

Edema is a symptom that results from an imbalance between capillary filtration and lymph drainage. Edema requires treatment of the underlying disorder that is precipitating tissue fluid excess. Precipitators can include cardiac, hepatic, renal, allergic, or hypoproteinic disease; venous obstruction; and medication complications[26] (see Table 16–1). Edema can develop into secondary lymphedema with sufficient lymphatic damage, such as in venous insufficiency or fractures of the lower extremities.[4,27,28]

### Lymphedema

A healthy lymphatic system helps regulate the tissue cellular environment, including collecting and returning plasma and proteins.[4] Daily, 20% to 50% of the total accumulating plasma proteins travel through 2 to 4 liters of lymph fluid in a healthy lymphatic system.[25] Lymphatics also remove cellular waste products, mutants, and debris; eliminate nonself antigens; and regulate local immune defense in the process of maintaining homeostasis[4] (Figure 16–1). Unidirectional vessels traverse from superficial to deep lymphatics through 600 to 700 lymph nodes, carrying lymph fluid to the venous system at the right or left venous angle of the anterior chest on either side of the neck (Figure 16–2). Lymph nodes purify lymph fluid, eliminating defective cells, toxins, and bacteria, explaining the increased risk of infection for patients with compromised lymphatics.[4] Lymphedema pathology signifies malfunction in any part of the process of collecting, transporting, and depositing lymph into the venous system. Lymphedema pathophysiology signifies disruption of these processes and is described in Table 16–1.

In brief, lymph fluid is transported initially from the interstitium by the initial lymphatic vessels, filtered through lymph nodes, then drained into the two large lymph collecting ducts, and finally returned to the venous bloodstreams via the left and right subclavian veins (Figure 16–3). Damage to any structures of the lymphatic system can lead to accumulation of lymph fluid in the affected area. Further, physiological variations in each individual's lymphatic system, such as numbers or sizes of lymph nodes, make it difficult to quantify each individual's risk for lymphedema.

Secondary lymphedema from cancer treatment is caused by trauma to the lymphatic system mainly from surgery and radiotherapy.[29,30] Surgery creates disruption to the lymphatic system by directly dissecting lymph vessels and removing lymph nodes.[11] Unfortunately, lymph nodes do not regenerate once dissected.[31] Formation of scar tissue and tissue fibrosis from surgery creates blockage to the lymphatic system. The disruption or blockage of the lymphatic system reduces its ability to transport and filter the lymph, resulting in a functional overload and insufficient capability of the lymphatic system to transport normal volume of lymph.[32] As a result, an abnormal accumulation of lymph fluid occurs, which leads to the swelling of the affected area.

Radiation exposure during radiotherapy is also traumatic to the lymphatic system. Radiation impairs the lymphatic system by causing tissue fibrosis surrounding the lymphatic vessels,[33] and it reduces lymphatic transport reserve by increasing long-term changes in basal lymph circulation and lymph flow in the affected area.[32] While lymphatic vessels are relatively insensitive to radiotherapy, lymph nodes are radiosensitive to conventional doses of radiotherapy.[30] The radiated lymph nodes respond first with lymphocyte depletion, followed by fatty replacement, then by fibrosis.[30] As a result, radiation hinders lymph nodes from properly filtering and transporting lymph and alters immune function. Research has not clarified the definite roles of chemotherapy in contributing to lymphedema.

Besides the definite risk from cancer treatment, certain personal risk factors such as weight gain or obesity (body mass index [BMI] >30) and immobility increase the risk for

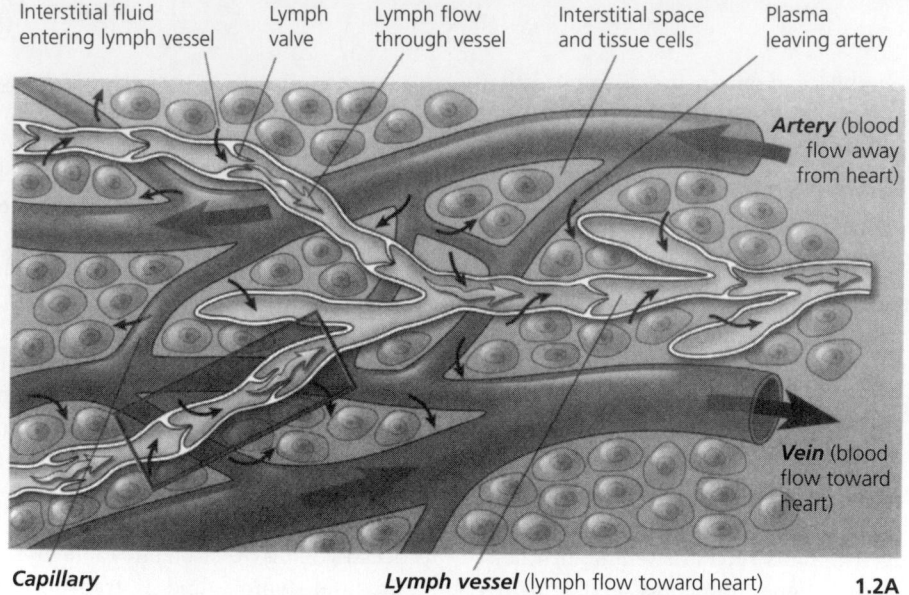

Interstitial fluid entering lymph vessel • Lymph valve • Lymph flow through vessel • Interstitial space and tissue cells • Plasma leaving artery

**Artery** (blood flow away from heart)

**Vein** (blood flow toward heart)

**Capillary**

**Lymph vessel** (lymph flow toward heart)

**1.2A**

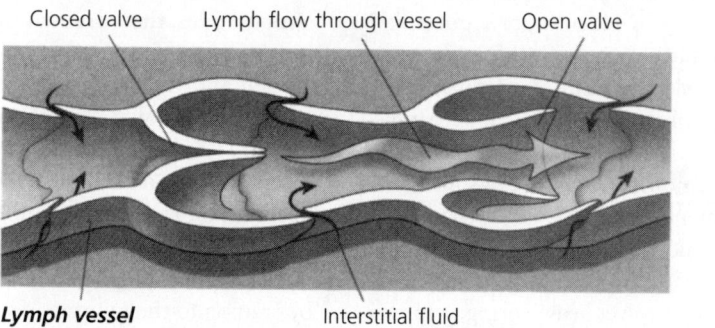

Closed valve • Lymph flow through vessel • Open valve

**Lymph vessel** • Interstitial fluid

**1.2B**

**Figure 16–1.** Lymphatic vessels and valves. *Source*: Reprinted, with permission, from the American Cancer Society. Lymphedema: Understanding and Managing Lymphedema After Cancer Treatment. Atlanta, GA: American Cancer Society; 2006, www.cancer.org/bookstore.

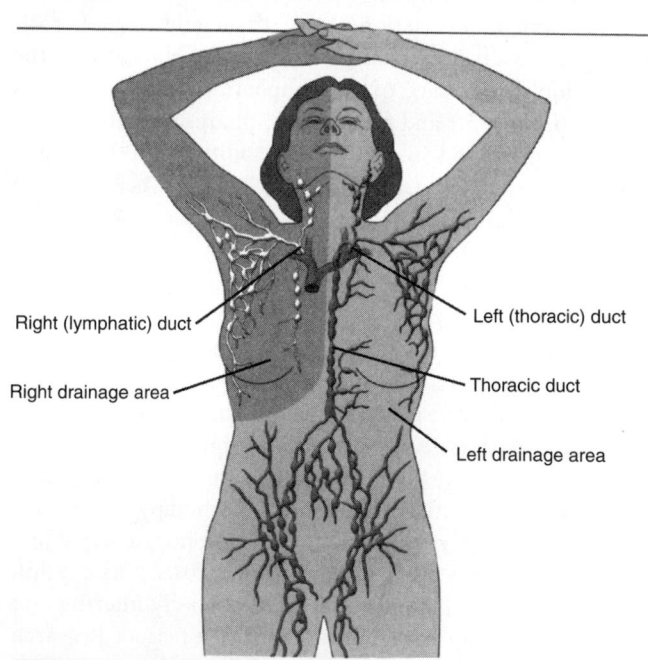

Right (lymphatic) duct

Right drainage area

Left (thoracic) duct

Thoracic duct

Left drainage area

**Figure 16–2.** Right (lymphatic) duct, left (thoracic duct), and drainage areas. *Source*: Reprinted, with permission, from the American Cancer Society. Lymphedema: Understanding and Managing Lymphedema After Cancer Treatment. Atlanta, GA: American Cancer Society; 2006, www.cancer.org/bookstore.

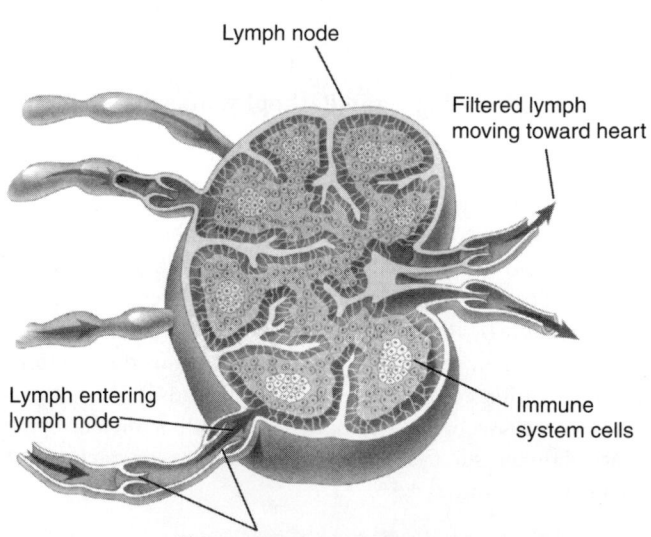

Lymph node

Filtered lymph moving toward heart

Lymph entering lymph node

Immune system cells

Valves allow lymph to move toward heart

**Figure 16–3.** Lymph node. *Source*: Reprinted, with permission, from the American Cancer Society. Lymphedema: Understanding and Managing Lymphedema After Cancer Treatment. Atlanta, GA: American Cancer Society; 2006, www.cancer.org/bookstore.

lymphedema.[16,17,34] Factors that trigger or stimulate development of lymphedema in an at-risk person have been identified, including: overuse of the affected limb; heavy lifting; infection; injury or burns to the affected limb; prolonged heat exposure; constriction; and traveling by air.[16,17,34]

## Assessment and Diagnosis

Early diagnosis is essential for prevention of complications and optimal management.[11,20] Diagnosing lymphedema remains a clinical challenge. Several factors contribute to the challenge: lack of universally recognized diagnostic criteria; failure to precisely evaluate symptoms; co-existing conditions; and lack of awareness of lymphedema among healthcare professionals.[35] To ensure accurate diagnosis, it is important to conduct a careful review of the patient's health history to rule out other medical conditions that may cause similar symptoms, such as recurrent cancer, deep vein thrombosis, chronic venous insufficiency, diabetes, hypertension, and cardiac and renal disease. These alternative diagnoses should be ruled out before establishing a diagnosis of lymphedema and referring the patient for lymphedema therapy. "Best Practice"[36] components of lymphedema nursing assessment are displayed in Table 16-2.

The first assessment priority is proper diagnosis. For example, assessment reveals that early symptoms of congestive heart failure are responsible for a suspected lymphedema in one elderly, frail patient referred for lymphedema assistance. When the results of the physical assessment and patient history are combined with dialogue, the patient reports that she has replaced her cardiac medication with several natural supplements in order to save money and avoid "toxic drugs." Edema then resolves within several days after she has resumed her cardiac medications. Some patients, especially those who are elderly, chronically ill, or significantly distressed, are not able to accurately provide a medical history. Requesting physician (physician assistant or nurse practitioner) dictations can provide excellent assessment information.

A patient health history questionnaire facilitates assessment. Useful health categories include: patient demographics; health history; etiology; signs and symptoms; complications; work and household responsibilities; support from significant others; spiritual health; and lymphedema goals.[36,37] Completion of the questionnaire before the initial assessment improves assessment accuracy and content and allows additional time for important nurse–patient dialogue.[38] Dialogue helps nurses to understand patients' perspective and gain essential patient knowledge: (1) patient's view of lymphedema, (2) patient's readiness for instruction and treatment, (3) patient's pertinent work and lifestyle, (4) spiritual concerns, (5) illness and adjustment issues, and (6) patient's desired goals. Often the patient's initial goal is cure, which is unattainable. In this situation, the patient needs time to adopt new goals. Nurses' awareness of patient quality-of-

---

**Table 16-2**
**Sequential Components of Lymphedema Assessment**

*Rule out or address immediate complications* (i.e., infection, thrombosis, severe pain, new or recurrent cancer, significant nonrelated disorders)

*History and physical examination*
   Routine physical assessments: vital signs, blood pressure, height and weight, body mass index
   Past and current health status, including medications and allergies (especially antibiotic allergies and history of infection, trauma, or surgery in affected area)
   Current activities of daily living (job, home responsibilities, leisure activities, sleep position, activities that aggravate lymphedema)
   Current psychological health, support people, view of lymphedema and health
   History of lymphedema etiology, presentation, duration, and progression

*Patient knowledge of and response to lymphedema, interest in assistance and goals*

*Third party payer status*

*Quantification of lymphedema status* (lymphedema signs and symptoms, volume, pain and other neurological symptoms, tissue status, range of motion of nearby joints, site-specific and overall patient function)

---

life goals[36] fosters collaboration and management success. Instruction, support, multidisciplinary referrals, goal-setting, assistance with self-care, complication avoidance, and long-term management are improved by nurses' and healthcare providers' understanding of patients' perspectives and knowledge.[36,39,40]

For example, a 58-year-old woman presented with large lower extremity primary lymphedema. She expressed a positive, easygoing life view; had a boyfriend, children, and grandchildren; cared for an elderly mother; and worked full-time, 50 miles away from home. She stated that her treatment goal was to "wear boots." If the nurse's goals were complete limb reduction and perfect compliance, both the nurse and the patient would be likely to experience frustration and failure. This failure *could* cause the nurse to conclude that the patient's poor outcome was caused by poor compliance. Alternatively, the nurse could incorporate the patient's life view, goals, and responsibilities into a workable treatment and self-care program.

An early lymphedema diagnosis is often determined solely from a history and physical examination,[39-41] especially if conservative management is planned and symptoms are not severe. Questionable clinical symptoms or etiology may require further evaluation. Lymphoscintigraphy (isotope lymphography) can ensure definite lymphedema diagnosis.[4] Lymphography (direct), is now rarely used in lymphedema patients[30] because of its potential to cause lymphatic injury and its inability to clarify function.[4]

Assessment for infection, thrombosis, or cancer metastasis (Figure 16–4) is required at every patient contact.[41,42] Although later signs of infection or thrombosis are well known, awareness and careful assessment allow early diagnosis and treatment. Lymphedema progression or treatment resistance may be the earliest sign of complication or may represent a lack of response to current treatment. Changes in pain or comfort, skin (color, temperature, condition), or mobility and range of motion are other possible early signs of major complications. Most infections develop subcutaneously, beneath intact skin. Cultures are not recommended, because they rarely document a bacterial source and can further increase the risk of infection.[31] Suspected thrombosis or new or recurring cancer requires appropriate diagnostic evaluation (e.g., Doppler ultrasonography, magnetic resonance imaging, positron emission tomography, computed tomographic scanning). Venous ultrasonography

is reported to be safer than venography for evaluation of suspected thrombosis in a limb with, or at high risk for, lymphedema.[43]

Figure 16–4 depicts ongoing complication assessment and decision-making. Basic treatment of complications is also included. Signs and symptoms of metastasis can include pain, neuropathies, new masses or lesions, skin/tissue color and texture changes, and treatment-resistant rashes. For thrombosis, signs can include distended veins, venous telangiectasis, and rapid edema progression beyond the affected limb.[27] Thrombosis requires anticoagulation, pain control, rest, and avoidance of use of external compression. Currently, no research clarifies the appropriate timing for use of compression after thrombosis, and the traditional 6-month delay until use of compression should be assumed.[40] Discussion of this issue with the physician is appropriate. Compression refers to the deliberate application of pressure

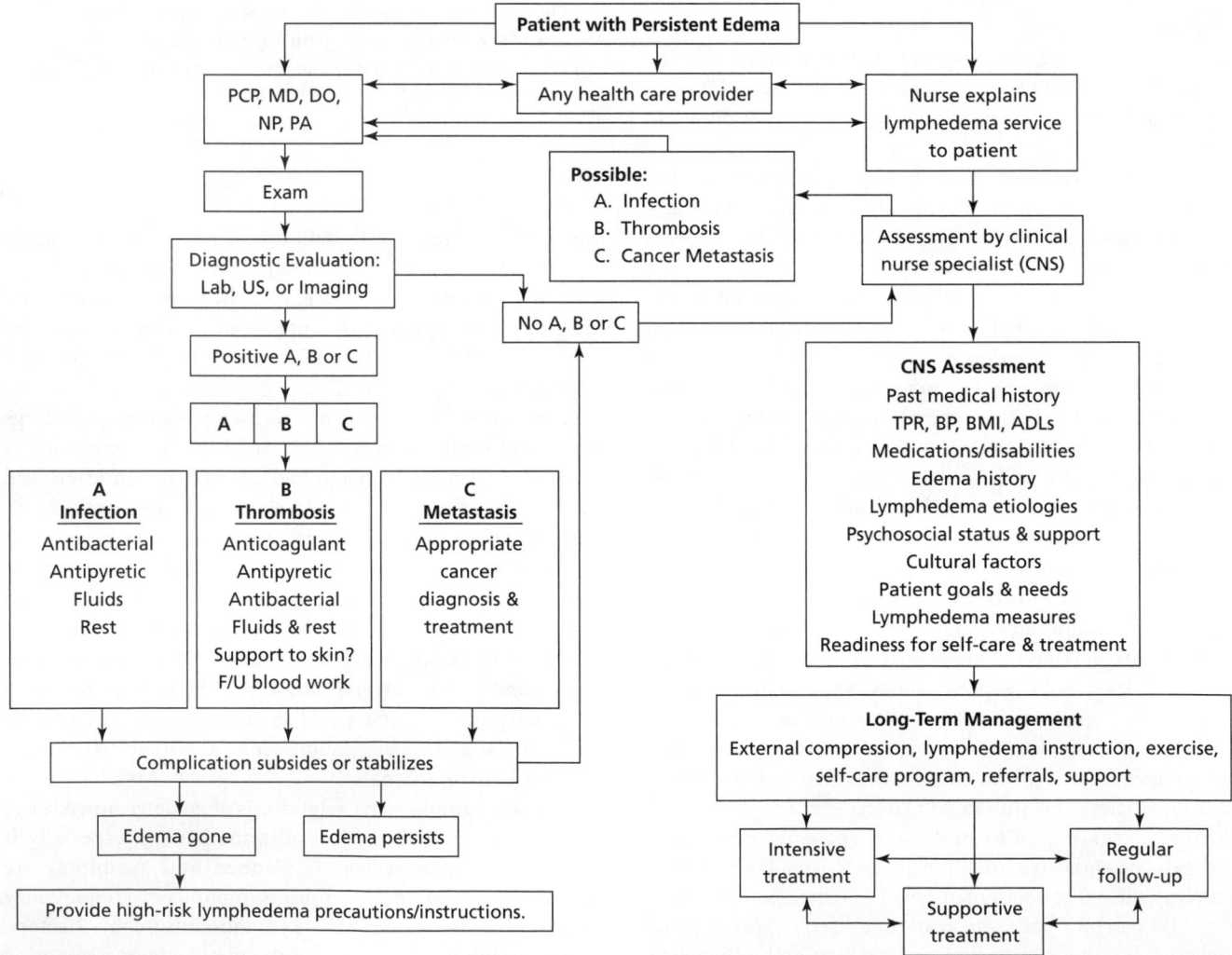

**Figure 16–4.** Assessment of complications in lymphedema management. ADLs, activities of daily living; BMI, body mass index; BP, blood pressure; DO, doctor of osteopathy; F/U, follow-up; MD, doctor of medicine; NP, nurse practitioner; PA, physician assistant; PCP, primary care physician; TPR, temperature, pulse, and respirations; US, ultrasonography.

to produce a desired clinical effect.[2] In contrast, some physicians recommend the use of limb support for several days or longer after painful thrombosis-related swelling, especially in the presence of metastatic cancer. Support signifies the retention and control of tissue without application of pressure.[2] Until research enables a practice standard, the physician must determine the use and timing of support and compression.

A diagnosis of early thrombosis was achieved for a 67-year-old patient with advanced metastatic lymphoma and leukemia when left leg thrombosis developed rapidly while the patient was hospitalized for a cancer complication. Thrombosis encompassed the entire leg. During anticoagulation, leg edema, pain, and signs of venous insufficiency continued to progress. Several weeks later, the patient was referred to the clinical nurse specialist for assistance. Excess edema volume in the affected leg (compared with the nonaffected leg) was 94% (4816 mL). A Tensoshape product (BSN Medical Ltd., Brierfield, England) was provided (with physician approval) for 1 week, and 9% limb reduction was achieved. Good product tolerance was reported. A demonstration of compression sleeve (lower extremity, full-leg product that uses high-low foam and a spandex compression sleeve; Peninsula Medical, Inc., Scotts Valley, CA) was then provided with instructions to use it as tolerated, reverting to the Tensoshape product whenever the compression sleeve was removed. One week later, follow-up assessment revealed edema reduction

of 43%, compared with the initial volume. Excess volume had decreased from 94% to 54% (2730 mL). The patient also agreed to referral to a lymphedema therapist to obtain daytime compression stockings and to undergo several sessions of lymphatic drainage massage. Five weeks after the initial assessment, the patient returned for follow-up wearing her new stockings, her "tight-legged" slacks, her wig, and a large smile. Pain level, skin color and condition, gait, and range of motion of the ankle, knee, and hip were significantly improved (Figure 16–5A). Edema reduction in the lymphedema limb was 81%; excess volume was 18% (926 mL). By 4¹/₂ months following the initial assessment, edema reduction had continued. Treatment included daytime stockings and compression sleeve usage several nights a week. Edema reduction at this time was 87%. Excess limb volume, compared to the contralateral leg, was 12% (634 mL). Figure 16–5B displays improvement from the initial assessment through the 4-month follow-up.

Lymphedema symptoms, such as heaviness, tightness, firmness, pain, numbness, or impaired mobility in the affected limb, may indicate a latent stage of lymphedema in which changes cannot be detected by objective measurements.[3,44] The latent stage of lymphedema may exist months or years before overt swelling occurs. Assessing lymphedema-related symptoms plays an important role in diagnosis until objective measurements capable of detecting latent stage of lymphedema are established in at-risk individuals.[45]

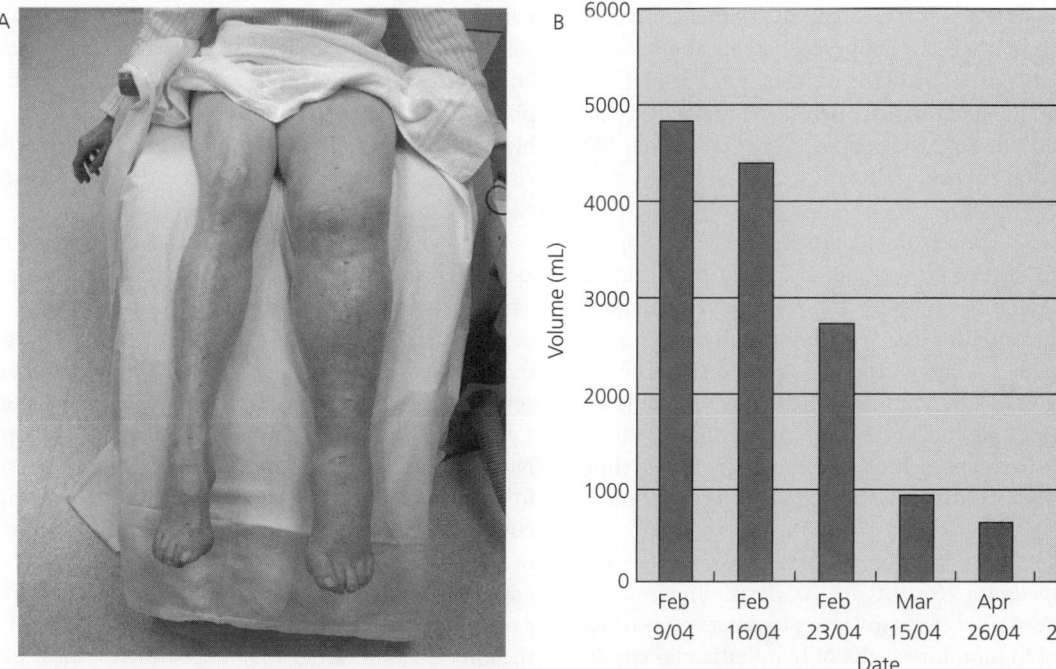

**Figure 16–5.** Metatstatic lymphoma patient with severe deep venous thrombosis in the left leg, showing excess edema volume (mL) in the affected compared with the unaffected leg. The graph shows the improvement in the lymphedema over time.

## Quantification of Lymphedema

A variety of measurement approaches make quantification of lymphedema a problem. Methods of measuring limb volume or circumference include sequential circumference limb measurement,[11] water displacement and infra-red perometry.[46] Bioelectrical impedance is emerging as a possible alternative. Unfortunately, lymphedema can also occur in the face, neck, shoulder, breast, abdomen, thoracic regions, and genital areas, which presents a challenge for quantifying lymphedema.

*Sequential Circumferential Arm Measurements.* Measuring limb volume and circumference are the most widely used diagnostic methods. A flexible non-stretch tape measure for circumferences is usually used to assure consistent tension over soft tissue, muscle, and bony prominences.[11] Measurements are done on both affected and non-affected limbs at the hand proximal to the metacarpals, wrist, and then every 4 cm from the wrist to axilla. The most common criterion for diagnosis has been a finding of $\geq$ 2 centimeters or $\geq$ 200 mL difference in limb volume as compared to the non-affected limb or 10% volume difference in the affected limb.[11,46]

*Water Displacement.* Although water displacement has been considered the "gold standard" for limb volume measurement and is identified as a sensitive and accurate measure in the laboratory setting, water displacement is seldom used in clinical settings because of spillover and hygienic concerns. Patients submerge the affected arm in a container filled with water and the overflow of water is caught in another container and weighed. This method does not provide data about localization of the edema or shape of the extremity.[47] The method is contraindicated in patients with open skin lesions. Patients may find it difficult to hold the position for the time needed for the tank overflow to drain.

*Infrared Perometry.* The Perometer 400T or S350, an optoelectronic device developed to meet the need for a quick, hygienic, and accurate method for volume calculation, works similar to computer-assisted tomography, but makes use of light instead of x-rays.[48] The volume and shape of the limb can be measured and volume changes can be calculated in seconds. Armer and colleagues[46] found perometry to be as reliable a measurement of limb volume change over time as circumferences in individuals undergoing breast cancer treatment.

*Bioelectrical Impedance (Imp XCA) Analysis.* Bioelectrical impedance has been used for many years to detect early onset lymphedema and to monitor results of lymphatic massage in clinical settings outside the United States.[49] The Imp XCA® (Impedimed, Brisbane, Australia), is a new generation impedance device for clinical assessment of unilateral lymphedema of the arm. The United States Food and Drug Administration approved the use of the Imp XCA® in clinical settings in March of 2007. The Imp XCA® measures impedance and resistance of the extracellular fluid using a single frequency below 30 kHz. The device uses the impedance ratio values between the unaffected and affected limb to calculate a *Lymphedema Index.* Measurement of limb takes less than five minutes when using the Imp-XCA® and results are immediately available to clinicians. Further research is needed to establish the reliability and validity of the device. The technique is currently of limited use in bilateral swelling (Figure 16–6).

## Lymphedema Risk Reduction

No research has demonstrated that "prevention" of lymphedema is possible. Rigid prevention measures may promote fears and frustration. The term "risk reduction" appears more accurate.[45] One essential risk reduction behavior is to achieve and maintain ideal body weight, because excess body weight is associated with decreased lymphatic function.[16,17,34]

Infection prevention is vital for lymphedema risk reduction;[16,17] infection is a significant risk factor and is the most frequent lymphedema complication.[20] Risk increases with breaches in skin integrity. Occasional drawing of blood, when no other reasonable option exists, is necessary for some patients. Patients can request an experienced phlebotomist and emphasize their increased infection risk. Subcutaneous, intramuscular, or intravenous injections can cause an allergic or inflammatory response and/or infection that compromises a weakened lymphatic system. These risks must be compared with the benefit and risk of use of a central venous catheter or suboptimal venipuncture site such as the lower extremity.[50] Diabetes potentially increases breast cancer patients' lymphedema risk when the affected limb is used for continual blood sticks or insulin injections. Patients with bilateral limb risk, especially of the upper extremities, face lifelong decisions regarding adherence to precautions.

Breast cancer disease and treatment factors are associated with increased lymphedema risk, including advanced cancer stage at diagnosis and radiation therapy to the axilla or supraclavicular area after a mastectomy. Benefits of early nurse interventions in decreasing lymphedema occurrence, severity of secondary lymphedema, and lymphedema symptoms in breast cancer survivors have been documented.[45,51] Nurses can assist high-risk patients by presenting or reinforcing prevention information and encouraging use of a compression sleeve at the earliest sign of edema. Emphasis on self-protection rather than rigid rules fosters patient empowerment.[20,45] For example, an empowered patient assumes responsibility for reminding staff to avoid use of the affected arm rather than expecting medical personnel to remember to do so.

Exercise restrictions have long been recommended for breast cancer survivors. However, a growing body of evidence

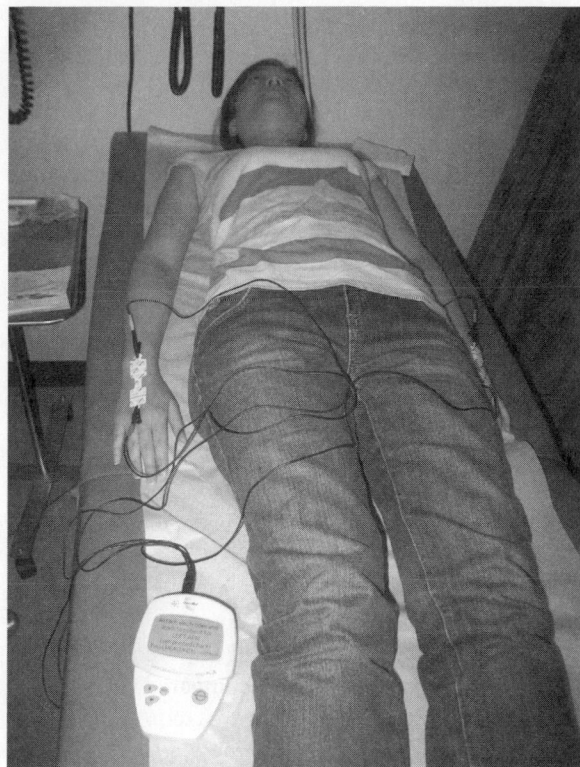

- The Imp SCA® (Impedimed, Brisbane, Australia) uses a single frequency below 30 kHz to measure impedance and resistance of the extracellular fluid.

- The device uses the impedance ratio values to calculate a *Lymphedema* Index [L-Dex], ranging from - 10 to +10.

□ **Advantages:**
✓ Time- and cost-efficient, hygienic
✓ Easy mastery of procedure
✓ Portable
✓ Reliability is established

□ **Limitations:**
✓ Further research is neeeded to establish validity and sensitivity of the device.

**Figure 16–6.** Bioelectrical Impedance Analysis (ImpXCA). *Source*: © copyright by Mei R. Fu. All rights reserved.

suggests that exercise does not necessarily increase lymphedema risk.[52,53] Although additional research is needed, preliminary research suggests that breast cancer survivors should be encouraged to carry out all postoperative exercises, resume normal precancer activities, and be as fit as possible, while regularly monitoring their high-risk or affected limb.[52–54] In addition to the importance of physical exercise in general health, weight control, and quality of life, physical exercise can promote lymph fluid drainage through large muscle movement. Individuals should be instructed to perform physical exercise according to the general exercise guildelines:[54,75] (1) initiate at lower intensity exercise; then graduate to increase exercise intensity; (2) exercise to the extent that the affected body part is not fatigued; (3) modify physical exercise to reduce the risk of trauma and injury; and (4) use a compression garment during exercise.

## Long-Term Management Versus Treatment

Edema usually subsides with proper treatment, whereas lymphedema requires long-term management.[20,36,55] Lymphedema is a lifelong and chronic condition. Long-term management focuses on daily activities and strategies undertaken to decrease the swelling, relieve symptom distress, and prevent acute exacerbations and infections.[20] Components of

| Table 16–3 |
| :--- |
| **Components of Long-Term Lymphedema Management** |
| History, physical examination, and ongoing assessment and support |
| Individualized and holistic care coordination |
| Multidisciplined referrals |
| Comprehensive initial and ongoing patient instruction |
| Ongoing psychosocial support |
| Promotion of ongoing optimal self-care management |
| Facilitation of appropriate evidence-based, individualized treatment |
| Patient and practice outcome measurement |
| Access and long-term follow-up and management |
| Communication and collaboration with related health care providers |

long-term lymphedema management are listed in Table 16–3 and described throughout the chapter. Long-term management is a process of fostering optimal physical, functional, psychosocial, and spiritual wellness. Spiritual care guidelines have been gradually evolving in nursing for several decades. Spiritual care supports patients' efforts to make meaning out of illness and to redefine themselves in their new state of being. Specific spiritual interventions can include: (1) support during the struggle with and exploration of life's ambiguities;

(2) acknowledgment of patients' real and potential losses and victories; and (3) guidance in patients' exploration of end-of-life issues and decisions.[37,56,57]

Long-term management requires quantification of ongoing patient, nurse, and program outcomes.[36,55-57] Limb size or volume has been commonly used in both research and practice to evaluate treatment effectiveness. Managing limb size or volume requires patients to initiate and maintain behaviors that promote lymph drainage and reduce triggering factors leading to severe lymphedema.[20] Other important outcomes include pain level, skin condition, range of motion of nearby joints, affected area and overall patient function, body mass index (BMI), incidence of infection, and other complications.[53,57-59] Patient's overall lymphedema-symptom experience such as psychological distress and fatigue are subjective outcomes which require supportive services from healthcare professionals such as psychologists or conditioning experts.[20,36]

Long-term management necessitates a multidisciplinary approach.[55] At each patient visit, nurses should assess for signs of infection, limb confirmation, and degree of swelling. Additional inquires need to be made as to any other symptoms patients may be experiencing because of the lymphedema. Nurses should assess self-care behaviors and encourage patients with lymphedema to wear their compression sleeves as prescribed, which includes during activities such as flying and exercise. All physicians or advance practice nurses should immediately refer patients with new onset or worsening lymphedema to certified lymphedema therapists for volume reduction treatment. They should also be prepared to prescribe antibiotics for infections. Certified lymphedema therapists should provide treatment for the swollen limb and provide individualized patient education about self-care practices (including recommended exercise and exercise progression based on individual lymphedema risk factors and level of fitness) and answer other questions, such as "Should a particular patient have massage in the limb by non-certified practitioners?" Collecting and reviewing outcomes with patients over time fosters ongoing instruction, complication prevention, sustained lymphedema improvement, and patient empowerment.[20,34,59]

### CASE STUDY
### *JoAnne, A Breast Cancer Survivor with Lymphedema*

JoAnne was diagnosed with breast cancer at age 55 years. Lymphedema manifested during radiation therapy several months after conservative breast surgery that included standard axillary node dissection. Lymphedema was accompanied by erythema and petechiae, which varied in intensity throughout each day. Antibiotic therapy did not provide benefit and was poorly tolerated. Edema volume in the surgical arm, compared with the nonaffected arm, was 29% (734 mL). No previous treatment had been available to JoAnne, who lived and received her breast cancer treatment a 2-hour car ride away from the lymphedema facility.

JoAnne was attentive and participatory during assessment and instruction. However, she was reluctant to use the recommended compression sleeve and gloves because of her belief of skin infection. She had a friend in whom this occurred. Acceptance and support of JoAnne's viewpoint validated her coping activities and fostered future self-care decision-making.[20,34] Patient readiness for, and acceptance of, treatment is crucial to successful chronic disease management and warrants nurses' patience.[34] JoAnne agreed to use demonstration nighttime compression products (a compression and Medi glove) for 6 to 8 hours at a time. Instruction was provided, including removal of the product (until she could speak with the clinical nurse specialist) if pain, numbness, tingling, infection, bleeding, or worrisome signs or symptoms occurred. One month later, she obtained her compression sleeve and assumed full responsibility for regular replacement.

JoAnne gradually increased her product-wearing time. Eight months after assessment, she had achieved 45% limb reduction. Excess limb volume, compared with the nonaffected arm, had decreased from 29% to 16% (405 mL). One year after assessment, JoAnne requested assistance in obtaining a compression sleeve and glove for daytime use. Over the next several months, daytime compression resulted in an 83% limb volume reduction compared with the initial pretreatment volume. Edema volume in the affected arm was reduced to 5% (124 mL). Patient self-reported satisfaction and compliance with management was consistently high, and no limb complications occurred. Asymptomatic mild erythema has continued. Follow-up is currently every 6 months.

## Edema Treatment

Edema treatment focuses on detection and intervention related to the causative factor or factors. Effective treatment stabilizes the interstitial fluid volume.[4] Tissue support and/or gentle compression can be useful in relieving edema that might progress to lymphedema.

## Lymphedema Treatment

Lymphedema treatment refers to therapies to help decrease or maintain swelling, including surgery, pharmacological therapy, and comprehensive decongestive physiotherapy.[20,61] Pharmacological therapy and surgery have limited proven effectiveness. Pharmacological therapy for lymphedema has included use of coumarin (a benzopyrone) and diuretics; however, coumarin and diuretics are not recommended for the treatment of lymphedema and are proven to be ineffective.[61,75]

Several surgical interventions include microsurgical anastomoses, debulking, and liposuction. Surgical procedures aimed at enhancing lymphatic function have been performed to try to remove excess fluid or tissue in the affected area;[62,75] these procedures have been shown to be only marginally effective. Surgery does not cure lymphedema, and follow-up use of compression is necessary.[79] Surgery has provided cosmetic improvement in eyelid or genital edema.[2,75] Potential complications may occur with surgical management of lymphedema, such as recurrence of swelling, poor wound healing, and infection; thus surgical treatment should only be considered when other treatments fail, and with careful consideration of the benefits to risks ratio.[63]

Liposuction has been performed on patients with long-standing, breast-cancer-related lymphedema.[82] It removes excess fat tissue and is considered only if the limb has not responded to standard conservative therapy.[75] Lack of response to conventional treatment resulted from formation of excess subcutaneous adipose tissue secondary to slow or absent lymph flow.[80-82] Liposuction has increased skin capillary blood flow and does not further impair already decreased lymph transport capacity in breast cancer patients with lymphedema.[81,82] Patients are able to maintain limb reductions with concordant use of compression garments after liposuction.[75,81,82] Liposuction does not correct inadequate lymph drainage and is not indicated when pitting is present. Liposuction has also been used for primary and secondary leg lymphedema with promising results.[75]

### Infection Prevention and Treatment

Infection is the most common lymphedema complication.[4] Lymph stasis, decreased local immune response, tissue congestion, and accumulated proteins and other debris foster infection.[64] Traditional signs and symptoms (fever, malaise, lethargy, and nausea) are often present. Decades of literature support prompt oral or intravenous antibiotic therapy.[4,61] Because streptococci and staphylococci are frequent precipitators, antibiotics must cover normal skin flora, as well as gram-positive cocci,[61,65] and have good skin penetration.[61,64,65] Early detection and treatment can help prevent the need for intravenous therapy and hospitalization.[65] Intravenous antibiotic therapy is recommended for systemic signs of infection or insufficient response to oral antibiotics.[65] Nursing activities include assisting patients in obtaining prompt antibiotic therapy, monitoring and reporting signs and symptoms, and providing instruction regarding high fluid intake, rest, elevation of the infected limb, and avoidance of strenuous activity. Garment-type compression is encouraged as soon as tolerable during infection.[66] Wound care or infectious disease specialists can be helpful in complicated cases. Infection prophylaxis has been highly effective for patients who experience repeated serious infections or inflammatory episodes.[66-69] Effective edema reduction and control may also help prevent lymphedema infection.[69]

The feet, which are especially susceptible to fungal infections in lower extremity lymphedema, can exhibit peeling, scaly skin, and toenail changes. Antifungal powders are recommended prophylactically. Antifungal creams should be used at the first sign of fungus. Diabetic-like skin care and use of cotton socks and well-fitted, breathable (leather or canvas), sturdy shoes are beneficial.[70]

## Pain Management

Approximately 30% to 60% patients with lymphedema post breast cancer treatment reported pain.[71,72] Causes of pain included infection, postoperative changes in the axilla, postmastectomy pain syndrome, brachial plexopathy, various arthritic conditions, peripheral entrapment neuropathies, vascular compromise, and cancer recurrence.[65,71,72] Sudden onset of pain requires careful assessment for complications (see Figure 16–4). Use of the 0-to-10 pain scale is recommended for cancer pain assessment.[72] Standard pain management principles are applicable for lymphedema-related pain.

### Self-Care

Optimal patient self-care typically includes adherence to risk reduction behaviors, use of compression, weight management, fitness and lymphedema exercises, optimal nutrition and hydration, healthy lifestyle practices, and seeking assistance for lymphedema-related problems. Patient empowerment for optimal self-care is a great impetus to long-term management success.[20,34,55]

For example, one female patient attended school, worked part-time, and was a single parent of two sons. She had experienced many lymphedema treatment failures after her initial presentation of lymphedema at age 5. Treatments had been painful, distressing, and unsuccessful. Emotional scars had resulted from having legs so different from those of her friends. Five years of intermittent support and encouragement were required to achieve patient treatment readiness. Achieving a successful treatment program required another year and included surgical repair of ingrown toenails. Use of outcomes provided concrete data that fostered excellent compression compliance (daytime garment and nighttime lower leg compression). Ultimately, external compression reduced pain and fatigue sufficiently to allow 3 extra hours of activity per day. Long-term treatment success included sustained reduction of lymphedema and pain, elimination of recurrent infections, excellent compression compliance and self-care, high treatment satisfaction, and minimal need for lymphedema assistance.

### Elevation

Elevation of the affected limb above the level of the heart is often recommended to reduce swelling.[3,75] Elevation promotes the drainage of lymph fluid by maximizing venous drainage and by decreasing capillary pressure and lymph production.

Elevation is considered the main treatment for early stage of lymphedema of an upper limb.[3] Anecdotal evidence suggests that limb elevation when the patient is sitting or in bed may be a useful adjunct to active treatment, but should not be allowed to impede function or activity.[75] Patients should be encouraged not to sleep in a chair but to go to bed at night to avoid the development of 'arm chair' legs or exacerbation of lower limb lymphedema. Patient avoidance of limb dependency is also appropriate risk-reduction strategy and ameliorates the symptoms of lymphedema.

### Exercise

Exercise or body movement is an integral part of lymphedema management and risk reduction. Exercise improves muscular strength, cardiovascular function, psychological well-being and functional capacity.[75] Gentle resistance exercise stimulates muscle pumps and increases lymph flow; aerobic exercise increases intra-abdominal pressure, which facilitates pumping of the thoracic duct.[54,65] A tailored exercise or body movement program that combines flexibility, resistance and aerobic exercise may be beneficial in reducing the risk of, and controlling, lymphedema.[75] General exercise guidelines include:[54,75]

- Start with low to moderate intensity exercise
- Walking, swimming, cycling and low impact aerobics are recommended
- Flexibility exercises should be performed to maintain range of movement
- Appropriate warming up and cooling down phases should be implemented as part of exercise to avoid exacerbation of swelling
- Heavy lifting and repetitive motion should be avoided
- Compression garments should be worn during exercise

### Skin Care

Skin care is important for lymphedema risk reduction and management, which optimizes the condition of the skin and prevents infection.[20,34,55,73] Diligent care is especially important for patients with lower extremity, genital, breast, head, neck, or late-stage lymphedema, additional skin alterations, or unrelated debilitating conditions. Lymphedema can cause skin dryness and irritation, which is increased with long-term use of compression products. Bland, non-scented products are recommended for daily cleansing and moisturizing.[73] Low pH moisturizers (e.g., AmLactin), which discourage infection, are recommended for advanced lymphedema, because skin and tissue changes increase infection risk. Water-based moisturizers, which are absorbed more readily, are less likely to damage compression products but are not suitable for all patients. Cotton clothing allows ventilation and is absorbent.

Advanced lymphedema can cause several skin complications, including lymphorrhea, lymphoceles, papillomas, and hyperkeratosis. Lymphorrhea is leakage of lymph fluid through the skin that occurs when skin cannot accommodate accumulated fluid. Nonadherent dressings, good skin care, and compression are used to alleviate leakage. Compression and good skin care also reduce the occurrence of lymphoceles, papillomas, and hyperkeratosis; these complications reflect skin adaptation to excess subcutaneous lymph.

### Bandages

Multi-layer lymphedema bandaging (MLLB) provides external compression. For some patients, MLLB may be used as part of long-term or palliative management. MLLB uses inelastic or low-stretch bandages to produce a massaging effect and stimulate lymph flow.[75] MLLB is especially important for patients with severe lymphedema, such as lymphedema with morbid obesity or neglected primary lymphedema. It is also important for patients who choose self or caregiver bandaging to enhance comfort or for use at night when they wear a compression garment during the day.[75] Foam or other padding is often used under bandages to improve edema reduction and foster limb uniformity. The time, effort, and dexterity required for bandaging can become burdensome or impossible for some patients, necessitating the use of an alternative compression method.[20] MLLB should be avoided for the following conditions: (1) Severe arterial insufficiency with an ankle/brachial index (ABI) of <0.5, although modified MLLB with reduced pressures can be used under close supervision; (2) Uncontrolled heart failure; and (3) Severe peripheral neuropathy.[1,75] Some components of the MLLB system can be washed and dried according to the manufacturer's instructions and reused. Over time, inelastic bandages will progressively lose their extensibility, which will increase their stiffness. Heavily soiled, cohesive and adhesive bandages should be discarded after use.[75]

### Compression Garments

Compression garments are recommended for patients with lymphedema of the extremities.[74,75] Compression garments can be used as initial management in patients who have mild upper or lower limb lymphedema (ISL stage I) with minor pitting, no significant tissue changes, no or minimal shape distortion, or palliative needs.[3,74,75] Physiological effects of compression include edema control or reduction, decreased accumulated protein, decreased arteriole outflow into the interstitium, improved muscle pump effect with movement and exercise of the affected area, and protection of skin. Gradient external pressure provides the greatest pressure distally and less pressure proximally; this is optimal for improved lymphatic transport.[74] Skin care, exercise or body movement, elevation and self-lymph drainage should be taught, along with self monitoring and proper application, removal and care of external compression garments.[20,75] Lower pressure compression garments can also relieve lymphedema symptoms for palliative care. Patients should be reviewed four to six weeks after initial fitting, and then at each garment renewal approximately every three to six months.[75]

Garment usage requires frequent laundering of products (daily to every other day), daily skin care and complication monitoring, and 2 replacements every 6 months. Various helpful products exist to assist patients in applying garments—an especially important task for elderly and disabled patients. Hand arthritis or neuropathy can hinder tolerance of garments. Garment removal is required if compression causes pain, neurological symptoms, or color or temperature changes. Readjustment and movement may remedy the problem; often, product replacement is required. Because a variety of products exist, staff and patient persistence is likely to result in good patient tolerance. Rubber gloves (dishwashing gloves) facilitate application of garments and extend their longevity. Timely garment replacement (usually every 6 months) is essential for good edema control.[74]

**Other Compression Products**

A growing number of alternative commercial compression products have become available. Semi-rigid products (e.g., ReidSleeve [Peninsula Medical, Inc., Scotts Valley CA], CircAid [CircAid, San Diego, CA]) use foam and Velcro straps to provide nonelastic compression designed to simulate bandaging while saving time and energy. JoVi (Innovative Medical Solutions, Inc., Selah, WA) and compression products use foam and an outer spandex compression sleeve. The compression sleeve allows adjustment for limb size changes, which can be ideal for limb reduction or increase or for weight changes affecting limb size. Distinct advantages of these products include ease and speed of application, overall comfort and tolerance, and product longevity. Haslett and Aitken[76] reported that the Tribute (LymphaCare, New York, NY) appeared to contribute to maintenance of previously achieved DLT reduction. Lund[77] reported that use of CircAid provided an acceptable substitute for bandaging. Research is needed to provide insight and direction regarding the use of these promising products.[78] Use of CircAid products on the lower extremities is currently contraindicated with ABI <0.5.[75,76]

**Decongestive Lymphatic Therapy and Lymph Drainage Massage**

Decongestive Lymphatic Therapy (DLT) evolved in Europe when Michael Foldi[31] combined Vodder's Manual Lymph Drainage (MLD) technique with bandaging, exercises, and specialized skin care. Dr. Foldi described his four-modality lymphedema treatment as "Complete Decongestive Therapy" (CDT). Complete Decongestive Therapy (CDT) comprised of manual lymph drainage (MLD), multi-layer, short-stretch compression bandaging, gentle remedial upper limb exercise, meticulous skin care, education in lymphedema self-management, and elastic compression garments, has become the standard of care for treating lymphedema.[60,61] In CDT, patients generally receive 2-hour treatments 5 days a week for 3 to 8 weeks. CDT requires patients to make a commitment to continue performing the exercise and skin care, as well as wearing the compression garments. Compliance with the prescribed treatment is difficult because even the most customized garments or sleeves sometimes are uncomfortable, unsightly, and laborious to put on.[62] A constellation of complex factors (e.g., physical, financial, aesthetic, time) can influence survivors' compliance with treatment. For treatment to be maximally effective, lymphedema needs to be treated by therapists with special training and experience in this field, as outlined by the National Lymphedema Network position paper on educational training for lymphedema therapists (http://www.lymphnet.org/pdfDocs/nlntraining.pdf) and the Lymphology Association of North America (LANA) (http://www.clt-lana.org/). These organizations have outlined training requirements for nurses, occupational therapists, physical therapists and assistants, physicians, and massage therapists to gain certification in this field.

**Pneumatic (Mechanical) Pumps**

Mechanical pumps use electricity to inflate a single-chamber or multichamber sleeve and produce external limb compression. A decreased tissue capillary filtration rate (documented by lymphoscintigraphy) produces tissue fluid reduction and, consequently, limb volume decrease.[83] Lymph formation decreases, but lymph transport, which would address lymphedema pathophysiology, is not affected. Badger and coworkers[60] initiated a Cochrane review of physical therapies used to treat lymphedema. Regarding pumps, she reported: (1) pumps are used as a way of both reducing lymphedema and controlling it; (2) opinion is divided on the use of pumps for lymphedema treatment; (3) pump use has reduced swelling, but concern exists regarding the way in which swelling is decreased as well as the rapid displacement of fluid elsewhere in the body; and (4) use of pumps does not eliminate the need for compression garments and may not provide more benefit than garments alone. Brennan and Miller[62] presented a consensus view of reservations related to tissue injury from improper pump prescription and use. Investigations have reported several pump complications, including lymphatic congestion and injury proximal to the pump sleeve, increased swelling adjacent to the pump cuff in up to 18% of patients,[84] lack of benefit in all but stage I (reversible) lymphedema, and development of genital lymphedema in up to 43% of patients with cancer-related lower extremity lymphedema.[84,85] After more than 50 years of pump use in lymphedema care and long-established Medicare reimbursement, no guidelines exist,

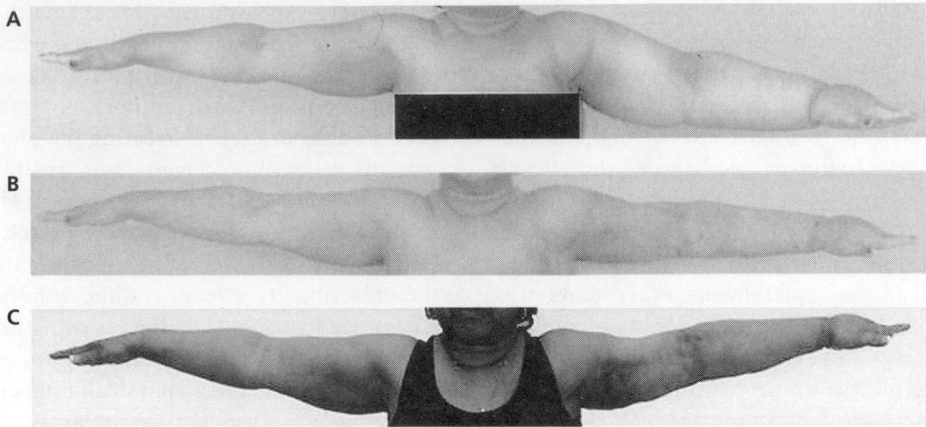

**Figure 16–7.** Photographs showing results of lymphedema treatment in a breast cancer survivor. A. Preoperative—2315 mL. B. Four weeks postoperative—100 mL. C. Three years postoperative—210 mL.

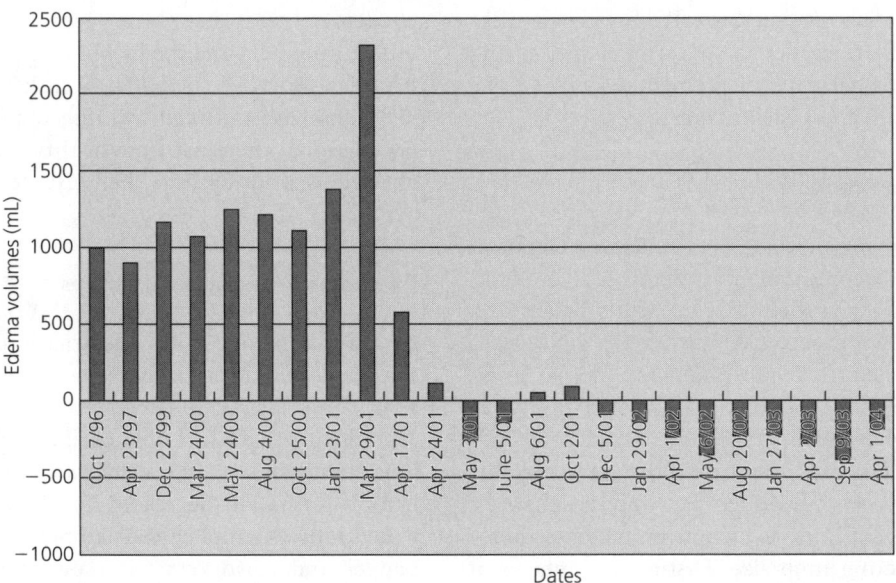

**Figure 16–8.** Affected arm excess edema volume, compared with nonaffected arm, over time. The patient, underwent liposuction of the affected arm in April 2001.

significant complications are reported, and research has not clarified benefit.

CASE STUDY

*Liz, A Breast Cancer Survivor with Resistant Lymphedema*

Liz, a California breast cancer survivor, developed lymphedema in 1988; she intermittently used garments and pumps for the next two decades. After relocating to New York in 2000, she was assisted by a Lymphedema Clinical Nurse Specialist. Over the next 3 years, Liz was referred for two courses of intensive DLT. The second course was provided at a well-known New York treatment center. Lymphedema gradually and continually progressed, in spite of good compliance to the use of compression products. The patient met liposuction surgery criteria and obtained third party payer approval for liposuction surgery in Sweden. Preoperatively, excess limb volume was 2315 mL; no pitting was present. The patient had agreed to lifelong use of compression and underwent liposuction surgery in April of 2004. The surgical aspirate contained 90% adipose tissue. One month after surgery, she had achieved 125% edema reduction.

Patient follow-up takes place at least every 6 months, and garments are replaced at each of these follow-ups. Three years after surgery, edema reduction was 119%. Hand edema subsequently returned. Liz has continued 100% compliance with use of compression products. She has also regained significant quality of life. In late 2007, Liz began using a compression sleeve at nighttime along with her Elvarex glove. She continues daytime use of the Elvarex sleeve and glove.

Table 16–4
**Lymphedema Secondary to Cancer of the Head and Neck**

Lymphedema secondary to head and neck cancer commonly presents following surgery and radiotherapy. Lymphedema is frequently found below the chin in the anterior neck. Difficult in swallowing and breathing are the major symptom distress from neck lymphedema. Mild swelling often progresses fairly rapidly to firm, non-pitting swelling; thus may often not be recognized or treated as lymphedema.

Quantification of neck edema can be achieved by measuring from the tip of one ear lobe to the tip of the contra-lateral ear lobe along the line of the chin, and then measuring this distance for every 2 cm (or 4 cm) interval down to the intersection of the neck and chest. Quantifiable outcome measurement over time fosters patient participation, improved long-term outcomes, and might be beneficial as substantiation for third-party payers.

The Epstein Facioplasty Support, made by BSN-Jobst, Inc., can be useful for neck lymphedema. This product provides gentle compression to the chin using two sets of long narrow Velcro straps that extend from the chin to the top of the head and to the back of the neck. This size-adjustable "chin strap" provides gentle, size-adjustable compression to the chin and neck. Patients are encouraged to use the product continually for at least several weeks or a month to achieve optimal edema reduction. Although life-long product use is encouraged for optimal lymph function, some patients have been able to transition to mainly nighttime product use and still maintain acceptable edema control.

Nursing interventions for head and neck lymphedema include:
- Help patients to make an informed decision in a supportive environment.
- Instruction and support in establishment of a life-long daily self-care regimen, including range of motion exercises, skin assessment and application of moisturizers; early, skilled patient complication assistance and use of safe external compression. A written self-care program may foster patient self-care adherence.
- Monitor external neck compression. External neck compression must provide sufficient pressure to stimulate lymphatic function without causing skin irritation/injury or impairment of breathing, eating or swallowing.
- Encourage the use of daily self care using Manual Lymph Drainage to further improve edema control.
- Document patient outcomes, including interval neck circumferences, skin integrity, pain level, and neck range of motion.

Greater than 100% edema reduction has been maintained. Liz reported relief at the variation between her daytime and nighttime products. Figures 16–7 and 16–8 display the results of lymphedema treatment used in a similar patient.

## Unusual Lymphedemas

Palliative care may require the management of unusual and challenging lymphedema sites, such as breast, head, neck, trunk, or genitals.[75] LDM, skin-softening techniques, foam chip pads, and external compression (if possible) are recommended.[2] External compression may be achieved with collars, vests, custom pants or tights, scrotal supports,[75] or spandex type exercise apparel. The assistance of occupational or physical therapists and a seamstress may be helpful. Nationally, instructional courses are available to provide guidance for managing these difficult lymphedemas, such as courses provided by the Lymphology Association of North America (LANA) (http://www.clt-lana.org/). Table 16–4 presents detailed information about neck lymphedema from head and neck cancer.

## Conclusion

Edema is a symptom usually relieved by addressing the causative factor. Lymphedema, often labeled as edema, is a chronic disorder that requires long-term management. Although external compression is essential to effective lymphedema management, third party payer reimbursement is inadequate and frustrating, patients are frequently fitted with products they cannot tolerate, and many patients have not been adequately prepared for compression products and therefore discontinue use when their product does not cure the lymphedema. Newer compression products, such as the CircAid, Legacy, and compression sleeve offer exciting product alternatives, but lack controlled research substantiation. Benefits of two commonly supported treatments, DLT and pneumatic compression pumps, have not been substantiated by randomized controlled clinical trials, according to several expert literature reviews. Controlled clinical trials are essential for establishing "gold standard" treatments and should be the basis for third party payer reimbursement. Research deficit has also precluded establishment of outcome and practice standards, allowing an "anything goes" treatment environment.

Nevertheless, over the last two decades, progress has been achieved in both lymphedema awareness and scientific research. Oncology nurses and other nurses have increasingly contributed to lymphedema management as they have improved cancer survivorship.[86] Nursing's unique focus and scope of practice is ideally suited to chronic illness management, both at entry and advanced practice levels. To meet the physical and psychological needs of patients, nurses and other healthcare professionals must make an effort to understand the pathophysiology and chronic nature of lymphedema, as well as its physical, functional, and psychosocial impact. Armed with such information, nurses can then engage patients in supportive dialogue about risk reduction and lymphedema management.[45,55] Combined with nurses' immense and diverse patient contact, enormous potential exists for nurses to dramatically improve both edema and lymphedema management.

### REFERENCES

1. Kelly DG. A Primer on Lymphedema. Upper Saddle River, NJ: Prentice-Hall, 2002.

2. Mortimer PS, Badger C. Lymphoedema. In Doyle D, Hanks GW, Cherny N, Calman K, eds. Oxford Textbook of Palliative Medicine. New York: Oxford University Press, 2004: 640–647.

3. International Society of Lymphology. The diagnosis and treatment of peripheral lymphedema. Consensus document of the International Society of Lymphology. Lymphology 2003;36:84–91.

4. Mortimer P. Lymphoedema. In: Warrell DA, Cox TM, Firth JD, eds. Oxford Textbook of Medicine (Vol 2) (2nd ed). Oxford: Oxford University Press, 2003:1202–1208.

5. Brorson H, Aberg M, Svensson H. Chronic lymphedema and adipocyte proliferation: Clinical therapeutic implications. The Lymphatic Continuum. National Institutes of Health, Bethesda, USA, 2002. Lymphat Res Biol 2003;1:88.

6. WHO: The World Health Report 2004—Changing History. Geneva: World Health Organization, 2004.

7. Ferrell R, Kimak M, Lawrence E, Finegold D. Candidate gene analysis in primary lymphedema. Lymphat Res Biol 2008;6:69–76.

8. Ghalamkarpour A, Morlot S, Raas-Rothschild A, et al. Hereditary Lymphedema type I associated with VEGFR3 mutation: The first de novo case and atypical presentation. Clin Genet 2006;70:330–335.

9. Spiegel R, Ghalamkarpour A, Daniel-Spiegel E, Vikkula M, Shalev S. Wide clinical spectrum in a family with hereditary lymphedema type I due to a novel Missense mutation in VEGFR3. J Human Genet 2006;51:846–850.

10. Moffatt CJ, Franks PJ, Doherty D, et al. Lymphoedema: An underestimated health problem. QJM 2003;96:731–38.

11. Armer J, Fu MR., Wainstock JM, Zagar E, Jacobs LK. Lymphedema following breast cancer treatment, including sentinel lymph node biopsy. Lymphology 2004;37:73–91.

12. Ozaslan C, Kuru B. Lymphedema after treatment of breast cancer. Am J Surg 2004;187;69–72.

13. Paskett ED, Naughton MJ, McCoy TP, Case LD, Abbott JM. The epidemiology of arm and hand swelling in premenopausal breast cancer survivors. Cancer Epidemiol Biomarkers Prev 2007;16:775–782.

14. Hong JH, Tsai CS, Lai CH, et al. Postoperative low pelvic irradiation for stage I-IIA cervical cancer patients with risk factors other than pelvic lymph node metastasis. Int J Radiat Oncol Biol Phys 2002;53:1284–1290.

15. Ryan M, Stainton MC, Slaytor EK, et al. Aetiology and prevalence of lower limb lymphoedema following treatment for gynaecological cancer. Aust N Z J Obstet Gynaecol 2003;43:148–151.

16. Johansson K, Ohlsson K, Ingvar C, Albertsson M, Ekdahl C. Factors associated with the development of arm lymphedema following breast cancer treatment: A match pair case-control study. Lymphology 2002;35:59–71.

17. Mak SS, Yeo W, Lee YM, Mo KF, Tse KY, Tse SM, Ho FP, Kwan, WH. Predictors of lymphedema in patients with breast cancer undergoing axillary lymph node dissection in Hong Kong. Nurs Res 2008;57:416–425.

18. Cheville AL, McGarvey CL, Petrek JA, Russo SA, Tylor ME, Tiadens SR. Lymphedema management. Semin Radiat Oncol 2003;13:290–301.

19. Vaqas B, Ryan TJ. Lymphoedema: Pathophysiology and management in resource-poor settings—relevance for lymphatic filariasis control programmes. Filaria J 2003;2:4.

20. Fu MR. Breast cancer survivors' intentions of managing lymphedema. Cancer Nurs 2005;28:446–457.

21. Fu MR. Women at work with breast cancer-related lymphoedema. J Lymphedema 2008;3:30–36.

22. Pyszel A, Malyszczak K, Pyszel K, Andrzejak R, Szuba A. Disability, psychological distress and quality of life in breast cancer survivors with arm lymphedema. Lymphology 2006;39:185–192.

23. Ruocco V, Schwartz RA, Ruocco E. Lymphedema: An immunologically vulnerable site for development of neoplasms. J Am Acad Dermat 2002;47:124–127.

24. Armer JM, Porock D. Self-reported fatigue among women with post-breast cancer LE. Lymph Link 2001;13(3):1,2,4.

25. Smith JK, Zobec A. Lymphedema management. In: Ferrell B, Coyle N, eds. The Oxford Textbook of Palliative Nursing. New York: Oxford University Press, 2001:92–203.

26. Firth J. Idiopathic oedema of women. In: Warrell DA, Cox TM, Firth JD, eds. Oxford Textbook of Medicine. Oxford: Oxford University Press, 2004:1209–1210.

27. Szuba A, Razavi M, Rockson SG. Diagnosis and treatment of concomitant venous obstruction in patients with secondary lymphedema. J Vasc Interv Radiol 2002;13:799–803.

28. Ganong WF. Dynamics of blood and lymph flow. In: Ganong WF, ed. Review of Medical Physiology. Chicago: Lange Medical Books, McGraw-Hill Medical Publishing Division, 2001:570–571.

29. Pressman PI. Surgical treatment and lymphedema. Cancer Suppl 1998;83:2782–2787.

30. Meek AG. Breast radiotherapy and lymphedema. Cancer Suppl 1998;83:2788–2797.

31. Foldi M, Foeldi E, Clodius L, Neu H. Complications of lymphedema. In Foeldi M, Foeldi E, Kubik S, eds. Textbook of Lymphology for Physicians and Lymphedema Therapists. Munchen: Urban & Fischer Verlag: Elsevier GmbH, 2003:267–275, English text revised by Biotext LLC, San Francisco.

32. Perbeck L, Celebioglu F, Svensson L, Danielsson R. Lymph circulation in the breast after radiotherapy and breast conservation. Lymphology 2006;39:33–40.

33. Kwan W, Jackason J, Dingee C, Mcgregor G, Olivotto I. Chronic arm morbidity after curative breast cancer treatment: Prevalence and impact on quality of life. J Clin Oncol 2005;20:4242–4248.

34. Soran A, D'Angelo G, Begovic M, Ardic F, Harlak A, Samuel Wieand H, Vogel VG, Johnson RR. Breast cancer-related lymphedema—what are the significant predictors and how they affect the severity of lymphedema? Breast J 2006;12: 536–543.

35. Fu MR, Ridner SH, Armer J. Post-breast cancer lymphedema: Impact and diagnosis. Am J Nurs March 2009;109:48–54.

36. Fu MR. Post-breast cancer lymphedema and management. Recent Adv Res Updates 2004;5:125–138.

37. Parran L. Spiritual care is elemental and fundamental to the heart. ONS News 2003;8(3):1,4,5.

38. Woods M. Using philosophy, knowledge and theory to assess a patient with lymphoedema. Int J Palliat Nurs 2002;8:176, 178–181.

39. Johansson K, Holmstrom H, Nilsson I, Ingvar C, Albertsson M, Ekdahl C. Breast cancer patients' experiences of lymphoedema. Scand J Caring Sci 2003;17:35–42.

40. Rymal C. Comprehensive decongestive therapy for lymphedema in patients with a history of cerebral vascular accident. Clin J Oncol Nurs 2003;7:677–678.

41. Szuba A, Rockson SG. Lymphedema: Classification, diagnosis and therapy. Vasc Med 1998;3:145–156.

42. Caban ME. Trends in the evaluation of lymphedema. Lymphology 2002;35:28–38.

43. Balzarini A, Millela M, Civelli E, Sigari C, De Conno F. Ultrasonography of arm edema after axillary dissection for breast cancer: A preliminary study. Lymphology 2001;34: 152–155.

44. Armer JM, Radina ME, Porock D, Culbertson SD. Predicting breast cancer-related lymphedema using self-reported symptoms. Nurs Res 2003;52:370–379.

45. Fu MR, Axelrod D, Haber J. Breast cancer-related lymphedema: Information, symptoms, and risk reduction behaviors. J Nurs Scholarsh 2008;40:341–348.

46. Armer JM, Stewart BR. A comparison of four diagnostic criteria for lymphedema in a post-breast cancer population. Lymphat Res Biol 2005;3:208–217.

47. Tierney S, Aslam M, Rennie K, Grace, P. Infrared optoelectronic volumetry, the ideal way to measure limb volume. Eur J Vasc Endovasc Surg 1996;12:412–417.

48. Petlund CF. Volumetry of limbs. In: Olszewski WI, ed. Lymph Stasis: Pathophysiology, Diagnosis and Treatment. Boston: CRC Press, 1991:444–451.

49. Cornish BH, Chapman M, Hirst C, Mirolo B, Bunce IH, Ward LC, Thomas BJ. Early diagnosis of lymphedema using multiple frequency bioimpedance. Lymphology 2001;34:2–11.

50. Venipuncture Policy. Penrose-St. Francis Health Services. Nursing Policy Committee, Colorado Springs, CO:2003.

51. Box RC, Reul-Hirche HM, Bullock-Saxton JE, Furnival CM. Physiotherapy after breast cancer surgery: Results of a randomised controlled study to minimise lymphedema. Breast Cancer Res Treat 2002;75:51–64.

52. Harris SR, Niesen-Vertommen S. Challenging the myth of exercise-induced lymphedema following breast cancer: A series of case reports. J Surg Oncol 2000;74:95–98.

53. Johannson K, Ohlsson K, Ingvar C, Albertsson M, Ekdahl C. Factors associated with the development of arm lymphedema following breast cancer treatment: A match pair case-control study. Lymphology 2002;35:59–71.

54. National Lymphedema Network (NLN). Position Paper on Lymphedema Risk Reduction Practices. Available at: http://www.lymphnet.org/lymphedemaFAQs/positionPapers.htm (accessed December 27, 2008).

55. Fu M.R, Ridner SH, Armer J. Post-breast cancer lymphedema: Risk-reduction and management. Am J Nurs 2009;109:34–41.

56. Highfield ME. Providing spiritual care to patients with cancer. Clin J Oncol Nurs 2000;4:115–120.

57. Taugher T. Helping patients search for meaning in their lives. CJON 2002;6:239–240.

58. Stanton AWB, Badger C, Sitzia J. Non-invasive assessment of the lymphedematous limb. Lymphology 2000;33:122–135.

59. Hoskins CL, Daugherty D. Disease management: Establishing standards of care for lymphedema treatment. Lymph Link 2003;15(4):5,26.

60. Badger C, Preston N, Seers K, Mortimer P. Physical therapies for reducing and controlling lymphoedema of the limbs. Cochrane Database Syst Rev 2004;(4):CD003141.

61. National Lymphedema Network (NLN). Position Paper on Treatment. Available at: http://www.lymphnet.org/lymphedemaFAQs/positionPapers.htm (accessed December 28, 2008).

62. Brennan M J, Miller LT. Overview of treatment options and review of the current role and use of compression garments, intermittent pumps, and exercise in the management of lymphedema. Cancer 1998;83:2821–2827.

63. Casley-Smith JR. Modern treatment of lymphoedema. Modern Med Australia 1992;5:70–83.

64. Regnard C, Allport S, Stephenson L. ABC of palliative care: Mouth care, skin care, and lymphoedema. Br Med J 1997;315:1004–1005.

65. Cohen SR, Payne DK, Tunkel RS. Lymphedema: Strategies for management. Cancer 2001;92(4 Suppl):980–987.

66. Macdonald JM. Wound healing and lymphedema: A new look at an old problem. Ostomy Wound Manage 2001;47(4): 52–57.

67. Mortimer P. Inflammation and infection in the lymphedema limb. Newsletter Lymphedema Assoc Aust 1997;15:3–4.

68. Olszewski W. Inflammatory changes of skin in lymphedema of extremities and efficacy of benzathine penicillin administration. NLN Newsletter 1996;8(4):1–3.

69. Ko DS, Lerner R, Klose G, Cosimi AB. Effective treatment of lymphedema of the extremities. Arch Surg 1998;133:452–458.

70. Williams AE, Bergl S, Twycross RG. A 5-year review of a lymphoedema service. Eur J Cancer Care 1996;5:56–59.

71. Foldi E. The treatment of lymphedema. Cancer 1998;83(12 Suppl American):2833–2834.

72. Serlin R, Mendoza T, Nakamura Y, Edwards KR, Cleeland CS. When is cancer pain mild, moderate or severe? Grading pain severity by its interference with function. Pain 1995;61: 277–284.

73. National Lymphedema Network (NLN). Position Paper on Risk Reduction. Available at: http://www.lymphnet.org/lymphedemaFAQs/positionPapers.htm (accessed December 28, 2008).

74. Rymal C. Compression modalities in lymphedema therapy. Innov Breast Cancer Care 1998;3(4):88–92.

75. Morgan PA, Moffat CJ. Lymphoedema Framework. Best Practice for the Management of Lymphoedema. International Consensus. London: MEP Ltd, 2006.

76. Haslett ML, Aitken MJ. Evaluating the effectiveness of a compression sleeve in managing secondary lymphoedema. J Wound Care 2002;11:401–404.

77. Lund E. Exploring the use of the CircAid legging in the management of lymphoedema. Int J Palliat Nurs 2000;6:383–391.

78. Cheville AJ. Lymphedema and palliative care. Lymph Link 2002;14(1):1–4.

79. Svensson H. Liposuction combined with controlled compression therapy reduces arm lymphedema more effectively than controlled compression therapy alone. Plast Reconstr Surg 1998;31:156–172.

80. Brorson H, Svensson H. Complete reduction of lymphoedema of the arm by liposuction after breast cancer. Scand J Plast Reconstr Surg Hand Surg 1997;31:137–143.

81. Brorson H. Liposuction in arm lymphedema treatment. Scand J Surg 2003;92:287–295.

82. Brorson H, Ohlin K, Olsson G, Langstrom G, Wiklund I, Svensson H. Quality of life following liposuction and conservative treatment of arm lymphedema. Lymphology 2006;39(1):8–25.

83. Miranda F Jr, Perez MC, Castiglioni ML, Juliano Y, Amorim JE, Nakano LC, de Barros N Jr, Lustre WG, Burinah E. Effect of sequential intermittent pneumatic compression on both leg lymphedema volume and on lymph transport as semi-quantitatively evaluated by lymphoscintigraphy. Lymphology 2001;34:135–141.

84. Lynnworth M. Greater Boston lymphedema support group pump survey. NLN Newsletter 1998;10(1):6–7.

85. Boris M, Weindorf S, Lasinski B. The risk of genital edema after external pump compression for lower limb lymphedema. Lymphology 1998;31:15–20.

86. Ferrell BR. The role of oncology nursing to ensure quality care for cancer survivors: A report commissioned by the National Cancer Policy Board and Institute of Medicine. Oncol Nurs Forum 2003;30(1):E1–E11.

# 17A

*Barbara M. Bates-Jensen*

# Skin Disorders: Pressure Ulcers—Prevention and Management

*I give her the pain medication before the dressing changes, but still she cries when I change the dressings, and the odor is intense. I don't know what else to do for her.—A treatment nurse caring for a patient with severe pressure ulcers at the end of life in a nursing home.*

*I always thought that be dsores came from neglect. I feel so guilty that I let this happen.—A patient's family member*

♦ **Key Points**
♦ *Palliative pressure ulcer care is not "lack of care," but care focused on comfort and limiting the extent or impact of the wound.*
♦ *Pressure ulcer prevention for palliative care includes use of flexible repositioning schedules with attention to adequate pain relief interventions before movement and use of pressure redistributing support surfaces for the bed and chair.*
♦ *Palliative care for pressure ulcers includes: attention to prevention measures; obtaining and maintaining a clean wound; management of pain, exudate, and odor; and prevention of complications such as wound infection.*
♦ *It is essential to involve the individual, family members, and caregivers in establishing goals of care, enacting a plan of care, and defining the individual's wishes.*

Palliative care for skin disorders is a broad area, encompassing prevention and care for chronic wounds such as pressure ulcers, management of malignant wounds and fistulas, and management of stomas. The goals of treatment are to reduce discomfort and pain, manage odor and drainage, and provide for optimal functional capacity. In each area, involvement of the caregiver and family in the plan of care is important. Management of skin disorders involves significant physical care as well as attention to psychological and social care. To meet the needs of the patient and family, access to the multidisciplinary care team is crucial, and consultation by an Enterostomal Therapy nurse, a certified Wound, Ostomy, Continence nurse, or a certified Wound Care nurse is highly desirable.

Because skin disorders are such an important issue in palliative nursing care, this chapter has been divided into two distinct parts. Part 17A addresses pressure ulcers in depth, and Part 17B addresses malignant wounds, fistulas, and stomas. While pressure ulcers are not the only wounds to occur at the end of life, they are the most common wound type to occur in patients receiving palliative care accounting for 40% to 50% of wounds.[1,2] Pressure ulcer prevalence in palliative care settings ranges from 9% to 38%[3-5] with incidence varying from 3% to 13%, the majority of which are stage I or stage II ulcers.[5,6] Pressure ulcers often occur in the two to three weeks prior to death and have been suggested as an indicator of failure of the skin as an organ.[7-9] This suggests that some pressure ulcers may be unavoidable in persons receiving palliative care. Contrary to many health care practitioner's beliefs, once a pressure ulcer develops healing is possible, with reports of wound healing in persons receiving palliative care ranging from 44% for those with cancer diagnoses to 78% for those with non-cancer diagnoses.[10] Thus, the emphasis on palliative wound care does not negate the potential for wound closure and healing even in those at the end of life.

## Definition

Pressure ulcers are areas of local tissue trauma that usually develop where soft tissues are compressed between bony prominences and external surfaces for prolonged periods. Mechanical injury to the skin and tissues causes hypoxia and ischemia, leading to tissue necrosis. Caring for the patient with a pressure ulcer can be frustrating for clinicians because of the chronic nature of the wound and because additional time and resources are often invested in the management of these wounds. Further, many family caregivers and health care providers view development of pressure ulcers as an indication of poor care or impending death. Pressure ulcers are painful, care is costly, and treatment costs increase as the severity of the wound increases. Additionally, not all pressure ulcers heal, and many heal slowly, causing a continual drain on caregivers and on financial resources. The chronic nature of a pressure ulcer challenges the health care provider to design more effective treatment plans.

Once a pressure ulcer develops, the usual goals are to manage the wound to support healing. However, some patients will benefit most from a palliative wound care approach. Palliative wound care goals are comfort and limiting the extent or impact of the wound, but without the intent of healing. Palliative care for chronic wounds, such as pressure ulcers, is appropriate for a wide variety of patient populations. Palliative care is often indicated for terminally ill patients, such as those with cancer or other diseases and those at the end of life. Institutionalized older adults with multiple comorbidities and older adults with severe functional decline at the end of life may also benefit from palliative care. Sometimes individuals with long-standing wounds and other life expectations benefit from a palliative care approach for a specified duration of time. For example, a wheelchair-bound young adult with a sacral pressure ulcer may make an informed choice to continue to be up in a wheelchair to attend school even though this choice severely diminishes the expectation for wound healing. The health care professional may decide jointly with the patient to treat the wound palliatively during this time frame.

The foundation for designing a care plan for the patient with a pressure ulcer is a comprehensive assessment. This is true even if the goals of care are palliative. Comprehensive assessment includes assessment of wound severity, wound status, and the total patient. Management of the wound is best accomplished within the context of the whole person, particularly if palliation is the outcome. Assessment is the first step in maintaining and evaluating a therapeutic plan of care. Without adequate baseline wound and patient assessment and valid interpretation of the assessment data, the plan of care for the wound may be inappropriate or ineffective—at the least, it may be disjointed and fragmented due to poor communication. An inadequate plan of care may lead to impaired or delayed healing, miscommunication regarding the goals of care (healing versus palliation), and complications such as infection.

## Pathophysiology of Pressure Ulcer Development

Pressure ulcers are the result of mechanical injury to the skin and underlying tissues. The primary forces involved are pressure and shear.[11–15] Pressure is the perpendicular force or load exerted on a specific area; it causes ischemia and hypoxia of the tissues. High-pressure areas in the supine position are the occiput, sacrum, and heels. In the sitting position, the ischial tuberosities exert the highest pressure, and the trochanters are affected in the side-lying position.[12,16]

As the amount of soft tissue available for compression decreases, the pressure gradient increases. Likewise, as the tissue available for compression increases, the pressure gradient decreases. For this reason, most pressure ulcers occur over bony prominences, where there is less tissue for compression.[16] This relationship is important to understand for palliative care, because most of the likely candidates for palliative care will have experienced significant changes in nutritional status and body weight, with diminished soft tissue available for compression and a more prominent bony structure. This more prominent bony structure is more susceptible to skin breakdown from external forces, because the soft tissue that is normally used to deflect physical forces (e.g., pressure, shear) is absent. Therefore, the tissues are less tolerant of external forces, and the pressure gradient within the vascular network is altered.[16]

Alterations in the vascular network allow an increase in the interstitial fluid pressure, which exceeds the venous flow. This results in an additional increase in the pressure and impedes arteriolar circulation. The capillary vessels collapse, and thrombosis occurs. Increased capillary arteriolar pressure leads to fluid loss through the capillaries, tissue edema, and subsequent autolysis. Lymphatic flow is decreased, allowing further tissue edema and contributing to the tissue necrosis.[13,15,17–19]

Pressure, over time, occludes blood and lymphatic circulation, causing deficient tissue nutrition and buildup of waste products due to ischemia. If pressure is relieved before a critical time period is reached, a normal compensatory mechanism, reactive hyperemia, restores tissue nutrition and compensates for compromised circulation. If pressure is not relieved before the critical time period, the blood vessels collapse and thrombose, causing tissue deprivation of oxygen, nutrients, and waste removal. In the absence of oxygen, cells utilize anaerobic pathways for metabolism and produce toxic byproducts. The toxic byproducts lead to tissue acidosis, increased cell membrane permeability, edema, and, eventually, cell death.[13,17]

Tissue damage may also be caused by reperfusion and reoxygenation of the ischemic tissues or by postischemic injury.[20] Oxygen is reintroduced into tissues during reperfusion after ischemia. This triggers oxygen-free radicals, known as superoxide anion, hydroxyl radicals, and hydrogen peroxide, which induce endothelial damage and decrease microvascular integrity. Ischemia and hypoxia of body tissues are produced when capillary blood flow is obstructed by localized pressure. The degree of pressure and the amount of time necessary for ulceration to occur have been a subject of study for many years. In 1930, Landis,[21] using single-capillary microinjection techniques, determined normal hydrostatic pressure to be 32 mm Hg at the arteriolar end and 15 mm Hg at the venular end. His work has served as a criterion for measuring occlusion of capillary blood flow. Generally, a range from 25 to 32 mm Hg is considered normal and is used as the marker for adequate relief of pressure on the tissues. In severely compromised patients, even this level of pressure may be too high.

During critical illness or at end of life (the period of time when a person is living with an illness that will often worsen and may eventually cause death), the skin, as with all organs, can and often does fail. This dysfunction of the skin as an organ occurs in varying degrees with resultant varying levels of injury. Dysfunction can occur at the tissue, cellular, or molecular level—all of which relate to decreased cutaneous perfusion leading to local hypoxia.[22,23] The end result is a reduced ability to use nutrients to maintain normal skin function. Thus, skin failure is a result of hypoperfusion, which creates an intense inflammatory reaction associated with severe dysfunction.[22] As the body faces critical illness, peripheral vasoconstriction may occur to shunt blood from the periphery and skin to the central vital organs. Much of the skin has collateral vascular supply, but some areas have a single vascular route. These areas include distal areas such as fingers and toes and the sacral coccygeal area which has no direct blood flow. The decrease in blood flow to the skin also results in reduced cutaneous metabolic processes, thus, minor forces can lead to major damage such as pressure ulcers. Both acute and chronic skin failure have been described.[23]

Pressure is greatest at the bony prominence and soft tissue interface and gradually lessens in a cone-shaped gradient to the periphery.[12,24,25] Therefore, although tissue damage apparent on the skin surface may be minimal, the damage to deeper structures can be severe. In addition, subcutaneous fat and muscle are more sensitive than the skin to ischemia. Muscle and fat tissues are more metabolically active and, therefore, more vulnerable to hypoxia with increased susceptibility to pressure damage. The vulnerability of muscle and fat tissues to pressure forces explains pressure ulcers, in which large areas of muscle and fat tissue are damaged, yet the skin opening is relatively small.[18] In patients with severe malnutrition and weight loss, there is less tissue between the bony prominence and the surface of the skin, so the potential for large ulcers with extensive undermining or pocketing is much higher.

There is a relationship between intensity and duration of pressure in pressure ulcer development. Low pressures over a long period of time are as capable of producing tissue damage as high pressures for a shorter period.[12] Tissues can tolerate higher cyclic pressures compared with constant pressure.[26] Pressures differ in various body positions. They are highest (70 mm Hg) on the buttocks in the lying position and in the sitting position can be as high as 300 mm Hg over the ischial

tuberosities.[12,16] These levels are well above the normal capillary closing pressures and are capable of causing tissue ischemia. If tissues have been compressed for prolonged periods, tissue damage will continue to occur even after the pressure is relieved.[22] This continued tissue damage relates to changes at the cellular level that lead to difficulties with restoration of perfusion (reperfusion injury). Initial skin breakdown can occur in 6 to 12 hours in healthy individuals and more quickly (less than 2 hours) in those who are debilitated.

More than 95% of all pressure ulcers develop over five classic locations: sacral/coccygeal area, greater trochanter, ischial tuberosity, heel, and lateral malleolus.[14] Correct anatomical terminology is important when identifying the true location of the pressure ulcer. For example, many clinicians often document pressure ulcers as being located on the patient's hip. The hip, or iliac crest, is actually an uncommon location for pressure ulceration. The iliac crest, located on the front of the body, is rarely subject to pressure forces. The area most clinicians are referring to is correctly termed the greater trochanter. The greater trochanter is the bony prominence located on the side of the body, just above the proximal, lateral aspect of the thigh, or "saddlebag" area. The majority of pressure ulcers occur on the lower half of the body. The location of the pressure ulcer may affect clinical interventions. For example, the patient with a pressure ulcer on the sacral/coccygeal area with concomitant urinary incontinence requires treatments that address the incontinence problem. Ulcers in the sacral/coccygeal area are also more at risk for friction and shearing damage due to the location of the wound. Figure 17A–1 shows the correct anatomical terminology for pressure ulcer locations. The most common locations for pressure ulcer development in palliative care patients are the sacral/coccygeal area and heels. Patients with contractures are at special risk for pressure ulcer development due to the internal pressure of the bony prominence and the abnormal alignment of the body and its extremities. Institutionalized older adults with severe functional decline are particularly susceptible to contractures due to immobilization for extended periods of time in conjunction with limited efforts for maintenance of range of motion.

❧

## Risk Factors for Pressure Ulcers

Pressure ulcers are physical evidence of multiple causative influences. Factors that contribute to pressure ulcer development can be thought of as those that affect the pressure force over the bony prominence and those that affect the tolerance of the tissues to pressure.

Mobility, sensory loss, and activity level are related to the concept of increasing pressure. Extrinsic factors including shear, friction, and moisture, as well as intrinsic factors such as nutrition, age, and arteriolar pressure, relate to the concept of tissue tolerance.[27] Several additional areas may influence pressure ulcer development, including emotional stress,

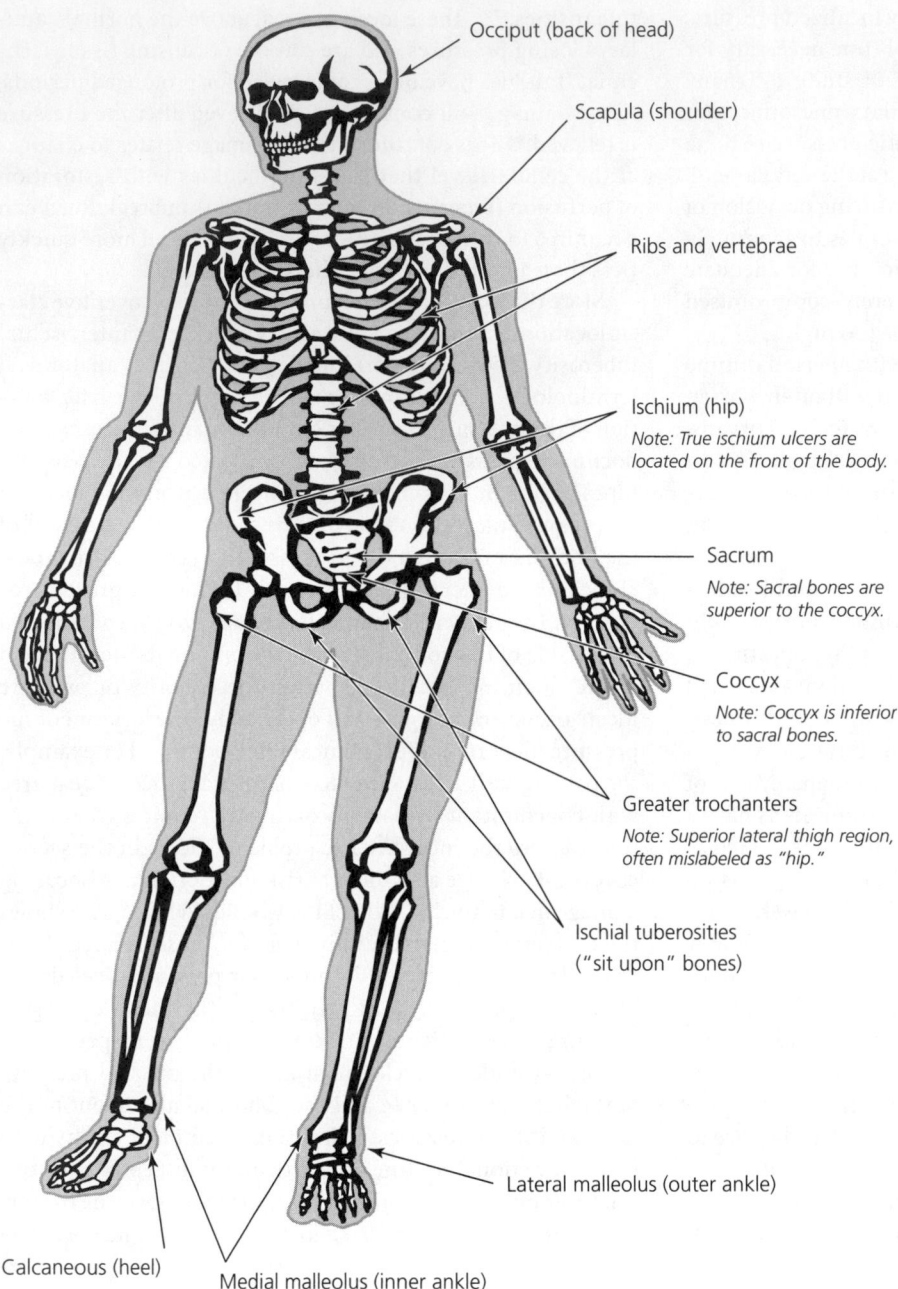

Occiput (back of head)

Scapula (shoulder)

Ribs and vertebrae

Ischium (hip)
*Note: True ischium ulcers are located on the front of the body.*

Sacrum
*Note: Sacral bones are superior to the coccyx.*

Coccyx
*Note: Coccyx is inferior to sacral bones.*

Greater trochanters
*Note: Superior lateral thigh region, often mislabeled as "hip."*

Ischial tuberosities
("sit upon" bones)

Lateral malleolus (outer ankle)

Calcaneous (heel)

Medial malleolus (inner ankle)

**Figure 17A–1.** Common anatomical locations of pressure ulcers.

temperature, smoking, and interstitial fluid flow.[28] Given their advanced illnesses and decreased functional capacity, patients receiving palliative care exhibit most or all of the risk factors for pressure ulcer development. Characteristics of palliative care patients that predict pressure ulcers include age, immobility, and physical inactivity.[29–31] Caregiver frailty in conjunction with patient risk factors increases the risk for pressure ulcer development.

### Immobility

Immobility, inactivity, and decreased sensory perception affect the duration and intensity of the pressure over the

bony prominence. Immobility or severely restricted mobility is the most important risk factor for all populations and a necessary condition for the development of pressure ulcers. Mobility is the state of being movable. The immobile patient cannot move, or facility or ease of movement is impaired. Closely related to immobility is limited activity.

### Inactivity

Activity is the production of energy or motion and implies an action. Activity is often clinically described by the ability of the individual to ambulate and move about. Those persons who are bed- or chair-bound, and thus inactive, are more at risk for pressure ulcer development.[32,33] A sudden change in activity level may signal significant change in health status and increased potential for pressure ulcer development.

### Sensory Loss

Sensory loss places patients at risk for compression of tissues and pressure ulcer development, because the normal mechanism for translating pain messages from the tissues is dysfunctional. Patients with intact nervous system pathways feel continuous local pressure, become uncomfortable, and change their position before tissue ischemia occurs. Spinal cord–injured patients have a higher incidence and prevalence of pressure ulcers.[34,35] Patients with paraplegia or quadriplegia are unable to sense increased pressure; if their body weight is not shifted, pressure ulceration develops. Likewise, patients with changes in mental status or functioning are at increased risk for pressure ulcer formation. They may not feel the discomfort from pressure, or be alert enough to move spontaneously. They may not remember to move, may be too confused to respond to commands to do so, or simply be physically unable to move. These risk factors are particularly evident in the palliative care population, in which individuals may be at the end of life.

### Shear

Extrinsic risk factors are those forces that make the tissues less tolerant of pressure. Extrinsic forces include shear, friction, and moisture. Whereas pressure acts perpendicularly to cause ischemia, shear causes ischemia by displacing blood vessels laterally and thereby impeding blood flow to tissues.[35–38] Shear is caused by the interplay of gravity and friction. Shear is a parallel force that stretches and twists tissues and blood vessels at the bony tissue interface; as such, it affects the deep blood vessels and deeper tissue structures. The most common example of shear is seen in the bed patient who is in a semi-sitting position with knees flexed and supported by pillows on the bed or by head-of-bed elevation. If the patient's skeleton slides down toward the foot of the bed, the sacral skin may stay in place (with the help of friction against the bed linen). This produces stretching, pinching, and occlusion of the underlying vessels, resulting in ulcers with large areas of internal tissue damage and less damage at the skin surface.

### Friction

Friction and moisture are not direct factors in pressure ulcer development, but they have been identified as contributing to the problem by reducing tolerance of tissues to pressure.[38] Friction occurs when two surfaces move across one another. Friction acts on tissue tolerance to pressure by abrading and damaging the epidermal and upper dermal layers of the skin. Additionally, friction acts with gravity to cause shear. Friction abrades the epidermis, which may lead to pressure

ulcer development by increasing the skin's susceptibility to pressure injury. Pressure combined with friction produces ulcerations at lower pressures than does pressure alone.[38] Friction acts in conjunction with shear to contribute to the development of sacral/coccygeal pressure ulcers on patients in the semi-Fowler position.

### Moisture

Moisture contributes to pressure ulcer development by removing oils on the skin, making it more friable, as well as interacting with body support surface friction. Constant moisture on the skin leads to maceration of the tissues. Waterlogging leads to softening of the skin's connective tissues. Macerated tissues are more prone to erosion, and once the epidermis is eroded, there is increased likelihood of further tissue breakdown.[39] Moisture alters the resiliency of the epidermis to external forces. Both shearing force and friction increase in the presence of mild to moderate moisture. Excess moisture may be caused by wound drainage, diaphoresis, or fecal or urinary incontinence.

### Incontinence

Urinary and fecal incontinence are common risk factors associated with pressure ulcer development. Incontinence contributes to pressure ulcer formation by creating excess moisture on the skin and by chemical damage to the skin. Fecal incontinence has the added detrimental effect of bacteria in the stool, which can contribute to infection as well as skin breakdown. Fecal incontinence is more significant as a risk factor for pressure ulceration because of the bacteria and enzymes in stool and their effects on the skin.[40] Inadequately managed incontinence poses a significant risk factor for pressure ulcer development, and fecal incontinence is highly correlated with pressure ulcer development.[32,41]

### Nutritional Risk Factors

There is some disagreement concerning the major intrinsic risk factors affecting tissue tolerance to pressure. However, most studies identify nutritional status as playing a role in pressure ulcer development. Hypoalbuminemia, weight loss, cachexia, and malnutrition are commonly identified as risk factors predisposing patients to pressure ulcer development.[42–45] Low serum albumin levels are associated both with having a pressure ulcer and with developing a pressure ulcer.

### Age

Age itself may be a risk factor for pressure ulcer development, with age-related changes in the skin and in wound healing increasing the risk of pressure ulcer development.[46] The skin and support structures undergo changes in the aging process. There is a loss of muscle, a decrease in serum albumin levels, diminished inflammatory response, decreased elasticity, and reduced cohesion between dermis and epidermis.[46,47] These changes combine with other changes related to aging to make the skin less tolerant of pressure forces, shear, and friction.

## Medical Conditions and Psychological Factors

Certain medical conditions or disease states are also associated with pressure ulcer development. Orthopedic injuries, altered mental status, and spinal cord injury are such conditions.[34,35,45,48,49] In palliative care populations, diagnoses of cancer and central nervous system disorders such as dementia are associated with higher incidence of pressure ulcer development.[2,31] Other psychological factors may affect risk for pressure ulcer development.[50–52] Self-concept, depression, and chronic emotional stress have been cited as factors in pressure ulcer development; the emerging role of cortisol levels in pressure ulcer development bears monitoring as well.

## Environmental Resources

Environmental resources include socioeconomic, psychosocial, health care system, and therapy resources. These factors are less understood than other risk factors; however, several of them play important roles in determining risk for pressure ulcer development and course of pressure ulcer care in patients receiving palliative care. Socioeconomic resources that may influence pressure ulcer development and healing are cost of therapy, type of payor (insurance type), and access to health care. In palliative care, cost of therapy becomes an important issue, particularly in long-term care facilities, where financial resources are limited and cost of therapy may hinder access to treatment.

Health care system resources are the type of health care setting and the experience, education level, and discipline of health care professionals. Patients receiving palliative care are often in long-term care facilities and dependent on the direct care practices of nurse aides with minimal education in health care, nursing and, especially, the needs of the palliative care patient. Therapy resources include topical treatments for wounds and systemic treatments. Palliative care patients often receive concomitant therapy that impairs mobility or sensory perception (e.g., pain medication) or normal healing mechanisms (e.g., steroids).

Psychosocial resources include adherence to the therapy plan, cultural values and beliefs, social support network (family and caregiver support), spiritual support, and alternative medicine use. The social support network is a key factor for palliative care. Patients receiving palliative care are often cared for in the home or in a long-term care facility. Home caregivers may be family members of the patient, often the spouse or significant other. If the patient is older and frail, it is typical to find that the caregiver is also older and frail, yet responsible for providing direct care 24 hours a day with minimal respite or support. Many times the nurse is dealing with two patients: the patient receiving palliative care and the patient's caregiver, who may also be frail and in need of services. The family member may be physically unable to reposition the patient or to provide other care services. In long-term care facilities, the problem may not be physical inability to perform the tasks but lack of staff, time or motivation. The availability of nurse attendants in the long-term care facility may be such that turning and repositioning of palliative care patients are not high-priority tasks.

In summary, environmental resources are not all well defined and, typically, are not included in formal risk-assessment tools for development of pressure ulcers. However, the importance of environmental resources in both the development and healing of pressure ulcers is clinically relevant in palliative care.

## Use of Risk-Assessment Scales

For practitioners to intervene in a cost-effective way, a method of screening for risk factors is necessary. Several risk-assessment instruments are available to clinicians. Screening tools assist in prevention by distinguishing those persons who are at risk for pressure ulcer development from those who are not. The only purpose in identifying patients who are at risk for pressure ulcer development is to allow for appropriate use of resources for prevention. The use of a risk-assessment tool allows for targeting of interventions to specific risk factors for individual patients. The risk-assessment instrument selected is based on its reliability for the intended raters, its predictive validity for the population, its sensitivity and specificity under consideration, and its ease of use including the time required for completion. The most common risk-assessment tools are the Braden Scale for Predicting Pressure Sore Risk[28] and the Norton Scale.[53] There is minimal information on the use of either instrument in palliative care patients, but both tools have been used in long-term care facilities, where many patients are assumed to be receiving palliative care. Two risk assessment tools specific to hospice patients have been developed and validated: the Hunters Hill Marie Curie Center Risk-Assessment tool[8] and the Hospice Pressure Ulcer Risk-Assessment Scale in use in Sweden.[4]

*Norton's Scale.* The Norton tool is the oldest risk-assessment instrument. Developed in 1961, it consists of five subscales: physical condition, mental state, activity, mobility, and incontinence.[54] Each parameter is rated on a scale of 1 to 4, with the sum of the ratings for all five parameters yielding a total score ranging from 5 to 20. Lower scores indicate increased risk, with scores of 16 or lower indicating "onset of risk" and scores of 12 or lower indicating high risk for pressure ulcer formation.[53]

*Braden Scale for Predicting Pressure Sores.* The Braden Scale was developed in 1987 and is composed of six subscales that conceptually reflect degrees of sensory perception, moisture, activity, nutrition, friction and shear, and mobility.[27,28] All subscales are rated from 1 to 4, except for friction and shear, which is rated from 1 to 3. The subscales may be summed for a total score ranging from 6 to 23.

Lower scores indicate lower function and higher risk for development of a pressure ulcer. The cutoff score for hospitalized adults is considered to be 16, with scores of 16 and lower indicating at-risk status.[28] In older patients, some have found cutoff scores of 17 or 18 to be better predictors of risk status.[15,30] Levels of risk are based on the predictive value of a positive test. Scores of 15 to 16 indicate mild risk, with a 50% to 60% chance of developing a stage I pressure ulcer; scores of 12 to 14 indicate moderate risk, with 65% to 90% chance of developing a stage I or II lesion; and scores lower than 12 indicate high risk, with a 90% to 100% chance of developing a stage II or deeper pressure ulcer.[44,45] The Braden Scale has been tested in acute care and long-term care with several levels of nurse raters and demonstrates high reliability with registered nurses.

Validity has been established by expert opinion, and predictive validity has been studied in several acute care settings, with good sensitivity and specificity demonstrated.[28,44] Some have shown that Braden Scale scores are highly correlated with Karnofsky/Palliative Performance Scale (PPS) scores ($r = .885$; $P < .001$),[55] which are prognostic performance status tools commonly used in palliative care settings.[56,57] The PPS is based on the Karnofsky performance scale, which is a tool to classify patients receiving cancer treatment according to their level of functional impairment. The PPS is scored 0 (death) to 100% (no limitation) in 10 unit increments.[56] Both the Karnofsky and PPS are scored similarly and used interchangeably in hospice settings. A score of 40% indicates that the patient spends most of his or her time in bed; a score of 30% indicates that the patient has increasing debility and requires total care. In the absence of a standardized risk assessment tool such as the Braden Scale, the PPS could be used as a proxy to determine risk for pressure ulcer development in hospice patients.[31,56,58] The Braden Scale is the model used in this chapter for prevention of pressure ulcers in patients requiring palliative care.

*Hunters Hill Marie Curie CenterRisk Assessment Tool.* The Hunters Hill Risk Assessment tool was developed in 2000 and is composed of seven subscales: sensation, mobility, moisture, activity in bed, nutrition/weight change, skin condition, and friction/shear.[8] Each factor is assessed on a four-point numerical scale with 1 indicating less risk and scores of 4 indicating highest risk for that factor. Individual factor scores can be summed for a total score which ranges from 7 signifying minimal risk to 28 demonstrating very high risk. The Hunters Hill tool was developed specifically for palliative care and validated in hospice patients using comparative analysis of the clinical judgement of experienced palliative care nurses.[8]

*The Hospice Pressure Ulcer Risk Assessment Scale.* The Hospice Pressure Ulcer Risk Assessment Scale was developed in 2003 after comparison of the Norton Scale and nine new scales derived from the Norton scale with various changes. Validity of the new scale was tested during development in 98 hospice patients. The items on the Hospice Pressure Ulcer Risk scale are physical activity, mobility, and age.[4]

Regardless of the instrument chosen to evaluate risk status, the clinical relevance is threefold. First, assessment for risk status must occur at frequent intervals. Assessment should be performed at admission to the health care organization (within 24 hours), at predetermined intervals (usually weekly), and whenever a significant change occurs in the patient's general health and status. The second clinical implication is the targeting of specific prevention strategies to identified risk factors. The final clinical implication is for those patients in whom prevention is not successful. For patients with an actual pressure ulcer, the continued monitoring of risk status may prevent further tissue trauma at the wound site and development of additional wound sites.

## Prevention of Pressure Ulcers

Prevention strategies are targeted at reducing risk factors and can be focused on eliminating specific risk factors. Early intervention for pressure ulcers is risk-factor specific and prophylactic in nature. The prevention strategies are presented here by risk factor, beginning with general information and ending with specific strategies to eliminate particular risk factors. Prevention is a key element for palliative care. If pressure ulcers can be prevented, the patient is spared tiresome, sometimes painful, and often overwhelming treatment. The Braden Scale is the basis for these prevention interventions. Prevention interventions that are appropriate to the patient's level of risk and specific to individual risk factors should be instituted. For example, the risk factor of immobility is managed very differently for the comatose patient compared with the patient with severe pain on movement with a single position of comfort or the patient who is still mobile even if bedbound. The comatose patient requires caregiver education and caregiver-dependent repositioning. The patient with severe pain on movement requires special support-surface intervention and minimal movement methods with a foam wedge. The patient who is still mobile but bedbound requires self-care education and may be able to perform self-repositioning. The interventions for the risk factor of immobility are very different for these patients.

### Immobility, Inactivity, and Sensory Loss

Patients who have impaired ability to reposition and who cannot independently change body positions must have local pressure alleviated by any of the following: passive repositioning by caregivers, pillow bridging, or pressure relief or reduction support surfaces for bed and chair.[33,48] In addition, measures to increase mobility and activity and to decrease friction and shear should be instituted. This is true for persons receiving palliative care until the terminal stage of the disease process. The difference for those receiving palliative care is the emphasis on providing adequate pain management as part of prevention interventions related to movement and repositioning.

Overhead bed frames with trapeze bars are helpful for patients with upper body strength and may increase mobility and independence with body repositioning. Wheelchair-bound patients with upper body strength can be taught and encouraged to do wheelchair pushups to relieve pressure and allow for reperfusion of the tissues in the ischial tuberosity region. For patients who are weak from prolonged inactivity, providing support and assistance for reconditioning and increasing strength and endurance may help prevent further decline. Mobility plans for each patient should be individualized, with the goal of attaining the highest level of mobility and activity possible in light of the goals of overall care. Caregivers in the home are often left to fend for themselves for prevention interventions and may be frail and have health problems themselves. A repeat demonstration of a repositioning procedure can be very informative to the nurse in terms evaluating caregiver's ability to perform the skill of repositioning patients. The nurse may need to coach, improvise, and think of creative strategies for caregivers to use in the home setting to meet the patient's needs for movement and tissue reperfusion.

*Passive Repositioning by Caregiver.* Turning schedules and passive repositioning by caregivers is the normal intervention response for patients with immobility risk factors. Typically, turning schedules are based on time or event. If time-based, turning is usually done every 2 hours for full-body change of position and more often for small shifts in position. Event-based schedules relate to typical events during the day (e.g., turning the patient after each meal). Full-body change of position involves turning the patient to a new lying position, such as from the right side-lying position to the left side-lying position or the supine position. If the side-lying position is used in bed, avoidance of direct pressure on the trochanter is essential. To avoid placing pressure on the trochanter, the patient is placed in a 30-degree, laterally inclined position instead of the commonly used 90-degree side-lying position, which increases tissue compression over the trochanter. The 30-degree, laterally inclined position allows for distribution of pressure over a greater area. Small shifts in position involve moving the patient but keeping the same lying position, such as changing the angle of the right side-lying position or changing the position of the lower extremities in the right side-lying position. Both strategies are helpful in achieving reperfusion of compressed tissues, but only a full-body change of position completely relieves pressure.

A foam wedge is very useful in positioning for frail caregivers and for patients with severe pain on movement. The foam wedge should provide a 30-degree angle of lift when fully inserted behind the patient, usually extending from the

shoulders to the hips/buttocks. Once it is in place, even the most frail of caregivers can easily pull the wedge out slightly every hour, providing for small shifts in position and tissue reperfusion. Even patients with pain on movement find the slight movement from the foam wedge tolerable. There are other techniques to make turning patients easier and less time-consuming. Turning sheets, draw sheets, and pillows are essential for passive movement of patients in bed. Turning sheets are useful in repositioning the patient to a side-lying position. Draw sheets are used for pulling patients up in bed; they help prevent dragging of the patient's skin over the bed surface.

The recommended time interval for a full change of position is every 2 hours, depending on the individual patient profile. Defloor and colleagues demonstrated that scheduled repositioning in conjunction with use of a non-powered, pressure-reducing mattress resulted in decreased pressure ulcer incidence.[59] In this study, stage II pressure ulcer incidence was significantly decreased in the group on pressure reduction surfaces and repositioned every 4 hours compared to all other groups (3% compared to 20%—on standard mattress with no turns, 14.3%—on standard mattress with 2 hr turning, 24.1%—on standard mattress with 3 hr turning, and 15.9%—on pressure reduction surface and 6 hr turning; $P = .002$).[59] Four-hour repositioning programs in conjunction with use of non-powered support surfaces may be beneficial for those receiving palliative care and for whom more frequent repositioning is too painful.

Similar approaches to repositioning are useful for patients in chairs. Full-body change of position involves standing the patient and then re-sitting the patient in a chair. Small shifts in position for those in chairs might involve changing the position of the lower extremities or inserting a small foam pillow or wedge. For the chair-bound patient, it is also helpful to use a foot stool to help reduce the pressure on the ischial tuberosities and to distribute the pressure over a wider surface. Attention to proper alignment and posture is essential. Individuals at risk for pressure ulcer development should avoid uninterrupted sitting in chairs, and clinical practice guidelines suggest repositioning every hour. The rationale behind the shorter time frame is the extremely high pressures generated on the ischial tuberosities in the seated position.[60] Those patients with upper-body strength should be taught to shift weight every 15 minutes, to allow for tissue reperfusion. Again, pillows may be used to help position the patient in proper body alignment. Physical therapy and occupational therapy can assist in body-alignment strategies with even the most contracted patient.

In many instances, patients receiving palliative care at home spend much of their time up in recliner chairs. The ability of recliner chairs to provide a pressure-reduction support surface is not known, and individual recliner chairs probably have various levels of pressure-reducing capability. Therefore, it is still prudent to institute a repositioning schedule for those using recliner chairs. Repositioning of patients in recliner chairs is more difficult due to the physical properties of the

**Table 17A–1**
**Selected Characteristics for Classes of Support Surface**

| Performance Characteristics | Powered Air Fluidized | Powered Low Air Loss | Powered Alternating Pressure Air | Non-powered Air, Water | Non-powered Foam | Standard Hospital Mattress |
|---|---|---|---|---|---|---|
| Increased support area | Yes | Yes | Yes | Yes | Yes | No |
| Low moisture retention | Yes | Yes | No | No | No | No |
| Reduced heat accumulation | Yes | Yes | No | No | No | No |
| Shear reduction | Yes | Yes | Yes | Yes | No | No |
| Pressure reduction | Yes | Yes | Yes | Yes | Yes | No |
| Dynamic | Yes | Yes | Yes | No | No | No |
| Cost per day | High | High/ Moderate | Moderate | Low | Low | Low |

chair and requires some creativity. The repositioning schedule should mimic the schedule for those in wheelchairs.

For patients with significant pain on movement, premedication 20 to 30 minutes before a scheduled large position change may make routine repositioning more acceptable for the patient and the family. In those close to death, repositioning schedules may be used solely for maintaining comfort, with few or no attempts to reposition as a strategy for preventing skin problems.

*Pillow Bridging.* Pillow bridging involves the use of pillows to position patients with minimal tissue compression. The use of pillows can help prevent pressure ulcers from occurring on the medial knees, the medial malleolus, and the heels. Pillows should be placed between the knees, between the ankles, and under the heels.

Pillow use is especially important for reducing the risk of development of heel ulcers regardless of the support surface in use.[33] The best prevention strategy for eliminating pressure ulcers on the heels is to keep the heels off the surface of the bed. Use of pillows under the lower extremities keeps the heel from making contact with the support surface of the bed. Pillows help to redistribute the pressure over a larger area, thus reducing high pressures in one specific area. The pillows should extend and support the leg from the groin or perineal area to the ankle. Use of donut-type or ring cushion devices is contraindicated. Donut ring cushions cause venous congestion and edema and actually increase pressure to the area of concern.[33]

*Use of Pressure Redistribution Support Surfaces.* There are specific guidelines for the use of support surfaces to prevent and manage pressure ulcers.[60–62,63] Regardless of the type of support surface in use, written repositioning and turning schedules remain essential. Support surfaces serve as adjuncts to strategies for positioning and careful monitoring of patients. The type of support surface chosen is based on a multitude of factors, including clinical condition of the patient, type of care setting, ease of use, maintenance, cost, and characteristics of the support surface. The primary concern should be the

therapeutic benefit to the palliative care patient. Table 17A–1 categorizes the types of support surfaces available and their general performance characteristics.[60] The National Pressure Ulcer Advisory Panel (NPUAP) categorizes support surfaces as non-powered and powered, and describes different pressure redistribution surfaces according to intensity of redistribution properties and physical characteristics.[64]

*Non-powered Support Surfaces.* Pressure redistributing devices that are non-powered (do not use electricity or batteries) include overlays (devices placed on top of a standard mattresss) and mattresses or beds composed of foam, air, or water. Generally, these devices lower tissue interface pressures but do not consistently maintain interface pressures below capillary closing pressures in all positions on all body locations. Non-powered support surfaces are indicated for patients who are at risk for pressure ulcer development, who can be turned, and who have skin breakdown involving only one sleep surface.[33] Patients with an existing pressure ulcer who are at risk for development of further skin breakdown should be managed on a non-powered support surface.

The difficulties with foam devices include retaining moisture and heat and not reducing shear. Air and water non-powered devices also have difficulties associated with retaining moisture and heat. Viscoelastic and elastic foam non-powered surfaces are both types of porous materials that conform in proportion to the applied weight and assist in reducing friction and shear.

One concern when using mattress overlays (non-powered or powered), is the "bottoming-out" phenomenon. Bottoming-out occurs when the patient's body sinks down, the support surface is compressed beyond function, and the patient's body lies directly on the hospital mattress. When bottoming-out occurs, there is no pressure reduction for the bony prominence of concern. Bottoming-out typically happens when the patient is placed on a static air mattress overlay that is not appropriately filled with air or when the patient has been on a foam mattress for extended periods. The nurse or caregiver can monitor for bottoming-out by inserting a flat, outstretched hand between the overlay and the patient's body part at risk. If the caregiver feels less than an inch of support material, the patient has bottomed-out. It is important to check for bottoming-out when the patient is in various body positions and to check at various body sites. For example, when the patient is lying supine, check the sacral/coccygeal area and the heels; and when the patient is side-lying, check the trochanter and lateral malleolus.[60]

*Powered Support Surfaces.* Powered support surfaces more consistently reduce tissue interface pressures to a level below capillary closing pressure in any position and in most body locations. A simple definition of a powered support surface is one that requires a motor or pump and electricity to operate. A powered support surface may have the ability to change it's load distribution properties. An example of a powered support surface is an alternating air mattress or bed. Alternating air mattresses provide pressure redistribution via cyclical changes in loading and unloading. Most of these devices use an electric pump to alternately inflate and deflate air cells or air columns, thus the term "alternating-air mattress." The key to determining effectiveness is the length of time over which cycles of inflation and deflation occur. Powered support surfaces may also have difficulties with moisture retention and heat accumulation. Powered devices may be preferable for palliative care patients, especially those with significant pain on movement, because they may help with tissue reperfusion when patients cannot be turned because of pain. Some patients have reported varying levels of comfort based on size of the cells in powered alternating-pressure air surfaces. When using powered devices, the caregiver must ensure that the device is functioning properly and that the patient is receiving pressure reduction.

Powered support surfaces are indicated for patients who are at high risk for pressure ulcer development and who cannot turn independently or have skin breakdown involving more than one body surface. High-end powered support surfaces include low air loss, fluidized air or high air loss, and kinetic or lateral rotation devices. These devices often assist with pain control as well as redistributing pressure.

Low air loss therapy devices use a bed frame with a series of connected air-filled pillows with surface fabrics of low-friction material. The amount of pressure in each pillow or zone can be controlled and calibrated to provide maximal pressure relief for the individual patient. These devices provide pressure redistribution in any position, and most models have built-in scales. Low air loss therapy devices that are placed on top of standard hospital mattresses may be of particular benefit for palliative care patients at home.

Fluidized air or high air loss therapy devices consist of bed frames containing silicone-coated glass beads and incorporate both air and fluid support. The beads become fluid when air is pumped through the device, making them behave like a liquid. High air loss therapy has bactericidal properties due to the alkalinity of the beads (pH 10), the temperature, and entrapment of microorganisms by the beads. High air loss therapy relieves pressure and reduces friction, shear, and moisture (due to the drying effect of the bed). These devices

cause difficulties when transferring patients because of the bed frame. The increased airflow can increase evaporative fluid loss, leading to dehydration. Finally, if the patient is able to sit up, a foam wedge may be required, limiting the beneficial effects of the bed on the upper back. In palliative care cases, use of high air loss therapy is typically not indicated for pressure ulcers alone but may be indicated for patients with significant pain as well as pressure ulcers.

*Support Surface Selection.* Determining which support surface is best for a particular patient can be confusing. The primary concern must always be the effectiveness of the surface for the individual patient's needs. There are no controlled trials indicating one specific support surface is superior to another. The Agency for Healthcare Research and Quality (AHRQ, formerly Agency for Health Care Policy and Research [AHCPR]) recommended the following criteria as guidelines for determining how to manage tissue loading and support surface selection, and these still provide guidance to clinicians making decisions about support surfaces.[33]

1. Assess all patients with existing pressure ulcers to determine their risk for developing additional pressure ulcers. If the patient remains at risk, use a pressure-reducing surface.
2. Use a static support surface if the patient can assume a variety of positions without bearing weight on an existing pressure ulcer and without "bottoming-out."
3. Use a dynamic support surface if the patient cannot assume a variety of positions without bearing weight on an existing pressure ulcer, if the patient fully compresses the static support surface, or if the pressure ulcer does not show evidence of healing.
4. If a patient has large stage III or stage IV pressure ulcers on multiple turning surfaces, a low air loss bed or a fluidized air (high air loss) bed may be indicated.
5. If excessive moisture on intact skin is a potential source of maceration and skin breakdown, a support surface that provides airflow can be important in drying the skin and preventing additional pressure ulcers.
6. Any individual who is at risk for developing pressure ulcers should be placed on a static or dynamic pressure-reducing support surface.

*Seating Support Surfaces.* Support surfaces for chairs and wheelchairs can be categorized similarly to support surfaces for beds. In general, providing adequate pressure relief for chair-bound or wheelchair-bound patients is critical. The patient at risk for pressure ulcer formation is at increased risk in the seated position because of the high pressures across the ischial tuberosities. Most pressure redistributing devices for chairs are non-powered overlays composed of foam, gel, air, or some a combination. Positioning of chair- or wheelchair-bound individuals must include consideration of individual anatomy and body contours, postural alignment, distribution of weight, balance, and stability, in addition to pressure redistribution.

## Reducing Friction and Shear

Measures to reduce friction and shear relate to passive or active movement of the patient. To reduce friction, several interventions are appropriate. Providing topical preparations to eliminate or reduce the surface tension between the skin and the bed linen or support surface assists in reducing friction-related injury. To lessen friction-induced skin breakdown, appropriate techniques must be used when moving patients so that skin is never dragged across the linens. Patients who exhibit voluntary or involuntary repetitive body movements (particularly movements of the heels or elbows) require stronger interventions. Use of a protective film such as a transparent film dressing or a skin sealant, a protective dressing such as a thin hydrocolloid, or protective padding, helps to eliminate the surface contact of the area and decrease the friction between the skin and the linens. Even though heel, ankle, and elbow protectors do nothing to reduce or relieve pressure, they can be effective aids against friction.

Most shear injury can be eliminated by proper positioning, such as avoidance of the semi-Fowler position and limited use of upright positions (i.e., positions more than 30 degrees inclined). Avoidance of upright positions may prevent sliding- and shear-related injuries. Use of foot boards and knee Gatch (or pillows under the lower leg) to prevent sliding and to maintain position is also helpful in reducing shear effects on the skin. Observation of the patient when sitting is also important, because the patient who slides out of the chair is at equally high risk for shear injury. Use of footstools and the foot pedals on wheelchairs, together with appropriate 90-degree flexion of the hip (which may be achieved with the use of pillows, special seat cushions, or orthotic devices) can help prevent chair sliding.

## Nutrition

Nutrition is an important element in maintaining healthy skin and tissues. There is a strong relationship between nutrition and pressure ulcer development.[42] The severity of pressure ulceration is also correlated with severity of nutritional deficits, especially low protein intake and low serum albumin levels.[42,44,45] Nutritional assessment is key in determining the appropriate interventions for the patient. A short nutritional assessment should be performed at routine intervals on all patients who are determined to be at risk for pressure ulcer formation.

Malnutrition may be diagnosed if the serum albumin level is lower than 3.5 mg/dL, the total lymphocyte count is less than 1800 cells/mm$^3$, or body weight has decreased by more than 15%.[60] Malnutrition impairs the immune system, and total lymphocyte counts are a reflection of immune competence. If the patient is diagnosed as malnourished, nutritional supplementation should be instituted to help achieve a positive nitrogen balance. Examples of oral supplements are assisted oral feedings and dietary supplements. Tube feedings have not been effective for patients with pressure ulcers. The goal of care is to provide approximately 30 to 35 calories per kilogram of weight per day and 1.25 to 1.5 g of protein per kilogram of weight per day.[60] It may be difficult for a pressure ulcer patient or an at-risk patient to ingest enough protein and calories necessary to maintain skin and tissue health. Oral supplements can be very helpful in boosting calorie and protein intake, but they are designed only to be an adjunct to regular oral intake. Monitoring of nutritional indices is helpful to determine the effectiveness of the care plan. Serum albumin, protein markers, body weight, and nutritional assessment should be performed every 3 months to monitor for changes in nutritional status if appropriate.

In palliative care, nutrition can be a major risk factor for pressure ulcer development. Nutritional supplementation may not be possible in all cases; however, if the patient can tolerate it, supplementation should be encouraged if it is in keeping with the overall goals of care. Involvement of a dietitian during the early assessment of the patient is important to the overall success of the plan. Maintenance of adequate nutrition to prevent pressure ulcer development and to repair existing pressure ulcers in palliative care patients is fraught with differing opinions. The issue is how to balance nutritional needs for skin care without providing artificial nutrition to prolong life. One of the problems in this area is the limited research available. The inadequate evidence base leaves clinicians to rely on expert opinion and their own clinical experience. Perhaps the best advice is to look at the whole clinical picture rather than focusing only on the wound. Viewing the pressure ulcer as a part of the whole, within the contextual circumstances of the patient, should provide some assistance in determining how aggressive to be in providing nutrition. The overriding concern in palliative care is to provide for comfort and to minimize symptoms. If providing supplemental nutrition aids in providing comfort to the patient and is mutually agreed upon by the patient, family caregivers, and health care provider, then supplemental nutrition (in any form) is very appropriate for palliative wound care. If the patient's condition is such that to provide supplemental nutrition (in any form) increases discomfort and the prognosis is expected to be poor and rapid, then providing supplemental nutrition should not be a concern and is not appropriate for palliative wound care. It is important to remember that little evidence exists for either of these viewpoints, yet expert opinions on the topic abound.

## Managing Moisture

The preventive interventions related to moisture include general skin care, accurate diagnosis of incontinence type, and appropriate incontinence management.

*General Skin Care.* General skin care involves routine skin assessment, incontinence assessment and management, skin hygiene interventions, and measures to maintain skin health. Routine skin assessment involves observation of the patient's skin, with particular attention to bony prominences. Reddened areas should not be massaged. Massage can further impair the perfusion to the tissues. Apply skin emollients liberally to maintain adequate skin moisture.

*Incontinence Management.* Volumes have been written about various incontinence management techniques. This discussion is meant to serve as a stepping-stone to those resources available to clinicians concerning management of incontinence. It does not include all management strategies and only briefly mentions several strategies that are most pertinent to palliative care patients at high risk of development of pressure ulcers. Management of incontinence is dependent on assessment and diagnosis of the problem (see Chapter 15).

*Incontinence Assessment.* Assessment of incontinence should include history of the incontinence, including patterns of elimination, characteristics of the urinary stream or fecal mass, and sensation of bladder or rectal filling. The physical examination is designed to gather specific information related to bladder or rectal functioning and therefore is limited in scope. A limited neurological examination should provide data on the mental status and motivation of the patient and caregiver, specific motor skills, and condition of back and lower extremities. The genitalia and perineal skin are assessed for signs of perineal skin lesions and perineal sensation.

The environmental assessment should include inspection of the patient's home or nursing home facility to evaluate for the presence of environmental barriers to continence. A voiding/defecation diary is very helpful in planning the treatment and management of incontinence. In cognitively impaired patients, the caregiver may complete the diary, and management strategies can be identified from the baseline data.

*Incontinence Management Strategies.* Palliative care patients who are at risk for pressure ulcer development may be candidates for behavioral management strategies for incontinence. Incontinence in palliative care patients may be successfully managed with scheduled toileting. Scheduled toileting is caregiver dependent and requires a motivated caregiver to be successful. Adequate fluid intake is an important component of a scheduled toileting program.

Scheduled toileting, or habit training, is toileting at planned time intervals. The goal is to keep the patient dry by assisting him or her to void at regular intervals. There can be attempts to match the interval to the individual patient's natural voiding schedule. There is no systematic effort to motivate patients to delay voiding or to resist the urge to void. Scheduled toileting may be based on the clock (e.g., toileting every 2 hours) or on activities (e.g., toileting after meals and before transferring to bed).

Underpads and briefs may be used to protect the skin of patients who are incontinent of urine or stool. These products are designed to absorb moisture, wick the wetness away from the skin, and maintain a quick-drying interface with the skin. Studies in both infants and adults demonstrate that products that are designed to present a quick-drying surface to the skin and to absorb moisture do keep the skin drier and are associated with a lower incidence of dermatitis.[65] The critical feature is the ability to absorb moisture and present a quick-drying surface, not whether the product is disposable or reusable.

Regardless of the product chosen, containment strategies imply the need for a check-and-change schedule for the incontinent patient, so that wet linens and pads may be removed in a timely manner. Underpads are not as tight or constricting as briefs. Kemp[39] suggested alternating use of underpads and briefs. This recommendation echoes the early work of Willis,[66] who studied warm-water immersion syndrome and found that the effects of water on the skin could be diminished by allowing the skin to dry out between wet periods. Use of briefs when the patient is up in a chair, ambulating, or visiting, and use of underpads when the patient is in bed, is one suggestion for combining the strengths of both products.[39]

External collection devices may be more effective with male patients. External catheters or condom catheters are devices applied to the shaft of the penis that direct the urine away from the body and into a collection device. Newer models of external catheters are self-adhesive and easy to apply. For patients with a retracted penis, a special pouching system, similar to an ostomy pouch, is available. A key concern with the use of external collection devices is routine removal of the product for inspection and hygiene of the skin.

There are special containment devices for fecal incontinence as well. A special indwelling fecal drainage tube (ActiFlo indwelling bowel catheter®, Hollister, Inc.) designed for prolonged use and made of soft flexible plastic can be inserted and will allow management of stool of varying consistencies as well as diarrhea. This device provides access to the bowel for colonic irrigation and permits delivery and retention of rectally administered medications. External collection devices also exist. Fecal incontinence collectors are composed of a self-adhesive skin barrier attached to a drainable pouch. Application of the device is somewhat dependent on the skill of the clinician. To facilitate success, the patient should be put on a routine for changing the pouch before leakage occurs. The skin barrier provides a physical obstacle to keep the stool away from the skin and helps to prevent dermatitis and associated skin problems. Skin barrier wafers without an attached pouch can be useful in protecting the skin from feces or urine.

Use of moisturizers for dry skin and use of lubricants for reduction of friction injuries are also recommended skin care strategies.[33] Moisture barriers are used to protect the skin from the effects of moisture. Although products that provide a moisture barrier are recommended, the reader is cautioned that the recommendation is derived from usual practice and clinical practice guidelines and is not research based. The success of the particular product is linked to how it is formulated and the hydrophobic properties of the product.[39] Generally, pastes are thicker and more repellent of moisture than ointments. As a quick evaluation, one can observe the ease with which the product can be removed with water during routine cleansing: if the product comes off the skin with just routine cleansing, it probably is not an effective barrier to moisture. Mineral oil may be used for cleansing some of the heavier barrier products (e.g., zinc oxide paste) to ease removal from the skin.

## Pressure Ulcer Assessment

The foundation for designing a palliative care plan for the patient with a pressure ulcer is a comprehensive assessment. Comprehensive assessment includes assessment of wound severity, wound status, and the total patient.

## Wound Severity

Assessment of wound severity refers to the use of a classification system for diagnosing the severity of tissue trauma by determining the tissue layers involved in the wound. Classification systems such as staging pressure ulcers provide communication regarding wound severity and the tissue layers involved in the injury.

Pressure ulcers are commonly classified according to grading or staging systems based on the depth of tissue destruction. The NPUAP staging classification system is most commonly used to describe depth of tissue damage. Staging systems measure only one characteristic of the wound and should not be viewed as a complete assessment independent of other indicators. Staging systems are best used as a diagnostic tool for indicating wound severity. Table 17A–2 presents pressure ulcer staging criteria according to the NPUAP. Pressure-induced skin damage that manifests as purple, blue, or black areas of intact skin may represent deep tissue injury (DTI). These lesions commonly occur on heels and the sacrum and

**Table 17A–2**
**Pressure Ulcer Staging Criteria**

| Pressure Ulcer Stage | Definition and Clinical Description |
| --- | --- |
| Stage I | Intact skin with non-blanchable redness of a localized area usually over a bony prominence. Darkly pigmented skin may not have visible blanching; its color may differ from the surrounding area. The area may be painful, firm, soft, warmer, or cooler as compared to adjacent tissue. Stage I may be difficult to detect in individuals with dark skin tones. May indicate "at risk" persons (a heralding sign of risk). |
| Stage II | Partial thickness loss of dermis presenting as a shallow open ulcer with a red pink wound bed, without slough. May also present as an intact or open/ruptured serum-filled blister. Presents as a shiny or dry shallow ulcer without slough or bruising.* This stage should not be used to describe skin tears, tape burns, perineal dermatitis, maceration, or excoriation. |
| Stage III | Full thickness tissue loss. Subcutaneous fat may be visible but bone, tendon, or muscle are not exposed. Slough may be present but does not obscure the depth of tissue loss. May include undermining and tunneling. The depth of a stage III pressure ulcer varies by anatomical location. The bridge of the nose, ear, occiput and malleolus do not have subcutaneous tissue and stage III ulcers can be shallow. In contrast, areas of significant adiposity can develop extremely deep stage III pressure ulcers. Bone/tendon is not visible or directly palpable. |
| Stage IV | Full thickness tissue loss with exposed bone, tendon, or muscle. Slough or eschar may be present on some parts of the wound bed. Often include undermining and tunneling. The depth of a stage IV pressure ulcer varies by anatomical location. The bridge of the nose, ear, occiput and malleolus do not have subcutaneous tissue and these ulcers can be shallow. Stage IV ulcers can extend into muscle and/or supporting structures (e.g., fascia, tendon, or joint capsule) making osteomyelitis possible. Exposed bone/tendon is visible or directly palpable. |
| Unstageable | Full thickness tissue loss in which the base of the ulcer is covered by slough (yellow, tan, gray, green, or brown) and/or eschar (tan, brown, or black) in the wound bed. Until enough slough and/or eschar is removed to expose the base of the wound, the true depth, and therefore stage, cannot be determined. Stable (dry, adherent, intact without erythema or fluctuance) eschar on the heels serves as "the body's natural (biological) cover" and should not be removed. |
| Suspected deep tissue injury | Purple or maroon localized area of discolored intact skin or blood-filled blister due to damage of underlying soft tissue from pressure and/or shear. The area may be preceded by tissue that is painful, firm, mushy, boggy, warmer, or cooler as compared to adjacent tissue. Deep tissue injury may be difficult to detect in individuals with dark skin tones. Evolution may include a thin blister over a dark wound bed. The wound may further evolve and become covered by thin eschar. Evolution may be rapid, exposing additional layers of tissue even with optimal treatment. |

*Source*: National Pressure Ulcer Advisory Panel (2007), http://www.npuap.org/pr2.htm. (accessed December 20, 2008).

signal more severe tissue damage below the skin surface. DTI lesions reflect tissue damage at the bony tissue interface and may progress rapidly to large tissue defects. Pressure ulcers that occur at the end of life may present with characteristics of DTI.

## Wound Status

Pressure ulcer assessment is the base for maintaining and evaluating the therapeutic plan of care. Assessment of wound status involves evaluation of multiple wound characteristics. Initial assessment and follow-up assessments at regular intervals to monitor progress or deterioration of the sore are necessary to determine the effectiveness of the treatment plan. Adequate assessment is important even when the goal of care is comfort, not healing. The assessment data enable clinicians to communicate clearly about a patient's pressure ulcer, provide for continuity in the plan of care, and allow evaluation of treatment modalities. Assessment of wound status should be performed weekly and whenever a significant change is noted in the wound. Assessment should not be confused with monitoring of the wound at each dressing change. Monitoring of the wound can be performed by less skilled caregivers, but assessment should be performed on a routine basis by health care practitioners. Use of a systematic approach with a comprehensive assessment tool is helpful.

There are few tools available that encompass multiple wound characteristics to evaluate overall wound status and healing. Two available tools are the Pressure Ulcer Scale for Healing (PUSH)[67] and the Bates-Jensen Wound Assessment Tool (BWAT, revised Pressure Sore Status Tool).[68]

The PUSH tool incorporates surface area measurements, exudate amount, and surface appearance. These wound characteristics were chosen based on principal component analysis to define the best model of healing.[67,69] The clinician measures the size of the wound, calculates the surface area (length times width), and chooses the appropriate size category on the tool (0 to 10). Exudate is evaluated as none (0), light (1), moderate (2), or heavy (3). Tissue type choices include closed (0), epithelial tissue (1), granulation tissue (2), slough (3), and necrotic tissue (4). The three subscores are then summed for a total score.[67]

The PUSH tool is best used as a method of prediction of wound healing. Therefore, it may not be the best tool for palliative care patients, because healing is not an expected outcome of care. Assessment of additional wound characteristics may still be needed, to develop a treatment plan for the pressure ulcer. The BWAT includes additional wound characteristics that may be helpful in designing a plan of care for the wound.

The BWAT, previously the Pressure Sore Status Tool (Figure 17A–2), developed in 1990 by Bates-Jensen[70] and revised in 2001, evaluates 13 wound characteristics with a numerical rating scale and rates them from best to worst possible. The BWAT is recommended as a method of assessment and monitoring of pressure ulcers and other chronic wounds. It is a pencil-and-paper instrument comprising 15 items: location, shape, size, depth, edges, undermining or pockets, necrotic tissue type, necrotic tissue amount, exudate type, exudate amount, surrounding skin color, peripheral tissue edema, peripheral tissue induration, granulation tissue, and epithelialization. Two items, location and shape, are nonscored. The remaining 13 are scored items, and each appears with characteristic descriptors rated on a scale of 1 (best for that characteristic) to 5 (worst attribute of the characteristic). It is recommended that wounds be scored initially for a baseline assessment and at regular intervals to evaluate therapy. Once a wound has been assessed for each item on the BWAT, the 13 item scores can be added to obtain a total score for the wound. The total score can then be monitored to determine "at a glance" the progress in healing or degeneration of the wound. Total scores range from 13 (skin intact but always at risk for further damage) to 65 (profound tissue degeneration). Appendix 17A–1 presents the instructions for use of the BWAT.

Reliability of the tool has been evaluated in an acute care setting with enterostomal therapy (ET) nurses (nurses with additional training in wound care)[71] and in long-term care with a variety of health care professionals and one ET nurse expert in wound assessment.[72] Interrater reliability ranged from $r = 0.915$ ($P = 0.0001$) for the ET nurses[71] to 0.78% agreement for the variety of health care professionals.[72] The BWAT is widely used in a variety of health care settings.

## Wound Characteristics

Adequate initial wound assessment should encompass a composite of wound characteristics, which forms a base for differential diagnosis, therapeutic intervention, and future reassessment comparisons.[73] The indices for wound assessment include all of the following: location, size of ulcer, depth of tissue involvement, stage or classification, condition of wound edges, presence of undermining or tunneling, necrotic tissue characteristics, exudate characteristics, surrounding tissue conditions, and wound healing characteristics of granulation tissue and epithelialization.[74–78] Wound characteristics of concern for the palliative care patient include wound edges, undermining and tunneling, necrotic tissue characteristics, exudate characteristics, and surrounding tissue conditions. These five characteristics, as well as healing attributes of granulation tissue and epithelialization, are discussed in the following sections.

*Edges or Margins.* Wound edge, or margin, includes characteristics of distinctness, degree of attachment to the wound base, color, and thickness. In pressure ulcers, as tissues degenerate, broad and indistinct areas, in which the wound edge is diffuse and difficult to observe, become shallow lesions with edges that are more distinct, thin, and separate. As tissue trauma from pressure progresses, the reaction intensifies with a thickening and rolling inward of the epidermis, so that the edge is well defined and sharply outlines the ulcer, with little or no evidence of new tissue growth. In long-standing pressure

**BATES-JENSEN WOUND ASSESSMENT TOOL**　　　　　NAME _____

Complete the rating sheet to assess wound status. Evaluate each item by picking the response that best describes the wound and entering the score in the item score column for the appropriate date.

**Location:** Anatomic site. Circle, identify right **(R)** or left **(L)** and use **"X"** to mark site on body diagrams:
____ Sacrum & coccyx　　____ Lateral ankle
____ Trochanter　　　　　____ Medial ankle
____ Ischial tuberosity　　____ Heel　　　　　Other Site ____

**Shape:** Overall wound pattern; assess by observing perimeter and depth.

Circle and date appropriate description:
____ Irregular　　　　　____ Linear or elongated
____ Round/oval　　　　____ Bowl/boat
____ Square/rectangle　　____ Butterfly　　　　Other Shape ____

| Item | Assessment | Date Score | Date Score | Date Score |
|------|-----------|-----------|-----------|-----------|
| **1. Size** | 1 = Length x width <4 sq cm<br>2 = Length x width 4–<16 sq cm<br>3 = Length x width 16.1–<36 sq cm<br>4 = Length x width 36.1–<80 sq cm<br>5 = Length x width >80 sq cm | | | |
| **2. Depth** | 1 = Non-blanchable erythema on intact skin<br>2 = Partial thickness skin loss involving epidermis &/or dermis<br>3 = Full thickness skin loss involving damage or necrosis of subcutaneous tissue; may extend down to but not through underlying fascia; &/or mixed partial & full thickness &/or tissue layers obscured by granulation tissue<br>4 = Obscured by necrosis<br>5 = Full thickness skin loss with extensive destruction, tissue necrosis or damage to muscle, bone or supporting structures | | | |
| **3. Edges** | 1 = Indistinct, diffuse, none clearly visible<br>2 = Distinct, outline clearly visible, attached, even with wound base<br>3 = Well-defined, not attached to wound base<br>4 = Well-defined, not attached to base, rolled under, thickened<br>5 = Well-defined, fibrotic, scarred or hyperkeratotic | | | |
| **4. Under-mining** | 1 = None present<br>2 = Undermining < 2 cm in any area<br>3 = Undermining 2–4 cm involving < 50% wound margins<br>4 = Undermining 2–4 cm involving > 50% wound margins<br>5 = Undermining > 4 cm or tunneling in any area | | | |
| **5. Necrotic Tissue Type** | 1 = None visible<br>2 = White/grey non-viable tissue &/or non-adherent yellow slough<br>3 = Loosely adherent yellow slough<br>4 = Adherent, soft, black eschar<br>5 = Firmly adherent, hard, black eschar | | | |
| **6. Necrotic Tissue Amount** | 1 = None visible<br>2 = < 25% of wound bed covered<br>3 = 25% to 50% of wound covered<br>4 = > 50% and < 75% of wound covered<br>5 = 75% to 100% of wound covered | | | |

**Figure 17A–2.** The Bates-Jensen Wound Assessment Tool (BWAT) for measuring pressure sore status.

ulcers, fibrosis and scarring result from repeated injury and repair, with the edges hyperpigmented, indurated, and firm,[79] and impairment in the migratory ability of epithelial cells.[80] Pressure ulcers in palliative care may show significant tissue damage, and the edges may indicate areas of full-thickness tissue loss with other areas of partial-thickness damage. In palliative care, pressure ulcers may be present for prolonged periods with no change in the wound; the wound edges often

| Item | Assessment | Date Score | Date Score | Date Score |
|------|-----------|------------|------------|------------|
| 7. Exudate Type | 1 = None<br>2 = Bloody<br>3 = Serosanguineous: thin, watery, pale red/pink<br>4 = Serous: thin, watery, clear<br>5 = Purulent: thin or thick, opaque, tan/yellow, with or without odor | | | |
| 8. Exudate Amount | 1 = None, dry wound<br>2 = Scant, wound moist but no observable exudate<br>3 = Small<br>4 = Moderate<br>5 = Large | | | |
| 9. Skin Color Surrounding Wound | 1 = Pink or normal for ethnic group<br>2 = Bright red &/or blanches to touch<br>3 = White or grey pallor or hypopigmented<br>4 = Dark red or purple &/or non-blanchable<br>5 = Black or hyperpigmented | | | |
| 10. Peripheral Tissue Edema | 1 = No swelling or edema<br>2 = Non-pitting edema extends <4 cm around wound<br>3 = Non-pitting edema extends  4 cm around wound<br>4 = Pitting edema extends < 4 cm around wound<br>5 = Crepitus and/or pitting edema extends  4 cm around wound | | | |
| 11. Peripheral Tissue Induration | 1 = None present<br>2 = Induration < 2 cm around wound<br>3 = Induration 2–4 cm extending < 50% around wound<br>4 = Induration 2–4 cm extending  50% around wound<br>5 = Induration > 4 cm in any area around wound | | | |
| 12. Granulation Tissue | 1 = Skin intact or partial thickness wound<br>2 = Bright, beefy red; 75% to 100% of wound filled &/or tissue overgrowth<br>3 = Bright, beefy red; < 75% & > 25% of wound filled<br>4 = Pink &/or dull, dusky red &/or fills  25% of wound<br>5 = No granulation tissue present | | | |
| 13. Epithelialization | 1 = 100% wound covered, surface intact<br>2 = 75% to <100% wound covered &/or epithelial tissue<br>    extends >0.5cm  into wound bed<br>3 = 50% to <75% wound covered &/or epithelial tissue<br>    extends to <0.5cm  into wound bed<br>4 = 25% to < 50% wound covered<br>5 = < 25%  wound covered | | | |
| **TOTAL SCORE** | | | | |
| **SIGNATURE** | | | | |

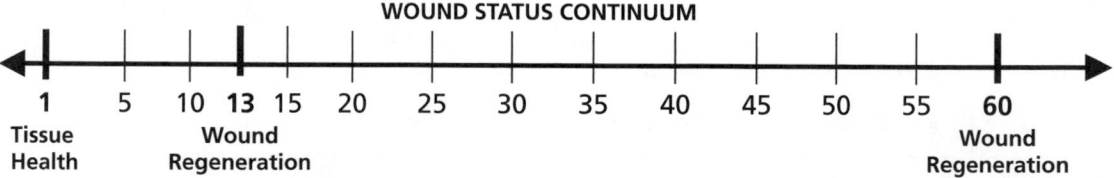

**WOUND STATUS CONTINUUM**

1    5    10  **13** 15    20    25    30    35    40    45    50    55    **60**

Tissue Health          Wound Regeneration                              Wound Regeneration

Plot the total score on the Wound Status Continuum by putting an **"X"** on the line and the date beneath the line.  Plot multiple scores with their dates to see-at-a-glance regeneration or degeneration of the wound.

**Figure 17A–2.** Continued.

exhibit hemosiderin staining or hyperpigmentation in conjunction with their rolled-under and thickened appearance.

When assessing edges, the nurse should look at the clarity and distinctness of the wound outline. With edges that are indistinct and diffuse, there are areas in which the normal tissues blend into the wound bed and the edges are not clearly visible. Edges that are even with the skin surface and the wound base are attached to the base of the wound. This means that the wound is flat, with no appreciable depth. Well-defined edges, on the other hand, are clear and distinct and can be outlined easily on a transparent piece of plastic. Edges that are not attached to the base of the wound imply a wound with some depth of tissue involvement. A crater or bowl or boat shape indicates a wound with edges that are not attached to the wound base. The wound has walls or sides. There is depth to the wound.

As the wound ages, the edges become rolled under and thickened to palpation. The edge achieves a unique hyperpigmented coloring due to hemosiderin staining. The pigment turns a gray or brown color in both dark- and light-skinned persons. Long-standing wounds may continue to thicken, with scar tissue and fibrosis developing in the wound edge, causing the edge to feel hard, rigid, and indurated. The wound edges are evaluated by visual inspection and palpation.

*Undermining and Tunneling.* The terms *undermining* and *tunneling* refer to the loss of tissue underneath an intact skin surface. Undermining, or pocketing, usually involves a greater percentage of the wound margins and more shallow length, compared with tunneling. Undermining usually involves subcutaneous tissues and follows the fascial planes next to the wound.

Wounds with undermining have more aerobic and anaerobic bacteria than do wounds that are in the process of healing with no undermining.[81] The degree and amount of undermining indicate the severity of tissue necrosis. As subcutaneous fat degenerates, wound pockets develop. Initially, deep fascia limits the depth of pocketing, encouraging more superficial internal spread of undermining. Once the fascia is penetrated, undermining of deeper tissues may proceed rapidly.[79] Internal dimensions of wound undermining are commonly measured with the use of cotton-tipped applicators and gentle probing of the wound. There are also premeasured devices that can be inserted under the wound edge and advanced into the deeper tissues to aid in determination of the extent of undermining.

Undermining and wound pockets should be assessed by inserting a cotton-tipped applicator under the wound edge, advancing it as far as it will go without using undue force, raising the tip of the applicator so that it may be seen or felt on the surface of the skin, marking the surface with a pen, and measuring the distance from the mark on the skin to the edge of the wound. This process is continued all around the wound. Then the percentage of the wound involved is determined with the help of a transparent metric measuring guide with concentric circles divided into quadrants. Another noninvasive method of assessment of wound pockets is the use of ultrasound to evaluate the undermined tissues. Ultrasonography provides a visual picture of the impaired tissues and can be repeated to monitor for improvement.

*Necrotic Tissue Type and Amount.* Necrotic tissue characteristics of color, consistency, adherence, and amount present in the wound must be incorporated into wound assessment. As tissues die during wound development, they change in color, consistency, and adherence to the wound bed. The level and type of tissue death influence the clinical appearance of the necrotic tissue. For example, as subcutaneous fat tissues die, a collection of stringy, yellow slough is formed. As muscle tissues degenerate, the dead tissue may be more thick or tenacious.

The characteristic "necrotic tissue type" is a qualitative variable, with most clinicians using descriptions of clinical observations of a composite of factors as a method of assessment. The characteristics of color, consistency, and adherence are most often used to describe the type of necrosis. Color varies, as necrosis worsens, from white/gray nonviable tissue, to yellow slough, and finally to black eschar. Consistency refers to the cohesiveness of the debris (i.e., thin or thick, stringy or clumpy). Consistency also varies on a continuum as the necrotic area deepens and becomes more dehydrated.

The terms *slough* and *eschar* refer to different levels of necrosis and are described according to color and consistency. A slough is described as yellow (or tan) and as thin, mucinous, or stringy, whereas eschar is described as black (or brown), and as soft or hard; eschar represents full-thickness tissue destruction. *Adherence* refers to the adhesiveness of the debris to the wound bed and the ease with which the two may be separated. Necrotic tissue tends to become more adherent to the wound bed as the level of damage increases. Clinically, eschar is more firmly adherent than is yellow slough.

Necrotic tissue is assessed for color, consistency, and adherence to the wound bed. The predominant characteristic present in the wound should be chosen for assessment. Necrotic tissue type changes as it ages in the wound, as debridement occurs, and as further tissue trauma causes increased cellular death. Slough usually is nonadherent or loosely adherent to the healthy tissues of the wound bed. By definition, nonadherent tissue appears scattered throughout the wound; it appears as if the tissue could easily be removed with gauze. Loosely adherent tissue is attached to the wound bed; it is thick and stringy and may appear as clumps of debris attached to wound tissue.

*Eschar Signifies Deeper Tissue Damage.* Eschar may be black, gray, or brown in color. It is usually adherent or firmly adherent to the wound tissues and may be soggy, soft or hard, or leathery in texture. A soft, soggy eschar is usually strongly attached to the base of the wound but may be lifting from (and loose from) the edges of the wound. A hard, crusty eschar is strongly attached to the base and edges of the wound. Hard eschars are often mistaken for scabs. Sometimes nonviable tissue appears before a wound is apparent. This can be seen as a white or gray area on the surface of the skin. The area usually demarcates within a day or two, when the wound appears and interrupts the skin surface.

Necrotic tissue retards wound healing because it is a medium for bacterial growth and a physical obstacle to epidermal resurfacing, wound contraction, and granulation. The greater the amount of necrotic tissue present in the wound bed, the more severe the insult to the tissue and the longer the time required to heal the wound. The amount of necrotic tissue usually affects the amount of exudate from the wound and causes wound odor, both of which are distressing to the patient and to caregivers. Because of the amount of necrotic tissue present, modifications of treatment and debridement techniques may be made. The depth of the wound cannot be assessed in the presence of necrosis that blocks visualization of the total wound.

The amount of necrotic tissue present in the wound is one of the easier characteristics to assess. The nurse visualizes the wound as a pie divided into four quadrants. The percentage of necrosis present is judged by evaluating each quadrant to determine the percent of the wound covered with necrosis. Alternatively, the length and width of the necrotic tissue may be measured to determine the surface area involved in the necrosis.

*Exudate Type and Amount.* Wound exudate (also known as wound fluid, wound drainage) is an important assessment feature, because the characteristics of the exudate help the clinician to diagnose signs of wound infection, to evaluate appropriateness of topical therapy, and to monitor wound healing. Wound infection retards wound healing, causes odor, and should be treated aggressively in most instances. Proper assessment of wound exudate is also important because it affirms the body's brief, normal inflammatory response to tissue injury. Accurate assessment and diagnosis of wound exudate and infection are critical components of effective wound management. One of the main goals of palliative wound care is to prevent infection and to control exudate, because these conditions lead to discomfort from the wound.

The healthy wound normally has some evidence of moisture on its surface. Healthy wound fluid contains enzymes and growth factors, which may play a role in promoting reepithelialization of the wound and provide needed growth factors for all phases of wound repair. The moist environment produced by wound exudate allows efficient migration of epidermal cells and prevents wound desiccation and further injury.[82,83]

In pressure ulcers, increased exudate is a response to the inflammatory process or infection. Increased capillary permeability causes leakage of fluids and substrates into the injured tissue. When a wound is present, tissue fluid leaks out of the open tissue. This fluid normally is serous or serosanguineous.

In the infected wound, the exudate may thicken, become purulent in nature, and continue to be present in moderate to large amounts. Examples of exudate character changes in infected wounds are the presence of *Pseudomonas*, which produces a thick, malodorously sweet-smelling, green drainage, or *Proteus* infection, which may have an ammonia-like odor. Wounds with foulsmelling drainage are generally infected or filled with necrotic debris, and healing time is prolonged as tissue destruction progresses.[81] Wounds with

significant amounts of necrotic debris often have a thick, tenacious, opaque, purulent, malodorous drainage in moderate to copious amounts. True wound exudate must be differentiated from necrotic tissue that sloughs off the wound as a result of debridement efforts. Exudate from sloughing necrotic tissue is commonly attached to or connected with the necrotic debris; frequently, the only method of differentiation is adequate debridement of necrotic tissue from the wound site. Liquefied necrotic tissue occurs most often as a result of enzymatic or autolytic debridement. Often, removal of the necrotic tissue reduces the amount and changes the character of wound exudate.

Exudate should be assessed for the amount and type of drainage that occurs. The type and color of wound exudate vary depending on the degree of moisture in the wound and the organisms present. Characteristics used to examine exudate are color, consistency, adherence, distribution in the wound, and presence of odor.

Estimating the amount of exudate in the wound is difficult due to wound size variability and topical dressing types. One problem with assessment of exudate amount is the size of the wound. What might be considered a large amount of drainage for a smaller wound may be considered a small amount for a larger wound, making clinically meaningful assessment of exudate difficult.

Certain dressing types interact with or trap wound fluid to create or mimic certain characteristics of exudate, such as color and consistency of purulent drainage. For example, both hydrocolloid and alginate dressings mimic a purulent drainage on removal of the dressing. Preparation of the wound site for appropriate assessment involves removal of the wound dressing and cleansing with normal saline to remove dressing debris in the wound bed, followed by evaluation of the wound for true exudate.

Although it is not a part of exudate assessment, evaluation of the wound dressing provides the clinician with valuable data about the effectiveness of treatment. Evaluation of the percentage of the wound dressing involved with wound drainage during a specific time frame is helpful for clinical management that includes dressings beyond traditional gauze. In estimating the percentage of the dressing involved with the wound exudate, clinical judgment must be quantified by putting a number to visual assessment of the dressing. For example, the clinician might determine that 50% of the hydrocolloid dressing was involved with wound drainage over a 4-day wearing period. Based on the data, the clinician might quantify the judgment for this type of dressing, length of dressing wear time, and wound cause as being a "minimal" amount of exudate. Clinical judgment of the amount of wound drainage requires some experience with expected wound exudate output in relation to phase of wound healing and type of wound, as well as knowledge of absorptive capacity and normal wear time of topical dressings.

Certain characteristics of exudate indicate wound degeneration and infection. If signs of cellulitis (erythema or skin discoloration, edema, pain, induration, purulent drainage) are present at the wound site, the exudate amount may be copious and seropurulent or purulent in character. The amount of exudate remains high or increases, and the character may change to frank purulence, with further wound degeneration. Wound infection must be considered in these cases.

Pressure ulcers manifest with a variety of wound exudate types and amounts. In partial-thickness pressure ulcers, the wound exudate is most likely to be serous or serosanguineous in nature and to be present in minimal to moderate amounts. In clean full-thickness pressure ulcers, the wound exudate is similar, with minimal to moderate amounts of serous to serosanguineous exudate. As healing progresses in the clean full-thickness pressure ulcer, the character of the exudate changes; it may become bloody if the fragile capillary bed is disrupted, and it lessens in amount.

For full-thickness pressure ulcers with necrotic debris, wound exudate is dependent on the presence or absence of infection and the type of therapy instituted. Exudate may appear moderate to large but, in fact, is related to the amount of necrotic tissue present and to liquefaction of the debris in the wound. Typically, the necrotic full-thickness pressure ulcer manifests with serous to seropurulent wound exudate in moderate to large amounts. With appropriate treatment, the wound exudate amount may temporarily increase, as the character gradually assumes a serous nature.

*Surrounding Tissue Condition.* The tissues surrounding the wound should be assessed for color, induration, and edema. The tissues surrounding the wound are often the first indication of impending further tissue damage and are a key gauge of successful prevention strategies. Color of the surrounding skin may indicate further injury from pressure, friction, or shearing. The tissues within 4 cm of the wound edge should be assessed. Dark-skinned persons show the colors "bright red" and "dark red" as a deepening of normal skin color or a purple or black hue. As full thickness wound healing occurs in dark-skinned persons, the new skin is pink and lacks pigmentation—thus, may never darken. In both light- and dark-skinned patients, new epithelium must be differentiated from tissues that are erythematous. To assess for blanchability in light-skinned patients, the nurse presses firmly on the skin with a finger, then lifts the finger and looks for "blanching," or sudden whitening, of the tissues followed by prompt return of color to the area. Non-blanchable erythema signals more severe tissue damage.

Edema in the surrounding tissues delays wound healing in the pressure ulcer. It is difficult for neoangiogenesis, or growth of new blood vessels into the wound, to occur in edematous tissues. Again, tissues within 4 cm of the wound edge are assessed. Nonpitting edema appears as skin that is shiny and taut, almost glistening. Pitting edema is identified by firmly pressing a finger down into the tissues and waiting for 5 seconds; on release of pressure, tissues fail to resume their previous position and an indentation appears. Crepitus is the accumulation of air or gas in tissues. The clinician should measure how far edema extends beyond the wound edges.

Induration is a sign of impending damage to the tissues. Along with skin-color changes, induration is an omen of further pressure-induced tissue trauma. Tissues within 4 cm of the wound edge are assessed. Induration is an abnormal firmness of tissues with margins. The nurse should palpate where the induration starts and where it ends by gently pinching the tissues. Induration results in an inability to pinch the tissues. Palpation proceeds from healthy tissue, moving toward the wound margins. It is usual to feel slight firmness at the wound edge itself. Normal tissues feel soft and spongy; induration feels hard and firm to the touch.

*Granulation Tissue and Epithelialization.* Granulation and epithelial tissues are markers of wound health. They signal the proliferative phase of wound healing and usually foretell wound closure. Granulation tissue is the growth of small blood vessels and connective tissue into the wound cavity. It is more observable in full-thickness wounds because of the tissue defect that occurs in such wounds. In partial-thickness wounds, granulation tissue may occur so quickly, and in concert with epithelialization, or skin resurfacing, that it is unobservable in most cases. The granulation tissue is healthy when it is bright, beefy-red, shiny, and granular with a velvety appearance. The tissue looks "bumpy" and may bleed easily. Unhealthy granulation tissue, resulting from poor vascular supply, appears pale pink or blanched to a dull, dusky red. Usually, the first layer of granulation tissue to be laid down in the wound is pale pink and, as the granulation tissue deepens and thickens, the color becomes bright, beefy red.

The percentage of the wound that is filled with granulation tissue and the color of the tissue are characteristics indicative of the health of the wound. The clinician makes a judgment as to what percent of the wound has been filled with granulation tissue. This is much easier if there is some past history with the wound. If the wound has been monitored by the same person over multiple observations, it is simple to judge the amount of granulation tissue present. If the initial observation was done by a different observer or if the data are not available, the clinician simply must use his or her best judgment to determine the amount of tissue present.

Partial-thickness wounds heal by epidermal resurfacing and regeneration. Epithelialization occurs via lateral migration at the wound edges and the base of hair follicles as epithelial cells proliferate and resurface the wound. Full-thickness wounds heal by scar formation: the tissue defect fills with granulation tissue, the edges contract, and the wound is resurfaced by epithelialization. Therefore, epithelialization may occur throughout the wound bed in partial-thickness wounds but only from the wound edges in full-thickness wounds.

Epithelialization can be assessed by evaluating the amount of the wound that is surrounded by new tissue and the distance to which new tissue extends into the wound base. Epithelialization appears as pink or red skin. Visualization of the new epithelium takes practice. A transparent measuring guide is used to help determine the percentage of wound involvement and the distance to which the epithelial tissue extends into the wound.

*Monitoring the Wound.* In palliative care, monitoring of the wound is important to continue to meet the goals of comfort and reduction in wound pain and wound symptoms such as odor and exudate. Evaluation of wound characteristics at scheduled intervals allows the nurse to revise the treatment plan as appropriate and often provides an indication of the overall health of the patient. In many cases, the pressure ulcer worsens as death approaches and as the patient's condition worsens. The skin may be the first organ to actually "fail," with other systems following the downward trend. Progressive monitoring is also important to determine whether the treatment is effectively controlling odor, managing exudate, preventing infection, and minimizing pain—the goals of wound care during palliative care.

**Total Patient Assessment**

Comprehensive assessment includes assessment of the total patient as well as of wound severity and wound status. Generally, diagnosis and management of the wound are best accomplished within the context of the whole person. Comprehensive assessment includes a focused history and physical examination, attention to specific laboratory and diagnostic tests, and a pain assessment. Table 17A–3 presents an overview of assessment for the patient with a pressure ulcer.

It is important to obtain a focused history and physical examination as part of the initial assessment. The patient history determines which relevant systems reviews are needed in the physical examination. The goals for treatment and the direction of care (e.g., curative with a goal of wound closure, palliative with a goal of reduced wound pain) can be determined with, at a minimum, the following patient history information: reason for admission to care facility or agency; expectations and perceptions about wound healing; psychological, social, cultural, and economic history; presence of medical comorbidities; current wound status; and previous management strategies.

The systems review portion of the patient history and physical examination provides information on comorbidities that may impair wound healing. Specific comorbidities such as diabetes,[84–87] vascular disease,[88,89] and immunocompromise[90–92] have been related to impaired healing. The individual's capacity to heal may be limited by specific disease effects on tissue integrity and perfusion, patient mobility, nutrition, and risk for wound infection. Therefore, throughout the patient history, systems review, and physical examination, the clinician considers host factors that affect wound healing.

Specific laboratory and diagnostic tests in a comprehensive assessment include data on nutrition, glucose management, and tissue oxygenation and perfusion. Nutritional parameters typically include evaluation of serum albumin. Serum albumin is a measure of protein available for healing; a normal level is greater than 3.5 mg/dL. Clinicians should

| Table 17A–3 |
|---|
| **National Pressure Ulcer Advisory Panel Recommended Palliative Care Pressure Ulcer Guidelines** |
| 1. Assess the risk for new pressure ulcer development by using a validated risk assessment tool. |
| 2. Reposition the individual at periodic intervals in accordance with the individual's wishes. |
| 3. Strive to maintain adequate nutrition and hydration compatible with the individual's condition and wishes. Adequate nutrition is often not attainable if the individual is unable or refuses to eat. |
| 4. Maintain skin integrity to the extent possible. |
| 5. Set treatment goals that are consistent with the values and goals of the individual. |
| 6. The goal for the palliative care individual with a pressure ulcer is often to enhance quality of life, even if the pressure ulcer cannot/does not lead to closure. |
| 7. Assess the individual initially and whenever there is a change in factors placing the individual at risk. |
| 8. Assess the pressure ulcer initially and weekly and document findings. Assess the pressure ulcer with each dressing change. |
| 9. Assess the impact of the pressure ulcer on quality of life of the patient and family. |
| 10. Manage the pressure ulcer and peri wound area on a regular basis. |
| 11. Control wound odor. |
| 12. Assess wound pain. |
| 13. Assess resources. |

evaluate laboratory values such as arterial blood gases to assess tissue perfusion and oxygenation abilities. Review of laboratory values is prudent to determine the level of diabetic control. Normal glucose levels are 80 mg/dL. Concentrations of 180 to 250 mg/dL or higher indicate that glucose levels are out of control. The nurse should look specifically for a fasting blood glucose concentration lower than 140 mg/dL and a glycosylated hemoglobin concentration (HgbA1C) lower than 7%. The HgbA1C helps to determine the level of glucose control the patient has had over the last 2 to 3 months.

The final aspect of the comprehensive assessment is pain assessment. Pain is an important factor in healing and pressure ulcers can lead to pain and disfigurement. Patients can quantify pressure ulcer pain and can differentiate pressure ulcer pain from pain due to other conditions.[93] Of those persons with pressure ulcers who are able to report pain, across nursing homes, home health and hospital settings, 87% report pain with dressing changes, 84% report pain at rest and 42% report pain both at rest and during dressing changes.[94] Further, 18% of those persons reporting dressing change wound pain report pain at the highest level (e.g., "excruciating"). Yet, only 6% of those persons reporting pressure ulcer pain receive any medication for pain.[94] The average Stage I and Stage II pressure ulcer pain has been reported at 4 cm and 3.5 cm on a 10 cm visual analogue scale, respectively. There is some evidence that a higher proportion of persons with stage

III or IV ulcers report ulcer pain compared to those persons with stage II ulcers and they report more severe pain than those with Stage II pressure ulcers with a mean numerical rating scale (0–100) of 54 for Stage III/IV and 48 for Stage II.[95] Persons with chronic wounds such as pressure ulcers experience procedural and non-procedural pain.[94] Procedural pain relates to pain associated with activities such as debridement, dressing changes, and repositioning. Non-procedural pain is the daily pain associated with having an open wound.

Wound pain can be assessed using numerical rating scales, the FACES scale, or a visual analogue scale.[96] Patients who are nonverbal should be observed for withdrawal, grimacing, crying out, or other nonverbal signs of pain. The Pain Detection Interview (PDI) may be helpful in screening for wound pain in persons with cognitive impairment. The PDI consists of four yes/no response questions:

1. Do you have wound pain now?
2. Do you have wound pain every day?
3. Does wound pain keep you from doing the activities you enjoy?
4. Does wound pain keep you from sleeping?

Affirmative responses to question 2 (wound pain every day) or to any two of the four questions indicates probable chronic wound pain and the patient should have a more extensive pain assessment conducted. Pain assessments should be done before and during wound procedures, such as dressing changes or debridement, and also at times when the dressing is intact and no procedures are in progress. The patient or caregiver should be encouraged to keep a pain diary, because the data may be valuable in evaluating changes in wound pain over time. The focused history, physical examination, evaluation of laboratory and diagnostic data, and pain assessment provide the context for the wound itself and, along with wound severity and wound status assessment, the basis for pressure ulcer treatment. Total patient assessment should also encompass evaluation of treatment appropriateness in light of the overall condition of the patient and the goals of palliative care.

## Pressure Ulcer Management

Pressure ulcer management should be based on clinical practice guidelines. While few guidelines for providing palliative care have been established, the existing guidelines are helpful in developing a palliative care plan. In the United States, most pressure ulcer care has been based on the 1994 AHRQ algorithms for treatment.[60] The AHRQ guidelines presented a general approach to use in developing a care plan for the patient with a pressure ulcer. Although they were published in 1994, the general principles of ulcer management remain similar; however, the evidence supporting many of the guidelines has improved. The NPUAP, in conjunction with the European Pressure Ulcer Advisory Panel, updated and revised the AHRQ pressure ulcer guidelines in 2009.[97] The

revised pressure ulcer clincial practice guidelines include specific guidelines for palliative care and pain management. Palliative pressure ulcer treatment is focused on:

- Repositioning the individual at periodic intervals in accordance with the individual's wishes.
- Striving to maintain adequate nutrition and hydration compatible with the individual's condition and wishes—with the understanding that adequate nutrition is often not attainable if the individual is unable or refuses to eat.
- Managing the pressure ulcer and peri-wound skin on a routine, regular basis.
- Controlling wound odor.
- Reducing wound pain.

*Repositioning and Management of Tissue Loads.* Repositioning and management of tissue loads refers to care related to those with pressure ulcers who are at risk for development of additional pressure ulcers. This is an important part of pressure ulcer treatment, because many individuals with a pressure ulcer are at risk for further pressure-induced tissue trauma. More information on support surfaces and management of tissue loads was presented in the earlier discussion of prevention of pressure ulcers. For persons who are unable or unwilling to be repositioned at regular intervals, a low-air-loss mattress or alternating air support surface are appropriate. Strive to reposition the individual every 4 hours on a pressure redistribution surface, but use a flexible repositioning schedule that is in accordance with the individual's preferences. Avoid positioning the patient directly on the pressure ulcer unless this is the single position of comfort for the individual. For individuals with pain on movement, pre-medicate 20–30 minutes prior to scheduled large position changes, as this may make routine repositioning more acceptable to the patient and family. However, comfort is of primary importance and may supersede prevention and wound care for those that are actively dying or have conditions causing them to have a single position of comfort. Observe individual choices after explaining the rationale for this intervention. It is important to understand that the goal of repositioning and managing tissue loads in the palliative care patient is to ease suffering and discomfort from the wound.

*Nutrition and Hydration Support.* Because many studies have linked malnutrition with pressure ulcers, adequate nutritional support is an important part of pressure ulcer management. Figure 17A–3 presents the nutritional assessment and support algorithm for pressure ulcer management from the original AHRQ guidelines. Prevention of malnutrition reduces the patient's risk for further tissue trauma related to pressure or impaired wound healing. As noted in the discussion of prevention, maintenance of adequate nutrition in the palliative care patient may not be possible. The palliative care pressure ulcer guidelines recommend nutrition and hydration support that is consistent with the palliative care patient's condition and wishes. This includes allowing the patient to consume

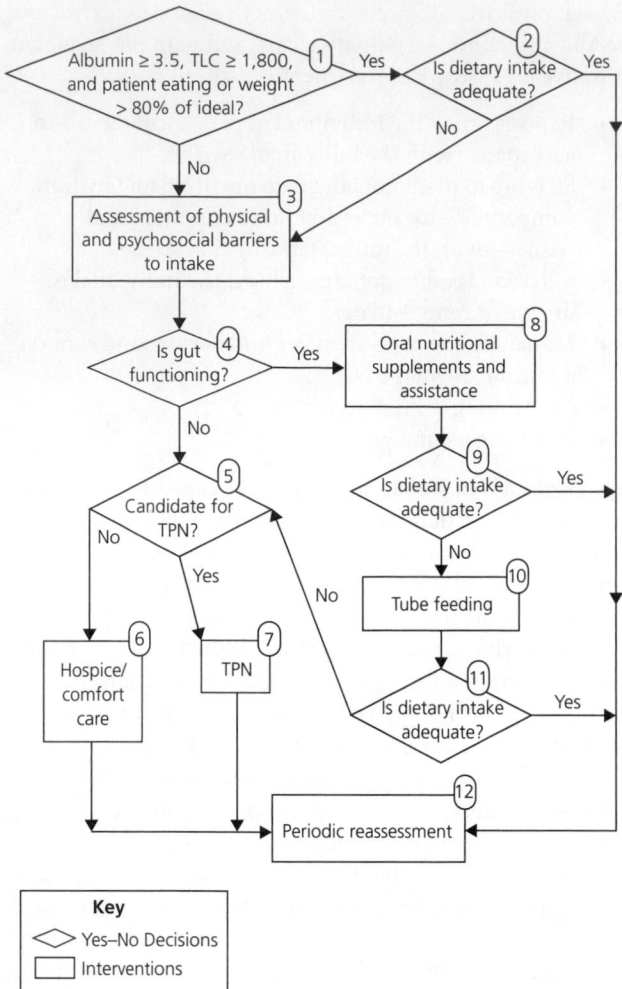

**Figure 17A–3.** Nutritional assessment and support algorithm from the United States Agency for Health Care Policy and Research (AHCPR). TLC, total lymphocyte count; TPN, total parenteral nutrition. *Source:* From Bergstrom et al. (1992), reference 42, with permission.

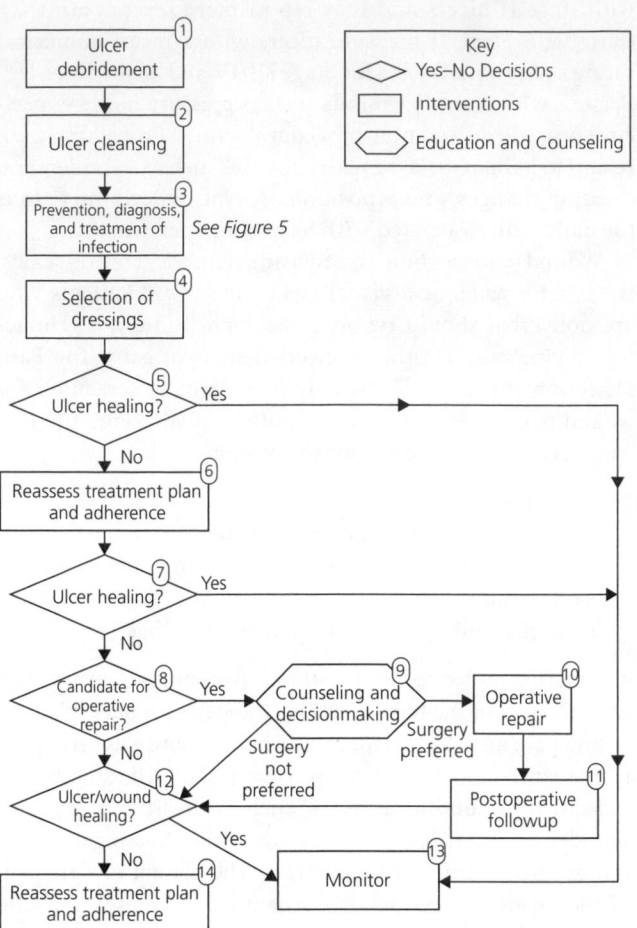

**Figure 17A–4.** Ulcer care algorithm from the United States Agency for Healthcare Research and Quality (AHRQ), formerly the Agency for Health Care Policy and Research (AHCPR). *Source:* From Bergstrom et al. (1992), reference 42, with permission.

foods and fluids of choice and allowing the patient to direct nutritional intake. Other recommendations include consuming multiple small meals throughout the day and offering nutritional supplements.

*Managing the Ulcer and Peri-Wound skin.* Direct-pressure ulcer care involves adequate debridement of necrotic material, management of bacterial colonization and infection, wound cleansing, management of odor and exudate, and selection of topical dressings. Figure 17A–4 presents an algorithm for general ulcer care.

*Ulcer Care: Debridement.* Adequate debridement of necrotic tissue is necessary for wound healing. Necrotic debris in the wound bed forms an obstacle to healing and provides a medium for bacterial growth. The patient's condition and the goals of care determine the method of debridement. In general, conservative methods of debridement may be more

appropriate for palliative care patients who may not tolerate sharp debridement. Conservative debridement methods including mechanical, enzymatic, biosurgical, or autolytic techniques may be used if there is no urgent need for drainage or removal of devitalized material from the wound. In the presence of advancing cellulitis, sepsis, or large and adherent amounts of necrotic debris, sharp debridement may be beneficial in promoting comfort and reducing wound symptoms of pain, exudate, and odor and should be performed. In palliative care, debridement is still important, because the removal of nonviable material decreases wound odor and exudate. In the case of the black eschar that forms on heels, debridement may not be necessary. Observation of the black heel with attention to the development of pathological signs such as erythema, drainage, odor, or bogginess of the tissues is necessary. If signs of erythema, drainage, odor, or bogginess appear, then debridement may be considered.

Mechanical debridement includes the use of wet-to-dry dressings at specific intervals, hydrotherapy, or wound irrigation. Of these three methods, wound irrigation is the most favorable for wound healing and most appropriate for palliative care. Wet-to-dry dressings are not advised because of the time and labor involved in performing the dressing technique correctly and the high potential for pain. Wet-to-dry dressings are not recommended for palliative care because of the frequency of dressing changes and the increased wound pain. Hydrotherapy or whirlpool treatments may be helpful for wounds with large amounts of necrotic debris adherent to healthy tissues. In these cases, hydrotherapy helps to loosen the material from the wound bed for easier removal with sharp debridement. Patients receiving palliative care may not tolerate the movement to and from the whirlpool tank, much less the sharp debridement. Wound irrigation may be performed using a pulsatile lavage device or a simple catheter and syringe.

Enzymatic debridement is performed by applying a topical agent containing an enzyme that destroys necrotic tissue. Enzymatic debridement may be an appropriate method for palliative care, because the frequency of dressing changes is usually once a day and the method is easy to use in conjunction with periodic sharp debridement by a certified wound care nurse or other health care professional with training in sharp debridement.

Biosurgical debridement is the application of maggots (disinfected fly larvae, *Phaenicia sericata*) to the wound, typically at a density of 5–8 per cm². Comparative controlled studies evaluating the use of maggot therapy for pressure ulcer debridement compared to standard debridement therapy reported maggot therapy to be more effective for debridement and granulation tissue formation.[98,99] However, biosurgery may not be acceptable to all patients and may not be available in all areas and there no studies specific to the palliative care population.

Autolytic debridement involves the use of moisture-retentive dressings to cover the wound and allow necrotic tissue to self-digest from enzymes normally found in wound fluid or exudate. Autolytic debridement may be used in conjunction with other debridement methods such as periodic sharp debridement or wound irrigation. Again, autolytic debridement may be particularly effective for palliative care. Autolytic debridement has the added benefits of decreased frequency of dressing changes (typically every 3 to 5 days) and odor containment, so the suffering associated with dressing changes is diminished.

*Ulcer Care: Bacterial Colonization and Infection.* Open pressure ulcers are colonized with microorganisms. In most cases, adequate debridement and wound cleansing prevent the bacterial colonization from proceeding to the point of clinical infection. Wound management can be enhanced in pressure ulcers by attention to debridement of necrotic debris and adequate wound cleansing. These two steps alone are often sufficient to prevent wound infection in pressure ulcers, because they remove the debris that supports bacterial growth.[60] Prevention of infection is an important goal for the palliative care patient. Use of prolonged silver-release topical dressings or cadexomer iodine dressings help control wound surface microorganisms and are effective against a broad range of pathogens, including methicillin-resistant *Staphylococcus aureus* (MRSA).

Identification of infection is best accomplished by clinical assessment. The common method of determining clinical infection is by assessing for presence of the classical clinical signs of erythema (rubor), edema (tumor), heat (calor), pain (dolor), and purulent exudate. In chronic wounds such as pressure ulcers, other signs and symptoms of wound infection include: increasing wound pain, wound breakdown including pocketing or undermining development at the base of the wound, friable granulation tissue, and foul odor.[100] Routine swab cultures should not be used to identify infection in most pressure ulcers. Swab cultures simply reflect the contamination on the surface of the wound and may not accurately identify the organisms causing tissue infection. Needle aspiration or tissue biopsy are the most accurate methods of identifying invading microorganisms, but these procedures are not easily accomplished in home care settings or nursing home settings. Further, these procedures may increase discomfort and suffering for the palliative care patient. If cultures are deemed essential in order to meet the goals of reducing wound pain, odor, and exudate, then an alternative method involves use of surface swabs. After cleansing the wound with normal saline to remove any dressing debris, the nurse swabs a 1 cm² area of the wound bed with the surface swab for 5 seconds, until tissue fluid is apparent on the swab, and then sends the swab directly to the laboratory. This technique may better reflect actual microorganism invasion of the wound tissues than do standard swab methods.[101]

Use of topical antimicrobial solutions is not indicated for clean pressure ulcers. Indeed, most topical antimicrobial solutions are toxic to the fibroblast, which is the cell responsible for wound healing and may cause a burning sensation, adding to the patient's discomfort. Topical antiseptics, such as povidone iodine, iodophor, sodium hypochlorite (Dakin's Solution), hydrogen peroxide, and acetic acid, do not significantly reduce the number of bacteria in wound tissue; however, they do harm the healthy wound tissues.[60,102] As such, these substances usually have no place in the treatment of clean pressure ulcers. In wounds with necrotic debris, antiseptic/antimicrobial solutions may be used for a short course of therapy (typically 2 weeks), to assist with decreasing surface bacteria and odor reduction, and then evaluated for further use.

*Ulcer Care: Wound Cleansing.* Cleansing of a wound assists healing because it removes necrotic tissue, excess wound exudate, dressing residue, and metabolic wastes from the wound bed. Wound healing is optimized, and the potential for wound infection is decreased when wound cleansing is a part of the treatment plan for pressure ulcers. Wound cleansing involves the selection of a solution for cleansing and a method of delivering the solution to the wound. Routine wound cleansing should be accomplished with minimal trauma to the wound bed. Wounds should be cleansed initially and at each dressing change. Minimal force should be applied when using gauze, sponges, or cloth to clean the wound bed. Skin cleansers and antimicrobial solutions are not indicated as solutions for cleaning pressure ulcers because they destroy the healthy wound tissues and are toxic to the fibroblast cell.[60] Normal saline is the preferred solution, because it is physiological and will not harm healing tissues. Additional alternatives include potable water and surfactant wound cleansers.

When wound irrigation is used to cleanse wounds, the irrigation pressure should fall within the range of 4 to 15 pounds per square inch (psi). Higher pressures may drive bacteria deeper into wound tissues or cause additional wound trauma. A 35-mL syringe with a 19-gauge angiocatheter delivers saline at 8 pounds psi and is an effective method for removing bacteria from the wound bed.

*Ulcer Care: Exudate and Topical Dressings.* In general, moisture-retentive wound dressings are the most appropriate dressing for pressure ulcers. For palliative care, they are the dressings of choice because of the decreased frequency of required changes (typically every 3 to 5 days). The goal of the wound dressing is to provide an environment that keeps the wound bed tissue moist and the surrounding, intact skin dry. Use of moist wound healing dressings supports a better rate of healing than use of dry gauze dressings;[60] more importantly in palliative care, moist wound healing dressings contain odor, absorb exudate, and minimize dressing change discomfort. Clinical judgment is needed to determine the best dressing for the wound. The appropriate dressing should keep the surrounding intact skin dry while controlling wound exudate and should provide a minimal amount of pain during dressing changes.

The clinician must be aware of the absorptive capacity and pain reduction properties of the major dressing types. In general, thin film dressings have no absorptive capacity and minimize pain by covering exposed nerve endings. Thin film dressings are adherent to the skin surrounding the wound and sometimes to the wound itself, making dressing removal more likely to be painful. Hydrocolloids, hydrogels, and foam dressings typically have a minimal to moderate absorptive capacity. Hydrocolloid dressings are occlusive and reduce pain by preventing exposure of the wound to air. They have adhesive properties and can cause pain if removed improperly. Foam dressings are moderately absorptive and nonadherent, resulting in reduced pain during dressing changes. Hydrogel dressings are cool and soothing and are particularly effective in wounds that induce a burning sensation. Hydrogel dressings also are nonadherent, reducing wound pain during dressing changes. Calcium alginates, alginate collagen dressings, and exudate absorbing beads, flakes, pastes, or powders absorb large amounts of drainage. Dressings with a large absorptive capacity reduce pain related to maceration of surrounding tissues and to pressure caused by the excess exudate. Calcium alginates and exudate-absorbing dressings are nonadherent and are easily removed from the wound during dressing changes. Soft silicone dressings absorb minimal amounts of drainage, but are nonadherent and reduce pain associated with dressing changes.

Wounds with small or minimal amounts of exudate can benefit from a variety of dressings, including hydrocolloids, hydrogels, thin film dressings, and foam dressings. Wounds with moderate amounts of exudate may require dressings with a higher absorptive capacity, such as hydrocolloids, foam dressings, hydrogel sheet dressings, or composite dressings (those including a combination of products, such as a thin film with a foam island in the center). Wounds with a large amount of drainage require dressings that are capable of absorbing it, such as calcium alginates, alginate collagen combinations, or specific beads, pastes, or powders designed to handle large amounts of drainage. Wounds with significant odor benefit from dressings formulated with charcoal, such as charcoal foam and dressings with a charcoal filter overlay.

If a wound shows a significant loss of tissue or if undermining or pockets are present, the wound cavities should be loosely filled with dressing to eliminate the potential for abscess formation. Eliminating the dead space helps to prevent premature wound closure with resulting abscess formation. Dressings such as calcium alginates, impregnated hydrogel gauze strips, or wound cavity fillers are useful for eliminating the dead space. Loose filling of the undermined areas also assists with exudate management, because these wounds tend to have large amounts of exudate.

Wounds in the sacral area require additional protection from stool or urine contamination. Because dressings near the anus may be difficult to maintain, the clinician must monitor dressings in this area more frequently. Some hydrocolloid dressings have been designed with specific shapes to improve their ability to stay in place over sacral/coccygeal wounds.

*Control Odor.* Wound odor results from bacterial overgrowth and necrotic tissue. Malodorous wounds are frequently polymicrobic, with both anaerobic and aerobic microorganisms present. Anaerobes release putrescine and cadaverine, both of which have been linked to ulcer smell.[103,104] The first step to controlling odor is to eliminate the cause if possible. Thus, adequate debridement of necrotic tissue is essential for odor control. Wound cleansing decreases microorganisms on the wound surface and also is helpful in reducing odor. Odor can also arise from infection. Use of topical antimicrobials including broad spectrum topical antibiotics, metronidazole, cadexomer iodine dressings or silver-release dressings all reduce odor by reducing bacterial burden. Topical metronidazole gel (0.77–1.0%) can be applied directly to the wound once a day for a week, or more often as needed, to control odor.[105] If the gel is not available, metronidazole tablets can be crushed and used topically.[106] Metronidazole acts by disrupting the DNA and protein synthesis of susceptible organisms. Wound dressings with activated charcoal can be used to reduce wound odor. Activated charcoal attracts and binds wound odor molecules. Once exudate leaks through activated charcoal dressings, odor control is lost—thus, these dressings are typically secondary dressings. For odorous pressure ulcers not anticipated to heal, moist dressings using povidone iodine or Dakin's solution (0.25%) can help reduce odor. Use of kitty litter, vinegar, coffee beans, or candles can help control odor in the patient's room by absorbing or filtering the odor.

*Reducing Wound Pain.* Wound pain must be managed with the same attention given to choice of wound dressings. In general, pain that is moderate to severe should be managed pharmacologically (see Chapters 6 and 7). The pressure ulcer alone may not require continuous pharmacological analgesia, but medication before procedures is essential. Lower levels of pain may be manageable with appropriate wound dressing choice and topical wound analgesia. Techniques useful for wound pain associated with procedures (e.g., debridement, dressing changes) include use of distraction (e.g., talking to the patient while performing the procedure), allowing the patient to call a "time-out" during the procedure, allowing the patient to control and participate in the procedure, providing opioids and/ or nonsteroidal anti-inflammatory drugs or acetominphen (preferred in elders) 30 minutes prior to procedures and afterwards, and administering topical anesthetics or topical opioids using hydrogels as a transport media. The lidocaine patch 5% (Lidoderm) blocks sodium channels and has been approved for postherpetic neuralgia.[107] It is effective for chronic neuropathic pain. Another option is EMLA cream (eutectic mixture of lidocaine 2.5% and prilocaine 2.5%), which reduces debridement pain scores in persons with venous leg ulcer and might have a vasoactive effect cutaneously.[108,109] Low-dose topical morphine (diamorphine in a hydrogel vehicle) can be used topically to reduce pressure ulcer pain.[110,111]

As evidenced by this discussion, attention to multiple wound characteristics helps to determine the most appropriate wound dressing. Evaluation of wound characteristics in follow-along assessments provides the basis for changes in topical dressings. For example, a wound that is heavily exudative may be treated topically with a calcium alginate dressing for several weeks; as the amount of wound exudate decreases, the wound dressing may appear dry at dressing changes. This indicates that use of a dressing with high absorptive capacity may not be needed any longer, and the wound dressing can be changed to one with minimal to moderate absorptive capacity, such as a hydrocolloid dressing. As the wound continues to heal and wound exudate becomes minimal or nonexistent, a thin film dressing may be used to provide protection from the environment.

## Patient and Caregiver Teaching Guidelines

Patient and caregiver instruction in self-care must be individualized according to specific pressure ulcer development risk factors, individual learning styles and coping mechanisms, and the ability of the patient or caregiver to perform procedures. In teaching prevention guidelines to caregivers, it is particularly important to use return demonstration to evaluate learning. Observing the caregiver perform turning maneuvers, repositioning, managing incontinence, and providing general skin care can be enlightening and provides a context in which the clinician supports and follows up education. In palliative care, it is important to include the reasons for specific actions, such as the continuation of some level of turning and repositioning to prevent further tissue damage and lessen discomfort from additional wounds. The patient and family should be informed about pressure ulcer development at the end of life and the information should be presented so there is understanding that not all pressure ulcers are avoidable. If a pressure ulcer develops, reminding the patient and caregiver of the care that has been provided and that the pressure ulcer is not a reflection of poor care is important to help allay caregiver's guilt.

## Summary

Poorly managed pressure ulcers can increase pain and suffering in those with a chronic debilitating illness. Although preventive measures in patients identified as at-risk for developing such pressure ulcers can be effective, some patients do develop pressure ulcers that require expert nursing management. Expert nursing management includes instituting preventive measures to preserve intact skin, obtaining and maintaining a clean wound, management of exudate and odor, and prevention of complications such as a superimposed wound infection. Because many dying and chronically ill, debilitated patients are cared for at home, educating family members about the development of pressure ulcers and involving family caregivers in the plan of care is critical. Many caregivers view pressure ulcers as a reflection of poor care; in reality, pressure ulcer development in persons at the end of life or in persons with certain comorbidites may be unavoidable even with the best care.

### REFERENCES

1. Tippett AW. Wounds at the end of life. Wounds 2005;17(4):91–98.
2. Maida V, Corbo M, Dolzhykov M, Ennis M, Irani S, Trozzolo L. Wounds in advanced illness: A prevalence and incidence study based on a prospective case series. Int Wound J 2008;5(2):305–314.
3. Hanson D, Langemo D, Olson B, Hunter S. Burd C. Evaluation of pressure ulcer prevalence rates for hospice patient post-implementation of pressure ulcer protocols. Am J Hosp Palliat Care 1994;11(6):14–19.
4. Henoch I, Gustafsson M. Pressure ulcers in palliative care: Development of a hospice pressure ulcer risk assessment scale. Int J Palliat Nurs 2003;9(11):474–484.
5. Galvin J. An audit of pressure ulcer incidence in a palliative care setting. Int J Palliat Nurs 2002;8(5):214–220.

6. Reifsnyder J, Hoplamazian LM, Maxwell T. Preventing and treating pressure ulcers in hospice patients. Caring 2004;30:30–37.

7. Brown G. Long-term outcomes of full-thickness pressure ulcers: Healing and mortality. Ostomy Wound Manage 2003;49(10):42–50.

8. Chaplin J. Pressure sore risk assessment in palliative care. J Tissue Viability 2000;10(1):27–31.

9. Hanson D, Langemo D, Olson B, Hunter S, Sauvage TR, Burd C, Cathcart-Silberberg T. The prevalence and incidence of pressure ulcers in the hospice setting: Analysis of two methodologies. Am J Palliat Care 1991;8(5):18–22.

10. McNees P, Meneses KD. Pressure ulcers and other chronic wounds in patients with and patients without cancer: A retrospective, comparative analysis of healing patterns. Ostomy Wound Manage 2007;53(2):70–78.

11. Daniel RK, Priest DL, Wheatley DC. Etiologic factors in pressure sores: An experimental model. Arch Phys Med Rehabil 1981;62:492–498.

12. Kosiak M. Etiology and pathology of ischemic ulcers. Arch Phys Med Rehabil 1959;40:62–69.

13. Reuler JB, Cooney TG. The pressure sore: Pathophysiology and principles of management. Ann Intern Med 1981;94:661.

14. Seiler WD, Stahelin HB. Recent findings on decubitus ulcer pathology: Implications for care. Geriatrics 1986;41:47–60.

15. Witkowski JA, Parish LC. Histopathology of the decubitus ulcer. J Am Acad Dermatol 1982;6:1014–1021.

16. Lindan O, Greenway RM, Piazza JM. Pressure distributor on the surface of the human body. Arch Phys Med Rehabil 1965;46:378.

17. Scales JT. Pressure on the patient. In: Kenedi RM, Cowden JM, eds. Bedsore Biomechanics. London: University Park Press, 1976:11–17.

18. Parish LC, Witkowski JA, Crissey JT. The Decubitus Ulcer. New York: Masson, 1983.

19. Slater H. Pressure Ulcers in the Elderly. Pittsburgh, PA: Synapse, 1985.

20. Parish LC, Witkowski JA, Crissey JT. The Decubitus Ulcer in Clinical Practice. Berlin: Springer, 1997.

21. Landis EM. Micro-injection studies of capillary blood pressure in human skin. Heart 1930;15:209.

22. Witkowski JA, Parish LC. The decubitus ulcer: Skin failure and destructive behavior. Int J Dermatol 2000;39(12):894–896.

23. Langemo DK, Brown G. Skin fails too: Acute, chronic and end-stage skin failure. Adv Skin Wound Care 2006;19(4):206–211.

24. Husain T. An experimental study of some pressure effects on tissues, with reference to the bedsore problem. J Pathol Bacteriol 1953;66:347–358.

25. Salcido R, Donofrio JC, Fisher SB, LeGrand EK, Dickey K, Carney JM, Schosser R, Liang R. Histopathology of decubitus ulcers as a result of sequential pressure sessions in a computer-controlled fuzzy rat model. Adv Wound Care 1994;7(5):40.

26. Kosiak M, Kubicek WG, Olsen ME. Evaluation of pressure as a factor in the production of ischial ulcers. Arch Phys Med Rehabil 1958;39:623.

27. Braden BJ, Bergstrom N. A conceptual schema for the study of etiology of pressure sores. Rehabil Nurs 1987;12:8–12.

28. Bergstrom N, Demuth PJ, Braden BJ. A clinical trial of the Braden Scale for Predicting Pressure Sore Risk. Nurs Clin North Am 1987;22:417–428.

29. Brink P, Smith TF, Linkewich B. Factors associated with pressure ulcers in palliative home care. J Palliat Med 2006;9(6):1369–1375.

30. Franks PJ, Winterberg H, Moffat CJ. Health-related quality of life and pressure ulceration assessment in patients treated in the community. Wound Rep Reg 2002;10(3):133–140.

31. Reifsnyder J, Magee HS. Development of pressure ulcers in patients receiving home hospice care. Wounds 2005;17(4):74–79.

32. Allman RM, Goode PS, Patrick MM, Burst N, Bartolucci AA. Pressure ulcer risk factors among hospitalized patients with activity limitations. JAMA 1995;273:865–870.

33. Panel for the Prediction and Prevention of Pressure Ulcers in Adults. Pressure Ulcers in Adults: Prediction and Prevention. Clinical Practice Guideline Number 3. Publication AHCPR 92–0047. Rockville, MD: Agency for Health Care Policy and Research, U. S. Department of Health and Human Services, 1992.

34. Curry K, Casady L. The relationship between extended periods of immobility and decubitus ulcer formation in the acutely spinal cord injured individual. J Neurosci Nurs 1992;24:185–189.

35. Hammond MC, Bozzacco VA, Stiens SA, Buhrer R, Lyman P. Pressure ulcer incidence on a spinal cord injury unit. Adv Wound Care 1994;7:57–60.

36. Reichel SM. Shearing force as a factor in decubitus ulcers in paraplegics. JAMA 1958;166:762–763.

37. Bennett L, Kavner D, Lee BY, Trainor FS, Lewis JM. Skin stress and blood flow in sitting paraplegic patients. Arch Phys Med Rehabil 1969;65:186–190.

38. Dinsdale SM. Decubitus ulcers: Role of pressure and friction in causation. Arch Phys Med Rehabil 1974;55:147–152.

39. Kemp MG. Protecting the skin from moisture and associated irritants. J Gerontol Nurs 1994;20:8–14.

40. Bates-Jensen B. Incontinence management. In: Parish LC, Witkowski JA, Crissey JT, eds. The Decubitus Ulcer in Clinical Practice. Berlin: Springer, 1997:189–199.

41. Maklebust J, Magnan MA. Risk factors associated with having a pressure ulcer: A secondary analysis. Adv Wound Care 1994;7:25–42.

42. Pinchcovsky-Devin G, Kaminsky MV Jr. Correlation of pressure sores and nutritional status. J Am Geriatr Soc 1986;34:435–440.

43. Bobel LM. Nutritional implications in the patient with pressure sores. Nurs Clin North Am 1987;22:379–390.

44. Bergstrom N, Braden B. A prospective study of pressure sore risk among institutionalized elderly. J Am Geriatr Soc 1992;40:747–758.

45. Allman RM, Laprade CA, Noel LB, Walker JM, Moorer CA, Dear MR, Smith CR. Pressure sores among hospitalized patients. Ann Intern Med 1986;105:337–342.

46. Jones PL, Millman A. Wound healing and the aged patient. Nurs Clin North Am 1990;25:263–277.

47. Eaglestein WH. Wound healing and aging. Clin Geriatr Med 1989;5:183.

48. Bergstrom N, Braden BJ, Boynton P, Bruch S. Using a research-based assessment scale in clinical practice. Nurs Clin North Am 1995;30:539.

49. Versluysen M. Pressure sores in elderly patients: The epidemiology related to hip operations. J Bone Joint Surg Br 1985;67:10–13.

50. Shannon ML. Pressure sores. In: Norris CM, ed. Concept Clarification in Nursing. Rockville, MD: Aspen, 1982.

51. Anderson TP, Andberg MM. Psychosocial factors associated with pressure sores. Arch Phys Med Rehabil 1979;60:341–346.

52. Vidal J, Sarrias M. An analysis of the diverse factors concerned with the development of pressure sores in spinal cord patients. Paraplegia 1991;29:261–267.

53. Norton D. Calculating the risk: Reflections on the Norton scale. Decubitus 1989;2:24–31.

54. Norton D, McLaren R, Exton-Smith NA. An Investigation of Geriatric Nursing Problems in Hospitals. London: National Corporation for the Care of Old People, 1962.

55. Maida V, Lau F, Downing M, Yang J. Correlation between Braden Scale and Palliative Performance Scale in advanced illness. Int Wound J 2008;5(4):585–590.

56. Morita T, Tsunoda J, Inoue S, Chihara S. Validity of the palliative performance scale from a survival perspective. J Pain Symptom Manage 1999;18(1):2–3.

57. Virik K, Glare P, Validation of the palliative performance scale for inpatients admitted to a palliative care unit in Sydney, Australia. J Pain Symptom Manage 2002;23(6):455–457.

58. Braden B, Bergstrom N. Clinical utility of the Braden Scale for Predicting Pressure Sore Risk. Decubitus 1989;2:44–51.

59. Defloor T, De Bacquer D, Grypdonck MH. The effect of various combinations of turning and pressure reducing devices on the incidence of pressure ulcers. Int J Nurs Stud 2005;42(1):37–46.

60. Bergstrom N, Bennett MA, Carlson CE, et al. Treatment of Pressure Ulcers. Clinical Practice Guideline Number 15. Publication AHCPR 95–0652. Rockville, MD: Agency for Health Care Policy and Research, U. S. Department of Health and Human Services, 1994.

61. McLean J. Pressure reduction or pressure relief: Making the right choice. J ET Nurs 1993;20:211–215.

62. Krouskop TA, Garber SL, Cullen BB. Factors to consider in selecting a support surface. In: Krasner D, ed. Chronic Wound Care. King of Prussia, PA: Health Management Publications, 1990:135–141.

63. National Pressure Ulcer Advisory Panel. Consensus statement. Adv Wound Care 1995;8:32–33.

64. National Pressure Ulcer Advisory Panel. Support surface standards initiative. Terms and Definitions. 2007. Available at: http://npuap.org/NPUAP_S3I_TD.pdf (accessed December 20, 2008).

65. Zimmerer RE, Lawson KD, Calvert CJ. The effects of wearing diapers on skin. Pediatr Dermatol 1986;3:95–101.

66. Willis I. The effects of prolonged water exposure on human skin. J Invest Dermatol 1973;60:166–171.

67. Thomas DR, Rodeheaver GT, Bartolucci AA, Franz RA, Sussman C, Ferrell BA, Cuddigan J, Stotts N, Maklebust J. Pressure Ulcer Scale for Healing: Derivation and validation of the PUSH tool. Adv Wound Care 1997;10:96–101.

68. Bates-Jensen BM, Vredevoe DL, Brecht ML. Validity and reliability of the Pressure Sore Status Tool. Decubitus 1992;5:20–28.

69. Stotts NA, Rodeheaver GT, Thomas DR, Frantz RA, Bartolucci AA, Sussman C, Ferrell BA, Cuddigan J, Maklebust J. An instrument to measure healing in pressure ulcers: Development and valdiation of the Pressure Ulcer Scale for Healing (PUSH). J Gerontol A Biol Sci Med Sic 2001;56(12):M795–M799.

70. Bates-Jensen B. New pressure ulcer status tool. Decubitus 1990;3:14–15.

71. Bates-Jensen BM, Vredevoe DL, Brecht ML. Validity and reliability of the Pressure Sore Status Tool. Decubitus 1992;5:20–28.

72. Bates-Jensen BM, McNees P. Toward an intelligent wound assessment system. Ostomy Wound Manage 1995;41(Suppl 7A):80–87.

73. Bates-Jensen B. The Pressure Sore Status Tool: An outcome measure for pressure sores. Top Geriatr Rehabil 1994;9:17–34.

74. Bates-Jensen BM. The Pressure Sore Status Tool a few thousand assessments later. Adv Wound Care 1997;10:65–73.

75. Cooper DM. Indices to include in wound assessment. Adv Wound Care 1995;8:28–15–28–18.

76. Lazarus GS, Cooper DM, Knighton DR, Mrgolis DJ, Pecorar RE, Rodeheaver G, Robson MC. Definitions and guidelines for assessment of wounds and evaluation of healing. Arch Dermatol 1994;130:489–493.

77. Van Rijswijk L. Wound assessment and documentation. In: Kane DP, Krasner D, eds. Chronic Wound Care: A Clinical Sourcebook for Healthcare Professionals (2nd ed). Wayne, PA: Health Management Publications, 1997:16–28.

78. Yarkony GM, Kirk PM, Carlson C, Roth EJ, Lovel L, Heinemann A, King R, Lee MY, Betts HB. Classification of pressure ulcers. Arch Dermatol 1990;126:1218–1219.

79. Shea JD. Pressure sores: Classification and management. Clin Orthop Rel Res 1975;112:89–100.

80. Seiler WD, Stahelin HB. Identification of factors that impair wound healing: A possible approach to wound healing research. Wounds 1995;6:101–106.

81. Sapico FL, Ginunas VJ, Thornhill-Hoynes M, Canawati HN, Capen DA, Klen NE, Khawa S, Montgomerie JZ. Quantitative microbiology of pressure sores in different stages of healing. Diagn Microbiol Infect Dis 1986;5:31–38.

82. Winter GD. Formation of the scab and the rate of reepithelialization of superficial wounds in the skin of the young domestic pig. Nature 1965;193:293–294.

83. Kerstein MD. Moist wound healing: The clinical perspective. Ostomy Wound Manage 1995;41(Suppl 7A):37S–44S.

84. Bagdade JD, Root RK, Bulger RJ. Impaired leukocyte function in patients with poorly controlled diabetes. Diabetes 1974;23:9–15.

85. Pecoraro RE, Ahroni JH, Boyko EJ, Stensel VL. Chronology and determinants of tissue repair in diabetic lower extremity ulcers. Diabetes 1991;40:1305–1313.

86. Goodson WH 3rd, Hunt TK. Studies of wound healing in experimental diabetes mellitus. J Surg Res 1977;22:221–227.

87. Yue DK, McLennan S, Marsh M, Mai YW, Spaliviero J, Delbridge L, Reeve T, Turtle JR. Effects of experimental diabetes, uremia, and malnutrition on wound healing. Diabetes 1987;36:295–299.

88. Coleridge Smith PD, Thomas P, Scurr JH, Dormandy JA. Causes of venous ulceration: A new hypothesis. BMJ 1998;296:1726–1727.

89. Falanga V. Growth factors and wound healing. Dermatol Clin 1993;11:667–674.

90. Barbul A, Lazarou SA, Efron DT, Wasserkrug HL, Efron G. Arginine enhances wound healing and lymphocyte immune responses in humans. Surgery 1990;108:331–336.

91. Kagan RJ, Bratescu A, Jonasson O, Matsuda T, Teodorescu M. The relationship between the percentage of circulating B cells, corticosteroid levels, and other immunologic parameters in thermally injured patients. J Trauma 1989;29:208–213.

92. Mosiello GC, Tufaro A, Kerstein M. Wound healing and complications in the immunosuppressed patient. Wounds 1994;6:83–87.

93. Dallam L, Smyth C, Jackson BS et al. Pressure ulcer pain: Assessment and quantification. J Wound Ostomy Continence Nurs 1995; 22(5):211–215; discussion 217–218.

94. Szor JK, Bourguignon C. Description of pressure ulcer pain at rest and at dressing change. J Wound Ostomy Continence Nurs 1999;26(3):115–120.

95. Roth RS, Lowery JC, Hamill JB. Assessing persistent pain and its relation to affective distress, depressive symptoms, and pain catastrophizing in patients with chronic wounds: A pilot study. Am J Phys Med Rehabil 2004;83(11):827–834.

96. Freeman K, Smyth C, Dallam L, Jackson B. Pain measurement scales: A comparison of the visual analogue and faces rating scales in measuring pressure ulcer pain. J Wound Ostomy Continence Nurs 2001;28(6):290–296.

97. National Pressure Ulcer Advisory Panel in collaboration with European Pressure Ulcer Advisory Panel . Pressure Ulcer Treatment Guideline Recommendations. Available at: http://pressureulcerguidelines.org/therapy/ (accessed December 20, 2008).

98. Sherman RA. Maggot versus conservative debridement therapy for the treatment of pressure ulcers. Wound Repair Regen 2002;10(4):208–214.

99. Steenvoorde P, Jacobi CE, Oskam J. Maggot Debridement Therapy: Free-Range or Contained? An In-vivo Study. Adv Skin Wound Care 2005;18(8):430–435.

100. Gardner SE, Frantz RA, Doebbeling BN. The validity of the clinical signs and symptoms used to identify localized chronic wound infection. Wound Repair Regen 2001;9(3):178–186.

101. Stotts NA. Determination of bacterial burden in wounds. Adv Wound Care 1995;8(4):suppl 46–52.

102. Sibbald RG, Orsted HL, Coutts PM, Keast DH. Best practice recommendations for preparing the wound bed. Update 2006. Wound Care Canada 2006;4(1):15–29.

103. Holloway S. Recognizing and treating the causes of chronic malodor wounds. Professional Nurse 2004;19(7):380–384.

104. Kalinski C, Schnepf M, Laboy D, Hernandez L, Nusbaum,J, McGrinder B, et al. Effectiveness of a topical formulation containing metronidazole for wound odor and exudate control. Wounds 2005;17(4):74–79.

105. Paul JC, Pieper BA. Topical metronidazole for the treatment of wound odor: A review of the literature. Ostomy Wound Manage 2008;54(3):18–27.

106. McDonald A, Lesage P. Palliative management of pressure ulcers and malignant wounds in patients with advanced illness. J Palliat Med 2006;9(2):285–295.

107. Argoff CE. New Analgesics for neuropathic pain: The lidocaine patch. Clin J Pain 2000;16(2 Suppl):S62–S66.

108. Briggs M, Nelson EA. Topical agents or dressings for pain in venous leg ulcers. Cochrane Database Syst Rev 2003;(1):CD001177.

109. Hafner HM, Thomma SR, Eichner M, Steins A, Junger M. The influence of EMLA cream on cutaneous microcirculation. Clin Hemorrheol Microcirc 2003;28:121–128.

110. Zeppetella G, Paul J, Ribeiro M. Analgesic efficacy of morphine applied topically to painful ulcers. J Pain Symptom Manage 2003;25:555–558.

111. Flock P. Pilot study to determine the effectiveness of diamorphine gel to control pressure ulcer pain. J Pain Symptom Manage 2003;25:547–554.

*Susie Seaman and Barbara M. Bates-Jensen*

# Skin Disorders: Malignant Wounds, Fistulas, and Stomas

*This constant drainage smells so bad, and my skin is so sore, life isn't worth living—I don't belong among people.—A palliative care patient*

♦ **Key Points**
♦ *Management of drainage and odor are key components of palliative care for malignant cutaneous wounds or tumor necrosis.*
♦ *Palliative care for the person with an ostomy is focused on maintenance of an efficient management plan and provision for optimal functional capacity.*
♦ *It is essential to involve caregivers and family members in the plan of care.*

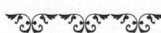

## MALIGNANT WOUNDS

### Definition

Malignant wounds, also known in the literature as fungating tumors, tumor necrosis, ulcerative malignant wounds, or fungating malignant wounds, present both a physical and an emotional challenge for the patient, caregiver, and clinician. These wounds are frequently associated with pain, odor, bleeding, and an unsightly appearance. They may be a blow to self-esteem and may cause social isolation just when the patient needs more time with loved ones. The goals in the care of patients with malignant wounds include managing wound exudate, odor, bleeding and pain, preventing infection, and promoting the emotional welfare of the patient and family.

Malignant cutaneous lesions occur in up to 5% of patients with cancer and 10% of patients with metastatic disease. To date, the largest study examining the incidence of cutaneous involvement of internal malignancies was performed by Lookingbill and colleagues,[1] who retrospectively reviewed data accumulated over a 10-year period from the tumor registry at Hershey Medical Center in Pennsylvania. Of 7,316 patients, 367 (5.0%) had cutaneous malignancies. Of these, 38 patients had lesions as a result of direct local invasion, 337 had metastatic lesions, and 8 had both. A secondary analysis from the same registry found that 420 patients (10.4%) of 4,020 with metastatic disease had cutaneous involvement.[2] In women, the most common origins of metastasis were breast carcinoma (70.7%) and melanoma (12.0%). In men, melanoma (32.3%), lung carcinoma (11.8%), and colorectal cancer (11.0%) accounted for the most common primary tumors. In a 10-year retrospective review of 677 patients with lung cancer, Ambrogi et al.[3] found that 26 (3.8%) patients had cutaneous metastasis. Mueller et al.[4] performed a meta-analysis of eight studies examining cutaneous metastasis of internal malignancies. Out of 81,618 primary visceral cancers, they identified 2,369 (2.9%) cases of metastasis to the skin. When they examined the percentage of cutaneous metastasis from genitourinary cancers, the incidence was 1.3%. Saeed et al.[5] found that of 77 patients with skin metastasis cared for over a 10-year period in a Veteran's Administration setting, the primary tumor sites were the lungs, skin (melanoma) and gastrointestinal tract. Although breast, lung, gastrointestinal tract, and melanoma account for the majority of cutaneous metastases, these lesions may arise from any type of malignant tumor.[6–9] In some cases, the tumor of origin may not be identified.[10]

## Pathophysiology of Malignant Wounds

Malignant wounds may occur from infiltration of the skin by local invasion of a primary tumor or by metastasis from another site.[11,12] Local invasion may initially manifest as inflammation with induration, redness, heat, tenderness, or some combination of these features. The skin may have a peau d'orange appearance and may be fixed to underlying tissue. As the tumor spreads and further tissue destruction occurs, the skin eventually ulcerates. The presentation differs in metastatic cutaneous infiltration. Tumor cells detach from the primary site and travel via blood or lymphatic vessels, or tissue planes, to distant organs, including the skin.[6,12–14] In general, cutaneous metastasis occurs in the region of the primary tumor, most commonly on the chest, head, neck, abdomen, and groin.[5,7,15] These lesions may initially manifest as an erythematous rash or plaque. More commonly, they present as well-demarcated, painless nodules ranging in size from a few millimeters to several centimeters. Their consistency may vary from firm to rubbery. Pigmentation changes may be noted over the lesions, from deep red to brown-black. Both locally invasive and metastatic lesions may initially be misdiagnosed as rashes, plaques, cellulitis, epidermal cysts, lipomas or other benign conditions. However, unlike many benign skin problems, these lesions will not resolve and over time may ulcerate, fungate, drain, and become very painful.

As these malignant lesions extend, changes in vascular and lymphatic flow lead to edema, exudate, and tissue necrosis.[11,16,17] The resulting lesion may be fungating, in which the tumor mass extends above the skin surface with a fungus or cauliflower-like appearance, or it may be erosive and ulcerative.[18] The wound bed may be pale to pink with very friable tissue, completely necrotic, or a combination of both. The surrounding skin may be erythematous, fragile, and exceedingly tender to touch. The skin may also be macerated in the presence of excessive wound exudate. The presence of necrotic tissue is an ideal culture medium for bacterial colonization, which may result in significant malodor.[19,20] The degree of pain experienced by the patient depends on wound location, depth of tissue invasion and damage, nerve involvement, and the patient's previous experience with pain and analgesia.[18]

## Assessment of Malignant Wounds

Ongoing comprehensive assessment of the patient and malignant wound facilitates formulation of an appropriate treatment plan, allows for adjustment of the treatment plan as findings change, and promotes recognition of wound complications. Specifically, wound location, size, appearance, exudate, odor, and condition of the surrounding skin guides local therapy. Associated symptoms should be noted so that appropriate measures can be taken to provide comfort. The potential for serious complications such as hemorrhage, vessel compression or obstruction, or airway obstruction should be noted so that the caregiver can be educated regarding their palliative management. Table 17B–1 presents highlights for the assessment of malignant wounds and associated rationale.

Haisfield-Wolfe and Baxendale-Cox[21] proposed a staging classification system for assessment of malignant cutaneous wounds. Use of wound classification may increase the effectiveness of communication among health care practitioners and make evaluation of treatment effectiveness consistent. In a pilot study with 13 wounds, they proposed a staging classification system that evaluates wound depth with clinical descriptors, predominant color of the wound, hydration status of the wound, drainage, pain, odor, and presence of tunneling or undermining. Use of this system provides a basis for a standard set of descriptors that nurses can use to both understand and assess malignant wounds.

Malignant wounds may change over time based on the aggressiveness of the cancer and whether the patient is undergoing palliative surgery, chemotherapy, or radiation. Although palliative treatment may result in regression or even disappearance of the cutaneous lesion, it can be expected to eventually recur.[22] Ongoing assessment allows the clinician to tailor the local wound management based on the current needs of the patient and wound.

## Management of Malignant Wounds

The goals of care for patients with malignant wounds include control of infection and odor, management of exudate, prevention and control of bleeding, and management of pain.[11,14,16,18,23–25] In determining the appropriate treatment regimen, the abilities of the caregiver must also be considered. There is limited published information on treatment effectiveness, which reflects the absence of evidence-based care in this area and the significant need for further research and dissemination of findings.[25] Many articles regarding malignant wounds are based on expert opinion and the personal experience of practitioners knowledgeable in palliative and hospice care. Although research-based treatment is the gold standard of care, anecdotal reports on successful treatment of these challenging wounds are helpful to nurses striving to provide the best care for their patients.

*Infection and Odor Control.* Control of infection and odor is achieved by controlling local bacterial colonization with

**Table 17B–1**
**Assessment of Malignant Wounds**

| Assessment | Rationale |
| --- | --- |
| **Wound location** | |
| Is mobility impaired? | Consider occupational therapy referral to facilitate activities of daily living |
| Located near wrinkled or flat skin? | Affects dressing selection |
| | Affects dressing fixation |
| **Wound appearance** | |
| Size: length, width, depth, undermining, deep structure exposure | Affects dressing selection, provides information on deterioration or response to palliative treatment |
| Fungating or ulcerative | Affects dressing selection and fixation |
| Percentage of viable vs. necrotic tissue | Need for cleansing/debridement |
| Tissue friability and bleeding | Need for nonadherent dressings and other measures to control bleeding |
| Presence of odor | Need for odor-reducing strategies |
| Presence of fistula | Possible need for pouching |
| Exudate amount | Affects dressing selection |
| Wound colonized or clinically infected | Need for local versus systemic care |
| **Surrounding skin** | |
| Erythematous | Infection or tumor extension |
| Fragile or denuded | Impacts dressing type and fixation |
| Nodular | Tumor extension/metastasis |
| Macerated | Need for improved exudate management |
| Radiation-related skin damage | Need for topical care of skin, affects dressing fixation |
| **Symptoms** | |
| Deep pain: aching, stabbing, continuous | Need to adjust systemic analgesia |
| Superficial pain: burning, stinging, may be associated only with dressing changes | Need for topical analgesia and rapid-onset, short-acting analgesics |
| Pruritus | Related to dressings? If not, may need systemic antipruritic medications |
| **Potential for serious complications** | |
| Lesion is near major blood vessels: potential for hemorrhage | Need for education of patient/family about palliative management of severe bleeding |
| Lesion is near major blood vessels: potential for vessel compression/obstruction | Need for education of patient/family about palliative management of severe swelling and pain, possible tissue necrosis |
| Lesion is near airway: potential for obstruction | Need for education of patient/family about palliative management of airway obstruction |

wound cleansing, wound debridement, and use of local antimicrobial agents. Because malignant wounds are frequently associated with necrotic tissue and odor, wound cleansing is essential to remove necrotic debris, decrease bacterial counts, and thus reduce odor. If the lesion is not very friable, the patient may be able to shower. This not only provides for local cleansing but also gives the added psychological benefit of helping the patient to feel clean. The patient should be instructed to allow the shower water to hit the skin above the wound and then run over the wound. If there is friable tissue (i.e., tissue that bleeds easily with minimal trauma) or the patient is not able to shower, the nurse or caregiver should gently irrigate the wound with normal saline or a commercial wound cleanser. Skin/incontinence cleansers, which contain mild soaps and antibacterial ingredients used in bathing, can be very effective at controlling local colonization and odor. As long as they do not cause burning, they may be sprayed directly on the wound. If pain and burning occur with use of skin cleansers in the wound, they should be used only on the surrounding skin. Topical antimicrobial agents such as hydrogen peroxide, Dakin's solution, and povidone iodine are recommended by some authors;[22] however, their use should be weighed against the potential negative effects of local pain, skin irritation, wound desiccation with subsequent pain and bleeding on dressing removal, and unpleasant odor associated with Dakin's and povidone iodine. In the authors' experience, the skin cleansers described provide cleansing and odor reduction without many of the negative effects of the topical antimicrobial agents.

The necrotic tissue in malignant wounds is typically moist yellow slough. Occasionally, in the absence of exudate, there may be dry black eschar, but this is less common. Debridement is best done with the use of autolytic and/or gentle mechanical methods, as opposed to wet-to-dry dressings, which are traumatic and can cause significant bleeding and pain upon removal. Autolytic debridement, which is the natural breakdown of necrotic tissue by enzymes and white cells present in wound fluid,[26] can be achieved with the use of dressings that support a moist wound environment,[26,27] but odor may be increased under occlusion and/or with the use of hydrogels. Local debridement may be performed by very gently scrubbing the necrotic areas with gauze saturated with skin or wound cleanser. Low-pressure irrigation with normal saline using a 35-mL syringe and a 19-gauge needle can be used to remove loose necrotic tissue and decrease bacterial counts. Care should be taken to avoid causing pain with either procedure. In addition, careful sharp debridement by clinicians trained in this procedure can be performed to remove loose necrotic tissue. Penetration of viable tissue should be avoided, because bleeding may be difficult to control. If necrotic tissue in the wound is extensive, surgical debridement may be indicated to promote infection control, odor reduction, and exudate management, if compatible with the palliative goals of care for the patient.

Local colonization and odor can be reduced with the use of topical antibacterial preparations. Odor is by far the most difficult management aspect of treating malignant wounds and is frequently the most distressing complaint that affected patients have. The literature supports use of topical metronidazole, which has a wide range of activity against anaerobic bacteria, to control wound odor.[28–34]

Topical therapy is available by crushing metronidazole tablets in sterile water and creating either a 0.5% solution (5 mg/mL) or a 1% solution (10 mg/mL).[28,29] This may be used as a wound irrigant, or gauze may be saturated with the solution and packed into wound cavities. Care must be taken not to allow the gauze packing to desiccate, because dressing adherence may lead to bleeding and pain.

An easy, effective alternative to metronidazole solution is metronidazole 0.75% gel, which is applied in a thin layer to the entire wound. Poteete[30] evaluated the use of metronidazole 0.75% gel in the treatment of 13 patients with malodorous wounds. Metronidazole gel was applied to the wounds daily and covered with either saline-moistened or hydrogel-saturated gauze. At the end of the 9-day observation period, no odor was detected in any wound after the dressings were removed. Finlay et al.[31] prospectively studied subjective odor and pain, appearance, and bacteriological response in 47 patients with malodorous wounds treated with daily application of metronidazole 0.75% gel. Ninety-five percent of the patients reported decreased odor at 14 days. Anaerobic colonization was discovered in 53% of patients and eliminated in 84% of these cases after treatment. Patients reported decreased pain at day 7, and both discharge and cellulitis were significantly decreased by day 14. Bale et al.[32] conducted a randomized controlled trial of the daily application of topical metronidazole gel vs. placebo gel in the treatment of 41 patients with malodorous wounds, including venous, arterial, and pressure ulcers, and other types of wounds. Based of subjective ratings of odor by the patient at start of therapy and days 1, 3, and 7, metronidazole gel eliminated odor faster than placebo gel. Interestingly, whereas all the patients treated with metronidazole gel noted odor elimination, 76% of placebo-gel-treated patients also noted odor elimination by the end of the study. The authors speculated that this good result in the placebo group may have been from daily wound attention and care. Kalinski et al.[33] conducted a prospective, uncontrolled trial of metronidazole 0.75% gel in 16 patients with malodorous, malignant fungating wounds. Metronidazole gel was applied to the wounds once or twice daily and covered with a non-adherent contact layer and a secondary gauze dressing. Using a subjective odor rating scale of 0–10, complete odor elimination was noted at day 1 in 10 patients, and significant improvement (> 3 units of improvement on rating scale) was noted in the other six patients. No adverse effects were seen with this regimen. Because metronidazole gel is now available generically, it is a simple, cost-effective method to reduce wound odor in patients with malignant wounds. Choice of dressing over metronidazole gel should be based on the amount of exudate. In low exudate wounds in which dressing adherence is a concern, the gel should be covered with a non-adherent contact layer, and then absorbent dressings such as gauze or ABD pads should be applied. In more heavily draining wounds, a non-adherent contact layer may not be necessary, and the absorbent dressings can be applied directly to the wound. For optimum odor control, dressings should be changed daily, and more often for high levels of exudate that soak through the bandage. In the United States, use of metronidazole gel is considered off-label use, but with significant support for its use in the literature, it can be considered an appropriate choice in the standard care of patients with malodorous malignant wounds.[34] Systemic use of metronidazole should only be used in patients with invasive infection, not those with local bacterial colonization.

Another topical antimicrobial agent is Iodosorb* gel (Smith & Nephew), 0.9% cadexomer iodine, which is iodine complexed in a starch copolymer. This product contains slow-release iodine and has been shown to decrease bacterial counts in wounds without cytotoxicity.[35] Cadexomer iodine is available in a 40-g tube and is applied to the wound in a one-eighth inch layer. An advantage of this product is exudate absorption: each gram absorbs 6 mL of fluid. Disadvantages include cost (comparable to metronidazole 0.75% gel) and possible burning on application.

There are dressings that may also help decrease bacterial colonization and odor in malignant wounds.[36] Charcoal dressings, which absorb and trap odor, are available as either primary or secondary bandages. Some products trap odor under the bandage, requiring application of a perfect seal around the dressing for effectiveness. This can be a disadvantage in that adhesive will have to be applied to fragile surrounding skin. Some charcoal products are complexed with absorptive ingredients such as alginates or hydrocolloids, which help to trap the odor in the dressings. Because these dressings vary in their application and performance, package inserts should be reviewed before use.

Any dressing that decreases bacterial counts in a wound has the potential to decrease odor. Silver has broad-spectrum activity against microorganisms found in wounds.[37] Silver-based dressings are available in multiple different types including alginates, hydrocolloids, hydrogels, hydrofibers, foams, contact layers, and mesh gauze.[38] Dressing type is chosen based on exudate level; for example, a silver-based alginate or hydrofiber might be used on a high exudating wound, whereas a silver-based contact layer and/or a silver-based hydrogel may be used on a low draining wound. Medical grade honey-based dressings and gels may also decrease wound odor as honey is naturally antibacterial.[36,39,40] It must be noted, however, that Cochrane Reviews of both honey as a topical treatment for chronic wounds, and silver dressings for treating infected wounds, failed to show significant evidence to provide recommendations for practice.[41,42] Data is not available on the use of these products in patients with malignant wounds.

Less conventional methods of odor management are also available. Topical application of yogurt to the wound may reduce wound odor,[43] but might be messy. Environmental deodorizers such as cat litter or charcoal briquettes can be placed under the bed to help reduce room odor for patients at home.[44] Use of peppermint oil or other aromatherapy products, applied below the nostril or near the bed may help mask the odor. Odor eliminating room sprays are more effective than room deodorant sprays and can be used before and after wound care to reduce the odor associated with wound exposure.

Although local colonization is treated with topical cleansing, debridement, and antibacterial agents, clinical infection, as evidenced by erythema, induration, increased pain and exudate, leukocytosis, and fever, should be treated with systemic antibiotics. Cultures should be used to identify infecting organisms once the wound is diagnosed with an infection based on clinical signs; cultures should not be used routinely to diagnose infection. Because of the local inflammatory effects of the tumor, wounds may have many of the same signs as infection, so the clinician must be discriminating in differentiating between the two. A complete blood count, assessing the white cell count and differential, may be helpful in guiding assessment and therapy. It is crucial to avoid treating patients with oral antibiotics if they are only colonized and not infected, to prevent side effects and emergence of resistant organisms.

*Management of Exudate.* Because of the inflammation and edema commonly associated with malignant wounds, there tends to be significant exudate. Dressings should be chosen to conceal and collect exudate and odor. This is essential because a patient who experiences unexpected drainage on clothing or bedding may suffer significant feelings of distress and loss of control. Specialty dressings, such as foams, alginates, or starch copolymers, are notably more expensive than gauze pads or cotton-based absorbent pads. However, if such dressings reduce the overall cost by reducing the need for frequent dressing changes, they may be cost-effective. Table 17B–2 summarizes dressing considerations with malignant wounds.

Non-adherent dressings are best utilized as the primary contact layer, because they minimize the trauma to the wound associated with dressing changes. Seaman[24] suggests using nonadherent contact layers, such as Vaseline gauze, for the primary dressing on the wound bed, and covering these with soft, absorbent dressings, such as gauze and ABD pads, for secondary dressings to contain drainage. The entire dressing should be changed once a day; the secondary dressing should be changed twice a day if drainage strikes through to the outside of the bandage. When applied over metronidazole gel, this dressing regimen is both clinically and cost effective. Many active patients may prefer to use menstrual pads as the secondary dressing, not only because of their excellent absorption, but also because the plastic backing blocks exudate and protects clothing. For patients with highly exudating wounds in which frequent bandage changes are required, an ostomy pouch may be used to contain the drainage. An appliance with a spout, such as urostomy pouch or wound management pouch, is applied to completely enclose the wound, and is changed twice a week. These devices are odor-proof as long as the seal is maintained; however, pouch deodorants may be used to decrease odor that will be noticed when the device is emptied. Partnering with a Certified Wound, Ostomy, Continence Nurse (CWOCN) when deciding whether to pouch a malignant wound is recommended.

Protection of the surrounding skin is another goal of exudate management. The skin around the malignant wound may be fragile secondary to previous radiation therapy, inflammation due to tumor extension, repeated use of adhesive dressings, and/or maceration. Although adhesive dressings may assist with drainage and odor control, their potential to strip the epidermis upon removal may outweigh their benefit. Using flat ostomy skin barriers on the skin surrounding the wound and then taping the dressings to the skin barriers is one method of protecting against excess drainage and skin stripping due to tape removal. The ostomy barriers are changed every 5 to 7 days. Another method of protecting the surrounding skin is to use a barrier ointment or skin sealant on the skin surrounding the ulcer. These barriers protect the fragile tissue from maceration and the irritating effects of the drainage on the skin. Avoid excessive use of skin barrier ointments though; they can actually cause or increase maceration if too much is used. Dressings can then be held in place with tape affixed to the skin barrier placed on healthy skin, flexible netting, tube dressings, sports bras, panties, briefs, snug tank tops, or tube tops.

*Controlling Bleeding.* The viable tissue in a malignant wound may be very friable, bleeding with even minimal manipulation. Prevention is the best therapy for controlling bleeding. Prevention involves use of a gentle hand in dressing removal and thoughtful attention to the use of non-adherent dressings or moist wound dressings. On wounds with a low amount of exudate, the use of hydrogel sheets, or amorphous hydrogels under a non-adherent contact layer, may keep the wound moist and prevent dressing adherence. Even highly

**Table 17B-2**
**Dressing Choices for Malignant Wounds**

| Type of Wound and Goals of Care | Dressing Choice |
| --- | --- |
| **Low exudate** | |
| Maintain moist environment | Nonadherent contact layers |
| Prevent dressing adherence and bleeding | • Adaptic (Johnson & Johnson) |
| | • Dermanet (DeRoyal) |
| | • Mepitel (MöInlycke) |
| | • Petrolatum gauze (numerous manufacturers) |
| | • Tegapore (3M Health Care) |
| | Amorphous hydrogels |
| | Sheet hydrogels |
| | Hydrocolloids: contraindicated with fragile surrounding skin, may increase odor |
| | Semipermeable films: contraindicated with fragile surrounding skin |
| **High exudate** | |
| Absorb and contain exudate | Alginates |
| Prevent dressing adherence in areas of lesion | Foams |
| with decreased exudate | Starch copolymers |
| | Gauze |
| | Soft cotton pads |
| | Menstrual pads (excessive exudate) |
| **Malodorous wounds** | |
| Wound cleansing (see text) | Charcoal dressings |
| Reduce or eliminate odor | Topical metronidazole (see text) |
| | Iodosorb Gel (Healthpoint): iodine-based, may cause burning |

exudating wounds may require a non-adherent contact layer to allow for atraumatic dressing removal. If dressings adhere to the wound on attempted removal, they should be soaked away with normal saline to lessen the trauma to the wound bed. If bleeding does occur, the first intervention should be direct pressure applied for 10 to 15 minutes. Local ice packs may also assist in controlling bleeding. If pressure alone is ineffective, several other options exist.[45,46] Application of an alginate dressing or sucralfate paste (1 g sucralfate tablet crushed in 5 mL water-soluble gel) may stop mild bleeding. Gauze soaked with 1:1000 epinephrine applied to the wound may control bleeding, but can lead to local tissue necrosis. Small bleeding points can be controlled with silver nitrate sticks. As an alternative, use of topical, absorbable hemostatic agents made from gelatin, collagen, and/or oxidized regenerated cellulose (e.g., Gelfoam*, Surgicel*, Promogran*) may be appropriate, but are costly. More aggressive therapy may be necessary in cases of significant bleeding,[46] including transcatheter embolization of the arteries feeding the tumor,[47] intraarterial infusion chemotherapy and radiotherapy,[48,49] or surgery if compatible with palliative care goals of the patient. Oral fibrinolytic inhibitors, such as tranexamic acid or aminocaproic acid have been used in the palliative management of cancer-associated bleeding[50] and have been used topically in patients with hemophilia.[51] Clinicians should not hesitate to consider these options if they will improve the quality of life in patients with malignant wounds.

*Pain Management.* Several types of pain are associated with tumor malignant wounds: deep pain, neuropathic pain, and superficial pain related to procedures.[18] Deep pain should be managed by pre-medication before dressing changes. Opioids for pre-procedural medication may be needed, and rapid-onset, short-acting analgesics may be especially useful for those already receiving other long-acting opioid medication. For management of superficial pain related to procedures, topical lidocaine or benzocaine may be helpful.[52] These local analgesics may be applied to the wound immediately after dressing removal, with wound care delayed until adequate local anesthesia is obtained. Ice packs used before or after wound care may also be helpful to reduce pain.

Another option for topical analgesia is the use of topical opioids, which bind to peripheral opioid receptors.[52-54] Back and Finlay[55] reported on the use of diamorphine 10 mg added to an amorphous hydrogel and applied to the wounds of three patients on a daily basis. Two of the patients had painful pressure ulcers, and the third had a painful malignant ulcer. All three were receiving systemic opioid therapy. The patients noted improved pain control on the first day of treatment. Zeppetella et al.[56] demonstrated efficacy of topically applied morphine sulfate 10 mg/mL in 8 g amorphous hydrogel in the treatment of five hospice patients with painful pressure ulcers. The results of this pilot study were later validated in a larger randomized controlled study.[57] Sixteen hospice inpatients with painful pressure or malignant wounds were randomized to receive topical morphine as described above or placebo (water for injection 1 mL in 8 g amorphous hydrogel) to their wounds. After 2 days of treatment, patients entered a 2-day washout period and then were crossed over to the opposite group for two more days. Patients assigned a numerical rating score to the analgesia that they obtained in each 2-day period, the lower score indicating better pain relief. Topically applied morphine provided significantly lower scores compared to pre-treatment and placebo ($P <$ 0.001) and was well tolerated. Lastly, Ballas[58] noted success in treating two patients with painful sickle cell ulcers using either topical crushed oxycodone or meperidine. Topical opioids may be a viable adjunct to systemic analgesia in the care of patients with malignant wounds.

### Adjunctive Therapies

Palliative care of the patient with a malignant wound may include surgical debulking of fungating masses and/or resection of new nodules, or chemotherapy, radiotherapy, and/or radiofrequency ablation for tumor shrinkage and pain control.[46,59–61] Topical chemotherapy regimens can also help to shrink the tumor and thus ease local care.[62] Although these interventions will not cure patients of their advanced cancers, they may extend life, ease pain and bleeding, and improve quality of life. Patients with malignant wounds should be referred for these treatments if compatible with the palliative goals of care.

### Promotion of Patient and Caregiver Welfare Through Education

Dealing with a cancer diagnosis is traumatic enough without the added physical and psychological burden of a malignant wound.[63] Lo et al.[64] interviewed ten patients with malignant fungating wounds to examine how this condition affected their lives. Central issues that negatively affected quality of life were pain, social isolation secondary to exudate and odor, and ignorance of both patients and health care providers regarding appropriate wound care. It was concluded that the key to improving quality of life for these patients was access to a wound care team or specialist who educated them on how to care for the wound with appropriate dressings, and how to control exudate and odor. Education must also focus on the psychosocial aspects of having a malignant wound. Patients may experience grief, anxiety, embarrassment, stigma and may withdraw from loved ones.[65,66] Caregivers may experience feelings of helplessness and fear about caring for the patient. The nurse can facilitate a trusting relationship with the patient and caregivers by reviewing the goals of care and by openly discussing issues that the patient may not have talked about with other providers. For example, it is helpful to acknowledge odor openly and then discuss how the odor will be managed. Attention to the cosmetic appearance of the wound with the dressing in place can assist the patient in dealing with body image disturbances. Use of soft flexible dressings that can fill a defect and protect clothing may help to restore symmetry and provide security for the patient.

Assisting the patient and the caregiver to cope with the distressing symptoms of the malignant wound such that odor and bleeding is managed, exudate is contained, and pain is alleviated, will improve the quality of life for these patients and contribute to the goal of satisfactory psychological well-being. Education must include realistic goals for the wound. In these patients, the goal of complete wound healing is seldom achievable; however, quality of life can be maintained even as the wound degenerates. Continual education and re-evaluation of the effectiveness of the treatment plan are essential to maintaining quality of life for those suffering from a malignant wound.

# FISTULAS

### Definition

A fistula is an abnormal passage or opening between two or more body organs or spaces. The most frequently involved organs are the skin and either the bladder or the digestive tract, although fistulas can occur between many other body organs and/or spaces. Often, the organs involved and the location of the fistula in difficult anatomic areas or open abdominal wounds influence management methods and complicate care. For example, fistulas involving the small bowel and the vaginal vault and those involving the esophagus and skin create extreme challenges in care related to both the location and the organs involved in the fistula. Although spontaneous closure occurs in at least 50% of all enteric or small-bowel fistulas, the time required to achieve closure is 4 to 7 weeks, so long-term treatment plans are required for all patients with fistulas. Ninety percent of those fistulas that close spontaneously do so within the 4- to 7-week time frame.[67] Therefore, if the fistula has not spontaneously closed with adequate medical treatment within 7 weeks, the goal of care may change to palliation, particularly if chances of closure are limited by other factors. Factors that inhibit fistula closure include complete disruption of bowel continuity, distal obstruction, presence of a foreign body in the fistula tract, an epithelium-lined tract contiguous with the skin, presence of cancer, previous radiation, and Crohn's disease. The presence of any of these factors can be deleterious for spontaneous closure of a fistula. The goals of management for fistula care involve containment of effluent, management of odor, comfort, and protection of the surrounding skin and tissues.

### Pathophysiology of Fistula Development

In cancer care, those with gastrointestinal cancers and those who have received irradiation to pelvic organs are at highest risk for fistula development. Fistula development occurs in 1% of patients with advanced malignancy.[67] In most cases of advanced malignancy, the fistula develops in relation to either obstruction from the malignancy or irradiation side effects. Radiation therapy damages the vasculature and underlying structures. In cancer-related fistula development, management is almost always palliative. However, fistula development is not limited to patients with cancer.

In addition to cancer and radiation therapy, postsurgical adhesions, inflammatory bowel disease (Crohn's disease), and small-bowel obstruction place an individual at high risk for fistula development. The number one cause of fistula development is postsurgical adhesions. Adhesions are scar tissues that cause fistula development by providing an obstructive process within the normal passageway. Enterocutaneous fistulas also arise as complications in 0.8%–2% of abdominal operations.[68] The incidence of fistula development as a result of abdominal surgery has declined due to techniques of modern wound management using plastic barriers to protect exposed viscera and topical negative pressure on the soft tissues in open abdominal wounds.[68–71] Further, the use of biological dressings like human acellular dermal matrix and fibrin glue to help seal the orifice of acute fistula has helped support early fistual closure.[72–74]. Unfortunately, once an enterocutaneous fistula develops, mortality remains 10%–30%.[68] Those with inflammatory bowel disease—Crohn's disease in particular—are prone to fistula development by virtue of the effects of the disease process on the bowel itself. Crohn's disease often involves the perianal area, with fissures and fistulas being common findings. Because Crohn's disease is a transmural disease, involving all layers of the bowel wall, patients are prone to fistula development. Crohn's disease can occur anywhere along the entire gastrointestinal tract, and there is no known cure. Initially, the disease is managed medically with steroids, immunotherapy, and metronidazole for perianal disease. If medical management fails, the patient may be treated with surgical creation of a colostomy, to remove the portion of bowel affected by the disease. In later stages of disease, if medical and surgical management have failed, multiple fistulas may present clinically, and the goal for care becomes living with the fistulas and palliation of symptoms.

Other factors contributing to fistula development include the presence of a foreign body next to a suture line, tension on a suture line, improper suturing technique, distal obstruction, hematoma/abscess formation, tumor or additional disease in anastomotic sites, and inadequate blood supply. Each of these can contribute to fistula formation by promoting an abnormal passage between two body organs. Typically, the contributing factor provides a tract for easier evacuation of stool or urine along the tract rather than through the normal route. Such is the case with a foreign body next to the suture line and with hematoma or abscess formation. In some cases, the normal passageway is blocked, as with tumor growth or obstructive processes. Finally, in many cases, the pathology relates to inadequate tissue perfusion, as with tension on the suture line, improper suturing, and inadequate blood supply.

**Fistula Assessment**

Assessment of the fistula involves assessment of the source, surrounding skin, output, and fluid and electrolyte status. Evaluation of the fistula source may involve diagnostic tests such as radiographs to determine the exact structures involved in the fistula tract. Assessment of the fistula source involves evaluation of fistula output, or effluent, for odor, color, consistency, pH, and amount. These characteristics provide clues to the origin of the output. Fistulas with highly odorous output are likely to originate in the colon or may be related to cancerous lesions. Fistula output with less odor may have a small-bowel origin. The color of fistula output also provides clues to the source: clear or white output is typical of esophageal fistulas, green output is usual of fistulas originating from the gastric area, and light brown or tan output may indicate small-bowel sources. Small-bowel output is typically thin and watery to thick and pasty in consistency, whereas colonic fistulas have output with a pasty to a soft consistency. The volume of output is often an indication of the source. For small-bowel fistulas, output is typically high, with volumes ranging from 500 to 3000 mL over 24 hours, for low-output and high-output fistulas, respectively. Esophageal fistula output may be as high as 1000 mL over 24 hours. Fistulas can be classified according to output, with those producing less than 500 mL over 24 hours classified as low output and those producing greater volumes classified as high output.[67]

The anatomical orifice location, proximity of the orifice to bony prominences, the regularity and stability of the surrounding skin, the number of fistula openings, and the level at which the fistula orifice exits onto the skin influence treatment options. Fistulas may be classified according to the organs involved and the location of the opening of the fistula orifice. Fistulas with openings from one internal body organ to another (e.g., from small bowel to bladder, from bladder to vagina) are internal fistulas; those with cutaneous involvement (e.g., small bowel to skin) are external fistulas.[67]

The location of the fistula often impedes containment of output. Skin integrity should be assessed for erythema, ulceration, maceration, or denudation from fistula output. Typically, the more caustic the fistula output, the more impaired the surrounding skin integrity. Multiple fistula tracts may also impede containment efforts.

Assessment of fluid and electrolyte balance is essential because of the risk of imbalance in both. In particular, the patient with a small-bowel fistula is at high risk for fluid volume deficit or dehydration and metabolic acidosis due to the loss of large volumes of alkaline small-bowel contents. Significant losses of sodium and potassium are common with small-bowel fistulas. Laboratory values should be monitored frequently. Evaluation for signs of fluid volume deficit is also recommended.

**Fistula Management**

Wherever anatomically possible, the fistula should be managed with an ostomy pouching technique. The surrounding skin should be cleansed with warm water without soap or antiseptics; skin barrier paste should then be used to fill uneven skin surfaces, so that a flat surface is created to apply the pouch. Pediatric pouches are often smaller and more flexible and may be useful for hard-to-pouch areas where flexibility is needed, such as the neck for esophageal fistulas. The type of pouch should be chosen based on the output of the fistula. For example, if the fistula output is watery and thin, a pouch with a narrow spigot or tube for closure is chosen; in contrast, a fistula with a thick, pasty output would be better managed with a pouch with an open end and a closure clamp. Pouches must be emptied frequently, at least when one-third to one-half full. There are several wound drainage pouching systems on the market that allow for visualization and direct access to the fistula through a valve or door that can be opened and closed. These wound management pouches are available in large sizes and often work well for abdominal fistulas. Pouching of the fistula allows for odor control (many fistulas are quite malodorous), containment of output, and protection of the surrounding skin from damage. Gauze dressings with or without charcoal filters may be used if the output from the fistula is less than 250 mL over 24 hours and is not severely offensive in odor. Colostomy caps (small closed-end pouches) can be useful for low-output fistulas that continue to be odorous.

There are specific pouching techniques that are useful in complex fistula management, including troughing, saddlebagging, and bridging. These techniques are particularly helpful when dealing with fistulas that occur in wounds, most commonly the small-bowel fistula that develops in the open abdominal wound. Troughing is useful for fistulas that occur in the posterior aspect of large abdominal wounds.[75] The skin surrounding the wound and fistula should be lined with a skin barrier wafer and the edge nearest the wound sealed with skin barrier paste. Then, thin film dressings are applied over the top or anterior aspect of the wound, down to the fistula orifice and the posterior aspect of the wound. Finally, a cut-to-fit ostomy pouch is used to pouch the opening in the thin film dressing at the fistula orifice. Wound exudate drains from the anterior portion of the wound (under the thin film dressing) to the posterior portion of the wound and out into the ostomy pouch, along with fistula output. The trough technique does not prevent fistula output from contaminating the wound site.

The bridging technique prevents fistula output from contaminating the wound site and allows for a unique wound dressing to be applied to the wound site. Bridging is appropriate for fistulas that occur in the posterior aspect of large abdominal wounds, where it is important to contain fistula output away from the wound site. Using small pieces of skin barrier wafers, the clinician builds a "bridge" by consecutively layering the skin barriers together until the skin barrier has the appearance of a wedge or bridge and is the same height as the depth of the wound.[67] With the use of a skin barrier paste, the skin barrier wedge is adhered to the wound bed (it does not harm the healthy tissues of the wound bed), next to the

fistula opening. An ostomy pouch is then cut to fit the fistula opening, using the wedge or bridge as a portion of intact surrounding skin to adhere the pouch.[67] The anterior aspect of the wound may then be dressed with the dressing of choice.

Saddlebagging is used for multiple fistulas, if it is important to keep the output from each fistula separated and the fistula orifices are close together. Two cut-to-fit ostomy pouches (or more for more fistulas) are used. The fistula openings are cut on the back of the pouch, off-center, or as far to the side as possible, and the second pouch is cut to fit the next fistula, off-center, or as far to the other side as possible. The skin is cleansed with warm water, and skin barrier paste is applied around the orifices. Ostomy pouches are applied and, where they contact each other (down the middle), they are affixed or adhered to each other in a "saddlebag" fashion. Multiple fistulas can also be managed with one ostomy pouching system that accommodates the multiple openings. Consultation with an enterostomal therapy (ET) nurse or ostomy nurse is extremely advantageous in these cases.

Another method of managing fistulas is by a closed suction wound drainage system. Jeter and colleagues[76] described the use of a Jackson-Pratt drain and continuous low suction in fistula management. After the wound is cleansed with normal saline, the fenestrated Jackson-Pratt drain is placed in the wound, on top of a moistened gauze that has been opened up to line the wound bed (primary contact layer); a second fluffed wet gauze is placed over the drain, and the surrounding skin is prepared with a skin sealant. Next, the entire site is covered with a thin film dressing, which is crimped around the tube of the drain where it exits the wound. The tube exit site is filled with skin barrier paste, and the drain is connected to low continuous wall suction; the connection site may need to be adjusted and may require use of a small "Christmas tree" connector or device and tape to secure it. Jeter and colleagues[76] advised changing the system every 3 to 5 days. Others have used a similar setup for pharyngocutaneous fistulas.[77]

Negative pressure wound therapy (NPWT) devices present an easier method of closed suction and have also been used for fistual management.[68-70] In certain circumstances, NPWT may help to promote healing in wounds with an enteric fistula. Candidates must have a fistula that has been examined/explored and the fistula opening must be readily visualized and accessible. The patient must be receiving nothing by mouth, on total parenteral nutrition with fistula effluent that is thin to viscous. In most cases, fistulas managed by NPWT occur in open abdominal wounds and use of NPWT assists with both fistula closure and wound healing.[68-70] Use of NPWT in open abdominal wounds with fistula formation should be used with caution, as there have been reports of new fistula formation after wound closure and an associated high mortality rate in these cases.

Pouches to contain the fistula output usually assist in containing odor as well. If odor continues to be problematic with an intact pouching system, internal body deodorants such as bismuth subgallate, charcoal compositions, or peppermint oil may be helpful.[78] Taking care to change the pouch in a well-ventilated room also helps with odor. If odor is caused by anaerobic bacteria, use of 400 mg metronidazole orally three times a day may be helpful. Management of high-output fistulas may be improved with administration of octreotide 300 mcg subcutaneously over 24 hours.[67]

Nutrition management and fluid and electrolyte maintenance are essential for adequate fistula care. Fluid and nutritional requirements may be greatly increased with fistulas, and there are difficulties with fistulas that involve the gastrointestinal system. As a general guideline, the intestinal system should be used whenever possible for nutritional support. If nutrition can bypass the fistula site, absorption and tolerance are better with use of the intestinal tract. For small-bowel fistulas, bypass of the fistula orifice is not always feasible. If the small-bowel fistula is located distally, enough of the intestinal tract may be available to adequately absorb nutrients before the fistula orifice is reached. If the fistula is located more proximally, there may not be enough intestinal tract available for nutrient absorption ahead of the fistula orifice. Many of these patients must be given intravenous hyperalimentation during the early stages of fistula management. The specific goals of fluid and electrolyte and nutritional support for fistula management must be discussed with the patient and family in view of the palliative nature of the overall care plan.

### Patient and Caregiver Education

Patient and caregiver teaching first involves adequate assessment of the self-care ability of the patient and of the caregiver's abilities. The patient and caregiver must be taught the management method for the fistula, including pouching techniques, how to empty the pouch, odor control methods, and strategies for increasing fluid and nutritional intake. Many of the pouching techniques used to manage fistulas are complicated and may require continual surveillance by an expert such as an ET nurse or ostomy nurse.

## PALLIATIVE STOMA CARE

The significance of palliative care for an individual with a stoma is to improve well-being during this critical time and to attain the best quality of life possible. In regard to the stoma, palliative care is achieved by restoring the most efficient management plan and providing optimal functional capacity. It is essential to involve the family in the plan of care and to provide care to the extent of the patient's wishes.

Management of the ostomy includes physical care as well as psychological and social care. To meet the needs of the patient and family, access to the multidisciplinary care team is crucial. This team may include the ET nurse, physicians such as the surgeon and oncologist, a nutritionist, and social service personnel. The urinary or fecal stoma can be managed (by the ET nurse) to incorporate the needs and goals of both the patient and the caregiver and to provide the highest quality of life possible.

### Pathophysiology

A stoma is an artificial opening in the abdominal wall that is surgically created to allow urine or stool to be eliminated by an alternative route. The most common indications for the creation of a stoma are as follows:

1. Cancers that interfere with the normal function of the urinary or gastrointestinal system.
2. Inflammatory bowel diseases such as Crohn's or ulcerative colitis.
3. Congenital diseases such as Hirschsprung's disease or familial adenomatous polyposis.
4. Trauma.

In planning the care of an individual with a stoma, it is necessary to understand the type of ostomy that was created, including the contents that will be eliminated.

### Types of Diversion

The three types of diversion created with a stoma as the outlet for urine or stool are the ileoconduit (urinary output), the ileostomy (fecal output), and the colostomy (fecal output). Construction of any of these diversions requires the person to wear an external appliance to collect the output.

*Ileoconduit.* Since the early 1950s, the Bricker ileoconduit has been the primary method for diverting urinary flow in the absence of bladder function. This procedure involves isolation of a section of the terminal ileum. The proximal end is closed, and the distal end is brought out through an opening in the abdominal wall at a site selected before surgery. The ileal segment is sutured to the skin, creating a stoma. The ureters are implanted into the ileal segment, urine flows into the conduit, and peristalsis propels the urine out through the stoma. An external appliance is worn to collect the urine; it is emptied when the pouch is one-third to one-half full, or approximately every 4 hours.

*Ileostomy.* The ileostomy is created to divert stool away from the large intestine, typically using the terminal ileum. The stoma is created by bringing the distal end of the ileum through an opening surgically created in the abdominal wall and suturing it to the skin. The output is usually a soft, unformed to semi-formed stool. Approximately 600 to 800 mL/day is eliminated. An external appliance is worn to collect the fecal material; it is emptied when the bag is one-third to one-half full, usually four to six times per day.

An ileostomy may be temporary or permanent. A temporary ileostomy usually is created when the colon needs time to heal or rest, such as after colon surgery or a colon obstruction. A permanent ileostomy is necessary if the entire colon, rectum, and anus has been surgically removed, such as in colorectal cancer or Crohn's disease.[78]

*Colostomy.* The colostomy is created proximal to the affected segment of the colon or rectum. A colostomy may be temporary or permanent. There are three sections of the colon: the ascending, transverse, and descending colon. The section of colon used to create the stoma determines in part the location and the consistency of output, which may affect the nutritional and hydration status of the individual at critical times. The ascending colon stoma usually is created on the right midquadrant of the abdomen, and the output is a semi-formed stool. The transverse stoma is created in the upper quadrants and is the largest stoma created; the output is usually a semi-formed to formed stool. The descending colon stoma most closely mirrors the activity of normal bowel function; it usually is located in the lower left quadrant.

The stoma is created by bringing the distal end of the colon through an opening surgically created in the abdominal wall and suturing it to the skin. An external appliance is worn to collect the fecal material; it is emptied when the bag is one-third to one-half full, usually one or two times per day. A second option for management is irrigation, to regulate the bowel. The patient is taught to instill 600 to 1000 mL of luke-warm tap water through the stoma, using a cone-shaped irrigation apparatus. This creates bowel distention, stimulating peristaltic activity and therefore elimination within 30 to 45 minutes. Repetition of this process over time induces bowel dependence on the stimulus, reducing the spillage of stool between irrigations. The elimination process after initial evacuation is suppressed for 24 to 48 hours.[79,80]

## Assessment

*Stoma Characteristics.* Viability of the stoma is assessed by its color. This should be checked regularly, especially in the early postoperative period. Normal color of the stoma is deep pink to deep red. The intestinal stomal tissue can be compared with the mucosal lining of the mouth. The stoma may bleed when rubbed because of the capillaries at the surface. Bleeding that occurs spontaneously or excessively from stoma trauma can usually be managed by the application of pressure. Bleeding that persists or that originates from the bowel requires prompt investigation, with the management plan based on the cause of the bleeding and the overall status of the individual.[79,80]

A stoma with a dusky appearance ranging from purple to black, or a necrotic appearance, indicates impairment of circulation and should be reported to the surgeon. A necrotic stoma may develop from abdominal distention that causes tension on the mesentery, from twisting of the intestine at the time of surgery, or from arterial or venous insufficiency. Necrotic tissue below the level of the fascia indicates infarction and potential intra-abdominal urine or stool leakage. Prompt recognition and surgical reexploration are necessary.

Stoma edema is normal in the early postoperative period as a result of surgical manipulation. This should not interfere with stoma functioning, but a larger opening will need to be cut in the appliance to prevent pressure or constriction of the stoma. Most stomas decrease by 4 to 6 weeks after surgery, with minor changes over 1 year. Teaching the individual to continue to measure the stoma with each change of appliance should alleviate the problem of wearing an appliance with an aperture too large for the stoma. The stoma needs only a space one-eighth of an inch in diameter to allow for expansion during peristalsis.

Stoma herniation occurs when the bowel moves through the muscle defect created at the time of stoma formation and into the subcutaneous tissue. The hernia usually reduces spontaneously when the patient lies in a supine position, as a result of decreased intraabdominal pressure. Problems associated with the formation of a peristomal hernia are increased difficulty with ostomy pouch adherence and possible bowel strangulation and obstruction. The peristomal hernia may be managed conservatively with the use of a peristomal hernia belt to maintain a reduction of the hernia. The belt is an abdominal binder with an opening to allow for the stoma and pouch. The belt is applied with the patient in a supine position, while the hernia is reduced, creating an external pressure that maintains the bowel in a reduced position. Aggressive treatment includes surgical intervention for correction of the peristomal hernia. However, this is usually reserved for emergency situations, such as obstruction or strangulation of the bowel. Colostomy patients who irrigate should be taught to irrigate with the hernia in a reduced position, to prevent perforation of the bowel.

Stoma prolapse occurs as a result of a weakened abdominal wall caused by abdominal distention, formation of a loop stoma, or a large aperture in the abdominal wall. The prolapse is a telescoping of the intestine through the stoma. Stoma prolapse may be managed by conservative or surgical intervention. Surgical intervention is required if there is bowel ischemia, bowel obstruction, or prolapse of excessive length and unreducible segment of bowel. Conservative management includes reducing the stoma while in a supine position to decrease the intraabdominal pressure, then applying continuous gentle pressure at the distal portion of the prolapse until the stoma returns to skin level. If the stoma is edematous, cold soaks or a hypertonic solution such as salt or sugar is applied to reduce the edema before stoma reduction is attempted. Once the stoma is reduced, a support binder is applied to prevent recurrence. In most cases, it is necessary to alter the pouching system by including a two-piece appliance and cutting the barrier size opening larger to accommodate changes in stoma size.

Retraction of the stoma below skin level can occur in the early postoperative period due to tension on the bowel or mesentery or related to breakdown at the mucocutaneous junction. Late retraction usually occurs as a result of tension on the bowel from abdominal distention, most likely as a result of intraperitoneal tumor growth or ascites. Stomal retraction is managed by modification of the pouching system—for example, by using a convex appliance to accommodate changes in skin contour. Stomas that retract below the fascia level require prompt surgical intervention.

Stenosis of the stoma can occur at the skin level or at the level of the fascia. Stenosis that interferes with normal bowel elimination requires intervention. Signs and symptoms of stenosis include change in bowel habits (e.g., decreased output, thin-caliber stools), abdominal cramping, abdominal distention, flank pain from urinary stomas, and nausea or vomiting. The stenotic area may be managed conservatively by dilatation or may require surgical intervention by local excision or laporatomy.[79,80] Many of the stoma problems discussed can occur from simple stretching and displacement of normal organs due to bulky tumors, as might occur in the end stages of some disease states.

*Peristomal Skin Problems.* Peristomal skin complications commonly include mechanical breakdown, chemical breakdown, rash, and allergic reaction. Mechanical breakdown is caused by trauma to the epidermal skin layer. This is most often related to frequent appliance changes that cause shearing or tearing to the epidermal skin. The result is denuded skin or erythematous, raw, moist, and painful skin. The use of pectin-based powder with or without a light coating of skin sealant aids in healing and protecting the skin from further damage, while allowing appliance adherence.

Chemical breakdown is caused by prolonged contact of urine or fecal effluent with the peristomal skin. Inappropriate use of adhesive skin solvents may also result in skin breakdown. The result of chemical breakdown is denudation of the peristomal skin that has been exposed to the caustic effects of the stool, urine, or adhesive solvents. Prompt recognition and management are essential. Modification of the pouching system, such as using a convex wafer instead of a flat wafer or adding protective skin products such as a paste (or both) can be used to correct the underlying problem. Instructing patients and caregivers to thoroughly cleanse the skin with plain water after using the skin solvent can eliminate the problem of denuded skin. Treatment of denuded skin is the same as described previously.

A peristomal fungal rash can occur as a result of excessive moisture or antibiotic administration that results in overgrowth of yeast in the bowel or, at the skin level, due to perspiration under a pouch or leakage of urine or stool under the barrier. The rash is characterized as having a macular, red border with a moist, red to yellow center; it is usually pruritic. Application of antifungal powder, such as nystatin powder, to the affected areas usually produces a prompt response. Blotting the powder with skin preparation or sealant may allow the pouching system to adhere more effectively.

Allergic reactions are most often caused by the barrier and tape used for the pouching system. Erythematous vesicles and pruritus characterize the area involved. Management includes removal of the offending agent. The distribution of the reaction can usually aid in defining the allergen. It may be necessary to perform skin testing if the causative agent is not clear. Patients with sensitive skin and those who use multiple products may respond to simple pouching techniques such as using water to clean the skin, patting the skin dry, and applying the wafer and pouch without the use of skin preparations. Changing to products from a different manufacturer may also eliminate the allergen. A nonadhesive pouching system may be used temporarily for patients with severe blistering and hypersensitivity, to allow healing and prevent further peristomal skin damage. Patients with severe blistering and pruritus may also require temporary use of systemic or topical antihistamines or corticosteriods.[79,80]

*Principles and Products for Pouching a Stoma.* The continuous outflow of urine or stool from the stoma requires the individual to wear an external appliance at all times. Ideally, the stoma protrudes one-half to three-fourths of an inch above the skin surface, to allow the urine or stool to drain efficiently into a pouch.[80] The objective of stoma management is to protect the peristomal skin, contain output, and control odor.

The skin around the stoma should be cleaned and thoroughly dried before the appliance is positioned over the stoma. An effective pouch should adhere for at least 3 days, although this is not always possible. If no leakage occurs, the same pouch may remain adhered to the skin for up to 10 days. It should then be changed for hygienic reasons and to observe the peristomal area. Today, there is an ever-changing supply of new appliances. Materials and design are being updated rapidly to provide the consumer with the best protection and easiest care.[81] Factors to consider when choosing a pouch include the consistency and type of effluent, the contour of the abdomen, the size and shape of the stoma, and the extent of protrusion, as a well as patient preferences.

Pouching systems are available as one-piece or two-piece systems. The one-piece system is constructed with the odor-proof pouch joined to a barrier ring that adheres to the skin. The barrier can be precut to the size of the stoma, or it can be customized with a cut-to-fit barrier. A two-piece system usually consists of an individual barrier with a flange ring and an odor-proof pouch, which attach (snap) together by matching the ring size of the barrier and pouch. The pouch barrier may be flat or convex and is chosen based on the contour of the abdomen and the extent of stoma protrusion. The colostomy pouch may be closed-ended or open-ended with a clip for closure. Some individuals choose to clean the pouch daily. The pouch of the one-piece system can be cleaned by instilling water into the pouch (with a syringe or turkey baster) and rinsing while preventing the water from reaching the stoma area. The pouch of the two-piece system can be cleaned daily by detaching and washing it in the sink with soap and water and drying it before reattaching it to the barrier.

The urinary pouch has a spout opening to allow for controlled emptying of the pouch. This end may also be attached to a bedside bag or bottle to collect urine. It typically holds up to 2000 mL of urine. The urinary system can be easily disassembled and cleaned with soap and water. After cleaning,

**Table 17B–3**
**Pouch Options**

| Type | Barrier | Odor-Proof Pouch |
|------|---------|------------------|
| 1-piece | Flat | Open end with clip (ileostomy with colostomy) |
| 2-piece | Convex | Closed end (colostomy) |
|  | Cut-to-fit | Spout opening (urostomy) |
|  | Precut |  |

a vinegar-and-water solution should be rinsed through the tubing and bag/bottle to prevent urine crystallization.

Skin barriers, skin sealants, powders such as Stomahesive powder or karaya powder, and pastes such as Stomahesive paste or karaya paste are available to protect the peristomal skin from the caustic affects of urine or stool. These products may also be used to aid in the healing of peristomal skin problems.

Belts and binders are available to assist in maintaining pouch adherence and for management of certain stoma problems.[80] Table 17B–3 presents an overview of pouching options for patients with fecal or urinary diversions.

## Interventions

*Prevention of Complications.* Stoma surgery performed as a palliative measure is not intended to provide a cure but, rather, to alleviate difficulties such as obstruction, pain, or severe incontinence. Unfortunately, at a difficult time in patients' and families' lives, the created stoma disrupts normal physical appearance, normal elimination of urine or stool, and control of elimination with, in some cases, loss of body parts and/or sexual function. The patient then has to learn to care for the stoma or allow someone else to care for them. Physically and psychologically, the patient has to come to terms with the presence of the stoma, its function, and care. This takes time and energy to cope emotionally, physically, and socially.[79,82]

Educating the patient and family regarding management issues related to ostomy care and palliation could assist in the physical and psychological adaptation to the ostomy. Additional therapies that may be required for treatment of the underlying disease or a new disease process, such as progressed or recurrent cancer, may affect the activity of the stoma or the peristomal skin. Additional therapies may include chemotherapy, radiation therapy, or analgesics for pain management.

Chemotherapy and radiation therapy may affect a fecal stoma by causing diarrhea. Associated symptoms include abdominal discomfort, larger quantities of loose or liquid stool produced per day, and potential dehydration and loss of appetite with prolonged diarrhea. The ostomy bag requires more frequent emptying, and the ostomy pouch seal needs to be monitored more closely for leakage. In addition, radiation therapy that includes the stoma in the radiation field

can cause peristomal skin irritation, particularly redness and maceration. The effects on the peristomal skin may be exacerbated by leakage of urine or stool, as described earlier.[79]

Analgesic use may result in constipation and ultimately bowel obstruction. It is necessary to coadminister stool softeners or laxatives for the prevention of constipation. Irrigation of the colostomy may also assist in treating constipation. The patient and family need to be instructed regarding these measures so that they can be used to treat and prevent constipation. The patient and family need to be aware that adequate pain relief and prevention of constipation can be achieved.[79,82]

Patients may become very tired or may experience anxiety, nausea, or pain as a result of their condition and palliative management. Patients often want to remain as independent as possible but may allow assistance from family and staff. For example, the patient may want to perform the actual pouch change but allow someone else to gather and prepare the supplies. This allows for conservation of energy during part of the task to be accomplished. The patient may also choose the time of day to perform such tasks—when he or she has the most energy and maximal pain and nausea control.[81]

*Nutrition and Hydration.* Anorexia and dehydration can be major problems for the patient with advancing disease or disease-related treatments such as chemotherapy and radiation therapy. Compromised ingestion, digestion, and absorption can have major influences on nutritional and hydration status.

*Anorexia* is the loss of appetite resulting from changes in gastrointestinal function, including changes in taste, changes in metabolism, psychological behaviors, and the effects of disease and treatment. Decreased oral intake and changes in metabolism, including decreased protein and fat metabolism, increased energy expenditure, and increased carbohydrate consumption, result in loss of muscle mass, loss of fat stores, and fatigue, leading to weight loss and malnutrition.[83]

Managing the underlying cause of poor nutritional and hydration status, such as controlling the cancer or disease, treating an infection, or slowing down the high-volume ileostomy output, can improve the nutritional state. However, despite effective treatment, other assistance may be necessary, such as small and more frequent meals, nutritional liquid supplements, appetite stimulants (e.g., megestrol acetate), corticosteroids, and parenteral or enteral support.[84] Foods and drinks need to be appealing to the patient. Strong odors and large-portion meals may result in appetite suppression. Promoting comfort before meals may also increase appetite; this may include administering antiemetics or analgesics, oral care, or resting for 30 minutes before mealtime.[84]

## Management Issues

Controlling odor, reducing gas, and preventing or managing diarrhea or constipation are management issues related to patients with a colostomy. Odor can be controlled by ensuring that the pouch seal is tight, that odor-proof pouches are used, and that a clean pouch opening is maintained. In addition, deodorants such as bismuth subgallate or chlorophyllin copper complex may be taken orally. Gas can be reduced by decreasing intake of gas-producing foods such as broccoli, cabbage, beans, and beer. Peppermint or chamomile tea may be effective in gas reduction.[79,82]

Diarrhea can be managed as in a patient with an intact rectum and anus. Diarrhea may be a result of viral illness or use of a chemotherapeutic agent. Management includes increased fluid intake, a low-fiber and low-fat diet, and administration of antidiarrhea medications such as loperamide (Imodium), bismuth subsalicylate (Pepto-Bismol), or diphenoxylate plus atropine (Lomotil) by prescription.[80,85] If the patient irrigates, it is necessary to hold irrigation until formed stools return. Constipation more commonly occurs in patients with advanced malignancies due to the affects of analgesic use, reduced activity level, and reduced dietary fiber intake. Management of constipation includes administration of laxatives such as milk of magnesia, mineral oil, or lactulose and initiation of a plan for prevention of constipation with use of stool softeners and laxatives as needed. Cleansing irrigation may be necessary for patients who normally do not irrigate. Cleansing irrigation is performed as described previously for individuals with a colostomy who irrigate for control of bowel movements.[80]

Skin protection, fluid and electrolyte maintenance, prevention of blockage, and modification of medications are management issues related to an ileostomy. Because of the high-volume liquid or loose stools, protecting the skin from this effluent is critical. Leakage of effluent can cause chemical skin breakdown and pain from the irritated skin. The ET nurse can work with the patient and family to determine the cause of the effluent leak. It may be necessary to modify the pouching system, to ensure a proper fit. The peristomal skin may need to be treated with a powder or skin sealant, or both, to aid in healing. The transit time of food and wastes through the gastrointestinal system and out through the ileostomy is rapid and potentially contributes to dehydration and fluid and electrolyte imbalance. Ensuring adequate fluid and electrolyte intake is essential and may be accomplished by ingestion of sports drinks or nutrition shakes. Patients with an ileostomy are instructed to include fiber in their diet, to bulk stools and promote absorption of nutrition and medications.

Food blockage occurs when undigested food particles or medications partially or completely obstruct the stoma outlet at the fascia level. It is necessary to instruct the patient and family about the signs of a blockage, including malodorous, high-volume liquid output or no output accompanied by abdominal cramping, distention, and/or nausea and vomiting. These symptoms should be reported as soon as they occur. Blockage is resolved by lavage or mini-irrigation performed by the physician or ET nurse. A catheter is gently inserted into the stoma until the blockage is reached, 30 to 60 mL of normal saline is instilled, and the catheter is removed to allow for the return. This process is repeated until the blockage has

resolved. Patient teaching should be reinforced regarding the need to chew food well before swallowing, to prevent food blockage. Time-release tablets and enteric-coated medications should be avoided because of inadequate or unpredictable absorption. Medications often come in various forms, including liquid, noncoated, patch, rectal suppository, and subcutaneous or intravenous administration. Choosing the most appropriate route that provides the greatest efficacy for the individual is essential. For example, a transdermal patch may be used for analgesia instead of a time-released pain tablet. For patients who have an intact rectum that is no longer in continuity with the proximal bowel, rectal administration of medications is effective.[85]

Management issues for an individual with an ileoconduit include prevention of a urinary tract infection, stone formation, peristomal skin protection, and odor control. Each of these issues is preventable by the maintenance of dilute and acidic urine through adequate fluid intake (1800 to 2400 mL/day). Vitamin C (500 to 1000 mg/day) and citrus fruits and drinks may assist in accomplishing acidic urine. Alkaline urine can cause encrustations on the stoma and peristomal skin damage with prolonged exposure. Acetic acid soaks may be applied three or four times per day to treat the encrustations until they dissolve. Adjustments in the pouching system may be necessary to prevent leakage of urine onto the skin, and the temporary addition of powder, paste, skin sealant, or some combination of these products may be needed to aid healing of the affected skin.[80]

### CASE STUDY
#### Wound Care in a Woman with Breast Cancer and a Fungating Ulcerative Lesion of Her Chest

A 64-year-old woman was referred to the wound clinic for assessment and management of wounds on the left anterior chest wall, shoulder, upper arm, and upper abdomen. She had a history of a left modified radical mastectomy for breast cancer, followed by local radiation therapy and chemotherapy six years prior. About two years prior to being referred to the wound clinic, she developed painless nodules on the left anterior chest. Biopsy revealed a local recurrence of breast cancer. She was started on a course of chemotherapy, but despite this, the lesions spread to her upper abdomen and left shoulder and upper arm. The left anterior chest wall eventually ulcerated and drained. Her main complaints to the nurse practitioner (NP) were exudate that leaked through her clothing during the day and her nightgown at night, and odor. She said that she had stopped meeting her girlfriends for their weekly lunch because of her embarrassment over this. She shared that she was quite disgusted by the lesions and was very afraid to touch them, so she would just lightly dab them with water to clean them and would cover the chest wounds with gauze in her bra, and tape gauze over the lesions on her abdomen. The nodules on the shoulder and upper arm were not draining, and she questioned whether or not she could have these surgically removed.

Assessment revealed a 12 x 8 cm irregularly shaped ulcerative lesion on the left chest wall with fungating tissue along the wound edges that was mildly friable. There was a moderate amount of serous exudate from this wound and mild to moderate odor. Surrounding skin was thin, mildly erythematous, and fragile. There were multiple nodules, some of which were coalesced, on her upper abdomen. Some had dry crust on their surface, but no apparent exudate. There were a few isolated, non-draining nodules on her left shoulder and upper arm.

She had continuous aching, vise-like pain in the left chest wall which she rated a 5–8 on a scale of 0–10. She only used acetaminophen for this, strongly refusing to take narcotics, stating that she did not want to get "hooked on drugs." Her husband, who accompanied her, was very concerned about his wife's uncontrolled pain, and he stated that he was available to help in any way that he could.

Goals of care included exudate and odor control, and pain management. A long discussion about palliative goals of care was undertaken. The nurse practitioner concentrated on what could be done (exudate, odor, pain control) vs. what could not be offered (permanent cure). The hope for quality of life with return to her social activities (which the patient stated she desired) was promoted. The patient's fears about touching the wound were also explored. With the NP's confidence that the patient could learn how to take care of the wound, she agreed to try. The patient was instructed regarding daily care:

1. Spray wound/incontinence cleanser on ulcerative wound and on surrounding skin.
2. Stand in shower and allow water to hit the skin above the wound and rinse over it.
3. Pat area dry with clean towel or paper towels or gauze.
4. Apply thin coat (the thinness of a dime) of metronidazole gel to the ulcerative wound on the chest.
5. Cover wound edges with petrolatum-impregnated contact layer (Adaptic™)
6. Cover wound area with two large ABD pads and secure with boy's-size tank top (this ended up being more comfortable than the bra). Small squares of paper tape were applied to a few areas of the ABD pad that contacted healthy skin.
7. Cover crusted abdominal lesions with ABD pad to protect from friction from clothing, and secure with paper tape.
8. No dressings were needed on the shoulder nodules and the patient preferred not to cover them with dressings. If she would have preferred coverage, soft gauze or an ABD pad could have been used.

The NP, patient, and husband had a long philosophical discussion about use of narcotics for pain management. The benefits of adequate pain management were discussed including the ability to enjoy activities, sleep better, and generally feel better. Misconceptions about opiate addiction vs. dependence were cleared up and the patient agreed to try some hydrocodone with acetaminophen, 5/500, 1–2 tabs every 4 hours as needed for pain.

The NP believed that it was entirely reasonable for the patient to have the discreet nodules on the left shoulder and upper arm removed. The patient was instructed that they might or might not return. She was referred back to her surgeon, who removed them, sutured the skin together, and she healed uneventfully.

The patient returned to the wound clinic two weeks later for a recheck. She was in better spirits and reported a complete cessation in the odor, good control of exudate, and much better pain control. She actually had plans to meet her friends for lunch, and because she was still concerned about exudate leakage, it was suggested that she use unscented menstrual pads over the chest wound instead of the ABD pads. She was grateful that the NP had "nagged" her about the pain management and acknowledged that she was sleeping better and feeling more rested. She appeared to have more hope that she could have some quality of life.

She was seen every month thereafter. At one point, her odor was so well controlled that she stopped the metronidazole gel and just used the skin cleanser with daily showers. This resulted in satisfactory odor control. She eventually started long-acting morphine for pain, and this led to a significant improvement in overall comfort.

The ulcer on the chest eventually eroded so that a rib was exposed. Six months after treatment started in the wound clinic, she had an episode of significant bleeding from the wound, which could not be stopped. She was sent to interventional radiology and underwent successful intra-arterial embolization of the artery feeding the tumor in her chest wall. At her next wound clinic visit, she was very afraid of further bleeding, and did complain of mild oozing from the wound edges. She and her husband were reassured and given written and verbal instructions regarding a stepwise approach for local control of bleeding:

1. Rest in a reclined position with the chest elevated.
2. Apply local pressure with water-moistened gauze for 10–15 minutes.
3. If still bleeding, apply collagen/oxidized regenerated cellulose dressing (Promogran*) to the area and hold pressure for 15 minutes.
4. If still bleeding, apply ice packs for 15–20 minutes.
5. May spot-treat bleeding areas with silver nitrate (the husband was competent to do this).
6. Contact wound clinic if these measures fail.
7. For severe bleeding, go to ER (this was compatible with the patient's wishes as she still wanted aggressive care).

Thereafter, the patient had mild episodes of bleeding but reported that she and her husband felt confident in their ability to control this with the instructions provided.

Although she did slow down in her remaining months, she remained fairly active until a week before her death, which occurred 11 months after first being seen at the wound clinic. She finally accepted hospice, and was able to die at home with her loved ones at her side. Her husband later called the NP and thanked her for helping them to cope with the wounds, stating that just knowing how to take care of them and what to expect had decreased their stress significantly and helped his wife have some quality and happiness in her last year of life.

༞༞

༞༞

## Summary

Skin disorders are both emotionally and physically challenging for patients and caregivers. Cutaneous symptoms may be the result of disease progression (e.g., malignant wounds, fistula development), complications associated with end-stage disease or the end of life (e.g., pressure ulcers), or simple changes in function of urinary or fecal diversions. All cutaneous symptoms require attention to basic care issues, creativity in management strategies, and thoughtful attention to the psychosocial implications of cutaneous manifestations. Palliative care intervention strategies for skin disorders reflect an approach similar to those for nonpalliative care. Although the goals of care do not include curing the condition, they always include alleviating the distressing symptomology and improving quality of life. The most distressing symptoms associated with skin disorders are odor, exudate, and pain. The importance of attention to skin disorders for palliative care is related to the major effect of these conditions on the quality of life and general psychological well-being of the patient.

REFERENCES

1. Lookingbill DP, Spangler N, Sexton FM. Skin involvement as the presenting sign of internal carcinoma. J Am Acad Dermatol 1990;22:19–26.
2. Lookingbill DP, Spangler N, Helm KF. Cutaneous metastases in patients with metastatic carcinoma: A retrospective study of 4020 patients. J Am Acad Dermatol 1993;29:228–236.
3. Ambrogi V, Nofroni I, Tonini G, Mineo TC. Skin metastasis in lung cancer: Analysis of a 10-year experience. Oncol Rep 2001;8:57–61.
4. Mueller TJ, Wu H, Greenberg RE, et al. Cutaneous metastases from genitourinary malignancies. Urology 2004;63:1021–1026.
5. Saeed S, Keehn CA, Morgan MB. Cutaneous metastasis: A clinical, pathological, and immunohistochemical appraisal. J Cutan Pathol 2004;31:419–430.
6. Brodland DG, Zitelli JA. Mechanisms of metastasis. J Am Acad Dermatol 1992;27:1–8.
7. Marcoval J, Moreno A, Peyri J. Cutaneous infiltration by cancer. J Am Acad Dermatol 2007;57:577–580.
8. Cormio G, Capotorto M, Di Vagno G, Cazzolla A, Carriero C, Selvaggi L. Skin metastases in ovarian carcinoma: A report of nine cases and a review of the literature. Gynecol Oncol 2003;90:682–685.
9. Pitman KT, Johnson JT. Skin metastases from head and neck squamous cell carcinoma: Incidence and impact. Head Neck 1999;21:560–565.
10. Carroll MC, Fleming M, Chitambar CR, Neuburg M. Diagnosis, workup, and prognosis of cutaneous metastases of unknown primary origin. Dermatol Surg 2002;28:533–535.
11. Ivetic O, Lyne PA. Fungating and ulcerating malignant lesions: A review of the literature. J Adv Nurs 1990;15:83–88.
12. Schwartz RA. Cutaneous metastatic disease. J Am Acad Dermatol 1995;33:161–182.
13. Cohen PR. Skin clues to primary and metastatic malignancy. Am Fam Physician 1995;51:1199–1204.
14. Wilson V. Assessment and management of fungating wounds: A review. Br J Community Nurs 2005;10(3):S28–S34.
15. Hu SC, Chen GS, Lu YW, Wu CS, Lan CC. Cutaneous metastases from different internal malignancies: A clinical and prognostic appraisal. J Eur Acad Dermatol Venereol 2008;22:735–740.
16. Grocott P, Cowley S. The palliative management of fungating malignant wounds: Generalising from multiple-case study data using a system of reasoning. Int J Nurs Stud 2001;38:533–545.
17. Collier M. The assessment of patients with malignant fungating wounds—a holistic approach: Part 1. Nurs Times 1997;93(suppl):1–4.
18. Naylor W. Assessment and management of pain in fungating wounds. Br J Nurs 2001;10(22 Suppl):S33–S36, S38, S40.
19. Clark J. Metronidazole gel in managing malodorous fungating wounds. Br J Nurs 2002;11(6 Suppl):S54–S60.
20. Bowler PG, Davies BJ, Jones SA. Microbial involvement in chronic wound malodour. J Wound Care 1999;8:216–218.
21. Haisfield-Wolfe ME, Baxendale-Cox LM. Staging of malignant cutaneous wounds: A pilot study. Oncol Nurs Forum 1999;26:1055–1064.
22. Van Leeuwen BL, Houwerzijl M, Hoekstra HJ. Educational tips in the treatment of malignant ulcerating tumours of the skin. Eur J Surg Oncol 2000;26:506–508.
23. Lazalle-Ali C. Psychological and physical care of malodorous fungating wounds. Br J Nurs 2007;16(15):S16–S24.
24. Seaman S. Management of malignant fungating wounds in advanced cancer. Semin Oncol Nurs 2006;22:185–193.
25. Adderly U, Smith R. Topical agents and dressings for fungating wounds. Cochrane Database Syst Rev April 18, 2007;(2):CD003948.
26. Doughty D. Dressings and more: Guidelines for topical wound management. Nurs Clin N Am 2005;40:217–231.
27. Seaman S. Dressing selection in chronic wound management. J Am Podiatr Med Assoc 2002;92:24–33.
28. Whedon MA. Practice corner: What methods do you use to manage tumor-associated wounds? Oncol Nurs Forum 1995;22:987–990.
29. Gomolin IH, Brandt JL. Topical metronidazole therapy for pressure sores of geriatric patients. J Am Geriatr Soc 1983;31:710–712.
30. Poteete V. Case study: Eliminating odors from wounds. Decubitus 1993;6(4):43–46.
31. Finlay IG, Bowszyc J, Ramlau C, Gwiezdzinski Z. The effect of topical 0.75% metronidazole gel on malodorous cutaneous ulcers. J Pain Symptom Manage 1996;11:158–162.

32. Bale S, Tebble N, Price P. A topical metronidazole gel used to treat malodorous wounds. Br J Nurs 2004;13(11):S4–S11.

33. Kalinski C, Schnepf M, Laboy D, et al. Effectiveness of a topical formulation containing metronidazole for wound odor and exudate control. Wounds 2005;17(4):84–90.

34. Paul JC, Pieper BA. Topical metronidazole for the treatment of wound odor: A review of the literature. Ostomy Wound Manage 2008;54(3):18–27.

35. Danielsen L, Cherry GW, Harding K, Rollman O. Cadexomer iodine in ulcers colonised by pseudomonas aeruginosa. J Wound Care 1997;6:169.

36. Hampton S. Malodorous fungating wounds: How dressings alleviate symptoms. Br J Community Nurs 2008;13(6):S31–S32, S34, S36, S38.

37. Lo SF, Hayter M, Chang CJ, Hu WY, Lee LL. A systematic review of silver-releasing dressings in the management of infected chronic wounds. J Clin Nurs 2008;17:1973–1985.

38. Ovington LG. The truth about silver. Ostomy Wound Manage 2004;50(9A Suppl):1S–10S.

39. Acton C, Dunwoody G. The use of medical grade honey in clinical practice. Br J Nurs 2008;17:S38–S44.

40. Molan PC. The evidence supporting the use of honey as a wound dressing. Int J Low Extrem Wounds 2006;5(1):40–54.

41. Jull AB, Rodgers A, Walker. Honey as a topical treatment for wounds. Cochrane Database Syst Rev October 8, 2008;(4):CD005083.

42. Vermeulen H, van Hattem JM, Storm-Versloot MN, Ubbink DT. Topical silver for treating infected wounds. Cochrane Database Syst Rev January 24, 2007;(1):CD005486.

43. Schulte MJ. Yogurt helps to control wound odor. Oncol Nurs Forum 1993;20:1262.

44. Cormier AC, McCann E, McKeithan L. Reducing odor caused by metastatic breast cancer skin lesions. Oncol Nurs Forum 1995;22:988–999.

45. McDonald A. Palliative management of pressure ulcers and malignant wounds in patients with advanced illness. J Palliat Med 2006;9:285–295.

46. Pereira J, Phan T. Management of bleeding in patients with advanced cancer. Oncologist 2004;9:561–570.

47. Tokunaga Y, Hosogi H, Nakagami M, Tokuka A, Ohsumi K. A case of chest wall recurrence of breast cancer treated with paclitaxel weekly, 5′-deoxy-5-fluorouridine, arterial embolization and chest wall resection. Breast Cancer 2003;10:366–370.

48. Murakami M, Kuroda Y, Sano A, et al. Validity of local treatment including intraarterial infusion chemotherapy and radiotherapy for fungating adenocarcinoma of the breast: Case report of more than 8-year survival. Am J Clin Oncol 2001;24:388–391.

49. Huang SF, Wu RC, Chang JT, et al. Intractable bleeding from solitary mandibular metastasis of hepatocellular carcinoma. World J Gastroenterol 2007;13:4526–4528.

50. Dean A, Tuffin P. Fibrinolytic inhibitors for cancer-associated bleeding. J Pain Symptom Manage 1997;13(1):20–24.

51. Coetzee MJ. The use of topical crushed tranexamic acid tablets to control bleeding after dental surgery and from skin ulcers in haemophilia. Hemophilia 2007;12:443–444.

52. Sawynok J. Topical and peripherally acting analgesics. Pharmacol Rev 2003;55:1–20.

53. Zeppetella G, Poraio G, Aielli F. Opioids applied topically to painful cutaneous malignant ulcers in a palliative cae setting. J Opioid Manag 2007;3(3):161–166.

54. Tran QN, Fancher T. Achieving analgesia for painful ulcers using topically applied morphine gel. J Support Oncol 2007;5:289–293.

55. Back IN, Finlay I. Analgesic effect of topical opioids on painful skin ulcers. J Pain Symptom Manage 1995;10:493.

56. Zeppetella G, Paul J, Ribeiro M. Analgesic efficacy morphine applied topically to painful ulcers. J Pain Symptom Manage 2003;25:555–558.

57. Zeppetella G, Ribeiro MD. Morphine in intrasite gel applied topically to painful ulcers. J Pain Symptom Manage 2005;29:118–119.

58. Ballas SK. Treatment of painful sickle cell leg ulcers with topical opioids. Blood 2002;99:1096.

59. vanSonnenberg E, Shankar S, Parker L, et al. Palliative radiofrequency ablation of a fungating symptomatic breast lesion. AJR Am J Roentgenol 2005;184:S126–S128.

60. Marchal F, Brunaud L, Baxin C, et al. Radiofrequency ablation in palliative supportive care: Early clinical experience. Oncol Rep 2006;15:495–499.

61. Fritz P, Hensley FW, Berns C, Harms W, Wannenmacher M. Long-term results of pulsed irradiation of skin metastases from breast cancer. Strahlenther Onkol 2000;176:368–376.

62. Leonard R, Hardy J, van Tienhoven G, et al. Randomized, double-blind, placebo-controlled, multicenter trial of 6% miltefosine solution, a topical chemotherapy in cutaneous metastases from breast cancer. J Clin Oncol 2001;19:4150–4159.

63. Goode ML. Psychological needs of patients when dressing a fungating wound: A literature review. J Wound Care 2004;13:380–382.

64. Lo S, Hu W, Hayter M, Chang S, Hsu M, Wu L. Experiences of living with a malignant fungating wound: A qualitative study. J Clin Nurs 2008;17:2699–2708.

65. Piggin C. Malodorous fungating wounds: Uncertain concepts underlying the management of social isolation. Int J Palliat Nurs 2003;9:216–221.

66. Lund-Nielsen B, Müller K, Adamsen L. Malignant wounds in women with breast cancer: Feminine and sexual perspectives. J Clin Nurs 2004;14:56–64.

67. Bryant RA. Management of drain sites and fistula. In: Bryant RA, ed. Acute and Chronic Wounds: Nursing Management. St. Louis: Mosby Year Book, 1992:248–287.

68. Wainstein DE, Fernandez E, Gonzalez D, Chara O, Berkowski D. Treatment of high-output enterocutaneous fistulas with a vacuum-compaction device. A ten-year experience. World J Surg 2008;32(3):430–435.

69. Becker HP, Willms A, Schwab R. Small bowel fistulas and the open abdomen. Scand J Surg 2007;96(4):263–271.

70. Goverman J, Yelon JA, Platz JJ, Singson RC, Turcinovic,M. The "Fistula VAC," a technique for management of enterocutaneous fistulae arising within the open abdomen: Report of 5 cases. J Trauma 2006;60(2):428–431; discussion 431.

71. Girard S, Sideman M, Spain DA. A novel approach to the problem of intestinal fistulization arising in patients managed with open peritoneal cavities. Am J Surg 2002;184(2):166–167.

72. Jamshidi R, Schecter WP. Biological dressings for the management of enteric fistulas in the open abdomen: A preliminary report. Arch Surg 2007;142(8):793–796.

73. Evenson AR, Fischer JE. Current management of enterocutaneous fistula. J Gastrointest Surg 2006;10(3):455–464.

74. Dearlove JL. Skin care management of gastrointestinal fistulas. Surg Clin North Am 1996;76(5):1095–1109.

75. Wiltshire BL. Challenging enterocutaneous fistula: A case presentation. J Wound Ostomy Cont Nurs 1996;23:297–301.

76. Jeter KF, Tintle TE, Chariker M. Managing draining wounds and fistula: New and established methods. In: Krasner D, ed. Chronic Wound Care. King of Prussia, PA: Health Management Publications, 1990:240–246.

77. Harris A, Komray RR. Cost-effective management of pharyngocutaneous fistulas following laryngectomy. Ostomy Wound Manage 1993;39:36–44.

78. McKenzie J, Gallacher M. A sweet smelling success. Nurs Times 1989;85:48–49.

79. Doughty D. Principles of fistula and stoma management. In: Berger A, Portenoy R, Weissman D, eds. Principles and Practice of Supportive Oncology. New York: Lippincott-Raven, 1998:285–294.

80. Erwin-Toth P, Doughty DB. Principles and procedures of stomal management. In: Hampton BG, Bryant RA, eds. Ostomies and Continent Diversions: Nursing Management. Philadelphia: Mosby Year Book, 1992:29–94.

81. Dodd M. Self-care and patient/family teaching. In: Yarbro C, Frogge M, Goodman M, eds. Cancer Symptom Management. Boston: Jones and Bartlett, 1999:20–32.

82. Breckman B. Rehabilitation in palliative care: Stoma management. In: Doyle D, Hanks G, MacDonald N, eds. Oxford Textbook of Palliative Medicine. New York: Oxford University Press, 1998:543–549.

83. Tait N. Anorexia–cachexia syndrome. In: Yarbro C, Frogge M, Goodman M, eds. Cancer Symptom Management. Boston: Jones and Bartlett, 1999:183–208.

84. Bruera E. ABC of palliative care: Anorexia, cachexia, and nutrition. BMJ 1997;315:1219–1222.

85. Martz C. Diarrhea. In: Yarbro C, Frogge M, Goodman M, eds. Cancer Symptom Management. Boston: Jones and Bartlett, 1999:522–545.

# 18 ❦ *Philip J. Larkin*

# Pruritis, Fever, and Sweats

*Those last days we were up all night changing the sheets, three, maybe four times a night. He was just soaked, drenched to the bone with the sweats. We were all exhausted.—A daughter's memory*

◆ **Key Points**
◆ *Pruritus, Fever, and sweats are complex and debilitating symptoms.*
◆ *The patients experience warrants a nursing response to care of the body.*
◆ *Comfort remains the key priority.*

It is a difficult task to accurately define the unique contribution of nursing to palliative care practice. Responding effectively to distressing symptoms is one core task of palliative nursing care.[1] The underpinnings of this response encompass a spectrum of philosophical constructs at the heart of modern concepts of palliative care; for example, hope, dignity, comfort, and empathy.[2–7] This chapter offers a clear example of the way in which good nursing care complements a biomedical approach to relieve symptom burden. At a fundamental level, a discussion of these complex and debilitating symptoms offers the opportunity to articulate how nursing has a responsibility to balance the science (rationale) and art (compassion) of caring. The patient's experience of pruritus, fevers and sweats warrants a nursing response to care of the body.[7] Efforts should be directed simultaneously toward both professional, objective management of symptoms and effective response to subjective patient experience. At its best, attention to the suffering and discomfort caused by these symptoms demonstrates what nursing intervention can truly contribute to palliative management.

In this chapter, although each of these symptoms will be addressed separately for clarity of explication, it is clear that patients may experience them in combination. For example, fever and sweating are frequently linked, and treating the former may well relieve both symptoms. A combined response to assessment and treatment would have mutual benefits overall, regardless of the root cause. However, as is often the case in palliative care, treatment of symptoms where there is a requirement to balance benefit over burden means that the implications of practice need to be considered. For example, treating fever with antibiotics can bring both benefit and burden to patients at end-of-life. This debate will be examined in the context of appropriate nursing responses, and the use of measures beyond the biomedical framework to alleviate the discomfort imposed by these symptoms. A case history will be used to focus the discussion around each symptom and its appropriate medical management. This will be followed by a review of the nursing response and care of the patient.

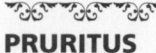

## PRURITUS

CASE STUDY
### The Impact of Itch on a Patient's Quality of Life

Eileen was a 58-year-old woman with advanced cancer of the pancreas admitted to the hospice for end-of-life care. On admission she complained of fatigue, nausea, and a generalized itch, which she rated at 8/10 on a linear scale of 0 = no discomfort to 10 = worst discomfort possible. Pain was relatively well controlled on opiates. Eileen also had evidence of mild to moderate jaundice on admission, indicative of malignant cholestasis. Despite medication, (chlorpheniramine nocte), the itch appeared to worsen, particularly at night and preventing sleep. She was unable to tolerate bedding on her body. Nursing records noted that Eileen's skin had been broken by constant scratching, particularly around her lower abdomen and back and shoulders. Even when sleep occurred with night sedation, Eileen would be restless in bed and scratching, which left her exhausted and frustrated.

Eileen was frail and weak and not a candidate for endoscopic stenting. Her chlorpheniramine nocte was supported by loratidine during the day, and a nursing management regimen of skin cleansing, moisturizing and cool bathing in the early evening was commenced. A short course of topical corticosteroids was prescribed for areas of persistent itch across her abdomen and front of her legs. A bout of nausea and vomiting associated with her clinical deterioration warranted the use of a 5-HT3 antagonist, Ondansatron. This was not only successful in the relief of vomiting, but also appeared to have a positive effect on the pruritus. A shift in rating scale from 8/10 to 4/10 was noted once Ondansatron therapy commenced. Although Eileen appeared to stabilize and endoscopic stenting was scheduled, a sudden and unexpected deterioration led to her death 10 days after admission.

## Interpreting Pruritus

Pruritus has been defined as "an unpleasant sensation that elicits either a conscious or reflex desire to scratch."[8] As a clinical problem, pruritus is prevalent in up to 12% of all palliative care patients.[9] Malignant cholestasis is only one example of the causes of pruritus experienced by palliative care patients. It does, however, give a clear picture of the presentation and impact of this symptom on well-being, and of the distress it engenders, as demonstrated through Eileen's case. Pruritus has been described as an "orphan" symptom[10] in that it has

received only limited research interest and remains poorly defined and understood. The evidence to explain the neurophysiology of pruritus remains weak and therefore management is problematic. This said, it is noted that pruritus should not be considered simply a skin disorder, but rather a systemic problem for which there are multiple causes.[11,12] There would appear to be some physiological synchronicity between pruritus and pain, given the fact that similar chemical messengers excite the unmyelinated C fibers. It may be that a specific subset of these fibers responds particularly to pruritus-inducing stimuli and mediators such as histamine and prostaglandins.[8,10] The ability to trace the neurological pathways of histamine through the dorsal horn and into the thalamus and sensorimotor cortex would appear to confirm this as the primary mediator of itch.[13,14] However, at a peripheral level, other peripheral mediators have been identified, including serotonin, prostaglandin, and dopamine.[8]

Pruritus associated with malignant choleostasis is specifically complex and poorly understood.[15,16] One possible theory suggests that excess bile salts that cannot be eliminated accumulate and interact with nerve endings in the skin.[17] Eileen's expression of the severity of pruritus associated with jaundice would not be uncommon. Sleep deprivation and broken skin from scratching are noted phenomena.[18]

For patients with pancreatic cancer, itching has been described as the worst symptom they experience.[11] Its subjective nature makes it both unrelenting and unpredictable, and although scratching behavior is observable and measurable, the burden experienced by the patient is not conducive to measurement.[19] Why scratching relieves an itch is not fully understood, but it has been postulated from the Melzak-Wall "gate theory" that scratching stimulates the large C fibers to open the "gate" and thereby inhibit the itch stimulus in the dorsal horn of the spinal cord.[11] However, where the physiological response is altered due to disease or damage, it may initiate a cycle of itching, localized histamine release, exacerbation of the itch and further scratching, so that the symptom is unrelieved. It is also noted that a psychological element as both cause and consequence of pruritus should not be discounted, particularly if the patient is anxious or fearful.

### Nursing Assessment and Differential Diagnosis

It is important to remember that pruritus may be both localized and generalized. There is a distinction between primary or idiopathic pruritus (where no cause can be determined) and secondary pruritus (related to systemic or localized disease).[20] General skin disorders such as eczema, psoriasis or infestation should be ruled out, or treated as necessary, before attributing the problem to an internal cause. However, systemic etiology may be present in up to 40% of all cases.[8] Therefore, in cases of non-specific generalized pruritus, it is important to monitor for the development of systemic disease over time. Table 18–1 lists some of the key causes of pruritus based on Bernhard's classification[21] with a specific focus on those causes seen in palliative care practice.

**Table 18–1**
**Key Causes of Pruritus**

| Bernhard's Classification | Overall Problem | Clinical Presentation |
|---|---|---|
| Dermatologic | Generalized skin problems | Psoriasis, eczema, urticaria, scabies, pediculosis, xerosis (dry skin) |
| | | Contact dermatitis, atopic dermatitis, allergy (e.g. nickel, bathing products) |
| | Medication (including hypersensitivity) | Opioids, amphetamines, acetlysalisylic acid, quinidine |
| | Blood dyscrasias (including hematological malignancy) | Iron deficiency anemia |
| | | Polycythemia rubra vera |
| | | Leukemias |
| | | Lymphomas |
| | | Hodgkins disease |
| Systemic | Organ failure | Liver failure (malignant cholestasis, primary biliary cirrhosis, hepatitis) |
| | | Renal failure (uremia, post dialysis dermatosis) |
| | Endocrine and metabolic dysfunction | Diabetes mellitus |
| | | Hyperthyroidism/hypothyroidism |
| | | Hyperparathyroidism/hypoparathyroidism |
| | | Zinc deficiency |
| | Connective tissue disorder | Systemic lupus erythematosus |
| | | Chronic graft versus host disease |
| Neuropathic/Neurogenic (including neuroanatomic and neurochemical disorders) | Chronic and potentially life-limiting disease | Neuroendocrine tumors |
| | | Paraneoplastic tumors |
| | | Multiple sclerosis |
| | | Stroke |
| | | Brain injury |
| | | Post herpes zoster infection |
| | | Syphilis |

---

Can a location for itch be specified?
Is there presence or absence of rash?
Is there evidence of a fungal or parasitic infection?
Is there evidence of broken or dry skin?
Is there bleeding or seepage of serous fluid?

**Figure 18–1.** Clinical assessment of pruritus.

## Pruritus and Opioids

Given the link between the physiological mechanisms of pain and pruritus, it is important here to make specific mention of the relationship of opioids and itch. It is known from animal studies that generalized pruritus is a side effect of morphine, particularly when administered centrally.[22] Like the theory of bile salt accumulation cited earlier,[11] a reaction to morphine salts has been suggested as one reason for morphine-induced pruritus.[20] The degranulation of mast cells by opiates stimulates histamine release, and this is considered the most likely causative factor for generalized pruritus in opioid-dependent patients. Evidence further suggests that this may be marked in the case of malignant cholestasis, and that opioid antagonists (such as Naloxone) reduce the itch of generalized pruritus associated with this symptom.[23,24] A recently reported case history of nine patients with chronic liver disease has suggested that the slow and careful intravenous administration of Naloxone followed by oral Naltrexone therapy can be beneficial, without risk of the opioid withdrawal phenomena commonly associated with opioid antagonists.[19] The complexity here is that one treatment possibility for pruritus may inhibit treatment for another, equally important symptom, pain. Therefore, careful monitoring of outcome and response is essential.

As in Eileen's case, it is important to quantify the level of discomfort imposed by itch. A thorough clinical assessment reflective of any systemic disease should include a consideration of the following (Figure 18–1):

If appropriate in the context of palliative stage of disease, laboratory blood tests may be useful in diagnosis. At the least, a complete blood count including urea and creatinine should be considered, as well as tests to rule out endocrine or metabolic dysfunction (for example, serum glucose, thyroxine, and bilirubin levels). The patient should also be questioned sensitively about his or her personal hygiene regime and use of specific deodorants, lotions and bath products. Associations with food, weather, and exposure to new environments (e.g. pets, new bedding or clothes) should also be explored.

### Medical Management of Pruritus

Due to the breadth of possible causes for pruritus, management needs to balance the response between intervention, patient perception of the problem, and clinical status. For example, endoscopic stenting, which is a first-line treatment option in malignant cholestasis, may well relieve jaundice and the concomitant itch. However, as with Eileen, the patient may not be well enough for the procedure. On admission, Eileen was weak and frail. The possibility of surgery, albeit palliative in nature, was not an initial treatment of choice for her or the palliative care team. Centrally acting antihistamine preparations such as Chlorpheniramine can be effective, but can be sedating and are therefore best administered at night. Since the symptom may be exacerbated at night, the sedative effect may not be a problem, and might even assist the patient in getting to sleep.

The benefit of drugs such as Cholestyramine, used to prevent reabsorption of bile salts, may be negligible. Evidence of a partial gastrointestinal obstruction limits the ability of the drug to bind and excrete salts.[11] Eileen found the drug unpalatable, and because she was exhausted from lack of sleep, she welcomed the sedating effect of Chlorpheniramine. However, for many patients, the use of a less sedating antihistamine such as Loratidine has been shown to be clinically effective.[11]

There is a wide array of medications that have been efficacious in the treatment of pruritus. The potential use of the antibiotic rifampicin has been noted in the literature.[17,18,25] Particularly where pruritus is considered opioid-induced and not responsive to antihistamine therapy, Rifampicin has been shown to achieve a rapid resolution of the symptom. In one case history report,[25] successful control of pruritus involved a switch in opioid management from morphine to methadone, which enabled Rifampicin to be discontinued with no recurrence of itch.[26,27]

Another medication that has been demonstrated as beneficial in the treatment of pruritus is Ondansatron, commonly used in the treatment of chemotherapy-induced nausea and vomiting. As a 5-HT3 serotonin antagonist, Ondansatron has shown a dramatic effect in reducing itch following intravenous infusion and regular oral administration in patients with malignant cholestasis, and has also been noted as effective in other patient populations.[28–30] Other potential choices of treatment would include local anesthetics[31] and antidepressants such as Mirtazapine, which has antiserotogenic effects at the 5-HT2 and 5-HT3 receptors, and offers benefits similar to those of Ondansatron. Gabapentin has also been utilized to good effect, as has buprenorphine with a very low dose of naloxone in combination.[25,32]

Topical and systemic corticosteroids have a place in treatment, although their use may be limited because of potential side effects.[33,34] Paroxetine has also been considered

effective.[35] However, it is important to note that most of the evidence available on the treatment of pruritus is limited to clinical reports, case histories and small-scale studies. Further research trials are needed to identify best treatment options.[36] In the palliative context, particularly where there may be multiorgan failure, systemic treatment choices may be very limited,[8] particularly if opiate use for optimal pain control is not stabilized. Therefore, a program of nursing management is an essential component of the approach to care.

### Nursing Management

Regardless of cause, the patient complaint focuses on the skin, and nursing management should endeavor to provide the highest standard of skin care to supplement medical intervention. Although topical treatment alone may have minimal benefit,[15] it may contribute to relieving the patient's discomfort. Skin cleansing is important, along with the prevention of xerosis (dry skin) which may exacerbate the pruritus. Bathing may assist hydration in the short term, but the essential need is to keep the skin moist. Emollient oils should be added to the bath near the end, as doing so at the beginning may have a drying effect.[11] A "soak and seal" method has been proposed that involves bathing, patting (not rubbing) the skin dry, and then adding an occlusive or moisturizer.[37] The choice of skin cleanser and moisturizer should ideally be pH neutral and free from fragrance and alcohol. Soap and talcum powder should be avoided due to their drying properties. The water content of the product should be relatively low, since it may evaporate quickly.[20]

Frequent application of moisturizer and the use of soft, cool clothing, preferably cotton, should be encouraged.[20] Topical antihistamine preparations, such as an oil-based calamine lotion, may soothe excoriated and scratched skin.[11] Cool packs, cool oatmeal baths, and loose, light bedding can be beneficial, particularly when settling the patient for sleep. An ambient room temperature (cooler rather than warmer) may be relaxing, although this is less easy to regulate if the patient is hospitalized. Although the evidence is dated, some nonpharmacological methods used for the relief of pain (e.g. TENS) can have a benefit in the treatment of pruritus.[38,39] The patient should be advised to keep nails short, and to rub or pat rather than scratch, if at all possible.[11] A physical examination for damage to skin or evidence of a secondary infection should be carried out regularly, and any damage or infection treated accordingly.

✱✱✱✱✱✱

## FEVER

✱✱

CASE STUDY
*Management of Fever in Relation to a Patient's Goals of Care*

Anthony, a 76-year-old man with a history of Alzheimer's disease, was admitted to the hospice with end-stage carcinoma of the bronchus. On admission he was frail, breathless on exertion, and tachypnoeic, complaining of a troublesome productive cough. He appeared flushed, diaphoretic, and was warm to the touch. Baseline measurements indicated a body temperature of 39.6°C (103.28°F). Blood bacterial cultures were undertaken and Anthony commenced on a broad spectrum antibiotic three times daily, as well as an antipyretic comfort program by nursing staff with particular emphasis on increased oral fluid intake and skin care. Results of the blood culture were inconclusive as to causative organism. Following a five-day course of treatment, Anthony appeared to improve and his body temperature returned to normal limits (37.2°C). However, prior to planned discharge, Anthony appeared to deteriorate clinically and "spiked" a further temperature of 38.9°C, rising to 40.1°C despite antipyretic measures. It was suggested that further blood bacterial cultures be undertaken, along with the administration of intravenous antibiotics. Hospice staff discussed the degree to which this infection should be treated aggressively, given Anthony's evident deterioration. Following a family meeting, a decision was made that further invasive blood culture testing was inappropriate but that a short trial of intravenous antibiotics might have some palliative benefit. However, prior to commencement, Anthony entered the terminal phase of his illness; his care plan was revised to comfort measures only, and he died peacefully.

※

## Interpreting Fever

Fever is defined as a rise in body temperature exceeding 38°C (100.4°F) from the norm (37°± 1°C) (98.78°F).[20,40] However, the degree to which a rise in temperature denotes "fever" would appear to vary widely in the literature[41,42] and it should be remembered that quantitative measurement of fever was only possible from the mid-19th century with the development of the thermometer.[43] Raised body temperature and fever occur as a response to an elevation in a thermal set-point regulated by the anterior hypothalamus.[20] Pathogens (viruses, bacteria, or fungi) may break down to release pyrogens, which may be both exogenous and endogenous. The most commonly noted endogenous pyrogens are interleukin-1 (IL-1), interleukin-6 (IL-6), tumor necrosis factor (TNFα), and interferon(INF).[20,44] The neurophysiological mechanism by which the thermal set-point is raised remains unclear, although cytokines and prostaglandins are considered to be partly influential.[43] Once the thermal set-point is raised, the hypothalamus continues to regulate body temperature, albeit around a higher set-point.

Table 18–2 outlines the many and varied causes of fever, most of which have direct relevance for palliative care patients. Notably, patients with advanced dementia (such as Anthony) may have fever as a common symptom of their end-of-life stage of illness, in this case exacerbated by malignant lung disease.[45] Further, older people may exhibit an altered febrile response, which makes the assessment of body temperature a limited diagnostic tool.[44]

The presentation of fever often manifests in three stages.[20,43] These have been described as chill, fever and flush.[44] In the chill phase, the body attempts to respond to the raised thermal set-point by vasoconstriction of the skin to prevent heat loss and muscle contraction to generate heat. This results in shivering and, in marked cases, rigors. The second phase is dominated by a sensation of warmth, flushed skin, lethargy, weakness and possibly dehydration, delirium and/or seizure. This occurs as the core body temperature rises to the new set-point. During fever, the basal metabolic rate is increased to meet new tissue and oxygenation requirements by up to 13% per 1°C increase.[20] In the third and final phase, the core temperature attempts to normalize with the new set-point through vasodilatation and sweating (diaphoresis). For the palliative care population, and particularly those with a cancer diagnosis that has led to episodes of neutropenia, infection and fever are not uncommon. As the patient becomes increasingly immunosuppressed, attack by pyrogens may lead to overwhelming sepsis and death if left untreated.[20] Again, the justification for aggressive intervention needs to be considered in relation to the patient's overall health status. The use of blood transfusions in palliative care is a debate in itself, but the risk of hemolytic reaction and associated fever is possible. Therefore, for many reasons,

**Table 18–2**
**Key Causes of Fever**

| Causative Factors | Causative Agent |
| --- | --- |
| Infection | Bacteria, fungi, viruses, parasites, tuberculosis, hepatitis, endocarditis, contaminated food. |
| Inflammation | Trauma, surgery, splenectomy heat, ulcerative colitis, pulmonary embolism, radiation, gastrointestinal bleeding. |
| Cancer treatment | Chemotherapeutic agents, blood products, immunosuppression, neutropenia, external devices for venous access, catheters. |
| Tumors | Hodgkin's and non-Hodgkin's disease, leukemia, carcinoma of the liver, lung and GU systems, adrenal cancer, Ewing's sarcoma, renal disease, tumors affecting the thermoregulatory system of the brain. |
| Autoimmune disease | Rheumatoid arthritis, connective tissue disorder, anaphylaxis, polymyalgia, HIV-AIDS. |
| Neurological disorder | Spinal/brain injury or infection, stroke. |
| Environmental | Allergens. |
| Other | Constipation, dehydration, medication. |

its benefit should be carefully evaluated. Given that bacterial infection can account for up to 90% of fevers,[20] anything that might introduce infection through damaged skin integrity (such as venous access and urinary catheters) also warrants aseptic practice and judicious use. Medications may also trigger a febrile response, most commonly penicillins, cephalosporins, antifungals (e.g. Amphotericin) and, of course, chemotherapy agents (e.g. bleomycin).[40,46]

### Nursing Assessment and Differential Diagnosis

The differential diagnosis of fever will determine realistic goals and the most appropriate plan of care. Clearly, a thorough physical examination and recent history are essential. Figure 18–2 identifies common diagnostic questions relevant to and inclusive of clinical examination. The list is not intended to be exhaustive, but rather to guide a holistic assessment in the context of increasing frailty and the likelihood of impending death.

### Medical Management of Fever

In the palliative context, the degree to which fever is treated aggressively raises the debate about burden over benefit—life quality versus the risk of prolonged dying. Clearly, as in Anthony's case, antibiotics can be beneficial and therefore have a place in palliative care practice. In one recent study, both physicians and family members rated antibiotics highly in terms of treatment options for their patient/relative, second only to opiates, and more highly than intravenous nutrition.[47] The challenge for palliative care is to decide how far to treat and when "enough is enough." This is not an easy discussion with family, and in Anthony's case it was complicated by the Alzheimer's disease that limited his ability to engage in the decision-making process. It is, however, a necessary discussion if the aim is to prevent undue suffering.

The complexity of the decision whether or not to use antibiotics is evidenced by the diversity of opinion within the

literature as to their value and efficacy. Some studies show that antibiotic therapy in palliative care patients can prolong survival, while others suggest bacterial infection has no real impact on the overall survival outcome of palliative care patients.[48,49] One study in particular has investigated fever in the context of Alzheimer's disease and found no significant change in overall outcome with antibiotic therapy.[45] A more recent study conducted in a large teaching hospital with end-of-life cancer patients identified a high rate of antibiotic prescription but a very poor rate of symptomatic improvement.[50] Whatever decision is made regarding antibiotics, it is important that a plan of care includes decisions on the conditions that would herald cessation of treatment. For Anthony, the decision about whether to proceed to intravenous antibiotics was avoided by his swift deterioration. It would seem that there is something of a general consensus that antibiotic use in the terminal phase is inappropriate. However, even if the patient's status is deemed "palliative," debate may arise about where active treatment ends and palliative care begins. A good principle on which to base the decision to treat actively is the degree of symptom burden to the patient, regardless of the clinical presentation.[44]

Acetaminophen has the benefit of offering relatively rapid response to pyrexia and is available in a variety of forms—tablet, suspension, or suppository. Aspirin, if tolerated, may also be effective. Corticosteroids also hold antipyretic properties, although their benefit needs to be weighed against the possible side effects.[20,51] It is also suggested that antipyretic medication be prescribed and administered regularly and not on a "PRN" basis, which may induce fluctuating patterns of fever and sweating.[43] More intensive management may be required depending on the cause of the fever. Fever related to tumor may be responsive to radiation, if the patient's condition is stable enough for treatment. Further, neuroleptic agents such as Chlorpromazine may be beneficial where the fever is centrally mediated.[20]

### Nursing Management of Fever

Using Anthony's case as an example, comfort should be the key priority in the palliative approach.[20] It is important to obtain a balance between "cooling" and "cold," the latter which may only exacerbate the discomfort caused by shivering and heat-generation. Bathing with tepid water, drying off gently and using light bedding may add to comfort, but cold packs and ice should be avoided. Cool fluids should be encouraged, and attention to mouth and skin care is imperative, particularly in cases where there is a risk of dehydration. Anthony was markedly cachexic, and his lethargy and lack of movement placed him at risk of decubitous ulcer formation, so an air mattress was used to good effect. A fan should be used to cool the ambient air and not be focused directly on the patient. Attention to these details in the evening may help to promote sleep. Even if there is no plan to revise the treatment plan, an occasional recording of temperature may help in deciding the timing and spacing of comfort care. Even

---

Is there evidence suggestive of a respiratory tract infection?
Is there evidence suggestive of a urinary infection?
How long has the patient been febrile?
What is the pattern of the fever (day or night, number of peaks of temperature over 24 hours)?
What medication or treatment is in progress or recently completed?
Has there been a recent blood transfusion?
Have there been any recent invasive procedures?
Blood tests?
Is there evidence of damage to the skin integument?
Are there any venous access devices or catheters?

**Figure 18–2.** Clinical assessment of fever.

though Anthony appeared well, and discharge planning was in progress, a random check of his temperature revealed a moderate elevation that within a few hours had progressed to an overall degeneration in his condition. Although it would not have influenced the final outcome, it did alert staff to the fact of a change in his condition and they were able to increase observation and respond accordingly as he became increasingly unwell during that day.

## SWEATS

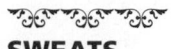

CASE STUDY
### Sweats with Both Disease Related and Emotions Related Components

Martin was a 74-year-old man with advanced cancer of the prostate, previously treated with hormone therapy. He was opiate-dependent but well controlled. He was admitted for respite care to the local hospice. During his first night, Martin experienced a drenching sweat that occurred without warning and required a full change of clothes and bed linen. He reported that this had happened on two other occasions at home, and was one of the reasons his wife had suggested respite care. He was embarrassed because he felt concern that other patients would think that he had been incontinent of urine, particularly given his diagnosis. He experienced a similar sweat on the second night, at which point his opioids were considered a causative factor and therefore reduced slightly, with minimal effect. A course of propranolol hydrochloride was found to be moderately beneficial, mainly attributed to the fact that Martin did not like to take medication. Although his sweating was presumed to be disease-related, Martin found some relief from the symptom through aromatherapy and relaxation sessions offered by the Complementary and Supportive Care Team, which suggested there was an emotional component to the problem. On discharge, nursing records indicated that for the last 10 days of his respite stay, Martin had experienced no episodes of sweating.

### Interpreting Sweats

Although sweats are considered one of the major problems experienced by patients,[52] research evidence for the management and treatment of sweats remains sparse. One epidemiological study identified severe sweating (described as drenching sweats that require bed clothing and linen to be changed) as a significant problem for patients admitted to hospice.[53] Evidently, there is a strong link between fever and sweating, although there is a distinction between the thermal diaphoresis described in the previous section, and controlled by the hypothalamus, and emotional

| Table 18-3 | |
| --- | --- |
| **Key Causes of Sweating** | |
| **Endocrine Disorders** | **Estrogen Deficiency, Hyperthyroidism, Hypoglycemia** |
| Malignancy | Lymphoma, breast cancer, prostate cancer, neuroendocrine tumors. |
| Chronic infection | Tuberculosis, lupus. |
| Medication (including withdrawal from) | Opioids, barbiturates. |
| Emotion | Stress, anxiety, fear. |

How often do you find yourself sweating?
How would you describe these sweats?
Are they a particular problem at night?
Do you have any other problems when you sweat [nausea, vomiting, feeling faint, anxious or fearful]?
Have you changed any medication recently?
Is your sweating all over your body, or confined to certain parts?
Have you identified anything that seems to make your sweating better or worse?
How much of a problem is this sweating for you?

**Figure 18–3.** Questions for care planning.

sweating that is controlled by the limbic system.[20] Age, gender, ambient temperature and exercise are all known to influence the amount of sweating that takes place, and that is usually greater from palms of the hands and soles of the feet.[20]

Hyperhidrosis (excessive sweating) may be directly related to disease or indeed, may have no evident cause. In each case, it can be localized or generalized.[44] It is noted in a variety of illnesses, including malignancy. Specifically, hormone treatment such as Martin was offered is known to influence hyperhidrosis through estrogen withdrawal.[20,44] This may present as "night sweats" as described above.[53]

### Nursing Assessment and Differential Diagnosis

Table 18–3 identifies the key causes of sweating.

An alternative description of hyperhidrosis is "hot flashes," related in particular to replacement hormone therapy. Notably, it is reported that this problem remains unaddressed for up to 75% of men in receipt of hormone therapy for their prostate disease.[21] Completely unpredictable, hot flashes interfere greatly with life quality and in particular, sleep. Figure 18–3 identifies some key questions that may be helpful when ascertaining the impact of the problem on life quality for the patient.

## Medical Management of Sweats

Unfortunately, drug therapy options to treat this problem are relatively limited and there is very little evidence beyond case reports and pilot trials to support the use of any specific treatment. Given the link to "menopausal" symptoms, a number of nonpharmacological preparations have been proposed, including evening primrose oil, phytoestrogens and herbs.[44,54] However, there is no definitive research evidence available for these preparations. Propranolol hydrochloride has been found efficacious in decreasing sympathetic symptoms,[21] and medications that work as antispasmodics and anticholinergics have also demonstrated some benefit.[20,44] A recently reported development has been the use of thalidomide in patients with advanced malignancy.[55,56] Although these have been small-scale studies and case reports, there appears to be a successful outcome on a moderate dose (50–100 mg) for the management of severe sweating. A further option is the use of Thioridazine, a phenothiazine, antipsychotic and anti-muscarinic agent.[57–59] One recent small-scale study demonstrated a significant improvement in nocturnal sweats and well-being for 7 out of 10 patients treated with a low dose between 10–25 mg.[55] In any case, the discomfort associated with this symptom indicates the need for sensitive and responsive nursing care.

## Nursing Management of Sweats

It is argued that the ethics of care begin with that which is most basic, and the care for the body is an example of that basic—but notably not simple—care.[7] Since the burden of sweats on the patient's quality of life would appear to be great, nursing care must include an approach that addresses the immediate discomfort and anxiety. Patients should be advised to have extra changes of nightwear (or day clothes if the symptoms are not restricted to the night) and additional bedding should be available. Just as in the fever type response, the patient may feel cold following diaphoresis, and so should be kept comfortable in an ambient temperature while washing and changing. Similar to the treatment of fever, cool (but not cold) fluids should be encouraged to avoid dehydration, since the risk of multiple sweats in one night is not uncommon.[20]

Patients may fear that their sweating indicates a deterioration or recurrence of disease. Night sweats may indicate this in the case of lymphoma.[20] Like Martin, the patient may be embarrassed by the symptom and withdraw from family and friends. Gentle discussion about the problem and reassurance that efforts are being made to find a solution may ease distress. Careful observation of factors relating to the sweats (time, duration, extent, patient response) may indicate a possible treatment pathway. Martin's distress led to his referral to the aromatherapist, and that intervention made a significant improvement in the symptom and Martin's response to it.

## Conclusions

Perhaps of all symptoms that palliative care patients endure, those of pruritus, fever and sweats most remind nurses of their fundamental grounding in caring for others. The care given to patients with these symptoms is reflective of skills learned and nurtured throughout the nursing career, and then specifically honed to meet end-of-life needs. The importance of comfort in palliative care has been well established.[3] Comfort remains the key priority, particularly where drug therapy may have limited effect. The "benefit-burden calculus"[44] should be uppermost in the mind with respect to the goals of treatment. As the medical team member with closest proximity to the patient, the nurse may need to voice his or her concerns, and the concerns of others, where an intervention appears to be unwarranted or even futile.

The attention to detail required in order to address these symptoms highlights the importance to palliative nursing of those philosophical constructs noted at the beginning of this chapter—hope, dignity, comfort and empathy.

REFERENCES

1. Payne S, Seymour J, Ingleton C, eds. Palliative Care Nursing Principles and Evidence for Practice. Berkshire: McGraw-Hill Open University Press, 2004:3.
2. Penz K. Theories of hope: Are they relevant for palliative care nurses and their practice? Int J Palliat Nurs 2008;14:408–412.
3. Currow DC, Ward AM, Plummer JL, Bruera E, Abernathy AP. Comfort in the last 2 weeks of life: Relationship to accessing palliative care services. Support Care Cancer 2008;16:1255–1263.
4. Chochinov HM. Dignity-conserving care—a new model for palliative care: Helping patients feel valued. JAMA 2002;287:2253–2260.
5. Degner LF, Gow CM, Thompson LA. Critical nursing behaviours in care for the dying. Cancer Nurs 1991;14:246–253.
6. Raudonis BM. The meaning and impact of empathetic relationships in hospice nursing. Cancer Nurs 1993;16:204–309.
7. Eugene B. Caring for the body at the end of life. Eur J Palliat Care 2005;12:212–214.
8. Summey BT. Pruritus. In: Walsh D, Caraceni AT, Fainsinger R, et al., eds. Palliative Medicine. Philadelphia PA: Saunders Elsevier, 2008:910–913.
9. Waller A, Caroline NL. Handbook of Palliative Care in Cancer. Woburn: Butterworth-Heinemann, 2000:115–124.
10. Mortimer PS. Management of skin problems. Sweating. In: Doyle D, Hanks GWC, MacDonald N. eds. Oxford Textbook of Palliative Medicine (2nd ed). Oxford: Oxford University Press, 1998:636–642.
11. Bosonnet L. Pruritus: Scratching the surface. Eur J Cancer Care 2003;12:162–165.
12. Karjnik M, Zylicz Z. Understanding pruritus in systemic disease. J Pain Symptom Manage 2001;21:151–168.
13. Jinks S, Carstens E. Superficial dorsal horn neurons identified by intracutaneous histamine. Chemonociceptive responses

and modulation by morphine. J Neurophysiol 2000;84: 616–627.

14. Mochizuki H, Tashiro M, Kano M, et al. Imaging of central itch modulation in the human brain using positron emission tomography. Pain 2003;105:339–346.

15. Jones EA, Bergasa NV. The pruritus of cholestasis: From bile acids to opiate agonists. Hepatology 1990;11:884–887.

16. Bain VG, Minuk GY. Jaundice, ascites and hepatic encephalopathy. In: Doyle D, Hanks GWC, MacDonald N, eds. Oxford Textbook of Palliative Medicine (1st ed). Oxford: Oxford University Press, 1993:34.

17. Price TJ, Patterson WK, Oliver IN. Rifampicin as treatment for pruritus in malignant cholestasis. Support Care Cancer 1998;6:533–535.

18. Raiford DS. Pruritus of chronic cholestasis. Quart J Med 1995;88:603–607.

19. Jones EA, Zylicz Z. Treatment of pruritus caused by cholestasis with opioid antagonists. J Palliat Med 2005;6:1290–1294.

20. Rhiner M, Slatkin NE. Pruritus, fever and sweats. In: Ferrell B, Coyle N, eds. Textbook of Palliative Nursing (2nd ed). Oxford: Oxford University Press, 2004:345–363.

21. Bernhard JD. Itch and pruritus: What are they, and how should itches be classified? Dermatol Ther 2005;18:288–291.

22. Thomas DA, Williams GW, Iwata K, Kenshalo Dr Jr, Dubner R. Effect of central administration of opioids on facial scratching in monkeys. Brain Res 1992;585:315–317.

23. Bergasa NV, Jones EA. The pruritus of cholestasis: Potential pathogenic and therapeutic implications of opioids. Gastroenterol 1995;108:1582–1588.

24. Jones EA, Bergasa NV. The pruritius of cholestasis. Hepatol 1999;29:1003–1006.

25. Mercadante S, Villari P, Fulfaro F. Rifampicin in opioid-induced itching. Supprt Care Cancer 2001;9:467–468.

26. Katcher J, Walsh D. Opioid induced-itching: Morphine sulphate and hydromorphone hydrochloride. J Pain Symptom Manage 1999;17:70–72.

27. Rogers A. Considering histamine release in prescribing opioid analgesics. J Pain Symptom Manage 1991;6:44–45.

28. Raderer M, Muller C, Scheithauser W. Ondansatron for pruritus due to cholestasis. N Engl J Med 1994;330:1540.

29. Schworer H, Ramadori G. Treatment of pruritus: A new indication for serotonin type 3 receptor antagonists. Clin Invest 1993;71:659–662.

30. Gross S, Overbaugh R, Jansen R. Ondansatron for treating itch in healing burns. Internet J Pain Symptom Cont Palliat Care 2006;5.4.

31. Pittlekow MR, Loprinzi CL. Pruritus and sweating. In: Doyle D, Hanks G, Cherny N, Calman K, eds. Oxford Textbook of Palliative Medicine (3rd ed). Oxford: Oxford University Press, 2004:573–587.

32. Winhoven S, Coulson I, Bottomley W. Brachioradial pruritus: Response to treatment with gabapentin. Br J Dermatol 2004;150:786.

33. Nicol NH, Baumeister LL. Topical corticosteroid therapy: Considerations for prescribing and use. Prim Care 1997;1:62–69.

34. Chaffman MO. Topical corticosteroids: A review of properties and principles in therapeutic use. Nurse Pract Forum 1999;10:95–105.

35. Zylicz Z, Krajnik M, Sorge AA, Costantini M. Paroxetine in the treatment of severe non-dermatological pruritus: A randomized controlled trial. J Pain Symptom Manage 2003;26:1105–1112.

36. Zylicz Z, Stork N, Krajnik M. Severe pruritus of cholestasis in disseminated cancer: Developing a rational treatment strategy. A case report. J Pain Symptom Manage 2005;29:100–103.

37. Nicol NH, Boguniewicz M. Understanding and treating atopic dermatitis. Nurse Pract Forum 1999;10:48–55.

38. Ostrawski MJ. Pain control in advanced malignant disease using transcutaneous nerve stimulation. Br J Clin Pract 1979;33:157–160.

39. OStrawski MJ, Dodd A. Transcutaneous nerve stimulation for relief of pain in advanced malignant disease. Nurs Times 1977;11:1233–1238.

40. Cleary JF. Fever and sweats. In: Berger AM, Portenoy RK, Weissman DE, eds. Principles and Practice of Palliative Care and Supportive Oncology (2nd ed). Philadelphia: Williams and Wilkins, 2002:154–167.

41. Mackowiak PA. Fever: Basic Mechanisms and Management (2nd ed). Philadelphia: Lippincott-Raven.

42. Thompson HJ. Fever: A concept analysis. J Adv Nurs 2005;51:484–492.

43. Styrt B, Sugarman B. Antipyresis and fever. Arch Intern Med 1990;150:1591–1597.

44. Bobb B, Lyckholm L, Coyne P. Fever and sweats. In: Walsh D, Caraceni AT, Fainsinger R, et al., eds. Palliative Medicine. Philadelphia: Saunders Elsevier, 2008:890–893.

45. Pinderhughes ST, Morrison RS. Evidence-based approach to management of fever in patients with end-stage dementia. J Palliat Med 2003;6:351–354.

46. Dalal S, Zhukovsky DS. Pathophysiology and management of fever. J Support Oncol 2006;4:9–16.

47. Oh DY, Kim JE, Lee CH, et al. Discrepancies among patients, family members and physicians in Korea in terms of values regarding the withholding of treatment form patients with terminal malignancies. Cancer 2004;100:1961–1966.

48. Fabiszewski KJ, Volicer B, Volicer L. Effect of antibiotic treatment on outcome of fevers in institutionalized Alzheimer patients. JAMA 1990;263:3168–3172.

49. Vitetta L, Kenner D, Sali A. Bacterial infections in terminally ill hospice patients. J Pain Symptom Manage 2000;20:326–334.

50. Oh DY, Kim JH, Kim et al. Antibiotic use during the last days of life in cancer patients. Eur J Can Care 2005;15:74–79.

51. Vargas R, Maneatis T, Bynum L, et al. Evaluation of the antipyretic effect of ketorolac, acetaminophen and placebo in endotoxin-induced fever. J Clin Pharmacol 1994;34:848–853.

52. De Lima L. The IAHPC list of essential medicines in palliative care. Palliat Med 2006;20:647–651.

53. Quigley CS, Baines M. Descriptive epidemiology of sweating in a hospice population. J Palliat Care 1997;13:22–26.

54. Quella SK, Loprinzi CL, Barton DL, et al. Evaluation of spy phytoestrogens for the treatment of hot flashes in breast cancer survivors: A North Central Cancer Group trial. J Clin Oncol 2000;18:1068–1074.

55. Deaner P. The use of Thalidomide in the management of severe sweating in patients with advanced malignancy. Palliat Med 2000;14:429–431.

56. Calder K, Bruera E. Thalidomide for night sweats in patients with advanced cancer. Palliat Med 2000;14:77.

57. Abbas SQ. Use of thioridazine in palliative care with troublesome sweating. J Pain Symptom Manage 2004;27:194–195.

58. Regnard C. Use of low dose thioridazine to control sweating in advanced cancer. Palliat Med 1996;10:78–79.

59. Cowap J, Hardy J. Thioridazine in the management of cancer related sweating. J Pain Symptom Manage 1998;33:199–204.

# 19 Judith A. Paice

# Neurological Disturbances

*The jerking was so awful as his pain exploded with each motion. I could not comfort him or hold him.—The wife of a patient with myoclonus*

◆ **Key Points**

◆ *Myoclonus, uncontrolled rhythmic jerking movements, is likely due to accumulation of opioid metabolites, particularly in patients with renal dysfunction, although other factors are implicated at the end of life.*

◆ *Headache is more common in those with primary or metastatic intracranial lesions, but can also develop after infection, vascular disorders or more acutely, from withdrawal of substances. Treatment includes pharmacologic and nonpharmacologic therapies, as well as attention to safety.*

◆ *Seizures may arise from central nervous system neoplasms, metabolic dysfunction, medications, stroke, and other causes. Aggressive management is indicated to reduce pain and exhaustion.*

◆ *Spasms, involving uncontrolled movement, rigidity, and hyperreflexia, can impair mobility and cause pain. Palliative care includes pharmacological and nonpharmacological management, along with safety measures.*

*Myoclonus* is frequently seen in palliative care settings, particularly during the final days of life. If left untreated, this neurological disturbance may progress to seizures. *Headache*, more common in those with intracranial tumors, can cause severe pain, as well as serious neurological changes. *Seizures* also may occur due to central nervous system (CNS) lesions, metabolic disorders, or medications. A fourth neurological disturbance, *spasticity*, involves involuntary movements that may produce discomfort and fatigue. Astute palliative care clinicians can prevent some of these disorders and treat those that cannot be prevented. Patient and family involvement is mandatory, since comfort and safety issues are prevalent in all three syndromes.

## Myoclonus

Myoclonus consists of sudden, uncontrollable, nonrhythmic jerking, usually of the extremities.[1] Frequently seen in the palliative care setting, myoclonus can be exhausting and can progress to more severe neurological dysfunction, including seizures. Early identification and rapid treatment are critical.

### Causes of Myoclonus

In the palliative care setting, myoclonus is most often associated with opioids. The prevalence of opioid-induced myoclonus ranges greatly, from 2.7% to 87%.[1] Nocturnal myoclonus is common, and often precedes opioid-induced myoclonus.[2] The precise cause of opioid-induced myoclonus is unknown; however, several mechanisms have been proposed.[3,4] High doses of opioids may result in the accumulation of neuroexcitatory metabolites. The best characterized are morphine-3-glucuronide and hydromorphone-3-glucuronide.[5,6] Serum and cerebrospinal fluid levels, as well as the ratios of these metabolites, are elevated in patients receiving morphine or hydromorphone for cancer and nonmalignant pain.[7] This is particularly true for patients with renal dysfunction.[8] However, clinical evidence of myoclonus does not consistently correlate with serum levels of morphine-3-glucuronide, and some patients may develop myoclonus with very low doses of opioids.[9] Hyperalgesia is particularly associated with these metabolites, although other opioids with no known metabolites have also produced myoclonus.[10] A variety of other metabolites of opioids exist, including morphine-6-glucuronide and hydromorphone-6-glucuronide, but these have been implicated in nausea and vomiting, as well as sedation, rather than myoclonus.

Opioids given in high doses may be more likely to result in myoclonus.[3] Bruera and Pereira[11] reported the development of acute confusion, restlessness, myoclonus, hallucinations, and hyperalgesia due to an inadvertant administration of 5000-mcg intravenous (IV) fentanyl (the patient had been receiving 1000 mcg/h subcutaneously). These symptoms were successfully treated with several doses of 0.1 to 0.2 mg of IV naloxone, followed by a continuous IV naloxone infusion of 0.2 mg/h. The patient did not demonstrate withdrawal symptoms initially, yet began to complain of return of pain after several hours (see Chapter 7 regarding the use of diluted naloxone to reverse adverse effects associated with opioids). Other opioids, including methadone,[12] meperidine,[13] and transdermal fentanyl[14] have been implicated in the development of myoclonus.

Other reported causes of myoclonus include beta-lactam antibiotics, both tricyclic and newer antidepressants, surgery to the brain,[15] placement of an intrathecal catheter,[16] AIDS dementia,[17] hypoxia,[18] chlorambucil,[19] and a paraneoplastic syndrome.[20] This paraneoplastic syndrome is rare, occurring in fewer than 1% of people with cancer. The etiology of the paraneoplastic syndrome can also be viral, and is believed to be immunologically mediated. Symptoms of this paraneoplastic (also called opsoclonus-myoclonus) syndrome include myoclonus, opsoclonus, ataxia, and encephalopathic features.[21] Treatment of the underlying tumor or infection and immunosuppression are possible options.[20,21]

### Assessment

An accurate history from the patient and family is essential. An analogy that can be used to help patients describe the symptoms is to compare the jerking to the feeling that often happens when one is close to falling asleep (a common condition called nocturnal myoclonus). The difference is that myoclonus associated with end-of-life care is usually continuous. Physical exam will reveal jerking of the extremities, which is uncontrolled by movement or other activities. Jerking can be induced by single or repeated tapping of a muscle group.

### Treatment

Opioid rotation is the primary treatment of myoclonus, particularly if the patient is receiving higher doses of an opioid and has renal dysfunction.[1] There is great variation in individual

response to opioids; thus, different agents may have a greater likelihood of producing myoclonus or other adverse effects. Presently, there are no tests that predict individual response, and trials are the only strategy for determining effectiveness as well as adverse effects. In addition, cross-tolerance is not complete; thus, lower equianalgesic doses of an alternate opioid may provide analgesia. Methadone has been successfully used as an alternative agent,[7] although other opioids may be easier to titrate, and methadone also has been reported to cause myoclonus.[12] Strategies that reduce the necessary amount of opioid, such as adding adjuvant analgesics, could reduce or eliminate myoclonus.

Little research is available regarding agents used to reduce myoclonic jerking. Benzodiazepines, including clonazepam, diazepam, and midazolam, have been recommended.[1,22] The antispasmodic baclofen has been used to treat myoclonus due to intraspinal opioid administration.[23] Dantrolene has been used, although it produces significant muscle weakness and hepatotoxicity.[24]

### Patient and Family Education

Safety measures are essential, as are interventions designed to reduce fatigue during myoclonus. Use padding around bed rails, and assistive devices if the patient is ambulatory. Provide a calm, relaxing environment. Pain assessment is critical as opioids are rotated, since equianalgesic conversions are approximations, and wide variability of response exists. Therefore, patients and family members are encouraged to track pain intensity as opioids are titrated to provide optimal relief.

✢

CASE STUDY
*Intractable Myoclonus Requiring Palliative Sedation*

A 46-year-old man had been diagnosed three years earlier with multiple myeloma. During the course of his treatment, he reported significant pain from vertebral body disease and other sites of pain. This was generally well managed with opioids and adjuvant analgesics. Despite aggressive therapy, the disease progressed, and one day while raising himself from a chair, his ulna fractured, leading to severe pain. He was immediately admitted to the palliative care unit, where an infusion of hydromorphone was initiated and titrated rapidly to obtain relief. He was also given corticosteroids and placed on an air-flow bed in an effort to relieve pain. Within 24 hours, he was comfortable. Unfortunately, he developed myclonic jerking, which resulted in severe pain with each jerk of his extremities. Hydration was increased, the opioid was rotated to morphine, and attempts were made to reduce the dose. Midazolam was started at a low infusion but was ineffective at reversing myoclonus until he was completely sedated. Because his renal status had deteriorated, it was thought he had only days to live, and palliative sedation was offered to him and his family. Per

**Table 19–1
Causes of Headache More Commonly Seen
in Palliative Care**

- Primary or metastatic brain tumors
- Central nervous system infection
- Vascular disorders
- Traumatic brain injury
- Adverse drug effects
- Withdrawal from drugs and other substances
- Fever

their request, palliative sedation was initiated by titrating midazolam to comfort. During this time his wife brought in photo albums of their life together, and friends and staff offered support. His wife commented that this time together, despite his inability to respond, helped prepare her for his death three days later.

## Headache

Headache can be a debilitating symptom resulting from a variety of etiologies common in palliative care, including intracranial tumors, vascular disorders, infection, or head trauma (Table 19–1). Although persistent headaches are more distressing, withdrawal from certain substances can occur in palliative care, which in turn can lead to acute onset of headache. These substances primarily include caffeine, cocaine, estrogen, marijuana, and opioids, and resolution of the headache occurs in 3–7 days. Additionally, fever due to systemic infection, which is prevalent in end-of-life, can produce headache. Although common throughout the general population, including those in palliative care, standard tension-type or migraine headaches will not be addressed here, but the reader is directed to several useful references.

More information is available regarding headaches associated with intracranial tumors or headache in HIV. The prevalence of headaches in patients with either primary or metastatic tumors in the brain is believed to be from 60% to 90%. In children, brain tumors are the most common solid tumor, and headache is the most common presenting sign. The mechanism of pain from intracerebral tumors is likely direct pressure on nerves, as well as distention and inflammation of surrounding vascular structures. In HIV-infected individuals, headache can occur from the virus itself, from antiviral therapy, from opportunistic infections, or from tumors in the central nervous system. Less is known about the prevalence of headache in patients who have experienced stroke, or other vascular or neurological disorders affecting the brain. It is estimated that up to 8% of people who have experienced stroke develop central pain syndromes, which may include headache. Patients who have had traumatic brain injury often experience

headache in the initial months after the injury, and for some, the headache persists with negative consequences on quality of life. Multiple sclerosis and other neurologic disorders have been associated with headache, yet little information exists about the experiences these patients face.

### Assessment

As with a general pain assessment, characteristics to evaluate in the patient with headache include intensity, location, quality, exacerbating and alleviating factors, the response to past and current therapies, and related symptoms. Most headaches experienced by individuals with intracerebral tumor are described as dull, poorly localized and of moderate intensity. Patients with metastases may experience pain on the same side as the lesion. Nausea, vomiting, photophobia, neck rigidity and other neurologic deficits may occur with headache, and some patients will progress to develop seizures and cognitive dysfunction. Patients may describe exacerbation of the headache by coughing, lifting heavier objects, or Valsalva's maneuver.

Physical assessment inlcudes palpation over the sites of pain to rule out possible sinus infection or non-malignant causes of headache. A careful neurological evaluation may reveal deficits that can identify the underlying site of tumor spread, as well as guide strategies for care. For example, metastases in the base of the skull, which occurs more frequently with breast, lung, and prostate cancers, can produce a wide variety of pain syndromes that vary with the tumor location. A specific case is orbital metastasis producing pain behind or above the eye, with possible blurred vision, double vision, and exophthalmos. Treatment should focus on pain control, as well as safety measures to prevent falls or other injuries.

### Management

Antitumor therapies, including surgery, radiotherapy, chemotherapy, and hormonal therapies may be indicated if this is consistent with the patient's goals of care. Analgesics include corticosteroids, opioids, anticonvulsants, and antidepressants. Dexamethasone is the most frequently employed corticosteroid in palliative care because of its availability in both oral and parenteral formulations, and it has less mineralocorticoid effect when compared with other agents. Because of the potential for steroid-induced myopathy, the lowest effective dose of dexamethasone should be used. (See next section on seizures for more information on dexamethasone, and Chapter 7 for more information about the use of analgesics in palliative care.)

### Patient and Family Education

Family members need significant support when caring for a loved one with severe, persistent headache. Not only is it devastating to witness pain, but the family may express feelings of loss and sadness as the patient develops cognitive and other neurological symptoms. Guilt, frustration, and exhaustion from providing care are common emotions that demand attention. Education regarding management of pain is crucial, as is information regarding safety measures tailored to the precise neurological deficits experienced by the patient. Positioning is important, as many people with headache from brain tumor experience less pain when the head of the bed is elevated. Patients and family members can be instructed on cognitive behavioral therapies, such as guided imagery, distraction, music, prayer, and other interventions.

## Seizures

Of the many neurological disorders that occur in advanced disease, seizures are the most frightening. This fear exists for the patient and for caregivers. Furthermore, seizures can be exhausting for the patient, eliminating the few energy reserves that might be better spent on quality activities. Therefore, seizures must be prevented whenever possible. When prevention is not feasible, all attempts should be made to limit the extent of the seizure and to ensure safety measures are in place to prevent trauma during these episodes.

Seizures occur when a large number of neurons discharge abnormally.[25] This abnormal discharge produces involuntary paroxysmal behavioral changes. There are two types of seizure, including primary (also called generalized) and focal (also called partial). Primary seizures involve large parts of the brain and include both grand mal and petit mal types. Focal seizures are isolated to specific regions of the brain, and symptoms reflect the area of disturbance.[25] For example, Jacksonian motor seizures result from abnormal discharge in the motor cortex. These patients may have involuntary twitching of muscle groups, usually on the contralateral side of the body. If the tumor is located in the left motor cortex (anterior to the central sulcus), the activity is seen on the right side of the body. Often, activity begins in one area and spreads throughout that side of the body as the abnormal discharge spreads to nearby cortical neurons. Patients generally remain conscious, unless the abnormal cortical discharge spreads to the opposite hemisphere. In the palliative care setting, there are many potential causes of seizure activity.

### Causes of Seizures

Careful consideration of the many causes of seizure activity must be included in the assessment of patients at the end of life, whether the patient has demonstrated seizure activity or not. This allows prevention whenever possible. Primary or metastatic neoplasms to the brain are common causes of seizures in palliative care, as are preexisting seizure disorders.[26] Medications, including phenothiazines, butyrophenones, and tricyclic antidepressants, can lower the seizure threshold.

| Table 19–2 |
| --- |
| **Causes of Seizures in Palliative Care** |
| Primary or metastatic neoplasm to the brain |
| Preexisting seizure disorder |
| Medications |
| • Lower seizure threshold |
| • Metabolites |
| • Preservatives, antioxidants, or other additives |
| • Abstinence |
| Metabolic disorders |
| Infection |
| Trauma |
| Strokes and hemorrhage |
| Paraneoplastic syndromes |

Other medication-related causes of seizures include metabolites (e.g., normeperidine), preservatives within these compounds (e.g., sodium bisulfite), or the abrupt discontinuation of certain drugs (e.g., benzodiazepines).[3,27] Additional causes of seizures at the end of life include metabolic disorders, infection, HIV, stroke, hemorrhage, oxygen deprivation, and some rare paraneoplastic syndromes (Table 19–2).[26,28,29]

*Primary or Metastatic Brain Tumors.* Brain tumors can result in either primary (generalized) or focal seizures. Seizures occur in approximately 25% of those with brain metastases.[30] Patients with malignancies known to metastasize to the brain, such as breast, lung, hypernephroma, and melanoma, should be considered at risk for seizures. Leukemias and lymphomas are also known to produce infiltrates in the brain. Multiple metastases, or brain and leptomeningeal disease, are more commonly associated with seizures.[30] The tumor location, size, and histology dictate whether seizures may result, and determine the symptoms associated with the seizure.

*Medications.* Medications can lead to seizures in the palliative care setting through several mechanisms. Medications such as the phenothiazines, butyrophenones, and tricyclic antidepressants can place patients at risk by lowering the seizure threshold. These agents should be used cautiously in patients with intracranial tumors or infection. There are reports of patients developing seizures due to fluoroquinolones, including ofloxacin and ifosfamide (more likely if serum creatinine is elevated and the patient has had prior treatment with cisplatin), as well as cephalosporins and monobactams.[31–35] In very high doses, any opioid can lead to seizures. Several opioids are associated with much higher risk due to their metabolites that cause seizures. Meperidine is converted to normeperidine during metabolism.[13] Individuals with renal dysfunction cannot excrete normeperidine efficiently; the metabolite then accumulates in the bloodstream and leads to seizures. Therefore, the clinical practice guidelines for cancer pain developed by the American Pain Society strongly discourage the use of meperidine in any patient, a practice long followed by those in palliative care.[36] These guidelines also discourage the use of propoxyphene (the weak opioid in Darvon) in persons with cancer, due to the metabolite norpropoxyphene.[36]

More recently, morphine and hydromorphone have been found to be metabolized by glucuronidation to morphine-3-glucuronide or hydromorphine-3-glucuronide, respectively. These metabolites may produce hyperalgesia (elevated pain intensity), myoclonus (see previous section), and seizure in patients unable to excrete them efficiently.[7,10] Clinically, patients respond acceptably to the opioid for the first day or two, then develop symptoms after the metabolite has accumulated. Alternately, the patient may have obtained good relief in the absence of opioid neurolotoxicity, until renal status diminishes, with concomitant difficulties in clearing the metabolite. Another opioid, tramadol, has been associated with seizure risk, especially when taken with other drugs that lower the seizure threshold.

Compounds added to medications to preserve the drug or prevent its breakdown (such as sodium bisulfite) are normally present in extremely small amounts. However, when high doses of a drug, usually opioids, are needed to treat severe pain, the concomitant dose of these additives increases. In this setting, there have been rare reports of seizures.[27] Using preservative-free solutions when administering high doses of any agent may prevent this activity. Hagen and Swanson[3] report a syndrome of opioid hyperexcitability that progressed to seizures in five patients with high-dose infusions. Parenteral midazolam infusion was used to treat the seizures, the patients were rotated to alternative opioids (including levorphanol and methadone), and aggressive supportive care was provided during the episodes.

Rapid cessation of various drugs can lead to seizure activity in the palliative care setting. Often, this occurs when staff are unaware that a patient uses certain medications and, as a result, these drugs are not provided when patients are hospitalized, or are unable to independently dispense their own drugs. Benzodiazepines, barbiturates, and baclofen are the most common drugs associated with seizures during abstinence.[25] This also can occur when the patient abuses these compounds or alcohol, and the staff or family is unaware. Alcohol abuse often is underrecognized in the palliative care setting.[37]

*Other Causes of Seizures in Palliative Care.* Infection within the brain, as may be seen in persons with human immunodeficiency virus (HIV) or acquired immunodeficiency syndrome (AIDS), can lead to seizure activity.[17,29] The syndrome of inappropriate antidiuretic hormone, associated with lung cancer and other malignancies, can result in increased water and sodium content within the cells.[38] The resultant swelling of neuronal cells within the brain causes increased intracranial pressure (ICP). Anoxia deprives the brain of needed nutrients, resulting in an inability to drive sodium out of neuronal tissue. Water follows into the cells, creating increased ICP. Hyponatremia (<130 mEq/L), especially when of rapid onset, can also lead to mental status changes and seizures.

## Assessment

Obtain a thorough history from the patient and caregiver to ascertain any symptoms existing with the onset of the seizure, the specific type of seizure activity, and whether there was any aura immediately before the seizure.[25] Headache, nausea, and projectile vomiting are associated with increased ICP and can occur immediately before seizure activity.[30] The family may relate a staring-type behavior, where the patient does not respond to stimuli for a brief moment.

The past medical history might reveal a seizure disorder. Review all drugs recently added to the plan of care for agents that might lower the seizure threshold or produce metabolites. Question whether the patient recently discontinued a drug, including recreational drugs. If the patient is currently taking anticonvulsants or corticosteroids for seizures and increased ICP, determine if there could be reasons that the drugs were not ingested or absorbed. These might include compliance issues, or nausea and vomiting.

Often, the clinician may not witness the seizure and must rely on the observation and memory of family members and caregivers. Assist family members in differentiating between seizures and myoclonus (see previous section) or altered level of consciousness due to other etiologies. A thorough examination is indicated, with attention to bruises and other signs of trauma. If these occur, additional teaching for family and caregivers regarding safety measures is warranted.

Measuring serum levels of anticonvulsants may be indicated to insure that the drug is adequately absorbed.[39] Dose adjustments may be implemented empirically, based on the patient's condition. Electroencephalography may be used to identify the site of abnormal discharge. Brain lesions may be scanned using computed tomography (CT) or magnetic resonance imaging (MRI). These tests should only be considered if they will provide information that will guide therapy, and if they are consistent with the patient's and family's goals of care.

## Treatment

Anticonvulsants are used when patients have demonstrated seizures (Table 19–3). The prophylactic use of anticonvulsants in patients who have not had a seizure is controversial. Prophylactic anticonvulsant therapy has demonstrated benefit only in the case of brain metastases from melanoma. Anticonvulsants are often used after craniotomy for brain tumor, with a reduction in postoperative seizure incidence, yet after one week there does not appear to be a benefit with long-term use of these drugs. The potential benefits must be weighed against the side effects associated with these agents.

The most common anticonvulsants used in the United States to prevent seizures are phenytoin, carbamazepine, valproate, and phenobarbital (see Table 19–3).[39] Newer anticonvulsants, such as gabapentin, pregabalin, vigabatrin, and lamotrigine, have not been extensively studied in the palliative care setting.[39,40] Agents used during a seizure include diazepam, lorazepam, midazolam, phenytoin, and phenobarbital (Table 19–4).

**Table 19–3**
**Prophylactic Pharmacological Management of Seizures**

| Drug | Adult Dose | Adverse Effects | Comments |
|---|---|---|---|
| Phenytoin (Dilantin)<br>• Tablets<br>• Capsules<br>• Suspension<br>• Parenteral | Loading dose: 5 mg/kg PO q3h × 3 doses (loading dose not to be used in patients with renal or hepatic disease). Maintenance: 5 mg/kg PO. | Nystagmus, ataxia, slurred speech, mental confusion, Stevens-Johnson syndrome.<br>Too rapid IV injection (>50 mg/min) can result in cardiac toxicity. | Usual serum level 10–20 mcg/mL (or 10–20 mg/L or 40–80 µmol/L) |
| Carbamazepine (Tegretol)<br>• Tablets<br>• Suspension | 400 mg/day:<br><br>Tablet: 200 mg bid<br>Suspension: 1 teaspoon qid<br>Maximum dose: 1600 mg/24 h. | Aplastic anemia, agranulocytosis Patients with known sensitivity to tricyclic antidepressants may be hypersensitive to carbamazepine. | Periodic blood counts and liver function tests indicated. Therapeutic plasma levels 4–12 mcg/mL. |
| Valproic acid (Depakene)<br>• Capsules<br>• Syrup | 15 mg/kg daily, increasing weekly in 5–10 mg increments. Syrup can be given rectally by a red rubber catheter 250–500 mg tid. | Hepatic failure, coagulopathies, nausea, vomiting, sedation. | Therapeutic plasma levels 50–100 mcg/mL. |
| Divalproex sodium (Depakote)<br>• Capsules<br>• Sprinkles<br>• Tablets | Same dosing for valproic acid and divalproex, although peaks and troughs may differ. | Chewing may produce irritation of the mouth and throat. | |
| Phenobarbital<br>• Tablets<br>• Elixir<br>• Parenteral | Oral: 60–200 mg/day.<br>Parenteral: 3–4-mg/kg q24h continuous SQ infusion. | Sedation, paradoxical excitation. | |
| Midazolam (Versed)<br>• Parenteral | 1–3 mg/h continuous SQ or IV infusion. | Sedation, respiratory depression if overdose. | Antagonist, flumazenil, can result in seizures. Use same extreme caution as when giving naloxone for suspected opioid overdose. |

SQ = subcutaneous; IV = intravenous.

**Table 19–4**
**Acute Treatment of Seizures**

| Drug | Dose |
|---|---|
| Diazepam (Valium) | 5–10 mg slow IV push (stop other infusions to prevent incompatibility problems) or 5–10 mg IM every 5–10 min if no IV access, can also use diazepam (Diastat) rectal gel, usually 10 mg per rectum. |
| Fosphenytoin (Cerebyx) | 15–20 mg phenytoin equivalents/kg IV loading dose. |
| Lorazepam (Ativan) | 1 mg/min up to 5 mg. |
| Midazolam (Versed) | 0.02–0.10 mg/kg continuous hourly infusion. |
| Phenobarbital | 20 mg/kg IV at a rate of 100 mg/min. |
| Phenytoin (Dilantin) | Acute treatment: 20 mg/kg IV infusion over 20–30 min.<br>An additional 5–10 mg/kg can be given if seizures persist. However, IV injections can cause severe local reactions, including edema, pain, and discoloration. |

A particular challenge in palliative care is the administration of these drugs when the patient is unable to take oral medications. The intramuscular route can be used for some (diazepam and phenobarbitol), but since this route is painful and absorption is unpredictable, its use should be reserved for situations when no other access is practical or possible. Diazepam is available in a rectal gel. Doses are 200 mcg/kg body weight, rounded down to the next available unit dose (10-mg, 15-mg, and 20-mg unit doses for adults) in debilitated patients. Phenobarbital is available in a solution for parenteral delivery, and pentobarbital (used more commonly in Canada and Europe) is available in rectal formulations. Intravenous phenytoin can lead to the purple-glove syndrome, a potentially serious local complication including edema, discoloration, and pain distal to the injection site.[41,42] Fosphenytoin, although more expensive, has an advantage in palliative care because it can be given subcutaneously (by either intermittent injection or infusion) for prevention or treatment of seizures. Dosing is based on phenytoin equivalents, generally 5- to 10-mg phenytoin equivalent/kg. Little research has compared the efficacy of these agents, particularly in the palliative care setting. The choice of agent is often based on the availability of the drug, comfort level of the practitioner, ability to use nonoral routes, and other factors. Because most medications are administered by nonprofessional caregivers in the home, often elderly spouses of aged patients, it is best to keep the drug regimen simple.

A recent review described tailoring anticonvulsant therapy based upon the comorbid conditions or symptoms experienced by the patient. For example, for patients with anxiety, gabapentin or pregabalin may provide benefit as a result of the anxiolytic properties of these agents. Since each anticonvulsant has different effects and drug profiles, careful consideration of the total needs of each patient must be given when these drugs are necessary components of the drug regimen.

Many patients with seizure disorders will also be taking dexamethasone. Dexamethasone is technically not an anticonvulsant, yet this compound is critical when intracranial lesions are present that might increase ICP.[39] Although many sources suggest four-times-a-day (qid) dosing, the long half-life of dexamethasone allows daily dosing with adequate serum levels maintained throughout the 24-hour period. Of additional concern is the interaction between phenytoin and dexamethasone. Phenytoin can decrease the bioavailability of dexamethasone by as much as 20%. Additionally, dexamethasone inhibits the metabolism of phenytoin, reducing the anticonvulsant effect of this drug. Thus, extreme care must be exercised when adding or titrating either drug when using combinations. Phenytoin can alter plasma levels of several drugs (Table 19–5). In the palliative care setting, if a patient decides to stop all corticosteroids, the professional must evaluate the likelihood of developing seizures. Prophylactic therapy must be considered.

Status epilepticus is a seizure that persists longer than five minutes, or repeated seizures without a return to consciousness between each episode.[43] This is considered a neuro-oncological emergency. Clear the airway, ensure adequate perfusion, give glucose (usually 50 mL of a 50% solution), evaluate electrolytes, and administer IV benzodiazepine (such as diazepam or lorazepam), followed by a loading dose of IV phenytoin. The Veterans Administration Cooperative Trial of Status Epilepticus revealed response rates during first-line treatment as follows: lorazepam 64.9%, phenobarbitol 58.2%, diazepam plus phenytoin 55.8%, and phenytoin alone 43.6%.[44] These results suggest that lorazepam should be the first drug of choice. If the seizure is not relieved in 5 to 7 minutes, add phenytoin or fosphenytoin. If recurrent, continuous infusion of phenobarbital or diazepam is indicated. In extreme cases, barbiturate anesthesia, neuromuscular blockade, and propofol may be indicated.[45]

## Patient and Family Education

Witnessing a seizure can be extremely frightening for family members and caregivers. Preparation is critical. Explain that restraining the patient or attempting to place objects in the mouth can lead to significant harm. Educate family members to move items out of the way that might cause trauma, and to get the patient to lie on one side if possible. Caregivers may be given information regarding the jaw-lift technique if the airway is compromised. Pillows placed around the bed, between the patient and the siderails (if a hospital-style bed is in use), and around the room can be quickly positioned to prevent trauma. Caution family members to refrain from feeding or providing fluids until the patient is fully alert and able to swallow. However, if the patient has grossly unstable blood sugar levels and is prone to developing hypoglycemia, candy, glucose, juice, or other sources of glucose can be given, but only if the patient is able to swallow. Glucagon can also be given subcutaneously. Inform family members that loss of continence is common during a seizure and does not imply that the patient is not able to control these functions at other times. Encourage them to assist the patient while being considerate of the patient's ability and dignity.

| Table 19–5 Drugs That Interact with Phenytoin |
| --- |
| **Drugs that may increase phenytoin serum levels** |
| Alcohol, amiodarone, choramphenicol, chlordiazepoxide, diazepam, dicumarol, disulfiram, estrongens, H₂ antagonists, halothane, isoniazide, methylphenidate, phenothiazines, phenylbutazone, salicylates, succinimides, sulfonamides, tolbutamide, trazodone. |
| **Drugs that may decrease phenytoin serum levels** |
| Carbamazepine, chronic alcohol abuse, reserpine, sucralfate, antacids with calcium (should not be taken with phenytoin but at a different time). |
| **Drugs that may have reduced efficacy due to phenytoin** |
| Corticosteroids (including dexamethasone), coumarin anticoagulants, digitoxin, doxycycline, estrogens, furosemide, oral contraceptives, quinidine, rifampin, theophylline, vitamin D. |

To help recovery after a seizure, the patient may benefit from reduced stimulation. Lower the lights, reduce the sound of televisions or radios, and speak softly and reassuringly. Assess for pain and treat accordingly. Relaxation exercises also may be helpful. Often, patients will sleep for several hours after the seizure.

## Spasticity

Spasticity is a movement disorder that results in a partial or complete loss of supraspinal control of spinal cord function. Patients may exhibit involuntary movement, abnormal posture, rigidity, and exaggerated reflexes. Spasticity may interfere with all aspects of life by limiting mobility, disturbing sleep, and causing pain.[46] Spasticity is often associated with advanced multiple sclerosis (MS), spinal cord trauma, tumors of the spinal cord, stroke, meningitis, and other infections.[47-49] In a study of 2104 patients with nontraumatic spasticity seen in a regional neuroscience center in the United Kingdom, 17.8% had MS, 16.4% had neoplasm, and 4.1% had motor neuron disease.[50]

### Assessment

Patients will describe a gradual onset of loss of muscle tone, followed by resistance and jerking when muscles are flexed. A recent history of urinary tract infection, decubitus ulcer, constipation, or pain may immediately predate the onset, or increased episodes, of spasticity.

Physical exam will yield resistance and spasticity when doing passive limb movement. The faster the passive movement, the more pronounced the effect. Reflexes may be hyperactive, particularly in the affected area. Bruises are common as patients inadvertently and uncontrollably move their limbs, resulting in trauma.

### Management

The standard therapies for reducing spasticity include oral baclofen, a gamma-aminobutyric acid-B agonist. Baclofen is generally started with lower doses, 5 to 10 mg/day, and titrated upward gradually, using three- or four-times-a-day dosing. Although effective for some patients, higher doses are often necessary and frequently result in cognitive changes and dizziness. For this reason, intrathecal baclofen has been administered with good results.[51] Those in palliative care must weigh the benefits of intrathecal baclofen therapy given the patient's prognosis, the availability of skilled clinicians to administer the therapy, cost, and other factors.

Muscle relaxants, such as dantrolene 50 to 100 mg/day, diminish the force of the contraction.[47] Start at 25 mg daily and increase by 25-mg increments in divided doses every 4 to 7 days. The contents can be mixed with liquids if the patient is unable to swallow capsules. Although this reduces spasticity, significant impairment in muscle strength can occur. Therefore, dantrolene is not recommended in ambulatory patients. Furthermore, dantrolene can cause hepatotoxicity. Marijuana, and its active ingredient delta-9-tetrahydrocannabinol (THC), has been described by patients as useful in the relief of spinal cord spasticity.[52] Newer synthetic compounds of THC have been shown to reduce spasticity associated with multiple sclerosis. Although not approved for this purpose, there is general agreement within the medical community that the treatment of spasticity may be a legitimate use of THC and related compounds.

### Patient and Family Education

Patients and their caregivers should be educated about factors that may worsen spasticity, including constipation, urinary tract infection, pressure ulcers, fatigue, and psychosocial concerns. Strategies to prevent and relieve these conditions should be clearly communicated, and early communication regarding their onset should be encouraged. When spasticity occurs, the patient and family members must understand the rationale for drug therapy. Nonpharmacological therapy also may be helpful. Family members may be encouraged to gently massage the affected extremities, although this may produce increased spasticity in some patients. Repositioning, heat, and range-of-motion exercises have been described by patients as being helpful. As with other neurological disorders, safety measures are imperative. Padding wheelchairs, bed rails, and any other furniture that might come in contact with spastic extremities, will reduce trauma.

## Conclusion

Neurological disorders, including myoclonus, headache, seizures, and spasticity, create fear, reduce energy levels, increase pain, and can complicate the course of a patient's illness. The goal in palliative care is prevention whenever possible. When not possible, early diagnosis and treatment are critical. Knowledge of pharmacotherapy is essential, including agents that might precipitate these disorders, drugs that are used to treat these syndromes, and drug interactions that might occur in the palliative care setting. As with all aspects of palliative care, the patient and family are the center of care. Nurses skilled in palliative care can empower them through education and support. The interdisciplinary approach exemplified by palliative care is key.

REFERENCES

1. Mercadante S. Pathophysiology and treatment of opioid-related myoclonus in cancer patients. Pain 1998;74:5–9.
2. Nunez-Olarte J. Opioid-induced myoclonus. Eur J Palliat Care 1995;2:146–150.

3. Hagen N, Swanson R. Strychnine-like multifocal myoclonus and seizures in extremely high-dose opioid administration: Treatment strategies. J Pain Symptom Manage 1997;14:51–58.

4. Hemstapat K, Monteith GR, Smith D, Smith MT. Morphine-3-glucuronide's neuro-excitatory effects are mediated via indirect activation of N-methyl-D-aspartic acid receptors: Mechanistic studies in embryonic cultured hippocampal neurones. Anesth Analg 2003;97:494–505, table of contents.

5. Smith MT. Neuroexcitatory effects of morphine and hydromorphone: Evidence implicating the 3-glucuronide metabolites. Clin Exp Pharmacol Physiol 2000;27:524–528.

6. Wright AW, Mather LE, Smith MT. Hydromorphone-3-glucuronide: A more potent neuro-excitant than its structural analogue, morphine-3-glucuronide. Life Sci 2001;69:409–420.

7. Sjogren P, Thunedborg LP, Christrup L, Hansen SH, Franks J. Is development of hyperalgesia, allodynia and myoclonus related to morphine metabolism during long-term administration? Six case histories. Acta Anaesthesiol Scand 1998;42:1070–1075.

8. Lee MA, Leng ME, Tiernan EJ. Retrospective study of the use of hydromorphone in palliative care patients with normal and abnormal urea and creatinine. Palliat Med 2001;15:26–34.

9. Klepstad P, Borchgrevink PC, Dale O, et al. Routine drug monitoring of serum concentrations of morphine, morphine-3-glucuronide and morphine-6-glucuronide do not predict clinical observations in cancer patients. Palliat Med 2003;17:679–687.

10. Gong QL, Hedner J, Bjorkman R, Hedner T. Morphine-3-glucuronide may functionally antagonize morphine-6-glucuronide induced antinociception and ventilatory depression in the rat. Pain 1992;48:249–255.

11. Bruera E, Pereira J. Acute neuropsychiatric findings in a patient receiving fentanyl for cancer pain. Pain 1997;69:199–201.

12. Sarhill N, Davis MP, Walsh D, Nouneh C. Methadone-induced myoclonus in advanced cancer. Am J Hosp Palliat Care 2001;18:51–53.

13. Kaiko RF, Foley KM, Grabinski PY, et al. Central nervous system excitatory effects of meperidine in cancer patients. Ann Neurol 1983;13:180–185.

14. Han PK, Arnold R, Bond G, Janson D, Abu-Elmagd K. Myoclonus secondary to withdrawal from transdermal fentanyl: Case report and literature review. J Pain Symptom Manage 2002;23:66–72.

15. Nishigaya K, Kaneko M, Nagaseki Y, Nukui H. Palatal myoclonus induced by extirpation of a cerebellar astrocytoma. Case report. J Neurosurg 1998;88:1107–1110.

16. Ford B, Pullman SL, Khandji A, Goodman R. Spinal myoclonus induced by an intrathecal catheter. Mov Disord 1997;12:1042–1045.

17. Maher J, Choudhri S, Halliday W, Power C, Nath A. AIDS dementia complex with generalized myoclonus. Mov Disord 1997;12:593–597.

18. Werhahn KJ, Brown P, Thompson PD, Marsden CD. The clinical features and prognosis of chronic posthypoxic myoclonus. Mov Disord 1997;12:216–220.

19. Wyllie AR, Bayliff CD, Kovacs MJ. Myoclonus due to chlorambucil in two adults with lymphoma. Ann Pharmacother 1997;31:171–174.

20. Pranzatelli MR, Tate ED, Kinsbourne M, Caviness VS, Jr, Mishra B. Forty-one year follow-up of childhood-onset opsoclonus-myoclonus-ataxia: Cerebellar atrophy, multiphasic relapses, and response to IVIG. Mov Disord 2002;17:1387–1390.

21. Batchelor TT, Platten M, Hochberg FH. Immunoadsorption therapy for paraneoplastic syndromes. J Neurooncol 1998;40:131–136.

22. Eisele JH, Jr., Grigsby EJ, Dea G. Clonazepam treatment of myoclonic contractions associated with high-dose opioids: Case report. Pain 1992;49:231–232.

23. Stayer C, Tronnier V, Dressnandt J, et al. Intrathecal baclofen therapy for stiff-man syndrome and progressive encephalomyelopathy with rigidity and myoclonus. Neurology 1997;49:1591–1597.

24. Mercadante S. Dantrolene treatment of opioid-induced myoclonus. Anesth Analg 1995;81:1307–1308.

25. Sirven JI. Classifying seizures and epilepsy: A synopsis. Semin Neurol 2002;22:237–246.

26. Lassman AB, DeAngelis LM. Brain metastases. Neurol Clin 2003;21:1–23, vii.

27. Gregory RE, Grossman S, Sheidler VR. Grand mal seizures associated with high-dose intravenous morphine infusions: Incidence and possible etiology. Pain 1992;51:255–258.

28. Steeghs N, de Jongh FE, Sillevis Smitt PA, van den Bent MJ. Cisplatin-induced encephalopathy and seizures. Anticancer Drugs 2003;14:443–446.

29. Romanelli F, Ryan M. Seizures in HIV-seropositive individuals: Epidemiology and treatment. CNS Drugs 2002;16:91–98.

30. Schaller B, Ruegg SJ. Brain tumor and seizures: Pathophysiology and its implications for treatment revisited. Epilepsia 2003;44:1223–1232.

31. Walton GD, Hon JK, Mulpur TG. Ofloxacin-induced seizure. Ann Pharmacother 1997;31:1475–1477.

32. Kushner JM, Peckman HJ, Snyder CR. Seizures associated with fluoroquinolones. Ann Pharmacother 2001;35:1194–1198.

33. Steinmann RA, Rickel MK. A 23-year-old with refractory seizures following an isoniazid overdose. J Emerg Nurs 2002;28:7–10.

34. Bassilios N, Restoux A, Vincent F, Rondeau E, Sraer JD. Piperacillin/Tazobactam inducing seizures in a hemodialysed patient. Clin Nephrol 2002;58:327–328.

35. Sugimoto M, Uchida I, Mashimo T, et al. Evidence for the involvement of GABA(A) receptor blockade in convulsions induced by cephalosporins. Neuropharmacology 2003;45:304–314.

36. Miaskowski C, Cleary J, Burney R, et al. Guideline for the Management of Cancer Pain in Adults and Children. APS Clinical Practice Guidelines Series, No. 3. Glenview, IL: American Pain Society, 2005.

37. Bruera E, Moyano J, Seifert L, Fainsinger RL, Hanson J, Suarez-Almazor M. The frequency of alcoholism among patients with pain due to terminal cancer. J Pain Symptom Manage 1995;10:599–603.

38. Daniels AC, Chokroverty S, Barron KD. Thalamic degeneration, dementia, and seizures. Inappropriate ADH secretion associated with bronchogenic carcinoma. Arch Neurol 1969;21:15–24.

39. Beydoun A, Passaro EA. Appropriate use of medications for seizures. Guiding principles on the path of efficacy. Postgrad Med 2002;111:69–82.

40. Kasteleijn-Nolst Trenite DG, Hirsch E. Levetiracetam: Preliminary efficacy in generalized seizures. Epileptic Disord 2003;5:S39–S44.

41. O'Brien TJ, Cascino GD, So EL, Hanna DR. Incidence and clinical consequence of the purple glove syndrome

in patients receiving intravenous phenytoin. Neurology 1998;51:1034–1039.

42. O'Brien TJ, Meara FM, Matthews H, Vajda FJ. Prospective study of local cutaneous reactions in patients receiving IV phenytoin. Neurology 2001;57:1508–1510.

43. Rosenow F, Arzimanoglou A, Baulac M. Recent developments in treatment of status epilepticus: A review. Epileptic Disord 2002;4:S41–S51.

44. Bleck TP. Management approaches to prolonged seizures and status epilepticus. Epilepsia 1999;40:S59–S63.

45. Golf M, Paice JA, Feulner E, O'Leary C, Marcotte S, Mulcahy M. Refractory status epilepticus. J Palliat Med 2004;7:85–88.

46. Gianino J, York M, Paice J. Intrathecal Drug Therapy for Spasticity and Pain. New York: Springer-Verlag, 1996: 67–76.

47. Ben-Zacharia AB, Lublin FD. Palliative care in patients with multiple sclerosis. Neurol Clin 2001;19:801–827.

48. Lorenz R. A causistic rationale for the treatment of spastic and myocloni in a childhood neurodegenerative disease: Neuronal ceroid lipofuscinosis of the type Jansky-Bielschowsky. Neuroendocrinol Lett 2002;23:387–390.

49. Watkins CL, Leathley MJ, Gregson JM, Moore AP, Smith TL, Sharma AK. Prevalence of spasticity post stroke. Clin Rehabil 2002;16:515–522.

50. Moore AP, Blumhardt LD. A prospective survey of the causes of non-traumatic spastic paraparesis and tetraparesis in 585 patients. Spinal Cord 1997;35:361–367.

51. Thompson E, Hicks F. Intrathecal baclofen and homeopathy for the treatment of painful muscle spasms associated with malignant spinal cord compression. Palliat Med 1998;12:119–121.

52. Fox SH, Kellett M, Moore AP, Crossman AR, Brotchie JM. Randomised, double-blind, placebo-controlled trial to assess the potential of cannabinoid receptor stimulation in the treatment of dystonia. Mov Disord 2002;17:145–149.

# 20

*Jeannie V. Pasacreta, Pamela A. Minarik, and Leslie Nield-Anderson*

# Anxiety and Depression

*I have nothing to live for—no hope, no future—only more pain to look forward to. I am no use to anyone, I am a burden to my family. Why can't I just die.—Palliative care patient*

♦ **Key Points**
♦ *The psychosocial issues in persons facing life-threatening illness are influenced by individual, sociocultural, medical, and family factors.*
♦ *Emotional turmoil may occur at times of transition in the disease course.*
♦ *Anxiety and depression are common symptoms in individuals facing chronic or life-threatening illness but should not be regarded as an inevitable consequence of advanced disease.*
♦ *These symptoms warrant evaluation and appropriate use of pharmacological and psychosocial interventions.*

This chapter provides information regarding the assessment and treatment of anxiety and depression among individuals faced with chronic or life-threatening illness, and delineates psychosocial interventions that are effective at minimizing these troubling symptoms. Practical guidelines regarding patient management, and identifying patients who may require formal psychiatric consultation, are offered.

CASE STUDY
### Mrs. Jones, A Patient with Depression

Mrs. Jones, a 38-year-old housewife and mother of two small children, was referred for consultation following segmental resection for stage IV breast cancer metastatic to the bone, with 15 positive nodes. On being told that she required chemotherapy, she refused, saying "It is hopeless—why bother?" Both her husband and oncologist persuaded her to discuss her decision with a psychiatric consultation-liaison nurse, and she reluctantly agreed. She was depressed and withdrawn, although moderately anxious. She wrung her hands throughout the interview, reporting intrusive thoughts of death that kept her from sleeping at night, and stated that she preferred that her children remembered her as she was. An early death would be preferable to the lingering debilitation she believed would be associated with chemotherapy. On further review, she described being 13 years old when her mother was diagnosed with breast cancer, and said that she had always feared it would happen to her, too. Her mother's mastectomy had been followed by painful bone metastasis despite chemotherapy. Mrs. Jones had distressing memories of her mother's suffering and had taken lengthy steps with her physicians to assure that mammograms and frequent breast exams would allow her to be diagnosed early should breast cancer develop. Several areas of calcification had been monitored for more than a year. She now had anger toward

425

her physician that her life was needlessly compromised by late diagnosis of something she had attempted to avoid for so long. The anger and hopelessness together were overwhelming, and she could not focus on anything else.

## Changes in Health Care That Have Accentuated Psychiatric Symptoms

Changes in health care delivery, and rapid scientific gains, are simultaneously increasing the number of individuals receiving or in need of palliative care at any given time, the longevity and course of chronic diseases, and the prevalence and intensity of the psychological symptoms that accompany them.[1,2] Furthermore, psychological distress is experienced within an increasingly complex, fragmented, and impersonal health care system that tends to intensify these symptoms. Despite these realities, psychological symptoms receive minimal attention, and health care providers often lack the needed education and support regarding assessment, treatment, and referral of these common problems.

Advances in science and technology have moved the crisis of a life-threatening medical diagnosis to the prediagnostic period, extending life expectancy and the number of treatment courses delivered over a lifetime. Individuals are being diagnosed earlier and living longer, with increasing opportunities to experience simultaneous, interrelated psychosocial and medical comorbidity. The human genome project has, theoretically and in some cases, practically, moved the psychosocial implications of chronic disease into the prediagnostic period. Concurrent treatment discoveries have increased quantity of life, albeit with ill-defined consequences to quality of life.[2,3] For example, an individual who learns of an inherited predisposition to cancer at age 25, is diagnosed at age 50, and receives intermittent treatment until death at age 79, incurs innumerable insults to her mental health and psychological well-being.

Soaring medical costs, managed-care arrangements, and the stigma associated with mental illness, have simultaneously placed a low priority on the recognition and treatment of psychosocial distress within our health care system. There is abundant documentation that psychiatric morbidity, particularly depression and anxiety, enhances vulnerability and creates formidable barriers to integrated health care.[3] Psychological factors have long been implicated as barriers to disease prevention, early diagnosis, and comprehensive treatment.[3,4] Lack of assessment and treatment of the common psychiatric sequelae to chronic disease have been linked to such problems as treatment-resistant depression and anxiety, family dysfunction, lack of compliance with prevention and treatment recommendations, potentiation of physical symptoms, and suicide, to name just a few.[3-6] These issues create long-term problems that drive up health care expenses and diminish access, quality, and efficiency of care. In health care settings, physical problems assume priority in the growing competition for scarce resources. Clinicians confronted with ambiguous symptoms are likely to interpret them within diagnostic paradigms most consistent to their specialty and theoretical orientation. As a consequence, the psychological symptoms that accompany life-threatening conditions may be interpreted and treated inappropriately, rendering care that is not comprehensive or cost effective.

We are at a critical juncture in the evolution of health care in this country. Systems are being overwhelmed by serious, often preventable, diseases that are not being treated comprehensively after diagnosis. Furthermore, in spite of cutting-edge therapies, a significant number of individuals experience unfavorable outcomes. As budget constraints limit the use of psychiatric specialists, these issues have intensified, and the importance of educating "front line" health providers to recognize and address psychiatric morbidity is compelling. In a health care system focused largely on pathogenesis, cure, and cost, psychological symptoms are all too often unrecognized and untreated in clinical settings, despite their insidious harm to patients As psychiatric consultation-liaison nurses, who work primarily in nonpsychiatric settings, the authors have been consistently struck by the limited knowledge of nursing and medical staff regarding key signs and symptoms that characterize depression and anxiety in the medically ill. Often, young patients with particularly poor prognoses, who elicit anxiety and sadness from staff, are referred for psychiatric evaluation, while their objectively depressed or anxious counterparts are not.

In dealing with depressed and/or anxious patients referred for evaluation, the decision to intervene with psychotherapy or pharmacological agents may be based largely on the philosophy, educational background, and past experience of individual clinicians. Not uncommonly, a diagnosis of clinical anxiety or depression is ruled out if the symptoms seem reactive and "appropriate" to the situation, or are viewed as organic in nature. Patients who exhibit depressive or anxious symptoms not considered severe enough to classify for "psychiatric" status are frequently not offered psychotherapeutic services, and the natural history of their symptoms is rarely monitored over time. The lack of attention to assessment and treatment of depression and anxiety among the medically ill may, for example, lead to ongoing dysphoria, family conflict, noncompliance with treatment, increased length of hospitalization, persistent worry, and suicidal ideation. Because depression and anxiety are common among individuals with chronic illness, recognition and management of these symptoms is extremely important, particularly because they are often responsive to treatment. Patients, family, and professional caregivers need to be informed of the factors that affect psychological adjustment, the wide range of psychological responses that accompany chronic and progressive disease, and the efficacy of various modes of intervention.

## The Clinical Course of Chronic Illness

Acute stress is a common response to the diagnosis of a life-threatening illness, and resurfaces at transitional points in the disease process (beginning treatment, recurrence, treatment failure, disease progression).[7] The response is characterized by shock, disbelief, anxiety, depression, sleep and appetite disturbance, and difficulty performing activities of daily living. Under favorable circumstances, these psychological symptoms should resolve within a short period.[7,8] The time period is variable, but consensus is that once the crisis has passed, and the individual knows what to expect in terms of a treatment plan, psychological symptoms diminish.[7,9] Patients who are diagnosed with late-stage disease, or have aggressive illnesses with no hope for cure, are often most vulnerable to psychological distress—particularly anxiety, depression, family problems, and physical discomfort.

### Diagnostic Phase

The period from time of diagnosis through initiation of a treatment plan is characterized by medical evaluation, the development of new relationships with unfamiliar medical personnel, and the need to integrate a barrage of information that, at best, is frightening and confusing. Patients and families frequently experience a heightened sense of responsibility, worry, and isolation during this period. They are particularly anxious and fearful when receiving initial information regarding diagnosis and treatment. Consequently, care should be taken by professionals to repeat information over several sessions and to inquire about patients' and families' understanding of the facts and treatment options. Weissman and colleagues described the first 100 days following a cancer diagnosis as the period of "existential plight."[8] Psychological distress varied according to patient diagnosis. Individuals with late-stage lung cancer were more distressed than individuals with early-stage disease, supporting the need for palliative care services directed toward psychological symptoms.

During the diagnostic period, patient concerns commonly focus on existential issues of life and death, rather than on concerns related to health, work, finances, religion, self, or relationships with family and friends. While it is unusual to observe extreme and sustained emotional reactions as the first response to diagnosis, it is important to assess the nature of early reactions because they are often predictive of later adaptation.[10,11] Early assessment by clinicians can help to identify individuals at risk for later adjustment problems or psychiatric disorders, and in the greatest need of ongoing psychosocial support.[7,12]

The initial response to diagnosis may be profoundly influenced by a person's prior association with a particular disease.[13] Those with memories of close relatives with the same illness often demonstrate heightened distress, particularly if the relative died or had negative treatment experiences.

During the diagnostic period, patients may search for explanations or causes for their disease and may struggle to give personal meaning to their experience. Since many clinicians are guarded about disclosing information until a firm diagnosis is established, patients may develop highly personal explanations that can be inaccurate and provoke intensely negative emotions. Ongoing involvement and accurate information will minimize uncertainty and the development of maladaptive coping strategies based on erroneous beliefs.

While the literature substantiates the devastating emotional impact of a life-threatening chronic illness, it also well documents that many individuals cope effectively. Positive coping strategies, such as taking action and finding favorable characteristics in the situation, have been reported to be effective.[14] Contrary to the beliefs of many clinicians, denial also has been found to assist patients in coping effectively,[15] unless sustained and used excessively to a point that it interferes with appropriate treatment. Health care practitioners play an important role in monitoring and supporting the patient's and family's psychosocial adjustment. With an awareness of the unique meaning the individual associates with the diagnosis, it is critical that practitioners keep patients informed and involved in their care. Even though patients may not be offered hope for cure, other hopes and goals to be achieved can be offered. Assisting the patient and family in maintaining comfort and control helps to facilitate adaptation and improved quality of life.

### Recurrence and Progressive Disease

Development of a recurrence after a disease-free interval can be especially devastating for patients and those close to them. The point of recurrence often signals a shift into a period of disease progression, and is clearly a time when palliative care services aimed at alleviating psychological symptoms are indicated. The medical workup may be difficult and anxiety-provoking;[16] psychosocial problems experienced at the time of diagnosis frequently resurface, often with greater intensity.[17,18] Shock and depression are not uncommon after relapse, and require individuals and their families to reevaluate the future. This period is a difficult one, during which patients may also experience pessimism, renewed preoccupation with death and dying, and feelings of helplessness and disenchantment with the medical system. Patients tend to be more guarded and cautious at this time, and feel as if they are in limbo.[18] Silverfarb and colleagues[18] examined emotional distress in a cross-sectional study of 146 women with breast cancer at three points in the clinical course (diagnosis, recurrence, stage-of-disease progression). The point of recurrence was found to be the most distressing time, with an increase in depression, anxiety, and suicidal ideation. As a disease progresses, the person frequently reports an upsetting scenario that includes frequent pain, disability, increased dependence on others, and diminished functional ability, which then potentiates psychological symptoms.[19] Investigators studying quality of life in cancer patients have demonstrated a clear relationship between an individual's perception of quality of life and the presence of discomfort.[20] As uncomfortable symptoms increase, perceived quality of life diminishes. Thus, an important goal in the psychosocial treatment of patients with advanced chronic illness focuses on symptom control.

An issue that repeatedly surfaces among patients, family members, and professional care providers deals with the use of aggressive treatment protocols in the presence of progressive disease. Often, patients and families request to participate in experimental protocols even when there is little likelihood of extending survival. Controversy continues about the efficacy of such therapies, and the role health professionals can play in facilitating patients' choices about participating. These issues become even more important because changes in the health care system may limit payment for costly and highly technical treatments, such as bone marrow transplants. It is essential for health care professionals to establish structured dialogue with patients, family members, and care providers regarding treatment goals and expectations. Despite the existence of progressive illness, certain individuals may respond to investigational treatment with increased hope. Efforts to separate and clarify values, thoughts, and emotional reactions of care providers, patients, and families to these delicate issues, is important if individualized care with attention to psychological symptoms is to be provided. Use of resources such as psychiatric consultation-liaison nurses, psychiatrists, social workers, and chaplains can be invaluable in assisting patients, family members, and staff to grapple with these issues in a meaningful and productive manner.

### Terminal Disease and Dying

Once the terminal period has begun, it is usually not the fact of dying but the quality of dying that is the overwhelming issue confronting the patient and family.[21,22] Continued palliative care into the terminal stage of cancer relieves physical and psychological symptoms, promotes comfort, and increases well-being. Patients and families who have received such services along the illness trajectory have been found to be more open and accepting of palliative efforts in the final stage of life.

Patients living in the final phase of any advanced chronic illness experience fears and anxiety related to uncertain future events, such as unrelieved pain, separation from loved ones, burden on family, and loss of control. Psychological distress is more likely in persons confronting diminished life span, physical debilitation associated with functional limitation, and/or symptoms associated with toxic therapies.[20,23] Therapeutic interventions should be directed toward increasing patients' sense of control and self-efficacy within the context of functional decline and increased dependence. In addition, if patients so desire, it is often therapeutic to let them know that there is help available to discuss the existential concerns that often accompany terminal illness. Personal values and beliefs, socioeconomic and cultural background, and religious belief systems influence patients' expectations

about quality of life and palliative care. Cultural affiliation can have a significant influence on perception of pain. Bates and colleagues[24] found that the best predictors of pain intensity are ethnic group affiliation and locus of control style. For example, an individual's stoic attitude, which serves to minimize or negate discomfort, may be related to a cultural value learned and reinforced through years of family experiences. Similarly, an individual's highly emotional response to routine events may become exaggerated during the terminal phase of illness and not necessarily signal maladjustment but, rather, a cultural norm. Awareness of the family system's cultural, religious, ethnic, and socioeconomic background is important to the understanding of their beliefs, attitudes, practices, and behaviors related to illness and death. Cultural patterns play a significant role in determining how individuals and families cope with illness and death.[25,26]

Delirium, depression, suicidal ideation, and severe anxiety are among the most common psychiatric complications encountered in terminally ill cancer patients.[27] When severe, these problems require urgent and aggressive assessment and treatment by psychiatric personnel, who can initiate pharmacological and psychotherapeutic treatment strategies. Psychiatric emergencies require the same rapid intervention as distressing physical symptoms and medical crises. In spite of the seemingly overwhelming nature of psychosocial responses along the chronic illness trajectory, most patients do indeed cope effectively. Periods of intense emotions, such as anxiety and depression, are not necessarily the same as maladaptive coping.

### Factors That Affect Psychological Adjustment

Psychological responses to chronic illness vary widely and are influenced by many individual factors. A review of the literature points to key factors that may impact psychological adjustment and the occurrence and expression of anxiety and depression. Three of the most important factors are: previous coping strategies and emotional stability, social support, and symptom distress. In addition, there are common medical conditions, treatments, and substances that may cause or intensify symptoms of anxiety and depression (Tables 20–1 and 20–2).

### Previous Coping Strategies and Emotional Stability

One of the most important predictors of psychological adjustment to chronic illness is the emotional stability and coping strategies used by the person prior to diagnosis.[28] Individuals with a history of poor psychological adjustment, and of clinically significant anxiety or depression, are at highest risk for emotional decompensation[29] and should be monitored closely throughout all phases of treatment. This is particularly true for people with a history of major psychiatric syndromes and/ or psychiatric hospitalization.[30]

**Table 20–1**
**Common Medical Conditions Associated with Anxiety and Depression**

| Anxiety | Depression |
|---|---|
| • Endocrine disorders: hyperthyroidism and hypothyroidism, hyperglycemia and hypoglycemia, Cushing's disease, carcinoid syndrome, pheochromocytoma<br>• Cardiovascular conditions: myocardial infarction, paroxysmal atrial tachycardia, angina pectoris, congestive heart failure, mitral valve prolapse, hypovolemia<br>• Metabolic conditions: hyperkalemia, hypertemia, hypercalcemia hypoglycemia, hyperthermia, anemia, hyponatremia<br>• Respiratory conditions: asthma, chronic obstructive pulmonary disease, pneumonia, pulmonary edema, pulmonary embolus, respiratory dependence, hypoxia<br>• Neoplasms: islet cell adenomas, pheochromocytoma<br>• Neurological conditions: akathisia, encephalopathy, seizure disorder, vertigo, mass lesion, postconcussion syndrome | • Cardiovascular: cardiovascular disease, congestive heart failure, myocardial infarct, cardiac arrhythmias<br>• Central nervous system: cerebrovascular accident, cerebral anoxia, Huntington's disease, subdural hematoma, Alzheimer's disease, human immunodeficiency virus (HIV) infection, dementia, carotid stenosis, temporal lobe epilepsy, multiple sclerosis, postconcussion syndrome, myasthenia gravis, narcolepsy, subarachnoid hemorrhage<br>• Autoimmune: rheumatoid arthritis, polyarteritis nodosa<br>• Endocrine: hyperparathyroidism, hypothyroidism, diabetes mellitus, Cushing's disease, Addison's disease<br>• Other: alcoholism, anemia, systemic lupus erythematosus, Epstein-Barr virus, hepatitis, malignancies, pulmonary insufficiency, pancreatic or liver disease, syphilis, encephalitis, malnutrition |

*Sources:* Stoudemire (1996), reference 77; Fernandez et al. (1995), reference 45; Kurlowicz (1994), reference 98; Wise & Taylor (1990), reference 19.

**Table 20–2**
**Common Medications and Substances Associated with Anxiety and Depression**

| Anxiety | Depression |
|---|---|
| Alcohol and nicotine withdrawal | Antihypertensives |
| Stimulants including caffeine | Analgesics |
| Thyroid replacement | Antiparkinsonian agents |
| Neuroleptics | Hypoglycemic agents |
| Corticosteroids | Steroids |
| Sedative–hypnotic withdrawal or paradoxical reaction | Chemotherapeutic agents |
| Bronchodilators and decongestants | Estrogen and progesterone |
| Cocaine | Antimicrobials |
| Epinephrine | L-dopa |
| Benzodiazepines and their withdrawal | Benzodiazepines |
| Digitalis toxicity | Barbiturates |
| Cannabis | Alcohol |
| Antihypertensives | Phenothiazines |
| Antihistamines | Amphetamines |
| Antiparkinsonian medications | Lithium carbonate |
| Oral contraceptives | Heavy metals |
| Anticholinergics | Cimetidine |
| Anesthetics and analgesics | Antibiotics |
| Toxins | |
| Antidepressants | |

*Sources:* Stoudemire (1996), reference 77; Fernandez et al. (1995), reference 45; Kurlowicz (1994), reference 98; Wise & Taylor (1990), reference 19.

## Social Support

Social support consistently has been found to influence a person's psychosocial adjustment to chronic illness.[31] The ability and availability of significant others in dealing with diagnosis and treatment can significantly affect the patient's view of him- or herself, and potentially the patient's survival.[32] Individuals diagnosed with all types of life-threatening chronic disorders experience a heightened need for interpersonal support. Individuals who are able to maintain close connections with family and friends during the course of illness are more likely to cope effectively with the disease than those who are not able to maintain such relationships.[33] This is especially true during the palliative care period.

## Symptom Distress

The effects of treatment for a variety of chronic diseases, as well as the impact of progressive illness, can inflict transient and/or permanent physical changes, physical symptom distress, and functional impairments in patients. It is a well-known clinical observation supported by research[34] that excessive psychological distress can exacerbate the side effects of cancer-treatment agents. Conversely, treatment side effects can have a dramatic impact on the psychological profiles of patients.[35] The potential for psychological distress, particularly anxiety and depression, appears to increase in patients with advanced illness,[36-39] especially when cure is not viable and palliation of symptoms is the issue. In a study that elicited information from oncology nurses regarding psychiatric symptoms present in their patients, almost twice as many patients with metastatic disease were reported to be depressed, in contrast to those with localized cancers.[40] Investigators studying quality of life in cancer patients have demonstrated a clear relationship between an individual's perception of quality of life, and the presence of discomfort.[20] As uncomfortable symptoms increase, perceived quality of life diminishes and psychiatric symptoms often worsen. The presence of increased physical discomfort, combined with a lack of control and predictability regarding the occurrence of symptoms, amplifies anxiety, depression, and organic mental symptoms in patients with advanced disease.

## Differentiating Psychiatric Complications from Expected Psychological Responses

Differentiating between symptoms related to a medical illness and symptoms related to an underlying psychiatric disorder is particularly challenging to health care practitioners. Anxiety and depression are normal responses to life events and illness, and occur throughout the palliative care trajectory. It is the intensity, duration, and extent to which symptomatology affects functioning that distinguishes an anxiety or depressive disorder from symptoms that individuals generally experience in the progression of an illness. Symptoms following stressful events in a person's life (employment difficulties, retirement, death of a family member, loss of a job, diagnosis of a medical illness/life-threatening illness) are expected to dissipate as an individual copes, with reassurance and validation from family and friends, and adapts to the situation. When responses predominantly include excessive nervousness, worry, and fear, diagnosis of an adjustment disorder with anxiety is applied. If an individual responds with tearfulness and feelings of hopelessness, he or she is characterized as experiencing an adjustment disorder with depressed mood. An adjustment disorder with mixed anxiety and depressed mood is characterized by a combination of both anxiety and depression.[41]

Referrals from primary care providers for psychiatric assistance with psychopharmacological treatment are indicated when symptoms continue, intensify, or disrupt an individual's life beyond a 6-month period, or when symptoms do not respond to conventional reassurance and validation by the primary care provider, and support from an individual's social network. Most patients develop transient psychological symptoms that are responsive to support, reassurance, and information about what to expect regarding a disease course and its treatment. There are some individuals, however, who require more aggressive psychotherapeutic intervention, such as pharmacotherapy and ongoing psychotherapy.

*Guidelines to help clinicians identify patients who exhibit behavior that suggests the presence of a psychiatric syndrome.* If the patient's problems become so severe that supportive measures are insufficient to control emotional distress, referral to a psychiatric clinician is indicated. Factors that may predict major psychiatric problems along the chronic illness trajectory include past psychiatric hospitalization; history of significant depression, manic-depressive illness, schizophrenia, organic mental conditions, or personality disorders; lack of social support; inadequate control of physical discomfort; history of or current alcohol and/or drug abuse; and currently prescribed psychotropic medication.

The need for psychiatric referral among patients receiving psychotropic medication deserves specific mention because it is often overlooked in clinical practice. Standard therapies used to treat major chronic diseases, such as surgery and chemotherapy, and/or disease progression itself can significantly change dosage requirements for medications used to treat major psychiatric syndromes such as anxiety, depression, and bipolar disorder. For example, dosage requirements for lithium carbonate, commonly used to treat the manic episodes associated with bipolar disorder and the depressive episodes associated with recurrent depressive disorder, can change significantly over the course of treatment for a number of chronic diseases. Therapeutic blood levels of lithium are closely tied to sodium and water balance. Additionally, lithium has a narrow therapeutic window, and life-threatening toxicity can develop rapidly. Treatment side effects such as diarrhea, fever, vomiting, and resulting dehydration warrant scrupulous monitoring of dosage and side effects.

Careful monitoring is also indicated during pre- and postoperative periods. Another common problem among patients treated with psychotropic medication is that medications may be discontinued at specific points in the treatment process, such as the time of surgery, and not restarted. This may produce an avoidable recurrence of emotionally disabling psychiatric symptoms, when the stress of a life-threatening chronic disease and its treatment is burden enough.

For some patients, psychological distress does not subside with the usual supportive interventions. Unfortunately, clinically relevant and severe psychiatric syndromes may go unrecognized by nonpsychiatric care providers.[41,42] Particularly, as a chronic illness progresses, anxiety and depression can occur in greater numbers of patients and with greater intensity.[43] One of the reasons that it may be difficult to detect serious anxiety and depression in patients is that several of the diagnostic criteria used to evaluate their presence, such as lack of appetite, insomnia, decreased sexual interest, psychomotor agitation, and diminished energy, may overlap with usual disease and treatment effects.[44]

Additionally, health care providers may confuse their own fears about chronic illness with the emotional reactions of their patients (e.g., "I too would be extremely depressed if I were in a similar situation").

## The Coexisting Nature of Psychiatric and Medical Symptoms

Depression and anxiety are appropriate to the stress of having a serious illness, and the boundary between normal and abnormal symptoms is often unclear. Even when diagnostic criteria are met for a major depressive episode or anxiety disorder, there is disagreement regarding the need for psychiatric treatment, as psychiatric symptoms may improve upon initiation of medical treatment. A major source of diagnostic confusion is the overlap of somatic symptoms associated with several chronic illnesses and their treatments, and those pathognomic to depression and anxiety themselves (e.g., fatigue, loss of appetite, weakness, weight loss, restlessness, agitation). Separating out whether a symptom is due to depression, anxiety, the medical illness and its treatment, or a combination of factors, is often exceedingly difficult.

Figure 20–1 diagrams the overlap between the symptoms of a chronic medical condition and/or its treatment effects, and the clinical manifestations of anxiety or depression. The symptoms of anxiety or depression may be intrinsic to the medical disorder or induced by certain treatment agents. Symptoms may cease when the medical disorder is treated or the medication is discontinued or decreased. Whether the psychiatric symptoms have a primary psychiatric etiology, occur following the medical diagnosis, or receive equal causal contributions from medical and psychiatric sources, neurovegetative symptoms are not reliable assessment parameters and treatment may be delayed or never started.

### Anxiety or Depression with a Medical or Pharmacological Etiology

During progressive or active treatment phases of a chronic disease, symptoms of anxiety or depression may recur at various intervals relative to a specific causative agent, the stress associated with the illness, or a combination of those and other factors. Diagnostic data from earlier points, both before the onset of the current illness and at various points along the

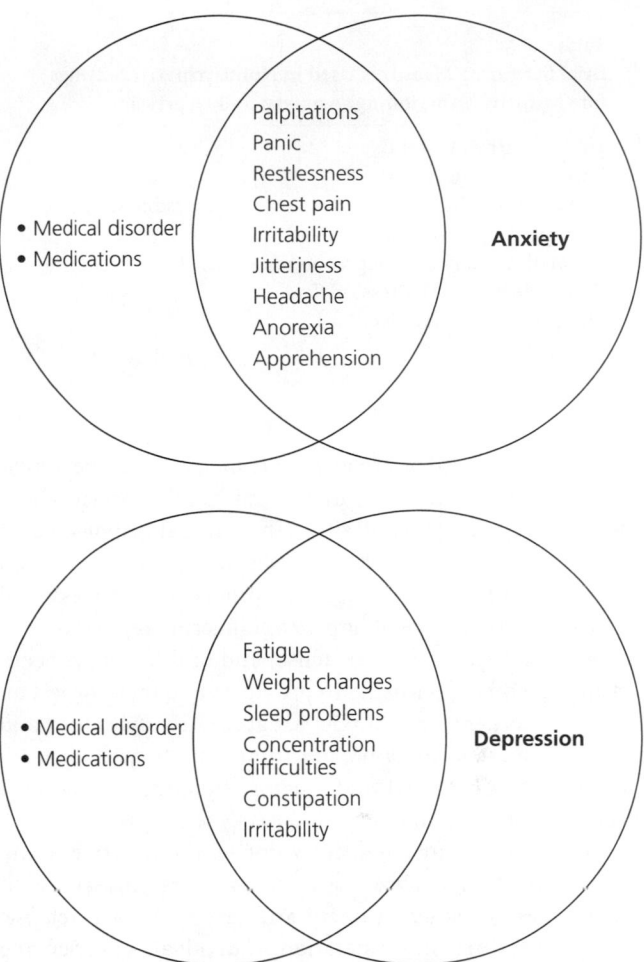

**Figure 20–1.** Symptoms of depression and anxiety with medical etiologies. *Source*: Adapted from Derogatis & Wise (1989), reference 102.

illness course, are important and should routinely be incorporated into the plan of care. As psychiatric symptoms become more prevalent within the context of the lengthening chronic illness trajectory, attention to the collection of this diagnostic information is an intrinsic aspect of quality comprehensive care. Physical and medication history, mental status, psychosocial and psychiatric histories (see Table 20–3 for screening instruments), electrocardiogram, comprehensive laboratory tests including toxicology screening, and relevant family information regarding available support systems, changes in lifestyle and functioning, all will promote accurate assessment and close monitoring throughout the palliative care trajectory. This information will assist the health care team in determining the etiology of anxiety and depressive symptoms and to treat and monitor them appropriately.

Some patients may have a primary psychiatric disorder that precedes the diagnosis of their chronic medical condition. This situation is encountered in primary care and chronic illness treatment settings. During the diagnostic phase, fear and anxiety are expected reactions to the diagnosis of a life-threatening or potentially life-threatening

---

**Table 20–3**

**Brief Screening Measures Used in Nonpsychiatric Settings for Cognitive Functioning, Anxiety, and Depression**

Folstein Mini-Mental Exam
Beck Depression Inventory
Center for Epidemiological Studies of Depression Scale
Geriatric Depression Scale
Hospital Anxiety and Depression Scale
Zung Self-Rating Depression Scale
Zung Self-Rating Anxiety Scale
PHQ9

---

disease. Heightened apprehension coincides with the anticipated course of treatment, uncertainty, and concerns about the potential impact on lifestyle. These initial responses usually resolve in a few weeks with the support of family and friends, use of personal resources, provision of professional care, and maintenance of hope.[45,46] Lingering reports of feeling weak, dizzy, worried, or tense, and of difficulty concentrating, are often confusing to providers and may suggest an anxiety disorder. When anxiety is accurately diagnosed and treated, somatic complaints may diminish. If symptoms are not correctly identified and treated, suffering can become needlessly prolonged.[39,41]

Depression occurs frequently during the recurrence and progressive disease phase. An illness course marked with recurrences engenders anxiety and fear with each relapse, as well as feelings of desperation. Individuals experiencing depression do not always present with a dysphoric effect, or report distressing feelings of hopelessness and helplessness.[47] Instead, they may present with somatic complaints such as dizziness, headaches, excessive fatigue, sleep disturbances, or irritability. Disturbances in appetite, sleep, energy, and concentration are hallmark symptoms of depression. However, in the medically ill, these symptoms are frequently caused by the medical illness.[48] Symptoms such as fearfulness, depressed appearance, social withdrawal, brooding, self-pity, pessimism, a sense of punishment, and mood that cannot be changed (e.g., cannot be cheered up, not smiling, does not respond to good news) are considered to be more reliable. It has been recommended that assessment of these affective symptoms provides more accurate diagnostic information for depression in medically ill patients than neurovegetative symptoms commonly used in healthy individuals.[48–51] Tables 20–4 and 20–5 list general criteria to diagnose an anxiety and depressive disorder in the medically ill.[41,50,51] Whenever symptoms are unremitting, or intensify and do not respond to conventional professional and family support, psychiatric evaluations for psychopharmacological and psychotherapeutic interventions are warranted.

Untreated or undertreated psychiatric disorders can be profoundly disabling and, as such, can precipitate or exacerbate the physical manifestations of chronic disease. The degree of anxiety and depression experienced by an

---

**Table 20–4**

**Symptoms Indicating an Anxiety Disorder in the Medically Ill in the Absence of Physiological Course**

Chronic apprehension, worry, inability to relax not related to illness or treatment
Difficulty concentrating
Irritability or outbursts of anger
Difficulty falling asleep or staying asleep not explained by illness or treatment
Trembling or shaking not explained by illness or treatment
Exaggerated startle response
Perspiring for no apparent reason
Chest pain or tightness in the chest
Fear of places, events, certain activities
Unrealistic fear of dying
Fear of "going crazy"
Recurrent and persistent ideas, thoughts, or impulses
Repetitive behaviors to prevent discomfort

*Sources*: Barraclough (1997), reference 46; Fernandex et al. (1995), reference 45; American Psychiatric Association (2000), reference 99.

---

**Table 20–5**

**Symptoms Indicating a Depressive Disorder in the Medically Ill in the Absence of Physiological Course**

Enduring depressed or sad mood, tearful
Marked disinterest or lack of pleasure in social activities, family, and friends not explained by pain or fatigue.
Feelings of worthlessness and hopelessness
Excessive enduring guilt that illness is a punishment
Significant weight loss or gain not explained by dieting, illness, or treatments
Hopelessness about the future
Enduring fatigue
Increase or decrease in sleep not explained by illness or treatment
Recurring thoughts of death or suicidal thoughts or acts
Diminished ability to think and make decisions

*Sources*: American Psychiatric Association (2000), reference 99; Cassem (1995), reference 43; Cavanaugh (1995), reference 44; Kurlowicz (1994), reference 98.

---

individual at any given point is influenced by the degree to which individuals and their families have been prepared for what to expect. These considerations include: physical and psychological manifestations of the illness; speed and extent of physical deterioration expected, including the likelihood of pain and other symptoms; available treatment options; and the individual's history of psychiatric illness.[40]

Anxiety and depression typically accompany difficult decisions regarding both the addition of comfort measures and the withdrawal of diagnostic procedures and aggressive medical treatments. Distress regarding separation from family and friends, worries about burdening caregivers, feeling overwhelmed with end-of-life decisions, and living in existential uncertainty are just a few of the issues that individuals and families confront during terminal phases of illness. Severe distress, thoughts of suicide, panic, and/or questions about assisted suicide may occur. Such responses require immediate attention and intervention. Suicide and assisted suicide are discussed at a later point in this chapter.

## Anxiety or Depression Precipitated by a Medical Disorder

In many cases, an anxiety or depressive disorder occurs secondary to the diagnosis of a chronic medical condition.[102] The stress of the medical illness itself typically induces anxiety or depression. Often these symptoms diminish when treatment is explained and initiated, and hope is offered. When a patient with a chronic illness experiences increasing physical dependence on others, prolonged pain, progressive loss of function and/or immobility, anxiety and depression can become severe and prolonged. Disease progression may affect body image, self-esteem, social relationships, employment, and family roles. The extent and speed at which disabling aspects of a chronic illness occur can impact an individual's ability to react and to integrate the changes and, subsequently, to develop adjustment skills. The development of adaptive coping mechanisms is influenced by many factors, particularly the patient's premorbid coping strategies and the availability of outside support.

Within the context of a chronic medical condition, anxiety and depression often occur simultaneously. In general, anxiety precedes depression, and depression is more likely to persevere in individuals who also have an anxiety disorder. When anxiety and depression coexist, assessment and treatment may be more challenging, underscoring the need for an aggressive, ongoing approach to assessment and treatment.

A common but erroneous assumption by clinicians is that the psychological distress that accompanies a medical condition, even when it is severe and unremitting, is natural, expected, and does not require or respond to treatment. This is thought to be particularly true when hope for a cure is unrealistic or the prognosis is grave. This attitude leads to underrecognition and undertreatment of high levels of suffering.[52] Receiving a life-threatening medical diagnosis and undergoing invasive treatment are potent catalysts for an acute stress response that is not typically expected, planned for, or routinely addressed in health care settings. Providers' dominant concerns are usually centered around treatment options, the pursuit of a cure or life-prolongation, improving prognosis, and relieving physical discomfort. Providers may also be desensitized to the intrusiveness of medical protocols and treatment environments. Most patients are not comfortable with, and are not encouraged to express to professional or family care providers, their feelings of helplessness, dependency, or fear. In fact, they frequently avoid such discussions in an attempt to decrease burden on others.

Untreated psychological symptoms can lead to a post traumatic stress disorder. Post traumatic stress disorders (PTSD), typically induced by exposure to extreme stress and/or trauma, are increasingly being linked in the literature to medical treatment situations. Providers are apt to confuse PTSD symptoms such as avoidance and withdrawal as nonpathological responses, e.g., acceptance adjustment. It is common for providers to hear "I do not remember anything about the hospitalization; it is a blur. I feel like I was in a daze...ask my wife/husband...my memory isn't so great." In the treatment of PTSD, psychopharmacological agents alone are inadequate and must be accompanied by aggressive psychotherapeutic interventions, education and support. PTSD is best treated by a professional skilled in treating this disorder. Routine psychiatric assessment and the availability of prompt treatment across the palliative care trajectory is needed to reduce the prevalence and morbidity of post traumatic stress disorders that occur in response to medical diagnosis and treatment.[35]

## Assessment and Screening Considerations

### Assessment of Anxiety

The experience of anxiety is virtually universal, especially when a person has a serious chronic illness. Anxiety is a vague, subjective feeling of apprehension, tension, insecurity, and uneasiness, usually without a known, specific cause identifiable by the individual. Normally, anxiety serves as an alerting response resulting from a real or perceived threat to a person's biological, psychological, or social integrity, including self-esteem, identity, or status. This alert occurs in response to actual happenings, or to thoughts about happenings in the past, present, or future. The greater the perceived threat, the greater the anxiety response.[26] A wide variety of signs and symptoms accompany anxiety along the continuum of mild, moderate, severe, and panic levels. Table 20–6 illustrates how anxiety affects attention, learning, and adaptation, all of which are essential to coping during the palliative care trajectory.[53] Anxiety responses can be adaptive, and anxiety can be a powerful motivating force for productive problem-solving. Talking, crying, sleeping, exercising, deep breathing, imagery, and relaxation techniques are adaptive anxiety-relief strategies. Responses to anxiety also can be maladaptive and may indicate psychiatric disorder, but not all distressing symptoms of anxiety indicate a psychiatric disorder. Table 20–4 lists anxiety symptoms that indicate a psychiatric disorder and call for psychiatric assessment and treatment. Skill in early recognition of anxiety is important so that care providers can intervene to alleviate symptoms, prevent escalation and loss of control, and enable adjustment and coping. Anxiety is interpersonally contagious. As a result, therapeutic effectiveness can be severely compromised when care providers fail to recognize and manage their own anxiety.

Table 20–6
Symptoms of Anxiety and Effects on Attention, Learning, and Adaptation

**Mild**

Awareness, alert attention, skill in seeing relationships or connections available for use

Notices more than previously, ability to observe improved

If the person has well-developed learning and adaptive skills, will be able to use all steps in the learning process, from observing and describing to analyzing, testing, and using what is learned

**Moderate**

Perceptual field is narrowed, ability to observe decreased, does not notice peripheral stimuli but can notice more if directed to do so (selective inattention)

If the person has well-developed learning and adaptive skills, will be able to use all steps in the learning process, from observing and describing to analyzing, testing, and using what is learned

**Severe**

Perceptual field is greatly reduced, focus on one detail or scattered details

May be able to notice what is pointed out by another person, but as anxiety escalates will be unable to attend

May dissociate to prevent panic (i.e., fail to notice what is happening in reference to self)

Even with well-developed learning and adaptive skills, behavior will orient toward getting immediate relief

Automatic (not requiring thought) behaviors used to reduce anxiety

**Panic**

Feelings of panic, awe, dread

Previous foci of attention "blown up" or scattering of details increased

Tendency to dissociate to prevent panic

Inability to focus attention even when directed by another person

Even with well-developed learning and adaptive skills, behavior will orient toward getting immediate relief

Automatic (not requiring thought) behaviors used to reduce anxiety

*Source*: Peplau (1963), reference 52.

## Assessment of Depression

Underrecognized and undertreated, depression has the potential to decrease immune response, decrease survival time, impair ability to adhere to treatment, and impair quality of life.[54] The assessment of depression in any setting depends on the provider's awareness of its potential to occur. In addition, providers must be cognizant of the risk factors associated with depression as well as its key signs, symptoms, and historical aspects. In addition to medical comorbidity, risk factors that favor the development of a depressive disorder include prior episodes of depression, family history of depression, prior suicide attempts, female gender, age under 40 years, postpartum period, lack of social support, stressful life events, personal history of sexual abuse, and current substance abuse.[55] The experience of chronic and progressive disease may increase dependence, helplessness, and uncertainty, and generate a negative, self-critical view. Cognitive distortions can easily develop, leading to interpretation of benign events as negative or catastrophic. Motivation to participate in care may be diminished, leading to withdrawal. Patients may see themselves as worthless and burdensome to family and friends. Family members may find themselves immobilized, impatient, or angry with the patient's lack of communication, cooperation, or motivation.[55]

### Cultural Considerations

Culture can be a powerful influence on the occurrence and presentation of psychiatric morbidity. In some cultures, anxiety and depression may be expressed through somatic symptoms rather than affective/behavioral symptoms such as guilt or sadness. Complaints of "nerves" and headaches (in Latino and Mediterranean cultures); of weakness, tiredness, or "imbalance" (in Chinese or Asian cultures); of problems of the "heart" (in Middle Eastern cultures); or of being "heartbroken" (among the Hopi) may be depressive equivalents. Cultures may differ in judgments about the seriousness of dysphoria; for example, irritability may be a greater concern than sadness or withdrawal. Experiences distinctive to certain cultures, such as fear of being hexed, or vivid feelings of being visited by those who have died, must be differentiated from actual hallucinations or delusions that may be part of a major depressive episode with psychotic features. However, a symptom should not be dismissed because it is seen as characteristic of a particular culture (see Table 20–5).[41,48,49,51]

### Conceptual and Diagnostic Considerations

The conceptualization of psychological distress is varied. Depression in particular has a variety of meanings, and has been used to describe a broad spectrum of human emotions and behaviors ranging from expected, transient, and nonclinical sadness following upsetting life events, to the clinically relevant extremes of suicidality and major depressive disorder. Depression is common among people with chronic illness. The term "depressive syndromes" refers to a specific constellation of symptoms that comprise a discrete psychiatric disorder. Examples are: major depression, dysthymia, organic affective disorder, and adjustment disorder with depressed features. Depressive symptoms describe varying degrees of depressed feelings not necessarily associated with psychiatric illness. Five major theoretical viewpoints have been used to understand and treat depression. In the psychoanalytic view, depression represents the introjection of hostility subsequent to the loss of an ambivalently loved object.[56] Cognitive views emphasize the mediating role that distorted and negative thinking plays in determining mood and behavior.[57] In the sociological view, depression is a social phenomenon in which a breakdown of self-esteem involves the loss of possessions such as status, roles and relationships, and life meaning.[58] Cultural and societal factors, including illness, increase vulnerability to depression. The biological view of depression emphasizes genetic vulnerability and biochemical alterations in neurotransmitters.[59] In studies of medically ill patients, depression is often equated with a crisis response, in which demands on the individual exceed the ability to respond.[60]

Conceptual viewpoints are important to the extent that they influence the understanding and subsequent treatment of the psychiatric symptoms experienced by patients with chronic physical illness. Diverse conceptualizations do not diminish the ability to plan and deliver effective care, and most often simply offer complementary ideas concerning the etiological significance of symptoms. In many health care settings, nurses have the most patient contact, and are likely to talk with individuals about their physical and emotional problems and thus to detect psychiatric symptoms and syndromes. Specific screening instruments, such as those listed in Table 20–3, may be used for assessment. In addition, direct questioning and clinical observation of mood, behavior, and thinking can be carried out concomitant with physical care. Questions related to mood may include the following: How have your spirits been lately? How would you describe your mood now? Have you felt sad or blue? Questions about behavior relate to sleeping patterns, appetite, activity level, and changes in energy: How are you sleeping lately? How much energy do you have now compared with 1 month or 6 months ago? Have you experienced recent changes in your appetite? Have you lost or gained weight? What do you usually do to cope with stress (talk to someone? go to a movie? work? exercise? drugs? alcohol?)? Questions related to cognition are as follows: What do you see in your future? What are the biggest problems facing you now? Are you as interested as usual in your family and friends, work, hobbies, etc.? Have you felt satisfied with yourself and with your life? Can you concentrate as well as you usually can? Do you have family or close friends readily available to help you? Do you feel able to call on them? As noted previously, disturbances in appetite, sleep, energy, and concentration may be caused by the illness and not necessarily indicative of depression.

## Screening for Anxiety and Depression

In chronic illness settings, the need for routine psychiatric screening has been well documented for identifying patients at high risk for psychiatric morbidity, as well as to identify those who can benefit from early-intervention programs. Patients may require different interventions based on their placement on the distress continuum. Researchers[61] concluded that newly diagnosed patients who are highly distressed can

benefit from evaluation and treatment for psychiatric consequences of illness, and that adaptation to the disease can be improved through the use of psychosocial interventions and close monitoring.

A number of tools have been developed to screen for psychological distress but have not been consistently incorporated into clinical care.[62,63] One tool that is easy to administer, reliable, and palatable to patients is the Distress Thermometer. This tool, developed by a team led by Dr. Jimmie Holland at Memorial Sloan Kettering Cancer Center, is similar to pain measurement scales that ask patients to rate their pain on a scale from 0 to 10, and consists of two cards. The first card is a picture of a thermometer, and the patient is asked to mark his or her level of distress. A rating of 5 or above indicates that a patient has symptoms indicating a need to be evaluated by a mental health professional and potential referral for services. The patient is then handed a second card and asked to identify which items from a six-item problem list relate to the patient's distress; that is, illness-related, family, emotional, practical, financial, or spiritual. This tool is part of the National Comprehensive Cancer Network (NCCN) distress-management practice guidelines in oncology. This interdisciplinary workgroup chose the term "distress management" because it was "more acceptable and less stigmatizing than psychiatric, psychosocial or emotional," and could be defined and measured by self-report.[64]

Again, striving for simplicity and clinical utility, Harvey Chochinov and colleagues compared the performance of four brief screening measures for depression in the terminally ill.[50] They found that asking the question "Are you depressed?" was reliable and valid for diagnosing depression and was extraordinarily useful in care of the terminally ill. Both the NCCN Practice Guidelines for distress management and the simple three-word screening sentence for depression can easily be incorporated into daily clinical practice.

## Addressing Deficits in Case-finding Strategies

Individuals are living longer with chronic illnesses, within the context of aggressive, physically and psychologically debilitating treatments. These trends promise to continue, and further study is needed to identify effective approaches to treatment. Available data clearly support a policy of routine psychological assessment in chronic-illness settings. Additional studies are needed to support intervention development that, at a minimum, will likely lead to improved quality of life for patients and cost savings at the systems level. In clinical settings, detection and case identification are particularly difficult. As mentioned, this is due to several factors, including: the high prevalence of clinically significant "subsyndromal" psychiatric symptoms in medically ill samples (symptoms not severe enough, or of sufficient duration, to be classified as a psychiatric disorder), and the overlapping nature of physical and neurovegetative symptoms such as fatigue, changes in appetite, sleep, and sex drive. Different clinical sites have their own unique limitations, including lack of knowledge, comfort, or time by health professionals to assess patients for these symptoms. Consequently, recognition of significant psychological distress (psychiatric morbidity) is seriously impeded in clinical settings.

Clinicians need to be trained to recognize the prognostic importance of comorbid medical illness and psychiatric symptoms, and to understand how the subtleties of case identification can affect treatment planning. The range in severity of psychiatric symptoms, and the often rapid change in both psychiatric and physical symptoms across the treatment trajectory, create both a great variance and the need to observe and record the dynamic interchange between physical and psychological phenomena over a small time span. The difficulties in case identification discussed may be highlighted by the severity of physical symptoms and the low prevalence of prior mood disorder. The presence of acute physical illnesses places the individual under severe physiological, psychological, and psychosocial stress. In addition, patients are often removed from their usual social support systems to receive treatment, and are exposed to psychosocial stressors unique to the treatment setting (e.g., dependency on hospital staff, unfamiliar and sometimes painful diagnostic and therapeutic procedures, altered eating, bathing, and sleep routines, and uncertain prognosis). Symptom assessments must strike a balance between overly inclusive (e.g., mistakenly treating the fatigue of cancer treatment as depression) and overly exclusive (e.g., erroneously dismissing the patient's mood symptoms as "understandable"). Case identification is a crucial first step. The approach to identifying psychiatric symptoms potentially confounded by medical illnesses must be defined explicitly. Choice of an inclusive approach avoids premature exclusion of relevant phenomena. The use of similar screening instruments across clinical sites would greatly facilitate comparisons of information and standardization of assessment and case-finding guidelines.

## Suicide

Suicide is the ninth leading cause of death in the United States. Five percent of suicides occur in patients with chronic medical illnesses, with spinal cord injuries, multiple sclerosis, cancer, and human immunodeficiency virus disease.[65] Because of underreporting, statistics underestimate the magnitude of suicide; intentional overdoses by the terminally ill and intentional car accidents are rarely labeled as suicides. The strongest suicide predictor is the presence of a psychiatric illness, especially depression and alcohol abuse, although a chronic deteriorating medical illness with perceived poor health, recent diagnosis of a life-threatening illness, and recent conflict or loss of a significant relationship also are considered to be predictive.[65] Being male, over age 45 years, and living alone and lacking a social support system are risk factors.[66] In one study, hopelessness was found to be more important than depression as a clinical marker of suicidal ideation in the terminally ill.[67] Individuals with progressive

chronic illness, particularly during the terminal stages, are at increased risk for suicide.[68] Other cancer-related risk factors include oral, pharyngeal, or lung cancer; poor prognosis; confusion and delirium; inadequately controlled pain; and the presence of deficits, such as loss of mobility, loss of bowel or bladder control, amputation, sensory loss, inability to eat or swallow, and exhaustion.[69] The highest-risk patients are those with severe and rapidly progressive disease producing rapid functional decline, intractable pain, and/or history of depression, suicide attempts, or substance abuse.[70]

### Physician-Assisted Suicide

Whereas suicide is the intentional ending of one's own life, physician-assisted suicide (PAS) refers to a physician acting to aid a person in the ending of his or her life.[71] Public demand for PAS has been fueled by burdensome, exhausting, and expensive dying in acute care settings.[72] It is highly controversial; the American Medical Association, the American Nurses Association, and the National Hospice and Palliative Care Organization have taken positions against it.[73,74] Implications for health care providers include the following: to be knowledgeable about the legal and moral/ethical aspects of PAS; to do a personal evaluation and prepare responses for situations with patients where the topic may arise; to improve education about pain management, symptom control, and related issues in the care of dying and seriously ill patients; to conduct rigorous research on the attitudes and practices of health care professionals with respect to assisted suicide; and to develop effective mechanisms to address conflicts.[72,74]

There is an ongoing debate about the legalization of PAS. Oregon was the first state in the United States where the majority of voters approved legalization of PAS.[75] However some fear that providing adequate pain relief might be seen as hastening the patient's death rather than controlling pain at end-of-life.[76] Events in Oregon highlight care as a priority and increase the understanding about the distinction between assisting suicide and honoring patient preferences for limiting life-sustaining treatment.[75] Patient concerns most often related to desire to hasten death are: unrelieved pain, poorly managed symptoms, depression, worries about loss of control, being a burden, being dependent on others for personal care, and loss of dignity.[76] Valente and Trainor[66] identified poor quality of life, failed requests for treatment withdrawal, and distressing treatments as typical reasons for suicide in the critically ill.

Patient requests for PAS are not rare, and some physicians are thought to provide such services, even where they are not legal.[77] Requests to physicians may also be indirect, as in the reported case of a patient asking for pain relief with the unspoken intent to cause death.[78] To further complicate the issue for health care providers, requests for suicide may appear to be rational and not simply a symptom of depression.[76] Rationality has been defined as the capacity to deliberate, to communicate in relationships, and to reflect on and to examine one's own values and purposes.[76] The accepted criteria for rational suicide among adults with terminal illness include the following: rational considerations, understandable motives, careful planning, review of alternatives, absence of coercion, and recognition of consequences.[76] The patient's decisional capacity may be impaired by agitation, disorientation, major depression, poor reality orientation, grief and loss, medications, effects of illness, and ambivalence. Particularly in these circumstances, a formal psychiatric evaluation is warranted. See Chapter 64, Palliative Care and Requests for Assistance in Dying, for a more in-depth review.

### Assessment of Suicide Risk

Assessment and treatment of depression, often overlooked in chronic-illness treatment settings, is a key suicide-prevention strategy. In addition, managing symptoms, communicating, and helping patients to maintain a sense of control are vitally important prevention strategies. An assessment of depression should always include direct questions about suicidal thinking, plans or attempts, despair or hopelessness, distress from poorly managed symptoms, and personal or family history of suicidal ideation, plans, or attempts.[76] When any indicator of suicide risk is recognized, there should be a thorough evaluation of risk factors, clues, suicidal ideation, level of depression, hopelessness and despair, and symptom distress, in order to estimate individual lethality. The rationality of the suicidal request or intent must also be evaluated. The nurse should interview the patient and family members to find out why the patient is thinking about suicide now.[76] Find out what method the patient is considering, and whether the means are available. Ask the patient what has prevented suicide before, and if he or she wants help or hopes someone else will decide.[76] Most people are relieved to be asked about suicidal thoughts because it opens communication. Initial and periodic evaluation of suicidal potential is necessary for patients with a history, thoughts, or risk factors of suicide.

### Recognition of Clues

Suicidal persons usually give verbal and/or behavioral clues, such as isolated or withdrawn behavior, or death wishes or death themes in art, writing, play, or conversation. Clues may be subtle or obvious; for example, joking about suicide, asking questions concerning death (e.g., "How many of these pills would it take to kill someone?"), comments with a theme of giving up, or statements that indicate hopelessness or helplessness. Keys to determining lethality are suicide plan, method, intended outcome (e.g., death or rescue), and availability of resources and ability to communicate.[74,76] Lethal means include guns, knives, jumping from heights, drowning, or carbon monoxide poisoning. Other potentially lethal means include hanging or strangulation (using strong pieces of twine, rope, electric cords, sheets), taking high doses of aspirin or Tylenol, being in a car crash, or undergoing exposure to extreme cold. Low to moderately lethal methods are wrist cutting and mild aspirin overdose.

### Suicide Interventions

Severely depressed and/or potentially suicidal patients must be identified as soon as possible to ensure a safe environment and appropriate treatment. Prompt action should be taken including provision of safety, supervision, and initiation of psychiatric evaluation. A patient with an immediate, lethal, and precise suicide plan needs strict safety precautions such as hospitalization and continuous or close supervision. The low-risk patient should not be underestimated. If circumstances change, risk could change. In all cases, notify the primary provider, and document the patient's behavior and verbatim statements, suicide assessment, and rationale for decisions, as well as the time and date the provider was notified.[76] If the provider is not responsive to the report of the patient's suicidal ideation, it is important to maintain observation and to pursue psychiatric consultation. The motivation for suicide can be reduced through palliative care interventions such as improved pain and symptom management; referral and treatment for depression or other psychiatric disorders; discussion of alternative interventions to improve quality of life; referral to spiritual, social, and psychiatric resources; and education and accurate facts about options for terminal care or end-of-life decision-making. Openness to talking about suffering, distress, death preferences, and decision-making in a sensitive and understanding manner, and advocacy to aid communication with others, are helpful for patients and their families.[76,77]

## Management of Anxiety and Depression

Psychosocial interventions can exert an important effect on the overall adjustment of patients and their families to chronic illness and treatment.[78] Several studies document the beneficial effect of counseling on anxiety, feelings of personal control,[79] depression, and generalized psychological distress.[80] Increased length of survival from time of diagnosis has highlighted the need for psychopharmacological, psychotherapeutic, and behaviorally oriented interventions to reduce anxiety and depression and to improve quality of life for patients diagnosed with a chronic illness.

### Pharmacological Interventions

Pharmacotherapy, as an adjunct to one or more of the psychotherapies, can be an important aid in bringing psychological symptoms under control.

*Pharmacological Management of Anxiety.* The prevalence of anxiety in medical illness is relatively high. As described in Figure 20–1, a variety of disorders have anxiety as a prominent symptom of the clinical presentation (see Tables 20–1 and 20–2), and many commonly used medications are associated with anxiety as a side effect. Studies have shown a high prevalence in cardiovascular, pulmonary, cerebrovascular, and gastrointestinal diseases, as well as cancer and diabetes. In addition, patients with a history of anxiety disorders have increased rates of diabetes, heart disease, arthritis, and physical handicaps compared to the general population. Pain, metabolic abnormalities, hypoxia, and drug withdrawal states can present as anxiety. Before instituting pharmacological treatment, any patient with acute or chronic symptoms of anxiety should be thoroughly evaluated, including a review of medications to assess the contribution of medical condition and/or medication-related etiologies for their complaints.

The following brief review of pharmacological treatment must be supplemented with other references concerning assessment, intervention, evaluation, and patient education (Table 20–7). Benzodiazepines are the most frequently used medications for anxiety in both medical and psychiatric settings. When longer-acting benzodiazepines, such as diazepam, are used in the elderly or in the presence of liver disease, dosages should be decreased and dosing intervals increased. They may suppress respiratory drive. Consultation-liaison services often use lorazepam in medically ill patients because its elimination half-life is relatively unaffected by liver disease, age, or concurrent use of selective serotonin reuptake inhibitors (SSRIs) or nefazodone. Drawbacks include amnestic

---

**Table 20–7**
**Selected Medications Commonly Used for the Treatment of Anxiety in the Medically Ill**

**Benzodiazepines**
Diazepam (Volium and others)
Alprazolam (Xanux)
Clonazepam (Klonopin)
Lorazepam (Ativan and others)
Oxazepam (Serax and others)

**Azapirones**
Buspirone (Buspar)

**Cyclic antidepressants**
Nortriptyline (Pamelor and others)

**Other antidepressents**
Fluoxetine (Prozac), an SSRI
Sertraline (Zoloft), an SSRI
Paroxetine (Paxil), an SSRI
Citalopram (Celexa) an SSRI
Escitalopram (Lexapro) an SSRI
Duloxetine (Cymbalta) an SNRI
Venlafaxine (Effexor), a serotonin/norepinephrine
    reuptake inhibitor
Mirtazapine (Remeron)

**Other medications selectively used for their anxiolytic effects**
β-Adrenergic blocking agents, such as propranolol
Neuroleptics (antipsychotics), such as Lanzapine
    (Zaffrapen), Quetrapine (Seroqud)

*Source*: Stoudemire (1996), reference 77.

---

episodes, and interdose anxiety caused by its short half-life. The latter can be remedied by more frequent dosing. If medically ill patients need a longer-acting benzodiazepine for panic disorder or generalized anxiety disorder, clonazepam is often used because it is not affected by concurrent use of SSRIs. Clonazepam may accumulate and result in oversedation and ataxia in the elderly; therefore, low doses are used. Temazepam is useful as a sedative-hypnotic.[35] Buspirone, used primarily for generalized anxiety disorder, is preferable for anxiety in the medically ill because of its lack of sedation, lack of negative effects on cognition, insignificant effect of age on elimination half-life, and limited effect of liver disease on half-life. Buspirone has almost no clinically significant interactions with drugs commonly used in general medicine. It may stimulate the respiratory drive, which makes it useful in patients with pulmonary disease or sleep apnea.[35]

Cyclic antidepressants are well established as anxiolytic agents, which are particularly effective in the treatment of panic disorder and in generalized anxiety disorder. If these drugs are used for anxiety in depressed medically ill patients, or used because of their sedating properties in patients with major depression or panic disorder, the side effects must be carefully considered. Potentially deleterious side effects in the medically ill are sedative, anticholinergic, orthostatic hypotensive, and quinidine-like. Liver disease and renal disease may affect metabolism and excretion of the drug and, therefore, require careful dosage titration.[34] Other drugs that may be used for anxiety include the β-adrenergic blocking agents, antihistamines, monoamine oxidase inhibitors, and neuroleptics. Beta-adrenergic blocking agents may be used for milder forms of generalized anxiety, but there are cautions and contraindications in the presence of pulmonary disease, diabetes, and congestive heart failure. Antihistamines are sometimes used, although the effects are largely nonspecific and sedative. Side effects, such as sedation and dizziness, can be significant for medically ill patients. Monoamine oxidase inhibitors are rarely used in the medically ill because of the precautions that must be taken to prevent drug interactions. Neuroleptics, such as haloperidol in low doses, are used for anxiety associated with severe behavioral agitation or psychotic symptoms.[34] When anxiety develops in the context of the terminal stages of cancer, it is often secondary to hypoxia and/or an untreated pain syndrome. Intravenous opiates, and oxygen if hypoxia is present, are usually an effective palliative treatment.[81] Anxiolytics are most effective when doses are scheduled; if given on an as-needed basis, anxiety may increase in patients already frightened and anxious. Anxiolytic medications help patients gain control over agonizing anxiety. Use of these medications may also assist the patient in psychotherapy, which can help control symptoms. All pharmacological treatments must be monitored for effectiveness and side effects. The effects of benzodiazepines are felt within hours, with a full response in days. Buspirone has no immediate effect, with a full response after 2 to 4 weeks. The sedating effects of benzodiazepines are associated with impaired motor performance and cognition. Benzodiazepines have dependence and abuse potential and the possibility of withdrawal symptoms when discontinued. Buspirone has no association with dependence or abuse.

*Pharmacological Management of Depression.* Patients with chronic illness commonly exhibit transient depressive symptoms at various points in the disease trajectory, particularly during the palliative care period when a hope for cure is no longer possible. As explained previously, depressive symptoms can be caused by the medical disorder itself, associated with medications used for treatment or symptom management, or caused or worsened by the stress related to coping with illness. Depression can also predate and recur with the medical illness. To further complicate matters, individuals with medical illness are often older, with potentially greater risk of adverse effects from both psychotropic and nonpsychotropic medications. Medical illnesses and the medications required to treat or manage symptoms may impose significantly modified prescribing regimens on the use of antidepressants. Therefore, it is necessary to evaluate the possible role of existing medical conditions and medications that could cause the depressive symptoms. Other general guidelines include: (1) use the medication with the least potential for drug–drug interactions and for adverse effects based on the patient's drug regimen and physiological vulnerabilities, and the greatest potential for improving the primary symptoms of the depression; (2) begin with low dosage, increase slowly, and establish the lowest effective dosage; and (3) reassess dosage requirements regularly.[81]

In the past, antidepressant drug selection was limited by the nearly sole availability of tricyclic antidepressants; but new drugs, such as the SSRIs, bupropion, and venlafaxine, have vastly simplified pharmacological treatment of depression in the medically ill.[82] No one medication is clearly more effective than another. The SSRIs have fewer long-term side effects than the tricyclic antidepressants and, in general, are the first line of pharmacological antidepressant treatment unless specific side-effect profiles associated with other classes of drugs are desired.

Psychostimulants such as dextroamphetamine and methylphenidate have been useful in the treatment of depression in medically ill patients.[83–85] Advantages include rapid onset of action and rapid clearance if side effects occur.[86] They can also counteract opioid-induced sedation and improve pain control through a positive action on mood.[87] Common side effects of psychostimulants include insomnia, anorexia, tachycardia, and hypertension,[83] although incremental dosage increases allow adequate monitoring of therapeutic versus side effects. In patients with cardiac conduction problems, stimulants may be the treatment of choice. In medically ill patients, a 1- to 2-month trial can provide remission from depression even after discontinuation of the drug. Different studies have shown a 48% to 80% improvement in depressive symptoms,[87] and this class of medication is often quite effective but underutilized in medical settings (Table 20–8).

Certain medications and treatment agents can produce severe depressive states. As reiterated throughout this chapter,

| Table 20–8 |
| --- |
| **Selected Medications Commonly used for the Treatment of Depression in the Medically Ill** |
| **Selective serotonin reuptake inhibitors** |
| Sertraline (Zoloft) |
| Paroxetine (Paxil) |
| Citalopram (Celexa) |
| Escitalopram (Lexapro) |
| **Serotonin/norepinephrine reuptake inhibitors** |
| Venlafaxine (Effexor) |
| Duloxetine (Cymbalta) |
| **Tricyclic antidepressants** |
| Amitriptyline (Elavil) |
| Desipramine (Norpramin) |
| Nortriptyline (Aventyl, Pamelor) |
| **Noradrenergic agonist** |
| Mirtazapine (Remeron) |
| **Psychostimulants** |
| Dextroamphetamine (Dexedrine) |
| Methylphenidate |
| Provigil (Modafinil) |
| **Dopamine reuptake blocking compounds** |
| Bupropion (Wellbutrin, Zyban) |
| *Source:* Beliles & Stoudemire (1998), reference 100. |

a diagnosis of major depression in medically ill patients relies heavily on the presence of affective symptoms such as hopelessness, crying spells, guilt, preoccupation with death and/or suicide, diminished self-worth, and loss of pleasure in most activities, for example, being with friends and loved ones. The neurovegetative symptoms that usually characterize depression in physically healthy individuals are not good predictors of depression in the medically ill, because disease and treatment can also produce these symptoms. A combination of psychotherapy and antidepressant medication will often prove useful in treating major depression in medically ill patients.[88] Peak dosages of antidepressants, regardless of drug class, are usually substantially lower than those tolerated by physically healthy individuals. Antidepressant medications may take 2 to 6 weeks to produce their desired effects. Patients may need ongoing support, reassurance, and monitoring before experiencing the antidepressant effects of medication. It is essential that patients are monitored closely by a consistent provider during the initiation and modification of psychopharmacological regimens. Patient education is essential in this area to decrease the possibility of nonadherence to the medication regimen.

## Psychotherapeutic Modalities

Psychosocial interventions are defined as systematic efforts applied to influence coping behavior through educational or psychotherapeutic means.[18] The goals of such interventions are to improve morale, self-esteem, coping ability, sense of control, and problem-solving abilities, and to decrease emotional distress. The educational approach is directive, using problem-solving and cognitive methods. It is important that the educational approach both clarify medical information that may be missed due to fear and anxiety, or misconceptions and/or misinformation regarding illness and treatment, and normalize emotional reactions throughout the illness trajectory. The psychotherapeutic approach uses psychodynamic and exploratory methods to help the individual understand aspects of the medical condition such as emotional responses and personal meaning of the disease. Psychotherapeutic interventions, as opposed to educational interventions, should be delivered by professionals with special training in both mental health and specific interventional modalities as applied to patients with chronic medical illnesses and palliative care needs. Psychotherapy with a patient who has cancer should maintain a primary focus on the illness and its implications, using a brief therapy and crisis-intervention model.[78] Expression of fears and concerns that may be too painful to reveal to family and friends is encouraged. Normalizing emotional distress, providing realistic reassurance and support, and bolstering existing strengths and coping skills are essential components of the therapeutic process. Gathering information about previous associations with the medical condition experienced through close relationships can also be instrumental in clarifying patients' fears and concerns, and establishing boundaries for and differences from the current situation.

Depending on the nature of the problem, the treatment modality may take the form of individual psychotherapy, support groups, family and marital therapy, or behaviorally oriented therapy such as progressive muscle relaxation and guided imagery. A primary role for clinicians is to facilitate a positive adjustment in patients under their care. Periodic emotional distress and coping problems can be expected during the palliative care trajectory, and monitored routinely. Emotional display is not the same as maladaptive coping. Understanding an individual's unique circumstances can assist nurses in supporting the constructive coping abilities that seem to work best for a particular patient.[78,89]

### Psychotherapeutic Interventions Targeted to Symptoms of Anxiety

Anxiety responses can be thought of as occurring along a continuum, from mild to moderate to severe to panic. Lazarus and Folkman's[92] differentiation of problem-focused coping and emotion-focused coping provides a framework for intervention strategies matched to the continuum of responses (Table 20–9). As a person moves along the continuum to moderate, severe, and panic levels of anxiety, the problem-causing distress is lost sight of, and distress itself becomes the focus of attention. Both preventive and treatment strategies can be used with patients and family members in a variety of settings. Before assuming that anxiety has a psychological basis,

consider the models of interaction and review the patient's history for recent changes in medical condition and/or medications. Asking whether the patient was taking medications for "nerves," depression, or insomnia will help to determine whether drugs were inappropriately discontinued, or whether anxiety symptoms predated the current illness. In addition, ask about over-the-counter medications, illegal drugs, alcohol intake, and smoking history. Documentation and communication of findings are essential to enhance teamwork among providers.

Frequently, patients can identify the factors causing their anxiety, as well as coping skills effective in the past, and when they do, their discomfort decreases. Anxiety may be greatly reduced by initiating a discussion of concerns that are painful, frightening, or shameful, such as being dependent or accepting help. Use open-ended questions, reflection, clarification, and/or empathic remarks, such as "You're afraid of being a burden?" to help the patient to identify previously effective coping strategies and to integrate them with new ones. Use statements such as "What has helped you get through difficult times like this before?" "How can we help you use those strategies now?" or "How about talking about some new strategies that may work now?" Encourage the patient to identify supportive individuals who can either help emotionally or with tasks.

### Preventive Strategies

Preventive strategies can help to maintain a useful level of anxiety, one that enhances rather than interferes with problem-solving (see Table 20–9). Effective preventive strategies that can be used by all providers involved with the patient follow:[26,90]

1. *Provide concrete, objective information.* Fear of the unknown, lack of recent prior experience, or misinterpretations about an illness, procedure, test, or medication, especially when coupled with a tendency to focus on emotional aspects of experiences, may be a source of anxiety. Help patients and families know what to expect, and focus attention by realistically describing the potentially threatening experience with concrete objective information. [91] Describe both the typical subjective (e.g., sensations and temporal features) and objective (e.g., timing, nature of environment) features of stressful health care events, using concrete terminology. Avoid qualitative adjectives, such as "terrible." Also known as mental rehearsal and stress inoculation, concrete information increases the patient's understanding of the situation, allows for preparation under less emergent and more supportive conditions, and facilitates coping. Encourage the patient to ask questions, and then match the detail of the preparatory information to the request. Since anxiety hinders retention, use of understandable terms and repetition is helpful. Too much information at once may increase anxiety.

**Table 20–9**
**Hierarchy of Anxiety Interventions**

| Anxiety Level | Interventions |
|---|---|
| **Level 1**<br>**Mild to moderate** | *Prevention strategies*<br>Provide concrete objective information.<br>Ensure stressful-event warning.<br>Increase opportunities for control.<br>Increase patient and family participation in care activities.<br>Acknowledge fears.<br>Explore near-miss events, past and/or present.<br>Control symptoms.<br>Structure uncertainty.<br>Limit sensory deprivation and isolation.<br>Encourage hope. |
| **Level 2**<br>**Moderate to severe** | *Treatment strategies*<br>Use presence of support person as "emotional anchor."<br>Support expression of feelings, doubts, and fears.<br>Explore near-miss events, past and/or present.<br>Provide accurate information for realistic restructuring of fearful ideas.<br>Teach anxiety-reduction strategies, such as focusing, breathing, relaxation, and imagery techniques.<br>Use massage, touch, and physical exercise.<br>Control symptoms.<br>Use antianxiety medications.<br>Delay procedures to promote patient control and readiness.<br>Consult psychiatric experts. |
| **Level 3**<br>**Panic** | *Treatment strategies*<br>Stay with the patient.<br>Maintain calm environment and reduce stimulation.<br>Use antianxiety medications and monitor carefully.<br>Control symptoms.<br>Use focusing and breathing techniques.<br>Use demonstration in addition to verbal direction.<br>Repeat realistic reassurances.<br>Communicate with repetition and simplicity.<br>Consult psychiatric experts. |

*Sources:* Minarik (1996), reference 17; Leavitt & Minarik (1989), reference 101.

2. *Ensure stressful event warning before the event.* For example, a person may experience magnetic resonance imaging as entrapping or traumatic, or the placement of a central line as painful and threatening. Giving time to anticipate and mentally rehearse coping with the experience helps the person to maintain a sense of control and endure the procedure.

3. *Increase opportunities for control.* Illness can seriously disrupt a person's sense of control and increase anxiety. Help the patient to make distinctions between what is controllable, partially controllable, or not controllable. Focus on what is controllable or partially controllable and create decision-making and choice opportunities that fit the patient's knowledge. Ask patients to make choices about scheduling the day of the visit and the readiness for, and timing of, procedures and interventions.

4. *Increase patient and family participation in care.* Participation in care helps directly in coping and can be taught to both the patient and family members. Participation may reduce helplessness and increase a sense of control. Patients and family members may vary in their interest in participating, and in their ability to do so. Often, female family members are more likely to be caregivers. Other factors influencing the ability to participate include family roles such as spouse, parent, and sibling; quality of relationships; presence or absence of conflicts; and other commitments, such as work or other family roles. Cultures also vary in expectations and the duty or obligation to caregiving based on gender or family position. Participation may also help with the resolution of ineffective denial when a person's condition is deteriorating. Family members who are

caring for a person may recognize and adjust to the deterioration.

5. *Encourage self-monitoring and the use of a stress diary.* Self-monitoring of stress is a cognitive-behavioral intervention. Ask the patient to record the situations, thoughts, and feelings that elicit stress and anxiety. The patient may record incidences of treatment-related stress, illness-related stress, or other, unrelated anxiety-provoking situations. Not only does this intervention provide assessment information, it also enhances collaboration with the patient and helps the patient understand the relationship between situations, thoughts, and feelings.

6. *Acknowledge fears.* Encourage and listen to the expression of feelings. Avoid denying the existence of problems or reassuring anxious people that "everything will be fine." Structure your availability. Refrain from avoiding anxious persons or their fears. Avoidance is likely to increase vulnerability, isolation, helplessness, and anxiety. Early structured intervention is more economical of time, and more effective.

7. *Explore near-miss events.* Past or current exposure to a near-miss event is a potent generator of extreme stress and anxiety, with heightened vigilance. A near-miss is a harrowing experience that overwhelms the ability to cope. It may be a one-time experience, such as a person's own near-death experience, the cardiac arrest of another person in similar circumstances, or something faced repeatedly, such as daily painful skin and wound care. Near-misses should be explored, fears acknowledged and realistically evaluated in view of the person's situation, and help given in developing coping strategies.

8. *Manage symptoms.* Managing symptoms such as pain, dyspnea, and fatigue is an essential part of promoting self-control. Symptoms such as pain signal threat, and may lead to worries about the meaning of the symptom and whether necessary treatments will be worse or more frightening. Ensure pain control, especially before painful or frightening procedures. Severe anxiety may increase the perception of pain and increase the requirement for analgesia. Symptom management reduces distress and allows for rest.

9. *Structure uncertainty.* Even when there are many unknowns, the period of uncertainty can be framed with expected events, procedures, updates, and meetings with providers.

10. *Reduce sensory deprivation.* Sensory deprivation and isolation can heighten attention to various signals in the environment. Without the means for the patient to accurately interpret the signals, to be reassured, and to feel in control, the signals take on frightening meanings, such as abandonment and helplessness. Feeling isolated and helpless increases the sense of vulnerability and danger.

11. *Build hope.* Provide information about possible satisfactory outcomes and means to achieve them. Hope also may be built around coping ability, sustaining relationships, revising goals such as pain-free or peaceful death, and determination to endure.[92] Many additional suggestions are provided in this text.

### Treatment Strategies

When it is evident that the person's anxiety level has escalated to the point of interfering with problem solving or comfort, the following strategies may be helpful.[26,90]

1. *Presence of supportive persons.* Familiar and supportive people, a family member, friend, or staff member can act as an "emotional anchor." Family and friends may need coaching to enable them to help in the situation without their own anxiety increasing.

2. *Expression of feelings, doubts, and fears.* Verbalizing feelings provides the opportunity to correct or restructure unrealistic misconceptions and automatic anxiety-provoking thoughts. Accurate information allows restructuring of perceptions and lends predictability to the situation. Aggressive confrontation of unrealistic perceptions may reinforce them, and is to be avoided.

3. *Use of antianxiety medications.* If medications are used, they should be given concurrently with other interventions and monitored. Use caution to avoid delirium from toxicity, especially in the older person.

4. *Promoting patient control and readiness.* If a patient is very frightened of a particular procedure, allow time for the patient to regain enough composure to make the decision to proceed. Forging ahead when a patient is panicked may appear to save time in the immediate situation, but it will increase the patient's sense of vulnerability and helplessness, possibly adding time over the long term.

5. *Management of panic.* When anxiety reaches panic, use presence and acknowledgment: "I know you are frightened. I'll stay with you." Communicate with repetition and simplicity. Guide the person to a smaller, quieter area away from other people and use quiet reassurance. Maintain a calm manner and reduce all environmental stimulation. Help the patient to focus on a single object (see below), and guide the patient in recognizing the physical features of the object while breathing rhythmically. Consider using prescribed anxiolytic medication.

6. *Massage, touch, and physical exercise.* For those who respond well to touch, massage releases muscle tension and may elicit emotional release. Physical exercise is a constructive way of releasing energy when direct problem-solving is impossible or ineffective, because it

reduces muscle tension and other physiological effects of anxiety.

7. *Relaxation techniques.* Relaxation techniques are likely to be effective for patients with mild to moderate anxiety who are able to concentrate and who desire to use them. Some techniques require learning and/or regular practice for effectiveness. Environmental awareness is reduced by focusing inward, with deliberate concentration on breathing, a sound, or an image, and suggestions of muscle relaxation. Progressive relaxation and autogenic relaxation are commonly used techniques, which require approximately 15 minutes. Relaxation and guided imagery scripts are readily available for use by clinicians.[26,93]

8. *Breathing techniques.* Simple and easy to learn, breathing exercises emphasize slow, rhythmic, controlled breathing patterns that relax and distract the patient while slowing the heart rate, thus decreasing anxiety. Ask the patient to notice his or her normal breathing. Then ask the patient to take a few slow, deep abdominal breaths and to think "relax" or "I am calm" with each exhalation. Encourage practice during the day. Some patients are helped by seeing photographs and drawings of lungs and breathing to visualize their actions.[94]

9. *Focusing techniques.* Useful for patients with episodes of severe-to-panic levels of anxiety, focusing repeatedly on one person or object in the room helps the patient to disengage from all other stimuli and promotes control. A combination of focusing, with demonstration and coaching of slow, rhythmic breathing (using a calm, low-pitched voice) is helpful. These techniques enhance the patient's self-control, which is desirable when the stress reaction is excessive and the stressful event cannot be changed or avoided. Both focusing and deep-breathing techniques can be used without prior practice and during extreme stress.

10. *Music therapy.* Soothing music or environmental sounds reduce anxiety by providing a tranquil environment and prompting recall of pleasant memories, which interrupt the stress response through distraction or direct sympathetic nervous system action.[95,96] Music most helpful for relaxation is primarily of string composition, low-pitched, with a simple and direct musical rhythm and a tempo of approximately 60 beats per minute,[95] although music with flute, a cappella voice, and synthesizer is also effective.

11. *Imagery and visualization techniques.* Imagery inhibits anxiety by invoking a calm, peaceful mental image, including memories, dreams, fantasies, and visions. Guided imagery is the deliberate, goal-directed use of the natural capacities of the imagination. Using all the senses, imagery serves as a bridge for connecting body, mind, and spirit.[76] Imagery, especially when combined with relaxation, promotes coping with illness by anxiety reduction, enhanced self-control, feeling expression, symptom relief, healing promotion, and dealing with role changes. Regular practice of imagery enhances success. Guided imagery for pain or anxiety reduction should not be attempted the first time during periods of extreme stress. Imagery in conversation is subtle and spontaneous. Often, without being aware of it, health care providers' questions and statements to patients include imagery. Easily combined with routine activities, the deliberate use of conversational imagery involves listening to and positively using the language, beliefs, and metaphors of the patient. Be aware of descriptors used for the effects of medications or treatments, because they affect the patient's attitude and response. Health care providers can enhance hope and self-control if they give empowering, healing messages that emphasize how the treatment will help.

## Psychotherapeutic Interventions Targeted to Symptoms of Depression

Depression is inadequately treated in palliative care, although many patients experience depressive symptoms. Goals for the depressed patient are (1) to ensure a safe environment, (2) to assist the patient in reducing depressive symptoms and maladaptive coping responses, (3) to restore or increase the patient's functional level, (4) to improve quality of life if possible, and (5) to prevent future relapse and recurrence of depression.

*Crisis Intervention.* Crisis intervention is appropriate treatment for a grief-and-loss reaction and when a patient feels overwhelmed. Effective strategies also include providing guidance on current problems, reinforcing coping resources and strengths, and enhancing social supports.[26]

*Cognitive Interventions.* Cognitive interventions (Table 20–10) are based on a view of depression as the result of faulty thinking. A person's reaction depends on how that person perceives and interprets the situation of chronic illness. Patterns of thinking associated with depression include self-condemnation, leading to feelings of inadequacy and guilt; hopelessness, which is often combined with helplessness; and self-pity, which comes from magnification or catastrophizing about one's problems. Cognitive approaches involve clarification of misconceptions and modification of faulty assumptions by identifying and correcting distorted, negative, and catastrophic thinking. Cognitive approaches are effective in treating forms of depression.[69] Therapy is usually brief, with the primary goal of reversing and decreasing the likelihood of recurrence of the symptoms of depression by modifying cognitions. It requires effort on the part of the patient. The effect is more powerful if homework and practice are included. Cognitive restructuring

**Table 20–10**
**Nonpharmacological Interventions for Treatment of Depression**

**Cognitive interventions**
Review and reinforce realistic ideas and expectations.
Help the patient test the accuracy of self-defeating assumptions.
Help the patient identify and test negative automatic thoughts.
Review and reinforce patient's strengths.
Set realistic, achievable goals.
Explain all actions and plans, seek feedback and participation in decision-making.
Provide choices (e.g., about the timing of an activity).
Teach thought stopping or thought interruption to halt negative or self-defeating thoughts.
Encourage exploration of feelings only for a specific purpose and only if the patient is not ruminating (e.g., constant repeating of failures or problems).
Direct the patient to activities with gentle reminders to focus as a way to discourage rumination.
Listen and take appropriate action on physical complaints, then redirect and assist the patient to accomplish activities.
Avoid denying the patient's sadness or depressed feelings or reason to feel that way.
Avoid chastising the patient for feeling sad.

**Interpersonal interventions**
Educate the patient about the physical and biochemical causes of depression and the good prognosis.
Enhance social skills through modeling, role playing, rehearsal, feedback, and reinforcement.
Build rapport with frequent, short visits.
Engage in normal social conversation with the patient as often as possible.
Give consistent attention, even when the patient is uncommunicative, to show that the patient is worthwhile.
Direct comments and questions to the patient rather than to significant others.
Allow adequate time for the patient to prepare a response.
Mobilize family and social support systems.
Encourage the patient to maintain open communication and share feelings with significant others.
Supportively involve family and friends and teach them how to help.
Avoid sharing with the patient your personal reactions to the patient's dependent behavior.
Avoid medical jargon, advice giving, sharing personal experiences, or making value judgments.
Avoid false reassurance.

**Behavioral interventions**
Provide directed activities.
Develop a hierarchy of behaviors with the patient and use a graded task assignment.
Develop structured daily activity schedules.
Encourage the at-home use of a diary or journal to monitor automatic thoughts, behaviors, and emotions; review this with the patient.
Use systematic application of reinforcement.
Encourage self-monitoring of predetermined behaviors, such as sleep pattern, diet, and physical exercise.
Focus on goal attainment and preparation for future adaptive coping.

**Specific behavioral strategies**
Observe the patient's self-care patterns, then negotiate with the patient to develop a structured, daily schedule.
Develop realistic daily self-care goals with the patient to increase sense of control.
Upgrade the goals gradually to provide increased opportunity for positive reinforcement and goal attainment.
Use a chart for monitoring daily progress; gold stars may be used as reinforcement; a visible chart facilitates communication, consistency among caregivers, and meaningful reinforcement (i.e., praise and positive attention from others).
Provide sufficient time and repetitive reassurance ("You can do it") to encourage patients to accomplish self-care actions.
Positively reinforce even small achievements.
Provide physical assistance with self-care activities, especially those related to appearance and hygiene, that the patient is unable to do.
Adjust physical assistance, verbal direction, reminders, and teaching to the actual needs and abilities of the patient; and avoid, increasing unnecessary dependence by overdoing.
Teach deep breathing or relaxation techniques for anxiety management.

**Complementary therapies**
Guided imagery and visualization
Art and music therapies
Humor
Aerobic exercise
Phototherapy
Phototherapy
Aromatherapy and massage

*Sources*: Minarik (1996), reference 17; Leavitt & Minarik (1989), reference 101.

is one of the strategies used in cognitive therapy. In this strategy, patients are aided in identifying and evaluating maladaptive attitudes, thoughts, and beliefs by self-monitoring and recording their automatic thoughts when they feel depressed. The patient is then helped to replace self-defeating patterns of

thinking with more constructive patterns. For example, "The treatment is not working. I can't cope; nothing works for me," could be replaced with a rational response such as "I can cope. I have learned how to help myself and I can do it." New self-statements and their associated feeling responses can also be written on the self-monitoring form. Over time, the patient learns to modify thinking, and learns a method for combating other automatic thoughts.[67]

Imagery rehearsal is a useful strategy for helping patients to cope with situations in which they usually become depressed. The first step is to anticipate events that could be problematic, such as a magnetic resonance procedure. The patient is helped to develop constructive self-statements; then, imagery is used to provide an opportunity for the patient to mentally rehearse how to think, act, and feel in the situation. The combination of imagery with cognitive restructuring increases the effectiveness.[67]

*Interpersonal Interventions.* Interpersonal interventions (see Table 20–10) focus on improved self-esteem, the development of effective social skills, and dealing with interpersonal and relationship difficulties. Interpersonal difficulties that could be a focus include role disruptions or transitions, social isolation, delayed grief reaction, family conflict, or role enactment. Psychotherapies include individual, group, and support groups led by a trained professional. Patient-led support groups or self-help groups are effective for the general chronic illness population, but are less able to address the needs of depressed persons.[68]

*Behavioral Interventions.* Behavioral interventions (see Table 20–10) are based on a functional analysis of behavior and on social learning theory. These interventions are often used in combination with cognitive interventions, such as self-monitoring and imagery rehearsal. The key to the behavioral approach is to avoid reinforcement of dependent or negative behaviors. Instead, provide a contingency relationship between positive reinforcement, and independent behavior and positive interactions with the environment. This approach suggests that, by altering behavior, subsequent thoughts and feelings are positively influenced. It is helpful to structure this approach using the following self-care functional areas: behavior related to breathing, eating, and drinking; elimination patterns; personal hygiene behavior; rest and activity patterns; and patterns of solitude and social interaction. The aim is to maintain involvement in activities associated with positive moods and, if possible, to avoid situations that trigger depression.[97] This approach has been effective at helping family members of terminally ill patients see and accept functional decline.

*Alternative and Complementary Therapies.* Complementary therapies may help reduce mild depressive symptoms, or they may be used as an adjunct to other therapies for more severe depressive symptoms.[68] Strategies described for anxiety, such as guided imagery and visualization, the use of drawings or photographs, and music therapy, also may be used for depression. Art therapy for creative self-expression, use of humor and laughter, aerobic exercise, and aromatherapy massage have been helpful for mild depressive symptoms.[68] Phototherapy, which is exposure to bright, wide-spectrum light, has shown promise in patients with cancer.[68] See Chapter 27, Complementary and Alternative Therapies in Palliative Care, for a more in-depth review.

## Conclusion

The psychosocial issues in persons facing life-threatening illness are influenced by individual, sociocultural, medical, and family factors. Most patients receiving palliative treatment, and their families, experience expected periods of emotional turmoil that occur at transition points, as is seen, for example, along the clinical course of cancer. Some patients experience anxiety and depressive disorders. This chapter has described the spectrum of anxiety and depressive symptoms during the palliative care trajectory; models useful for understanding the interaction of psychiatric and medical symptoms and for designing appropriate treatments; guidelines for referral to trained psychiatric clinicians; and a range of treatments for anxiety and depression. Supportive psychotherapeutic measures, such as those described in this chapter, should be used routinely because they minimize distress, and enhance feelings of control and mastery over self and environment. Assessment and treatment of psychosocial problems, including physical symptoms, psychological distress, caregiver burden, and psychiatric disorders, can enhance quality of life throughout the palliative care trajectory.

This was reflected in Mrs. Jones's outcome. Following clarification that she would be receiving chemotherapy to halt disease progression, plus awareness that her reason for refusing was based on memories of her mother and, thus, assumptions about her own outcome, led the patient to reconsider and accept treatment recommendations. A low-dose anxiolytic was suggested for use at bedtime, which the patient received on a short-term basis. Mrs. Jones was still well at the 1-year follow-up.

REFERENCES

1. Zabora J, Brintzenhofeszoc K, Curbow B, Hooker C, Piantadosi S. The prevalence of psychological distress by cancer site. Psychooncology 2001;10:19.
2. Richardson JL, Zamegar Z, Bisno B, Levine A. Psychosocial status at initiation of cancer treatment and survival. J Psychosom Res 1990;34:189.
3. Wellisch DK, Centeno J, Guzman J, Belin T, Schiller GJ. Bone marrow transplantation vs high-dose cytorabine-based consolidation chemotherapy for acute myelogenous leukemia: A long-term follow-up study of quality-of-life measures of survivors. Psychosomatics 1996;37:144.
4. Syrjala KL, Chapko MK, Vitaliano PP, et al. Recovery after allogenic marrow transplantation: A prospective study of predictors of long-term physical and psychosocial functioning. Bone Marrow Transplant 1993;11:319.
5. Tschuschke V, Hertenstein B, Arnold R, et al. Associations between coping and survival time of adult leukemia patients

receiving allogeneic bone marrow transplantation: Results of a prospective study. J Psychosom Res 2001;50:277.

6. Steinhauser KE, Christakis NA, Clipp EC, et al. Factors considered important at the end of life by patients, family, physicians, and other care providers. JAMA 2000;284:2476.

7. Holland J. Clinical course of cancer. In: Holland JC, Rowland JH, eds. Handbook of Psychooncology: Psychological Care of the Patient with Cancer. New York: Oxford University Press, 1989:75–110.

8. Weissman A, Worden JW. The existential plight in cancer: significance of the first 100 days. Int J Psychiatry Med 1976;7:1.

9. Endicott J. Measurement of depression in patients with cancer. In: Proceedings of the Working Conference on Methodology in Behavioral and Psychosocial Cancer Research. American Cancer Society, St. Petersburg Beach, FL, April 21–23, 1983;2243–2247.

10. Graydon JE. Factors that predict patients' functioning following treatment for cancer. Int J Nurs Stud 1988;25:117–124.

11. Richardson JL, Zamegar Z, Bisno B, Levine A. Psychosocial status at initiation of cancer treatment and survival. J Psychosom Res 1990;34:189.

12. Vickberg SMJ, Duhamel KN, Smith MY, et al. Global meaning and psychological adjustment among survivors of bone marrow transplant. Psychooncology 2001;10:29.

13. Pasacreta JV, Pickett M. Psychosocial aspects of palliative care. Semin Oncol Nurs 1998;26:77–92.

14. Watson M, Greer S, Blake S, Sharpnell K. Reaction to a diagnosis of breast cancer: Relationship between denial, delay, and rates of psychological morbidity. Cancer 1984;53:2008–2012.

15. Molassiotis A, Van Den Akker OBA, Milligan DW, Goldman JM. Symptom distress, coping style and biological variables as predictors of survival after bone marrow transplantation. J Psychosomatic Res 1997;42:275.

16. Bope E. Follow-up of the cancer patient: Surveillance for metastasis. Prim Care 1987;14:391–401.

17. Minarik P. Psychosocial intervention with ineffective coping responses to physical illness: Anxiety-related. In: Barry PD, ed. Psychosocial Nursing: Care of Physically Ill Patients and Their Families. New York: Lippincott-Raven, 1996:301–322.

18. Silverfarb PM, Maurer LH, Crouthamel CS. Psychosocial aspects of neoplastic disease: I. Functional status of breast cancer patients during different treatment regimens. Am J Psychiatry 1980;137:450–455.

19. Wise MG, Taylor SE. Anxiety and mood disorders in medically ill patients. J Clin Psychiatry 1990;51(Suppl 1):27–32.

20. Breitbart W. Identifying patients at risk for and treatment of major psychiatric complications of cancer. Support Care Cancer 1995;3:45–60.

21. McGrath P. End-of-life care for hematological malignancies: the "technological imperative" and palliative care. J Palliat Care 2002;18:39.

22. Steinhauser KE, Christakis NA, Clipp EC, et al. Factors considered important at the end of life by patients, family, physicians, and other care providers. JAMA 2000;284:2476.

23. Emanuel EJ, Emanuel LL. The promise of a good death. Lancet 1998;351:21.

24. Bates MS, Edwards WT, Anderson KO. Ethnocultural influences on variation in chronic pain perception. Pain 1993;52:101–112.

25. Pickett M. Cultural awareness in the context of terminal illness. Cancer Nurs 1993;16:102–106.

26. Tang ST, McCorkle R. Determinants of place of death for terminal cancer patients. Cancer Invest 2001;19:165.

27. Roth AJ, Breitbart W. Psychiatric emergencies in terminally ill cancer patients. Hematol Oncol Clin North Am 1996;10:235–259.

28. Minarik P. Psychosocial intervention with ineffective coping responses to physical illness: Depression-related. In: Barry PD, ed. Psychosocial Nursing: Care of Physically Ill Patients and Their Families. New York: Lippincott-Raven, 1996:323–339.

29. Levenson J, Lesko LM. Psychiatric aspects of adult leukemia. Semin Oncol Nurs 1990;6:76–83.

30. Pasacreta JV, Pickett M. Psychosocial aspects of palliative care. Semin Oncol Nurs 1998;14:110–120.

31. Bloom JR. Social support, accommodation to stress and adjustment to breast cancer. Soc Sci Med 1982;16:1329–1338.

32. Molassiotis A, Van Den Akker OBA, Boughton BJ. Perceived social support, family environment and psychosocial recovery in bone marrow transplant long-term survivors. Soc Sci Med 1997;44:317.

33. Andrykowski MA, Brady MJ, Henslee-Downey PJ. Psychosocial factors predictive of survival after allogenic bone marrow transplantation for leukemia. Psychosom Med 1994;56:432.

34. Molassiotis A, Van Den Akker OBA, Milligan DW, Goldman JM. Symptom distress, coping style and biological variables as predictors of survival after bone marrow transplantation. J Psychosom Res 1997;42:275.

35. Burish TG, Lyles JN. Effectiveness of relaxation training in reducing adverse reactions to cancer chemotherapy. J Behav Med 1981;4:65–78.

36. Worden JW. Psychosocial screening of cancer patients. J Psychosoc Oncol 1983;1:1–10.

37. Derogatis LR, Morrow GR, Fetting J, et al. The prevalence of psychiatric disorders among cancer patients. JAMA 1983;249:751–757.

38. Massie MJ, Gagnon P, Holland JC. Depression and suicide in patients with cancer. J Pain Symptom Manage 1994;9:325–340.

39. Pasacreta JV, Massie MJ. Psychiatric complications in patients with cancer. Oncol Nurs Forum 1990;17:19–24.

40. Pasacreta JV, Massie MJ. Nurses' reports of psychiatric complications in patients with cancer. Oncol Nurs Forum 1990;3:347–353.

41. Pasacreta JV, McCorkle R. Psychosocial aspects of cancer. In: McCorkle R, Grant M, Stromborg MF, Baird S, eds. Cancer Nursing: A Comprehensive Textbook (2nd ed). Philadelphia: WB Saunders, 1991:1074–1090.

42. McDaniel JS, Messelman DL, Porter MR, Reed DA, Nemeroff CB. Depression in patients with cancer. Diagnosis, biology and treatment. Arch Gen Psychiatry 1995;52:89–99.

43. Cassem EH. Depressive disorders in the medically ill. Psychosomatics 1995;36:S2–S10.

44. Cavanaugh S. Depression in the medically ill. Psychosomatics 1995;36:48–59.

45. Fernandez R, Levy JK, Lachar BL, Small GW. The management of depression and anxiety in the elderly. J Clin Psychiatry 1995;56(Suppl 2):20–29.

46. Barraclough J. ABC of palliative care: Depression, anxiety, and confusion. BMJ 1997;315:1365–1368.

47. Morse JM, Doberneck B. Delineating the concept of hope. Image: J Nurs Scholarsh 1995;27:277–285.

48. Loge JH, Abrahamsen AF, Ekeberg O, Kaasa S. Fatigue and psychiatric morbidity among Hodgkin's disease survivors. J Pain Symptom Manage 2000;19:91.

49. McCoy, D.M. Treatment considerations for depression in patients with significant medical comorbidity. J Fam Pract 1996;43(Suppl):S35–S44.

50. Chochinov HM, Wilson KG, Enns M, Lander S. Depression, hopelessness, and suicidal ideation in the terminally ill. Psychosomatics 1998;39:366–370.

51. Wettergren L, Langius A, Bjorkholm M, Bjorvell H. Post-traumatic stress symptoms in patients undergoing autologous stem cell transplantation. Acta Oncol 1999;38:475.

52. Peplau H. A working definition of anxiety. In: Burd SF, Marshall MA, eds. Some Clinical Approaches to Psychiatric Nursing. New York: Macmillan, 1963;323–327.

53. Sarna L, McCorkle R. Living with lung cancer: a prototype to describe the burden of care for patient, family and caregivers. Cancer Pract 1996;4:245–251.

54. McCorkle R, Yost LS, Jespon C, et al. A cancer experience: Relationship of patient psychosocial responses to caregiver burden over time. Psychooncology 1993;2:21.

55. Robinson LA, Berman JS, Neimeyer RA. Psychotherapy for the treatment of depression: A comprehensive review of controlled outcome research. Psychol Bull 1990;108:30–49.

56. Beck AT, Rush AJ, Shaw BF, et al. Cognitive Therapy of Depression. A Treatment Manual. New York: Guilford Press, 1979.

57. Beck AT. Cognitive therapy: A 30-year retrospective. Am Psychol 1991;46:368–375.

58. Johnson J, Weissman MM, Klerman GL. Service utilization and social morbidity associated with depressive symptoms in the community. JAMA 1992;267:1478–1483.

59. Koenig HG, George LK, Peterson BL, Pieper CF. Depression in medically ill hospitalized older adults: Prevalence characteristics, and course of symptoms according to six diagnostic schemes. Am J Psychiatry 1997;154:1376–1383.

60. Holland J, Massie MJ, Straker N. Psychotherapeutic interventions. In: Holland JC, Rowland JH, eds. Handbook of Psychooncology: Psychological Care of the Patient with Cancer. New York: Oxford University Press, 1989: 455–469.

61. DiMatteo MR, Lepper HS, Croghan TW. Depression is a risk factor for noncompliance with medical treatment: Meta-analysis of the effects of anxiety and depression on patient adherence. Arch Intern Med 2000;160:2101–2107.

62. Barg F, Cooley M, Pasacreta JV, Senay B, McCorkle R. Development of a self-administered psychosocial cancer screening tool. Cancer Pract 1994;2:288–296.

63. Roth AJ, Kornblith AB, Batel-Copel L, Holland J. Rapid screening for psychologic distress in men with prostate carcinoma. Cancer 1998;82:1904–1908.

64. Pasacreta JV, McCorkle R, Jacobsen P, Lundberg J, Holland JC. Distress management training for oncology nurses: Description of an innovative and timely new program. Cancer Nurs 2008;31:485–490.

65. Hall RCW, Platt DE. Suicide risk assessment: A review of risk factors for suicide in 100 patients who made severe suicide attempts: Evaluation of suicide risk in a time of managed care. Psychosomatics 1990;40:18–27.

66. Valente SM, Trainor D. Rational suicide among patients who are terminally ill. AORN J 1998;68:252–264.

67. Eisendrath SJ. Psychiatric problems. In: Bongard FS, Sue DY, eds. Current Critical Care Diagnosis and Treatment. Norwalk, CT: Appleton and Lange, 1994:233–244.

68. Back AL, Wallace JI, Starks HE, Pearlman RA. Physician-assisted suicide and euthanasia in Washington State. Patient requests and physician responses. JAMA 1996;275:919–925.

69. Scanlon C. Euthanasia and nursing practice—right question, wrong answer. N Engl J Med 1996;344:1401–1402.

70. Daley BJ, Berry D, Fitzpatrick JJ, Drew B, Montgomery K. Assisted suicide: Implications for nurses and nursing. Nurs Outlook 1997;45:209–214.

71. St John PD, Man-Son-Hing M. Physician-assisted suicide: The physician as an unwitting accomplice. J Palliat Care 1999;15:56–58.

72. Tilden VP, Tolle SW, Lee MA, Nelson CA. Oregon's physician-assisted suicide vote: Its effect on palliative care. Nurs Outlook 1996;44:80–83.

73. Fawzy FL, Fawzy NW, Arndt LA, Pasnau RO. Critical review of psychosocial interventions in cancer care. Arch Gen Psychiatry 1995;52:100.

74. Thomas C Jr., Petry T, Goldman JR. Comparison of cognitive and behavioral self-control treatments of depression. Psychol Rep 1987;60:975–982.

75. Robinson LA, Berman, JS Neimeyer RA. Psychotherapy for the treatment of depression: A comprehensive review of controlled outcome research. Psychol Bull 1990;108:30–49.

76. Eisenberg L. Treating depression and anxiety in primary care: Closing the gap between knowledge and practice. N Engl J Med 1992;326:1080–1084.

77. Stoudemire A. Epidemiology and psychopharmacology of anxiety in medical patients. J Clin Psychiatry 1996;57(Suppl 7):977–986.

78. Bailey K. Lippincott's Need-to-Know Psychotropic Drug Facts. Philadelphia: Lippincott Williams & Wilkins, 1998.

79. Stuber ML, Reed GM. "Never been done before": Consultative issues in innovative therapies. Gen Hosp Psychiatry 1991;13:337.

80. Koenig HG, Breitner JCS. Use of antidepressants in medically ill older patients. Psychosomatics 1990;31:22–32.

81. Frank L, Revicki DA, Sorensen SV, Shih YC. The economics of selective serotonin reuptake inhibitors in depression: a critical review. CNS Drugs 2001;15:59–83.

82. Katzelnick DJ, Kobak KA, Jefferson JW. Prescribing pattern of antidepressant medications for depression in a HMO. Formulary 1996;31:374–388.

83. Shuster JL, Stern TA, Greenberg DB. Pros and cons of fluoxitine for the depressed cancer patient. Oncology 2002;11:45–55.

84. Reich MG, Razavi D. Role of amphetamines in cancerology: A review of the literature. Bull Cancer 1996;83:891–900.

85. Hyma SE, Arana GW. Other agents: psychostimulants, beta adrenergic blockers and clonidine. In: Hyman SE, Arana GW, eds. Handbook of Psychiatric Drug Therapy. Boston: Little, Brown and Co., 1997:134–152.

86. Vigano A, Watanabe S, Bruera E. Methylphenidate for the management of somatization in terminal cancer patients. J Pain Symptom Manage 1995;10:167–170.

87. Woods SW, Tesar GE, Murray GB. Psychostimulant treatment of depressive disorders secondary to medical illness. J Clin Psychiatry 1996;47:12–15.

88. American Psychiatric Association. Practice guidelines for major depressive disorder in adults. Am J Psychiatry 1993;150:1–21.

89. Anderson CM, Griffin S, Rossi A. A comparative study of the impact of education vs process groups for families of patients with affective disorders. Fam Process 1986;25:185–204.

90. Gallagher DE, Thompson LW. Treatment of major depressive disorder in older adult outpatients with brief psychotherapies. Psychother Theory Res Practice 1982;19:482–490.

91. Persons JB, Burns DD, Perloff JM. Predictors of dropout and outcome in cognitive therapy for depression in a private practice setting. Cognit Ther Res 1998;12:557–574.

92. Lazarus RS, Folkman S. Stress, Appraisal and Coping. New York: Springer, 1984.

93. Christman NJ, Kirchhoff KT, Oakley MG. Concrete objective information. In: Bulechek GM, McCloskey JC, eds. Nursing Interventions: Essential Nursing Treatments (2nd ed). Philadelphia: WB Saunders, 1992.

94. Morse JM, Doberneck B. Delineating the concept of hope. Image: J Nurs Scholarsh 1995;27:277–285.

95. Dossey BM. Imagery: Awakening the inner healer. In: Dossey BM, Keegan L, Guzzetta CE, Kolkmeier LG, eds. Holistic Nursing: A Handbook for Practice. Rockville, MD: Aspen, 1988.

96. White JM. Music therapy: An intervention to reduce anxiety in the myocardial infarction patient. Clin Nurse Spec 1992;6:58.

97. Tommassini N. The client with a mood disorder (depression). In: Antai-Otong D, ed. Psychiatric Nursing: Biological and Behavioral Concepts. Philadelphia, PA: WB Saunders, 1995:178–189.

98. Kurlowicz LH. Depression in hospitalized medically ill edlers; evoluation of the concept. Arch Psychiatric Nurs 1994;7:124–136.

99. American Psychiatric Association. Diagnostic and Statistical Manual of Mental Disorders, Text Revision (DSM-IV-TR) (4th ed). Washington DC: APA, 2000.

100. Beliles K, Stoudemire A. Psychopharmacologic treatment of depression in the medically ill. Psychosomatics 1998;39: S2–S19.

101. Leavitt M, Minarik PA. The agitated, hypervigilant response. In: Rigel B, Ehrenreich D, eds. Psychological Aspects of Critical Care Nursing. Rockville, MD: Aspen, 1989:49–65.

102. Derogatis LR, Wise TN. Anxiety and Depressive Disorders in the Medical Patient. Washington, DC: American Psychiatric Press, 1989.

# 21

*Debra E. Heidrich and Nancy English*

# Delirium, Confusion, Agitation, and Restlessness

*I thought I was in a bad dream. Everyone was trying to hurt me...I was afraid to talk because talking might make the dream real.—R.M., a patient describing an experience with delirium.*

♦ **Key Points**

♦ *Delirium, confusion, and agitation are common symptoms in the palliative care setting and are extremely distressing to both patient and family.*

♦ *Identifying patients at risk of developing these symptoms can lead to early recognition and prompt treatment.*

♦ *The etiology of these symptoms is frequently multi-factorial; some causes are reversible and others not.*

♦ *Patient and family education regarding the reasons for these mental changes and how they will be managed is essential.*

CASE STUDY—PART 1
### Introduction to Mr. H, A Patient with Delirium

Mr. H, an 82-year-old man, has moderate dementia and heart failure with a left ventricular ejection fraction of 45%. He was discharged from the hospital to a skilled nursing facility two weeks ago after surgical repair of a fractured hip. Mr. H was doing well with his physical therapy and able to walk short distances with a walker. He was found on the floor at the skilled care facility and brought to the emergency department with a change in mental status and a fever of 102° Fahrenheit. His right leg was noted to be internally rotated and he moaned when turned and repositioned. He was lethargic but aroused with gentle shaking of his shoulder and verbal stimulation. He was oriented to person only, did not recognize his family members, and mumbled incoherently. A medical work-up revealed a urinary tract infection, probable pneumonia, mild dehydration, and a dislocated hip. A urinary catheter was inserted, antibiotics and intravenous fluids initiated, and Mr. H was admitted to a medical–surgical unit. The following day, Mr. H recognized family members, was easily aroused, but was still sleeping most of the day. He denied pain when asked, yet continued to moan when repositioned. The orthopedic surgeon attempted a closed reduction of the dislocated hip, but it was not successful and plans were made for surgery when medically stable. He had an order for morphine 2 to 4 mg intravenous for pain every 4 hours as needed.

On day 3 of admission, Mr. H was afebrile, electrolytes were normal, and the white blood cell count was decreasing. He continued to be drowsy, but his family attributed this to reports from the night shift that he was awake off and on all night. Because of his drowsiness, Mr. H had not received any pain medication in the past 24 hours out of fear that it would make him more lethargic. His family was concerned because when they awakened him, he seemed very confused; they

449

reported he imagined a cat on his bed and pool of blood on the floor, and was very upset by these "events." He ate only a few bites of food from his breakfast tray, and drifted off to sleep while they were trying to feed him lunch. Mr. H's family reported that while he had short-term memory problems from his dementia, he usually loved to talk and watch sports on television, had a great appetite, and had not previously shown any worsening of confusion at bedtime or problems sleeping through the night.

Later on day 3, the personal care assistant reported that Mr. H was combative, swore at her when she provided personal care, and was attempting to get out of bed. Mr. H's family were both frightened and embarrassed by his behavior. The nurse notified the physician about the patient's change of behavior and received an order for lorazepam 0.5 mg intravenous every 4 hours. A vest restraint was placed on the patient to prevent him from climbing out of bed, as well as mitts to prevent him from pulling out his intravenous line. Over the next 12 hours, Mr. H received 3 doses of lorazepam; he slept for about one hour after each dose, then became increasingly restless and agitated.

It is likely that Mr. H became delirious at the skilled facility due to infection, fever, and dehydration; this change in mental status may have led to the fall. The initial improvement in his mental status had been due to appropriate treatment with hydration and antibiotics. But, what made his symptoms worse?

Delirium is a common neuropsychiatric disorder seen in all health care settings, and is frequently under-diagnosed, mis-diagnosed, and poorly managed. Often, patients are labeled as "confused" and no further evaluation is performed to determine the cause of this confusion. This is particularly an issue with the elderly, whose confusion is often dismissed as dementia. Patients at highest risk for delirium include those who are elderly, in intensive care units, or post-operative, as well as those with advanced illnesses. This syndrome is associated with significant morbidity and mortality, leading to increased length of hospital and nursing home stays, and risk of earlier death. The experience of delirium is frightening to both patients and their significant others; it impairs quality of living—and quality of dying. Prompt recognition and treatment are essential to improve patient outcomes, especially in the final stages of an illness. This chapter will discuss the prevalence of delirium, its associated symptoms, factors that contribute to delirium, assessment for delirium, interventions to prevent or lessen the severity of delirium, and important patient/family teaching points.

## Prevalence and Outcomes

Delirium is considered the most common and serious cognitive disorder in hospitals and in the palliative care setting.[1,2] Delirium is reported to be found in 14% to 56% of hospitalized elderly, 60% to 80% of mechanically ventilated medical and surgical ICU patients, 50% to 70% of non-ventilated medical ICU patients, 40% to 80% of cancer inpatients, 29% of palliative care inpatients, and up to 90% of cancer patients in the dying phase of the illness.[1,3-12] However, the true incidence of delirium is unknown because it often goes undetected or misdiagnosed. Kishi, et al. found that the diagnosis of delirium was missed by the referring service in 46% of hospitalized medical patients referred for psychiatric consultations.[13] Likewise, Fang and colleagues found that the overall detection rate for delirium by the palliative care team was 44.9%, with the detection rate of only 20.5% for the hypoactive form of delirium.[10] A systematic review of the literature revealed that nurse recognition of delirium ranged from 26% to 83%.[14] Factors that contribute to a missed diagnosis include the following:[13-16]

- History of a past psychiatric diagnosis, such as dementia, to which the symptoms may be attributed.
- The presence of pain.
- Transient and fluctuating nature of symptoms.
- Imprecise and overlapping use of terminology, such as delirium, acute confusion, and terminal restlessness.
- Inconsistencies in use of and types of assessment tools used to diagnose delirium.

Delirium is associated with adverse physical, cognitive, and psychological outcomes. One prospective study of hospitalized medical patients reported that those with delirium had a two-fold increase in mortality, an average increase of eight days in the length of hospital stay, worse physical and cognitive recovery at six and 12 months, and increased need for long-term care after hospitalization.[17]

While not everyone remembers their experience of delirium, those who do report having distressing feelings during the experience, including fear, anxiety, and feeling threatened.[18,19] Visual hallucinations of people or animals in the room intertwine with the people who are actually present, to create a confusing and frightening experience. Misinterpretations of real sensory experiences also lead to fear, anxiety, or the sense of being trapped in the experience, as illustrated by the quote at the beginning of this chapter. Procedures like injections may be interpreted as attempts to do harm; and interventions to reorient or reassure delirious patients may be met with suspicion and the fear that everyone is lying to them.[19,20] Irritation, aggression, and combative behavior may result from feeling threatened.[20] And, the delirious patient may try to escape from the experience, putting him or her at risk for wandering behavior and falls. After the episode of delirium, persons report feeling humiliated and ashamed of their behavior while delirious. They also report a fear of experiencing delirium again in the future.[20] Interestingly, those who have the most severe symptoms are the least likely to remember their delirium experience.[18] O'Malley and associates speculate that this may be due to greater use of antipsychotic medications in patients with the most severe symptoms, and suggest that a more proactive approach to detecting and treating delirium may reduce severity and later recall of the event.[19]

Family members and professional staff also experience distress related to delirium. The major predictors of family member distress were hyperactive delirium and poor functional status, whereas the strongest predictors of nurse distress were severe delirium and perceptual disturbances.[18] When delirium occurs at the end of life, the behaviors may be interpreted as pain, mental distress, or anxiety about death.[21,22] Therefore, treatment of the patient's distress can decrease the distress of family caregivers. Family members need not only optimal treatment of the patient's symptoms, but also information to help them understand the delirium and how best to care for the patient with delirium.

In the palliative care setting, delirium is often the harbinger of impending death and is viewed by some as a natural part of the dying process.[1,23] Some clinicians make a distinction between terminal restlessness and delirium, viewing terminal restlessness as the whole spectrum of unsettled behaviors commonly seen in the last few days of life that overlaps with, but does not fit the specific diagnostic criteria of delirium.[23,24] Others feel that what is labeled terminal restlessness is actually delirium.[25] Whether viewed as separate syndromes or not, it is important to assess the dying patient to ensure that reversible causes of delirium and restlessness are addressed.[24,25]

Given the increased length of stays in hospital and nursing homes associated with delirium, it is clear that delirium carries a financial burden as well as the negative physical and psychological impacts of the syndrome. As noted earlier, the length of stay for patients with delirium in the acute care setting is, on average, eight days longer.[17] According to data from the national Healthcare Costs and Utilization Project, the median charge to Medicare for a median hospital stay of 4.0 days in 2006 was $17,916.[26] Although actual costs of hospitals stays are quite different from charges, and the per-day cost at the end of a hospital stay are usually less than the initial days, it is still clear that the additional length of stay caused by delirium increases costs significantly. A study examining one-year health care costs associated with delirium in the elderly, estimated the total cost attributable to delirium to be $16,303 to $64,421 per patient, implying that the national burden of delirium on the health care systems ranges from $38 billion to $152 billion each year.[27] Studies looking at the cost of multimodality interventions to prevent and treat delirium in hospitalized elderly support that these interventions at minimum improved quality of life without increasing overall costs of care, and may even decrease these overall costs.[28,29]

### Definition and Key Features of Delirium

Understanding the many symptoms, syndromes, and diagnoses associated with cognitive changes in persons with an advanced illness can be difficult at best. Terms such as confusion, acute confusion, delirium and terminal restlessness are often used to describe changes in mental status without clear definitions or use of standard psychiatric classifications. The use of imprecise terminology can lead to mislabeling of behaviors,

---

**Box 21–1**
**Diagnostic Criteria for Delirium**

- Disturbance of consciousness with reduced ability to focus, sustain, or shift attention.
- Change in cognition or the development of a perceptual disturbance.
- Disturbance develops in a short period of time and fluctuates over the course of the day.
- History, physical examination, and laboratory findings show that delirium can be a physiological consequence of general condition; caused by intoxication; caused by medication; and caused by more than one etiology.

*Source*: Adapted from American Psychiatric Association (1994), reference 30.

---

miscommunication among health care professionals, and misdiagnoses of cognitive changes. Therefore, the potential for the mismanagement of any cognitive change is extremely high.

The fourth edition of the Diagnostic and Statistical Manual of Mental Disorders (DSM–IV) criteria for delirium are listed in Box 21–1.[30] These criteria focus on disordered attention and cognition. Additional clinical features associated with delirium include restlessness, anxiety, easy distractibility, increased or decreased psychomotor activity, disturbances in the sleep-wake cycle, affective symptoms (emotional lability, sadness, anger, or euphoria), altered perceptions (misperceptions, illusions, delusions, and hallucinations), disorganized thinking and incoherent speech, disorientation to time, place, or person, and memory impairment.[1,31] There are no diagnostic tests for delirium; the diagnosis is primarily clinical, based on careful observation and awareness of the key features. The wide range of abnormal behaviors that may indicate delirium partly explains why the diagnosis is frequently missed.[1,31] Because the presentation of symptoms can sometimes be subtle, and symptoms fluctuate throughout the day, nurses, who have more frequent and continuous contact with patients, are key to the early recognition of delirium.[32] However, without education about delirium, and use of tools to assist in identifying it, nurses often miss the diagnosis.[14,16]

*Disturbance of consciousness* refers to impairments in attention and in the ability to be aware of and sustain attention to the environment. These changes can be highly variable and range from an agitated or aggressive state to one of lethargy or stupor.[33] Patients may be slow to respond, unable to maintain eye contact, or may fall asleep between stimuli, requiring an increased amount of stimuli (touch, calling name) to elicit a response. Conversely, patients may be hyperalert, overreact to stimuli, and exhibit signs of agitation. This is a feature that can help distinguish delirium from dementia, as dementia occurs in individuals who are alert with relatively little clouding of consciousness.[34]

*Changes in cognition* in delirium include memory deficit, disorientation, language disturbances, and perceptual disturbances.[30,33] Disruptions in orientation usually manifest as disorientation to time or place, with time disorientation being the first to be affected. Short-term memory deficits are the most evident memory impairments. Patients may not remember conversations, television shows, or verbal instructions. For example, the person experiencing cognitive changes may remember the nurse visiting, but not anything the nurse said or did. Disorganized thought is evidenced by incoherent or jumbled speech or an illogical presentation of ideas.[33] There may be long pauses in the conversation or use of repetitive phrases by the patient. Perceptual disturbances may include misinterpretations, illusions, or hallucinations. Visual misperceptions and hallucinations are most common, but auditory, tactile, gustatory, and olfactory misperceptions or hallucinations can also occur. As illustrated by the quote at the beginning of this chapter, the delirious patient may have the delusional conviction that the hallucination is real. Aggressive or combative behavior occurs if the patient misperceives caregivers' actions as intent to harm.

*Development over a short time and fluctuation during the course of the day* are important considerations in both identifying delirium and in differentiating it from dementia. In dementia, short-term memory problems occur progressively over months versus over hours or days with delirium. Obtaining a history of memory issues from the family is vital to establishing the patient's baseline. A change from the baseline may be indicative of delirium. The waxing and waning nature of delirium, alternating with periods of lucidity and reversal of symptoms, can be deceiving.[33] Thus, assessment throughout the course of the day is essential to identify delirium.

*Additional clinical features* of delirium that are not included in the diagnostic criteria but are frequently present include psychomotor agitation, paranoid delusions, sleep-wake cycle disruption, and emotional lability.[3,33,35,36] Again, some of these features help in differentiating delirium from dementia, as persons with dementia do not typically have delusions or hallucinations. Sleep-wake cycle disruptions are more pronounced in persons with delirium and are of new onset. "Sundowning," or increased confusion and agitation at night, should be viewed as a potential sign of delirium unless this behavior has been present for weeks to months in the person with dementia.

## Subtypes of Delirium

There are three clinical subtypes of delirium based on arousal disturbance and psychomotor behavior: hyperactive, hypoactive, and mixed.[33,37] There are some variations in the definitions of these subtypes from one author to another, but in general, hyperactive delirium is associated with hypervigilance, restlessness, and agitation; the hypoactive subtype is characterized by confusion and somnolence; and the mixed subtype has alternating features of hyperactive and

hypoactive delirium. Although psychotic features, such as delusions or hallucinations, are most often associated with hyperactive delirium, Stagno and colleagues demonstrated that these symptoms are present in more than half of patients with hypoactive delirium.[38] And, the psychotic features of delirium are clearly correlated with patient, spouse, and caregiver distress.[18,38]

Hyperactive delirium is identified more often than the other subtypes because of the recognizable symptoms of hypervigilence, restlessness and agitation. However, the hypoactive form appears to be the most prevalent, accounting for up to 86% of palliative care patients with delirium.[11] The hypoactive form of delirium is much less noticeable, or may be misdiagnosed as depression or fatigue unless appropriate screening tools are used to identify all types of delirium. The hypoactive and mixed subtypes of delirium tend to have the worst prognoses.[38,39] Prompt recognition and management is essential.

## Terminal Restlessness, Nearing Death Awarenesss, and Terminal Anguish

A variety of terms, such as terminal restlessness, terminal delirium, terminal agitation, pre-terminal restlessness, and terminal psychosis, have been used in the literature to describe a clinical spectrum of unsettled behaviors in the final days of life.[24] In the 1997 clinical practice protocol from Hospice and Palliative Nurses Association, terminal restlessness is described as a common, observable syndrome often seen in the final days of life. It is characterized by (1) frequent, nonpurposeful motor activity, (2) inability to concentrate or relax, (3) disturbances in sleep/rest patterns, (4) fluctuating levels of consciousness, cognitive failure, and/or anxiety, and (5) potential progression to agitation.[40] These characteristic behaviors overlap with the diagnositic criteria for delirium and, as mentioned previously, some clinicians feel terminal restlessness is a synonym for delirium.[25] It is vital that restless behaviors in the dying patient are not labeled as simply "part of the dying process," because reversal of delirium may be possible. Lawlor and colleagues found that delirium was reversable in 49% of terminally ill cancer patients.[25] Importantly, this means that delirim was not reversable in 51% of the patients in the study, necessitating appropriate interventions to address the distress that accompanies delirium for both patients and their caregivers.

The concept of "nearing death awareness" was defined by two hospice nurses as a special knowledge about the process of dying that may reveal what dying is like, or what is needed to die peacefully.[41] Callanan and Kelley emphasize that the symbolic communications of nearing death awareness should not be labeled as confusion or hallucinations. Themes of nearing death awareness include describing a place, talking to or being in the presence of someone who is not alive, knowledge of when death will occur, choosing the time of death, needing reconciliation, preparing for travel or change, being held back, and symbolic dreams. It may be helpful to discuss the concept of nearing death awareness with patients and their caregivers to normalize these experiences. Often, these communications are spiritually and emotionally comforting. Some clinicians cite the pleasantness or comforting nature of the experiences as a way to distinguish between nearing death awareness and delirium, while others believe these experiences, pleasant or not, are signs of delirium. However, even among clinicians who feel patients that have these experiences are delirious, there is controversy as to whether or not pleasant hallucinations should be treated with neuroleptics at the end of life.[1]

"Terminal anguish" is another term sometimes seen in the palliative care literature that does not have a broadly accepted definition. Twycross and Lichter described terminal anguish as a tormented state of mind related to long-standing unresolved emotional problems, interpersonal conflicts, or suppressed unpleasant memories that the dying patient is now too weak to address.[42] Signs and symptoms of terminal anguish include restlessness, thrashing, moaning, and crying out. A more general understanding of terminal anguish is suffering from any cause (physical, emotional, or spiritual) that is so severe that even very aggressive interventions are not sufficient to address the extreme distress (i.e., the symptom is refractory).[43] Patients experiencing terminal anguish may require sedation in order to achieve some level of comfort.

## Pathophysiology and Etiology of Delirium

The pathophysiology of delirium is not clearly understood. Disturbances in cerebral oxygenation or blood flow, neurotransmitters, cytokine production, and plasma esterase activity have all been identified as potential contributing factors. Diminished blood flow and decreased oxygenation are seen with aging, hypotension, hypoxia, and sepsis,[44–47] and may explain the long-term cognitive changes seen with prolonged delirium.[48,49] Acetylcholine deficiency, gamma-aminobutyric acid (GABA) deficiency, and dopamine excess are three of several neurotransmitter disturbances associated with delirium; neurotransmitter changes help to explain delirium associated with the use of medications such as anticholinergics and benzodiazepines, withdrawal from opioids and alcohol, organ system failure, sleep deprivation, and insults to the brain, such as ischemia.[31,47,50–54] Elevated levels of various cytokines have been shown in patients with delirium associated with sepsis, and severe physical stresses such as hip fracture and surgery.[50,55–59] A decrease in the activity of plasma esterases, important drug metabolizing enzymes, has been found in delirium and explains, in part, the mechanism behind medication-induced delirium.[31] These various theories to explain delirium are complementary, and it is likely an interconnection of several pathological mechanisms that leads to delirium.[31,47]

Delirium usually develops due to the interrelationship between patient vulnerability (predisposing factors) and

| Table 21–1 Predisposing and Precipitating Factors for Delirium | |
|---|---|
| **Predisposing Factors** | **Precipitating Factors** |
| *Demographic characteristics* | *Drugs* |
|   Age of 65 years or older |   Sedative hypnotics |
|   Male sex |   Narcotics |
| *Cognitive status* |   Anticholinergic drugs |
|   Dementia |   Treatment with multiple |
|   Cognitive impairment |     drugs |
|   History of delirium |   Alcohol or drug withdrawal |
|   Depression | *Primary neurologic diseases* |
| *Functional status* |   Stroke, particularly non- |
|   Functional dependence |     dominant hemispheric |
|   Immobility |   Intracranial bleeding |
|   Low level of activity |   Meningitis or encephalitis |
|   History of falls | *Intercurrent illnesses* |
| *Sensory impairment* |   Infections |
|   Visual impairment |   Iatrogenic complications |
|   Hearing impairment |   Severe acute illness |
| *Decreased oral intake* |   Hypoxia |
|   Dehydration |   Shock |
|   Malnutrition |   Fever or hypothermia |
| *Drugs* |   Anemia |
|   Treatment with multiple |   Dehydration |
|     psychoactive drugs |   Poor nutritional status |
|   Treatment with many |   Low serum albumin level |
|     drugs |   Metabolic derangements |
|   Alcohol abuse |     (e.g., electrolyte, |
| *Coexisting medical* |     glucose, acid–base) |
|   *conditions* | *Surgery* |
|   Severe illness |   Orthopedic surgery |
|   Multiple coexisting |   Cardiac surgery |
|     conditions |   Prolonged cardiopulmonary |
|   Chronic renal or hepatic |     bypass |
|     disease |   Noncardiac surgery |
|   History of stroke | *Environmental* |
|   Neurologic disease |   Admission to an intensive |
|   Metabolic derangements |     care unit |
|   Fracture or trauma |   Use of physical restraints |
|   Terminal illness |   Use of bladder catheter |
|   Infection with human |   Use of multiple procedures |
|     immunodeficiency |   Pain |
|     virus |   Emotional stress |
| | *Prolonged sleep deprivation* |

*Source:* Adapted from Inouye (2006), reference 3.

noxious insults (precipitating factors).[33,60,61] Table 21–1 identifies some of the common predisposing and precipitating factors for delirium. While a single precipitating factor in the predisposed patient may be enough to lead to delirium (for example, a single dose of an anticholinergic medication in a patient with dementia), there are often multiple factors involved in the development of delirium. Addressing only a single factor likely will not aid in improving delirium; an approach that addresses as many predisposing and precipitating factors as possible is needed for resolution.[33]

**Table 21–2**
**Differentiating Delirium from Dementia**

|  | Delirium | Dementia |
|---|---|---|
| Onset | Acute or subacute, occurs over a short period of time (hours–days). | Insidious, often slow and progressive. |
| Course | Fluctuates over the course of the day, worsens at night. Resolves over days to weeks. | Stable over the course of the day; is progressive. |
| Duration | If reversible, short term. | Chronic and nonreversible. |
| Consciousness | Impaired and can fluctuate rapidly. Clouded, with a reduced awareness of the environment. | Clear and alert until the later stages. May become delirious, which will interfere. |
| Cognitive defects | Impaired short-term memory, poor attention span. | Poor short-term memory; attention span less affected until later stage. |
| Attention | Reduced ability to focus, sustain, or shift attention. | Relatively unaffected in the earlier stages. |
| Orientation | Disoriented to time and place. | Intact until months or years with the later stages. May have anomia (difficulty recognizing common objects) or agnosia (difficulty recognizing familiar people). |
| Delusions | Common, fleeting, usually transient and poorly organized. | Often absent. |
| Hallucinations | Common and usually visual, tactile, and olfactory. | Often absent. |
| Speech | Often uncharacteristic, loud, rapid, or slow (hypoactive). | Difficulty in finding words and articulating thoughts; aphasia. |
| Affect | Mood liability. | Mood liability. |
| Sleep–wake cycle | Disturbed; may be reversed. | Can be fragmented. |
| Psychomotor activity | Increased, reduced, or unpredictable; variable depending on hyper/hypo delirium. | Can be normal; may exhibit apraxia. |

*Sources*: Adapted from Arnold (2005), reference 35; Milisen et al. (2006) reference 36.

Cognitive impairment and dementia are the leading predisposing factors for delirium;[33,61–63] and persons with dementia are vulnerable to delirium at lower levels of medical acuity than non-demented persons.[62,64] One study showed that persons with dementia had poorer functional and nutritional status than those in the same age group who did not have dementia.[65] As both poor functional status and malnutrition are additional predisposing factors for delirium (see Table 21–1), this higher risk of delirium with dementia is not surprising. There likely are other factors (e.g., changes in levels of neurotransmitters and cerebral blood flow) in persons with dementia that also contribute to this increased vulnerability. Nurses must be aware of the increased risk of delirium in patients with dementia, carefully assess for signs of delirium, and work to eliminate or decrease precipitating factors that can be controlled. Too often, changes in behavior are dismissed as signs of the individual's dementia instead of being identified as signs of delirium. Table 21–2 identifies the factors that help in differentiating dementia from delirium.

Several studies have identified key factors that increase the risk of delirium in subsets of populations. Despite an incidence rate of 40% to 80% in persons with cancer, delirium is rarely appreciated as a source of symptom distress in oncology settings.[1,10,18,66] Table 21–3 outlines the cancer-specific considerations as they relate to the risk factors for delirium, illustrating that persons with cancer have many predisposing risk factors and are exposed to multiple precipitating factors for delirium. A study of patients undergoing urologic surgery showed that preoperative cognitive deficits, preexisting depression, impaired vision, and operative time were associated with an increased risk of delirium.[64] Inouye and colleagues identified five risk factors for persistent delirium at discharge from the hospital: dementia, vision impairment, functional impairment, high comorbidity, and use of physical restraints during delirium.[67] These studies reinforce the increased vulnerability of persons with underlying dementia or cognitive impairments.

## Assessment

Comprehensive and ongoing assessment is necessary to identify patients at risk for delirium and for early detection of delirium. During routine assessments, nurses often observe behavior changes that are signs of delirium, but often do not "put the pieces together" to recognize this syndrome. Standardized assessment tools for delirium administered by

**Table 21–3**
**Cancer-Specific Risk Factors for Delirium**

| Type of Physiologic Risk Factor | Cancer-Specific Considerations |
|---|---|
| **Nutritional deficiencies**<br>B vitamins<br>Vitamin C<br>Hypoproteinemia | • Symptom distress: nausea, emesis, mucositis, diarrhea, pain, and anorexia or cachexia syndrome<br>• Surgical alteration of the head and neck region or gastrointestinal tract<br>• Non-oral feeding routes: gastrostomy feeding tube and use of total parenteral nutrition |
| **Cardiovascular abnormalities**<br>Decreased cardiac output states: myocardial infarction, dysrythmias, congestive heart failure, and cardiogenic shock<br>Alterations in peripheral vascular resistance: increased and decreased states<br>Vascular occlusion: emboli and disseminated intravascular coagulopathy | • Septic shock syndrome<br>• Hypercoagulopathy and hyperviscosity<br>• Anthracycline-related cardiomyopathy<br>• Central line occlusion<br>• Thrombi associated with immobility and paraneoplastic syndromes<br>• Disseminated intravascular coagulopathy |
| **Cerebral disease**<br>Vascular insufficiency: transient ischemic attacks, cerebral vascular accidents, and thrombosis<br>Central nervous system infection: acute or chronic meningitis, brain abscess, and neurosyphylis<br>Trauma: subdural hematoma, contusion, concussion, and intracranial hemorrhage | • Intracerebral bleed caused by thrombocytopenia<br>• Meningeal carcinomatosis<br>• Central nervous system edema secondary to brain malignancy or whole-brain radiation therapy<br>• Fall risk<br>• Malignancy: primary or metastatic involving brain and cranial irradiation |
| **Endocrine disturbance**<br>Hypothyroidism<br>Diabetes mellitus<br>Hypercalcemia<br>Hyponatremia<br>Hypopituitarism | • Mantle field radiation therapy<br>• Steroid induced<br>• Related to bone metastases<br>• Syndrome of inappropriate antidiuretic hormone, rigorous hydration, and dehydration<br>• Brain tumor in or adjacent to pituitary gland |
| **Temperature regulation fluctuation**<br>Hypothermia<br>Hyperthermia | • Absence of customary warm clothes<br>• Fever |
| **Pulmonary abnormalities**<br>Inadequate gas-exchange states: pulmonary disease and alveolar hypoventilation<br>Infection: pneumonia | • Hypoxemia<br>• Anemia<br>• Lung metastases<br>• Bleomycin-induced pulmonary fibrosis<br>• Radiotherapy to chest<br>• Chest tubes<br>• Neutropenia and immobility |
| **Systemic infective process (acute or chronic)**<br>Viral<br>Fungal<br>Bacterial: endocarditis, pyelonephritis, and cystitis | • Prominence of neutropenia<br>• Steroids<br>• Hypogammaglobunemia |
| **Metabolic disturbance**<br>Electrolyte abnormalities: hypercalcemia, hypo- and hypernatremia, hypo and hyperkalemia, hypo- and hypercalcemia, and hyperphosphatemia<br>Acidosis and alkalosis<br>Hypo- and hyperglycemia<br>Acute and chronic renal failure<br>Volume depletion: hemorrhage, inadequate fluid intake, diuretics, and diarrhea<br>Hepatic failure | • Syndrome of inappropriate antidiuretic hormone<br>• Bone metastases<br>• Diabetes secondary to steroids<br>• Renal malignancy<br>• Dehydration and diarrhea secondary to pelvic radiotherapy or chemotherapy<br>• Liver primary or metastases with ascites or encephalopathy<br>• Tumor lysis syndrome |
| **Drug intoxication (therapeutic or substance abuse)**<br>Misuse of prescribed medications<br>Side effects of therapeutic medications<br>Drug–drug interactions<br>Drug and herb interactions<br>Improper use of over-the-counter medications<br>Alcohol intoxication or withdrawal | • Polypharmacy with drugs having anticholinergic or central nervous system effects<br>• Inadequate knowledge about geriatric-specific pharmacokinetic considerations in dosing<br>• Self-medication with over-the-counter or herbal remedies in the absence of healthcare professional awareness<br>• Alcohol withdrawal perioperatively in patients with head and neck cancer |

*Source*: Boyle (2006), reference 66. Used with permission.

healthcare providers trained in using these tools improves the identification of delirium in the clinical setting.[14,68–70] Assessment tools include those designed to screen for delirium symptoms, make a formal diagnosis of delirium, and rate the severity of delirium.

The Mini-mental State Examination (MMSE) is a 20-item screening tool that provides a clinical evaluation of cognitive function, but is not specifically designed to assess for delirium and does not differentiate between dementia and delirium.[71–73] It assesses orientation, attention, recall, and language function. The MMSE is widely used in practice and research, and data support the scoring system to identify the severity of cognitive impairment. The length of this examination and the writing and drawing questions included in it may be cumbersome and difficult to perform in a palliative care population.[73] Fayers and colleagues reported that a subset of four items from the MMSE is adequate to screen for delirium and cognitive impairment: current year, date, backward spelling, and copy a design.[73] Additional research would be required to support the validity of using only these four items for screening. Whether using the full MMSE or a modification, it may be best to view it as a predictive instrument that directs the clinician to use a delirium assessment instrument for additional information.

Table 21–4 provides an overview of the instruments used to assess delirium. These instruments are reviewed because they distinguish delirium from dementia, and assess at least several of the multiple features of delirium. While all of these instruments require further study to determine application across varied settings and among different patient populations, the following have shown good reliability and validity in identifying delirium in selected populations.[74]

- The Memorial Delirium Assessment Scale (MDAS) is a 10-item tool based on the DSM–IV criteria that is designed to quantify the severity of delirium.[75,76] It takes about 10 minutes to administer. The MDAS requires minimal training for use and is appropriate for both clinical practice and research.
- The Delirium Rating Scale (DRS) is a 10-item scale intended to be used by clinicians with psychiatric training. It looks at symptoms over a 24-hour period and may be used to assess severity of delirium.[77,78] No publications are available on the use of the DRS by nurses.[74]
- The Confusion Assessment Method (CAM) is based on the DSM–IV criteria for delirium, and is designed for use by a trained interviewer to assess cognitive functioning in elderly patients on a daily scheduled basis.[79] While sometimes described as being difficult to use, Waszynski and Petrovic found that with proper education and support, the CAM can be incorporated by nurses into routine assessment of patients.[74,80,81]
- Nurses designed the NEECHAM Confusion Scale (NCS) for rapid and unobtrusive assessment and monitoring of acute confusion in hospitalized elderly.[74,82] It contains nine scaled items divided into three subscales and takes about 10 minutes to complete. The NCS has been studied in many populations, including nonintubated patients in intensive care units.[83]
- The Bedside Confusion Scale (BCS) consists of observation of the level of consciousness and timed recitation of the months of the year in reverse order starting with December, and is designed for use in the palliative care setting.[84,85] It requires minimal training and only about 2 minutes to complete. The BCS was

**Table 21–4**
**Overview of Delirium Assessment Tools**

|  | MDAS | DRS | CAM | NCS | BCS | DOS | Nu-DESC |
|---|---|---|---|---|---|---|---|
| **DSM–IV criterion** | | | | | | | |
| Acute onset |  | × | × |  |  | × | × |
| Fluctuating nature |  | × | × |  |  | × | × |
| Physical disorder |  | × | × |  |  |  |  |
| Consciousness | × |  | × |  | × | × | × |
| Attention/concentration | × |  | × | × | × | × |  |
| Thinking | × | × | × | × | × | × | × |
| Disorientation | × |  | × | × |  | × | × |
| Memory | × | × | × | × | × | × |  |
| Perception | × | × | × |  |  | × | × |
| **Purpose** | | | | | | | |
| Screening/diagnosis |  | × | × | × | × | × | × |
| Symptom severity | × | × |  |  |  |  |  |
| **Number of items** | 10 | 10 | 9 | 9 | 2 | 13 | 5 |
| **Time to complete (minutes)** | 10 | Not specified | <5 | 10 | <2 | 5 | 1 |

MDAS, Memorial Delirium Assessment Scale; DRS, Delirium Rating Scale; CAM, Confusion Assessment Method; NCS, NEECHAM Confusion Scale; BCS, Bedside Confusion Scale; DOS, Delirium Observation Scale; Nu-DESC, Nursing Delirium Screening Scale.

found to correlate with the CAM, but it is subject to bias or inappropriate interpretation, and has a limited capacity to assess the multiple cognitive domains influenced by delirium.[86]

- The Delirium Observation Scale (DOS) is based on the DSM–IV criteria and is designed to assist nurses in the early recognition of delirium during regular care.[74,87] The original version of the scale has 25 items. After studies on geriatric and hip fracture patients, the scale was reduced to 13 items that can be rated as present or absent in less than 5 minutes.[87,88]

- The Nursing Delirium Screening Scale (Nu-DESC) is an observational 5-item instrument designed to be completed in about one minute at the beside.[89] It has been shown to have validity and sensitivity comparable to the MDAS in oncology populations and is a sensitive test in the recovery room to detect delirium.[89,90]

Given the fluctuating nature of delirium, every-shift assessments in hospital and nursing home settings, using a simple screening tool such as the BCS, DOS or Nu-DESC, are appropriate, especially for high risk populations. There are no published recommendations on the frequency with which delirum assessment tools should be used in outatient and home care settings. Too-frequent evaluation for delirium in persons at low risk is burdensome to both the patient and the clinician. It makes sense to complete a baseline evaluation on all patients, and then base the frequency of follow-up assessments on the number of risk factors present for delirium.

## Management of Delirium

Nurses can promote excellent care by implementing a standard of care for all patients who are admitted to palliative care settings. This involves identifying those patients who are at high risk for developing delirium, and taking steps to eliminate as many of the precipitating factors for delirium as possible; closely monitoring for changes in the cognitive and behavioral status of all patients to promote early identification of delirium; working collaboratively with the interdisciplinary team to address the suspected causes of delirium; and advocating for and using prescribed pharmacological interventions as appropriate to relieve the physical symptoms and emotional distress of delirium. Educating patients, families, and staff about the possibility of a delirium episode is a key role for nurses. Integrating complementary interventions in conjunction with pharmacological management is often of value. Figure 21–1 provides an algorithm for the management of delirium.

### Risk Prevention

The ideal strategy to manage delirium is to prevent it before it develops. Given the correlation between the number of risk factors and the incidence of delirium, prompt intervention to reduce as many of these factors as possible is essential. A systematic review of randomized controlled trials, evaluating any interventions to prevent delirium in hospitalized patients, concluded that research evidence on effectiveness of interventions to prevent delirium is sparse.[91] While more research is needed to support the effectiveness of preventive interventions, there have been some good, controlled trials of targeted multifactorial interventions that show as many as 30% to 40% of cases of delirium may be preventable.[34,92–96] Pitkala, et al, showed this type of program improved overall health-related quality of life without increasing overall costs of care.[96] The Hospital Elder Life Program (HELP) developed by Inouye and colleagues serves as a model for the types of interdisciplinary interventions that may significantly decrease episodes of delirium.[97,98] HELP directs care toward engaging patients in meaningful conversation, providing frequent orientation cues, encouraging socialization, and promoting daily exercise. Attention is also given to promoting sleep using nonpharmacological methods, assuring that appropriate vision and hearing adaptations and equipment are available, and providing assistance and companionship during meals to encourage optimal hydration and nutrition.[97,98] It is often the simple task of replacing hearing aid batteries or cleaning glass lenses that can help patients remain cognizant of their surroundings. All patients in the palliative care setting, not just the elderly, may benefit from the suggested targeted interventions of this type of program. Families, patients, and ancillary staff can also be instructed on the importance of a target fluid intake, as well as on monitoring bowel elimination. This is especially important in older patients where problems of dehydration and constipation are common.

A review of the patient's medications is an important component of risk reduction. As noted in Table 21–1, sedative hypnotics, opioids, medications with anticholinergic effects, and the use of multiple medications are precipitating factors for delirium. Patients with many different specialists involved in their care over the course of an illness are at particular risk of being on many different medications. Often, some of these medications are no longer necessary or appropriate. An interdisciplinary review may help to streamline the medication list. Note that many of the medications required for symptom control in palliative care settings are medications that increase the risk of delirium. Therefore, a comprehensive assessment is needed to determine the best treatment options. Patients with pain and delirium, for example, may require upward or downward titration of opioids depending on the type of pain, the relief the patient gets from the current regimen, and the evidence that the delirium is related to the opioid versus some other cause.

### Monitoring of Patients at Risk

Studies have identified a specific profile of persons at highest risk for developing delirium during a hospitalization.

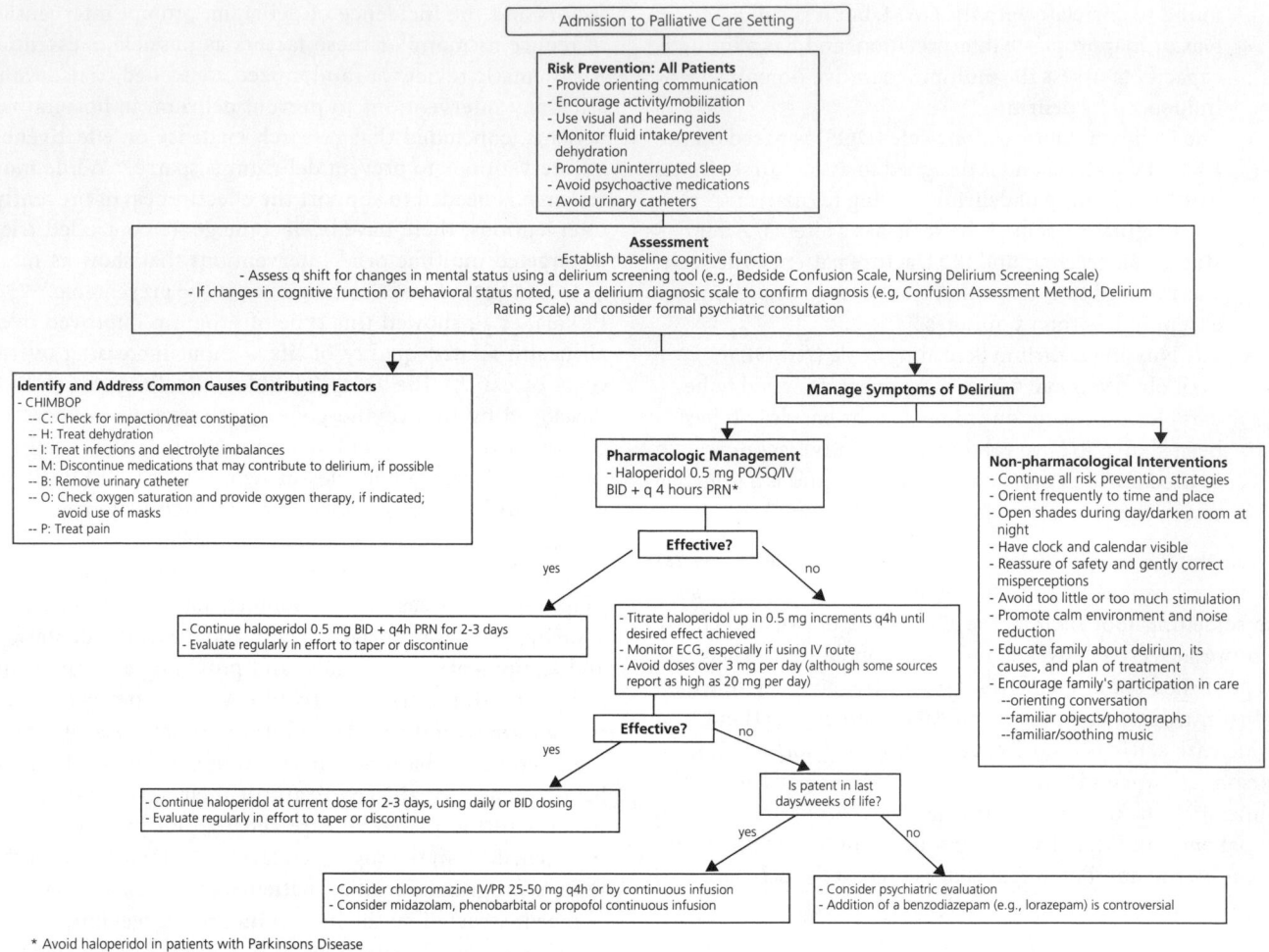

**Figure 21–1.** Delirium algorithm. *Sources*: Adapted from Inouye (2006), reference 3; Shuster et al (2008), reference 113.

Patients who are over 70 years old, have vision deficits, are dehydrated at admission, have an acute illness, and have had a previous episode of acute confusion are at especially high risk of developing delirium.[99] These risk factors alert the palliative care staff to closely monitor cognitive and behavioral status, as well as to implement other preventive measures in these patients' care.

Frequent assessments of mental status may be helpful in early detection of changes in cognition. This is especially important in the diagnosis of the hypoactive type of delirium. The use of a brief delirium screening tool, such as the Bedside Confusion Scale or the Nursing Delirium Screening Scale, can monitor for cognitive and behavior changes over time.[84,85,89] This type of screen provides the care team with a graphic record of the subtle changes that occur days before delirium is recognized and diagnosed. Use of a screening tool also provides an opportunity for the nurse to educate the patient and family about the causes and incidence of delirium. In the home setting, a numerical tool can easily be taught to family caregivers. Hallenbeck suggests that by preparing the family for a possible episode of delirium, their

confidence in caring for the patient is increased when and if the patient develops delirium.[100]

In the inpatient palliative care setting, assessment of a patient's cognitive and behavioral status should begin on admission and be recorded every shift. The first step in assessing patients is to obtain information about baseline cognitive and behavioral status. If the patient is confused upon admission, a psychiatric consultation can be requested and a diagnosis of delirium confirmed; if necessary, a differential diagnosis of dementia or depression can also then be evaluated. If this first step of assessment is not completed, a diagnosis of delirium is often overlooked until symptoms escalate.[3]

When a patient is unable to sleep, restless, irritable or emotionally labile, the first tendency is to increase doses of, or prescribe new, medications. Additional medications can worsen confusion or agitation. If delirium is suspected, new medications should not be given until a diagnosis of delirium is either confirmed or ruled out.[101] A nonpharmacologic sleep protocol consisting of a back rub, warm drink, and relaxation tapes, was found to significantly decrease the use of sedative–hypnotic medications, and is included in the HELP model described previously.[98,102]

## Nursing Care of the Patient with Delirium

When signs and symptoms of delirium are present, the goals of care are to identify the cause of the delirium, treat the cause whenever possible and appropriate, and administer the appropriate medications to treat the symptoms of delirium. A differential diagnosis by the interdisciplinary team of the potential etiology of delirium should be formulated, and appropriate actions taken.[1] In the palliative care setting, diagnostic studies should be performed only when the test will confirm the suspected etiology of delirium *and* guide the treatment plan. For example, if a metastatic brain lesion is suspected, but the patient would not be a candidate for therapies to treat it, brain imaging is not appropriate.

White and Hammond reported using the acronym CHIMBOP to assist staff to identify seven of the easily reversible causes of delirium in the palliative care setting.[103] While this tool does not address all of the potentially reversible causes of delirium, it does provide a framework for nurses to use to initiate nursing interventions. The examples of nursing interventions below are used *when appropriate* for the setting and the patient's condition:

- C = Constipation—check for impaction; administer prescribed bowel stimulants and laxatives.
- H = Hypovolemia, hypoglycemia—encourage oral intake or provide parenteral fluids; treat hypoglycemia.
- I = Infection—evaluate for signs and symptoms of infection; contact the physician or advance practice nurse (APN) for anti-infective medication.
- M = Medications—review the patient's medications for those known to contribute to delirium; discuss discontinuation or minimizing use of these medications with the physician or APN.
- B = Bladder catheter, bladder outlet obstruction—avoid the use of/remove urinary catheters; check for bladder distension and insert catheter (straight or indwelling) if required.
- O = Oxygen deficiency—check oxygen saturation or signs of hypoxia and administer oxygen.
- P = Pain—evaluate for and treat pain.

Additional nursing measures include providing safe surroundings for the patient, supporting the family, and creating an environment that is quiet and comforting. If the patient is in an area of high activity, either in the home or hospital, moving the patient to a quiet location may help.[21] Eliminate extraneous noises such as televisions and intercoms that page into the room to help calm the overactive mind. The voice of a family member/significant other, or the touch of their hand, can communicate understanding and reassurance to the patient.[41,103]

Physical restraints should be avoided whenever possible. The use of physical restraints is a recognized independent risk factor for delirium and for its persistence at discharge.[3,67] Only when a patient poses a clear risk of harm to self or others should restraints be used. A better alternative is to arrange for one-on-one observation of the patient to assure the patient's safety. Not only does one-on-one observation promote safety, the presence of a trusted person may also reduce the patient's anxiety and provide orientation cues; i.e., this person becomes part of the treatment plan for delirium, not simply a "sitter."

The nurse in palliative care can offer support to the patient and family while educating family and caregivers regarding the following:

- Symptoms of delirium are temporary.
- Symptoms are usually related to the patient's disease and/or treatment.
- The patient may or may not be aware of his/her behavior or actions.
- The cognitive and behavioral changes will fluctuate from morning to night.
- Frequent repetition of time, place, and person, as well as telling the patient they are safe and taken care of, is important. However, if the patient becomes more agitated when attempts to reorient are made, wait for a period of time before attempting to reorient again.
- Memory loss is due to the delirium.

## Nursing Care of Patient with Delirium at the End of Life

As discussed earlier, terminal restlessness and delirium may or may not be separate syndromes, but it is recognized that restlessness or agitation can occur in over 70% of patients as they approach death.[21,104,105] In the final days of life, the goals of care change to preparing the family for impending death and planning for ways to provide the patient with a dignified and respectful death. It is important to do a comprehensive assessment to determine if there is a reversible cause for the restless behavior. Again, review the common causes of delirium and take steps to eliminate or minimize them, paying special attention to the effect of the many medications that are used for symptom control, but are associated with delirium.[24] Careful listening to patients' words and descriptions of "hallucinations" may reveal a symbolic theme associated with nearing death awareness. Phrases such as "I will be home soon," "I am sorry," and "Please open the door," can be interpreted as a patient's preparation or transition to death. The nurse can help the family understand how to respond to the patient by acknowledging the patient's experiences and modeling/encouraging responses such as, "I know you are ready," "I forgive you," "We love you," and "Thank you."[41,106] The nurse and spiritual caregiver may facilitate the experience as a sacred passage for the patient, where family and loved ones are offered a time to heal and say goodbye.

## Caring for the Patient with Terminal Anguish

The extreme agitation associated with refractory physical, emotional or spiritual issues is very distressing for patients and caregivers. Palliative sedation (discussed in the pharmacology section below) is often the only approach that is effective in managing this suffering. Families may help by offering insights to any unresolved emotional or spiritual issues. Acknowledging the patient's fear, and addressing longstanding guilt and shame with the assistance of a spiritual caregiver, may provide some solace to the patient and family. However, because these issues may have festered in the mind for many years, it is often difficult to address the core issues in the final days and hours of life.

## Integrating Complementary Therapies in the Plan of Care

Fear and anxiety are often experienced by patients during an episode of delirium.[18,100] Familiar sounds, smells and touches may provide a sense of safety and security and, therefore, assist in relieving some of the distress. Aromatherapy massage is used in many palliative care settings and is one of the most widely used complementary therapies in nursing practice. Essential plant oils are added to massage oils and then applied in the form of a massage. The benefits are attributed to the double effect of inhalation and touch. Two essential oils have been shown to have therapeutic properties that promote relaxation: lavender *(lavandula angustifolia)* and sandalwood.[107] A gentle aromatherapy massage to the hands and/or feet may be of value in reducing anxiety and promoting sleep.

The sound of familiar music can also quiet the restless mind. Ask the family or caregiver about the patient's favorite music, and encourage its use. Integrating the use of poems, sacred readings, and prayer may be of value to the patient and family, depending on their usual spiritual practices. Knowledge of rituals used in various cultures, along with individual/family belief systems, is essential.

## Pharmacological Interventions for the Management of Delirium

Nonpharmacological approaches and interventions to treat or lessen risk factors causing delirium are the first-line treatments for this syndrome.[33] No medications have been approved by the U.S. Food and Drug Administration (FDA) for the treatment of delirium, but when pharmacological agents are required, antipsychotic agents are the medications of choice.[1,23,108–113] However, the use of antipsychotics for the treatment of delirium is not without controversy. Some clinicians feel that pharmacological management should be used only for those who have severe agitation that interferes with medical treatments, or in patients that pose a danger to themselves.[3,33] This approach means that those with hypoactive delirium rarely receive antipsychotics. Others suggest that pharmacological interventions should be considered in all patients with delirium, especially those who have agitation, paranoia, hallucination, or altered sensorium because of the distressing nature of these symptoms.[1,18,19,38,114] Additional support for using antipsychotics for more than the severely agitated is that these medications have been shown to improve both arousal disturbance and impaired cognitive functioning in patients with hypoactive delirium.[115] Clinicians who choose to take a "wait-and-see" approach before using antipsychotics for the delirious patient who is not agitated or having distressing hallucinations should be prepared to act quickly, as the hypoactive, somnolent patient can become agitated very quickly.[1] What is clear from the literature is that there is a wide range of prescribing patterns in the use of antipsychotics to manage delirium.[116]

Haloperidol is the most widely studied and used antipsychotic for delirium.[3,33,108,112] After review of the literature, Jackson and Lipman concluded that there is not enough evidence to draw any conclusions about the role of pharmacology in terminally ill patients with delirium, but that perhaps haloperidol is the most suitable drug therapy for delirium treatment near the end of life.[111] Haloperidol has fewer anticholinergic side effects, is less sedating, and has fewer active metabolites than other typical antipsychotics. There are little data to support the optimal dose or route of administration of haloperidol for delirium, and little is known about the optimal duration of treatment. Starting doses of 1 to 2 mg every 2 to 4 hours are suggested, with the added comments that lower doses (0.25 to 0.5 mg every 4 hours) may be sufficient in the elderly, and higher doses may be required for severely agitated patients.[3,108,113] One approach is to use a scheduled dose plus an as-needed dose until symptoms are controlled, such as 1 mg IV every 6 hours plus 1 mg IV every hour as needed.[107] When symptoms are controlled, twice- or three-times-a-day dosing may be sufficient. Doses above 20 mg per day are not recommended, but have been used.[108] A systematic review of the literature concluded that doses greater than 4.5 mg per day were associated with more adverse side effects than the atypical antipsychotics.[112] Generally, after 2 to 3 days on an effective regimen, the medication can be weaned while evaluating for return of symptoms. Ideally, during this time other interventions to address the underlying cause(s) of delirium are also used.

Haloperidol can be given by the oral, sublingual, rectal, subcutaneous, intramuscular, or intravenous routes.[113] Oral administration is associated with more frequent extrapyramidal side effects than the intravenous route.[108,110] However, the intravenous route is not without problems. Haloperidol can prolong the QT interval and has been associated with Torsades de Points (TdP), especially when given intravenously or in higher doses than recommended. In 2007, the FDA issued an alert warning that cases of sudden death, TdP and QT prolongation have been reported even in the absence of predisposing factors; this warning included a reminder that haloperidol is not approved for intravenous administration, and recommended ECG monitoring if it is given

**Table 21–5**
**Pharmacological Treatment of Delirium**

| Class & Drug | Usual Starting Dose | Comments |
|---|---|---|
| **Typical antipsychotic** | | |
| • Haloperidol | 0.5–2 mg PO/SL/SQ/IM/ IV every 2–12 hr, ATC or PRN | • Most commonly used and studied medication for delirium<br>• EPS, especially if dose is > 3 mg per day<br>• Monitor QT interval<br>• Due to long half-life may be able to dose once daily after effective dose established |
| • Chlorpromazine | 12.5–50 mg PO/SL/PR/ IM/IV every 4–8 hr ATC or PRN | • Useful if a more sedating agent is desired<br>• Higher risk of EPS than with haloperidol<br>• Monitor blood pressure for orthostatic hypotension<br>• If using IV route, give by slow push or infusion over 10–15 minutes |
| **Atypical antipsychotic** | | **Class characteristics:**<br>• EPS equivalent to or slightly less than those of haloperidol<br>• Prolonged QT interval<br>• More expensive than typical antipsychotics |
| • Olanzapine | 2.5–5 mg PO daily | • Available in orally disintegrating tablets |
| • Risperidone | 0.25–1 mg PO twice daily | • Available in orally disintegrating tablets<br>• Monitor blood pressure for orthostatic hypotension |
| • Quetiapine | 25 mg PO twice daily | • Most sedating of this class<br>• Preferred agent in patients with Parkinson's Disease<br>• Monitor blood pressure for orthostatic hypotension |
| **Benzodiazepine** | | |
| • Lorazepam | 0.5–1mg PO/IV every 4 hr PRN | • Often worsens delirium<br>• Sedating, but can see paradoxical excitation<br>• Medication of choice in patients with delirium associated with sedative or alcohol withdrawal or those with neuroleptic malignant syndrome<br>• Second-line agent for delirium in patients with Parkinson's Disease |

PO, oral; SL, sublingual; PR, rectal; SQ, subcutaneous; IV, intravenous; ATC, around the clock; PRN, as needed; EPS, extrapyramidal symptoms
*Sources*: Inouye (2006), reference 3; Breitbart & Alici (2008), reference 23; Shuster et al. (2008), reference 113.

intravenously.[117] In nonterminal patients, QT intervals should be monitored regularly.[23] And, consideration should be given to switching to a different route as soon as possible, recognizing the potential for increased extrapyramidal symptoms with the oral route.

Chlorpromazine is another typical antipsychotic that may be used to treat delirium. Doses of 12.5 mg to 50 mg by the oral, sublingual or parenteral route may be used.[113] Chlorpromazine is associated with more extrapyramidal side effects, orthostatic hypotension, and sedation than haloperidol. Therefore, it is usually used only when the additional sedation will be of benefit and haloperidol has not been completely effective; i.e., in patients described as experiencing terminal anguish or refractory delirium.

The newer, atypical antipsychotics have the advantage of fewer extrapyramidal side effects, less effect on QT interval, and less frequent administration (once or twice daily).[109,112,114,118,119,120] Starting doses are outlined in Table 21–5. None of these medications are FDA approved for the treatment of delirium, and all of them are more expensive than haloperidol. The authors of a systematic review of the literature concluded that haloperidol (in doses less than 3.5 mg per day), risperidone, and olanzapine were equally effective in treating delirium with few adverse events, based on only three studies that satisfied the selection criteria.[112] Other atypical antipsychotics that are reported to be effective in treating delirium include aripiprazole and quetiapine.[113,114,118,119,121]

Cholinesterase inhibitors have been studied for the treatment of delirium based on the understanding that disruption of the cholinergic system may be one of the underlying mechanisms of this syndrome. However, there is currently no evidence from controlled trials that the cholinesterase inhibitors are effective in the treatment of delirium.[120]

Benzodiazepines are not recommended for treatment of delirium, except for delirium associated with alcohol or sedative-hypnotic drug withdrawal.[23,34,108,109,122] This class of medications tends to cause oversedation and exacerbate confusion, potentially making delirium worse.[115] However, when antipsychotics alone do not control the symptoms of delirium, a sedative agent such as a benzodiazepine, propofol, or opioids may be added.[23] Refractory delirium is often cited as an indication for palliative sedation, accounting for between

5% to 57% of the patients requiring palliative sedation for comfort.[123,124] Midazolam is the most frequently used medication for palliative sedation.[123] While sedation may decrease severe agitation, it decreases the capacity to communicate.[124] Clinicians should periodically lighten the sedation to reassess delirium and to allow communication with family and staff, if possible.[23]

## Patient Family Teaching

Patient and family education is the cornerstone of comprehensive end-of-life care. Through proper education and support, cognitive disorders may be avoided, recognized early, or shortened. When a cognitive disorder leads to distress, appropriate education and support can decrease the severity of symptoms by providing open and adequate communication to lessen the stimuli that exacerbate symptoms. Teaching activities associated with cognitive disorders at the end of life involve prevention, identification, intervention, and supportive care issues.

*Preventing Delirium in the Dying.* As medications are the most common reversible and preventable cause of delirium, patients and families require education on the proper dosing and scheduling of all medications.[3,33] Delirium can be caused by taking too much medication (leading to toxicity) or too little (causing discomfort or potential withdrawal). It is important for nurses who care for patients in home care and clinic settings to review all medications with the patient and primary caregiver. Ideally, patients and family caregivers will recognize both the generic and trade names of their medications. Patients and family caregivers need to know the schedule for each medication, the side effects of each to report to their clinicians, and what to do if they should lose or run out of a medication. Medication charts, pillboxes, and medication information cards or sheets may be useful tools.

Patients and families also need to understand that any discomfort that is not adequately addressed can lead to complications, such as feeling nervous, confused, or worse. Thus, education for managing symptoms such as pain, nausea, constipation, and insomnia, is an important component of the teaching plan to prevent delirium.

Knowing that sensory deprivation, sensory overload, and unfamiliar or threatening surroundings may contribute to the development of delirium, it becomes evident that patient and family education should include evaluating the patient's sensory environment and developing strategies to provide appropriate levels of sensory stimulation. For some patients, this may mean encouraging interactions with caregivers and others (e.g., hospice volunteers), having the television or radio at a level pleasing to the patient, being sure the patient can see out a window to sense day and night cues, encouraging touch (e.g., massage or range-of-motion exercises), and assuring that the patient uses any needed sensory aids, such as eyeglasses or hearing aids.

Conversely, the patient who is in an environment where sensory overload is a potential requires education on decreasing sensory stimuli. Acute care settings are well known for the potential for sensory overload. However, many times, the potential for sensory overload in the home is not assessed. The combination of noises from vacuums, mixers, dishwashers, televisions, radios, conversations, and patient equipment (e.g., oxygen concentrators) can be overwhelming. In the susceptible patient, it may be helpful to close room doors, to run dishwashers or other equipment at different times of the day, to turn off or turn down televisions and radios when conversing, or to unplug the telephone at certain times of the day.

Being in a strange or threatening environment can contribute to delirium. Should a patient need to be admitted to an acute care or extended care setting, it is important to make that environment as familiar as possible. Encourage the patient and family to bring in familiar photographs or objects, establish a plan for familiar persons to visit regularly, teach family to greet their loved one at eye level, and encourage the use of touch, since this is very reassuring to the patient.

*Early Identification of the Symptoms of Delirium.* The prodromal symptoms of delirium may be easily overlooked. It is not uncommon for persons with advanced diseases to feel restless, anxious, depressed, irritable, angry, or emotionally labile. These symptoms may go unnoticed, only to be recalled later in family interviews.[108] Therefore, it is important to teach the patient and family to report any new feelings of uneasiness, anxiety, restlessness, or mood changes.

*Lessening the Severity of the Symptoms of Delirium.* The individual experiencing delirium may be very frightened about what is happening. Clinicians need to provide reassurance that delirium is usually temporary, and that the symptoms are part of a medical condition.[108] This intervention may significantly decrease fear and anxiety. The purpose of all supportive measures needs to be explained to both the patient and the family.

The family should be informed regarding the fluctuating nature of delirium, to prepare them for the changes in behavior and to prevent them from misinterpreting these frequent changes. Reorienting the patient to time, place, and persons in the environment may assist him or her to stay oriented. Repetition is important to compensate for memory impairment.[43] Thus, the family should be taught to correct the patient's orientation errors gently and regularly. If, however, correcting orientation errors leads to increased distress in the patient, this strategy should be discontinued.

The delirious patient is at risk for misinterpreting the environment. The family should be encouraged to evaluate the patient's environment for over- or undersensory stimulation. Interventions to correct the potential for sensory deprivation or overload, as mentioned above, may be appropriate.

Behaviors associated with delirium can be distressing for family caregivers to observe, and may lead to fears that their loved one has "gone crazy."[43,108] The family needs to hear that delirium is the result of a biological disorder and that the symptoms are generally temporary. The family should also be included in discussions of current, predicted, or resolving delirium in the patient.

*Teaching Following an Episode of Delirium.*  Follow-up teaching will include a discussion with the patient about the apparent cause of delirium, so that both the patient and family are aware of risk factors. The individual may or may not recall events that occurred during delirious episodes. Some individuals have frightening recollections of the delirious episode. Thus, it is important to assess the presence of any distressing memories. Extra psychotherapeutic support to work through the experience may be appropriate.[108]

⁓❧⁓

CASE STUDY—PART 2
*Mr. H (continued)*

The nurse recognized the patient's behavior as fitting the DSM–IV criteria for delirium: disturbed level of consciousness (somnolence to agitation), change in cognition (confusion and hallucinations), fluctuating nature of the symptoms, and multiple potential medical causes of delirium. Using the Nursing Delirium Screening Scale, Mr. H's score was evaluated as 9 out of maximum of 10. Mr. H had many predisposing factors for delirium—age over 65, dementia, history of falls, cardiac disease, and fracture—putting him at high risk for delirium. On admission, Mr. H had dehydration and infection as precipitating factors that contributed to the delirium initially seen. Those two factors had been addressed. However, Mr. H still had other risk factors for delirium, including pain (no morphine was given in the past 24 hours), use of urinary catheter, use of restraints, change of environment, sensory overload, and sleep deprivation. Mr. H also received several doses of lorazepam, which can worsen confusion and is not helpful for delirium. And, the nurse noted that Mr. H had not had a bowel movement since admission.

While waiting for a return call from the physician to discuss the concerns about delirium, the nurse initiated a plan to address as many of the factors contributing to delirium as possible. Pain was addressed using the prescribed opioid, monitoring for pain behaviors, and using appropriate turning techniques and supportive devices. The urinary catheter was removed and the patient offered a urinal regularly while monitoring for incontinence. The vest restraint was removed while the family was in the room monitoring the patient, but the mitt continued to preserve the intravenous site. The family was encouraged to talk to the patient about familiar topics to orient him gently to place, time, and the reason for admission to the hospital. A sitter was requested for the night shift, so that the patient could be monitored closely without disturbing

his sleep by keeping the door open and staff going in and out of the room frequently. Care activities such as vital signs, turning, and bathing were grouped together to minimize disruptions. And, the lorazepam was held. Haloperidol 1 mg intravenous every 8 hours plus 1 mg every 2 hours as needed, and a bowel protocol that included a softener and laxative, were ordered by the physician.

Over the course of the next 24 hours, Mr. H received a total of 4 mg of IV haloperidol. It is now day 5 of Mr. H's admission. The night shift reported he slept through the night when not disturbed, but was easily aroused for care activities. Mr. H was oriented to person and place on this day. His family reported that he recognized them, carried on conversations between naps, and did not appear to be having any hallucinations. Mitt restraints were no longer required. He did not ask for the urinal, but was agreeable to using it when offered. Mr. H ate only bites of meals despite encouragement. His Nu-DESC score improved to 2 out of the maximum of 10. His haloperidol was switched to 1 mg by mouth every 12 hours plus 1 mg by mouth as needed, and the intravenous morphine was changed to oxycodone 5 mg/acetaminophen 325 mg by mouth every 4 hours as needed. He was given a bisacodyl suppository with good results, and the bowel regimen continued.

The following morning (day 6 of admission), Mr. H's right foot was dusky with poor pedal pulses. Testing shows a massive deep vein thrombosis. He was again drowsy, aroused easily but drifted back to sleep when not stimulated. He was incontinent of urine and did not seem to understand instructions when offered a urinal. He recognized family, but reported the year was 1952 and that he was in a different city. The Nu-DESC score on this morning was 6 out of the maximum of 10. After review of the patient's overall status by the palliative medicine specialist, orthopedic surgeon, cardiologist and hospitalist, there was agreement that Mr. H was at high risk for complications from surgery and from anticoagulant therapy. The family was informed of the medical concerns, the pros and cons of inferior vena cava filter to prevent pulmonary embolus, and the team's recommendation to focus on comfort care. A referral was made for home care hospice. Haloperidol and oxycodone/acetaminophen were switched to oral solutions for ease of use at home, and continued on the current regimen. Two weeks later, Mr. H died at home with the support of a hospice team.

⁓❧⁓

Mr. H initially improved significantly with the aggressive nursing and pharmaceutical interventions, illustrating that an assessment of delirium risk factors and implementation of a comprehensive plan to eliminate or minimize these risks, along with appropriate use of antipsychotics, are effective in managing delirium. This case also illustrates that one additional uncontrollable event in a high-risk patient is all it takes to worsen delirium. In this situation, the worsening of the delirium was, indeed, the harbinger of impending death.

REFERENCES

1. Breitbart W, Chochinov H, Passik S. Psychiatric symptoms in palliative care. In: Doyle D, Hanks G, Cherny N, Calman K, eds. Oxford Textbook of Palliative Medicine (3rd ed). Oxford: Oxford University Press, 2004:746–771.

2. Young J, Leentjens A, George J, et al. Systematic approaches to the prevention and management of patients with delirium. J Psychosom Res 2008;65:267–272.

3. Inouye S. Delirium in older persons. N Engl J Med 2006;354:1157–1165.

4. Siddiqi N, House A, Holmes J. Occurrence and outcome of delirium in medical in-patients: A systematic literature review. Age Ageing 2006;35:350–364.

5. Kirshner H. Delirium: A focused review. Curr Neurol Neurosci Rep 2007;7:479–482.

6. Balas M, Deutschman C, Sullivan-Marx E, et al. Delirium in older patients in surgical intensive care units. J Nurs Scholarsh 2007;39:147–154.

7. Pandharipande P, Costabile S, Cotton B, et al. Prevalence of delirium in surgical ICU patients. Crit Care Med 2005;33:A45.

8. Micek S, Anand N, Laible B, et al. Delirium as detected by the CAM–ICU predicts restraint use among mechanically ventilated medical patients. Crit Care Med 2005;33:1260–1265.

9. Thomason J, Sintani A, Peterson J, et al. Intensive care unit delirium is an independent predictor of longer hospital stay: A prospective analysis of 261 non-ventilated patients. Crit Care 2005;9:R375–R381.

10. Fang C, Chen H, Liu S, Lin C, Tsai L, Lai Y. Prevalence, detection, and treatment of delirium in terminal cancer patients: A prospective survey. Jpn J Clin Oncol 2008;38:56–63.

11. Spiller J, Keen J. Hypoactive delirium: Assessing the extent of the problem for inpatient specialist palliative care. Palliat Med 2006;20:17–23.

12. Agar M, Lawlor P. Delirium in cancer patients: A focus on treatment-induced psychopathology. Curr Opin Oncol 2008;20:360–366.

13. Kishi Y, Kato M, Okuyama T, et al. Delirium: Patient characteristics that predict a missed diagnosis at psychiatric consultation. Gen Hosp Psychiatry 2007;29:442–445.

14. Steis M, Fick D. Are nurses recognizing delirium? A systematic review. J Gerontol Nurs 2008;34:40–48.

15. Inouye S, Schlesinger M, Lydon T. Delirium: A symptom of how hospital care is failing older persons and a window to improve quality of hospital care. Am J Med 1999;106:565–573.

16. Fick D, Hodo D, Lawrence F, et al. Recognizing delirium superimposed on dementia: Assessing nurses' knowledge using case vignettes. J Gerontol Nurs 2007;33:40–49.

17. McCusker J, Cole M, Dendukuri N, et al. The course of delirium in older medical inpatients. J Gen Intern Med 2003; 18:696–704.

18. Breitbart W, Gibson C, Tremblay A. The delirium experience: Delirium recall and delirium-related distress in hospitalized patients with cancer, their spouses/caregivers, and their nurses. Psychosomatics 2002;43:183–194.

19. O'Malley G, Leonard M, Meagher D, et al. The delirium experience: A review. J Psychosom Res 2008;65:223–228.

20. Fagerberg I, Jonhagen M. Temporary confusion: A fearful experience. J Psychiatr Ment Health Nurs 2002;9:339–346.

21. Namba M, Morita T, Imura C, et al. Terminal delirium: Families' experience. Palliat Med 2007;21:587–594.

22. Brajtman S, Higuchi K, McPherson C. Caring for patients with terminal delirium: Palliative care unit and home care nurses' experiences. Int J Palliat Nurs 2006;12:150–156.

23. Breitbart W, Alici Y. Agitation and delirium at the end of life: "We couldn't manage him." JAMA 2008;300:2898–2910.

24. White C, McCann M, Jackson N. First do no harm…terminal restlessness or drug-induced delirium. J Palliat Med 2007;10:345–351.

25. Lawlor P, Gagnon B, Mancini I, et al. Occurrence, causes, and outcomes of delirium in patients with advanced cancer: A prospective study. Arch Intern Med 2000;160:786–794.

26. Healthcare Cost and Utilization Project. Available at: http://hcupnet.ahrq.gov/HCUPnet.jsp (accessed February 14, 2009).

27. Leslie D, Marcantonio E, Zhang Y, et al. One-year health costs associated with delirium in the elderly population. Arch Intern Med 2008;168:27–32.

28. Pitkala K, Laurila J, Strandberg T, et al. Multicomponent geriatric intervention for elderly inpatients with delirium: Effects on costs and health-related quality of life. J Gerontol A Biol Sci Med Sci 2008;63:56–61.

29. Leslie D, Zhang Y, Bogardus S, et al. Consequences of preventing delirium in hospitalized older adults on nursing home costs. J Am Geriatr Soc 2005;53:405–409.

30. American Psychiatric Association. Diagnostic and Statistical Manual of Mental Disorders (4th ed). Washington DC: American Psychiatric Association, 1994.

31. Young J, Inouye S. Delirium in older people. BMJ 2007;334:842–846.

32. Inouye S, Foreman M, Mion L, et al. Nurses' recognition of delirium and its symptoms: Comparison of nurse and researcher ratings. Arch Intern Med 2001;161:2467–2473.

33. Fearing M, Inouye S. Delirium. In: Blazer D, Steffens D, eds. The American Psychiatric Publishing Textbook of Geriatric Psychiatry (4th ed). Washington, DC: American Psychiatric Publishing, 2009:229–241.

34. Gibson C, Lichtenthal W, Berg A, et al. Psychologic issues in palliative care. Anesthesiology Clin N Am 2006;24:61–80.

35. Arnold E. Sorting out the 3 D's: Delirium, dementia, depression: Learn how to sift through overlapping signs and symptoms so you can help improve an older patient's quality of life. Holist Nurs Pract 2005;19:99–104.

36. Milisen K, Braes T, Fick D, et al. Cognitive assessment and differentiating the 3 Ds (dementia, depression, delirium). Nurs Clin North Am 2006;41:1–22.

37. Lipowski Z. Delirium: Acute Confusional State. Oxford: Oxford University Press, 1990.

38. Stagno D, Gibson C, Breitbart W. The delirium subtypes: A review of prevalence, phenomenology, pathophysiology, and treatment response. Palliat Support Care 2004;2:171–179.

39. Kiely D, Jones R, Bergmann M, et al. Association between psychomotor activity delirium subtypes and mortality among newly admitted post-acute facility patients. J Gerontol A Biol Sci Med Sci 2007;62:174–179.

40. Kuebler K. Hospice and Palliative Clinical Practice Protocol: Terminal Restlessness. Pittsburgh: Hospice and Palliative Nurses Association, 1997.

41. Callanan C, Kelley P. Final Gifts. New York: Poseidon Press, 1992:67–71.

42. Twycross R, Lichter I. The terminal phase. In: Doyle D, Hanks G, MacDonald N, eds. Oxford Textbook of Palliative Medicine. Oxford: Oxford University Press, 1993:658–659.

43. Furst C, Doyle D. The terminal phase. In: Doyle D, Hanks G, Cherny N, Calman K, eds. Oxford Textbook of Palliative Medicine (3rd ed). Oxford: Oxford University Press, 2004:1117–1134.

44. Yokota H, Ogawa S, Kurokawa A, et al. Regional cerebral blood flow in delirium patients. Psychiatry Clin Neurosci 2003;57:337–339.

45. Fong T, Bogardus S, Daftary A, et al. Cerebral perfusion changes in older delirious patients using 99mTc HMPAO SPECT. J Gerontol A Biol Sci Med Sci 2006;61:1294–1299.

46. Gottesman R, Hillis A, Grega M, et al. Early postoperative cognitive dysfunction and blood pressure during coronary artery bypass graft operation. Arch Neurol 2007;64:1111–1114.

47. Maldonado J. Pathoetiological model of delirium: A comprehensive understanding of the neurobiology of delirium and an evidence-based approach to prevention and treatment. Crit Care Clin 2008;24:789–856.

48. Gunther M, Jackson J, Ely E. Loss of IQ in the ICU: Brain injury without the insult. Med Hypotheses 2007;69:1179–1182.

49. Jackson J, Gordon S, Hart R, et al. The association between delirium and cognitive decline: A review of the empirical literature. Neuropsychol Rev 2004;14:87–98.

50. Gunther M, Morandi A, Ely E. Pathophysiology of delirium in the intensive care unit. Crit Care Clin 2008;24:45–65.

51. Hshieh T, Fong T, Marcantonio E, et al. Cholinergic deficiency hypothesis in delirium: A synthesis of current evidence. J Gerontol A Biol Sci Med Sci 2008;63:764–772.

52. Trzepacz P. Is there a common neural pathway in delirium? Focus on acetylcholine and dopamine. Semin Clin Neuropsychiatry 2000;5:132–148.

53. Kreek M, Zhou Y, Butelman E, et al. Opiate and cocaine addiction: From bench to clinic and back to the bench. Curr Opin Pharmacol 2009;9:74–80.

54. Segal M, Avital A, Rusakov A, et al. Serum creatine kinase activity differentiates alcohol syndromes of dependence, withdrawal and delirium tremens. Eur Neuropsychopharmacol 2009;19:92–96.

55. Pfister D, Siegemund M, Dell-Kuster S, et al. Cerebral perfusion in sepsis-associated delirium. Crit Care 2008;12:R63. Available at: http://ccforum.com/content/12/3/R63 (accessed March 9, 2009).

56. Siami S, Annane D, Sharshar T. The encephalopathy in sepsis. Crit Care Clin 2008;24:67–82.

57. deRooij S, vanMunster B, Korevaar J, et al. Cytokines and acute phase response in delirium. J Psychosom Res 2007;62:521–525.

58. vanMunster B, Korevaar J, Zwinderman A, et al. Time-course of cytokines during delirium in elderly patients with hip fractures. J Am Geriatr Soc 2008;56:1704–1709.

59. Beloosesky Y, Hendel D, Weiss A, et al. Cytokines and C-reactive protein production in hip-fracture-operated elderly patients. J Gerontal A Biol Sci Med Sci 2007;62:420–426.

60. Inouye S, Charpentier P. Precipitating factors for delirium in hospitalized elderly persons. Predictive model and interrelationship with baseline vulnerability. JAMA 1996;20:852–858.

61. Inouye S. Current concepts: Delirium in older persons. N Engl J Med 2006;354:1157–1165.

62. Margiotta A, Bianchetti A, Ranieri P, et al. Clinical characteristics and risk factors of delirium in demented and not demented elderly medical inpatients. J Nutr Health Aging 2006;10:535–539.

63. Cole M. Delirium in elderly patients. Am J Geriatr Psychiatry 2004;12:7–21.

64. Hamann J, Bickel H, Schwaibold H, et al. Postoperative acute confusional state in typical urologic population: Incidence, risk factors, and strategies for prevention. Urology 2005;65:449–453.

65. Zekry D, Herrmann F, Grandjean R, et al. Demented versus non-demented very old inpatients: The same comorbidities but poorer functional and nutritional status. Age Ageing 2008;37:83–89.

66. Boyle D. Delirium in older adults with cancer: Implications for practice and research. Oncol Nurs Forum 2006;33:61–78.

67. Inouye S, Zhang Y, Jones R, et al. Risk factors for delirium at discharge: Development and validation of a predictive model. Arch Intern Med 2007;167:1406–1413.

68. Devlin J, Fong J, Schumaker G, et al. Use of a validated delirium assessment tool improves the ability of physicians to identify delirium in medical intensive care unit patients. Crit Care Med 2007;35:2721–2724.

69. Ryan K, Leonard M, Guerin S, et al. Validation of the confusion assessment method in the palliative care setting. Palliat Med 2009;23:40–45.

70. Gaudreau J, Gagnon P, Harel F, et al. Impact on delirium detection of using a sensitive instrument integrated into clinical practice. Gen Hosp Psychiatry 2005;27:194–199.

71. Folstein M, Folstein S, McHugh P. Mini-mental state: A practical method for grading the cognitive state of patients for the clinician. J Psychiatr Res 1975;12:189–198.

72. Hjermstad M, Loge J, Kaasa S. Methods for assessment of cognitive failure and delirium in palliative care patients: Implications for practice and research. Palliat Med 2004;18:494–506.

73. Fayers P, Hjernstad M, Ranhoff A, et al. Which mini-mental state exam items can be used to screen for delirium and cognitive impairment? J Pain Symptom Manage 2005;30:41–50.

74. Schuurmans M, Deschamps P, Markham S, et al. The measurement of delirium: Review of scales. Res Theory Nurs Pract 2003;17:207–224.

75. Breitbart W, Rosenfeld B, Roth A, et al. The Memorial Delirium Assessment Scale. J Pain Symptom Manage 1997;13:128–137.

76. Bosisio M, Caraceni A, Grassi L, et al. Phenomenology of delirium in cancer patients as described by the Memorial Delirium Assessment scale (MDAS) and the Delirium Rating Scale (DRS). Psychosomatics 2006;47:471–478.

77. Trzepacz P. The Delirium Rating Scale: Its use in consultation-liaison research. Psychosomatics 1999;40:193–204.

78. Trzepacz P, Mittal D, Tores R, et al. Validation of the Delirium Rating Scale-revised-98: Comparison with the delirium rating scale and the cognitive test for delirium. J Neuropsychiatry Clin Neurosci 2001;13:229–242.

79. Inouye S. The Confusion Assessment Method (CAM): Training manual and coding guide. New Haven: Yale University School of Medicine, 2003. Available at: http://elderlife.med.yale.edu/pdf/The_Confusion_Assessment_Method.pdf (accessed March 8, 2009).

80. Lemiengre J, Nelis T, Joosten E, et al. Detection of delirium by beside nurses using the confusion assessment method. J Am Geriatr Soc 2006;54:685–689.

81. Waszynski C, Petrovic K. Nurses' evaluation of the Confusion Assessment Method: A pilot study. J Gerontol Nurs 2008;34:49–56.

82. Neelon V, Champagne M, Carlson J, et al. The NEECHAM Confusion Scale: Construction, validation, and clinical testing. Nurs Res 1996;45:324–330.

83. Van Rompaey B, Schuurmans M, Shortridge-Baggett L, et al. A comparison of the CAM–ICU and the NEEDHAM Confusion Scale in intensive care delirium assessment: An observational study in non-intubated patients. Crit Care 2008;12:R16. Available at:http://ccforum.com/content/12/1/R16 (accessed March 8, 2009).

84. Stillman M, Rybicki L. The bedside confusion scale: Development of a portable bedside test for confusion and its application to the palliative medicine population. J Palliat Med 2000;3:449–456.

85. Sarhill N, Walsh D, Nelson K, et al. Assessment of delirium in advanced cancer: The use of the bedside confusion scale. Am J Hosp Palliat Care 2001;18:335–341.

86. Zama I, Maynard W, Davis M. Clocking delirium: The value of the clock drawing test with case illustrations. Am J Hosp Palliat Care 2008;25:385–388.

87. Schuurmans M, Shortridge-Baggett L, Duursma S. The Delirium Observation Screening Scale: A screening instrument for delirium. Res Theory Nurs Pract 2003;17:31–50.

88. Gemert van L, Schuurmans M. The NEECHAM confusion scale and the delirium observation screening scale: Capacity to discriminate and ease of use in clinical practice. BMC Nurs 2007;6:3. Available at: http://www.biomedcentral.com/content/pdf/1472-6955-6-3.pdf (accessed March 8, 2009).

89. Gaudreau J, Gagnon P, Harel F, et al. Fast, systematic, and continuous delirium assessment in hospitalized patients: The nursing delirium screening scale. J Pain Symptom Manage 2005;29:368–375.

90. Radtke R, Franck M, Schneider M, et al. Comparison of three scores for delirium in the recovery room. 2008;101:338–343.

91. Siddiqi N, Stockdale R, Britton A, et al. Interventions for preventing delirium in hospitalised patients. Cochrane Database of Systematic Reviews 2007, Issue 2. Art. No.: CD005563. DOI: 10.1002/14651858.CD005563.pub2. Available at: http://www.mrw.interscience.wiley.com/cochrane/clsysrev/articles/CD005563/pdf_standard_fs.html (accessed March 14, 2009).

92. Bergmann M, Murphy K, Kiely D, et al. A model for management of delirious post-acute care patients. J Am Geriatr Soc 2005;53:1817–1825.

93. Caplan G, Coconis J, Board N, et al. Does home treatment affect delirium? A randomized controlled trial of rehabilitation of elderly and care at home or usual treatment (The REACH-OUT trial). Age Ageing 2006;53:53–60.

94. Lundstrom M, Edlund A, Karisson S, et al. A multifactorial intervention program reduces the duration of delirium, length of hospitalization, and mortality in delirious patients. J Am Geriat Soc 2005;53:622–628.

95. Naughton B, Saltzman S, Ramadan F, et al. A multifactorial intervention to reduce prevalence of delirium and shorten hospital length of stay. J Am Geriatr Soc 2005;35:18–23.

96. Pitkala K, Laurila J, Strandberg T, et al. Multicomponent geriatric intervention for elderly inpatients with delirium: A randomized, controlled trial. J Gerontol A Biol Sci Med Sci 2006;61:176–181.

97. Inouye S, Bogardus S, Charpentier P, et al. A multicomponent intervention to prevent delirium in hospitalized older patients. N Engl J Med 1999;340:669–676.

98. Inouye S. The Hospital Elder Life Program (HELP), 2007. Available at: http://www.hospitalelderlifeprogram.org (accessed March 14, 2009).

99. Caraceni A. Delirium in palliative medicine. Eur J Palliat Care 1995;2:62–67.

100. Hallenbeck J. Palliative care in the final days of life: "They were expecting it at any time." JAMA 2005;293:2265–2271.

101. Gaudreau J, Gagnon P, Harel F, et al. Psychoactive medications and risk of delirium in hospitalized cancer patients. J Clin Oncol 2005;23:6712–6718.

102. McDowell J, Mion L, Lydon T, et al. A nonpharmacolgic sleep protocol for hospitalized older patients. J Am Geriatr Soc 1998;46:700–705.

103. White J, Hammond L. Delirium assessment tool for end of life: CHIMBOP. J Palliat Med 2008;11:1069.

104. Caraceni A, Grassi L, eds. Acute Confusional States in Palliative Medicine. Oxford: Oxford University Press, 2003:172–179.

105. Buss M, Vanderwerker L, Inouye S, et al. Associations between caregiver-perceived delirium in patients with cancer and generalized anxiety in their caregivers. J Palliat Med 2007;10:1083–1092.

106. Byock I. Dying Well: The Prospect for Growth at the End of Life. New York: Riverhead Books, 1997:43–45.

107. Kyle G. Evaluating the effectiveness of aromatherapy in reducing levels of anxiety in palliative care patients: Results of a pilot study. Complement Ther Clin Pract 2006;12:148–155.

108. American Psychiatric Association. Practice guideline for the treatment of patients with delirium. Am J Psychiatry 1999;156(Suppl 5):1–20.

109. Del Fabbro E, Dalal S, Bruera E. Symptom control in palliative care—part III: Dyspnea and delirium. J Palliat Med 2006;9:422–436.

110. Lacasse H, Perreault M, Williamson D. Systematic review of antipsychotics for the treatment of hospital-associated delirium in medically or surgically ill patients. Ann Pharmacother 2006;40:1966–1973.

111. Jackson K, Lipman A. Drug therapy for delirium in terminally ill patients. Cochrane Database Syst Rev 2004, Issue 2. Art. No.: CD004770. DOI: 10.1002/14651858.CD004770. Available at: http://www.mrw.interscience.wiley.com/cochrane/clsysrev/articles/CD004770/pdf_fs.html (accessed March 14, 2009).

112. Lonergan E, Britton AM, Luxenberg J. Antipsychotics for delirium. Cochrane Database Syst Rev 2007, Issue 2. Art. No.: CD005594. DOI: 10.1002/14651858.CD005594.pub2. Available at: http://www.mrw.interscience.wiley.com/cochrane/clsysrev/articles/CD005594/pdf_fs.html (accessed March 14, 2009).

113. Shuster J, Thrower M, Redden J. Delirium. In Grauer P, Shuster J, Protus B, eds. Palliative Care Consultant: A Reference Guide for Palliative Care (3rd ed). Dubuque, IA: Kendall/Hunt Publishing Co., 2008:78–85.

114. Alici-Evcimen Y, Breitbart W. An update on the use of antipsychotics in the treatment of delirium. Palliat Support Care 2008;6:177–182.

115. Breitbart W, Marotta R, Platt M, et al. A double-blind trial of haloperidol, chlorpromazine, and lorazepam in the treatment of delirium in hospitalized AIDS patients. Am J Psychiatry 1996;153:231–237.

116. Tropea J, Slee J, Holmes A, et al. Use of antipsychotic medications for the management of delirium: An audit of current practice in the acute care setting. Int Psychogeriatr 2008;5:1–8.

117. U.S. Food and Drug Administration. Information for healthcare professionals: Haloperidol (marketed as Haldol, Haldol Decanoate and Haldol Lactate). U.S. Food and Drug Administration. 2007. Available at: http://www.fda.gov/Drugs/DrugSafety/PostmarketDrugSafetyInformationforPatientsand

Providers/DrugSafetyInformationforHeathcareProfessionals/ucm085203.htm (accessed March 14, 2009).

118. Ozbolt L, Paniagua M, Kaiser R. Atypical antipsychotics for the treatment of delirious elders. J Am Med Dir Assoc 2008;9:18–28.

119. Straker D, Shapiro P, Muskin P. Aripiprazole in the treatment of delirium. Psychosomatics 2006;47:385–391.

120. Overshott R, Karim S, Burns A. Cholinesterase inhibitors for delirium. Cochrane Database Syst Rev 2008, Issue 1. Art. No.: CD005317. DOI: 10.1002/14651858.CD005317.pub2. Available at: http://mrw.interscience.wiley.com/cochrane/clsysrev/articles/CD006379/pdf_fs.html (accessed March 14, 2009).

121. Rea R, Battistone S, Fong J, et al. Atypical antipsychotics versus haloperidol for treatment of delirium in acutely ill patients. Pharmacotherapy 2007;27:588–594.

122. Lonergan E, Luxenberg J, Areosa Sastre A, Wyller TB. Benzodiazepines for delirium. Cochrane Database Syst Rev 2009, Issue 1. Art. No.: CD006379. DOI:10.1002/14651858.CD006379.pub2. Available at: http://mrw.interscience.wiley.com/cochrane/clsysrev/articles/CD006379/pdf_fs.html (accessed March 14, 2009).

123. Claessens P, Menten J, Schotsmans P, et al. Palliative sedation: A review of the research literature. J Pain Symptom Manage 2008;36:310–333.

124. Mercadante S, Intravaia G, Villari P, et al. Controlled sedation for refractory symptoms in dying patient. J Pain Symptom Manage 2009;37:771–779.

# 22

*Laura Bourdeanu, Marjorie J. Hein, and Pamela R. Tryon*

# Insomnia

*A ruffled mind makes a restless pillow.—Charlotte Brontë*

◆ **Key Points**
◆ *Insomnia is a symptom characterized as inconsistent or ineffective sleep patterns which can significantly impact a person's quality of life.*
◆ *There remains a lack of knowledge specifically related to assessing and managing insomnia in cancer patients. Many pharmacological and nonpharmacological therapies are available that can be helpful.*
◆ *All nurses in all settings can play an important role in advancing the knowledge and skills related to addressing insomnia.*

Insomnia is a prevalent health complaint, with an estimated 64 million Americans suffering from insomnia on a regular basis each year.[1] Insomnia is predominant among the elderly, those with chronic medical illness, and those with anxiety or depressive disorders.[2-4] Unchecked, insomnia can lead to various adverse sequelae in psychiatric, neurocognitive and medical domains, as well as significant reduction in quality of life.[5-8] In addition, insomnia can lead to daytime dysfunction, such as daytime sleepiness, irritability, depressive or anxious mood and accidents.[9]

Sleep is a "highly structured and well-organized activity following a circadian periodicity that is regulated by the interplay of internal biological processes and environmental factors."[10] According to the International Classification of Sleep Disorders and DSM–IV, insomnia is a "heterogeneous complaint that may involve difficulties falling asleep, difficulty maintaining sleep with more than 30 minutes of nocturnal awakenings, early-morning awaking with inability to resume sleep, or a complaint of nonrestorative sleep with corresponding sleep efficiency less than 85%."[11,12]

In patients with cancer, insomnia is reported to be a common problem. The prevalence of insomnia and associated symptoms in cancer patients, either newly diagnosed or recently treated patients, was reported to be 23%–61%.[13,14,10] However, insomnia was present in 23%–44% of patients 2–5 years after treatment.[15,16,10] The causes for insomnia in patients with cancer may be related to psychological factors (anxiety or depression), pain, treatment-related toxicity, or other comorbid medical conditions. Further, insomnia was linked with increased rates of depression, decreased quality of life, and increased fatigue in other patient populations.[17]

Though it is a common symptom noted by cancer patients, especially those undergoing aggressive forms of treatment, research regarding insomnia in cancer patients is scarce. This chapter will apply as a model for assessment and treatment of insomnia to cancer patients; however, these principles can also be considered for patients without cancer.

CASE STUDY
*Andrew, A Man with the Go-Fight-Win Spirit...Most of the Time*

Andrew, a 51-year-old executive producer of a major sports network and newly married, has metastatic gastric cancer. He was initially diagnosed in May of 2007, after experiencing worsening abdominal pain that he thought was "bad heartburn." After being deemed surgically untreatable, Andrew is now in the midst of his fourth line of aggressive chemotherapy. As a consequence of aggressively fighting for his life with toxic therapy, Andrew's quality of life has been compromised with chronic nausea, vomiting, neuropathies, fatigue, syncopal episodes, deep vein thrombosis, pain, and poor oral intake. As a result of his gastric cancer, Andrew has become TPN dependent, requiring his faithful wife to diligently connect him to an infusion pump for at least sixteen hours a day. Between routine physical exams, home infusions, chemotherapy, taking medication, and maintaining his routine activities of daily living, Andrew states that he is having problems with insomnia. He is able to sleep for 1–2 hours at a time in the evening, but then awakens and is unable to sleep the rest of the night. He is napping throughout the day and constantly feels fatigued. He reports that his multiple physical symptoms are well controlled with his current medications, which include Compazine, Zofran, Ativan, Scopolamine patches, Remeron, Marinol, MS Contin 30 mg twice daily, Restoril, and Ambien for insomnia. The nurse conducts a thorough assessment of this latter symptom by speaking with Andrew and his wife in order to identify the tangible causes contributing to his insomnia, including how many hours a day he naps, if any, and an assessment of the effectiveness of his medications to control his other symptoms. In addition, a thorough physical exam is performed, including a neurological evaluation.

Through the assessment, the nurse discovers that Andrew currently leads a sedentary lifestyle, sitting on the couch or remaining in bed between administrations of his medications throughout the day. Although he is able, he does not feel motivated to exercise or continue working. He also admits to an emotional component, with bouts of anxiety and depression. After discussing Andrew's care with the physician, the nurse reviews both nonpharmacological and pharmacological approaches to combat insomnia, including dietary recommendations, decreasing nap frequency, using the bed only for sleeping, and incorporating a routine exercise regimen. The nurse also outlines, with both Andrew and his wife, an ideal time interval for each medication he takes—especially Restoril and Ambien—and Andrew is motivated to follow these recommendations. The nurse also suggests a consultation with ancillary services including dietary, psychiatry, and palliative medicine, explaining that both altered emotional and physical states can snowball the effects of insomnia. After seeing the above specialists,

Andrew is now on Restoril alone, with Ritalin during the day to combat the sedative effects of his anti-emetics and pain medication. He has consolidated his intravenous infusions to a set time in the evening, tries to coordinate all his medical appointments to a day or two per week, and has incorporated a diet and exercise regimen that he is able to tolerate. Within less than one month, Andrew states that he is able to get 5–6 hours of restful sleep each evening and no longer feels that insomnia is a major complaint.

## Factors Related to Insomnia

Insomnia is among one of the most prevalent, distressing, and under-managed symptoms experienced by patients with cancer. Insomnia is associated with adverse outcomes and should be proactively targeted for intervention.[18] A. J. Spielman, in the late 1980s, created a model of insomnia in terms of predisposing, precipitating, and perpetuating factors.[19] Precipitating factors of developing insomnia are likely to be genetic and neurobiologic factors, such as psychosocial, medical, or psychiatric.[19] The process of sleep and wakefulness is an active and tightly regulated process, and differs among individuals who have different susceptibilities to exogenous influence.[19]

Often, sleep disturbances are associated with situational stresses such as illness, aging, and drug treatments.[10] However, in patients with cancer, the physical illness, pain, hospitalization, and cancer treatment drugs, along with the psychological impact of the disease, may disrupt sleeping patterns of the individual. A history of poor sleep patterns will adversely affect the individual's daytime mood and performance. Among the general population, an individual with complaints of persistent insomnia has been associated with an increased risk of developing anxiety or depression. Complaints of sleep disturbances and a pattern of sleep–wake cycle reversals may be an early sign of a developing delirium.[20]

Paraneoplastic syndromes may exacerbate sleep disturbances if they are associated with increased steroid production, and if the patient has symptoms associated with tumor invasion such as draining lesions, gastrointestinal and genitourinary changes, pain, fever, cough, dyspnea, pruritus, and fatigue. Moreover, medications used by patients to control symptoms of the disease, or side effects of treatment, may cause insomnia. For example, medications such as vitamins, corticosteroids, neuroleptics for nausea and vomiting, and sympathomimetics to relieve dyspnea may negatively impact sleep patterns.[20] Frequently, hospitalized patients are likely to have their sleep interrupted by treatment schedules, routine hospital procedures, and other patients sharing the room. All of these factors may either singularly or collectively alter the sleep–wake cycle. Other considerations influencing the sleep–wake cycles of patients with cancer include age, comfort, pain, and anxiety; and environmental noise, and temperature.[21]

There are four major categories of sleep disorders according to the Sleep Disorders Classification Committee of the American Academy of Sleep Medicine:

1. Disorders of initiating and maintaining sleep (insomnias).
2. Disorders of the sleep–wake cycle.
3. Dysfunctions associated with sleep, sleep stages, or partial arousals (parasomnias).
4. Disorders of excessive somnolence.[22]

According to the DSM-IV-TR (Diagnostic and Statistical Manual of Mental Disorders: Fourth edition text revision), sleep disorders are organized into four major categories according to the etiology of the sleep disorder[11]:

1. *Primary sleep disorders* consist of all other etiologies other than the ones listed below. Primary sleep disorders are assumed to develop from endogenous abnormalities in sleep–wake patterns, accompanied by conditioning factors.
   a. *Dyssomnias* are abnormalities in the amount, quality, or timing of sleep.
   b. *Parasomnias* are abnormal behavioral or physiological events.
2. *Sleep disorder related to another mental disorder* resulting from a diagnosable mental disorder, usually mood or anxiety disorder, but severe enough to receive clinical attention.
3. *Sleep disorder due to a general medical condition* resulting from the effects of a physiological medical condition.
4. *Substance-induced sleep disorder* resulting from concurrent use or a recent discontinuation of a drug.[11]

Insomnia may also be caused by medications commonly used in the treatment of cancer. The sustained use of central nervous system (CNS) stimulants such as, amphetamines, caffeine, and diet pills (including some dietary supplements that promote weight loss and appetite suppression); sedatives and hypnotics (e.g., glutethimide, benzodiazepines, pentobarbital, chloral hydrate, secobarbital sodium, and amobarbital sodium); cancer chemotherapeutic agents (especially antimetabolites); anticonvulsants (e.g., phenytoin); adrenocorticotropin; oral contraceptives; monoamine oxidase inhibitors; methyldopa; propranolol; atenolol; alcohol; and thyroid preparations can cause insomnia.[22] In addition, withdrawal from CNS depressants (e.g., barbiturates, opioids, glutethimide, chloral hydrate, methaqualone, ethchlorvynol, alcohol, and over-the-counter and prescription antihistamine sedatives), benzodiazepines, major tranquilizers, tricyclic and monamine oxidase inhibitor antidepressants, and illicit drugs (e.g., marijuana, cocaine, phencyclidine) can cause insomnia.[20]

Hypnotics that are commonly prescribed to patients with cancer can interfere with rapid eye movement (REM) sleep, resulting in irritability, apathy, and decreased mental alertness. An abrupt withdrawal of hypnotics and sedatives may cause nervousness, jitteriness, seizures, and REM rebound.

REM rebound is a "marked increase in REM sleep with increased frequency and intensity of dreaming, including nightmares."[23] The increased physiologic arousal that occurs during REM rebound may be dangerous for patients with peptic ulcers or a history of cardiovascular problems.

## Pathophysiology

Normal sleep consists of two phases: rapid eye movement (REM) sleep and non-rapid eye movement (NREM) sleep.[24] The brain is active during REM sleep or dream sleep. NREM sleep is the quiet or restful phase of sleep. NREMs divided into four stages of progressively deepening sleep based on electroencephalogram findings. Sleep occurs in stages of a repeated pattern, or cycle, of NREM followed by REM, in which each cycle lasts approximately 90 minutes. The cycle is repeated four to six times during a 7- to 8-hour sleep period.[25]

A biological clock, or circadian rhythm, dictates the sleep-wake cycle. A disruption in an individual's sleep pattern may disturb the circadian rhythm and impair the sleep cycle.[26] Exogenous influences such as caffeine, light, and stress have been indicated in recent studies to be influenced by genetic factors. An example in one study found that differences in the adenosine 2A receptor gene (ADORA2) determine the differential sensitivity to caffeine's effect on sleep. The ADORA2A c. 1083T>C genotype determines how closely the caffeine-induced changes in brain electrical activity (increased beta activity) during sleep resemble the alterations observed in patients with insomnia.[19] A patient with a history of chronic insomnia may have a mutation in the gene (GABAa beta3) that is believed to affect an individual's ability to handle stress or make them more susceptible to depression.[20]

Patients with chronic insomnia (in clinical trials) were noted to have increased brain arousal. Demonstrations of fast-frequency activity during NREM sleep, an EEG sign of hyper-arousal, and evidence of reduced deactivation in key sleep/wake regions during NREM sleep, were noted in patients with chronic primary insomnia. Also, patients with insomnia were noted to have higher day and night body temperatures, urinary cortisol, adrenaline secretion, and adrenocorticotropic hormone ACTH, than patients with normal sleep. Evidence demonstrated that sleep deprivation was not a factor in the differences found between individuals with insomnia and normal sleepers. Studies have indicated that only a small percentage of patients with medical and psychiatric conditions develop insomnia, which suggests that some patients have an inherent susceptibility (whether psychosocial, medical, or psychiatric) to develop insomnia in the context of a stressful event.[20]

## Perpetuating Factors

Cognitive and behavioral mechanisms perpetuate insomnia, regardless of how insomnia is triggered. Patients have misconceptions about what are normal sleep requirements, and then develop excessive worry about not having adequate sleep. This often causes the patient to become obsessive about sleep. The patient develops a dysfunctional belief, often worsening the disruptive sleep behavior—for example taking daytime naps or "sleeping in late"—which in turn reduces the natural homeostatic drive to sleep at a normal bedtime.[20]

Patients develop a conditioned arousal to stimuli that would normally be associated with sleep (i.e., heightened anxiety and ruminations about going to sleep once they are in the bedroom). The patient then develops a cycle in which the more they strive to sleep, the more agitated they become, and the less they are able to fall asleep. Also, the patient may have ruminative thoughts or clock-watching behavior as they try to fall asleep in the bedroom. Therefore, conditioned environmental stimuli cause insomnia to develop from the continued association of sleeplessness with situations and behaviors that are typically related to sleep.[20]

## Treatment

Insomnia in cancer patients may be due to a variety of disease-related factors, cancer treatment, or psychological factors. The initial strategy to treat insomnia in cancer patients is to address the underlying physical and psychological factors contributing to the sleep disturbance. If the precipitating factors are not fully manageable, then pharmacological or behavioral interventions, or both, should be used to treat both acute and chronic insomnia. Pharmacological interventions are more commonly used in cancer patients who seek help for their insomnia; however, long-term pharmacotherapy is not desirable.[27–29] Hence, the treatment for insomnia in cancer patients must be multimodal and should include both pharmacologic and nonpharmacologic interventions.

### Pharmacologic Interventions

Pharmacologic interventions, particularly hypnotics, have historically played a prominent role in the management of insomnia in cancer patients, despite the lack of controlled trials. Pharmacological agents approved by the U.S. Food and Drug Administration for the treatment of insomnia include: benzodiazepine gamma-aminobutyric acid (GABA$_A$) agonists, nonbenzodiazepine GABA$_A$ agonists, and melatonin-receptor agonists (Table 22–1).[30]

*Benzodiazepine Receptor Agonists.* Benzodiazepines are still frequently used in the management of insomnia because of their undisputed efficacy and relative safety compared to other agents such as barbiturates. Benzodiazepines facilitate the GABA-mediated inhibition of cell firing by occupying the subunits of the GABA receptor complex present throughout the brain, including the ventral lateral preoptic

| Table 22–1 Pharmacologic Agents Approved by FDA | |
|---|---|
| Benzodiazepine receptor agonists | Clonazepam |
| | Lorazepam |
| | Oxazepam |
| | Estazolam |
| | Flurazepam |
| | Temazepam |
| | Triazolam |
| | Quazepam |
| Nonbenzodiazepines receptor agonists | Zaleplon |
| | Zolpidem |
| | Zopiclone |
| Melatonin receptor agonists | Ramelteon |

area that controls sleep. The sleep architecture is altered by suppressing sleep stages 3 and 4, and prolonging stages 1 and 2 of sleep, thereby increasing total sleep time.[31] Although benzodiazepines are effective agents, they have several unwanted side effects, such as daytime drowsiness, dizziness or lightheadedness, cognitive impairments, motor incoordination, tolerance, dependence, rebound insomnia, and daytime anxiety.[10]

*Nonbenzodiazepine Receptor Agonists.* Nonbenzodiazepines are the most widely used medications because they can induce sleep with fewer side effects than benzodiazepines. Nonbenzodiazepines inhibit neuronal firing by binding selectively to the alpha-1 subunit of the omega-1 receptor of the GABA receptor complex.[32] Although both nonbenzodiazepines and benzodiazepines exert their effect on the GABA receptor complex, nonbenzodiazepines do not disturb the architecture of sleep.[10] Nonbenzodiazepines have fewer residual side effects, including a lower risk for abuse and dependence, less psychomotor impairment, amnesia, and daytime somnolence.[33]

*Melatonin-Receptor Agonists.* Melatonin-receptor agonists are an emerging class of drugs that can be used to treat insomnia. Melatonin-receptor agonists bind to the MT1 and MT2 receptors in the suprachiasmatic nucleus. These receptors are thought to be involved in the maintenance of the circadian rhythm underlying the normal sleep–wake cycle.[34] Melatonin-receptor agonists have the advantage of having minimal side effects and no potential for abuse or dependence.[35] Presently, the only melatonin-receptor agonist approved for the treatment of insomnia by the FDA is ramelteon (Rozerem).

*Others.* Other classes of drugs have been used to treat insomnia in cancer patients, including antidepressants, antihistamines, atypical antipsychotic agents, and neurolepics. Antidepressants are increasingly used for the management of insomnia.[36] Specifically, tricyclic antidepressants such as amitripyline or doxepin, trazadone, and mirtazapine, may provide sedation in patients who are not depressed, as well as those who are depressed. Antihistamines such as diphenhydramine and hydroxyzine are used for their sedative properties as well as for their anticholinergic properties to treat insomnia and help relieve nausea and vomiting. Atypical antipsychotics such as danzapine have been used for their sedating effects and their ability to improve appetite and relieve opioid-induced nausea. Neuroleptics, such as thioridazine, have been found to promote sleep, especially in patients with insomnia associated with organic mental syndrome and delirium.[37]

## Nonpharmacologic Intervention

Several nonpharmacologic interventions have been used for the treatment of insomnia in healthy patients, but more intervention studies are needed to address insomnia in patients with cancer. Currently there are four categories of nonpharmacologic interventions for insomnia: cognitive–behavioral therapies (CBT), complementary therapies (CT), psychoeducation and information, and exercise.

*Cognitive–Behavioral Therapies.* Cognitive–behavioral therapies involve a variety of behavioral and psychological treatments aimed at changing negative thought processes, attitudes, and behaviors related to a person's ability to fall asleep, stay asleep, get enough sleep, and function during the day. Cognitive–behavioral therapies that have been tested in patients with cancer include stimulus control, sleep restriction, relaxation therapy, sleep hygiene, profile-tailored CBT, and cognitive restructuring strategies. These therapies have been shown to produce significant improvement sleep quality, longer duration, higher sleep efficiency.[38–42]

*Complimentary Therapies.* Complimentary therapies are interventions that are not considered to be part of conventional medicine. In patients with cancer, several complimentary therapies have been tested: aromatherapy, expressive therapy, expressive writing, healing, autogenic training, massage, muscle relaxation, mindfulness-based stress reduction, and yoga. These therapies have resulted in improvement in sleep quality, duration and efficiency, use of fewer medications, and less daytime dysfunction.[43–55]

*Psychoeducation.* Psychoeducation includes the use of structured education provided to patients with specific information regarding treatments and side effects. Two studies evaluated the effect of psychoeducation on the severity of the side effects from radiation and chemotherapy.[55,56] Kim and colleagues (2002) found that educational information tapes increased sleep duration in men receiving radiation for localized prostate cancer. Williams and Schreier[56] found no change in sleep disturbances after using informational audiotapes in women with breast cancer undergoing chemotherapy. The results suggest that patients who receive more detailed, user-friendly information about their treatment may benefit from this form of assistance for their insomnia. Further studies are necessary to explore the benefit of psychoeducation in insomnia in patients with cancer and other diseases.

*Exercise Interventions.* Exercise interventions involve any planned, structured, and repetitive bodily movement that is performed for the purpose of conditioning any part of the body, improving health, or maintaining fitness. Several studies evaluated the efficacy of exercise intervention for the treatment of insomnia in patients with cancer and they reported less difficulty sleeping and improved sleep patterns and quality.[57–59]

*Sleep Hygiene.* Sleep hygiene involves changing current health practices and environmental factors to new behaviors that will promote improved quantity and quality of sleep.[17] Included in the sleep hygiene interventions are curtailing time in bed, eliminating the bedroom clock, exercising in the late afternoon or early evening, avoiding alcohol, caffeine and nicotine, regularizing the bedtime, eating a light bedtime snack, exploring napping, avoiding use of sleeping pills, limiting liquids before bed, taking hot baths, leaving the bed if awake, eliminating noise from the bedroom, and regulating the temperature in the bedroom.[10,60,61] Sleep hygiene is a promising behavioral approach to aid sleep in patients with cancer and other diseases.

## Nursing Interventions

One of the key components of oncology nurses' and palliative care nurses' scope of practice is symptom management. These nurses are often the first-line providers and thus are responsible for understanding the consequences of insomnia on quality of life, and for recognizing the relationships between patient insomnia and disease-related treatments (Table 22–2). Nurses are often in a position to influence decisions regarding interventions to promote optimal sleep, both pharmacologic and nonpharmacologic. Educational programs for nurses that offer information about insomnia and interventions are therefore important and should be introduced at the graduate and undergraduate level.[62]

---

**Table 22–2**
**Potential Consequences of Insomnia in the Context of Cancer**

**Psychologic and behavioral consequences**
Fatigue
Cognitive impairments (e.g., memory, concentration)
Mood disturbances and psychiatric disorders

**Psychological and health consequences**
Health problems and physical symptoms (e.g., pain)
Longevity
Immunosuppression

*Source:* Data from Savard & Morin (2001), reference 10.

## Conclusion

Insomnia remains a common and distressing complaint in patients with cancer, in cancer survivors, and in those with chronic debilitating diseases. Insomnia has been linked to psychological and/or physiological malfunction. The importance of healthy sleep in patients who are chronically ill cannot be overestimated.

Effective management of insomnia begins with a thorough assessment that will include the exploration of predisposing factors such as insomnia prior to diagnosis, usual sleep patterns, emotional status, exercise and activity level, and other disease-related symptoms and medications. Tools such as The Clinical Sleep Assessment for Adults and Children may be used to screen for insomnia.[63] Typically, insomnia is treated with hypnotic drugs; however, more recent findings support the use of cognitive–behavioral therapies, complementary therapies, psychoeducation and information, and exercise to treat insomnia.

The challenge for palliative care nurses is to adequately provide patients with education regarding healthy sleep patterns. Nurses need to acquire a better understanding of the multidimensionality of sleep and to be aware that patients may not relate their symptoms to sleep issues. Unfortunately, insomnia in patients with cancer and other debilitating chronic diseases has only recently received attention from cancer researchers. Studies aimed to determine the etiology of insomnia in this population, and the appropriate treatment, is much needed.

REFERENCES

1. Department of Health & Human Services. Insomnia. Available at: www.hhs.gov (accessed November 12, 2008).
2. Bixler EO, Kales A, Soldatos CR, Kales JD, Healey S. Prevalence of sleep disorders in the Los Angeles metropolitan area. Am J Psychiatry 1979;136(10):1257–1262.
3. Ford DE, Kamerow DB. Epidemiologic study of sleep disturbances and psychiatric disorders. An opportunity for prevention? JAMA 1989;262(11):1479–1484.
4. Mellinger GD, Balter MB, Uhlenhuth EH. Insomnia and its treatment. Prevalence and correlates. Arch Gen Psychiatry 1985;42(3):225–232.
5. Agargun MY, Kara H, Solmaz M. Sleep disturbances and suicidal behavior in patients with major depression. J Clin Psychiatry 1997;58:249–251.
6. Benca RM. Consequences of insomnia and its therapies. J Clin Psychiatry 2001;62:33–38.
7. McCall WV. A psychiatric perspective on insomnia. J Clin Psychiatry 2001;62:27–32.
8. Roth T, Ancoli-Israel S. Daytime consequences and correlates of insomnia in the United States: Results of the 1991 National Sleep Foundation Survey II. Sleep Med Rev 1999;22:S354–S358.
9. Dinges DF, Pack F, Williams K. Cumulative sleepiness, mood disturbance, and psychomotor vigilance performance decrements during a week of sleep restricted to 4–5 hours per night. Sleep Med Rev 1997;20:267–277.
10. Savard J, Morin CM. Insomnia in the context of cancer: A review of a neglected problem. J Clin Oncol 2001;19:895–908.
11. American Psychiatric Association. Diagnostic and Statistical Manual of Mental Disorders (4th ed). Washington, DC: American Psychiatric Association, 2000.
12. American Sleep Disorders Association. The International Classification of Sleep Disorders: Diagnostic and Coding Manual. Rochester, MN: American Sleep Disorders Association, 1997.
13. Fortner BV, Stepanski EJ, Wang SC, Kasprowicz S, Durrence HH. Sleep and quality of life in breast cancer patients. J Pain Symptom Manage 2002;24(5):471–480.
14. Kaye J, Kaye K, Madow L. Sleep patterns in patients with cancer and patients with cardiac disease. J Psychol 1983;114(1st Half):107–113.
15. Couzi RJ, Helzlsouer KJ, Fetting JH. Prevalence of menopausal symptoms among women with a history of breast cancer and attitudes toward estrogen replacement therapy. J Clin Oncol 1995;13:2737–2744.
16. Lindley C, Vasa S, Sawyer WT, Winer EP. Quality of life and preferences for treatment following systemic adjuvant therapy for early-stage breast cancer. J Clin Oncol 1998;16:1380–1387.
17. Stepanski EJ, Wyatt JK. Use of sleep hygiene in the treatment of insomnia. Sleep Med Rev 2003;7:215–225.
18. Kozachik SL, Bandeen-Roche K. Predictors of patterns of pain, fatigue, and insomnia during the first year after a cancer diagnosis in the elderly. Cancer Nurs 2008;31(5):334–344.
19. Passaro E. Insomnia. eMedicine from WebMD. 2008. Available at: http://emedicine.medscape.com (accessed September 23, 2008).
20. National Cancer Institute. Sleep Disorders (PDQ). U.S. National Institutes in Health, 2009. Available at: http://www.cancer.gov/cancertopics/pdq/supportivecare/sleepdisorders/HealthProfessional (accessed February 9, 2009).
21. Sivertsen B, Omvik S, Pallesen S, et al. Cognitive behavioral therapy vs. zopiclone for treatment of chronic primary insomnia in older adults: A randomized controlled trial. JAMA 2006;295(24):2851–2858.
22. Schutte-Rodin S, Broch L, Buysse D, Dorsey C, Sateia M. Clinical guideline for the evaluation and management of chronic insomnia in adults. J Clin Sleep Med 2008;4(5):487–504.
23. Edinger JD, Wohlgemuth WK, Radtke RA, Coffman CJ, Carney CE. Dose-response effects of cognitive–behavioral insomnia therapy: A randomized clinical trial. Sleep 2007;30(2):203–212.
24. Strine TW, Chapman DP, Ahluwalia IB. Menstrual-related problems and psychological distress among women in the United States. J Womens Health (Larchmt) 2005;14(4):316–323.
25. Morin CM, Bootzin RR, Buysse DJ, Edinger JD, Espie CA, Lichstein KL. Psychological and behavioral treatment of insomnia: Update of the recent evidence (1998–2004). Sleep 2006;29(11):1398–1414.
26. Walsh JK, Krystal AD, Amato DA, et al. Nightly treatment of primary insomnia with eszopiclone for six months: Effect on sleep, quality of life, and work limitations. Sleep 2007;30(8):959–968.
27. Buysse DJ. Rational pharmacotherapy for insomnia: Time for a new paradigm. Sleep Med Rev 2000;4:521–527.
28. Derogatis LR, Feldstein M, Morrow G. A survey of psychotropic drug prescriptions in an oncology population. Cancer 1997;44:1919–1929.
29. Kripke D. Hypnotic drugs: Deadly risks, doubtful benefits. Sleep Med Rev 2000;4:5–20.

30. Kryger M, Roth T, Dement W. Principles and Practice of Sleep Medicine. Philadelphia: Elsevier, Inc., 2005.

31. Eszopiclone. A new hypnotic. Med Lett Drugs Ther 2005; 47:17–19.

32. Greenblatt DJ. Pharmacology of benzodiazepine hypnotics. J Clin Psychiatry 1992;53(Suppl 6):7–13.

33. Neubauer DN. Pharmacological approaches for the treatment of chronic insomnia. Clin Cornerstone 2003;5:16–27.

34. Uchikawa O, Fukatsu K, Tokunoh R. Synthesis of a novel series of tricyclic indan derivatives as melatonin receptor agonists. J Med Chem 2002;45:4222–4239.

35. Erman M, Seiden D, Zammit G, Sainati S, Zhang J. An efficacy, safety, and dose-response study of ramelteon in patients with chronic primary insomnia. Sleep Med 2006;7:17–24.

36. Walsh JK, Schweitzer PK. Ten-year trends in the pharmacological treatment of insomnia. Sleep 1999;22:371–375.

37. National Cancer Institute (NCI). Sleep Disorders (PDQ) Health Professional Version. NCI, 2002. Available at: http://www.cancer.gov/cancertopics/pdq/supportivecare/sleepdisorders (accessed December 1, 2008).

38. Allison PJ, Edgar L, Nicolau B, Archer J, Black M, Hier M. Results of a feasibility study for a psycho-educational intervention in head and neck cancer. Psychooncology 2004;13:482–485.

39. Allison PJ, Nicolau B, Edgar L, Archer J, Black M, Hier M. Teaching head and neck cancer patients coping strategies: Results of a feasibility study. Oral Oncol 2004;40:538–544.

40. Davidson JR, Waisberg JL, Brundage MD, MacLean AW. Nonpharmacologic group treatment of insomnia: A preliminary study with cancer survivors. Psychooncology 2001;10:389–397.

41. Quesnel C, Savard J, Simard S, Ivers H, Morin CM. Efficacy of cognitive–behavioral therapy for insomnia in women treated for nonmetastatic breast cancer. J Consult Clin Psychol 2003;71:189–200.

42. Savard J, Simard S, Ivers H, Morin CM. Randomized study on the efficacy of cognitive–behavioral therapy for insomnia secondary to breast cancer, part I: Sleep and psychological effects. J Clin Oncol 2005;23:6083–6096.

43. Cannici J, Malcolm R, Peek LA. Treatment of insomnia in cancer patients using muscle relaxation training. J Behav Ther Exp Psychiatry September 1983;14(3):251–256.

44. Carlson LE, Garland SN. Impact of mindfulness-based stress reduction (MBSR) on sleep, mood, stress and fatigue symptoms in cancer outpatients. Int J Behav Med 2005;12(4):278–285.

45. Carlson LE, Speca M, Patel KD, Goodey E. Mindfulness-based stress reduction in relation to quality of life, mood, symptoms of stress, and immune parameters in breast and prostate cancer outpatients. Psychosom Med 2003;65(4):571–581.

46. Carlson LE, Speca M, Patel KD, Goodey E. Mindfulness-based stress reduction in relation to quality of life, mood, symptoms of stress and levels of cortisol, dehydroepiandrosterone sulfate (DHEAS) and melatonin in breast and prostate cancer outpatients. Psychoneuroendocrinology 2004;29(4):448–474.

47. Cohen L, Warneke C, Fouladi RT, Rodriguez MA, Chaoul-Reich A. Psychological adjustment and sleep quality in a randomized trial of the effects of a Tibetan yoga intervention in patients with lymphoma. Cancer 2004;100(10):2253–2260.

48. de Moor C, Sterner J, Hall M, et al. A pilot study of the effects of expressive writing on psychological and behavioral adjustment in patients enrolled in a Phase II trial of vaccine therapy for metastatic renal cell carcinoma. Health Psychol 2002;21(6):615–619.

49. Fobair P, Koopman C, DiMiceli S, et al. Psychosocial intervention for lesbians with primary breast cancer. Psychooncology 2002;11(5):427–438.

50. Shapiro SL, Bootzin RR, Figueredo AJ, Lopez AM, Schwartz GE. The efficacy of mindfulness-based stress reduction in the treatment of sleep disturbance in women with breast cancer: An exploratory study. J Psychosom Res 2003;54(1):85–91.

51. Simeit R, Deck R, Conta-Marx B. Sleep management training for cancer patients with insomnia. Support Care Cancer 2004;12(3):176–183.

52. Soden K, Vincent K, Craske S, Lucas C, Ashley S. A randomized controlled trial of aromatherapy massage in a hospice setting. Palliat Med 2004;18(2):87–92.

53. Weze C, Leathard HL, Grange J, Tiplady P, Stevens G. Evaluation of healing by gentle touch in 35 clients with cancer. Eur J Oncol Nurs 2004;8(1):40–49.

54. Wright S, Courtney U, Crowther D. A quantitative and qualitative pilot study of the perceived benefits of autogenic training for a group of people with cancer. Eur J Cancer Care (Engl) 2002;11(2):122–130.

55. Kim Y, Roscoe JA, Morrow GR. The effects of information and negative affect on severity of side effects from radiation therapy for prostate cancer. Support Care Cancer 2002;10:416–421.

56. Williams SA, Schreier AM. The role of education in managing fatigue, anxiety, and sleep disorders in women undergoing chemotherapy for breast cancer. Appl Nurs Res 2005;18:138–147.

57. Coleman EA, Coon S, Hall-Barrow J, Richards K, Gaylor D, Stewart. Feasibility of exercise during treatment for multiple myeloma. Cancer Nurs 2003;26:410–419.

58. Mock V, Dow KH, Meares CJ, et al. Effects of exercise on fatigue, physical functioning, and emotional distress during radiation therapy for breast cancer. Oncol Nurs Forum 1997;24:991–1000.

59. Young-McCaughan S, Mays MZ, Arzola SM, et al. Research and commentary: Change in exercise tolerance, activity and sleep patterns, and quality of life in patients with cancer participating in a structured exercise program. Oncol Nurs Forum 2003;30:441–454.

60. Jones R, Beck S. Decision Making in Oncology Nursing. Philadelphia: B.C. Decker, Inc., 1996.

61. McNally J, Stair J, Somerville E. Guidelines for Cancer Nursing Practice. Orlando: Grune and Stratton, Inc., 1998.

62. Lee KA, Landis C, Chasens ER, et al. Sleep and chronobiology: Recommendations for nursing education. Nurs Outlook 2004;52:126–133.

63. Lee KA, Ward TM. Critical components of a sleep assessment for clinical practice settings. Issues Ment Health Nurs 2005;26:739–750.

# 23

*Marianne Matzo*

# Sexuality

*I am a single woman but have been in a serious relationship for the past two years. My boyfriend has been very understanding and supportive during my diagnosis and treatment for Hodgkin's disease. Sex is a very important part of our relationship. We have lived together for the past year. I was admitted to the hospital several days ago. The nurses, doctors, and others come and go all day long. I wanted a private room but really couldn't afford the extra expense. One night, just before visiting hours were over, we decided to try to have a 'quickie.' We thought my roommate was asleep and tried to be very quiet. We pulled the curtains around the bed and turned off the lights. All of a sudden, the light went on and the curtain was pulled back. Come to find out my room-mate heard the noise I was making and thought I was having difficulty breathing. She had put on her call light for the nurse. We were so embarrassed. My boyfriend left quickly and I'm afraid I won't see him again. I think this is just too much for a 28-year-old guy.—A 26-year-old woman with Hodgkin's disease*

◆ **Key Points**
◆ *Sexuality is an integral part of the human experience.*
◆ *Health care providers often overlook the sexual needs of those receiving palliative care.*
◆ *Communication, privacy, and practical solutions to physical changes may have a positive impact on sexual health for the palliative care patient.*

Terminal illness and end-of-life care can interfere with sexual health and physical sexual functioning in many ways. These include: physiological changes; tissue damage; other organic manifestations of the disease; attempts to palliate the symptoms of advancing disease, such as fatigue, pain, nausea and vomiting; and psychological sequelae such as anxiety, depression, and body-image changes. The complexities of human sexuality are broad, especially for people coping with life-threatening illness and those who are facing the end of their lives.

The Sexual Health Model[1] (Figure 23–1) reflects these complexities by identifying ten broad components posited to be essential domains of healthy human sexuality: talking about sex; culture and sexual identity; sexual anatomy and functioning; sexual health care and safer sex; overcoming challenges to sexual health; body image; masturbation/fantasy; positive sexuality, intimacy and relationships; and spirituality and values.[1] A patient's experiences, symptoms and concerns throughout the course of his or her illness are dynamic and complex, and are represented in the model as potentially impacting sexual health and, ultimately, quality of life. This chapter is organized according to each component of the Sexual Health Model.[1]

## Talking About Sex

A cornerstone of the Sexual Health Model is the ability to talk comfortably and explicitly about sexuality, especially one's own sexual values, preferences, attractions, history, and behaviors.[1] This communication is necessary for one to effectively express needs to a partner, and to discuss with a health care provider the alterations in sexual health that have

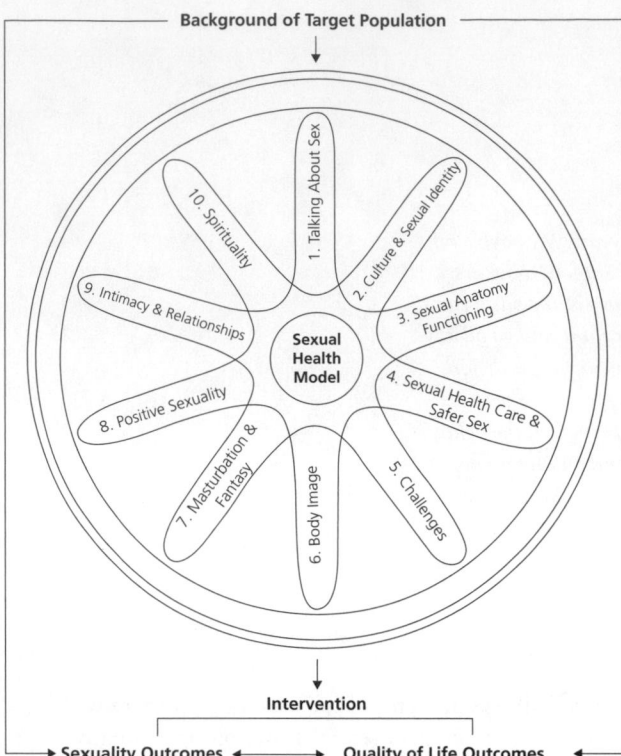

**Figure 23–1.** Sexual Health Model. *Source*: Robinson BBE, et al. (2002), reference 1. Used with permission.

resulted from illness. This is a valuable skill that must be learned and practiced.

An Institute of Medicine[2] report that addresses cancer care for the whole patient states that, in order to ensure appropriate psychosocial health, health care practitioners should facilitate effective communication. One study of an oncology population documented that 28% of the patients indicated their physicians do not pay attention to anything other than their medical needs.[3] Psychologic distress that patients or their partners experiences during diagnosis and treatment of malignancy can impair a healthy sexual response cycle.[4]

## Culture and Sexual Identity

Culture influences one's sexuality and sense of sexual self. It is important that individuals examine the impact of their particular cultural heritage on their sexual identities, attitudes, behaviors, and health.[1] The cultural meaning of sexual behaviors needs to be taken into account, because that meaning may impact a person's willingness or interest in maintaining sexual intimacy while receiving palliative care.

The patient and family are at the center of palliative care. A patient's desire or interest in maintaining physical sexual relations is highly variable. Some may find expression of physical love an important aspect of their life right up to death, while others may relinquish their "sexual being" early in the

end-of-life trajectory. Each individual's identity is influenced, in part, by his or her sexual identity. Roles between spouses or sexual partners are additionally defined by the sexual intimacy between them.

Sexual integrity can be both altered and compromised during the course of an incurable disease, deleteriously affecting both the identity and the role fulfillment of the affected person. Health care providers should not make assumptions about the level of interest or capacity a couple has for physical intimacy. Sexuality goes far beyond "sexual intercourse." Sexuality may encompass physical touch of any kind, as well as experiences of warmth, tenderness, and the expression of love.

The importance of physical intimacy vacillates throughout a relationship, and may be diminished or rekindled by a superimposed illness. Long-term palliative care providers may see sexual desire and expression ebb and flow between couples throughout the course of care. The patient may view sexual expression as an affirmation of life, a part of being human, a means to maintain role relationships, or the expression of passion in and for life itself.

Part IX of this book includes an international perspective on palliative care. There exists tremendous diversity of cultural, religious, and spiritual beliefs in relation to sexual intimacy and death. Culture often guides interactions between people, and even the mores within sexual interactions. Culturally competent health care providers should take into consideration the effect of culture on sexual expression. For example, do both members of the couple possess the same cultural identity? If not, are their identities similar in respect to beliefs about intimacy? What are the couple's health, illness, and sexual beliefs and practices? What are their customs and beliefs about intimacy, illness, and death? Issues such as personal space, eye contact, touch, and permissible topics to discuss with health care providers and/or members of the opposite sex may influence one's ability to intercede within the realm of intimate relations.

A cultural assessment is vital to determining whether these factors are an issue. Variations in sexual orientation must also be considered within the area of cultural competence. The beliefs, actions, and normative actions of homosexual and bisexual couples are important considerations when providing palliative care to a couple with alternate sexual expression.[5-7] Gay and lesbian couples may be offended by the assumption that they are heterosexual.[8] An example demonstrating the need for acknowledging and respecting individual sexuality follows.

CASE STUDY
*A 67-Year-Old Man with Prostate Cancer*

A 67-year-old man dying of prostate cancer once stated, "I am gay but I was married years ago and have three grown children. I have maintained a close supportive relationship with my ex-wife and children. However, for the past 17 years

I've been in a homosexual relationship with Todd. We are very close emotionally, spiritually, and physically. We have been very forthright about our sexual orientation with our families and friends, but it is difficult when I'm admitted to the hospital. Both my ex-wife and my partner visit me regularly. The staff acknowledges my ex-wife, but seem to think Todd is my business partner because I first introduced him as 'my partner.' From the onset, this was an embarrassing assumption on their part, and one I felt awkward in correcting. I have Todd accompany me more often than my ex-wife, but they see him as a friend who gives me rides. I know I should just come right out and explain the nature of my relationship; the problem is, I see so many different providers. I feel like I would have to keep going over this again and again. I don't want to be put in this position repeatedly. Todd is very frustrated by this misunderstanding, and I hate to see him upset. It is difficult enough to be going through the terminal cancer experience without adding another layer of embarrassment and confusion."

## Sexual Anatomy and Functioning

Sexual health assumes a basic knowledge, understanding, and acceptance of one's sexual anatomy, sexual response, and sexual functioning, as well as freedom from sexual dysfunction and other sexual problems.[1] Physical sexual expression is a basic aspect of human life, seen by many as fundamental to "being human." It is a complex phenomenon that basically comprises the greatest intimacy between two humans. The ability to give and to receive physical love is very important for many individuals, throughout the trajectory of an incurable illness.[9,10] The ability to maintain close sexual relations can be viewed as maintaining an essential part of one's "self."

Sexuality can affirm love, relieve stress and anxiety, and distract one from the emotional and physical sequelae of an eventually terminal chronic illness. Sexual expression can foster hope and accentuate spirituality. Health care providers in all clinical settings where palliative care is provided can be pivotal in facilitating the expression of sexuality in the terminal stages of life. Holistic palliative care throughout the trajectory of an incurable illness should include the promotion of sexual expression and assistance in preventing or minimizing the negative effects of disease progression on a couple's intimacy. Sexual partners' caring can comfortably include sexual expression if both parties are interested and able.

## Sexual Health Care and Safer Sex

As a component of the Sexual Health Model, physical health includes, but is not limited to, practicing safer sex behaviors,

knowing one's body, obtaining regular exams, and responding to physical changes with appropriate medical interventions.[1] The promotion or restoration of sexual health begins with a sexual assessment. Interventions to address alterations in sexual health cannot be adequately planned without thorough assessment.

Assessment should include the patient as well as his or her partner. Securing permission to include the sexual partner is necessary. For the nurse to perform this assessment, she or he must be comfortable with the topic of sexuality. Comfort with one's own sexuality conveys comfort to others. Additionally, the nurse's values, beliefs, and attitudes regarding sexuality greatly influence the capacity to discuss these issues in a nonjudgmental way.[11]

Perceived insufficient knowledge on the part of the health care provider is often an obstacle to frank sexual discussions. Additional sexual education and consistent assessment and counseling approaches will allay this discomfort. Education can be gained informally via discussions with colleagues and through consultation with experts in the area of human sexuality. Formal training is gained through in-service education offerings, workshops, and sexual-attitude reassessment programs. Knowledge can also be fostered by keeping abreast of new developments within the field by attending conferences, and reviewing journals and professional information via the Internet.[12]

Assessment of sexuality begins with a sexual history, and is then supplemented by data regarding the patient and partner's physical health as it influences intimacy, psychological sequelae of the chronic illness, sociocultural influences, and possible environmental issues.[13] Sexual health varies from person to person, so it is essential to determine if the couple is satisfied with their current level of sexual functioning.[14] Celibacy, for example, may have been present in the relationship for years. However, the trajectory of palliative care may have forced celibacy on an otherwise sexually active couple.[15] Determining the couple's need for interventions and assistance in this area is vital to determining appropriate interventions. The health care provider has many interventions available to prevent or minimize the untoward effects that palliative care may impose on sexual health.[13]

Obtaining a sexual history and performing a subsequent sexual assessment can be augmented using several communication techniques—assuring privacy and confidentiality; allowing for ample, uninterrupted time; and maintaining a nonjudgmental attitude. Addressing the topic of sexuality early in the relationship with a palliative care patient legitimizes the issue of intimacy.[16] It delivers the message that this is an appropriate topic for concern within the professional relationship, and is often met with relief on the part of the patient and couple. Often, sexuality concerns are present but unvoiced.[4]

Incorporating several techniques of therapeutic communication enhances the interview. These techniques include asking open-ended questions ("Some people who have an incurable illness are frustrated by their lack of private time with their spouse/sexual partner. How is this experience for you?"); using questions that refer to frequency as opposed to occurrence ("How often do you have intimate relations with your wife/husband/partner?" as opposed to "Do you have intimate relations with your wife/husband/partner?"); and "unloading" the question ("Some couples enjoy oral sex on a regular basis, while others seldom or never have oral sex. How often do you engage in oral sex?"). This last technique legitimizes the activity and allows the patient to feel safe in responding to the question in a variety of ways.[13]

Gender and age may also play a part in the patient's comfort with sexual discussions. An adolescent boy may feel more comfortable discussing sexual concerns with a male health care provider, whereas an elder woman may prefer to discuss sexual issues with a woman closer to her own age. Assessment of these factors may include statements like the following: "Many young men have questions about sexuality and the effect their illness may have on sexual functioning. This is something we can discuss or, if you'd be more comfortable, I could have one of the male nurses talk to you about this. Which would you prefer?"[13]

If the sexual history reveals a specific sexual problem, a more in-depth assessment is warranted. This would include the onset and course of the problem, the patient's or couple's thoughts about what caused the problem, any solutions that have been attempted, and potential solutions and their acceptability to the patient/couple. For example, use of a vibrator in the case of male impotence may be entirely acceptable to some couples but abhorrent to others. Determining what is and is not acceptable regarding potential solutions is part of the logical next step in sexual assessment.

Finally, documentation in the patient's chart should reflect the findings of the sexual assessment. Many institutions have a section for sexual assessment embedded within their intake form. This can be completed, and more thorough notes added to the narrative section on the chart. Findings, suggestions for remediation, and desired outcomes should be documented. This will prevent duplication of efforts, enhance communication within the health care team, and support continuity of care within the realm of sexual health.

## Challenges: Overcoming Barriers to Sexual Health

Challenges to sexual health include previous sexual history, developmental issues, privacy, and physical symptoms or side effects of symptom management.[7] Previous sexual history such as sexual abuse, substance abuse, compulsive sexual behavior, sex work, harassment, and discrimination are critical in any discussion of sexual health. This is particularly true in the context of interventions for cultural and sexual minorities, many of whom are disproportionately affected by these issues.[1] It is not uncommon to see our patients only as they present to us, without full appreciation of their previous life histories.

### Developmental Issues

There are a number of developmental issues that may play a part in the patient's ability to maintain intimacy during palliative care.[17] Often, health care providers assume sexual abstinence in the elderly and, to some degree, in adolescents and unmarried young adults.[18] However, intimacy may be a vital part of these individuals' lives.[19]

Chronological age may or may not be a determination of sexual activity.[20] For underage patients, parental influence may interfere with the ability to express physical love. Likewise, older adults may be inhibited by perceived societal values and judgments about their sexuality.[19–25] Maintaining an open, nonjudgmental approach to patients of all ages, sexual orientations, and marital status when assessing sexual health may foster trust and facilitate communication.

### Privacy

One of the main external challenges to maintaining intimate relations during palliative care is the lack of privacy. In Part VI of this book, the various settings in which end-of-life care may take place, and the concomitant issues raised within each setting, are addressed. In the acute care setting, privacy is often difficult to achieve. However, this obstacle can be removed or minimized by recognizing the need for intimacy and making arrangements to ensure quiet, uninterrupted time for couples. Private rooms are, of course, ideal. However, if this is not possible, arranging for roommates and visitors to leave for periods of time is necessary. A sign could be posted on the door that alerts health care providers, staff, and visitors that privacy is required. Finally, many rooms in the acute care setting have windows as opposed to walls, requiring the use of blinds and/or curtains to assure privacy. The nurse should offer such strategies rather than expecting patients to request privacy.

Similar issues may arise in the long-term care environment.[23] If privacy is a scarce commodity, assisting couples to maintain desired intimate relations is crucial in providing holistic care. Nurses in long-term care settings can initiate strategies to offer privacy. Such privacy may be more important than in acute care settings because the stay in long-term care is usually quite extended.[26] In both the acute care and long-term care settings, nurses can play a vital role in setting policy to facilitate the expression of intimacy and the maintenance of sexual health.

Home care may present an array of different obstacles for maintaining intimate relations, such as the ongoing presence of a health care provider other than the sexual partner. The home setting is often interrupted by professional visits as well as visits from family, friends, and clergy, which may be unplanned or unannounced. The telephone itself may be an unwelcome interruption. Often, when receiving home hospice care, the patient may have been moved from a more private bedroom setting to a more convenient central location, such as a den or family room, to aid caregiving and to enable the patient to maintain an integral role in family life. However, this move does not provide the privacy usually sought for intimate activity. There may not be a door to close; proximity of the patient's bed to the main rooms of the house may inhibit a couple's intimate activities, and they may need to schedule private time together. Necessary steps to maintain sexual relations include scheduling "rest periods" when one will not be disturbed; turning the ringer of the phone off; asking health care providers, friends, and clergy to call before visiting; and having family members respect periods of uninterrupted time.

CASE STUDY
*Privacy Issues at the End of Life*

My husband and I have been married for over 50 years. When I was diagnosed with ovarian cancer 9 months ago, it was devastating for both of us. The nights I spent in the hospital after my exploratory surgery were some of the roughest times in my life. Before then, I could count on one hand how many nights since our marriage we had not spent together in the same bed. Now it seems that number is growing exponentially. I wish we could have some time alone together. Now that the doctors have said the chemotherapy isn't working, there seems to be a steady stream of people through our house, both night and day. Our three grown children live in the area and often drop by to see us. Along with them come their spouses and grandchildren. Hospice has started paying daily visits, and friends and neighbors come by often. I long for just a little privacy with my husband. Just to hold each other, maybe snuggle and kiss or even just fall asleep in each other's arms would mean the world to me.—A patient with end-stage ovarian cancer

### Fatigue

Fatigue may be secondary to many factors. In Chapter 8, the etiology and management of fatigue were thoroughly addressed. Fatigue may render a patient unable to perform sexually. If fatigue is identified as a factor in the patient's ability to initiate or maintain sexual arousal, several strategies may be suggested to diminish these untoward effects.[27] Minimizing exertion during intimate relations may be necessary. Providing time for rest before and after sexual relations is often a sufficient strategy to overcome the detrimental effects of fatigue. Likewise, avoiding the stress of a heavy meal, alcohol consumption, or extremes in temperature may be helpful. Experimenting with positions that require minimal patient exertion (male-patient, female astride; female-patient, male astride) is often helpful. Finally, timing should be taken into consideration. Sexual activity in the morning upon awakening may be preferable over relations at the end of a long day. Planning for intimate time may replace spontaneity, but this can be a beneficial tradeoff.

### Pain

Sexual health can be impaired by the presence of pain, as well as the use of pain medication (especially opiates) which can interfere with sexual arousal.[28] In Chapters 6 and 7, the issues of pain assessment and management are comprehensively discussed. The goal of pain therapy is to alleviate or minimize discomfort; however, attaining that goal may result in an alteration in sexual responsiveness (i.e., libido or erectile function). Temporarily adjusting pain medications, or experimenting with complementary methods of pain management, should be explored. For example, using relaxation techniques and/or romantic music may decrease discomfort through distraction and relaxation, while enhancing sexual interest.

Physical sexual activity itself can be viewed as a form of distraction and subsequent relaxation. The couple should be encouraged to explore positions that offer the most comfort. Traditional positions may be abandoned for more comfortable ones, such as sitting in a chair or taking a side-lying position. Pillows can be used to support painful limbs or to maintain certain positions. A warm bath or shower before sexual activity may help pain relief and be seen as preparatory to intimate relations. Massage can be used as both an arousal technique and a therapeutic strategy for minimizing discomfort. Finally, suggesting the exploration of alternate ways of expressing tenderness and sexual gratification may be necessary if the couple's traditional intimacy repertoire is not feasible due to discomfort.

### Nausea and Vomiting

Nausea and vomiting are common during the palliative care trajectory and negatively impact sexual health. Chapter 10 discusses the etiology and treatment of these symptoms. There are many medications that suppress nausea; however, they may interfere with sexual functioning due to their sedative effects. If the patient complains of sexual difficulties secondary to treatment for nausea and vomiting, assess which antiemetics are prescribed and try another medication and/or use alternate nonpharmacological methods to control nausea and vomiting. As with fatigue, timing may be an important consideration for intimate relations. If the patient/couple notes that nausea is more prevalent during a certain time of the day, planning for intimacy at alternate times may circumvent this problem.[27]

### Neutropenia and Thrombocytopenia

Neutropenia and thrombocytopenia, per se, do not necessarily interfere with intimacy, but they do pose some potential problems. Sexual intimacy during neutropenic phases may jeopardize the compromised patient, because severe neutropenia predisposes the patient to infections. Close physical contact may be inadvisable if the sexual partner has a communicable disease, such as an upper respiratory infection or influenza. Specific sexual practices, such as anal intercourse, are prohibited during neutropenic states due to the likelihood of subsequent infection. The absolute neutrophil count, if available, is a good indicator of neutropenic status and associated risk for infection. Patient and partner education about the risks associated with neutropenia is essential.

Thrombocytopenia and the associated risk of bleeding, bruising, or hemorrhage should be considered when counseling a couple about intimacy issues. Again, anal intercourse is contraindicated due to risk for bleeding. Likewise, vigorous genital intercourse may cause vaginal bleeding. Indeed, even forceful or energetic hugging, massage, or kissing may cause bruising or bleeding. Preventative suggestions might include such strategies as gentle lovemaking, with minimal pressure on the thrombocytopenic patient, or having the patient assume the dominant position to control force and pressure.

### Dyspnea

Dyspnea is an extremely distressing occurrence in the end-of-life trajectory. In Chapter 14, the management of this symptom is reviewed. Dyspnea, or even the fear of initiating dyspnea, can impair sexual functioning.[29] General strategies can be employed to minimize dyspnea during sexual play. These can include using a waterbed to accentuate physical movements, raising the dyspneic patient's head and shoulders to facilitate oxygenation, using supplementary oxygen and/or inhalers before and during sexual activity, performing pulmonary hygiene measures before intimacy, encouraging slower movements to conserve energy, and modifying sexual activity to allow for enjoyment and respiratory comfort.[30,31]

### Neuropathies

Neuropathies can be a result of disease progression or complication of prior aggressive treatment. Neurological disturbances are discussed in depth in Chapter 19. Neuropathies can manifest as pain, paresthesia, and/or weakness. Depending on the location and severity of the neuropathy, sexual functioning can be altered or completely suppressed. Management or diminution of the neuropathy may or may not be feasible. If not, creative ways to evade the negative sequelae of this occurrence are necessary. Such strategies might include creative positioning, use of pillows to support affected body parts, or alternate ways of expressing physical love. The distraction of physical sexual expression may temporarily minimize the perception of the neuropathy.

### Mobility and Range of Motion

Mobility issues and compromised range of motion may interfere with sexual expression. Similar to issues related to fatigue, a decrease in mobility can inhibit a couple's customary means of expressing physical love.[32] A compromise in range of motion can result in a similar dilemma. For example, a female patient may no longer be able to position herself

in such a way as to allow penile penetration from above due to hip or back restrictions. Likewise, a male patient may have knee or back restrictions that make it impossible for him to be astride his partner. Regardless of the exact nature of the range-of-motion/mobility concern, several suggestions can be offered. Anti-inflammatory medication before sexual activity, experimenting with alternate positions, employing relaxation techniques before sexual play, massage, warm baths, and exploring alternative methods of expressing physical intimacy should be encouraged.[33]

### Erectile Dysfunction

Erectile dysfunction can be caused by physiological, psychological, and emotional factors.[34] These factors include vascular, endocrine, and neurological causes; chronic diseases, such as renal failure[35] and diabetes; and iatrogenic factors, such as surgery and medications. Surgical severing of the small nerve branches essential for erection is often a side-effect of radical pelvic surgery, radical prostatectomy, and aortoiliac surgery.[6] Vascular and neurological causes may not be reversible, although endocrine causes may be minimized. For example, the use of estrogen in advanced prostate cancer may be terminated in palliative care, which may result in the return of erectile function.

Many medications decrease desire and erectile capacity in men. The most common offenders are antihypertensives, antidepressants, antihistamines, antispasmodics, sedatives or tranquilizers, barbiturates, sex hormone preparations, narcotics, and psychoactive drugs.[36] Often, these medications cannot be discontinued to permit the return of erectile function; for those patients, penile implants may be an option.[37]

The use of sildenafil (Viagra), vardenafil HCl (Levitra), tadalafil (Cialis), and yohimbine (Yohimbine) have not been researched with patients receiving palliative care. These medications are classified as selective enzyme inhibitors. They relax smooth muscle, increase blood flow, and facilitate erection.[38] If a vascular component is part of the underlying erectile dysfunction, the use of one of these medications may correct the problem.[39] Contraindications such as underlying heart disease and other current medications should be taken into consideration.[40] Otherwise, if acceptable to the couple, digital or oral stimulation of the female partner or use of a vibrator can be suggested.[41]

### Dyspareunia

Dyspareunia, like erectile dysfunction, can be caused by physiological, psychological, and emotional factors. These factors include vascular, endocrine, and neurological causes as well as iatrogenic factors such as surgery and medications.[42] Vascular and neurological causes may not be reversible; endocrine causes may be minimized. For example, the use of estrogen replacement therapy (ERT), vaginal estrogen creams, or water-soluble lubricants may be helpful in diminishing vaginal dryness, which can cause painful intercourse. Gynecological surgery and pelvic irradiation may result in physiological changes that prevent comfortable intercourse.[43]

Post-irradiation changes, such as vaginal shortening, thickening, and narrowing, may result in severe dyspareunia.[44] For women, as with male patients, many medications decrease desire and function. These drugs include antihypertensives, antidepressants, antihistamines, antispasmodics, sedatives or tranquilizers, barbiturates, sex hormone preparations, narcotics, and psychoactive drugs. Often, these medications cannot be discontinued in order to facilitate the return of sexual health. For those patients, digital or oral stimulation of the male partner may be suggested, if acceptable. Additionally, intrathigh and intramammary penetration may be suggested to women who find vaginal intercourse too painful.

### Anxiety and Depression

Anxiety and depression related to the incurable and terminal aspects of the disease may interfere with sexual desire and response.[45] As two of the most common affective disorders during end-of-life care, they are thoroughly discussed in Chapter 20. Both anxiety and depression have profound effects on sexual functioning. Decreases in sexual desire, libido, and activity are common sequelae of these affective disorders. However, some interventions, especially pharmacological management, can further compromise sexual functioning.

A thorough assessment of the patient's psychological state and an evaluation of the medications currently prescribed for this condition may reveal the source of the problem. Anxiolytics and antidepressants are often prescribed for these conditions and have the potential for interfering with sexual functioning. Patients may choose symptom management and sacrifice sexual function. However, relaxation techniques, imagery, and biofeedback may lower anxiety to a tolerable level. Additionally, the release of sexual tension may itself resolve anxiety.

If desire is maintained and function alone is compromised for male patients, the couple may explore alternate ways of pleasing each other. For female patients, use of water-soluble lubricants can offset the interference with arousal, if interest remains intact. Open communication between the partners and with the health care provider allows for frank discussions and the presentation of possible alternatives to expressing physical affection.

### Body Image

In a culture with so many sexual images focused on a type of physical beauty unattainable for many, body image is an important aspect of sexual health. Challenging one, narrow standard of beauty and encouraging self-acceptance is relevant to all populations, and should be carried out in a culturally sensitive manner.[1] An incurable illness and concomitant end-of-life care can alter one's physical appearance. Additionally, past treatments for disease often irrevocably alter body appearance and function. Issues such as alopecia, weight loss, cachexia, the presence of a stoma, or amputation of a body part, to name a few, can result in feelings of sexual inadequacy and/or disinterest.[46,47]

End-of-life care can focus on the identification and remediation of issues related to body image changes. Although an altered appearance may be permanent, counseling and behavior modification, as well as specific suggestions to minimize or mask these appearances, can improve body image to a level compatible with positive sexual health. The use of a wig, scarf, or headbands can mask alopecia. Some patients, rather than try to conceal hair loss, choose to emphasize it by shaving their heads. Weight loss and cachexia can be masked through clothing and the creative use of padding.

The presence of an ostomy can significantly alter body image and negatively affect sexual functioning.[48,49] Specific interventions for minimizing the effect that the presence of an ostomy has on sexual functioning depend, in part, on the particular type of ostomy. Some patients are continent, while others need an appliance attached at all times.

If the patient has a continent ostomy, timing sexual activity can allow for removal of the appliance and covering the stoma. If the ostomy appliance cannot be safely removed, the patient should be taught to empty the appliance before intimate relations and to use a cover or body stocking to conceal the appliance. Alternate positions may also be considered, and in the event of a leak, sexual activity can continue in the shower. The United Ostomy Association (http://www.uoa.org) publishes four patient information booklets on sexuality and the ostomate.

### Masturbation and Fantasy

The topics of masturbation and fantasy are saddled with a myriad of historical myths associated with sin, illness, and immaturity that would need to be confronted in order to normalize masturbation. Encouraging masturbation as a normal adjunct to partnered sex can decrease the pressures on people to engage in penetrative sex with their partners more frequently than they have desire and arousal for.[1]

Some patients may view sexual expression as an essential aspect of their being, while others may see it as ancillary or unimportant. Some may have an established sexual partner; some may lose a partner through separation, divorce, or widowhood; others may begin a relationship during the course of their illness trajectory. Some patients may have several sexual partners; some couples may be gay or lesbian; others, without a sexual partner, may gain pleasure by erotic thoughts and masturbation. All of these scenarios are within the realm of the palliative care provider's patient base. Understanding the various forms of sexual expression and pleasure is paramount in providing comprehensive care.

## Intimacy and Relationships

Intimacy is a universal need that people try to meet through their relationships.[1] A sexual partner's interest and ability to maintain sexual relations throughout the palliative care trajectory can also be affected by many variables. Sexual expression may be impeded by the partner's mood state (anxiety, depression, grief, or guilt), exhaustion from caregiving and assuming multiple family roles, and misconceptions about sexual appropriateness during palliative care. Anxiety and depression have profound effects on sexual functioning. Decreases in libido and sexual activity can result from depressive and anxious states.[50,51]

A partner may feel that the patient is "too ill" to engage in sexual activity. In turn, the partner may feel remorse or guilt for even thinking about their loved one in a sexual capacity during this time. Partners may fear that they may injure their loved one during sexual activity due to the loved one's perceived or actual weakened state or appearance. The partner may have difficulty adjusting to the altered physical appearance of the patient (cachexia, alopecia, stomatitis, pallor, amputation, etc.). The role of caregiver may seem incompatible with that of sexual partner.

As the ill partner's health deteriorates, the well partner may assume caretaking roles that may seem incompatible with those of a lover. The myriad of responsibilities sequentially assumed by the well partner may leave him or her exhausted, which can interfere with sexual health and impede sexual performance. The partner may harbor misconceptions about sexual relations with a terminally ill partner, including diminishing the patient's waning energy reserves or causing the illness to progress more rapidly.

## Spirituality and Values

Sexual health assumes congruence between one's ethical, spiritual, and moral beliefs and one's sexual behaviors and values. In this context, spirituality may or may not include identification with formal religions, but it addresses moral and ethical concerns. Exposure to multiple cultural traditions (e.g., Native American storytelling, African American church activism, etc.) is important, especially in those traditions that have a positive and life-affirming view of sexuality.[1]

Individual, family, and cultural factors influence the development of healthy sexuality in adolescents. One factor that is less often considered, but may play a role, is religion/spirituality. Attitudes or beliefs about having sex before marriage, decisions about the timing of coital debut, or contraceptive practices may be shaped by their religious/spiritual belief system, or the cultural/religious context in which they were raised.[52] These values may influence the decisions that an adolescent with a life-limiting disease may make regarding sexual experiences that they choose to engage in before they die.

## Interventions

The specific sexual needs and concerns of the patient and couple determine the approach and type of intervention. The intervention can address current needs, or focus on potential future needs in the form of anticipatory guidance. False assumptions about intimacy during palliative care can be addressed, and anticipatory guidance regarding what to expect as a result of advancing disease and palliative treatment is included in this discussion.

Specific suggestions should go beyond limited information, and be explicit, to help the patient and their partner attain a mutually stated goal. Specific suggestions usually pertain to communication, symptom management, and alternate physical expression. Open communication between the couple and their health care practitioner regarding sexual health is essential for successful symptom management. Candid discussions regarding their emotional responses to this phase of their relationship, their fears and concerns, and their hopes and desires are included in these interactions.

Symptom management is essential to optimizing sexual expression. Alternate expressions of physical intimacy may be necessary if sexual disruption is due to organic changes. If intercourse is difficult, painful, or impossible, the couple may be counseled regarding how to expand their sexual repertoire. A thorough discussion of the couple's values, attitudes, and preferences should be done before suggesting alternatives. Using language that is understandable to the patient/partner is essential. However, the use of slang or street language may be uncomfortable to the health care practitioner—defining terms early in the discussion will alleviate this potential problem.

There are many ways of giving and receiving sexual pleasure; genital intercourse is only one way of expressing physical love. The nurse can encourage the couple to expand their sexual expression to include hugging, massage, fondling, caressing, cuddling, kissing, hand-holding, and masturbation, either mutually or singularly. Sexual gratification may be derived from manual, oral, and digital stimulation. Intrathigh, anal, and intramammary intercourse are also options if the female partner is unable to continue vaginal penetration.

## Summary

Incurable illness and end-of-life care may result in compromising a couple's intimacy. To prevent or minimize this, health care practitioners should assume a leading role in the assessment and remediation of potential or identified alterations in sexual functioning. Not all couples will be concerned about their sexual health at this point of their life together. However, if sexual health is desired, all attempts should be made to facilitate this important aspect of life. People may find that being physically close to the one they love is life-affirming and comforting.

As patients draw close to the end of life, their needs, hopes, and concerns remain intact as in any other stage of their life. Assessment of sexual health should occur for all patients to determine if these needs and hopes include maintenance of their sexual health. The health care practitioner's offer of information and support can make a significant difference in a couple's ability to adjust to the changes in sexual health during end-of-life care. The realm of sexual health and intimacy during end-of-life care remains an area in which further research is warranted. Incorporating intimacy research into end-of-life care research is a natural and much-needed area of inquiry.

## REFERENCES

1. Robinson BBE, Bockting WO, Simon Rosser BR, Miner M, Coleman E. The Sexual Health Model: Application of a sexological approach to HIV prevention. Health Educ Res 2002;17(1):43–57.

2. Institute of Medicine. Cancer Care for the Whole Patient: Meeting Psychosocial Health Needs. Washington, DC: The National Academies Press, 2007.

3. Young P. Caring for the whole patient: The Institute of Medicine proposes a new standard of care. Community Oncol 2007;4(12):748–751.

4. Krychman ML, Pereira L, Carter J, Amsterdam A. Sexual oncology: Sexual health issues in women with cancer. Oncology 2006;71(1–2):18–25.

5. Alfano CM, Rowland JH. Recovery issues in cancer survivorship: A new challenge for supportive care. Cancer J 2006;12(5):432–443.

6. Galbraith ME, Crighton F, Galbraith ME, Crighton F. Alterations of sexual function in men with cancer. Semin Oncol Nurs 2008;24(2):102–114.

7. Shell JA, Shell JA. Sexual issues in the palliative care population. Semin Oncol Nurs 2008;24(2):131–134.

8. Dibble SL, Eliason MJ, Christiansen MAD. Chronic illness care for lesbian, gay, & bisexual individuals. Nurs Clin North Am 2007;42(4):655–674.

9. Hordern AJ, Currow DC. A patient-centered approach to sexuality in the face of life-limiting illness. Med J Aust 2003;179(6 Suppl):S8–S11.

10. Rice A. Sexuality in cancer and palliative care 1: Effects of disease and treatment. Int J Palliat Nurs 2000;6(8):392–397.

11. Krebs LU. Sexual assessment: Research and clinical. Nurs Clin North Am 2007;42(4):515–529.

12. Hordern A, Street A. Communicating about patient sexuality and intimacy after cancer: Mismatched expectations and unmet needs. MJA 2007;186(5):224–227.

13. Sadovsky R, Nusbaum M. Sexual health inquiry and support is a primary care priority. J Sex Med 2006;3(1):3–11.

14. Higgins A, Barker P, Begley CM. Sexuality: The challenge to espoused holistic care. Int J Nurs Pract 2006;12(6):345–351.

15. Sanders S, Pedro LW, Bantum EO, Galbraith ME. Couples surviving prostate cancer: Long-term intimacy needs and concerns following treatment. Clin J Oncol Nurs 2006;4:503–508, 21–23.

16. Huber C, Ramnarace T, McCaffrey R. Sexuality and intimacy issues facing women with breast cancer. Oncol Nurs Forum 2006;33(6):1163–1167.

17. Stausmire JM. Sexuality at the end of life. Am J Hosp Palliat Med 2004;21(1):33–39.

18. Stroberg P, Hedelin H, Bergstrom AB. Is sex only for the healthy and wealthy? J Sex Med 2007;4(1):176–182.

19. Hurd Clarke L. Older women and sexuality: Experiences in marital relationships across the life course. Can J Aging 2006;25(2):129–140.

20. Lindau ST, Schumm LP, Laumann EO, Levinson W, O'Muircheartaigh CA, Waite LJ. A study of sexuality and health among older adults in the United States. N Engl J Med 2007;357:762–774.

21. Lesser J, Hughes S, Kumar S. Sexual dysfunction in the older woman. Complex medical, psychiatric illnesses should be considered in evaluation and management. Psychiatr Consult 2005;60(8):18–22.

22. Loehr J, Verma S, Seguin V. Issues of sexuality in older women. J Womens Health 1997;6(4):451–457.

23. Malatesta VJ. Sexual problems, women and aging: An overview. J Women Aging 2007;19(1–2):139–154.

24. Scott LD. Sexuality & older women. Exploring issues while promoting health. AWHONN Lifelines 2002;6(6):520–525.

25. Robinson JG, Molzahn AE. Sexuality and quality of life. J Gerontol Nurs 2007;33(3):19–29.

26. Everett B, Everett B. Supporting sexual activity in long-term care. Nurs Ethics 2008;15(1):87–96.

27. Stead ML. Sexual function after treatment for gynecological malignancy. Curr Opin Oncol 2004;16:492–495.

28. Abs R, Verhelst J, Maeyaert J, et al. Endocrine consequences of long-term intrathecal administration of opioids. J Clin Endocrinol Metab 2000;85(6):2215–2222.

29. Vincent EE, Singh SJ. Review article: Addressing the sexual health of patients with COPD: The needs of the patient and implications for health care professionals. Chron Respir Dis 2007;4(2):111–115.

30. Hardin S. Cardiac disease and sexuality: Implications for research and practice. Nurs Clin North Am 2007;42(4):593–603.

31. Goodell TT. Sexuality in chronic lung disease. Nurs Clin North Am 2007;42(4):631–638.

32. Newman AM. Arthritis and sexuality. Nurs Clin North Am 2007;42(4):621–630.

33. Kautz DD. Hope for love: Practical advice for intimacy and sex after stroke…including commentary by Secrest J. Rehabil Nurs 2007;32(3):95–103, 32.

34. Resendes LA, McCorkle R. Spousal responses to prostate cancer: An integrative review. Cancer Invest 2006;24:192–198.

35. Katz A. What have my kidneys got to do with my sex life?: The impact of late-stage chronic kidney disease on sexual function. AJN, Am J Nurs 2006;106(9):81–83.

36. Karadeniz T, Topsakal M, Aydogmus A, et al. Erectile dysfunction under age 40: Etiology and role of contributing factors. Scientific WorldJournal 2004;4(Suppl 1):171–174.

37. Mulcahy JJ, Wilson SK, Mulcahy JJ, Wilson SK. Current use of penile implants in erectile dysfunction. Curr Urol Rep 2006;7(6):485–489.

38. Ali ST, Ali ST. Effectiveness of sildenafil citrate (Viagra) and tadalafil (Cialis) on sexual responses in Saudi men with erectile dysfunction in routine clinical practice. Pak J Pharm Sci 2008;21(3):275–281.

39. Hartmann U, Burkart M. Erectile dysfunctions in patient–physician communication: Optimized strategies for addressing sexual issues and the benefit of using a patient questionnaire. J Sex Med 2007;4(1):38–46.

40. Ezzell A, Baum N, Ezzell A, Baum N. When Viagra doesn't work. Treating erectile dysfunction. Diabetes Self Manag 2008;25(2):29–30.

41. Bruner DW, Calvano T. The sexual impact of cancer and cancer treatments in men. Nurs Clin North Am 2007;42(4):555–580.

42. Stead ML, Stead ML. Sexual function after treatment for gynecological malignancy. Curr Opin Oncol 2004;16(5):492–495.

43. Carmack Taylor CL, Basen-Engquist K, Shinn EH, et al. Predictors of sexual functioning in ovarian cancer patients. J Clin Oncol 2004;22(5):881–889.

44. Yamamoto R, Okamoto K, Ebina Y, Shirato H, Sakuragi N, Fujimoto S. Prevention of vaginal shortening following radical hysterectomy. BJOG 2000;107(7):841–845.

45. Brandberg Y, Sandelin K, Erikson S, et al. Psychological reactions, quality of life, and body image after bilateral prophylactic mastectomy in women at high risk for breast cancer: A prospective 1-year follow-up study. [see comment]. J Clin Oncol 2008;26(24):3943–3949.

46. Alfano CM, Rowland JH, Alfano CM, Rowland JH. Recovery issues in cancer survivorship: A new challenge for supportive care. Cancer J 2006;12(5):432–443.

47. Hinsley R, Hughes R, Hinsley R, Hughes R. 'The reflections you get': An exploration of body image and cachexia. Int J Palliat Nurs 2007;13(2):84–89.

48. Penson RT, Gallagher J, Gioiella ME, et al. Sexuality and cancer: Conversation comfort zone. Oncologist 2000;5(4):336–344.

49. Kilic E, Taycan O, Belli AK, et al. The effect of permanent ostomy on body image, self-esteem, marital adjustment, and sexual functioning. Turk Psikiyatri Dergisi 2007;18(4):302–310.

50. Barton-Burke M, Gustason CJ. Sexuality in women with cancer. Nurs Clin North Am 2007;42(4):531–554.

51. Stead ML, Brown JM, Fallowfield L, Selby P. Communication about sexual problems and sexual concerns in ovarian cancer: A qualitative study. West J Med 2002;176(1):18–19.

52. Cotton S, Berry D, Cotton S, Berry D. Religiosity, spirituality, and adolescent sexuality. Adolesc Med 2007;18(3):471–483.

# 24

*Patrick J. Coyne, Thomas J. Smith, and Laurel J. Lyckholm*

# Clinical Interventions, Economic Impact, and Palliative Care

*You Ain't Seen Nothing Yet.—Bachman Turner Overdrive*

♦ **Key Points**
♦ *The scope of nursing and nursing education has expanded to include multiple domains, many of which overlap other disciplines such as wellness, disease prevention, and health services administration.*
♦ *Economic outcome is an area in which nursing plays an essential role in providing efficient, cost-effective, and appropriate palliative care.*
♦ *Health services research regarding economic outcomes, while limited, may help create a framework for addressing how to make palliative care available to everyone in an ethical, economic, and effective manner.*
♦ *Most nurses have major a influence in clinical interventions, yet often do not consider the economic impact.*

## Why Are Economic Outcomes Important?

- Health care spending and health care quality are major challenges in the United States, with health care spending reaching $2.3 trillion or $7,600 per person, a number expected to triple in the next 10 years. By several measures, health care spending continues to rise at the fastest rate in history. By 2007, there was an annual increase of 6.9%, In 2007, employer health insurance premiums increased by 6.1 percent—two times the rate of inflation. The annual premium for an employer health plan covering a family of four averaged nearly $12,100, and the annual premium for single coverage averaged over $4,400.[1,2] Drug costs and rising hospital expenses fueled much of this spending.[1-7]

- The financial costs of cancer are great, for both the individual and for society as a whole. The economic burden is likely to increase as the population ages, the absolute number of people treated for cancer increases, and newer technologies and expensive treatments are adopted as standards of care.[5] Already in the year 2004, the National Institutes of Health estimated overall annual costs for cancer to be $189.8 billion, with direct medical costs totaling $69.4 million, and indirect costs from lost productivity to be $16.9 billion due to illness and $103.5 billion due to premature death.[4] The United States spends more on health care than other industrialized nations, and those countries provide health insurance to all their citizens.[3] Nearly 47 million Americans are uninsured, primarily because of the high cost of health insurance coverage.[5]

- Rising health care costs correlate to reductions in health insurance coverage.[4] According to the 2003 National Health Interview Survey data, nearly 27% of Americans between the ages of 18 and 24, and 20% of Americans between the ages of 25 and 44 reported not having a regular source of health care.[4] Additionally, 17% of Americans under age 65 have no health insurance, and about one third of older individuals have Medicare coverage only.[6]

- We spend too much money on care near the end of life. Nearly one third of all Medicare dollars are spent on patients in their last year of life.[8,9] Although it is not a zero-sum situation, there is good evidence that the more is spent on high-technology care for the elderly, the less funds are available for preventive services or treatment of chronic disease conditions for the same population.[10] In addition, 16%–20% of solid tumor patients receive chemotherapy within two weeks of their death. Such treatment is unlikely to benefit them, but is likely to increase toxicity and costs[10]. The drain on health care-directed funds is likely to increase, due to heightened demands from an educated elderly population, more elderly long-term survivors, new and expensive technologies, new diseases, and demands for cost cutting.

Cost effectiveness of interventions must be continually assessed. Whatever is spent must be both appropriate to the patient's goals and maximize the resources available.[11,12] The question of when, where, and why to use high-tech and high-cost interventions at least partially drives this debate and must be carefully explored.

There are substantial concerns about the quality of palliative care in our current system. The Study to Understand Prognoses and Preferences for Outcomes and Risks of Treatment (SUPPORT) showed that half of all dying patients had unnecessary pain and suffering in their final days of life while in the hospital.[13] Cleeland and colleagues found that nearly half of all patients suffer unnecessary pain, even when cared for by oncologists.[14] Experts agree that our health care system has inefficiencies, excessive administrative expenses, inflated prices, poor management, and in some cases inappropriate care, waste and fraud. These problems significantly increase the cost of medical care and health insurance for employers and workers, and affect the financial security of families. Palliative care can help decrease costs while improving the care received. A recent report on multiple health care systems indicated that provision of palliative care saves money for society, in amounts ranging from several hundred to several thousand dollars per admission.[15,16]

The neglected area of cancer care quality and costs is under scrutiny. Active efforts are underway to improve both areas.[16] The relationship of volume to quality is striking,[17] as revealed in the following reports: (1) a significant (5% to 10%) overall survival advantage at a breast cancer specialty center versus community hospitals;[18,19] (2) better survival for testicular cancer patients treated at specialist centers;[20] (3) better survival and fewer complications for ovarian cancer surgery performed by specialist gynecological oncologists rather than general surgeons or gynecologists;[21] and (4) better survival for prostate cancer patients at high-volume centers.[21–23] Clearly, there is a need for additional research to address these questions of quality care. In addition, nurses must be knowledgeable about health care outcomes, in particular those issues related to palliative care: the patient/family unit of care, quality of life, and decision making around end-of-life care. Unfortunately, many nurses are largely unaware and/or uninformed about these issues. Those that are aware may not have a voice within their institutions. Greater knowledge may empower nurses to take a more prominent, collaborative place at the table when such issues are being discussed and decisions are being made.

We have identified some important questions about economic outcomes and palliative care, which are listed in Tables 24–1 and 24–2.

## The Ethics of Adding Economic Outcomes

In the modern arena of health care, nonmedical concerns, such as cost control, oversight and audit, utilization review,

**Table 24–1**
**Types of Needed Health and Service Research Studies**

| Type of Study | Question Posed |
|---|---|
| Policy analysis | What outcomes justify treatment? Who should make those decisions? |
| Type of care: chemotherapy vs. best or other types of supportive care | Does chemotherapy save money compared to best supportive care when all costs are considered? |
| Site of service | Is home site more effective and less costly compared to hospital? |
| Structural and process changes in care | Can costs be reduced by changing how care is delivered, e.g., by inpatient hospice or at home? |
| Hospice vs. nonhospice | Does hospice improve quality of life and/or reduce costs of care? |
| Advance directives and do-not-resuscitate orders | Do advance directives influence medical treatment decisions and/or change costs? |
| Nursing ability to impact cost at end of life | Can skilled palliative care nurses effectively palliate patients and effect a savings of resources? |

Table 24–2
Outcomes that Justify a Medical Intervention

| Justify | Do Not Justify |
|---|---|
| Improved overall survival | False hope that survival will be improved |
| Improved disease-free survival | |
| Improved quality of life | |
| Less toxicity | |
| Improved cost effectiveness | Cost alone |

and decreasing liability risk, have assumed a significant role. Almost all authorities have argued that such management tools are ethical.[23] While quality care is the primary goal of hospice and palliative medicine, cost control is an important consideration. Nursing and medicine aspire to promoting health and providing comfort and relief of suffering in a just manner. Cost control through aggressive disease management, or "critical paths," may actually promote these goals by making more and/or better care available. However, the current systems reward/pay for hi-tech interventions but fail to reimburse effective low-tech treatments.[24,25] An example of this discrepancy is that some insurance will reimburse a patient-controlled analgesia pump but will not reimburse oral analgesics.

Cost control must be differentiated from profit motivation and entrepreneurship, which have not traditionally been considered the goals of medicine. These activities in the context of health care are unethical in that they may make medical care more expensive and difficult to access, especially for those who are socially disadvantaged. They may also create further conflicts of interest in already precarious fiduciary relationships between clinicians and their patients. A code of ethics that covers all professionals, rather than medicine alone, might be useful.[26–31]

If palliative care can be improved and/or made less costly without sacrificing quality, it should be done in the service of promoting the values of beneficence, compassion, and respect for autonomy. Palliative care has emerged as a national movement, with the advent of several important initiatives (e.g., Oncology Nursing Society; Hospice and Palliative Nurses Association; Education for Physicians on End-of-Life Care (EPEC); and the End of Life Nursing Consortium (ELNEC)). Other well established national resource educational programs include the National Palliative Care Resource Center; City of Hope, CA; the Center to Improve Care of the Dying at George Washington University; and the Center to Advance Palliative Care at Mount Sinai Hospital in New York). In addition, palliative care programs continue to develop all over the world.

The Healthcare Finance Administration's approval of an International Classification of Diseases 9 code (ICD-9) for palliative care was a start in the effort to obtain data on the impact of palliative care in the health care system. It is to be expected that both hospice and palliative care will undergo careful scrutiny in the next several years.[26]

Some have argued that budgets should not be balanced with penalty to one group, such as the elderly or those on Medicare.[28] Many health care goods are rationed justly (benefit versus risk) according to age, such as transplants, coronary bypass, and hemodialysis. This rationing is based on the theory of equality of opportunity according to ability to benefit from such procedures.[29] However, palliative care is different in that age does not determine whether a person stands to benefit. In this circumstance, the ethic of distributive justice supports the concept that medical and social needs dictate who stands to benefit most from palliative care. Daniels[30] reported that "it does not seem reasonable to postulate that the medical needs of the elderly terminally ill are any less than those of younger patients, and indeed they may be greater because of multiple additional pathologies associated with aging." Sidgwick's[31] argument that each moment of life is equally valuable, no matter when it occurs, is most poignant in the instance of palliative care. This would also apply to extending palliative care to neonates expected to live only a short time after birth.

Patients may view benefit and toxicity in ways very different from their health care providers and from those who are well. Data from multiple studies show that many dying cancer patients would undergo almost any treatment toxicity for a 1% chance of short-term survival, while their doctors and nurses would not; and these decisions were not changed after patients experienced the toxicity of treatment.[32,33] A study of palliative radiotherapy for brain tumor patients showed little survival, modest functional benefit, and a substantial decrease in intellectual function; but most patients and families would still want it.[34,35] A study of hospice patients compared to those who continued on chemotherapy showed better survival, consistent with less toxicity if chemotherapy is avoided.[36] This is a complex appraisal that needs further study.

## What Is the Right Amount to Spend on Health Care?

How much to spend on health care cannot be determined without knowing the economic and cultural particulars of a country or even a health system. Blanket statements about a percentage of the gross national product (GNP) may be misleading if a comparison country spends a higher percentage on social safety net programs but less on direct medical care costs. Comments about health care spending as a percent of the GNP may also reflect opinions about alternative uses; for example, "We should stop spending money on defense and spend it on health care." In the United States, the amount spent on education has declined from 6% to 5% of the GNP, while the amount spent on health care (especially for the elderly) has risen from 6% to about 14%.[37] Clearly, in all countries, the

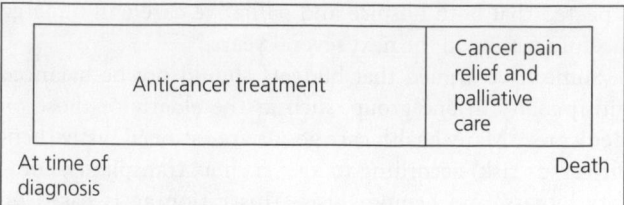

**Figure 24–1.** Present allocation worldwide of cancer resources. Palliative care must receive more of these resources. *Source*: World Health Organization (1990), reference 87. Reproduced by permission of WHO.

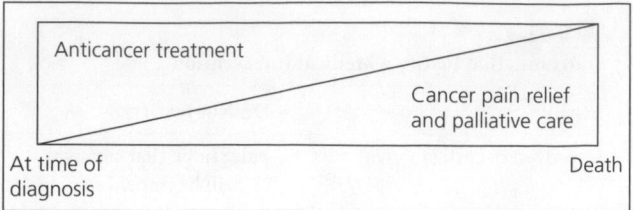

**Figure 24–2.** Proposed allocation of cancer resources in developed countries. Curative and palliative care are not mutually exclusive. Resources should be dispensed to allow the greatest benefits for the majority of individuals. *Source*: World Health Organization (1990), reference 87. Reproduced by permission of WHO.

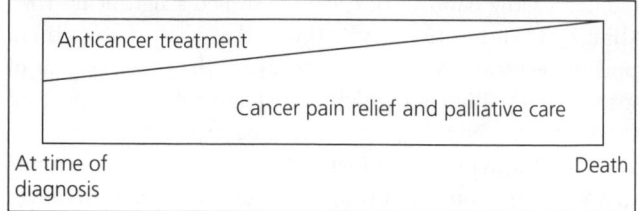

**Figure 24–3.** Proposed allocation of cancer resources in developing countries. As developing countries are the least likely to prevent, detect, and cure cancers, the distribution of resources should be further tailored to best meet the needs of their population. (It is a great ethical dilemma: do you cure one to allow 1000 more to suffer?) *Source*: World Health Organization (1990), reference 87. Reproduced by permission of WHO.

entire system of health care needs to be explored with policies designed to ensure that palliative care is a component of the overall health care system (Figure 24–1).[38] A common threshold is the World Health Organization's recommended 3-times per-capita GNP per quality-adjusted life year; in the U.S. that would be about $140,100 in 2008 U.S. dollars.[39]

## Should There Be Special Economic or Policy Considerations for Palliative Care?

We believe that, in general, there should be no special considerations for palliative care. Most health care policy analysts and economists would argue that all care should be evaluated equally. For example, a therapy that gains 1 week for 52 patients should be valued as much as a therapy of equivalent cost that gains 52 weeks for 1 patient.[40] Some health economists have argued that time given to those who are most at risk should be valued more (e.g., time added in the last 6 months of life should be given triple value).[41] The analogy was made to food and hunger: a sandwich given to a starving person would be of more intrinsic value than one given to a person who already had many sandwiches. Such discussions, while interesting, are outside the scope of this chapter; but many of the ethical concepts applied to these global discussions have relevance to decisions about palliative care.

The World Health Organization (WHO) has listed priorities for health care. In cancer care, palliative care has always been included in the same category as curative therapy. In part, this was done because most palliative care is relatively inexpensive, as well as clinically appropriate.

Current allocation of resources greatly favors curative care with less support for palliative care. As Figures 24–2 and 24–3 illustrate, WHO advocates a more equal distribution of resources in developed countries, and an even greater support of palliative care in developing countries, where most of the population will experience advanced disease rather than cure or long-term survival.

One approach to funding treatments has been based on cost-effectiveness ratios.[41] Laupacis and colleagues[42] in Canada proposed explicit funding criteria: (1) treatments that work better and are less expensive should be adopted; (2) treatments

with cost-effectiveness ratios of less than C$20,000 per additional life year (LY) gained should be accepted, with the recognition that they cost additional resources; (3) treatments with cost-effectiveness ratios of $20,000 to C$100,000/LY should be examined on a case-by-case basis with caution; (4) and treatments with cost-effectiveness ratios of greater than C$100,000/LY should be rejected. These criteria are valid in a system where all resources are shared equally; it is not clear how they apply to other health care systems, where resources may not be shared.[43] Alternatively, patients might be allowed to purchase additional insurance for expensive treatments or pay for them out of pocket. In the United States, there has been no accepted answer, but most authorities have agreed on an implicitly defined benchmark of $35,000 to $50,000/LY saved.[40] For example, an individual with a pathological fracture of a femur is sent to the operating room for pinning. This surgery will aid in relieving pain, improving function, and probably decreasing other potential complications, such as decubitus ulcer and deep venous thrombosis. In addition, home care may become a viable option.

## What Are Important Economic Outcomes?

Economic and clinical outcomes are closely related. Cost should always be considered along with clinical benefit.

Table 24–3
**Standard Definitions for Economic Outcome Analysis**

| Term | Definition | Comment |
|------|-----------|---------|
| Resource utilization | Number of units used (e.g., 9 hospital days) | Best collected prospectively, using a combination of clinical research forms, hospital bills, and patient diaries for outpatient or off-site events. |
| Charge | What is billed to the patient | May be fair representation of the cost of service. Can be accurately converted to costs using ratio of charges to cost.[92] |
| Cost | What it costs society to provide the service | This is different from the charge because many services cost more or less than what is billed. |
| Direct medical cost | Costs of standard medical interventions | Usual "cost-drivers" include hospital days, professional fees, diagnostic tests, pharmacy fees, other (e.g., blood products, operating room, emergency services). |
| Direct nonmedical cost | Costs of medical interventions not usually captured but directly caused | Includes transportation, time lost from work, caregiver costs, etc. Most are not covered by insurance and may be "out-of-pocket" costs. |
| Perspective | The viewpoint of the analysis | Should be explicitly stated. Most analyses are done from the perspective of society (valuing this intervention vs. other uses of the same money) or a health care system (valuing this intervention against other local health care needs). The perspective of the individual patient or provider may give less attention to the needs of others.[36] |
| Discounting | Adjusts value of intervention for future benefit to present-time amount | Health effects and costs should normally be discounted at 3% per year. Health benefits in the present are worth more than those in the future. |

*Source:* Smith (1993), reference 40. Copyright © 1993, American Medical Association. All right reserved.

However, making decisions is not easy. For example, the American Society of Clinical Oncology (ASCO),[43] could not define the lowest amount of benefit that justified an intervention; for example, two weeks of quality survival. They did, however, recommend,that the benefit be weighed against the toxicity and costs.[44]

The economic data necessary to make decisions about treatment may be collected in much the same way as clinical information, and within standard formats for collection and analysis.[45–47] Some standard definitions are listed in Table 24–3.

It is important to organize data in a way that balances clinical and cost information side by side, as shown in Table 24–3. Cost effectiveness is the amount of money someone must pay to gain additional months or years of life. The usual benchmark is "life years gained" or LYs. The standard cost-effectiveness question is $\Delta C/\Delta E = (C_2 - C_1)/(E_2 - E_1)$ where $C$ = costs and $E$ = effectiveness of treatment measured in time. To adjust for quality of life, when the quantity does not change, the concept of utility is used. Utility is the value placed on time in a particular state of health. Perfect health would be assigned a utility value of 1.0 and death a value of 0.0. When utility, or the time × the utility value, is added, the equation becomes $\Delta C/\Delta U$ where $\Delta U = U_2 - U_1$. For example, a therapy that does not improve survival but increases utility by 10% will increase U by (1 year) × (0.10) = 0.1 year. If this treatment costs an additional \$10,000/year, then the cost-utility ratio is:

$$\Delta C = C_2 - C_1 = \$10,000 = \$100,000/QALY.$$

$$\Delta U = U_2 - U_1 = 0.10$$

Such values can be compared to other medical interventions, as shown in Table 24–4. Some countries such as Canada and the United Kingdom use such tables to make decisions on what can be afforded. The decision making process is never easy, since as it always means withholding some desired care.

## Chemotherapy and Palliative Care

Chemotherapy may be an appropriate treatment decision in palliative care as long as the transition to palliative care is made while resources and quality time are still available to the patient and family.[49,50] It is possible to give palliative chemotherapy with cost effectiveness within accepted limits[51–54] (Table 24–5). Lung cancer chemotherapy with older regimens improved survival by a few months, and relieved symptoms, at a reasonable cost to society. For example, chemotherapy

**Table 24-4**
**Ways to Balance Clinical Evaluation and Cost Studies**

| Type of Study | Advantages and Disadvantages |
|---|---|
| Clinical outcomes only | Ignore costs. Easy to choose among clearly superior therapies such as cisplatin for testicular cancer; harder among all others that give lesser benefits at high costs. |
| Cost only (e.g., cost of treating febrile neutropenia) | Ignores clinical outcomes. Does not help choose among clinical strategies. The cost of colony-stimulating factor (CSF) mobilization of stem cells may be higher than that of bone marrow collection, but it saves money later by reducing hospital stay.[35] |
| Costs and clinical outcomes together | |
|    Cost minimization | Assumes that two strategies are equal; lowest cost strategy is preferred. |
|    Cost effectiveness | Compares two strategies; assigns dollar amount per additional year of life (life year [LY]) saved by strategy. Example: at present, CSFs have not improved survival, so cost must be lower for therapy to be cost-effective. |
|    Cost utility | Compares two strategies; assigns dollar amount per additional LY saved by strategy, then estimates the quality of that benefit in cost per quality adjusted LY. No data show significant improvement in quality of life or utilities in patients who have received CSFs, so they are unlikely to have major impact. |
|    Cost benefit | Compares two strategies but converts the clinical benefits to money (e.g., a year of life is worth $100,000). This is possible but is rarely done due to difficulty in assigning monetary value to benefit; requires assigning a monetary value to human life. |

**Table 24-5**
**Chemotherapy vs. Best Palliative Care or Alternative Treatments**

| Topic | Conclusion |
|---|---|
| Lung cancer | |
|    Chemotherapy vs. best supportive care in non-small-cell lung cancer.[44,46] | Chemotherapy gained 8–13 weeks compared to best supportive care.[44] |
| | Chemotherapy generally saved money for the province of Ontario, from a savings of $8000 to an additional cost of $20,000 depending on assumptions. Similar results were found for vinorelbine and cisplatin.[46] |
|    Combined modality including chemotherapy vs. radiation or surgery for stage III non-small-cell lung cancer.[47–49] | Chemotherapy in combination with radiation or surgery adds clinical benefit; for chemotherapy plus radiation, 1- and 5-year survival rates are increased from 40% to 54% and from 6% to 17%, respectively. The addition of chemotherapy to IIIB patients added cost of $15,866, and addition of chemotherapy to IIIB patients added $8912. The cost per year of life gained was well within accepted bounds at $3348 to $14,958 CAN. |
|    Alternating chemotherapy for small-cell lung cancer[84] | The alternating chemotherapy arm cost more, but because it was more effective, the marginal cost effectiveness was only $4560/year of life. |
| Gastrointestinal cancer | |
|    Chemotherapy vs. best supportive care followed by chemotherapy for gastrointestinal cancer patients[50] | Chemotherapy added 5 months median survival if given early rather than late, with symptom palliation for 4 months. The additional cost of about $20,000 per life year was within accepted bounds. |
| Prostate cancer | |
|    Palliative chemotherapy with mitoxantrone plus prednisone vs. prednisone[51,52] | Mitoxantrone did not improve survival but did improve quality of life as measured by several indices, and the mitoxantrone strategy cost less than prednisone supportive care. |
| Breast cancer | |
|    High-dose chemotherapy for limited metastatic disease vs. standard chemotherapy[56] | High-dose chemotherapy added 6 months at a cost of $58,000, or $116,000 per life year; this is palliative care because this treatment has not been shown to be curative. |
| Other | |
|    Acute myelogenous leukemia[58] | Chemotherapy, compared to supportive care, added additional cost, but the cost effectiveness was $18,000/life year, within acceptable limits. |

with cisplatin and vinorelbine, compared to vinorelbine alone or cisplatin and vindesine, added substantial clinical benefit to the patient[54-56] at a reasonable cost effectiveness of C$15,000 to C$17,000/LY.[55] Such studies are in critical need of updating with drugs such as bevacizumab, which can cost $100,000 a year but adds two months of survival.[56]

Chemotherapy for metastatic prostate cancer improves survival by about 2.4 months; the cost effectiveness ratio of £33,000 ($49,000 US) for year of life added is within usual societal accepted values. Because of this, chemotherapy for metastatic prostate cancer has been approved in Great Britian by the National Institute for Clinical Effectivnesss (NICE) program.[57] However, in the United States, several different types of chemotherapy may be offered to the patient when only one has known efficacy. The cost effectiveness of all but docetaxol is likely to be exceedingly high.

## Models of Care and Cost

The less expensive the setting, the less costly the intervention, as shown in Table 24–6. Home opioid infusions had lower total costs. This was associated with the lower cost of home care despite higher drug equipment and nursing costs.[58] Outpatient administration of chemotherapy was less expensive than inpatient administration.[59,60] Home chemotherapy compared to outpatient chemotherapy was usually well accepted by patients, with only two of 424 patients electing to discontinue home treatment. The total costs were equivalent, with an average cost of $50 as compared to $116 in the hospital, and equal total costs.[59]

Disease-management strategies have shown some modest improvements, with better quality of care, less cost, and high patient satisfaction. The available studies are shown in Table 24–7.

Coordinated care may be one of the most economically successful disease-management strategies. The Medicare Hospice Benefit requires nurse coordination, team management, easy access to low per diem hospital beds for respite or temporary care, and expanded drug coverage.[61,62] Adding a nurse coordinator for terminally ill patients in England did not change disease outcomes. The patients still died, and most still had some unrelieved symptoms. However, patient and family satisfaction did improve slightly.[63] Total costs were reduced from £8814 to £4414. The cost savings were associated with decreased number of hospital days. The cost savings of 41% was seen regardless of diagnosis. Home nursing care was associated with more patients dying at home, and hospice patients who did not continue with chemotherapy appear to have lived longer than those who stayed on chemotherapy.

Recent randomized studies show that a modified palliative care presence (with lower costs than full hospice care per diem charges), and control over the clinical care of the patient, is associated with fewer hospitalizations, fewer ICU hospital days, and lower costs. Brumley et al. studied patients in the Kaiser Permanente health maintenance organization, 161 in the Palliative Care Program and 139 in the comparison group.[63-66] Palliative care patients had significantly fewer emergency department visits, hospital days, skilled nursing facility days, and physician visits. There was a 45% decrease in costs as compared to usual care patients. A randomized study showed increased satisfaction when palliative care was added to usual care. There were fewer emergency room visits, and lower costs (mean cost for patients enrolled in the

| Table 24–6 Site of Service | |
|---|---|
| Topic | Conclusion |
| Opioids in home infusion | Per diem costs were higher for home patients, but total costs were lower, with equivalent palliation.[59] |
| Inpatient or outpatient | Outpatient administration was less expensive, $184 vs. $223US.[60] |
| Home or inpatient/clinic chemotherapy | Home chemotherapy was safe, well accepted, and cost less per treatment.[61] |

| Table 24–7 Process or Structural Changes in Care | |
|---|---|
| Topic | Conclusion |
| Reducing uncontrolled pain admissions | A system-wide intervention of focus on pain management, a supportive-care consultation team, and a pain resource center. This was associated with a reduction in admissions from 255/5772 (4.4%) to 121/4076 (3.0%), at a project cost savings of $2,719,245.[66] |
| Presence of nursing care for end of life | Nursing care availability allowed more patients to die at home, consistent with the wishes of most patients.[65] |
| Clinical practice guidelines for supportive care: antiemetics, treatment of febrile neutropenia, treatment of pain | A division changed practice to standardized oral antiemetics and once-daily ceftriaxone and gentamicin. Cost savings were estimated at $250,000 for each intervention, yearly.[63,85,88,89] |

palliative care group was $12,670, compared with $20,222 for usual care).[67,68] The palliative care approach has been adopted by many other Kaiser Permanente groups as part of routine care for patients with advanced illness.

Teaching staff about choices for intensive care unit (ICU) use can improve economic outcomes. In one setting, an ethicist in the surgical ICU addressed the issues of patient choice about dying, and the ethics of futile care. This was associated with a decrease in length of stay from 28 to 16 days, and a decrease in surgical intensive care days from 2028 to 1003, far greater than observed in other parts of the hospital. Cost savings were estimated at $1.8 million.[69] In a similar project, Dowdy and colleagues[70] did proactive ethics consultations for all mechanically ventilated patients beyond four days, and showed improved length of stay (less use of the ICU, either by discontinuing futile care or transferring the patient to lesser-intensity units) and a decrease in costs.

Clinical practice guidelines for supportive care may decrease costs, but formal data have not been published.[71] While there have been significant anecdotal data and clinical opinion that hospice provides improved quality and decreased cost, the available research data do not show that hospice improves care or saves money, as shown in Table 24–8.[70–72] A large, randomized controlled trial of hospice versus standard care showed that hospice did not improve quality of care by any measured benchmark (pain, ability to perform activities of daily living). Patients still used many hospital days (48 for

controls, and 51 for hospice), but more of the hospice patients were hospitalized on the hospice unit. There was no difference in diagnostic procedures or total costs (about $15,000 per patient).[73]

Other data suggest that hospice care can be cost saving.[16,66,67] For example, several studies have demostrated that utilizing palliative care improves quality while reducing cost.[11,15,25,68] In the 1992 Medicare files, those cancer patients who elected hospice cost less than those who did not elect hospice. For those who enrolled in hospice in the last month of life, Medicare saved $1.65 for each $1 spent. However, those who elected hospice tended to use more resources in the months from diagnosis until about three months before death, so the total disease-management savings were close to zero. Similar findings were reported previously.[72] Database studies have shown similar results. In a retrospective study of 12,000 patients at 40 centers, Aiken[73] found that hospice patients were more likely to receive home nursing care and to spend less time in the hospital than conventional care patients. Of the three models of care evaluated, conventional care was the least expensive when overall disease-management costs were calculated, but hospital-based hospice ($2270) and home care hospice ($2657) were less expensive than conventional care ($6100) in the last month of life.

Advanced directives, such as "do-not-resuscitate" (DNR) orders, have been advocated to allow patients to make autonomous choices about their care at the end of life, and possibly

**Table 24–8**
**Hospice vs. Nonhospice Care**

| Topic | Conclusion |
| --- | --- |
| Randomized controlled trial of hospice vs. nonhospice care in Veterans Hospital | Hospice did not improve or worsen quality of care by any measured benchmark (pain, ability to perform activities of daily living). There was no difference in diagnostic procedures. Total costs were $15,000 per patient, with no difference in the arms.[87] |
| Hospice election vs. standard care, Medicare beneficiaries, 1992 | Medicare saved $1.65 for each $1 spent on hospice programs; most of the savings occurred during the last month of life.[72] |
| Hospice election vs. standard care, Medicare beneficiaries, 1988 | Medicare saved $1.26 for each $1 spent on hospice programs; most of the savings occurred during the last month of life.[74] |
| Total costs from databases | No significant difference in total costs from diagnosis to death, but significant cost savings of 39% for hospice patients who were in hospice more than 2 weeks.[88] |
| Total disease-management costs comparing those who elected hospice to those who did not | No different or slightly higher costs among Medicare beneficiaries who elected hospice. Within the hospice period, average 27 days, costs were slightly lower for those who elected hospice.[63] |
| Home care | Home care provided by relatives is not much different ($4563 for each 3-month period) from costs in a nursing home or similar setting. The sicker the patient became, the more the cost to the family regardless of diagnosis. Costs were lowest when the patient and caregiver lived in the same household.[89,90] |
| Matching resource use to the dying patient | Hospice patients were likely to receive more home nursing and to spend less time in the hospital than conventional care patients. Conventional care was the least expensive when overall disease management costs were calculated, but hospital-based hospice ($2270) and home care hospice ($2657) were less. |

**Table 24–9**
**Use of Advanced Directives, Do-Not-Resuscitate (DNR) Orders**

| Study | Conclusion |
| --- | --- |
| California durable power of attorney for health care placed on chart[78] | No effect on treatment charges, types of treatment, or health status. |
| DNR[94] | Average of $57,334 for those without DNR orders, compared to $62,594 for those with DNR orders. |
| Advance directives in SUPPORT hospitals[77] | No cost savings with advance directives. Before the SUPPORT intervention, there was a 23% reduction in cost associated with presence of advance directives ($21,284 versus $26,127). |
| | Intervention patients were more likely to have advance directives documented. |
| | Average cost was $24,178 for those without advance directives, $28,017 for those with advance directives on the intervention arm. |

to reduce costs by preventing futile care. However, as reviewed by Emanuel and Emanuel,[74,75] there has been no cost saving associated with the use of either advance directives or DNR orders (Table 24–9). These findings were confirmed in the SUPPORT study.[76]

End-of-life or advance planning is clearly a part of palliative care and care of the dying. Levinsky[27] has questioned whether end-of-life planning has become an economic strategy as much as a way to respect a patient's wishes: "Confusion between advance planning as a method to find out what the patient wants, and advance planning as a mechanism to reduce medical care and thereby contain costs, represents a clear danger to the goals of informed consent and autonomy for patients." In a randomized study of 204 patients with life-threatening diseases, it was found that in those who executed an advance directive, there was no significant positive or negative effect on well-being, health status, medical treatments, or medical treatment charges.[77]

Studies show that a palliative care presence is associated with fewer hospitalizations, fewer ICU hospital days, and lower costs. As palliative care continues to expand and develop, obtaining and assessing the data will allow the true impact of this field to be known.

❧

## Nursing Issues

Nurses play a large role in the decisions patients, families, and other health care providers make, and those decisions drive the cost of care. Role utilization and its potential influence will vary within each setting.[78] For example, a complete interdisciplinary palliative care team may be necessary to meet the needs of the population in a large university-based hospital, yet a specially trained nurse with interdiciplinary support. may be adequate in a small community hospital. Such coupling of services should be examined from the standpoint of quality of care and cost effectiveness.[79] The Advanced Practice nurse may play a significant role in identifying and coordinating the needs of patients/families requiring palliation. Advanced Practice Nurses are

perfectly positioned to fill such a critical need for this population in the hospital, hospice, and nursing home.[80–83]

A factor not fully examined is the out-of-pocket cost that the patient's significant others bear in caring for them. These include lost work hours, expended resources, and simple care hours not reimbursed through insurance or government assistance. Also to be determined is the increased health care costs of those caregivers, who frequently neglect their own health while caring for others.[83,84]

Nursing as a profession needs to continue to advocate for this population while supporting effective quality care, and fair utilization of resources. The use of advanced technology, especially expensive diagnostic tests, may be accepted as routine in an acute care hospital, regardless of cost and goals of care.[85] Consider the following examples:

1. An 82-year-old man with end-stage chronic obstructive pulmonary disease requests removal from a respirator and comfort measures only. He is deemed competent, yet it is questionable whether he will be able to survive off the respirator. His wishes are followed, and he is extubated. While adamantly refusing any discussion regarding reintubation, he continues to have arterial blood gases sampled every 2 to 3 hours around the clock. Clearly, use of such sampling is impractical, wasteful and potentially harmful because the patient refuses reintubation. In addition, he is kept in the ICU, which he no longer requires as the level of monitoring has changed in accordance with his wishes for comfort care only.

2. A 32-year-old man with widely metastatic colon cancer arrives in your facility with a bowel obstruction related to his disease. He has been in the local hospice program. After evaluation, his prognosis is confirmed to be approximately six weeks. He has a nasogastric tube placed to relieve persistent nausea, vomiting, and abdominal discomfort. After four days of nasogastric decompression, the tube is clamped and he is given subcutaneous octreotide, which alone controls the nausea and vomiting. The local hospice refuses to accept this patient, as the octreotide is too costly.

3.  A 29-year-old woman with acquired immunodeficiency syndrome (AIDS) is admitted for severe debilitating neuropathic pain, unresponsive to typical adjunctive analgesic agents. The patient is losing her ability to ambulate and perform activities of daily living, due to the pain. She is given a trial of epidural opioids with local anesthetic, which offers almost complete pain relief and significantly improved function. An intrathecally implanted pump, at a cost of over ten thousand dollars, is placed. While the initial cost is staggering, the long-term benefits are considerable, including measurable improved functional status, decreased occurrence of depression, decrease in required skilled and nonskilled nursing care hours, and improved quality of life for both the patient and her significant others.

4.  A 60-year-old woman with refractory, late stage multiple myeloma is admitted with an adjusted serum calcium level of 17.9 g/dL. Intravenous fluids, diuretics, bisphosphonate, and calcitonin are administered, and serum calcium is drawn every 12 hours. The patient's disease is irreversible. The prescribed interventions will perhaps delay an inevitable outcome by a few days, but they will cost thousands of dollars while marginally, if at all, improving her quality of life.

5.  A 36-year-old man with a self-inflicted gunshot wound arrives in the emergency department of a financially struggling inner-city hospital. The neurosurgical team determines the injury to the brain is devastating and that the prognosis is grave. The family requests all measures to keep him alive "no matter what." They demand ongoing ventilator and nutritional support. His primary nurse wonders what his role should be in this situation. How will he advocate for the patient while still advocating for ethical and just utilization of resources?

6.  A 68-year-old previously healthy woman has suffered a traumatic subdural hematoma, with significant brain damage. She only opens her eyes to verbal stimuli and does not follow commands two weeks after her injury. She has been receiving nasogastric feedings. The patient has a living will that clearly states no artificial nutrition if her condition becomes irreversible. The social worker informs the medical team that she cannot place this patient in a nursing home unless she becomes "skilled," which a gastrostomy feeding tube would accomplish. The hospital could lose considerable revenue if the patient is not placed in a nursing home.

## Summary

Economic outcomes are increasingly important for all types of health care, including palliative care. There are substantial opportunities for improvement by using disease management strategies. Chemotherapy for some cancers (non-small-cell lung cancer, prostate cancer, and gastrointestinal cancer) is reasonably effective and has acceptable cost-effectiveness ratios. Coordination of palliative care shows no major clinical benefit but does show major cost savings. Directed, ethically-motivated interventions about futile care appear to produce significant cost savings. The use of advance directives or hospice care may be good medical care, but have not been shown to produce major economic benefit. Most recently, integrated palliative care teams have been shown to reduce hospital and end-of-life care costs for seriously ill patients.

The cost of care is rising due to the increasing age of the population, more cancer cases and chronic diseases, increased demand for treatment, and new and expensive technologies. Our limited resources must be rationed wisely so that we can provide both curative and palliative care. The ethical implications of using economic and management outcomes rather than traditional health outcomes include shifting emphasis from helping at all cost to helping at a cost society can afford, as well as how much society is willing to pay. The value of care to the dying versus those with curable illnesses, and tolerance of suboptimal care, are ethical and societal issues.

From the perspective of economics or health service research, the outcomes of palliative care do not differ from those of other cancer treatment or treatment of other chronic illnesses. For treatment to be justified, there must be some demonstrable improvement in disease-free or overall survival, toxicity, quality of life, or cost effectiveness. Palliative care usually does not change survival, and it does not have a measurable cost-effectiveness ratio since it does usually not gain years of life.

Only a few studies have assessed the economic outcomes of palliative therapy. The major areas of interest include the following: (1) palliative chemotherapy versus best supportive care; (2) supportive care for cancer symptoms; (3) the process and structure of care; (4) follow-up; (5) cost savings; and (6) hospice care. Palliative first-line chemotherapy for stage III and IV non-small-cell lung cancer, mitoxantrone for prostate cancer, and fluorouracil-based chemotherapy for gastrointestinal cancer have acceptable cost-effectiveness ratios. Supportive care effectiveness and cost for infections, nausea, and pain can be improved. Research outside of cancer is scant. Hospice care does not increase costs or worsen survival. Integrated palliative care appears to improve care and reduce overall costs. Nurses clearly have the ability to impact the care and cost for this population and should be at the forefront of these issues.

## Acknowledgments

This work is based on a chapter published in *Topics in Palliative Care, Vol. 5*, edited by R.K. Portenoy, and E. Bruera: *Economic outcomes and palliative care*, by Thomas J. Smith and Laurie Lyckholm. New York: Oxford University Press, 2001:157–175.

## REFERENCES

1. Poisal JA, et al. Health spending projections through 2016: Modest changes obscure part D's impact. Health Aff February 21, 2007:W242–W253.
2. The Henry J. Kaiser Family Foundation. Employee Health Benefits: 2007 Annual Survey. Available at: http://www.kff.org/insurance/7672/index.cfm (accessed September 11, 2006).
3. California Health Care Foundation. Health Care Costs 101—2005.Available at: http://www.chcf.org/ (accessed March 2, 2005).
4. Centers for Medicare and Medicaid Services. Projections of National Health Expenditures, Methadology and Model Specifications. Available at: http://www.cms.hhs.gov/NationalHealthExpendData/downloads/projections-methodology.pdf (accessed January 10, 2009).
5. National Cancer Institute. Cancer Progress Report: 2007 Update. Available at: http://progressreport.cancer.gov (accessed January 10, 2009).
6. American Cancer Society. Cancer Facts & Figures 2005. Atlanta: Author, 2005.
7. National Heart, Lung and Blood Institute. Fact Book Fiscal Year 2003. Available at: http://www.nhlbi.nih.gov/about/03factbk.pdf (accessed January 10, 2009).
8. Lubitz JD, Riley GF. Trends in Medicare payments in the last year of life. N Engl J Med 1993;328:1092–1096.
9. Lubitz J, Beebe J, Baker C. Longevity and medicare expenditures. N Engl J Med 1995;332:999–1003.
10. Harrington SE, Smith TJ. The role of chemotherapy at the end of life: "When is enough, enough?" JAMA June 11, 2008;299(22):2667–2678.
11. Smith TJ, Cassel JB. Economics of palliative care. In: Hanks G, Cherny NI, Christakis NA, Fallon M, Kaasa S, Porteney R.K, eds. Oxford Textbook of Palliative Medicine, (4th ed). Oxford: Oxford University Press, 2008:151–163.
12. Brunner D. Cost effectiveness of palliative care. Semin Oncol Nurs 1998;14:164–167.
13. SUPPORT Principal Investigators. A controlled trial to improve care for seriously ill hospitalized patients. The Study to Understand Prognoses and Preferences for Outcomes and Risks of Treatments (SUPPORT). JAMA 1995;274:1591–1598.
14. Cleeland CS, Gonin R, Hatfield AK, et al. Pain and its treatment in outpatients with metastatic cancer. N Engl J Med 1994;330:592–596.
15. Morrison RS, Penrod JD, Cassel JB, Caust-Ellenbogen M, Litke A, Spragens L, Meier DE; Palliative Care Leadership Centers' Outcomes Group. Cost savings associated with US hospital palliative care consultation programs. Arch Intern Med September 8, 2008;168(16):1783–1790.
16. Smith T, Coyne P, Cassel B, Penberthy L, Hopson A, Hager M. A high-volume specialist palliative care unit and team may reduce in-hospital end-of-life care costs. J Palliat Med 2003;6:699–705.
17. Bevan G. Taking equity seriously: A dilemma for government from allocating resources to primary care groups. BMJ 1998;316:39–43.
18. Hillner BE, Smith TJ. Hospital volume and patient outcomes in major cancer surgery: A catalyst for quality assessment and concentration of cancer services. JAMA 1998; 280:1784.
19. Gillis CR, Hole DJ. Survival outcome of care by specialist surgeons in breast cancer: A study of 3786 patients in the west of Scotland. BMJ 1996;312:145–148.
20. Feuer EJ, Frey CM, Brawley OW, et al. After a treatment breakthrough: A comparison of trial and population-based data for advanced testicular cancer. J Clin Oncol 1994;12:368–377.
21. Nguyen HN, Averette HE, Hoskins W, Penalver M, Sevin B, Steren A. National survey of ovarian carcinoma, Part V. The impact of physician's specialty on patient's survival. Cancer 1993;72:3663–3670.
22. Desch CE, Penberthy L, Newschaffer C, ct al. Factors that determine the treatment of local and regional prostate cancer. Med Care 1996;34:152–162.
23. Smith R. An ethical code for everybody in health care: A code that covered all rather than single groups might be useful. BMJ 1997;315:1633–1634.
24. Olson V, Coyne P, Smith V, Hudson C. Critical pathway improves outcomes for patients with sickle-cell disease. Oncol Nurs Forum 1997;24:1682.
25. Khatcheressian J, Cassel JB, Lyckholm L, Coyne P, Hagenmuller A, Smith T. Improving palliative and supportive care in cancer patients. Oncology September 2005;19(10):1365–1376.
26. Berger JT, Rosner F. The ethics of practice guidelines. Arch Intern Med 1996;156:2051–2056.
27. Levinsky NG. The purpose of advance medical planning—autonomy for patients or limitation of care? N Engl J Med 1996;335:741–743.
28. Callahan D. Controlling the costs of health care for the elderly—fair means and foul. N Engl J Med 1996;335:744–746.
29. Randall F. Palliative Care Ethics: A Good Companion. New York: Oxford University Press, 1996.
30. Daniels N. Just Health Care. New York: Cambridge University Press, 1985.
31. Sidgwick H. The Methods of Ethics. London: McMillan, 1907.
32. Matsuyama R, Reddy S, Smith TJ. Why do patients choose chemotherapy near the end of life? A review of the perspective of those facing death from cancer. J Clin Oncol July 20, 2006;24(21):3490–3496.
33. Slevin ML, Stubbs L, Plant HJ, et al. Attitudes to chemotherapy: Comparing views of patients with cancer with those of doctors, nurses, and general public. BMJ 1990;300:1458–1460.
34. Davies E, Clarke C, Hopkins A. Malignant cerebral glioma—I: Survival, disability, and morbidity after radiotherapy. BMJ 1996;313:1507–1512.
35. Davies E, Clarke C, Hopkins A. Malignant cerebral glioma—II: Perspectives of patients and relatives on the value of radiotherapy. BMJ 1996;313:1512–1516.
36. Connor SR, Pyenson B, Fitch K, Spence C, Iwasaki K. Comparing hospice and nonhospice patient survival among patients who die within a three-year window. J Pain Symptom Manage March 2007;33(3):238–246.
37. Lamm RD. The ghost of health care future. Inquiry 1994;31:365–367.
38. Coyne P. International efforts in cancer pain relief. Semin Oncol Nurs 1997;13:57–62.
39. Central Intelligence Agency. The World Factbook. United States. Available at: https://www.cia.gov/library/publications/the-world-factbook/geos/us.html (accessed November 20, 2008).
40. Smith TJ, Hillner BE, Desch CE. Efficacy and cost-effectiveness of cancer treatment: Rational allocation of resources based on decision analysis. J Natl Cancer Inst 1993;85:1460–1474.

41. Waugh N, Scott D. How should different life expectancies be valued? BMJ 1998:1140–1316.

42. Laupacis A, Feeny D, Detsky AS, Tugwell PX. How attractive does a new technology have to be to warrant adoption and utilization? Tentative guidelines for using clinical and economic evaluation. Can Med Assoc J 1992;146:473–481.

43. Smith TJ. Which hat do I wear? JAMA 1993;270:1657–1659.

44. Brown M, Glick H, Harrell F, et al. Integrating economic analysis into cancer clinical trials: The National Cancer Institute–American Society of Clinical Oncology Economics Workbook, 1998.

45. Brown M, Glick H, Harrell F, et al. Integrating economic analysis into cancer clinical trials: The National Cancer Institute–American Society of Clinical Oncology Economics Workbook, 1998:151–163.

46. Cassel J. Measurement issues for palliative care programs. In: Panke J, Coyne P, eds. Conversations in Palliative Care (2nd ed). Dubuque, IA: Kendall/Hunt Publishing Co., 2006.

47. Temel JS, Jackson VA, Billings JA, et al. Phase II study: Integrated palliative care in newly diagnosed advanced non-small-cell lung cancer patients. J Clin Oncol 2007;25: 2377–2382.

48. Martoni AA, Tanneberger S, Mutri V. Cancer chemotherapy near the end of life: The time has come to set guidelines for its appropriate use. Tumori 2007;93:417–422.

49. Steinbrook R. Saying no isn't NICE—the travails of Britain's National Institute for Health and Clinical Excellence. N Engl J Med 2008;359:1977–1981.

50. Smith TJ, Hillner BE, Schmitz N, et al. Economic analysis of a randomized clinical trial to compare filgrastim-mobilized peripheral blood progenitor cell transplantation and autologous bone marrow transplantation in patients with Hodgkin and non-Hodgkin lymphoma. J Clin Oncol 1997;15:5–10.

51. Smith TJ, Desch CE, Hillner BE. Ways to reduce the cost of oncology care without compromising the quality. Cancer Invest 1994;12:257–265.

52. Le Chevalier T, Brisgand D, Douillard JY, et al. Randomized study of vinorelbine and cisplatin versus vindesine and cisplatin versus vinorelbine alone in advanced non-small cell lung cancer: Results of a European multicenter trial including 612 patients. J Clin Oncol 1994;12:360–367.

53. Evans WK, Will BP, Berthelot JM, et al. Cost of combined modality interventions for stage III non-small cell lung cancer. J Clin Oncol 1997;15:3030–3048.

54. Evans WK, Will BP. The cost of managing lung cancer in Canada. Oncology (Huntingt) 1995;2(Suppl 11):147–153.

55. Evans WK, Will BP, Berthelot JM, Wolfson MC. The economics of lung cancer management in Canada. Lung Cancer 1996;14:13–17.

56. Smith TJ, Hilner BE, Neighbors DM, McSorley PA, Le Chevalier T. An economic evaluation of a ramdominized clinical trial comparing vinorelbine, vinorelbine plus cisplatin and vindesine plus cisplatin for non-small cell lung cancer. J Clin Oncol 1995;13:2166–2173.

57. Sandler A, Gray R, Perry MC, Brahmer J, Schiller JH, Dowlati A, Lilenbaum R, Johnson DH. Paclitaxel-carboplatin alone or with bevacizumab for non-small-cell lung cancer. N Engl J Med December 14, 2006;355(24):2542–2550.

58. Collins R, Fenwick E, Trowman R, Perard R, Norman G, Light K, Birtle A, Palmer S, Riemsma R. Health Technol Assess January 2007;11(2):iii–iv, xv–xviii, 1–179. Review.

59. Ferris FD, Wodinsky HB, Kerr IG, Sone M, Hume S, Coons C. A cost-minimization study of cancer patients requiring a narcotic infusion in hospital and at home. J Clin Epidemiol 1991;44:313–327.

60. Wodinsky HB, DeAngelis C, Rusthoven JJ, et al. Re-evaluating the cost of outpatient cancer chemotherapy. Can Med Assoc J 1987;137:903–906.

61. Lowenthal RM, Piaszczyk A, Arthur GE, O'Malley S. Home chemotherapy for cancer patients: Cost analysis and safety. Med J Aust 1996;165:184–187.

62. Harris NJ, Dunmore R, Tscheu MJ. The Medicare hospice benefit: Fiscal implications for hospice program management. Cancer Manage 1996;May/June:6–11.

63. Smith TJ. End of Life Care: Preserving Quality and Quantity of Life in Managed Care. Alexandria, VA. ASCO: Education Book 33rd Annual Meeting, 1997:303–307.

64. Raftery JP, Addington-Hall JM, MacDonald LD, et al. A randomized controlled trial of the cost-effectiveness of a district coordinating service for terminally ill cancer patients. Palliat Med 1996;10:151–161.

65. McWhinney IR, Bass MJ, Orr V. Factors associated with location of death (home or hospital) or patients referred to a palliative care team. Can Med Assoc J 1995;152:361–370.

66. Gade G, Venohr I, Conner D, et al. Impact of an inpatient palliative care team: A randomized control trial. J Palliat Med 2008;11:180–190.

67. Brumley R, Enguidanos S, Cherin D. Effectiveness of a home-based palliative care program for end-of-life. J Palliat Med 2004;6:715–724.

68. Brumley R, Enguidanos S, Jamison P, Seitz R, Morgenstern N, Saito S, McIlwane J, Hillary K, Gonzalez J. Increased satisfaction with care and lower costs: Results of a randomized trial of in-home palliative care. J Am Geriatr Soc July 2007;55(7):993–1000.

69. Twaddle ML, Maxwell TL, Cassel JB, Liao S, Coyne PJ, Usher BM, Amin A, Cuny J. Palliative care benchmarks from academic medical centers. J Palliat Med February 2007;10(1):86–98.

70. Holloran SD, Starkey GW, Burke PA, Steele G Jr, Forse RA. An educational intervention in the surgical intensive care unit to improve ethical decisions. Surgery 1995;118:294–298.

71. Dowdy MD, Robertson C, Bander JA. A study of proactive ethics consultation for critically and terminally ill patients with extended lengths of stay. Crit Care Med 1998;26:252–259.

72. Smith TJ. End of Life Care: Preserving Quality and Quantity of Life in Managed Care. Alexandria, VA. ASCO: Education Book 33rd Annual Meeting, 1997:303–307.

73. Kidder D. The effects of hospice coverage on Medicare expenditures. Health Serv Res 1992;27:195–217.

74. Aiken LH. Evaluation and research and public policy: Lessons learned from the National Hospice study. J Chronic Dis 1986;39:1–4.

75. Emanuel EJ. Cost savings at the end of life. What do the data show? JAMA 1996;275:1907–1914.

76. Emanuel EJ, Emanuel LL. The economics of dying. The illusion of cost savings at the end of life. N Engl J Med 1994;330:540–544.

77. Teno J, Lynn J, Connors AF, Jr, et al. The illusion of end-of-life resource savings with advance directives. SUPPORT Investigators: Study to Understand Prognoses and Preferences for Outcomes and Risks of Treatment. J Am Geriatr Soc 1997; 45:513–518.

78. Schneiderman LJ, Kronick R, Kaplan RM, Anderson JP, Langer RD. Effects of offering advance directives on medical treatments and costs. Ann Intern Med 1992;117:599–606.

79. Cassel J. Measurement issues for palliative care programs. In Panke J, Coyne P, eds. Conversations in Palliative Care (2nd ed). Dubuque, IA: Kendall/Hunt Publishing Co., 2006:231–236.

80. Coyne P, Ratliff B, Smith T. Frequently Asked Questions (FAQ's) about palliative care financing. In: Panke J, Coyne P, eds. Conversations in Palliative Care (2nd ed). Dubuque, IA: Kendall/Hunt Publishing Co., 2006.

81. Coyne PJ. Evolution of the advanced practice nurse within palliative care. J Palliat Med 2003;6:767–768.

82. Reb A. Palliative and end of life care: Policy analysis. Oncol Nurs Forum 2003;30:35–50.

83. Coyne P, Dahlin C, Campbell M, Lentz J, Lynch M, Stahl D. Value of advanced practice nurse in palliative care: An HPNA position statement. J Hospice Palliative Nurs 2007;9(2):72–73.

84. Cawthone V. Resource utilization. In: Panke J, Coyne P, eds. Conversations in Palliative Care (2nd ed). Dubuque, IA: Kendall/Hunt Publishing Co., 2006:223–230.

85. Levine C. The loneliness of the long-term care giver. N Engl J Med 1999;340:1587–1590.

86. Coyne P. A bridge to where? J Hospice Palliative Nurs 2007; 9(5):231–232.

87. World Health Organization. Cancer Pain Relief and Palliative care. Technical Report Series 304. Geneva:Author, 1990.

88. Smith TJ. Reducing the costs of supportive care. 1: Antibiotics for febrile neutropenia. Clin Oncol Alert 1996;11:47–49.

89. Smith TJ. Reducing the costs of supportive care. 11: Antiemetics. Clin Oncol Alert 1996;11:62–64.

90. Kane PL, Berstein L, Whales J, Leibowitz A, Kaplan S. A randomized control trial of hospice care. Lancet 1984;1:890–894.

91. Brooks CH, Smyth-Staruch K. Hospice home care cost savings to third party insurers. Mes Care 1984;22:691–703.

92. Stommel M, Given CW, Given BA. The cost of cancer home care to families. Cancer 1993;71:1867–1874.

93. Given BA, Given CW, Stommel M. Family and out-of-pocket costs for women with breast cancer. Cancer Pract 1994;2:187–193.

# 25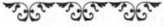

*Barton T. Bobb*

# Urgent Syndromes at the End of Life

*I really need to have this bed at home to stay comfortable, since I can't move my legs. This bed has made a huge difference.—Joe, a patient with probably only a few weeks left to live and malignant spinal cord compression that rapidly progressed from causing weakness to paraplegia, in spite of aggressive treatment; he is explaining, prior to discharge from the palliative care unit, why he needs the same specialty bed at home*

*Syndromes Covered in This Chapter Include:*
- *Superior vena caval obstruction*
- *Pleural effusion*
- *Pericardial effusion*
- *Hemoptysis*
- *Spinal cord compression*
- *Hypercalcemia*

Hallmarks of palliative care are skilled assessment and rapid evaluation and management of symptoms that impact negatively on patient and family quality of life. This chapter addresses select syndromes that unless recognized and treated promptly will cause unnecessary suffering for the patient and family.

## SUPERIOR VENA CAVAL OBSTRUCTION

CASE STUDY
*Mr. B, A Patient with Non-Small Cell Lung Cancer*

Mr. B, a 56-year-old bricklayer, was diagnosed with small-cell lung cancer three months ago and has been receiving chemotherapy. He is going to receive radiation therapy in the future. He has tried to continue working as much as possible. He comes in to see his oncologist for scheduled follow-up today, and during his nursing assessment he complains, "I've been having more shortness of breath the past few days. I've also got this funny dry cough and get a little dizzy every now and then. Come to think of it, my face and upper right arm look a little puffy. What do you think? Should I be worried about this?"

- *Key Points*
- *Superior vena caval obstruction can cause distressing symptoms that are amenable to palliation.*
- *The common presenting symptoms are dyspnea, facial swelling, and feeling of fullness in the head.*
- *The patient's swollen and distorted facial features can be highly upsetting to the patient and family.*
- *The diagnosis of vena caval syndrome can usually be made on clinical grounds.*

## Definition

Superior vena caval obstruction (SVCO) is a disorder produced by obstruction of blood flow in the superior vena cava, which results in impairment of blood flow through the superior vena cava into the right atrium. Severity of the syndrome depends on rapidity of onset, location of the obstruction, and whether or not the obstruction is partial or complete. Obstruction may occur acutely or gradually, and symptoms may be severe and debilitating.[1,2]

## Epidemiology

The patient most likely to experience SVCO is a 50- to 70-year-old man with a primary or metastatic tumor of the mediastinum. More than 90% of SVCO cases have been due to cancer, most commonly, endobronchial tumors.[2,3] More recent research indicates that the percentage of SVCO cases due to nonmalignant causes, primarily due to the higher use of intravascular devices, has probably risen.[4] In the majority of patients, the presence of SVCO is not a poor prognostic indicator of survival.[5] The prognosis of patients with SVCO strongly correlates with the prognosis of underlying disease.

Two types of obstruction may cause SVCO: (1) intrinsic obstruction, and (2) extrinsic obstruction.[1] Intrinsic obstruction is usually caused by primary tracheal malignancies that invade the airway epithelium, that is, squamous cell carcinoma and adenoid cystic carcinoma, as well as other benign and malignant tumors. Extrinsic obstruction occurs when airways are surrounded and compressed by external tumors or enlarged lymph nodes, that is, lymphoma, and locally advanced thyroid, lung, or esophageal cancers. Obstruction may be caused by a tumor arising in the right main or upper-lobe bronchus or by large-volume lymphadenopathy in the right paratracheal or precarinal lymph node chains.[6]

Thrombosis of the superior vena cava (SVC) is also associated with insertion of indwelling intracaval catheters and central-venous access devices, which are thought to damage the intima of vessels. Both adults and children may experience thrombosis of the SVC. More than compression or tumor, thrombosis is likely to cause acute and complete obstruction of the SVC.[7] Cancer patients are also at greater risk of experiencing hypercoagulopathies, which increase the risk of experiencing thrombosis and SVCO. Other less common nonmalignant causes associated with SVCO are mediastinal fibrosis from histoplasmosis and iatrogenic complications from cardiovascular surgery.[7,8]

## Pathophysiology

The superior vena cava is located in the rigid thoracic cavity and is surrounded by a number of structures, including the sternum, trachea, right bronchus, aorta, pulmonary artery, and several lymph node chains. There is little room for structures to move or expand within this cavity, thus the superior vena cava is vulnerable to any space-occupying lesion in its vicinity. Venous drainage from the head, neck, upper extremities, and upper thorax collects in the SVC on its way to the right atrium. The SVC has a thin wall, and normally, blood flows through the vessel under low pressure. When the vessel is compressed, blood flow is slowed, fluid pressure is increased, and occlusion may occur.[9]

When venous collateral circulation has time to develop, the symptoms of SVCO are likely to develop insidiously.[10] The presence of collateral circulation, tumor growth rate, and extent and location of the blockage are factors in determining how rapidly SVCO develops.[11]

## Signs and Symptoms

The onset of symptoms is often insidious. Patients may report subtle signs that include venous engorgement in the morning hours after awakening from sleep, difficulty removing rings from fingers, and an increase in symptoms when bending forward or stooping, all of which may not be noticed initially.[1,9,12,13] The most common symptom of the syndrome is dyspnea.[12,14,15] Swelling of the neck and face is seen in 50% of patients. Other common symptoms are cough (54%), arm swelling (18%), chest pain (15%), and dysphagia (9%).[7] Physical findings include venous distention of the neck (66%), venous distention of the chest wall (54%), facial edema (46%), plethora, a very ruddy facial complexion (19%), and cyanosis (19%). Patients may experience tachypnea, hoarseness, nasal stuffiness, periorbital edema, redness and edema of the conjunctivae, and, rarely, paralyzed vocal cord.[16]

In severe or rapid cases, where collateral circulation has not yet made accommodation for increased blood flow, symptoms may be immediately life-threatening. Patients may experience orthopnea, stridor, respiratory distress, headache, visual disturbances, dizziness, syncope, lethargy, and irritability. As the condition further progresses, significant mental status changes occur, including stupor, coma, seizures, and, ultimately, death.[17]

## Diagnostic Procedures

Plain chest x-ray films are the least invasive diagnostic modality.[7] Computed tomography (CT) is the most widely available and used modality to elucidate the location, extent of obstruction or stenosis, presence and extent of thrombus formation, and status of collateral circulation,[18–20] and can be performed unless the patient is so debilitated that no further treatment is indicated or desired by the patient.[21] Magnetic resonance imaging (MRI) is another diagnostic tool that can confirm the diagnosis of SVC[21] and distinguish between tumor mass or thrombosis.

## Palliation of Symptoms

The effectiveness of palliation of symptoms of SVCO in patients who have persistent or recurrent small-cell lung cancer (SCLC) has been reviewed.[5] Chemotherapy or mediastinal radiation therapy were found to be very effective as initial treatment for patients who have SCLC and SVCO at first presentation, as well as in those with recurrent or persistent disease. It was recommended that radiation therapy be used in those patients who have been previously treated with chemotherapy. However, due to side effects, large fractions should be avoided.[5] When comparing the treatment modalities used to treat SVCO, including chemotherapy alone, chemotherapy and radiation therapy, and radiation therapy alone, none has proved superior.[6] Adverse prognostic indicators are dysphagia, hoarseness, and stridor.

## SVC Stenting

Current American College of Chest Physicians (ACCP) guidelines state that lung cancer patients with symptomatic SVCO can be treated with a combination of chemotherapy, radiation therapy, and/or insertion of an SVC stent.[22] Patients with severe symptoms are often best treated initially by SVC stenting, especially if a tissue diagnosis has not been made yet. However, the decision should be made on a case by case basis, as many patients with lung cancer respond very quickly to radiation or chemotherapy.[1] Although there are no controlled studies comparing radiation therapy with SVC stenting, several reviews and nonrandomized studies indicate that this procedure can relieve edema, promote improved superficial collateral vein drainage, and improve neurological impairment. It can also relieve dyspnea, provide greater relief of obstruction, create few or minor complications,[1,6,17,23-26] and allow for the full use of chemotherapy and radiation therapy,[17] thus providing more rapid relief in a higher proportion of patients.[6] Complications associated with SVC stenting procedures include bleeding due to anticoagulation, arrhythmia, septic episodes, thrombosis, fibrosis, and migration of the stent.

## Thrombolytic Therapies

Thrombolytic therapy has often been successful in the lysing of SVC thrombi.[27] Another alternative, percutaneous angioplasty with or without thrombolytics, may open SVC obstructions. Documented thrombi may be treated with tissue plasminogen activators (TPS).

## Drug Therapy

Steroids have been one of the standard therapies for treatment of SVCO, in spite of the lack of research-based evidence to support their use. Prednisone and methylprednisolone have both been used to reduce inflammation in the treatment of SVCO, but the typical regimen is generally 4 mg of dexamethasone every 6 hours.[2]

Diuretics, such as furosemide, may be given to promote diuresis, thus decreasing venous return to the heart, which reduces pressure in the SVC. However, caution must be exercised to avoid dehydration.[28]

## Nursing Management

The primary nursing goals are to identify patients at risk for developing SVC syndrome, to recognize the syndrome if it does occur, and to relieve dyspnea and other symptoms. Reduction of anxiety is another important nursing goal. The patient and family may experience significant distress not only because of physical symptoms experienced, but also because of an altered physical appearance, including a ruddy, swollen, distorted face and neck.

The nurse monitors the patient for side effects of treatment and provides symptom management. For example, if the patient is receiving radiation therapy, be alert for signs of dyspnea (which may indicate presence of tracheal edema), pneumonitis, dysphagia, pharyngitis, esophagitis, leukopenia, anemia, skin changes, and fatigue. If the patient is receiving chemotherapy, be alert for signs of stomatitis, nausea and vomiting, fatigue, leukopenia, anemia, and thrombocytopenia. If the patient is receiving steroid therapy, educate the patient and family about the potential for developing proximal muscle weakness, mood swings, insomnia, oral candida, and hyperglycemia. Aspects of palliative nursing care that are always of primary importance are: early recognition and management of symptoms, educating the patient and

family about these symptoms and what to report, and providing reassurance that these symptoms, if they occur, will be controlled.

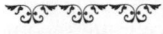

# PLEURAL EFFUSION

CASE STUDY
*Mr. D, A Patient with Pancreatic Cancer*

Mr. D, a 46-year-old father of three, was diagnosed with pancreatic cancer six months ago, and the disease has progressed in spite of surgery and multiple regimens of chemotherapy. He has bone and lung metastases. He presents to the emergency room with progressive dyspnea and some chest pain. He says, "I've been getting more shortwinded the past couple weeks, mainly when I would walk for longer distances at first, but it's gotten so bad that I can barely go to the bathroom without losing my breath. I have to prop my head up on three pillows at night to get some sleep. My chest hurts a little, too. I feel terrible. I'm sure it's the cancer's fault and I know it can't be cured, but can you help me feel better?" Examination reveals decreased breath sounds on the right base, dullness to percussion, as well as decreased tactile fremitus. He is tachypneic with a respiratory rate of 32 and he is also splinting.

- ◆ *Key Points*
- ◆ *The treatment of pleural effusion is palliative and symptomatic.*
- ◆ *The treatment approach depends on clinical circumstances, the patient's general condition, and nearness to death.*
- ◆ *Preemptive pain management is a critical nursing function when patients undergo invasive procedures.*

## Definition

Pleural effusion is defined as a disparity between secretion and absorption of fluid in the pleural space secondary to increased secretion, impaired absorption, or both, resulting in excessive fluid collection.[29-32]

## Epidemiology

More than 150,000 pleural effusions (PE) are diagnosed each year in the United States.[32] Parapneumonic disease is the most common cause of pleural effusions, followed by malignant disease. Breast, ovarian, and lung cancer plus lymphomas account for over 75% of all malignant pleural effusions (MPE),[34] followed by ovarian cancer and gastric cancer, in order of descending frequency.[35] Almost half of patients with metastatic disease will experience a pleural effusion sometime during the course of their disease.[36-40]

Pleural effusions occur in 7% to 27% of hospitalized human immunodeficiency virus (HIV) patients.[41] The three leading causes of PE in those with HIV disease are parapneumonic infection, pulmonary Kaposi's sarcoma (KS), and tuberculosis.[42-44] The overall mortality rate associated with pleural effusion in HIV patients is 10% to 40%.[44] Unfortunately, the presence of malignant pleural effusion is usually associated with widespread disease and poor clinical prognosis, particularly in those with malignancy or AIDS. The overall mean survival for cancer patients who have MPE is 4 to 12 months.[34,45,46] Lung cancer patients usually die within 2 to 3 months, breast cancer patients within 7 to 15 months, and ovarian cancer patients within 9 months.[47-49] The mean survival period of those with pulmonary KS and MPE is 2 to 10 months; for those who have lymphoma and MPE, it is about 9 months.[50-52] Nearly all patients who have malignant pleural effusion are appropriate candidates for hospice care.[47]

## Pathophysiology

Each lung is covered with a serous membrane called the *pleura*. A closed cavity is located between the pleura and the surface of each lung, called the pleural cavity. Under normal circumstances, it is bathed with 10 to 120 mL of almost protein-free fluid that continuously flows across the pleural membrane. The fluid moves from the systemic circulation into the pleural cavity and then into the pulmonary circulation.[53] Osmotic and hydrostatic pressure act to ensure that equilibrium is maintained between absorption and production of fluid in the pleural space. When this equilibrium is disturbed, fluid can accumulate in the pleural cavity.[54-56]

A number of factors may disturb this equilibrium: (1) metastatic implants or inflammation that cause increased hydrostatic pressure in pulmonary circulation; (2) inflammatory processes that increase capillary permeability and increase oncotic fluid pressure in the pleural space; (3) hypoalbuminemia that decreases systemic oncotic pressure; (4) tumor obstruction or lung damage that creates increased negative intrapleural pressure; (5) impaired absorption of lymph when channels are blocked by tumor; and (6) increased vascular permeability caused by growth factors expressed by tumor cells.[29-31,57,58] Patients with large pleural effusions have demonstrated left-ventricular diastolic collapse and cardiac tamponade, which resolved with thoracentesis.[59,60]

## Diagnostic Procedures

A chest x-ray will usually establish the presence of the pleural effusion, and should also differentiate the presence of free versus loculated pleural fluid.[61] CT can show pleural or lung masses, adenopathy, pulmonary abnormalities such as infiltrates or atelectasis, or distant disease.[62-64] Chest ultrasound may differentiate between pleural fluid and pleural-thickening disease.[65,66]

In some cases, once evidence of the effusion has been established and obvious nonmalignant causes have been ruled out, a diagnostic thoracentesis may be helpful in establishing the diagnosis. Sonographic guidance can avoid problems associated with performing "blind" thoracentesis.[32]

## Signs and Symptoms

Dyspnea is the most common symptom of pleural effusion and occurs in about 75% of patients.[32,33,35-37,67] Its onset may be insidious or abrupt, and depends on how rapidly the fluid accumulates.[47] It is almost always related to collapse of the lung from the increase of pleural fluid pressure on the lung.[57]

The patient's inability to expand the lung leads initially to complaints of exertional dyspnea. As the effusion increases in volume, resting dyspnea, orthopnea, and tachypnea develop. The patient may complain of a dry, nonproductive cough, and an aching pain or heaviness in the chest. Pain is often described as dull or pleuritic in character.[68] Generalized systemic symptoms associated with advanced disease may also be present: malaise, anorexia, and fatigue.[30,34,66]

Physical examination reveals the presence of dullness to percussion of the affected hemithorax, decreased breath sounds, egophony, decreased vocal fremitus, whispered pectoriloquy, and decreased or no diaphragmatic excursion.[30,69,70] A large effusion may cause mediastinal shift to the side of the effusion; tracheal deviation may be present. Cyanosis and plethora, a ruddy facial complexion that occurs with partial caval obstruction, may also be present.[30,70]

## Medical and Nursing Management

Overall medical management of malignant pleural effusion depends on multiple factors, including the history of the primary tumor, prior patient history and response to therapy, extent of disease and overall medical condition, goals of care, and severity of symptom distress. In some cases, systemic therapy, hormonal therapy, or mediastinal radiation therapy may provide control of pleural effusions.[64] Symptomatic management of symptoms with pharmacotherapy includes the use of opioids to manage both pain and dyspnea, as well as anxiolytics to control concomitant anxiety.[32]

If the patient is to have a chest tube placed, or other invasive procedures to drain the fluid or to prevent fluid reaccumulation, the nurse must aggressively manage the patient's pain and anxiety. Educating the patient about what to expect, being present during the procedure, and medicating the patient preemptively are important aspects of palliative nursing care. Use of patient-controlled analgesia (PCA) for pain management is appropriate. Unfortunately, pain assessment and management is frequently not recognized as a priority when patients undergo these procedures.

## Thoracentesis Alone

Thoracentesis has been shown to relieve dyspnea associated with large pleural effusions.[64] When thoracentesis is undertaken, relief of symptoms may rapidly occur, but fluid reaccumulates quickly, usually within 3 to 4 days, and in 97% of patients within 30 days.[71] The decision to perform repeated thoracenteses should be tempered by the knowledge that risks include empyema, pneumothorax, trapped lung from inadequate drainage and/or loculated fluid, and the possibility of increasing malnutrition as a result of the removal of large amounts of protein-rich effusion fluid.[57]

Repeated thoracenteses rarely provide lasting control of malignant effusions.[72–74] There are no studies that compare repeated thoracenteses to other management approaches.[2] Instead of a second thoracentesis, a thoracostomy with pleurodesis should be considered.[47] It can be used to reduce adhesions, draw off fluid, and initiate drainage, all at the same time.

## Tube Thoracostomy and Pleurodesis

Palliative treatment, especially for those with a life expectancy of months rather than weeks, is best accomplished by performing closed-tube thoracoscopy, using imaging guidance with smaller bore tubes.[47] The goal of this therapy is to drain the pleural cavity completely, expand the lung fully, and then to instill the chemical agent into the pleural cavity. However, if there is a large effusion, only 1000 mL to 1500 mL should be drained initially.[47] Too-rapid drainage of a large volume of fluid can cause reexpansion pulmonary edema, and some patients have developed large hydropneumothoraces following rapid evacuation of fluid.[47] The thoracoscopy tube should then be clamped for 30 to 60 minutes. Approximately 1000 mL can be drained every hour until the chest is completely empty, but a slow rate of drainage is recommended.[64,75] The chest tube is then connected to a closed-drainage device. To prevent reexpansion pulmonary edema, water-seal drainage alone and intermittent tube clamping should be used to allow fluid to drain slowly.

Complications of chest tube placement include bleeding and development of pneumothorax, which occurs when fluid is rapidly removed in patients who have an underlying noncompliant lung. Patients who have chest tubes inserted should receive intrapleural bupivacaine or epidural and intravenous (IV) conscious sedation, as the procedure can be moderately to severely painful.[74,76–81]

## Pleurodesis

Chest radiography is used to monitor the position of the thoracostomy tube after thoracostomy is completed. It is thought that tube irritation of the pleural cavity may encourage loculations, which can lessen the effectiveness of potential sclerosing agents.[57] Current evidence indicates that it is not necessary to wait for drainage to fall below a certain level, and that the sclerosing agent can be injected as soon as the lung is fully reexpanded.[76] If the lung fails to expand and there is no evidence of obstruction or noncompliant lung, additional chest tube placement may be considered. Fibrinolysis with urokinase or streptokinase may improve drainage in those cases where fluid is still present or is thick

or gelatinous.[82] Intrapleural instillation of urokinase 100,000 units in 100-mL 0.9% saline can be attempted, and the chest tube clamped for 6 hours, with suction then being resumed for 24 hours. Once the pleural fluid has been drained and the lung is fully expanded, pleurodesis may be initiated. This can usually take place the day after chest tube insertion.[36,74,83–85]

The purpose of pleurodesis is to administer agents that cause inflammation and subsequent fibrosis into the pleural cavity to produce long-term adhesion of the visceral and parietal pleural surfaces. The goal of this procedure is to prevent reaccumulation of pleural fluid.[35,72] Various sclerosing agents are used to treat MPE. They include bleomycin, doxycycline, and sterilized asbestos-free talc. There is some research indicating that talc should be the agent of choice based on its success rate in preventing recurrence, and overall effectiveness.[34,86]

## Pleuroperitoneal Shunt

This procedure is useful for patients who have refractory MPE despite sclerotherapy.[29,72,73,87–89] Two catheters are connected by a pump to a chamber between the pleural cavity and the peritoneal cavity. Manually pushing the pumping chamber moves fluid from the pleural cavity to the peritoneal cavity. Releasing the compression moves the fluid from the pleural cavity into the chamber.

The major advantage of this device is that it can be used on an outpatient basis and allows the patient to remain at home. Its disadvantages include obstruction risk, infection, and tumor seeding; general anesthesia is needed for placement, and the device requires motivation and ability on the part of the patient to operate it. Most patients with advanced disease are unable to physically overcome the positive peritoneal pressure required to pump the device. Pumping is required hundreds of times a day, and therefore this device is not likely to be useful in those who are close to death.[90]

## Pleurectomy

Surgical stripping of the parietal pleura, with or without lung decortication (if the underlying lung is trapped), is more than 90% effective, but it has a high complication rate[67,72] and should be reserved for only those who have a reasonable life expectancy and physical reserve to withstand surgery.[29,32] Video-assisted thoracoscopy (VATS) and pleurectomy have been performed successfully in small, selected groups of patients.[91] However, it is likely to be an inappropriate choice in the palliative care patient at end of life.

## Indwelling Pleural Catheters

Indwelling pleural catheters can be placed under local anesthesia.[34] Those who meet criteria for ambulatory therapy—that is, those with symptomatic, unilateral effusions, and who have a reasonable performance status—may benefit from this therapy. It has been suggested that tunneled pleural catheters may permit long-term drainage and control of MPE in more than 80% to 90% of patients.[36,92] These catheters can be used to treat trapped lungs and large locules. Spontaneous pleurodesis eventually occurred in over 40% of catheter insertions (103 out of 240) in one study.[93]

Small-bore tubes attached to gravity drainage bags or vacuum drainage have been reported to be successful on an outpatient basis.[47] Rare complications include tumor seeding, obstruction, infection, cellulitis of tract site, and pain during drainage. If spontaneous pleurodesis does not occur, then continuing drainage may present management challenges. This treatment offers the potential for better quality of life and reduction in overall health care costs.

## Subcutaneous Access Ports

In this procedure a fenestrated catheter is placed in the pleural cavity. It can be accessed for repeated drainage without risk of pneumothorax or hemothorax.[47] Complications include occlusion, kinking, and wound infection.

## Nursing Management

Dyspnea and anxiety are primary symptoms experienced by the patient who has a pleural effusion. When invasive diagnostic procedures are being considered, these choices should be guided by the stage of disease, prognosis, the risk/benefit ratio of tests or interventions, pain-management considerations, and the desires of the patient and family.[94] The nurse can educate the patient and family about each procedure, including its purpose, how it is carried out, how pain will be addressed, and possible side effects or complications that may occur. This not only allows for informed consent but also may help to reduce anxiety and thus decrease dyspnea.[94]

A variety of nonpharmacological techniques can relieve the patient's dyspnea and pain, and can be used in combination with opioids and anxiolytics, as well as concurrently with medical treatment. These approaches include positioning the patient to comfort, using relaxation techniques, and providing oxygenation as appropriate.[94] Aggressive pain assessment and monitoring are particularly important for patients who receive invasive procedures.

# PERICARDIAL EFFUSION

CASE STUDY
*Mr. F, A Patient with Lymphoma*

Mr. F, a 62-year-old retired dentist, has undergone multiple rounds of chemotherapy for lymphoma and he has recently received experimental chemotherapy since he has not responded significantly to any other treatments. He realizes that all treatment is palliative at this point, and has already elected to have a DNR/DNI code status. He comes in to

the oncology clinic for follow-up, and during the nurse's assessment he mentions, "I've been gradually getting more short of breath recently, especially when I lie down at night. My chest has been feeling a little uncomfortable, too. It may not be anything, but I thought I would mention it." On exam, his lungs are clear to auscultation and percussion, but his heart sounds seem to be a little muffled.

- ◆  *Key Points*
- ◆  *Malignant pericardial effusions occur in less than 5% of patients with cancer, but the incidence may be nearer to 20% in patients with lung cancer.*
- ◆  *Effusions usually develop in patients with advanced disease and are usually a poor prognostic sign.*
- ◆  *The clinical features depend on the volume of pericardial fluid, the rate of accumulation of fluid, and the underlying cardiac function.*
- ◆  *Dyspnea is the most common presenting symptom.*

## Definition

A pericardial effusion is defined as an abnormal accumulation of fluid or tumor in the pericardial sac.[95] Pericardial effusions can lead to life-threatening sequelae. They can be caused by malignancies and their treatment, and by nonmalignant conditions. Pericardial effusions can lead to cardiac tamponade, which, if not treated, will cause cardiovascular collapse and death.[95]

## Epidemiology

Malignant disease is the most common cause of pericardial effusions.[96] Pericardial effusion is most commonly associated with lung and breast cancer, leukemia, and lymphoma.[96] Twenty-five percent to 50% of all patients who require surgical pericardial drainage have malignant pericardial involvement.[96] Metastatic spread or local extension from esophageal tumors and from sarcomas, melanomas, and liver, gastric, and pancreatic cancers can also occur.[97–100] Many pericardial effusions are asymptomatic and are discovered only on autopsy.[101] Up to 40% of cancer patients who have a symptomatic pericardial effusion will have a benign cause of the effusion.[57] Nonmalignant causes of pericardial effusions include pericarditis, congestive heart failure, uremia, myocardial infarction, and autoimmune disease, such as systemic lupus erythematosus. Other causes are infections, fungi, virus, tuberculosis, hypothyroidism, renal and hepatic failure, hypoalbuminemia, chest trauma, aneurysm, and complications of angiographic and central venous catheter procedures.[102,103]

A treatment-related cause of pericardial effusion is radiation therapy to the mediastinal area of more than 4000 cGy, which can lead to pericarditis and possible cardiac tamponade.[99,104,105] The anthracycline-based chemotherapies, such as doxorubicin, can also cause pericardial effusions.[106]

## Pathophysiology

The heart is covered by a thin sac called the pericardium. There are usually 15 to 50 mL of fluid between the pericardium and the heart itself.[57] Pericardial fluid originates in lymphatic channels surrounding the heart and is reabsorbed and drained by the lymph system into the mediastinum and into the right side of the heart.[10,11] This fluid minimizes friction, provides a barrier against inflammation, supports the chambers of the heart, and maintains the heart's position in the chest against accelerational and gravitational forces.[107–110] A pericardial effusion occurs when there is excessive fluid in this space. This fluid causes increased pressure to build in the pericardial sac, and the heart cannot fill or pump adequately. A pericardial effusion refers to the increased fluid or tumor in the pericardial sac. Cardiac tamponade is the physiological hemodynamic response of the heart to the effusion.[9]

Malignancies can cause effusions in the pericardial space by: (1) blocking lymph and blood drainage and preventing their resorption, (2) producing excess fluid in the space, (3) bleeding into the space, and (4) growing tumor into the space. The pericardial sac can hold up to 1800 mL of fluid before the heart begins to decompensate.[111,112] Thus, volume of fluid and distensibility will affect the impact of effusion on intrapericardial pressure.

Cardiac tamponade occurs when the heart cannot beat effectively because of excess pressure being exerted on its muscle.[99,102] As the pressure of fluid in the pericardial sac increases, the heart chambers are compressed. First, the right side of the heart, including the right atrium and right ventricle, is compressed. Less blood volume returns to the right side of the heart, thus increasing venous pressure. As the ventricles are further compressed, the heart cannot fill adequately, which leads to decreased stroke volume and cardiac output, and poor perfusion throughout the body. The body attempts to compensate by activating the adrenergic nervous system to keep the heart stimulated and its chambers filled with circulating blood volume. Heart rate increases, veins constrict, and the kidneys increase sodium and fluid retention. The heart ultimately is overwhelmed due to increased fluid, decreased filling, and decreased cardiac output, which leads to hypotension and circulatory collapse.[10,110,111]

Pericardial effusion can develop gradually over a period of weeks or months. The pericardium becomes more compliant, stretching to accommodate as much as 2 liters or more of fluid, with minimal effect on pericardial pressure. This is known as the "stress relaxation" phenomenon. Unfortunately, patients with chronic pericardial effusions may not exhibit physical signs of cardiac tamponade until compression of the heart and surrounding structures occurs, leading to sudden, life-threatening cardiac decompensation.[113–115]

## Signs and Symptoms

Pericardial tamponade that results from metastatic disease has a gradual onset that may be chronic and insidious.[9,107,114] Vague symptoms may be reported. Early in the decompensation process it may be difficult to differentiate symptoms of cardiac dysfunction from the effects seen in advancing cancer. The severity of symptoms is related to volume of the effusion, rate of accumulation, and the patient's underlying cardiac function.[10,99,111,116] Generally, rapid accumulation of fluid is associated with more severe cardiac tamponade. The most powerful predictor of the development of cardiac tamponade is the size of the pericardial effusion.[117]

Dyspnea is the most common presenting symptom.[118,119] The patient may complain of the inability to catch his or her breath, which progresses from dyspnea on exertion to dyspnea at rest. In advanced stages, the individual may be able to speak only one word at a time. Chest heaviness, cough, and weakness are also symptoms.[57] Pressure on adjacent structures, that is, the esophagus, trachea, and lung may increase.[120]

Tachycardia occurs as a response to decrease in cardiac output. A narrowing pulse pressure (difference between systolic and diastolic blood pressure) may be seen when blood backs up in the venous system, causing the systolic blood pressure to decrease and the diastolic blood pressure to increase.[9,120] Compression of the mediastinal nerves may lead to cough, dysphagia, hoarseness, or hiccups.[11] Increased venous pressure in the chest may lead to gastrointestinal (GI) complaints, such as nausea.[121,122] Retrosternal chest pain that increases when the patient is supine and decreases when he is leaning forward may occur, but is often not present.[110,120] Engorged neck veins, hepatomegaly, edema, and increased diastolic blood pressure are late signs of effusion. Anxiety, confusion, restlessness, dizziness, lightheadedness, and agitation related to hypoxemia may be present as the process progresses.[10,13,99,110,118,123] Poor cardiac output will lead to complaints of fatigue and weakness.

As the effusion increases and the heart begins to fail, symptoms worsen and dyspnea and orthopnea progress. Increasing venous congestion leads to peripheral edema. As cerebral perfusion worsens and hypoxemia increases, confusion increases. Ultimately, there is cardiovascular collapse, anuria, and decreased tissue perfusion, which causes obtundation, coma, and death.[10] Patients with chronic symptomatic pericardial effusions will often exhibit tachycardia, jugular venous distension, hepatomegaly, and peripheral edema.[120]

When examining the patient, one should listen for early signs of cardiac tamponade: (1) muffled heart sounds and perhaps a positional pericardial friction rub, and weak apical pulse; (2) presence of a compensatory tachycardia; (3) abdominal venous congestion and possible peripheral edema; and (4) a fever.[13,110,118,120,124] The signs and symptoms of pericardial effusion and cardiac tamponade may be mistaken for those of other pulmonary complications or pleural effusions. Many cancer patients have both pleural and pericardial effusions.[110,118] Unfortunately, symptoms of cardiac tamponade may be the first indication of the presence of pericardial effusion.

The triad of hypotension, increased jugular venous pressure, and quiet heart sounds that are diagnostic for pericardial effusion occurs in less than a third of patients.[125] If clear lung fields are present, this can help the clinician differentiate between pericardial effusion and congestive heart failure.[125] Pulsus paradoxus is a cardinal sign of cardiac tamponade. It occurs in 77% of those with acute tamponade and in only about 30% of those with chronic pericardial effusion.[114,125] However, its absence does not rule out pericardial effusion. Pulsus paradoxus is a fall in systolic blood pressure of greater than 10 mmHg with inspiration. Normally, blood pressure lowers on inspiration, but when the heart is compressed it receives even less blood flow. The resulting lowered volume and output result in a greater decrease in blood pressure.[110,121,126] Hepatojugular reflux is a late sign of cardiac tamponade.[10,123]

Late in the process of deterioration, diaphoresis and cyanosis are also present. The patient develops increasing ascites, hepatomegaly, peripheral edema, and central venous pressure. Decreased renal flow progresses to anuria. Further impairment in tissue perfusion leads to loss of consciousness, obtundation, coma, and death.[9,10,13,99,110,118]

### Diagnostic Procedures

Initially, a standard chest x-ray is likely to show a change in the size or contour of the heart and clear lung fields.[57] A pleural effusion may be evident in up to 70% of patients. Chest x-ray can also demonstrate mediastinal widening or hilar adenopathy. This diagnostic tool is cost-effective, minimally invasive, readily available, and may detect tamponade before the patient becomes symptomatic. However, when used alone, it is not specific enough to diagnose pericardial effusions and does not indicate the level of heart decompensation.[10,121] 2-D echocardiogram (2-D echo) is the most sensitive and precise test to determine if pericardial effusion or cardiac tamponade is present.[118] It can be used at the bedside and is noninvasive.

Some cancer patients may have both pericardial effusions and pleural effusions.[110,118] Pleural effusions can mimic the signs and symptoms of pericardial tamponade, causing symptoms of dyspnea and respiratory distress. Chest x-ray may hide or mimic the presence of pericardial tamponade, so depending on the goals of care, a 2D-echo should be performed to differentiate between these phenomena and to detect decompensation of the heart.

Other tests, including MRI and CT, can be used to detect effusions, pericardial masses and thickening, and cardiac tamponade. However, these tests do not indicate how well the heart is functioning, and they have limited use due to safety and comfort concerns in very ill patients.[118,120] If echocardiography is not available, a cardiac catheterization, which will detect depressed cardiac output and pressure levels in all four chambers of the heart, may be considered on a case-by-case basis.[120]

### Medical and Nursing Management

Options for medical management include pericardiocentesis with or without catheter drainage, pericardial sclerosis, percutaneous balloon pericardiotomy, pericardiectomy, pericardioperitoneal shunt, tunneled pericardial catheters, radiation therapy and chemotherapy, and aggressive symptom management without invasive procedures.

### Pericardiocentesis

The most simple, safe, and effective (97%) treatment is echocardiography-guided pericardiocentesis, with a procedural morbidity of 2% to 4% and mortality of 0%.[127–130] Since more than 50% of pericardial effusions reoccur, it is recommended that a 60-cm pigtail catheter (6 to 8 French) be threaded over the needle to allow for drainage of fluid over time.[120,127,131] The procedure can be performed emergently at the bedside, blindly, or with ECG guidance, but it should not be attempted in this manner except in extreme emergencies.[132] Adverse complications of the blind procedure include myocardial laceration, myocardial "stunning," arrhythmias, pneumothorax, abscess, and infection.[95,133] The failure rate of this procedure is 10% to 20% because of posterior pericardial loculation or catheter obstruction.

### Pericardial Sclerosis

Patients who experience pericardial tamponade face a 50% rate of recurrence when the underlying disease is not effectively treatable.[120] Pericardial sclerosis should be considered in those patients whose disease is not being actively or effectively treated. Pericardial sclerosis is defined as the instilling of chemicals through an indwelling catheter into the pericardial sac for the purpose of causing inflammation and fibrosis, to prevent further fluid reaccumulation. Doxycycline and bleomycin are the most common drugs instilled into the pericardial space.[126] Twenty-two patients were treated with bleomycin in one study, 95% of them successfully.[134] A common side effect of sclerosing therapy is severe retrosternal chest pain, especially with talc administration, and sometimes with bleomycin therapy.[126] A preemptive pain management plan is essential for the well-being of the patient. Arrhythmias, catheter occlusion, and transient fever of up to 38°C without associated bacteremia are also associated complications, primarily of talc and bleomycin therapy.[114,135,136] While sclerosing therapy may initially be "successful," that is, with evidence of disappearance of effusion or absence of tamponade symptoms for more than 30 days, multiple instillations may be necessary for true success.[120] The use of thiotepa has been recommended for pericardial instillation because it can be instilled into the drained space, is not associated with severe pain, and is reasonably effective.[126] A major complication is pericardial constriction. A serious discussion of risks, benefits, side effects of the therapy, and its impact on quality of life should take place in the context of end-of-life decision-making.

### Percutaneous Balloon Pericardiotomy

This is a safe, nonsurgical method that can be used to relieve the symptoms of chronic recurrent pericardial effusions.[120] It is performed in a cardiac catheterization lab under fluoroscopic guidance using IV conscious sedation and local anesthesia. A guidewire is inserted into the pericardial space, and a small pigtail catheter is inserted over the wire. The wire is removed and some pericardial fluid is withdrawn. Next, the pigtail catheter is removed and replaced with a balloon-dilating catheter that is advanced into the pericardial space and inflated. A pericardial drainage catheter is left in place and is removed when there is less than 100 mL of drainage daily.[137] Patients have reported experiencing severe pain during and after this procedure. A plan for aggressive pain management must be in place before this procedure and rapidly implemented if pain occurs.

Fever and pneumothorax are the most common complications.[137] Pleural effusion has also been associated with the procedure. It is suggested that percutaneous balloon pericardiotomy can be used in place of surgical drainage in patients with malignancy and a short life expectancy.[138]

## Surgical Pericardiectomy

Another option is to surgically create a pericardial "window" (partial pericardiectomy), a small opening in the pericardium and suture it to the lung. This allows pericardial fluid to drain out of the pericardial cavity, especially loculated effusions.[126] One study observed a 6.4% morbidity and 2.1% mortality rate after pericardial window surgery as the definitive method of treatment for malignant pericardial effusion.[139] When other procedures fail and the patient is expected to have long-term survival and good quality of life, partial or complete pericardiectomy may be considered.[120]

## Video-Assisted Thoracoscopic Surgery

Video-assisted thoracoscopic surgery (VATS), a minimally invasive procedure, can be used to manage chronic pericardial effusions. In this case, a thoracoscope is introduced into the left or right chest and a pericardial window is performed under thoracoscopic vision.[139,140] The pleura and pericardium can be visualized, tissue diagnosis can be obtained, and loculated effusions can be drained.[141] It has a 100% long-term success rate, and there is no significant morbidity or mortality associated with its use.[120]

## Radiation Therapy and Chemotherapy

In some cases, radiation therapy can be used to treat chronic effusions after the pericardial effusion has been drained,[120] and when tamponade is not present. It can be effective in radiosensitive tumors such as leukemias and lymphomas, but is less so in solid tumors.[114] Systemic chemotherapy can be considered if the malignancy is chemotherapy sensitive.[119]

Chronic pericardial effusions and their management can be challenging. Treatment of symptomatic chronic pericardial effusions will depend on patient prognosis, extent of symptoms, presence of concurrent medical conditions, and general condition. In many cases, treatment may be planned and carried out in a less urgent manner, keeping in mind the long-term benefits and side effects of interventions. Optimal treatment should focus on relieving symptoms caused by pressure on adjacent structures and, in the case of underlying malignancy, the first priority should be the promotion of comfort. When choosing a plan, the ability to treat the underlying cause, the long-term prognosis, and patient comfort should be of greatest importance.[120]

## Nursing Management

The priority goals in managing this condition are to provide comfort, to promote pain relief, and to reduce anxiety. The nurse should know both early and late signs of cardiac tamponade. Early recognition of these signs and their implications is most important because early intervention may prevent life-threatening sequelae.[9]

Aggressive symptom management includes the administration of opioids and anxiolytics to reduce pain and anxiety. If invasive cardiac procedures are carried out in an emergency at the bedside, the nurse should be present to provide support to the patient and family, to control pain and anxiety, and to monitor vital signs as indicated.[9]

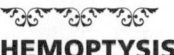

# HEMOPTYSIS

CASE STUDY
*Mrs. B, A Patient with Non-Small Cell Lung Cancer*

Mrs. B, a 67-year-old retired widow without children, was diagnosed with non-small cell lung cancer nine months ago and the disease has progressed rapidly in recent weeks despite aggressive treatment. She has recently started complaining of more dyspnea as well as some hemoptysis, but she has been reluctant to talk to her oncologist because she is afraid of what this may mean. The hemoptysis has been getting gradually worse and she finally goes to the emergency room. A CT scan reveals that a tumor appears to be eroding into an intrapleural vessel. The ER physician briefly tells her the CT scan results but instructs her to see her oncologist for further discussion. She asks the nurse taking care of her, "What does this mean? What's going to happen to me? I'm home alone most of the time and afraid....what happens if the bleeding gets worse?"

- ◆ *Key Points*
- ◆ *Hemoptysis occurs commonly in patients with advanced cancer and is most commonly due to malignant infiltration or infection.*
- ◆ *Hemoptysis should be distinguished from gastrointestinal and nasopharyngeal bleeding.*
- ◆ *Hemoptysis frequently provokes considerable anxiety.*
- ◆ *Massive hemoptysis, while rare, is a life-threatening crisis for patient, family, and staff. Massive hemoptysis occurs in fewer than 5% of cases, but the mortality rate is 85% if surgery is not feasible.*

(continued)

◆ *Skilled palliative nursing intervention includes provision of 24-hour psychological support and guidance.*

### Definition

Hemoptysis is defined as blood that is expectorated from the lower respiratory tract. Hemoptysis can be classified according to the amount of blood expectorated: (1) mild—less than 15 to 20 mL in a 24-hour period; (2) moderate—greater than 15 to 20 mL but less than 200 mL in a 24-hour period; and (3) massive—greater than 200 mL to 600 mL in a 24-hour period.[142] The primary risk to the patient is asphyxiation from blood-clot formation obstructing the airway, rather than from exsanguination. Massive hemoptysis carries a high mortality rate if not treated.

### Epidemiology

Tuberculosis is the most common worldwide cause of hemoptysis.[143] The most common causes of hemoptysis in the United States are bronchitis, bronchiectasis, and bronchogenic carcinoma.[143] Other nonmalignant causes of hemoptysis are lung abscess, sarcoidosis, mycobacterium invasion, emphysema, fungal diseases, and AIDS. There is no underlying cause found in 15% to 30% of hemoptic episodes.[143–145]

Metastatic lung disease caused by other primary tumors is associated with nonfatal hemoptysis.[146] Tumors in the trachea usually cause obstructive symptoms rather than massive bleeding.[147] Massive hemoptysis occurs in fewer than 5% of cases, but the mortality rate is 85% if surgery is not feasible.[148,149] Bleeding occurs most often from proximal endobronchial tumors that are not amenable to surgical intervention. Prognosis is usually grim in the case of end-stage lung disease and in the setting of massive hemoptysis.

### Pathophysiology

Each lung is supplied with blood by way of two circulatory systems. Pulmonary circulation delivers blood under low pressure from the right ventricle to the alveolar capillaries, where oxygen and carbon dioxide are exchanged. Bronchial circulation arises from the systemic circulation that branches off the aorta, which delivers blood to the lungs under high pressure. These systems anastomose in precapillary pulmonary arterioles and pulmonary veins.[146]

The bronchial venous system returns blood to the heart by two pathways: (1) blood is returned to the right atrium by way of the azygous, hemiazygous, or intercostal veins, and (2) blood is returned to the left ventricle by way of the pulmonary veins. The second pathway carries the bulk of bronchial venous return to the heart.[146]

In the setting of inflammation, tumor, or infection, the bronchial vasculature develops new vascularization pathways. Bronchial blood flow increases as the result of increases in both size and number of these collateral vessels. When these vessels are damaged by inflammation, malignancy, or other injury, blood flow is increased and this raises pulmonary vascular pressure. Hemoptysis occurs in the setting of multiple collateral vessels, high vascular pressure, and damaged, enlarged, and diseased airways.[146,150,151]

In patients who have HIV disease, bacterial pneumonia and infections cause 63% of episodes of hemoptysis. Kaposi's sarcoma causes 10% of episodes, and pulmonary embolism causes 4% of episodes.[152] Patients on anticoagulant or thrombolytic therapy may also experience hemoptysis.[149,153]

### Diagnostic Procedures

Flexible fiberoptic bronchoscopy is initially the quickest and surest way to visualize the source of bleeding in the upper lung lobes and to localize it in the lower respiratory tract.[143] This procedure can be done at the bedside without putting the patient under general anesthesia, and it can also visualize distal airways.[146] If there is brisk bleeding, the rigid bronchoscope can suction more efficiently, remove clots and foreign bodies, allow for better airway control, and can be used to obtain material for diagnostic purposes.[154] In some cases, bronchoscopy may locate the area of bleeding but not the direct source of bleeding. In this case, the segment of affected tissue may be purposely suctioned until it collapses.[43] Bronchoscopy should not be undertaken if there is evidence of pulmonary embolism, pneumonia, or bronchitis, or when the patient's condition is so poor or unstable that no further intervention would be undertaken no matter what the results.[151]

If treatment is to be initiated, the combination of bronchoscopy and high-resolution CT can identify the cause of hemoptysis in 81% of patients. It is also quick, noninvasive, and less costly than other modalities.[143] If pulmonary embolism is suspected and therapy is to be initiated, a ventilation-perfusion scan may be warranted.[155]

### Signs and Symptoms

Respiratory complaints that raise suspicion of bleeding into the lungs may include cough, dyspnea, wheezing, chest pain, sputum expectoration, and systemic clues, such as fever, night sweats, and weight loss. Clues to nasopharyngeal bleeding as the possible source include frequent nosebleeds, throat pain, tongue or mouth lesions, dysphonia, and hoarseness.[156] Clues to GI bleeding as the possible source include the presence of dyspepsia, heartburn, and/or dysphagia. Coffee-grounds-colored vomitus and blood in vomitus does not rule out hemoptysis, because blood from respiratory sources can be swallowed. Patients and family members should be asked to describe the color of blood, and should be asked about any changes in color and pattern of bleeding in vomitus and stool.[156]

During an active bleeding episode, a focused examination should be performed as quickly as possible. If possible, the nasopharynx, larynx, and upper airways should be thoroughly visually examined to rule out an upper airway source of bleeding.[143,154,156] If bleeding is brisk and views are obstructed, examination may best be accomplished with bronchoscopy. The patient may be coughing or vomiting blood, and may be short of breath. If possible, sputum, blood and vomitus should be examined.[143,151] Some patients may not yet have a diagnosis of malignancy. In these cases one should note clubbing of fingernails and presence of cervical or supraclavicular adenopathy. This may indicate the presence of a malignancy.[156]

Massive bleeding may take place in the lung without the presence of hemoptysis, so listening to lung sounds is very important. Auscultation of the lungs may reveal localized wheezing, an indication of possible airway obstruction.[156] Fine diffuse rales and asymmetric chest excursion may indicate the presence of an infectious or consolidative process.[156] If petechiae and ecchymosis are present, then there should be strong suspicion that a bleeding diathesis is present.[156]

### Medical and Nursing Management

If the episode of bleeding is severe and the goal is active treatment or prolongation of life, then the primary focus is to maintain an adequate airway. This will usually require endotracheal intubation, which may have to be performed immediately at the bedside, and oxygenation. If bleeding can be localized and controlled quickly, a short period of intubation may be considered if it will allow for improved quality of life.[146]

Specific methods of treatment include radiation therapy, laser coagulation therapy, bronchial arterial embolization, endobronchial balloon tamponade, epinephrine injection, iced saline lavage, and, in very rare cases, surgical resection.

### Radiation Therapy

External-beam radiation therapy can stop hemoptysis in more than 80% of cases, especially in those patients who have unresectable lung cancers.[157,158] The goal is to provide therapy in the shortest time period possible, at the lowest dose to achieve symptom control while minimizing side effects. Complications of therapy are radiation fibrosis, and, unfortunately, massive hemoptysis.[159]

Endobronchial brachytherapy has been effective in some patients who have failed previous external-beam radiation attempts.[160] Brachytherapy and bronchoscopy laser therapy have also resulted in resolution of hemoptysis. Results have not been as favorable in patients who have failed previous external-beam radiation therapy, or when combined with laser therapy.[161] Side effects associated with brachytherapy, particularly high-dose brachytherapy, include mucositis, fistula formation, and fatal hemoptysis.[162,163] The benefits of this treatment should be carefully weighed against potential side effects and their impact on quality of life, particularly in those patients who have short-term prognoses.

### Endobronchial Tamponade

In this procedure, flexible bronchoscopy is used to find the bleeding site after the site has been lavaged with iced saline.

A balloon catheter attached to the tip of the bronchoscope is placed on the site and is then inflated and left on the bleeding site for 24 to 48 hours.[164] In the case of life-threatening hemoptysis, a rigid bronchoscope should be used. This is not a uniformly successful procedure, and should be considered a temporizing measure only.[143] A different approach to endobronchial tamponade that was recently utilized involved the placement of two self-expanding bronchial stents which stopped the bleeding permanently and allowed the patient to be extubated and continue treatment.[165]

### Laser Coagulation Therapy

In the case of obstructing tracheal tumors, Nd-YAG photocoagulation may control bleeding from endobronchial lesions, and it has a response rate of 60%.[166] Anecdotal reports of the effectiveness of electrocautery to control hemoptysis have been reported; argon plasma coagulation has led to resolution of hemoptysis for at least a 3-month followup. However, highly vascular tumors are at risk for bleeding when exposed to laser therapy.[165]

### Bronchial Arterial Embolization

When an endoscopically visualized lung cancer is the source of bleeding, bronchial artery embolization is effective as a palliative intervention. It stops bleeding in 77% to 93% of cases.[154,167] Bronchial artery embolization, preceded by bronchoscopy, involves injecting a variety of agents angiographically into the bronchial artery to stop blood flow.[151,168] Thirty percent of patients will rebleed within the first or later months, and repeated embolizations may be required.[168,169]

There are major risks associated with this procedure, including transverse myelitis, paraplegia, ischemic colitis, severe pneumonia, esophagobronchial fistula formation, and temporary severe retrosternal pain.[170] Superselective catheterization now reduces the chance of inadvertently catheterizing the spinal cord branch of the bronchial artery, which has led to spinal cord paraplegia in the past.[171] The risks of rebleeding and the prospect of having repeated embolizations should be carefully reviewed and discussed with the patient and family before carrying out this therapy.

### Endobronchial Epinephrine Injections

A 1:10,000 epinephrine solution may be instilled on visualized lesions to constrict veins and reduce bleeding. Vasopressin and chlorpromazine have also been used in this procedure, which is performed in patients who are not candidates for surgery and when bronchial artery embolization is not available.[143,154]

### Iced Saline Lavage

Iced saline solution lavage has been used as a temporary non-standard measure to provide improved visualization and localization of the bleeding site. It does not appear to improve outcomes.[143,154]

## Surgery

In rare cases, some patients who continue to have life-threatening hemorrhage after receiving other therapies may be considered as candidates for surgical intervention. Only those whose life expectancy, condition, ability to tolerate major surgery, and ability to maintain an airway make them suitable candidates should be considered. It is important to remember that most lung cancers are well advanced at diagnosis and that undertaking this procedure may not meet quality-of-life goals for those with short-term prognoses.[143]

## Palliative Care

When a decision has been made to forego aggressive treatment measures, then promotion of comfort for the patient is the primary goal. Death from massive hemoptysis is usually rapid, occurring within minutes. However, even when the family has been carefully "prepared" for this possibility and coached in a step-by-step manner in what to do, family members inevitably remain unprepared and distraught if a massive hemorrhage does occur, especially in the home without medical personnel around. Preemptive planning includes anxiolytic and opioids readily available in the home, a 24-hour palliative care number to call for immediate guidance and support, and dark-colored towels to reduce the visibility of blood and thus make it less overwhelming.

# SPINAL CORD COMPRESSION

CASE STUDY
*Mrs. S, A Patient with Multiple Myeloma*

Mrs. S is a 73-year-old woman diagnosed with multiple myeloma two months ago. Chemotherapy has not helped so far, and she has been found to have several spinal metastases which cause mild back pain. This has been well-controlled by 10 mg of Oxycodone IR two or three times a day. She is admitted directly to the palliative care unit by her oncologist after she called, complaining, "I've been having more and more back pain the past few days, especially when I'm lying in bed at night, and the pain medicine isn't really helping anymore, even though I'm taking it as often as I can. I'm also having this weird numbness and tingling in my legs that I've never had before." On exam, Mrs. S is found to have slight weakness in both legs, but no other focal findings.

- ◆ *Key Points*
- ◆ *Pain is the primary presenting symptom of spinal cord compression. It may be present long before neurological dysfunction occurs.*
- ◆ *The pain is classically worse when lying flat and improved when upright.*

- ◆ *In a patient with cancer, increasing back pain that is worse when lying flat and improved when standing is presumed to be cord compression until proven otherwise.*
- ◆ *Early detection and treatment may prevent permanent loss of function. It is therefore considered a medical emergency.*
- ◆ *The use of steroids and radiation therapy in patients with far advanced cancer can decrease the pain and usually preserve function. Steroids alone can usually decrease pain and preserve function in those who are close to death and do not want to undergo radiation therapy, even in truncated form.*

## Definition

Spinal cord compression (SCC) is compression of the thecal sac at the level of the spinal cord or cauda equina. Spinal cord injury may cause progressive and irreversible neurological damage and requires immediate intervention to prevent disability. SCC in the presence of malignancy often carries a poor prognosis, with a median life expectancy of 3 to 6 months.[2,172] Prognostic factors for longer survival include: only one site of cord compression, ability to ambulate pre- and post-treatment, bone metastases only, and tumor that is responsive to radiation.[172]

## Epidemiology

Compression of the spinal cord and cauda equina is a major cause of morbidity in patients with cancer. It occurs in approximately 5% to 10% of patients with malignant disease,[173,174] and is most commonly associated with metastatic disease from tumors of the breast, lung, and prostate. Less than 50% of patients will regain functional losses due to SCC.[10,174–176]

Compression of the spine in 85% to 90% of cases is caused by direct hematological extension of solid tumor cells into a vertebral body.[150,177–180] A less common pathway is by direct extension of tumor from adjacent tissue through the intervertebral foramina. Tumor cells can also enter the epidural space directly by circulating in the cerebral spinal fluid (CSF). Paraneoplastic syndromes, leptomeningeal disease, and toxicity of chemotherapy drugs can cause spinal cord syndromes.[181]

Nonmalignant causes of SCC include benign tumors, degenerative, inflammatory, and infectious diseases that affect the spinal column, and from trauma, herniated disks, osteoporosis, or other structural diseases.[22,181]

## Pathophysiology

There are 26 vertebrae in the vertebral column: 7 cervical, 12 thoracic, 5 lumbar, 1 sacral, and 1 coccygeal. Inside this flexible protective vertebral column is the spinal cord, which is an elongated mass of nervous tissue covered and protected by membranes called *meninges*. The outermost layer is the dura mater, the middle layer is the arachnoid membrane, and the innermost layer closest to the spinal cord is the pia mater. The epidural space is located between the outer layer of the dura mater and the vertebral column.[10]

The spinal cord begins where it is attached to the medulla oblongata in the brain and descends through the foramen magnum of the skull until it ends at the level of the first lumbar vertebra. Lumbar and sacral nerve roots then descend below the distal tip of the vertebral column, and spread to the lumbar and sacral areas. These long nerve roots resemble a horse's tail that is called the *cauda equina*. Thirty-one pairs of spinal nerves exit from the spinal cord.[176,182,183] Transmission of nerve impulses travels the length of the spinal cord to and from the brain in ascending and descending tracts. Impulses from the spinal cord to the brain travel through the anterior spinothalamic tracts, and impulses from the brain to the spinal cord travel through the lateral corticospinal tracts. Injury to these nerves, or to the cord itself, can result in sensory-motor and autonomic impairment.[176]

Eighty-five percent of SCCs are extradural in nature.[9,10,174,184] That is, they originate outside the cord itself. Extradural metastatic tumors may be osteolytic, where lesions invade the marrow of the vertebrae and cause absorption of bone tissue, which leads to bone destruction. They may also be osteoblastic, where lesions invade the bone marrow and cause bone development, tumor invasion, and collapse of the vertebral body, which then pushes tumor or bone fragments into the spinal cord.[10,182,184] Neurological deficits caused by SCC include direct compression on the cord or cauda equina, vascular supply interruption, or pathological fracture, causing vertebral collapse. When nerve tissue dies, neurological regeneration is not always possible. Function may be quickly and irreversibly lost.

## Diagnostic Procedures

Plain spinal x-rays are an excellent screening tool and can determine the presence of tumor and the stability of the spine.[181] They can identify lytic or blastic lesions in up to 85% of vertebral lesions. However, false negatives can occur due to poor visualization, mild pathology, or poor interpretation.[177] More than 50% collapse and pedicle erosion must be present before x-ray can detect SCC.[185,186] Epidural spread of tumor through the foramina might not always be visualized using plain x-rays. A bone scan may detect vertebral abnormalities when plain films are negative.[187–189]

MRI is the imaging choice for emergent SCC.[186] It is non-invasive and does not require injection with contrast material. It has an advantage over CT because it can image the entire spine, thus detecting multiple areas of compression.[173,181,190] Decisions about diagnostic testing will be tempered by a number of factors, including the potential for treatment, prognosis, patient's condition, and the patient's and/or family's wishes for treatment.

## Signs and Symptoms

The presence of increasing back pain, worse on lying flat and improved on standing, with or without signs of bowel and bladder impairment, in a patient with a history of cancer, should presumed to be SCC until proven otherwise. Neurological function before initiation of therapy is the single most important prognostic factor in SCC.[16] Misdiagnosis of SCC has been attributed to poor history, inadequate examination, and insufficient diagnostic evaluation.[191] Patients who have only localized back pain and a normal neurological examination may have more than 75% of the spinal cord compressed. Upper motor neuron weakness may occur above the L1 vertebral body in 75% of patients with SCC at diagnosis. Sensory changes occur in about half of patients at presentation. Sensory change without pain complaint is extremely rare.

A thorough history should pay special attention to the onset of pain, its location, its intensity, duration, quality, and what activities increase or decrease the pain.[180,184,192] A history of sensory or motor weakness and autonomic dysfunction should be evaluated and should include onset and degree of weakness; heaviness or stiffness of limbs; difficulty walking; numbness in arms, hands, fingers, toes, and trunk; and change in temperature or touch. Specific questions about bowel, bladder, and sexual function should be asked directly, because patients may not volunteer these symptoms, such as difficulty in passing urine or stool, incontinence of bowel or bladder, loss of sphincter control, and ability to obtain and maintain an erection. Constipation usually precedes urinary retention or incontinence.[184]

Physical examination includes observation of the spine, muscles, extremities and skin, and palpation and gentle percussion of vertebrae. Spinal manipulation to elicit pain responses should be carried out cautiously because it may cause muscle spasm or further injury.[181] Mental status, cranial nerves, motor function, reflexes, sensation, coordination, strength, and gait should be evaluated (where appropriate to the patient's status and closeness to death). Focused examination may include performing straight leg raises until the patient feels pain, then dorsiflexing the foot. If this action increases pain down the back of the leg, this suggests that nerve root compression is present. Testing of reflexes will indicate the presence and impact of nerve root compression on motor ability. Cord compression may cause hyperactive deep-tendon reflexes, while nerve-root compression may cause decreased deep-tendon reflexes. A positive Babinski sign and sustained ankle clonus indicate motor involvement.[184]

Sensory function should be tested by assessing pain (sharp, dull), temperature (hot, cold), touch (light), vibration (tuning fork test), and position senses (fingers and toes). Examination may reveal a demarcated area of sensory loss and brisk or absent reflexes.[184] The mapping of positive sensation can be used to pinpoint the level of SCC, usually one or two levels below the site of compression.[184] Bladder percussion and digital rectal examination will elicit retention and laxity of sphincter control, a late sign of SCC.

Pain may be reported for weeks to months before any obvious neurological dysfunction.[173] Pain may be local initially (in the central back, for example), then progress to a radicular pattern that follows a particular dermatome.[175,181] Local pain may be caused by stretching of bone periosteum by tumor or vertebral collapse, and is usually described by the patient as constant, dull, aching, and progressive in nature. Radicular pain is caused by pressure of tumor along the length of the nerve root.[10,123,176] The patient who reports radicular pain will describe it as shooting, burning, or shocklike in nature and will state that it is worsened by movement, sneezing, straining, neck flexion, or by lying down.

A classic sign of cord compression is if pain is relieved by sitting up or standing and is worsened by lying flat. Also, if pain increases at night when the patient is lying down to sleep, one should be suspicious of SCC rather than degenerative or disk disease.[173] Radicular pain is present in 90% of lumbosacral SCC, 79% in cervical SCC, and in 55% of thoracic SCC.[193] Radicular pain is typically bilateral in thoracic lesions, and is often described as a tight band around the chest or abdomen, but it may also be experienced in only part of one dermatome.[173,177] Nonradicular referred pain may also be associated with vague paresthesias and point tenderness.[173,177,181] Vigilance is called for when these radicular symptoms occur: (1) shoulder tip pain from C7/T1 metastases; (2) anterior or abdominal, flank, or hip pain from T12–L2 metastases; or (3) lateral or anterior rib pain from thoracic metastases.[181]

The sequence of neurological symptoms usually progresses in the following manner: first there is pain, then motor weakness that progresses to sensory loss, then motor loss, and finally, autonomic dysfunction.[9] The patient will initially complain of heaviness or stiffness in the extremities, loss of coordination, and ataxia.[194,195] Sensory complaints include paresthesias and numbness, and loss of heat sensation. Dysfunction begins in the toes and ascends in a stocking-like pattern to the level of the lesion.[173] Loss of proprioception, deep pressure and vibration are late signs of sensory loss.[10,22,123,176] When the cauda equina is affected, sensory loss is bilateral; the dermatome that follows the perianal area, posterior thigh, and lateral aspect of the leg is involved. Late signs of SCC are motor loss and paralysis. Loss of sphincter control is associated with poor return to functionality.[10,22,176]

## Medical and Nursing Management

The focus of management of SCC should be the relief of pain and preservation or restoration of neurological function. Rapid intervention is required to prevent permanent loss of function and concomitant quality of life. The patient status (e.g., goals of care and closeness to death), rate of neurological impairment, and prior radiation therapy experience are other factors to consider.[184] Corticosteroids, surgical decompression, radiation therapy, and adjuvant chemotherapy or hormonal therapy are the standard treatments for SCC.[13,184,196]

## Corticosteroids

Corticosteroids decrease vasogenic edema and inflammation and thus relieve pain and neurological symptoms, and may have some oncolytic effect on tumor.[192] Dexamethasone is the preferred corticosteroid because it is less likely to promote systemic edema caused by other steroids, or to cause cognitive and behavioral dysfunction, and it improves overall outcomes after specific therapy.[173]

There has been controversy about dosage and scheduling of dexamethasone therapy in the management of SCC.[172,173,185] In animal studies, neurological status has improved more rapidly with high dose steroid therapy.[177,178,198–201] A recent Cochrane review examining interventions for metastatic extradural SCC was, however, unable to demonstrate any evidence-based differences in benefit from high-dose versus low-dose corticosteroids. The review did however, conclude that the incidence of adverse side effects was greater with high-dose compared to low-dose steroid therapy.[197] One suggested approach would be to administer high-dose therapy for patients who are no longer ambulatory or have rapidly increasing motor deficits, and low-dose therapy for those patients who can walk and do not have significant/worsening motor deficits.[172]

Currently, high-dose therapy regimens recommend administering a 100-mg IV bolus of dexamethasone, followed by 24 mg dexamethasone orally QID for 3 days, then tapering the dose over 10 days. High-dose therapy may increase analgesia but, as mentioned, can also increase side effects that are significant. These include GI bleeding, hyperglycemia, depression and psychosis, myopathy, osteoporosis, and acute adrenal insufficiency with abrupt withdrawal.[182] Low-dose dexamethasone regimen recommends administering a 10 mg IV bolus of dexamethasone, followed by 4 mg IV QID for 3 days, then tapering the dose over 14 days.[173] Rapid IV push of corticosteroids causes severe burning pain in the perineum, and the patient needs to be warned that this will occur but does not signify that anything is wrong. Corticosteroids are metabolized by the cytochrome P-450 system, and there are implications for interactions with other medications, particularly anticonvulsants.

## Decompressive Surgery

The goals of surgery are to decompress neural structures, resect tumor if possible, establish local disease control, achieve spinal stability, restore the ability to ambulate, treat pain, and improve quality of life. Surgery for SCC has been used to (1) establish a diagnosis when tissue is required for histologic analysis; (2) halt rapidly deteriorating function; (3) achieve cure for primary malignancy; (4) treat those with previously irradiated radio-resistant tumor and who have continuing symptomatic progressive loss of function; (5) rule out infection or hematoma; (6) alleviate respiratory paralysis caused by high cervical spinal cord lesions; and (7) decompress and stabilize spine structure.[10,13,22,184] Benefits and burden of surgery to the patient in a palliative care setting must be carefully weighed so that the patient and family can make an informed decision.

## Radiation Therapy

Fractionated external-beam radiation therapy (XRT) to the spine is given to inhibit tumor growth, restore and preserve neurological function, treat pain, and improve quality of life.[9,202] It has been the primary treatment for SCC.[173] The standard treatment regimen is 30 Gy over the course of 10 fractions, but hypofractionation (e.g. 8 Gy once or 4 Gy over 5 fractions) may be used in patients with limited expected survival.[158] Only symptomatic sections of the spine are treated. Seventy percent of patients who are ambulatory at the start of treatment will retain their ability to walk. Thirty-five percent of paraparetic patients will regain their ability to walk, while only 5% of completely paraplegic patients will do so.[16,203] Primary side effects of radiation therapy include skin alterations of erythema, dry or moist desquamation, pigmentation changes, as well as generalized fatigue.

## Nursing Management

The goal of nursing management is to identify patients at high risk for cord compression, to educate the patient and family regarding signs and symptoms to report, to detect early signs of SCC, and to work as a member of the palliative care team in managing symptoms. In those patients who have far advanced disease, palliative care efforts focus on promoting comfort, relieving pain and providing family support.

# HYPERCALCEMIA

CASE STUDY
### Mrs. R, A Patient with Breast Cancer

Mrs. R, a 45-year-old mother of two and businesswoman, has been fighting breast cancer for the past three years, and she currently has multiple sites of bony metastasis. She has been taking oral chemotherapy as well as radiation therapy. She is very stoic and determined to "beat this cancer." Her job requires a lot of concentration, but she has recently had some difficulty focusing on tasks and is having some memory lapses as well. Her co-workers and family finally convince her to call her oncologist's office, and she talks to his nurse. During this conversation she also lists constipation, loss of appetite, and fatigue as new issues. Mrs. R is instructed to come in to the office for an exam and to have blood drawn.

- **Key Points**
- *Hypercalcemia occurs in 8% to 10% of patients with cancer, with an incidence of 40% in patients with breast cancer and multiple myeloma.*
- *Common presenting signs are fatigue, lethargy, nausea, polyuria, and confusion.*
- *The combination of nausea and polyuria can lead to dehydration and worsening of hypercalcemia.*
- *Severity of symptoms depends on the level of free ionized calcium and the speed with which the level rises.*
- *The serum calcium level is adjusted according to the serum albumin in patients with significant hypoalbuminemia.*

- *All patients with hypercalcemia who are symptomatic warrant a trial of therapy.*
- *Control of hypercalcemia will not affect prognosis but may greatly improve symptoms and quality of life in these patients.*

## Definition

Hypercalcemia is an excessive amount of ionized calcium in the blood.[204,205] If hypercalcemia is left untreated, the patient may experience irreversible renal damage, coma, or death. Mortality from untreated hypercalcemia approaches 50%.

## Epidemiology

About 10% to 20% of cancer patients will develop hypercalcemia at some time during their illness.[204,206–208,210] Carcinomas of the breast and lung, multiple myeloma, and squamous cell carcinomas of the head, neck, and esophagus are the most common malignancies associated with hypercalcemia. Incidence ranges from 30% to 40% for breast cancer with bone metastases, 20% to 40% for multiple myeloma, 12.5% to 35% for the squamous cell lung carcinomas, and 2.9% to 25% for head and neck malignancies.[204] Hypercalcemia is rare in prostate cancer, GI cancers, and cancers of the biliary tract.[204]

Primary hyperparathyroidism as a cause of hypercalcemia is more common in the ambulatory and asymptomatic population.[209,211,216] Other conditions associated with hypercalcemia include lithium therapy, Addison's disease, Paget's disease, granulomatous disease, vitamin D intoxication, hyperthyroidism, vitamin A intoxication, and aluminum intoxication.[205,212]

## Pathophysiology

Calcium helps the body to maintain its acid-base balance, maintain permeability of cell membranes, promote coagulation, and maintain proper nerve and muscle function.[213] Under normal circumstances, bone resorption and bone formation are in a steady state and are regulated by three hormones—parathyroid hormone (PTH), calcitriol (1,25 dihydroxyvitamin D, a metabolite of vitamin D), and calcitonin.[205] These hormones act at bone sites, in the intestine, and in the kidney. PTH directly increases resorption of calcium from the bone and calcium resorption in the renal tubule. Calcitriol stimulates absorption of calcium in the intestine. It enhances bone resorption and increases renal resorption. Calcitonin is excreted by the thyroid gland and inhibits bone resorption and increases excretion of calcium.

Bone undergoes constant remodeling in the human body. Osteoblasts form bone and osteoclasts resorb bone. About 99% of the body's calcium is found in bone. The remaining 1% circulates in the blood or is found inside cells. Half of plasma calcium is bound to either protein (albumin) or to other ions, such as phosphate, carbonate, or citrate. The remaining calcium circulates as free ions. Since free calcium is biologically active, its level is maintained in a narrow range in the normal physiological state.

Hypercalcemia in malignant disease is primarily due to increased mobilization of calcium from bone. Increased renal tubular calcium resorption is also a factor in hypercalcemia of malignancy. There are three major mechanisms that contribute to the development of malignant hypercalcemia.[206] First, higher levels of PTHrP (parathyroid hormone-related protein) are found in hypercalcemic patients who have solid tumors, particularly squamous cell carcinomas. The presence of elevated PTHrP levels is associated with more advanced cancer, a worse prognosis, and a poor response to bisphosphonate therapy. Approximately 80% of cases of malignant hypercalcemia are related to the presence of this protein.

Second, osteolysis of bone is caused by the release of tumor and other cell mediators. When this mechanism is operating, hypercalcemia occurs late in disease and is usually associated with extensive osteolytic bone metastases. Third, the increased production of calcitriol by lymphoma tumor cells, for example, leads to increased resorption of calcium in the gut. Hypercalcemia induced by calcitriol usually responds to corticosteroid therapy.

The kidney normally adapts to disturbances in calcium homeostasis. However, in the presence of malignancy, patients may experience treatment or disease-related side effects including vomiting, mucositis, anorexia, dysphagia, and fever, all of which can lead to volume depletion.[204] This imbalance signals the kidney to reabsorb sodium to correct extracellular volume depletion. Calcium and sodium resorption are closely linked in the body; when sodium is resorbed, calcium is also resorbed. As calcium ions are resorbed in the kidney, the tubules lose their ability to concentrate urine, leading to high-output polyuria and further dehydration. Poor renal perfusion, reduced glomerular filtration and compromised excretion of calcium lead to a further increase of calcium in the blood. Ultimately, renal failure will occur.

A high calcium level can alter the patient's mental status significantly, which, in turn, can greatly affect the patient's ability to drink fluids. Cellular dehydration and resulting hypotension are exacerbated by decreased proximal renal tubule reabsorption of sodium, magnesium, and potassium. Bone loss due to immobilization, lack of physical exercise, inappropriate use of thiazide diuretics, poor diet, and general physiological wasting will also increase the amount of free calcium ions in the circulation, further increasing calcium levels.

### Diagnostic Tests and Procedures

The ionized calcium concentration is the most important laboratory test to use in the diagnostic workup for hypercalcemia. It is the most accurate indicator of the level of calcium in the blood. (There is only a fair correlation between the total serum calcium level and ionized calcium.) When ionized calcium cannot be used as a diagnostic tool, the total serum calcium value may be used, but it must be corrected for serum albumin. A rule of thumb is to add 0.8 for each 1 g/dL the albumin has dropped below the normal range (3.7 to 5 g/dL).[204,205]

### Signs and Symptoms

Symptoms of hypercalcemia, their severity, and how quickly they appear will vary from patient to patient. The extent of metastatic bone disease is not associated with hypercalcemia levels.[208,209,210,214] It is important to remember that patients, especially the elderly and the debilitated,[204,209,212,215] may experience severe symptoms even when serum calcium is not extremely elevated.[204] Symptoms of hypercalcemia, such as vomiting, nausea, anorexia, weakness, constipation, and impaired mental status, may be mistakenly attributed to the disease or effects of treatment. Factors that will influence patients' response to hypercalcemia include age,[212] performance status, renal or hepatic failure, and sites of metastatic disease.

Patients with a corrected serum calcium level less than 12 mg/dL who are asymptomatic can be considered to have mild hypercalcemia. Patients who have a serum calcium level between 12 and 14 mg/dL should be closely monitored and may require urgent intervention, depending on goals of care in the palliative setting. Those patients with a calcium level greater than 14 mg/dL will require urgent treatment, again depending on goals of care in the palliative setting.[206]

The patient may complain of numerous symptoms that can mimic symptoms of advanced malignancy.[204] These include GI symptoms of nausea, vomiting, anorexia, constipation, obstipation and even complete ileus. Polydipsia and polyuria may also be present. Muscle weakness, fatigue, and difficulty climbing stairs or getting out of a car, are musculoskeletal symptoms that can progress to profound weakness, hypotonia, and fracture. Neuropsychological symptoms can begin with confusion, personality change, restlessness, and mood alterations, and can progress to slurred speech, psychotic behavior, stupor, and coma. These are also symptoms that must be evaluated. The patient may also complain of bone pain, although the precise mechanism of bone-pain hypercalcemia is unknown.

Early signs of delirium in the hypercalcemic patient are associated with multiple factors that include electrolyte imbalance, metabolic disturbance, and renal failure, among others. If recognized early, treatment of the condition can alleviate and possibly reverse the symptoms.[216] Management of confusion includes both pharmacotherapy and a reassuring and calm environment.

### Medical and Nursing Management

Regardless of the goals of care, active treatment goals are to promote alleviation of distressing symptoms. All patients with hypercalcemia who are symptomatic warrant a trial of therapy. When the goal is to reverse the hypercalcemia, this is accomplished by replenishing depleted intravascular volume, promoting diuresis of calcium, shutting down osteoclast activity in the bone, inhibiting renal tubular reabsorption of calcium, and promoting patient mobilization to the extent it is possible.[205,206]

Hydration is the first step in treatment. The purpose of hydration is to increase urinary calcium excretion, which improves renal function.[207] One to 2 liters of isotonic saline is administered over 1 to 4 hours, and the patient's fluid intake and urinary output are closely monitored. The rate of fluid administration depends on the clinical estimate of the extent of hydration, patient's cardiovascular function, and renal excretion capacity.[206]

Electrolytes and other laboratory values are closely monitored in appropriate patients. These include serum calcium (ionized or corrected), potassium, magnesium, as well as other electrolytes, and albumin and bicarbonate levels. Renal function tests, including BUN and creatinine, are monitored. In rare cases, dialysis may be considered. In most patients, cardiac effects of hypercalcemia are minimal and outcomes are not usually affected, so cardiac monitoring is not usually necessary.

## Bisphosphonate Therapy

Most hypercalcemic patients are treated with bisphosphonate therapy. It is an effective therapy for a number of cancers.[218-221] Bisphosphonate therapy inhibits bone resorption by osteoclasts, thus reducing the amount of calcium released into the bloodstream. Several IV bisphosphonates and amino-bisphosphonates are available for use in patients.[222,223] Pamidronate and etidronate are the oldest ones available in the United States.[208,217,224,225] The newer agents include risedronate sodium, ibandronate, and zoledronic acid.[226]

Pamidronate has been the most frequently used bisphosphonate, but zoledronate is becoming more widely used in the outpatient setting due to its much more rapid infusion time (30 minutes versus 2–6 hours for pamidronate). Pamidronate is usually given as 60 mg to 90 mg IV approximately every 3 to 4 weeks. In general, there is a 60% response to a 60-mg dose and a 100% response to a 90-mg dose.[211] Zoledronate, usually given as 4 mg IV, has been shown to have a higher rate and duration of control of hypercalcemia compared to pamidronate.[227] Pamidronate, and especially zoledronate, can cause renal toxicity (thus making evaluation and continued monitoring of kidney function essential prior to/during administration). Biphosphonates can cause osteonecrosis of the jaw, especially in patients with myeloma who have been treated with pamidronate and zoledronate for a long period of time, as well as patients with dental problems.[227]

Since hypercalcemia tends to recur, pamidronate or zoledronate must be given approximately every 4 weeks. Immediate side effects of pamidronate therapy include low-grade fever appearing within 48 hours of treatment, redness, induration, and swelling at the site of catheter. Hypomagnesia and hypocalcemia may also occur. Rapid administration of IV bisphosphonates can cause significant pain and this practice should be avoided. Subcutaneous administration of clodronate has been found to be an efficient treatment for malignant hypercalcemia.[228] This route may be particularly useful in hospital, home, and hospice settings and spares the patient discomfort and the costs associated with transportation and IV administration in the hospital environment.

## Calcitonin

Calcitonin inhibits resorption of calcium and can rapidly restore normocalcemia, often within 2 to 4 hours of administration. It is much less effective than pamidronate. Its role in managing hypercalcemia is limited to short-term use, usually of only 2 to 3 days' duration. Side effects are usually mild and include nausea and vomiting, skin rashes, and flushing. Calcitonin can be an alternative for treatment in patients with kidney failure (where pamidronate and zoledronate are contraindicated).[227]

## Gallium Nitrate and Plicamycin

Gallium nitrate is an effective bone resorptive agent. Its mechanism of action is unknown.[229] Its main disadvantages are that it has potential to cause nephrotoxicity, and it must be given as a continuous IV infusion over 5 days.[205,217] Plicamycin is an antitumor antibiotic.[230,231] Its mechanism is unknown. It has a hypocalcemic effect that occurs within 48 hours of administration and that lasts for 3 to 7 days, but it exhibits marrow, hepatic, and renal toxicities.[205] Individual response variations make this drug unpredictable, and it must be administered repeatedly.

## Corticosteroids

Corticosteroids have a limited role in the treatment of hypercalcemia.[206]

## Dialysis

The use of dialysis has been reserved for those patients who have severe hypercalcemia, renal failure, congestive heart failure, and cannot be given saline hydration.[232,233] The decision to offer this therapy is made on a case-by-case basis, but, in general, dialysis is not offered in the palliative care arena.

## Palliative Nursing Care

Hypercalcemia can cause significantly painful and distressing symptoms, including bone pain, agitation and confusion, severe constipation, and delirium. Treatment of hypercalcemia can reduce pain and other symptoms, improve quality of life, and reduce hospitalizations. At end of life, the promotion of comfort and management of symptoms are the primary goals of the palliative nursing care. If hypercalcemia cannot be reversed, or the patient decides that the burden of interventions is greater than the benefit, the patient should be given the option of discontinuing such treatment. Ongoing management of symptoms, including sedation if desired, must be guaranteed to the patient and their family.

## Conclusion

This chapter addressed a group of syndromes, which, unless recognized and treated promptly, will cause unnecessary suffering for the patient and family. Emphasis has been given to the epidemiology and basic pathophysiology of each syndrome, as well as diagnostic assessment. Providing this information, although by necessity limited in detail, enables the palliative care nurse to explain to the patient and/or family why particular symptoms are occurring and why a particular management approach is being suggested. Treatment advice and decisions are always couched within the framework of "Is the underlying cause reversible or not?"; "What is the benefit/ burden ratio of the treatment and how does that fit in with the patient's values and goals?"; "What is the likely outcome if the syndrome is not treated?"; "How will resultant symptoms be managed?"; "Is palliative sedation available to a patient at end of life if desired?"; and "Will the site of care impact on treatment decisions?"

## Acknowledgment

The author wishes to thank Ashby Watson for her outstanding first version (in the 2nd edition) of this chapter that made the task of updating it so much easier. Unfortunately, she could not be reached to get her feedback and retain her as first author.

REFERENCES

1. Wilson LD, Detterbeck FC, Yahalom J. Superior vena cava syndrome with malignant causes. N Engl J Med 2007;356:1862–1869.

2. Walji N, Chan AK, Peake DR. Common acute oncological emergencies: Diagnosis, investigation and management. Postgrad Med J 2008;84:418–427.

3. Ostler PJ, Clarke DP, Watkinson AF. Superior vena cava obstruction: A modern management strategy. Clin Oncol 1997;9:83–89.

4. Rice TW, Rodriguez RM, Light RW. The superior vena cava syndrome: Clinical characteristics and evolving etiology. Medicine 2006;85:3742.

5. Chan RH, Dar AR, Yu E, et al. Superior vena cava obstruction in small-cell lung cancer. Int J Radiat Oncol Biol Phys 1997;38:513–520.

6. Rowell NP, Gleeson FV. Steroids, radiotherapy, chemotherapy and stents for superior vena caval obstruction in carcinoma of the bronchus: A systematic review. Clin Oncol 2002;14:338–351.

7. Yaholom J. Superior vena cava syndrome. In: Devita VT, Hellman S, Rosenberg SA, eds. Cancer Principles and Practice of Oncology (6th ed). Philadelphia: Lippincott Williams & Wilkins, 2001:2609–2616.

8. Beeson MS. Superior Vena Cava Syndrome. Available at: http://www.emedicine.medscape.com/article/760361-overview (accessed December 1, 2008).

9. Flounders JA. Oncology emergency modules: Spinal cord compression. Oncol Nurs Forum 2003;30:E17–E23.

10. Schafer S. Oncologic complications. In: Otto S, ed. Oncology Nursing (3rd ed). St. Louis: Mosby, 1997:406–476.

11. Uaje C, Kathsen K, Parish L. Oncology emergencies. Crit Care Nurs Q 1996;18:26–34.

12. Armstrong BA, Perez CA, Simpson JR. Role of irradiation in the management of superior vena cava syndrome. Int J Radiat Oncol Biol Phys 1987;13:531–539.

13. Hunter J. Structural emergencies. In: Itano J, Taoka K, eds. Core Curriculum for Oncology Nursing (3rd ed). Philadelphia: W.B. Saunders, 1998:340–354.

14. Parish JM, Marschke RF, Dines DE. Etiologic considerations in superior vena cava syndrome. Mayo Clin Proc 1981;56:407–413.

15. Bell DR, Woods RL, Levi JA. Superior vena caval obstruction: A 10-year experience. Med J Aust 1986;145:566–568.

16. Falk S, Fallon M. ABC of palliative care: Emergencies. BMJ 1997;315:1525–1528.

17. Urruticoechea A, Mesia R, Dominquez J, et al. Treatment of malignant superior vena cava syndrome by endovascular stent insertion: Experience on 52 patients with lung cancer. Lung Cancer 2004;43:209–214.

18. Yedlicka JW, Schultz K, Moncada R. CT findings in superior vena cava obstruction. Semin Roentgenol 1989;24:84–90.

19. Quinadli SD, El Heajjam M, Bruckert F. Helical CT phlebography of the superior vena cava: Diagnosis and evaluation of venous obstruction. Am J Roentgen 1999;172:1327–1333.

20. Moncada R, Cardella R, Demos TC. Evaluation of superior vena cava syndrome by axial CT and CT phlebography. Am J Roentgen 1984;143:731–736.

21. Silvestri GA, Tanoue LT, Margolis ML. The noninvasive staging of non-small cell lung cancer: The guidelines. Chest 2003;123:147S–156S.

22. Alberts WM. Diagnosis and management of lung cancer executive summary: ACCP evidence-based clinical practice guidelines (2nd ed). Chest 2007;132:1–19.

23. Sasano S, Onuki T, Mae M. Wallstent endovascular prosthesis for the treatment of superior vena cava syndrome. Jpn J Thorac Cardiovasc Surg 2001;49:165–170.

24. Tanigawa N, Sawada S, Mishima K. Clinical outcome of stenting in superior vena cava syndrome associated with malignant tumors: Comparison with conventional treatment. Acta Radiologica 1998;39:669–674.

25. Nicholson AA, Ettles DF, Arnold A. Treatment of malignant superior vena cava obstruction: Metal stents or radiation therapy. J Vasc Intervent Radiol 1997;8:781–788.

26. Irving JD, Dondelinger RF, Reidy JF. Gianturco self-expanding stents: Clinical experience in the vena cava and large veins. Cardiovasc Intervent Radiol 1992;15:328–333.

27. Gauden SJ. Superior vena cava syndrome induced by bronchogenic carcinoma: Is this an oncological emergency? Australas Radiol 1993;37:363–366.

28. National Cancer Institute (NCI). Cancer Information Service: Physicians Desk Query Supportive Care Guideline: Superior Vena Cava Syndrome. Available at: http://www.nci.nih.gov/cancertopics/pdq/supportivecare/cardiopulmonary/HealthProfessional/page6 (accessed December 2, 2008).

29. Fiocco M, Krasna MJ. The management of malignant pleural and pericardial effusions. Hematol Oncol Clin North Am 1997;11:253–265.

30. Hausheer FH, Yarbro JW. Diagnosis and management of malignant pleural effusions. Semin Oncol 1985;12:54–75.

31. Andrews CO, Gora ML. Pleural effusions: Pathophysiology and management. Ann Pharmacother 1994;28:894–903.

32. Neragi-Miandoab S. Malignant pleural effusion, current and evolving approaches for its diagnosis and management. Lung Cancer 2006;54:1–9.

33. American Thoracic Society. Management of malignant pleural effusions. Am J Resp Crit Care Med 2000;162:1987–2001.

34. Heffner JE, Klein JS. Recent advances in the diagnosis and management of malignant pleural effusion. Mayo Clin Proc 2008;83:235–250.

35. Sahn SA. Malignancy metastatic to the pleura. Clin Chest Med 1998;19:351–361.

36. Pollak JS. Malignant pleural effusions: Treatment with tunneled long-term drainage catheters. Curr Opin Pulm Med 2002;8:302–307.

37. Grossi F, Pennucci MC, Tixi L, et al. Management of malignant pleural effusions. Drugs 1998;55:47–58.

38. Tattersall DJ. Management of malignant pleural effusion. Aust N Z J Med 1998;28:394–396.

39. Baker GL, Barnes HJ. Superior vena cava syndrome: Etiology, diagnosis, and treatment. Am J Crit Care 1992;1:54–64.

40. Kreamer K. Superior vena cava syndrome. In: Gross J, Johnson BL, eds. Handbook of Oncology Nursing (2nd ed). Boston: Jones and Bartlett, 1994:628–638.

41. Afessa B. Pleural effusions and pneumothoraces in AIDS. Curr Opin Pulm Med 2001;7:202–209.

42. Armbruster C, Schalleschak J, Vetter N, et al. Pleural effusions in human immunodeficiency virus-infected patients: Correlation with concomitant pulmonary diseases. Acta Cytol 1995;39:698–700.

43. Joseph J, Strange C, Sahn SA. Pleural effusions in hospitalized patients with AIDS. Ann Intern Med 1993;118:856–859.

44. Soubani AO, Michelson MK, Karnik A. Pleural fluid findings in patients with the acquired immunodeficiency syndrome: Correlation with concomitant pulmonary disease. South Med J 1999;92:400–403.

45. Burrows CM, Mathews WC, Colt HG. Predicting survival in patients with recurrent symptomatic malignant pleural effusions: An assessment of the prognostic values of physiologic, morphologic, and quality of life measures of extent of disease. Chest 2000;117:73–78.

46. Heffner J, Nietert P, Barbieri C. Pleural fluid pH as a predictor of survival for patients with malignant pleural effusions. Chest 2000;117:79–86.

47. American Society of Clinical Oncology (ASCO). Optimizing cancer care—the importance of symptom management (Vol II): Malignant pleural effusions. ASCO Curriculum 2001. Dubuque, IA: Kendall/Hunt Publishing Company, 2001:1–27.

48. Chernow B, Sahn SA. Carcinomatous involvement of the pleura. Am J Med 1977;63:695–702.

49. Yano S, Herbst RS, Shinohara H, et al. Production of experimental malignant pleural effusion of human lung adenocarcinoma by inhibition of vascular endothelial growth factor receptor tyrosine kinase phosphorylation. Clin CA Res 2000;6:957–965.

50. Light RW, MacGregor MI, Luchsinger PC, et al. Pleural effusions: The diagnostic separation of transudates and exudates. Ann Intern Med 1972;77:507–513.

51. Gill PS, Akil B, Colletti P, Rarick M, Loweiro C, Bernstein-Singer M. Pulmonary Kaposi's sarcoma: Clinical findings and results of therapy. Am J Med 1989;87:57–61.

52. Levine AM. Acquired immunodeficiency syndrome-related lymphoma: Clinical aspects. Semin Oncol 2000;27:442–453.

53. Milne ENC, Pistolesi M. Pleural effusions: Normal physiology, pathophysiology, and diagnosis. In: Patterson S, ed. Reading the Chest Radiograph: A Physiologic Approach. St. Louis: Mosby, 1993:120–163.

54. Black LF. The pleural space and pleural fluid. Mayo Clin Proc 1972;47:493–506.

55. Meyer PC. Metastatic carcinoma of the pleura. Thorax 1966;21:437–443.

56. Leff A, Hopewell PC, Costello J. Pleural effusion from malignancy. Ann Intern Med 1978;88:532–537.

57. Ruckdeschel JC, Robinson LA. Management of pleural and pericardial effusions. In: Berger AM, Portenoy RK, Weissman DE, eds. Principles and Practice of Palliative Care and Supportive Oncology (2nd ed). Philadelphia: Lippincott Williams & Wilkins, 2002:389–412.

58. Wailer A. Caroline NL. Handbook of Palliative Care in Cancer. Boston: Butterworth-Heineman, 1996:217.

59. Vaska K, Wann LS, Sagar KK, et al. Pleural effusion as a cause of right ventricular collapse. Circulation 1992;86:609–617.

60. Kaplan LM, Epstein SK, Schwartz SL, et al. Clinical, echocardiographic, and hemodynamic evidence of cardiac tamponade caused by large pleural effusions. Am J Resp Crit Care Med 1995;151:904–908.

61. Woodring JH, Loh FK, Kryscio RJ. Mediastinal hemorrhage: An evaluation of radiographic manifestations. Radiology 1984;23:393–397.

62. Doust BD, Baum JK, Maklad NF. Ultrasonic evaluation of pleural opacities. Radiology 1975;114:135–140.

63. Ravin CE, Chotas HC. Chest radiography. Radiology 1997;204:593–600.

64. Nemchek AA. Management of malignant pleural effusions. J Vasc Interv Radiol 1998;9:115–120.

65. Gryminski J, Krakowka P, Lypacewicz G. The diagnosis of pleural effusion by ultrasonic and radiologic techniques. Chest 1976;70:83–87.

66. Bartter T, Santarelli R, Akers S, et al. The evaluation of pleural effusion. Chest 1994;106:1209–1214.

67. Martini N, Eisenberg B, Baisden CE. Indications for pleurectomy in malignant effusion. Cancer 1975;35:734–738.

68. Nally AT. Critical care of the patient with lung cancer. AACN Clin Issues: Adv Practice Acute Crit Care 1996;7:79–94.

69. Chernecky C, Shelton B. Pulmonary complications in patients with cancer: Diagnostic and treatment information for the noncritical care nurse. AJN 2001;101:24A, 24E, 24G–24H.

70. Ruckdeschel JC. Management of malignant pleural effusion: An overview. Semin Oncol 1988;15:24–28.

71. Anderson CB, Philpott GW, Ferguson TB. The treatment of malignant pleural effusions. Cancer 1974;33:916–922.

72. Light RW. Malignant pleural effusions. In: Light RW, ed. Pleural Diseases (3rd ed). Baltimore: Williams and Wilkins, 1995:94–116.

73. Belani CP, Patz EF. Malignant pleural effusion: Advances in management. Pittsburgh: University of Pittsburgh Medical Center, 1995, monograph.

74. Antunes G, Neville E. Management of malignant pleural effusions. Thorax 2000;55:981–983.

75. Ratliff JL, Chavez CM, Majchuk A. Re-expansion pulmonary edema. Chest 1973;64:654–656.

76. DeCamp MM, Mentzer SJ, Swanson SJ. Malignant effusive disease of the pleura and pericardium. Chest 1997;112 (Suppl):291S–295S.

77. Clarke K. Effective pain relief with intrapleural analgesia. Nurs Times 1999;95:49–50.

78. Short K, Scheeres D, Mlakar J, et al. Evaluation of intrapleural analgesia in the management of blunt traumatic chest wall pain: A clinical trial. Am Surg 1996;62:488–493.

79. Reigler FX. Pro: Intrapleural anesthesia is useful for thoracic analgesia. Con: Unreliable benefit after thoracotomy—epidural is a better choice. J Cardiothorac Vasc Anesth 1996;10:429–431.

80. McIlvaine WB. Intrapleural anesthesia is useful for thoracic analgesia. Pro: Intrapleural anesthesia is useful for thoracic analgesia. J Cardiothorac Vasc Anesth 1996;10:425–428.

81. Gaeta RR, Marcario A, Brodsky JB, et al. Pain outcomes after thoracotomy: Lumbar epidural hydromorphone versus intrapleural bupivacaine. J Cardiothorac Vasc Anesth 1995;9:534–537.

82. Robinson LA, Mouton AL, Fleming WH, et al. Intrapleural doxycycline control of malignant pleural effusions. Am Thorac Surg 1993;55:1115–1122.

83. Piehler JM, Pluth JR, Schaff HV, et al. Surgical management of effusive pericardial disease: Influence of extent of pericardial resection on clinical course. J Thorac Cardiovasc Surg 1985;90:506–516.

84. Gilkeson RC, Silverman P, Haaga JR. Using urokinase to treat malignant pleural effusions. Am J Roent 1999;173:781–783.

85. Lee KA, Harvey JC, Reich H, et al. Management of malignant pleural effusions with pleuroperitoneal shunting. J Am Coll Surg 1994;178:586–588.

86. Tan C, Sedrakyan A, Brown J, et al. The evidence on the effectiveness of management for malignant pleural effusion: A systematic review. Eur J Cardiothorac Surg 2006;29:829–838.

87. Petrou M, Kaplan D, Goldstraw P. Management of recurrent malignant pleural effusions: The complementary role of talc pleurodesis and pleuroperitoneal shunting. Chest 1995;75:801–805.

88. Woodruff R. Palliative Medicine (2nd ed). Melbourne: Asperula Pty Ltd., 1996:143.

89. Sherman S, Raviskrishnan KP, Patel AS. Optimum anesthesia with intrapleural lidocaine during chemical pleurodesis with tetracycline. Chest 1988;94:533–536.

90. Leslie WK, Kinasewitz GT. Clinical characteristics of the patient with nonspecific pleuritis. Chest 1988;94:603–608.

91. Harvey JC, Erdman CB, Beattie EJ. Early experience with videothorascopic hydrodissection pleurectomy in the treatment of malignant pleural effusion. J Surg Onc 1995;59:243–245.

92. Pollak JS, Burdge CM, Rosenblatt M, et al. Treatment of malignant pleural effusions with tunneled long-term drainage catheters. J Vasc Interv Radiol 2001;12:201–208.

93. Tremblay A, Michaud G. Single-center experience with 250 tunnelled pleural catheter insertions for malignant pleural effusion. Chest 2006;129:362–368.

94. Dudgeon DJ, Lertzman M, Askew GR. Physiological changes and clinical correlates of dyspnea in cancer outpatients. J Pain Symptom Manage 2001;21:373–379.

95. Braunwald E. Cardiac tampanade. In: Braunwald E, ed. Heart Disease: A Textbook of Cardiovascular Medicine. Philadelphia: W.B. Saunders, 1997:1446–1496.

96. Weinberg BA, Conces DJ Jr, Waller BF. Cardiac manifestations of noncardiac tumors. Part 1: Direct effects. Clin Cardiol 1989;12:289–296.

97. Palatianos GM, Thurer RJ, Pompeo MQ, Kaiser GA. Clinical experience with subxiphoid drainage of pericardial effusions. Ann Thorac Surg 1989;48:381–385.

98. Mills SA, Graeber GM, Nelson MG. Therapy of malignant tumors involving the pericardium. In: Roth J, Ruckdeschel JC, Weisenburger T, eds. Thoracic Oncology (2nd ed). Philadelphia: W.B. Saunders, 1995:492–513.

99. Knoop T, Willenberg K. Cardiac tamponade. Semin Oncol Nurs 1999;15:168–175.

100. McAllister H, Hall R, Cooley D. Tumors of the heart and pericardium. Curr Prob Cardiol 1999;24:57–116.

101. National Hospital Discharge Summary: Annual Survey 1993. U.S. Department of Health and Human Services, Public Health Service. Centers for Disease Control and Prevention, National Center for Health Statistics. Hyattsville, MD, 1993, DHHS Publication No. (PHS) 93–1775.

102. Bullock B. Altered cardiac function. In: Bullock B, Henze R, eds. Focus on Pathophysiology. Philadelphia: Lippincott Williams & Wilkins, 2000:455–502.

103. Lawler P. Effusions. In: Yarbro C, Frogge M, Goodman M, eds. Cancer Symptom Management (2nd ed). Boston: Jones and Bartlett, 1999:419–433.

104. Chabner B, Myers C. Antitumor antibiotics. In: DeVita V, Hellman S, Rosenberg S, eds. Cancer Principles and Practice of Oncology (4th ed). Philadelphia: J. B. Lippincott, 1993:374–384.

105. Harken A, Hammond G, Edmunds L. Pericardial diseases. In: Edmunds L, ed. Cardiac Surgery in the Adult. New York: McGraw Hill, 1997:1303–1317.

106. Smeltzer S, Bare B. Oncology: Nursing the patient with cancer. In: Smeltzer S, Bare B, eds. Brunner and Suddarth's Textbook of Medical-Surgical Nursing (8th ed). Philadelphia: Lippincott-Raven, 1996:309–316.

107. Spodick DH. Effective management of congestive cardiomyopathy: Relation to ventricular structure and function. Arch Intern Med 1982;4:689–692.

108. Miller RR, McGregor DH. Hemorrhage from carcinoma of the lung. Cancer 1980;46:200–205.

109. Pories WJ, Gaudiani VA. Cardiac tamponade. Surg Clin N Am 1975;55:573–589.

110. Beauchamp K. Pericardial tamponade: An oncologic emergency. Clin J Oncol Nurs 1998;2:85–95.

111. Spodick DH. Pericardial windows are suboptimal. Am J Cardiol 1983;51:607.

112. Ruckdeschel JC. Preoperative paclitaxel plus carboplatin for patients with intermediate-risk non-small cell lung cancer. Semin Oncol 1996;23:62–67.

113. Freeman GL, LeWinter MM. Pericardial adaptations during chronic cardiac dilation in dogs. Circ Res 1984;54:294–300.

114. Press OW, Livingston R. Management of malignant pericardial effusion and tamponade. JAMA 1987;8:1088–1092.

115. Fowler NO, Gabel M. The hemodynamic effects of cardiac tamponade: Mainly the result of atrial, not ventricular, compression. Circulation 1985;71:154–157.

116. Posner J. Neurologic Complications of Cancer. Philadelphia: F.A. Davis, 1995.

117. Buck M, Ingle JN, Giulani ER, Gordon JR, Therneau TM. Pericardial effusion in women with breast cancer. Cancer 1987;60:263–269.

118. Shepherd F. Malignant pericardial effusion. Curr Opin Oncol 1997;9:170–174.

119. Vaitkus PT, Herrmann HC, LeWinter MM. Treatment of malignant pericardial effusion. JAMA 1994;272:59–64.

120. Stouffer GA, Sheahan RG, Lenihan DJ, et al. Diagnosis and management of chronic pericardial effusions. Am J Med Sci 2001;322:79–87.

121. Mangan C. Malignant pericardial effusions: Pathophysiology and clinical correlates. Oncol Nurs Forum 1992;19:1215–1223.

122. Nguyen DM, Schrump DS. Malignant pleural and pericardial effusions. In: DeVita V, Hellman S, Rosenberg S, eds. Cancer Principles and Practice of Oncology (7th ed). Philadelphia: Lippincott Williams & Wilkins, 2005:2381–2392.

123. Dietz K, Flaherty A. Oncologic emergencies. In: Groenwald S, Frogge M, Goodman M, Yarbro C, eds. Cancer Nursing (3rd ed). Boston: Jones and Bartlett, 1993:800–839.

124. Bickley L. Bates' Guide to Physical Examination and History Taking (7th ed). Philadelphia: Lippincott Williams & Wilkins, 1999.

125. Gueberman B, Fowler N, Engel P. Cardiac tamponade in medical patients. Circulation 1987;64:633–640.

126. Keefe D. Cardiovascular emergencies in the cancer patient. Semin Oncol 2000;27:244–255.

127. Kopecky SL, Callahan JA, Tajik AJ, Seward JB. Percutaneous pericardial catheter drainage: Report of 42 consecutive cases. Am J. Cardiol 1986;7:633–635.

128. Tsang TS, Freeman WK, Sinah LJ, Seward JB. Echocardiographically guided pericardiocentesis: Evolution and state-of-the-art technique. Mayo Clin Proc 1998;73:647–652.

129. Callahan JA, Seward JB, Tajik AJ. Cardiac tamponade: Pericardiocentesis directed by two-dimensional echocardiography. Mayo Clin Proc 1985;60:344–347.

130. Tsang TS, Barnes ME, Hayes SN, Freeman WK, Dearani JA, Butler SL. Clinical and echocardiographic characteristics of significant pericardial effusions following cardiothoracic surgery and outcomes of echo-guided pericardiocentesis for management: Mayo Clinic experience, 1979–1998. Chest 1999;116:322–331.

131. Tsang TS, Seward JB, Barnes ME, Bailey KR, Sinah LJ, Urban LH. Outcomes of primary and secondary treatment of pericardial effusion in patients with malignancy. Mayo Clin Proc 2000;73:248–253.

132. Chong HH, Plotnick GD. Pericardial effusion and tamponade: Evaluation, imaging, modalities, and management. Compr Ther 1995;21:378–385.

133. Shepherd F. Malignant pericardial effusion. Curr Opin Oncol 1997;9:170–174.

134. Maruyama R, Yokohama H, Seto T, et al. Catheter drainage followed by the instillation of bleomycin to manage malignant pericardial effusion in non-small cell lung cancer: A multi-institutional phase II trial. J Thorac Oncol 2007;2:65–68.

135. Lissoni P, Barni S, Ardiozzoia A. Intracavitary administration of interleukin-2 as palliative therapy for neoplastic effusion. Tumori 1992;78:118–120.

136. Maher EA, Shepherd FA, Todd T Jr. Pericardial sclerosis as the primary management of malignant pericardial effusion and cardiac tamponade. J Thorac Cardiovasc Surg 1996;112:637–643.

137. Ziskind AA, Pearce AC, Lemmon CC, et al. Percutaneous balloon pericardiotomy for the treatment of cardiac tamponade and large pericardial effusions: Descriptions of technique and report of the first 50 cases. J Am Coll Cardiol 1993;21:1–5.

138. Jackson G, Keane D, Mishra B. Percutaneous balloon pericardiotomy in the management of recurrent malignant of recurrent malignant pericardial effusions. Br Heart J 1992;68:613–615.

139. Gross JL, Younes RN, Deheinzelin D, et al. Surgical management of symptomatic management of pericardial effusion in the patient with solid malignancies. Ann Surg Oncol 2006;13:1732–1738.

140. Hurley JP, McCarthy J, Wood AE. Retrospective analysis of the utility of video-assisted thoracic surgery in 100 consecutive procedures. Eur J Cardiothorac Surg 1994;8:589–592.

141. Liu H, Chang C, Lin P, et al. Thoracoscopic management of effusive pericardial disease: Indication and technique. Ann Thorac Surg 1994;58:1695–1697.

142. Lewis MM, Read CA. Hemoptysis, part 1: Identifying the cause. J Resp Dis 2000;21:335–341.

143. Corder R. Hemoptysis. Emerg Med Clinics N Am 2003;21:421–435.

144. Harries ML, Morrison M. Management of unilateral vocal cord paralysis by injection medialization with Teflon paste—quantitative results. Ann Otol Rhinol Laryngol 1998;107:332–336.

145. Schwartz AR, Smith PL, Kashima HK, et al. Respiratory function of the upper airways. In: Murray JF, Nadel JA, eds. Respiratory Medicine. Philadelphia: W.B. Saunders, 1994:1451–1470.

146. Lipchik RJ. Hemoptysis. In: Berger AM, Portenoy RK, Weissman DE, eds. Principles and Practice of Palliative Care and Supportive Oncology (2nd ed). Philadelphia: Lippincott Williams & Wilkins, 2002:372–377.

147. Rizzi A, Rocco G, Robustellini M, et al. Results of surgical management of tuberculosis: Experience in 206 patients undergoing operation. Ann Thorac Surg 1995;59:896–900.

148. Chan C, Elazar-Popovic E, Farver C, et al. Endobronchial involvement in uncommon diseases. J Bronch 1996;3:53–63.

149. Levine MN, Raskob G, Landefeld S, et al. Hemorrhagic complications of anticoagulant treatment. Chest 1995;108:276S–290S.

150. Levine MN, Goldhaber SZ, Gore JM, et al. Hemorrhagic complications of thrombolytic therapy in the treatment of myocardial infarction and venous thromboembolism. Chest 1995;108:291S–301S.

151. Corey R, Hla KM. Major and massive hemoptysis: Reassessment of conservative management. Am J Med Sci 1987;294:301–309.

152. Luce K, O'Donnell EE, Morton AR. A combination of calcitonin and bisphosphonate for the emergency treatment of severe tumor-induced hypercalcemia. Calcif Tissue Int 1993;52:70–71.

153. Boyars M. Current strategies for diagnosing and managing hemoptysis. J Crit Ill 1999;14:148–156.

154. Lewis MM, Read CA. Hemoptysis, part 2: Treatment options. J Resp Dis 2000;21:392–394.

155. Saltzman HA, Alavi A, Greespan RH. Value of the ventilation/perfusion scan in acute pulmonary embolism: Results of the prospective investigation of pulmonary embolism diagnosis. JAMA 1990;263:2753–2759.

156. Colice GL. Hemoptysis: Three questions that can direct management. Postgrad Med 1996;100:227–236.

157. Awan AM, Weichselbarum RR. Palliative radiotherapy. Hematol Oncol Clin North Am 1990;4:1169–1181.

158. Kwok Y, DeYoung C, Garofalo M, et al. Radiation oncology emergencies. Hematol Oncol Clin North Am 2006;20:505–522.

159. Makker HK, Barnes PC. Fatal hemoptysis from the pulmonary artery as a late complication of pulmonary irradiation. Thorax 1991;46:609–610.

160. Villaneuva AG, Lo TCM, Beamis JF. Endobronchial brachytherapy. Clin Chest Med 1995;16:445–454.

161. Sutedgja G, Baris G, Schaake-Koning C, et al. High dose rates brachytherapy in patients with local recurrences after radiotherapy of non-small cell lung cancer. Int J Radiat Oncol Biol Phys 1992;24:551–553.

162. Hatlevoll R, Karlsen KO, Skovlund E. Endobronchial radiotherapy for malignant bronchial obstruction or recurrence. Acta Oncol 1999;38:999–1004.

163. Khanavkar B, Stern P, Alberti W, et al. Complications associated with brachytherapy alone or with laser in lung cancer. Chest 1991;99:1062–1065.

164. Aurora R, Milite F, Vander Els N. Respiratory emergencies. Semin Oncol 2000;27:256–269.

165. Brandes JC, Schmidt E, Yung R. Occlusive endobrachial stent placement as a novel management approach to massive hemoptysis from lung cancer. J Thorac Oncol 2008;3:1071–1072.

166. Schray MF, McDougall JC, Martinez A, et al. Management of malignant airway compromise with laser and low dose brachytherapy: The Mayo Clinic experience. Chest 1988;93:264–269.

167. Hayakawa K, Tanaka F, Torizuka T, et al. Bronchial artery embolization for hemoptysis: Immediate and long-term results. Cardiovasc Intervent Radiol 1992;15:154–158.

168. Adelman M, Haponik E, Bleeker E, et al. Cryptogenic hemoptysis. Ann Intern Med 1985;102:829–834.

169. Mal H, Rullon I, Mellot F, et al. Immediate and long-term results of bronchial artery embolization for life-threatening hemoptysis. J Crit Ill 1999;14:148–156.

170. Brinson G, Noone P, Mauro M, et al. Bronchial artery embolization for the treatment of hemoptysis in patients with cystic fibrosis. Am J Resp Crit Care Med 1998;157:1951–1958.

171. Hirscherg B, Biran I, Glazer M, et al. Hemoptysis: Etiology, evaluation, and outcome in a tertiary referral hospital. Chest 1997;112:440–444.

172. Cole JS, Patchell RA. Metastatic epidural spinal cord compression. Lancet Neurol 2008;7:459–466.

173. Quinn J, DeAngelis L. Neurologic emergencies in the cancer patient. Semin Oncol 2000;27:311–321.

174. Byrne TN. Metastatic epidural spinal cord compression. In: Black P, Loeffler J, eds. Cancer of the Nervous System. London: Blackwell Scientific, 1997:664–673.

175. Byrne TN. Spinal cord compression from epidural metastases. N Engl J Med 1992;327:614–619.

176. Wilkes G. Neurological disturbances. In: Yarbro C, Frogge M, Goodman M, eds. Cancer Symptom Management (2nd ed). Boston: Jones and Bartlett, 1999:344–381.

177. Posner J. Neurologic Complications of Cancer. Philadelphia: F.A. Davis, 1995:111–142.

178. Portenoy RK. Chronic nociceptive pain syndromes: Cancer pain. In: North RB, Levy RM, eds. Neurosurgical Management of Pain. New York: Springer-Verlag, 1997:62–74.

179. Perrin RG, Janjan NA, Langford LA. Spinal axis metastases. In: Levin VA, ed. Cancer in the Nervous System. New York: Churchill Livingstone, 1996:259.

180. Caraceni A, Martini C, Simonetti F. Neurological disturbances in advanced cancer. In: Doyle D, Hanks G, Cherny N, Calman K, eds. Oxford Textbook of Palliative Medicine. Oxford: Oxford University Press, 2004:702–726.

181. Weinstein SM. Management of spinal cord and cauda equina compression. In: Berger AM, Portenoy RK, Weissman DE, eds. Principles and Practice of Palliative Care and Supportive Oncology (2nd ed). Philadelphia: Lippincott Williams & Wilkins, 2002:532–543.

182. Belford K. Central nervous system cancers. In: Groenwald S, Frogge M, Goodman M, Yarbro C, eds. Cancer Nursing (4th ed). Boston: Jones and Bartlett, 1997:721–741.

183. Henze R. Traumatic and vascular injuries of the central nervous system. In: Bullock B, Henze R, eds. Focus on Pathophysiology. Philadelphia: Lippincott Williams & Wilkins, 2000:938–978.

184. Bucholtz J. Metastatic epidural spinal cord compression. Semin Oncol Nurs 1999;15:150–159.

185. Fuller BG, Heiss JD, Oldfield EH. Spinal cord compression. In: Devita VT, Hellman S, Rosenberg SA, eds. Cancer Principles and Practice of Oncology (6th ed). Philadelphia: Lippincott Williams & Wilkins, 2001:2617–2632.

186. Hewitt DJ, Foley KM. Neuroimaging of pain. In: Greenberg JO, ed. Neuroimaging. New York: McGraw-Hill, 1995:41.

187. Frank JA, Ling A, Patronas NJ. Detection of malignant bone tumors: MRI imaging vs. scintigraphy. Am J Roentgenol 1990;155:1043–1048.

188. Algra PR, Bloem JL, Tissing H. Detection of vertebral body metastases: Comparison between MR imaging and bone scintigraphy. Radiograph 1991;11:219–232.

189. St. Amour TE, Hodges SC, Laakman RW, et al. MRI of the Spine. New York: Raven, 1994:435.

190. Sze G. Magnetic resonance imaging in the evaluation of spinal tumors. Cancer 1991;67:1229–1241.

191. Burger EL, Lindeque BG. Sacral and non-spinal tumors presenting as a backache: A retrospective study of 17 patients. Acta Orthoped Scand 1994;65:344–346.

192. Abrahm JL. Management of pain and spinal cord compression in patients with advanced cancer. Ann Intern Med 1999;131:37–46.

193. Gilbert RW, Kim JH, Posner JB. Epidural spinal cord compression from metastatic tumor: Diagnosis and treatment. Ann Neurol 1978;3:40–51.

194. Hainline B, Tuzynski MH, Posner JB. Ataxia in epidural spinal cord compression. Neurol 1992;42:2193–2195.

195. Gudesblatt M, Cohen JA, Gerber O. Truncal ataxia presumably due to malignant spinal cord compression. Ann Neurol 1987;21:511–512.

196. Patchell R, Tibbs PA, Regine WF, et al. A randomized trial of direct decompressive surgical resection in the treatment of spinal cord compression caused by metastasis. Proc Am Soc Clin Oncol 2003;22(abstract 2):1.

197. George R, Jeba J, Ramkumar G, et al. Interventions for the treatment of metastatic extradural spinal cord compression in adults. Cochrane Database Syst Rev 2008;Issue 4. Art. No.:CD006716. DOI:10.1002/14651858.CD006716.pub2.

198. Greenberg HS, Kim JH, Posner JB. Epidural spinal cord compression from metastatic tumor: Results from a new treatment protocol. Ann Neurol 1980;8:1–366.

199. Delattre JY, Arbit E, Thaler HT. A dose response study of dexamethasone in a model of spinal cord compression caused by epidural tumor. J Neurosurg 1989;70:920–925.

200. Loblaw D, Laperriere N. Emergency treatment of malignant extradural spinal cord compression: An evidence-based guideline. J Clin Oncol 1998;16:1613–1624.

201. Grant R, Papadopoulos SM, Greenberg HS. Metastatic epidural spinal cord compression. Neurol Clin 1991;9:825–841.

202. Flower CDR, Jackson JE. The role of radiology in the investigation and management of patients with hemoptysis. Clin Radiol 1996;51:391–400.

203. Sitton E. Nursing implications of radiation therapy. In: Itano J, Toaka K, eds. Core Curriculum for Oncology Nursing (3rd ed). Philadelphia: W.B. Saunders, 1998:616–629.

204. Clayton K. Cancer-related hypercalcemia: How to spot it, how to manage it. AJN 1997;97:42–48.

205. Morton AR, Ritch PS. Hypercalcemia. In: Berger AM, Portenoy RK, Weissman DE, eds. Principles and Practice of Palliative Care and Supportive Oncology (2nd ed). Philadelphia: Lippincott Williams & Wilkins, 2002:493–507.

206. Warrell RP. Metabolic emergencies. In: Devita VT, Hellman S, Rosenberg SA, eds. Cancer Principles and Practice of Oncology (6th ed). Philadelphia: Lippincott Williams & Wilkins, 2001:2633–2645.

207. Bajorunas D. Clinical manifestations of cancer-related hypercalcemia. Semin Oncol 1990;17:16–24.

208. Mundy GR. Pathophysiology of cancer-associated hypercalcemia. Semin Oncol 1990;17:10–15.

209. Ralston SH. Pathogenesis and management of cancer-associated hypercalcemia. In: Rubens RD, Fogelman I, eds. Bone Metastases: Diagnosis and Treatment. New York: Springer Verlag, 1991:149–169.

210. Gaich G, Burtis WJ. The diagnosis and treatment of malignancy-associated hypercalcemia. N Engl J Med 1992;326:1196–1203.

211. Nussbaum SR. Pathophysiology and management of severe hypercalcemia. Endocrinol Metab Clin North Am 1993;2:343–362.

212. Kovacs CS, MacDonald SM, Chik CL, et al. Hypercalcemia of malignancy in the palliative care patient: A treatment strategy. J Pain Symptom Manage 1995;10:224–232.

212a. Lange B, D'Angio G, Ross AJ, et al. Oncologic emergencies. In: Pizzo PA, Poplack DG, eds. Principles and Practice of Pediatric Oncology. Philadelphia: J.B. Lippincott, 1989:799–819.

213. King PA. Oncologic emergencies: Assessment, identification, and interventions in the emergency department. J Emerg Nurs 1995;21:213–218.

214. Burtis WJ. Parathyroid hormone-related protein: Structure, function, and measurement. Clin Chem 1992;38:2171–2183.

215. Mercadante S. Malignant bone pain: Pathophysiology and treatment. Pain 1997;69:1–18.

216. Kuebler KK. Palliative nursing care for the patient experiencing end-stage renal failure. Urol Nurs 2001;21:167–168, 171–178.

217. Flombaum CD. Oncologic emergencies: Metabolic emergencies. Semin Oncol 2000;27:322–334.

218. Djulbvegovic B, Wheatley K, Ross J, et al. Bisphosphonates in multiple myeloma. Cochrane Database Syst Rev 2002;3:CD0031188.

219. Pavlakis N, Schmidt RL, Stockler PN. Bisphosphonates for breast cancer. Cochrane Database Syst Rev 2005;3. Available at: http://www.cochrane.org/reviews/en/ab003474.html (accessed December 22, 2008).

220. American Society of Clinical Oncology (ASCO). Optimizing cancer care—the importance of symptom management: Malignant pleural effusions. ASCO Curriculum. Dubuque, IA: Kendall/Hunt Publishing Company, 2001:1–27.

221. Wong RKS, Wiffen PJ. Bisphosphonates for the relief of pain secondary to bone metastases. Cochrane Library, 2003, Available at: http://www.cochrane.org/reviews/en/ab002068.htm (accessed December 22, 2008).

222. Ralston SH, Gallacher SJ, Patel U, et al. Comparison of three intravenous bisphosphonates in cancer-associated hypercalcemia. Lancet 1989;2:1180–1182.

223. Gallacher SJ, Ralston SH, Fraser WD. A comparison of low versus high dose pamidronate in cancer-associated hypercalcemia. Bone Miner 1991;15:249–256.

224. Gucalp R, Theriault R, Gill I, et al. Comparative study of pamidronate disodium and etidronate disodium in the treatment of cancer-related hypercalcemia. J Clin Oncol 1992;10:134–142.

225. Purohit OP, Radstone CR, Anthony C, et al. A randomized double-blind comparison of intravenous pamidronate and clodronate in the hypercalcemia of malignancy. Br J Cancer 1995;72:1289–1293.

226. Major P, Lortholary A, Hon J, et al. Zoledronic acid is more effective than pamidronate for hypercalcemia of malignancy. Evid based Oncol 2001;2:159–162.

227. Lumachi F, Brunello A, Roma A, Basso U. Medical treatment of malignancy-associated hypercalcemia. Curr Med Chem 2008;15:415–421.

228. Roemer-Becuwe C, Vigano A, Romano F, et al. Safety of subcutaneous clodronate and efficacy in hypercalcemia of malignancy: A novel route of administration. J Pain Symptom Manage 2003;26:843–848.

229. Warrell RP Jr, Bockman RS, Coonley CJ, et al. Gallium nitrate inhibits calcium resorption from bone and is effective treatment for cancer-related hypercalcemia. J Clin Invest 1984;73:1487–1490.

230. Smith IE, Powles TJ. Mithramycin for hypercalcemia associated with myeloma and other malignancies. BMJ 1975;1:268–269.

231. Mundy GR. Mechanisms of bone metastasis. Cancer 1997;80:1546–1556.

232. Koo WS, Jeon DS, Ahn SJ, et al. Calcium-free dialysis for the management of hypercalcemia. Nephron 1996;72:424–428.

233. Leehey DJ, Ing TS. Correction of hypercalcemia and hypophosphatemia by hemodialysis using a conventional, calcium-containing dialysis solution enriched with phosphorus. Am J Kidney Dis 1997;29:288–290.

# 26

## Sedation for Refractory Symptoms and Terminal Weaning

*Patti Knight and Laura A. Espinosa*

*I can't bear the thought of my dad dying like this; he is such a good man.—Daughter watching her father suffer with bone pain while dying of cancer*

*It's not the withdrawal of care that's the hard part; it's the infliction of care when—when there's no need for it. It's not going to make any difference. All you're going to do is make somebody suffer longer. Why? I'd rather let somebody die.—ICU Nurse*

◆ **Key Points**
◆ *Palliative sedation is sedation used to control refractory and intolerable symptoms at the end of life when control of these symptoms is not possible and the person remains awake and alert.*
◆ *Proportionality is a concept that implies that a patient's consciousness is reduced just enough to relieve refractory symptoms.*
◆ *Determining refractoriness of symptoms and closeness to death can be difficult and requires assessment by a skilled practitioner.*
◆ *Patient/family/proxy involvement is central in decisions concerning use of palliative sedation or terminal weaning. Clear communication with significant others, precise documentation, and informed consent are necessary.*
◆ *Most hospital deaths involve a decision to withhold or withdraw some form of life support.*

In the United States, approximately 2.5 million people die each year, with greater than 60% of deaths occurring in hospitals.[1] These statistics are alarming and underscore the public's concern about how well the dying are cared for. The results of a survey by the Last Acts Coalition, funded by the Robert Wood Johnson Foundation, indicated that many of the general public feel that deaths in hospitals are not well managed. Ninety-three percent of respondents stated that it was "very important" or "somewhat important" to improve how the health care system cares for dying Americans.[2] This survey also demonstrated that patients and their family members wanted to be involved in decision-making and to be comfortable at the end of life with well-managed symptoms, and care that does not exhaust life savings.

Oregon's Death with Dignity Act has been in effect since 1997. This Act allows terminally ill Oregonians to end their lives through the voluntary self-administration of medications prescribed by a physician for that purpose. Before the law was passed, opponents argued that good palliative and hospice care would largely replace the need for such a law. In the first 10 years after the law was passed, 341 patients chose to end their lives under the protection of the Death with Dignity Act. The Oregon Department of Health Services (ODHS) is required to collect information about patients and physicians who participate in the process. The 2007 ODHS report states that 33% of participating patients mentioned concern about pain (up from 26% in past years) as one reason for seeking a prescription for lethal medications. ODHS also reports that 100% of patients mentioned loss of autonomy as the main reason for seeking a prescription, and 86% cited decreasing ability to participate in enjoyable activities, as well as loss of dignity, as highly significant in their decision. In 2008, the state of Washington passed a Death with Dignity Act modeled after the Oregon law.[3] Obviously, this is an issue with which patients and the public are concerned. With this in mind, both nurses and physicians need to develop skills in assessing why a particular patient is requesting a hastened death, so that appropriate interventions can be initiated.

Palliative care providers are faced with the challenge of managing a multitude of complex symptoms in terminally ill patients. Although many of these symptoms respond to skilled palliative management, others can remain refractory to treatment.[4-9] Suffering at the end of life involves physical, psychological, social, and spiritual distress. In most situations, multidisciplinary palliative interventions provide effective comfort,[7-9] but in some instances suffering becomes refractory and intolerable.[7,10]

This chapter explores the use of palliative sedation and terminal weaning in the hospital setting. It presents case studies involving palliative sedation and withholding or withdrawing life support, discusses several definitions of palliative sedation, frequency of palliative sedation , reasons for palliative sedation, medications used, guidelines for nursing care, time-to-death issues, ethical considerations, informed consent, and the role of the nurse-caregiver.

The following two cases provide examples of clinical situations in which decisions regarding sedation and terminal weaning were required.

### CASE STUDY 1

Mr. C is a 63-year-old man with a 3-month-old diagnosis of bladder cancer that metastasized to his ribs, spine, pelvis, right clavicle, and right femur and humerus. He was admitted to the Acute Palliative Unit by his primary oncologist for management of uncontrolled pain, depressed mood, and difficulty coping with the cancer diagnosis. His primary oncologist is offering palliative treatment, but is not ruling out curative therapy if Mr. C's overwhelming symptom burden is brought under control. Mr. C, who is divorced, is accompanied by his two children and three siblings. While his family is supportive, they are also having difficulty coping with the cancer diagnosis and with watching their loved one suffer uncontrolled pain. Mr. C was initially started on a hydromorphone infusion (patient-controlled analgesia) for immediate pain relief. Palliative radiation therapy for the tumor in his femur was also started. Adopting a multidisciplinary approach, the primary oncologist asked a psychiatrist to assess Mr. C's depressed mood, an orthopedic surgeon to assess options for femur stabilization, and an anesthesia pain specialist to evaluate the feasibility of a nerve block or other interventions to provide added pain relief. Shortly after admission, Mr. C's femur fractured upon transfer to radiation therapy. Consultants from the orthopedic and pain services felt he was not a candidate for surgery for multiple reasons, including coagulopathies related to his renal cancer. The psychiatrist who evaluated Mr. C diagnosed an adjustment disorder stemming from the stress associated with his cancer diagnosis, and multiple family issues that required immediate attention. The patient and family's distress were compounded by his escalating pain and his dependency and need for daily care. His pain was initially managed by escalating his hydromorphone dose and adding steroids to his regimen. With increasing doses of hydromorphone and the addition of steroids, he developed a delirium; Haloperidol was added to his regimen and he was rotated to methadone. The patient's sensorium cleared, his pain remained difficult to control while he remained awake and alert, and he stated that he did not want further cancer-focused treatment. He acknowledged that his death was near and that he wanted to be sedated in his dying.

### CASE STUDY 2

Mrs. M, a 74-year-old woman with end-stage heart failure, was admitted to the coronary care unit (CCU) for respiratory support. She was a widow with three adult daughters, ages 23, 30, and 34. Mrs. M was awake and alert but on a ventilator. Once stabilized and diuresed she was able to be extubated. Her physician asked if she would want to be reintubated in the case of a recurrence of respiratory failure. Mrs. M stated that she did not want to be reintubated—all she wanted was to be home for Thanksgiving. The two older daughters agreed to honor their mother's decision. An interdisciplinary team meeting was held including a hospice nurse, and a plan was developed to get the patient home the day before Thanksgiving. The patient would receive home hospice care once discharged. Morphine was to be used for any respiratory distress, and glycopyrrolate for excessive secretions.

## Definitions

### From Terminal Sedation to Palliative Sedation

Numerous efforts have been made to standardize a definition for terminal sedation (this phrase was first used by Enck after a reviewing series of cases where physical symptoms were treated with sedation at the end of life),[11] and to separate sedation at end of life from sedation used in other medical settings.[5-8,12-14] Terms used for sedation at end of life include "palliative sedation,"[5,7,8,13] "terminal sedation,"[9] "total sedation,"[15] "sedation for intractable symptoms,"[16] and "sedation for distress in the imminently dying."[5] Palliative sedation has been termed "slow euthanasia."[17] This is not a widely accepted definition of palliative sedation, as the intent of sedation at end of life is to relieve suffering and not to hasten death. In this chapter the term "palliative sedation" will be used for sedation at end of life. It is defined as the monitored use of medications to induce sedation as a means to control refractory and unendurable symptoms near the end

---

**Table 26–1**
**Palliative Sedation Definitions**

**Existential suffering (sometimes referred to as terminal anguish):** Refractory psychological symptoms.

**Imminent death:** Death that is expected to occur within hours to days based on the person's condition, disease progression, and symptom constellation.

**Intent:** The purpose or state of mind at the time of an action. Intent of the patient/proxy and health care provider is a critical issue in ethical decision-making regarding palliative sedation. Relief of suffering, not hastening or causing death, is the intent of palliative sedation.

**Palliative sedation:** The monitored use of medications intended to provide relief of refractory symptoms by inducing varying degrees of unconsciousness, but not death, in terminally ill patients (Hospice and Palliative Nurses Association [2003], reference 53). *Levels of sedations:* Mild (somnotence): The patient is awake with a lowered level of consciousness.

**Intermediate (stupor):** the patient is asleep but can be awakened to communicate briefly. Deep (coma): The patient is unconscious and unresponsive (Beel et al. (2002), reference 6).

**Double effect:** In terminal sedation, an act with more than one potential effect (one good and one bad) is ethical if (1) the intended end (relief of distressing symptoms) is a good one, (2) the bad effect (death) is foreseen but not intended, (3) the bad effect is not the means of bringing about the good effect (death is not what relieves the distress), and (4) the good effect outweighs the bad effect (in a dying patient, the risk of hastening death for the benefit of comfort is appropriate) (Thorns [2002], reference 54).

**Refractory symptom:** A symptom that cannot be adequately controlled in a tolerable time frame despite the aggressive use of usual therapies and that seems unlikely to be adequately controlled by further invasive or noninvasive therapies without excessive or intolerable acute or chronic side effects.

**Terminal weaning (slow withdrawal):** Removal of mechanical ventilation, which is performed by gradually reducing the fraction of inspired oxygen ($FIO_2$) and/or mandatory ventilator rate, leading to the development of hypoxemia and hypercarbia, when the patient is not expected to survive.[21]

**Terminal extubation (abrupt withdrawal):** Removal of an endotracheal tube.[22]

---

of life. The intent is to control symptoms, not hasten death. The acceptance of the term "palliative sedation" over "terminal sedation" has evolved to emphasize the difference between management of refractory symptoms at end of life, and euthanasia. Table 26–1 lists common terms used in relation to palliative sedation and terminal weaning.

The goal of palliative sedation is the relief of suffering, and includes the concept of proportionality. Proportionality, in this setting, implies that the patient's consciousness is reduced just enough to relieve refractory suffering. Depending on the patient's situation, the level of sedation that is required may be light or deep. The endpoint that is sought is the relief of suffering. This range in depth of sedation is captured in a proposed definition of palliative sedation at the end of life as the "intentional administration of sedative drugs in dosages and combinations as required to reduce the consciousness of a terminally ill patient as much as necessary to relieve one or more refractory symptoms."[18] This definition reflects proportionality and clearly separates out palliative sedation at end of life from euthanasia.

## "Terminal Wean"

The term "terminal wean" is used when mechanical ventilation is withdrawn and the patient is not expected to survive.[19,20] A frequent approach to a terminal wean is to gradually reduce the fraction of inspired oxygen ($FIO_2$) and/or mandatory ventilator rate. This may lead to the development of hypoxemia or

hypocarbia or both.[21] Another commonly used term is "terminal extubation," which refers to removal of the patient's endotracheal tube. The decision to remove the endotracheal tube during or after a terminal weaning process is practitioner-dependent at this time.[22] Grenvik, in 1983, was the first to describe a systematic approach to ventilator withdrawal, suggesting a gradual reduction in ventilator settings over the course of several hours.[20] Some practitioners prefer a more abrupt withdrawal from ventilator support. In a 1992 survey of Society of Critical Care Medicine physicians about general ICU patients in need of extubation, 33% preferred terminal weaning, 13% preferred extubation, and the remainder used both.[23] Surgeons and anesthesiologists were more likely to use terminal weaning, and internists and pediatricians were more likely to use terminal extubation. While both methods include administration of sedatives and analgesics as indicated, the primary advantage of terminal weaning cited is that patients do not develop signs of upper airway obstruction during the withdrawal process. Terminal weaning can be viewed as less abrupt and disruptive than terminal extubation, reducing the anxiety of family and caregivers. On the other hand, terminal extubation can be viewed as not prolonging the dying process, and allowing a natural death and peace for the patient.

## Frequency of Palliative Sedation

Because the definition of palliative sedation is so varied, it is difficult to determine how often palliative sedation at end of life occurs in practice. Estimates range from 10% to 52%, varying by definition and practice sites.[5-8,24,25]

## Withholding or Withdrawing Life Supports

Approximately one-half of patients who die in hospitals have been cared for in an ICU within the previous 3 days, and one-third of these patients spend at least 10 days in ICU during their final hospitalization.[26] In the United States, approximately 22% of all hospital deaths occur in an ICU.[27] The majority of ICU deaths involve withholding or withdrawing life-sustaining treatments, although there are wide geographic variations.[28,29] A 1997 survey of the American Thoracic Society's critical care section revealed that 96% of the physicians who responded reported that they had withheld or withdrawn some form of life support.[29] A survey by Luce and Prendergast demonstrated wide geographical variations in the proportion of deaths in ICUs that are preceded by withdrawal of life support (0% to 79%) and the proportion of deaths that are preceded by a do-not-resuscitate (DNR) order (0% to 83%).[29,30]

## Reasons for Palliative Sedation

Deep sedation is a usual and accepted standard of practice prior to surgery or an extremely painful or highly distressing procedure. However, sedation at end of life has not the same level of acceptance.[14,17,31-33] Common symptoms at the end of life include pain, dyspnea, delirium, nausea, and vomiting, as well as feelings of hopelessness, remorse, anxiety, and loss of meaning.[5,6] Palliative sedation is most commonly used and accepted for the relief of refractory physical symptoms. Claessens and colleagues, in a literature review of palliative sedation, found that the majority of practitioners listed physical symptoms as the reasons for sedation at end of life, with a smaller number indicating existential suffering as the reason for sedation. The most common physical symptoms were listed as delirium, dyspnea, and pain. The nonphysical symptoms were feelings of meaninglessness, being a burden, dependency, death anxiety, and wishing to control the timing and manner of death.[18] Fainsinger and associates, in a multicenter international study, found that 1% to 4% of terminally ill patients needed sedation for pain, 0% to 6% for nausea and vomiting, 0% to 13% for dyspnea, and 9% to 23% for delirium.[34] Multiple physical and psychological symptoms are common.[13] Chater and colleagues surveyed a number of palliative care experts and asked a series of questions regarding symptoms and palliative sedation in their patients, These clinical experts reported that half of their patients had more than one symptom and that 34% received sedation for nonphysical symptoms such as anguish, fear, panic, anxiety, terror, and emotional, spiritual or psychological distress.[9]

Various factors that may affect varying standards of practice for palliative sedation include the physician's philosophy of what constitutes a "good death," personal and/or professional experiences, religious beliefs, and level of fatigue or burnout.[34,35] Although there is no consensus on the use of palliative sedation for existential suffering, literature suggests that its use in these circumstances may be increasing.[24,34] Ganzini and colleagues reviewed Oregon physician's perceptions of reasons for patients request for a hastened death and found avoidance of dependency on others and wanting to control the timing and manner of their death frequently cited.[36] In the ICU setting, reasons for palliative sedation are related to both refractory symptom management and terminal weaning from a ventilator.

## Medications and Monitoring

Drugs most commonly used for palliative sedation outside the ICU setting are benzodiazepines, neuroleptics, barbiturates, and anesthetics.[7,8,13,16] Midazolam is the most commonly used of these drugs.[7,37,38] The drug and route chosen vary based on the route available, location of the patient, and cost, as well as the preference of the provider.[7] Usually in inpatient settings the medications are given intravenously or subcutaneously and continuously. In general, the chosen medication is started at a low dose and titrated upward rapidly until the symptom is controlled and the patient does not evidence signs of distress. Classes of medications used and routes of administration are presented in Table 26–2. Dose ranges are highly variable and determined by the patient's weight, renal and hepatic function, state of hydration, concurrent medication use, and other variables. The right dose is the dose that results in the patient resting comfortably without showing evidence of distress.[6] It is recommended that doses be started low and titrated at approximately 30% an hour until sedation is achieved and the desired Richmond Agitation–Sedation Scale (RASS) level is reached[39] (Table 26–3). The type of medication that can be administered by nurses may be influenced by state regulatory rules. The drugs used for refractory symptoms and terminal weaning in the ICU include opiates, benzodiazepines, neuroleptics, and anesthetics.[2,19,21,22,40-42] These drugs can be continually infused and titrated until the patient appears comfortable. Morphine or other opioids are used to provide analgesia and reduce dyspnea. Propofol is a general anesthetic but can be used at sedative doses for ICU patients. Propofol is a good drug of choice because of its rapid onset and rapid offset. Haloperidol is used in the treatment of delirium, and can be combined with opiates and sedative agents to manage acute agitation or to protect against delirium in vulnerable patients.[22] The drugs of choice for deep sedation are usually classified as anesthesia medications, and therefore can only be used in monitored settings. Copies of protocols and sample orders for palliative sedation from a major Cancer Center are included in Appendices 26–1 through 26–3.

If the patient is on a neuromuscular-blocking agent this should be discontinued before the patient is removed from the ventilator.[42,43] Neuromuscular blockades make it

**Table 26–2**
**Management of Distressing Physical Symptoms**

| Symptom | Considerations Before Defining a Symptom as Refractory |
|---------|--------------------------------------------------------|
| Agitation and confusion | Discontinue all nonessential medications. Change required medications to ones less likely to cause delirium. Check for bladder distention and rectal impaction. Evaluate for undiagnosed or undertreated pain. Review role of hydration therapy. Consider evaluation and therapy for potentially reversible processes, such as hypoxia, hyponatremia, and hypercalcemia. |
| Pain | Maximize opioid, nonopioid, and adjuvant analgesics including agent, route, and schedule. Consider other therapies, including invasive/neurosurgical procedures, environmental changes, wound care, physical therapy, and psychotherapy. Anticipate and aggressively manage analgesic side effects. |
| Shortness of breath | Provide oxygen therapy. Maximize opioid and anxiolytic therapy. Review the role of temporizing therapy, including thoracentesis, stents, and respiratory therapy. |
| Muscle twitching | Differentiate from seizure activity. Remember the use of opioid rotation, clonidine, and benzodiazepines if muscle twitching is caused by high-dose opioids. |

*Source:* Cowan and Palmer (2002), reference 7.

**Table 26–3**
**Medications Used for Palliative Sedation**

| Medication | Dose and Route | Comments |
|------------|----------------|----------|
| Benzodiazepines/ midazolam | Loading dose of 0.5–5.0 mg, followed by 0.5–10 mg/h continuously infused IV or SQ | Monitor for paradoxical agitation with all benzodiazepines |
| Lorazepam | 0.5–5.0 mg every 1–2 h PO, SL, or IV | — |
| Neuroleptics/haloperidol | Loading dose of 0.5–5.0 mg PO, SL, SC, or IV, followed by an IV bolus of 1–5 mg every 4 h or 1–5 mg/h continuously infused IV or SQ | Monitor for extrapyramidal side effects |
| Chlorpromazine | 12.5–25.0 mg every 2–4 h PO, PR, or IV | More sedating than haloperidol |
| Barbiturates/ pentobarbital | 60–200 mg PR every 4–8 h; loading dose of 2–3 mg/kg bolus IV, followed by 1–2 mg/kg/h continuously infused IV | Do not mix with other drugs when given IV |
| Phenobarbital | Loading dose of 200 mg, followed by 0.5 mg/kg/h continuously injected SQ or IV | — |
| Anesthetics/propofol | Begin with 2.5–5.0 μg/kg/min and titrate to desired effect every 10 min by increments of 10–20 mg/h | — |

IV, intravenously; SQ, subcutaneously; PO, per os; SL, sublingually, PR, per rectum.
*Source:* Lynch (2003), reference 8.

extremely difficult to assess a patient's comfort level because their use prevents spontaneous movement. The patients may be experiencing pain, respiratory distress, and/or anxiety, but may be unable to communicate their distress. Because neuromuscular blockade can take several days to clear, ventilator support is occasionally withdrawn despite the presence of a neuromuscular blockade. This is not common practice. In such a situation death is expected to be rapid and certain after removal of the ventilator. A practitioner skilled in palliative sedation and vent withdrawal must be present at all vent withdrawals, and if possible a respiratory therapist also skilled in this area should be present.

## Assessment Tools to Measure Sedation and Agitation

Assessment tools to measure sedation and agitation are important in assessing and managing levels of consciousness in patients undergoing palliative sedation. The Richmond Agitation–Sedation Scale (RASS) has demonstrated validity and reliability in medical and surgical, ventilated and nonventilated patients, and in sedated and nonsedated adult ICU patients.[39] The RASS assessment scale is also being used in some Palliative Care Units to assess and monitor patients undergoing mild or intermediate sedation.

## Guidelines for Palliative Sedation

Institutional guidelines are important for palliative sedation and vent withdrawal so that there is a consistent standard of care and essential education for all involved practitioners can be provided.[7,25] Table 26–4 is a sample checklist for palliative sedation. Table 26–5 is a sample checklist used in an ICU setting for terminal weaning. Four factors need to be present for a patient to be considered for palliative sedation. First, the patient is terminally ill; second, the patient has severe symptoms that are refractory to treatment and intolerable to the patient, and a palliative care expert agrees that the symptoms are intractable; third, a DNR order is in effect; and fourth, death is imminent (within hours to days), although this can be challenging to determine.[7,8] If the first three conditions exist, sedation may be appropriate for a patient in severe distress who has been unresponsive to skilled palliative interventions. Ethics consultations or patient advocate services have been found to be useful if there is conflict about goals of care and appropriate care of someone near to death, especially in the ICU setting.[44]

## Palliative Sedation Checklist

A major role of the palliative care team is to assist families in making the transition in treatment goals from cure to comfort. Refractory symptoms and the distress they cause can create a very difficult and abrupt need for this transition phase. Use of the interdisciplinary team to both plan for treatment options and participate in family meetings is critical to the success of the team. The social worker plays an important role in assessing caregiver stress and family dynamics, and coordinating family meetings. The chaplain and other psychosocial professionals provide spiritual assistance and counseling and support the decision-makers through anticipatory and actual grief. The nurse is a consistent presence and skilled resource to the patient and family.

## Nursing Care: Back to Basics

### Communication

An important role of the nurse in the end of life process is to facilitate communication and establish trust between the patient, family members, and health care providers.[45] Communication is vital to developing a relationship of trust and avoiding conflict during any illness, but it becomes even more important when dealing with end of life issues. The team

---

**Table 26–4**
**Palliative Sedation Checklist**

**Part A. Background**
— Confirm patient has
  • Irreversible advanced disease.
  • Apparent imminent death within hours, days, or weeks.
  • A "do not attempt resuscitation" order.
— Confirm that symptoms are refractory to other therapies that are acceptable to the patient and have a reasonable/practical potential to achieve comfort goals.
— Consider obtaining a peer consultation to confirm that the patient is near death with refractory symptoms.
— Complete informed consent process for palliative sedation (PS).
— Discontinue interventions not focused on comfort.
  • Discontinue routine laboratory and imaging studies.
  • Review medications, limit to those for comfort, and adjust for ease of administration (timing and route).
  • Discontinue unnecessary cardiopulmonary and vital sign monitoring.
  • Review the role of cardiac support devices (e.g., pacemaker) and disable functioning implanted defibrillators.
  • Integrate a plan to discontinue ventilator support with PS.
— Develop a plan for the use or withdrawal of nutrition and hydration during PS.
— Identify a location and an environment acceptable for providing PS.
— Use providers familiar with PS and the use of sedatives.

**Part B. Treatment/care of the patient**
— Institute and maintain aspiration precautions.
— Provide mouth care and eye protection.
— Use oxygen only for comfort, not to maintain a specific blood oxygen saturation.
— Provide medications primarily by IV or SQ route.
— Maintain bowel, bladder, and pressure point care.
— Continue, do not taper, routine opioids.
— Provide sedating medication:
  • Around the clock.
  • Titrate to symptom control not level of consciousness, using frequent re-evaluation.
  • Limit vital sign monitoring to temperature and respiratory rate for dyspnea.
— Choose sedating medication based on provider experience, route available, and patient location.
  *Home initial dosing (choose one):*
  • Chlorpromazine, 25 mg suppository or 12.5 mg IV infusion every 4–6 h.
  • Midazolam, 0.4 mg/h by continuous IV or SQ infusion.
  • Lorazepam, 0.5–2.0 mg IV sublingually every 4–6 h.
  *Hospital initial dosing (choose one):*
  • Chlorpromazine, 12.5–25.0 mg every 4–6 h.
  • Midazolam, 0.4 mg/h by continuous IV or SQ infusion.
  • Amobarbital or thiopental, 20 mg/h by continuous IV infusion.
  • Propofol, 2.5 mg/kg/min by continuous IV infusion.

*Source:* Lynch, (2003), reference 8.

**Table 26–5**
**Checklist for Intensive Care Unit Personnel End-of-Life Criterion**

| Assessment | MET | NOT MET |
|---|---|---|
| 1. Determine that primary physician, critical care physician, family and possibly patient are in agreement with discontinuation of life sustaining treatment. | ___ | ___ |
| 2. Assist family in preparation or fulfillment of familial or religious predeath rituals. | ___ | ___ |
| 3. Place, "do not resuscitate" orders on chart. | ___ | ___ |
| 4. Turn off neuromuscular blockade agents (e.g., paralytics). | ___ | ___ |
| 5. Provide a calm, quiet, restful atmosphere free of medical devices and technology for the patient and family, including dimming the lights in the room. | ___ | ___ |
| 6. Turn off arrhythmia detection and turn off or decrease all auditory alarms at bedside and central station. | ___ | ___ |
| 7. Remove all monitoring equipment from patient and patient's room except for the electrocardiograph (ECG). | ___ | ___ |
| 8. Remove all devices unless the removal of the device would create discomfort for the patient (e.g., sequential compression device, nasogastric tube). | ___ | ___ |
| 9. Remove or discontinue treatments that do not provide comfort to the patient. | ___ | ___ |
| 10. Obtain orders to discontinue test and laboratory studies. | ___ | ___ |
| 11. Liberalize visitation. | ___ | ___ |
| 12. Notify respiratory therapist of end-of-life care. | ___ | ___ |
| 13. Notify chaplain and social worker of end-of-life care; obtain grief packet from chaplain. | ___ | ___ |
| 14. Determine that family participants in the end-of-life process are present, if appropriate; place sufficient chairs in the patient's room for family members. | ___ | ___ |
| 15. Maintain the patient's personal comfort and dignity with attention to hygiene, hairstyle, and providing moisturizers for lips and eyes. | ___ | ___ |
| 16. Gather ordered sedation and analgesics. Frequent assessment of the patient's condition assists in titrating medications per end-of-life protocol and level of patient discomfort. | ___ | ___ |
| 17. Document the patient's signs and symptoms that indicate discomfort, including but not limited to the following: | ___ | ___ |

| | |
|---|---|
| Agitated behavior | Grimacing |
| Altered cognition | Increased work of |
| Anxiety | breathing |
| Autonomic hyperactivity | Irritation |
| Confusion | Moaning |
| Coughing | Pain |
| Dyspnea | Perspiration |
| Restlessness | Tachypnea |
| Self-report of symptoms | Tension |
| Splinting | Trembling |
| Stiffness | |
| Tachycardia | |

| Assessment | MET | NOT MET |
|---|---|---|
| 18. Remain at bedside to<br>a. assess patient for comfort/discomfort.<br>b. promptly administer sedation, analgesics.<br>c. provide emotional support to patient and family.<br>d. ask patient/family if additional comfort measures are needed. | | |
| 19. Obtain physician orders for additional or alterations in pain and sedation medications if the end-of-life protocol medications are ineffective in controlling the patient's discomfort. | ___ | ___ |
| 20. Respiratory therapist should remain in room until ventilator is function at minimal capacity or patient is extubated and the ventilator is removed from the room. | ___ | ___ |
| 21. Support and educate the patient's family regarding interpretation of the clinical signs and symptoms the patient may experience during the end of life. | ___ | ___ |
| 22. Assess the family's need to be alone with the patient during and after the death process. | ___ | ___ |
| 23. Assess the family to determine the amount of support they require during the end-of-life process. | ___ | ___ |
| 24. Assist the family in meeting its needs and the patient's needs for communication, final expressions of love and concern (e.g., holding a hand, talking with the patient, remembering past events). | ___ | ___ |

*(continued)*

**Table 26–5**
**Checklist for Intensive Care Unit Personnel End-of-Life Criterion** (*continued*)

| Assessment | MET | NOT MET |
|---|---|---|
| 25. Discuss signs of death and how the physician will pronounce the patient; the family will be asked to leave the room while the physician examines the patient. | ___ | ___ |
| 26. If the patient is transferred to the general care floors during end-of-life care, provide the accepting nurse a verbal report and discuss the dosage of IV medications and the signs and symptoms for medication titration. Suggest to the critical care physician or attending physician a patient referral to or consultation with palliative care services. | ___ | ___ |
| 27. Notify intensive care unit physician to pronounce patient. An ECG strip of a straight line or asystole is not needed to document patient death. | ___ | ___ |
| 28. Notify primary care physician. | ___ | ___ |
| 29. Assist family with decisions regarding need for autopsy. | ___ | ___ |
| 30. Notify clinical nurse specialist Monday through Friday before 3 P.M. to complete death paperwork. | ___ | ___ |
| 31. Notify in-house administrator after 3 P.M. and on weekends to complete death paperwork. | ___ | ___ |
| 32. Notify chaplain, if chaplain not present. | ___ | ___ |
| 33. If the patient is to have an autopsy, leave all tubes in place; if no autopsy, remove all tubes (IV lines may be clamped instead of removed). | ___ | ___ |
| 34. Permit family visitation after the patient has been cleaned and tubes removed. | ___ | ___ |
| 35. Prepare patient for the morgue, shroud etc. | ___ | ___ |

MET, Indicates that the individual is prepared, follows suggested steps in appropriate sequence, and demonstrates minimal safe practice; NOT MET, Indicates that the individual is unprepared, needs repeated assistance or suggestions in order to proceed, and or omits necessary steps.
*Source:* M.D. Anderson Cancer Center, Houston, Texas. Reprinted with permission.

has to build a trusting relationship with patients and families as they make difficult decisions together. If the patient or family members do not trust the health care team, conflict is likely. Communication includes: (1) being honest and truthful; (2) letting the patient and family members know they will not be abandoned; (3) including them in care decisions; (4) helping the patient and family explore all options; (5) asking them to clearly define what they need from the team; (6) working to ensure that the entire team knows and understands the plan; and, most important, (7) practicing active listening when talking to the patient and family members.[45] In a qualitative study examining nurses' perceptions of palliative sedation, two factors made nurses more comfortable with their role in the dying process. The first was how well the nurse knew the patient as a person, and the second was the interdisciplinary team collaboration.[46]

When the decision is made to use either palliative sedation or terminal weaning, caring and thoughtful communication make a tremendous difference in the family's experience with the death of their loved one. The patient and/or family health care agent are central in this decision, and need ongoing reassurance that the decision made is the right one. They may need frequent confirmation that the person is dying of their disease, and that the intent of the sedation is to ensure a peaceful death but not to hasten death. The concept of "presence" with the patient and family during the death vigil is difficult to quantify, but critical during periods of extreme distress.[47,48] Untreated symptoms cause families and staff to be traumatized by a "horrible death." The family may fear that this "final event" will be equally traumatic. They don't want their loved one to suffer any more. They need constant

explanations and reassurance about what to expect, what is happening, and the opportunity to express their grief.[7]

**Physical care**

As the patient becomes more sedated, protective reflexes decrease. The ability to clear secretions decreases. This can be anticipated, and appropriate medication should be given proactively. Suctioning is kept to a minimum and only done if really necessary. The blink reflex also decreases and eyes can become dry, requiring frequent eye drops (artificial tears). Bowel and bladder management needs to be carefully monitored to maintain comfort. A urinary catheter is often appropriate to minimize the need for frequent changing and cleaning, and to prevent skin breakdown. General nursing care for immobilized patients is especially important; mattress pads that decrease pressure, excellent skin care, and attention to positioning are all needed. Allowing the family to participate in the basic comfort care of their loved one at end of life, such as bathing, brushing the hair, and applying a lubricant to the lips, can be quite meaningful to some family members. Other family members may prefer not do help with physical care and they should be reassured that their presence alone, even if in spirit only, is equally important.

**Terminal Weaning**

**Special Considerations in the Intensive Care Unit**

Conversations with the family prior to the weaning process are essential so they know what to expect and can be present for the weaning if they so chose. In addition, friends may want to visit to say their goodbyes before the terminal weaning takes place. Immediately before terminal weaning, the physician and nurse should again briefly review the procedure and answer any questions the patient and/or family members may have. In some institutions a respiratory therapist is always present for terminal weans; their presence is part of the institutional protocol. If a family member wants to be present during the terminal weaning process, a social worker and or nurse should be present solely to take care of the family. Chaplaincy may also be present if that is appropriate for this particular family. Members of the interdisciplinary team should be familiar with the terminal weaning process, so that they can be consistent in the information that they give to the family, to reassure the family that the patient will not suffer, and that medication will be immediately administered if there is any sign of distress.

Before beginning the weaning process, physiological monitoring alarms should be deactivated and unnecessary tubes or equipment removed. Unnecessary medications (i.e. those not related to symptom control) should also be discontinued. Each step should be explained to the family, questions answered, and reassurance given. Before extubation, appropriate medications are administered to ensure symptom control and the necessary level of sedation. Frequently opioids are used for dyspnea, and benzodiazepines for anxiety. The need for additional medications must be anticipated and readily available if needed. Oxygen is frequently set at 21%. The patient is constantly monitored for any signs of distress and medicated accordingly. The nurse's presence is critical in this monitoring process.

Once the patient appears comfortable, if the patient is to be extubated, the physician removes the endotracheal tube. Throughout this process, the nurse should allow space for the patient's family at the bedside. The decision to stay at the bedside or not is a personal decision, and it is important that the nurse validates and supports whatever decision is made by each family member. The family, if appropriate, and with coaching beforehand, can be encouraged to assist with the patient's care by wiping the patient's forehead, holding the patient's hand, and/or talking softly to the patient reassuring them that they are there. Chaplaincy and or other psychosocial support should be available to the family throughout the process. After the patient dies, the family should be allowed adequate time with their loved to say their goodbyes and move to the next phase in the grieving process.

Debriefing following the patient's death allows the family to go over what happened, have their questions answered once more, and be supported by those who were present during the terminal wean. Ensuring ongoing bereavement support for the family is an important nursing role.

## Time to Death

### Palliative Sedation

One of the concerns many people have with palliative sedation is that it might hasten death. Part of this concern stems from the difficulty in predicting the time of death. Several studies using different methodologies have examined effects of sedation on survival rates.[49,50] The mean time-to-death in a large 4-country study ranged from 1.9 to 3.2 days,[34] and the median time to death in a Taiwanese study was 5 days.[51] A study of patients in Japanese hospices indicated that sedating medications did not shorten lifespan.[49] However, because of ethical considerations none of these studies were controlled trials, so it is not possible to determine whether sedation may or may not result in hastening the death. In situations of unbearable distress, sedation remains an appropriate option to relieve suffering.

## Ethical Considerations Concerning Palliative Sedation and Terminal Weaning

Palliative sedation is a medical therapy for the imminently dying when pain and suffering are intolerable, and other interventions have proved inadequate. Intent is the critical issue, and separates palliative sedation at end of life from assisted dying and euthanasia. With sedation the intent is to produce somnolence and relieve suffering, not hasten death. In assisted dying—where the intent is to produce death to relieve suffering—the agent is the patient. In euthanasia—the intent is to produce death to relieve suffering—the agent is another. The ethical and legal principles that apply to palliative sedation are patient autonomy (patient's choice), beneficence (do good), nonmaleficence (do no harm), and the principle of double effect.[7,16,52–56] The reader is referred to Chapter 62 for a more in-depth discussion on ethical principles and issues in palliative care and end of life care.

In 1997, the U.S. Supreme Court ruled unanimously that "there is no constitutional right to physician-assisted suicide" but "terminal sedation is intended for symptom relief and not assisted suicide...and is appropriate in the aggressive practice of palliative care."[57,58] The American Nurses Association and the Oncology Nursing Society have Position Papers opposed to physician-assisted suicide.[59,60] Although neither of the Position Papers address the exact issue of palliative sedation or terminal weaning, both support the risk of hastening death through treatments aimed at alleviating suffering or controlling symptoms, as ethically and legally acceptable. The Hospice and Palliative Nurses Association has issued a Position Paper in support of palliative sedation.[53] The use of palliative sedation for existential suffering remains controversial.[5]

The ethical principles that apply to withdrawal of mechanical ventilation are patient autonomy, nonmaleficence, and beneficence. However, terminal weaning can be disturbing for those who do not understand the principles that guide caregivers' actions, which includes respect for the patient's right to discontinue unwanted treatment including ventilator withdrawal. In addition, the terminal weaning process can be more difficult for the caregiver if the patient is awake and alert enough to participate in the decision to withdraw life support, but the guiding principles remain the same.

## Informed Consent

Informed consent is always a process. A patient's symptoms may have been difficult to control over time and may have escalated as the patient's disease has progressed. Patients (or their agents when they cannot speak for themselves) must always be involved in these decisions. Palliative sedation involves an important trade-off between symptom control and alertness, and different patients will weigh this differently. The need for sedation may be a palliative care emergency to relieve distress, and consent would be similar to obtaining consent in any other emergency situation. A family meeting to discuss the situation would then follow.

A family meeting includes a well planned, compassionate, and clear discussion with the patient and family about the patient's goals and values in the setting of end of life care. The bedside nurse is an important participant in these meetings to provide insight into the care and support needed by the family. It is important to plan these meetings carefully if at all possible, to ensure that the appropriate family members are present. Allowing the designated decision-maker to invite significant people to the planned meeting allows key participants to hear the information at the same time. A religious or spiritual representative can be helpful at these meetings, if the family so desires.

The primary physician usually begins the family meeting with a brief, clear report on the current condition of the patient. Supporting documentation of the current condition, such as recent laboratory data or other diagnostic test results, may be helpful to some families. The patient and or family should be provided all the time necessary to raise concerns, clarify information, and have their questions answered. The same questions may be raised time and time again to different team members, and need to be answered with consistent information to reduce uncertainty. Next, the treatment options should be discussed. When discussing terminal sedation options, it is important to assess the patient's and family's cultural and religious beliefs and concerns. Documentation in the chart should include the parties present, the reason for sedation (symptom distress), and the primary goal (patient comfort), as well as patient terminal status, notation of any professional consultations, documentation that the patient is near death and has refractory symptoms, planned discontinuance of treatments not focused on comfort, plan regarding hydration and nutrition, and anticipated risks or burdens of sedation.[7] Either at the end of the family meeting, or the next day in nonemergency cases, some institutions require that an informed consent document is signed by the patient, family, or health care agent. Because it usually is not possible to communicate verbally with the sedated patient, it is important to make sure that the patient and family are given time to talk with each other and say their goodbyes, if that is possible, prior to proceeding with sedation. A well-planned family meeting decreases miscommunication and supports the family during a difficult decision-making time by allowing all pertinent parties to hear the same information at the same time. The decision for palliative sedation or terminal wean is a patient/agent/family decision (whoever is the decision-maker) with guidance from the palliative care team.

In the ICU setting, there should also be a succinct description of the terminal weaning process. One of the most common reasons for withholding or withdrawing life support is that the patient has a very poor prognosis and is unlikely to improve.[61] Although there are published guidelines for withholding and withdrawing life support, the actual implementation of such measures is often difficult for the health care team members as well as the patient and family. Physicians may have a difficult time discussing such interventions with patients and families, and this in turn may lead to the continuation of treatments that are medically inappropriate, increase suffering, or are futile. The patient and family members must be allowed sufficient time to reach a consensus about whether to discontinue life support. It is their decision. This is a process that is made easier by the provision of consistent, compassionate, accurate information about the patient's prognosis and likely course. Ongoing nurse–physician communication is essential so that the patient, where possible, and the family, is given consistent information about the patient's status. Clear documentation as indicated earlier is also essential so that all members of the team and others involved in the patient's care are clear about the goals of care and treatment plan.

## The Nurse Caregiver

In a literature review examining the experience of nurses caring for terminally ill patients in ICU settings, several barriers related to provision of terminal care were identified. These included: (1) lack of involvement in the plan of care and comfort; (2) disagreement among physicians and other health care team members; (3) inadequacy of pain relief; (4) unrealistic expectations of families; (5) personal difficulty coping; (6) lack of experience and education; (7) staffing levels; and (8) environmental circumstances.[62] In a Japanese study of 2607 nurses involved in palliative sedation, 37% reported they wanted to leave their current jobs because of the burden of palliative sedation; 12% reported that their involvement in palliative sedation made them feel helpless; and 11% would avoid a patient who is being treated with palliative sedation if possible. This study concluded that a significant number of nurses felt serious emotional burdens related to palliative sedation.[63]

Nurses who work with patients requiring palliative sedation and terminal weaning are at increased risk of burnout if not intimately involved with the team decision-making process.

In addition, if left out of decision-making processes such as the team planning and family conferences, they are denied the information needed for effective counseling at the patient's bedside.[64] A formal and informal support system for nurses as well as education in end of life care, spiritual support, and individual support are essential.

An interdisciplinary team meeting after the death of the patient can function as both a learning experience and a debriefing session. Working in an environment that recognizes the need for support and education of staff, and one that recognizes the importance of mentors and advance practice nurses, allows nurses to face these challenges as they arise.

## Conclusion

Although nurses and other health care practitioners may disagree about what a "good death" is, there is general agreement about what is a "bad death." Palliative sedation and terminal weaning are a necessary option for a small number of patients with refractory and intolerable symptoms and suffering at end of life. These options are part of the spectrum of palliative care and are ethically and legally supported. However, the ability to determine refractoriness of symptoms can be complicated and is largely dependent on the skills of the practitioner and the tools available to manage complex symptoms. Nurses have a central role in ensuring that a dying patient undergoing palliative sedation or ventilator withdrawal has his or her symptoms well controlled, and that the family members are well supported. Education of palliative care nurses in these areas is essential.

REFERENCES

1. Miller PA, Forbes S, Boyle DK. End-of-life care in the intensive care unit: A challenge for nurses. Am J Crit Care 2001;10:230–237.
2. Robert Wood Johnson Foundation. Survey results: What Americans think about the American way of death, 2002. Available at: http://www.rwjf.org/news/special/meansSummary.html (accessed April 14, 2004).
3. Aungst H. 'Death with dignity'. The first decade of Oregon's physician-assisted death act. Geriatrics 2008;63:20–24.
4. Ventafridda V, Ripamonte C, De Conno F, Tamburini M, Cassileth BR. Symptom prevalence and control during cancer patients' last days of life. J Palliat Care 1990;6:7–11.
5. Wein S. Sedation in the imminently dying patient. Oncology 2000;14:585–601.
6. Beel A, McClement S, Harlos M. Palliative sedation therapy: A review of definitions and usage. Int J Palliat Nurs 2002;8:190–199.
7. Cowan JD, Palmer TW. Practical guide to palliative sedation. Curr Oncol Rep 2002;4:242–249.
8. Lynch M. Palliative sedation. Clin J Oncol Nurs 2003;7:653–667.
9. Chater S, Viola R, Paterson J, Jarvis V. Sedation for intractable distress in the dying: A survey of experts. Palliat Med 1998;12:255–269.
10. Volker DL. Assisted dying and end of life symptom management. Cancer Nurs 2003;26:392–399.
11. Enck RE. Drug-induced terminal sedation for symptom control. Am Hospice Palliat Care 1991;84:332–337.
12. Cherny NI, Portenoy RK. Sedation in the management of refractory symptoms: Guidelines for evaluation and treatment. J Palliat Care 1994;10:31–38.
13. Cowan JD, Walsh D. Terminal sedation in palliative medicine: Definition and review of literature. Support Cancer Care 2001;9:403–407.
14. Morita T, Tsuneto S, Shima Y. Proposed definitions of sedation for symptom relief: A systematic literature review and a proposal of operation criteria. J Pain Symptom Manage 2002;24:447–453.
15. Peruselli C, Di Giulio P, Toscani F, Gallucci M, Brunelli C, Costantini M, Tamburini M, Paci E, Miccinesi G, Addington-Hall JM, Higginson U. Home palliative care for terminal cancer patients: A survey on the final week of life. Palliat Med 1999;13:233–241.
16. Krakauer EL, Penson RT, Troug RD, King LA, Chabner BA, Lynch TJ Jr. Sedation for intractable distress of a dying patient: Acute palliative care and the principle of double effect. Oncologist 2000;5:53–62.
17. Billings JA, Block SD. Slow euthanasia. J Palliat Care 1996;12:21–30.
18. Claessens P, Menten J, Schotsmans P, Broeckaert B. Palliative Sedation: A review of the research literature. J Pain Symptom Manage 2008;36(3):310–333.
19. 19..Campbell ML, Carlson RW. Terminal weaning from mechanical ventilation: Ethical and practical considerations for patient management. Am J Crit Care 1992;1:52–56.
20. Grenvik A. "Terminal weaning": Discontinuance of life-support therapy in the terminally ill patient. Crit Care Med 1983;11:394–395.
21. Truog RD, Cist AF, Brackett SF, Burns JP, Curley MAQ, Danis M, DeVita MA, Rosenbaum SH, Rothenberg DM, Sprung CL, Webb SA, Wlody GS, Hurford WE. Recommendations for end-of-life care in the intensive care unit: The Ethics Committee of the Society of Critical Care Medicine. Crit Care Med 2001;29:2332–2348.
22. Troug RD, Campbell M, Curtis JR, Hass CE, Luce J, Rubenfeld GD, Rushton CH, Kaufman DC. Recommendations for end-of-life care in the intensive care unit: A consensus statement by the American College of Critical Care Medicine. Crit Care Med 2008;36:953–963.
23. Faber-Langendoen K. The clinical management of dying patients receiving mechanical ventilation: Survey of physician practice. Chest 1994;106:880–888.
24. Cherney N. Sedation for the care of patients with advanced cancer. Nat Clin Pract Oncol 2006;3(9):492–500.
25. Rousseau P. Existential suffering and palliative sedation: A brief commentary with a proposal for clinical guidelines. Am J Hosp Palliat Care 2001;18:151–153.
26. Curtis JR, Patrick DL. How to discuss death and dying in the ICU. In: Curtis JR, Rubenfeld GD, eds. Managing Death in the ICU. New York: Oxford University Press, 2001:85–102.
27. Angus DC, Barnato AE, Linde-Zwirble WT, Weissfeld LA, Watson RS, Rickert T, Rubenfeld GD. Use of intensive care at the end of life in the United States: An epidemiologic study. Crit Care Med 2004;32(3):638–643.
28. Rocker GM, Curtis JR. Caring for the dying in the intensive care unit: In search of clarity. JAMA 2003;290:820–822.
29. Prendergast TJ, Luce JM. Increasing incidence of withholding and withdrawal of life support from the critically ill. Am J Respir Crit Care Med 1997;155:15–20.

30. Luce JM, Prendergast TJ. The changing nature of death in the ICU. In: Curtis JR, Rubenfeld GD, eds. Managing Death in the Intensive Care Unit. New York: Oxford University Press, 2001:19–29.

31. Sykes N, Thorns A. Sedative use in the last week of life and the implications for end of life decision making. Arch Intern Med 2003;163:341–344.

32. Jansen LA, Sulmasy DP. Sedation, alimentation, hydration, and equivocation: Careful conversation about care at the end of life. Ann Intern Med 2002;136:845–849.

33. Hallenbeck JL. Terminal sedation: Ethical implications in different situations. J Palliat Med 2000;3:313–320.

34. Fainsinger RL, Waller A, Bercovici M, Bengtson K, Landman W, Hosking M, Nunez-Olarte JM, deMoissac D. A multicentre international study of sedation for uncontrolled symptoms in terminally ill patients. Palliat Med 2000;14:257–265.

35. Breitbart W, Bruera E, Chochinov H, Lynch M. Neuropsychiatric syndromes and psychological symptoms in patients with advanced cancer. J Pain Symptom Manage 1995;10:131–141.

36. Ganzini L, Dobscha SK, Heintz RT, Press N. Oregon physicians' perceptions of patients who request assisted suicide and their families. J Palliat Med 2003:6:381–390.

37. De Graeff A, Dean M. Palliative sedation therapy in the last weeks of life: A literature review and recommendations for standards. J Palliat Med 2007;10(1):67–87.

38. Cheng C, Roemer-Becuwe C, Pereira J. When midazolam fails. J Pain Symptom Manage 2002;23:256–265.

39. Sessler CN, Jo Grap M, Ramsay MA. Evaluating and monitoring analgesia and sedation in the intensive care unit. Crit Care 2008;12 Suppl 3:15.

40. Hospice & Palliative Care Federation of Massachusetts. Palliative Sedation Protocol: A report of the Standards and Best Practice Committee Hospice & Palliative Care Federation of MA, 2004.

41. Truog RD, Berde CB, Mitchell C, Grier HE. Barbiturates in the care of the terminally ill. N Engl J Med 1992;327:1678–1681.

42. Truog RD, Burns JP, Mitchell C, Johnson J, Robinson W. Sounding board: Pharmacological paralysis and withdrawal of mechanical ventilation at the end of life. N Engl J Med 2000;342:508–511.

43. Rushton CH, Terry PB. Neuromuscular blockade and ventilator withdrawal: Ethical controversies. Am J Crit Care 1995;4:112–115.

44. Schneiderman LJ, Gilmer T, Teetzel HD, Dugan DO, Blustein J, Cranford R, Briggs KB, Komatsu GI, Goodman-Crew P, Cohn F, Young EWD. Effects of ethics consultations on nonbeneficial life-sustaining treatments in the intensive care setting. JAMA 2003;209:1166–1172.

45. Matzo ML, Sherman DW, Sheehan DC, Ferrell BR, Penn B. Communication skills for end of life nursing care. Nurs Educ Perspect 2003;24:176–183.

46. Beel AC, Hawranik PG, McClement S, Daeninck P. Palliative sedation: Nurses' perceptions. Int J Palliat Nurs 2006;12(11):510–518.

47. . Pitorak EF. Care at the time of death: How nurses can make the last hours of life a richer, more comfortable experience. Am J Nurs 2003;103:42–53.

48. Walsh SM, Hogan NS. Oncology nursing education: Nursing students' commitment of "presence" with the dying patient and the family. Nurs Educ Perspect 2003;24:86–90.

49. Morita T, Tsunoda J, Inoue S, Chihara S. Effects of high-dose opioids and sedatives on survival in terminally ill cancer patients. J Pain Symptom Manage 2001;21:282–289.

50. Rousseau P. The ethical validity and clinical experience of palliative sedation. Mayo Clin Proc 2000;75:1064–1069.

51. Chiu TY, Hu WY, Lue BH, Cheng SY, Chen CY. Sedation for refractory symptoms of terminal cancer patients in Taiwan. J Pain Symptom Manage 2001;21:467–472.

52. A report by the National Ethics Committee of the Veterans Health Administration. The Ethics of Palliative Sedation, 2006.

53. Hospice and Palliative Nurses Association. Position paper: Palliative sedation at the end of life. J Hosp Palliat Nurs 2003;5:235–237.

54. Hayes C. Ethics in end of life care. J Hosp Palliat Nurs 2004;6:36–43.

55. Gallagher A, Wainwright P. Terminal sedation: Promoting ethical nursing practice. Nurs Stand 2007;21(34):42–46.

56. Quill TE, Dresser R, Brock DW. The rule of double effect: A critique of its role in end of life decision making. N Engl J Med 1997;337:1768–1771.

57. Orentlicher D. The Supreme Court and physician-assisted suicide: Rejecting assisted suicide but embracing euthanasia. N Engl J Med 1997;337:1236–1239.

58. Burt RA. The Supreme Court speaks: Not assisted suicide but a constitutional right to palliative care. N Engl J Med 1997;337:1234–1236.

59. American Nurses Association. Code of Ethics for Nurses with Interpretive Statements. Washington, DC: American Nurses Association, 2001.

60. Oncology Nursing Society. Position statement on the nurse's responsibility to the patient requesting assisted suicide, 2001. Available at: http//www.ons.org/publications/positions/AssistedSuicide.shtml (accessed January 6, 2005).

61. Keenan SB, Busche KD, Chen LM, McCarthy L, Inman KJ, Sibbald WJ. A retrospective review of a large cohort of patients undergoing the process of withholding or withdrawal of life support. Crit Care Med 1997;25:1324–1321.

62. Espinosa L, Young E, Walsh T. Barriers to ICU nurses providing terminal care: An integrated literature review. Crit Care Nurse 2008;31:83–93.

63. Morita T, Miyashita M, Kimura R, Adachi I, Shima Y. Emotional burden of nurses in palliative sedation therapy. Palliat Med 2004;18:550–557.

64. Frederich ME, Strong R, von Gunten CF. Physician-nurse conflict: Can nurses refuse to carry out doctor's orders? J Palliat Med 2002;5:155–158.

APPENDIX 26–1
## End-of-life Protocol

### Introduction

The Intensive Care Unit (ICU) healthcare team provides complex medical and nursing interventions to stabilize and improve the physical status of critically ill patients. However, there are frequent situations in which the patient cannot be stabilized, their status cannot be improved or continued life-sustaining interventions would be medically inappropriate.

The end-of-life Protocol is a guide and educational tool for the ICU healthcare team. Consequently the patient will benefit from expert, competent, compassionate, consistent end of life care.

The end-of-life Protocol should be initiated subsequent to a patient care conference and a written DNR order.

### Definitions

*ICU healthcare team*—The ICU healthcare team is multidisciplinary and the participants vary according to the needs of the patient or family. Members may include: physicians, nurses, social worker, respiratory therapist, ethicist, dietician, physical therapy, pharmacist, chaplain, and others depending on the patient's physical and mental status.

*Intensive care physician*—The Intensive Care Physician supervising the initiation of the end of life Protocol will sign the End-of Life Orders and will be readily available to consult with the nurse and family during the patient's end of life care.

*Contact alternate physician*—If the Intensive Care Physician is unavailable during the patient's end-of-life care, the Intensive Care Physician will indicate a physician that will assume supervision of the patient's care. This physician will be known as the Alternate Physician Contact and will be identified on the end of life Orders by name and pager number.

*Comfort measures*—Comfort measures are interventions that ease the patient's discomfort. Comfort measures may include: regulation of hypothermia or hyperthermia, oral care, basic hygiene, music therapy, control of pain and sedation.

*Family*—Family includes spouse, mother, father, sibling, guardian, or any significant other to the patient.

*Patient care conference*—The family and or patient meets with the Intensive Care Physician, Attending Physician, nurse, social worker and other appropriate members from the ICU healthcare team to discuss the patient's medical status. The goal for the Patient Care Conference is to develop a plan of care that may include the end of life Protocol.

*Plan of care*—The plan of care gives direction and prioritizes the care the patient receives.

*Signs and symptoms of discomfort*—Signs and symptoms of discomfort include, but are not limited to: agitated behavior, altered cognition, anxiety, autonomic hyperactivity, confusion, coughing, dyspnea, grimacing, increased work of breathing, irritation, moaning, pain, restlessness, tachycardia, splinting, tenseness, self-report of discomfort, perspiration, stiffness, trembling and tachypnea.

*When appropriate*—The terms "when appropriate" or "appropriate" in reference to the end of life Protocol defines a time when the patient, family and ICU healthcare team are present and prepared to initiate the steps outlined in the Protocol. The timing for Protocol initiation will accommodate the needs of the patient and family.

### Purpose

The purpose for the end of life Protocol is to guide the ICU healthcare team, promote consistency of care, and improve the quality of care provided during the patient's end of life.

### Goal

The goal for the end of life Protocol is to maximize patient comfort and dignity without prolongation of life, extension of the dying process or hastening the dying process.

### Objectives

The end of life Protocol and care may include the following actions:

- Create a quiet, calm, restful atmosphere with minimal medical devices and technology in the patient's room.
- Remove or discontinue treatments that do not provide comfort for the patient.
- Provide controlled and comfortable end of life care for the patient.
- Promote patient comfort with a variety of approaches including medications.
- Provide physical, psychological, social, emotional, and spiritual resources for the patient and family.
- Educate and support the patient's family regarding the progression of end of life care and the interpretation of the clinical signs and symptoms the patient may experience.
- Assist the family in meeting their needs and the patient's needs for communication, final expressions of love, and concern.
- Assist the family in fulfilling familial, cultural or religious death rituals.

# Institutional Policies

**Volume XI**
**Book J Division of Nursing Procedures**
**Chapter 24 Palliative Care**
Policy XI.J.24.01

## NURSING ADMINISTRATION OF MIDAZOLAM AND PROPOFOL TO NON-INTUBATED PATIENTS FOR PALLIATION OF SEVERE INTRACTABLE SYMPTOMS FOR TERMINALLY ILL CANCER PATIENTS ON THE PALLIATIVE CARE UNIT

**PURPOSE**    To establish an institutional standard for administering and monitoring sedation using midazolam and/or propofol for palliation of severe intractable symptoms for terminally ill cancer patients on the Palliative Care unit (PCU). This protocol does not address the use of midazolam or propofol or other benzodiazepines for conscious sedation or anesthesia.

**GENERAL**
**INFORMATION**    Administration of anesthetic agents by RNs to non-intubated patients be practiced in accordance with the following guidelines. These are systematically developed recommendations that will provide nurses with criteria for making decisions about the administration of anesthetic agents that are consistent with evidence-based practice guidelines and the position statement of the <u>Texas Board of Nurse Examiners on Anesthesia by RNs</u>.

**SCOPE**    The Texas Board of Nurse Examiners states: "The clinical effects for patients receiving anesthetic agents may vary widely within a negligible dose range. Because of the danger of unintended deep sedation and/or general anesthesia with pharmacologic agents classified as "anesthetic" agents, the Board advises caution for registered nurses who are not qualified anesthesia providers in administering such agents in non-intubated patients. Both nurses and facilities should consider evidence-based practice guidelines put forth by the respective specialty group(s) for a given practice area in developing the appropriate guidance for the RN in the specific practice setting."

The procedure covers the administration of midazolam or propofol continuous infusion for the purposes of palliation of severe and unendurable symptoms, such as agitated delirium, severe dyspnea, or active severe bleeding. This procedure applies to terminally ill cancer patients under the care of the Palliative Care service. These symptoms can be a source of great distress to the patient and family. Sedation is a widely used intervention by Palliative Care providers, in the U.S. and internationally, to control symptoms in these rare circumstances. The practice is widely supported by the Palliative Care Literature. Midazolam is the most frequently reported agent in use. Propofol is also an agent of choice due to its speed of onset, easy titration and easy reversibility. See also "Palliative Sedation Policy for the Symptom Control and Palliative Care Service".

**DEFINITIONS**

**Palliative sedation** (previously known as terminal sedation) is defined as the monitored use of medications (midazolam or propofol) that induce sedation to control refractory and unendurable symptoms near the end of life when the control of these symptoms is not possible using less aggressive measures.
The purpose is to control symptoms and not to hasten death.

**Refractory Symptoms** are defined as those symptoms that cannot be adequately relieved or controlled despite aggressive use of usually effective therapies (e.g. medications, other interventions), and seem unlikely to respond to further invasive or non-invasive therapies in a timely way without excessive or intolerable side effects/complications.

**Continuous infusion administration** is defined as the administration of medication directly into an intravenous or subcutaneous site continuously by measured and metered dosage using an infusion pump.

**Midazolam** is a very short acting benzodiazepine (onset of action within 3-5 minutes after intravenous injection with peak effect seen in 20-60 minutes), used most frequently as an induction agent for general anesthesia or to provide conscious sedation during brief invasive diagnostic procedures. The drug is given by IV/SQ infusion with starting dose of 0.5-1mg/Hr.

**Propofol** is an intravenous sedative hypnotic agent useful in the induction and maintenance of general anesthesia, and in sedation of mechanically ventilated patients. The onset of action is given by continuous infusion with a staring dose of 0.15mg/kg/Hr.

## ORDERING/ADMINISTERING PROCEDURES

**PRIVILEGES**

1. The Department of Palliative Care and Rehabilitation Medicine will recommend the award of privileges for Palliative Care Staff physicians for palliative sedation on the PCU using midazolam and propofol. This privilege covers evaluation of terminally ill patients for the need for the procedure, and the issuance of orders for palliative sedation.

2. Nurses who have successfully completed the Palliative Sedation Competency may administer palliative sedation as described by the Palliative care physician.

3. If ordered for palliative sedation, each of the following criteria must be met in order for midazolam or propofol to be administered.

Irreversible advanced disease with death appearing imminent (within days to weeks).

Severe unendurable symptoms.

Refractory symptoms to conventional interventions.

Anti cancer therapies have been discontinued and all interventions are tailored to patient comfort.

DNR order in place.

Meets medical necessity criteria based on medical judgment of a palliative care physician.

**CONSENT**

4. If ordered for palliative sedation, the patient and/or family receive education about the goal of palliative sedation, which is to control intractable symptoms rather than hasten death. Efforts are made to develop consensus among family members concerning the goal of this intervention. Informed consent is obtained prior to the procedure and documented in the patient medical records. If the patient is disoriented or comatose, the consent may be obtained from the individual having Medical Power of Attorney. A final review by members of the Clinical Ethics Service may be offered to the patient and/or family prior to implementation,

These medications have the potential to induce conscious sedation and/or general anesthesia, and must be monitored accordingly. "Palliative Sedation Policy for the Symptom Control and Palliative Care Service".

**PROTOCOL**

5. a. Midazolam or propofol continuous infusions, administered by subcutaneous or intravenous routes, may be used for the control of refractory symptoms in the PCU (Palliative Care Unit) using Palliative Sedation Physician Orders.

b. If midazolam or propofol continuous infusion is being considered for the management of refractory symptoms, a palliative care consultation should be established and if considered appropriate the patient will be moved to the palliative care unit where less aggressive symptom management trials may be attempted by the palliative care team. The decision to institute sedation using continuous IV midazolam or propofol should be made by the palliative care attending and documented in the patient medical records.

c. An intravenous (IV) or subcutaneous (SQ) line is established prior to the administration of midazolam continuous infusion. An intravenous line is established before starting propofol.

d. Assess and document vital signs prior to administration of drug.

e.   Maintain aspiration precaution, provide mouth and eye care, maintain bowel and bladder care and avoid pressure sores by turning the patient regularly from side to side.

f.   Continue opioids, oxygen and other medications as needed for comfort measures.

g.   A patient receiving a midazloam or propofol by continuous infusion is monitored for respiratory depression and sedation. Patient monitoring requires assessment of level of consciousness and respiratory rate as medically appropriate using the Palliative Sedation record

h.   Midazolam or propofol is never pushed or bolused. Administer at a continuous rate only in the Palliative Care Unit, with titration (increases or decreases in dose) no more frequently than q1h.

**STARTING ANALGESIA**   6.   a.   For Midazolam start at a dose of 0.5-1mg/hr by continuous IV or subcutaneous infusion

b.   Use propofol at a starting dose of 0.15mg/kg/hr by continuous IV infusion.

c.   Keep flumazenil 0.2 mg IV handy for immediate reversal of respiratory depression from infusion.

**MONITORING**   7.   a.   The registered nurse managing the care of the patient receiving IV or SQ palliative sedation shall have no other responsibilities that would leave the patient unattended until the medication is titrated to adequate symptom control. The RN will check respiratory rate as medically appropriate.

b.   Use the smallest effective dose to control symptoms.

c.   The order for palliative sedation should be reviewed daily by a Palliative Care physician and renewed if necessary.

REFERENCES:
1. Fainsinger RL, Waller A, Bercovici M, Bengtson K, Landman W, Hosking M, Nunez-Olarte JM, deMoissac D. A multicentre international study of sedation for uncontrolled symptoms in terminally ill patients. Palliative Med 2000; 14:257-265.

2. Cowan JD, Walsh D. Terminal sedation in palliative medicine - definition and review of the literature. Support Care Cancer, 2001; 9:403-407.

3. Gremaud G, Zulian GB. Letter, Indications and limitations of intravenous and subcutaneous Midazolam in a palliative care center. J Pain Symptom Manag

1998; 15:331-333.

4. Chater S, Viola R, Paterson J, Jarvis V. Sedation for intractable distress in the dying - a survey of experts. Palliative Med 1998; 12:255-269.

5. Cherny NI, Coyle N, Foley KM. The treatment of suffering when patients request elective death. J Palliat Care 1994; 10:71-79.

6. Fainsinger RL. Use of sedation by a hospital palliative care support team. J Palliat Med 1998; 14:51-54.

7. Glover ML, Kodish E, Reed MD. Continuous propofol infusion for relief of treatment-resistant discomfort in a terminally ill pediatric patient with cancer. J Pediatr Hematol+ Oncol 1996; 18:377-380.

8. Mercadante S, De Conno F, Ripamonti C. Propofol in terminal care. J Pain Symptom Manage 1995; 10:639-642.

9. Moyle J. The use of propofol in palliative medicine. J Pain Symptom Manage 1995; 10:643-646.

10. Ramani S, Karnad AB. Long-term subcutaneous infusion of midazolam for refractory delirium in terminal breast cancer. South Med J 1996; 89:1101-1103.

11. Stone P, Phillips C, Spruyt O, Waight C. A comparison of the use of sedatives in a hospital support team and in a hospice. Palliat Med 1997; 11:140-144.

12. Vainio A, Auvinen A. and members of the Symptom Prevalence Group. Prevalence of symptoms among patients with advanced cancer: an international collaborative study. J Pain Symptom Manage 1996; 12:3-10.

**APPENDIX 26-3**
## Sample ICU end of life Orders

Date Printed:
**09/24/2004**

THE UNIVERSITY OF TEXAS
**MD ANDERSON
CANCER CENTER**

**Inpatient
Physician Orders**

**ICU End of Life Orders**

MRN:

Pt Name:

**Attending Physician:** _____

DOB: _____    Sex: _____

**Height:** _____ cm    **Weight:** _____ Kg

**Primary Diagnosis:** _____    Admitting Diagnosis _____

**Allergies:** _____

*Provider's signature indicates all orders with boxes checked are activated.*

☐ Verify that physician determination of resuscitation status is consistent with a plan to optimize patient comfort.
☐ Titrate medications to alleviate the patient's signs and symptoms of discomfort.
☐ Contact Chaplain of family's choice for spiritual support.

**Transitional Care:**
☐ Discontinue neuromuscular blockade agents prior to weaning ventilator.
☐ Discontinue all tests and laboratory studies.
☐ Remove all monitoring equipment from the patient and patient's bedside except for the ECG.
☐ Suspend arrhythmia detection at bedside and central station.
☐ Suspend or decrease all auditory alarms at bedside and central station.
☐ Discontinue medications and fluids when appropriate:
    ☐ Hydration    ☐ Vasoactive medication    ☐ other _____
☐ Discontinue mechanical support devices:
    ☐ Dialysis    ☐ IABP    ☐ other _____
☐ Assess and monitor the patient for signs and symptoms of discomfort.
☐ Liberalize visitation

**Medications:**
☐ Morphine drip at _____ mg/hr **or** ☐ Fentanyl drip at _____ mcg/hr.
☐ Lorazepam drip at _____ mg/hr **or** ☐ Midazolam drip at _____ mg/hr.
☐ Other medication drips (i.e. benzodiazepine, barbiturate, propofol):
    ☐ _____ mg/mcg/kg/hr    ☐ _____ mg/mcg/Kg/hr
    ☐ _____ mg/mcg/kg/hr    ☐ _____ mg/mcg/Kg/hr
☐ For signs of patient discomfort give IV bolus of medication equal to drip rate every 3 minutes until patient is comfortable.
☐ To **maintain** patient comfort, increase drip rate up to 50 % of prior rate.
☐ Contact physician and charge nurse regarding patient status.

**Ventilator:**
☐ Initiate ventilator wean once patient appears comfortable.
☐ Oscillatory Ventilation converted to conventional ventilator.
☐ Initial Ventilator setting: $F_iO_2$ _____ Bilevel – High PEEP _____    Low PEEP _____
    PS _____    IMV _____    PEEP _____
☐ Reduce all ventilator alarms to minimum settings.
☐ Transition $F_iO_2$ to 0.21 and PEEP to zero.
☐ Assess for signs and symptoms of patient discomfort while decreasing the tidal volume and rate.
☐ When the patient is comfortable on minimal ventilator support, select one:
    ☐ extubate to room air    ☐ T-piece    ☐ remain on ventilator

**Signature / Credentials / ID Code:** _____

**Pager:** _____    **Date:** _____    **Time:** _____

FAX COMPLETED ORDERS TO PHARMACY
File under: Physician Order                    Page 1 of 1                    POS ICU 00032 V2 10/25/04

# 27 Kate Kravits and Susan Berenson

# Complementary and Alternative Therapies in Palliative Care

*I was a number one skeptic, but I was so desperate because the doctor threatened to put me in the hospital again. I decided I would try anything once.—L.W., bone marrow transplant patient*

♦ **Key Points**
♦ *Complementary therapies improve quality of life in patients with advanced cancer.*
♦ *Complementary therapies reduce physical, psychosocial, and spiritual symptoms and provide comfort.*
♦ *Complementary therapies offer the patient an opportunity to develop enhanced feelings of self-efficacy.*
♦ *Nurses bring hope and empower patients and families by providing education and guidance in the safe utilization of complementary therapies.*

## Introduction to Complementary and Alternative Therapies

There is worldwide use of complementary and alternative medicine (CAM) by cancer patients for many reasons (Table 27-1), but many oncologists and nurses that provide care for cancer patients have limited or no knowledge of these therapies or their benefits and risks. Complementary medicine has become an important aspect of palliative and supportive cancer care.[1] The management of debilitating physical symptoms, particularly in terminally ill patients, is integral to good palliative care. When curative treatment is no longer an option, the emphasis of care shifts to palliation and symptom management. Comfort measures become the main focus.[2]

Many patients in the advanced stages of cancer seek treatments outside conventional medicine in hopes of a cure and better management of debilitating physical symptoms. Some CAM therapies can improve quality of life, such as management of pain, dyspnea, nausea and vomiting, fatigue, anxiety, depression, insomnia, and peripheral neuropathy, whereas others may be potentially harmful or useless. It is difficult, if not impossible, for most people to distinguish between reputable treatments and promotions of unproven alternatives pushed by vested interests. Understanding CAM is complicated because of its unfamiliar terminology, large numbers of available therapies, and the abundance of controversial anecdotal stories versus good research studies. It is confusing for patients, families, doctors and nurses to find their way through to the most effective and safest choices.

In this chapter, the focus is on the most helpful complementary therapies. Cancer is used as a model of chronic progressive disease. Most of the literature and research on CAM is related to cancer but can be expanded to cardiac, liver, and lung disease, diabetes, and other illnesses. Evidence-based complementary therapies are shown to affect patients'

| Table 27–1 Reasons for Use of Complementary and Alternative Medicine |
| --- |
| Poor prognosis |
| Focus of care is comfort not cure |
| Desire to be more active in one's own health care |
| Reduce side effects of treatment |
| Reduce side effects of the disease |
| Desire to cover all the options |
| Suggestions by family/friends/society to try it |
| Philosophical or cultural orientation |
| Less expensive than conventional medicine |
| Easier access to health food store than physician |
| Dissatisfaction with or loss of trust in conventional medicine |
| Desire to treat the disease in a "natural" way |
| Hope of altering the disease progression |
| Decrease the feelings of helplessness and hopelessness |
| Improve the immune system |
| Improve overall health |
| Improve the quality of one's life |

**Table 27–2**
**Evidence-based Complementary Medicine Therapies for Symptom Control and Quality of Life**

| Physical | Cognitive |
| --- | --- |
| Acupuncture | Art therapy |
| Acupressure | Biofeedback |
| Aromatherapy | Creative visualization |
| Chiropractic medicine | Focused breathing |
| Exercise | Guided imagery |
| Massage | Hypnosis |
| Nutrition | Meditation |
| Polarity | Music therapy |
| Qi gong | Progressive muscle relaxation |
| Reflexology | |
| Reiki | |
| Shiatsu | |
| Therapeutic touch | |
| Yoga | |

physical, emotional, and spiritual well-being, in safe ways. Individuals who can participate in their care in the last stages of their illnesses are often more hopeful and positive than those who are passive participants. Patients in the advanced stages of their disease can participate in their care by knowing that they have options to promote comfort and quality of life. It is the role of nurses to educate themselves, their patients and families, to assist in critical decision-making related to CAM.

The goals of this chapter are (1) to define terms related to CAM; (2) to list, define, and describe the benefits and risks of the most common CAM therapies; (3) to emphasize the most beneficial, evidenced-based complementary therapies along with the supportive research; and (4) to describe the role of the nurse as educator, researcher, and clinical practitioner in the CAM setting. Patients look to their nurses to guide them to make informed and safe complementary therapy choices. Nurses can bring hope and a sense of empowerment to their patients and families by teaching, supporting, and encouraging the use of safe complementary therapies when indicated.

## Definitions

The National Center for Complementary and Alternative Medicine defines CAM as "...a group of diverse medical and health care systems, practices, therapies, and products that are not presently considered to be part of conventional medicine."[3]

"They range from adjunctive modalities that effectively enhance quality of life and promising antitumor herbal remedies now under investigation, to bogus therapies that claim to cure cancer and that harm not only directly, but also indirectly by encouraging patients to avoid or postpone effective cancer care."[4] The list of what is considered to be CAM changes continually, as therapies that are proven to be safe and effective are adopted into conventional health care.

Although they are grouped together, complementary and alternative therapies are very different. Complementary therapies are used together with conventional care. They are not promoted as cancer cures but are used as soothing, noninvasive therapies to provide comfort and enhance the quality of life for patients (Table 27–2). The goals of complementary cancer care are to promote relaxation, reduce stress and anxiety, relieve pain and other symptoms, reduce adverse effects of conventional therapies, and improve sleep.[1] An example of a complementary therapy is the use of reflexology to help to lessen a patient's anxiety as he or she awaits a painful procedure.

In contrast, alternative therapies are used in place of surgery, chemotherapy, and radiation therapies. They are invasive, biologically active, and unproven, and are promoted as viable cures and alternatives to be used in place of mainstream cancer treatments.[5] Some examples of alternative therapies are Laetrile, dietary cancer cures, oxygen therapy, and biomagnetics. There is not a single alternative intervention (as opposed to mainstream therapies) that has been demonstrated to constitute an effective cure for cancer. Alternative therapies can misguide, raise false hopes, and financially exploit patients, and may be associated with significant risks. They may prevent patients from seeking known, helpful medical oncological interventions.[6]

Integrative oncology medicine promotes the use of evidence-based complementary therapies along with mainstream cancer treatments. At a major comprehensive cancer center, Memorial Sloan-Kettering Cancer Center (MSKCC) in New York City, Integrative Medicine practitioners of massage, reflexology, Reiki, meditation, acupuncture, art therapy, and music therapy work with inpatients who have been self-referred or referred by doctors, nurses, or other hospital professionals. Outpatients are offered these same therapies along with nutritional counseling, yoga, Tai chi, Qi gong, and other exercise classes.

## History

The history of medicine is filled with descriptions of persons using herbs, potions, and physical and spiritual manipulations to heal the sick. Traditional medicine came into being in the United States in the late 1890s when physicians began to develop the science of medicine, with a focus on cure. Anything other than the allopathic physician using science-based diagnosis and prescribing tested medicines began to be considered quackery.[7] The healer became passé. Recently, however, there has been a resurgence of interest in the use of herbal and other CAM therapies that fall outside mainstream medicine. People are living longer with chronic diseases, cancer being one of them. Patients look to CAM therapies to help with quality of life, to allow them to participate in their own self-care, and to provide a glimmer of hope and maybe a cure.

The increasing use of CAM by Americans prompted the United States Congress to establish in 1992 the Office of Alternative Medicine (OAM) as part of the National Institutes of Health (NIH). In 1998, the name was changed to the National Center for Complementary and Alternative Medicine (NCCAM), and a larger budget was assigned. NCCAM's mission is to explore complementary and alternative healing practices in the context of rigorous science, to train CAM researchers, and to inform the public and health professionals about the results of CAM research studies.

## Prevalence

### General Population

The use of CAM by the general population in the United States is common, widespread, and on the rise. In a national health interview survey conducted by the Centers for Disease Control and Prevention (CDC) in 2002, use of CAM therapies among U.S. adults was 36% when prayer was excluded, and 62% when prayer for health reasons was included.[8] Some publications cite prayer as a CAM therapy. It is excluded from further discussion as a CAM therapy in this chapter. Other findings of the CDC study were that women are more likely than men to use CAM, black adults more likely than white or Asian adults, persons with higher educations more likely than those with lower education, and those who have been hospitalized in the past year more likely than those who have not been hospitalized.

### Cancer Population

Among cancer patients, rates of CAM use are usually higher than in the general population. Ernst and Cassileth,[9] in 1998, found that the average use in 26 surveys from 13 countries was 31.4%, ranging from 7% to 64%. They believed that lack of specificity and inconsistent definitions of CAM to have contributed to this variability. For example, some studies included counseling, group therapy, prayer, wellness regimens, and self-help efforts as CAM, whereas others counted these as mainstream therapies. Molassiotis et al. reported in 2005 the results of their study of 14 European countries. In that study, they found that 35.9% of the cancer patients used some form of CAM therapy.[10] Another study reported 63% use of CAM therapies by adult cancer patients enrolled in an National Cancer Institute (NCI) clinical trial.[11] Higher use among women and among patients with higher education was also observed. Sixty-two percent of the patients in this study reported that they would have liked to talk to their physicians about the use of these therapies, but 57% said that their physicians did not ask them about CAM therapies.

### Rural Cancer Population

One study looked only at the use of complementary therapies in a rural cancer population.[12] Eighty-seven percent of the patients were using at least one complementary therapy, most commonly prayer, humor, support group, and relaxing music and visualization. Again, women were found to be more interested in CAM, but education and income did not seem to make a difference in this population.

### Comprehensive Cancer Center

In an outpatient clinic in a comprehensive cancer center, 83% of the patients had used at least one CAM therapy.[13] When psychotherapy and spiritual practices were eliminated, 68.7% had used at least one other CAM therapy. Use of multiple CAM therapies with conventional treatment was widespread, disclosure of CAM to the physician was low, and seeking information about CAM was high.

### Breast Cancer Patients

The prevalence of CAM among breast cancer patients varies. In one study conducted in the United States, it is reported to range from 48–70%.[14] New use of CAM after surgery in patients with early-stage breast cancer (28.1%) was thought to be a marker for greater psychosocial distress and worse quality of life.[15] It was suggested that physicians take note of such usage and evaluate patients for anxiety, depression, and physical symptoms. The prevalence of CAM use among breast cancer survivors in Ontario, Canada, was 66.7% and was mostly associated with the hope of boosting the immune system.[7,16] Women with breast cancer tended to use more

CAM, compared to patients with other malignancies (63% versus 83%, respectively).[7,17] In the largest patient cohort to date (500 women with breast and gynecological cancers), 48% of the breast cancer patients used CAM therapies, and the number increased to 58% after patients who had recurrent disease were included.[18] It is not possible from these studies to infer the reasons for the use of CAM therapies. Higher percentages may be indicative of the patients' levels of distress, but they may also indicate the seeking of hope and attempts to control their situations.

## Pediatric Population

The 2007 National Health Interview Survey reports on the use of CAM therapies by adults and children. The results of this survey indicate that 12% of children use some form of CAM therapy with 23.9% using CAM therapies if their parents are using them as well.[19] A 2003 study of CAM usage by pediatric cancer patients reported that 47% of the patients survey had used CAM therapies since diagnosis.[20] This study also reported that the most commonly used therapies were faith healing, vitamins, massage, herbal medicines, and relaxation.[20]

Relaxation techniques and imagery were used to reduce chemotherapy side effects in children and adolescents.[21] In one well controlled, randomized, non-blinded study, imagery was used with 73 pediatric patients to manage post-operative pain and anxiety. A significant reduction in both were reported.[22] In another randomized, controlled clinical trial of hypnosis in 80 pediatric patients undergoing lumbar puncture, the results indicated that the participants experienced less pain and anxiety.[23]

Creative arts therapies, music therapy, art therapy, and movement therapy are used with the pediatric population, but due to the lack of well designed clinical studies, it is difficult to assess the impact of these therapies on the participants.[24]

Health care providers have a responsibility to provide education to families that are using or considering the use of complementary and alternative therapies. A comprehensive health assessment should include a discussion of other therapies used to manage illness, especially in light of the data suggesting a growing popularity of these therapies. There is some evidence from letters published in the *New England Journal of Medicine*[25] that some parents choose alternative approaches where evidence of efficiency is lacking, rather than conventional evidence-based therapies. Use of conventional and alternative therapies simultaneously is also of concern, because there could be a harmful reaction between the two. The possibility that a patient is using CAM therapies calls for education and discussion with the patient and family in a nonjudgmental and collaborative manner about known risks and potential benefits of such therapies. Involving the health care team in these discussions through effective communication and documentation of dialogues can benefit the patient and family and lead to the use of these therapies in a safe and rational manner.[26]

## Culture and Ethnicity

There appears to be a relationship between ethnicity and CAM use. The 2007 National Health Interview Survey reports that 50.3% of American Indians/Alaska Natives had used CAM therapies within the last 12 months as compared to 43.1% of white adults, 39.9% of Asian adults, and 25.5% of black adults. Variations in use of CAM therapies by Hispanic populations were reported as Mexican adults 18.2%, Puerto Rican 29.7%, Mexican American 27.4%, Dominican 28.2%, and South American 23.4%.[19]

In a diverse population in Hawaii, CAM use was highest among Filipino and Caucasian patients, intermediate among the Native Hawaiians and Chinese, and significantly lower among Japanese patients.[27] The preferences were as follows: Filipinos, religious healing or prayer; Japanese, vitamins and supplements; Chinese, herbal therapies; Native Hawaiians, religious healing, prayer, vitamins, supplements, massage, and bodywork; and Caucasians, vitamins and supplements along with support groups and homeopathy. A study by Lee and associates[28] on the use and choices of CAM by women with breast cancer in four ethnic populations revealed that blacks most often chose spiritual healing, Chinese chose herbal remedies, Latinas chose dietary therapies and spiritual healing, and whites chose dietary methods and physical methods such as massage and acupuncture.[28] Another study of Navajo patients revealed that 62% used native healers but did not see a conflict between the use of a native healer and use of conventional medicine.[29] These studies suggest that culture can influence CAM choices and should be considered when caring for patients.

## Elderly

Older adults are challenged by the physical consequences of the aging of their bodies. The United States, as well as many other countries around the world, is experiencing an aging population. It is important to understand how older adults use all of the types of health care resources available to them. Recent studies indicate that older adults use CAM therapies to manage their health care issues.[19,30–33]

In results reported in the 2002 National Health Interview Survey, Arcury and colleagues used logistic regression models to determine the impact of ethnicity, sex, age, education, and health conditions on the use of CAM therapies. Their results indicated that 27.7% of older adults use CAM therapies, with the highest levels of use by Asians (48.6%).[30] CAM therapy use by Hispanics reached a rate of 31.6%, Whites 27.7%, and Blacks 20.5%. Older adults living in New York City were surveyed and their use of CAM therapies was reported as 58%. The factors associated with CAM use in this population were gender (female), education, thyroid disease, and arthritis.[31]

In a survey of rural Caucasian and African American adults, results indicate use of CAM therapies by both groups with Caucasians using more CAM therapies than African Americans.[32] Other reasons cited for the use of CAM therapies by older adults include pain relief, improved quality of life, self-care and fitness.[33] Older adults *are* using CAM therapies—education about CAM therapies is essential for promoting safe and effective use of these strategies. Health care providers have the responsibility to open a dialogue with all their patients about CAM therapies, so that appropriate consultation and education may take place.

## Cost

Most insurance companies do not reimburse for CAM. In the United States in 1997, it is estimated that individuals spent between $36 billion and $47 billion on CAM therapies. Of this amount, between $12 billion and $20 billion were paid out-of-pocket, with $5 billion spent on herbal products alone.[3] The cost of CAM may prevent many patients from receiving these therapies. There is movement within the U.S. Congress to begin to acknowledge the value of these therapies and to reimburse for them. It is suggested that patients check with their insurance companies to see whether use of CAM can be reimbursed. There is hope that reimbursement will be soon forthcoming.

### CASE STUDY

*Fred, A 51-year-old Gentleman 100 Days after Bone Marrow Transplant for Leukemia*

Fred is an active professional person who describes himself as a workaholic. He is thin and slightly unsteady on his feet. He is the father of three daughters between the ages of 33 and 18. His oldest daughter has severe health problems. Fred has been married for 25 years. He states that his social support comes from his wife, co-workers, and church community.

Fred reports that he experienced a long period of frequent, apparently minor illnesses prior to being diagnosed with leukemia. He states that he made frequent visits to his health care provider with aching joints, cold-like symptoms, loss of weight, and a perception of losing strength. At the final hospital visit prior to his diagnosis, Fred insisted on staying in the hospital until he was told what was wrong with him. Ultimately, he was diagnosed with pneumonia and leukemia. Fred states that "It was a relief to know."

Fred was treated with a bone marrow transplant. Following the bone marrow transplant, Fred's recovery progressed as expected except that Fred continued to experience loss of appetitie, nausea, and vomiting. He lost 2–3 pounds per week following discharge from the hospital. He was unable to participate in family activities such as joining them for meals. In order to cope with his nausea and vomiting, Fred began to isolate himself in his home office.

Fred's condition was monitored by his physician, who could not find an organic reason for the continued nausea and vomiting. Fred had lost 25 pounds by this time, and reported that he felt profoundly weak. The physician considered putting Fred in the hospital in order to manage his weight loss, nausea and vomiting. However, the physician was made aware of an opportunity for Fred to receive hypnosis for nausea control, and offered that option to Fred since nothing else they had tried seemed to have an impact. According to Fred, he was desperate to stay out of the hospital and was willing to try anything once, but he did not believe that the hypnosis would have any effect on his symptoms. He was referred to a nurse trained in providing hypnosis and an appointment was scheduled.

During the initial session, the nurse and Fred took some time to explore his illness, treatment and recovery. Fred stated, "I feel useless." He reported that images of food on TV and even thoughts of food triggered episodes of nausea and gagging. He described his eating habits, clearly stating he could eat easily in the morning, having cereal, fruit, or other cold foods. However, he could not eat meat at all—and if he allowed too long a period to pass between attempts to eat, he would not be able to eat.

The nurse assessed the intentsity of his symptoms during the first session by asking Fred to complete a Visual Analog Scale rating distress, anxiety, appetite, and nausea. On a 0–10 scale with 0 = no symptoms and 10 = the worst possible symptoms, Fred rated his pre-intervention distress as 5, anxiety as 3.2, lack of appetite as 8.5, and nausea as 5.8.

The nurse described hypnosis, and clarified for Fred the benefits and risks associated with the intervention. Fred's questions and concerns were answered before beginning the intervention. The nurse, in collaboration with Fred, conducted a 20-minute guided hypnotic intervention using the metaphor of "sanctuary" as a foundation for creating relaxation and safety. A suggestion was given for deep breathing and repeating the word "sanctuary" to help restore a sense of relaxation and to decrease nausea. Following the intervention, Fred rated his symptoms using the visual analog scale with anxiety rated at 2.5, lack of appetite at 8.7, and nausea at 2.7.

Fred returned in one week for a second session. He denied any episodes of vomiting and stated that he had been able to eat a meal with his family. His feelings of progress were reinforced at his doctor's visit, as his weight had remained stable during this week. This was Fred's first week without weight loss since discharge from the hospital. A hypnotic intervention was conducted in session two, and Fred was given an audiotape to listen to at bedtime.

Session three was conducted a month after session two, and was the last face-to-face session. Fred's weight remained stable and he was beginning to work with a personal trainer. He reported that, while he was able to eat, cooking odors still bothered him. The intervention was adjusted to include suggestions addressing the distress related to aromas. He reported using the the audiotape and finding it helpful.

### FOLLOW-UP

Seven months following the final interview, Fred has returned to work. He has regained weight and is no longer suffering with nausea and vomiting. He reports that he has developed his own way of using the techniques that he learned. He goes to a quiet, private space and turns on soft jazz music. He then guides himself through the hypnotic intervention. He reports that it is very effective for him and that now he uses it to promote relaxation and reduce stress at the end of his work day.

After reading this chapter, the reader should begin to understand the rationale for the choices that Fred made in response to his symptom distress.

## Overview of Complementary and Alternative Therapies

CAM therapies have been grouped into five major domains by the National Center for Complementary and Alternative Medicine: (1) alternative medical systems (traditional Chinese medicine, ayurvedic medicine, homeopathic medicine, naturopathic medicine, Native American medicine, and Tibetan medicine); (2) mind–body interventions (meditation, focused breathing, progressive muscle relaxation, guided imagery, creative visualization, hypnosis, biofeedback, music therapy, and art therapy); (3) biologically based therapies, nutrition, and special diets (e.g., macrobiotics, megavitamin and orthomolecular therapies, metabolic therapies, individual biological therapies such as shark cartilage) and herbal medicine; (4) manipulative and body-based methods (massage, aromatherapy, reflexology, acupressure, Shiatsu, polarity, chiropractic medicine, yoga, and exercise); and (5) energy therapies (Reiki, Qi gong, and therapeutic touch). The currently popular therapies are discussed in the following sections. Many of these methods are not proven, whereas others have been documented as helpful complementary therapies.

Counseling, group therapy, prayer, and spirituality, which we already know to be very helpful to cancer patients, are not included in this chapter because many view them as part of mainstream therapies.

### Alternative Medical Systems

Instead of disease-oriented therapies, ancient systems of healing were based on attributing health, illness, and death to an invisible energy or life force, and the suggestion of an interaction between the human body, humankind, the spirit world, and the universe. In the earliest of times, there seemed to be a link between religion, magic, and medicine. This is in contrast to modern Western medicine, which is focused on the cause and curing of the disease. These alternative medicine systems are briefly discussed in this chapter because they are followed by many people today. The best known examples of alternative medical systems are traditional Chinese medicine (TCM), India's ayurvedic medicine, homeopathic medicine,

naturopathic medicine, Native American medicine, and Tibetan medicine. Ancient healing systems tend to remain unchanged, unlike modern medicine, which keeps growing and expanding on a regular basis. A common feature across alternative medical systems is an emphasis on working with internal natural forces to achieve a harmonic state of mind and body, which can promote a sense of well-being and comfort. This idea, although outmoded and unscientific, has great appeal for many in the general public and especially for cancer patients dealing with advanced disease.

### Traditional Chinese Medicine

The cornerstone concept in Chinese medicine is *qi* (life force), which is energy that flows through the body along pathways known as meridians. TCM views people as ecosystems in miniature.[34] Any imbalance or disruption in the circulation of Chi or qi (pronounced "chee") is thought to result in illness. Restoration of one's health is therefore dependent on returning the balance and flow of the life force. A TCM diagnosis is based on examination of the person's complexion, tongue, radial pulse, and detection of scents in bodily materials. Treatment is geared toward correcting imbalances or disruptions of the qi, primarily with herbal formulas and acupuncture.[34]

Acupuncture is one of the best known forms of CAM. It is one component of TCM. It is based on the belief that qi, the life force, flows through the human body in vertical energy channels known as meridians. There are 12 main meridians, which are believed to be dotted with acupoints that correspond to every body part and organ. To restore the balance and flow of qi, very fine disposable needles are inserted into the acupoints just under the skin. Other stimuli can be used along with acupuncture, such as heat (moxibustion), suction (cupping), external pressure (acupressure), and electrical currents (electroacupuncture). The biological basis of qi or meridians has not been found, but is thought that acupuncture needling releases endorphins and other neurotransmitters in the brain.[35] There is good evidence in the oncology literature that acupuncture helps control pain and nausea and vomiting. There is current research on its possible effectiveness for fatigue and dyspnea. Risks associated with acupuncture include mild discomfort or, occasionally, a drop of blood and/or a small bruise at the site of the insertion, but they can include more serious problems, such as an infection or (in the most extreme case) a pneumothorax, which is rare, and depends on the training and experience of the acupuncturist.

### Ayurvedic Medicine

The term *ayurveda* comes from Sanskrit words *ayur* (life) and *veda* (knowledge) and is about 5000 years old. Ayurvedic medicine is based on the idea that illness is the absence of physical, emotional, and spiritual harmony.[36] Many of the basic principles are similar to those of Chinese medicine.

Ayurveda is a natural system of medicine that uses diet, herbs, cleansing and purification practices, meditation, yoga, astrology, and gemstones to bring about healing. It sees causation of disease as an accumulation of toxins in the body and an imbalance of emotions. It prescribes individualized diets, regular detoxification, cleansing from all orifices, meditation, and yoga as some of the therapies. There is no scientific evidence that ayurvedic healing techniques cure illness.

## Homeopathic Medicine

Homeopathy is a medical system that was devised by Samuel Hahnemann 200 years ago, when the causes of diseases, bacteria and viruses were unknown, and little was understood about the workings of the bodily organs. The thinking was that symptoms of ill health represent expressions of disharmony within the person, and attempts of the body to heal itself and return to a state of balance. It is the person, not the disease, that needs treatment. The treatment of disease is based on the principle, "Like cures like." Homeopathic medicines are made by taking original substances from plants, animals, and minerals, and highly diluting them. It is believed that the body's own healing ability is stimulated by these medicines. Homeopathic medicines are sold over the counter without prescription. They are so dilute that they are thought to have no side effects, and at the same time to be ineffectual for medical conditions, including cancer-related conditions.

## Naturopathic Medicine

Naturopathy is more of a philosophical approach to health than a particular form of therapy. It is an alternative medical system that attempts to cure disease by harnessing the body's own natural healing powers, and restoring good health and preventing disease. Rejecting synthetic drugs and invasive procedures, it stresses the restorative powers of nature, the search for the underlying causes of disease, and the treatment of the whole person. It takes very seriously the motto, "First, do no harm." Naturopathic medicine began as a quasispiritual "back to nature" movement in the 19th century. European founders advocated exposure to air, water, and sunlight as the best therapy for all ailments and recommended such spa treatments as hot mineral baths as virtual cure-alls. This system relies on natural healing approaches such as herbs, nutrition, and movement or manipulation of the body. Most naturopathic remedies are considered harmless by conventional practitioners.[36]

## Traditional Healing Systems of American Indians/Alaska Natives

It is difficult to characterize a traditional healing system of American Indian/Alaska Native (AI/AN) peoples, as there are 562 federally recognized tribes speaking over 270 different languages.[37] American Indian/Alaska Native (AI/AN) traditional healing methods are rooted in the culture of the people. Traditional healing methods are themselves an expression of cultural identity.[38]

Despite the diversity of tribal beliefs, shared concepts that influence health behaviors can be identified. A significant belief that underlies many traditional healing systems is that all things are interconnected and composed of a spiritual essence.[39] Spirituality is a critical component of most AI/AN traditional healing methods. Therefore, traditional healing is an expression of a cultural identity that is informed by a rich tradition of spirituality.[38]

## Wellness and Illness

Wellness is another important concept in AI/AN traditional healing systems. Wellness is an expression of balance and harmony in individual, family, and community systems. Many tranditional healing methods focus on restoring balance and harmony to one or more of these elements.[38] Concepts of illness and its causes vary among tribal groups. However, beliefs in the spiritual reality of life often serve to provide a framework for understanding illness. Even seemingly accidental causes of injury may be viewed as having occurred to someone who may be living out of balance and harmony with traditional ways of being, as defined by the group's spiritual belief systems. Therefore, illness is often attritubted to the violation of spiritual norms.[38]

Healing is often viewed by American Indians/Alaska Natives as the restoration of harmony and balance. Healing may be facilitated by traditional healers, who may be called many things and take many forms depending upon the native group. Rituals, herbs, and purification processes are used by traditional healers to restore balance and harmony in a manner consistent with the values and beliefs of their people. Traditional healers are considered respected leaders within and outside of their communities.[38]

## Pluralistic Practice

It is common for AI/AN to incorporate multiple healing systems into their lives. Both traditional healing systems and the biomedicine of European-American society may be employed. Contributions to European-American biomedicine have been made by the traditional healing systems of AI/AN. The most important evidence of Native American influence on traditional American medicine is the fact that >200 indigenous medicines used by one or more tribes have been listed in the Pharmacopeia of the United States of America.[40]

## Tibetan Medicine

Tibetan medicine views the human body as an ecological system, a microcosm directly related to the macrocosm of the world. It attempts to investigate the root causes of illness. The belief is that all of the material that makes up our universe is based on the qualities of five basic elements (earth, water, fire, wind, and space). It is understood through experience that natural environmental forces can influence the functioning of the human organism. The Tibetan doctor bases his practice of diagnosis on his own spiritual practice, intellectual training, and intuition. The Tibetan medical diagnosis is a result of the patient interview, observation of the urine, taking of the 12 pulses, looking at the sclera and surface of the tongue, and feeling for sensitivity on certain parts of the body. The treatment is similar to that used in Chinese medicine.

## Mind–Body Interventions

Mind/Body Therapies (MBT) are defined by the National Center for Complementary and Alternative Medicine as, "…a variety of techniques designed to enhance the mind's ability to affect bodily function and symptoms."[3] There is a long history of the use of interventions currently categorized as Mind/Body Therapies such as distraction, breathing, relaxation, imagery, and hypnosis.[41] Frequently used outside of formal Western medical contexts, they have become accepted as useful by the public at large. One study indicates that as of 2002 approximately 17% of the adult U.S. population used some type of Mind/Body Therapy, and when including prayer as an MBT, 53% of the population use or have used some form of MBT.[42] The National Health Interview Survey conducted in 2007 reports that the use of deep breathing, meditation, and yoga increased from 2002 to 2007.[19]

According to one study, Mind/Body Therapies are most often used by the public to treat medical conditions (59%).[43] Other reasons cited for the use of MBTs include wellness/prevention, and lifestyle.[43] The majority of MBTs are used as self-guided therapies by lay users. Only 12% of the users were shown to seek care from a health care and/or MBT providers.[42] One reason cited in the literature for the prevalence of self-guided Mind/Body Therapies over practitioner-guided therapies is availability of health care providers who have received training in, and are competent to provide, Mind/Body Therapies.[44]

The ability to influence health with the mind is an extremely appealing concept for many individuals. One of the benefits of self-guided Mind/Body Therapies is the ability to support and affirm feelings of self-efficacy. Since there is emerging evidence of the effectiveness of meditation, guided imagery, hypnosis, progressive muscle relaxation, biofeedback, and yoga for stress reduction, and as adjunct therapies for the management of pain, nausea and vomiting, fatigue, anxiety and disease related distress, it is important for nurses and other health care providers to be well educated about these therapies . While the evidence supports the ability of these therapies to control stress, to reduce selected symptoms and to improve the response to cardiac rehabilitation , there are no reliable, well controlled studies to support the idea that these therapies can cure disease.[3,45] A word of caution: some patients may feel guilty, responsible and a failure when their

disease continues to progress despite the use of mind–body interventions.

## Meditation

Meditation is the intentional self-regulation of attention. It enhances concentration and awareness as the individual focuses systematically and intentionally on particular aspects of inner or outer experience. It allows one to stay present in the moment, and without judgment.[46] Historically, most meditation practices were developed within a spiritual or religious context with the goal of spiritual growth, personal transformation, or transcendental experience.[45]

There are two categories of meditation: concentration and mindfulness. Concentrative methods cultivate one-pointedness of attention and start with mantras (sounds, words, or phrases repeated), as in Transcendental Meditation (TM). Mindfulness-based stress reduction (MBSR) practices start with the observation, without judgment, of thoughts, emotions, and sensations as they arise in the field of awareness.[46] "Meditation can help individuals connect with what is deepest and most nourishing in themselves, and to mobilize the full range of inner and outer resources available to them."[46] Meditation has been helpful for terminally ill cancer patients. It has shown to be helpful in the relief of physical and emotional pain when integrated into a palliative care program. Many dying cancer patients discover that the calmness and quiet of meditation promotes a profound feeling of acceptance, well-being, and inner peace.[46] Walking meditation is appealing to those that cannot sit still. The focus might be on taking one step at a time, smelling the fresh air, taking in one breath at a time, or listening to the birds as one walks.

## Relaxation Techniques

Relaxation techniques are those simple techniques that, when learned by the patient, can promote relaxation. They include progressive muscle relaxation (contracting and relaxing muscle groups one at a time from head to toe), passive progressive muscle relaxation (no contraction of muscles, but focusing in the mind on sequentially relaxing groups of muscles),[47] focused breathing (counting of breaths as one exhales, which can be used by itself or as an introduction to guided imagery).

## Guided Imagery

Imagery is the formation of mental images. Guided imagery is the intentional formation of mental images in response to verbal suggestion for the purpose of achieving a specific therapeutic result.[41,48–54] Some investigators categorize guided imagery and hypnosis as part of the same continuum of experience, with imagery playing a particular role in inducing a state of relaxation necessary for therapeutic intervention.[55] Imagery is a natural phenomenon in our lives that occurs all day long. For example, when we wake in the morning we might imagine our day, where we will be going, what we will wear, what we will eat. This is a form of self-guided visualization and imagery. There is strong evidence that guided imagery is useful as an adjunct therapy in cardiac rehabilitation for the promotion of relaxation, in the management of cancer symptoms, and in reduction of procedure/surgery-related pain.[45] There are minimal risks associated with guided imagery. Due to the requirement for focused attention, it is contraindicated in patients with severe cognitive impairments and/or thought disorders. It is important that those providing guided imagery are well trained and conform to the ethical standards of practice of their profession. Guided imagery should be taught to nurses so that they may assist patients and family members to develop skills in self-guided imagery that will allow them to enhance their quality of life.[47]

## Hypnosis

As the technology for understanding the mechanisms underlying the experience known as hypnosis becomes more advanced, more precise and accurate definitions of the phenomenon are created. At present, hypnosis is defined as "…a natural state of aroused, attentive focal concentration coupled with a relative suspension of peripheral awareness."[45] Activation of the anterior cingulate cortex, the thalamus, and the anterior basal ganglia, along with alterations in the orbital frontal cortex, support the state of hypnosis.[56,57] One study using fMRI has identified the neural processes underlying the mechanism for hypnotic pain reduction. This study determined that the hypnotic state prevents nociceptive inputs from reaching the cortical structures.[56] These findings support the concept that there are specific neural processes underlying hypnosis that are responsible for its clinical affect. Hypnosis does not have the same mechanism of action as distraction, but has similar mechanisms to meditation.[58]

Some evidence is available supporting the use of hypnosis for the management of cancer symptoms (pain, nausea and vomiting, fatigue, anxiety and distress) and the promotion of positive surgical outcomes (decreased pain, nausea and vomiting, medication usage, recovery time, and anxiety).[45] Hypnosis may be practiced as a facilitated experience or a self-guided experience. It is not uncommon for practitioners of hypnosis to begin with a facilitated experience that transitions to a self-guided practice through the use of supportive tools such as audiotapes/cds.

The hypnotic state is achieved by using a variety of strategies to induce a state of profound relaxation and focused attention, including deep breathing, relaxation and imagery. The process of inducing the hypnotic state is known as the induction. Once a sufficient state of relaxation and focused concentration is achieved, suggestions may be used to achieve therapeutic goals. These suggestions, identified as therapeutic suggestion, are suggestions for behaving, thinking and/or feeling in a particular way with a specific outcome in mind (i.e., pain reduction).[59,60] The suggestion may be direct or indirect depending upon the needs of the client and the skills and preferences of the provider.[60]

Minimal risks are associated with hypnosis. One risk is the unintentional stimulation of emotionally laden memories that may be upsetting. Careful exploration of the patient's life experiences prior to using hypnosis minimizes the chance these memories will accidentally be triggered.[59] Due to the requirement for focused attention, it is contraindicated in patients with severe cognitive impairments and/or thought disorders. It is recommended that only those individuals with licensure in a health care profession, and who have received formal training in hypnosis, be allowed to provide this service.

## Biofeedback

Biofeedback involves the use of devices that amplify physiological processes (e.g., blood pressure, muscle activity, skin temperature, perspiration, pulse, respiratory rate, and electroencephalography) that ordinarily cannot be perceived without amplification. Patients are guided through relaxation and imagery exercises and are instructed to alter their physiological processes using as a guide the provided biofeedback (typically visual or auditory data). The primary objective of biofeedback is to promote relaxation. It is a noninvasive procedure. It has been shown to be effective for anxiety and headaches.[45]

## Music Therapy

Music therapy in the palliative care setting is essential. Music can break the cyclic nature of pain, alter mood, promote relaxation, and improve communication.[61] Music can facilitate the participation of the patient with family and hospital staff. Music therapists apply psychotherapeutic skills in the setting of music as they care for patients with advanced cancer. Music therapy interventions consist of use of precomposed songs (reflecting messages or feelings that are foremost in the patient's thoughts), improvisation (offering opportunities for spontaneous expression and discovery), chanting and toning (use of vocalization to promote attentiveness and relaxation), imagery (exploration of images and feelings that arise in the music), music listening techniques (which facilitate reminiscence and build self-esteem through reflection on accomplishments), and taping of the music session as a gift for the family.[61] Music therapy may help to facilitate a life review for the patient. It can also help in management of the most common symptoms of advanced cancer: pain,[62] anxiety and depression,[63] nausea and vomiting,[64] shortness of breath,[65] and sleeplessness.[64] Live music has been shown to be more effective than taped music.[66]

## Art Therapy

Art therapy is a form of psychotherapy. Art therapists are trained professionals. Art therapy focuses on assisting patients to express, explore, and transform sensations, emotions, and thoughts connected with physical and psychological suffering.[61] In art therapy, the art therapist and the art materials (e.g., paper, colored markers, oil pastels, cut-up images from magazines) help patients get in touch with their feelings, their fears, and their hopes, and put them out onto the paper, thus helping patients process their experience of illness. It can easily be accommodated to hospitalized inpatients as well as to outpatient art groups or individuals. Art therapy can assist patients with advanced-stage cancer in the management of pain, fatigue, and stress.[67] Art images can serve to help the dying patient with issues of anger, bereavement, and loss. The art therapist may help dying patients find "personal symbols" to express something so powerful and so mysterious as the end of life.[67]

## Biologically Based Therapies

Alternative diets have an ancient history, both medical and cultural, of plants and herbs as the first medicines. The example of vitamin C curing scurvy reinforces the idea of foods being medicines and curing illness. Some of the ancient medicine systems are still being practiced today; for example, ayurvedic medicine uses special diets, herbs, and cleansings to treat illness and promote health.

Today's food pyramid recommends fiber, grains, fruits and vegetables, and less protein, meat, and dairy products than was emphasized in earlier U.S. Department of Agriculture government guidelines. It emphasizes balance. Changes in guidelines are based on carefully controlled scientific studies. Many alternative and fad diets, herbs, and supplements are either not scientifically validated or are marketed despite having been found worthless or harmful.

### Nutrition

Some alternative practitioners believe that dietary treatments can prevent cancer or even go a step further to believe that foods or vitamins can cure cancer. The American Cancer Society Guidelines on Nutrition form the basis for a healthful diet that emphasizes vegetables, fruits, legumes, and whole grains; low-fat or nonfat dairy products; and limited amounts of red meat (lean preferred). Special dietary problems should be discussed with the doctor and an oncology-registered dietitian. It should be emphasized to the patient and family that the doctor should be informed before the patient takes any vitamin, mineral, or herb.

### Special Diets

*Macrobiotics.* The philosophy of the macrobiotic diet is curing through diet. It was developed in the 1930s by a Japanese philosopher, George Ohsawa. Originally, the diet consisted of brown rice with very little liquid. It was nutritionally deficient. Today it consists of 50% to 60% whole grains, 25% to 30% vegetables, and the remainder beans, seaweeds, and soups. Soybean foods are encouraged, and a small amount of fish is allowed. In-season foods are preferred. Proponents of this diet believe that it cures cancer. There is no evidence that the macrobiotic diet is beneficial for cancer patients.

*Megavitamin and Orthomolecular Therapy.* Some alternative practitioners believe that huge doses of vitamins can cure cancer. Linus Pauling coined the term *orthomolecular*, meaning large quantities of minerals and other nutrients. His claim that large doses of vitamin C could cure cancer was disproved. There was no evidence in 1979 that megavitamin or orthomolecular therapy was effective in treating any disease.[68] In 1985, Moertel and colleagues[69] showed that vitamin C was ineffective against advanced malignant cancer. There are side effects to the overdosing of vitamins and minerals.[36] A nutritionally healthy diet is recommended for overall good health. Some people have special needs and may require supplements. Patients should not attempt to treat themselves with megadoses of vitamins or minerals, but should seek professional attention for nutritional advice.

*Metabolic Therapies.* Metabolic therapies are based on the theory that disease is caused by the accumulations of toxic substances in the body. The goal of treatment is to eliminate the toxins. Metabolic therapies usually include a special diet; high-dose vitamins, minerals, or other dietary supplements; and detoxification with coffee enemas or irrigation of the colon. Colon detoxification is not used in mainstream medicine, and there are no data to support the claims that dried food and toxins remain stuck in the walls of the colon. The development of metabolic therapy is attributed to Max Gerson, a physician who emigrated from Germany in 1936. Today, cancer is the most common illness treated with metabolic therapies. Research does not substantiate the beliefs and practices of metabolic therapies, and patients may lose valuable time during which they could be receiving treatments with proven benefits.

*Individual Biological Therapy.* Advocates of shark and bovine cartilage therapy claim that it can reduce tumor size, slow or stop the growth of cancer, and help reverse bone diseases such as osteoporosis. More importantly, shark and bovine cartilage are thought to play a role in angiogenesis, which involves halting the blood supply to cancer cells. There is no firm evidence that cartilage treatment is effective against cancer.

### Herbal Medicine

Herbs have been used as medicines going back to ancient times. Belief in the magic of herbs for the treatment of cancer exists today, especially in the face of advanced cancer and few or no options. There is a romance about herbs, in that they are natural and come from the earth and therefore must be pure, safe, and harmless. A major concern exists that patients are using herbs indiscriminately on a routine basis without knowledge that these herbs interact with drugs, can interfere with the efficacy of anticancer drugs, and can cause death.[70] There is a lack of knowledge that most herbal remedies have not been tested in carefully designed clinical studies.[71] Currently, some herbal remedies are being studied for their ability to induce or extend a cancer remission. We must remember and teach our patients that herbs have potency comparable to that of pharmaceuticals.[72] They can cause medical problems such as allergic reactions, toxic reactions, adverse effects, drug interactions, and drug contamination.[34]

An important aspect of cancer care is to recognize that herbs can be toxic to cancer patients and should be discussed with the doctor and other qualified practitioners. MSKCC advises patients to avoid taking any herbs for 2 weeks before any cancer therapy and to refrain from using supplements while in the hospital. Some herbs, such as St. John's wort,[73] may interfere with the effectiveness of chemotherapy. Garlic may alter clotting times in a surgical candidate. Dong qui may make the skin more sensitive to burns during radiation. The active ingredients in many herbs are not known. In the United States, herbal and other dietary supplements are not regulated by the U.S. Food and Drug Administration (FDA) as drugs. This means that they do not have to meet the same standards as drugs and over-the-counter medications for proof of safety and effectiveness. Identifying the active ingredients and understanding how they affect the body are important areas of research being done by NCCAM. Differences have been found in some cases between what is listed on the label and what is in the bottle, and some contaminants have been identified as heavy metals, microorganisms, or unspecified prescription drugs and adulterants. Standardization and authentication of herbs is important. An excellent resource to obtain information about herbs can be found on MSKCC's website for Integrative Medicine,[74] and in a resource book by Cassileth and Lucarelli on herb-drug interactions.[75] The website has pages written for consumers as well as a professional section; both are available to all at no cost. None of these resources make any medical recommendations about herbs; the website is specifically for information.

Mikail and colleagues[76] found in a study of medical residents that they had a knowledge deficit concerning herbal medicines. Ninety percent of them wanted to learn more about herbal medicine, including uses of herbs, contraindications, and drug interactions, as well as being able to talk to patients about their use. As the prevalence of herbal remedy use grows, equipping nurses and doctors with information and vocabulary will help them discuss with, and offer their patients information about proper precautions. Patients should be encouraged to talk to their doctors and nurses about the herbs they are taking. It is important to listen with patience, and then to respond without judgment. This approach promotes open, ongoing communication between the patient and the doctor or nurse.

## Manipulative and Body-Based Methods

Touch is the first sense to develop, and it is our primary way of experiencing the world, starting with infancy up until the moment of the last breath.[77] It is critical to growth and development. Infants, the elderly, the ill, and animals that do not receive regular touch fail to thrive and eventually die. In ancient times, the "laying on of hands" was an early practice of healing by touch. Medicine consisted of touch before the advent of pharmaceutical therapies. Today drugs, technology, paperwork, and heavy patient loads keep the doctor and nurse from the bedside. Patients comment, "I don't get touched very much any more. If I do, it is a medical touch and it can hurt. My family and friends don't seem to touch either, maybe out of fear." Touch is a healing agent, but is underutilized by healing practitioners. Touch is our most social sense and implies a communication between two people. Cultural differences in touching are essential to keep in mind, so as to always be respectful.

### Massage

Massage therapy is one of the oldest health care practices in use. Chinese medical texts referred to it more than 4000 years ago. It is one of the most widely accepted forms of complementary therapies today. Massage employs the manual techniques of rubbing, stroking, tapping, or kneading the body's soft tissues to influence the whole person. Simms[2] suggested that touch is a fundamental element in patient care that can encourage better communication and promote comfort and well-being. The concern of the medical profession and patients has been that massage would spread cancer cells. There is no evidence that this is the case, because the stimulation caused by massage is no more than everyday exercise.[78] The benefits of massage are many and include improving circulation, relaxing muscles and nerve tissue, releasing tension, reducing pain, decreasing anxiety and depression, energizing, and promoting an overall sense of well-being. Massage is contraindicated under some circumstances: over metastatic bones (for risk of bone fracture or breakage), if the platelet count is <35,000 to 40,000/mm³ (for risk of bruising), over sites of blood clots (for risk of promoting movement of a thrombus in the circulation), and over surgical sites or rashes. Medical massage for the cancer patient, and especially for the end-stage cancer patient, uses light pressure. Deep tissue massage is not appropriate and is potentially harmful.

### Aromatherapy

Aromatherapy is the controlled use of plant essences for therapeutic purposes. Essential oils are the aromatic essences of plants in the form of oil or resin, which has been extracted in a highly concentrated solution.[79] The history of medicinal use of plant oils goes back to ancient Egypt, China, and Renaissance Europe. Essential oils are thought to have different mechanisms of action: antiviral, antiseptic, antibacterial, anti-inflammatory, fungicidal, sedative, and easing congestion. Aromatherapy is often practiced with massage and has been found to de-stress, empower, and promote communication and a sense of security.[80] Aromatherapy is a delightful tool in enhancing yoga.[81] Recent randomized, controlled studies of aromatherapy have not demonstrated a significant, lasting, positive effect.[82–84] Aromatherapy should be administered only by a certified practitioner. Essential oils should not be administered orally or applied undiluted to the skin. Possible contraindications to the use of essential oils are contagious disease, venous thrombosis, open wounds, and recent surgery. Possible adverse events are photosensitivity, allergic reactions, nausea, and headache. Many essential oils have the potential to enhance or reduce the effects of prescribed medications.[85]

### Reflexology

Reflexology is touch therapy that goes back 5000 years to ancient Egypt. It is based on the assumption that the body contains energy flowing through it. Reflexology is an art and a science that is based on the principle that there are reflex points and areas in the ears, hands, and especially the feet that correspond to every gland, organ, and part of the body. By skillful stimulation of these areas and points with hand, finger, and thumb techniques, the body systems are facilitated to greater balance.[86] Reflexology should be done to the tolerance of the patient; it should not hurt. Reflexology is generally used to reduce stress, to promote relaxation and sleep, to improve circulation, to energize, to diminish symptoms of pain, anxiety, nausea, and peripheral neuropathy, and to promote an overall sense of well-being. It can be made special and pleasant when preceded by an aroma foot bath. It is contraindicated if blood clots, infection, skin rash, bruising, or wounds are present on the extremities. Reflexology can be performed anywhere, requires no special equipment, is noninvasive, and does not interfere with the patient's privacy. It can easily be taught to the family to empower them to provide comfort to their loved one.

### Acupressure

Acupressure is the pressing of a single point or specific acupuncture point to relieve pain and stress in a particular area or part of the body. It is acupuncture without the needles. It involves placing the finger firmly on an acupoint. More than 300 acupoints dot the lengths of the hypothesized meridians (channels) that run vertically head to toe. The acupoint to be pressed is determined by the energy channel that is blocked and is causing the problem.[36] Acupressure promotes relaxation and comfort. It should be done to the tolerance of the patient. It need not be painful. It should not be applied near areas of fractures or broken bones, or near blood clots, wounds, sores, or bruises.

### Shiatsu

Shiatsu is a modern outgrowth of ancient acupressure. It is a Japanese body therapy that works on the energetic pathways (meridians) and points of access to acupuncture points in order to harmonize the energy flow (qi). The philosophy is rooted in TCM, which views illness as being caused by energy imbalances. Shiatsu, a touch therapy, was developed from an ancient form of Japanese massage into the use of pressure with thumbs, palms, elbows, and knees and stretching, applied to these meridians and to the specific acupoints that are located on these pathways. The focus is on prevention and healing. Shiatsu is contraindicated with widespread bone metastases, pulmonary emboli, and deep vein thromboses. The benefits are relaxation, higher energy levels, improved physical capability, and enhanced symptom control. Light touch is suggested for the palliative care patient.[87]

### Polarity

Polarity views good health as a balance among internal energies, such as earth, air, fire, water, and space. When these energies are blocked due to stress or other factors, physical and emotional problems follow. The therapist provides a series of gentle stretching, light rocking, and holding of pressure points until the body's energy is brought into balance. Most often patients report a deep sense of relaxation.

### Chiropractic

The hands-on joint manipulation known as chiropractic is particularly helpful for lower back pain. Chiropractic medicine is a system of therapy based on the premise that the relationship between structure (primarily the spine) and function (as coordinated by the nervous system) in the human body is a significant health factor. Disease is considered to be the result of irregular or misaligned vertebrae and abnormal functioning of the nervous system. Back pain is one of the most frequent health problems, although neck, shoulder, head, and carpal tunnel syndrome are frequently treated by chiropractors. The normal transmission and expression of nerve energy are essential to the restoration and maintenance of health. Chiropractic medicine emphasizes the inherent recuperative power of the body to heal itself without the use of drugs or surgery. The method of treatment usually involves manipulation of the spinal column and other body structures to realign or readjust joints. Research evidence does not support chiropractic claims that cancer can be cured with spinal manipulation. Chiropractic is not recommended for patients with advanced cancer.

### Yoga

Yoga is the Sanskrit word for union or oneness. It is a centuries-old Eastern philosophy, science, and art form that can be used as a tool to achieve inner peace and freedom. Through mental (meditation) and physical (movement and simple poses with deep breathing) techniques, pathways lead into the yoga state of oneness.[81] Yoga helps align the body, promotes relaxation, and reduces fatigue. There are different types of yoga: hatha yoga (physical posturing), pranayama (yoga breathing), mantra yoga (sacred sound symbols in the sound of a chant designed to awaken the left hemisphere of the brain to rational thinking and clarity), and yantra yoga (visualizing symbols and energy patterns). Yoga can be accommodated to any patient, in any position, at any stage of their cancer. It should be guided by an accredited yoga teacher and done to the tolerance of the patient, starting out very slowly and simply.

### Exercise

Patients with cancer often experience lack of energy and loss of physical performance and strength.[88] Researchers have found that exercise can alleviate patients' fatigue and improve their physical performance and psychological outlook.[89] A pilot study demonstrated that myeloma patients with bone lesions were able to do a home-based exercise program, once taught, without supervision and without injury.[88] Another pilot study supported the suitability of exercise for the palliative care population who were given an exercise program, which included 5-minute walks, arm exercises with a resisted rubber band in a chair, marching on a spot, or dancing to their favorite music.[90] All patients expressed a sense of satisfaction in attaining their activity levels. Individuals who knowingly and actively participate in their care have a more positive outlook than those who are passive participants.[91] Patients with advanced cancer should be assessed first by a medical professional and then given an individualized exercise program that they can gradually work into.

### Energy Therapies

NCCAM has classified Reiki, Qi gong, and Therapeutic Touch (TT) as biofield therapies. Biofield therapies are defined as those therapies intended to affect energies that purportedly surround and interpenetrate the human body. They are thought to be able to rebalance the biofield. Some believe that these therapies can remove the subtle causes of illness and enhance overall resilience. The existence of such fields has not yet been scientifically proven.

### Reiki

Reiki is a vibrational or subtle energy most commonly facilitated by light touch. *Rei* means universal or highest energy, and *ki* means subtle energy. Reiki therapy is thought to balance the biofield and to strengthen the body to heal itself. Reiki is offered to a fully clothed individual and involves placement of hands on the head and front and back; it may include placement of hands on the site of discomfort, if desired. The gentle touch is soothing to patients and promotes deep relaxation. A single study of Reiki use for the management of pain in cancer patients showed a reduction in the report of pain intensity without an associated decrease in opoid use.[92] Further research is required to understand the role of this therapy.

### Qi gong

Qi gong is a component of traditional Chinese medicine that combines movement, meditation, and regulation of breathing to enhance the flow of qi (vital energy) in the body, to improve circulation, and to enhance immune function. With practice, qi gong can lower stress levels, reduce anxiety, and provide increased well-being and peace of mind. It is important to note that there is no evidence that qi gong exercises can increase resistance to illness or cure existing disease.[36]

### Therapeutic Touch

Therapeutic Touch (TT), as described by Dolores Kreiger,[93] is "the conscious, intentional act of directing universal energy with the intent to help and heal." It is defined by Nurse Healers Professional Associates[94] as an intentionally directed process of energy exchange during which the practitioner uses the hands as a focus to facilitate the healing process. TT was developed by Kreiger and Dora Kunz in the 1970s from studying techniques of ancient healing practices. It is believed that healing is promoted when the body's energies are in balance. The hands are usually passed over the patient so that the practitioner can detect energy imbalances and facilitate rebalancing. It is believed to affect a profound relaxation response and to help with pain.[95] The effectiveness of TT was evaluated in a meta-analytic review.[96] The results seemed to indicate that TT has a positive and medium effect on physiological and psychological variables, although the studies had significant methodological issues. In another randomized, double-blind, three-group experimental study of TT, the results indicated that there was a significant positive impact on behavioral symptoms of dementia; specifically, manual manipulation and vocalization were diminished.[97] More research needs to be done.

### Pre-therapy Nursing Assessment

The nurse needs to assess the patient first, before any therapy is given or ordered.

### Current Medical History

The practitioner should determine the diagnosis, extent of disease, location of tumors, sites of metastatic disease, medications, CAM therapies (including vitamins, supplements, and herbs), site of blood clots, surgical site, site of radiation, and blood counts. He or she should determine which positions are most comfortable for the patient. All information must be obtained from the chart, doctor, or patient and family before doing a touch therapy.

## Symptoms

Ask patients what symptoms they are currently experiencing. Ask patients to rate their symptoms on a scale of 0 to 10 as an estimate of their level of distress. This is necessary to select the most appropriate and the most effective CAM therapy. If the patient has pain, medicate first, before therapy is provided; the patient is much more likely to enjoy it. Have patients rate their individual symptoms after the chosen therapy, to make clear to the patient and medical staff the benefit of the therapy.

## Religious/Cultural Background

What is the patient's cultural background? What therapies were used at home? Are there any cultural taboos? For example, it is not acceptable for a Hasidic Jewish man to be touched by a woman. It is important that the patient's cutural beliefs are respected and incorporated into the plan of care as long as there is no evidence-based reason to exclude them.

## Previous Use

What do the patients know about these therapies? Have they had previous experiences? Were they positive or negative experiences? Do they have any fears or reticence?

## Patient's Requests

Who is asking for these therapies? Is it the patient or the family? What would the patient like to try?

## Remember:

- Do not massage on bones where there is metastatic disease, because bones are at risk for fracture or breakage; if the platelet count is <35,000 to 40,000/mm,[3] because there is risk for bruising; on a site of current radiation, due to increased fragility of the skin; or where there are blood clots, due to the risk of setting a clot free to travel.
- There is no deep tissue massage given especially in a patient with advanced disease. Gentle light massage is most appropriate.

## Symptom Management with Evidence-Based Complementary Therapies

Dying patients experience a heavy symptom burden, including pain, nausea and vomiting, anxiety, depression, fatigue,

dyspnea, insomnia, and peripheral neuropathy. When some of these symptoms are treated with medicines such as opioids, additional problematic side effects, such as sedation, delirium, and constipation can occur. Complementary therapies have fewer, if any, side effects and may be more consistent to the patient's and family's culture and health care beliefs.[50]

## Complementary Therapies for Control of Pain

A multicenter trial of seriously ill hospitalized patients with diverse diagnoses documented that 50% of patients who died in the hospital had moderate to severe pain during the last few days before death.[98] Pain is highly prevalent for the patient with advanced-stage cancer. Cancer pain can be very difficult to control; analgesic drugs do not always completely relieve it. Pain can isolate the patient from everything and everyone as it completely takes over, preventing communication between the patient and family. It can prevent a peaceful good-bye. The following adjuvant complementary therapies can provide much-needed extra help for pain control: acupuncture, massage, hypnosis, relaxation, guided imagery, music therapy, and TENS.[99] They can be chosen based on the nurse's assessment and the patient's wishes.

Control of pain is a well known use of acupuncture. Randomized trials support the use of acupuncture for acute pain, in dental surgery,[100] and for chronic pain such as migraine headaches.[101] In one study, pain control was achieved for at least 1 month in all of the patients with mild to moderate pain and in 72% of those with severe pain[102]; 48% of the patients in another study reported pain relief for 3 days and an increase in mobility.[103] Auricular acupuncture has demonstrated analgesic effects for cancer pain.[104] One very interesting study with pediatric patients, ages 6 to 18 years, successfully used acupuncture and hypnosis for chronic pain.[105] Acupuncture was also easily integrated into an outpatient clinic, where it provided 71% relief of pain.[106]

Massage therapy and aromatherapy can provide immediate pain relief and a sense of well-being in cancer patients experiencing pain.[107–109] Ferrell-Torry and Glick[110] reported that massage reduced pain perception by an average of 60%. Of note is a study by Walach and colleagues,[111] which found that pain improvement lasted until the 3-month follow-up visit. According to a review article published by the Cochrane Library, the evidence that currently exists for the use of aromatherapy and massage is mixed. Some immediate benefits are seen, but further studies are indicated.[112] NCCAM recommends massage for treatment of refractory cancer pain. Reflexology has a significant effect on the symptom of pain.[108,110,113,114] It is a relatively simple nursing intervention and can be quite effective in <10 minutes. Relaxation and imagery can provide some pain relief.[115,116] Marcus and associates[132] suggested numbing parts of the body where there is pain through the use of hypnosis. These therapies require that the patient be alert and not in too much pain to concentrate.

In palliative care, music therapists provide services to treat pain.[65] Music increases the patient's comfort, is soothing, and creates a safe environment to ease the dying process. Reiki, which is safe and noninvasive, facilitates relaxation and decreases pain. Hartford Hospital, which has a hospital Reiki program, reports that Reiki provides significant pain relief for surgery patients.[117] Reiki, because it is a light holding touch, can be given to any patient. Art therapy may be used to help patients communicate the painful side of their illness in such a way that they can feel understood and respected.[118] This intervention, with the guidance of a trained art therapist, uses a "body outline" that allows the patient to draw the location and type of physical pain and express the feelings around it without guilt or shame. This may be the starting point for some patients who seem to be verbally unreachable and might benefit from communicating their physical and emotional pain with the result of lessening their distress.

## Complementary Therapies for Control of Nausea and Vomiting

Nausea and vomiting can greatly compromise patients' quality of life. The causes may be multiple, including a reaction to medications (chemotherapy, antibiotics, opiates), bad taste in the mouth, or bowel obstruction. Nausea and vomiting can be so severe that patients would rather discontinue their chemotherapy, or wish to die. Acupuncture, relaxation techniques, acupressure, reflexology, massage, music, imagery, hypnosis, art therapy and meditation are effective therapies for nausea and vomiting and can be used alongside pharmacotherapy.

Acupuncture can be used along with antiemetics. There is clear evidence that needle acupuncture is efficacious for adult postoperative and chemotherapy-related nausea and vomiting.[119] There is often an element of anxiety with nausea and vomiting; progressive muscle relaxation has been shown to be very effective in decreasing nausea and vomiting as well as anxiety.[120] In a small pilot study, finger acupressure decreased nausea in women undergoing chemotherapy for breast cancer.[121] They were taught to apply pressure to the anterior surface of the forearm (P6) and the back of the knee (ST36), an intervention that is easy to learn and use. Reflexology was effective in promoting relaxation, which improved nausea.[113] Music therapy distracts patients by having them pick their own music, listen to live music, sing, or play an instrument, resulting in decreased nausea.[122] Music therapy is easy to implement. Guided imagery encourages patients to focus on past pleasant images to distract from the negative experience of nausea.[123,124] Art therapy can be used as a distraction intervention to reduce nausea and vomiting.[125] Meditation can also distract from the unpleasant sensation of nausea.

## Complementary Therapies for Control of Anxiety

People with advanced stages of cancer may live with chronic anxiety and pain. The most common causes of anxiety in cancer patients with advanced disease are situational anxiety, previous history of anxiety, poorly controlled pain, abnormal metabolic states (e.g., hypoxia, sepsis, delirium), and side effects of medications (e.g., corticosteroids, neuroleptics).[126] The complementary therapies that are effective for the control of anxiety are massage, reflexology, meditation, relaxation, hypnosis, guided imagery, Reiki, music therapy, and exercise.[99,127]

Massage promoted relaxation and significantly reduced the perception of pain and anxiety.[110] Meek[128] reported that her hospice patients, who were in the terminal stage of illness, received a slow stroke back massage and were provided comfort and induced relaxation. Cassileth and Vickers[129] have demonstrated a 52.2% reduction in anxiety with massage. In bone marrow transplant patients, the strongest effects were seen immediately after massage, with a reduction in diastolic blood pressure, anxiety, and nausea.[130] A significant reduction in anxiety 3 months after massage was seen by Walach and colleagues.[111] Family members can be taught to provide slow massage strokes to soothe the patient. Reflexology reduced anxiety in a randomized trial of patients with breast or lung cancer.[114] Gambles and associates[131] found that hospice patients reported 91% relief from tension and anxiety after a course of six reflexology sessions.

"Many dying patients find that the calmness and silence of meditation bring profound feelings of acceptance, well-being and inner peace."[46] Cancer patients frequently experience anxiety as they anticipate entering the final stages of life. Hypnotic relaxation has been found to significantly reduce terminal anxiety.[132] Relaxation training reduced treatment-related anxiety.[133] Imagery work can be a distraction that removes the patient from the stressor of the present. Reiki, which is a light touch therapy, promotes stress reduction and relaxation.[117] Music therapy reduced mood disturbance in cancer patients during hospitalization for autologous bone marrow transplantation.[63] Live music was found to be more effective than taped recorded music.[66] Music therapy was found to be more effective than quiet time in decreasing anxiety in ventilator-dependent patients.[134] Exercise is an intervention that may assist in the reduction of anxiety.[135]

## Complementary Therapies for Control of Depression

The National Comprehensive Cancer Network (NCCN), in their Guidelines of 2003, chose to focus on the patient's distress management. They recognized that distress extends along a continuum, ranging from feelings of vulnerability, sadness, and fear to disabling conditions such as clinical depression, anxiety, panic, isolation, and existential or spiritual crisis.[136] An estimated 20% to 25% of cancer patients experience depression at some time during their illness. In the advanced stages of cancer, the incidence of major depressive syndromes increases to 58%.[137] Factors that place patients at greater risk for depression are history of depression, advanced stage of cancer, poorly controlled pain, and medications. The following complementary therapies are effective for the relief of depression: mind–body therapies (hypnosis, relaxation and guided imagery), massage, and music.[138,139]

Depression was significantly reduced with the use of progressive muscle relaxation together with guided imagery in patients with advanced cancer.[139] MBSR was effective in reducing anxiety and depression in cancer outpatients.[140] Massage therapy achieved major reduction in pain, fatigue, nausea, anxiety, and depression at a major cancer center.[129] Music therapy reduced mood disturbance in patients hospitalized for autologous stem cell transplantation.[63] "Music therapy is an invaluable resource for diminishing suffering in advanced cancer"; and can help the patient link to inner strengths, restore a sense of identity, and open doorways during times of pain and loss.[62] Music can help the patient begin a life review and facilitate finding meaning and purpose in life.[64]

## Complementary Therapies for Control of Fatigue

Fatigue is a common symptom among patients with advanced cancer. A multivariate analysis found that fatigue severity in advanced cancer was significantly associated with pain and dyspnea.[141] Portenoy and Itri[142] reported that fatigue can profoundly undermine the quality of life of patients with cancer. There are some nonpharmacological interventions for cancer-related fatigue, and the following complementary therapies are recommended: acupuncture, exercise, massage, reflexology, mind–body therapies, and music.

MSKCC reported a 31.1% reduction in fatigue with acupuncture in a population of cancer patients with postchemotherapy fatigue.[143] Decreased physical activity, regardless of the reason, leads to decreased energetic capacity. A pilot study provided an exercise program for advanced cancer patients, resulting in increased energy and decreased fatigue.[90] There is a chair-aerobics exercise class in the Integrative Medicine department at MSKCC that is run by an oncology clinical nurse specialist and personal trainer. This class is a fitness program targeted to help breathlessness and fatigue, and to improve physical and psychological well-being of cancer patients. There are currently several stage IV patients in this class, who report that it is hard to get to class because of fatigue, but that after class they feel energized and proud to have accomplished something. Nail[144] summarized a number of nonpharmacological interventions for fatigue, including aerobic exercises and attention-restoring exercises. Coleman and colleagues[88] suggested tailoring exercise to the patients' capabilities as they move through the disease continuum, so that they do not get discouraged. Massage and reflexology can be very stimulating as well as relaxing. Imagery can include visualization of oneself as being very active. Patients can be very stimulated by listening to energetic music or by playing an instrument, especially drums.

## Complementary Therapies for Control of Dyspnea

Breathlessness is an extremely distressing and frightening symptom that can completely dominate a patient's life. It can cause physical disability, high anxiety, dependence, and loss of self-esteem. The following complementary therapies are recommended for dyspnea: relaxation techniques, Reiki, reflexology, gentle massage, music, specific exercise, acupuncture, and hypnosis.

Lung cancer patients using breathing retraining, simple relaxation techniques, activity pacing, and psychosocial support were able to reduce breathlessness from 73% to 27%.[145] Reiki has been shown to reduce anxiety,[146] as have reflexology, gentle massage, and music. Reduction of anxiety aids in the reduction of perceived breathlessness. Chair aerobics exercise helps decrease breathlessness, control panic, and improve muscle tone. Acupuncture was shown to promote quality of life in patients with chronic obstructive asthma.[147] For patients with active, progressive, or far advanced disease, and for those with a short life expectancy, hypnosis can provide reduction of dyspnea and enhance coping.[132]

## Complementary Therapies for Control of Insomnia

Insomnia is a prevalent problem in cancer. Studies conducted among heterogeneous samples of cancer patients suggest that between 30% and 50% of cancer patients have sleep difficulties.[148] The contributing factors, especially for advanced cancer, are hypoxia, pain, anxiety, delirium, medications, or withdrawal from medications. The causes need to be treated, but, in addition, therapies that promote stress reduction and relaxation can be considered. The following complementary therapies can be helpful in the management of insomnia: mind–body therapies (relaxation and imagery), massage, reflexology, Reiki, exercise, and music.

Mind–body therapies such as relaxation, imagery, meditation, and biofeedback may be chosen to reduce body tension and anxiety and promote sleep.[45] Massage, reflexology, and Reiki, being touch therapies, can promote relaxation. Exercise is an intervention that can help reduce anxiety and improve quality of life in cancer patients.[91,149] Music can promote relaxation for sleep.

## Complementary Therapies for Control of Peripheral Neuropathy

Peripheral neuropathy is a common problem for cancer patients receiving certain chemotherapies and for those with diabetes. It is a difficult problem to treat, and its severity and recovery can vary with each patient. It can be so severe that the oncologist may have to stop the chemotherapy. It may be described by patients as numbness, tingling, or burning. Cisplatin is known to induce sensory peripheral neuropathy, and paclitaxel causes sensory and motor neuropathy. Neurological toxicity eventually decreases the patient's ability to perform physical functions necessary for activities of daily living, and thus can interfere with quality of life.[150]

One study looked at the prevalence and patterns of use of CAM therapies in a group of outpatients with peripheral neuropathy.[151] Reportedly, 43% of the patients used CAM for peripheral neuropathy. The following complementary therapies can be helpful in the management of peripheral neuropathy: reflexology and acupuncture.

## Support for the Family

Caregivers of patients with cancer experience stress. They must learn to participate in complicated medical regimens, assist patients in daily activities of living, drive or accompany them to clinics or treatments, and perhaps at the same time be responsible for finances, running of the household, and preparing for the death.[152,153] Perception of discomfort in the dying patient may be another stress factor for the relatives.[154] Family members have difficulty dealing with patients' pain, dyspnea, appetite loss,[155] and delirium.[156] Caregivers of cancer patients undergoing autologous hematopoietic stem cell transplantation were enrolled in a study to receive massage therapy. Massage significantly reduced anxiety, depression, and fatigue; it reduced motivation fatigue and emotional fatigue.[152]

A program of care for family members is offered at MSKCC. Family members are offered massage, reflexology, meditation, yoga, and other evidence-based complementary therapies for stress reduction. "Touch Therapy for the Caregiver" is a monthly program offered to family members, who are taught how to give light upper back and neck massage to provide comfort to the patient. They are instructed to check with the patient's doctor to determine where it will be safe to do gentle massage.

## Complementary and Alternative Therapies for the Nurse

Stress and burnout in oncology is well documented.[157–161] Stress and burnout are particularly relevant in oncology nursing, where nurses work closely with patients and families and bear witness to suffering and dying on a daily basis.

MSKCC's Integrative Medicine Service offers massage to the nursing staff as well as reflexology, meditation, and yoga classes to provide a program of care for nurses. MSKCC is invested in their nurses and knows the great benefit these therapies can offer them. Programs are offered in which nurses are taught Reiki, as well as very simplified versions of gentle upper body massage and reflexology, which they can integrate into their nursing practice after reviewing the indications and contraindications. These skills are a necessary part of any palliative care program.

## Summary

It is a privilege to work with patients who have advanced debilitating illness and are in their last days of life. Gone are the days when a patient or a family might be told, "There is nothing more we can do." There remain many treatment options, including complementary therapies, that patients can choose and receive as a part of palliative care.

Nurses can educate patients and families about the safe choices of evidence-based complementary therapies that can affect their quality of life. But first, they need to educate themselves about CAM—what these therapies are, what are their specific benefits and risks, and which ones are safe—before guiding patients. Nurses want to be respectful of the patient's desire to seek out CAM in the setting of advanced disease. Nurses must listen to the patient and then give suggestions of effective complementary therapies for comfort. Palliative care nurses are exposed to an abnormal amount of suffering and death, and need to take care of themselves in order to give to others. Use of complementary therapies for themselves will benefit all.

Nurses can help patients live their lives to the last with hope. One patient said, "I didn't mind returning to the hospital, because I knew Integrative Medicine would be there for me." Another inpatient reported, after her reflexology session, "You have made me want to stay alive longer, I feel so good." And yes, there is Mary, our case history, who always looked for us in her hospital doorway and called us her angels. We cannot change the course of patients' terminal illnesses, but we can accompany them on the last days of their journey with gentle touch.

REFERENCES

1. Ernst E. Complementary therapies in palliative cancer care. Cancer 2001;91:2181–2185.
2. Sims S. The significance of touch in palliative care. Palliat Med 1998;2:58–61.
3. National Center for Complementary and Alternative Medicine. The use of complementary and alternative medicine in the United States. NCCAM News and Events, 2008.
4. Cassileth BR. Evaluating complementary and alternative therapies for cancer patients [review]. CA Cancer J Clin 1999;49:362–375.
5. Schraub S. Unproven methods in cancer: A worldwide problem. Support Care Cancer 2000;8:10–15.
6. Vickers A, Cassileth BR. Unconventional therapies for cancer and cancer-related symptoms. Lancet Oncol 2001;2:226–232.
7. Morris T, Johnson N, Homer L, Walts D. A comparison of complementary therapy use between breast cancer patients and patients with other primary tumor sites. Am J Surg 2000;179:407–411.
8. Barnes P, Powell-Griner E, McFann K, Nahin R. Complementary and alternative medicine use among adults: United States, 2002. U.S. Department of Health and Human Services, Centers for Disease Control and Prevention, National Center for Health Statistics. CDC Advance Data Reprt No. 343. May 27, 2004.
9. Ernst E, Cassileth BR. The prevalence of complementary/alternative medicine in cancer. Cancer 1998;83:777–782.
10. Molassiotis A, Fernadez-Ortega P, Pud D, et al. Use of complementary and alternative medicine in cancer patients: A European survey. Ann Oncol 2005;16:655–663.
11. Sparber A, Bauer L, Curt G, Eisenberg D, Levin T, Parks S, Steinberg SM, Wootton J. Use of complementary medicine

by adult patients participating in cancer clinical trials. Oncol Nurs Forum 2000;27:623–630.

12. Bennet M, Lengacher C. Use of complementary therapies in a rural cancer population. Oncol Nurs Forum 1999;26:1287–1294.

13. Richardson MA, Sanders S, Palmer J, et al. Complementary/alternative medicine use in a comprehensive cancer center and the implications for oncology. J Clin Oncol 2000;18:2505–2514.

14. Nahleh Z, Tabbara IA. Complementary and alternative medicine in breast cancer patients. Palliat Support Care 2003;1:267–273.

15. Burstein H, Gelber S, Guadagnoli E, Weeks J. Use of alternative medicine by women with early-stage breast cancer. N Engl J Med 1999;340:1733–1739.

16. Boon H, Stewart M, Kennard MA, Gray R, Sawka C, Brown JB, McWilliam C, Gavin A, Baron RA, Aaron D, Haines-Kamka T. Use of complementary/alternative medicine by breast cancer survivors in Ontario: Prevalence and perceptions. J Clin Oncol 2000;18:2515–2521.

17. DiGianni L, Garber J, Winer E. Complementary and alternative medicine use among women with breast cancer. J Clin Oncol 2002;20:34s–38s.

18. Navo M, Phan P, Vaughan C, Palmer J, Michaud L, Jones K, Bodurka D, Basen-Engquist K, Hortobagyi G, Kavanagh J, Smith J. An assessment of the utilization of complementary and alternative medication in women with gynecologic or breast malignancies. J Clin Oncol 2004;22:671–677.

19. Barnes PM, Bloom B, Nahin RL. Complementary and alternative medicine use among adults and children: United States, 2007. US Department of Health and Human Services, Centers for Disease Control and Prevention, and National Center for Health Statistics 2007;12:1–24.

20. McCurdy EA, Spangler JG, Wofford MM, Chauvenet AR, McLean TW. Religiosity is associated with the use of complementary medical therapies by pediatric oncology patients. J Pediatr Hematol Oncol 2003;25:125–129.

21. McQuaid E, Nassau J. Empirically supported treatments of disease-related symptoms in pediatric psychology: Asthma, diabetes, and cancer. J Pediatr Psychol 1999;24:333–334.

22. Huth MM, Broome ME, Good M. Imagery reduces children's post-operative pain. Pain 2004;110:439–448.

23. Liossi C, Hatira P. Clinical hypnosis versus cognitive behavioral training for pain management with the pediatric cancer patients undergoing bone marrow aspirations. Int J Clin Exp Hypn 1999;47:104–116.

24. Tsao JCI, Zeltzer LK. Complementary and alternative medicine approaches for pediatric pain: A review of the state-of-the-science. eCAM 2005;2:149–159.

25. Coppes M, Anderson R, Egeler R, Wolff J. Alternative therapies for the treatment of childhood cancer. N Engl J Med 1998;339:846–847.

26. Fernandez C, Pyesmany A, Stutzer C. Alternative therapies in childhood cancer. N Engl J Med 1999;340:569–570.

27. Maskarinec G, Shumay D, Kakai H, Gotay C. Ethnic differences in complementary and alternative medicine use among cancer patients. J Altern Complement Med 2000;6:531–538.

28. Lee M, Lin S, Wrensch M, Adler S, Eisenberg D. Alternative therapies used by women with breast cancer in four ethnic populations. J Natl Cancer Inst 2000;92:42–47.

29. Kim C, Kwok Y. Navajo use of native healers. Arch Intern Med 1998;158:2245–2249.

30. Arcury TA, Suerken CK, Grzywacz JG, Bell RA, Lang W, Quandt SA. Complementary and alternative medicine use among older adults: Ethnic variation. Ethn Dis 2006;16:723–731.

31. Cherniack EP, Senzel RS, Pan CX Correlates of use of alternative medicine by the elderly in an urban population. J Altern Complement Med 2001;7:277–280.

32. Cuellar N, Aycock T, Cahill B, Ford J. Complementary and alternative medicine (CAM) use by African American (AA) and Caucasian American (CA) older adults in a rural setting: A descriptive, comparative study. BMC Complement Altern Med 2003;3(8):1–7.

33. Williamson AT, Fletcher PC, Dawson KA. Complementary and alternative medicine, use in an older population. J Gerontol Nurs 2003;29(5):20–28.

34. Cassileth BR, Deng G. Complementary and alternative therapies for cancer. Oncologist 2004;9:80–89.

35. Kaptchuk T. Acupuncture: Theory, efficacy, and practice. Ann Intern Med 2002;136:374–383.

36. Cassileth BR. The Alternative Medicine Handbook: The Complete Reference Guide to Alternative and Complementary Therapies. New York: WW Norton, 1998.

37. Bureau of Indian Affairs. Indian entities recognized and eligible to receive services from the United States. Fed Regist 2002;67:46328–46333.

38. Johnston SL. Native American traditional and alternative medicine. Ann Am Acad Pol Soc Sci 2002;583:195–213.

39. Unger JB, Soto C, Thomas N. Translation of health programs for American Indians in the United States. Eval Health Prof 2008;31:124–144.

40. Vogel V. American Indian Medicine. The Civilization of the American Indian Series. Norman, OK: University of Oklahoma Press, 1970.

41. Redd WH, Montgomery GH, DuHamel KN. Behavioral intervention for cancer treatment side effects. J Natl Cancer Inst 2001;93:810–823.

42. Barnes PM, Powell-Griner E, McFann K, Nahin RL. Complementary and alternative medicine use among adults. United States, 2002. Adv Data 2004;343:1–20.

43. Wolsko PM, Eisenberg DM, Davis RB, Phillips RS. Use of mind–body medical therapies: Results of a national survey. J Gen Intern Med 2004;19:43–50.

44. Halcon LL, Chlan LL, Kreitzer MJ, Leonard BJ. Complementary therapies and healing practices: Faculty/student beliefs and attitudes and the implications for nursing education. J Prof Nurs 2003;9:387–397.

45. Astin JA, Shapiro SL, Eisenberg DM, et al. Mind–body medicine: State of the science, implications for practice. J Am Board Fam Pract 2003;16:131–147.

46. Kabat Zinn J, Massion A, Hebert J, Rosenbaum E. Meditation. In: Holland J, ed. Psycho-oncology. Oxford: Oxford University Press, 1998:767–779.

47. Berenson S. The cancer patient. In: Zhourek R, ed. Relaxation and Imagery: Tools for Therapeutic Communication and Intervention. Philadelphia: WB Saunders, 1988:168–191.

48. Giedt JF. Guided Imagery: A psychoneuroimmunological intervention in holistic nursing practice. J Holist Nurs 1997;15:112–127.

49. Jacobsen PB, Jim HS. Psychosocial interventions for anxiety and depression in adult cancer patients: Achievements and challenges. CA Cancer J Clin 2008;58:214–230.

50. Pan CX, Morrison S, Ness J, Fugh-Berman A, Leipzig RM. Complementary and alternative medicine in the management

of pain, dyspnea, and nausea and vomiting near the end of life: A systematic review. J Pain Symptom Manage 2000;20:374–387.

51. Deng G, Cassileth BR. Integrative oncology: Complementary therapies for pain, anxiety, and mood disturbance. CA Cancer J Clin 2005;55:109–116.

52. Menzies V, Taylor AG, Bourguignon C. Effects of guided imagery on outcomes of pain, functional status, and self-efficacy in persons diagnosed with fibromyalgia. J Altern Complement Med 2006;12:23–30.

53. Reed T. Imagery in the clinical setting: A tool for healing. Nurs Clin North Am 2007;42:261–277.

54. Roffe L, Schmidt K, Ernst E. A systematic review of guided imagery as an adjuvant cancer therapy. Psychooncology 2005;14:607–617.

55. Bakke AC, Purtzer MA, Newton P. The effect of hypnotic-guided imagery on psychological well-being and immune function in patients with prior breast cancer. J Psychosom Res 2002;53:1131–1137.

56. Schulz-Stubner S, Krings T, Meister IG, Rex S, Thron A, Rossaint R. Clinical hypnosis modulates functional magnetic resonance imaging signal intensities and pain perception in a thermal stimulation paradigm. Reg Anesth Pain Med 2004;29:549–556.

57. Rainville P, Hofbauer RK, Bushnell MK, Duncan GH, Price DD. Hypnosis modulates activity in brain structures involved in the regulation of consciousness. J Cogn Neurosci 2002;14:887–901.

58. Grant JA, Rainville P. Hypnosis and meditation: Similar experiential changes and shared brain mechanisms. Med Hypotheses 2005;65:625–626.

59. Hammond DC. Formulating hypnotic and post-hypnotic suggestions. In: Hammond DC, ed. Handbook of Hypnotic Suggestions and Metaphors. New York: W.W. Norton & Company, 1990:11–23, 323.

60. Rossi EL, Rossi KL. What is a suggestion? The neuroscience of implicit processing heuristics in therapeutic hypnosis and psychotherapy. Am J Clin Hypn 2007;49:67–281.

61. Magill L, Luzzatto P. Music therapy and art therapy. In: Berger A, Portenoy R, Weissman D, eds. Principles and Practice of Palliative Care and Supportive Oncology (2nd ed). Philadelphia: Lippincott Williams & Wilkins, 2002:993–1005.

62. Magill L. The use of music therapy to address the suffering in advanced cancer pain. J Palliat Care 2001;17:167–172.

63. Cassileth BR, Vickers A, Magill L. Music therapy for mood disturbance during hospitalization for autologous stem cell transplantation. Cancer 2003;98:2723–2729.

64. Halstead M, Roscoe S. Restoring the spirit at the end of life: Music as an intervention for oncology nurses. Clin J Oncol Nurs 2002;6:332–336.

65. Hilliard R. Music therapy in pediatric care: Complementing the interdisciplinary approach. J Palliat Care 2003;19:127–132.

66. Bailey L. The effects of live music versus tape-recorded music on hospitalized cancer patients. Music Ther 1983;3:17–28.

67. Luzzatto P, Gabriel B. Art therapy. In: Holland J, ed. Psycho-oncology. Oxford: Oxford University Press, 1998:743–757.

68. Creagan ET, Moertel CG, O'Fallon JR, Schutt A, O'Connell M, Rubin J, Frytak S. Failure of high-dose vitamin C (ascorbic acid) therapy to benefit patients with advanced cancer: A controlled study. N Engl J Med 1979;301:687–690.

69. Moertel CG, Fleming TR, Creagan ET, Rubin J, O'Connell M, Ames M. High-dose vitamin C versus placebo in the treatment of patients with advanced cancer who have had no prior chemotherapy: A randomized double-blind comparison. N Engl J Med 1985;312:137–141.

70. Sparreboom A, Cox M, Acharya M, Figg W. Herbal remedies in the United States: Potential adverse interactions with anti-cancer agents. J Clin Oncol 2004;22:2489–2503.

71. Cassidy A. Are herbal remedies and dietary supplements safe and effective for breast cancer patients? Breast Cancer Res 2003;5:300–302.

72. Cassileth BR, Vickers A. Complementary and alternative cancer therapies. In: Holland J, Frei E, eds. Cancer Medicine (Vol 1). Hamilton, Ontario: BC Decker, 2003:1101–1111.

73. Barone G, Gurley B, Ketel B, Lightfoot M, Abul-Ezz S. Drug interaction between St John's wort and cyclosporine. Ann Pharmacother 2000;34:1013–1016.

74. Integrative Medicine Service at Memorial Sloan-Kettering Cancer Center, New York. Available at: http://www.mskcc.org/integrativemedicine (accessed January 6, 2005).

75. Cassileth BR, Lucarelli C. Herb-Drug Interactions in Oncology. Hamilton, Ontario: BC Decker, 2003.

76. Mikail C, Hearney E, Nemesure B. Increasing physician awareness of the common uses and contraindications of herbal medicines: Utility of a case-based tutorial for residents. J Altern Complement Med 2003;9:571–576.

77. Field T. Touch. Cambridge, MA: MIT Press, 2001.

78. Kassab S, Stevensen C. Common misunderstandings about complementary therapies for patients with cancer. Complement Ther Nurs Midwifery 1996;2:62–65.

79. Betty P, Andrusia D. Essential Beauty: Using Nature's Essential Oils to Rejuvenate, Replenish, and Revitalize. Los Angeles: Keats Publishing, 2000.

80. Dunwoody L, Smyth A, Davidson R. Cancer patients' experiences and evaluations of aromatherapy massage in palliative care. Int J Palliat Nurs 2002;8:497–504.

81. Cummins S. Peaceful Journey: A Yogi's Travel Kit. Hauppauge, NY: Barrons, 2001.

82. Cooke B, Ernst E. Aromatherapy: A systematic review. Br J Gen Pract 2000;50:493–496.

83. Graham PH, Browne L, Cox H, Graham J. Inhalation aromatherapy during radiotherapy: Results of a placebo-controlled, double-blind, randomized trial. J Clin Oncol 2003;21:2372–2376.

84. Soden K, Vincent K, Craske S, Lucas C, Ashley S. A randomized, controlled trial of aromatherapy massage in a hospice setting. Palliat Med 2004;18:87–92.

85. Perez C. Clinical aromatherapy. Part I: An introduction into nursing practice. Clin J Oncol Nurs 2003;7:595–598.

86. Norman L. Feet First: A Guide to Foot Reflexology. New York: Simon & Schuster, 1988.

87. Cheesman S, Christian R, Cresswell J. Exploring the value of shiatsu in palliative care day services. Int J Palliat Nurs 2001;7:234–239.

88. Coleman E, Hall-Barrow J, Coon S, Stewart C. Facilitating exercise adherence for patients with multiple myeloma. Clin J Oncol Nurs 2003;7:529–534.

89. Dimeo F. Effects of exercise on cancer-related fatigue. Cancer 2001;92:1689–1693.

90. Porock D, Kristjanson L, Tinnelly K, Duke T, Blight J. An exercise intervention for advanced cancer patients experiencing fatigue: A pilot study. J Palliat Care 2000;16:30–36.

91. Wall L. Changes in hope and power in lung cancer patients who exercise. Nurs Sci Q 2000;13:234–242.

92. Olson K, Hanson J, Michaud M. A phase II trial of reiki for the management of pain in advanced cancer patients. J Pain Symptom Manage 2003;26:990–997.

93. Kreiger D. The Therapeutic Touch: How to Use Your Hands to Help or to Heal. Englewood Cliffs, NJ: Prentice-Hall, 1979.

94. Nurse Healers Professional Associates International. Available at: http://www.therapeutic-touch.org (accessed January 6, 2005).

95. Samarel N, Fawcett J, Davis M, Ryan F. Effects of dialogue and therapeutic touch on preoperative and postoperative experiences of breast cancer surgery: An exploratory study. Oncol Nurs Forum 1998;25:1369–1376.

96. Peters R. The effectiveness of therapeutic touch: A meta-analytic review. Nurs Sci Q 1999;12:52–61.

97. Woods DL, Craven RF, Whitney J. The effect of therapeutic touch on behavioral symptoms of persons with dementia. Altern Ther Health Med 2005;11:66–74.

98. SUPPORT Principal Investigators. A controlled trial to improve care for seriously ill hospitalized patients: The Study to Understand Prognoses and Preferences for Outcomes and Risks of Treatments (SUPPORT). JAMA 1995;274:1591–1598.

99. Mansky PJ, Wallerstedt DB. Complementary medicine in palliative care and cancer symptom management. Cancer J 2006;12:425–431.

100. Lao L, Bergman S, Langenberg P, Wong R, Berman B. Efficacy of Chinese acupuncture on postoperative oral surgery pain. Oral Surg Oral Med Oral Pathol 1995;79:423–428.

101. Melchart D, Linde K, Fisher P, White A, Allais G, Vickers A, Berman B. Acupuncture for recurrent headaches: A systematic review of randomized controlled trials. Cephalalgia 1999;19:779–786.

102. Xu S, Liu Z, Li Y. Treatment of cancerous abdominal pain by acupuncture on Zusanli (ST36): A report of 92 cases. J Tradit Chin Med 1995;15:189–191.

103. Filshie J, Redman D. Acupuncture and malignant pain problems. Eur J Surg Oncol 1985;11:389–394.

104. Alimi D, Rubino C, Leandri E, Brule S. Analgesic effects of auricular acupuncture for cancer care. J Pain Symptom Manage 2000;19:81–82.

105. Zeltzer L, Tsao J, Stelling C, Powers M, Levy S, Waterhouse M. A phase I study on the feasibility and acceptability of an acupuncture/hypnosis intervention for chronic pediatric pain. J Pain Symptom Manage 2002;24:437–446.

106. Johnstone P, Polston G, Niemtzow R, Martin P. Integration of acupuncture into the oncology clinic. Palliat Med 2002;16:235–239.

107. Gray R. The use of massage therapy in palliative care. Complement Ther Nurs Midwifery 2000;6:77–82.

108. Weinrich S, Weinrich M. The effect of massage on pain in cancer patients. Appl Nurs Res 1990;3:140–145.

109. Wilkinson S, Aldridge J, Salmon I, Cain E, Wilson B. An evaluation of aromatherapy massage in palliative care. Palliat Med 1999;13:409–417.

110. Ferrell-Torry A, Glick O. The use of therapeutic massage as a nursing intervention to modify anxiety and the perception of cancer pain. Cancer Nurs 1993;16:93–101.

111. Walach H, Guthlin C, Konig M. Efficacy of massage therapy in chronic pain: A pragmatic randomized trial. J Altern Complement Med 2003;9:837–846.

112. Fellowes D, Barnes K, Wilkinson SSM. Aromatherapy and massage for symptom relief in patients with cancer. Cochrane Database Syst Rev 2008(4). CD002287.

113. Grealish L, Lomasney A, Whiteman B. Foot massage: A nursing intervention to modify the distressing symptoms of pain and nausea in patients hospitalized with cancer. Cancer Nurs 2000;23:237–243.

114. Stephenson N, Weinrich S, Tavakoli A. The effects of foot reflexology on anxiety and pain in patients with breast and lung cancer. Oncol Nurs Forum 2000;27:67–72.

115. Fleming U. Relaxation therapy for far-advanced cancer. Practitioner 1985;229:471–475.

116. Syrjala K, Donaldson G, Davis M, Kippes M, Carr J. Relaxation and imagery and cognitive-behavioral training reduce pain during cancer treatment: A controlled clinical trial. Pain 1995;63:189–198.

117. Miles P, True G. Reiki—review of a biofield therapy: History, theory, practice, and research. Altern Ther 2003;9:62–72.

118. Luzzatto P, Sereno V, Capps R. A communication tool for cancer patients with pain: The art therapy technique of the body outline. Palliat Support Care 2003;1:135–142.

119. Shen J, Wenger N, Glaspy J, Hays R, Albert P, Choi C, Shekelle P. Electroacupuncture for control of myeloablative chemotherapy-induced emesis. JAMA 2000;284:2755–2761.

120. Arakawa S. Relaxation to reduce nausea, vomiting, and anxiety induced by chemotherapy in Japanese patients. Cancer Nurs 1997;20:342–349.

121. Dibble S, Chapman J, Mack K, Shih A. Acupressure for nausea: Results of a pilot study. Oncol Nurs Forum 2000;27:41–47.

122. Bender C, McDaniel R, Murphy-Ende K, Pickett M, Rittenberg C, Rogers M, Schneider S, Schwartz R. Chemotherapy-induced nausea and vomiting. Clin J Oncol Nurs 2002;6:94–102.

123. King C. Nonpharmacologic management of chemotherapy-induced nausea and vomiting. Oncol Nurs Forum 1997;24:41–48.

124. Van Fleet S. Relaxation and imagery for symptom management: Improving patient assessment and individualizing treatment. Oncol Nurs Forum 2000;27:501–510.

125. Gabriel B, Bromberg E, Vandenbovenkamp J, Walka P, Komblith A, Luzzatto P. Art therapy with adult bone marrow transplant patients in isolation: A pilot study. Psychooncology 2001;10:114–123.

126. Massie MJ. Anxiety, panic, and phobias. In: Holland JC, Rowland JH, eds. Handbook of Psychooncology: Psychological Care of the Patient with Cancer. Oxford: Oxford University Press, 1990:300–309.

127. Sadat H, Drummond-Lewis J, Maranets I, Kaplan D, Saadat A, Wang SM, Kain ZN. Hypnosis reduces preoperative anxiety in adult patients. Anesth Analg 2006;102:1394–1396.

128. Meek S. Effects of slow stroke back massage on relaxation in hospice clients. IMAGE: J Nurs Schol 1993;25:17–21.

129. Cassileth BR, Vickers A. Massage therapy for symptom control: Outcome study at a major cancer center. J Pain Symptom Manag 2004;28:244–249.

130. Ahles T, Tope D, Pinkson B, Walch S, Hann D, Whedon M, Dain B, Weiss J, Mills L, Silberfarb P. Massage therapy for patients undergoing autologous bone marrow transplantation. J Pain Symptom Manage 1999;18:157–163.

131. Gambles M, Crooke M, Wilkinson S. Evaluation of a hospice based reflexology service: A qualitative audit of patient perceptions. Eur J Oncol Nurs 2002;6:37–44.

132. Marcus J, Elkins G, Mott F. The integration of hypnosis into a model of palliative care. Integr Cancer Ther 2003;2:365–370.

133. Luebblert K, Dahme B, Hasenbring M. The effectiveness of relaxation training in reducing treatment related symptoms

and improving emotional adjustment in acute non-surgical cancer treatment: A meta-analytical review. Psychooncology 2001;10:490–502.

134. Wong H, Lopez–Nahas V, Molassiotis A. Effects of music therapy on anxiety in ventilator-dependent patients. Heart Lung 2001;30:376–387.

135. Blanchard C, Courynea K, Laing D. Effects of acute exercise on state anxiety in breast cancer survivors. Oncol Nurs Forum 2001;28:1617–1621.

136. National Comprehensive Cancer Network. Distress management: Clinical practice guidelines. J Natl Compr Canc Netw 2003;1:344–374.

137. Breitbart W. Identifying patients at risk for, and treatment of major psychiatric complications of cancer. Support Care Cancer 1995;95(3):45–60.

138. Iglesias A. Hypnosis and existential psychotherapy with end-stage terminally ill patients. Am J Clin Hypn 2004;46:201–214.

139. Sloman R. Relaxation and imagery for anxiety and depression control in community patients with advanced cancer. Cancer Nurs 2002;25:432–435.

140. Speca M, Carlson L, Goodey E, Angen M. A randomized, wait-list controlled clinical trial: The effect of a mindfulness meditation-based stress reduction program on mood and symptoms of stress in cancer outpatients. Psychosom Med 2000;62:613–622.

141. Stone P, Hardy J, Broadley K, Tookman A, Kurowska A, A'Hern R. Fatigue in advanced cancer: A prospective controlled cross-sectional study. Br J Cancer 1999;79:1479–1486.

142. Portenoy R, Itri L. Cancer-related fatigue: Guidelines for evaluation and management. Oncologist 1999;4:1–10.

143. Vickers A, Straus D, Fearon B, Cassileth BR. Acupuncture for post-chemotherapy fatigue: A phase II study. J Clin Oncol 2004;22:1731–1735.

144. Nail L. CLIR: Center for Leadership, Information, and Research/Continuing Education: Fatigue in patients with cancer. Oncol Nurs Forum 2002;29:537–546.

145. Hately J, Laurence V, Scott A, Baker R, Thomas P. Breathlessness clinics within specialist palliative care settings can improve the quality of life and functional capacity of patients with lung cancer. Palliat Med 2003;17:410–417.

146. Wardell D, Engebretson J. Biological correlates of Reiki touch healing. J Adv Nurs 2001;33:439–445.

147. Maa SH, Sun MF, Hsu KH, Hung TJ, Chen HC, Yu CT, Wang CH, Lin HC. Effect of acupuncture or acupressure on quality of life of patients with chronic obstructive asthma: A pilot study. J Altern Complement Med 2003;9:659–670.

148. Savard J, Morin C. Insomnia in the context of cancer: A review of a neglected problem. J Clin Oncol 2001;19:895–908.

149. Courneya K. Exercise in cancer survivors: An overview of research. Med Sci Sports Exerc 2003;35:1846–1852.

150. Almadrones L, McGuire D, Walczak J, Florio C, Tian C. Psychometric evaluation of two scales assessing functional status and peripheral neuropathy associated with chemotherapy for ovarian cancer: A gynecologic oncology group study. Oncol Nurs Forum 2004;31:615–623.

151. Brunelli B, Gorson K. The use of complementary and alternative medicines by patients with peripheral neuropathy. J Neurol Sci 2004;218:59–66.

152. Rexilius S, Mundt C, Megel M, Agrawal S. Therapeutic effects of massage therapy and healing touch on caregivers of patients undergoing autologous hematopoietic stem cell transplant. Oncol Nurs Forum 2002;29:E35–E34.

153. Mok E, Chan F, Chan V, Yeung E. Family experience caring for terminally ill patients with cancer in Hong Kong. Cancer Nurs 2003;26:267–275.

154. Bruera E, Sweeney C, Willey J, Palmer J, Strasser F, Strauch E. Perception of discomfort by relatives and nurses in unresponsive terminally ill patients with cancer: A prospective study. J Pain Symptom Manage 2003;26:818–826.

155. Ogasawara C, Kume Y, Andou M. Family satisfaction with perception of and barriers to terminal care in Japan. Oncol Nurs Forum 2003;30:763–766.

156. Brajtman S. The impact on the family of terminal restlessness and its management. Palliat Med 2003;17:454–460.

157. Kushnir T, Rabin S, Azulai S. A descriptive study of stress management in a group of pediatric oncology nurses. Cancer Nurs 1997;20:414–421.

158. Kash K, Holland JJ, Breitbart B, Berenson S, Dougherty J, Ouellette-Kobasa S, Lesko L. Stress and burnout in oncology. Oncology (Huntingt) 2000;14:1621–1633.

159. Penson R, Dignan F, Canellos G, Picard C, Lynch TJ Jr. Burnout: Caring for the caregivers. Oncologist 2000;5:425–434.

160. Grunfeld E, Whelan T, Zitzelsberger L, Willan AR, Montesanto B, Evans WK. Cancer care workers in Ontario: Prevalence of burnout, job stress and job satisfaction. CMAJ 2000;163:166–169.

161. Medland J, Howard-Ruben J, Whitaker E. Fostering psychosocial wellness in oncology nurses: Addressing burnout and social support in the workplace. Oncol Nurs Forum 2004;31:47–54.

# 28 Withdrawal of Life-Sustaining Therapies: Mechanical Ventilation, Dialysis, and Cardiac Devices

*Margaret L. Campbell, Linda M. Gorman, and Peggy Kalowes*

*I don't want to live on machines—Patient*

♦ *Key Points*
♦ *Any form of life-sustaining therapy or treatment can be withheld or withdrawn.*
♦ *Distress can be anticipated and treated during withdrawal of life supports.*
♦ *Death follows life support withdrawal along varying trajectories characteristic of the organ or organs in failure.*

## MECHANICAL VENTILATION

CASE STUDY
*Ventilator Withdrawal in an Elderly Man After Clarification of Goals of Care*

Steven Brown, an 83-year-old man, tripped over a scatter rug in his home and fell, fracturing his left hip. On hospital admission a hip replacement was planned, but the high-morbidity procedure was discussed in detail with Mr. Brown and his wife, since Mr. Brown had advanced stage COPD and heart failure; they agreed to proceed with surgery understanding the high risk of postoperative complications.

As predicted, the postoperative course was complicated by ventilator dependence, exacerbation of heart failure, and a urinary tract infection. On postoperative day #9 the surgical team met with Mr. Brown and his wife to discuss treatment alternatives in the face of refractory ventilator dependence: (1) placement of a tracheostomy and gastrostomy tube with transfer to a long-term acute facility, or (2) withdrawal of ventilation and likely subsequent death from respiratory failure. Mr. Brown wrote a note stating "I don't want to live on a machine." His wife asked clarifying questions about the clinical team's certainty about refractory respiratory failure and the benefits/burdens of continued treatment at a long-term care facility with tracheostomy and enteral feedings.

After a day of reflection and visits from their children, the Browns reported a wish for ventilator withdrawal. The hospital chaplain came and led prayers, and the family gathered around the bedside. Mr. Brown was pre-medicated with morphine 5 mg and lorazepam 2 mg, and a continuous morphine infusion was initiated at 2 mg/hr. Rapid terminal weaning was conducted by the surgeon with the ICU nurse and respiratory therapist, with minor adjustments in morphine during the weaning. After 20 minutes Mr. Brown was breathing spontaneously with no signs of respiratory distress. He was extubated and a nasal cannula with room air flowing at 2 liters/minute was placed. His family remained at the bedside throughout. Over the next hour his breathing pattern slowed and 2 hours after ventilator withdrawal Mr. Brown died.

## Benefits and Burdens of Mechanical Ventilation

Mechanical ventilation (MV) has been used for decades to support breathing when patients experienced acute or chronic respiratory failure. Mechanical ventilation is of benefit when the patient, for a number of reasons, cannot maintain normal ventilation as evidenced by increasing carbon dioxide and respiratory acidosis; invasive and noninvasive modalities are employed. Invasive MV is accomplished after the establishment of an artificial airway such as an endotracheal tube or tracheostomy. Noninvasive MV is applied over the nose or nose and mouth via a tight-fitting face mask.

Invasive MV is employed after cardiopulmonary arrest, during general anesthesia, to treat respiratory failure that is not responsive to noninvasive ventilation, or for patients who are ventilator dependent. Endotracheal intubation is used for periods of <2 weeks of ventilation; continued ventilation after 2 weeks is supported by tracheostomy. When respiratory failure occurs during an exacerbation of chronic pulmonary disease, noninvasive ventilation is often useful as a first response.[1] Patients with obstructive sleep apnea, COPD, and ALS often use noninvasive ventilation at night or when breathing is difficult during the day.

Patients often experience discomfort during MV. With noninvasive modalities the tight-fitting mask may produce generalized pressure-associated discomfort, feelings of suffocation, and pressure lesions on the bridge of the nose. Endotracheal intubation causes gagging, coughing, drooling, and leaves the patient unable to verbalize since the tube passes through the vocal cords. In many cases of endotracheal intubation and some cases of noninvasive ventilation, the patient requires mechanical restraints or sedation to maintain the integrity of the life-saving treatment and to ensure ventilator synchrony.

Ventilator-dependent patients experience fewer burdens since they are routinely ventilated through a tracheostomy. Nonetheless, chronic ventilator dependence limits patient mobility and contributes to the development of immobility complications such as pressure ulcers, deep venous thrombosis and pneumonia.

Ventilator withdrawal is considered as a treatment option when the treatment is more burdensome than beneficial, such as when the patient has a terminal illness or is unconscious or when the patient makes an informed, capable decision to cease treatment because her/his quality of life is poor.[2] In critical care units (adult, pediatric and neonatal), ventilator withdrawal is usually undertaken because the

---

| Table 28–1 |
| --- |
| **Legal Consensus About Foregoing Treatment[5]** |

- Competent patients have a common-law and constitutional right to refuse treatment.
- Incompetent patients have the same rights as competent patients; however, the manner in which these rights are exercised is, of necessity, different.
- No right is absolute, and societal interests impose limitations on the right to refuse treatment.
- The decision-making process should generally occur in the clinical setting without recourse to the courts.
- In making decisions for incompetent patients, surrogate decision makers should apply, in descending order of preference, the subjective standard, the substituted judgment standard, and the best interests' standard.
- In ascertaining an incompetent patient's preferences, the attending physician and surrogate may rely on a patient's "advance directive."
- Artificial nutrition and hydration is a medical treatment and may be withheld or withdrawn under the same conditions as any other form of medical treatment.
- Active euthanasia and assisted suicide are morally and legally distinct from foregoing life-sustaining treatment.

*Source*: Reprinted with permission. American Association of Critical Care Nurses, Campbell, ML. Foregoing life-sustaining therapy: How to care for the patient who is near death. Alisa Viejo, CA, 1998, Table 1.3, p.4.

---

patient is not expected to survive and/or to regain functional consciousness.[3,4]

Clinical standards, policies, and procedures about foregoing life-sustaining therapy, including MV, are in wide use and reflect broad agreement about the underlying principles regarding these decisions; a legal consensus is also evident (See Table 28–1).

Although withdrawal of ventilation occurs on a frequent basis across settings of care, there is little empiric evidence to guide the process. A review of the evidence to guide a ventilator withdrawal process[6] demonstrated that small samples and largely retrospective chart reviews characterize the body of evidence about processes for ventilator withdrawal.[7–14]

The cited research is not conclusive to make recommendations in all cases of ventilator withdrawal. However, a number of suggested processes may be useful in this clinical context, along with a team approach to the procedure, and patient care to address anticipated symptoms.

Patients are ventilated because of respiratory failure and an inability to exchange respiratory gases without mechanical support. Dyspnea arises from increased inspiratory effort, hypercarbia, and/or hypoxemia; dyspnea is anticipated during and after ventilator withdrawal. Prevention and alleviation of dyspnea or respiratory distress becomes the focus of care. Some patients, if awake, may experience fear or anxiety before or during ventilator withdrawal which will require attention if present. Adult patients may experience barotrauma to the trachea from the pressure in the cuff. This can lead to tracheomalacia, fistulae, and laryngeal edema or spasm after extubation.

## Ventilator Withdrawal Processes: Advance Preparation

The Centers for Medicare and Medicaid services has enacted guidelines for consistent processes around organ donation.[15] Hospital staff must notify their state Organ Procurement Organization (OPO) when decisions about ventilator withdrawal are being considered. The OPO will collaborate with the hospital staff to identify if the patient is a donor candidate, and to seek consent from the next of kin. This evaluation by the OPO must be completed before ventilation is withdrawn.

Timing to conduct the withdrawal process is generally negotiated with the patient's family and the health care team. This timing will depend on which team members will be present, including support personnel such as a chaplain. The time needs to be communicated to all clinical team members, and ideally the assigned nurse should have a reduced assignment to be able to spend 1:1 time with the patient and family.

Not all family members want to be present at the bedside during withdrawal. Another room nearby can be arranged with adequate seating, tissues, water and access to a telephone. Religious observances or family-specific rituals need to be accommodated and completed before beginning the withdrawal process. Patient and/or family questions about what to expect can be addressed before beginning the process.[16,17] When ventilation is withdrawn from a small child, infant, or neonate, it is customary for a parent to hold the child on his/her lap during the process.[18]

## Measuring Distress

Dyspnea, also known as breathlessness, is a nociceptive phenomenon defined as "a subjective experience of breathing discomfort that consists of qualitatively distinct sensations that vary in intensity. The experience derives from interactions among multiple physiological, psychological, social and environmental factors, and may induce secondary physiological and behavioral responses."[19] Dyspnea can be perceived and verified only by the person experiencing it. Many patients who are undergoing ventilator withdrawal are cognitively impaired or unconscious as a result of underlying neurologic lesions or hemodynamic, metabolic, or respiratory dysfunction, that produce cognitive impairment or unconsciousness.[3] Respiratory distress is an observable (behavioral) corollary to dyspnea; the physical and emotional suffering that results from the experience of asphyxiation is characterized by behaviors that can be observed and measured.[20,21]

Neuromuscular blocking agents (NMBA) are being used with less frequency in the ICU; however, when in use it is impossible to assess the patient's comfort. Thus, the NMBA should be discontinued with evidence of patient neuromuscular recovery before ventilator withdrawal is undertaken.[22–24] In some cases the duration of action of these agents is prolonged, such as when the patient has liver or renal failure and impaired clearance. Therefore, although controversial, withdrawal can proceed with careful attention to ensuring patient comfort if an unacceptable delay in withdrawing MV occurs because of protracted effects of NMBA.[24]

A common measure of dyspnea or respiratory distress should be identified and used across clinicians to guide the initiation and escalation of opioids or sedatives, such as noting the presence of behaviors specific to respiratory distress, including tachypnea, tachycardia, accessory muscle use, paradoxical breathing pattern, fearful facial expression, and nasal flaring.[21] Patients with coma are unlikely to demonstrate distress—aside, perhaps, from tachypnea and tachycardia.[9] Infants and neonates often display nasal flaring, grunting at end-expiration and sternal retraction.[18] Brain-dead patients by definition will not show distress, cough, gag, or breathe during or following ventilator withdrawal, and sedation or analgesia is not indicated.

Most patients undergoing ventilator withdrawal will be unable to provide a self-report about any dyspnea experienced, particularly patients who are unconscious, severely cognitively impaired, or infants and neonates. Attempts to elicit a self-report should be made if the patient is conscious. Skill is required to detect nuances of behaviors, particularly when the patient is unable to validate the nurse's assessment. Investigation of the reliability and validity of a Respiratory Distress Observation Scale for adult patients suggests that there may be common behaviors displayed by patients in response to hypercarbia, hypoxemia or inspiratory effort.[25,26] Some would argue that routine pre-medication with opioids and sedatives will prevent distress during ventilator withdrawal; however, many clinicians fear hastening patient death and are reluctant to medicate without clear evidence of patient distress.[27] Initiation and escalation of sedatives and opioids should be guided by patient behaviors.

## Pre-medication for Anticipated Distress

As is the standard with pain management, opioids should be initiated to signs of distress and the advice to "start low and titrate slowly" is sage. For the opioid-naïve adult, an initial bolus of 3 or 5 mg of morphine followed by initiation of a continuous infusion at 50% the bolus is recommended. Thus, a patient may get a 5 mg bolus and an infusion at 2.5 mg/hr to begin. Pediatric dosing is usually initiated at 0.1 to 0.2 mg/kg.[28] Anticipatory pre-medication is a sound practice if distress is already evident and if distress can be anticipated. There is no justification for medicating a brain-dead patient, and one could argue that the patient in coma with only minimal brainstem function is also unlikely to experience distress. Doses that correspond to customary dosing for the treatment of dyspnea should guide dosing during ventilator withdrawal. Documentation of the signs of distress and rationale for dose escalation is important to ensure continuity across professional caregivers, and to prevent overmedication and the appearance of hastening death.

## Weaning Method

Terminal extubation is characterized by ceasing ventilatory support and removing the endotracheal tube in one step. Terminal weaning is a process of stepwise, gradual reductions in oxygen and ventilation, terminating with placement of a t-piece or with extubation. There are no known investigations comparing one method to another.[6]

With no comparative evidence to support one method over another, it is difficult to make a recommendation. Rapid terminal weaning may afford the clinician with the most control because it allows for careful, sequential adjustments to the ventilator with precise titration of medications to ensure patient comfort.[9] Continuous patient monitoring with readily accessible opioids and sedatives will afford the patient and family with comfort regardless of method employed.

## Extubation Considerations

Patients who are ventilator dependent are generally ventilated through a tracheostomy tube. After ventilator withdrawal a tracheostomy mask with humidified room air or low-flow oxygen can be placed. Patients experiencing acute respiratory failure are ventilated through a nasal or oral endotracheal tube. Adult tubes have a cuff to maintain tube placement and occlude the trachea to prevent air leaking and loss of tidal volume; neonatal tubes are cuffless.

Removal of the endotracheal tube should be performed whenever possible because of patient comfort and the aesthetic appearance of the patient. However, in some cases airway compromise can be anticipated, such as when the patient has a swollen, protuberant tongue, or has no gag or cough reflexes. In cases of airway compromise, the disconcerting noises may be more distressing to the attendant family than the presence of the tube. Medication with dexamethasone may reduce airway edema, permitting extubation when patients are at high risk for post-extubation laryngeal edema, but dosing would need to start 12 hours before withdrawal if the timing permits. Aerosolized racemic epinephrine is a useful intervention to reduce stridor after extubation. Family counseling about usual noises that can be expected, and cause no distress to the patient, should take place prior to extubation.

Across studies of adults the duration of survival ranged from 2 minutes to 9 days after ventilator withdrawal. Median survival across studies ranged from 35 minutes[10] to 7.5 hours.[8] The median survival time in a study of infants undergoing ventilator withdrawal was 20 minutes.[28] Campbell and colleagues reported no relationship between duration of survival and use of sedation/analgesia, Glasgow Coma Scale, or $PaO_2/FiO_2$ but there was a significant inverse correlation with illness severity; in other words the sickest patients died most rapidly.[9]

# DIALYSIS DISCONTINUATION

CASE STUDY
*Discontinuing Dialysis When the Burden of Treatment Outweighed the Benefit*

Marcella Whitney, an 80-year-old woman with a 3-year history of multiple myeloma, was started on hemodialysis when the myeloma advanced to kidney involvement; she had been tolerating treatment for the myeloma including chemotherapy. She was in early stage of Alzheimer's dementia but continued to be able to make medical decisions with the support of her daughter. Recent history was characterized by weakness, anorexia, exhibiting some signs of aspiration, and increased anxiety. Mrs. Whitney was admitted to the hospital with aspiration pneumonia and new onset of bone pain. She began crying when the transporter came to take her to the dialysis unit; she said she did not want to go to dialysis. Her daughter and the physicians were unsure if the patient understood that she would die without dialysis; they questioned her decision-making capacity. Mrs. Whitney's daughter agreed to meet with the palliative care team to help her make decisions about continued dialysis. The daughter acknowledged that the patient's quality of life had been declining over the past year due to the dementia and the myeloma. Based on past conversations over the years, the daughter felt her mother would not want her life prolonged in the face of dementia but wanted to wait a little longer before making the decision to stop dialysis. The palliative care team recommended an analgesic and anxiolytic regimen with a trial of continued dialysis. The patient stopped complaining of pain, but continued to express fear and distress when moved to dialysis. Mrs. Whitney missed several dialysis treatments due to anxiety when she refused to go to treatment or would not cooperate in the dialysis unit. Her daughter decided that the anxiety was creating too much suffering, and her mother's life should not be prolonged with further dialysis. A discharge home with hospice was arranged and dialysis was discontinued. Mrs. Whitney had no signs of discomfort and no anxiety during her first four days at home; she ate small amounts of her favorite foods and continued to be anuric. The hospice team prepared the daughter for what to expect, and had medications available to treat any potential symptoms of pain, dyspnea, nausea, pooling secretions, itching and anxiety. Mrs. Whitney required no additions to her analgesia regimen until the 6th day without dialysis, when treatment for increased pain, nausea and itching was started. Sublingual methadone, hyoscyamine for secretions, and lorazepam for itching were given with good effect. She lapsed into a coma on the 8th day after the last dialysis and died peacefully at home with family around her on the 9th day.

### Benefits and Burdens of Dialysis

Dialysis was introduced as a treatment for end stage renal disease in 1962. In the early years the number of patients receiving dialysis was limited by the small number of dialysis machines available, and only individuals less than 40 years of age, family breadwinners, and those without severe medical problems like diabetes were considered.[29] In 1973, Medicare established universal entitlement for chronic dialysis; currently over 300,000 Americans receive dialysis.[30] Chronic kidney disease (CKD) Stage 5, also called End Stage Renal Disease (ESRD), is defined as a glomerular filtration rate of less than 15 ml/minute (normal ≥ 90 ml/minute). The most common causes include diabetes mellitus, heart failure, hypertension, and glomerulonephritis. Acute renal failure, commonly seen in the critically ill, is often treated with dialysis and is caused by dehydration, sepsis, hypotension, and/or trauma.

In the last 10 years the dialysis population has changed. The current dialysis population is older with more comorbidities, higher symptom burden, and a higher mortality rate.[31] Patients older than 80 years now constitute the fastest-growing segment of this population and have a 46% mortality rate in the first year of dialysis.[32] These patients are not transplant candidates, so they will remain on dialysis until they die or until it is discontinued. A decision to stop dialysis is a frequent occurrence, especially in a frail elderly population. The field of nephrology has been moving to address improved quality of life, and incorporating advances from the palliative care field. Several national initiatives including the ESRD Workgroup are addressing the growing needs of the dialysis population because this population has shortened life expectancy and also carry a very high symptom burden.[33-36]

Symptoms of uremia are usually controlled quickly with dialysis; paradoxically, dialysis produces one of the highest symptom burdens as well as hospitalization rates of any chronic illness population.[37] Jablonski found an average of 5.67 uncomfortable symptoms,[38] while other investigators reported 9 uncomfortable symptoms experienced by dialysis patients.[39] Davison and Jhangri found over 50% of dialysis patients complain of chronic pain and 41% have moderate to severe pain.[40] Other common discomforts with dialysis include fatigue, pruritus, constipation, anorexia, anxiety, and sleep disturbances. The frail elderly with multiple comorbidities receiving dialysis are particularly vulnerable to a high symptom burden.[41] Therefore, although life may be prolonged with dialytic management of uremia, the patient's quality of life will often not improve. Thus, a trial of dialysis may be offered to elderly patients to see if dialysis will improve symptoms, although this will require a vascular access.

### Discontinuing Dialysis

In the early years of dialysis, it was rarely withdrawn unless there was loss of vascular access which made dialysis impossible.[29] Today 20–25% of patients receiving dialysis have it discontinued each year;[30] this number is expected to increase as more frail elderly are receiving dialysis. Stopping dialysis remains the 2nd leading cause of death in this population.[30] In 1991, an Institute of Medicine report identified the need to develop guidelines to address patient wishes to stop dialysis.[42] In 2003, Cohen, Germain, & Poppel published guidelines for nephrology professionals to address these issues[43] (see Table 28–2).

The most common reasons for stopping dialysis include: unacceptable quality of life including symptom burden; pain; acute complication such as infection; technical problems with dialysis; dementia; stroke; and cancer.[44-47] Additionally, some patients become too unstable to complete the dialysis session. Peritoneal dialysis patients may be too sick to carry out exchanges and need to obtain vascular access for hemodialysis. Inserting new access lines may cause the patient to reconsider discontinuing dialysis. A thorough assessment of symptoms is important to address patient suffering. Addressing symptom burden, including psychological symptoms, is an important consideration before making the decision to discontinue dialysis. Patients on dialysis often struggle with depression, changes in body image, sexual dysfunction, loss of control, and dependency issues. Irritability, weakness, and progressive debility can all contribute to a patient's distress and wish to consider stopping dialysis. A thorough psychosocial

---

**Table 28–2**
**Guidelines for Making Dialysis Discontinuation Decisions**[43]

- Identify patients who may benefit from discontinuation including those patients with poor prognosis, poor quality of life, pain that is poorly responsive to treatment, progressive untreatable disease, technically difficult dialysis.
- Discuss goals with patient/family.
- Discuss quality of life.
- Discuss possible symptoms and their palliation.
- Clarify that dialysis discontinuation is an option, as part of review of treatment modalities, when educating patients who are new to dialysis.
- Provide reassurance of a peaceful death.
- Allow time for discussion.
- Make the recommendation to stop dialysis and request family assent.
- Provide reassurance that the decision is reversible.

assessment and interventions to address these issues should be part of any treatment plan when discontinuing dialysis is being considered.

When patients make their own decisions, stopping dialysis can be a freeing, almost euphoric experience. The patient usually has a few days before uremic symptoms begin, and this time can include eating favorite, formerly forbidden foods and opportunities to say good-bye to loved ones. This allows a patient to maintain some sense of control over his/her life and the dying process. Choosing the date of the last dialysis, where he/she wants to be for the last days, choosing what foods to eat, all can enhance a sense of control. Family members may struggle with accepting the patient's choice. Loved ones need to be prepared that the patient may become cognitively impaired suddenly as the creatinine rises.

When the patient is unable to participate in decision-making because of dementia, delirium, or critical illness, families and/or surrogates often struggle with making this literally life-and-death decision. But if the patient's suffering with dialysis has been evident, it can be easier for them to make the decision to stop.

### Treating Symptoms after Discontinuation

Death after discontinuation of dialysis generally occurs in 8–12 days, though patients with many comorbidities may die sooner, and patients who make urine will live longer. Nearly all patients discontinuing dialysis die within 1 month.[47] Principles for treating uremic symptoms follow in Table 28–3.

Frequent pain assessment and aggressive analgesia is important, as symptoms can develop quickly. Uremia itself is painless but patients may experience pain from their general medical condition.[47] Morphine should be avoided due to its metabolite morphine-6-glucuronide, which increases in kidney failure making the patient at risk for myoclonus; fentanyl or methadone are better choices.[47,49] Hydromorphone and oxycodone can be used but with caution. Hydromorphone does have a metabolite that can accumulate, and oxycodone has not been well studied in this population.[47,49] Myoclonus can be treated with benzodiazepines if it occurs. As the patient becomes obtunded near death, swallowing a pill may become difficult. Methadone elixir given sublingually or into the buccal space will gradually trickle into the pharynx and be swallowed.

Delirium, confusion, and somnolence are expected as part of the uremic syndrome. A more severe form of delirium called uremic encephalopathy occurs infrequently. It is characterized by extreme agitation and hallucinations. Haloperidol, clonazepam, or lorazepam are useful if the patient becomes agitated and the dose is not dependent on renal function.

Dyspnea can occur from fluid retention and pleural effusion. Anticholinergics to reduce oral secretions, opioids for dyspnea and low-flow oxygen may be helpful. Stopping artificial hydration and nutrition will minimize fluid retention. Pulmonary edema is a palliative care emergency that may arise from volume overload. Diuresis is not possible but

| **Table 28–3**<br>**Treatment Principles When Discontinuing Dialysis**[29,33,45,47,48] |
| --- |
| • Avoid volume overload including hydration and artificial nutrition.<br>• Utilize symptom management medications not metabolized via the kidneys.<br>• Discontinue all non-symptom management medications to reduce risk of toxicities.<br>• Involve a pharmacist consultation early to ensure no medications given are metabolized via kidneys.<br>• Anticipate common symptoms and have appropriate medications available as symptoms can occur suddenly.<br>• Prepare patient and family for what to expect, especially addressing common unfounded fears of drowning in fluid.<br>• Move quickly to offer supportive services and maximize symptom management strategies, as time frame to death is brief. As part of the treatment plan for discontinuation of dialysis, address the role of hospice, patient/family wishes on location of death, early.<br>• The most common symptoms that should be assessed and treated include pain, delirium, dyspnea, nausea, and itching.<br>• Less commonly, patients may exhibit retained upper airway secretions. |

systemic vasodilation may provide relief; nitroglycerin paste every 6 hours is recommended. Ultrafiltration through the dialysis access, if patent, and if the patient is still in the hospital, will also relieve volume overload.

Nausea may be an effect of uremia as well as delayed gastric emptying that is common in ESRD; haloperidol is a useful antiemetic in this context. The liberty to eat previously forbidden foods may contribute to the onset of nausea and vomiting, and the patient will need to be counseled about moderation. Pruritis is another effect of uremia and responds well to benzodiazepines and diphenhydramine, along with lanolin based skin creams.[50]

Last days and hours are characterized by hypersomnolence followed by coma. Death from uremia is often described as a painless and peaceful death. Cohen and colleagues found that the majority of families whose loved ones died after withdrawal of dialysis rated the death as good to very good.[51]

### Role of Palliative Care and Hospice

Dialysis centers are encouraged to develop a palliative care approach to address their patients' needs, which may include advance care planning for timing of discontinuation of dialysis. Hospice care can also be appropriate both for dialysis patients with comorbidities and patients who are considering discontinuing dialysis; however, hospice has historically been underutilized in this population.[33,47,52,53] (See Table 28–4 for a list of barriers to hospice utilization.) Patients may qualify for

Table 28–4
**Barriers to Use of Hospice in ESRD Patient Population[33,47,52,53]**

Financial disincentives and confusion about coverage and eligibility.

Hospice agencies often do not have relationships with local dialysis centers.

Nephrology professionals not addressing end-of-life issues with patients.

Dialysis staff may have inaccurate information about hospice care.

Patients/families with lack of awareness of life-limiting nature of ESRD.

Hospice not offered when dialysis is being discontinued due to brief life expectancy.

hospice while continuing on dialysis due to their poor prognosis and comorbidities. Making a referral to hospice early in the discussion period about stopping dialysis may increase access earlier. Hospice can help these patients remain at home after dialysis is stopped, and manage symptoms effectively.

# DEACTIVATION OF CARDIAC IMPLANTABLE DEVICES

CASE STUDY
*The Impact of Delayed Deactivation of an ICD at End-of-Life*

Carol Mayer, 76, had an Implantable Cardioverter Defibrillator (ICD) inserted four years after her first episode of ventricular fibrillation. As her heart failure progressed to stage IV, the episodes of ventricular fibrillation increased. While at home one afternoon, Carol's defibrillator shocked her several times and she was admitted to the hospital. Carol went in and out of consciousness and was hemodynamically unstable for the next 72 hours. After a long family conference, her family and cardiologist decided that no further aggressive treatments would be continued and that Carol's care would focus on palliation. During the night Carol's ICD shocked her 15 times, while her nurse tried desperately to contact someone to deactivate her ICD. Finally at 3:00 a.m. the cardiologist came in and deactivated the ICD, and Carol died 2 hours later.

## Benefits and Burdens of Cardiac Assist Devices

Implantable cardioverter defibrillators (ICDs), pacemakers, ventricular assist devices (VADs), and even a totally artificial replacement heart used for many patients with advanced cardiac disease, represent advanced life-sustaining technology. The number of adult patients with implantable cardiac devices is rising sharply; in fact, nearly 600,000 implants were performed in 2007 in the U.S. alone, making it among the most common cardiovascular devices used in contemporary clinical practice.[54–56] Because these devices reduce the incidence of sudden death, patients with implantable defibrillators are more likely to die of other nonarrhythmic causes such as cancer, lung disease, advanced dementia, and congestive heart failure.[57,58]

## Discussions for Deactivation of ICDs/Pacemakers/VADs

Prior to insertion of an ICD/Pacemaker/VAD a general discussion should occur with the patient/and family regarding the possibility that the device may be deactivated at a future point in time if therapy is ineffective, no longer needed, or not desired. During the informed consent process, information is provided to the patient about the device, indications, how it works, the expected benefits, the risks, required follow-up, device maintenance (e.g. battery changes) and the possibility that the device may be deactivated in the future. A statement such as the following introduces the topic: "A time may come in the future when the device may not work as we had anticipated, or you may decide that you no longer want it. If that time comes we will talk about deactivating the device." When having end-of-life "discussions with patients and their families facing the last chapter, it is easier if they have heard previously of the potential circumstances for turning the defibrillation off."[59]

Grassman reported, "We had a patient who went home with hospice care. The ICD was never turned off. As a result, the wife told us that the patient died in her arms while the defibrillator jolted him 33 times before the battery ran down."[60] Thus, not addressing deactivation of the ICD can not only cause unnecessary suffering for the patient, but also distress for the patient's family. A number of anecdotal reports attest to the increasing burden of active ICDs during the dying process.[61–63] Even when death is expected and discussions have occurred regarding resuscitation and other end of life care, the topic of deactivating the ICD is not routinely discussed.[62]

## Deactivation Procedures

### Pacemakers

A pacemaker is intended to correct an abnormal heart rate or rhythm. Some patients are only mildly reliant on the device; others are totally dependent to the extent that if the pacemaker is deactivated, discomfort secondary to complete heart block or bradycardia can occur. Sudden death at the time of disabling the pacemaker is unlikely, unless the patient is pacemaker dependent.

Trained personnel should interrogate the pacemaker with the pacemaker programmer. Prepare the patient and family for a rapid death after deactivation if the patient is pacemaker dependent. Adjust the pacemaker settings (e.g. rate and output) so pacing does not occur; this can be done gradually or all at once. The patient can be pre-medicated with an anxiolytic or sedative if desired, particularly if a relatively sudden death can be anticipated and the patient is capable of experiencing distress.

## ICDs

Defibrillators are intended only to convert a lethal ventricular arrhythmia. Deactivation of an ICD will not degrade quality of life or create discomfort. Conversely, as illustrated previously, ICD firing while the patient is dying can be distressing to both the patient and family.

Deactivation should be done by trained personnel; this may also include the presence of the company representative, using the programmer for either device. A pacemaker magnet can be placed over the ICD generator, palpable under the skin, to deactivate when an ICD programmer is unavailable. However, it will not deactivate the backup pacing function of the ICD; this can only be done by an ICD programmer. The funeral director will need to be informed about the presence of the device if cremation is planned.

## VADs

VADs are mechanical pumps surgically implanted to improve the performance of the damaged left (LVAD), right (RVAD), or both (BiVAD) ventricles. VADs can be used short term as a bridge to recovery or transplantation, or as destination therapy that is an alternative to transplantation.[64] Short-term support is indicated for patients who develop cardiogenic shock in which recovery is anticipated, with devices outside the body attached to large consoles. The average duration of VAD support for these critically ill patients is a week, but the units are capable of providing support for up to a month. Prolonged support is associated with coagulopathy, thrombocytopenia, thromboembolism, and hemolysis. When VADs are inserted as destination therapy, it is expected that the patient will need the VAD the rest of his/her life; thus, the VAD is considered a final treatment. Technological advances have made VADs compact and portable, allowing freedom for patients to be discharged home from the hospital, with high-level home health follow-up. "VADs are a treatment, not a cure, and mortality on device support remains high. The risk of death is highest immediately following implantation, followed by a mortality of 16% at one month, 32% at six months, and 45% at one year, regardless of the device used or intention to treat."[65]

Trained personnel should stop the VAD after patient and family preparation, and silencing the device alarms. The patient may experience distress from heart failure and may benefit from pre-medication with a diuretic and an anxiolytic. After deactivation the patient will require close monitoring and treatment of heart failure until death occurs.

## Summary

Withdrawal of mechanical ventilation, discontinuation of dialysis, and deactivation of cardiac devices are procedures that occur with relative frequency. The benefits of these therapies, when initiated, are to replace failing organs, extend life, and improve quality of life by relieving symptom distress associated with organ failure. When the burdens exceed the benefits, or when the patient is near death or unresponsive, decisions may be made to cease these therapies.

In some cases, such as ICD deactivation, no distress is anticipated. In others, such as discontinuing dialysis or withdrawing MV, measures to palliate anticipated distress must be applied. A peaceful death after cessation of life-prolonging therapies can be provided.

REFERENCES

1. Levy M, Tanios MA, Nelson D, et al. Outcomes of patients with do-not-intubate orders treated with noninvasive ventilation. Crit Care Med 2004;32:2002–2007.
2. Campbell ML, Carslon RW. Terminal weaning from mechanical ventilation: Ethical and practical considerations. Am J Crit Care 1992;1:52–56.
3. Campbell ML, Thill MC. Impact of patient consciousness on the intensity of the do-not-resuscitate therapeutic plan. Am J Crit Care 1996;5(5):339–345.
4. Prendergast TJ, Luce JM. Increasing incidence of withholding and withdrawal of life support from the critically ill. Am J Respir Crit Care Med 1997;155(1):15–20.
5. Meisel A. The legal consensus about foregoing life-sustaining treatment: Its status and its prospects. Kennedy Inst Ethics J 1993;2:309–335.
6. Campbell ML. How to withdraw mechanical ventilation: A systematic review of the literature. AACN Adv Crit Care 2007;18(4):397–403.
7. Ankrom M, Zelesnick L, Barofsky I, Georas S, Finucane TE, Greenough WB 3rd. Elective discontinuation of life-sustaining mechanical ventilation on a chronic ventilator unit. J Am Geriatr Soc 2001;49(11):1549–1554.
8. Mayer SA, Kossoff SB. Withdrawal of life support in the neurological intensive care unit. Neurology 1999;52(8):1602–1609.
9. Campbell ML, Bizek KS, Thill M. Patient responses during rapid terminal weaning from mechanical ventilation: A prospective study. Crit Care Med 1999;27(1):73–77.
10. Chan JD, Treece PD, Engelberg RA, et al. Narcotic and benzodiazepine use after withdrawal of life support: Association with time to death? Chest 2004;126:286–293.
11. Daly BJ, Thomas D, Dyer MA. Procedures used in withdrawal of mechanical ventilation. Am J Crit Care 1996;5:331–338.

12. Faber-Langendoen K, Bartels DM. Process of forgoing life-sustaining treatment in a university hospital: An empirical study. Crit Care Med 1992;20(5):570–577.

13. O'Mahony S, McHugh M, Zallman L, Selwyn P. Ventilator withdrawal: Procedures and outcomes. J Pain Symptom Manage 2003;26:954–961.

14. Rocker GM, Heyland DK, Cook DJ, Dodek PM, Kutsogiannis DJ, O'Callaghan CJ. Most critically ill patients are perceived to die in comfort during withdrawal of life support: A Canadian multicentre study. Can J Anesth 2004;51:623–630.

15. Hospital conditions of participation about organ/tissue donation. Available at: http://www.cms.gov/manuals/downloads/som107ap_a_hospitals.pdf (accessed November 6, 2008).

16. Kirchhoff KT, Conradt KL, Anumandla PR. ICU nurses' preparation of families for death of patients following withdrawal of ventilator support. Appl Nurs Res 2003;16(2):85–92.

17. Kirchhoff KT, Faas AI. Family support at end of life. AACN Adv Crit Care 2007;18(4):426–435.

18. Catlin A, Carter B. Creation of a neonatal end-of-life palliative care protocol. J Perinatol 2002;22(3):184–195.

19. American Thoracic Society. Dyspnea. Mechanisms, assessment, and management: A consensus statement. American Thoracic Society. Am J Respir Crit Care Med 1999;159(1):321–340.

20. Campbell ML. Terminal dyspnea and respiratory distress. Crit Care Clin 2004;20(3):403–417.

21. Campbell ML. Fear and pulmonary stress behaviors to an asphyxial threat across cognitive states. Res Nurs Health 2007;30(6):572–583.

22. Rushton C, Terry PB. Neuromuscular blockade and ventilator withdrawal: Ethical controversies. Am J Crit Care 1995;4:112–115.

23. Truog RD, Burns JP. To breathe or not to breathe. J Clin Ethics 1994;5(1):39–42.

24. Truog RD, Campbell ML, Curtis JR, et al. Recommendations for end-of-life care in the intensive care unit: A consensus statement by the American College of Critical Care Medicine. Crit Care Med 2008;36(3):953–963.

25. Campbell ML. Psychometric testing of a respiratory distress observation scale. J Palliat Med 2008;11(1):44–50.

26. Campbell ML, Templin T, Walch J. Psychometric testing of a revised respiratory distress observation scale. J Palliat Med 2009;10:881–884.

27. Campbell ML. Treating distress at the end of life: The principle of double effect. AACN Adv Crit Care 2008;19(3):340–344.

28. Partridge JC, Wall SN. Analgesia for dying infants whose life support is withdrawn or withheld. Pediatrics 1997;99(1):76–79.

29. Germain MJ, Cohen LM, Davison SN. Withholding and withdrawal from dialysis: What we know about how our patients die. Semin Dial 2007;20(3):195–199.

30. USRDS 2008 Annual Data Report: Atlas of End-Stage Renal Disease in the United States. National Institutes of Health, National Institute Diabetes and Digestive and Kidney Diseases, 2008. Available at: www.usrds.org/adr.htm (accessed November 20, 2008).

31. Davison SN, Jhangri GS, Holley JL, Moss AH. Nephrologists' reported preparedness for end-of-life decision-making. Clin J Am Soc Nephrol 2006;1(6):1256–1262.

32. Kurella M, Covinsky KE, Collins AJ, Chertow GM. Octogenarians and nonagenarians starting dialysis in the United States. Ann Intern Med 2007;146(3):177–183.

33. Cohen LM, Moss AH, Weisbord SD, Germain MJ. Renal palliative care. J Palliat Med 2006;9(4):977–992.

34. Dinwiddie LC. Insight into the ESRD Workgroup Final Report Summary on end-of-life care. Nephrol Nurs J 2003;30(1):58.

35. Final Report Summary on End of Life Care: Recommendations to the Field. Promoting Excellence, 2002. Available at: www.promotingexcellence.org (accessed November 1, 2008).

36. Holley JL, Davison SN, Moss AH. Nephrologists' changing practices in reported end-of-life decision-making. Clin J Am Soc Nephrol 2007;2(1):107–111.

37. Germain MJ, Cohen LM. Maintaining quality of life at the end of life in the end-stage renal disease population. Adv Chronic Kidney Dis 2008;15(2):133–139.

38. Jablonski A. Level of symptom relief and the need for palliative care in the hemodialysis population. J Hosp Palliat Nurs 2007;9(1):50–60.

39. Weisbord SD, Fried LF, Arnold RM, et al. Prevalence, severity, and importance of physical and emotional symptoms in chronic hemodialysis patients. J Am Soc Nephrol 2005;16(8):2487–2494.

40. Davison SN, Jhangri GS. The impact of chronic pain on depression, sleep, and the desire to withdraw from dialysis in hemodialysis patients. J Pain Symptom Manage 2005;30(5):465–473.

41. Murtagh FE, Addington-Hall J, Higginson IJ. The prevalence of symptoms in end-stage renal disease: A systematic review. Adv Chronic Kidney Dis 2007;14(1):82–99.

42. Rettig RA, Levinsky NG. Kidney Failure and the Federal Government. Washington, D.C.: National Academy Press, 1991.

43. Cohen LM, Germain MJ, Poppel DM. Practical considerations in dialysis withdrawal: "To have that option is a blessing". JAMA 2003;289(16):2113–2119.

44. Cohen LM, Germain M, Poppel DM, Woods A, Kjellstrand CM. Dialysis discontinuation and palliative care. Am J Kidney Dis 2000;36(1):140–144.

45. Levy J. End of life. In: Chambers EJ, Germain M, Brown E, eds. Supportive Care for the Renal Patient. New York: Oxford University Press, 2004:247–261.

46. McDade-Montez EA, Christensen AJ, Cvengros JA, Lawton WJ. The role of depression symptoms in dialysis withdrawal. Health Psychol 2006;25(2):198–204.

47. Moss AH. Kidney failure. In: Emanuel LL, Librach SL, eds. Palliative Care: Core Skills and Clinical Competencies. Philadelphia: Saunders Elsevier, 2007:355–369.

48. Holley JL. A single-center review of the death notification form: Discontinuing dialysis before death is not a surrogate for withdrawal from dialysis. Am J Kidney Dis 2002;40(3):525–530.

49. Dean M. Opioids in renal failure and dialysis patients. J Pain Symptom Manage 2004;28(5):497–504.

50. Gorman L. Renal. In: Coyne P, ed. Compendium of Treatment of End Stage Non-cancer Diagnoses. Dubuque, IA: Kendall/Hunt Publishing Company, 2005:19–20.

51. Cohen LM, Poppel DM, Cohn GM, Reiter GS. A very good death: Measuring quality of dying in end-stage renal disease. J Palliat Med 2001;4(2):167–172.

52. Holley JL. Palliative care in end-stage renal disease: Illness trajectories, communication, and hospice use. Adv Chronic Kidney Dis 2007;14(4):402–408.

53. Murray AM, Arko C, Chen SC, Gilbertson DT, Moss AH. Use of hospice in the United States dialysis population. Clin J Am Soc Nephrol 2006;1(6):1248–1255.

54. Lewis WR, Luebke DL, Johnson NJ, Harrington MD, Costantini O, Aulisio MP. Withdrawing implantable

defibrillator shock therapy in terminally ill patients. Am J Med 2006;119(10):892–896.

55. McCullough LB, Richman BW, Jones JW. Withdrawal of life-sustaining low-burden care. J Vasc Surg 2005;42(1):176–177.

56. Saul L. Cardiac resynchronization therapy. Crit Care Nurs Q 2007;30(1):58–66.

57. Bramstedt KA. Elective inactivation of total artificial heart technology in non-futile situations: Inpatients, outpatients and research participants. Death Stud 2004;28(5):423–433.

58. Lipman HI. Deactivation of advanced lifesaving technologies. Am J Geriatr Cardiol 2007;16(2):109–111.

59. Stevenson LW, Desai AS. Selecting patients for discussion of the ICD as primary prevention for sudden death in heart failure. J Card Fail 2006;12(6):407–412.

60. Grassman D. EOL considerations in defibrillator deactivation. Am J Hosp Palliat Care 2005;22(3):179; author reply, 80.

61. Braun TC, Hagen NA, Hatfield RE, Wyse DG. Cardiac pacemakers and implantable defibrillators in terminal care. J Pain Symptom Manage 1999;18(2):126–131.

62. Nambisan V, Chao D. Dying and defibrillation: A shocking experience. Palliat Med 2004;18(5):482–483.

63. Quill TE, Barold SS, Sussman BL. Discontinuing an implantable cardioverter defibrillator as a life-sustaining treatment. Am J Cardiol 1994;74(2):205–207.

64. Nemeh HW, Smedira NG. Mechanical treatment of heart failure: The growing role of LVADs and artificial hearts. Cleve Clin J Med 2003;70(3):223–226, 9–33.

65. MacIver J, Ross HJ. Withdrawal of ventricular assist device support. J Palliat Care 2005;21(3):151–156.

# III
# Psychosocial Support

# 29

*Mary Ersek and Valerie T. Cotter*

# The Meaning of Hope in the Dying

*Every time life asks us to give up a desire, to change our direction or redefine our goals; every time we lose a friend, break a relationship, or start a new plan, we are invited to widen our perspectives and to touch, under the superficial waves of our daily lives, the deeper currents of hope.—Henri Nouwen[1]*

♦ **Key Points**
♦ *Hope is a key factor in coping with and finding meaning in the experience of lifethreatening illness.*
♦ *People with life-threatening illness and their families do not invariably lose hope; in fact, hope can increase at the end of life.*
♦ *Nurses can implement evidence-based practices to foster and sustain hope for patients and families at the end of life.*
♦ *Nurses need to understand and respect individual variations in hope processes to provide sensitive, effective care to patients and their families at the end of life.*

Hope has long been recognized as fundamental to the human experience. Many authors have contemplated hope, extolling it as a virtue and an energy that brings life and joy.[2–4] Fromm[3] called hope "a psychic commitment to life and growth." Some authors assert that life without hope is impossible.[4]

Despite its positive connotations, hope is intimately bound with loss and suffering. As the French philosopher Gabriel Marcel[2] observed, "Hope is situated within the framework of the trial." It is this paradox that manifests itself so fully at the end of life.

Indeed, the critical role that hope plays in human life takes on special meaning as death nears. The ability to hope often is challenged, and it can elude patients and families during terminal illness. Hope for a cure is almost certainly destroyed, and even a prolonged reprieve from death is unlikely. Many patients and families experience multiple losses as they continue an illness trajectory that is marked by increasing disability and pain.

Even when hope appears to be strong within the dying person or the family, it can be problematic if hopefulness is perceived to be based on unrealistic ideas about the future.[5,6] Tension grows within relationships as people become absorbed in a struggle between competing versions of reality. Important issues may be left unresolved as individuals continue to deny the reality of impending death.

Despite these somber realities and the inevitable suffering, many people do maintain hope as they die, and families recover and find hope even within the experience of loss. How can this be? Part of the reason lies in the nature of hope itself—its resiliency and capacity to coexist with suffering. As witnesses to suffering and hope, palliative care nurses must understand these complexities and be confident and sensitive in their efforts to address hope and hopelessness in the people for whom they care.

To assist palliative care nurses, this chapter explores the many dimensions of hope and identifies its possible influence on health and quality of life. Nursing assessment and strategies to foster hope are described. In addition, specific issues such as "unrealistic hopefulness" and cultural considerations in the expression and maintenance of hope are discussed. The goals of the chapter are to provide the reader with an understanding about this complex but vital phenomenon; to offer guidance in the clinical application of this concept to palliative nursing care; and to explore some of the controversies about hope that challenge clinicians.

## Definitions and Dimensions of Hope

Hope is an important concept for many disciplines, including philosophy, theology, psychology, nursing, and medicine. Many authors have attempted to define hope and describe its attributes.[7-9] Some authors are more successful than others in capturing its complexity. A classic nursing theory of hope, developed by Karin Dufault[8,10] and based on qualitative research involving elderly people with cancer, is particularly notable in its comprehensiveness. Dufault[8] described hope as "a multidimensional, dynamic life force characterized by a confident yet uncertain expectation of achieving a future good which, to the hoping person, is realistically possible and personally significant." Dufault also theorized that hope has two interrelated spheres: particularized and generalized. *Particularized hope* is centered and dependent on specific, valued goals or hope objects. An example is the hope of a terminally ill patient to live long enough to celebrate a particular holiday or event. In contrast, *generalized hope* is a broader, nonspecific sense of a more positive future that is not directly related to a particular goal or desire. Dufault likened this sphere to an umbrella that creates a diffuse, positive glow on life.

Dufault postulated six dimensions of hope: affective, spiritual, relational, cognitive, behavioral, and contextual. The *affective* dimension of hope encompasses a myriad of emotions. Of course, hope is accompanied by many positive feelings, including joy, confidence, strength, and excitement. The full experience of hope, however, also includes uncertainty, fear, anger, suffering, and, sometimes, despair.[2,11-14] The philosopher Gabriel Marcel, for example, argued that in its fullest sense hope could only follow an experience of suffering or trial.[2] Marcel's thesis is corroborated by the experiences described by people with cancer who see their disease as "a wake-up call" that has opened their eyes to a greater appreciation for life and an opportunity for self-growth—in other words, an event that has forced them to confront their mortality while also inspiring hope.[15] The *spiritual* dimension is a central component of hope.[16-19] Hopefulness is associated with spiritual well-being,[18,20,21] and qualitative studies have shown that spirituality and spiritual practices provide a context in which to define hope and articulate hope-fostering activities.[7,8,22-24] These activities include religious beliefs and rituals but extend to broader conceptualizations of spirituality that encompass meaning and purpose in life, self-transcendence, and connectedness with a deity or other

life-force.[19,25] Although spirituality is almost always viewed as a hope-fostering influence, serious illness and suffering can challenge one's belief and trust in a benevolent deity, or be viewed as punishment from God; either interpretation of suffering can result in hopelessness.[26]

*Relationships* with significant others are another important dimension of hope. Interconnectedness with others is cited as a source of hope in virtually every study, and physical and psychological isolation from others is a frequent threat to hope.[7,27-29] Hope levels are positively associated with social support.[30-33] In addition to family members and friends, patients also have identified nurses as having a significant influence on hope.[34,35] Harris et al.[29] reported that the HIV peer-counseling relationships inspired hope in both the counseling recipients and their counselors. Despite being vital sources of hope, other people can threaten a patient's hope by distancing themselves from the patient, showing disrespect, discounting the patient's experiences, disclosing negative information, or withholding information.[36,37]

The *cognitive* dimension of hope encompasses many intellectual strategies, particularly those involving specific goals that require planning and effort to attain. Identifying goals can motivate and energize people, thereby increasing hope.[38,39] When identifying goals, people assess what they desire and value within a context of what is realistically possible. They appraise the resources necessary to accomplish their goals against the resources that are available to them. They then take action to secure the resources or meet the goals, and they decide on a reasonable time frame in which to accomplish the goals.[38,39] Active involvement in one's situation and attainment of goals increases the sense of personal control and self-efficacy, which, in turn, increases hope.[38,40] If a person repeatedly fails to attain valued goals, hopelessness and passivity can result.[38,39]

The *behavioral*, goal-focused thoughts and activities that foster hope are similar to the problem-focused coping strategies originally described by Lazarus and Folkman.[41] This similarity is not surprising, because hope is strongly associated with coping.[31,42] Hope has been identified as a foundation or mediator for successful coping, a method of coping, and an outcome of successful coping.[31,42] Many strategies that people use to maintain hope have been previously identified as coping methods, and models of maintaining hope overlap substantially with models of coping.[5,7,38,39] Strategies to maintain hope include problem-focused coping methods (e.g., setting goals, actively managing symptoms, getting one's affairs in order) and emotion-focused strategies (e.g., using distraction techniques, appraising the illness in nonthreatening ways).[5,7,38]

*Contextual* dimensions of hope are the life circumstances and abilities that influence hope—for example, physical health, financial stability, and functional and cognitive abilities. Common threats to hope include acute, chronic, and terminal illness; cognitive decline; fatigue; pain; and impaired functional status.[43-46] These factors, particularly physical illness and impairment, do not inevitably decrease hope if people are able to overcome the threat through cognitive, spiritual, relational, or other strategies.

## Influence of Hope and Hopelessness on Adaptation to Illness

Hope influences health and adaptation to illness. Empirical evidence indicates that diminished hope is associated with poorer quality of life,[47,48] increased severity of suicidal intent,[44,48] and higher incidence of suicide.[44,48,49] Hopelessness also increases the likelihood that people will consider physician-assisted death as an option for themselves.[50,51] If hopelessness occurs, anxiety and depression can result.[45,47,30] Lower levels of hope also are associated with lower self-esteem.[32,33,52]

In addition to its influence on psychological states and behaviors, there is some evidence to suggest that hope affects physical states as well. Researchers have found associations between hope and neuro-endocrine function.[53–55] Berg et al.[56] reported that hope was positively associated with pain tolerance. Decreased hope is associated with a worse prognosis in several patient populations.[57–59]

## Variations in Hope Among Different Populations

The preceding description of hope is derived from studies involving diverse populations, including children, adolescents, older adults, and adults with early-stage dementia. In addition, research has been conducted in inpatient, outpatient, and community settings with well persons and those with a variety of chronic and life-threatening illnesses. The experiences of families also have been described. Over these diverse populations and settings, many core concepts have been identified that transcend specific groups. However, some subtle but important differences exist. For this reason, hopefulness in selected populations is addressed in the following sections.

### Hope in Children and Adolescents

A few investigators have examined hope in pediatric populations. In an early study, Wright and Shontz[60] studied hope in children with chronic disabilities, and in the significant adults in their lives (e.g., parents, teachers, physical therapists). Both the children and the adults were interviewed, allowing for the identification of differences between the two samples. The investigators found that hope for the children in their study was two-dimensional. Hoping involved (1) an awareness of the positive and (2) a sense of time orientation. For younger children, hope was present-focused, whereas hope in older children had a future orientation. Younger children also saw adults as being in control of a situation, and were less concerned about assessing how realistic their particular hopes were. In contrast, adults actively assessed the realities of the present and possibilities for the future.

Artinian[61] explored hope in older children, aged 10 to 20 years, who underwent bone marrow transplantation. The findings suggested that ways to reduce stress and instill hope among younger patients and their parents include managing physical discomforts, making children and parents feel cared for, being nonjudgmental when children and parents vent anger, preventing boredom, and assisting with making and altering plans.

A program of research by Hinds and colleagues elucidated the experience of hoping in adolescents.[9,34,62–64] These investigators conducted studies in well adolescents, adolescents undergoing inpatient treatment for substance abuse, and adolescents with cancer. Based on qualitative studies, Hinds defined adolescent hopefulness as "the degree to which an adolescent possesses a comforting or life-sustaining, reality-based belief that a positive future exists for self and others."[9] Interestingly, inclusion of the phrase "and others" arose from the sample of adolescent cancer patients. Hinds found that only in this sample did adolescents express a concern and articulate their hopes for others. Examples of this attribute included such hopes as "My parents will be O.K. if I die," and "There will be a cure soon so patient 'X' will not die."[9] This ability to go beyond oneself and hope for others may be influenced by the adolescents' sense of mortality that accompanies the cancer diagnosis.[9]

Despite the stress of life-threatening illness, many adolescents are able to remain hopeful. Ritchie[52] examined hopefulness and self-esteem in 45 adolescents with cancer. She found that the average hopefulness and self-esteem scores for her sample were as high as those for healthy adolescents. Moreover, high self-esteem was an important predictor of hopefulness. These results suggest that teens are able to respond to serious illness with intact self-esteem and hope.

### Hope and Older Adults

Numerous studies have examined hope in ill and healthy older adults.[10,21,22,43,65,66] Findings from these studies suggest that certain hope-related themes and factors take on special significance for this age group. For example, religious beliefs and spiritual well-being are strongly associated with hope in elders;[21] these factors also were prominent themes in qualitative studies.[10,43,66] Common health-related factors, such as impaired physical functioning, poor physical health, decreased mobility, fatigue, and cognitive impairment, are negatively associated with hope in older adults.[43,46,66,67] Although chronic illness that impairs physical functioning is linked with decreased hope, diagnosis of a life-threatening disease, such as cancer, is not associated with low levels of hope.[68] This finding may reflect an attitude among older adults that the quality of life that remains matters more than the quantity.

Among younger European American adults, hope tends to be tied to being productive; personal and professional achievements figure prominently in one's ability to nurture and maintain hope. In contrast, older adults are more likely to focus on spirituality, relationships, leaving a legacy focused on others, and other factors that are not linked with accomplishment.[22,66,69] Hope-fostering activities include reminiscing, participating in purposeful volunteer activities, religious activities, and connecting with others.

## Hope in People with Dementia

Studies of people in the moderate and severe stages of dementia suggest that hope can still exist and thrives within the context of a caring relationship.[65,70] Cutcliffe and Grant have drawn attention to the importance of the interpersonal aspects of hope in dementia, and suggest that nurses inspire and instill hope through humanistic practice, pragmatic knowledge, interpersonal relations, organization, and planning.[65] Hope is central to the adjustment process in early-stage dementia when trying to maintain a sense of normalcy, and in developing cognitive, social and behavioral strategies to improve confidence.[71,72] Religion or spirituality provides solace by inspiring feelings of hope, strength, security, or guidance to help cope with the effects of early stage dementia.[6] Hope in the afterlife and a renewal of spiritual interests and influences can be important resources for people with Alzheimer's disease (AD).[6] Ostwald, Duggleby, and Hepburn[73] found that hope surfaced when individuals were talking about their own deaths, concerns about the quality of remaining life, and the effects of the disease on family. Hoping for a cure or medication that would stabilize dementia is self-protective, and attempts to maintain a sense of self and normality.[74,75] Uncertainty about the future produces faith that ongoing research and new treatments could provide alternative futures.[76] Not being "pessimistic," and seeking a perspective about dementia that focuses on abilities as well as impaired abilities, maximizes coping strategies.[77,72] Hope is evident in the coping process when individuals make comparisons to others with dementia in the later stages and recognize that there will be inevitable decline in the future.[71,78]

Individuals with early stage dementia develop specific strategies, such as diaries, calendars, lists, notes, written instructions, reminders on sticky-backed notes, colored labels, alarms, and systematic files of correspondence—not to eradicate the problems, but to offer some hope.[71] Rather than focusing on how the disease will get worse, individuals and caregivers look for ways to be useful, and find support from participating in research and community activities.[71,73,79,80] Finding adaptations to daily living and developing strategies and new activities builds hope for the future.[71,77]

CASE STUDY
### Dr. L, A Patient with Early Stage AD

Dr. L, a 56-year-old married man and a well respected physician, was diagnosed nine months ago with early stage AD by a neurologist at a teaching institution. For several months, he had experienced difficulty calculating drug doses and relied heavily on a trusted nurse for assistance with his patients. His wife noticed personality changes and suspected depression. Six months ago he reluctantly retired from his medical practice at the urging of his neurologist and his wife. He and his wife reached out to the Alzheimer's Association for information and support and joined an eight-week specialized support group program for individuals with early-stage dementia and their caregivers.

Dr. L's hope developed as he became aware of the impact of the diagnosis on his identity as a physician and husband. With his profound sense of loss, he was active in making changes, sought feedback, and verbalized his anger and negative feelings within the small support group and among his family. Dr. L's hope was influenced by his anticipation that a cure was possible for AD. He positively influenced his own hope by organizing a team of 25 individuals who participated in the Alzheimer's Association Memory Walk to raise thousands of dollars for research and education. He and his wife adapted by finding new activities for him while she worked as a teacher, such as more involvement with running the household and auditing a community college course. The specialized support group assisted the couple with strategies to compensate and adapt to daily living, and enabled them to reappraise and reconstruct their individual self-concepts and their identity as a couple.

## Hope from the Family Caregiver's Perspective

Family caregivers are an integral component in palliative care. Patients and families influence each other's hope, and nursing interventions must focus on both groups. Often, the physical and psychological demands placed on family caregivers are great, as are threats to hope.[81–83] Threats to hope in caregivers include isolation from support networks, questioning of one's spiritual beliefs; concurrent losses, including loss of significant others, health, and income; and inability to control the patient's symptoms. Holtslander and Duggleby[84] reported that difficulties in communicating with health care providers, feelings of depersonalization, and receipt of "too many negative messages" also eroded caregivers' hope. Caregivers with poor health status, high fatigue, multiple losses, and sleep disturbances were significantly less hopeful than caregivers without these problems.[83]

Herth[83] reported that as death became imminent, the need "to do" for the patient was replaced by a wanting simply "to be" with the patient. In addition, little emphasis was placed on the "future" in caregivers' descriptions of hope.[83]

Strategies to maintain hope in family caregivers are similar to those found in patients, with a few differences. Spending time with others in the support network was very important for caregivers. In addition, being able to reprioritize demands helped caregivers conserve much-needed energy. Caregivers also maintained hope through engaging in relaxing activities, such as listening to or playing music, or gardening.[83] Obtaining respite from the caregiving role also promoted hope.[84]

## Hope in Terminally Ill Patients: Is Hope Compatible with Death?

Research demonstrates that many people are able to maintain hope during acute and chronic illness. Hope also can thrive during the terminal phase of an illness, despite the realization that no cure is possible. In one study, the hope in terminally ill patients and their caregivers actually increased over time as death neared.[24,83]

Although hope levels may not decrease, the nature of hope often is altered through the dying process. Hope tends to be defined more in terms of "being" rather than "doing."[35,85] Other changes in hope at the end of life include an increased focus on relationships and trusting in others, as well as a desire to leave a legacy and to be well remembered.[10,22,86] Spirituality also increases in importance during the terminal phases of illness. In a study of 160 terminally ill patients, decreased spiritual well-being was significantly associated with hopelessness.[87] People also adopt specific strategies to foster hope at the end of life.[24,39,86,88] Many of these approaches are summarized in Table 29–1.

Although hope tends to change in people with terminal illness, maintaining a delicate balance between acceptance of death and hope for a cure often remains an important task up until the time of death, even when people acknowledge that cure is virtually impossible.[39,86] The dying person also needs to envision future moments of happiness, fulfillment, and connection. For example, Benzein and colleagues[86] reported that people with life-threatening illness needed to dream about possibilities and situations even if the imagined events and goals were unlikely to occur. As one of their participants related,[86]

> Sometimes I let myself imagine that I'll live until Christmas and sometimes in the night I lie and think about where to put the tree. I know it's silly but it feels good to think about myself sitting there by the tree with everyone...a lovely picture.

## Multicultural Views of Hope

Over the past three decades, understanding of the clinical phenomenon of hope has increased dramatically through theoretical discourse and empirical investigation. Although knowledge regarding the components, processes, and outcomes of hope has grown dramatically, progress in multicultural research on hope has been limited. The samples in many studies that examine hope or hopelessness are ethnically homogeneous,[22,23,31] or their ethnic composition is

---

**Table 29–1**

**Sources of Hope/Hope-Fostering Strategies in Terminally Ill Adults**

- Having one or more meaningful, shared relationships in which one feels a sense of "being needed" or "being a part of something."
- Maintaining a feeling of lightheartedness; feeling delight, joy, or playfulness and communicating that feeling; using humor.
- Recalling joyous, meaningful events.
- Having one's individuality acknowledged, accepted, and honored; having one's worth affirmed by others.
- Identifying positive personal attributes such as courage, determination, serenity.
- Having spiritual beliefs and engaging in spiritual practices that provide a sense of meaning for their suffering.
- Focusing attention and effort on the short-term future.
- Thinking about and directing efforts at specific, short-term attainable aims (earlier in terminal illness).
- Thinking about global, positive aims that are focused on others (e.g., support for the bereaved, happiness for their children) (later in terminal illness).
- Desiring serenity, inner peace, eternal rest (last days and weeks of life).

*Source:* Adapted from Herth (1990), reference 24.

---

unknown.[38,86] The studies that do include ethnically diverse samples are small,[89–91] precluding any comparisons or generalization of findings.

Several excellent European studies have contributed greatly to the general understanding of hope.[11,13,86,92–96] However, many of these investigations use frameworks and instruments developed by U.S. researchers whose work is founded on homogeneous samples. Moreover, it may be that hopefulness for Europeans is more similar to that of middle-class Americans than it is different.

Some descriptive research using translations of instruments developed by North American investigators has been conducted in Korean and Taiwanese cancer patients.[45,94,97–99] Although findings from these studies generally are consistent with those conducted in the United States and Canada, discrete differences may reflect cultural dissimilarities. For example, Lin and associates[98] hypothesized that cultural differences in physicians' willingness to disclose a cancer diagnosis may have contributed to changes in hope levels in Taiwanese cancer patients.

Farone and colleagues[100] examined the associations among locus of control, negative affect, hope, and self-reported health in 109 older Mexican-American women with cancer. They found that hope and internal locus of control both showed significant associations with better health outcomes. Although these findings are similar to those for white, nonHispanic samples, the authors cautioned that they were unable to explore the characteristics of control that may be unique to Latina populations. They recommended that future research include attribution of control based on religious beliefs and the concept of *fatalismo* (fatalism).

Despite the growing body of research in diverse samples, existing research may not adequately reflect the experience of hope for people from nonEuropean cultures. Several known cultural differences could certainly limit the applicability of current conceptualizations of hope, especially within the palliative care context. Three issues that theoretically could have a major impact on multicultural views of hope are time orientation, truth-telling, and one's beliefs about control.

Time orientation is identified as a cultural phenomenon that varies among cultural groups. Some cultural groups, particularly those within the Euro-American culture, tend to be future oriented. Within these groups, people prefer to look ahead, make short- and long-term plans, and organize their schedules to meet goals.[101] Because hope is defined as being future-oriented, with hopeful people more likely to identify and take action to meet goals, members of these future-oriented cultures may possibly appear more hopeful than people who are predominantly present-focused. On the other hand, people who are more focused on the present may be better able to sustain hope at the end of life, when the ability to create long-range goals is hindered by the uncertainty surrounding a terminal diagnosis. Additional research is needed to clarify these relationships.

The value for truth-telling in Western health care systems also may affect hope. Current ethical and legal standards require full disclosure of all relevant health care information to patients.[102] Informed consent and patient autonomy in medical decision-making, two eminent values in American health care, are impossible without this disclosure.[102] Although few would advocate lying to patients, truth-telling is not universally viewed as helpful or desirable.[103,104] In some cultures, it is believed that patients should be protected from burdensome information that could threaten hope. Truthful, but blunt, communication may also be seen as rude and disrespectful in some cultures, and the feeling of being devalued and disrespected has a negative impact on hope. In addition to the threats to hope that frank discussion is believed to engender, people who prefer nondisclosure of threatening information may be seen as attempting to cling to unrealistic hopes by refusing to listen to discouraging facts about their condition.

A third cultural concept that may affect hope is one's feeling of being in control. As described earlier, control is a core attribute in many conceptualizations of hope. Although control can be relinquished to others, including health care providers or a transcendent power, personal control often is central to the hoping process. In Euro-American cultures, applying one's will and energy to alter the course of an illness or to direct the dying process seems natural and desirable. Advance directives are one culturally sanctioned way in which members of these societies exert control over the dying process.[105] However, this desire for and belief in personal control

is not a common feature in many other cultures. In cultures where death is viewed as part of the inherent harmony of living and dying, attempts to exert any influence over the dying process may seem unnatural or inappropriate.[106] People from diverse cultures who take a more passive role in their health care, or who do not espouse a desire to control their illness or the dying process, may be viewed as less hopeful than people who manifest a "fighting spirit" and active stance.

More research is needed to test theories of hope in multicultural groups, both to ensure the appropriate application of current conceptualizations to diverse cultural groups, and to develop new theories that are relevant for these groups. Until this work is done, palliative care clinicians must be cautious in applying current hope theories, and sensitive to the possible variations in diverse populations.

## Models of Maintaining Hope for People with Life-Threatening Illnesses

Many investigators have identified factors that foster hope, and strategies that enable people to sustain hope despite life-threatening or chronic illness. Although there is considerable concordance across these studies regarding many of the major themes, various models emphasize different styles and strategies that demonstrate the diversity in hope-fostering approaches.

As described previously, many people with terminal illness turn to activities and coping strategies that cultivate generalized hope rather than an emphasis on achievement and control. These strategies reflect a sense of peace and acceptance of death, and center on "being" rather than "doing." These strategies are described in Table 29–1.

In contrast, some models focus more on active, goal-oriented or problem-solving strategies. One model[15,23] emphasizes that maintaining hope requires a dynamic interplay, or dialectic, between two types of hope-sustaining strategies: "Dealing With It" and "Keeping It In Its Place." "Dealing With It" is defined as the process of confronting the negative possibilities inherent in the illness experience, including death, and allowing the full range of thoughts, behaviors, and emotions resulting from the recognition. "Keeping It In Its Place" is defined as the process of managing the impact of the disease and its treatment by controlling one's response to the disease, prognosis, and therapy (Table 29–2). This model underscores the complex and sometimes contradictory nature of sustaining hope through serious illness. People use multiple strategies that allow them to confront and to avoid the negative aspects of illness and death. Although the strategies used to manage the threat of death often seem to predominate, these activities occur within a background of recognition and acknowledgment of the possibility of death. This process of negotiating between acknowledgment and management of these fears has been identified in other studies of people with life-threatening illnesses.[11,14,40]

**Table 29–2**
**Structure of "Keeping It In Its Place": Hope-Maintaining Strategies in People with Life-Threatening Illness**

I. **Appraising the illness in a nonthreatening manner**
  A. Seeing the disease/treatment as a challenge or a test
  B. Seeing the disease/treatment as a positive influence
    1. Reprioritizing one's life
    2. Becoming altruistic
    3. Looking at the bright side

II. **Managing the cognitions related to the illness experience**
  A. Joking about it
  B. Avoiding thinking or talking about the negative
  C. Keeping distracted
  D. Forgetting about it
  E. Not dwelling on it
  F. Focusing on loved ones

III. **Managing the emotional response to the illness experience**
  A. Limiting the emotional response
  B. Severing the cognitive from the emotional response
  C. Shifting from one emotion to another
  D. Translating emotional pain into physical pain

IV. **Managing the sense of control**
  A. Maintaining control
    1. Getting information/staying informed
    2. Restraining the disease through exercise, diet, and stress management
    3. Decisional control—making decisions about treatment or other aspects of life to exert control
  B. Relinquishing control
    1. To a deity
    2. To the medical and nursing staffs
    3. To medical science

V. **Taking a stance toward the illness and treatment**
  A. Fighting the illness
    1. "Go down fighting"
    2. Imagining the illness as the enemy or an evil being
  B. Accepting the illness
    1. "It's God's will"
    2. "It's just part of the process"
    3. Expecting the disease/death

VI. **Managing uncertainty**
  A. Minimizing the uncertainty
    1. "Knowing" the future
    2. "Having to believe"
  B. Maximizing the uncertainty
    1. "They (the physicians) could always be wrong"
    2. "I'm not a statistic!"—beating the odds

VII. **Managing the focus on the future**
  A. Living day to day
  B. Focusing on long-term goals
    1. Making mutable goals
    2. Establishing interim goals
    3. Using previously met goals as a source of hope
    4. Using unmet goals as a source of hope

VIII. **Managing the view of the self in relation to the illness**
  A. Minimizing the illness and the treatment
    1. "It (the disease) is just a flaw in my system"
    2. "It (the therapy) is just a temporary inconvenience"
  B. Maximizing personal strength
    1. Identifying personal attributes of strength
    2. Making downward comparisons with others (e.g., "At least I don't have AIDS")
    3. Focusing on successful others
    4. Identifying a history of personal strength

*Source*: Adapted from Ersek (1991), reference 15, and Ersek (1992), reference 23, with permission.

Gum and Snyder[39] elaborated a model of hoping that emphasizes the need for people to set goals and take action to achieve them. Although some people continue to search for a cure after receiving a terminal diagnosis, most people eventually accept their prognosis and mourn the loss of their original goals. At this point, they need to develop and pursue alternative goals that are possible in light of their diminished physical function, end-of-life symptoms, and loss of energy.

These different approaches for maintaining hope are important to describe and understand because they assist the palliative care nurse in designing effective strategies to foster hope. They increase clinicians' awareness regarding the various ways that people respond to chronic and terminal illness, and guide clinicians in their interactions with patients and families to sustain hope. They also help palliative care providers understand difficult or troubling responses, such as unrealistic hopefulness.

## The Issue of Unrealistic Hopefulness

Reality surveillance is a feature of many conceptualizations of hope. Often, clinicians, researchers, and theorists believe that mentally healthy people should choose and work toward realistic goals. In these frameworks, adhering to unrealistic hopes or denying reality is a sign of maladaptive cognitions that could lead to negative health outcomes. Therefore, denial and unrealistic hopes and ideas are discouraged and treated as pathological.[5,6]

Clinical examples of unrealistic hopes that cause consternation are numerous and diverse. For instance, one patient with advanced cancer might hope that his persistent severe sciatica is from exercise and overuse rather than spinal metastases. The nurse working with this patient may continually contradict his theory, asserting that his denial of the probable malignant cause of the pain will delay effective treatment. Another patient might insist that a new cure for her illness is imminent, causing distress for the nurse, who believes that the patient's unrealistic hopes will hinder acceptance of and preparation for death.

Despite these concerns, however, some investigators argue that the nurses' fears may be unfounded. This perspective is based on studies conducted over the past few decades, which have led social psychologists to question the view that denial and unrealistic hopes are always maladaptive. Instead, these researchers argue that human interpretation of information from the environment is inherently biased and inaccurate.[6,39,40]

Shelley Taylor and colleagues developed this idea further in their theory of positive illusions, which is based on an extensive program of research spanning more than two decades.[55,107-109] They describe positive illusions as general, and enduring cognitive patterns involving error and/or bias, that provide a foundation for successful adaptation to many threatening events, including serious illness. Especially important are unrealistically positive evaluations of the self, exaggerated perceptions of control, and unrealistic optimism about the future.[110] They support their theory with empirical evidence that denial and positive illusions often are associated with positive outcomes, such as better psychological adjustment to illness, less physical and emotional distress, and even decreased mortality.[40,55,109,111]

Snyder and colleagues[112] also take issue with the idea that "false hopes" are maladaptive. They argue that people should not be discouraged from striving for goals that seem "too lofty." Citing numerous studies, Snyder et al. provide evidence that hopeful people with ambitious goals (1) are motivated and engerized to achieve them; this activity may protect against discouragment and depression; (2) often demonstrate flexibilty in their thinking, finding new ways to achieve the goal; and (3) may be able to endure increased stress.

In addition to promoting positive outcomes, unrealistic hopes need to be assessed within the context of uncertainty. For instance, people frequently respond to dire prognostic news with the observation that they can always "beat the odds." Given that no one can predict the future with absolute certainty, it is impossible to predict which individuals with a 2% chance of remission or recovery will actually be cured. So, if a person hopes for something in the future that appears highly unlikely, can it be known for certain that it will not occur? Patients and families often need to focus on this uncertainty to sustain hope.[14,23] Research supports the idea that patients' and families' hopes and goals are effective coping strategies, even when the likelihood of obtaining them seems remote.[112]

A third argument against aggressive "reality orientation" for all patients and families is the evidence that unrealistic hopes and illusions often are abandoned over time and without intensive intervention from professionals.[10,109,110] In other words, most people acknowledge and accept distressing information, but need to do so on their own schedules.

The preceding discussion may seem to imply that clinicians should not be concerned about unrealistic hopefulness. Of course, that is not the case. Despite their adaptive

| Table 29–3 |
| --- |
| **Assessing Unrealistic Hopes** |
| 1. Is the focus of the unrealistic hope broad or severe (e.g., complete denial of a disease that has been documented)? |
| 2. Is the persistence of the unrealistic hope severe, i.e., does it persist despite multiple pieces of information from multiple sources (e.g., family, physicians, nurses) that the hope is unlikely to be realized? |
| 3. Is the person's adherence to the unrealistic hope *complete*, or does the person admit at times that there are limitations and acknowledge negative possibilities? Does the person continually use words such as "knowing" what will happen, rather than acknowledging that what he or she hopes for might *not* occur? |
| 4. Does the hope cause the person to engage in reckless behaviors? |
| 5. Does the hope cause the person to ignore warning signs (e.g., angina, increased pain) that should be treated promptly? |
| 6. Does the hope cause great distress for family members and significant others? |
| 7. Has the person become isolated from others, either to avoid their challenges to the unrealistic hope or because others are uncomfortable in responding to the person? |
| 8. Does it appear that adhering to the hope actually is causing distress and anxiety for the person (who may tacitly doubt or disbelieve in the illusion or hope, but is afraid to discuss that possibility with others)? |
| 9. Is death imminent, and the unrealistic hopefulness is hindering efforts to get affairs in order, say good-bye, or receive emotional support? |

potential, illusions and denial may result in adverse outcomes. For example, unrealistic hopes may lead parents to insist on aggressive, futile therapy that increases their child's suffering without curing or controlling the disease. Similarly, a person who denies that his illness is terminal may isolate himself from his family to protect his beliefs and avoid contradictory opinions. Unfortunately, in these cases and others, there is insufficient research to inform clinicians fully regarding situations that are potentially maladaptive, and even less guidance about appropriate therapeutic strategies. However, evidence exists that some situations should be viewed with caution and may indicate a need for gentle interventions, such as offering alternative hopes or providing skillful counseling. Table 29–3 lists several questions regarding unrealistic hopes. If the answer to any of these question is "Yes," then further assessment and possible intervention may be necessary.

## Assessing Hope

As in all nursing care, thorough assessment of physical and psychosocial factors must precede thoughtful planning and implementation of therapeutic strategies. Therefore, consistent and comprehensive evaluations of hope should be included in the palliative nursing assessment. Some conceptual elements of hope, such as those focusing on meaning and purpose in life, are included in a spiritual assessment. Rarely, however, are comprehensive guides to assessing hope included in standardized nursing assessment forms.

The guidelines produced by Farran, Wilken, and Popovich[113] for the clinical assessment of hope appropriately use the acronym HOPE to designate the major areas of evaluation: The areas are Health, Others, Purpose in Life, and Engaging Process. The term "engaging process" refers to identifying goals, taking actions to achieve goals, sense of control over one's situation, and identifying hope-inspiring factors in one's past, present, and future. In Table 29–4, this framework has been adapted and applied to terminally ill patients. It includes examples of questions and probes that can be used to assess hope.

Like pain, hope is a subjective experience and assessment should focus on self-report. However, behavioral cues can also provide information regarding a person's state of hope or hopelessness. Hopelessness is a central feature of depression; therefore, behaviors such as social withdrawal, flat affect, alcohol and substance abuse, insomnia, and passivity may indicate hopelessness.

As discussed earlier, the patient's terminal illness affects the hope of family caregivers, who, in turn, influence the hope of the patients. Therefore, the hope of the patient's family caregivers and other significant support people also should be assessed.

Over the past decades, researchers from several disciplines have developed instruments to measure hope and hopelessness. The theoretical and empirical literature documents the comprehensiveness and face validity of these tools. Advances in psychometric theory and methods have allowed the evaluation of multiple dimensions of validity and reliability. The development and use of well-designed and well-tested tools has contributed greatly to the science of hope. Although a thorough discussion of these measures is beyond the scope of this chapter, Table 29–5 provides a brief description of several widely used and tested instruments. More complete descriptions and evaluations of these scales can be found elsewhere.[114,115]

## Nursing Interventions to Maintain Hope at End of Life

Clinicians, theorists, and researchers recognize that nurses play an important role in instilling, maintaining, and restoring hope in people for whom they care. Researchers have identified many ways in which nurses assist patients and families to sustain hope in the face of life-threatening illness. Table 29–6 provides a summary of nursing approaches to instill hope. A brief perusal of this table reveals an important point about these strategies: For the most part, nursing care to maintain patients' and families' hope fundamentally is about providing excellent physical, psychosocial, and spiritual palliative care. There are few unique interventions to maintain hope, and yet there is much nurses can do. Because hope is inextricably connected to virtually all facets of the illness experience—including physical pain, coping, anxiety, and spirituality—improvement or deterioration in one area has repercussions in other areas. Attending to these relationships reminds clinicians that virtually every action they take can influence hope, negatively or positively.

Another vital observation about hope-inspiring strategies is that many approaches begin with the patient and family. The experience of hope is a personal one, defined and determined by the hoping person. Although others greatly influence that experience, ultimately the meanings and effects of words and actions are determined by the person experiencing hope or hopelessness. Many approaches used by people with life-threatening illness to maintain hope are strategies initiated with little influence from others. For example, some people pray; others distract themselves with television watching, conversation, or other activities; and many patients use cognitive strategies, such as minimizing negative thoughts, identifying personal strengths, and focusing on the positive. For many patients and families, careful observation and active support of an individual's established strategies to maintain hope will be most successful.

A final point is to remind the reader that family caregivers and other support people should be included in these approaches. Ample evidence exists that patients and people within their support systems reciprocally influence one another's hope. In addition, family and significant others are always incorporated into the palliative care plan and considered part of the unit of care. Maintenance of hope also is a goal after death, in that hope-restoring and -maintaining strategies must be an integral part of bereavement counseling.[116,117]

## Specific Interventions

The framework for the following discussion is adapted from Farran, Herth, and Popovich,[7] who articulated four central attributes of hope: experiential, spiritual/transcendent, relational, and rational thought. These areas encompass the major themes found in the literature, and although they are not mutually exclusive, they provide a useful organizing device. This section also includes a brief discussion of ways in which nurses need to explore and understand their own hopes and values in order to provide palliative care that fosters hope in others.

### Experiential Process Interventions

The experiential process of hope involves the acknowledgment and acceptance of suffering, while at the same time using the imagination to move beyond the suffering and find hope.[91] Included in these types of strategies are methods to decrease physical suffering and cognitive strategies aimed at managing the threat of the terminal illness.

**Table 29-4**
**Guidelines for the Clinical Assessment of Hope in Palliative Care**

| Interview Question/Probe | Rationale |
|---|---|
| **Health (and symptom management)** | |
| 1. Tell me about your illness. What is your understanding of the probable course of your illness? | Explore the person's perceptions of seriousness of his or her illness, and possible trajectories |
| 2. How hopeful are you right now, and how does your illness affect your sense of hope? | Determine the person's general sense of hope and the effect of the terminal illness on hope |
| 3. How well are you able to control the symptoms of your illness? How do these symptoms affect your hope? | Uncontrolled end-of-life symptoms have been found to negatively influence hope |
| **Others** | |
| 1. Who provides you with emotional, physical, and spiritual support? | Identify people in the environment that provide support and enhance hope |
| 2. Who are you most likely to confide in when you have a problem or concern? | Identify others in whom the person has trust |
| 3. What kinds of difficulty experiences have you and your family/partner/support network had to deal with in the past? How did you manage those experiences? | Explore experiences of coping with stressful situations |
| 4. What kinds of things do family, support people, health care providers do that make you more hopeful? Less hopeful? | Identify specific behaviors that affect hope and recognize that other people can also decrease hope |
| **Purpose in life** | |
| 1. What gives you hope? | Identify relationships, beliefs, and activities that provide a sense of purpose and contribute positively to hope |
| 2. What helps you make sense of your situation right now? | Identify the ways in which the person makes meaning of difficult situations. |
| 3. Do you have spiritual or religious practices or support people who help you? If "yes", what are these practices people? | Identify if and how spirituality acts as a source of hope |
| 4. Has your illness caused you to question your spiritual beliefs? If "yes," how? | Terminal illness can threaten the person's basic beliefs and test one's faith |
| 5. How can we help you maintain these practices and personal connections with spiritual support people? | Identify ways in which clinicians and others can support spiritual practices that enhance hope |
| **Goals** | |
| 1. Right now, what are your major goals? | Identify major goals and priorities |
| | Examine whether these goals are congruent with the views of others |
| 2. What do you see are the chances that you will meet these goals? | Explore how realistic the person thinks the goals are; if the goals are not perceived as being attainable, assess the impact on hope |
| 3. What actions can you take to meet these goals? | Identify specific actions the person can take to meet the goals |
| 4. What actions have you already taken to meet these goals? | Identify how active the person has been in attaining the goals |
| 5. What resources do you have for meeting these goals? | Determine other resources to which the person has access for the purpose of attaining goals |
| **Sense of control** | |
| 1. Do you feel that you have much control over your current situation? | Determine if the person feels any ability to control or change the situation |
| | Explore whether the person wants to have more control |
| 2. Are there others that you feel have some control over your current situation? If "yes," who are they and in what ways do they have control? | Determine if the person feels as though trusted others (e.g., health-care providers, family, deity) can control or change the situation |
| **Sources of hope over time** | |
| 1. In the past, what or who has made you hopeful? | Identify sources of hope from the person's past that may continue to provide hope during the terminal phase |
| 2. Right now who and what provides you with hope? | Identify current sources of hope |
| 3. What do you hope for in the future? | Assess generalized and specific hopes for the future |

*Source*: Adapted from Farran, Wilken, and Popovich (1992), reference 113; Farran, Herth and Popovich (1995), reference 7.

**Table 29–5**
**Descriptions of Selected Instruments to Measure Hope and Hopelessness**

| Instrument Name | Brief Description | Selected References |
|---|---|---|
| Beck Hopelessness Scale | • 20-item, true-false format | 44, 49, 129, 130 |
| | • Based on Stotland's definition of hopelessness: system of negative expectancies concerning oneself and one's future | 87 |
| | • Developed to assess psychopathological levels of hopelessness; correlates highly with attempted and actual suicide | 131–135 |
| Herth Hope Index | • 12-item, 4-point Likert scale; total score is sum of all items; range of scores 12–48 | 136 |
| | • Designed for well and ill populations | 16, 24, 45, 83, 92, 97, 125, 137–141 |
| | • Assesses three overlapping dimensions: (1) cognitive-temporal, (2) affective-behavioral, (3) affiliative-behavioral | 142 |
| | • Spanish, Thai, Chinese, Swedish translations available | |
| Hopefulness Scale for Adolescents (Hinds) | • 24-item visual analog scale | 143 |
| | • Assesses the degree of the adolescent's positive future orientation | 63 |
| | • Assesses only the relational and rational thoughts processes of hope | 52 |
| | • Tested in several populations of adolescents: well, substance abusers, adolescents with emotional and mental problems, cancer patients | 64, 144 |
| Miller Hope Scale | • 40-item scale, 5-point Likert scale | 145 |
| | • Assesses 10 elements: (a) mutuality/ affiliation, (b) avoidance of absolutizing, (c) sense of the possible, (d) psychological well-being and coping, (e) achieving goals, (f) purpose and meaning in life, (g) reality surveillance-optimism, (h) mental and physical activation, (i) anticipation, (j) freedom | 92 |
| | | 33 |
| | | 146 |
| | | 147 |
| | | 32 |
| | • Chinese and Swedish versions | 148 |
| Snyder Hope Scale | • 12-item, 4-point Likert scale | 115, 128, 149–154 |
| | • Based on Stotland's definition of hope; focus is on goals identification and achievement | |
| | • Tested in healthy adults, and adults with psychiatric illness | |
| | • Also has developed tool to measure hope in children | |

Uncontrolled symptoms, such as pain, fatigue, dyspnea, and anxiety, cause suffering and challenge the hopefulness of patients and caregivers. Timely and adept symptom prevention and management is central to maintaining hope. In home-care settings, teaching patients and families the knowledge and skills to manage symptoms confidently and competently also is essential.

Other ways to help people find hope in suffering is to provide them a cognitive reprieve from their situation. One powerful strategy to achieve this temporary suspension is through humor. Humor helps put things in perspective and frees the self, at least momentarily, from the onerous burden of illness and suffering. Making light of a grim situation brings a sense of control over one's response to the situation, even when one has little influence over it. Of course, the use of humor with patients and families requires sensitivity as well as a sense of timing. The nurse should take cues from the patient and family, observe how they use humor to dispel stress, and let them take the lead in joking about threatening information and events. In general, humor should be focused on oneself or on events outside the immediate concerns of the patient and family.

Other ways to move people cognitively beyond their suffering is to assist them in identifying and enjoying that which is joyful in life. Engagement in aesthetic experiences, such as watching movies or listening to music that is uplifting, can enable people to transcend their suffering. Sharing one's own hope-inspiring stories also can help.

Another strategy is to support people in their own positive self-talk. Often people naturally cope with stress by comparing themselves with people they perceive to be less fortunate or by identifying attributes of personal strength that help them find hope.[29,118] For example, an elderly, married woman with advanced breast cancer may comment that, despite the seriousness of her disease, she feels luckier than another woman with the same disease who is younger or without social support. By comparing herself with less fortunate others, she can take solace in recognizing that "things could be worse." Similarly, a person can maintain hope by focusing on particular talents or previous accomplishments that indicate an ability to cope with illness. In one study, a woman asserted that her ability to survive an abusive marriage gave her hope that she could cope with and manage her illness and treatment.[15] People may also cite their high level of motivation as a reason to feel hopeful about the future. Acknowledgment and validation of these attributes supports hope and affirms self-worth for patients and families.

**Table 29–6**
**Nursing Actions to Foster Hope**

**Experiential processes**
- Prevent and manage end-of-life symptoms
- Use lightheartedness and humor appropriately
- Encourage the patient and family to transcend their current situation
- Encourage aesthetic experiences
- Encourage engagement in creative and joyous endeavors
- Suggest literature, movies, and art that are uplifting and highlight the joy in life
- Encourage reminiscing
- Assist patient and family to focus on present and past joys
- Share positive, hope-inspiring stories
- Support patient and family in positive self-talk

**Spiritual/transcendent processes**
- Facilitate participation in religious rituals and spiritual practices
- Make necessary referrals to clergy and other spiritual support people
- Assist the patient and family in finding meaning in the current situation
- Assist the patient/family to keep a journal
- Suggest literature, movies, and art that explore the meaning of suffering

**Relational processes**
- Minimize patient and family isolation
- Establish and maintain an open relationship
- Affirm patients' and families' sense of self-worth
- Recognize and reinforce the reciprocal nature of hopefulness between patient and support system
- Provide time for relationships (especially important in institutional settings)
- Foster attachment ideation by assisting the patient to identify significant others and then to reflect on personal characteristics and experiences that endear the significant other to the patient
- Communicate one's own sense of hopefulness

**Rational thought processes**
- Assist patient and family to establish, obtain, and revise goals without imposing one's own agenda
- Assist in identifying available and needed resources to meet goals
- Assist in procuring needed resources; assist with breaking larger goals into smaller steps to increase feelings of success
- Provide accurate information regarding patient's condition and treatment in a skillful and sensitive manner
- Facilitate reality surveillance as appropriate
- Help patient and family identify past successes
- Increase patients' and families' sense of control when possible

## Spiritual Process Interventions

Several specific strategies can foster hope while incorporating spirituality. These strategies include providing opportunities for the expression of spiritual beliefs and arranging for involvement in religious rituals and spiritual practices.

Assisting patients and families to explore and make meaning of their trials and suffering is another useful approach. Encouraging patients and families to keep a journal of thoughts and feelings can help people in this process. Suggesting books, films, or art that focuses on religious or existential understanding and transcendence of suffering is another effective way to help people make sense of illness and death.

Palliative care nurses also should assess for signs of spiritual distress and make appropriate referrals to clergy and other professionals with expertise in counseling during spiritual and existential crises. Other spiritual and existential strategies are described in Chapters 30, 31 and 32 of this text.

### Relational Process Interventions

To maximize hope, nurses should establish and maintain an open relationship with patients and members of their support network, taking the time to learn what their priorities and needs are and then addressing those needs in timely, effective ways. Demonstrating respect and interest, and being available to listen and be with people—that is, affirming each person's worth—are essential.

Fostering and sustaining connectedness among the patient, family, and friends can be accomplished by providing time for uninterrupted interactions, which is especially important in institutional settings. Nurses can increase hope by enlisting help from others to help achieve goals. For example, recruiting friends or arranging for a volunteer to transport an ill person to purchase a gift for a grandchild can cultivate hope for everyone involved. It is important to help others realize how vital they are in sustaining a person's hope.

### Rational Thought Process Interventions

The rational thought process is the dimension of hope that specifically focuses on goals, resources, personal control and self-efficacy, and action. Interventions related to this dimension include assisting patients and families in devising and attaining goals. Providing accurate and timely information about the patient's condition and treatment helps patients and families decide which goals are achievable. At times, gentle assistance with monitoring and acknowledging negative possibilities helps the patient and family to choose realistic goals. Helping to identify and procure the resources necessary to meet goals also is important.

Often, major goals need to be broken into smaller, shorter-term achievements. For example, a patient with painful, metastatic lung cancer might want to attend a family event that is 2 weeks away. The successful achievement of this goal depends on many factors, including adequate pain control, transportation, and ability to transfer to and from a wheelchair. By breaking the larger goal into several smaller ones, the person is able to identify all the necessary steps and resources. Attainment of a subgoal, such as being able to transfer with minimal assistance, can empower patients and families and help energize them to reach more difficult and complex goals.[112]

Supporting patients and families to identify those areas of life and death in which they do have real influence can increase self-esteem and self-efficacy, thereby instilling hope. It also helps to review their previous successes in attaining important goals.

This domain also includes ways in which clinicians balance the need to communicate "bad news" while sustaining patients' and families' hope. The difficulties inherent in delivering negative information to patients and families does not release us from our duty to communicate openly and honestly; however, it does require that palliative care nurses and other clinicians communicate skillfully in ways that assist patients and families to sustain hope. There are many articles describing empirically-derived methods for delivering bad news sensitively and communicating in ways that maintain hope.[119-122] More information about communication can be found in Chapter 5.

## Programs to Enhance Hopefulness

In addition to discrete actions that individual nurses take to foster hope, several investigators have developed and tested programs to enhance hope in people with life-threatening illness.

Herth[91,123] designed and tested a Hope Intervention Program (HIP), which she evaluated in a sample of people with recurrent cancer. Based on her empirically-derived theory of hope, the intervention consisted of eight sessions delivered in a nurse-facilitated group setting. Six sessions focused on strategies that specifically addressed the four hope processes: experiential, relational, spiritual/transcendent, and rational thought. During the final session, participants developed an individual plan with strategies to maintain and foster hope. When Herth tested this intervention, she found significantly increased hope levels in the treatment group compared with two control groups. These significant differences persisted at the 3-, 6-, and 9-month follow-up measurements.[123]

Recently, Cantrell and Conte[124] adapted the HIP for internet use and conducted a pilot test with six female survivors of childhood cancer. This innovative delivery method showed promise as a strategy to bridge geographic distances, and may appeal to individuals who are more comfortable communicating online.

Duggleby and colleagues[125] evaluated the effectiveness of the *Living with Hope Program* (LWHP), a brief intervention designed for older adults with advanced cancer receiving home-based palliative care services. Grounded in their earlier research,[22] the LWHP is a one-week intervention consisting of a visit from a trained assistant, a copy of the film "Living with Hope," and a choice of one of three hope-focused activities. The investigators found that compared to the control group, LWHP participants reported greater hope and existential quality of life one week following the intervention. The LWHP also has been pilot-tested in a sample of 10 family caregivers, and results suggest that the program may increase hope and quality of life in this group.[126]

Hinds and colleagues developed a Psychosocial Research–Translation Team to integrate evidence-based hope intervention guidelines into the cancer care department at St. Jude Children's Hospital.[127] Using this innovative approach, the multidisciplinary team reviewed the literature on hope and interviewed experts on the topic. The team used this information to develop its own definition of hope and to identify potential projects aimed at translating the evidence-based guidelines on hope into practice. These projects included (1) adding information about hope to the parent handbook; (2) developing patient, parent, and staff educational sheets about hope; (3) developing a telephone hotline that allows for the efficient and personal delivery of messages of hope to callers; and (4) designing and launching websites about hope. This program demonstrates the creative and diverse approaches that health care providers can use to support and promote hope among patients and families facing life-threatening illnesses.

## Ensuring the Self-Knowledge Necessary to Provide Palliative Care

Providing holistic palliative care requires a broad range of skills. Astute management of physical symptoms and a solid command of technical skills must be matched with an ability to provide psychosocial and spiritual care for patients and families at a time of great vulnerability. To nurture these latter skills, nurses should continually reflect on and evaluate their own hopes, beliefs, and biases and identify how these factors influence their care. In an intriguing study, investigators examined the relationship between nurses' hope and their comfort in caring for and communicating with dying children and their families. They found that, after controlling for number of years in nursing, nurses' hope and hours of palliative care education both were significantly associated with comfort in caring for dying children and their families.[128] These findings underscore the importance of education as well as self-reflection in delivering compassionate, skilled palliative care. In providing high quality care, nurses also should evaluate how they are affected by patients' and families' responses and strategies to maintain hope. For example, does it anger or frustrate the nurse that the patient seems to refuse to acknowledge that his or her disease is incurable? Is this anger communicated nonverbally or verbally to the patient or family? In addition to self-reflection, it is important for palliative care nurses to remain hopeful while working with dying patients by engaging in self-care activities.

## Summary

Hope is central to the human experience of living and dying, and it is integrally entwined with spiritual and psychosocial well-being. Although terminal illness can challenge and even temporarily diminish hope, the dying process does not inevitably bring despair. The human spirit, manifesting its creativity and resiliency, can forge new and deeper hopes at the end of life. Palliative care nurses play important roles in supporting patients and families with this process by providing expert physical, psychosocial, and spiritual care. Sensitive, skillful attention to maintaining hope can enhance quality of life and contribute significantly to a "good death" as defined by the patient and family. Fostering hope is a primary means by which palliative care nurses accompany patients and families on the journey through terminal illness.

REFERENCES

1. Nouwen H, Gaffney W. Aging. New York: Image Books, 1990.
2. Marcel G. Homo viator: Introduction to the metaphysic of hope. New York: Harper and Row, 1962.
3. Fromm E. The Revolution of Hope. New York: Bantam Books, 1968.
4. Menninger K. Hope. Bull Menninger Clin 1987;51(5):447–462.
5. Ersek M. Examining the process and dilemmas of reality negotiation. Image J Nurs Sch 1992;24(1):19–25.
6. Snyder CR, Rand KL. The case against false hope. Am Psychol 2003;58(10):820–822; authors' reply 823–824.
7. Farran CJ, Herth KA, Popovich JM. Hope and Hopelessness: Critical Clinical Constructs. Thousand Oaks, CA: Sage Publications, 1995.
8. Dufault K, Martocchio B. Hope: Its spheres and dimensions. Nurs Clin North Am 1985;20:379–391.
9. Hinds PS. Adolescent hopefulness in illness and health. Adv Nurs Sci 1988;10(3):79–88.
10. Dufault K. Hope of Elderly Persons with Cancer [Unpublished dissertation]. Cleveland: Case Western Reserve University, 1981.
11. Kylma J, Vehvilainen-Julkunen K, Lahdevirta J. Hope, despair and hopelessness in living with HIV/AIDS: A grounded theory study. J Adv Nurs 2001;33(6):764–775.
12. Morse JM, Penrod J. Linking concepts of enduring, uncertainty, suffering, and hope. Image J Nurs Sch 1999;31(2):145–150.
13. Kylma J, Vehvilainen-Julkunen K, Lahdevirta J. Dynamically fluctuating hope, despair and hopelessness along the HIV/AIDS continuum as described by caregivers in voluntary organizations in Finland. Issues Ment Health Nurs 2001;22(4):353–377.
14. De Graves S, Aranda S. Living with hope and fear—the uncertainty of childhood cancer after relapse. Cancer Nurs July-August 2008;31(4):292–301.
15. Ersek M. The Process of Maintaining Hope in Adults with Leukemia Undergoing Bone Marrow Transplantation [Doctoral dissertation]. Seattle: University of Washington, 1991.
16. Herth KA. The relationship between level of hope and level of coping response and other variables in patients with cancer. Oncol Nurs Forum 1989;16(1):67–72.
17. Cutcliffe J, Herth K. The concept of hope in nursing 2: Hope and mental health nursing. Br J Nurs 2002;11(13):885–889.
18. Gibson LM. Inter-relationships among sense of coherence, hope, and spiritual perspective (inner resources) of African-American and European-American breast cancer survivors. Appl Nurs Res 2003;16(4):236–244.
19. Haase JE, Britt T, Coward DD, Leidy NK, Penn PE. Simultaneous concept analysis of spiritual perspective, hope, acceptance and self-transcendence. Image J Nurs Sch 1992;24(2):141–147.
20. Carson V, Soeken KL, Shanty J, Terry L. Hope and spiritual well-being: Essentials for living with AIDS. Perspect Psychiatr Care 1990;26(2):28–34.
21. Fehring RJ, Miller JF, Shaw C. Spiritual well-being, religiosity, hope, depression, and other mood states in elderly people coping with cancer. Oncol Nurs Forum 1997;24(4):663–671.
22. Duggleby W, Wright K. Transforming hope: How elderly palliative patients live with hope. Can J Nurs Res June 2005;37(2):70–84.
23. Ersek M. The process of maintaining hope in adults undergoing bone marrow transplantation for leukemia. Oncol Nurs Forum 1992;19(6):883–889.
24. Herth K. Fostering hope in terminally-ill people. J Adv Nurs 1990;15(11):1250–1259.
25. Fanos JH, Gelinas DF, Foster RS, Postone N, Miller RG. Hope in palliative care: From narcissism to self-transcendence in amyotrophic lateral sclerosis. J Palliat Med April 2008;11(3):470–475.
26. Borneman T, Brown-Saltzman K. Meaning in illness. In: Ferrell B, Coyle N, eds. Textbook of Palliative Nursing. New York: Oxford University Press, 2001:415–424.
27. Cutcliffe JR, Herth K. The concept of hope in nursing 1: Its origins, background and nature. Br J Nurs 2002;11(12):832–840.
28. Crothers MK, Tomter HD, Garske JP. The relationships between satisfaction with social support, affect balance, and hope in cancer patients. J Psychosoc Oncol 2005;23(4):103–118.
29. Harris GE, Larsen D. HIV peer counseling and the development of hope: Perspectives from peer counselors and peer counseling recipients. AIDS Patient Care STDS 2007;21(11):843–859.
30. Johnson JG, Alloy LB, Panzarella C, Metalsky GI, Rabkin JG, Williams JBW, Abramson LY. Hopelessness as a mediator of the association between social support and depressive symptoms: Findings of a study of men with HIV. J Consult Clin Psychol 2001;69(6):1056–1060.
31. Ebright PR, Lyon B. Understanding hope and factors that enhance hope in women with breast cancer. Oncol Nurs Forum 2002;29(3):561–568.
32. Foote AW, Piazza D, Holcombe J, Paul P, Daffin P. Hope, self-esteem and social support in persons with multiple sclerosis. J Neurosci Nurs 1990;22(3):155–159.
33. Piazza D, Holcombe J, Foote A, Paul P, Love S, Daffin P. Hope, social support and self-esteem of patients with spinal cord injuries. J Neurosci Nurs 1991;23(4):224–230.
34. Hinds PS. Fostering coping by adolescents with newly diagnosed cancer. Semin Oncol Nurs 2000;16(4):317–327; discussion 328–336.
35. Herth KA, Cutcliffe JR. The concept of hope in nursing 3: Hope and palliative care nursing. Br J Nurs 2002;11(14):977–983.
36. Schmid Mast M, Kindlimann A, Langewitz W. Recipients' perspective on breaking bad news: How you put it really makes a difference. Patient Educ Couns September 2005;58(3):244–251.
37. Dias L, Chabner BA, Lynch TJ, Jr, Penson RT. Breaking bad news: A patient's perspective. Oncologist 2003;8(6):587–596.
38. Nekolaichuk CL, Jevne RF, Maguire TO. Structuring the meaning of hope in health and illness. Soc Sci Med 1999;48(5):591–605.
39. Gum AS, C.R. Coping with terminal illness: The role of hopeful thinking. J Palliat Med 2002;5(6):883–894.

40. Taylor SE, Kemeny ME, Reed GM, Bower JE, Gruenewald TL. Psychological resources, positive illusions, and health. Am Psychol 2000;55(1):99–109.

41. Lazarus RS, Folkman S. Stress, Appraisal, and Coping. New York: Springer Publishing, 1984.

42. Wineman NM, Schwetz KM, Zeller R, Cyphert J. Longitudinal analysis of illness uncertainty, coping, hopefulness, and mood during participation in a clinical drug trial. J Neurosci Nurs 2003;35(2):100–106.

43. Bays CL. Older adults' descriptions of hope after a stroke. Rehabil Nurs 2001;26(1):18–20.

44. Patten SB, Metz LM. Hopelessness ratings in relapsing-remitting and secondary progressive multiple sclerosis. Int J Psychiatry Med 2002;32(2):155–165.

45. Lin CC, Lai YL, Ward SE. Effect of cancer pain on performance status, mood states, and level of hope among Taiwanese cancer patients. J Pain Symptom Manage 2003;25(1):29–37.

46. Harwood DG, Sultzer DL. "Life is not worth living": Hopelessness in Alzheimer's disease. J Geriatr Psychiatry Neurol 2002;15(1):38–43.

47. Evangelista LS, Doering LV, Dracup K, Vassilakis ME, Kobashigawa J. Hope, mood states and quality of life in female heart transplant recipients. J Heart Lung Transplant 2003;22(6):681–686.

48. Sullivan MD. Hope and hopelessness at the end of life. Am J Geriatr Psychiatry 2003;11(4):393–405.

49. Beck AT, Brown G, Steer RA. Prediction of eventual suicide in psychiatric inpatients by clinical ratings of hopelessness. J Consult Clin Psychol 1989;57(2):309–310.

50. Wilson KG, Scott JF, Graham ID, et al. Attitudes of terminally ill patients toward euthanasia and physician-assisted suicide. Arch Intern Med 2000;160(16):2454–2460.

51. Breitbart W, Rosenfeld B, Pessin H, et al. Depression, hopelessness, and desire for hastened death in terminally ill patients with cancer. JAMA 2000;284(22):2907–2911.

52. Ritchie MA. Self-esteem and hopefulness in adolescents with cancer. J Pediatr Nurs 2001;16(1):35–42.

53. Segerstrom SC, Taylor SE, Kemeny ME, Fahey JL. Optimism is associated with mood, coping, and immune change in response to stress. J Pers Soc Psychol 1998;74(6):1646–1655.

54. Bower JE, Kemeny ME, Taylor SE, Fahey JL. Cognitive processing, discovery of meaning, CD4 decline, and AIDS-related mortality among bereaved HIV-seropositive men. J Consult Clin Psychol 1998;66(6):979–986.

55. Taylor SE, Lerner JS, Sherman DK, Sage RM, McDowell NK. Are self-enhancing cognitions associated with healthy or unhealthy biological profiles? J Pers Soc Psychol 2003;85(4):605–615.

56. Berg CJ, Snyder CR, Hamilton N. The effectiveness of a hope intervention in coping with cold pressor pain. J Health Psychol September 2008;13(6):804–809.

57. Watson M, Haviland JS, Greer S, Davidson J, Bliss JM. Influence of psychological response on survival in breast cancer: A population-based cohort study. Lancet 1999;354(9187):1331–1336.

58. Barefoot JC, Brummett BH, Helms MJ, Mark DB, Siegler IC, Williams RB. Depressive symptoms and survival of patients with coronary artery disease. Psychosom Med 2000;62(6):790–795.

59. Stern SL, Dhanda R, Hazuda HP. Hopelessness predicts mortality in older Mexican and European Americans. Psychosom Med 2001;63(3):344–351.

60. Wright BA, Shontz FC. Process and tasks in in hoping. Rehabil Lit 1968;29(11):322–331.

61. Artinian BM. Fostering hope in the bone marrow transplant child. Matern Child Nurs J 1984;13(1):57–71.

62. Hinds PS, Martin J, Vogel RJ. Nursing strategies to influence adolescent hopefulness during oncologic illness. J Assoc Pediatr Oncol Nurses 1987;4(1–2):14–22.

63. Hinds PS, Stoker HW. Adolescents' preferences for a scaling format: A validity issue. J Pediatr Nurs 1988;3(6):408–411.

64. Hinds PS, Quargnenti A, Fairclough D, et al. Hopefulness and its characteristics in adolescents with cancer. West J Nurs Res 1999;21(5):600–616; discussion 617–620.

65. Cutcliffe JR, Grant G. What are the principles and processes of inspiring hope in cognitively impaired older adults within a continuing care environment? J Psychiatr Ment Health Nurs 2001;8(5):427–436.

66. Herth K. Hope in older adults in community and institutional settings. Issues Ment Health Nurs 1993;14(2):139–156.

67. Farran CJ, McCann J. Longitudinal analysis of hope in community-based older adults. Arch Psychiatr Nurs 1989;3(5):272–276.

68. Esbensen BA, Swane CE, Hallberg IR, Thome B. Being given a cancer diagnosis in old age: A phenomenological study. Int J Nurs Stud 2008;45:393–405.

69. Herth KA, Cutcliffe JR. The concept of hope in nursing 4: Hope and gerontological nursing. Br J Nurs 2002;11(17):1148–1156.

70. Spector A, Orrell M. Quality of life (QoL) in dementia: A comparison of the perceptions of people with dementia and care staff in residential homes. Alzheimer Dis Assoc Disord 2006;20(3):160–165.

71. Clare L. We'll fight it as long as we can: Coping with the onset of Alzheimer's disease. Aging Ment Health May 2002;6(2):139–148.

72. Werczak L, Stewart N. Learning to live with early dementia. Can J Nurs Res 2002;34:67–85.

73. Ostwald SK, Duggleby W, Hepburn KW. The stress of dementia: View from the inside. Am J Alzheimers Dis Other Demen 2002;17(5):303–312.

74. Clare L. Managing threats to self: Awareness in early stage Alzheimer's disease. Soc Sci Med 2003;57:1017–1029.

75. Lindstrom HA, Smyth KA, Sami SA, et al. Medication use to treat memory loss in dementia: Perspectives of persons with dementia and their caregivers. Dementia 2006;5:27–50.

76. Pearce A, Clare L, Pistrang N. Managing sense of self: Coping in the early stages of Alzheimer's disease. Dementia 2002;1:173–192.

77. Pratt R, Wilkinson H. A psychosocial model of understanding the experience of receiving a diagnosis of dementia. Dementia 2003;2(2):181–199.

78. Harman G, Clare L. Illness representations and lived experience in early-stage dementia. Qual Health Res 2006;16(4):484–502.

79. Beard RL. In their voices: Identity preservation and experiences of Alzheimer's disease. J Aging Stud 2004;18:415–428.

80. Clare L, Roth I, Pratt R. Perceptions of change over time in early-stage Alzheimer's disease: Implications for understanding awareness and coping style. Dementia 2005;4(4):487–520.

81. Benzein EGB, A.C. The level of and relation between hope, hopelessness and fatigue in patients and family members in palliative care. Palliat Med 2005;19:234–240.

82. Borneman T, Stahl C, Ferrell BR, Smith D. The concept of hope in family caregivers of cancer patients at home. J Hosp Palliat Nurs 2002;4(1):21–33.

83. Herth K. Hope in the family caregiver of terminally ill people. J Adv Nurs 1993;18(4):538–548.

84. Holtslander LF, Duggleby W, Williams AM, Wright KE. The experience of hope for informal caregivers of palliative patients. J Palliat Care Winter 2005;21(4):285–291.

85. Nekolaichuk CL, Bruera E. On the nature of hope in palliative care. J Palliat Care 1998;14(1):36–42.

86. Benzein E, Norberg A, Saveman BI. The meaning of the lived experience of hope in patients with cancer in palliative home care. Palliat Med 2001;15(2):117–126.

87. McClain CS, Rosenfeld B, Breitbart W. Effect of spiritual well-being on end-of-life despair in terminally ill cancer patients. Lancet 2003;361(9369):1603–1607.

88. Herth K. Contributions of humor as perceived by the terminally ill. Am J Hosp Care 1990;7(1):36–40.

89. Herth K. Hope from the perspective of homeless families. J Adv Nurs 1996;24(4):743–753.

90. Herth K. Hope as seen through the eyes of homeless children. J Adv Nurs 1998;28(5):1053–1062.

91. Herth KA. Development and implementation of a hope intervention program. Oncol Nurs Forum 2001;28(6):1009–1016.

92. Benzein E, Berg A. The Swedish version of Herth Hope Index—an instrument for palliative care. Scand J Caring Sci 2003;17(4):409–415.

93. Kylma J, Vehvilainen-Julkunen K, Lahdevirta J. Dynamics of hope in HIV/AIDS affected people: An exploration of significant others' experiences. Res Theory Nurs Pract 2003;17(3):191–205.

94. Lee EH. Fatigue and hope: Relationships to psychosocial adjustment in Korean women with breast cancer. Appl Nurs Res 2001;14(2):87–93.

95. Rustoen T, Hanestad BR. Nursing intervention to increase hope in cancer patients. J Clin Nurs 1998;7(1):19–27.

96. Rustoen T, Wiklund I, Hanestad BR, Moum T. Nursing intervention to increase hope and quality of life in newly diagnosed cancer patients. Cancer Nurs 1998;21(4):235–245.

97. Hsu TH, Lu MS, Tsou TS, Lin CC. The relationship of pain, uncertainty, and hope in Taiwanese lung cancer patients. J Pain Symptom Manage 2003;26(3):835–842.

98. Lin CC, Tsai HF, Chiou JF, Lai YH, Kao CC, Tsou TS. Changes in levels of hope after diagnostic disclosure among Taiwanese patients with cancer. Cancer Nurs 2003;26(2):155–160.

99. Chen ML. Pain and hope in patients with cancer: A role for cognition. Cancer Nurs 2003;26(1):61–67.

100. Farone DW, Fitzpatrick TR, Bushfield SY. Hope, locus of control, and quality of health among elder latina cancer survivors. Soc Work Health Care 2008;46(2):51–70.

101. Purnell L, Paulanka B. The Purnell Model for cultural competence. In: Purnell L, Paulanka B, eds. Transcultural Health Care: A Culturally Competent Approach (3rd ed). Philadelphia: F.A. Davis, 2008:8–39.

102. Beauchamp TL, Childress JF. Principles of Biomedical Ethics (6th ed). New York: Oxford University Press, 2009.

103. Shaw S. Exploring the concepts behind truth-telling in palliative care. Int J Palliat Nurs July 2008;14(7):356–359.

104. Oliffe J, Thorne S, Hislop TG, Armstrong EA. "Truth telling" and cultural assumptions in an era of informed consent. Fam Community Health January–March 2007;30(1):5–15.

105. Ersek M, Kagawa-Singer M, Barnes D, Blackhall L, Koenig BA. Multicultural considerations in the use of advance directives. Oncol Nurs Forum 1998;25(10):1683–1690.

106. Hepburn K, Reed R. Ethical and clinical issues with Native-American elders. End-of-life decision making. Clin Geriat Med 1995;11(1):97–111.

107. Taylor SE. Adjustment to threatening events: A theory of cognitive adaptation. Am Psychol 1983;38:1164–1171.

108. Taylor SE, Lichtman RR, Wood JV. Attributions, beliefs about cancer, and adjustment to breast cancer. J Pers Soc Psychol 1984;46:489–502.

109. Taylor SE. Positive Illusions: Creative Self-Deception and the Healthy Mind. New York: Basic Books, 1989.

110. Taylor SE, Brown JD. Illusion and well-being: A social psychological perspective on mental health. Psychol Bull 1988;103(2):193–210.

111. Gana K, Alaphilippe D, Bailly N. Positive illusions and mental and physical health in later life. Aging Ment Health 2004;8(1):58–64.

112. Snyder CR, Rand KL, King EA, Feldman DB, Woodward JT. "False" hope. J Clin Psychol 2002;58(9):1003–1022.

113. Farran CJ, Wilken C, Popovich JM. Clinical assessment of hope. Issues Ment Health Nurs 1992;13(2):129–138.

114. Stoner M. Measuring hope. In: Frank-Stromborg M, Olsen S, eds. Instruments for Clinical Health–Care Research (3rd ed). Boston: Jones and Bartlett, 2004:215–228.

115. Edwards LM, Rand KL, Lopez SJ, Snyder CR. Understanding hope: A review of measurement and construct validity research. In: Ong AD, Van Dulmen MHM, eds. Oxford Handbook of Methods of Positive Psychology. New York: Oxford University Press, 2007:83–95.

116. Holtslander L, Duggleby W. An inner struggle for hope: Insights from the diaries of bereaved family caregivers. Int J Palliat Nurs October 2008;14(10):478–484.

117. Holtslander LF. Caring for bereaved family caregivers: Analyzing the context of care. Clin J Oncol Nurs June 2008;12(3):501–506.

118. Taylor SE, Lobel M. Social comparison under threat: Downward comparisons and upward contacts. Psychol Rev 1989;96:569–575.

119. Casarett DJ, Quill TE. "I'm not ready for hospice": Strategies for timely and effective hospice discussions. Ann Intern Med March 20 2007;146(6):443–449.

120. Curtis JR, Engelberg R, Young JP, et al. An approach to understanding the interaction of hope and desire for explicit prognostic information among individuals with severe chronic obstructive pulmonary disease or advanced cancer. J Palliat Med 2008;11(4):610–620.

121. Barclay JS, Blackhall LJ, Tulsky JA. Communication strategies and cultural issues in the delivery of bad news. J Palliat Med 2007;10(4):958–977.

122. Robinson TM, Alexander SC, Hays M, et al. Patient-oncologist communication in advanced cancer: Predictors of patient perception of prognosis. Support Care Cancer 2008;16(9):1049–1057.

123. Herth K. Enhancing hope in people with a first recurrence of cancer. J Adv Nurs 2000;32(6):1431–1441.

124. Cantrell MA, Conte T. Enhancing hope among early female survivors of childhood cancer via the internet: A feasibility study. Cancer Nurs 2008;31(5):370–379.

125. Duggleby WD, Degner L, Williams A, et al. Living with hope: Initial evaluation of a psychosocial hope intervention for older palliative home care patients. J Pain Symptom Manage 2007;33(3):247–257.

126. Duggleby W, Wright K, Williams A, Degner L, Cammer A, Holtslander L. Developing a living with hope program for caregivers of family members with advanced cancer. J Palliat Care 2007;23(1):24–31.

127. Hinds PS, Gattuso JS, Barnwell E, et al. Translating psychosocial research findings into practice guidelines. J Nurs Adm 2003;33(7–8):397–403.

128. Feudtner C, Santucci G, Feinstein JA, Snyder CR, Rourke MT, Kang TI. Hopeful thinking and level of comfort regarding providing pediatric palliative care: A survey of hospital nurses. Pediatrics 2007;119(1):e186–e192.

129. Beck AT, Steer RA, Kovacs M, Garrison B. Hopelessness and eventual suicide: A 10-year prospective study of patients hospitalized with suicidal ideation. Am J Psychiatry 1985;142(5):559–563.

130. Beck AT, Weissman A, Lester D, Trexler L. The measurement of pessimism: The hopelessness scale. J Consult Clin Psychol 1974;42(6):861–865.

131. Mystakidou K, Parpa E, Tsilika E, Gennatas C, Galanos A, Vlahos L. How is sleep quality affected by the psychological and symptom distress of advanced cancer patients? Palliat Med 2009;23(1):46–53.

132. Bayat M, Erdem E, Gul Kuzucu E. Depression, anxiety, hopelessness, and social support levels of the parents of children with cancer. J Pediatr Oncol Nurs 2008;25(5):247–253.

133. Ellis J, Lin J, Walsh A, et al. Predictors of referral for specialized psychosocial oncology care in patients with metastatic cancer: The contributions of age, distress, and marital status. J Clin Oncol December 29, 2008;27:699–705.

134. McMillan D, Gilbody S, Beresford E, Neilly L. Can we predict suicide and non-fatal self-harm with the Beck Hopelessness Scale? A meta-analysis. Psychol Med 2007;37(6):769–778.

135. Dyce JA. Factor structure of the Beck Hopelessness Scale. J Clin Psychol 1996;52(5):555–558.

136. Herth K. Development and refinement of an instrument to measure hope. Sch Inq Nurs Pract 1991;5(1):39–51; discussion 53–36.

137. Buckley J, Herth K. Fostering hope in terminally ill patients. Nurs Stand 2004;19(10):33–41.

138. Herth K. Abbreviated instrument to measure hope: Development and psychometric evaluation. J Adv Nurs 1992;17(10):1251–1259.

139. Phillips-Salimi CR, Haase JE, Kintner EK, Monahan PO, Azzouz F. Psychometric properties of the Herth Hope Index in adolescents and young adults with cancer. J Nurs Meas 2007;15(1):3–23.

140. Sanatani M, Schreier G, Stitt L. Level and direction of hope in cancer patients: An exploratory longitudinal study. Support Care Cancer 2008;16(5):493–499.

141. Utne I, Miaskowski C, Bjordal K, Paul SM, Jakobsen G, Rustoen T. The relationship between hope and pain in a sample of hospitalized oncology patients. Palliat Support Care 2008;6(4):327–334.

142. Rustoen T, Wahl AK, Hanestad BR, Lerdal A, Miaskowski C, Moum T. Hope in the general Norwegian population, measured using the Herth Hope Index. Palliat Support Care 2003;1(4):309–318.

143. Hinds PS, Gattuso JS. Measuring hopefulness in adolescents. J Pediatr Oncol Nurs 1991;8(2):92–94.

144. Cantrell MA, Lupinacci P. A predictive model of hopefulness for adolescents. J Adolesc Health 2004;35(6):478–485.

145. Miller JF, Powers MJ. Development of an instrument to measure hope. Nurs Res 1988;37(1):6–10.

146. Jakobsson A, Segesten K, Nordholm L, Oresland S. Establishing a Swedish instrument measuring hope. Scand J Caring Sci 1993;7(3):135–139.

147. Canty-Mitchell J. Life change events, hope, and self-care agency in inner-city adolescents. J Child Adolesc Psychiatr Nurs 2001;14(1):18–31.

148. Brackney BE, Westman AS. Relationships among hope, psychosocial development, and locus of control. Psychol Rep 1992;70(3 Pt 1):864–866.

149. Snyder CR, Hoza B, Pelham WE, et al. The development and validation of the Children's Hope Scale. J Pediatr Psychol 1997;22(3):399–421.

150. Snyder CR, Harris C, Anderson JR, et al. The will and the ways: Development and validation of an individual-differences measure of hope. J Pers Soc Psychol 1991;60(4):570–585.

151. Rand KL. Hope and optimism: Latent structures and influences on grade expectancy and academic performance. J Pers 2009;77(1):231–260.

152. Cramer KM, Dyrkacz L. Differential prediction of maladjustment scores with the Snyder Hope subscales. Psychol Rep 1998;83(3 Pt 1):1035–1041.

153. Snyder CR, Sympson SC, Ybasco FC, Borders TF, Babyak MA, Higgins RL. Development and validation of the State Hope Scale. J Pers Soc Psychol 1996;70(2):321–335.

154. Brouwer D, Meijer RR, Weekers AM, Baneke JJ. On the dimensionality of the Dispositional Hope Scale. Psychol Assess 2008;20(3):310–315.

# 30    *Inge B. Corless*

# Bereavement

*What is it like to know you are dying? I will tell you. I just want to go—just to go out in a flash like a light. This knowing that the end is coming and of all I will leave behind is killing me. How do you say goodbye, let go? —A patient*

♦ ***Key Points***
♦ *Bereavement is the state of having lost a significant other.*
♦ *Loss is a generic term indicating the absence of a current or future possession or relationship.*
♦ *Grief is the emotional response to loss.*
♦ *Mourning encompasses the death rituals engaged in by the bereaved.*

On December 20, 2008, a young woman, a wife and mother, died after a lengthy illness. She had a two-year, apparently illness-free, period that was punctuated by metasteses to liver and lung. That is not the important part of her story, although it accounts for her demise. The important part of her story is how beloved she was not only by her immediate and extended family, but by the community of those she had met throughout her life and the community in which she lived. The vivid grief expressed by those in attendance at her funeral is in sharp contrast to the more restained expression of grief typical at white Anglo-Saxon funerals. Not that all in attendance were Caucasian—the mourners at this funeral represented multiple ethnic groups. Those who were most expressive in their grief were those who, culturally, would have been expected to have a stiff upper lip. Would such a response have occurred had the deceased lived her four score years and ten? How do we account for this response to bereavement? In the following pages we will examine some of the factors that might help us understand this expression of grief.

Bereavement takes many forms. It is influenced first and foremost by culture. In Victorian times, bereaved women in the northeastern United States wore black for a year and used black-edged stationery, while men wore a black armband for a matter of days before resuming their regular activities. Bereavement is also influenced by religious practice, the nature of the relationship with the deceased, the age of the deceased, and the manner of death. In this chapter, the impact of social and cultural forces on the form of bereavement are examined.

Changes have occurred in what is considered "appropriate" to the expression of grief. The wearing of black by a widow ("widow's weeds") for the remainder of her life, and the presumption that grief will be "resolved" within a year, are no longer societal or professional expectations. There are other expectations, however, that color the expressions of bereavement, loss, mourning, and grief. Given that greater emphasis is placed upon the discussion of bereavement and grief, it behooves us to define these terms and examine their related elements.

## A Matter of Definition

### Bereavement

With the pronouncement of death, those who have the closest blood or legal connections to the deceased are considered *bereaved*. Stated simply, "bereavement is defined as the state of having experienced the death of a significant other."[1] Bereavement confers a special status on the individual, entailing both obligations and special rights. The obligations concern disposition of the body and any attendant ceremonies, as well as disposal of the worldly goods of the deceased, unless indicated otherwise in a legal document such as a last will and testament. The rights include dispensation from worldly activities such as work and, to a lesser degree, family roles for a variable period of time. Before an expanded discussion of bereavement is undertaken, it is important to distinguish the concept of bereavement from such related terms as loss, mourning, and grief.

### Loss

Loss is a generic term that signifies absence of an object, position, ability, or attribute. More recently it also has been applied to the death of an animal or person. Absence or loss of the same entity has different implications, depending on the strength of the relationship to the owner. For example, loss of a dog with which there was an indifferent relationship results in less emotional disruption for the owner than the loss of a dog that was cherished. The term is often applied to the death of an individual, and it is the bereaved person who is considered to have experienced a loss. Robinson and McKenna[2] noted three critical attributes of loss:

1. Loss signifies that someone or something one has had, or ought to have had in the future, has been taken away.
2. That which is taken away must have been valued by the person experiencing the loss.
3. The meaning of loss is determined individually, subjectively, and contextually by the person experiencing it.

As is evident from the example of the loss of a dog, the individual determination of meaning indicates that the second attribute suggested by Robinson and McKenna— namely, that what was lost was valued—is not necessarily congruent with the third attribute, which indicates individual evaluation and is in fact superfluous. A loss occurs, and its meaning is determined by the person who sustained the loss. The attributes of loss can be reformulated as follows:

1. Loss signifies the absence of a possession or future possession.
2. Each loss is valued differently and ranges from no or little value to great value.
3. The meaning of the loss is determined primarily by the individual sustaining it.

This suggests that it is wiser not to make assumptions about loss, but to query further as to its meaning to the individual. This is all the more relevant in instances of ambiguous loss. Lee and Whiting employ the theory of ambiguous loss to discuss the situation of foster children, whose caregivers may be physically present but psychologically absent, physically absent but psychologically present, or in transient relationships. Feelings of confusion, hopelessness, and ambivalence may accompany ambiguous loss (p. 418). Mourning and grief under these circumstances may not receive the recognition that is warrented.

### Mourning

Mourning has been described in various ways. Kagawa-Singer[3] described mourning as "the social customs and cultural practices that follow a death." This definition highlights the external manifestations of the process of separation from the deceased and the ultimate reintegration of the bereaved into the family and, to varying degrees, society. Durkheim,[4] one of the founders of sociology, stated that "mourning is not a natural movement of private feelings wounded by a cruel loss; it is a duty imposed by the group." (p. 443). This duty is participation in the customary rituals appropriate to membership in a given group. Participation in such rituals has meaning for the mourner and group.[5] These rituals and behaviors acknowledge that a loss has occurred for the individual and the group, and that the individual and the group are adjusting their relationships so as to move forward without the presence of the deceased individual.

DeSpelder and Strickland[6] highlighted two important aspects of mourning. They stated that mourning is "the process of incorporating the experience of loss into our ongoing lives" and also "the outward acknowledgment of loss" (p. 207). That outward acknowledgment consists of participation in various death and bereavement rituals. As noted, these vary by religious and cultural traditions as well as by personal preferences. Martinson[7] described the variation in practices in eastern Asia due to the influences of folk practices, Confucianism, Buddhism, and Christianity.

Whereas ancestor worship is important to varying degrees in Asia, Latin cultures believe in "the interdependence between life and death," a belief that reflects "the value that is placed on the continuity of relationships between the living and the dead.[8] This relationship is considered sacred and is expressed openly in some of the ritual practices dedicated to the dead."[8,9] These practices have many functions, including signifying respect for the deceased and providing a mechanism for the expression of feelings by the bereaved.

Mourning is also expressed in the symbolism entailed in funerals and burials. Burial grounds contain the expressions of what was considered appropriate in each time period for the memorialization of the deceased. These memorials may be above or below ground, in cemeteries or memorial parks, as part of individual graves or mausoleums, or various permutations. The availability of space for burials influences the manner in which burials and memorials are constructed. Bachelor[10] examines the various reasons for the visit to cemeteries by mourners including: to fulfill obligations, to help achieve independence from the deceased; and to seek solace (p. 408).

## Grief

Grief has been defined as "a person's emotional response to the event of loss,"[5] as the "state of mental and physical pain that is experienced when the loss of a significant object, person, or part of the self is realized,"[6] and as "the highly personal and subjective set of responses that an individual makes to a real, perceived, or anticipated loss."[11] And, as we saw in the opening paragraph of this chapter, grief can vary in the manner in which it is expressed. There are numerous definitions of grief, and these are illustrative of variations on a theme. The process of grief has been studied and reformulated, phases identified, types proposed (anticipatory, complicated, disenfranchised), and expressions of grief described.

Given that nurses work largely with individuals and families, but in some cases also with communities, several sections of this chapter focus on grief as it relates to these different entities. However, even in those sections that putatively deal with associated topics, the subject of grief is related and may be interwoven. With these preliminary definitions as a basis, bereavement, grief, and mourning can now be addressed in greater depth.

## The Process of Bereavement

The process and meaning of bereavement vary depending on a number of factors, including age, gender, ethnicity, cultural background, education, and socioeconomic status. For African-American widows, storytelling was the means by which the bereavement experience was described.[12] The themes identified in a study of these widows included awareness of death, caregiving, getting through, moving on, changing feelings, and financial security. These themes describe well the concerns of bereavement.

To measure core bereavement phenomena, Burnett and colleagues[13] identified 17 items that they considered central to the process of bereavement. They categorized these items under three subscales, namely images and thoughts (e.g., "Do you think about 'X'?"), acute separation (e.g., "Do you find yourself missing 'X'?"), and grief (e.g., "Do reminders of 'X,' such as photos, situations, music, or places, cause you to cry about 'X'?").[13] Although the purpose of this scale is to "assess the intensities of the bereavement reaction in different community samples of bereaved subjects," the bereavement reaction that is being addressed is grief.

The impact of grief affects the health outcomes of bereavement, notably the physical and mental health of the bereaved. These outcomes have been examined by Stroebe, Schut, and Stroebe.[14] In a review of the literature, they found that there is an increase in mortality from a variety of causes for the bereaved, including changes in personal habits and social activities, and psycholgical distress; that psycholgical distress can take the form of grief or depression.

The distinction between grief and depression in the bereaved is an important one.[15] As Middleton and associates[16] concluded, "The bereaved can experience considerable pain and yet be coping adaptively, and they can fulfill many depressive criteria yet at the same time be experiencing phenomena that are not depressive in nature." Even in individuals with a history of "sadness or irritability" before bereavement, although they may have more intense expressions of grief, the rate of recovery is the same as for those without such a history.[17] Other authors are not as sanguine, and caution that subsyndromal symptomatic depressions are "frequently seen complications of bereavement that may be chronic and often are associated with substantial morbidity."[18] Nortriptyline and psychotherapy have been found efficacious in the treatment of bereavement-related major depressive episodes.[19]

Boelen and coworkers[20] pointed out that traumatic grief is distinct from bereavement-related depression and anxiety. Identifying these differences clinically is essential for appropriate treatment. A Bereavement Risk Questionnaire with 19 possible factors for identifying complicated bereavement was distributed to 508 hospice bereavement coordinators; of these, 262 (52%) responded. Significant risk factors for caregivers included lack of social support, caregiver history of drug or alcohol abuse, poor coping skills, history of mental illness, and "patient is a child."[21]

Bereavement-related grief was conceptualized by Rubin and Schecter[22] into two pathways: "a dimension concerned with how the bereaved individual functions following loss" and "a dimension concerned with the nature of that individual's relational bond to the deceased." They observed further that loss involves disruption of multiple spheres of the individual's life. The two-track model of bereavement was developed as a means of understanding and addressing the bereavement process and its outcome: "Track I focuses on the physiological, somatic, affective, cognitive, social and behavioral factors that are affected by loss—and Track II examines ways of transforming the bereaved's attachment to the deceased and establishing new forms of ongoing relationship to the memories of that person."[22,23] In essence, bereavement involves adjusting to a world without the physical, psychological, and social presence of the deceased.

Although Bernard and Guarnaccia[24] found differences between husbands and daughters of breast cancer patients, ultimately the family role relationship affected bereavement adjustment. The quality of the family relationship, with greater expression of family affect and cohesion, was found to be predictive of the expression of fewer grief symptoms over time.[25] Pre-bereavement mental distress such as depression and anxiety, as well as a high level of perceived burden with lack of support, were predictive of a poor bereavement outcome.[26]

Bereavement becomes complicated (in the literature and in life) when adjustment is impeded, as in posttraumatic stress disorder.[27] Whether such bereavement occurs as a result of vehicular accident, war, or natural disaster, the suddenness or overwhelming nature of the event dislodges the sense that all is well with the world. Even in instances in which an elective medical procedure such as abortion occurs, the emotional response may not become evident until many years later.

Death before its time, as in children and young and middle-aged adults, not only affects the bereaved directly, but also affects the social roles of the survivors that require read-justment. The idea that parental outcomes are worse when a child's death is by suicide was not confirmed empirically, however.[28] Another myth is that divorce is more common among bereaved couples than in the general population. The empirical evidence is insufficient either to substantiate or dis-confirm this myth.[28] The issues occasioned by the death of a child with intellectual disabilities has much in common with disenfranchised grief.[29] The need for post-bereavement support in such cases was underscored in this paper and others.[29,30] Disenfranchised grief is compounded by stigma for children with a father on death row, who must contend first with the loss of having an incarcerated parent and then with his death by execution.[31] More will be said about disen-franchised grief shortly.

Hutton and Bradley,[32] in their study of the bereaved sib-lings of babies who were casualties of sudden infant death, were uncertain as to whether these siblings actually exhib-ited more behavioral problems, or were thought to be doing so by mothers whose perceptions were distorted. The need for greater attention to children who are bereaved was underscored by Mahon,[33] who observed that most of the literature in this area concerns "parental impressions of children's grief and studies of adolescent bereavement." The hesitancy of children to exhibit their own sadness so as not to upset their parents requires that professionals encourage parents to give their children permission to be sad when that is how they feel. By taking care of their parents, chil-dren may not receive the attention they require. In a study that sought to identify those factors that helped or hindered adolescent sibling bereavement, a youngster stated: "What helped me the most was my mother, who was totally honest with me from the time Sarah got sick through her death. My mother took the time to listen to how I felt as well as under-stand and hug me."[34]

Situations where individuals are expected to "get on with it" may pose difficulties for those who are bereaved. Individuals such as university faculty members who have demanding work responsibilities may not receive the sup-port required as a result of the need to remain productive.[35] Work factors may be compounded by the personality of the bereaved. Personality correlates were found to influence bereavement narratives, with those testing high in consci-entiousness providing brief, factual narratives, those high in neurotocism being self-focused, and those high in extraver-sion giving naratives associated with social reasons.[36]

Cognitive processing and finding meaning can be helpful to a variety of clients. However, older persons have been noted to be more reluctant to express their feelings.[37] Nurses can be helpful to these clients by encouraging them to express their feelings and being available when needed. Further, Maddocks[38] observed that routine bereavement care can be helpful in identifying people at risk for complicated grieving. Given that the best therapy is prevention, palliative care teams who identify caregivers at risk for bereavement maladjustment can intervene early to prevent long term difficulties.[39]

Aside from such proactive approaches for all bereaved per-sons, Sheldon[40] reported the following predisposing factors for a poor bereavement outcome: ambivalent or dependent relationship; multiple prior bereavements; previous mental illness, especially depression; and low self-esteem. Billings[41] added prior physical health problems to these predisposing factors. Sheldon[40] identified the following factors at the time of death: sudden and unexpected death, untimely death of a young person, preparation for the death, stigmatized deaths (e.g., AIDS, suicide, culpable death), sex of the bereaved per-son (e.g., elderly male widower), caring for the deceased per-son for >6 months, and inability to carry out valued religious rituals. The impact of trauma characterized by violence on bereavement was found by Kaltman and Bonanno to lead to posttraumatic stress disorder symptoms beyond those of nor-mal grief.[42]

Penultimately, after the death, such factors as level of perceived social support, hardiness, lack of opportunities for new interests, and stress from other life crises—as well as dysfunctional behaviors and attitudes appearing early in the bereavement period, consumption of alcohol and drugs, smoking, morbid guilt, and the professional caregiver's gut feeling that this patient will not do well—are predictive of poor outcomes.[40,41,43] Knowledge of and alertness to such predisposing factors are useful for the provision of help, both lay and professional, early in the course of the bereavement so as to prevent further debilitating events. As well as social support, health care policy can have a profound affect on the experience of bereavement as part of the context in which care is provided.[44]

## The Nature of Grief

Rando[45] observed that, although Freud was not the first per-son to examine the effects of bereavement, he nonetheless is taken as an important point of departure. The observation that grief is a normal process and that "a lost love object is never totally relinquished" are congruent with current thinking.[45] The notion that one needs to totally "let go" of the beloved, ascribed to Freud on the basis of some of his work, has influenced professionals to the current day.

The initiation of the modern study of death and dying, however, especially in America, is often attributed to Erich

Lindemann, a physician at Massachusetts General Hospital, who responded to the survivors of a fire in Boston's Coconut Grove nightclub. Five hundred persons died as a result of the fire, which took place on Thanksgiving eve, 1942. Lindemann, a psychiatrist, was interested at the time in the emotional reaction of patients to body disfigurement and plastic surgery.[46] With this medical interest, "Lindemann was struck by the similarity of responses between his patients' reactions to facial disfigurement or loss of a body part and the reactions of the survivors of the fire" (p. 105).[46]

This observation led Lindemann to a study of 101 patients including (1) psychoneurotic patients who lost a relative during the course of treatment, (2) relatives of patients who died in the hospital, (3) bereaved disaster victims (Coconut Grove fire) and their close relatives, and (4) relatives of members of the armed forces.[47] Based on the study of these patients, he determined the five indicators that are "pathognomonic for grief[47]: (1) sensations of somatic distress, such as tightness in the throat, choking and shortness of breath; (2) intense preoccupation with the image of the deceased; (3) strong feelings of guilt; (4) a loss of warmth toward others with a tendency to respond with irritability and anger; and (5) disoriented behavior patterns. Lindemann coined the term "grief work" to describe the process by which individuals attempt to adjust to their loss.[46]

Various theorists have developed a series of stages and phases of grief work.[48-51] The best known of these to the general public are the stages formulated by Elizabeth Kübler-Ross. Proposed for those facing a death, these stages have also been applied to those experiencing a loss. Kübler-Ross[52] identified five stages: denial and isolation, anger, bargaining, depression, and acceptance. The commonality among all theorists of the stages of grief is that the individual moves through (1) notification and shock, (2) experience of the loss emotionally and cognitively, and (3) reintegration. Rando,[53] for example, used the terms avoidance, confrontation, and reestablishment for these three phases. Building on the work of Worden,[54] Corr and Doka[55] propose the following tasks:

1. To share acknowledgment of the reality of death.
2. To share in the process of working through to the pain of grief.
3. To reorganize the family system.
4. To restructure the family's relationship with the deceased and to reinvest in other relationships and life pursuits.

With regard to the last task, some dispute has arisen concerning the degree to which separation from the deceased must occur. Klass and associates[56] made the compelling argument that such bonds continue. They advocated that "survivors hold the deceased in loving memory for long periods, often forever," and that maintaining an inner representation of the deceased is normal rather than abnormal. Winston's study of African-American grandmothers demonstrated that they maintained strong bonds with the deceased.[57]

The second area of dissension and new consensus is the expectation that grief must be resolved within a year This is not to say that the expected trajectory of grieving is one in which grief continues at an intense pitch for years.

A third area of discussion concerns whether the concept of recovery, or some other term, best connotes what occurs after coming to terms with a death and getting on with one's life.[58,59] It has been suggested that recovery is a term more appropriate to an illness, and that death is a normal process of life. Balk,[60] however, argues for a term that incoporates the potential for transformative growth.

A fourth area of debate is the isuue of the medicalization of the grief process.[61] Given that death is a normal part of the cycle of living, grief too is considered a normal process. As shall be observed in the following sections of this chapter, grief, although considered normal, may also become "complicated." As such, interventions may be needed. A medical diagnosis provides legitimacy to those engaged in the treatment encounter, including funding for those who are engaged in providing treatment.

A fifth area of vigorous discussion concerns the efficacy of grief counseling. Larson and Hoyt[62] provide a compelling argument that the basis of the pessimistic view of the value of grief counseling is unfounded. The question of continuing bonds and the length of the grief process are addressed again at the close of this chapter. The reader is invited to consider all of these questions in light of their own experience and reading of the literature . In this next section, types of grief are examined.

## Types of Grief

The types of grief examined in this section are not exhaustive of all types of grief, but rather encompass the major categories. Different terms may be used for some of these same phenomena such as "common grief" and "chronic grief."[63]

### Anticipatory Grief

Anticipatory grief shares similarities with other forms of grief. It is also different. The onset may be associated with the receipt of bad news.[5] Anticipatory grief must be distinguished from the concept of forewarning. An example of forewarning is learning of a terminal diagnosis. Anticipatory grief is an unconscious process, whereas forewarning is a conscious process. With forewarning of a terminal diagnosis, the question is, "What if we do?" With a death, that question becomes, "What if we had done?" With the former question, there is the potential for hope; with the latter query, there may be guilt.

Stephenson[5] described a roller-coaster experience of hope followed by negative experience countered by hope. Even with forewarning, preparation for loss may not occur, given that this may be perceived to be a betrayal of the terminally ill person. There also have been instances of family members unconsciously preparing for the death of an individual and going through the grieving process, only to have that person recover to find no place in the lives of his or her loved ones. This is an example of anticipatory grief.

The question of the utility of forewarning is one of how this time is used. If it is used to make some preparation for role change, such as becoming familiar with the intricacies of the role the terminally ill person plays in the family (e.g., mastering a checking account or other financial responsibilities of the family), such time may be used to the benefit of all concerned. On the other hand, anticipatory grieving that results in reinvestment of emotional energy before the death of the terminally ill person is detrimental to the relationship.

Byrne and Raphael[64] found that "widowers who were unable to anticipate their wife's death, even when their wife had suffered a long final illness, had a more severe bereavement reaction." (The term "anticipate" is used by Byrne and Raphael in the sense of forewarning.) Family members and friends are "warned" when their loved one is diagnosed with certain disease entities such as cancer with metastases. If the primary problem is Alzheimer's disease, there may be a long decline in which, ultimately, familiar figures are no longer recognized. In either situation, the death of the ill person may be experienced both with sadness and with a sense of relief that the caregiving burden is no more. The price of that relief is that the patient is no more.

The sense of relief experienced by caregivers is often a source of guilt feelings about wishing the patient dead. It is important to clarify for the family member or significant other that feelings of relief in being freed of the caregiver burden are not equivalent to wishing someone dead. A woman who experienced relief from not having to care for her bulky husband was assisted to examine this distinction, and consequently was able to grieve uncomplicated by feelings of guilt. Further, persons who have cared for a dying person may experience a sense of accomplishment, knowing that they have done everything they could for their loved one.[65] Schultz and associates[66] pointed out that bereavement is "not only a phenomenon that affects caregivers after the death but also... one that affects many caregivers before the death occurs" (p. 8).

Duke,[67] in a qualitative study of anticipatory grief, enlarged the understanding not so much of anticipatory grief but of the status changes of widowhood. She interviewed five spouses in the second year of their bereavement. Although the findings may have been biased by the distortion of hindsight, they provide much food for thought. The research identified four areas of change: role change from spouse to caregiver during the illness, followed by loss of those roles in bereavement and needing to be cared for; relationship changes from being with spouse to being alone; coping changes from being in suspense to being in turmoil; and the change from experiencing and gathering memories to remembering and constructing memories.[67] It is interesting that these findings reflect the general changes that occur over a terminal illness and not the experience of anticipatory grief. Anticipatory grief, as noted

previously, is unconscious preparation for status change and not a conscious, deliberative process. It should be noted here that the term "premature grief" has also been given to this process.[68] In the following section, anticipatory grief is contrasted with what is termed uncomplicated grief.

## Uncomplicated Grief

Uncomplicated grief, or normal grief, was described by Cowles[69] as dynamic, pervasive, highly individualized, and a process. Worthington[70] depicted a linear model of grief based on adjustment. In this model, an individual in a normal emotional state experiences a loss that causes a reaction and an emotional low; subsequently, the individual begins a recovery to his or her former state. This process of recovery is occasioned by brief periods of relapse, but not to the depths experienced previously. Ultimately, the individual moves to adjustment to the loss. Although this description simplifies the turmoil that may be experienced, discussion of expressions of grief later in this chapter capture the physical, psychological, behavioral, and social upset that characterizes even uncomplicated grief.

Niemeyer[71] offered a new perspective by focusing on meaning reconstruction. He developed a set of propositions to capture adaptation to loss:

1. Death as an event can validate or invalidate the constructions that form the basis on which we live, or it may stand as a novel experience for which we have no constructions.
2. Grief is a personal process, one that is idiosyncratic, intimate, and inextricable from our sense of who we are.
3. Grieving is something we do, not something that is done to us.
4. Grieving is the act of affirming or reconstructing a personal world of meaning that has been challenged by loss.
5. Feelings have functions and should be understood as signals of the state of our meaning-making efforts.
6. We construct and reconstruct our identities as survivors of loss in negotiations with others.

Niemeyer[71] viewed meaning reconstruction as the central process of grief. The inability to make meaning may lead to complications.

## Complicated Grief

In her discussion of complicated mourning, Rando[45] made observations applicable to complicated grief. She observed that, after a suitable length of time, the mourner is attempting to "deny, repress, or avoid aspects of the loss, its pain, and its implications and... to hold onto, and avoid relinquishing, the lost loved one. These attempts, or some variants thereof, cause the complications in mourning." These complications have also been noted to occur pre-death in the caregivers of cancer patients.[72]

Researchers have identified the diagnostic criteria for complicated grief disorder.[73] These criteria include "the current experience (>1 year after a loss) of intensive intrusive thoughts, pangs of severe emotion, distressing yearnings, feeling excessively alone and empty, excessively avoiding tasks reminiscent of the deceased, unusual sleep disturbances, and maladaptive levels of loss of interest in personal activities." Other researchers have underscored the need for the specification of complicated grief as a unique disorder, and have developed an inventory of complicated grief to measure maladaptive symptoms of loss.[74-76] The Inventory of Complicated Grief is composed of 19 items with responses ranging from "Never" to "Rarely," "Sometimes," "Often," and "Always." Examples of items include, "I think about this person so much that it's hard for me to do the things I usually do"; "Ever since she (or he) died it is hard for me to trust people"; "I feel that it is unfair that I should live when this person died"; and "I feel lonely a great deal of the time ever since she (or he) died."[76] This inventory may be helpful to health care practitioners because it differentiates between complicated grief and depression.[77] Finally, it is the severity of symptomatology and the duration that distinguishes abnormal and complicated responses to bereavement.[78,79] Ruminative coping as an avoidance of grief work as been proposed as a variant of complicated chronic grief.[80]

The Inventory of Complicated Grief was used by Ott[63] with 112 bereaved participants in a study in which those identified as experiencing complicated grief were compared with those who were not.[81] Those with complicated grief both identified more additional life stressors, and felt they had less social support, than the other bereaved individuals in the study. The perspective of complicated grief as a stress response syndrome has been explicated by Shear and colleagues.[81] It is important to observe that the characteristics of complicated grief have not been found to vary by race or by the violence of the loss.[82,83]

It should be noted that there is some concern among professionals that what is a normal process is being medicalized by health care practitioners.[61] Complicated grief, however, may require professional intervention.[62] Approaches to therapy have included cognitive–behavioral therapy, presented face-to-face as well as over the internet, and supportive counseling.[84,85] More is said about this later in the chapter. Bearing this in mind, disenfranchised grief poses different but potentially related problems.

## Disenfranchised Grief

Doka[86] defined disenfranchised grief as "the grief that persons experience when they incur a loss that is not or cannot be openly acknowledged, publicly mourned, or socially supported." Doka continued, "The concept of disenfranchised grief recognizes that societies have sets of norms—in effect, grieving rules—that attempt to specify who, when, where, how, how long, and for whom people should grieve" (p. 272).[86] In addition, these norms suggest who may grieve publicly and expect to receive support.

Those who are grieving the loss of relationships that may not be publicly acknowledged—for example, with a mistress or with a family conceived outside a legally recognized union, or in some cases with stepfamilies, colleagues, or friends—are not accorded the deference and support usually afforded the bereaved. Further nonsanctioned relationships, either heterosexual or homosexual, may result in the exclusion of individuals not legitimated by blood or legal union. Individuals in homosexual relationships of long standing who care for their partners throughout their last illness, may find themselves barred both from the funeral and from the home that was shared.[87] A recent study underscores the finding of less social support for the bereaved spouses of same-sex couples.[88] For some time, infection with HIV was hidden from the community, thereby depriving both the infected and their caregivers of support. The AIDS quilt has done much to provide a public mourning ritual, but has not alleviated the disenfranchised status of homosexual or lesbian partners. The result is what has been termed "modulated mourning."[87] This response to stigmatization constrains the public display of mourning by the griever. In this situation, the griever is not recognized.

There are other instances in which a loss has not been legitimized. Loss resulting from miscarriage or abortion has only recently been recognized. In Japan, a "cemetery" is devoted to letters written by families each year telling miscarried or aborted children about the important events that occurred in the family that year, and also expressing continued grief at their loss. Grieving in secret is a burden that makes the process more difficult to complete. Disenfranchised grief may also be a harbinger of unresolved grief.

## Unresolved Grief

Unresolved grief is a failure to accomplish the necessary grief work. According to Rando,[53] a variety of factors may give rise to unresolved grief, including guilt, loss of an extension of the self, reawakening of an old loss, multiple loss, inadequate ego development, and idiosyncratic resistance to mourning (pp. 64–65). In addition to these psychological factors, such social factors as social negation of a loss, socially unspeakable loss, social isolation and/or geographic distance from social support, assumption of the role of the strong one, and uncertainty over the loss (e.g., a disappearance at sea) may be implicated in unresolved grief (pp. 66–67). By helping significant others express their feelings and complete their business before the death of a loved one, unresolved grief and the accompanying manifestations can be prevented to some extent.

Eakes and coworkers[89] questioned whether "closure" is a necessary outcome. They explored the concept of "chronic sorrow" in bereaved individuals who experienced episodic bouts of sadness related to specific incidents or significant dates. These authors suggested the fruitfulness of maintaining an open-ended model of grief. With this in mind, grief is always unresolved to some degree; this is not considered pathological but rather an acknowledgment of a death.

## Expressions of Grief

### Symptoms of Grief

In some of the earlier sections of this chapter, various manifestations of grief were mentioned. In this section, expressions of grief that are within the range considered normal in this society are described. It is important to note that what is considered appropriate in one group may be considered deviant or even pathological in another. It also bears repeating that the manifestations of grief and bereavement are influenced by culture.[90]

In Table 30–1, physical, cognitive, emotional, and behavioral symptoms of grief are presented. Table 30–1 is not exhaustive of all of the potential symptoms, but rather is illustrative of the expressions and manifestations of grief. What distinguishes so-called normal grief is that it is usually self-limited. Although manifestations of grief at 1, 3, and 15 months after the death are not the same in intensity, a recent paper may change our assumptions about grief. The widows in the study by Kowalski and Bondmass,[91] while experiencing a decline in symptomatology, also continued experiencing symptoms for up to five years—the limit of the bereavement experience of the research participants.

A potentially useful bereavement assessment tool links the questions to be asked to the needs in the Maslow Hierarchy, thereby attempting to assess the level of need.[92] The five questions address physiological, safety, belongingness, esteem, and self-actualization needs. The author provides no clinical or research data on the use of the hierarchy. Nonetheless, this approach merits further investigation. Meriting further discussion are the outward manifestations that are the expressions of mourning.

### Mourning

O'Gorman[93] contrasted death rituals in England with those in Ireland. She recalled the "Protestant hushed respectfulness which had somehow infiltrated and taken over a Catholic community."[93] The body was taken from the home by the funeral director. Children continued with school and stayed with relatives; they were shielded from the death. By way of contrast, in an Irish wake, "The body, laid out by a member of the family in order to receive a 'special blessing,' would be in the parlour of a country house surrounded by flowers from the garden and lighted candles." The children, along with the adult members of the family, viewed the corpse. "When visitors had paid their last respects they would join the crowd in the kitchen, who would then spend all night recounting stories associated with the dead person."[93] O'Gorman noted the plentiful availability of alcohol and stated, "By the end of the night, to the uninitiated the event would appear to be more like a party than a melancholy event." Although O'Gorman initially found this distasteful, she "now believes that rituals like the Irish wake celebrate death as a happy occasion and bestow grace upon those leaving life and upon a community of those who mourn them."[93]

The Irish wake, like the reception held in a church basement, hall, restaurant, or private home, serves not only for the expression of condolences but also as an opportunity to reinforce the connections of the community. Anyone familiar with such events knows that a variety of social and business arrangements are made by mourners both within and outside the immediate family. And although some gatherings are more reserved and others lustier, giving the deceased a good send-off ("good" being defined by the group) is central to each. The good send-off is part of the function of the funeral as a piacular rite—that is, as a means of atoning for

---

**Table 30–1**
**Manifestations of Grief**

| Physical | Cognitive | Emotional | Behavioral |
|---|---|---|---|
| Headaches | Sense of depersonalization | Anger | Impaired work performance |
| Dizziness | Inability to concentrate | Guilt | Crying |
| Exhaustion | Sense of disbelief and confusion | Anxiety | Withdrawal |
| Muscular aches | Idealization of the deceased | Sense of helplessness | Avoiding reminders of the deceased |
| Sexual impotency | Search for meaning of life and death | Sadness | Seeking or carrying reminders of |
| Loss of appetite | Dreams of the deceased | Shock | the deceased |
| Insomnia | Preoccupation with image of deceased | Yearning | Overreactivity |
| Feelings of tightness | Fleeting visual, tactile, olfactory, | Numbness | Changed relationships |
| or hollowness | auditory hallucinatory experiences | Self-blame | |
| Breathlessness | | Relief | |
| Tremors | | | |
| Shakes | | | |
| Oversensitivity to noise | | | |

*Source:* Adapted from Doka, (1989), reference 12.

the sins of the mortal being, and as preparation for life in the afterworld.[94] Fulton[94] noted two other functions of funerals, namely integration and separation. The former concerns the living; the latter refers to separation from the loved one as a mortal person. The value of the Irish wake, which in the United States may look more like the Protestant burial O'Gorman describes, is the time spent together sharing stories and feelings.

In the United States, funeral services are held not only in religious establishments such as churches or synagogues, but also in funeral homes. These services, frequently under the aegis of a clergyperson, may also be conducted by a staff member of the funeral home. More recently these services have also taken on the earmarks of a memorial service, accompanied by pictures of the deceased and the bereaved and remarks by selected close family members and friends of the deceased.

In the Irish wake as practiced in Ireland, one is not alone with one's feelings but in the company of others who are devoting the time to mourning (integration). This devotion of time to mourning is also found in the Jewish religion, where the bereaved "sit shiva," usually for 7 days.[95] In Judaism, the assumption is that the bereaved are to focus on their loss and the grieving of that loss. They are to pay no attention to worldly considerations. This period of time of exemption from customary roles may facilitate the process. Certainly having a "minion," in which 10 men and women (10 men for Orthodox Jews) say prayers each evening, reinforces the reality of the death and the separation. For the Orthodox, the mourning period is one year.

A very different pattern is practiced by the Hopi in Arizona. The Hopi have a brief ceremony with the purpose of completing the funeral as quickly as possible so as to get back to customary activities.[95] The fear of death and the dead, and of spirits, induces distancing by the Hopi from nonliving phenomena. Stroebe and Stroebe[95] contrasted Shinto and Buddhist mourners in Japan with the Hopi. Both Shinto and Buddhist mourners practice ancestor worship; as a result, the bereaved can keep contact with the deceased, who become ancestors. Speaking to ancestors as well as offering food is accepted practice. In contrast to this Japanese practice, what occurs in the United States is that those bereaved who speak with a deceased person do so quietly, hiding the fact from others, believing others will consider it suspect or pathological. It is, however, a common occurrence. Bringing food to the ancestor, or (e.g., to celebrate the Day of the Dead) to the cemetery, is part of the mourning practice in Hispanic and many other societies.

Practices, however, change with time, although one can often find the imprint of earlier rituals. The practice of saving a lock of hair or the footprint of a deceased newborn may have evolved from the practice in Victorian times of using hair for mourning brooches and lockets. As a salesperson of these items commented, "They liked to be reminded of their dead in those days. Now it's out of sight, out of mind."[96] These mourning practices provide continuing bonds with the deceased and offer a clue to the answer to the question posed for the last section of this chapter: When is it over? Before addressing this question, another needs to be raised, and that is the question of support.

## A Question of Support

### Formal Support

Many of the mourning practices noted previously provide support by the community to the bereaved (Table 30–2). Formal support in the Jewish tradition is exemplified by the practice of attending a minion for the deceased person. The minion expresses support for the living. It is formal in that it is prescribed behavior on the part of observant Jews and incorporates a prayer service.

Other examples of formal support include support groups such as the widow-to-widow program and the Compassionate Friends, Inc. for families of deceased children. The assumption underlying the widow-to-widow program is that grief and mourning are not in and of themselves pathological, and that laypersons can be helpful to one another. The widow-to-widow program provides a formal mechanism for sharing one's emotions and experience with individuals who have had a similar experience. The Widowed Persons Service offers support for men and women via self-help support groups and a variety of educational and social activities. The Compassionate Friends, Inc., also a self-help organization, seeks to help parents and siblings after the death of a child. Other support groups may or may not have the input of a professional to run the group.

| Table 30–2 Bereavement Practices | |
| --- | --- |
| Lay | Professional |
| 1. Friendly visiting | 1. Clergy visiting |
| 2. Provision of meals | 2. Clergy counseling |
| 3. Informal support by previously bereaved | 3. Nurse, M.D., psychologist, social worker, psychiatrist counseling |
| 4. Lay support groups | 4. Professionally led support groups |
| 5. Participation in cultural and religious rituals | 5. Organization of memorial services by hospice and palliative care organizations |
| 6. A friendly listener | 6. A thoughtful listener |
| 7. Involvement in a cause-related group | 7. Referral to individuals with similar cause-related concerns |
| 8. Exercise | 8. Referral to a health club |
| 9. Joining a new group | 9. Referral to a bereavement program |

Formal programs for children's bereavement support include peer support programs and art therapy programs. Institutions with bereavement programs, whether for children or adults, often send cards at the time of a patient's death, on the birthday of the deceased, and at 3, 6, 12, and 24 months after the death.[97] Pamphlets with information about grief, a bibliography of appropriate readings, and contact numbers of support groups are also helpful.[97] Family bereavement programs have been found to lead to improved parenting, coping, and caregiver mental health.[98]

Attention to bereavement support has been given by institutional trauma programs, in emergency departments, and in critical care departments.[1,99–101] Brosche[102] provides a description of a grief team within a health care system. This attention to the grief of health care providers empowers those involved to express their grief rather than to suppress it. All of these programs, whether for health care providers or family and significant others, maintain contact with the bereaved so as to provide support and make referrals to pastoral care personnel and other professionals as needed.

A variety of approaches have been used in working with the bereaved. Indeed, the combination of "religious psychotherapy" and a cognitive–behavioral approach was observed to be helpful to highly religious bereaved persons.[103] Religious psychotherapy for a group of Malays who adhered to the religion of Islam consisted of discussion and reading of verses of the Koran and Hadith, the encouragement of prayers, and a total of 12 to 16 psychotherapy sessions.[103] Targeting of the follow-up approach to the characteristics of the population eschews the notion that "one size fits all."

A bereavement support group intervention was demonstrated to have a significant impact on the grief of homosexual men who were or were not seropositive for the human immunodeficiency virus (HIV-1).[104] The need for support was found to be all the more necessary for bereaved women living with HIV, who "may be at increased risk for bereavement complicated with psychiatric morbidity and thoughts of suicide" (Summers et al., p. 225).[105,106] Cognitive processing and finding meaning were found to have immunologic and health benefits independent of the baseline health status of bereaved HIV-positive homosexual men.[107] The risk reduction sequelae of a community bereavement support program for HIV-positive individuals was demonstrated by a community support program in Ontario, Canada.[108] These outcomes have implications for the approaches nurses use with other bereaved clients.

Support groups may be open-ended (i.e., without a set number of sessions), or they may be closed and limited to a particular set of individuals. Support groups with a set number of sessions have a beginning and end, and are therefore more likely to be closed to new members until a new set of sessions begins. Open-ended groups have members who stay for varying lengths of time and may or may not have a topic for each session. Lev and McCorkle[109] cited the finding that short-term programs of two to seven sessions, or meeting as needed, were the most effective.

Other formal support entails working with a therapist or other health care provider (bereavement counseling). Arnold[110] suggested that the nurse should follow a process to assess the meaning of loss, the nature of the relationship, expressions and manifestations of grief, previous experience with grief, support systems, ability to maintain attachments, and progression of grief. Further, Arnold underscored the importance of viewing grief as a healing process (Table 30–3). She gave the following example of a patient situation and two different approaches to diagnosis:[110]

A newly widowed woman feels awkward about maintaining social relationships with group of married couples with whom she had participated with her husband.

- Grief as a pathological diagnosis: social isolation.
- Grief as a healthy diagnosis: redefinition of social support.

In addition to conventional talking therapy, such techniques as letter writing, empty chair, guided imagery, and journal writing can be used (Table 30–4).[111] In letter writing, the empty chair technique, and guided imagery, the bereaved are encouraged to express feelings about the past or about

---

**Table 30–3**
**Assessment of Grief**

The bereaved often are weary from caring for the deceased. During this period they may not have looked after themselves. An assessment should include:

1. A general health checkup and assessment of somatic symptoms
2. A dental visit
3. An eye checkup as appropriate
4. Nutritional evaluation
5. Sleep assessment
6. Examination of ability to maintain work and family roles
7. Determination of whether there are major changes in presentation of self
8. Assessment of changes resulting from the death and the difficulties with these changes
9. Assessment of social networks

The health care worker needs to bear in mind that there is no magic formula for grieving. The key question is whether the bereaved is able to function effectively. Cues to the need for assistance include:

1. Clinical depression
2. Prolonged deep grief
3. Extreme grief reaction
4. Self-destructive behavior
5. Increased use of alcohol and/or drugs
6. Preoccupation with the deceased to the exclusion of others
7. Previous mental illness
8. Perceived lack of social support

**Table 30–4**
**Counseling Interventions**

It must be emphasized that grief is not a pathology. It is a normal process that is expressed in individual ways. The following techniques may prove helpful to the individual who is experiencing guilt about things not said or done. This list is not exhaustive, merely illustrative.

| | |
|---|---|
| 1. Letter writing | The bereaved writes a letter to the deceased expressing the thoughts and feelings that may or may not have been expressed. |
| 2. Empty chair | The bereaved sits across from an empty chair on which the deceased is imagined to be sitting. The bereaved is encouraged to express his or her feelings. |
| 3. Empty chair with picture | A picture of the deceased is placed on the chair to facilitate the expressions of feelings by the bereaved. |
| 4. Therapist assumes role of the deceased | In this intervention, the therapist helps the bereaved to explore his or her feelings toward the deceased by participating in a role play. |
| 5. Guided imagery | This intervention demands a higher level of skill than, for example, letter writing. Guided imagery can be used to explore situations that require verbalization by the bereaved to achieve completion. Imagery can also be used to recreate situations of dissension with the goal of achieving greater understanding for the bereaved. |
| 6. Journal writing | This technique provides an ongoing vehicle for exploring past situations and current feelings. It is a helpful intervention to many. |
| 7. Drawing pictures | For the artistically and not so artistically inclined, drawing pictures and explaining their content is another vehicle for discussing feelings and concerns. |
| 8. Analysis of role changes | Helping the bereaved obtain help with the changes secondary to the death, such as with balancing a checkbook or securing reliable help with various home needs; assists with some of the secondary losses with the death of a loved one. |
| 9. Listening | The bereaved has the need to tell his or her story. Respectful listening and concern for the bereaved is a powerful intervention that is much appreciated. |
| 10. Venting anger | The professional can suggest the following: <br><br> • Banging a pillow on the mattress. If combined with screaming, it is the best to do with the windows closed and no one in the home. <br> • Screaming—at home or parked in a car in an isolated spot with the windows closed. <br> • Crying—at home, followed by a warm bath and cup of tea or warm milk. |
| 11. Normality barometer | Assuring the bereaved that the distress experienced is normal is very helpful to the bereaved. |

what life is like without the deceased. These techniques can be helpful as the "wish I had said" becomes said. A journal is also a vehicle for recording ongoing feelings of the lived experience of bereavement.

Another part of bereavement counseling is the instillation or reemergence of hope. As Cutcliffe[112] concluded, "There are many theories of bereavement counseling, with commonalities between these theories. Whilst the theories indicate implicitly the re-emergence of hope in the bereft individual as a result of the counseling, they do not make specific reference to how this inspiration occurs." Cutcliffe saw the clear need to understand this process.

In her exposition of the concept "hope," Stephenson[113] noted the association made by Frankl[114] between hope and meaning. Stephenson stated, "Frankl equated hope with having found meaning in life, and lack of hope as [having] no meaning in life."[114] Meaning-making appears key to the emergence of hope, and hope has been associated with coping.[115]

In hospice programs, health care providers encourage dying persons and their families to have hope for each day. This compression of one's vision to the here and now may also

be useful for the person who is grieving the loss of a loved one. Hope for the future and a personal future is the process that Cutcliffe[112] wished to elucidate. It may be a process that is predicated on hope for each day and having found meaning for the past.

Sikkema and colleagues[106] compared the effectiveness of individual and group approaches by evaluating individual psychotherapy and psychiatric services-on-demand with a support group format. The strategies employed in dealing with grief included establishing a sense of control and predictability, anger expression and management, resolution of guilt, promotion of self-mastery through empowerment, and development of new relationships. Those assigned to individual therapy may or may not have taken advantage of the option. It is proposed that future research examine three groups: those receiving individual counseling, those receiving group therapy, and those assigned no specific intervention but given information about various options for counseling and support in a pamphlet.

A therapist provides a vehicle for ongoing discussion of the loss that informal caregivers may be unable to provide. A support group of bereaved individuals, or periodic contact by an institutional bereavement service, may also prove useful. What is helpful depends on the individual and his or her needs and also on the informal support that is available.

## Informal Support

Informal support that is perceived as supportive and helpful can assist the bereaved to come to terms with life after the death of the beloved. Strategies evaluated as being helpful included "—presence ('being there'), expressing the willingness to listen, and expressing care and concern, whereas the least positively evaluated strategies included giving advice, and minimization of other's feelings" (p. 419).[116] Whether the bereaved is isolated, or is part of a family or social group, is of tremendous import to the physical, psychological, and social welfare of the individual. Community in a psychosocial sense and a continuing role in the group are key factors in adjustment.

In societies where the widow has no role without her husband, she is figuratively if not literally disposed of in one way or another. It is for this reason that the woman who is the first in her group to experience widowhood has a much more difficult social experience than a woman who is in a social group where several women have become widows. In the former there is no reference group; in the latter there is.[117]

The presence of family and friends takes on added significance after the initial weeks following the funeral. In those initial weeks, friendly visiting occurs with provision of a variety of types of foods considered appropriate in the group. After the initial period, friendly visiting is likely to decrease, and the bereaved individuals may find themselves alone or the objects of financial predators. The counsel by the health care provider or by family and friends, not to make life-altering decisions (e.g., moving) at this time unless absolutely necessary, continues to be valuable advice. On the other hand, the comment that "time makes it easier" is a half-truth that is not perceived as helpful by the bereaved.[117,118]

What is helpful is being listened to by an interested person. Having family members with whom to grieve has been shown to be significant to the process of grief processing, and may enhance family bonding.[118] Quinton[119] disliked the term "counseling" in that it implies the availability of a person with good counsel to confer. What Quinton considered important was "lots of listening to what the victim wants to off-load." She observed, "The turning point for me was realizing that I had a right to feel sad, and to grieve and to feel miserable for as long as I felt the need."[119] By owning the grieving process, Quinton provided herself with the most important support for her recovery from a devastating experience—her mother's murder in a massacre by the Irish Republican Army in 1987. The lesson is applicable, however, to any bereaved person regardless of whether the death was traumatic or anticipated. Quinton's turning point is another clue to answering the question of the last section of this chapter: When is it over?

## When is it Over?

To use the colloquial phrase, it's not over until it's over. What does this mean? As long as life and memory persist, the deceased individual remains part of the consciousness of family and friends. When is the grieving over? Unfortunately, there is no easy answer and the only reasonable response, is "It depends." Lindemann's concept of grief work,[46,47] mentioned earlier in this chapter, is applicable. Sooner or later that work needs to be accomplished. Delay protracts the time when accommodation is made. And grief work is never over, in the sense that there will be moments in years to come when an occasion or an object revives feelings of loss. The difference is that the pain is not the same acute pain as that experienced when the loss initially occurred. How one arrives at the point of accommodation is a process termed "letting go."

### Letting Go

The term "letting go" refers to acknowledgment of the loss of future togetherness—physical, psychological, and social. There is no longer a "we," only an "I" or a "we" without the deceased. Family members speak of events such as the first time a flower or bush blooms, major holidays, birthdays, anniversaries, and special shared times. Corless[120] quoted Jacqueline Kennedy, who spoke about "last year" (meaning 1962–1963) as the last time that her husband, John Kennedy, experienced a specific occasion:

> On so many days—his birthday, an anniversary, watching his children running to the sea—I have thought, "but this day last year was his last to see that." He was so full of love and life on all those days. He seems so vulnerable now, when you think that each one was a last time.

Mrs. Kennedy also wrote about the process of letting go, although she didn't call it that:[87]

> Soon the final day will come around again—as inexorably as it did last year. But expected this time. It will find some of us different people than we were a year ago. Learning to accept what was unthinkable when he was alive changes you.

Finally, she addressed an essential truth of bereavement:[120]

> I don't think there is any consolation. What was lost cannot be replaced.

Letting go encompasses recognizing the uniqueness of the individual. It also entails finding meaning in the relationship and experience. It does not require cutting oneself off from memories of the deceased.

## Continuing Bonds

Klass and associates[56] contributed to the reformulation of thinking on the nature of accommodating to loss. Although theorists postulated that the grief process should be completed in one year, with one's emotional energies once again invested in the living, the experience of the bereaved suggested otherwise. Bereaved persons visit the grave for periodic discussions with the deceased. They gaze at a picture and seek advice on various matters. They maintain the presence of the deceased in their lives in a variety of different ways—some shared and some solitary. Such behavior is not pathological. The provocative thesis that those with higher scores on the Continuing Bonds Scale experience elevated grief suggests not only an additional tool for assessment, but that grief is the price that is exacted in the dissolution of close relationships.[121]

It is a common expectation that teachers in the educational system will have an influence on their students. The students progress and may or may not have continuing contact with those educators. Given that assumption about education, how could we not expect to feel the continuing influence and memory of those informal teachers in our lives, our deceased family members and friends? Integration of those influences strengthens the individual at any point in his or her life.

A Turkish expression in the presence of death is, "May you live."[122] That indeed is the challenge of bereavement.

REFERENCES

1. Warren NA. Bereavement care in the critical care setting. Crit Care Nurs Q 1997;20:42.
2. Robinson DS, McKenna HP. Loss: An analysis of a concept of particular interest to nursing. J Adv Nurs 1998;27:782.
3. Kagawa-Singer M. The cultural context of death rituals and mourning practices. ONF 1998;25:1752.
4. Durkheim E. The Elementary Forms of Religious Life. New York: Collier, 1961.
5. Stephenson JS. Grief and mourning. In: Fulton R, Bendikson R, eds. Death and Identity (3rd ed). Philadelphia: Charles Press, 1994:136–176.
6. DeSpelder LA, Strickland AL. The Last Dance (2nd ed). Mountain View, CA: Mayfield Publishing, 1987:207.
7. Martinson IM. Funeral rituals in Taiwan and Korea. ONF 1998;25:1756–1760.
8. Chidester D. Patterns of Transcendence: Religion, Death and Dying. Belmont, CA: Wadsworth, 1990.
9. Munet-Vilaro F. Grieving and death rituals of Latinos. ONF 1998;25:1761.
10. Bachelor P. Practical bereavement. Health Soc Rev 2007;16: 405–414.
11. Doka K. Grief. In: Kastenbaum R, Kastenbaum B, eds. Encyclopedia of Death. Phoenix, AZ: Oryx Press; 1989:127.
12. Rodgers L. Meaning of bereavement among older African-American widows. Geriatr Nurs 2004;25:10–16.
13. Burnett P, Middleton W, Raphael B, Martinek N. Measuring core bereavement phenomena. Psychol Med 1997;27:49–57.

14. Stroebe M, Schut H, Stroebe W. Health outcomes of bereavement. Lancet 2007;370:1960–1973.
15. Zisook S, Kendler KS. Is bereavement-related depression different then non-bereavement-related depression? Psychol Med 2007;37:779–794.
16. Middleton W, Franzp MD, Raphael B, Franzp MD, Burnett P, Martinek N. Psychological distress and bereavement. J Nerv Ment Dis 1997;185:452.
17. Hays JC, Kasl S, Jacobs S. Past personal history of dysphoria, social support, and psychological distress following conjugal bereavement. J Am Geriatr Soc 1994;42:712–718.
18. Zisook S, Shuchter SR, Sledge PA, Paulus M, Judd ll. The spectrum of depressive phenomena after spousal bereavement. J Clin Psychiatry 1994;55(suppl):35.
19. Reynolds CF, Miller MD, Pasternak RE, et al. Treatment of bereavement-related major depressive episodes in later life: A controlled study of acute and continuation treatment with nortriptyline and interpersonal psychotherapy. Am J Psychiatry 1999;156:202–208.
20. Boelen PA, van den Bout J, de Keijser J. Traumatic grief as a disorder distinct from bereavement-related depression and anxiety: A replication study with bereaved mental health care patients. Am J Psychiatry 2003;160:1339–1341.
21. Ellifritt J, Nelson, KA, Walsh D. Complicated bereavement: A national survey of potential risk factors. Am J Hosp Palliat Care 2003;20:114–120.
22. Rubin SS, Schecter N. Exploring the social construction of bereavement: Perceptions of adjustment and recovery in bereaved men. Am J Orthopsychiatry 1997;67:280.
23. Rubin SS, Malkinson R, Witzum E. Trauma and bereavement: Conceptual and clinical issues revolving around relationships. Death Stud 2003;27:667–690.
24. Bernard LL, Guarnaccia CA. Two models of caregiver strain and bereavement adjustment: A comparison of husband and daughter caregivers of breast cancer hospice patients. Gerontologist 2003;43:808–816.
25. Traylor ES, Hayslip B Jr, Kaminski PL, York C. Relationships between grief and family system characteristics: A cross-lagged longitudinal analysis. Death Stud 2003;27:575–601.
26. Schults R, Herbert R, Boerner K. Bereavement after caregiving. Geriatrics 2008;63:20–22.
27. Stewart AE. Complicated bereavement and posttraumatic stress disorder following fatal car crashes: Recommendations for death notification practice. Death Stud 1997;23:289–321.
28. Murphy SA, Johnson JL, Lohan J. Challenging the myths about parents' adjustment after the sudden violent death of a child. J Nurs Scholarsh 2003;35:359–364.
29. Todd S. Silenced grief: Living with the death of a child with intellectual disabilities. J Intellect Disabil Res 2007;51:637–648.
30. Reilly DE, Hastings RP, Vaughan FL, Huws JC. Parental bereavement and the loss of a child with intellectual disbilities: A review of the literature. Intellect Dev Disabil 2008;46:27–43.
31. Beck E, Jones SJ. Children of the condemned: Grieving the loss of a father to death row. Omega 2008;56:191–215.
32. Hutton CJ, Bradley BS. Effects of sudden infant death on bereaved siblings: A comparative study. J Child Psychol Psychiat 1994;55:723–732.
33. Mahon MM. Childhood bereavement after the death of a sibling. Holistic Nurs Pract 1995;9:16.
34. Hogan NS, DeSantis L. Things that help and hinder adolescent sibling bereavement. West J Nurs Res 1994;16:137.

35. Fitzpatrick, TR. Bereavement among faculty members in a university setting. Soc Work Health Care 2007;45:83–109.

36. Baddeley Jl, Singer JA. Telling losses: Personality correlates and functions of bereavement narratives. J Res Pers 2008;42:421–438.

37. Anderson KL, Dimond MF. The experience of bereavement in older adults. J Adv Nurs 1995;22:308–315.

38. Maddocks I. Grief and bereavement. Med J Aust 2003;179 (6 Suppl):S6–S7.

39. Rossi Ferrario S, Cardillo V, Vicarfio F, Balzarini E, Zotti AM. Advanced cancer at home: Caregiving and bereavement. Palliat Med 2004;18:129–136.

40. Sheldon F. ABC of palliative care—Bereavement. BMJ 1998;316:456.

41. Billings JA. Useful predictors of poor outcomes in bereavement. In: JA Billings, coordinator. Palliative Care Role Model Course. Boston, MA: Massachusetts General Hospital, 1999.

42. Kaltman S, Bonanno GA. Trauma and bereavement: Examining the impact of sudden and violent deaths. J Anxiety Disord 2003;17:131–147.

43. Matthews LL, Servaty-Seib HL. Hardiness and grief in a sample of bereaved college students. Death Stud 2007;183–204.

44. Holtslander LF. Caring for bereaved family caregivers: Analyzing the context of care. Clin J Onc Nurs 2008;510–506.

45. Rando TA. Grief and mourning: Accommodating to loss. In: Wass H, Neimeyer RA, eds. Dying—Facing the Facts. Philadelphia: Taylor and Francis; 1995:211–241.

46. Fulton R, Bendikson R. Introduction—Grief and the Process of Mourning. In: Fulton R, Bendicksen R, eds. Death and Identity (3rd ed). Philadelphia: Charles Press Publishers, 1994:105–109.

47. Lindemann E. Symptomatology and management of acute grief. Am J Psychiatry (Sesquicentennial Suppl) 1994;151(6):156.

48. Gorer G. Death, Grief and Mourning. London: Cresset Press, 1965.

49. Kavanaugh R. Facing Death. Baltimore: Penguin Books, 1974.

50. Raphael B. The Anatomy of Bereavement. New York: Basic Books, 1983.

51. Weizman SG, Kamm P. About Mourning: Support and Guidance for the Bereaved. New York: Human Sciences Press, 1985.

52. Kübler-Ross E. On Death and Dying. New York: Macmillan, 1969.

53. Rando TA. Grief, Dying and Death—Clinical Interventions for Caregivers. Champaign, IL: Research Press Company, 1984.

54. Worden JW. Grief Counseling and Grief Therapy: A Handbook for the Mental Health Practitioner (2nd ed). New York: Springer, 1991.

55. Corr CA, Doka KJ. Current models of death, dying and bereavement. Crit Care Nurs Clin North Am 1994;6:545–552.

56. Klass D, Silverman P, Nickman S. Continuing Bonds. Philadelphia: Taylor and Francis Publishing, 1996.

57. Winston CA. African American grandmothers parenting AIDS orphans: Concomitant grief and loss. Am J Orthopsychiatry 2003;73:91–100.

58. Shapiro ER. Whose recovery of what? Relationships and environments promoting grief and growth. Death Stud 2008;40–58.

59. Rosenblatt PC. Recovery following bereavement: Metaphor, phenomenology, and Culture. Death Stud 2008;6–16.

60. Balk DE. A modest proposal about Bereavement and recovery. Death Stud 2008;84–93.

61. Breen LJ, O'Connor M. The fundamental paradox in the grief literature: A critical reflection. Omega 2007;199–218.

62. Larson DG, Hoyt WT. What has beome of grief counseling? An evaluation of the empirical foundations of the new pessimism. Prof Psychol Res Pract 2007;347–355.

63. Ott CH. The impact of complicated grief on mental and physical health at various points in the bereavement process. Death Stud 2003;27:249–272.

64. Byrne GJA, Raphael B. A longitudinal study of bereavement phenomena in recently widowed elderly men. Psychol Med 1994;23:411–421.

65. Koop PM, Strang V. Predictors of bereavement outcomes in families of patients with cancer: A literature review. Can J Nurs Res 1997;29:33–50.

66. Schultz R, Mendelsohn AB, Haley WE, Mahoney D, Allen RS, Zhang S, Thompson L, Belle SH. End-of-Life care and the effects of bereavement on family caregivers of persons with dementia. N Engl J Med 2003;349:1936–1942.

67. Duke S. An exploration of anticipatory grief: The lived experience of people during their spouses' terminal illness and in bereavement. J Adv Nurs 1998;28:829–839.

68. Grassi L. Bereavement in families with relatives dying of cancer. Curr Opin Support Palliat Care 2007;43–49.

69. Cowles KV. Cultural perspectives of grief: An expanded concept analysis. J Adv Nurs 1996;23:287–294.

70. Worthington RC. Models of linear and cyclical grief—Different approaches to different experiences. Clin Pediatr 1994;33:297–300.

71. Neimeyer RA. Meaning reconstruction and the experience of chronic loss. In: Doka KJ, Davidson J, eds. Living with Grief: When Illness Is Prolonged. Philadelphia: Taylor and Francis; 1997:159–176.

72. Tomarken A, Holland J, Schachter S, et al. Factors of complicated grief pre-death in caregivers of cancer patients. Psycho-Oncology 2008;17:105–111.

73. Horowitz MJ, Siegel B, Holen A, Bonanno GA, Milbrath C, Stinson CH. Diagnostic criteria for complicated grief disorder. Am J Psychiatry 1997;154:904–910.

74. Prigerson HG, Frank E, Kasl SV, et al. Complicated grief and bereavement-related depression as distinct disorders: Preliminary empirical validation in elderly bereaved spouses. Am J Psychiatry 1995;152:22–30.

75. Prigerson HG, Bierhals AJ, Kasl SV, et al. Complicated grief as a disorder distinct from bereavement-related depression and anxiety: A replication study. Am J Psychiatry 1996;153:1484–1486.

76. Prigerson HG, Maciejewski PK, Reynolds CF III, et al. Inventory of complicated grief: A scale to measure maladaptive symptoms of loss. Psychiatry Res 1995;59:65–79.

77. Ogrodniczuk JS. Differentiating symptoms of complicated grief and depression among psychiatric outpatients. Can J Psychiatry 2003;48:87–93.

78. Krigger KW, McNeely JD, Lippmann SB. Dying, death and grief: Helping patients and their families through the process. Postgrad Med 1997;101:263–270.

79. Boelen PA, van den Bout J. Complicated grief and uncomplicated grief are distinguishable constructs. Psychiatry Res 2008;157:311–314.

80. Stroebe M, Boelen PA, van den Hout M, Stroebe W, Salemink E, van den Bout J. Ruminative coping as avoidance: A reinterpretation of its function in adjustment to bereavement. Eur Arch Psychiatry Clin Neurosci 2007;257:462–472.

81. Shear K, Monk T, Houck P, et al. An attachment-based model of complicated grief including the role of avoidance. Eur Arch Psychitry Clin Neurosci 2007; 257:453–461.

82. Cruz M, Scott J, Houck P, Reynolds CF, Frank E, Shear MK. Clinical presentation and treatment outcome of African Americans with complicated grief. Psychiatr Serv 2007;58:700–702.

83. Boelen PA, van den Bout J. Examination of proposed criteria for complicated grief in people confronted with violent or nonviolent loss. Death Stud 2007;31:155–164.

84. Boelen PA, de Keijser J, van den Hout M, van den Bout J. Treatment of complicated grief: A comparison between cognitive-behavioral therapy and supportive counseling. J Counsel Clin Psychol 2007;75: 277–284.

85. Wagner B. Maercker A. A 1.5 –year follow-up of an internet–based intervention for complicated grief. J Trauma Stress 2007;20:625–629.

86. Doka KJ. Disenfranchised grief. In: DeSpelderf LA, Strickland AL, eds. The Path Ahead. Mountain View, CA: Mayfield; 1995:271–275.

87. Corless IB. Modulated mourning: The grief and mourning of those infected and affected by HIV/AIDS. In: Doka KJ, Davidson J, eds. Living with Grief: When Illness Is Prolonged. Philadelphia: Taylor and Francis; 1997:108–118.

88. Boswell C. A phenomenological study of the experience of grief resulting from spousal bereavement in heterosexual and homosexual men and women. A dissrtation presented to the Faculty of the College of Education University of Houston. 2007.

89. Eakes GG, Burke ML, Hainsworth MA. Chronic sorrow: The experiences of bereaved individuals. Illness Crisis Loss 1999;7:172–182.

90. HardyBougere M. Cultural manifestations of grief and bereavement: A clinical perspective. J Cult Divers 2008;15:66–69.

91. Kowalski SD, Bondmass MD. Physiological and psychological symptoms of grief in widows. Res Nurs Health 2008;31:23–30.

92. Love AW. Progress in understanding grief, complicated grief, and caring for the bereaved. Contemp Nurse 2007;27:73–83.

93. O'Gorman SM. Death and dying in contemporary society: An evaluation of current attitudes and the rituals associated with death and dying and their relevance to recent understandings of health and healing. J Adv Nurs 1998;2:1127–1135.

94. Fulton R. The funeral in contemporary society. In Fulton R, Bendiksen R, eds. Death and Identity (3rd ed). Philadelphia: Charles Press; 1994:288–312.

95. Stroebe W, Stroebe MS. Is grief universal? Cultural variations in the emotional reaction to loss. In Fulton R, Bendiksen R, eds. Death and Identity (3rd ed). Philadelphia: Charles Press; 1994:177–207.

96. Byatt AS. Possession—A Romance. New York: Vintage Books, 1990:6.

97. Coolican MB. Families facing the sudden death of a loved one. Crit Care Nurs Clin North Am 1994;6:607–612.

98. Sandler IN, Ayers TS, Wolchik SA, et al. The family bereavement program: Efficacy evaluation of a theory-based prevention program for parentally bereaved children and adolescents. J Consult Clin Psychol 2003;71:587–600.

99. Coolican MB, Pearce T. After care bereavement program. Crit Care Nurs Prog North Am 1995;7:519–527.

100. Snyder J. Bereavement protocols. J Emerg Nurs 1996;22:39–42.

101. LeBrocq P, Charles A, Chan T, Buchanan M. Establishing a bereavement program: Caring for bereaved families and staff in the emergency department. Accid Emerg Nurs 2003;11:85–90.

102. Brosche TA. A grief team within a healthcare system. Dimens Crit Care Nurs 2007;26:21–28.

103. Azhar MZ, Varma SL. Religious psychotherapy as management of bereavement. Acta Psychiatry Scand 1995;91: 233–235.

104. Goodkin K, Blaney NT, Feaster DJ, Baldewicz T, Burkhalter JE, Leeds B. A randomized controlled clinical trial of a bereavement support group intervention in human immunodeficiency virus type 1-seropositive and -seronegative homosexual men. Arch Gen Psychiatry 1999;56:52–59.

105. Summers J, Zisook S, Sciolla AD, Patterson T, Atkinson JH, San Diego HIV Neurobehavioral Research Center (HNRC) Group. Gender, AIDS, and bereavement: A comparison of women and men living with HIV. Death Stud 2004;28:225–241.

106. Sikkema KJ, Hansen NB, Kochman A, Tate DC, Difranceisco W. Outcomes from a randomized controlled trial of a group intervention for HIV positive men and women coping with AIDS-related loss and bereavement. Death Stud 2004; 28:187–209.

107. Bower JE, Kemeny ME, Taylor SE, Fahy JL. Cognitive processing, discovery of meaning, CD4 decline, and AIDS-related mortality among bereaved HIV-seropositive men. J Consult Clin Pscyhol 1998;66:979–986.

108. Leaver CA, Perreault Y, Demetrakopoulos A,; AIDs Bereavement Project of Ontarios' Survive and Thrive Working Group. Understanding AIDS-related bereavement and multiple loss among long-term survivors of HIV in Ontario. Can J Hum Sex 2008:17:37–52.

109. Lev EL, McCorkle R. Loss, grief and bereavement in family members of cancer patients. Semin Oncol Nurs 1998;4:145–151.

110. Arnold J. Rethinking—Nursing implications for health promotion. Home Healthc Nurse 1996;14:779–780.

111. Rancour P. Recognizing and treating dysfunctional grief. ONF 1998;25:1310–1311.

112. Cutcliffe JR. Hope, counselling, and complicated bereavement reactions. J Adv Nurs 1998;28:760.

113. Stephenson C. The concept of hope revisited for nursing. J Adv Nurs 1991;16:1456–1461.

114. Frankl V. Man's Search for Meaning: An Introduction to Logotherapy. New York: Simon and Schuster, 1959.

115. Herth KA. The relationship between level of hope and level of coping and other variables in patients with cancer. ONF 1989;16:62–72.

116. Rack JJ, Burleson BR, Bodie GD, Holmstrom AJ, Servaty-Seib H. Bereaved adults' evaluations of grief management messages: Effects of message person centeredness, recipient individual differences, and contextual factors. Death Stud 2008;32:399–427.

117. Watson MA. Bereavement in the elderly. AORN J 1994;59:1084.

118. Pressman DL, Bonanno GA. With whom do we grieve? Social and cultural determinants of grief processing in the United States and China. J Soc Pers Relat 2007;24:729–746.

119. Quinton A. Permission to mourn. Nurs Times 1994;90:31–32.

120. Corless IB. And when famous people die. In: Corless IB, Germino BA, Pittman MA, eds. A Challenge for Living—Dying, Death, and Bereavement. Boston: Jones & Bartlett Publishers; 1995:398.

121. Field NP, Gal-Oz E, Bonanno GA. Continuing bonds and adjustment at 5 years after the death of a spouse. J Consult Clin Psychol 2003;71:110–117.

122. [Commentary by newscaster on Turkish earthquake.] ABC News, 1999.

Betty Davies and Rose Steele

# 31

# Supporting Families in Palliative Care

*Our personal relationships have changed because of her illness...because of the severity of her illness and the rapid decline in her mobility and her bodily functions. We have to adjust to those things. She has a lot of adjustment to make, and so do I, and so do our children. We each have to adjust—but so does our family, and it's not always easy to do that. But, our relationship is growing and blossoming even further.—Husband of 60-year-old woman with cancer*

♦ **Key Points**
♦ *Family-centered care is a basic tenet of palliative care philosophy, which recognizes that terminally ill patients exist within the family system. The patient's illness affects the whole family, and, in turn, the family's responses affect the patient. Supporting families in palliative care means that nurses must plan their care with an understanding not only of the individual patient's needs but also of the family system within which the patient functions.*
♦ *Families with a member who requires palliative care are in transition. Families have described this as a "transition of fading away," characterized by seven dimensions that help nurses to understand families' experiences and to support them.*
♦ *Level of family functioning also plays a role in family experience, and serves to guide nursing interventions for families with varying levels of functioning.*

## Family-Centered Palliative Care

Recognizing the importance of a family focus necessitates clearly defining what is meant by "family." Most often, families in palliative care do consist of patients, their spouses, and their children. But in today's world of divorce and remarriage, step-relatives must also enter into the family portrait. In other instances, people unrelated by blood or marriage may function as family.[1] Therefore, the definition of family must be expanded. The family is a group of individuals inextricably linked in ways that are constantly interactive and mutually reinforcing. Family can mean direct blood relatives, relationships through an emotional commitment, or the group or person with which an individual feels most connected.[2] Moreover, family in its fullest sense embraces all generations—past, present, future; those living, those dead, and those yet to be born. Shadows of the past and dreams of the future also contribute to the understanding of families.

Palliative care programs are based on the principle that the family is the unit of care. In practice, however, the family is often viewed as a group of individuals who can either prove helpful or resist efforts to deliver care. Nurses and other health professionals must strive to understand the meaning of the palliative experience to the family.[3] If quality care is to be provided, nurses need to understand how all family members perceive their experience, how the relationships fit together, and that a multitude of factors combine to make families what they are. However, only recently has research gone beyond focusing on the needs of dying patients for comfort and palliation, to addressing issues relevant to other family members. Much of this research has focused on the family's perceptions of their needs[4]; experiences and challenges faced[4–9]; adaptation and coping skills required for home care[4,10–12]; the supportiveness of nursing behaviors[13] or physician behaviors[14]; and satisfaction with care.[15,16] Most research has focused on families of patients with cancer, though recent reports extend to end-of-life care for other diagnostic populations, such as Parkinson's disease,[5] cardiac disease,[6] and dementia.[17,18] Findings make it clear that family members look to health professionals to provide quality care to the patient. Family members also expect health professionals to meet their own needs for information, emotional support, and assistance with care.[15]

Much of the research that purports to address the impact of cancer on the family is based on the perceptions of individuals—either the patient or adult family members (usually the spouse). As well, many of the studies were conducted retrospectively, that is, after the patient's death. But even studies conducted during the palliative period frequently exclude the patient—the one who is at the center of the palliative care situation. Examining the palliative experience of the family unit has been rare.

As a basis for offering optimal support to families in palliative care, this chapter focuses on describing the findings of a research program that prospectively examined the experiences of such families.[19] The research evolved from nurses' concerns about how to provide family-centered palliative care. Nurses in a regional cancer center constantly had to attend to the needs of not only patients but also patients' families, particularly as they moved back and forth between hospital and home. In searching the literature for guidelines about family-centered care, they found that many articles were about the needs of patients and family members, about levels of family members' satisfaction with care, and about family members' perceptions of nurses, but nothing really described the families' experiences as they coped with the terminal illness of a beloved family member. Research involving families included patients with advanced cancer, their spouses, and at least one of their adult children (>18 years of age). Since the completion of the original research, families with AIDS, Alzheimer's disease, and cardiac disease have provided anecdotal validation of the findings for their experiences. In addition, families of children with progressive, life-threatening illness have provided similar validation. Therefore, it seems that the conceptualization has relevance for a wide range of families in palliative care. The findings from this research program form the basis for the description that follows; references to additional research studies are also included to supplement and emphasize the ongoing development of knowledge in the field of family-centered end-of-life care.

## The Transition of Fading Away

The common view is that transitions are initiated by changes, by the start of something new. However, as Bridges[20] suggests, most transitions actually begin with endings. This is true for families living with serious illness in a loved one. The nurses' research findings generated a theoretical scheme that conceptualized families' experiences as a transition—a transition that families themselves labeled as "fading away." The transition of fading away for families facing terminal illness began with the ending of life as they knew it. They came to realize that the ill family member was no longer living with cancer but was now dying from cancer.

Despite the fact that family members had been told about the seriousness of the prognosis, often since the time of diagnosis, and had experienced the usual ups and downs associated with the illness trajectory, for many the "gut" realization that the patient's death was inevitable occurred suddenly: "It struck me hard—it hit me like a bolt. Dad is not going to get better!" The awareness was triggered when family members saw, with "new eyes," a change in the patient's body or physical capacity, such as the patient's weight loss, extreme weakness, lack of mobility, or diminished mental capacity. Realizing that the patient would not recover, family members began the transition of fading away. As one patient commented, "My body has shrunk so much—the other day, I tried on my favorite old blue dress and I could see then how much weight I have lost. I feel like a skeleton with skin! I am getting weaker. . . . I just can't eat much now, I don't want to. I can see that I am fading. . . . I am definitely fading away."

The transition of fading away is characterized by seven dimensions: redefining, burdening, struggling with paradox, contending with change, searching for meaning, living day by day, and preparing for death. The dimensions do not occur in linear fashion; rather, they are interrelated and inextricably linked to one another. Redefining, however, plays a central role. All family members experience these dimensions, although patients, spouses, and children experience each dimension somewhat differently.

## Redefining

Redefining involves a shift from "what used to be" to "what is now." It demands adjustment in how individuals see themselves and each other. Patients maintained their usual patterns for as long as possible, and then began to implement feasible alternatives once they realized that their capacities were seriously changing. Joe, a truck driver, altered his identity over time: "I just can't do what I used to. I finally had to accept the fact that the seizures made it unsafe for me to drive." Joe requested to help out at his company's distribution desk. When he could no longer concentrate on keeping the orders straight, Joe offered to assist with supervising the light loading. One day, Joe was acutely aware he didn't have the energy to even sit and watch the others: "I couldn't do it anymore," Joe sighed. "I had reached the end of my work life and the beginning of the end of my life." Another patient, Cora, lamented that she used to drive to her son's home to babysit her toddler-aged grandchildren; then her son dropped the children off at her house to preserve the energy it took for her to travel; and now, her son has made other child care arrangements. He brings the children for only short visits because of her extreme fatigue.

Both Joe and Cora, like the other patients, accepted their limitations with much sadness and a sense of great loss. Their focus narrowed, and they began to pay attention to details of everyday life that they had previously ignored or overlooked.

Joe commented, "When I first was at home, I wanted to keep in touch with the guys at the depot; I wanted to know what was going on. Now, I get a lot of good just watching the grandkids out there playing in the yard."

Patients were eager to reinforce that they were still the same on the inside, although they acknowledged the drastic changes in their physical appearance. They often became more spiritual in their orientation to life and nature. As Joe said, "I always liked being outside—was never much of an office-type person. But, now, it seems I like it even more. That part of me hasn't changed even though it's hard for some of the fellas (at work) to recognize me now." When patients were able to redefine themselves as Joe did, they made the best of their situation, differentiating what parts of them were still intact. Joe continued, "Yeah, I like just being outside, or watching the kids. And, you know, they still come to their Grandpa when their toy trucks break down—I can pretty much always fix 'em." Similarly, Cora commented: "At least, I can still make cookies for when my family comes, although I don't make them from scratch anymore." Patients shared their changing perceptions with family members and others, who then were able to offer understanding and support.

Patients who were unable to redefine themselves in this way attempted to maintain their regular patterns despite the obvious changes in their capacity to do so. They ended up frustrated, angry, and feeling worthless. These reactions distanced them from others, resulting in the patients feeling alone and, sometimes, abandoned. Ralph, for example, was an educational administrator. Despite his deteriorating health, he insisted that he was managing without difficulty. "Nothing's wrong with me, really. . . . We are being accredited this year. There's a lot to do to get ready for that." Ralph insisted on going into the office each day to prepare the necessary reports. His increasing confusion and inability to concentrate made his reports inaccurate and inadequate, but Ralph refused to acknowledge his limitations or delegate the work. Instead, his colleagues had to work overtime to correct Ralph's work after he left the office. According to Ralph's wife, anger and frustration were commonplace among his colleagues, but they were reluctant to discuss the issue with Ralph. Instead, they avoided conversations with Ralph, and he complained to his wife about his colleagues' lack of interest in the project.

For the most part, spouses took the patient's physical changes in stride. They attributed the changes to the disease, not to the patient personally, and as a result, they were able to empathize with the patient. Patients' redefining focused on themselves, the changes in their physical status and intrapersonal aspects; spouses' redefining centered on their relationship with the patient. Spouses did their best to "continue on as normal," primarily for the sake of the patient. In doing so, they considered alternatives and reorganized their priorities.

Sherman[21] described the "reciprocity of suffering" that family members experience, which results from the physical and emotional distress that is rooted in their anguish of dealing with the impending death of the loved one, and in their attempt to fill new roles as caregivers. The degree to which family members experienced this phenomenon varied according to patients' redefining. When patients were able to redefine themselves, spouses had an easier time. Such patients accepted spouses' offers of support; patients and spouses were able to talk about the changes that were occurring. Spouses felt satisfied in the care that they provided. But when patients were less able to redefine, then spouses' offers of support were rejected or unappreciated. For example, Ralph's wife worried about his work pattern and its impact on his colleagues. She encouraged him to cut back, but Ralph only ignored her pleas and implied that she didn't understand how important this accreditation was to the future of his school. Even when Ralph was no longer able to go to the office, he continued to work from home, frequently phoning his colleagues to supervise their progress on the report. His wife lamented, "For an educated man, he doesn't know much. I guess it's too late to teach an old dog new tricks."

In such situations, spouses avoided talking about or doing anything that reminded the patient of the changes he or she was experiencing but not acknowledging. The relationship between the spouse and patient suffered. Rather than feeling satisfied with their care, spouses were frustrated and angry, although often they remained silent and simply "endured" the situation. The ill person contributed significantly to the caregiver's ability to cope. Indeed, the ill person was not simply a passive recipient of care but had an impact on the experience of the caregiving spouse. Similarly, in their study of factors that influence family caregiving of persons with advanced cancer, Strang and Koop[22] found that the ill person contributed significantly to the capacity of the spouse to continue to provide care despite their experience of overwhelming emotional and physical strain. Caregivers drew strength from the dying person when the ill person accepted the impending death, had an understanding of the caregivers' needs, and had attitudes, values, and beliefs that sustained their caregivers.

Adult children also redefined the ill family member; they redefined their ill parent from someone who was strong and competent to someone who was increasingly frail. Children felt vulnerable in ways they had not previously experienced. Most often, children perceived that the changes in their ill parent were the result of disease and not intentional: "It's not my father doing this consciously." Younger adult children were particularly sensitive to keeping the situation private, claiming they wanted to protect the dignity of the patient, but seemed to want to protect their own sense of propriety. For example, one young woman in her early twenties was "devastated" when her father's urinary bag dragged behind him as he left the living room where she and her friends were visiting. It was difficult for some young adults to accept such manifestations of their parent's illness. Adolescents in particular had a difficult time redefining the situation. They preferred to continue on as if nothing was wrong and to shield themselves against any information that would force them to see the situation realistically.

When the ill parent was able to redefine to a greater degree, then children were better able to appreciate that death is part of life. They recognized their own susceptibility and vowed to take better care of their own health; older children with families of their own committed to spending more quality time with their children. Joe talked, although indirectly, with his son about the situation: "I won't be here forever to fix the kids' toys." Together, Joe and his son reminisced about how Joe had always been available to his son and grandchildren as "Mr. Fix-it." Joe's son valued his dad's active participation in his life and promised to be the same kind of father to his own sons. In contrast, when the ill parent was unable to redefine, then children tended to ignore the present. They attempted to recreate the past to construct happy memories they never had. In doing so, they often neglected their own families. Ralph's daughter described her dad as a "workaholic." Feeling as if she had never had enough time with her dad, she began visiting her parents daily, with suggestions of places she could take him. He only became annoyed with her unfamiliar, constant presence: "It's okay she comes over every day, but enough is enough."

The extent to which spouses and adult children commented on the important contribution made by the dying family member is a provocative finding that underscores the importance of relationships among and between family members in facilitating their coping with the situation of terminal illness.

## Burdening

Feeling as if they are a burden for their family is common among patients. If patients see themselves as purposeless, dependent, and immobile, they have a greater sense of burdening their loved ones. The more realistically patients redefined themselves as their capacities diminished, the more accurate they were in their perceptions of burdening. They acknowledged other family members' efforts, appreciated those efforts, and encouraged family members to rest and take time to care for themselves. Patients who were less able to redefine themselves did not see that they were burdening other family members in any way. They denied or minimized the strain on others. As Ralph said during the last week of his life, "I can't do much, but I am fine really. Not much has changed. It's a burden on my wife, but not much. It might be some extra work. . . . She was a nursing aide, so she is used to this kind of work."

Most spouses acknowledged the "extra load" of caring for their dying partner, but indicated that they did not regard the situation as a "burden." They agreed that it's "just something you do for the one you love." Spouses did not focus on their own difficulties; they managed to put aside their own distress so that it would not have a negative impact on their loved one. They sometimes shared stories of loneliness and helplessness, but also stories of deepening respect and love for their partner. Again, spouses of patients who were able to redefine were energized by the patient's acknowledgment of their efforts

and were inspired to continue on. Spouses of patients who were not able to redefine felt unappreciated, exhausted, and confessed to "waiting for the patient to die."

The literature provides a comprehensive description of the multidimensional nature of the burden experienced by family caregivers, but no attention has been given to the burdening felt by patients or adult children specifically. Caregiver burden, usually by spouses, has been described in terms of physical burden, which includes fatigue and physical exhaustion, sleeplessness, and deterioration of health.[3,8,10,23] Social burden encompasses limited time for self and social stress related to isolation.[8,10,23] Regardless of the type of burden, however, most caregivers, including the ones in the fading away studies, expressed much satisfaction with their caregiving.[3,8,10] Despite feeling burdened, most caregivers would repeat the experience: "Yes, it was difficult and exhausting, and there were days I didn't think I could manage one more minute. But, if I had to do it over again, I would. I have no regrets for what I am doing."

Children, too, experienced burdening, but the source stemmed from the extra responsibilities involved in helping to care for a dying parent, superimposed on their work responsibilities, career development, and their own families. As a result, adult children of all ages felt a mixture of satisfaction and exhaustion. Their sense of burdening was also influenced by the ill parent's redefining—if the ill parent acknowledged their efforts, they were more likely to feel satisfaction. However, children's sense of burdening was also influenced by the state of health of the well parent. If that parent also was ill or debilitated, the burden on children was compounded. If children were able to prioritize their responsibilities so that they could pay attention to their own needs as well as helping both their parents, they felt less burdened. Children seemed less likely than their well parents to perceive caregiving as something they themselves would do. Of course, they did not have the life experience of a long-term relationship that motivated the spouses to care for their partners.

Finding effective ways to support family caregivers is critical, because an increase in the proportion of elderly people in the population means growing numbers of people with chronic, life-threatening, or serious illness require care. The responsibility for the care of such individuals is increasingly being placed on families. Respite care is often suggested as a strategy for relieving burden in family caregivers.[4,5,10] Respite and other resources or services should be offered to families, but each family must decide what will actually be helpful for them. For some families, inpatient respite services during the last year of life may help relieve their burden, while other caregivers may experience feelings of guilt and increased stress because of worrying about the quality of care provided.[24] Caregivers may be supported in their role simply by knowing there are other resources and support readily available, even if they do not make use of them.[4]

Another potential factor influencing the success of respite care may be the dynamics within the family, in particular between the patient and family caregivers. Respite must be assessed in conjunction with the role of redefining in burdening. Support for this suggestion comes from a study,[11] based in the Netherlands, of the experiences of caregivers, which showed that support from informal and professional caregivers was not sufficient to balance the stresses of caregiving and the missing element may be internal to the family. These findings encourage greater exploration into respite care and its meaning to caregivers. In one study of home-based family caregiving, caregivers differentiated between cognitive and physical breaks.[12] They valued cognitive breaks during which they remained within the caregiving environment, but physical separation from the caregiving environment was valuable only if it contributed in some meaningful way to the caregiving.

## Struggling with Paradox

Struggling with paradox stems from the fact that the patient is both living and dying. For patients, the struggle focuses on wanting to believe they will survive and knowing that they will not. On "good days," patients felt optimistic about the outcome; on other days, they succumbed to the inevitability of their approaching demise. Often, patients did not want to "give up" but at the same time were "tired of fighting." They wanted to "continue on" for the sake of their families but also wanted "it to end soon" so their families could "get on with their lives." Patients coped by hoping for miracles, fighting for the sake of their families, and focusing on the good days. As Joe said, "I like to think about the times when things are pretty good. I enjoy those days. But, on the bad days, when I'm tired, or when the pain gets the best of me, then I just wonder if it wouldn't be best to just quit. But you never know—maybe I'll be the one in a million who makes it at the last minute." He then added wryly, "Hmmm, big chance of that."

Spouses struggled with a paradox of their own: they wanted to care for and spend time with the patient, and they also wanted a "normal" life. They coped by juggling their time as best they could, and usually put their own life on hold. Spouses who managed to find ways of tending to their own needs usually were less exhausted and reported fewer health problems than spouses who neglected their own needs. For years, Joe and his wife had been square dancers. They hadn't been dancing together for many months when his wife resumed going to "dance night as a sub" or to prepare the evening's refreshments. "Sometimes, I feel guilty for going and leaving Joe at home, but I know I need a break. When I did miss dance night, I could see I was getting really bitchy—I need to get out for a breather so I don't suffocate Joe."

Children struggled with hanging on and letting go to a greater extent than their parents. They wanted to spend time with their ill parent and also to "get on with their own lives." Feeling the pressure of dual loyalties (to their parents and to their own young families), the demands of both compounded the struggle that children faced.

## Contending with Change

Those facing terminal illness in a family member experience changes in every realm of daily life—relationships, roles, socialization, and work patterns. The focus of the changes differed among family members. Patients faced changes in their relationships with everyone they knew. They realized that the greatest change of their life was underway, and that life as they knew it would soon be gone. They tended to break down tasks into manageable pieces, and increasingly they focused inward. The greatest change that spouses faced was in their relationship with the patient. They coped by attempting to keep everything as normal as possible. Children contended with changes that were more all-encompassing. They could not withdraw as their ill parent did, nor could they prioritize their lives to the degree that their well parent could. They easily become exhausted. As Joe's son explained, "It's a real challenge coming by this often—I try to come twice a week and then bring the kids on the weekends. But I just got a promotion at work this year, so that's extra work too. Seems like I don't see my wife much—but she's a real trooper. Her dad died last year so she knows what it's like."

## Searching for Meaning

Searching for meaning has to do with seeking answers to help in understanding the situation. Patients tended to journey inward, reflect on spiritual aspects, deepen their most important connections, and become closer to nature: "The spiritual thing has always been at the back of my mind, but it's developing more. . . . When you're sick like that, your attitude changes toward life. You come not to be afraid of death."

Spouses concentrated on their relationship with the patient. Some searched for meaning through personal growth, whereas others searched for meaning by simply tolerating the situation. Some focused on spiritual growth, and others adhered rigidly to their religion with little, if any, sense of inner growth or insight. Joe's wife commented, "Joe and I are closer than ever now. We don't like this business, but we have learned to love each other even more than when we were younger—sickness is a hard lesson that way." In contrast, Ralph's wife said with resignation, "He's so stubborn—always has been. I sometimes wonder why I stayed. But, here I am." Spouses and patients may attribute different meanings to other aspects of their experience as well. For example, when seeing their loved one in pain, many spouses felt helpless and fearful. Once the pain was controlled, they felt peaceful and relaxed and interpreted this as an indication that the couple would return to their old routines. The patient's meaning of the experience, however, often focused on future consequences of the pain.[7] The meaning attributed to the patient's experience also influenced spousal bereavement. For example, spouses who witnessed the patient die a painful death, and who believed that physician negligence was the cause of the pain, experienced elevated anger and much distress after the death.[25]

Children tended to reflect on and reevaluate all aspects of their lives: "It puts in perspective how important some of our goals are. . . . Having financial independence and being able to retire at a decent age. . . . Those things are important, but not at the expense of sacrificing today."

### Living Day to Day

Not all families reached the point of living day to day. If patients were able to find some meaning in their experience, then they were better able to adopt an attitude of living each day. Their attitude was characterized by "making the most of it." As one patient described it, "There's not much point in going over things in the past; not much point in projecting yourself too far into the future either. It's the current time that counts." Patients who were unable to find much meaning in their experience, or who didn't search for meaning, focused more on "getting through it." As Ralph said with determination, "Sure, I am getting weaker. I know I am sick. . . . But I will get through this!"

Spouses who searched for meaning focused on "making the best of it" while making every effort to enjoy the time they had left with their partner. Other spouses simply endured the situation without paying much attention to philosophizing about the experience. Children often had difficulty concentrating on living day to day, because they were unable to defer their obligations and therefore were constantly worrying about what else needed to be done. However, some children were still able to convey an attitude of "Live for today, today—worry about tomorrow, tomorrow."

### Preparing for Death

Preparing for death involved concrete actions that would have benefit in the future, after the patient died. Patients had their family's needs uppermost in their minds and worked hard to teach or guide family members with regard to various tasks and activities that the patient would no longer be around to do. Patients were committed to leaving legacies for their loved ones, not only as a means of being remembered but also as a way of comforting loved ones in their grief. Joe spent time "jotting down a few Mr. Fix-it pointers" for his wife and son. Ralph's energy was consumed by focusing on the work he still had to do, so he was unable to consider what he might do for his wife and daughter.

Spouses concentrated on meeting the patient's wishes. Whatever the patient wanted, spouses would try to do. They attended to practical details and anticipated their future in practical ways. Children offered considerable help to their parents with legal and financial matters. They also prepared their own children for what was to come. A central aspect was reassuring the dying parent that they would take care of the surviving parent. Children also prepared for the death by envisioning their future without their parent: "I think about it sometimes . . . about how my children will never have a grandfather. It makes me so sad. That's why the photos we have been taking are so important to me. . . . They will show our children who their grandfather was."

※※

## Palliative Care for Diagnoses Other Than Cancer

Traditionally, palliative care practice and discussions have focused on families of cancer patients. At the same time, care of the patient with cardiac disease, for example, has traditionally focused on restoring health and enabling a return to normal life. So, the idea of providing a patient with aggressive versus palliative treatment has, until recently, not been a well-discussed issue in the treatment of the patient with heart disease. For most patients with heart disease, and particularly for those with heart failure, the decline in functional status is slower than for patients diagnosed with cancer.[6] However, if palliative care is considered only after disease-related care fails or becomes too burdensome, the opportunity for patients to achieve symptom relief, and for patients and family members to engage in the process of fading away, may be lost. Consequently, following a model of care wherein issues of treatment and end-of-life care are discussed early and throughout the illness trajectory facilitates patient and family coping, and enables nurses to optimally support families.

Varying disease trajectories for other conditions, such as dementia, also influence the nature of support that nurses provide patients and families. For example, in a comparative study of staff's assessment of support needed by families of dementia and cancer patients, staff in dementia care stressed significantly more the need for forming support groups for families, offering respite care, educating families, and trying to relieve families' feeling of guilt. In the cancer-care group, staff assigned greater importance to being available to listen, creating a sense of security, and supporting the family after death.[17]

### Family Involvement According to Location of Care

Over the past century, nursing homes and hospitals increasingly have become the site of death. A landmark national study evaluated the U.S. dying experience at home and in institutional settings.[26] Family members of 1578 deceased individuals were asked via telephone survey about the patient's experience at the last place of care at which the patient spent >48 hours. Results showed that two thirds (67.2%) of patients were last cared for in an institution. Family members reported greater satisfaction with patient's symptom management, and with emotional support for both the patient and family, if they received care at home with hospice services. Families have greater opportunities for involvement in the care if home care is possible. Family involvement in hospital care also makes for better outcomes. Among geriatric patients receiving end-of-life care in a hospital setting, family involvement before death reduces the use of technology and increases the use of comfort care as patients die.[27]

Nurses, therefore, must consider how best to include families in the care of their dying loved ones, regardless of the location of care.

Large variations exist in the provision of home-based palliative and terminal care across the United States, although the development of hospice home services has enabled increasing numbers of seriously ill patients to experience care at home. However, dying at home can present special challenges for family members.[28] Lack of support and lack of confidence have been found to be determinants contributing to hospital admissions and the breakdown of informal caregiving for people with a life-threatening illness. A lack of support from the health care system is given as the reason many caregivers have to admit their loved one to the hospital.[23] They also report that fragmentation of services and lack of forward planning jeopardizes the success of home care.[29,30]

Moreover, the decision for home care has a profound effect on family members.[3,23,31,32] In an ethnographic study investigating palliative care at home,[33,34] caregiver decisions for home care were characterized in three ways. Some caregivers made uninformed decisions, giving little consideration to the implications of their decision: "I made the decision just like that. . . . There wasn't much thought that went into it." Such decisions were made early in the patient's disease trajectory or when the patient was imminently dying, and they were often influenced by the unrealistic portrayal in the media about dying at home. Indifferent decisions occurred if caregivers felt they had little choice. The patient's needs and wishes often drove decisions, with caregivers paying little attention to their own needs. Negotiated decisions for home care typically occurred if caregivers and patients were able to talk openly about dying, and had done so throughout the disease trajectory. For some families, a home death can bring additional burdens, worries, and responsibilities,[28] so it is important that open discussion is facilitated.

Family members' decisions were influenced by three major factors: making promises to care for the loved one at home, the desire to maintain as much as possible a "normal" life for the patient and themselves, and negative experiences with institutional care. Of interest, family members did not think of themselves as the target of professional interventions. They were reluctant to ask for help or to let their needs be known. Consequently, when working with caregiving families, health care providers could mediate discussions with the aim of coming to a mutually acceptable decision about home care. Such discussions could facilitate the sharing of perspectives, to allow for decisions that would work well for all concerned. Ideally, such discussions should begin early in the disease trajectory.

Importantly, ongoing attention should be paid to improving hospital end-of-life care so that families feel they have a meaningful alternative to home care. A small-scale study to develop and evaluate care pathways for the last days of life in a community setting was developed and tested in the United Kingdom, based on the pioneering work of Ellershaw.[35] The plan outlines the expected course of a patient's trajectory; brings together all the anticipated aspects of care, particularly with regard to symptom management and caregiver support; and encourages forward planning to avoid crisis admission to the hospital.[36] It serves as a model for how home care can be optimally delivered to those with terminal illness, echoing Doyle's[37] observation that good palliative care is an exercise in anticipation.

Clinicians must recognize the emotional impact of providing palliative care at home, and must be sensitive to the sometimes overwhelming task that caregiving imposes on family caregivers. Acknowledging that availability and access to service is important, Stajduhar and Davies[38] specified that care must be provided within a team context so that families can benefit from a whole set of services needed to support death at home. Clinicians must work with the dying patients, with family caregivers, and with each other as equal partners in the caregiving process.

Clinicians must be available to families, offering anticipatory guidance and support throughout the caregiving experience. Health care professionals must assist family members as they traverse the maze of treatment and care decisions, ranging from whether to give particular "as needed" medications, or what food to make for the patient to eat, to whether or not to seek hospice care, to sign "do-not-resuscitate" documents, or to terminate treatment. It is critical that palliative care professionals continually engage with caregivers in forward planning, interpretation, and monitoring of the inevitable decline and dying process of the ill person, so as to facilitate the feeling in caregivers that they are secure and supported in their physically and emotionally exhausting work. Families need to know whom to call and when, and how to reach them.

Some simple guidelines for families can serve to encourage their coping. For example, caregivers should be told to keep a small notebook handy for jotting down questions and answers. The pages may be divided in half lengthwise, using the column on the left for questions and the other column for answers. Or, the left-sided page may be used for questions and the opposite page for the answers. They should be advised to have the notebook with them whenever they talk with a member of the palliative care team. Family members should be reassured that nothing is trivial. All questions are important, and all observations are valuable. They should be encouraged to say when they do not understand something, and to ask for information to be repeated as necessary. Palliative care professionals can help by spelling words that family members do not understand or by jotting down explanations. They should reassure family members that asking for help is not a sign of failure, but rather a sign of good common sense. Following such simple guidelines helps keep families from feeling overwhelmed. And, if they do feel "out of control," such guidelines, simple as they may seem, give family members some concrete action they can take to help with whatever the situation may be.

Clinicians must also remember that their own attitudes are critical; if families feel they are a "nuisance" to health care providers, they tend to be more anxious and to shy away from asking for help. Furthermore, clinicians are in ideal positions to advocate with politicians and policy makers to expand resources for home-based palliative care programs so that families can adequately and humanely be supported in their caregiving work.

## Caregiving at a Distance

Not all caregiving is provided by family members who live with, or are geographically close to, the patient. Distant caregiving, the provision of instrumental and/or emotional support to an ill loved one who lives a long distance from the caregiver, is prevalent in today's changing society. Adult children often live far from their parents and find themselves caregiving from a distance. Millions of Americans are distant caregivers[39] and the number is expected to reach approximately 14 million by the year 2012[40] as baby boomers and their parents age. An estimated 15% of adult children are caregiving parents from a distance.[41] These adult children are dealing with the added challenges and stressors associated with living at a distance, such as lack of nearby family support. There is some indication that stress related to the distant caregiving is reported by about 79% of these caregivers.[42] Otherwise, little is known about their experiences, yet most interventions have been designed to support local caregivers. Clinicians must remember that interventions to decrease caregiver burden and improve caregiver well-being may not be as applicable to distant caregivers, who may need extra flexibility and accommodations, such as increased telephone communication, in order to meet their needs.

## Guidelines for Nursing Interventions

Respect for persons requires that clinicians understand diversity and are able to manage issues that may arise when caring for people with varied backgrounds. The cultural and spiritual backgrounds of families, as well as those of the clinician, need to be taken into account because cultural or spiritual beliefs may be important in assisting families to cope.[43] All nursing interventions should be provided with respect to an individual's background. However, despite differences across cultures, it is important to remember that similarities exist in regards to basic needs for support, dignity, and connections with others.[44]

Much of the nursing literature, which provides guidelines for nursing care, addresses the importance of four major interventions that have relevance for all members of the palliative care team:

1. *Maintain hope* in patients and their family members. As families pass through the illness trajectory, the nature of their hope changes from hope for cure, to hope for remission, to hope for comfort, to hope for a good death. Offering hope during fading away can be as simple as reassuring families that everything will be done to ensure the patient's comfort. Talking about the past also can help some families by reaffirming the good times spent together and the ongoing connections that will continue among family members. Referring to the future beyond the immediate suffering and emotional pain can also sustain hope. For example, when adult children reassure the ill parent that they will care for the other parent, the patient is hopeful that the surviving spouse will be all right.

2. *Involve families* in all aspects of care. Include them in decision-making, and encourage active participation in the physical care of the patient. This is their life—they have the right to control it as they will. Involvement is especially important for children when a family member is very ill. The more children are involved in care during the terminal phase, and in the activities that follow the death, the better able they are to cope with bereavement.[45]

3. *Offer information*. Tell families about what is happening in straightforward terms and about what they can expect to happen, particularly about the patient's condition and the process their loved one is to undergo. Doing so also provides families with a sense of control. Initiate the discussion of relevant issues that family members themselves may hesitate to mention. For example, the nurse might say, "Many family members feel as if they are being pulled in two or more directions when a loved one is very ill. They want to spend as much time as possible with the patient, but they also feel the pull of their own daily lives, careers, or families. How does this fit with your experience?"

4. *Communicate openly*. Open and honest communication with nurses and other health professionals is frequently the most important need of families. They need to be informed; they need opportunities to ask questions and to have their questions answered in terms that they can comprehend. Open communication among team members is basic to open communication with the families.

It is not an easy task for families to give up their comfortable and established views of themselves as death approaches. The challenge for members of the health care team is to help family members anticipate what lies ahead, without violating their need to relinquish old orientations and hopes at a pace they can handle. These four broad interventions assist health care providers in providing good palliative care; the following guidelines offer further direction. They are derived from the direct accounts of patients, spouses, and children about the strategies they used to cope with the dimensions of fading away.

## Redefining

Supporting patients and other family members with redefining requires that health care providers appreciate how difficult it is for family members to relinquish familiar perceptions of themselves and adopt unfamiliar, unwelcome, and unasked-for changes to their self-perceptions. Disengagement from former perceptions and the adoption of new orientations occur over time. Nurses and other care providers are challenged to help family members anticipate and prepare for what lies ahead, while not pushing them at a pace that threatens their sense of integrity. Each family member redefines at his or her own pace; interventions must be tailored according to the individual needs of each. At the same time, health care providers must support the family as a unit by reassuring family members that their varying coping responses and strategies are to be expected.

Provide opportunities for patients to talk about the losses incurred due to the illness, the enforced changes, the adaptations they have made, and their feelings associated with these changes. Reinforce their normal patterns of living as long as possible and as appropriate. When they can no longer function as they once did, focus on what patients still can do, reinforcing those aspects of self that remain intact. Acknowledge that roles and responsibilities may be expressed in new and different ways, and suggest new activities appropriate to the patient's interest and current capabilities.

The focus with spouses and children centers on explaining how the disease or treatment contributes to changes in the patient physically, psychologically, and socially. Provide opportunities for spouses to talk about how changes in the patient affect their marital relationship. Help children appreciate their parent from another perspective, such as in recalling favorite memories or identifying the legacies left. Discuss how they can face their own vulnerability by channeling concerns into positive steps for self-care. Reinforce the spouse's and children's usual patterns of living for as long as possible and as appropriate; when former patterns are no longer feasible, help them to consider adjustments or alternatives.

Provide opportunities for spouses to discuss how they may reorganize priorities in order to be with and care for the patient to the degree they desire. Consider resources that enable the spouse to do this, such as the assistance of volunteers, home support services, or additional nursing services. Teach caregiving techniques if the spouse shows interest. With the children, discuss the degree to which they want to be open or private about the patient's illness with those outside the family. Acknowledge that family members will vary in their ability to assimilate changes in the patient and in their family life.

## Burdening

Palliative care professionals can help patients find ways to relieve their sense of burden, and can provide patients with opportunities to talk about their fears and concerns and to consider with whom they want to share their worries. In this way, patients may alleviate their concern for putting excessive demands on family members. Explain the importance of a break for family members, and suggest that patients accept

assistance from a volunteer or home-support services at those times to relieve family members from worry. Explain that when patients affirm family members for their efforts, this contributes to family members feeling appreciated and reduces their sense of burden.

Nurses and all members of the interdisciplinary team can assist spouses with burdening by supporting the spouse's reassurances to the patient that he or she is not a burden. Acknowledge spouses' efforts when they put their own needs on hold to care for the patient; help them to appreciate the importance of taking care of themselves as a legitimate way of sustaining the energy they need for the patient. Talk with spouses about how they might take time out, and consider the various resources they might use. Acknowledge the negative feelings spouses may have about how long they can continue; do not negate their positive desire to help.

For children, acknowledge the reorganization and the considerable adjustment in their daily routines. Explain that ambivalent feelings are common—the positive feelings associated with helping, and the negative feelings associated with less time spent on careers and their own families. Acknowledge that communicating regularly with their parents by telephoning or visiting often is part of the "work" of caring; the extra effort involved should not be underestimated. Encourage children to take time out for themselves, and support them in their desire to maintain involvement in their typical lives.

## Struggling with Paradox

Facing the usual business of living and directly dealing with dying is a considerable challenge for all members of the family. The care provider's challenge is to appreciate that it is not possible to alleviate completely the family's psychosocial and spiritual pain. Team members must face their own comfort level in working with families who are facing paradoxical situations and the associated ambivalent feelings. Like family members, nurses, social workers, physicians, and all team members may also sometimes want to avoid the distress of struggling with paradox. They may feel unprepared to handle conversations in which no simple solution exists, and strong feelings abound.

Care providers can support patients and other family members by providing opportunities for all family members to ventilate their frustrations and not minimizing their pain and anguish. On the good days, rejoice with them. Listen to their expressions of ambivalence, and be prepared for the ups and downs and changes of opinion that are sure to occur. Reassure them that their ambivalence is a common response. Encourage "time out" as a way to replenish depleted energy.

## Contending with Change

Palliative care team members must realize that not all families communicate openly or work easily together in solving problems. Nurses in particular can support patients and family members to contend with change by creating an environment in which families explore and manage their own concerns and feelings according to their particular coping style. Providing information so that families can explore various alternatives helps them to determine what adjustments they can make. Make information available not only verbally but also in writing. Or, tape-record informative discussions so that families can revisit what they have been told.

Rituals can be helpful during periods of terminal illness. A family ritual is a behavior or action that reflects some symbolic meaning for all members of the family and is part of their collective experience. A ritual does not have to be religious in nature. Rituals may already exist, or they can be newly created to assist the family in contending with change. For example, the writing of an "ethical will," whereby one passes on wisdom to others or elaborates on his or her hopes for their loved ones' future, can help ill family members communicate what they might not be able to verbalize to their loved ones. Developing new rituals can help with the changes in everyday life; for example, one woman had always been the sounding board for her children on their return from school. It was a pattern that continued as her children entered the work force. Cancer of the trachea prevented her participation in the same way. Instead, she requested her young adult children to sit by her side, hold her hand, and recount their days. Instead of words, the mother responded with varying hand squeezes to let them know she was listening. The altered daily ritual served both mother and children in adapting to the changes in their lives.

### Searching for Meaning

Palliative care professionals help families search for meaning by enabling them to tell their personal stories and make sense of them. It is essential that team members appreciate the value of storytelling—when a family talks about its current situation and recollections of the past, it is not just idle chatter. It is a vital part of making sense of the situation and coping with it. Professional team members must appreciate that much of the search for meaning involves examining spiritual dimensions, belief systems, values, and relationships within and outside the family. Nurses can be supportive by suggesting approaches for personal reflection, such as journal writing or writing letters.

### Living Day to Day

In living day to day, families make subtle shifts in their orientation to living with a dying family member. They move from thinking that there is no future to making the most of the time they have left. This is a good time to review the resources available to the family, to ensure that they are using all possible sources of assistance so that their time together is optimally spent.

### Preparing for Death

In helping families prepare for death, nurses in particular must be comfortable talking about the inevitability of death, describing the dying process, and helping families make plans for wills and funerals. It is important not to push or force such issues; it is equally important not to avoid them because of the nurse's personal discomfort with dying and death. Encourage such discussions among family members while acknowledging how difficult they can be. Affirm them for their courage to face these difficult issues. Encourage patients to attend to practical details, such as finalizing a will and distributing possessions. Encourage them to do "last things," such as participating in a special holiday celebration.

Provide information to spouses and children about the dying process. If the plan is for death at home, provide information about what procedures will need to be followed and the resources that are available. Provide opportunities for family members to express their concerns and ask questions. Encourage them to reminisce with the patient as a way of saying "good-bye," and acknowledge the bittersweet quality of such remembrances. Provide information to the adult children about how they can help their own children with the impending death.

The foregoing guidelines are intended to assist nurses and all members of the palliative care team in their care of individual family members. The guidelines are summarized in Table 31–1. In addition, family-centered care also means focusing on the family as a unit. Health care providers must appreciate that the family as a whole has a life of its own that is distinct, but always connected to the individuals who are part of it. Both levels of care are important.[19] The families in the "fading away" study also provided insights about how family functioning plays a role in coping with terminal illness in a family member.

### Family Functioning and Fading Away

Families experienced the transition of fading away with greater or lesser difficulty, depending on their level of functioning according to eight dimensions: integrating the past, dealing with feelings, solving problems, utilizing resources, considering others, portraying family identity, fulfilling roles, and tolerating differences. These dimensions occurred along a continuum of functionality; family interactions tended to vary along this continuum rather than being positive or negative, good or bad.

Some families acknowledged the pain of past experience with illness, loss, and other adversity, and integrated previous learning into how they were managing their current situation. These families expressed a range of feelings, from happiness and satisfaction, through uncertainty and dread, to sadness and sorrow. Family members acknowledged their vulnerabilities and their ambivalent feelings. All topics were open for discussion. There were no clearcut rights and wrongs, and no absolute answers to the family's problems. They applied a flexible approach to problem-solving and openly exchanged all information. They engaged in

**Table 31–1**
**Dimensions of Fading Away: Nursing Interventions for Family Members**

**Redefining**

Appreciate that relinquishing old and comfortable views of themselves occurs over time and does not necessarily occur simultaneously with physical changes in the patient

Tailor interventions according to the various abilities of family members to assimilate the changes

Reassure family members that a range of responses and coping strategies is to be expected within and among family members

Provide opportunities for patients to talk about the illness, the enforced changes in their lives, and the ways in which they have adapted; for spouses to talk about how changes in the patient affect their marital relationship; and for children to talk about their own feelings of vulnerability and the degree to which they want to be open or private about the situation

Reinforce normal patterns of living for as long as possible and as appropriate. When patterns are no longer viable, consider adjustments or alternatives

Focus on the patient's attributes that remain intact, and acknowledge that roles and responsibilities may be expressed differently. Consider adjustments or alternatives when former patterns are no longer feasible

Help spouses consider how they might reorganize priorities and consider resources to help them do this

Help children appreciate their parent from another perspective, such as in recalling favorite stories or identifying legacies left

**Burdening**

Provide opportunities for patients to talk about fears and anxieties about dying and death, and to consider with whom to share their concerns

Help patients stay involved for as long as possible as a way of sustaining self-esteem and a sense of control

Assist family members to take on tasks appropriate to their comfort level and skill and share tasks among themselves

Support family members' reassurances to patient that he or she is not a burden. Explain that when patients reaffirm family members for their efforts, this contributes to their feeling appreciated and lessens the potential for feeling burdened

Explain the importance of breaks for family members. Encourage others to take over for patients on a regular basis so family members can take a break

Acknowledge the reorganization of priorities and the considerable adjustment in family routines and extra demands placed on family members. Acknowledge the "work" of caring for all family members

Realize that family members will vary in their ability to assimilate the changes and that a range of reactions and coping strategies is normal

**Struggling with paradox**

Appreciate that you, as a nurse, cannot completely alleviate the psychosocial-spiritual pain inherent in the family's struggle

Assess your own comfort level in working with people facing paradoxical situations and ambivalent feelings

Provide opportunities for family members to mourn the loss of their hopes and plans. Do not minimize these losses; help them modify their previous hopes and plans and consider new ones

Listen to their expressions of ambivalence, and be prepared for the ups and downs of opinions

Ensure effective symptom management, because this allows patients and family members to focus outside the illness

Explain the importance of respite as a strategy for renewing energy for dealing with the situation

**Contending with change**

Create an environment in which family members can explore and manage their own concerns and feelings. Encourage dialogue about family members' beliefs, feelings, hopes, fears, and dilemmas so they can determine their own course of action

Recognize that families communicate in well-entrenched patterns and their ability to communicate openly and honestly differs

Normalize the experience of family members and explain that such feelings do not negate the positive feelings of concern and affection

Provide information so families can explore the available resources, their options, and the pros and cons of the various options. Provide information in writing as well as verbally

Explain the wide-ranging nature of the changes that occur within the patient's immediate and extended family

**Searching for meaning**

Appreciate that the search for meaning involves examination of the self, of relationships with other family members, and of spiritual aspects.

Realize that talking about the current situation and their recollections of past illness and losses is part of making sense of the situation

Encourage life reviews and reminiscing. Listen to the life stories that family members tell

Suggest approaches for self-examination such as journal writing, and approaches for facilitating interactions between family members such as writing letters

**Living day to day**

Listen carefully for the subtle shifts in orientation to living with a dying relative and gauge family members' readiness for a new orientation

Ensure effective control of symptoms so that the patient can make the most of the time available. Assess the need for aids

Without minimizing their losses and concerns, affirm their ability to appreciate and make the most of the time left

Review resources that would free family members to spend more time with the patient

**Preparing for death**

Assess your own comfort level in talking about the inevitability of death, describing the dying process, and helping families make plans for wills and funerals

Provide information about the dying process

Discuss patients' preferences about the circumstances of their death. Encourage patients to discuss these issues with their family. Acknowledge how difficult such discussions can be

Encourage patients to do important "last things," such as completing a project as a legacy for their family

Provide opportunities for spouses and children to express their concerns about their future without the patient. Provide them with opportunities to reminisce about their life together. Acknowledge such remembrances will have a bittersweet quality

*Source:* Davies et al. (1995), reference 19.

**Table 31–2**
**Dimensions of Family Functioning: Examples of the Range of Behaviors**

| More Helpful | Less Helpful |
|---|---|
| **Integrating the past** | |
| Describe the painful experiences as they relate to present experience | Describe past experiences repeatedly |
| Describe positive and negative feelings concerning the past | Dwell on painful feeling associated with past experiences |
| Incorporate learning from the past into subsequent experiences | Do not integrate learning from the past to the current situation |
| Reminisce about pleasurable experiences in the past | Focus on trying to "fix" the past to create happy memories which are absent from their family life |
| **Dealing with feelings** | |
| Express a range of feelings including vulnerability, fear, and uncertainty | Express predominantly negative feelings, such as anger, hurt, bitterness, and fear |
| Acknowledge paradoxical feelings | Acknowledge little uncertainty or few paradoxical feelings |
| **Solving problems** | |
| Identify problems as they occur | Focus more on fault finding than on finding solutions |
| Reach consensus about a problem and possible courses of action | Dwell on the emotions associated with the problem |
| Consider multiple options | Unable to clearly communicate needs and expectations |
| Open to suggestions | Feel powerless about influencing the care they are receiving |
| Approach problems as a team rather than as individuals | Display exaggerated response to unexpected events |
| | Withhold or inaccurately share information with other family members |
| **Utilizing resources** | |
| Utilize a wide range of resources | Utilize few resources |
| Open to accepting support | Reluctant to seek help or accept offers of help |
| Open to suggestions regarding resources | Receive help mostly from formal sources rather than from informal support networks |
| Take the initiative in procuring additional resources | |
| Express satisfaction with results obtained | Express dissatisfaction with help received |
| Describe the involvement of many friends, acquaintances, and support persons | Describe fewer friends and acquaintances who offer help |
| **Considering others** | |
| Acknowledge multidimensional effects of situation on other family members | Focus concern on own emotional needs |
| Express concern for well-being of other family members | Fail to acknowledge or minimize extra tasks taken on by others |
| Focus concern on patient's well-being | |
| Appreciate individualized attention from health care professionals, but do not express strong need for such attention | Display inordinate need for individualized attention |
| Direct concerns about how other family members are managing rather than with themselves | |
| Identify characteristic coping styles of family unit and of individual members | Describe own characteristic coping styles rather than the characteristic way the family as a unit coped |
| Demonstrate warmth and caring toward other family members | Allow one member to dominate group interaction |
| Consider present situation as potential opportunity for family's growth and development | Lack comfort with expressing true feelings in the family group |
| Value contributions of all family members | Feign group consensus where none exists |
| Describe a history of closeness among family members | Describe few family interactions prior to illness |
| **Fulfilling roles** | |
| Demonstrate flexibility in adapting to role changes | Demonstrate rigidity in adapting to role changes and responsibilities |
| Share extra responsibilities willingly | Demonstrate less sharing of responsibilities created by extra demands of patient care |
| Adjust priorities to incorporate extra demands of patient care and express satisfaction with this decision | Refer to caregiving as a duty or obligation |
| | Criticize or mistrust caregiving provided by others |
| **Tolerating differences** | |
| Allow differing opinions and beliefs within the family | Display intolerance for differing opinions or approaches of caregiving |
| Tolerate different views from people outside the family | Demonstrate critical views of friends who fail to respond as expected |
| Willing to examine own belief and value systems | Adhere rigidly to belief and value systems |

*Source:* Davies, et al. (1994), reference 49. Reprinted with permission.

**Table 31–3**
**Family Functioning: Guidelines for Interventions in Palliative Care**

## Assessing family functioning

*Use dimensions of family functioning to assess families.* For example: Do members focus their concern on the patient's well-being and recognize the effect of the situation on other family members, or do family members focus their concerns on their own individual needs and minimize how others might be affected? Putting your assessment of all the dimensions together will help you determine to what degree you are dealing with a more cohesive family unit or a more loosely coupled group of individuals, and hence what approaches are most appropriate.

*Be prepared to collect information over time and from different family members.* Some family members may not be willing to reveal their true feelings until they have developed trust. Others may be reluctant to share differing viewpoints in the presence of one another. In some families, certain individuals take on the role of spokesperson for the family. Assessing whether everyone in the family shares the viewpoints of the spokesperson, or whether different family members have divergent opinions but are reluctant to share them, is a critical part of the assessment.

*Listen to the family's story and use clinical judgment to determine where intervention is required.* Part of understanding a family is listening to their story. In some families, the stories tend to be repeated and the feelings associated with them resurface. Talking about the past is a way of being for some families. It is important that the nurse determine whether family members are repeatedly telling their story because they want to be better understood or because they want help to change the way their family deals with the situation. Most often the stories are retold simply because family members want the nurse to understand them and their situation better, not because they are looking for help to change the way their family functions.

## Solving problems

*Use your assessment of family functioning to guide your approaches.* For example, in families where there is little consensus about the problems, rigidity in beliefs, and inflexibility in roles and relationships, the common rule of thumb—offering families various options so they may choose those that suit them best—tends to be less successful. For these families, carefully consider which resource provides the best possible fit for that particular family. Offer resources slowly, perhaps one at a time. Focus considerable attention on the degree of disruption associated with the introduction of the resource, and prepare the family for the change that ensues. Otherwise, the family may reject the resource as unsuitable and perceive the experience as yet another example of failure of the health care system to meet their needs.

*Be aware of the limitations of family conferences and be prepared to follow up.* Family conferences work well for more cohesive family units. However, where more disparity exists among the members, they may not follow through with the decisions made, even though consensus was apparently achieved. Though not voicing their disagreement, some family members may not be committed to the solution put forward and may disregard the agreed-upon plan. The nurse needs to follow up to ensure that any trouble spots are addressed.

*Be prepared to repeat information.* In less-cohesive families, do not assume that information will be accurately and openly shared with other family members. You may have to repeat information several times to different family members and repeat answers to the same questions from various family members.

*Evaluate the appropriateness of support groups.* Support groups can be a valuable resource. They help by providing people with the opportunity to hear the perspectives of others in similar situations. However, some family members need more individualized attention than a support group provides. They do not benefit from hearing how others have experienced the situation and dealt with the problems. They need one-to-one interaction focused on themselves with someone with whom they have developed trust.

*Adjust care to the level of family functioning.* Some families are more overwhelmed by the palliative care experience than others. Understanding family functioning can help nurses appreciate that expectations for some families to "pull together" to cope with the stress of palliative care may be unrealistic. Nurses need to adjust their care according to the family's way of functioning and be prepared for the fact that working with some families is more demanding and the outcomes achieved are less optimal.

*Source*: Davies et al. (1995), reference 19.

mutual decision-making, considering each member's point of view and feelings. Each family member was permitted to voice both positive and negative opinions in the process of making decisions. They agreed on the characteristics of their family and allowed individual variation within the family. They allocated household and patient care responsibilities in a flexible way. These families were often amenable to outside intervention and were comfortable in seeking and using external resources. Such families were often appealing to palliative care nurses and other personnel, because they openly discussed their situation, shared their concerns, and accepted help willingly.

Other families were more challenging for palliative care professionals. These were families who hung on to negative past experiences and continued to dwell on the painful feelings associated with past events. They appeared to avoid the feelings of turmoil and ambivalence, shielding themselves from the pain, often indicating that they did not usually express their feelings. These families approached problems by focusing more on why the problem occurred and who was at fault, rather than generating potential solutions. They often were unable to communicate their needs or expectations to each other or to health care professionals, and were angry when their wishes were not fulfilled. They expressed discrepant views only in individual interviews, not when all members were present, and tended not to tolerate differences. Varying approaches by health care workers were not generally well tolerated, either. These families did not adapt easily to new roles, nor did they welcome outside assistance. Such families showed little concern for others. They used few resources, because family members were often unable or reluctant to seek help from others. Such families often presented a challenge for nursing care. Nurses must realize that expecting such families to "pull together" to cope with the stresses of palliative care is unrealistic. It is essential not to judge these families, but rather to appreciate that the family is coping as best it can under very difficult circumstances. These families need support and affirmation of their existing coping strategies, not judgmental criticisms.

Palliative care clinicians are encouraged to complete assessments of level of family system functioning early in their encounters with families.[46,47] This is the best time to begin to develop an understanding of the family as a whole, as a basis for the services to be offered. In fact, the value of focusing on patterns of family functioning has been demonstrated by a clinical approach that screens for families, rather than individuals, at high risk.[48] Assessment of family functioning provides a basis for effective interactions to ensure a family-focused approach in palliative care. The eight dimensions of family functioning provide a guideline for assessment. Table 31–2 summarizes these dimensions and gives examples of the range of behaviors evident in each dimension. The table summarizes those behaviors that on one end of the continuum are more helpful, and on the other end are less helpful to families facing the transition of fading away.

Understanding the concept of family functioning enhances the nurse's ability to assess the unique characteristics of each family. An assessment of family functioning enables the nurse to interact appropriately with the family and help them solve problems more effectively (Table 31–3). For example, in families where communication is open and shared among all members, the nurse can be confident that communication with one family member will be accurately passed on to other members. In families where communication is not as open, the nurse must take extra time to share the information with all members. Or, in families who dwell on their negative past experiences with the health care system, nurses must realize that establishing trust is likely to require extra effort and time. Families who are open to outside intervention are more likely to benefit from resource referrals; other families may need more encouragement and time to open their doors to external assistance.

Nurses, and all palliative care providers, must remember that each family is unique and comes with its own life story and circumstances; listening to the story is central to understanding the family. There may be threads of commonality, but there will not be duplicate experiences. Nurses must assist family members to recognize the essential role they are playing in the experience, and to acknowledge their contributions. Most importantly, nurses must realize that each family is doing the best it can. Nurses must sensitively, creatively, and patiently support families as they encounter one of the greatest challenges families must face—the transition of fading away.

REFERENCES

1. Panke JT, Ferrell BR. Emotional problems in the family. In: Doyle D, Hanks G, Cherny N, Calman K, eds. Oxford Textbook of Palliative Medicine (3rd ed). Oxford: Oxford University Press; 2004:895–991.

2. Field MJ, Cassell CK, eds. Approaching Death: Improving Care at the End of Life. Washington, DC: National Academy Press, 1997.

3. Andershed B. Relatives in end-of-life care—part 1: A systematic review of the literature the past five years, January 1999–February 2004. J Clin Nurs 2006;15:1158–1169.

4. Stajduhar KI, Martin WL, Barwich D, Fyles G. Factors influencing family caregivers' ability to cope with providing end-of-life cancer care at home. Canc Nurs 2008;31:77–85.

5. Goy ER, Carter JH, Ganzini L. Parkinson disease at the end of life: Caregiver perspectives. Neurology 2007;69:611–612.

6. Barnes S, Gott M, Payne S, et al. Characteristics and views of family carers of older people with heart failure. Int J Palliat Nurs 2006;12:380–389.

7. Mehta A, Ezer H. My love is hurting: The meaning spouses attribute to their loved ones' pain during palliative care. J Palliat Care 2003;19:87–94.

8. Stajduhar K, Davies B. Palliative care at home: Reflections on HIV/AIDS family caregiving experiences. J Palliat Care 1998;14:14–22.

9. Riley J, Fenton G. A terminal diagnosis: The carers' perspective. CPR 2007;7:86–91.

10. Jo S, Brazil K, Lohfield L, Willison K. Caregiving at the end of life: Perspectives from spousal caregivers and care recipients. Pall Support Care 2007;5:11–17.

11. Proot IM, Abu-Saad HH, Crebolder HF, Goldsteen M, Luker KA, Widdershoven GA. Vulnerability of family caregivers in terminal palliative care at home: Balancing between burden and capacity. Scand J Caring 2003;17:113–121.

12. Strang V, Koop P, Peden J. The experience of respite during home-based family caregiving for persons with advanced cancer. J Palliat Care 2003;18:97–104.

13. Benzein EG, Saveman B. Health-promoting conversations about hope and suffering with couples in palliative care. Int J Palliat Nurse 2008;14:439–445.

14. Cantor J, Blustein J, Carlson MJ, Gould D. Next-of-kin perceptions in physician responsiveness to symptoms of hospitalized patients near death. J Palliat Med 2003;6:531–539.

15. Rhodes RL, Mitchell SL, Miller SC, Connor SR, Teno JM. Bereaved family members' evaluation of hospice care: What factors influence overall satisfaction with care? J Pain Sympt Manage 2008;35:365–371.

16. Baker R, Wu AW, Teno JM, et al. Family satisfaction with end-of-life care in seriously ill hospitalized patients: Findings of the SUPPORT program. J Am Geriatr Soc 2000;48:S61–S69.

17. Albinsson L, Strang P. Differences in supporting families of dementia patients and cancer patients: A palliative perspective. Palliat Med 2003;17:359–367.

18. Caron CD, Griffith J, Arcand M. End-of-life decision making in dementia: The perspective of family caregivers. Dementia 2005;4:113–136.

19. Davies B, Chekryn Reimer J, Brown P, Martens N. Fading Away: The Experience of Transition in Families with Terminal Illness. Amityville, NY: Baywood, 1995.

20. Bridges W. Transitions: Making Sense of Life's Changes. Reading, MA: Addison-Wesley, 1980.

21. Sherman DW. Reciprocal suffering: The need to improve family caregivers' quality of life through palliative care. J Palliat Care 1998;1:357–366.

22. Koop P, Strang V. The bereavement experience following home-based family caregiving for persons with advanced cancer. Clin Nurs Res 2003;12:127–144.

23. Perreault A, Fothergill-Bourbonnais F, Fiset V. The experience of family members caring for a dying loved one. Int J Palliat Nurs 2004;10:133–143.

24. Skilbeck JK, Payne SA, Ingleton MC, Nolan M, Carey I, Hanson A. An exploration of family carers' experience of respite services in one specialist palliative care unit. Pall Med 2005;19:610–618.

25. Carr D. A "good death" for whom? Quality of spouse's death and psychological distress among older widowed persons. J Health Social Behav 2003;44:215–232.

26. Teno JM, Clarridge BR, Casey V, et al. Family perspectives on end-of-life care at the last place of death. JAMA 2004;291:88–93.

27. Tschann JM, Kaufman SR, Micco GP. Family involvement in end-of-life hospital care. J Am Geriatr Soc 2003;51:835–840.

28. Brazil K, Howell D, Bedard M, Krueger P, Heidebrecht C. Preferences for place of care and place of death among inforaml caregivers of the terminally ill. Pall Med 2005;19:492–499.

29. Beaver K, Luker K, Woods S. Primary care services received curing terminal illness. Int J Palliat Nurs 2000;6:220–227.

30. Thomas K. Out-of-hours palliative care: Bridging the gap. Eur J Palliat Care 2000;7:22–25.

31. Addington-Hall J, Karlsen S. Do home deaths increase distress in bereavement? Palliat Med 2000;14:161–162.

32. Aranda SK, Hayman-White K. Home caregivers of the person with advanced cancer: An Australian perspective. Cancer Nurs 2001;24:300–307.

33. Stajduhar KI. Examining the perspectives of family members involved in the delivery of palliative care at home. J Palliat Care 2003;19:27–35.

34. Stajduhar KI, Davies B. Variations in and factors influencing family members' decisions for palliative home care. Palliat Med 2005;19:21–32.

35. Ellershaw J, Foster A, Murphy D, Shea T, Overill S. Developing an integrated care pathway for the dying patient. Eur J Palliat Care 1997;4:203–207.

36. Pooler J, McCrory F, Steadman Y, Westwell H, Peers S. Dying at home: A care pathway for the last days of life in a community setting. Int J Palliat Nurs 2003;9:258–264.

37. Doyle D. Palliative medicine in the home: An overview. In: Doyle D, Hanks G, MacDonald N, eds. Oxford Textbook of Palliative Care (2nd ed). Oxford: Oxford University Press; 2004:1097–1114.

38. Stajduhar K, Davies B. Death at home: Challenges for families and directions for the future. J Palliat Care 1996;14:8–14.

39. Wagner, D. Caring across the miles: Findings of a survey of long-distance caregivers. Final Report for the National Council on the Aging. Washington, D.C.: National Council on the Aging, 1997.

40. National Council on Aging. Nearly 7 million long-distance caregivers make work and personal sacrifices. Washington, D.C.: Author. 1997. Retrieved December 5, 2008, from https://www.ncoa.org/content.cfm?sectionID=105&detail=49

41. National Alliance for Caregiving & AARP. Caregiving in the U.S. 2004. Retrieved December 5, 2008, from http://www.caregiving.org/data/04finalreport.pdf

42. Koerin B, Harrigan M. P.S. I love you: Long distance caregiving. J Social Work 2002;40:63–81.

43. Torke AM, Garas NS, Sexson W, Branch WT Jr. Medical care at the end of life: Views of African American patients in an urban hospital. J Pall Med, 2005;8:593–602.

44. Diver F, Molassiotis A, Weeks L. The palliative care needs of ethnic minority patients attending a day-care centre: A qualitative study. Int J Pall Nurs, 2003;9:389–396.

45. Davies B. Environmental factors affecting sibling bereavement. In: Davies B. Shadows in the Sun: Experiences of Sibling Bereavement in Childhood. Philadelphia: Brunner/Mazel; 1999:123–148.

46. Jassak P. Families: An essential element in the care of the patient with cancer. Oncol Nurs Forum 1992;19:871–986.

47. Gulla J. Family assessment and its relation to hospice care. Am J Hospice Palliat Care 1992 (July/August):30–34.

48. Kissane DW, McKenzie M, McKenzie DP, Forbes A, O'Neill I, Block S. Psychosocial morbidity associated with patterns of family functioning in palliative care: Baseline data from the Family Focused Grief Therapy controlled trial. Palliat Med 2003;17:527–537.

49. Davies B, Reimer J, Martens N. Family functioning and its implications for palliative care. J Palliat Care 1994;10:35–36.

# 32 ❧❧❧
*Patricia Berry and Julie Griffie*

# Planning for the Actual Death

*My "little sister's" pancreatic cancer had weighed on my sister and her family for the last two years. Her life partner never communicated well with our family, so she has lived in relative isolation from us for the last 25 years. Now, as she is very close to death, there are problems with this person and the hospice staff, as he can be volatile and threatening. Consequently, they established a contract with him to assure everyone's safety.*

*So I was apprehensive over what I would encounter on my first visit. I hadn't seen her since they had struggled with her physicians over the hospice decision. I found her gently confused, such that I was her brother, but not sure which one. I was able to speak from my heart and tell her how much I loved her. Later the nurse took me aside to talk privately and she told me what they were doing for my sister, the goals for her care, and most importantly assuring me she was comfortable and treated with dignity.*

*I came away knowing that my sister would be okay. The relationship between our family, my sister, and her partner suddenly seemed to be a non-issue. We will probably continue to have issues in the last days of her life, and probably after her death, but are all finally agreeing on the important things, and the hospice staff is giving all of us an opportunity to finally say and do some very long-overdue things.—"The older brother"*

- ♦ **Key Points**
- ♦ *The care of patients and families near to death and afterward is a important nursing function—arguably one of the most important. There are often no dress rehearsals; nurses and other health care professionals often only have one chance to "get it right."*
- ♦ *Assessment and aggressive management of symptoms remains a priority, especially as death approaches.*
- ♦ *As the dying person nears death, the goals of care often change with patient and family needs, desires, and perspectives, providing a different experience for everyone.*
- ♦ *Care of the body after death, including honoring rituals and individual requests, can clearly communicate to the family that the person who died was indeed important and valued.*

Issues and needs at the time of death are exceedingly important and, at the same time, exceedingly personal. Although the physiology of dying may be the same for most expected deaths, the psychological, spiritual, cultural, and family issues are as unique and varied as the patients and families themselves. As death nears, the goals of care must be discussed and appropriately redefined. Some treatments may be discontinued, and symptoms may intensify, subside, or even appear anew. Physiological changes as death approaches must also be defined, explained, and interpreted to the patient whenever possible, as well as to the patient's family, close others, and caregivers. The nurse occupies a key position in assisting patients' family members at the time of death by supporting or suggesting death rituals, caring for the body after death, and facilitating early grief work. Most of the focus on death and dying in the past has been on dying in general, making the need for a chapter focused specifically on the actual death even more important.

Terminally ill persons are cared for in a variety of settings, including home settings with hospice care or traditional home care, hospice residential facilities, nursing homes, assisted living facilities, hospitals, intensive care units, prisons, and group homes. Deaths in intensive care settings may present special challenges, such as restrictive visiting hours and lack of space and less privacy for families—shortcomings that can be addressed by thoughtful and creative nursing care. Likewise, death in a nursing home setting may also offer unique challenges. Regardless of the setting, anticipating and managing pain and symptoms can minimize distress and maximize quality of life. Families can be supported in a way that optimizes use of valuable time, and lessens distress during the bereavement period. Like it or not, health professionals only have one chance to "get it right" when caring for dying persons and their families as death nears. In other words, there is no dress rehearsal for the time surrounding death; extensive planning ensures the least stressful and best possible outcome for all involved.

The patient's family is especially important as death nears. Family members may become full- or part-time caregivers; daughters and sons may find themselves in a position to "parent" their parents; and family issues, long forgotten or ignored, may surface. Although "family" is often thought of in traditional terms, a family may take on several forms and configurations. For purposes of this chapter, the definition of family recognizes that many patients have nontraditional families and may be cared for by a large extended entity, such as a church community, a group of supportive friends, or the staff of a health care facility. Family is defined broadly to include not only persons bound by biology or legal ties, but also those whom the patient defines or who define themselves as "close others" or who function for the patient in as a family member would, including nurturance, intimacy, and economic, social, and psychological support in times of need; support in illness (including dealing with those outside the family); and companionship.

The occurrence of symptoms at end-of-life is temporal in nature; that is, there is a constellation of symptoms common throughout the course of end-stage disease, and symptoms that appear during the period immediately preceding death, most often 2–3 days prior. As death nears, symptoms can escalate and new ones appear. While there is much known about the assessment and management of symptoms as death nears, most research demonstrates that many people experience a death with symptoms not well controlled. It is estimated that up to 52% of patients have refractory symptoms at the very end of life that at times require palliative sedation.[3] Within a few days of death, many patients experience a higher frequency of noisy and moist breathing, urinary incontinence and retention, restlessness, agitation, delirium, and nausea and vomiting.[4–6] Symptoms that occur, but with less frequency, include sweating and myoclonus, with myoclnus sometimes occurring as a reversible toxic effect of morphine.[7–9] In most studies, symptoms requiring maximum diligence in assessment, prevention, and aggressive treatment during the final day or two before death are respiratory tract secretions (with a prevalence of 23–92%), pain, dyspnea, and agitated delirium (with a prevalence of 80–90%).[10] In most studies, symptoms requiring maximum diligence in assessment, prevention, and aggressive treatment during the final day or two before death were respiratory tract secretions, pain, dyspnea, restlessness, and agitation.[3,10,11]

For some patients, the pathway to death is characterized by progressive sleepiness leading to coma and death. For others, the pathway to death is marked by increasing symptoms, including restlessness, confusion, hallucinations, sometimes seizure activity, and then coma and death.[11] Some authors have emphasized that persons with cognitive impairment require specific attention to symptoms, especially as death nears.[10] In any case, the nurse plays a key role in anticipating symptoms and educating family members and other caregivers about the assessment, treatment, and continual evaluation of these symptoms.

Regardless of individual patient and family needs, attitudes, and "unfinished business," the nurse's professional approach and demeanor at the time near death is crucial and worthy of close attention. Patients experience total and profound dependency at this stage of their illness. Families are often called upon to assume total caregiving duties, often disrupting their own responsibilities for home, children, and career. Although there may be similarities, patients and families experience this time through the unique lens of their own perspective, and form their own unique meaning.

Some authors suggest theories and guidelines as the bases for establishing and maintaining meaningful, helpful, and therapeutic relationships with patients or clients and their families. One example is Carl Rogers' theory of helping relationships, in which he proposed that the characteristics of a helping relationship are empathy, unconditional positive regard, and genuineness.[12] These characteristics, defined later as part of the nurse's approach to patients and families, are essential in facilitating care at the end of life. To this may be added "attention to detail," because this additional characteristic is essential for quality palliative care.[13,14] Readers are urged to consider the following characteristics in the context of their own practices, as a basis for facilitating and providing supportive relationships:

- *Empathy:* the ability to put oneself in the other person's place, trying to understand the patient or client from his or her own frame of reference; it also requires the deliberate setting aside of one's own frame of reference and bias.
- *Unconditional positive regard:* a warm feeling toward others, with a nonjudgmental acceptance of all they reveal themselves to be; the ability to convey a sense of respect and esteem at a time and place in which it is particularly important to do so.
- *Genuineness:* the ability to convey trustworthiness and openness that is real rather than a professional facade; also the ability to admit that one has limitations, makes mistakes, and does not have all the answers.
- *Attention to detail:* the learned and practiced ability to think critically about a situation and not make assumptions. The nurse, for example, discusses challenging patient and family concerns with colleagues and other members of the interdisciplinary team. The nurse considers every "what if" before making a decision and, in particular, before making any judgment. Finally, the nurse is constantly aware of how his or her actions, attitudes, and words may be interpreted—or misinterpreted—by others.[13]

The events and interactions—positive as well as negative—at the bedside of a dying person set the tone for the patient's care and form lasting memories for family members. The time of death and the care received by both the individual who has died, and the family members who are present, are predominant aspects of the survivors' memories of this momentous event. Approaching patients and families with a genuine openness characterized by empathy and positive regard eases the way in making this difficult time meaningful, individualized, and deeply profound.

This chapter discusses some key issues surrounding the death itself, including advance planning, the changing focus of care as death nears, common signs and symptoms of nearing death and their management, and care of the patient and family at time of death. It concludes with two case examples illustrating the chapter's content.

## Advance Planning: Evolving Choices and Goals of Care

Health care choices related to wellness are generally viewed as clearcut or easy. We have an infection, we seek treatment, and the problem resolves. Throughout most of the lifespan, medical treatment choices are obvious. As wellness moves along the health care continuum to illness, choices become less clear and consequences of choices have a significantly greater impact.

Many end-of-life illnesses manifest with well-known and well-documented natural courses. Providing the patient and family with information on the natural course of the disease at appropriate intervals is a critical function of health care providers such as nurses. Providing an opening for discussion, such as, "Would you like to talk about the future?" "Do you have any concerns that I can help you address?" or "It seems you are not as active as you were before," may allow a much-needed discussion of fears and concerns about impending death. Family members may request information that patients do not wish to know at certain points in time. With the patient's permission, discussions with the family may occur in the patient's absence. Family members may also need coaching to initiate end-of-life discussions with the patient. End-of-life goal setting is greatly enhanced when the patient is aware of the support of family.

End-of-life care issues should always be discussed with patients and family members. The patient who is capable of participating in and making decisions is always the acknowledged decision-maker. The involvement of family ensures maximal consensus for patient support as decisions are actually implemented. Decisions for patients who lack decision-making capacity should be made by a consensus approach, using family conference methodology. If documents such as a durable power of attorney for health care or a living will are available, they can be used as a guide for examining wishes that influence decision-making and goal-setting. The decision-maker, usually the person named as health care power of attorney (HCPOA), or the patient's primary family members, should be clearly identified. This approach may also be used with patients who are able to make their own decisions.

To facilitate decision-making, a family conference is initiated that involves the decision makers (decisional patient, family members, and the HCPOA), the patient's phyisican or provider, nurse, chaplain, and social worker. A history of how the patient's health care status evolved from diagnosis to the present is reviewed. The family is presented with the natural course of the disease. Choices on how care may proceed in the future are reviewed. Guidance or support for those choices is provided based on existing data and clinical experience with the particular disease in relation to the current status of the patient. If no consensus for the needed decisions occurs, decision-making is postponed. Third-party support by a trusted individual or consultant may then be enlisted. Personal fundamental values of the patient, family, and physician should be recognized and protected throughout this process.[15]

Decisions by patients and families cross the spectrum of care range from continuing treatment for the actual disease, such as undergoing chemotherapy or renal dialysis or utilization of medications, to initiating cardiopulmonary resuscitation (CPR). The health care provider may work with the patient and family, making care decisions for specific treatments and timing treatment discontinuance within a clear and logical framework. A goal-setting discussion may determine a patient's personal framework for care, such as

- Treatment and enrollment in any clinical studies for which I am eligible.
- Treatment as long as statistically there is a greater than 50% chance of response.
- Full treatment as long as I am ambulatory and able to come to the clinic or office.
- Treatment only of "fixable" conditions such as infections or blood glucose levels.
- Treatment only for controlling symptomatic aspects of disease.

Once a goal framework has been established with the patient, the appropriateness of interventions such as CPR, renal dialysis, or intravenous antibiotics is clear. For instance, if the patient states a desire for renal dialysis as long as transportation to the clinic is possible without the use of an ambulance, the endpoint of dialysis treatment is quite clear. At this point, the futility of CPR would also be apparent. Allowing a patient to determine when the treatment is a burden that is unjustified by his or her value system, and communicating this determination to family and caregivers, is perhaps the most pivotal point in management of the patient's care. Table 32–1 suggests a format for an effective and comprehensive family conference.

## Changing the Focus of Care as Death Nears

### Vital Signs

As nurses, we derive a good deal of security in performing the ritual of measurement of vital signs, one of the hallmarks of

**Table 32–1**
**Family Conference**

I. Why: Clarify goals in your own mind.

II. Where: Provide comfort, privacy, circular seating.

III. Who: Include legal decision maker/health care power of attorney; family members; social support; key health care professionals, patient if capable to participate.

IV. How:

    A. Introduction

        1. Introduce self and others.

        2. Review meeting goals: State meeting goals and specific decisions.

        3. Establish ground rules: Each person will have a chance to ask questions and express views; no interruptions; identify legal decision-maker, and describe importance of supportive decision-making.

        4. If new to patient/family, spend some time getting to know him or her as a person.

    B. Determine what the patient/family knows.

    C. Review medical status

        1. Review current status, plan, and prognosis.

        2. Ask each family member in turn for any questions about current status, plan, and prognosis.

        3. Defer discussion of decision until the next step.

        4. Respond to emotions.

    D. Family discussion with decisional patient

        1. Ask patient, "What decision(s) are you considering?"

        2. Ask each family member, "Do you have questions or concerns about the treatment plan? How can you support the patient?"

    E. Family discussion with nondecisional patient

        1. Ask each family member in turn, "What do you believe the patient would choose if he (or she) could speak for himself (or herself)?"

        2. Ask each family member, "What do you think should be done?"

        3. Leave room to let family discuss alone.

        4. If there is consensus, go to V; if no consensus, go to F.

    F. When there is no consensus:

        1. Restate goal: "What would the patient say if he or she could speak?"

        2. Use time as ally: Schedule a follow-up conference the next day.

        3. Try further discussion: "What values is your decision based on? How will the decision affect you and other family members?"

        4. Identify legal decision-maker.

        5. Identify resources: minister/priest; other physicians; ethics committee.

V. Wrap-up

        1. Summarize consensus, decisions, and plan.

        2. Caution against unexpected outcomes.

        3. Identify family spokesperson for ongoing communication.

        4. Document in the chart who was present, what decisions were made, follow-up plan.

        5. Approach discontinuation of treatment as an interdisciplinary team, not just as a nursing function.

        6. Continuity: Maintain contact with family and medical team; schedule follow-up meetings as needed.

VI. Family dynamics and decisions

        1. Family structure: Respect the family hierarchy whenever possible.

        2. Established patterns of family interaction will continue.

        3. Unresolved conflicts between family members may be evident.

        4. Past problems with authority figures, doctors, and hospitals affect the process; ask specifically about bad experiences in the past.

        5. Family grieving and decision-making may include

          • Denial: False hopes.

          • Guilt: Fear of letting go.

          • Depression: Passivity and inability to decide; or anger and irritability.

*Source:* Adapted from Ambuael & Weissman (2005), reference 38. Copyright ©2005, Medical College of Wisconsin, Inc.

nursing care. When death is approaching, we need to question the rationale for measuring vital signs. Are interventions going to change if it is discovered that the patient has experienced a drop in blood pressure? If the plan of care no longer involves intervening in changes in blood pressure and pulse rate, the measurements should cease. The time spent taking vital signs can then be channeled to assessment of patient comfort and provision of family support. Changes in respiratory rate are visually noted and do not require routine monitoring of rates, unless symptom management issues develop that could be more accurately assessed by measurement of vital signs. The measurement of body temperature using a noninvasive route should continue on a regular basis until death, allowing for the detection and management of fever, a frequent symptom that can cause distress and may require management.

Fever often suggests infection. As death approaches, goal-setting should include a discussion of the nontreatment of infection. Indications for treatment of infection are based on the degree of distress and patient discomfort.[16] Pharmacological management of fever includes antipyretics, including acetaminophen, and nonsteroidal antiinflammatory drugs. In some cases, treatment of an infection with an anitbiotic may increase patient comfort. Ice packs, alcohol baths, and cooling blankets should be used cautiously, because they often cause more distress than the fever itself.[16]

Fever may also suggest dehydration. As with the management of fever, interventions are guided by the degree of distress and patient discomfort. The appropriateness of beginning artificial hydration for the treatment of fever is based on individual patient assessment.

## Cardiopulmonary Resuscitation

Patients and family members may need to discuss the issue of the futility of CPR when death is expected from a terminal illness. Developed in the 1960s as a method of restarting the heart in the event of sudden, unexpected clinical death, CPR was originally intended for circumstances in which death was unexpected or accidental. It is not indicated in certain situations, such as cases of terminal irreversible illness where death is not unexpected; resuscitation in these circumstances may represent an active violation of a person's right to die with dignity.

Over the years, predictors of the success of CPR have become apparent, along with the predictors of the burden of CPR. In general, a poor outcome of CPR is predicted in patients with advanced terminal illnesses, patients with dementia, and patients with poor functional status who depend on others for meeting their basic care needs. Poor outcomes or physical problems resulting from CPR include fractured ribs, punctured lung, brain damage if anoxia has occurred for too long, and permanent unconsciousness or persistent vegetative state.[17–19] Most importantly, the use of CPR negates the possibility of a peaceful death. This is considered the gravest of poor outcomes.

## Medically-administered Fluids

The issue of medically administered or "artificial" hydration is emotional for many patients and families because of the role that giving and consuming fluids plays in our culture. When patients are not able to take fluids, concern surfaces among caregivers. A decision must be reached regarding the appropriate use of fluids within the context of the patient's framework of goals. Beginning artificial hydration is a relatively easy task, but the decision to stop is generally much more problematic given its emotional implications. Ethical, moral, and most religious viewpoints state that there is no difference between withholding and withdrawing a treatment such as artificial hydration. However, the emotional response attached to withdrawing a treatment adds a world of difference to the decision to suspend. It is therefore much less burdensome to not begin treatment, if this decision is acceptable in light of the specific patient circumstances.[20]

Most patients and families are aware that, without fluids, death will occur quickly. The literature suggests that fluids should not be routinely administered to dying patients, nor automatically withheld from them. Instead, the decision should be based on careful, individual assessment. Zerwekh[21] suggested consideration of the following questions when the choice to initiate or continue hydration is evaluated:

- Is the patient's well-being enhanced by the overall effect of hydration?
- Which current symptoms are being relieved by artificial hydration?
- Are other end-of-life symptoms being aggravated by the fluids?
- Does hydration improve the patient's level of consciousness? If so, is this within the patient's goals and wishes for end-of-life care?
- Does hydration appear to prolong the patient's survival? If so, is this within the patient's goals and wishes for end-of-life care?
- What is the effect of the infusion technology on the patient's well-being, mobility, and ability to interact and be with family?
- What is the burden of the infusion technology on the family in terms of caregiver stress, finance? Is it justified by benefit to the patient?

Research suggests that, although some dying patients may actually benefit from dehydration, others may experience increased discomfort such as confusion, agitated delirium, or opioid toxicity that can be corrected or prevented by hydration.[22] In any case, the uniqueness of the individual situation, the goals of care, the benefits and burdens of the proposed treatment, and the comfort of the patient must always be considered.[23]

Terminal dehydration refers to the process in which the dying patient's condition naturally results in a decrease in fluid intake. A gradual withdrawal from activities of daily living may occur as symptoms such as dysphagia, nausea, and fatigue become more obvious. Families commonly ask whether the patient will be thirsty as fluid intake decreases. The arguments are complex, but several studies have demonstrated that, although patients reported thirst, there was no correlation between thirst and hydration, resulting in the assumption that artificial hydration to relieve symptoms may be futile.[22] Medically, hydration has the potential to result in fluid accumulation, resulting in distressful symptoms such as edema, ascites, nausea and vomiting, and pulmonary congestion.

Does medically adminstered hydration prolong life? There is no evidence that rehydration actually prolongs life.[22] Health care providers need to assist patients and family members to refocus on the natural course of the disease and the notion that the patient's death will be caused by the disease, not by dehydration, which is a natural occurrence in advanced illness and dying. Nurses may then assist families in dealing with symptoms caused by dehydration.

Dry mouth, a consistently reported distressing symptom of dehydration, can be relieved with sips of beverages, ice chips, or hard candies. Another simple comfort measure for dry mouth is spraying normal saline into the mouth with a spray bottle or atomizer. (Normal saline is made by mixing one teaspoon of table salt in a quart of water.) Meticulous mouth care must be administered to keep the patient's mouth clean. Family members can be instructed to anticipate this need. The nurse can facilitate this care by ensuring that the necessary provisions are on hand to assist the patient.

## Medications

Medications unrelated to the terminal diagnosis are generally continued as long as their administration is not burdensome. When swallowing pills becomes too difficult, the medication may be offered in a liquid or other form if available, considering patient and family comfort. Continuing medications, however, may be seen by some patients and families as a way of normalizing daily activities and therefore should be supported. Considerable tact, kindness, and knowledge of the patient and family are needed in assisting them to make decisions about discontinuing medications.

Medications that do not contribute to daily comfort should be evaluated on an individual basis for possible discontinuance. Medications such as antihypertensives, replacement hormones, vitamin supplements, iron preparations, hypoglycemics, long-term antibiotics, antiarrhythmics, and laxatives, unless they are essential to patient comfort, can and should be discontinued unless doing so would cause symptoms or discomfort. Accordingly, special consderation should be given to the use of diuretics with patients with end-stage heart disease and corticosteroids in patients with neuropathic pain or for the treatment of increased intracranial pressure. The control or prevention of distressing symptoms should be the guiding principle in the use of medications, especially in the final days of life. Resumption of the drug at any point is always an option that should be offered to the patient and family if the need becomes apparent. Customarily, the only drugs necessary in the final days of life are analgesics, anticonvulsants, antiemetics, antipyretics, anti-secretories, and sedatives.[24]

## Implantable Cardioverter Defibrillator

Implantable cardioverter defibrillators (ICDs) are used to prevent cardiac arrest due to ventricular tachycardia or ventricular fibrillation. Patients with ICDs who are dying of another terminal condition or are withdrawn from anti-arrythmic medications may choose to have the defibrillator deactivated, or turned off, so that there will be no interference from the device at the time of death.

Patients with ICDs are instructed to carry a wallet identification card at all times that provides the model and serial number of the implanted device. The identification card will also have the name of the physician to contact for assistance. Deactivating the ICD is a simple, noninvasive procedure and usually overseen by an ICD specialist. The device is tested after it is turned off to ensure that it is no longer operational, and the test result is placed in the patient record. Patients who are at peace with their impending death find this procedure important to provide assurance that death indeed will be quiet and easy, when it does occur.[25]

## Renal Dialysis

Renal dialysis is a life-sustaining treatment, and as death approaches it is important to recognize and agree on its limitations. Discontinuation of dialysis should be considered in the following cases:

- Patients with acute, concurrent illness, who, if they survive, will be burdened with a great deal of disability as defined by the patient and family.
- Patients with progressive and untreatable disease or disability.
- Patients with dementia or severe neurological deficit.

There is general agreement that dialysis should not be used to prolong the dying process.[26] The time between discontinuing dialysis and death varies widely, from a matter of hours or days (for patients with acute illnesses, such as those described earlier) to days, or a week or longer if some residual renal function remains.[26,27] Opening a discussion about the burden of treatment, however, is a delicate task. There may be competing opinions among the patient, family, and even staff about the tolerability or intolerability of continuing treatment. The nurse who sees the patient and family on a regular basis may be the most logical person to recognize the discrete changes in status. Gently validating these observations may open a much-needed discussion regarding the goals of care.

The discussions and decisions surrounding discontinuation or modification of treatment are never easy. Phrases such as, "There is nothing more that can be done" or "We have tried everything" have no place in end-of-life discussions with patients and families. Always reassure the patient and family members—and be prepared to follow through—that you will stand by them and do all you can to provide help and comfort. This is essential to ensure that palliative care is not interpreted as abandonment.

## Common Signs and Symptoms of Imminent Death and Their Management

There usually are predictable sets of processes that occur during the final stages of a terminal illness due to gradual hypoxia, respiratory acidosis, metabolic consequences of renal failure, and the signs and symptoms of hypoxic brain function.[3,11,28] These processes account for the signs and symptoms of imminent death and can assist the nurse in helping the family plan for the actual death.

The following signs and symptoms provide cues that death is only days away[2,3,11,28,29]:

- Profound weakness (patient is usually bedbound and requires assistance with all or most care).
- Gaunt and pale physical appearance (most common in persons with cancer if corticosteroids have not been used as treatment).
- Drowsiness and/or a reduction in awareness, insight, and perception (often with extended periods of drowsiness, extreme difficulty in concentrating, severely limited attention span, inability to cooperate with caregivers, disorientation to time and place, or semicomatose state).
- Increasing lack of interest in food and fluid with diminished intake (only able to take sips of fluids).
- Increasing difficulty in swallowing oral medications.

During the final days, these signs and symptoms become more pronounced, and, as oxygen concentrations drop, new symptoms also appear. Measurement of oxygen concentration in the dying person is not advocated, because it adds discomfort and does not alter the course of care. However, knowledge of the signs and symptoms associated with decreasing oxygen concentrations can assist the nurse in guiding the family as death nears.[28] As oxygen saturation drops below 80%, signs and symptoms related to hypoxia appear. As the dying process proceeds, special issues related to normalizing the dying process for the family, symptom control, and patient and family support present themselves. Table 32–2 summarizes the physiological process of dying and suggests interventions for both patients and families.

As the imminently dying person takes in less fluid, third-spaced fluids, clinically manifested as peripheral edema, acites, or pleural effusions, may be reabsorbed. Breathing may become easier, and there may be less discomfort from tissue distention. Accordingly, as the person experiences dehydration, swelling is often reduced around tumor masses. Patients may experience transient improvements in comfort, including increased mental status and decreased pain. The family needs a careful and compassionate explanation regarding these temporary improvements and encouragement to make the most of this short but potentially meaningful time.

There are multiple patient and family educational tools available to assist families in interpreting the signs and symptoms of approaching death (Figure 32–1). However, as with all aspects of palliative care, consideration of the individual perspective and associated relationships of the patient or family member, the underlying disease course trajectory, anticipated symptoms, and the setting of care is essential for optimal care at all stages of illness, but especially during the final days and hours.[30]

## Care at the Time of Death, Death Rituals, and Facilitating Early Grieving

At the time of death, the nurse has a unique opportunity to provide information helpful in making decisions about organ and body donation and autopsy. In addition, the nurse can support the family's choice of death rituals, gently care for the body, assist in funeral planning, and facilitate the early process of grieving.

Family members' needs around the time of death change, just as the goals of care change. During this important time, plans are reviewed and perhaps refined. Special issues affecting the time of death, such as cultural influences, decisions regarding organ or body donation, and the need for autopsy, are also reviewed.

Under U.S. federal law, if death occurs in a hospital setting, staff must approach the family decision-maker regarding the possibility of organ donation.[31] Although approaching family at this time may seem onerous, the opportunity to assist another is often comforting. Some hospital-based palliative care programs include information about organ donation in their admission or bereavement information. Readers are urged to review their own organizations' policies and procedures.

In any case, it is important to clarify specifically with family members what their desires and needs are at the time of death. Do they wish to be present? Do they know of others who wish to now say a final goodbye? Have they said everything they wish to say to the person who is dying? Do they have any regrets? Are they concerned about anything? Do they wish something could be different? Every person in a family has different and unique needs that, unless explored, can go unmet. Family members recall the time before the death and immediately afterward with great acuity and detail. As mentioned earlier, there is no chance for a dress rehearsal—we only have the one chance to "get it right" and make the experience an individualized and memorable one.

Although an expected death can be anticipated with some degree of certainty, the exact time of death is often not predictable. Death often occurs when no health care professionals are present. Frequently, dying people seem to determine the time of their own death—for example, waiting for someone to

**Table 32–2**
**Symptoms in the Normal Progression of Dying and Suggested Interventions**

| Symptoms | Suggested Interventions |
|---|---|
| **Early stage sensation/perception**<br>• Impairment in the ability to grasp ideas and reason; periods of alertness along with periods of disorientation and restlessness are also noted. | • Interpret the signs and symptoms to the patient (when appropriate) and family as part of the normal dying process; for example, assure them the patient's "seeing" and even talking to persons who have died is normal and often expected.<br>• Urge family members to look for metaphors for death in speech and conversation (e.g., talk of a long journey, needing maps or tickets, or in preparing for a trip in other ways) and using these metaphors as a departure point for conversation with the patient.<br>• Urge family to take advantage of the patient's periods of lucidity to talk with patient and ensure nothing is left unsaid.<br>• Encourage family members to touch and speak slowly and gently to the patient without being patronizing.<br>• Maximize safety; for example, use bedrails and schedule people to sit with the patient. |
| • Some loss of visual acuity. | • Keep sensory stimulation to a minimum, including light, sounds, and visual stimulation; reading to a patient who has enjoyed reading in the past may provide comfort. |
| • Increased sensitivity to bright lights while other senses, except hearing, are dulled. | • Urge the family to be mindful of what they say "over" the patient, because hearing remains present; also continue to urge family to say what they wish not to be left unsaid. |
| **Cardiorespiratory**<br>• Increased pulse and respiratory rate.<br>• Agonal respirations or sounds of gasping for air without apparent discomfort.<br>• Apnea, periodic, or Cheyne-Stokes respirations.<br>• Inability to cough or clear secretions efficiently, resulting in gurgling or congested breathing (sometimes referred to as the "death rattle"). | • Normalize the observed changes by interpreting the signs and symptoms as part of the normal dying process and ensuring the patient's comfort.<br>• Assess and treat respiratory distress as appropriate.<br>• Assess use and need for parenteral fluids, tube feedings, or hydration. (It is generally appropriate to either discontinue or greatly decrease these at this point in time.)<br>• Reposition the patient in a side-lying position with the head of the bed elevated.<br>• Suctioning is rarely needed, but when appropriate, suction should be gentle and only at the level of the mouth, throat, and nasal pharynx.<br>• Administer anticholinergic drugs (transdermal scopolamine, hyoscyamine) as appropriate, recognizing and discussing with the family that they will not decrease already existing secretions. |
| **Renal/Urinary**<br>• *Decreasing urinary output, sometimes urinary incontinence or retention.* | • Insert catheter and/or use absorbent padding.<br>• Carefully assess for urinary retention, because restlessness can be a related symptom. |
| **Musculoskeletal**<br>• Gradual loss of the ability to move, beginning with the legs, then progressing. | • Reposition every few hours as appropriate.<br>• Anticipate needs such as sips of fluids, oral care, changing of bed pads and linens, and so on. |
| **Late stage sensation/perception**<br>• Unconsciousness.<br>• Eyes remain half open, blink reflex is absent; sense of hearing remains intact and may slowly decrease. | • Interpret the patient's unconsciousness to the family as part of the normal dying process.<br>• Provide for total care, including incontinence of urine and stool.<br>• Encourage family members to speak slowly and gently to the patient, with the assurance that hearing remains intact. |

*(continued)*

Table 32–2
**Symptoms in the Normal Progression of Dying and Suggested Interventions** *(continued)*

| Symptoms | Suggested Interventions |
|---|---|
| **Cardiorespiratory** <br>• Heart rate may double, strength of contractions decrease; rhythm becomes irregular. <br>• Patient feels cool to the touch and becomes diaphoretic. <br>• Cyanosis is noted in the tip of the nose, nail beds, and knees; extremities may become mottled (progressive mottling indicates death within a few days); absence of a palpable radial pulse may indicate death within hours. | • Interpret these changes to family members as part of the normal dying process. <br>• Frequent linen changes and sponge baths may enhance comfort. |
| **Renal/Urinary** <br>• A precipitous drop in urinary output. | • Interpret to the family the drop in urinary output as a normal sign that death is near. <br>• Carefully assess for urinary retention; restlessness can be a related symptom. |

arrive, for a date or event to pass, or even for family members to leave—even if the leave-taking is brief. For this reason, it is crucial to ask family members who wish to be present at the time of death whether they have thought about the possibility they will not be there. This opens an essential discussion regarding the time of death and its unpredictability. Gently reminding family members of that possibility can assist them in preparing for any eventuality.

### Determining That Death Has Occurred

Death often occurs when health professionals are not present at the bedside or in the home. Regardless of the site of death, a plan must be in place for who will be contacted, how the death pronouncement will be handled, and how the body will be removed. This is especially important for deaths that occur outside a health care institution.

Death pronouncement procedures vary from state to state, and sometimes from county to county within a state. In some states, nurses can pronounce death; in others, they cannot. In inpatient settings, the organization's policy and procedures are followed. In hospice home care, generally the nurse makes a home visit, assesses the lack of vital signs, contacts the physician, who verbally agrees to sign the death certificate, and then contacts the funeral home or mortuary. Local customs, the ability of a health care agency to ensure the safety of a nurse during the home visit, and provision for "do-not-resuscitate" orders outside a hospital setting, among other factors, account for wide variability in the practices and procedures surrounding pronouncement of death in the home. Although practices vary widely, the police or coroner may need to be called if the circumstances of the death were unusual, were associated with trauma (regardless of the cause of the death), or occurred within 24 hours of a hospital admission.

The practice of actual death pronouncement varies widely and is not often taught in medical school or residencies. The customary procedure is to first identify the patient, then note the following[32]:

- General appearance of the body.
- Lack of reaction to verbal or tactile stimuli.
- Lack of pupillary light reflex (pupils will be fixed and dilated).
- Absent breathing and lung sounds.
- Absent carotid and apical pulses (in some situations, listening for an apical pulse for a full minute is advisable).

Documentation of the death is equally important and should be thorough and clear. The following guidelines are suggested.[32]

- Patient's name and time of call.
- Who was present at the time of death and at the time of the pronouncement.
- Detailed findings of the physical examination.
- Date and time of death pronouncement (either pronouncement by the nurse, or the time at which the physician either assessed the patient or was notified).
- Who else was notified and when—for example, additional family members, attending physician, or other staff members.
- Whether the coroner was notified, rationale, and outcome, if known.
- Special plans for disposition and outcome (e.g., organ or body donation, autopsy, special care related to cultural or religious traditions).

### Care of the Body After Death

Regardless of the site of death, care of the body is an important nursing function. In gently caring for the body, the nurse can continue to communicate care and concern for the patient and family members, and model behaviors that may be helpful as the family members continue their important grief work.

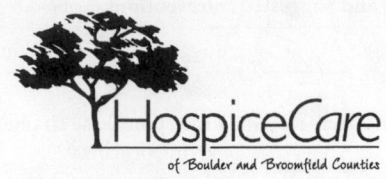

## SIGNS AND SYMPTOMS OF APPROACHING DEATH

This list of symptoms and what to do about them may appear frightening, but knowing what to expect may reduce some of your anxiety about the approaching death.

Each person approaches death in their own way, bringing to this last experience their own uniqueness. Our list of "Symptoms and What To Do" is a map to the goal of a peaceful death. Like all maps, there are many different routes to the same destination.

You may see all of these symptoms or none. Death will come in its own time, and its own way to each of us. It is important to remember that <u>dying</u> <u>is</u> <u>a</u> <u>natural</u> <u>process</u>.

| | | |
|---|---|---|
| 1. | <u>Withdrawal</u> - Physical and emotional, and increased sleep. | Natural process of withdrawing from everything outside of one's self, looking inward, reviewing one's self and one's life. Your loved one may turn inward, withdraw physically and emotionally. This occurs in an attempt to cope with the many changes that are occurring. |
| 2. | Reduced food and fluid intake. | Decreased <u>need</u> because body will naturally begin to conserve energy. Dehydration is a <u>natural</u> <u>comfort</u> <u>measure</u>, since the body systems can't process fluids effectively. At no time should food/fluids be <u>forced.</u> |
| 3. | Confusion/Agitation can vary from mild to end stage agitation which may include trying to get out of bed, picking at covers, seeing things that are not apparent to us. | Talk calmly and assuredly. Keep lights on, use times when patient is alert for meaningful conversation. Music can be very calming. Medication often used to control this symptom. |

*(continued)*

**Figure 32–1.** Sample handout for families responsible for end-of-life care. *Source*: Courtesy of Hospice Care of Boulder and Broomfield Counties, Colorado, June 2004.

Caring for the body after death also calls for an understanding of the physiological changes that occur. By understanding these changes, the nurse can interpret and dispel any myths and explain these changes to the family members, thereby assisting the family in making their own personal decisions about the time immediately following death and funeral plans.

A classic article regarding postmortem care emphasized that, although postmortem care may be a ritualized nursing

| 4. | Change in breathing patterns. | This is common. You may see irregular breathing: very rapid, very slow, and/or 10 to 30 seconds of no breathing at all (called apnea). These symptoms are very common and indicative of a decrease in circulation. It does not mean that your loved one is uncomfortable or struggling. |
|----|----|----|
| 5. | Oral secretions collect in back of throat causing noisy respiration. | Swallowing reflex may be absent. Patient may be breathing through the secretions.<br>• This may be more uncomfortable for us as observers than patient experiencing it.<br>• Elevate head of bed or turn patient on side. |
| 6. | Incontinence of urine and stool. | Reduced intake results in reduced output with darker color. Bedpads and diapers can be used to protect bed linens. Cleanse patient and change linens frequently to maintain comfort and protect skin. |
| 7. | Changes in skin temperature and color. | Decreased circulation can cause coolness and discoloration of skin. Use light covers, turn side to side frequently to maintain comfort and prevent skin breakdown (bedsores). Heating pads and electric blankets NOT recommended. |

Hearing is the last sense to be lost, so the patient can hear all that is being said. This is a good time to say good-bye, reassure them that you will be all right even though you will miss them greatly. (You may tell them it's OK to "let go".) This permission is often helpful for a peaceful death.

How would you know death has occurred?
1.  No breathing
2.  No heartbeat or pulse

If you believe that death has occurred, call Hospice at 449-7740. **Do not call 911 or the physician.** We will come to your home to help you. (You may want to use the time until we arrive to say your last good-byes.)

signs & symptoms death: 7/04

**Figure 32–1.** *(continued)*

procedure, the scientific rationale for the procedure rests on the basics of the physiological changes that occur after death.[33] These changes occur at a regular rate depending on the temperature of the body at the time of death, the size of the body, the extent of infection (if any), and the temperature of the air. The three important physiological changes—rigor mortis, algor mortis, and postmortem decomposition—are discussed along with the relevant nursing implications in Table 32–3.

**Table 32–3**
**Normal Postmortem Physiological Changes and Their Implications for Nursing**

| Change | Underlying Mechanisms | Nursing Implications |
|---|---|---|
| Rigor mortis | Approximately 2 to 4 hours after death, adenosine phosphate (ATP) ceases to be synthesized due to the depletion of glycogen stores. ATP is necessary for muscle fiber relaxation, so the lack of ATP results in an exaggerated contraction of the muscle fibers that eventually immobilizes the joints. Rigor begins in the involuntary muscles (heart, gastrointestinal tract, bladder, arteries) and progresses to the muscles of the head and neck, trunk and lower limbs. After approximately 96 hours, however, muscle chemical activity totally ceases, and rigor passes. Persons with large muscle mass (e.g., body builders) are prone to more pronounced rigor mortis. Conversely, frail elderly persons and persons who have been bed bound for long periods are less subject to rigor mortis.[37] | The guiding principle is to understand rigor mortis is a natural and temporary post-mortem change and immediate positioning of the deceased does not impact the appearance of the body long term. After death position the person in a relaxed and peaceful manner as is possible. For example, close the eyes, prop the jaw closed and fold the hands. If rigor mortis does occur, it can often be "massaged out" by the funeral director.[37] Finally, by understanding this physiology, the nurse can also reassure the family about the myth that due to rigor mortis, muscles can suddenly contract and the body can appear to move. |
| Algor mortis | After the circulation ceases and the hypothalamus stops functioning, internal body temperature drops by approximately 1° C or 1.8° F per hour until it reaches room temperature. As the body cools, skin loses its natural elasticity. If a high fever was present at death, the changes in body temperature are more pronounced and the person may appear to "sweat" after death. Body cooling may also take several more hours.[37] | The nurse can prepare family members for the coolness of the skin to touch or the increased moisture by explaining the changes that happen after death. The nurse may also suggest kissing the person on their hair instead of their skin. The skin, due to loss of elasticity, becomes fragile and easily torn. If dressings are to be applied, it is best to apply them with either a circular bandage or paper tape. Handle the body gently as well, being sure to not place traction on the skin. |
| Postmortem decomposition or "liver mortis" | Discoloration and softening of the body are caused largely by the breakdown of red blood cells and the resultant release of hemoglobin that stains the vessel walls and surrounding tissue. This staining appears as a mottling, bruising, or both in the dependent parts of the body as well as parts of the body where the skin has been punctured (e.g., intravenous or chest tube sites).[37] Often this discoloration becomes extensive in a very short time. The remainder of the body has a gray hue. In cardiac-related deaths, the face often appears purple in color regardless of the positioning at or after death.[37] | As the body is handled (e.g., while bathing and dressing), the nurse informs the family member about this normal change that occurs after death. Prop the body up with pillows under the head & shoulders or raise the head of the bed approx 30°. Remove heavy blankets & clothing & cover the deceased with a light blanket of sheet.[37] |

Care of and respect for the body after death by nursing staff should clearly communicate to the family that the person who died was indeed important and valued. Often, caring for the body after death provides the needed link between family members and the reality of the death, recognizing that everyone present at the time of death and soon after will have a different experience and a different sense of loss. Many institutions no longer require nursing staff to care for patients after death or perform postmortem care. Further, there are few resources related to postmortem care, and those available are largely found in the British nursing literature and do not reflect a thorough knowledge of post-mortem changes.[34–36]

A kind, gentle approach and meticulous attention to detail grounded in knowledge of the physiology of dying and death is imperative.

Rituals that family members and others present find comforting should be encouraged. Rituals are practices within a social context that facilitate and provide ways to understand and cope with the contradictory and complex nature of human existence. They provide a means to express and contain strong emotions, ease feelings of anxiety and impotence, and provide structure in times of chaos and disorder. Rituals can take many forms—a brief service at the time of death, a special preparation of the body, as in the Orthodox Jewish tradition, or an Irish wake, where, after paying respect to the person who has died, family and friends gather to share stories, food, and drink. Of utmost importance, however, is to ensure that family members see the ritual as comforting and meaningful. It is the family's needs and desires that direct this activity—not the nurse's. There are, again, no rules that govern the appropriateness of rituals; rituals are comforting and serve to begin the process of healing and acceptance.

To facilitate the grieving process, it is often helpful to create a pleasant, peaceful, and comfortable environment for family members who wish to spend time with the body, according to their desires and cultural or religious traditions. The nurse should consider engaging family members in after-death care and ritual by inviting them to either comb the hair or wash the person's hands and face, or more, if they are comfortable. Parents can be encouraged to hold and cuddle their baby or child. Including siblings or other involved children in rituals, traditions, and other end-of-life care activities according to their developmental level is also essential. During this time, family members should be invited to talk about their family member who has died, and encouraged to reminisce—valuable rituals that can help them begin to work through their grief.[35]

The family should be encouraged to touch, hold, and kiss the person's body, as they feel comfortable. Parents may wish to clip and save a lock of hair as a keepsake. The nurse may offer to dress the person's body in something other than a hospital gown or other nightclothes. Babies may be wrapped snugly in a blanket. Many families choose to dress the body in a favorite article of clothing before removal by the funeral home. It should be noted that, at times, when a body is being turned, air escapes from the lungs, producing a "sighing" sound. Informing family members of this possibility is wise. Again, modeling gentle and careful handling of the body can communicate care and concern on the part of the nurse and facilitate grieving and the creation of positive and long-lasting memories.

Postmortem care also includes, unless an autopsy or the coroner is involved, removal of any tubes, drains, and other devices. In home care settings, these can be placed in a plastic bag and given to the funeral home for disposal as medical waste or simply double-bagged and placed in the family's regular trash. Placing a waterproof pad, diaper, or adult incontinence brief on the patient often prevents soiling and odor as the patient's body is moved and the rectal and urinary bladder sphincters relax. Packing of the rectum and vagina is considered unnecessary, because not allowing these areas to drain increases the rate of bacterial proliferation that naturally occurs.[37]

Occasionally families, especially in the home care setting, wish to keep the person's body at home, perhaps to wait for another family member to come from a distance and to ensure that everyone has adequate time with the deceased. If the family wishes the body to be embalmed, this is best done within 12 hours. If embalming is not desired, the body can remain in the home for approximately 24 hours before further decomposition and odor production occur. The nurse should suggest to the family that they adjust the temperature in the immediate area to a comfortable but cooler level and remove heavy blankets or coverings [37] Be sure, however, to inform the funeral director that the family has chosen to keep the body at home a little longer. Finally, funeral directors are a reliable source of information regarding postdeath changes, local customs, and cultural issues.

The care of patients and families near the time of death and afterward is an important nursing function—arguably one of the most important. As the following case studies are reviewed, consider how the nurse interceded in a positive manner, mindful of the changing tempo of care and the changing patient and family needs, desires, and perspectives.

CASE STUDY
*Harold, An 88-Year-Old Gentleman with Pneumonia*

Harold is an 88-year-old retired farmer who lived with his wife of 68 years in their rural home. They have two adult sons. The youngest son recently retired from farming, and is married and lives close by. The oldest son is developmentally disabled and lives with Harold and his wife. Harold has a history of multiple chronic illnesses: diabetes, cardiovascular disease, arthritis, and minimal kidney function. Ten years ago, a pacemaker was placed. After acquiring winter colds that developed into pneumonia, both he and his wife were admitted to the hospital for treatment. They were placed together in a semiprivate room, and began IV antibiotic treatment.

> *Goals and framework of care:* Their family physician hoped to that 2–3 days of IV antibiotics and fluids would assist both Harold and his wife in getting through what was hoped was a treatable pneumonia. "Let's start treatment and see. Hopefully we'll have them both home in 3–4 days."

Initially, having the husband and wife in the same room was believed a good idea. Within 24 hours of the admission, the staff soon realized that Harold was sicker and weaker than his wife. Because his wife was in the same room, he would ask her to get out of bed to help him with personal care, and would not allow the nursing staff to assist him. The nursing staff decided to separate the Harold and his wife, which was upsetting to both of them. By the end of the second day, it was obvious that Harold was not responding as hoped to the IV antibiotics and was developing respiratory distress and markedly increased anxiety. Because of the concern about Harold's changing respiratory status, he was moved to the intensive care unit.

> *Goals and framework of care:* Watchful waiting continued. Support efforts for Harold' wife and family were facilitated. Could she visit in the ICU when she might still be contagious to others? Arrangements were made for other family members to visit and report to her, and she was allowed to visit once a day, when appropriate precautions for all could be maintained.

By the third day, it was obvious that Harold's wife was recovering. She was placed on oral antibiotics and arrangements were made for her to move to the in-hospital rehabilitation unit so that she could remain close by. Harold's condition remained unstable and intubation was discussed with his wife and sons. Harold had never discussed with his family his wishes for such intervention, and they were unsure of what he would desire. Harold declined discussion about the topic, saying he was too anxious. The physician handling his care had known Harold for many years, and the physician's father and Harold had been friends since childhood. Their families had neighboring farm land and shared membership in a local church. The physician recognized that their long-term ties, at times, clouded the difficult treatment decisions for his friend. Before a consensus decision with the family "not to intubate" could be reached, Harold's condition further deteriorated, and he was intubated emergently.

> *Goals and framework of care:* With saddened emotions, Harold's family suddenly was faced with trying to decide, "What would Harold want if he could speak and tell us?" It was agreed to allow Harold to 'rest' for 24 hours on the ventilator, and then come together.

The family gathered and wanted to talk privately. Nursing staff assisted the family by contacting their minister, who arrived shortly. The family did not want other staff to join them. When the nurse brought the minister to the family, she asked Harold's wife to tell her sons the stories about how they had met, his recollection of their early marriage, and some of his most pleasant memories. "Maybe it will make things clearer for all of you to think about what Harold could tell you if he were able to." She quietly left the room, as the reminiscing began.

Shortly after the meeting ended, Harold's wife came to the nurse and asked to have the physician called. The family message was…"one more day. If he's not better tomorrow, we'd like you to remove the ventilator." The family gathered the next morning with their minister. Harold's youngest son stayed with him as the ventilator was removed. Harold died peacefully an hour later, with the entire family at his side.

### Critical Points

- Death can suddenly become an expectation of a hospital admission for a perceived treatable process. Nurses who note a patient's downhill trajectory early can begin sharing objective observations to the family that will help prepare them if the trajectory does not change.
- Elderly patients with multiple chronic illnesses are frequently overlooked for discussions with their physicians about end-of-life goals.
- When advance directives are completed, both primary and secondary decision-makers should be made aware of the patient's wishes, especially in elderly patients with multiple chronic illnesses.

- Life-extending procedures such as pacemaker placement should be looked upon as an opportunity to open conversations with patient and health care providers about goals for end-of-life care.

CASE STUDY
### Elaine G, A 28-Year-Old Woman with Breast Cancer

Elaine was breast feeding her first child, who was 8 months old, when she noted a mass in her breast. She immediately saw her physician, who was not certain of the mass's relationship to lactation but ordered an ultrasound of the breast to be "on the safe side." The ultrasound was completed and was soon followed by a mammogram, biopsy, and diagnosis of Stage II breast cancer with one positive lymph node. Elaine underwent a staging workup, surgery, and started chemotherapy within 3 weeks of noticing the breast lump. It was difficult for her to see past the positive lymph node; all discussions seemed to come back to it, and the meaning of one positive node. Her anxiety was apparent during her interactions with care providers. Program staff worked to provide extra time for her, and strong emotional support. Family and friends were present and expressed the desire to be ready to help at any time.

> *Goals and framework of care:* Despite Elaine's positive lymph node, the cancer was still considered 'early' and very treatable. Elaine successfully completed chemotherapy and radiation therapy and was set up for routine surveillance. She was encouraged to use the program's psychosocial resources to help her with any questions, and particularly when her fears of recurrence and a dismal future seemed to immobilize her.

Elaine openly talked of what would happen if her cancer did reoccur. Who would assist her husband in raising her child? What would be important for her to leave her child? She was encouraged to think these things through, so she could have the appropriate discussions with her husband and then move forward as best she could. Slowly, she was able to do this.

Elaine focused on regaining her past lifestyle. She returned to community work on a part time basis, and often talked of the value of her work in helping others. She had a great sense of 'giving back.' Life seemed to settle for her, until one day when she called reporting a sudden onset of back pain. Bone scan and CT showed bone and early lung metastasis. Elaine and her husband received imaging results together in the clinic, and then opted to return the next day to speak with the medical oncologist.

> *Goals and framework of care:* Together with her medical oncologist, Elaine and her husband mapped out a plan for initial treatment. Although she was not eligible for clinical trials, she was interested in looking for

any opportunity that would give her the best chance of quality time. She clearly stated her goal "to receive treatment that would buy as many days of 'quality time' that were available, defining quality time as being present, participating, and enjoying her son's daily life." Her goal had been well thought out.

Elaine started on chemotherapy. She responded well for 9 months, and had an "almost normal" life. When the second-line chemotherapy failed to control her disease, she agreed to the third-line chemotherapy. Although she tolerated the third line well, her disease progressed in spite of the treatment. Scans and lab work were not necessary to tell the staff that her liver function was rapidly declining. Ascites from her new liver metastasis complicated her comfort level and functional status. She agreed to hospitalization for symptomatic evaluation.

*Goals and framework of care:* During her admission to the hospital, Elaine was offered a fourth-line chemotherapy regimen. After a quick discussion with her husband, she refused. She asked only that a plan for management of her discomfort be addressed, and that hospice arranged for her.

Elaine said her good-byes to the staff. She was discharged with a home hospice program, stating she simply wanted to have the freedom to have her son with her to hug and cuddle without any restrictions or expectations. She died at home, surrounded by prepared, loving and caring family and friends, 48 hours later.

### Critical Points

- Patients will often process their disease trajectory with minimal help other than the supportive, listening ears of their care providers.
- Patient fears are based in their reality and we as care providers must not minimize or dismiss them.
- Patients who set clearly defined goals and are given the opportunity to share them with their care providers are generally observed to have a higher quality death experience for themselves, their family members, and the staff who care for them.

## Summary

Assisting and walking alongside dying patients and their families, especially near and after death, is an honor and privilege. Nowhere else in the practice of nursing are we invited to be companions on such a remarkable journey as that of a dying patient and his or her family. Likewise, nowhere else in the practice of nursing are our words, actions, and guidance more remembered and cherished. Caring for dying patients and families is indeed the essence of nursing. Take this responsibility seriously, understanding that although it may be stressful and difficult at times, it comes with personal and professional satisfaction beyond measure. Listen to your patients and their families. They are the guides to this remarkable and momentous journey. Listen to them with a positive regard, empathy, and genuineness, and approach their care with an acute attention to every detail. They—in fact, all of us—are counting on you.

### REFERENCES

1. SUPPORT Study Principal Investigators. A controlled trial to improve care for seriously ill hospitalized patients: A Study to Understand Prognoses and Preferences for Outcomes and Risks of Treatments (SUPPORT). JAMA 1995;274:1591–1598.
2. Ellershaw J, Ward C. Care of the dying patient: The last hours or days of life. BMJ 2003;326:30–34.
3. Fürst CJ, Doyle D. The terminal phase. In: Doyle D, Hanks G, Cherny NI, Calman K, eds. Oxford Textbook of Palliative Medicine (3rd ed). Oxford: Oxford University Press; 2005:1119–1133.
4. Wildiers H, Menten J. Death rattle: Prevalence, prevention and treatment. J Pain Symptom Manage 2002;23:310–317.
5. Klinkenberg M, Willems DL, van der Wal G, Deeg DJ. Symptom burden in the last week of life. J Pain Symptom Manage 2004;27:5–13.
6. Potter J, Hami F, Bryan T, Quigley C. Symptoms in 400 patients referred to palliative care services: Prevalence and patterns. Palliat Med 2003;17(4):310–4.
7. McNicol E, Horowicz-Mehler N, Fisk RA, et al. Management of opioid side effects in cancer-related and chronic noncancer pain: A systematic review. Pain 2003;4(5):231–56.
8. Glare P, Walsh D Sheehan D. The adverse effects of morphine: a prospective survey of common symptoms during repeated dosing for chronic pain. Am J Hosp Palliat Care 2006;23(3):229–35.
9. Ventafridda V, Ripamonti C, De Conno F, Tamburini M, Cassileth BR. Symptom prevalence and control during cancer patients' last days of life. J Palliat Care 1990;6:7–11.
10. Hall P, Schroder C, Weaver L. The last 48 hours of life in long-term care: A focused chart audit. J Am Geriatr Soc 2002;50:501–506.
11. Ferris F. Last hours of living. Clin Ger Med 2004; 20:641–67.
12. Rogers C. On Becoming a Person: A Therapist's View of Psychology. Boston: Houghton Mifflin, 1961.
13. Twycross R. Symptom Management in Advanced Cancer (2nd ed). Oxan, UK: Radcliffe Medical Press, 1997.
14. Du Boulay S. Cicely Saunders: Founder of the Modern Hospice Movement. London: Hodder and Stoughton, 1984.
15. Karlawish HT, Quill T, Meier D (for the ACP-ASIM End of Life Care Consensus Panel). A consensus-based approach to providing palliative care to patients who lack decision making capacity. Ann Intern Med 1999;130:835–840.
16. Osenga K, Cleary JF. Fever and sweats. In: Berger AM, Shuster JL, Von Roenn JH. Principles and Practice of Palliative Care and Supportive Oncology (3rd ed). New York: Lippincott Williams & Wilkins; 2007:105–116.

17. Peberdy MA, Kaye W, Ornato JP, et al. Cardiopulmonary resuscitation of adults in the hospital: A report of 14,720 cardiac arrests from the National Registry of Cardiopulmonary Resuscitation. *Resuscitation* 2003;58 297–308.

18. Ebell MH, Becker LA, Barry HC, Hagen M. Survival after in-hospital cardiopulmonary resuscitation: A meta-analysis. *J Gen Int Med* 1998;13(12):805–16.

19. Reisfield GM, Wallace SK, Munsell MF, Webb FJ, Alvarez ER, Wilson GR. Survival in cancer patients undergoing in-hospital cardiopulmonary resuscitation: a meta-analysis. *Resuscitation* 2006;71:152–160.

20. Dunn H. Hard Choices for Loving People: CPR, Artificial Feeding, Comfort Care and the Patient with a Life-Threatening Illness (4th ed). Herndon, VA: A & A Publishers, 2001.

21. Zerwekh J. Do dying patients really need IV fluids? Am J Nurs 1997;97:26–31.

22. Bavin L. Artifical rehydration in the last days of life: Is it beneficial? Int J Palliat Nurs 2007;13(9):445–9.

23. Hospice and Palliative Nurses Association. HPNA Position Statement: Withholding and/or Withdrawing Life Sustaining Therapies. Pittsburgh: Hospice and Palliative Nurses Association, 2008.

24. Working Party on Clinical Guidelines in Palliative Care. Changing Gear—Guidelines for Managing the Last Days of Life. London: National Council for Hospice and Specialist Palliative Care Services, 2006.

25. Harrington MD, Luebke DL, Lewis WR, Aulisio MP, Johnson NJ. Fast Fact and Concept #112: Implantable Defibrillator (ICD) at End of Life. 2004. Available at: http://www.eperc.mcw.edu/FastFactPDF/Concept%20112.pdf (accessed January 5, 2009).

26. Davison, SN, Rosielle DA. Fast Fact and Concept #207: Withdrawal of Dialysis: Decision-Making. 2008. Available at http://www.eperc.mcw.edu/FastFactPDF/Concept%20207.pdf (accessed January 5, 2009).

27. Davison, SN, Rosielle DA. Fast Facts and Concepts #208: Clinical Care Following Withdrawal of Dialysis. 2008. Available at http://www.eperc.mcw.edu/FastFactPDF/Concept%20208.pdf (accessed January 5, 2009).

28. Kelly C, Yetman L. At the end of life. Can Nurse 1987;83: 33–34.

29. Quill TE, Hollaway RG, Shah MS, Caprio TV, Storey P. Primer of Pallaitive Care (4th ed). Glenview, IL: American Academy of Hospice and Palliative Medicine, 2007.

30. Kehl KA, Kirchoff KT, Finster MP, Cleary JF. Materials to prepare hsopice families for dying in the home. J Palliat Med 2008;11(7):969–972.

31. Department of Health and Human Services, Health Care Financing Administration. Medicare and Medicaid Programs; Hospital Conditions of Participation; Identification of Potential Organ, Tissue, and Eye Donors and Transplant Hospitals' Provision of Transplant-Related Data. Final rule. 63 Federal Register 119 (1998) (codified at 42 CFR §482.45).

32. Weissman DE, Heidenreich CA. Fast Fact and Concept #004: Death Pronouncement (2nd ed). 2005. Available at http://www.eperc.mcw.edu/FastFactPDF/Concept%20004.PDF (accessed January 5, 2009).

33. Pennington EA. Postmortem care: More than ritual. Am J Nurs 1978;75:846–847.

34. Beattie S. Hands-on-help: Post-mortem care. RN 2006;69(10):24ac1–4.

35. Higgins D. Clinical practical programs: Carrying out last offices, Part 1—Preparing for the procedure. Nurs Times 2008;104(37):20–1.

36. Higgins D. Clinical practical programs: Carrying out last offices, Part 2—Preparation of the body. Nurs Times. 2008;104(38):24–5.

37. Starks, J. Licensed Funeral Director, Starks Funeral Parlor, Salt Lake City, UT, personal communication, January, 2009.

38. Ambuel B, Weissman D. Fast Fact and Concept #016: Conducting a Family Conference (2nd ed). 2005. Available at http://www.eperc.mcw.edu/FastFactPDF/Concept%20016.PDF (accessed January 5, 2009).

# IV
# Spiritual Care

# 33 Spiritual Assessment

*Elizabeth Johnston Taylor*

*Everything we do affects the patient's spirit! Approaching a patient with empathy, caring, an open mind, making good eye contact, touch, active listening, all the things a nurse does. If you skip or shortchange any of these things, you are not only shortchanging the patient, you are cheating yourself out of enjoying the art of nursing.*

*Always, always, always listen. People love to share and communicate their stories Just be patient and willing to listen. The information learned is invaluable!—Registered nurses responding to a survey about providing spiritual care*

♦ **Key Points**
♦ *Spiritual assessment precedes effective spiritual caregiving. Because palliative care patients and their family members use spiritual coping strategies, and spiritual well-being can buffer the distress of dying, spiritual care is integral to palliative care.*
♦ *Numerous typologies identifying the dimensions of spirituality exist and provide guidance for what to address in a spiritual assessment.*
♦ *A two-tiered approach to spiritual assessment allows the nurse to first conduct a superficial assessment to screen for spiritual problems or needs.*
♦ *If needed, a more comprehensive spiritual assessment should be conducted by a competent professional, typically a chaplain.*
♦ *Most experts recommending a spiritual screening question agree that it is first important to assess how important or relevant spirituality is to the patient.*
♦ *Other salient spiritual screening questions include: "How does your spirituality help you to live with your illness?" and "What can I/we do to support your spiritual beliefs and practices?"*
♦ *Spiritual assessment strategies include spiritual histories, life stories, pictorial depictions of spiritual experience, as well as the traditional verbal probing.*
♦ *Although spirituality should be assessed near the time of admission to palliative care service, the process of assessment should be ongoing.*
♦ *Spiritual assessment data should be documented to at least some extent.*

To solve any problem, one must first assess what the problem is. Consequently, the nursing process dictates that the nurse begin care with an assessment of the patient's health needs. Although palliative nurses are accustomed to assessing patients' pain experiences, hydration status, and so forth, they less frequently participate in assessing patients' and family members' spirituality.

Because spirituality is an inherent and integrating, and often extremely valued, dimension for those who receive palliative nursing care, it is essential that palliative care nurses know to some degree how to conduct a spiritual assessment. This chapter reviews models for spiritual assessment, presents general guidelines on how to conduct a spiritual assessment, and discusses what the nurse ought to do with data from a spiritual assessment. These topics are prefaced by arguments supporting the need for spiritual assessments, descriptions of what spirituality "looks like" among the terminally ill, and risk factors for those who are likely to experience spiritual distress. But first, a description of spirituality is in order.

## What Is Spirituality?

Numerous recent analyses of the concept of spirituality have identified key aspects of this ethereal and intangible phenomenon.[1] Conceptualizations of spirituality often include the following as aspects of spirituality: the need for purpose and meaning, forgiveness, love and relatedness, hope, creativity, and religious faith and its expression. A well-accepted definition for spirituality authored by Reed[2] proposed that spirituality involves meaning-making through intrapersonal, interpersonal, and transpersonal connection. A more recent definition that incorporates themes found in nursing literature is Narayanasamy's[3] description of spirituality as "the essense of our being and it gives meaning and purpose to our existence" (p. 140). Narayanasamy accepts that spirituality is a "guiding force," an "inner source of power," and "source of wisdom": "It drives us to search for meaning and purpose, and establish positive and trusting relationships with others. There is a mysterious nature to our spirituality and it gives peace and tranquility through our relationship with 'something other' or things we value as supreme" (p. 140).

Usually, spirituality is differentiated from religion—the organized, codified, and often institutionalized beliefs and practices that express one's spirituality.[1] Or to use Narayansamy's[3] metaphor: "Spirituality is more of a journey and religion may be the transport to help us in our journey" (p. 141). Definitions of spirituality typically include transcendence—that is, spirituality explains persons' needs to transcend the self, often manifested in a recognition of an Ultimate Other, Sacred Source, Higher Power, divinity, or God. Although these definitions allow for an open interpretation of what a person considers to be sacred or Transcendent, some have argued that such a definition for spirituality is inappropriate for atheistics, humanists, and those who do not accept a spiritual reality.[4] Indeed, a pluralistic definition of spirituality (however "elastic" and vague it is) is necessary for ethical practice, and hence a spiritual assessment process that is sensitive to the myriad of world views is essential—if it is even appropriate for those who reject a spiritual reality.[5]

The spiritual assessment methods introduced in this chapter are all influenced inherently by some conceptualization of spirituality. Some, however, have questioned whether spiritual assessment is possible, given the broad, encompassing definition typically espoused by nurses.[5,6] Bash contended that spirituality is an "elastic" term that cannot be universally defined. Because a patient's definition of spirituality may differ from the nurse's assumptions about it, Bash argued that widely applicable tools for spiritual assessment are impossible to design. It is important to note, therefore, that the literature and methods for spiritual assessment presented in this chapter are primarily from the United States and United Kingdom, influenced most by Western Judeo-Christian traditions and peoples. Hence, they are most applicable to these people.

## Why is it Important for a Palliative Care Nurse to Conduct a Spiritual Assessment?

Spiritual awareness increases as one faces an imminent death.[8–12] Although some may experience spiritual distress or "soul pain," others may have a spiritual transformation or experience spiritual growth and health.[13] There is mounting empirical evidence to suggest that persons with terminal illnesses consider spirituality to be one of the most important contributors to quality of life.[14,15] For example, Taylor[16] observed that spiritual well-being functioned to protect terminal cancer patients against end-of-life despair. The author found spiritual well-being to have moderately strong inverse relationships with the desire for a hastened death, hopelessness, and suicidal ideations. Religious beliefs and practices

(e.g., prayer, beliefs that explain suffering or death) are also known to be valued and frequently used as helpful coping strategies among those who suffer and die from physical illness.[15–19] Family caregivers of seriously ill patients also find comfort and strength from their spirituality that assists them in coping.[18–23] Over a decade ago, a national telephone survey of 1200 adults also confirmed that Americans project that their spiritual beliefs (e.g., beliefs in an afterlife, beliefs about life belonging to God, and being "born again") will be important sources of comfort when they are dying.[24]

The above themes from research imply that attention to the spirituality of terminally ill patients and their caregivers is of utmost importance. That is, if patients' spiritual resources assist them in coping, and if imminent death precipitates heightened spiritual awareness and concerns, and if patients view their spiritual health as most important to their quality of life, then spiritual assessment that initiates a process promoting spiritual health is vital to effective palliative care.[9,10]

Underscoring these theoretical reasons for spiritual assessment is a very pragmatic one: the mandate of the Joint Commission to conduct a spiritual assessment for clients entering an approved facility.[25] Until recently, the Joint Commission mandated that a spiritual assessment should, at least, "determine the patients denomination, beliefs, and what spiritual practices are important." Now they stipulate that the institution define the scope and process of the assessment, and who completes it. But why should palliative care nurses be conducting spiritual assessments? Hunt and colleagues[26] accepted that although chaplains are the spiritual care experts, all members of a hospice team participate in spiritual caregiving. In surveying hospice team members, Millison and Dudley[27] found nurses are often the ones responsible for completing spiritual assessments. Other authors imply that nurses are pivotal in the process of spiritual assessment.[1,28–30] Considering nurses' frontline position, coordination role, and intimacy with the concerns of patients, the holistic perspective on care, and even their lack of religious cloaking, nurses can be the ideal professionals for completing an initial spiritual assessment if they have some preparation for doing so.

However, nurses must recognize that they are not specialists in spiritual assessment and caregiving; they are generalists. Most oncology and hospice nurses perceive that they do not receive adequate training in spiritual assessment and care.[31,32] In fact, it is this lack of training, accompanied by role confusion, lack of time, and other factors that nurses often cite as barriers to completing spiritual assessments.[33,34] A study of 71 British hospital nurses, nearly half of whom failed to document patient spirituality, reported that they were noncompliant mostly because they did not think the spiritual assessment was necessary or thought the assessment question was intrusive.[30] Only 23% of the 30 noncompliant nurses identified lack of time as an obstacle. Three-quarters of these nurses agreed that knowing what the spiritual assessment data would be used for and receiving more education about how to assess and care for spiritual distress would improve their performance. When a nurse's assessment indicates need for further sensitive assessment and specialized care, a referral to a specialist (e.g., chaplain, clergy, patient's spiritual director) is in order.

## How Does Spirituality Manifest Itself?

To understand how to assess spirituality, the palliative care nurse must know what to look for. What subjective and objective observations would indicate spiritual disease or health? To approach an answer, it is helpful to consider two research studies exploring qualitatively what are clients' perceptions of spiritual need. Hermann[35] interviewed 19 hospice patients to determine what specifically their spiritual needs were. The 29 resulting spiritual needs were categorized under the following themes: need for involvement and control, need for companionship, need to finish business, need to experience nature, need for a positive outlook, as well as need for religion. Taylor[20] interviewed 28 cancer patients and family caregivers, some for whom death was imminent, and identified eight categories of spiritual need. These spiritual needs included the need to:

- Relate to God or an Ultimate Other (e.g., the need to believe God will or has healed, the need to remember God's providence, the need to remember that "there is Someone out there looking out for me")
- Have gratitude and optimism (e.g., the need to keep a positive outlook, to count one's blessings, or just enjoy life)
- Love others (e.g., to forgive or "get right" with others, to return others' kindnesses, to make the world a better place, to protect family members from witnessing the suffering from cancer)
- Receive love from others (e.g., the need to feel valued and appreciated by family, to know others are praying for you, or just being with others considered to be family)
- Review spiritual beliefs (e.g., wondering if religious beliefs are correct, thinking about the unfairness of personal circumstances, or asking "why?" questions)
- Create meaning, find purpose for cancer and for life (e.g., the need to "get past" asking "why me?" and becoming aware of positive outcomes from illness, lessening the frustration of not being able to do meaningful work, or sensing that there is a reason for being alive)
- Sustain religious experience (e.g., reading spirit-nurturing material, having quiet time to reflect, or receiving a sacrament from a religious leader)
- Prepare for death (e.g., balancing thoughts about dying with hoping for health, cognitively creating a purpose for death, or making sure personal business is in order).

Dudley and colleagues[36] found hospice spiritual assessment forms often include more specific spiritual problems, such as fear of death or abandonment, spiritual emptiness, unresolved grief, unresolved past experiences, confusion or doubts about beliefs, and the need for reconciliation, comfort, or peace.

Although the terminology "spiritual need" may suggest a problem, spiritual needs can also be of a positive nature. For example, patients can have a need to express their joy about sensing closeness to others, or have a need to pursue activities that allow expression of creative impulses (e.g., artwork, music making, writing). Although the following models for conducting a spiritual assessment will provide more understanding of how spirituality manifests, the reader is referred to Galek and colleagues,[37] Taylor,[1] Highfield and Cason's[38] seminal article for further concrete indicators of spiritual need.

## Spiritual Assessment Models

Health-care professionals from multiple disciplines offer models for spiritual assessment. The most useful models from chaplaincy, medicine, social work, and nursing will be presented here. Although some assessment models have been published during the past few years, many were developed in the 1990s, when the research about spiritual care began to proliferate. Although some were developed by clinicians caring for the terminally ill, others—easily adapted or used with those at the end of life—were developed for general use for those with an illness.

Many advocate a two-tiered approach to spiritual assessment.[1,7,26,39] That is, a brief assessment for screening purposes is conducted when a patient enters a health care institution for palliative care. If the screening assessment generates an impression that there are spiritual needs, then spiritual care can only be planned if further information is collected. The second tier of assessment allows for focused, in-depth assessment. Some chaplains further distinguish a spiritual assessment from a spiritual history, an indepth review of one's spiritual journey through life (best done by a trained chaplain or spiritual care expert). After reviewing recommended spiritual screening questions, more comprehensive models or approaches to spiritual assessment will be presented.

### Screening

To appreciate the spiritual plurality within society, that some persons may not experience a spiritual reality, Pesut and colleagues[5] suggest that an initial screening must therefore assess for this basic orientation. Others assume spirituality is universal and posit that a spiritual screening should check for the significance of the beliefs and practices to the present illness circumstances and ascertain how the patient may want spiritual support from the health care team. Various clinical authors profer single questions for broaching the topic of spirituality with a patient. For example:

- How important is spirituality or religion to you?[40] Kub and colleagues,[41] in their research with 114 terminally ill persons, found that a single question about the importance of religion to be more discriminating than a question about frequency of attendance at religious services—a question that has often been the sole "spiritual assessment" in some institutions.
- What do you rely on in times of illness?[42]
- Are you at peace? This question was found to correlate highly with spiritual and emotional well-being in large a study of terminally ill patients.[43]

Two other screening approaches that are very concise have been proposed by physicians Lo and colleagues,[44] who suggested the following questions for use in palliative care settings:

- Is faith/religion/spirituality important to you in this illness? Has faith been important to you at other times in your life?
- Do you have someone to talk to about religious matters? Would you like to explore religious matters with someone?

Striving to have an even more streamlined spiritual assessment, Matthews and colleagues[45] proposed initial spiritual assessments could be limited to asking "Is your religion (or faith) helpful to you in handling your illness?" and "What can I do to support your faith or religious commitment?"

Several clinicians have devised mnemonic tools for use in spiritual assessment (see Table 33–1).[46–50] Although some of these are fairly comprehensive, some of them are designed so as to collect superficial information—to screen. The most widely cited tool is Pulchaski's[46] FICA tool. FICA prompts the clinician to assess to what *faith* and beliefs the patient has (F), how *important* or *influential* this faith is (I), what faith community or spiritual support group they participate in (C), and how the client would like the health/hospice care team to *address* their spiritual needs (A). This mnemonic is easy to recall, and provides a bit more information than would the single screening items above.

Hodge[51] essentially proposed the same content for his brief assessment, arguing that it well meets The Joint Commission requirement. Hodge's assessment questions include:

- "I was wondering if spirituality or religion is important to you?
- Are there certain spiritual beliefs and practices that you find particularly helpful in dealing with problems?
- I was wondering if you attend a church or some other type of spiritual community?
- Are there any spiritual needs or concerns I can help you with?" (p. 319)

The non-intrusive tone with which these questions are worded is exemplary.

A German medical researcher, using basically the same content (i.e., Would you describe yourself—in the broadest sense of the term—as a believing/spiritual/religious person? What is the place of spirituality in your life? How integrated are you in a spiritual community? What role would you like to assign to your health care team with regard to spirituality?), found that these questions were helpful for both patients and physicians.[52]

Anandarajah and Hight[47] developed a simpler mnemonic for remembering aspects of a spiritual assessment: HOPE. "H" reminds the clinician to assess for sources of **h**ope, strength, comfort, meaning, peace, love, and connection. "O" refers to the patient's **o**rganized religion, while "P" stands for **p**ersonal spirituality and **p**ractices. "E" prompts the clinician to assess for spirituality **e**ffects on medical care and **e**nd-of-life decisions. Although the mnemonic may be stretched, the parsimony of the assessment strategy is appreciated.

LaRocca-Pitts[53] offered another mnemonic, FACT, for a spiritual screening, advocating that a tool that incorporates a response to an assessment is needed. FACT reminds the clinician to assess for: F (faith)—or spiritual beliefs; A (availability/accessibility/applicability)—or how well spiritual support can be accessed; C (coping/comfort)—or how faith functions to help comfort and cope; and T (treatment)—what spiritual care is needed given FAC.

Table 33–2 provides a prototype for a spiritual screening tool. This tool can be adapted to meet the unique needs of any palliative care context. It can be completed by either the patient or with the assistance of a nurse. Because it is unknown how well family can serve as proxies for measurements of spiritual health, and because responses may be easily swayed by social desireability, it is best to not have family complete such a tool. Such a tool can be inserted in the patient chart and guide ongoing spiritual assessment and care. This tool is purposefully concise to accommodate the palliative care patient who is often weak and suffering from symptom distress.

## Comprehensive Models

If the screening assessment, or subsequent observation, provides preliminary evidence that a spiritual need exists that might benefit from spiritual care from a member of the palliative care team, then a more comprehensive assessment is in order. Depending on the situation, a more indepth assessment regarding the specific spiritual need or a grand tour assessment that covers multiple aspects of the patient's spirituality, will provide the evidence upon which to plan appropriate spiritual care.[1] For example, if a nurse observes a terminally ill patient's spouse crying and stating, "Why does God have to take my sweetheart?," then the nurse would want to understand further what factors are contributing to or may relieve this spiritual pain. To focus the assessment on the pertinent topic, the nurse would then ask questions that explore the spouse's "why" questions, beliefs about misfortune, perceptions of God, and spiritual coping strategies.

When should clinicians probe more deeply? Hodge[51] suggested four criteria for determining whether to move on to

**Table 33–1**
**Mnemonics to Guide a Spiritual Assessment**

| Author/s | Components (Mnemonic) | Illustrative Questions |
|---|---|---|
| Maugens[48] | • S (spiritual belief system)<br>• P (personal spirituality)<br>• I (integration with a spiritual community)<br>• R (ritualized practices and restrictions)<br>• I (implications for medical care)<br>• T (terminal events planning) | • What is your formal religious affiliation?<br>• Describe the beliefs and practices of your religion or spiritual system that you personally accept. What is the importance of your spirituality/religion in daily life?<br>• Do you belong to any spiritual or religious group or community? What importance does this group have to you? Does or could this group provide help in dealing with health issues?<br>• Are there specific elements of medical care that you forbid on the basis of religious/spiritual grounds?<br>• What aspects of your religion/spirituality would you like me to keep in mind as I care for you? Are there any barriers to our relationship based on religious or spiritual issues?<br>• As we plan for your care near the end of life, how does your faith impact on your decisions? |
| Anandarajah & Hight[47] | • H (sources of hope)<br>• O (organized religion)<br>• P (personal spirituality or spiritual practices)<br>• E (effects on medical care and/or end-of-life issues) | • What or who is it that gives you hope?<br>• Are you a part of an organized faith group? What does this group do for you as a person?<br>• What personal spiritual practices, like prayer or meditation, help you?<br>• Do you have any beliefs that may affect how the healthcare team cares for you? |
| Puchalski[46] | • F (faith)<br>• I (import or Influence)<br>• C (community)<br>• A (address) | • Do you have a faith belief? What is it that gives your life meaning?<br>• What importance does your faith have In your life? How does your faith belief influence your life?<br>• Are you a member of a faith community? How does this support you?<br>• How would you like for me to integrate or address these issues in your care? |
| LaRocca-Pitts[53] | • F (faith)<br>• A (availability/accessibility/applicability)<br>• C (coping/comfort)<br>• T (treatment) | • What spiritual beliefs are important to you now?<br>• Are you able to find the spiritual nurture that you would like now?<br>• How comforting/helpful are your spiritual beliefs at this time?<br>• How can I/we provide spiritual support? |
| Skalla & McCoy[49] | • M (moral authority)<br>• V (vocational)<br>• A (aesthetic)<br>• S (social)<br>• T (TRANSENDENT) | • What guides you to decide what is right or wrong for you?<br>• What mission or role do you fell passionate about?<br>• How are you able to express your creativity? How do you deal with boredom?<br>• What people or faith community do you sense you belong with most?<br>• Is there an Ultimate Other (an entity that is sacred, for example)? If so, how do you relate to It? |
| McEvoy (pediatric context)[50] | • B (belief system)<br>• E (ethics or values)<br>• L (lifestyle)<br>• I (involvement in spiritual community)<br>• E (EDUCATION)<br>• F (near future events of spiritual significance for which to prepare the child) | • What religious or spiritual beliefs, if any, do members of your family have?<br>• What standards/values/rules for life does your family think important?<br>• What spiritual habits or activities does your family commit to becausee of spiritual beliefs? (e.g. Any sacred times to observe or diet you keep?)<br>• How connected to a faith community are you? Would you like us to help you reconnect with this group now?<br>• Are you receiving any form of religious education? How can we help you keep up with it?<br>• Are there any upcoming religious ceremonies that you are getty ready for? |

**Table 33–2**
**Self (or Nurse-Assisted) Spiritual Screening Assessment for Palliative Care Patients**

Dear_____,

Your palliative care team wants to make sure you receive the physical, emotional, and spiritual care and comfort you need. Typically, persons receiving palliative care find themselves becoming more aware of their spirituality. This form will allow us to understand what are your spiritual care and comfort needs.

Directions: Place an "X" on the lines to show the answer that comes closest to describing your experience.

1. How important is spirituality and/or religion to you now?

/_____/

Not at all important                                        Very important

2. Recently, my spirits have been…

/_____/

Awful--.... low.... okay.... good.... great--

What can a nurse do that would help to nurture or boost your spirits? (check all that apply)

— spend quiet time with you
— have prayer with you
— help you meditate
— allow time and space for your private prayer or meditation
— let you know nurse(s) are praying privately for you
— read spiritually helpful literature to you
— bring art or music to you that nurtures your spirit
— bring you literature that you feel is spiritually helpful
— help you to stay connected to your spiritual community
— help you to observe religious practices
— listen to your thoughts about certain spiritual matters
— help you to remember how you have grown from previous difficult life experiences
— help you to tell your life story
— help you to face painful questions, doubts, or suffering
— just be with you, not necessarily talking with you
— just show a genuine and personal interest in you

Please list anything else the nurses can do to support you spiritually: _____
_____

I would also like help in boosting my spirits from:

— my friends and family
— other health care professionals—please specify who:
— a chaplain at this institution                    _____
— my faith community—please identify tradition and congregation or group: _____
_____
— my own clergy or spiritual mentor—please provide name and any contact information:_____
_____

Is there anything else about your spiritual beliefs or practices that the palliative care team should know about? (e.g., diet or lifestyle proscribed by your religion? beliefs guiding your preparation for death?) Please write here (or on the back side) or tell your nurse.

a more comprehensive assessment. First, consider patient autonomy. The patient must give informed consent. A comprehensive assessment may drill into inner depths the patient does not wish to expose to a clinician. Second, consider the competency of the clincian with regard to discussing spiritual matters. Is the clinician culturally sensitve and aware of how a personal worldview might conflict with the patient's? Might the clinician suffer from religious counter transference and inappropriately relate to the patient from personal biases? Third, consider if the spiritual issue identified is relevant to the present health care situation. If not, it may not be in nurses' purview. For patients at the end of life, however, many past and diverse spiritual struggles can resurface; although they may

seem tangential to present health caregiving, they may benefit from spiritual expertise which aids them to address these issues before death. Finally, consider the importance of spirituality to the patient. The extreme illustration of this would be if a patient states spirituality is personally irrelevant, then a comprehensive spiritual assessment would be inappropriate.

Although a comprehensive spiritual assessment may well be beneficial to many patients at the end of life, it is likely that few palliative care nurses are competent or able to conduct such an assessment.[5] The screening models presented thus far are most relevant for palliative care nurses. By reviewing more comprehensive models, however, nurses can extend their knowledge and gain appreciation for the territory that spiritual care experts may travel with patients. Nurses are in a pivotal position to refer patients to chaplains or other spiritual care specialists who can conduct a comprehensive assessment.

In a groundbreaking and still cited article, Stoll[54] suggested four areas for spiritual assessment:

- The patient's concept or God or deity
- Sources of hope and strength
- Religious practices
- The relationship between spiritual beliefs and health.

These areas continue to be included in more contemporary assessments. A quarter of a century later, British nurse Narayanasamy[3] synthesizes the categories of spiritual need found in the nursing literature and recommends a spiritual assessment guide that includes questions or observations that address patient meaning and purpose, sources of strength and hope, love and relatedness, self-esteem, fear and anxiety, anger, and relation between spiritual beliefs and health.

Likewise, family physician T.A. Maugens[48] offers the mnemonic SPIRIT for remembering six components to cover during a spiritual assessment. "Spiritual belief system" refers to religious affiliation and theology. "Personal spirituality" refers to the spiritual views shaped by life experiences that are unique to the individual and not necessarily related to one's religion. "Integration and involvement with a spiritual community" reminds the clinician to assess for a patient's membership and role in a religious organization or other group that provides spiritual support. "Ritualized practices and restrictions" are the behaviors and lifestyle activities that influence one's health. "Implications for medical care" reminds the nurse to assess how spiritual beliefs and practices influence the patient's desire and participation in health care. "Terminal events planning" reminds the clinician to assess end-of-life concerns. These components of a spiritual assessment are most appropriate for use in palliative care settings; the mnemonic may be helpful for remembering them.

Fitchett,[55] a chaplain developed the "7-by-7" model for spiritual assessment with a multidisciplinary group of health professionals. In addition to reviewing seven dimensions of a person (medical, psychological, psychosocial, family system, ethnic and cultural, societal issues, and spiritual dimensions), Fitchett advances seven spiritual dimensions to include in an assessment:

- beliefs and meaning (i.e., mission, purpose, religious and nonreligious meaning in life);
- vocation and consequences (what persons believe they should do, what their calling is);
- experience (of the divine or demonic) and emotion (the tone emerging from one's spiritual experience);
- courage and growth (the ability to encounter doubt and inner change);
- ritual and practice (activities that make life meaningful);
- community (involvement in any formal or informal community that shares spiritual beliefs and practices); and

- authority and guidance (exploring where or with whom one places trusts, seeks guidance).

Skalla and McCoy[49] proposed the "Mor-VAST" model for guiding spiritual assessments with cancer patients. This model suggests the clinician query patients regarding their:

- Moral authority (e.g., "Where does your sense of what to do come from?")
- Vocation (e.g., What gives your life purpose? What work is important to you?)
- Aesthetic (e.g., What brings beauty or pleasure to your life now?)
- Social (e.g., Do you belong to a community that nourishes you spiritually?)
- Transcendent (e.g., Who or what controls what happens in life? Who/what supports you when you are ill?)

The authors of this model (a nurse and a chaplain) remind the user that the questions are a guide, and not prescriptive; they can be threaded into the natural course of a conversation.[49]

The Royal Free Interview Schedule developed in the United Kingdom by King, Speck, and Thomas[56] is a 2½-page self-report questionnaire. The tool showed acceptable reliability and various forms of validity when it was tested among 297 persons, who were primarily hospital employees and church members. Questionnaire items assess both spiritual and religious "understanding in life" (1 item), religious/spiritual beliefs (8 items), religious/spiritual practices (3 items), and "intense" spiritual or "near death" experiences (6 items). Response options for items include Likert scales, categorical options, and space for answering open-ended questions.

Other paper and pencil type questionnaires for measuring spirituality for research purposes abound. Although discussion of such questionnaires is beyond the scope of this chapter, it is possible that some of them could be used for clinical assessments. For example, the often used FACIT-Sp is a short, valid instrument that assesses both religious and existential/spiritual well-being in persons with cancer.[57] Other brief tools that measure daily spiritual experience and religious commitment can be found in a compendium of instruments measuring spirituality and religiosity in healthcare settings.[58]

CASE STUDY
*Mr. S, Entering Hospice Service with Parkinson's Disease*

Mr. S, is a 76-year-old Protestant gentleman who was diagnosed about 13 years ago with Parkinson's disease. Until 8 months ago, he lived alone. When he realized he could no longer safely live alone, he moved to an assisted living facility. Now his condition has deteriorated further, requiring his admission to a skilled nursing facility. This facility has obtained hospice services for Mr. S. He is receiving anti-parkinsonian and anti-depressive medications.

Mr. S is divorced from his third wife and estranged from his only son and a stepson. The son lives 7 hours away (by car), and usually reenters Mr. S's life when he needs financial assistance. The only family that appears to show interest in supporting Mr. S is a niece and her husband, who live 2 hours away. Since Mr. S's divorce 10 years ago, he has been befriended by a middle-aged woman, Sally, who has entered several business ventures with Mr. S's money.

The following are excerpts from conversations the author had with Mr. S:

"My dad was a doctor. He practiced until he was 91! He was very respected and well-known. He loved to yacht; he won the Trans-Pac race one year. I was a teen then, and could only travel with him if I was the crew's cook. So my mom taught me to peel potatoes....!

I wanted to be a doctor. I just couldn't get the grades, got kicked out of college...never could have gotten into med school. So I sold cookware instead. But they said I could sell snow in Alaska—I was good at selling....

I was born and raised in the church. Went to Christian schools all the way through college. I was an elder at my little church before I moved down here. I've got the church even in my will....

I know Sally is using me, but I love her. I would marry her if I could. [She was married.] My head says one thing, but my heart says another....

I remember once making love to a woman and her reaction was, 'Oh my God!' I guess that was a spiritual experience I helped her have!

There's not much for me to do here. Just a bunch of old people around here. Sometimes I wonder, 'Why? Why keep going?'.... I don't have anymore money to give.... My body doesn't work anymore....

[During a phonecall when Mr. S related he felt anxious:] I'm having a hard time...really worried about how its all going to end. How will it?...[When asked, "How at peace do you feel inside?":] Not at all. [When asked, "Is there anything you can think of that would bring comfort to you now?":] No, nothing."

### Assessment (using FICA):

F (faith)—verbalized about some indicators of adherence to a faith tradition; inward (or intrinsic) faith is fundamentally challenged as he faces his end; his faith appears to lean toward an extrinsic faith (e.g., attendance at services, donating money).

I (importance)—states it is important.

C (community)—until institutionalized, was a leader in a local Seventh-day Adventist congregation; desires to continue to attend.

A (address)—readily responds positively to query regarding having local pastor visit him; also accepts offer of loaned spiritual viewing materials (e.g., videos of dramatized Gospels) and musical CDs. When asked

how the staff can spiritually support, he states, "No, they don't need to butt into this part of my life."

### Assessment (using Mor-VAST):

Moral authority—He states the Bible is the guide for what is right or wrong. He admits struggling about how to morally relate to Sally and yearns to reconnect with his sons.

Vocational—He excelled as a salesman during mid-adult years. More recently, his business ventures have failed. During his youth, he aspired to be a physician, yet failed to attain that goal. His life seems to have been lived in the shadow of his fathers, perhaps challenging his sense of worth. His financial failure also seems to challenge his sense of success and purposefulness.

Aesthetic—Loves "cars, motorcycles, and beautiful women!" His disease now prevents his ability to enjoy these interests, as he can no longer drive or attract women for a date. He does enjoy eating and listening to jazz.

Social—until institutionalized, was a leader in a local Seventh-day Adventist congregation; desires to continue to attend as he enjoys the opportunity to see old friends and meet people there.

Transcendent—says he prays before each meal and at bedtime, and then at times when he is very distressed, but reports that "sometimes it feels like the prayers don't go anywhere." Never describes a time in his life when there was an affective experience of God; rather, his descriptions of religious experience seem cerebral and proscribed. He does describe several times in his life when he believes his life was spared, and interprets these events as showing God intervening in his life.

Note: Comparing the two assessments above reveals that different data were generated. Other assessment approaches could be taken. Each would offer yet other emphases or angles for making sense of assessment data. It should be remembered, therefore, that each approach to spiritual assessment is one lens and may fail to address other important areas of spirituality (e.g., spiritually comforting practices are and preparation for death are omitted from the above FICA and Mor-VAST approaches).

## Summary of Spiritual Assessment Models

The above summaries of various models for spiritual assessment identify spiritual dimensions that may be included in a spiritual assessment. Many of the dimensions identified in one model are observed (often using different language) in other models. Except for Hodge's[40] diagramatic methods, these assessment approaches generally require the professional to make observations while asking questions and listening for the patient's response. The vast majority of questions recommended for use in following such a model are open-ended. Several of the questions—indeed, the dimensions of spirituality—identified in this literature use "God language" or assume a patient will have belief in some transcendent divinity. All these models are developed by professionals who are influenced predominantly by Western, Judeo-Christian ways of thinking.

※⊗⊗

## General Observations and Suggestions for Conducting a Spiritual Assessment

### What Approach to Use

Whereas researchers often assess individuals' spirituality quantitatively with "paper and pencil" questionnaires, health care professionals generally assess spirituality using qualitative methods (e.g., participant observations, semistructured interviews). However, it is possible to use questionnaires during the clinical spiritual-assessment process.[1,28] This approach to conducting a spiritual assessment allows for identification, and possibly, measurement, of how one believes, belongs, and behaves. This type of tool, however, should not "stand alone" in the process of spiritual assessment; rather, it can be the springboard for a more thorough assessment and deeper encounter with a patient, as appropriate. A quantitative tool should never replace human contact, instead, it should facilitate it. Although a quantitative spiritual self-assessment form provides an opportunity for health care teams to glean substantial information when screening for spiritual beliefs and practices, without spending any professional's time, it also is limited by its mechanistic, rigid, and nonindividualized nature.[59]

A group of nurse educators[29] developed an approach to spiritual assessment for their undergraduate students that provides checklists of indicators of spiritual integrity and distress, as well as open questions to prompt further assessment. One checklist on the tool prompts the student to look for objects in the environment and non-verbal indicators that might reveal information about a patient's spiritual health. Another checklist allows the student to tick off positive or negative indications about spiritual health that a patient has expressed verbally or demontrated (e.g., appreciation for nature, requests for special diet or clergy, loneliness). Although designed for students, this quasi-quantitative, semi-structured format may provide nurses in palliative care settings an appropriate "crutch" when completing a spiritual assessment is a new or challenging task. (Note: This tool also includes items to tick off for spiritual diagnosis and plans for spiritual care.) An example of a tool that can be completed by either the nurse or patient is offered in Table 33–2.

Other approaches to spiritual assessment have been described in addition to the interview and questionnaire techniques. LeFavi and Wessels[60] described how life reviews can become, in essence, spiritual assessments. Life reviews are especially valuable for persons who are dying, as they allow patients to make sense of and reconcile their life story.[61] By doing a life review with a terminally ill patient, the nurse can assess many dimensions of spirituality (e.g., world views, commitments, missions, values) in a natural, noncontrived manner.

Life reviews can be prompted by questions about the significant events, people, and challenges during the lifespan. A life review can also occur when inquiring about personal objects, pictures, or other memorabilia the patient wants to share.

Hodge[40] identified several creative approaches to collecting information about client spirituality. As a social worker, Hodge is well aware that some patients are not verbal or are not comfortable expressing their spirituality in words. Thus, he explained more visual ways for a patient to describe their spiritual experiences. These methods for assessments include:

- Spiritual lifemaps, or a pictoral depiction of where the patient has been spiritually, where the patient is presently, and where the patient expects to go. It can be a simple pencil drawing on a large piece of paper; words and illustrations can be used to convey the spiritual story—the spiritual highs and lows, blessings and burdens, and so forth.
- Spiritual genogram, like a standard genogram, depicts the issues and influences over one to three generations. Sources of spiritual influence from certain relationships (including those external to the family) can be drawn. Words that identify key spiritual beliefs and practices that were transmitted via relationships, and significant spiritual events that contribute to the patient's spiritual life can noted around this spiritual family tree.
- Spiritual ecomaps, rather than focusing on past spiritual influences, directs the patient to consider present spiritual experience. In particular, the patient can diagram (with self portrayed in the center) the relationship with God or transcendent other/value, rituals, faith community, and encounters with other spiritual entities.
- Spiritual ecograms allow the patient to diagram present perspectives on both family and spiritual relationships; it is a fusion of the spiritual genogram and ecomap.[40]
- Other strategies include having clients draw a spiritual timeline that includes significant books, experiences, events, and so forth. Another unusual approach involves sentence completion. For example, a client may fill in the blank of sentences like "My relation to God…" or "What I would really like to be…" or "When I feel overwhelmed…." Having verbally oriented assessment strategies as well as these nonverbal methods provides clinicians with a "toolbox" for assessing spirituality, allowing the clinician to choose an approach that fits the patient personality, circumstances, and purpose for assessment.

### When to Assess

Typically, palliative care settings has at least one question about spirituality in their admission questions. Many hospices have spiritual carers who complete an assessment sometime after admission.[62] However, most experts agree that spiritual assessment should also be an ongoing process.[1,63,64] The nurse does not complete a spiritual assessment simply by asking some questions about religion or spirituality during an intake interview. Instead, spiritual assessment should be ongoing throughout the nurse–patient relationship. A nurse tuned to know how spiritual health is manifested will be able to see and hear patient spirituality as it is embedded in and suffuses the everyday encounter.[65]

Stoll,[54] recognizing the significance of timing when asking patients questions about spirituality, suggested that spiritual assessment be separated from a sexual assessment because both topics are so sensitive and intimate. However, both spiritual and sexual assessment should occur during the general assessment for the purposes of screening for problems. Several authors remind their readers that spiritual assessments can only be effectively completed if the health-care professional has first established trust and rapport with the patient.[7,54,62]

### Gaining Entrée

Spiritual needs are complex and often difficult to acknowledge, and more so, to describe with words. Furthermore, the patient may not yet feel comfortable divulging such intimate information to a nurse with whom rapport has not been established. Indeed, some patients may not want to share such inner, heart-touching experience. Two studies provide evidence regarding what patients are looking for in a clinician if they are going to talk openly about their spirituality.[66,67]

Survey responses from cancer patients and family caregivers ($n$ = 224) about what requisites they would want in a nurse who provided spiritual care revealed that relationship (i.e., "show me kindness and respect" and "get to know me first") were ranked highest, with a nurse's training in spiritual care or sharing similar beliefs as the patient being less important.[68] Likewise, a small qualitative study of chronically and terminally ill patients observed that these informants viewed relational characteristics (e.g., caring, honor and respect, rapport/trust) as prerequisites for discussing spirituality with a physician.[69] Ellis and Campbell's study identified other factors that patients perceive facilitate spiritual assessment by a physician: a condusive setting, sharing life priorities or values, perceived receptivity of physician to spiritual questions, and sensing that spiritual health was considered by the physician to be integral to health.[69]

Because spirituality and religiosity are sensitive and personal topics (as are most other topics nurses assess), it is polite for a nurse to preface a spiritual assessment with an acknowledgment of the sensitivity of the questions and an explanation for why such an assessment is necessary.[1,48] For example, Maugens[48] suggested this preface: Many people have strong spiritual or religious beliefs that shape their lives, including their health and experiences with illness. If you are comfortable talking about this topic, would you please share any of your beliefs and practices that you might want me to know as your physician (p. 12).

Such a preface undoubtedly will help both the patient and the clinician to feel at ease during the assessment.

### Assessing Nonverbal Indicators of Spirituality

Although this discussion of spiritual assessment has thus far focused on how to frame a verbal question and allow a patient to verbalize a response, the nurse must remember that most communication occurs nonverbally. Hence, the nurse must assess the nonverbal communication and the environment of the patient[29,70] Does the patient appear agitated or angry? What does the body language convey? What is the speed and tone of voice?[65] Assessment of the patient's environment can provide clues about spiritual state.[1,29,70] Are there religious objects on the bedside table? Are there religious paintings or crucifixes on the walls? Get-well cards or books with spiritual themes? Are there indicators that the patient has many friends and family providing love and a sense of community? Are the curtains closed and the bedspread pulled over the face? Many of the factors a palliative care nurse usually assesses will provide data for a spiritual assessment as well as the psychosocial assessment.

### Language: Religious or Spiritual Words?

One barrier to spiritual assessment is the nurse's fear of offending a nonreligious patient by using religious language. However, when one remembers the nonreligious nature of spirituality, this barrier disappears. Patient spirituality can be discussed without God language or reference to religion. Also, using the terms "need" or "distress" immediately after "spiritual" could be denograting for a patient. Especially with spirituality, patients may be upset when they hear others consider them to be with need. Nurses can easily avoid such jargon.[63]

To know what language will not be offensive during a spiritual assessment, the nurse must remember two guidelines. First, the nurse can begin the assessment with questions that are general and unrelated to religious assumptions. For example, "What is giving you the strength to cope with your illness now?" or "What spiritual beliefs and practices are important to you as you cope with your illness?" Second, the nurse must listen for the language of the patient, and use the patient's language when formulating more specific follow-up questions. If a patient responds to a question with "My faith and prayers help me," then the nurse knows "faith" and "prayer" are words that will not offend this patient. If a patient states that the "Great Spirit guides," then the sensitive nurse will not respond with, "Tell me how Jesus is your guide."

### Asking Questions

Because asking a patient questions is an integral part of most spiritual assessments, it is good to remember some of the basics of formulating good questions. Asking close-ended questions that allow for short factual or yes/no responses is helpful when a nurse truly has no time or ability for further

**Table 33–3**
**A Collection of Nonreligious Questions to Broach Topic of Spirituality with Palliative Care Patients**

You've gone through so much lately. Where do you get your inner strength and courage to keep going?

What is helping you to cope?

What comforts are most satisfying for you now?

As you think about your future, what worries you most?

Some people seem more to live while they are dying, while others seem to die while they are living. Which way is it for you? What makes it that way?

What kind of person do you see yourself as? (Note: Chaplains suggest that how one views self parallels how one views their Creator or God.)

What do you see as the purpose for your life now, given your body isn't allowing you to do all you used to do?

What hopes and dreams do you have for your future? For your family?

What legacy would you like to leave? How can we make sure that that happens?

As I've gotten to know you, I've noticed you speak often of (spiritual theme [e.g., betrayal, yearning for love]). How do you think this theme has influenced your life, or will influence your future? How happy with your life's theme are you?

Tell me about times during your life where faced a huge challenge. What got you through? Is that resource still available to you now?

assessment. Otherwise, to appreciate the uniqueness and complexity of an individual's spirituality, the nurse must focus on asking open-ended questions. The best open-ended questions begin with how, what, when, who, or phrases like "Tell me about..." Generally, questions beginning with "why" are not helpful; they are often mixed with a sense of threat or challenge (e.g., "Why do you believe that?").[65] A few questions you may want to memorize while you are honing your spiritual assessment skill are presented in Table 33–3.

### Listening to the Answers

Although it is easy to focus on and to worry about what to say during an assessment, the palliative care nurse must remember the importance of listening to the patient's responses. Discussion of active listening is beyond the scope of this chapter, yet a few comments are in order. Remember that silence is appropriate when listening to a patient's spiritual and sacred story; silence has a work. Remain neutral, nonjudgmental. View the patient as a fellow sojourner on the journey of life. Recognize that you are not the authority or savior for the patient expressing spiritual pain. Rather you are a companion, or a supporter if so privileged. Listen for more than words; listen for metaphors, listen for a spiritual theme that keeps reemerging throughout life stories, listen for where the patient places energy, listen for emotion in addition to cognitions.[65] The nurse will do well to listen to his or her own inner response. This response will mirror the feelings of the patient.

### Overcoming the Time Barrier

Health-care professionals may believe that they do not have enough time to conduct a spiritual assessment. Indeed, Maugens[45] observed that completing his spiritual history with patients took about 10 to 15 minutes. Although this is much less time than Maugen and his colleagues expected it to take, it is still a considerable amount of time in today's health-care context. One response to this time barrier is to

remember that spiritual assessment is a process that develops as the nurse gains the trust of a patient. The nurse can accomplish the assessment during "clinical chatterings."[45] Furthermore, data for a spiritual assessment can be simultaneously collected with other assessments or during interventions (e.g., while bathing or completing bedtime care). And finally, it can be argued that nurses do not have time to not conduct a spiritual assessment, considering the fundamental and powerful nature of spirituality.

### Overcoming Personal Barriers

Nurses can encounter personal barriers to conducting a spiritual assessment. These barriers can include feelings of embarrassment or insecurity about the topic, or can result from projection of unresolved and painful personal spiritual doubts or struggles. Every nurse has a personal philosophy or world view that influences his or her spiritual beliefs. These beliefs can color or blind the nurse's assessment techniques and interpretation. Hence, an accurate and sensitive spiritual assessment presumably correlates with the degree of the nurse's spiritual self-awareness. Put another way, your ability to hear your own spiritual story is directly related to your ability to hear a patient's spiritual story.[65] Nurses can increase their comfort with the topic and their awareness of their spiritual self if they ask themselves variations of the questions they anticipate asking patients. For example, "What gives my life meaning and purpose?" "How do my spiritual beliefs influence the way I relate to my own death?" "How do I love myself and forgive myself?" Recognizing how one's spiritual beliefs motivate one's vocation as a nurse is also extremely helpful.

### Concluding Cautions

Although the presented models and evidence supporting spiritual assessment imply that it is an unproblematic and simple process, it would be naïve to leave this impression.

Several experts suggest potential problems associated with spiritual assessment. These include:

- The process of taking spiritual assessment data to make a spiritual diagnosis pathologizes what may be a normal process of spiritual growth.[59] Assessment tools often assume that spiritual well-being correlates with feeling good; spiritual health and suffering cannot coexist.[5] (A more appropriate way to evaluate spirituality may be to ask how harmful one's spirituality is to self and others.)

- A "tick box" approach to spiritual assessment could freeze patient spirituality to the time when the assessment was completed; spiritual assessment would be considered complete and fail to continue in an ongoing manner.[59]

- A fairly prescribed assessment tool could have the unintended outcome of disempowering a patient. That is, the clinician controls (overpowers) the agenda by determining what spiritual matters are discussed.[61] A tool used for assessment could end up limiting and controlling patient expression.[10]

- A spiritual assessment to some degree will reflect the assumptions influencing the clinician (a major one being that spirituality is universal). Thus, a spiritual worldview will be imposed to some degree on a vulnerable patient. An ethical spiritual assessment would be non-alienating, non-discriminating, engage and respect the patient.[64,71]

Thus, a spiritual assessment tool—if a tool is needed—should be able to generate helpful data for guiding patient care, encourage patient participation, be flexible, easy to use, take little clinician time, be non-intrusive, allow for a patient's unique story to be understood to some degree, and be simple and clear.[71] A tall ask? Perhaps. But important to strive toward.

## Assessing Special Populations

### Assessing Impaired Patients

Although verbal conversation is integral to a typical spiritual assessment, some terminally ill patients may not be able to speak, hear, or understand a verbal assessment. Patients who are unable to communicate verbally may feel unheard. In such situations, the nurse again must remember alternative sources of information. The nurse can consult with the family members and observe the patient's environment and nonverbal communications. For example, Telos[72] proposed that for some patients, terminal restlessness was a manifestation of spiritual distress. Ruling out other causes, and relying on previous spiritual assessment opportunities that have revealed unresolved spiritual issues, supports the palliative care team to draw this conclusion. (Hence, the importance of proactively conducting spiritual assessments for those with terminal illness.)[72]

Alternative methods for "conversing" can also be used. For patients who can write, paper-and-pencil questionnaires can be very helpful. Always be patient and be unafraid of the tears that can follow. Questions that demonstrate concern for their innermost well-being may release their floodgates for tears.

For persons with dementia or other cognitive impairments, it is helpful to recognize that communication can still occur on an emotional or physical level if not intellectually. Their disjointed stories will still offer you a window to their world. Even if you cannot sew the pieces together, trying will help you to remain curious and engaged.[65]

### Assessing Children

Several strategies can be employed to assess the spirituality of children. The clinician must remember, however, that building trust and rapport with children is essential to completing a helpful spiritual assessment. Children are especially capable of ascertaining an adult's degree of authenticity. Children also are less likely to be offended by a question about religion. If a nurse creates a comfortable and nonjudgmental atmosphere in which a child can discuss spiritual topics, then the child will talk. Never underestimate the profoundness of a child's spiritual experience, especially a dying child's.

In addition to asking assessment questions verbally, the nurse can use play interviews, picture drawings, observations, and informal interviews.[73,74] The nurse may need to be more creative in formulating questions if the child's vocabulary is limited. For example, instead of asking the child about helpful religious rituals, the nurse may need to ask questions about what they do to get ready to sleep or what they do on weekends. When asking, "Does your mommy pray with you before you go to sleep?" or "What do you do on Sunday or Sabbath mornings?" the nurse can learn whether prayer or religious service attendance are a part of this child's life. An assessment question that Sexson's[74] colleague Patricia Fosarelli found to be particularly helpful with 6- to 18-year-olds was: "If you could get God to answer one question, what one question would you ask God?"

Understanding the family's spirituality is pivotal to understanding the child's. Structured interviews or unstructured conversations with parents and even older siblings will inform the health care team about the child's spirituality.[74,75] Barnes and colleagues[76] suggested the following questions as guides for assessing how a family's spirituality affects illness experience:

- How does the family understand life's purpose and meaning?
- How do they explain illness and suffering?
- How do they view the person in the context of the body, mind, soul, spirit, and so forth?
- How is the specific illness of the child explained?
- What treatments are necessary for the child?
- Who is the qualified person to address these various treatments for the various parts of the child's healing?
- What is the outcome measurement that the family is using to measure successful treatment (good death)?

While assessing children, it is vital to consider their stage of cognitive and faith development.[73,74] Questions must be framed in age-appropriate language (a 4-year-old will likely not understand what "spiritual belief" means!). Toddlers and preschoolers talk about their spirituality in very concrete terms, with an egocentric manner. School-aged and adolescent children should be addressed straightforwardly about how they see their illness. Inquiring about the cause of their illness is especially important, as many children view their illness and impending death as punishment.[73]

## Assessing Diverse Spiritualities

Spiritual assessment methods must be flexible enough to obtain valid data from persons with diverse spiritual and religious backgrounds. Although the questions and assumptions presented in this chapter will be helpful for assessing most patients living in Western, Euro-American cultures, they may not be for some patients who do not share these presuppositions. For example, some may believe it is wrong to discuss their inner spiritual turmoil as they face death and will refuse to fully engage in the process of spiritual assessment. (Whereas some Buddhists and Hindus may believe they must be in a peaceful state to be reincarnated to a better state, African-American Christians may think it is sinful to express doubts or anger towards God.) Framing spiritual assessment in a positive tone may overcome this type of barrier (e.g., "Tell me about how you are at peace now.") Others may assume they are void of spirituality and therefore decline any questions regarding their "spirituality." This barrier to assessment can be overcome with questions that are void of such language (e.g., "What gives your life meaning?" or "How is your courage?").

For patients who are religious, it is important to remember that no two members of a religious community or family are exactly alike. For example, one orthodoxly religious person may believe he should never consume any mind-altering drugs, such as morphine, while a less conservative member of the same denomination may understand that such drugs are a gracious Godly gift. Although having a cursory understanding of the world's major religious traditions provides nurses with some framework for inquiry, remaining open to the variation of religious experience and expression is essential.

## The Next Step: What To Do with a Spiritual Assessment

Making Sense of Information from a Spiritual Assessment
Even a spiritual screening can generate a lot of information. This information must be processed to identify what, if any, spiritual need exists and plan spiritual care. Several points can be considered while processing the data. These include:

- What patients tell you at first reflects not how well you have asked a good question; rather it shows how safe and respected the patient feels with you.

- Consider what incongruities exist. Do the affect, behavior, and communication (ABCs) line up?
- Consider the level of concreteness or abstractness in the patient's talk about spiritual matters. Healthy spirituality straddles between these opposites.
- Consider how defensive or threatened the patient is by talk about spirituality. Did the patient change the topic? Give superficial answers? Become competitive? Intellectual feelings?
- Keep in mind that crisies (e.g., illness) expose the gaps in a patient's spiritual development. Did significant events earlier in life in effect stunt the patient's spiritual growth?
- Remember that religion offers a lens for interpreting life. Likewise, when patients tell meaningful stories, legends, or passages from their holy scripture, they are telling you about themselves.
- Reflect on how helpful versus harmful are a patient's spiritual beliefs and practices. Do they create inner anxiety? Do they limit the patient from using other helpful coping strategies?[65]

Although an in-depth analysis is beyond the scope of most palliative care nurses, having an awareness of these various ways to evaluate what a patient says will help the nurse to begin to make sense of the data.

## Documentation

Although assessments of physiological phenomenon are readily documented in patient charts, assessments and diagnoses of spiritual problems are less frequently documented. However, for many reasons, spiritual assessments and care should be documented to at least some degree. These reasons include: (1) to facilitate the continuity of patient care among palliative care team members and (2) to document for the monitoring purposes of accrediting bodies, researchers, quality improvement teams, and so forth. Power[59] recognized that the data collected during spiritual assessments is often very private, sensitive material; to document such may breach confidentiality and thus pose an ethical dilemma. As with other sensitive charted information, nurses must treat spiritual assessment data with much respect and observe applicable privacy codes.

Formats for documenting spiritual assessments and diagnoses can vary. Some institutions encourage staff to use SOAP (Subjective, Objective, Assessment, Plan) or similar formatting in progress notes shared by the multidisciplinary team. Others have developed quick and easy checklists for documenting spiritual and religious issues. Perhaps an assessment format that allows for both rapid documentation and optional narrative data is best. However, merely documenting one's religious affiliation and whether one desires a referral to a spiritual care specialist certainly does not adequately indicate a patient's spiritual status and need.

A summary of assessment forms created by professionals at hospices is reported by Dudley, Smith, and Millison.[36]

These researchers synthesized the spiritual assessment forms from 53 hospices, finding questions about religious affiliation and rituals, religious problems or barriers, and questions about spiritual (nonreligious) topics, that is, questions void of overtly religious language. Although Dudley and colleagues summarize the content of these forms, they do not review the format for documentation on these forms.

~✖~

## Summary

Spirituality is an elemental and pervading dimension for persons, especially those for whom death is imminent. Spiritual assessment is essential to effective and sensitive spiritual care. Indeed, spiritual assessment is the beginning of spiritual care. While the nurse questions a patient about spirituality, the nurse is simultaneously assisting the patient to reflect on the innermost and most important aspects of being human. The nurse is also indicating to the patient that grappling with spiritual issues is normal and valuable. The nurse also provides spiritual care during an assessment by being present and witnessing what is sacred for the patient.

REFERENCES

1. Taylor EJ. Spiritual Care: Nursing Theory, Research, and Practice. Upper Saddle River, NJ: Prentice Hall, 2002.
2. Reed PG. An emerging paradigm for the investigation of spirituality in nursing. Res Nurs Health 1992;15:349–357.
3. Narayansamy A. The puzzle of spirituality for nursing: A guide to practical assessment. Br J Nurs 2004;13(19):1140–1144.
4. Paley J. Spirituality and secularization: nursing and the sociology of religion. J Clin Nurs 2008;17:175–186.
5. Pesut B, Fowler M, Reimer-Kirkham S, Taylor EJ, Sawatzky R. Particularizing spirituality in points of tension Nurs Inquiry (in press).
6. Bash A. Spirituality: The emperor's new clothes? J Clin Nurs 2004;13:11–16.
7. McSherry W, Ross L. Dilemmas of spiritual assessment: Considerations for nursing practice. J Adv Nurs 2002;38:479–488.
8. Williams AL. Perspectives on spirituality at the end of life: A meta-summary. Palliat Support Care 2006;4:407–417.
9. Brown AE, Whitney SN, Duffy JD. The physician's role in the assessment and treatment of spiritual distress at the end of life. Palliat Support Care 2006;4:81–86.
10. Byrne M. Spirituality in palliative care: What language do we need? Learning from pastoral care. Int J Palliat Nurs 2007;13(3):118–121.
11. Chio CC, Shih FJ, Chiou JF, Lin HW, Hsiao FH, Chen YT. The lived experiences of spiritual suffering and the healing process among Taiwanese patients with terminal cancer. J Clin Nurs 2008;17:735–743.
12. Tamura K, Ichihara K, Maetake E, Takayama K, Tanisawa K, Ikenaga M. Development of a spiritual pain assessment sheet for terminal cancer patients: Targeting terminal cancer patients admitted to palliative care units in Japan. Palliat Support Care 2006;4:179–188.
13. McGrath P. Spiritual pain: A comparison of findings from survivors and hospice patients. Am J Hosp Palliat Care 2003;20(1):23–33.
14. Taylor EJ. Spiritual quality of life. In: King CR, Hinds PS, eds. Quality of Life: From Nursing and Patient Perspectives (3rd ed). Sudbury, MA: Jones and Bartlett, in press.
15. Taylor EJ. Spiritual complementary therapies in cancer care. Sem Oncol Nurs 2005;21(3):159–163.
16. Taylor EJ. Spiritual responses to cancer (Chapter 73). In: Yarbro CH, Wujcik D, Gobel BH, eds. Cancer Nursing: Principles and Practice (7th ed). Sudbury, MA: Jones & Bartlett (in press).
17. Tatsumura Y, Maskarinec G, Shumay DM, Kakai H. Religious and spiritual resources, CAM, and conventional treatment in the lives of cancer patients. Altern Ther Health Med 2003;9:64–71.
18. Nolan MT, Hodgin MB, Olsen SJ, et al. Spiritual issues of family members in a pancreatic cancer chat room. Oncol Nurs Forum 2006;33:239–244.
19. Steele RG, Fitch MI: Coping strategies of family caregivers of home hospice patients with cancer. Oncol Nurs Forum 1996;23:955–960.
20. Taylor EJ. Spiritual needs of cancer patients and family caregivers. Cancer Nurs 2003;26:260–266.
21. Taylor EJ. Prevalence of spiritual needs among cancer patients and family caregivers. Oncol Nurs Forum 2006;33(4):729–735.
22. Steele RG, Fitch MI. Coping strategies of family caregivers of home hospice patients with cancer. Oncol Nurs Forum 1996;23:955–960.
23. Nolan MT, Hodgin MB, Olsen SJ, et al. Spiritual issues of family members in a pancreatic cancer chat room. Oncol Nurs Forum 2006;33:239–244.
24. Spiritual Beliefs and the Dying Process: Key Findings. New York: Nathan Cummings Foundation and Fetzer Institute, October 1997.
25. The Joint Commission. Spiritual assessment. Available at http://www.jointcommission.org/AccreditationPrograms/HomeCare/Standards/09_FAQs/PC/Spiritual_Assessment.htm (accessed December 31, 2008).
26. Hunt J, Cobb M, Keeley VL, Ahmedzai SH. The quality of spiritual care—developing a standard. Int J Palliat Nurs 2003;9:208–215.
27. Millison M, Dudley JR. Providing spiritual support: A job for all hospice professionals. Hospice J 1992;8:49–65.
28. O'Brien ME. Spirituality in Nursing: Standing on Holy Ground (2nd ed). Sudbury, MA: Jones and Bartlett, 2003.
29. Hoffert D, Henshaw C, Mvududu N. Enhancing the ability of nursing students to perform a spiritual assessment. Nurse Educator 2007;32(2):66–72.
30. Swift C, Calcutawalla S, Elliot R. Nursing attitudes towards recording of religious and spiritual data. Br J Nurs 2007;16:1279–1282.
31. Taylor EJ, Highfield MF, Amenta MO. Predictors of oncology and hospice nurses' spiritual care perspectives and practices. Appl Nurs Res 1999;12:30–37.
32. Highfield MEF, Taylor EJ, Amenta MO. Preparation to care: The spiritual care education of oncology and hospice nurses. J Hosp Palliat Nurs 2000;2:53–63.
33. Kuuppelomaki M. Spiritual support for families of patients with cancer: A pilot study of nursing staff assessments. Cancer Nurs 2002;25:209–218.

34. Kristeller JL, Zumbrun CS, Schilling RF. "I would if I could": How oncology nurses address spiritual distress in cancer patients. Psycho-Oncol 1999;8:451–458.

35. Hermann CP. Spiritual needs of dying patients: A qualitative study. Oncol Nurs Forum 2001;28:67–72.

36. Dudley JR, Smith C, Millison MB. Unfinished business: Assessing the spiritual needs of hospice clients. Am J Hospice Palliat Care 1995;12:30–37.

37. Galek K, Flannelly KJ, Vane A, Galek RM. Assessing a patient's spiritual needs: A comprehensive instrument. Holist Nurs Pract 2005;19(2):62–69.

38. Highfield MF, Cason C. Spiritual needs of patients: Are they recognized? Cancer Nurs 1983;6:187–192.

39. Massey K, Fitchett G, Roberts P. Assessment and diagnosis in spiritual care. In: Mauk KL, Schmidt NK, eds. Spiritual Care in Nursing Practice. Philadelphia, PA: Lippincott Williams & Wilkins, 2004.

40. Hodge D. Developing a spiritual assessment toolbox: A discussion of the strengths and limitations of five different assessment methods. Health Social Work 2005;10:314–323.

41. Kub JE, Nolan MT, Hughes MT, et al. Religious importance and practices of patients with a life-threatening illness: Implications for screening protocols. Appl Nurs Res 2003;16:196–200.

42. Lawrence RT, Smith DW. Principles to make a spiritual assessment work in your practice. J Fam Pract 2004;53:625–631.

43. Steinhauser KE, Voils CI, Clipp EC, Bosworth HB, Christakis NA, Tulsky JA. "Are you at peace?": One item to probe spiritual concerns at the end of life. Arch Intern Med 2006;166(1):101–105.

44. Lo B, Quill T, Tulsky J. Discussing palliative care with patients. Ann Intern Med 1999;130:744–749.

45. Matthews DA, McCullough ME, Larson DB, Koenig HG, Swyers JP, Milano MG. Religious commitment and health status: A review of the research and implications for family medicine. Arch Fam Med 1998;7:118–124.

46. Puchalski, C, Romer, AL. Taking a spiritual history allows clinicians to understand patients more fully. J Palliat Med 2000;3:129–138.

47. Anandarajah G, Hight E. Spirituality and medical practice: Using the HOPE questions as a practical tool for spiritual assessment. Am Fam Physician 2001;63:81–89.

48. Maugens TA. The SPIRITual history. Arch Fam Med 1996;5:11–16.

49. Skalla KA, McCoy JP. Spiritual assessment of patients with cancer: The moral authority, vocational, aesthetic, social, and transcendent model. Oncol Nurs Forum 2006;33:745–751.

50. McEvoy M. An added dimension to the pediatric health maintenance visit: The spiritual history. J Ped Health Care 2000;14:216–220.

51. Hodge D. A template for spiritual assessment: A review of the JCAHO requirements and guidelines for implementation. Social Work 2006;51:317–326.

52. Frick E, Riedner C, Fegg MJ, Hauf S, Borasio GD. A clinical interview assessing cancer patients' spiritual needs and preferences. Eur J Cancer Care (Engl) 2006;15:238–243.

53. LaRocca-Pitts M. A spiritual history tool: FACT. Available at http://www.professionalchaplains.org/uploadedFiles/pdf/FACT%20spiritual% (accessed December 29, 2008, from Association of Professional Chaplains' website.)

54. Stoll RI. Guidelines for spiritual assessment. Am J Nurs 1979;79:1574–1577.

55. Fitchett G. Assessing Spiritual Needs: A Guide for Caregivers. Minneapolis, MN: Fortress Press, 1993.

56. King M, Speck P, Thomas A. The royal free interview for spiritual and religious beliefs: development and validation of a self-report version. Psychol Med 2001;31:1015–1023.

57. Peterman A, Fitchett, G, Brady MJ, Hernandez L, Cella D. Measuring spiritual well-being in people with cancer: The Functional Assessment of Chronic Illness Therapy-Spiritual Well-Being Scale (FACIT-Sp). Ann Behav Med 2002;24(1):49–58.

58. Fetzer Institute. Multidimensional measurement of religiousness/spirituality for use in health research: A report of the Fetzer Institute/National Institute on Aging Working Group. Kalamazoo, MI: Fetzer, 1999.

59. Power J. Spiritual assessment: Developing an assessment tool. Nurs Older People 2006;18(2):16–18.

60. LeFavi RG, Wessels MH. Life review in pastoral care counseling: Background and efficacy for the terminally Ill. J Pastoral Care Council 2003;57:281–292.

61. Pronk K. Role of the doctor in relieving spiritual distress at the end of life. Am J Hospice Palliat Med 2005;22:419–425.

62. O'Connor TS, O'Niell K, Van Staalduinen G, Meakes E, Penner C, Davis K. Not well known, used little and needed: Canadian chaplains' experiences of published spiritual assessment tools. J Pastoral Care Counsel 2005;59(1–2):97–107.

63. Taylor EJ. Nurses caring for the spirit: Patients with cancer and family caregiver expectations. Oncol Nurs Forum 2003;30:585–590.

64. Rumbold BD. A review of spiritual assessment in health care practice. Med J Austr 2007;186(10):S60–S62.

65. Taylor EJ. What do I say? Talking with patients about spirituality. Philadelphia, PA: Templeton Press, 2007.

66. Taylor, EJ, Mamier I. Spiritual Care Nursing: What Cancer Patients and Family Caregivers Want. J Adv Nurs 2005;49(3):260–267.

67. Kvale K. Do cancer patients always want to talk about difficult emotions? A qualitative study of cancer inpatients communication needs. Eur J Oncol Nurs 2007;11(4):320–327.

68. Taylor EJ. Client perspectives about nurse requisites for spiritual caregiving. App Nurs Res 2007;20(1):44–46.

69. Ellis MR, Campbell JD. Patients' views about discussing spiritual issues with primary care physicians. South Med J 2004;97:1158–1164.

70. Carson VB. Spirituality: Identifying and meeting spiritual needs. In: Carson VB, Koenig HG, eds. Spiritual dimensions of nursing practice (rev ed). West Conshohocken, PA: Templeton Foundation Press, 2008.

71. Timmins F, Kelly J. Spiritual assessment in intensive and cardiac care nursing. Nurs Crit Care 2008;13(3):124–131.

72. Telos N. Proactive: Spiritual care for terminal restlessness. Palliat Support Care 2005;3:245–246.

73. Hart D, Schneider D. Spiritual care for children with cancer. Semin Oncol Nurs 1997;13:263–270.

74. Sexson SB. Religious and spiritual assessment of the child and adolescent. Child Adolesc Psychiatr Clin N Am 2004;13:35–47.

75. Heilferty CM. Spiritual development and the dying child: The pediatric nurse practitioner's role. J Pediatr Health Care 2004;18:271–275.

76. Barnes LP, Plotnikoff GA, Fox K, Pendleton S. Spirituality, religion, and pediatrics: Intersecting worlds of healing. Pediatrics 2000;104:899–908.

# 34 ❧❧❧ *Rev. Pamela Baird*

# Spiritual Care Interventions

- ◆ *Key Points*
- ◆ *Recognizing and addressing patients' spiritual needs is fundamental to palliative care.*
- ◆ *Spiritual care addresses issues of religion, existential suffering and humanity.*
- ◆ *Nurses provide spiritual care through deep listening, presence, bearing witness and compassion.*

Spiritual care is, perhaps, the most mysterious and often misunderstood part of palliative care. There is much discussion about what constitutes good spiritual care, and to date there is no agreed upon definition of terms. The misunderstanding is caused, in part, by this lack of agreement. It is important to establish clear definitions to demystify spiritual care. For the purposes of this chapter the terms are defined as follows:

- *Spirituality:* Our relationship with ourselves, others, nature, and the transcendent.[1]
- *Religion:* An organization that has a set of rites, rules, practices, values, and beliefs that prescribe how individuals should live their lives and respond to God.[2]
- *Spiritual Care:* Allowing our humanity to touch another's by providing presence, deep listening, and compassion.[3]
- *Compassion:* The ability to be empathetically present to another while he or she is suffering and is trying to find meaning.[4,5]
- *Existential:* Relating to human existence and experience.[6]

Although the literature is trending toward defining them separately, some use the terms "spiritual" and "religious" interchangeably, implying they are the same. It is sometimes assumed that spiritual care is only about a person's religious traditions and beliefs. Using the definitions above, not everyone would describe him- or herself as religious, but everyone is spiritual.[7] In fact, these definitions can determine the care given to patients. If a person does not identify as "religious" and the spiritual care offered is only about religious issues, then the person is denied this care, which could, in fact, provide compassion, peace, and comfort in the midst of the fear, pain, and chaos of illness. There is much spiritual care that can be given to support a person's relationship with him- or herself, others, nature, and the transcendent even when religion is not a factor.

*A 45-Year-Old Man Dying of Colon Cancer*

A 45-year-old man and hospice patient was dying alone in his apartment after he had alienated his ex-wife and three grown children. His entire adult life had been consumed by alcohol and gambling. Although he was receiving care from the hospice team, he had refused a chaplain because he said he was an atheist and did not want or need one. He had agreed to check into a skilled nursing facility with hospice care when he could no longer take care of himself at home. The day came. It was a day of many deaths and emergencies, and the hospice agency and the patient's nurse, social worker, and home health aide were all otherwise unavailable. The chaplain was sent to the patient's home to prepare him, to gather his things, and to wait for the ambulance to arrive for transport. She sat with him, at home, for a couple of hours—listening, talking. When he was moved to the nursing home, she followed and made sure that he was introduced to the facility and the staff and that he felt as comfortable as possible in his new surroundings. When he was finally settled, the chaplain told him she was going to leave. That is when he asked, "What is it you do again?" She told him, "I'm the chaplain." He replied, "I'm an atheist. I don't believe in God." The chaplain said to him, "It doesn't matter to me if you believe in God or not. That's not why I'm here. I'm here to offer support." He took her hand, looked into her eyes and said, "You've done that." He died the next day.

## What is Spiritual Care?

Spiritual care is simply meeting the other person, human to human, providing compassionate presence, and being available for whatever comes up. In the aforementioned case study, not only was it unnecessary to talk about God, or seemingly spiritual or religious things, it would have been inappropriate and perhaps harmful to this patient, risking further alienation from yet another person. The spiritual interchange took place just by being with the person, understanding where he was—emotionally and spiritually—and taking care of what was important to him.[8]

At other times, with other people, spiritual care might include saying prayers, reading from Holy Texts, or talking about God and the mysteries of the universe. It is not for us to decide what the spiritual care looks like. On some level, what we do to provide spiritual care is less important than *who* we bring to the room. Good spiritual care requires that the person who walks into the room put aside his/her own expectations and agenda and, instead, focus on the patient—doing whatever is needed, at the time, for the person receiving the care.

| Table 34–1 |
|---|
| **The Essential Elements of Spiritual Care** |
| **Spiritual care encompasses:** |
| • Authenticity |
| • Kindness |
| • Compassion |
| • Respect |
| • Dignity |
| • Humanity |
| • Vulnerability |
| • Service |
| • Honesty |
| • Empathy |

At its core, spiritual care is about being honest, being authentically human, and allowing our own humanity to touch the humanity of another[9] (Table 34–1). In the course of offering spiritual care, God and religious beliefs and ideas may emerge, but they do not have to. Religion is one way, one very important and significant way, that we express our spirituality. But religion is not a prerequisite. Spirituality can be expressed in a million ways: sitting quietly by the side of the road, taking food to a friend, watching a toddler learn to walk, working in the garden, praying, or crying with a man whose wife just died.

Rachel Naomi Remen speaks to the essence of spiritual care when she writes about the difference between "helping" and "serving." When we "help" someone, we assume they are broken and need fixing—they are weak, we are stronger, and we have the answers. But when we go to the bedside not to help or fix, but to serve, we allow our humanness, our wholeness, our brokenness, our compassion, and our vulnerability to be present and forefront. When we "help" or "fix" patients, they are in our debt. Service requires no payment. Service is mutually beneficial. When we serve, we create a space where healing can occur, both for the served and the server.[10]

## "I'm only the nurse. What do I know about providing spiritual care?"

Spiritual care is in the purview of everyone: the medical staff, the palliative care team, and the patient's family and friends.[11] Given the mystery and misunderstanding surrounding spiritual care, it is understandable that many people feel unqualified and uncomfortable to provide spiritual interventions. Many feel that because they, themselves, are not religious, they could not possibly be of spiritual support to anyone. Others, although defining themselves as religious, do not feel comfortable to pray out loud or with someone else, or they think they do not know the Bible or the Quran, or any of the holy books, well enough. Here again, the religious

**Table 34–2**
**Questions Requiring Chaplain Referral**

- What have I done to deserve this?
- I pray but I'm still sick.
- I used to believe in God, but now I'm not so sure.
- How will my family get along without me?
- What did my life mean?
- I'm scared.

**Table 34–3**
**Spiritual Interventions**

- Compassionate presence and listening deeply
- Bearing witness
- Compassion at work

interventions are only a part of spiritual care, and they are often best handled by the chaplain or professional spiritual caregiver. If patients are asking questions about God, expressing concerns, or ruminating over existential issues, then an appropriate intervention would be to make a referral to the chaplain (Table 34–2).[12] Chaplains are trained to address spiritual and existential concerns, both the religious and non-religious. However, a chaplain referral is not the only spiritual intervention that can, or should, be made.

Because nurses are at the bedside 24/7 and, generally, are the medical professionals who spend the most time with patients and their families, it is important for nurses to know how to provide spiritual care and to do it well. It does not require a special degree, but it does take awareness of oneself, and the other, and it takes effort and a strong commitment. As stated earlier, at its core spiritual care is about being human and allowing our humanity to touch the humanity of another. Our humanity is expressed, in part, by providing presence, deep listening, bearing witness, and putting our compassion into action.[13] This is the foundation of spiritual care (Table 34–3).[14]

## Compassionate Presence and Deep Listening

It is not possible for the medical community to promise that a patient will never experience pain or suffering or to guarantee a calm and peaceful death. But it is possible to promise to accompany the patient for the journey. This does not mean that an individual nurse should promise to always be at the patient's side, but it does mean the medical team can assure the patient it will do everything possible to alleviate pain and suffering and that the patient and family will not be abandoned.[15]

Being present has been described by Gardner in two ways: "physical and psychological, 'being there' and 'being with.'"[16] Physical presence refers to being in touchable proximity to another. Psychological presence entails work and effort on the part of the caregiver. Kindness, deep listening, and empathy are required for psychological or compassionate presence.[17]

Providing compassionate presence is more than just showing up or walking into a room. There is a quality to the presence that gives the message, "There is no where else I would rather be at this moment than here with you." It is not just about being physically in the room with another, but being present in that room—body, mind, and spirit. It is about "exhibiting empathy and focused attention."[18–21] Presence does not take any more time than just showing up, but it does take a lot more effort, energy, and intention, and it makes an enormous difference to the person who is the recipient. A nurse can go into a patient's room, walk directly to the IV pole, hang the medication, turn, and walk out. Or, that same nurse can go into the patient's room, walk over to the patient, make eye contact, smile, gently touch the patient's hand, walk to the IV pole, hang the medication, look directly into the patient's eyes once again, smile, turn, and walk out the door.

Human beings have a need to be seen and heard. "When dying patients are seen, and know that they are seen, as being worthy of honour and esteem by those who care for them, dignity is more likely to be maintained."[22] Spiritual care is about preserving dignity and truly seeing the other person. It is also about hearing the spirit of the message. It is not enough just to see the body or to hear the words. Spiritual care is about connecting to the heart and mind and soul because that connection says, "I see you. I hear your concerns. You matter. You are important. You are not alone. I care."

A woman and her family were going though hard times. There were children to feed, a mortgage, and all the usual expenses that go along with supporting a family of six. The woman and her husband owned a business that had been floundering for 4 years, and they were close to losing everything. They had $2.48 in the bank, creditors calling, and no guarantee of when the next money would arrive. The woman was in her minister's office, embarrassed, telling her story, crying, and feeling terrified by life. As she was pouring her heart out, someone walked by the minister's door, caught the attention of the cleric, and the pastor immediately stood up and waved and said, "Oh, hello!" and began talking to the passerby. The woman never again shared anything of importance or consequence with her minister.

To deeply listen means hearing what is being said and what is not being said and trying to understand the emotions and feelings behind the words. It means to "tune in" to another person so that we understand who that person really is on a deep, authentic level.[23] Listening deeply also requires the ability to hold the pain and suffering of another. When someone trusts us enough to be vulnerable in our presence and then goes even further, explaining the circumstances of the pain and suffering, he/she has offered us a gift. It is our responsibility to embrace and protect that gift and treat it with the utmost respect, care, and deference.

The minister dismissed the woman's pain and trivialized her suffering by allowing herself to be distracted when being present was so crucial. It could have been a time of healing. Although the minister could not change the woman's circumstances, she had the opportunity to be truly present, thereby offering a human connection to the woman who was in such despair. The minister missed the moment and ensured that she would never again be given the chance to connect with her parishioner in such an intimate way.

Talking, listening, and telling our stories are all part of the human experience. In a study conducted by Mako, Galek, and Poppito to investigate spiritual pain, they found that patients were more likely to request someone to sit and talk and be with them than they were to ask for religious interventions. "Patients asked that the chaplain 'stay with me as long as possible,' and 'stop by every now and then and talk to me.'"[24] Listening deeply and being "psychologically" or compassionately present are spiritual interventions that anyone can learn. But it takes time, practice, effort, willingness, and intention to be truly available to another human being. For many receiving palliative care, they have been told that there is no cure for them. A cure may not be possible, but the opportunity for healing is. Healthcare professionals can be the conduit to healing simply by being present and listening deeply.

## Bearing Witness

The term "bearing witness" may seem a foreign concept to some, but it is integral to spiritual care and a part of our experience as human beings. A friend is diagnosed with cancer, a coworker dies, an airplane crashes. These sad, life-changing events, and those that are happy and joyous as well, generally stimulate a response. That response is to tell the story of what happened. We feel the need to share our experiences, and we feel compelled to hear other people's stories. To bear witness is to be present to the events and the emotions of another's life and experience. We find strength and comfort in knowing that other human beings bear witness to the significant events of our lives—the good and the bad.

It may seem that bearing witness is a passive event, such as just watching and observing. But, indeed, beneficially bearing witness takes focus and intention just like compassionate presence and deep listening. Bearing witness is not "fixing," "helping," or imparting answers or platitudes. Platitudes are seldom healing and "answers" can function to alienate the one we seek to serve. People seek medical attention looking for answers. There are some things in medicine that have definitive answers and some that do not. In the spiritual/existential realm there are very few, if any, absolutes. Two people asking the question, "Why did I get sick?" will most likely have two different answers, if they can find answers at all. Our spiritual/existential answers are our own, revealed

to us through years of living life through our own lens and experience. Nurses and healthcare providers might find it a relief to know that they do not have to have the answers to patients' spiritual questions. Furthermore, offering an answer to another's spiritual questions, or providing meaning, is not in the purview of healthcare professionals and generally is not helpful or beneficial.[25] We cannot know the answers to others' questions, so to assume we do and to assert those "answers" might be harmful to the patient or, at the very least, stop them from their own process of finding meaning.

So what does it really mean to bear witness? Bearing witness means compassionate presence, deep listening, watching, observing—being with. "Your job is to offer not only compassion but also to accompany as best as you can those dying on their journey."[26] Bearing witness means to compassionately accompany another.

Like presence and listening, bearing witness does not mean taking away the person's pain or suffering. Bearing witness means being present to the pain and suffering. In fact, if our primary goal is to take away the suffering, then that itself can interfere with our ability to be present in the moment.[27] Bearing witness is the ability to sit in the midst of whatever is happening. We often betray our own discomfort while listening to the stories of patients' suffering when we jump up to get a tissue for their tears. We tell ourselves that the tissue is for the one who is crying, to make him/her more comfortable, when in fact it can say more about our own desire to step back and move away from the pain. The message we risk sending is, "Stop crying. I don't want to hear anymore. I need you to stop crying now."

When someone is sharing an intense story, if we are truly present in the moment, then we can find ourselves almost not breathing, listening to, or attending to the other. When we move, we break the moment and it can stop the process, the story, and the tears. Something as simple as reaching over and touching a person while he/she is telling the emotion-filled story can stop the flow and interrupt the process. When these interruptions occur, there is a good chance that the story, which was so important to tell, might never again find the opportunity to be told. It takes time, experience, and thoughtful awareness to learn when to speak, or move, or get tissues.

Bearing witness means being comfortable enough in our own pain and suffering that we can just sit quietly, be with another human being who is suffering, and not run. It also means being aware of our own grief and being in touch with that grief so that it does not spill over and leak out onto the patients and families we serve.

CASE STUDY

*A 65-Year-Old Female Patient Dying in the Hospital From Breast Cancer*

A chaplain was asked to see Mrs. F because the hospital staff said she would probably be dying in the next few weeks and she had not, to anyone's knowledge, talked with her grown daughter about her impending death. The chaplain was warned that Mrs. F, avoided talking about her prognosis and would probably be "resistant." The chaplain later reported that she, herself, was struggling with some personal grief issues and found herself unusually anxious about going to see this patient. The chaplain made her way into the patient's room, introduced herself, and felt her own anxiety level soar. There was not much of a conversation, as there was not room for the patient to "comply," or be "resistant," because the chaplain's own anxiety caused her to talk faster and faster, fearful the patient's grief would touch her own. The patient was polite and pleasant and, not surprisingly, did not want to talk at all, about anything. The chaplain's grief filled the room. Because she had not dealt with her own grief before she saw the patient, not only was she unable to serve Mrs. F, but the chaplain may have done harm in allowing her own grief to be such a strong presence in the room.

It is not easy for caregivers to manage both their own grief and the grief of their patients. But to ensure that professional caregivers are providing the best care for their patients and are caring for themselves as well, it is incumbent upon them to be aware of, work with, and reconcile their own grief.[28] This will be addressed more fully later in the chapter.

## Compassion at Work

Being present, listening deeply, and bearing witness require a commitment from the one who serves. After these interventions, the next step in providing good spiritual care is action based on compassion. Is there anything missing? Is there something more to be done? Deep listening can reveal a patient's hopes, desires, and longing. Sometimes what is needed is very simple but it can make a huge difference in the quality of the patient's life.

For many, healthcare professionals and laypersons alike, being unsure of what to say can cause discomfort at the thought of spending any quality time with one who is dying. Empathy is vital to spiritual care. The capacity to put ourselves in the place of another is paramount. We can never know what another person is really feeling, but we can, in our own mind, imagine what it might be like for us to be in the patient's situation. "How would I feel if I was the one who was dying?" "What would I want?" "What would I want someone to say...or not say?" "What would feel supportive?"

To ask ourselves these kinds of questions is the first step in being attuned to the other person's suffering and pain. Although we can only guess what a patient might or might not want to talk about, we can ask some open-ended, leading questions that will give the patient the opportunity to express his/her feelings if he/she chooses. If we ask a question or two and the patient seems reticent or reluctant to talk, then we can assume that either this is not a good time or it is not something he/she wants to talk about with us. It does not

mean we never ask another question but that we take our cues from the patient, listening carefully for a time when he/she might be open and willing to talk.

We often hear "Mrs. White just does not want to talk about it." This may or may not be true. When we are experiencing pain and suffering, it is not uncommon for us to be very particular with whom we share our feelings and innermost thoughts. We want to make sure that the person we tell will have some understanding of what we are going through and will respect our feelings and care for them. So, although Mrs. White "does not want to talk about it" with just anyone, she might be willing, even eager, to talk if the right person walked into her room—a person who would listen deeply, be present, and bear witness to her deepest fears and concerns. This would likely also be a person who would know when to honor the silence and say nothing and then would know what to say at the appropriate time.

How do we know what to say? This is something we can learn with time and experience. It is vital to be observant when we are with other people, listening to what they say, when they say it, and how the message is delivered. Watching to see what "works" and what "does not" can be a wonderful way for us to learn how to listen and communicate effectively, especially in sensitive circumstances. To learn this skill requires that we be acutely aware—aware of our own responses and the responses, verbally and non-verbally, of the ones we are observing.

It is almost always appropriate to ask a person to tell us more about the story. "How did you feel when that happened?" "What happened next?" "Tell me more about that." There are times when we are so touched or overwhelmed by a story that we honestly do not know what to say. It is an authentic response and it is not inappropriate to say, "I have no idea what to say at this moment." Because it is genuine and honest, people usually respond well to a statement that bears such candor. It is certainly preferable to making a casual remark that runs the risk of trivializing the person's feelings or the situation.

Even when a person is open and wants to talk about his/her experience and feelings, it can be difficult to know just how far to take the conversation. What questions are appropriate to ask? Questions that inquire about a person's feelings or experience are generally welcomed (Table 34–4). If a

---

**Table 34–4**
**Spiritual Care Questions**

Are you scared?
What makes life worth living?
Is there anything you haven't done that you need to do?
What do you hope for?
What are you most afraid of?
Is there anything worse than death?
What are you most proud of in your life?
Do you have regrets?

question is asked that a patient does not want to talk about, then he/she usually finds a way to "talk around" the question without actually giving an answer. Listening carefully to what is "not" said is crucial. It can tell us that he/she, at this moment, does not want to go there.

Sometimes talking and listening are not enough. What a patient has to say may reveal that he or she needs more: a chaplain referral, a phone call to a family member, prayer, a walk in the garden, or a feeling of urgency to leave the hospital and go home. Just as advocating for patients is a standard component of nursing care, it is also a vital element of spiritual care and is a spiritual care intervention.

CASE STUDY

*A 75-Year-Old Woman, Living With Her Husband, Dying at Home, on Hospice*

Whenever the chaplain visited, the patient's husband took center stage and monopolized the conversation. He did not seem to be able to hear his wife's concerns when she talked about feeling weaker and getting worse. He would respond with, "Just keep praying, dear. God answers prayer." One day in October, the nurse called the chaplain to say, "We've got a problem. She's worse. She's crying but her husband just keeps telling her she'll be fine...just pray." The nurse suggested that when the chaplain arrived he would take the patient's husband into the kitchen and leave the patient and chaplain to talk. When the woman and the chaplain were finally alone, it was apparent the woman was weaker...and afraid. After a few minutes, the patient said she needed to see her daughters. It was very obvious how important this was to her. The chaplain knew the daughters, who lived 500 miles away, were planning to come for Thanksgiving. When the chaplain reminded the patient of her daughters' upcoming visit, the woman started to cry. "You're not going to be here at Thanksgiving are you?" the chaplain asked. And the woman shook her head "no." After clearing the plan with the patient, the chaplain called the husband back into the room and explained to him the conversation she and his wife had just had. She gently told him that what his wife needed most right now was for him to understand she didn't have much longer, and she needed him to call their daughters and explain how important it was for them to come immediately. It was difficult for the husband to hear—but he did—and he called their daughters that night. They arrived the next day. They were able to make several trips to be with their mother and father in the next 4 weeks. The woman died a week before Thanksgiving.

Presence, deep listening, and bearing witness were important and vital, but in this case more was needed. Sometimes just engaging in life review—telling the story of one's life—is what brings a sense of peace, and there is nothing more to be done. In other cases, it is not enough to just be with, be present, and listen. Sometimes, as with this patient, the situation calls for action, for doing something more.

Patients often give us specific information when we engage them in conversation, but it is not the only way we discover who patients are and what is important to them. Sometimes the clues are more subtle. They can be as simple as noticing a rosary on the bed or pictures of grandchildren on the wall. Sometimes just being aware of who visits the patient can provide insight about his/her spirituality. Noticing that a rabbi visited the patient can be a perfect entrée to asking about a person's spiritual/religious beliefs. "I noticed a rabbi came to see you this morning. It made me wonder if you're Jewish, and if you are, if there is anything we can do here in the hospital to support you in your faith?" It is important to ask and not just assume that because a rabbi was in the room that the person is Jewish. But it does give the healthcare provider a place to start in an effort to determine what kind of spiritual care, if any, the person may want or need.

One man had been hospitalized for the better part of a year, and it had been extremely difficult for him and his family. He was a bone marrow transplant patient, which meant he could not have plants or flowers in his room and could not go outside for much of that year he was in the hospital. Only after the "spiritual intervention" from his daughter did the staff discover that he was quite a gifted rose gardener. It was somewhat ironic because the hospital was known for its huge rose gardens. Unfortunately, not being allowed outside meant this patient was not able to enjoy them. However, his daughter had the idea of photographing the roses in his yard as well as some on the hospital grounds. She took beautiful, close-up pictures of individual roses in all stages of unfolding, had the prints enlarged, cut around each one of them, and taped those hundreds of roses all over the walls of his room. It was beautiful! It gave enjoyment to not only the patient and his family but to the medical staff as well. Moreover, it told something significant about the man and generated conversation with him, as a person, apart from his identity as a patient. It made him more than just another body in a bed, with no particular identity other than his diagnosis. He was the one in the hospital who loved to be outside and knew how to grow beautiful roses. It gave the staff another way to connect with him, besides just his illness.

A week before Christmas, the chaplain was paged back to the hospital shortly after leaving for the night. A 35-year-old patient was about a week away from dying and her mother and father, who were at her bedside, requested the chaplain come pray with them. The patient, who for medical reasons could no longer speak, was not particularly interested in a prayer, but she did want to sing Christmas carols. She couldn't make a sound to talk but was able to make a little noise when she tried to sing. The words were completely unintelligible, but some of the tune made itself known. The patient, her mother, and the chaplain sang for the better part of the evening, one carol after another, frequently joined by a nurse, phlebotomist, or other healthcare professionals as they entered the room to give care. Before leaving for the night, the chaplain rushed out to buy Christmas CDs, which the family played all night according to the parents' report the next day.

An elderly woman, dying at home with hospice care, told the hospice team that years before, she and her husband had raised English Setters. She spoke longingly about that time in their lives. The chaplain had a friend who had an English Setter. He and his dog, Sarah, were a part of the local hospital's pet team. Sarah was very comfortable being with people who were sick in bed. With the patient and her husband's consent, the chaplain made arrangements for Sarah to visit and lie beside the woman in her last days. The pleasure and the memories were apparent on the patient's face as she hugged and petted Sarah.

Some patients clearly verbalize what they need physically, mentally, emotionally, and spiritually and are eager to talk and share their feelings. Try as we might, others just do not express who they are, and what they need, quite so obviously. But when we do discover something that will provide comfort, or a way for a person to more fully express his/her spirituality, it is important to do whatever we can to make it available. The clues, and the outcomes, do not have to be dramatic. One patient told everyone who would listen about her favorite nurse. The reason the nurse was so special? Whenever she went into the room to provide care, she sang the patient a song. These signs are merely ways to start a conversation about what is meaningful in a person's life.

The nurse does not have to be the only one to provide spiritual interventions. The nurse may be the one to learn what is needed, but sometimes another member of the healthcare team might be better suited to make it happen. If a patient wants someone to come and pray, perhaps, the chaplain would be the best person to provide the intervention. If the patient's goal is to complete a will or advance directive, then maybe the social worker would be best to call. Sometimes it takes more than one person to help the patient achieve his/her goal. The nurse discovered that the patient did not want further medical treatment and really just wanted to go home to die. The nurse offered spiritual intervention when she advocated for the patient by informing the physician and the medical team, who made it possible for the patient to leave the hospital and go home.

Spiritual care means finding a way to make a connection, discovering any needs or desires that might improve quality of life, and then advocating and making arrangements for the fulfillment of those needs and desires. The job of a spiritual caregiver is always to be open (absent an agenda), listen, observe, and, when in doubt, ask questions. Assuming anything, without asking, leaves open the possibility that we will get it wrong. We never can be certain what is inside someone else's mind and heart. To ask is always best.[29]

## The Use of Rituals in Spiritual Care

Often when we think of rituals we speak of religious traditions that have been practiced and passed down for hundreds

or thousands of years. Some of the most obvious rituals are: Holy Communion; Anointing of the Sick; prayer; and Scripture reading, chanting, singing, or saying the rosary.

But rituals do not have to be religious in nature and can be created spontaneously, in the moment, to meaningfully acknowledge a person, event, or circumstance in our lives. Angeles Arrien stated, "Ritual is recognizing a life change, and doing something to honor and support the change."[30] We engage in non-religious, yet spiritual, rituals everyday when we bake a birthday cake for a friend and sing "Happy Birthday," read a bedtime story to our children each night, or even read the newspaper over a cup of coffee in the morning.

When patients are receiving palliative care they have often been sick for a long time and sometimes forget who they were before the illness began. Many times, the disease becomes the descriptor by which they identify themselves. For patients to avoid losing their identity to the disease, it can be especially helpful to maintain as much normalcy as possible, particularly when they have been confined to the hospital for long periods of time. Birthday cakes, bedtime stories, and reading the morning paper with a cup of coffee are simple rituals that can remind us of what we held dear before the onset of the disease.

In a cancer hospital where bone marrow transplants require patients to be hospitalized for weeks—even months—at a time, a group of patients created a ritual that served them well. Every evening after dinner they met in a lounge area and played cards. This ritual was the highlight of their hospital stay. They looked forward to an activity that under "normal" circumstances might seem ordinary and routine. But under these circumstances, this ritual afforded them the opportunity to not only get out of their rooms but allowed them to be with other people (people who had a good understanding of what they were going through) and to forget they had cancer for a while, to participate in an activity that felt "normal" again, to socially engage with other people... and the list goes on. The nursing staff was incredibly supportive, adjusting the schedules of what needed to be done so that these patients could be free in the evenings to participate in their nightly ritual.

Nurses can be invaluable in suggesting, and supporting, "rituals" for patients. When professional caregivers are aware of their patients as unique individuals with distinct wants, needs, and desires, then caregivers can offer meaningful suggestions for rituals that might be supportive to the patient's life and experience. Listening to music during unpleasant treatments might be soothing to a musician or a teenager who loves music. Getting a patient dressed early each morning, before breakfast, might be a practice that helps the person feel more able to take on the day. Sitting at the bedside to hear a patient's stories could be important to a young mother who wants to talk about the time she spent with her children who visited earlier in the day. The list of rituals is endless.

Although religious rituals are fewer in number, they can be equally important and beneficial. Caregivers cannot be expected to know all the religious rituals people practice, so it can be beneficial for the nurse, and others, to ask patients about any traditions or rituals that may be meaningful or important to them. Although the healthcare professional may not be involved with the rituals themselves, they can play a vital role in making sure the patient has some time alone, uninterrupted, so that the ritual will have the opportunity to be fully expressed and experienced. Rituals are a part of each of our lives. Nurses can be the conduit through which palliative care patients can find support and meaning by recognizing the importance of ritual and by facilitating their expression.

## Spiritual Care Near the Time of Death

As death draws near, it is even more important that professional caregivers attend to patients and their families with kindness, authenticity, and deep awareness. This awareness hears what is being said, and not said, and sees the visual signs of want, need, desire, and distress. Even those families who cannot begin to entertain the possibility of death are aware, on some level, that life is changing. So it is a great kindness to be especially insightful and responsive to their wants, needs, desires, feelings, and fears. Patients may not be able, or willing, to ask for what they want, but if nurses and other healthcare professionals are attentive and perceptive, clues are frequently obvious and reveal what is needed. When providing spiritual care for those who are imminently dying, the three most important things to remember are: don't wait; intently watch and listen; and trust your instincts.

A grandmother, who was in relatively good health until 3 weeks prior, fell and broke a hip, was bedridden at home on hospice, and declining rapidly. Some days she was alert and oriented; other days, she was wildly confused. This particular morning began with her mind and memory cloudy. While sleeping, her breathing pattern changed and it caught the attention of her granddaughter. The elderly woman was being cared for around the clock by her three daughters and a granddaughter who also worked as a hospice chaplain. Becoming aware of the subtle changes, the granddaughter instinctively felt they should call the rest of the family to the bedside. They did just that, and within a couple of hours there were dozens of grandchildren, great-grandchildren, family members, and friends assembled in the old woman's tiny house. When the family began to arrive the grandmother perked up and became much more alive and alert than she had been in weeks. This woman, who loved her family deeply but was never one to hug or kiss or show affection of any kind—and certainly had never been described as having a sense of humor—blossomed and came to life in front of her family. She was affectionate, chatty, warm, and funny, and her family saw a side of her no one there had witnessed, ever, in the grandmother's 90 years. The day was filled with stories and great humor. She lived another 10 days. They were quiet days, and she was withdrawn and frequently confused. Although

the family never again experienced the joy, affection, and laughter of that Friday, the family continues to describe it as the best time they ever had with her, and they are exceedingly grateful for the gift. Had the granddaughter ignored the almost imperceptible signs of decline and neglected to call in the family, who knows if they would have ever had another opportunity to experience their loved one in such a significant way?

It is easy to doubt and question ourselves, or dismiss signs and clues that are often barely visible and unclear. Good spiritual care, especially for the dying, requires caregivers to hone their skills in assessing these subtleties. Don't wait; intently watch and listen; and trust your instincts. To not do these things risks missing the moment and the opportunity that, literally, might never come again for the one who is dying.

## Healthcare Professional Grief and Well-Being

Everyday, healthcare professionals deal with their patients' grief, but that does not make the caregivers immune to their own. The death of a loved one or friend is not the only kind of grief we experience. All people who are alive and aware experience grief, whether or not they have ever known someone who has died. When someone is disrespectful and rude to us, when we do not get the job we want, or when we are transferred to another part of the country, we experience grief. Grief can be the belief that we are not enough or that we failed, or the realization that life is changing and our hopes and dreams will never be realized.[31] When a loved one dies or when we experience extreme disappointment and loss, the grief never completely goes away, but with time and effort, it is possible to come to terms with the loss, establish a new relationship with the deceased, or circumstance, and move on.[28]

Although time does have its own way of easing suffering, it is not the only thing required to heal our grief. Grief is not an event. Grief is not linear. It is a process and it takes not only time, but effort, energy, work, and intention. It is most often a sequence of "two steps forward, one step back." Individual grief therapy or grief support groups can be useful tools in teaching us how to deal with our grief.

It is also important for us to be patient and mercy for ourselves.[32] There is no set time frame for grief. It takes as long as it takes. One man's wife died and he felt it took about 3 years to reconcile the loss. Another woman died and her husband did not feel like he had moved forward at all, even after 5 years.

Many hospices, which have served to educate our society on the importance of the grief process, give their employees only 3 days paid bereavement—and then only for very immediate family members. Very often the person has not been buried, or a service conducted, in those 3 days, and the shock of the death can delay active grieving for some time. Three days is not enough time to face the world after a painful loss and then be expected to act as though everything is just fine. Just being familiar with death and grief does not guarantee understanding, or ease, in dealing with the process. Healthcare professionals can have just as much difficulty as their patients—maybe more—given the frequency with which they come face to face with dying, death, and grief. It can be difficult to care for someone who is grieving when the caregiver is in the midst of his/her own grief journey. A caregiver's grief can be triggered just by being in the presence of a patient who is also grieving. It is sometimes challenging for a busy caregiver to distinguish between the patient's grief and his/her own. For the well-being of all concerned, it is essential for healthcare professionals to be aware of and deal with their own grief and loss. Nurses and others are better able to serve when they have acknowledged their own pain and have made the effort to work through their own grief process.[31]

## Nurses Providing Spiritual Care

Deep listening, presence, bearing witness, and compassion at work are all simple ideas. Although simple, these interventions are not easy. To provide these interventions in a way that invites healing requires, from the caregiver, a willingness to learn, the ability to be without agenda, and the commitment to be ever vigilant and self-introspective. Nurses, who are called upon to provide these interventions, are at the forefront of patient care. They are asked, everyday, to deal with the medical, emotional, social, and spiritual crises and burdens of others' lives. They are expected to ease suffering whenever, and wherever, possible. At best, nursing is difficult work. We seem to be asking almost superhuman acts from nurses, who want deeply to provide all that is asked of them. Fortunately, quality spiritual care does not require superhuman acts. It does require human kindness, compassion, and caring.

REFERENCES

1. Halifax J. Project on Being with Dying Training for Health Care Professionals. Santa Fe, New Mexico, 2001.
2. Thoresen EC. Spirituality and health: Is there a relationship? J Health Psychol 1999;4(3):409–431.
3. Bryson KA. Spirituality, meaning, and transcendence. J Palliat Support Care 2004;2:321–328.
4. Bryson KA. Spirituality, meaning, and transcendence. J Palliat Support Care 2004;2:321–328.
5. Post SG. Unlimited love: Altruism, compassion and service. Philadelphia, PA: Templeton Foundation Press: 2003.
6. www.macmillandictionary.com/dictionary/american/existential (accessed October 6, 2009).
7. Wright MC. The essence of spiritual care: A phenomenological enquiry. J Palliat Med 2002;16:125–132.
8. Chochinov HM, Cann BJ. Interventions to enhance the spiritual aspects of dying. J Palliat Med 2005;8(S-1):S-103–S-115.
9. Bryson KA. Spirituality, meaning, and transcendence. J Palliat Support Care 2004;2:321–328.
10. Remen RN. In the service of life. Noetic Sciences Review, Spring 1996;37:24–25.
11. Hanson LC, Dobbs D, Usher BM, Williams S, Rawlings J, Daaleman TP. Providers and types of spiritual care during serious illness. J Palliat Med 2008;11(6):907–914.
12. Strang S, Strang P. Questions posed to hospital chaplains by palliative care patients. J Palliat Med 2002;5(6):857–864.
13. Halifax J. Project on Being with Dying Training for Health Care Professionals. Santa Fe, New Mexico, 2001.
14. Halifax J. Project on Being with Dying Training for Health Care Professionals. Santa Fe, New Mexico, 2001.
15. Byock I. The meaning and value of death. J Palliat Med 2002;5(2):279–288.
16. Gardner D. Presence. In: Bulechek G, McCloskey J, eds. Nursing Interventions: Treatments for Nursing Diagnosis. Philadelphia, PA: Saunders; 1985:316–324.
17. Neff KD. Self-compassion: An alternative conceptualization of a healthy attitude toward oneself. Self Identity 2003;2:85–102.
18. McDonough-Means S, Kreitzer MJ, Bell I. Fostering a healing presence and investigating its mediators. J Altern Complement Med 2004;10(S1):S-25–S-41.
19. Christensen JF, Levinson W, Colligan JL, Dunn PM, Jones SR, Morgenstern A. A one-day communication workshop for internal medicine residents. J Med Educ 1987;62:687–690.
20. Frankel RM. Emotion and the physician–patient relationship. Motiv Emotion 1995;19:163–173.
21. Fossum B, Arborelius E, Theorell T. How do patients experience consultations at an orthopedic out-patient clinic? Eur J Public Health 1998;8:59–65.
22. Chochinov HM, Cann BJ. Interventions to enhance the spiritual aspects of dying. J Palliat Med 2005;8(S-1):S-103–S-115.
23. Slater V. What does "spiritual care" now mean to palliative care? Eur J Palliat Care 2007;14(1):32–34.
24. Mako C, Galek K, Poppito SR. Spiritual pain among patients with advanced cancer in palliative care. J Palliat Med 2006;9(5)1106–1113.
25. Sulmasy DP. Spiritual issues in the care of dying patients: "…it is okay between me and god." JAMA 2006;296(11):1385–1392.
26. Halifax J. personal communication December 12, 2008.
27. Millspaugh D. Assessment and response to spiritual pain: Part II. J Palliat Med 2005;8(6):1110–1117.
28. Klaus D, Silverman PR, Nickman SL. Continuing Bonds: New Understandings of Grief. Philadelphia, PA: Taylor & Francis, 1996.
29. Pronk K. Role of the doctor in relieving spiritual distress at the end of life. Am J Hosp Palliat Med 2005;22(6):419–425.
30. Arrien A. The Four-fold Way. San Francisco, CA: Harper San Francisco, 1993.
31. Levine S, Levine O. The grief process. Boulder, CO: Sounds True: 1999.
32. Levine S, Levine O. The grief process. Boulder, CO: Sounds True: 1999.

# 35

*Tami Borneman and Katherine Brown-Saltzman*

# Meaning in Illness

*But there is something about cancer that helps people to change. It gives momentum for transformation—Cancer patient*

*…Um I thought I was doing fine on [meds] otherwise until this happened but then I don't know what to expect. What do I, run around laughing? I mean that's what I asked my husband one night, I says is it supposed to show that you have a good attitude, are you supposed to walk around with a big smile on your face and say 'Oh gee, I've been diagnosed with cancer but that's okay.' You know and I wonder sometimes am I gonna go cuckoo about this or what?—Cancer patient*

*In the driest whitest stretch*
*Of pain's infinite desert*
*I lost my sanity*
*And found this rose*
*—Galal al-Din Rumi; Persia, 1207–1273*

♦ **Key Points**
♦ *Finding meaning in illness is an important issue when facing the end of life.*
♦ *The process of finding meaning in illness involves a journey through sometimes very difficult transitions.*
♦ *A terminal illness can greatly impact the patient–caregiver relationship.*
♦ *It is essential for nurses to experience their own journey regarding the dying process and bring with them a willingness to be transformed by it.*

Is it possible to adequately articulate and give definition to meaning in illness? Or is meaning in illness better described and understood through using symbolism and metaphors such as the above poem? To try to define that which is enigmatic and bordering on the ineffable seems almost sacrilegious. The unique individual journey of finding meaning in illness experienced by each patient facing the end of life and their family caregiver would seem to be diminished by the very process that seeks to understand through the use of language.

Is it that we seek to find meaning in illness or is it that we seek to find meaning in the life that is now left and in those relationships and things we value? Do we seek to find meaning in illness itself as an isolated event or that which is beyond the illness, such as how to live out this newly imposed way of life? Terminal illness often forces us to reappraise the meaning and purpose of our life. If we allow space in our lives for the process of meaning in illness to unfold, we then move from the superficial to the profound.

Terminal illness also forces us at some point to look directly at death, yet we resist getting in touch with the feelings that arise. Everything in us seeks life. Everything in us hopes for life. Everything in us denies death. There is something very cold, very unmoving, and very disturbing about it all. Does the end of one's human existence on Earth need to be the sole metaphor for death?

Although end-of-life issues have progressed nearer to the forefront of health care, the dying patient is still the recipient of an impersonal, detached, and cure-focused system, thereby exacerbating an already catastrophic situation. As necessary as it is for nurses to use the nursing process, it is not enough. The patient's illness odyssey beckons us to go beyond assessment, diagnosis, intervention, and evaluation to a place of vulnerability, not in an unprofessional manner but, rather, in a way that allows for a shared connectedness unique to each patient–nurse relationship. We need to be willing to use feelings appropriately as part of the therapeutic process. Separating ourselves from touching and feeling to protect ourselves only serves to make us more vulnerable, because we have then placed our emotions in isolation. Nurses can be a catalyst for helping the patient and family find meaning in the illness and, in the process, can help themselves define or redefine their own meaning in life, illness, and death.

## Meaning Defined

Johnston-Taylor[1] presents several definitions for meaning (Table 35–1). In the dictionary,[2] one finds meaning defined simply as "something that is conveyed or signified" or as "an interpreted goal, intent, or end." But it is the etymology of the word "mean" that helps nursing come to understand our potential for supporting patients in the process of finding

**Table 35–1**
**Definitions of Meaning**

| | |
|---|---|
| Meaning | "refers to sense, or coherence....A search for meaning implies a search for coherence. 'Purpose' refers to intention, aim, function....however, 'purpose' of life and 'meaning' of life are used interchangeably"[37] |
| | "a structure which relates purposes to expectations so as to organise actions....Meaning...makes sense of actions by providing reasons for it"[39] |
| [Search for] meaning | "is an effort to understand the event: why it happened and what impact it has had...[and] attempts to answer the question(s), What is the significance of the event?...What caused the event to happen?...[and] What does my life mean now?"[40] |
| | "is an attempt to restore the sense that one's life orderly and purposeful"[41] |
| Personal search for meaning | "the process by which a person seeks to interpret a life circumstance. The search involves questioning the personal significance of a life circumstance, in order to give the experience purpose and to place it in the context of a person's total life pattern. The basis of the process is the interaction between meaning in and of life and involves the reworking and redefining of past meaning while looking for meaning in a current life curcumstance."[42] |

meaning in their lives, even as they face death. Mean comes from the Old English *maenan*, "to tell of." One does not find meaning in a vacuum; it has everything to do with relationships, spirituality, and connectedness. While the process of finding meaning depends greatly on an inward journey, it also relies on the telling of that journey. The telling may use language, but it may also be conveyed by the eyes, through the hands, or just in the way the body is held. Frankl[3] reminds us that the "will to meaning" is a basic drive for all of humanity and is unique to each individual. A life-threatening illness begs the question of meaning with a new urgency and necessity.

Cassell[4] tells us that "all events are assigned meaning," which entails judging their significance and value. Meaning cannot be separated from the person's past; it requires the thought of future and ultimately influences perception of that future (p. 67). Finding meaning is not a stagnant process; it changes as each day unfolds and the occurrences are interpreted. As one patient reflected upon his diagnosis, "Even though I have this I am still a whole person my thoughts are different, my ambitions are a little different because I want to spend as much time as I can with my grandkids."[5] Coming face to face with one's mortality not only defines what is important but also the poignancy of the loss of much that has been meaningful.

One's spirituality is often the key to transcending those losses and finding ways to maintain those connections, whether it is the belief that one's love, work, or creativity will remain after the physical separation or the belief that one's spirit goes on to an afterlife or through reincarnation. Meaning in life concerns the individual's realm of life on Earth. It has to do with one's humanness, the temporal, and the composites of what one has done in life to give it meaning. Meaning of life has more to do with the existential. It is looking beyond one's earthly physical existence to an eternal, secure, and indelible God or spiritual plane. The existential realm of life provides a sense of security whereby one can integrate experiences.[6]

Spirituality has been defined as a search for meaning.[7,8] One of the Hebrew words for meaning is *biynah* (bee-naw), which is understanding, knowledge, meaning, and wisdom. It comes from the root word *biyn* (bene), which means to separate mentally or to distinguish.[9] How is it that one can come to knowledge and understanding? Patients receiving palliative care often describe a sense of isolation and loneliness. They frequently have endless hours available, while at the same time experiencing a shortening of their life. It is here that nursing has a pivotal role as the listener, for when the ruminations of the dying are given voice, there is an opportunity for meaning. Important life themes are shared, and the unanswerable questions are at least asked. As the stranger develops intimacy and trust, meaning takes hold.

Suffering creates one of the greatest challenges to uncovering meaning. For the dying patient, suffering comes in many packages: physical pain, unrelenting symptoms (nausea, pruritus, dyspnea, etc.), spiritual distress, dependency,

**Table 35–2**
**Summary of Hypotheses and Theses from the Literature on Meaning**

| Hypothesis/Thesis | Authors |
|---|---|
| The search for meaning is a basic human need. | Frankl 1959.[3] |
| Meaning is necessary for human fulfillment. | Steeves and Kahn 1987.[43] |
| Finding meaning fosters positive coping and increased hopefulness. | Ersek 1991;[44] Steeves and Kahn 1987;[43] Taylor 1983.[41] |
| One type of meaning-making activity in response to threatening events is to develop causal attributions. | Gotay 1983;[45] Haberman 1987;[46] Steeves and Kahn 1987;[43] Taylor 1983;[41] Chrisman and Haberman 1977.[47] |
| Meaning making can involve the search for a higher order. | Ersek 1991;[44] Ferrell et al. 1993;[48] Steeves and Kahn 1987.[43] |
| Making meaning often involves the use of social comparisons. | Ferrell et al. 1993;[48] Taylor 1983;[41] Ersek 1991;[44] Haberman 1987.[46] |
| Meaning can be derived through construing benefits from a negative experience. | Ersek 1991;[44] Haberman 1987;[46] Taylor 1983.[41] |
| Meaning sometimes focuses on illness as challenge, enemy, or punishment. | Barkwell 1991;[49] Ersek 1991;[44] Lipowski 1970.[50] |
| Pain and suffering often prompt a search for meaning. | Frankl 1959;[3] Steeves and Kahn 1987;[43] Taylor 1983.[41] |
| Uncontrolled pain or overwhelming suffering hinder the experience of meaning. | Steeves and Kahn 1987.[43] |
| One goal of care is to promote patients' and caregivers' search for and experiences of meaning. | Ersek 1991;[44] Ferrell et al. 1993;[48] Steeves and Kahn 1987;[43] Haberman 1988.[51] |

multiple losses, and anticipatory grieving. Even the benefits of medical treatments given to provide hope or palliation can sometimes be outweighed by side effects (e.g., sedation and constipation from pain medication), inducing yet further suffering. The dictionary defines suffering in this way: "To feel pain or distress; sustain loss, injury, harm, or punishment."[2] But once again, it is the root word that moves us to a more primitive understanding—the Latin sufferer, which comprises sub, "below" and ferre, "to carry." The weight and isolation of that suffering now becomes more real at the visceral level. Cassell[4] reminds us that pain itself does not foreordain suffering; it is, in fact, the meaning that is attributed to that pain that determines the suffering. In his clinical definition, "Suffering is a state of severe distress induced by the loss of the intactness of person, or by a threat that the person believes will result in the loss of his or her intactness" (p. 63). Suffering is an individual and private experience and will be greatly influenced by the personality and character of the person; for example, the patient who has needed control during times of wellness will find the out-of-control experience of illness as suffering.[4] In writing about cancer pain and its meaning, Ersek and Ferrell[10] provide a summary of hypotheses and theses from the literature (Table 35–2).

Although not always recognized, it is the duty of all who care for patients to alleviate suffering and not just treat the physical dimensions of the illness. This is no small task, as professionals must first be free from denial and the need to self-protect to see the suffering of another. Then, they must be able to attend to it without trying to fix it or simplify it. The suffering needs to be witnessed; in the midst of suffering, presence and compassion become the balm and hope for its relief.

## The Process of Finding Meaning in Illness

From years of working with terminally ill patients and their families, the authors have found that the process of finding meaning in illness invokes many themes. The title given to each theme is an attempt to represent observed transitions that many terminally ill patients seem to experience. Not all patients experience the transitions in order, and not all transitions are experienced. However, we have observed that these transitions are experienced by the majority of patients. Issues faced by family caregivers and health-care professionals are discussed in later sections. The themes shared in this section are the imposed transition, loss and confusion, dark night of the soul, randomness and absence of God, brokenness, and reappraisal. In experiencing some or all of these transitions, one can perhaps find meaning in this difficult time of life.

### The Imposed Transition

Being told that you have a terminal illness can be like hearing the sound of prison doors slam shut. Life will never be the same. The sentence has been handed down, and there is no reversing the verdict. Terminal illness is a loss, and there is nothing we can do to change the prognosis even though we may be able to temporarily delay the final outcome. The essence of our being is shaken, and our souls are stricken with a panic unlike any other we have ever felt. For the first time, we are faced with an "existential awareness of nonbeing."[11] For a brief moment, the silence is deafening, as if suspended between two worlds, the known and the unknown. As one "regains consciousness," so to speak, the pain and pandemonium of thoughts and emotions begin to storm the floodgates of our faith, our coping abilities, and our internal fortitude, while simultaneously the word "terminal" reverberates in our heads. There is no easy or quick transition into the acceptance of a terminal diagnosis.

Facing the end of life provokes questions. The self-reflective questions include both the meaning *of* life and the meaning *in* life. Whether we embrace with greater fervor the people and things that collectively give us meaning in life or we view it all as now lost, the loss and pain are real. Nothing can be done to prevent the inevitable. There is a sense of separation or disconnectedness in that while I am the same person, I have also become permanently different from you. Unless you become like me, diagnosed with a terminal illness, we are in this sense separated. In a rhetorical sense, the meanings we gain in life from relationships and the material world serve to affirm us as participants in these meanings.[11] When these meanings are threatened by a terminal diagnosis, we fear the loss of who we are as functioning productive human beings. The affirmations we received from our meanings in life are now at a standstill.

A 65-year-old retired military man, although accepting of his prognosis, fought to delay the inevitable for as long as possible. As a military man, he was not afraid of dying. The relationship with one of his grown children was very good and he adored his grandchildren. They were the reason he was fighting the cancer. He felt that life was most enjoyable when he spent time with them. His concern about dying was that because the grandchildren were young, there would not be enough time with them for them to remember him after he died. "My grandkids are more important you know so cause they got to remember their grandpa. I want them to think about me, what grandparents did you know?"[12] When we discussed ways that he might be able to leave them a legacy, he began to understand that he saw himself and his remaining time in limited ways. He feared losing what had come to define his life. Encouraging him to redefine his life in terms of meaning through leaving a legacy for his grandchildren gave him new insights and provided a practical way to spend the rest of his days.

In addition to questioning meaning *in* life, those facing the end of life also question the meaning *of* life. A life-threatening illness makes it difficult to maintain an illusion of immortality.[13] What happens when we die? Is there really a God? Is it too late for reconciliation? For those believing in life after death, the questions may focus on uncertainty of eternal life, fear of what eternal life will be like, or the possibility of this being a test of faith. No matter what the belief system, the existential questions are asked. We reach out for a connection with God or something beyond one's self to obtain some sense of security and stability. Then, in this ability to transcend the situation, ironically, we somehow feel a sense of groundedness. Frankl[3] states, "It denotes the fact that being human always points, and is directed, to something or someone, other than oneself—be it a meaning to fulfill or another human being to encounter." There is an incredibly strong spiritual need to find meaning in this new senseless and chaotic world.

## Loss and Confusion

One cancer patient stated, "Our lives are like big run-on sentences and when cancer occurs, it's like a period was placed at the end of the sentence. In reality, we all have a period at the end of the sentence, but we don't really pay attention to it."[14] With a terminal diagnosis, life is changed forever, for however long that life may be. Each day life seems to change as one is forced to experience a new aspect of the loss. There is a sense of immortality that pervades our lust for life, and when we are made to look at our mortality, it is staggering. With all of the many losses, coupled with the fear of dying, one can be left feeling confused from the infinite possibilities of the unknown. The panorama of suffering seems to be limitless.

The pain of loss is as great as the pleasure we derived from life.[15] The pain is pure and somewhat holy. The confusion comes not only from one's world having been turned upside down but also from those who love us and care about us. It is not intentional; nevertheless, its impact is greatly felt. In trying to bring encouragement or trying to help one find meaning, the loss and pain are sometimes minimized by comparing losses, attempting to save God's reputation by denying the one hurting the freedom to be angry at God, or by immediately focusing on the time left to live. The hurting soul needs to feel the depth of the loss by whatever means it can. The pain from loss is relentless, like waves from a dark storm at sea crashing repeatedly against rocks on the shoreline.

A 55-year-old woman with terminal lung cancer experienced further physical decline each day. She was supported by a husband who lovingly doted on her. She was one who loved life and loved her family. Many losses were experienced because of her comorbid conditions along with the cancer. The fact that her family wanted her to focus on life and not her disease or death added to these losses. Her husband informed us that they knew she was going to die but felt that her quality of life would be better if these issues were not discussed. The patient had many thoughts and feelings to sort through and wanted to talk, but no one was listening. Her loss was not just physical; it also was an imposed emotional loss caused by a loving family trying to do the right thing. Many times the patient ended up in tearful frustration. The communications with her family were different, constantly reminding her that nothing was the same and, in turn, reminded her of her losses and impending death.

## Dark Night of the Soul

The descent of darkness pervades every crack and crevice of one's being. One now exists in the place of Nowhere surrounded by nothingness that is void of texture and contour. One's signature is seemingly wiped away, taking with it the identification of a living soul.[15] Job states, "And now my soul is poured out within me; days of affliction have seized me. At night it pierces my bones within me, and my gnawing pains take no rest…My days are swifter than a weaver's shuttle, and come to an end without hope."[16] "One enters the abyss of emptiness—with the perverse twist that one is not empty of the tortured feeling of emptiness."[17] This is pain's infinite desert.

Darkness looms as one thinks about the past, full of people and things that provided meaning in life, that will soon have to be given up. Darkness looms as one thinks about the future, because death precludes holding on to all that is loved and valued. Darkness consumes one's mind and heart like fire consumes wood. It makes its way to the center with great fury, where it proceeds to take possession, leaving nothing but a smoldering heap of ashes and no hope of recovering any essence of life.[18]

A woman with fairly young children relapsed after several years free of colon cancer. She received several months of treatment with an experimental protocol. She suffered greatly, not only from the effects of the chemotherapy but also from the long periods of time not being able to "be there" for her children. When it became clear that the chemo was not working as expected, she became tortured by the thought of abandoning her children at a time when they so greatly needed a mother and the fact that she had gambled with the little time she had left and had lost. Now in her mind, her children had the double loss of months of quality time she could have had with them and her impending death. She became inconsolable because of this darkness. Time to intervene was very limited. Allowing her the room for suffering and being "present" to this suffering as a nurse was essential. In addition, moving back into her mothering role and providing for her children by helping to prepare them for her death became the pathway through the darkness and into meaning.

Although one might try, there are no answers—theological or otherwise—to the "whys" that engulf one's existence. Death moves from an "existential phenomenon to a personal reality."[19] All our presuppositions about life fall away and we are left emotionally naked. There is neither the physical, the emotional, nor the spiritual strength to help our own fragility. The world becomes too big for us and our inner worlds are overwhelming.[15] The enigma of facing death strips order from one's life, creating fragmentation and leaving one with the awareness that life is no longer tenable.

## Randomness and the Absence of God

The pronouncement of a terminal diagnosis provokes inner turmoil and ruminating thoughts from dawn to dusk. Even in one's chaotic life, there was order. But order does not always prevail. A young athlete being recruited for a professional sport is suddenly killed in a tragic car accident. A mother of three small children is diagnosed with a chronic debilitating disease that will end in death. An earthquake levels a brand new home that a husband and wife had spent years saving for. A playful young toddler drowns in a pool. There seems to be no reason. It would be different if negligence were involved.

For example, if the young athlete were speeding, or driving drunk, although the loss is still quite devastating, a "logical" reason could be assigned to it. But randomness leaves us with no "logical" explanation.[17]

The word "random" comes from the Middle English word *radon*, which is derived from the Old French word *randon*, meaning violence and speed. The word connotes an impetuous and haphazard movement, lacking careful choice, aim, or purpose.[2] The feeling of vulnerability is overwhelming. In an effort to find shelter from this randomness, meaning and comfort is sought from God or from something beyond one's self, but how do we know that God or something beyond ourselves is not the cause of our loss? Our trust is shaken. Can we reconcile God's sovereignty with our loss?[17] Can we stay connected to and continue to pull or gain strength and security from something beyond ourselves that may be the originator of our pain? There is a sense of abandonment by that which has been our stronghold in life. Yet to cut ourselves off from that stronghold out of anger would leave us in a state of total disconnection. A sense of connection is a vital emotion necessary for existence, no matter how short that existence may be. But facing death forbids us to keep our existential questions and desires at a distance. Rather, it seems to propel us into a deeper search for meaning as the questions continue to echo in our minds.

## Brokenness

Does one come to a place of acceptance within brokenness? Is acceptance even attainable? Sometimes. Sometimes not. Coming to a place of acceptance is an individual experience for each person. In a wonderful analogy of acceptance, Kearney[20] states, "Acceptance is not something an individual can choose at will. It is not like some light switch that can at will be flicked on or off. Deep emotional acceptance is like the settling of a cloud of silt in a troubled pool. With time the silt rests on the bottom and the water is clear"(p. 98). Brokenness does, however, open the door to relinquishing the illusion of immortality. Brokenness allows the soul to cry and to shed tears of anguish. It elicits the existential question "why?" once again, only this time not to gain answers but to find meaning.

A woman in her mid-60s, dying of lung cancer, shared how she came to a place of acceptance. When she was first diagnosed, the cancer was already well advanced. Her health rapidly declined, and she was more or less confined to bed or sitting. Out of her frustration, anger at God, sadness, and tears came the desire to paint again. It was her way of coping, but it became more than that. It brought her to a place of peace in her heart. She had gotten away from painting because of busyness and was now learning to be blessed by quietness. She was very good at creating cards with her own designs in watercolor, leaving the insides blank to be filled in by the giver. She would give these cards away to many people as her gesture of love and gratitude.

If we go back to the poem at the beginning of this chapter, it wasn't until "sanity" was lost that the rose was found.

A gradual perception occurs, whereby we realize that the way out is by no longer struggling.[20] When we come to the end of ourselves and the need to fight the inevitable that is death, we give space for meaning to unfold. It is not that we give up the desire but that we relinquish the need to emotionally turn the situation around and to have all our questions answered. Sittser,[17] a minister who experienced a sudden loss of several immediate family members, states, "My experience taught me that loss reduces people to a state of almost total brokenness and vulnerability. I did not simply feel raw pain; I was raw pain" (p. 164). Pain and loss are still profound, but in the midst of these heavy emotions there begins to be a glimmer of light. Like the flame of a candle, the light may wax and wane. It is enough to begin to silhouette those people and things that still can provide meaning.

**Reappraisal**

It is here where one begins to realize that something positive can come from even a terminal diagnosis and the losses it imposes. The good that is gained does not mitigate the pain of loss but, rather, fosters hope—hope that is not contingent on healing but on reconciliation, on creating memories with loved ones, on making the most of every day, on loving and being loved.[21] It is a hope that transcends science and explanations and changes with the situation. It is not based on a particular outcome but, rather, focuses on the future, however long that may be. Despair undermines hope, but hope robs death of despair.[22]

A male patient in his late 30s, facing the end of life after battling leukemia and having gone through a bone marrow transplant, shared that he knew he was going to die. It took him a long time to be able to admit it to himself. The patient recalled recently visiting a young man who had basically given up and did not want his last dose of chemotherapy. He talked a while with this young man and encouraged him to "go for it." He told him that there is nothing like watching the last drop of chemo go down the tube and into his body, and the sense of it finally being all over. The patient shared with the young man that when he received his own last dose of chemotherapy, he stayed up until three in the morning to watch the last drop go down the tube. Although the chemotherapy did not help him to the extent that he wanted, he wanted to encourage the young man to hope and not give up. Life was not yet over. He had tears in his eyes when he finished the story.

Facing end of life with a terminal diagnosis will never be a happy event. It will always be tragic because it causes pain and loss to everyone involved. But at a time unique to each person facing death, a choice can be made as to whether one wants to become bitter and devalue the remaining time or value the time that is left as much as possible.

An important choice to be made during this time is whether to forgive or to be unforgiving—toward oneself, others, God, or one's stronghold of security in life. Being unforgiving breeds bitterness and superficiality. As we face the end of life, we need both an existential connection and a connection with others. Being unforgiving separates us from those connections, and it is only through forgiveness that the breech is healed. Forgiveness neither condones another's actions nor does it mean that this terminal diagnosis is fair. Rather, forgiveness is letting go of expectations that one somehow will be vindicated for the pain and loss. Whether by overt anger or by emotional withdrawal, in seeking to avoid vulnerability to further pain and loss, we only succeed in making ourselves more vulnerable. Now we have chosen a deeper separation that goes beyond facing the death of the physical body—that of the soul.[17] Positive vulnerability through forgiveness provides a means of healing and, when possible, reconciliation with others. It always provides healing and reconciliation with one's God or one's stronghold of security. Forgiveness allows both physical and emotional energy to be used for creating and enjoying the time left for living.

A 30-year-old woman was admitted to the hospital with advanced metastatic breast cancer. She was unknown to the hospital staff but had a good relationship with her oncologist. During the admissions assessment, the young woman could not give the name of anyone to contact in the event of an emergency. When pressed, she stated that she was alienated from her family and chose not to be in touch. She agreed that after her death her mother could be called, but not before. A social worker was summoned in the hope that something could be done to help with some unification. However, the social worker came out of the room devastated by the woman's resolve. The chaplain also found no way to reconnect this woman's family. The nursing staff experienced moral distress as they watched this woman die, all alone in the world. One of the authors worked with the staff to help them realize that they had become trusted and in a sense were her substitute family. One may not always be able to fix the pain of life's fractures or bring people to a place of forgiveness, but it is important not to underestimate what is happening in the moment. Healing for this patient came through the relationship with her doctors and nurses, and she died not alone but cared for.

There are many emotions and issues with which those facing death must contend. It is not an easy journey and the process is wearing; nevertheless, the rose can be found.

## Impact of the Terminal Illness on the Patient–Caregiver Relationship

Each of us comes to new situations with our life's experiences and the meanings we have gained from them. It is no different when being confronted with illness and the end of life. However, in this special episode of life, there are often no personal "reruns" from which to glean insight. Patient and family come together as novices, each helping the other through this unknown passage. Because different roles and relationships exist, the impending loss will create different meanings for each person involved.

Facing the loss of someone you love is extremely difficult. For the family caregiver, the process of finding meaning is influenced by the one facing death. One example experienced by one of the authors of this chapter involved a wife's discussion with her terminally ill husband over several months regarding his outlook on life. As Christians, they knew where death would take them, but she was curious as to what that meant to him and how he was handling the unknown. She felt strong in her own faith but also felt like she was giving lip service to it at times. He described life as having even more meaning in that although he loved her very much and the life they had together, he could now "cherish" every moment of that time. He was sad knowing that he would eventually die from the cancer, but until that time came, he just wanted to enjoy life with her. She shared that while what he said seemed obvious when he said it, for some reason this time it really spoke to her soul and she felt peace.

In another example, a woman helped her family create meaning for themselves from the picture she had painted of herself sitting on the beach as a little girl next to a little boy. She explained that the little boy had his arm around her as they stared out at the sea. Each time the waves covered the surface of the beach and then retreated, the sea would carry with it bits and pieces of her fears and disease. The birds circling overhead would then swoop down to pick up and carry off any pieces not taken by the sea. The little boy's arm around her signified all the loving support she had received from others. When the time would come for her to die, she would be ready because she had been able to let go of life as she knew it. She had let the waves slowly carry that which was of life out to sea and yet had learned to hold on to the meaning that that life had represented. In doing so, she enabled her family to hold on to the meaning of their relationship with her and enabled them to remain symbolically connected after her death.

A final, poignant story offers a different perspective. A 60-year-old woman with stage IV ovarian cancer was very angry at her husband and perplexed at God. She had troubles finding any positive meaning in anything in life. She was upset that life would be cut short, and she would not live to see her grandchildren grow. She blamed her husband for not wanting to have children after the surgeon told her that never having children increased the risk for ovarian cancer. She resented the fact that she had lived in a difficult marriage and now "this" was happening to her. She felt horrible for having these feelings because she didn't like feeling this way. She also dealt with an obsessive compulsive disorder (OCD) regarding cleanliness that made life miserable for herself and those around her. This presented problems for the family in trying to care for her because as the cancer got worse, she needed more physical care but the OCD presented a barrier not easily maneuvered around, leaving family members exhausted and frustrated. The family felt like they could give her much better care but were prevented from doing so. This was extremely difficult for her family. When the patient died, the relationships were very good, but the family had spent a lot of time talking about what all of this meant to them. They were able to talk about the positives and negatives and realized that they did the best they could given the imposed limitations by the patient.

These actual patient stories were presented to exemplify how the patient's meaning in illness affects the meaning held or created by family members. Differing or divergent meanings can be detrimental in a relationship, or they can be used to strengthen it, thereby increasing the quality of time left together. That is not to imply that the patient is responsible for the meaning created by family members; rather, they are responsible for how one affects the other. Germino, Fife, and Funk[23] suggest that the goal is not merely converging meanings within the patient–family dyad but, rather, encouraging a sharing of individual meanings so that all can learn, and relationships can be deepened and strengthened.

There are many issues that family caregivers face in caring for a loved one nearing the end of life. They are discussed at length in the literature. There is one issue, however, that warrants more attention: the loss of dreams. The loss of dreams for a future with the person is in addition to the loss of the person. It is the loss of the way one used to imagine life and how it would have been with that person. It is the loss of an emotional image of oneself and the abandonment of chosen plans for the future and what might have been.[24]

For a child and the surviving parent, those losses of dreams will be played out each time Mother's or Father's Day arrives and important life-cycle events, such as graduations, weddings, or the birth of the first grandchild. As her mother lay dying, one child expressed that loss in the simple statement, "Mommy, you won't be here for my birthday!" The mother and child wept, holding and comforting each other. Nothing could change the loss, but the comforting would remain forever.

The loss of dreams is an internal process, spiritual for some, and seldom recognized by others as needing processing.[14,24–26] Nurses have a wonderful opportunity at this point to verbally recognize the family caregivers' loss of dreams and to encourage them in their search to find meaning in the loss. The ability to transcend and connect to God or something greater than one's self helps the healing process.

## Transcendence: Strength for the Journey That Lies Ahead

Transcendence is defined as lying beyond the ordinary range of perception; being above and independent of the material universe. The Latin root is *trans-*, "from or beyond," plus *scandere*, "to climb."[2] The images are many: the man in a pit climbing his way out one handhold at a time; the story of Job as he endured one defeat after another and yet found meaning; the climber who reaches the mountaintop, becoming closer to the heavens while still having the connection to the earth; or the dying patient who, in peace, is already seeing into another reality. The ability to transcend truly is a gift of the human spirit and often comes after a long struggle and out of suffering. It is often unclear which comes first—does meaning open the door for transcendence, or, quite the opposite, does the act of transcendence bring the meaning? More than likely, it is an intimate dance between the two, one fueling the other. In the Buddhist tradition, suffering and being are a totality, and integrating suffering in this light becomes an act of transcendence.[27]

Transcendence of suffering can also be accomplished by viewing it as reparation for sins while still living—preparing the way for eternity, as in the Islamic tradition. In other traditions, transcendence is often relationship-based, the connection to others, and sometimes to a higher power.[3] For example, the Christian seeing Christ on the cross connects one to the relationship and endurance of God and the reality that suffering is a part of life. For others, it is finding meaning in relating to others, even the act of caring for others. And for some, that relationship may be with the Earth, a sense of stewardship and leaving the environment a better place. It is rare that patients reach a state of transcendence and remain there through their dying. Instead, for most it is a process in which there are moments when they reach a sense of expansion that supports them in facing death. The existential crisis does not rule, because one can frame the relationship beyond death; for example, "I will remain in their hearts and memories forever, I will live on through my children, or my spirit will live beyond my limited physical state."

### Nursing Interventions

If one returns to the root word of meaning, *maenan*, or "to tell of," this concept can be the guide that directs the nurse toward interventions. Given the nature of this work, interventions may not be the true representation of what is needed. For intervention implies action that the nurse has an answer and she can direct the course of care by intervening. It is defined as "To come, appear, or lie between two things. To come in or between so as to hinder or alter an action."[2] But finding meaning is process-oriented; while finely honed psychosocial skills and knowledge can be immensely helpful, there is no bag of tricks. One example would be of a chaplain who walks in the room and relies only on offering prayer to the patient, preventing any real discourse or relationship-building. The patient's personhood has been diminished, and potentially, more harm than good has been done.

So let us revisit "to tell of." What is required of the professional who enters into the healing dimension of a patient's suffering and search for meaning? It would seem that respect may be the starting point—respect for that individual's way of experiencing suffering and attempts of making sense of the illness. Second, allow for an environment and time for the telling. Even as this is written, the sighs of frustration are heard, "We have no time!" If nursing fails at this, if nurses turn their backs on their intrinsic promise to alleviate suffering, then nursing can no longer exist. Instead, the nurse becomes simply the technician and the scheduler—the nurse becomes a part of the problem. She has violated the Code for Nurses that states, "Nursing care is directed toward the prevention and relief of the suffering commonly associated with the dying process…and emphasizes human contact."[28]

If patients in the midst of suffering receive the message, nonverbally or directly, that there is no time, energy, or compassion, they will, in their vulnerability, withdraw or become more needy. Their alienation becomes complete. On the other hand, if privacy and a moment of honor and focused attention are provided, this allows for the tears to spill or the anguish to be spoken. Then the alienation is broken, and the opportunity for healing one dimension is begun. The terminally ill are a vulnerable population. They die and do not complete patient satisfaction surveys; their grievances and their stories die with them. But the violation does not, for each nurse now holds that violation, as does society as a whole. The wound begets wounds, and the nurse sinks further into the protected and unavailable approach, alienated. The work holds no rewards, only endless days and demands. He or She has nothing left to give. The patient and family are ultimately abandoned. In the work of Kahn and Steeves,[29] one finds a model for the nurse's role in psychosocial processes and suffering. It represents the dynamic relationship of caring, acted out in caregiving as well as in the patient's coping, which transform each other.

For the nurse to provide this level of caregiving, he/she must understand the obstructions that may interfere. It is essential that the nurse undergo his/her own journey, visiting the intense emotions around the dying process and the act of witnessing suffering. We can serve the suffering person best if we ourselves are willing to be transformed through the process of our own grief as well as by the grief of others.[30] Presence may, in fact, be our greatest gift to these patients and their families. Still, imagine charting or accounting for presence on an acuity system! Presence "transcends role obligations and acknowledges the vulnerable humanness of us all…to be present means to unconceal, to be aware of tone of voice, eye contact, affect, and body language, to be in tune with the patient's messages."[30] Presence provides confirmation, nurturing, and compassion and is an essential transcendent act.

Touch becomes one of the tools of presence. Used with sensitivity, it can be as simple as the holding of the hand or as powerful as the holding of the whole person. Sometimes, because of agitation or pain, direct touch becomes intrusive; even then touch can be invoked, by the touching of a pillow or the sheet or the offering of a cold cloth. Healing touch takes on another level of intention through the directing energy of prayer.

If a key aspect of meaning is to tell, then one might be led to believe that the spoken word would be imperative. However, over and over, it is silence that conveys the meaning of suffering, "a primitive form of existence that is without an effective voice and imprisoned in silence." Compassionate listeners in respect and presence become mute themselves.[30] They use the most intuitive skills to carry the message. This may also be why other approaches that use symbols, metaphors, and the arts are the most potent in helping the patient to communicate and make sense of meaning. The arts, whether writing, music, or visual arts, often help the patient not only gain new insight but convey that meaning to others. There are many levels on which this is accomplished. Whether it is done passively, through reading poetry, listening to music, or viewing paintings, or actively through creation, thoughts can be inspired, feelings moved, and the sense of connectedness and being understood can evolve. What once was ubiquitous can now be seen outside of one's soul, as feelings become tangible. It can be relational, because the act of creation can link one to the creator, or it can downplay the role of dependency, as the ill one now cares for others with a legacy of creational gifts.[31]

Meditation is another act of transcendence that can be extremely powerful for the dying.[32,33] Even those who have never experienced a meditational state can find that this new world in many ways links them to living and dying. The relaxation response allows the anxious patient to escape into a meditative state, experiencing an element of control while relinquishing control. Many patients describe it as a floating state, a time of great peace and calm. Some who have never had such an experience can find the first time frightening, as the existential crisis, quelled so well by boundaries, is no longer confined. Most, given a trusting and safe teacher, will find that meditation will serve them well. The meditation can be in the form of prayer, guided imagery, breathing techniques, or mantras.

Prayer is well-documented in the literature[34,35] as having meaning for patients and families; not only does it connect one to God, but it also again becomes a relational connection to others. Knowing that one is prayed for not only by those close at hand but by strangers, communities, and those at a great distance can be deeply nurturing. Often forgotten is the role in which the patient can be empowered, that of praying for others. One of the authors experienced her patient's prayers for her as the tables were turned, and the patient became the healer. The patient suddenly lost the sense of worthlessness and glowed with joy.

Leaving a legacy may be one of the most concrete ways for patients to find meaning in this last stage of their lives.[36] It most often requires the mastering of the existential challenges, in which patients know that death is at hand and choose to direct their course and what they leave behind. For some patients, that will mean going out as warriors, fighting until the end; for others, it will mean end-of-life planning that focuses on quality of life. Some patients will design their funerals, using rituals and readings that reveal their values and messages for others. Others will create videos, write letters, or distribute their wealth in meaningful ways. Parents who are leaving young children sometimes have the greatest difficulty with this aspect. On one hand, the feelings of horror at "abandoning" their children are so strong that they have great difficulty facing their death. Still, there is often a part of them that has this need to leave a legacy. The tug-of-war

between these two willful emotions tends to leave only short windows of opportunity to prepare. The extreme can be observed in the young father who began to push his toddler away, using excuses for the distancing. It was only after a trusting relationship had been established with one of the authors that she could help him to see how this protective maneuver was, in fact, harming the child. The father needed not only to see what he was doing but to see how his love would help the child and how others would be there for the child and wife in their pain and grief. With relief, the father reconnected to his young son, creating living memories and a lifetime protection of love.

Another courageous parent anticipating the missed birthdays, bought cards, and wrote a note in each one, so that the child would be touched not only by the individual messages, but the knowledge that the parent found a way to be there for him with each new year. A mother wrote a note for her young daughter so that if she should ever marry, she would have a gift to be opened on her wedding day. The note described the mother's love, wisdom about marriage, and her daughter's specialness, already known through a mother's eyes. An elderly person may write or tape an autobiography or even record the family tree lest it be lost with the passing of a generation. The nurse can often be the one who inspires these acts, but it must always be done with great care so as not to instill a sense of "should" or "must," which would add yet another burden.

Helping patients to reframe hope is another important intervention. Recently, Dr. William Brietbart, Chief of the Psychiatry Services at Memorial Sloan-Kettering Cancer Center in New York City, designed and conducted research on a meaning-centered psychotherapeutic intervention to help terminally ill patients with cancer maintain hope and meaning as they face the end of their lives.[37] This research was inspired by the works of Dr. Victor Frankl, a psychiatrist and Holocaust survivor. Cancer patients attended an 8-week, group-focused, standardized course of experiential exercises that addressed constructs of despair at the end of life, such as hopelessness, depression, loss of meaning, suicidal ideation, and desire for a hastened death. The study revealed that the patient's spiritual well-being, loss of meaning in part, was more highly correlated to the components that made up despair at the end of life than either depression or hopelessness alone. As a result, if the patient could manipulate or reframe his/her sense of meaning and spiritual well-being, this would positively affect the foundational elements of despair at the end of life. When patients are able to do this, their hope is sustained because they have been able to reframe the focus of their hope.

## The Health-Care Professional

Although the health-care professional can be educated about death and grieving, like the patient and family, it is in living out the experience that understanding is reached. It is a developmental process, and given the demands of the work, the nurse is at great risk for turning away from her feelings. There is often little mentoring that accompanies the first deaths, let alone formal debriefing or counseling. How can it be that we leave such important learning to chance? And what about cumulative losses and the years of witnessing suffering? Healthcare needs healing rituals for all of its health-care professionals to support and guide them in this work. Individual institutions can develop programs that address these needs.

At one institution, "Teas for the Soul" (sponsored by the Pastoral Care Department) provide respite in the workplace on a regular basis, as well as after difficult deaths or traumas. A cart with cookies and tea, as well as soft music, are provided as physical nurturance and nurture the emotions of the staff and legitimize the need to come together in support. Another support is a renewal program, the "Circle of Caring." This retreat supports health-care professionals from a variety of institutions in a weekend of self-care that integrates spirituality, the arts, and community building. The element of suffering is a focal point for a small-group process that unburdens cumulative effects of the work and teaches skills and rituals for coping with the ongoing demands.

Clearly, there is much that can be done in this area to support nurses individually and to support organizations. There are many opportunities for assisting nurses in their own search for meaning and for enhancing the care of patients and families. When the nurse takes the time to find meaning in this work, he/she is finding a health restorative practice that will protect him/her personally and professionally. Like the patient, he/she will need to choose this journey and find pathways that foster and challenge him/her.

> As long as we can love each other,
> And remember the feeling of love we had,
> We can die without ever really going away.
> All the love you created is still there.
> All the memories are still there.
> You live on – in the hearts of everyone you have
> Touched and nurtured while you were here.
> —Morrie Schwartz[38]

## REFERENCES

1. Taylor EJ. Whys and wherefores: Adult patient perspectives of the meaning of cancer. Semin Oncol Nurs 1995;11(1):32–40.
2. Dictionary. The American Heritage Dictionary. Boston, MA: Houghton Mifflin, 2008.
3. Frankl VE. Man's Search for Meaning: An Introduction to Logotherapy. Boston: Beacon, 1959.
4. Cassell EJ. The relationship between pain and suffering. Adv Pain Res Ther 1989;11:61–70.
5. Personal. Personal interview; May 22, 2007.
6. Koestenbaum P. Is There an Answer to Death? Englewood Cliffs, NJ: Prentice-Hall, 1976.
7. Puchalski C. Spirituality. In Berger A, Shuster J, Roenn JV, eds. Principles and Practice of Palliative Care and Supportive Oncology (3rd ed). Philadelphia, PA: Lippincott Williams & Wilkins; 2007:633–644.
8. Vachon ML. Meaning, spirituality, and wellness in cancer survivors. Semin Oncol Nurs 2008;24(3):218–225.
9. Concordance. Strong's Exhaustive Concordance. Peabody, MA: Hendrickson Publishers, 2007.
10. Ersek M, Ferrell BR. Providing relief from cancer pain by assisting in the search for meaning. J Palliat Care 1994;10(4):15–22.
11. Tillich P. The Courage To Be. New Haven, CT: Yale University Press, 1952.
12. Personal communication; May 22, 2007.
13. Benson H. Timeless Healing. New York, NY: Simon and Schuster, 1997.
14. Putnam C. Personal Communication; September 26, 1999.
15. O'Donohue J. Eternal Echoes. New York, NY: HarperCollins Publishers, 1999.
16. Bible. New American Standard Bible. Grand Rapids, MI: World Publishing, 1995.
17. Sittser G. A Grace Disguised. Grand Rapids, MI: Zondervan Publishing House, 1995.
18. Cross SJ. Dark Night of the Sourl. Kila, MT: Kessinger Publishing Company, 1959.
19. Kritek P. Reflections on Healing. Boston, MA: Jones and Bartlett Publishers, 2003.
20. Kearney M. Mortally Wounded. New York, NY: Simon and Schuster, 1996.
21. Martins L. The silence of God: The absence of healing. In: Fundis GCaR, ed. Spiritual, Ethical and Pastoral Aspects of Death and Bereavement. Amityville, NY: Baywood Publishing Company; 1992:25–31.
22. Pellegrino E, Thomasma D. The Christian Virtues in Medical Practice. Washington, DC: Georgetown University Press, 1996.
23. Germino BB, Fife BL, Funk SG. Cancer and the partner relationship: What is its meaning? Semin Oncol Nurs 1995;11(1):43–50.
24. Bowman T. Facing loss of dreams: A special kind of grief. Int J Palliat Nurs 1997;3(2):76–80.
25. Garbarino J. The spiritual challenge of violent trauma. Am J Orthopsychiatry 1996;66(1):162–163.
26. Rando TA. Treatment of Complicated Mourning. Champaign, IL: Research Press, 1993.
27. Kallenberg K. Is there meaning in suffering? An external question in a new context. Paper presented at: Cancer Nursing Changing Frontiers, 1992, Vienna.
28. ANA. American Nurses Association Code for Nurses with Interpretive Statements. Washington, DC: American Nurses Publishing, 2001.
29. Kahn DL, Steeves RH. The significance of suffering in cancer care. Semin Oncol Nurs 1995;11(1):9–16.
30. Byock I. When suffering persists. J Pall Care 1994;10(2):8–13.
31. Bailey SS. The arts in spiritual care. Semin Oncol Nurs 1997;13(4):242–247.
32. Baldacchino D, Draper P. Spiritual coping strategies: A review of the nursing research literature. J Adv Nurs 2001;34(6):833–841.
33. Sellers SC. The spiritual care meanings of adults residing in the midwest. Nurs Sci Q 2001;14(3):239–248.
34. Albaugh JA. Spirituality and life-threatening illness: A phenomenologic study. Oncol Nurs Forum 2003;30(4):593–598.
35. Taylor EJ. Nurses caring for the spirit: Patients with cancer and family caregiver expectations. Oncol Nurs Forum 2003;30(4):585–590.

36. Kaut K. Religion, spirituality, and existentialism near the end of life. Am Behav Sci 2002;46(2):220–234.

37. Breitbart W. Reframing hope: Meaning-centered care for patients near the end of life. Interview by Karen S. Heller. J Palliat Med 2003;6(6):979–988.

38. Albom M. Tuesdays With Morrie. New York, NY: Doubleday, 1997.

39. Yalom ID. Existential Psychotherapy. New York, NY: Basic Books, 1980.

40. Marris P. Loss and Change (2nd ed). London, England: Routledge and Kegan Paul, 1986.

41. Taylor SE. Adjustment to threatening events: A theory of cognitive adaptation. Am Psychol 1983;38:1161–1173.

42. O'Connor AP, Wicker CA, Germino BB. Understanding the cancer patient's search for meaning. Cancer Nurs 1990;13(3):167–175.

43. Steeves RH, Kahn DL. Experience of meaning in suffering. Image J Nurs Sch 1987;19(3):114–116.

44. Ersek M. The process of maintaining hope in adults with leukemia undergoing bone marrow transplantation [Unpublished doctoral dissertation]. Seattle, University of Washington; 1991.

45. Gotay CC. Why me? Attributions and adjustment by cancer patients and their mates at two stages in the disease process. Soc Sci Med 1985;20(8):825–831.

46. Haberman MR. Living with leukemia: The personal meaning attributed to illness and treatment by adults undergoing bone marrow transplantation [Unpublished doctoral dissertation]. Seattle, University of Washington, 1987.

47. Chrisman H. The health seeking process: An approach to the natural history of illness. Cult Med Psychiatry 1977;1(4):351–377.

48. Ferrell BR, Taylor EJ, Sattler GR, Fowler M, Cheyney BL. Searching for the meaning of pain: Cancer patients', caregivers', and nurses' perspectives. Cancer Pract 1993;1(3):185–194.

49. Barkwell DP. Ascribing meaning: A critical factor in coping and pain attenuation in patients with cancer-related pain. J Palliat Care 1991;7(3):5–10.

50. Lipowski Z. Physical illness, the individual and their coping processes. International J Psychiatr Med 1970;1(9):101.

51. Haberman MR. Psychosocial aspects of bone marrow transplantation. Semin Oncol Nurs 1988;4(1):55–59.

# V
# Special Patient Populations

# 36 Caring for Those with Chronic Illness

*Terri L. Maxwell*

*I have had COPD for 20 years but I have been living with COPD. Now I'm dying with COPD.*
*I just don't want to suffocate. I think this is worse than cancer.—48-year-old woman*

- ◆ **Key Points**
- ◆ *Patients with advanced chronic conditions frequently have an uncertain illness trajectory and many live for years in chronically poor health marked by declining functional status and intermittent disease exacerbations.*
- ◆ *Communication about end-of-life issues is particularly challenging in the chronically ill population because of prognostic uncertainty, poor understanding among patient and family members about the terminal nature of the condition, and lack of recognition of the benefits of palliative or hospice care.*
- ◆ *Patients with chronic conditions experience myriad symptoms that diminish the quality of life and require a combination of pharmacological and nonpharmacological approaches.*
- ◆ *The provision of hospice and palliative care should be based on patient need, especially with regards to symptom management and declining functional status.*
- ◆ *Individuals with chronic progressive illness and their families benefit from an interdisciplinary palliative approach to care, and as the disease advances, hospice care should be considered.*

## Introduction

Although hospice programs were initally developed to care for cancer patients, cancer represents less than a quarter of all deaths in the United States.[1] Individuals suffering from life-limiting illnesses, such as end-stage cardiac or pulmonary disease, advanced dementia, and other neurological conditions, also need palliative care. For many with progressive chronic illness, the dying process has become so prolonged that it is sometimes viewed as a distinct stage of life.[2] The health-care system and society are confronted with the challenge of providing cost-effective, high-quality, compassionate care for the rising numbers of individuals whose deaths occur after months of gradual debilitation resulting from chronic illness.

Recognizing the growing needs among those with chronic illness and their families, palliative care programs have sprung up across the county, and the hospice industry has gone beyond primarily caring for those with cancer to include all patients with life-limiting illness. The number of patients enrolling in hospice with non-cancer diagnoses has been steadily climbing; in 2007, non-cancer diagnoses accounted for more than half of all hospice admissions (58.7%).[3] The top five non-cancer diagnoses in hospice as a percent of admissions are heart disease (11.8%), debility unspecified (11.2%), dementia (10.1%), and lung disease/chronic obstructive lung disease (7.9%).

Despite the growing number of patients with non-cancer conditions accessing hospice and palliative care, there are numerous barriers leading to their underutilization among the chronic care population. According to Medicare and Medicaid requirements for admission to hospice, patients must have a diagnosed terminal illness with a limited life expectancy and written certification by a physician of a life expectancy of 6 months or less. However, determining a 6-month prognosis or determining when someone is terminal is difficult for those with life-limiting diseases such as end-stage cardiac, hepatic, pulmonary, renal, or neurological diseases. Individuals with these conditions have prognoses that are commonly much more difficult to predict than for those with advanced cancer. Patients with cancer generally experience a more precipitous decline in the weeks and months before their death, whereas those with non-cancer conditions often have a much less predictable course and may have a long period of survival, including survival with a reasonable quality of life. Individuals with non-cancer diseases also commonly die suddenly or unexpectedly from other causes, such as multiple organ failure or persistent recurrent infection, rather than directly from their primary diagnosis. Also, some elderly persons have multiple medical problems, none of which individually amount to a terminal diagnosis but, when taken together, create a terminal condition that is difficult to prognosticate or identify as in need of hospice or palliative care.

Recognizing these challenges, the National Hospice and Palliative Care Organization (NHPCO) published medical guidelines for determining prognosis in selected non-cancer diseases to aid clinicians with prognostication.[4] These guidelines are based on the premise that the prognosis of terminal illness depends on clinical judgment combined with the following: objective assessment of the natural history of the disease; treatments and response to date; performance status; thorough physical assessment, including neurological and orthopedic; and knowledge of the psychological and sociological factors of the patient, family, and physician. Alternatively, others[2] have suggested using the question "Do you think the patient is likely to die within the next year?" as a marker for determining if palliative or hospice care might be appropriate. This chapter reviews the palliative management of common non-cancer conditions.

## Heart Failure

Heart failure is a clinical syndrome that results from an underlying disease that causes structural or functional damage to the heart so that the heart's pumping function grows weaker and the heart is unable to deliver a sufficient supply of oxygenated blood to meet the body's demands. It is estimated that between 2 and 3 million Americans have heart failure with about 400,000 new cases annually,[5] and the numbers are rising among the growing population of elderly persons with comorbid conditions. Among elderly patients admitted to the hospital for heart failure, 1-year mortality is over 60%, which is higher than with most cancers.[6] Heart failure has a devastating effect on patients' quality of life and functional status, yet both hospice and palliative care are underutilized in this population.

The American College of Cardiology (ACC) and the American Heart Association (AHA) published a new staging system for heart failure in 2001[7] (Table 36–1). The first

| Table 36–1 |
| --- |
| **ACC/AHA Classification System**[7] |
| Stage A: High risk for heart failure, no structural disorder present, no symptoms |
| Stage B: Structural heart disorder present, no symptoms |
| Stage C: Current or previous heart failure symptoms associated with structural heart disease |
| Stage D: Advanced heart failure with symptoms occurring at rest despite maximal medical therapy |

two stages (A and B) identify persons at risk to develop heart failure. Stage C designates patients with current or previous symptoms of heart failure that represent the bulk of the heart failure population. Stage D denotes persons with advanced heart failure whose symptoms progress despite maximal medical therapy with diuretics, angiotensin-converting enzyme (ACE) inhibitors, β-blockers, and possibly digoxin. Stage D patients should be evaluated for specialized therapies such as cardiac transplantation, inotropic infusions, mechanical circulatory support, and/or palliative or hospice care.[7]

Heart failure is a consequence of cardiac damage from a number of underlying diseases, such as coronary artery disease, myocardial infarction, hypertension, dilated cardiomyopathy, valvular heart disease, and so forth. The heart attempts to compensate for the damage through a process called remodeling. Remodeling leads to enlargement of the heart and/or hypertrophy of the ventricles, resulting in decreased cardiac output and an increase in afterload. The abnormal loading induces dilatation of the ventricles that changes the shape of the ventricle, decreasing the pumping ability of the heart and contributing to symptoms despite treatment.[8]

Heart failure can be characterized based on ventricular involvement. Systolic dysfunction is the most common, whereas diastolic dysfunction is estimated to occur in 20% to 50% of cases.[9] Patients with preserved systolic function have normal ejection fractions but have abnormal ventricular filling, leading to pulmonary congestion, dyspnea, and symptoms of anorexia, fatigue, and depression; whereas those with right-sided (systolic) dysfunction present with symptoms of weight gain, edema, dsypnea, and early satiety. Persons with diastolic heart failure are typically elderly, generally female, usually obese, and have hypertension and diabetes.[9]

Patients with heart failure have an uncertain illness trajectory, and many live for years in chronically poor health marked by declining functional status and unpredictable episodes of heart failure exacerbations. Although models have been developed to predict mortality in patients with advanced heart disease, they lack specificity, making determining prognosis very difficult. This variability in prognosis was illustrated by the Study to Understand Prognoses and Preferences for Outcomes and Risks of Treatment (SUPPORT), in which over half of those with heart failure had an estimated 6-month survival prognosis within 3 days of

| Table 36–2 |  |
|---|---|
| **Symptoms of Advanced Heart Failure** |  |
| Fatigue/weakness | Pain |
| Decreased appetite | Depressed mood |
| Shortness of breath | Anxiety |
| Lower extremity edema | Difficulty sleeping |
| Ascites | Decreased sexual interest |
| Cough |  |

death.[10] In addition, patients with heart failure have an array of treatments available, and they become accustomed to good treatment responses to exacerbations, making the decision to accept a palliative approach only more difficult.[11] Because of these challenges, patients with heart failure frequently lack access to specialist palliative care services and may end up being discharged alive from hospice.

Persons with advanced heart failure usually have a number of disabling symptoms. Complications of heart failure include pulmonary congestion, evidenced by lung symptoms, congestive heart failure, cor pulmonale, arrhythmias, and cardiac arrest. Common symptoms of advanced heart failure are listed in Table 36–2. The SUPPORT described symptoms in patients hospitalized with heart failure at the end of life. Severe dsypnea was experienced by 63% of patients, and 41% had severe pain within the last 3 days of life. During the last month of life, 70% of patients with heart failure perceived their quality of life as poor.[10]

## Management

There is an array of pharmacological and nonpharmacological therapy options for heart failure. The primary goals of therapy are to improve survival, slow disease progression, minimize risk factors, and reduce symptoms. Early recognition of signs and symptoms of heart failure can decrease hospitalizations and improve quality of life.

The 2005 ACC/AHA guidelines outline treatment options based on heart failure stage.[8] Patients with structural disease and previous or current symptoms (stage C) should be prescribed ACE inhibitors and β-blockers, diruretics, digoxin, sodium-restricted diet, and exercise as appropriate. ACE inhibitors and β-blockers have demonstrated improvements in survival, morbidity, ejection fraction, remodeling, quality of life, rate of hospitalization, and incidence of sudden death. They are generally recommended for all patients, even those entering hospice.[9,11] Diuretics help to control volume overload and enhance urinary sodium excretion. Loop diuretics, such as furosemide, are generally the drugs of choice. Digoxin has been shown to reduce the risk of heart failure-associated hospitalizations. Aldosterone antagonists, such as spironolactone, have demonstrated improvements in symptoms and reductions in death and hospitalization in some patients with advanced heart failure. According to ACC/AHA guidelines, patients with advanced disease should be considered for cardiac resynchronization devices such as implantable cardioverter-defibrillators (ICDs) to prevent sudden death from conduction defects, inotropic therapy to manage refractory symptoms, and ventricular assist devices (VADs), or cardiac transplantation as indicated.[8]

Patient education is also a central component of heart failure management. The importance of adhering to their medication regimen should be underscored with all patients. They should be placed on a moderate sodium-restricted diet, and some patients with advanced disease may benefit from restricting fluids. Patients should be encouraged to monitor their weight daily so that volume changes can be identified before symptoms occur. Patients should also be taught to avoid nonsteroidal anti-inflammatory agents (NSAIDs). NSAIDs worsen or exacerbate heart failure symptoms and are associated with heart failure hospitalizations.[12]

### Symptom Management

Symptom management in patients with advanced heart disease begins with optimal treatment with ACE inhibitors or angiotensin- receptor blockers (ARBs) and β-blockers, as described above.[11] Less-than-optimal treatment may result in premature referrals to hospice or palliative care programs.

Pain is commonly experienced by those with advanced heart disease because of immobility, edema, or ischemia. Patients may also have comorbidities such as arthritis, diabetic neuropathy, or other conditions that cause discomfort. Nitrates and opioids are indicated for anginal pain. As described earlier, NSAIDs should be avoided because of the possibility of worsening kidney function and subsequent fluid retention. Other than avoiding NSAIDs, nonopioids and opioids should be prescribed according to guidelines used for other chronic conditions.

Dyspnea is a prominent symptom among those with severe heart failure (*see* Chapter 14). Nonpharmacological therapies such as creating a calm environment, employing techniques to manage anxiety, and using a fan to improve air circulation may reduce symptoms of dyspnea. Supplemental oxygen therapy may be helpful in those with ischemic symptoms but does not necessarily decrease the sensation of breathlessness among non-hypoxemic patients and is associated with hemodynamic deterioration in severe heart failure.[13] The primary treatment of dyspnea involves managing fluid status with cardiac medications. Oral and parenteral opioids have demonstrated substantial benefit in reducing the feeling of breathlessness in patients with advanced disease of any cause,[14] but they are often overlooked for use in those with heart failure. In fact, opioids should be considered a first-line therapy for those with advanced heart disease as they have been proven safe and effective.[15] Although the exact mechanism by which opioids alleviate dyspnea is unknown, one popular theory is that they decrease respiratory distress by altering the perception of breathlessness, as well as by decreasing ventilatory response to declining oxygen and rising $CO_2$ levels. Contrary to popular belief, opioids do not improve dyspnea through inhibition of the respiratory drive; in fact, opioids improve dyspnea without causing significant deterioration in respiratory function.[16] Although the efficacy of opioids in managing dyspnea has been demonstrated in clinical studies, the optimal dosing and route of administration is highly debated. Most clinicians agree that it is best to initiate therapy with a low dose and increase the dose slowly as needed, because respiratory drive suppression can occur if serum opioid levels rise quickly. Morphine is the opioid most studied in the treatment of dyspnea; other opioids, such as hydromorphone or codeine, are also effective. The usual dose of morphine in the opioid-naïve patient is 5 mg orally (preferred route) every 4 hours, which can be titrated upward in 25%- to 50%-increments until symptoms are controlled.[17] Nebulized morphine has been used to relieve dyspnea with some success, but at this time, evidence to support its use is weak and it should not be used in place of oral or parenteral dosing.[14] If dyspnea causes anxiety, the addition of a short-acting benzodiazepine such as lorazepam may be beneficial.

Benzodiazepines may also help manage symptoms of anxiety or insomnia commonly experienced by patients with heart failure. Depression is also a common but frequently unrecognized comorbidity among those with advanced heart failure. Depression can be treated with selective serotonin reuptake inhibitors (SSRIs); however, they should be carefully titrated, as they can elevate blood pressure and worsen tachycardia. Tricyclic antidepressants should be avoided because they are poorly tolerated in the elderly and have negative effects on cardiac rhythms. Fatigue, often accompanied by depression, can have a profound effect on quality of life. Fatigue usually results from the heart failure itself, although the clinician should carefully assess for reversible causes or the need for more diuretic. Patients should be encouraged to be as active as possible and to reset goals of physical activity to accommodate changes in energy levels.

Patients with advanced heart failure frequently experience early satiety and nausea resulting from pressure from an enlarged, congested liver or as a result of gastric stasis. Patients with a congested liver should be treated with a loop diuretic or spironolactone and may require inotropic support. Metoclopramide may be effective in patients with gastroparesis. Patients may also benefit from antiemetics such as haloperidol or procholoperazine.

## Specialized Interventions for Refractory Heart Failure

Intotropic and vasoactive agents such as neosynephrine, dobutamine, or milrinone work by forcing the contractility of the myocardium, thereby improving patient symptoms. They are frequently initiated with the expectation that brief support during a period of decompensation will enhance diuresis and accelerate hospital discharge. However, some patients cannot be weaned without clinical deterioration and progressive

renal dysfunction. Unfortunately, there are no approved oral versions of inotropic agents and the routine use of intermittent inotropic infusions administered in outpatient clinics has not been supported by clinical trials,[18] and survival on home inotropic infusions is poor.[19] Symptom improvement associated with the provision of inotropic therapy is believed to result primarily from the increased clinical contact that could be accomplished in less resource intensive ways. Most hospices do not support the use of inotropic therapy because of cost considerations.[11]

Implantable cardioverter-defibrillators (ICDs) are implanted to prevent sudden cardiac death. The mortality benefit of these devices has been demonstrated by a number of clinical trials.[20] ICDs do not slow progression of heart failure, so increasing numbers of patients are approaching end of life with these devices in place and are at risk to have painful shocks delivered during the dying process. Therefore, discussion of ICD deactivation should happen when the device is placed; unfortunately, this rarely occurs.[21]

Fewer than 5% of patients with advanced heart failure are eligible for cardiac transplantation, which is partially limited by the number of organs available.[19] Some patients awaiting transplantation, or select patients who are ineligible or choose not to undergo transplant, may opt for a left VAD. A VAD is a surgically implanted mechanical pump to improve ventricular functions. Although originally used as a bridge to transplantation, now that VADs are more compact and portable, they are increasingly used as destination therapy for patients with end-stage heart disease.[22] Despite increases in survival, the morbidity and mortality associated with the use of a VAD is high, mainly because of infection or mechanical failure of the device.[23] Before placing the device, clinicians should discuss scenarios with the patient and family to determine under what circumstances they would want the device deactivated.[24]

## Advance Care Planning/Communication Challenges

There is also a notable lack of advanced care planning and dialogue between heart failure patients and their providers regarding end-of-life care. Communication is particularly challenging prognostic uncertainty because of the unpredictable nature of the disease trajectory, poor understanding among patient and family members about the disease itself, and lack of recognition that heart failure is a terminal condition. To enhance end-of-life decision making and the provision of palliative care, the 1995 ACC/AHA practice guidelines recommend: *(a)* ongoing patient and family education regarding prognosis for functional capacity and survival: *(b)* patient and family education about options for formulating and implementing advanced directives; *(c)* discussion regarding the option of inactivating ICDs; *(d)* continuity of medical care between inpatient and outpatient settings; *(e)* components of hospice care to relieve suffering, including opiates; and *(f)* examination of and work toward improving approaches to palliative care.[8]

## Hospice Eligibility Criteria and Referral

Hospice is underutilized by patients with advanced heart failure for a number of reasons. The inability to predict actual time to death and the patient's preference for resuscitation orders compared to cancer patients are important barriers to hospice referral. Physicians may be reluctant to engage in end-of-life discussions with their patients or may lack the skills to do so. Furthermore, there is still a misconception among many health-care providers that hospice care is for cancer patients and they are unaware of the benefits of hospice for patients with heart failure.[25] Although helpful, NHPCO guidelines for determining hospice eligibility for patients with heart failure do not adequately predict short-term prognosis, so patients may be on hospice service for a long time.[26] It is important to remember that those who stabilize while on hospice care can be discharged and readmitted when their condition deteriorates. In addition to hospice, interdisciplinary palliative care should be more available to patients during hospitalization and thereafter. Doing so may improve quality-of-life outcomes for patients and families and reduce hospitalizations and costs.

## Chronic Obstructive Pulmonary Disease

Chronic Obstructive Pulmonary Disease (COPD) is a respiratory disorder characterized by chronic airway obstruction and lung hyperinflation resulting from chronic bronchitis and emphysema. During the last 30 years, the death rate for COPD has doubled.[27] It is the fourth leading cause of chronic morbidity and mortality in the world, largely as a result of the cumulative exposure to tobacco smoke.[28] From COPD increases with age and occurs more often in men, although death rates for women have been rising since the 1970s. COPD is a progressive illness, and even with treatment, lung function generally worsens over time.

The severity of COPD is based on the patient's level of symptoms, severity of spirometric abnormality, and the presence of comorbidities than can lead to complications. The Global Initiative for Chronic Obstructive Lung Disease (GOLD) guidelines describe four stages of COPD characterized by worsening airflow limitation (Table 36–3).[29]

### Symptoms

Reductions in airflow, as evidenced by declining $FEV_1$ readings, primarily results from inflammation, fibrosis, and exudates in small airways. As air gets trapped, the lungs hyperinflate and alveoli are destroyed. Hyperinflation results in decreased inspiratory capacity and increased functional residual capacity, causing dyspnea. Gas exchange abnormalities bring about hypoxemia and rising $CO_2$ levels. Some patients, especially those with chronic bronchitis, have a chronic productive cough. Patients with advanced COPD are at risk to develop pulmonary hypertension that may progress

| Table 36–3 |
| --- |
| **Stages of COPD** |
| Stage I: Mild COPD: $FEV_1/FVC < 0.70$; $FEV1 \geq 80\%$ predicted. Patient unaware lung function is abnormal. |
| Stage II: Moderate COPD: $FEV_1/FVC < 0.70$; $50\% \leq FEV_1 < 80\%$ predicted. Patient typically seeks medical attention because of pulmonary symptoms. |
| Stage III: Severe COPD: $FEV_1/FVC < 0.70$; $30\% \leq FEV_1 < 50\%$ predicted. Greater shortness of breath, reduced exercise tolerance, decreased quality of life. |
| Stage IV: Very severe COPD: $FEV_1/FVC < 0.70$; $30\% \leq FEV1 < 50\%$ predicted *plus* the presence of chronic respiratory failure. May have signs of cor pulmonale. |

*Source*: Adapted from GOLD Guidelines[29].

to right ventricular hypertrophy and cor pulmonale (right-sided heart failure). In addition to respiratory symptoms, persons with COPD frequently have systemic features such as weight loss and skeletal muscle wasting and are at risk for osteoporosis, myocardial infarction, respiratory infection, depression, sleep disorders, diabetes, and glaucoma.[29]

### Management

The primary goals of COPD management are to relieve symptoms, ameliorate disease progression, improve exercise tolerance and health status, and prevent and treat complications and disease exacerbations. Treatment varies based on the impact of symptoms on the patient's quality of life and degree of disability.

The comprehensive management of COPD consists of a combination of pharmacotherapeutic and non-pharmacotherapeutic interventions, although it should be noted that none of the existing therapies have been shown to modify the long-term decline in lung function associated with COPD.[29] Patients should be counseled to stop smoking and to monitor their symptoms for signs of exacerbation. Nonpharmacological therapies include pulmonary rehabilitation/exercise training as tolerated and nutritional counseling. Patients with very severe (stage IV) disease may benefit from oxygen therapy, which has been shown to increase survival and may prevent progression of pulmonary hypertension.[30] Oxygen therapy also improves alertness and may have positive effects on quality of life, including mood. The GOLD guidelines recommend oxygen treatment for at least 15 hours or more per day provided from a fixed oxygen concentrator with piping to allow the patient to move throughout their home.[29]

In patients with advanced COPD, various medications are used to prevent and control symptoms and to reduce the frequency and severity of exacerbations. These medications are generally added as the disease and symptoms worsen. By the time a patient's disease is advanced, they will likely be prescribed a long-acting and short-acting bronchodilator such as albuterol; anticholinergics such as ipratropium bromide or tiotropium;

methylxanthines such as aminophylline or theophylline; and combination inhaled therapies such as formoterol/budesonide. Whereas regular treatment with inhaled glucocorticosteroids reduces exacerbations and improves health status, long-term treatment with oral corticosterioids is not recommended because of lack of benefit and high risk of adverse effects.[29]

Other pharmacological treatments include yearly inoculation with influenza vaccines and antitussives to control cough. Mucolytic agents and prophylactic, continuous use of antibiotics has not been shown to be effective; antibiotics should be reserved to treat infectious exacerbations and other bacterial infections only. Oral and parenteral opioids are used to treat dyspnea in patients with advanced COPD, but clinical trials are limited and study results are mixed. One small study of the administration of long-acting morphine for dyspnea actually worsened exercise tolerance, did not improve breathlessness, and was associated with adverse effects such as nausea, constipation, and drowsiness;[31] whereas a larger, more adequately powered study by Abernethy and colleagues[15] demonstrated improved dsypnea and sleep scores for those prescribed sustained release oral morphine . Nebulized opioids have not demonstrated a reduction in breathlessness in patients with COPD[32] and should not be used in place of oral or parenteral routes. Anxiolytics may be helpful in managing anxiety that can accompany severe dyspnea.

Decisions about the use of invasive ventilation are frequently based on the patient's prognosis, which can be difficult to determine. In patients where invasive ventilation is not deemed to be in the best interest of the patient, noninvasive ventilation (NIV) is being used first line to treat acute respiratory failure among patients with COPD. NIV devices rhythmically blow air into the lungs through a mask attached over the nose and mouth. Whereas the benefits of NIV for acute exacerbations is known, its value among those with stage IV (very severe) COPD has not been demonstrated[29] although it may have a time-limited role for some patients at the end of life.

### End-of-life Issues

Similarly to other chronic conditions, prognosis in patients with COPD is difficult to predict. The provision of palliative care should be based on patient need, especially with regards to symptom management and declining functional status. Pulmonologists and palliative care teams should work together to improve communication at the end of life, especially related to goals of care and advanced care planning. Hospice should be considered for stage IV patients who prefer a palliative approach to care.

### End-Stage Renal Disease

End-stage renal disease (ESRD) is the most feared consequence of kidney disease. ESRD results when kidney function deteriorates to the point where it is no longer adequate to sustain life. Patients with kidney function less than 10% of normal are considered to have ESRD, usually following a long history of chronic kidney failure.[33] Diabetes and hypertension are the most common causes of ESRD, with African-Americans disproportionately affected.[34] The rising incidence of ESRD parallels an increase in the prevalence of and the rising median age of the dialysis population.[35] The ESRD population is expected to grow to 650,000 by 2010. Patients with ESRD have a high percentage of comorbities such as coronary artery disease, congestive heart failure, peripheral vascular disease, and malnutrition. Dialysis and kidney transplantation are the only treatments for ESRD.

Signs of ESRD include oliguria, high BUN and serum creatinine levels, severe anemia, and electrolyte imbalances. Common symptoms include fatigue/lack of energy, drowsiness, numbness/tingling, dry mouth, pruritis, and pain. In addition to these physical symptoms, emotional symptoms include worrying, anxiety, feeling sad, and feeling irritable.[36] The addition of other comordities heightens the symptom burden and makes prognosis even more uncertain. All anuric postdialysis patients die within days, but those who produce even small amounts of urine may have residual renal function that can enable them to live for weeks or, in rare cases, months. However, 6-month survival is extremely rare.

### Palliative and Hospice Care Services

Although palliative and hospice care have the potential to improve the quality of life of ESRD patients and their families, access to these services is limited. In fact, patients with kidney disease comprised only 2.6% of hospice admissions in 2007.[3] The underutilization of hospice services by patients with ESRD has been attributed to the Medicare payment structure; however, it does not explain the underutilization of palliative care services among this group.[37] Patients with ESRD who elect hospice are required to forgo dialysis treatment; however, patients receiving care for a terminal condition not related to ESRD may receive covered services under both the ESRD benefit and hospice benefit.[38] All patients who are discontinuing dialysis for ESRD or those with ESRD who refuse to initiate dialysis should be considered for hospice.

Over 60% of patients with advanced kidney disease die in the hospital.[35] Recognizing the need for improved palliative care, some dialysis clinics and hospitals are developing palliative care initiatives with the goal of integrating palliative care into routine nephrology practice.[39]

### Palliative Management

The primary components of palliative care in ESRD are outlined in Table 36–4.

### Communication and Care Planning

Advance care planning is an important consideration in ESRD because patients are likely to face important treatment

**Table 36–4**
**Components of Palliative Care in ESRD**

Advance care planning
Symptom management
Psychosocial and spirtual support
Ethical issues in dialysis decision-making

*Source*: Adapted from Poppel et al. 2003.

**Table 36–5**
**Guidelines for Discussing Dialysis Withdrawal[41]**

1. Identify patients who may benefit from withdrawal.
   a. Very limited prognosis
   b. Poor quality of life
   c. Pain unresponsive to treatment
   d. Progressive untreatable disease
   e. Dialysis technically difficult
2. Discuss goals of care with patient and family.
3. Discuss quality of life.
4. Discuss possible symptoms and their management.
5. Clarify that dialysis withdrawal is an option.
6. Reassure that it can result in a peaceful death.
7. Make recommendation to stop dialysis and request family support.
8. Provide reassurance that the decision is reversible.

decisions as their disease progresses, including potentially deciding to forego dialysis. Although most dialysis patients discuss their end-of-life wishes, far fewer complete advance directives.[40] Similarly to others with progressive conditions, discussions of advance care planning should focus should on health states that the patient would deem unacceptable, rather than on treatment interventions.

## Withdrawal of Dialysis

The goal of dialysis goes beyond life prolongation to include quality-of-life benefits. However, when the burdens associated with treatment outweigh the benefits or if dialysis is only serving to prolong a patient's death, discontinuation of dialysis should be considered. Once considered a form of suicide, stopping dialysis is now an accepted practice with a sound ethical basis. Today, approximately 25% of patients with ESRD decide to withdraw dialysis.[41]

Patients and families who are considering stopping dialyisis should be informed that the average survival time following dialysis withdrawal is 8 to 10 days but, depending on reserve renal status, could be weeks.[42] Table 36–5 describes guidelines for discussion about dialysis withdrawal. Uremic death is usually peaceful and is typically preceded by progressive encephalopathy. Symptoms that may be experienced in the last 24 hours of life include confusion/agitation, nausea, pain, anxiety, pruritis, and edema.[43]

## Symptom Management

Pain is a common and severe symptom in ESRD and is undertreated in 75% of patients.[44] Pain should be managed similarly to other chronic conditions, but opioids that are metabolized by the kidneys such as morphine, propoxyphene, codeine, and meperidine should be avoided. Morphine use can lead to the accumulation of active metabolites that are neurotoxic, and chronic use can lead to myoclonus. Fentanyl and methadone are safe and effective in patients with renal insufficiency, whereas hydromorphone and oxycodone should be used with caution.[45]

Delirium resulting from uremic encephalopathy frequently manifests itself as mild confusion. Haloperidol is effective and will help to manage nausea and vomiting as well. Pruritis is treated with diphenhydramine or benzodiazepines, in addition to nonpharmacological approaches.

Tube feedings and hydration should be avoided as they may contribute to peripheral edema and excessive secretions. Dyspnea should be managed with opioids, and anticholingeric medications such as atropine will help to control secretions.

## Alzheimer's Disease/Dementia

Alzheimer's dementia is an irreversible, progressive brain disease that slowly destroys memory and thinking skills. Alzheimer's disease accounts for approximately half of all dementias. Other types of dementia are listed in Table 36–6. Typical of other progressive chronic illnesses, the course of dementia is one of continuing gradual decline. The median survival after diagnosis of Alzheimer's disease is 4 to 6 years.[46] The incidence of Alzheimer's disease is rising and it is now the courth leading cause of death in persons over age 65. Approximately 4.5 million people in the United States are estimated to have Alzheimer's disease; by the year 2050, this number may reach 16 million.[46]

There are a number of causes of dementia, including neurodegenerative changes in the brain, strokes, head injuries, drugs, and nutritional deficiencies. In Alzheimer's disease, abnormal protein deposits in the brain destroy cells that control mental functions and memory. Vascular dementia is caused by atherosclerosis in the brain, leading to multiple strokes. Lewy body dementias are caused by abnormal deposits of Lewy body protein in the brain. Patients with Lewy body dementia have symptoms similar to patients with Parkinson's disease, including tremor and muscle rigidity, and are more likely to experience delirium and hallucinations. The diagnosis of dementia is not straightforward and is largely established by a combination of clinical findings and confirmed by physiological changes in the brain seen on MRI or on autopsy.

| Table 36-6 |
| --- |
| Dementia Subtypes and Prevalence |
| Alzheimer's Disease 40%–75% |
| Cerebrovascular dementia 15%–30% |
| Lewy Body dementia 10%–15% |
| Frontotemporal dementia <1% |

| Table 36-7 |
| --- |
| Clinical Presentation of Severe Dementia |
| Neurocognitive |
| -Progressive worsening of: |
| • Memory |
| • Confusion/disorientation |
| • Combativeness |
| • Inability to communicate |
| • Incoherent and unresponsive |
| • Inability to recognize self |
| Functional |
| • Loss of ability to walk or maintain posture |
| • Totally dependent on others for care |
| Nutritional |
| • Progressive loss of appetite |
| • Loss of ability to recognize food |
| • Loss of capacity to swallow |
| Miscellaneous |
| • Bowel and bladder incontinence |
| • Fevers and infections |
| • Decubitus ulcers |
| • Development of contractures |

*Source*: Data from Ouldred E, Bryant C. Dementia care. Part 3: end-of-life care for people with advanced dementia. Br J Nurs 2008;17(5):308–314.

## Symptoms

Alzheimer's disease progresses slowly, and its symptoms are variable depending on the area of the brain affected. One of the first areas to be affected is the hippocampus, located in the temporal lobe. The hippocampus plays an essential role in processing new memories and in spatial navigation. Areas of the brain responsible for reasoning, emotional responses, language, and memory are also commonly involved, whereas the occipital lobe, which is responsible for visual processing, as well as primary sensory and motor neurons, are usually spared. Once the dementia has reached the severe stage, most memory is lost and patients experience incontinence, eating difficulties, and motor impairment. In the advanced/terminal stage, patients are usually bedfast, mute, and dysphagic and suffer from infections. At this stage, patients usually die from complications such as pneumonia, urinary tract infections, hip fractures, or as a consequence of malnutrition. Table 36-7 lists the clinical presentation of severe dementia.

## Symptom Management

### Behavioral Symptoms

Patients with dementia frequently exhibit behavioral symptoms such as agitation, depression, delirium, and, in some cases, hallucinations and psychosis. The management of these behaviors is important to the quality of life of the patient and his/her caregiver.[47]

In the mid-1990s, a group of medications called cholinesterase inhibitors (e.g., glanatamine, donepezil, and rivastigmine) were FDA-approved for the treatment of mild-to-moderate Alzheimer's disease. More recently, donepezil was approved for use in patients with moderate-to-severe disease. These agents may improve neuropsychiatric symptoms such as agitation, hallucinations, depression, nighttime behaviors, and appetite disorders and may delay disease progression in some patients.[48] The clinical significance of cholinesterase inhibitors is debated and they are estimated to benefit only about half of those who take them, although a small percentage of patients may benefit dramatically.[49] Memantine, a N-methyl-D-aspartic acid (NMDA) receptor antagonist was FDA-approved in 2003 to help slow progression of symptoms in the severe stages of illness.[50] Because of a lack of data describing the value of these medications in patients with disease advanced enough to meet hospice eligibility criteria, clinicians generally rely on clinical experience and patient/ family preferences to evaluate whether to recommend continuing or discontinuing these therapies in hospice patients. A study of a large national hospice pharmacy database indicated that 21% of patients were prescribed either a cholinesterase inhibitor or NMDA receptor antagonist at the time of hospice enrollment.[51] In addition to questionable efficacy, the high cost is likely an additional deterrent to their use in hospice.

### Agitation and Delirium

Agitation is an imprecise term that refers to restlessness accompanied by mental tension. Patients who are agitated are often seen pacing or may pull off their clothes or have vocal outbursts. Common causes of agitation in dementia patients include untreated or mismanaged pain, urinary retention, or social isolation. Agitation can be confused with delirium, which is an acute symptom characterized by disturbances in attention, cognition, and perception.[52] Delirium frequently goes unrecognized and has many underlying causes. It is often difficult to differentiate between dementia and delirium as they share common clinical features, such as impaired memory or thinking. Patients experiencing delirium have a fluctuating level of consciousness, altered attention span, and disturbed sleep–wake cycle, whereas dementia is characterized by little to no clouding of consciousness; chronic, progressive symptoms; and less impaired sleep–wake cycle. Resolution of delirium depends on the resolution (when possible) of the underlying cause. Nonpharmacological approaches, such as providing sensory stimulation, reorientation, and reassurance, are important. When a pharmacological approach is needed, a benzodiazepine such as lorazepam is generally used to manage agitation. Although not approved for this indication, antipsychotic agents such as haloperidol or risperidone are frequently used to treat delirium or psychosis in dementia patients. These medications should be used judiciously, as recent meta-analyses have revealed that treatment with either typical or atypical antipsychotics increase the risk of death in patients, especially among those taking higher than conventional doses.[53] Despite these warnings, when used appropriately, antipsychotic drugs can have quality-of-life benefits in patients with advanced dementia and should be prescribed based on the goals of care and at the discretion of the prescriber after sharing the potential risk with the caregiver. It is important to recognize that patients with Lewy Body dementia can be very sensitive to the effects of neuroleptic and anticholinergic medications, and they should be avoided in this patient population. Quetiapine is the first-line atypical antipsychotic agent for these patients or for those with Parkinson's disease; however, it should be used with caution and only when benefits clearly outweigh risks.

## Depression

Depression is prevalent in approximately 20% to 25% of persons with dementia, although because of the difficulties associated with assessing depression, it may be underreported.[54] Depression may also be confused with apathy, which is commonly seen in Alzheimer's disease, especially in more advanced stages. In addition to nonpharmacological approaches such as providing social interaction and activity, pharmacological management might be indicated. The medications of choice for depression are SSRIs because of their low side effect profile and reasonable tolerability in the elderly. If the patient has a poor prognosis, then a trial of a psychostimulant is recommended. Because of the risk for adverse effects in the elderly, start with the lowest dose and slowly titrate upward.

## Pain

Patients with dementia tend to be older and are at risk to experience chronic pain commonly associated with aging. In addition to pain from comorbid conditions, patients with advanced disease may have pain resulting from immobility or as a consequence of complications such as urinary tract infections or decubitus ulcers. Pain perception and pain thresholds of persons with dementia are thought to be similar to that of the cognitively intact older adult.[55] Cognitively impaired persons are at increased risk for undertreatment of their pain.[56] Persons with dementia might not be able to report pain because of reduced verbal capacity and thinking, so pain assessment in this population can be especially challenging. Although some patients with dementia are able to self-report, for those who are unable, a variety of assessment strategies should be employed. These include searching for potential causes of pain or discomfort or monitoring behaviors indicative of pain.[57] Pain in advanced dementia may present as agitation or social withdrawal and may be accompanied by vocalizations, grimacing, or bracing. There are a number of validated observation scales to assess pain in persons with dementia, such as the Pain Assessment in Advanced Dementia (PAIN-AD) tool. The PAIN-AD scale consists of five items: negative vocalization, facial expression, body language, consolability, and a scale that allows the practitioner to assign a score to a particular behavior in a standardized manner. Each element of the scale can be scored from 0 to 2, for a total score of 0 to 10 (maximal pain).[58] However, the lack of specificity when observing pain behaviors remains a challenge; therefore, pain experts recommend an empirical analgesic trial if pain is suspected.[59] Furthermore, patients who require opioids should not have them withheld because of concerns about worsening confusion as this concern is not supported by the literature.[60]

## End-Stage Issues

In the advanced stage of dementia, the patient becomes totally dependent on others for care and is at risk for developing complications such as urinary tract infections, pneumonia, fractures, and swallowing difficulties. When possible, advanced care planning should take place early in the disease course, and a surrogate decision-maker should be appointed to make treatment decisions when the patient loses decisional capacity.

## Nutrition and Hydration

One of the more challenging end-stage concerns for family members relates to the problem of nutrition and hydration. Persons in the advanced stages of dementia experience a progressive loss of appetite, loss of ability to swallow, and increased aspiration risk. Eventually, they resist or become indifferent to eating, have difficulty handling food in their mouths, and are at high risk for choking when swallowing.[61] The use of artificial nutrition and hydration in the final stages of dementia is controversial. Various studies have demonstrated that feeding tubes are not associated with good outcomes; specifically, they have not been demonstrated to prevent malnutrition, pressure ulcers, or aspiration pneumonia nor do they provide comfort or prolong survival.[61] Caregivers are encouraged to hand-feed as long as possible and to use a variety of strategies to improve food intake. Caregivers need to be reassured that patients with end-stage dementia can be kept comfortable without the use of feeding tubes.

## Treatment of Infections

Infections are common among persons with end-stage dementia. Similarly to other end-of-life management issues, the use of antibiotics to treat infections is not without controversy.

A recent study showed that antibiotics are frequently used in patients with advanced dementia, particularly in the last 2 weeks of life.[62] However, in addition to public health concerns about the spread of antimicrobial-resistant bacteria, the provision of antibiotics can be burdensome and may not promote comfort any better than good palliative care would.[62]

## Hospice Care for Dementia

As the dementia approaches the end-stage, hospice should be considered, as hospice enrollment is associated with improved patient and caregiver outcomes compared to routine care.[63,64] Given the shifts in disease prevalence and benefits of hospice, it is not surprising that dementia now represents the third most common non-cancer diagnosis for hospice services. In 2007, dementia accounted for 10.1% of hospice admissions, compared to only 6.9% in 2001.[3,65]

Similarly to other chronic illnesses, patients with Alzheimer's disease or other subtypes of dementia meet Medicare hospice eligibility requirements once they have a predicted life expectancy of 6 months or less and have decided not to continue cure-focused therapies. According to NHPCO guidelines, hospice-eligible patients with dementia are those who are unable to walk, unable to dress or bathe without assistance, have urinary and fecal incontinence, and cannot speak more than five intelligible words daily (FAST stage 7c). In addition to these functional limitations, hospice eligibility requirements include the presence of coexisting medical complications such as aspiration pneumonia, urinary tract infections, sepsis, decubitus ulcers, or weight loss.[66] Caregivers of dementia patients endure many losses throughout the disease process and require a great deal of support.

## Neurodengerative Diseases: Amyotrophic Lateral Sclerosis and Parkinson's Disease

### Amyotrophic Lateral Sclerosis

Amyotrophic Lateral Sclerosis (ALS) is a progressive neurodegenerative disease with no known cure that affects both upper and lower motor neurons. Although rare, it is estimated that up to 30,000 Americans have ALS at any given time. ALS is more common among males and usually develops between the ages of 40 and 70 years, although cases can develop in younger persons.[67] Development of ALS is usually sporadic, although 5% to 10% of cases are familial.[68] The course and prognosis of ALS is variable and may depend on whether patients opt for therapies that can prolong survival, such as mechanical ventilation. Median survival is approximately 3 years, although patients may live 15 years or longer with long-term mechanical ventilation.[68] Respiratory failure resulting from progressive respiratory muscle weakness is the most common cause of death from ALS.

| Table 36–8 Symptoms of ALS | |
|---|---|
| **Direct** | **Indirect** |
| Progressive muscle weakness and atrophy | Depression Anxiety Sleep disturbances |
| Fasciculations and muscle cramps | Thick secretions and/or drooling Pain/muscle aches |
| Spasticity | Symptoms of chronic |
| Slurred or slowed speech | hypoventilation (morning headache, anorexia, weight |
| Pathological laughter or crying | loss, depression/anxiety, dyspnea, severe fatigue) |
| Dyspnea Dysphagia | |

ALS usually presents with arm or leg weakness. Over time, the weakness increases in severity and affects more areas of the body until only sphincter control and eye movements are spared.[68] Although cognition usually remains intact, cognitive impairment and dementia has been noted to occur in close to one-third of individuals with ALS.[69] There is no definitive diagnostic test for ALS, and it is frequently a diagnosis of exclusion, which may take months. Currently, riluzole, a glutamate antagonist is the only FDA-approved treatment for ALS. Riluzole prolongs survival by 3 to 6 months in some patients but does not improve functional status.[70]

Individuals with ALS suffer numerous symptoms that are directly or indirectly related to the disease (Table 36–8). An interdisciplinary approach, preferably at a specialized ALS center, is helpful in addressing the myriad of issues that patients with ALS and their families face.[68] Physical and occupational therapists assist patients in performing activities of daily living by improving mobility, reducing spasticity, and providing adaptive equipment. Speech therapists help to facilitate communication. Symptomatic treatments include anticholinergics such as atropine drops to reduce drooling,[71] quinine sulfate or carbamazine for muscle cramps, baclofen for spasticity, and tricyclic antidepressants such as amitriptyline to help reduce uncontrollable laughing or crying. Depression, insomnia, and anxiety are also common and should be treated accordingly. As swallowing problems emerge, patients may benefit from placement of a percutaneous endoscopic gastrostomy tube.[72] When breathing difficulties develop, patients require some type of ventilatory support. Most patients opt for bilevel positive airway pressure support that has been found to improve symptoms of hypoventilation, quality of life, and survival.[73] Fewer patients agree to the use of mechanical ventilation because of concerns about prolonged immobilization, limited communication, and family burden.[68] Home hospice can provide much -needed physical, psychological, and spiritual support and should be discussed before lung capacity considerably declines.

## Parkinson's Disease

Parkinson's disease is a degenerative motor system disorder that results from the progressive loss of dopamine-producing brain cells. Without dopamine, the nerve cells cannot properly transmit messages, resulting in loss of muscle function. Hallmark symptoms include trembling of hands, arms, legs, jaw and face, stiffness of the arms, legs and trunk, slowness of voluntary movement, and poor balance and coordination. As symptoms progress, individuals with Parkinson's disease may develop depression, sleep disorders, difficulty swallowing or speaking, delayed gastric emptying, constipation, bladder dysfunction/incontinence, pain, psychosis, and dementia. There is no specific test to diagnose dementia; diagnosis depends on the presence of at least two of three major signs: tremor at rest, rigidity, and bradykinesia in the absence of secondary causes such as dopamine-depleting medications. Parkinson's disease prevalence increases with age and it usually has a long, chronic course.

Currently, there are numerous treatments that improve motor function and quality of life; however, there is no known cure for Parkinson's disease, and persons affected with the disease become increasingly disabled over time. Patients sometimes need to be cared for in long-term care settings as they become increasingly functionally disabled.[74] Parkinson's disease is treated with a variety of drugs such as carbidopa/levodopa, dopamine agonists, and MAO-B inhibitors.[75] Unfortunately, long-term levodopa use results in dyskinesias, such as writhing, twisting, and shaking. Dyskinesias are a dose-limiting effect of these agents over time. Some patients are candidates for deep-brain stimulation to block electrical signals in the brain that cause Parkinson's disease symptoms. When effective, patients treated with deep-brain stimulation experience significant improvements in motor function and quality of life without troubling side effects associated with medical therapy.[76] Once the patient becomes increasingly disabled despite optimal therapy, goals of care may shift more towards palliation. Patients usually die as a result of complications of the disease, such as from pneumonia or other infections. Similarly to caring for those with ALS, patients with Parkinson's disease require a multidisciplinary approach to address the debilitating and distressing aspects of the disease.

Good nursing care, including skin care, oral hygiene, positioning, incontinence and constipation management, and support for end-of-life decision making is an important part of care for a patient with Parkinson's disease. Pain is a common problem arising from restricted movement, rigidity, or spasms and should be treated with analgesics in a fashion similar to other chronic diseases. Psychosis or hallucinations are traditionally treated by reducing the dose or eliminating dopaminergic or anticholinergic drugs used to treat Parkinson's disease, even if motor symptoms worsen as a consequence.[74] If an antipsychotic is required, then quetiapine is preferred because the use of risperidone or olanzapine or haloperidol is associated with worsening of Parkinsonian symptoms,[77] although its efficacy is limited.[78]

## Conclusion

The prevalence of chronic illness is increasing as the population ages. Despite differences in illness trajectories and difficulty estimating prognosis, patients with chronic non-cancer conditions experience similar symptoms and have common needs as the illness progresses. Individuals with chronic progressive illness and their families benefit from an interdisciplinary palliative approach to care, and as the disease advances, hospice care should be considered.

REFERENCES

1. Centers for Disease Control. National Vital Statistics System. June 16 2008; Available from http://www.cdc.gov/nchs/data/dvs/LCWK9_2005.pdf
2. Lynn J, Schuster JL, Kabcenell A. Improving Care for the End of Life: A Sourcebook for Healthcare Managers and Clinicians. New York: Oxford University Press, 2000.
3. National Hospice and Palliative Care Organization. NHPCO Facts and Figures: Hospice Care in America. 2008 [cited December 7 2008]; Available from http://www.nhpco.org/files/public/Statistics_Research/NHPCO_facts-and-figures_2008.pdf.
4. National Hospice Organization. Medical Guidelines for Determining Prognosis in Selected Non-cancer Diseases. Arlington, VA: National Hospice Organization, 1995.
5. American Heart Association Heart Disease and Stroke Statistics—2008 [cited 2008 Dec 23]; Available from http://www.americanheart.org/presenter.jhtml?identifier=1200026.
6. Jong P, Vowinckel E, Liu P, Gong Y, Tu JV. Prognosis and determinants of survival in patients newly hospitalized for heart failure: A population-based study. Arch Intern Med 2002;162:1689–1694.
7. Hunt SA, Baker DW Chin MH, et al. ACC/AHA guidelines for the evaluation and management of chronic heart failure in the adult: Executive summary: A report of the American College of Cardiology/American Heart Association Task Force on Practice Guidelines. J Am Coll Cardiol 2001;38:2101–2113.
8. Hunt SA, Abraham WT, Chin MH, et al. Chronic Heart Failure in the Adult: ACC/AHA 2005 guidelines for the evaluation and management of chronic heart failure in the adult: Executive summary: A report of the American College of Cardiology/American Heart Association Task Force on Practice Guidelines. (Committee to revise the 1995 Guidelines for the Evaluation and Management of Heart Failure) J Am Coll Cardiol 2005;46:1116–1143.
9. Jessup M, Bronza S. Heart failure. N Engl J Med 2003;348:2007–2018.
10. Levenson JW, McCarthy EP, Lynn J, Davis RB, Phillips RS. The last six months of life for patients with congestive heart failure. J Am Geriatr Soc 2000;48(5 Suppl):S101–S109.
11. Stuart B. Palliative care and hospice in advanced heart failure. J Pall Med 2007;10(2):210–228.
12. Page J, Henry, D. Consumption of NSAIDs and the development of congestive heart failure in elderly patients: An under recognized public health problem. Arch Intern Med 2000;160:777–784.

13. Haque WA, Boehmer J, Clemson BS, Leuenberger UA, Silber DH, Sionway LI. Hemodynamic effects of supplemental oxygen in congestive heart failure. J Am Coll Cardiol 1996:27:353–357.

14. Jennings AL, Davies AN, Higgins JPT, Gibbs JSR, Broadley KE. A systematic review of the use of opioids in the management of dyspnoea. Thorax. 2002;57(11):939–944.

15. Abernethy AP, Currow DC, Frith P, Fazekas BS, McHugh A, Bui C. Randomised, double blind, placebo controlled crossover trial of sustained release morphine for the management of refractory dyspnoea. Br Med J 2003;327(7414):523–528.

16. Hallenbeck JL. Non-pain symptom management: Dyspnea. In: Hallenbeck JL, ed. Palliative Care Perspectives. New York: Oxford University Press; 2003.

17. Williams CM. Dyspnea. Cancer J. 2006;12(5):365–373.

18. Cuffe MS, Califf RM, Adams KF Jr, et al. Outcomes of a Prospective Trial of Intravenous Milrinone for Exacerbations of Chronic Heart Failure (OPTIME_CHF) Investigators. JAMA 2002;287:1541–1547.

19. Nohria A, Lewis E, Stevenson LW. Medical management of advanced heart failure. JAMA 2002;287(5):628–640.

20. Moss AJ, Hall WJ, Cannom DS, et al.; for the Multicenter Automatic Defibrillator Implantation Trial Investigators. Improved survival with an implanted defibrillator in patients with coronary artery disease at high risk for ventricular arrhythmia. N Engl J Med 1996;335:1933–1940.

21. Kelley AS, Mehta SS, Reid MC. Management of patients with ICDs at the end of life (EOL): A qualitative study. Am J Hosp Pall Med 2009;25:440–446.

22. Renlund DG, Kfoury AG. When the failing, end stage heart is not end stage. N Engl J Med 2006;355:1922–1925.

23. Rose EA, Gelijns AC, Moskowitz AJ, et al. Long-term use of a left ventricular assist device for end-stage heart failure. N Engl J Med 2001;345:1435–1443.

24. Weigand DLM, Kalowes PG. Withdrawal of cardiac medications and devices. AACN Adv Crit Care 2007;18:415–425.

25. Hauptman PJ, Havanek EP. Integrating palliative care into heart failure care. Arch Int Med 2005;165: 374–378.

26. Stuart B, Alexander C, Arenella C, et al. Medical guidelines for determining prognosis in selected non-cancer diseases (2nd ed). Arlington BA. National Hospice Organization, 1996.

27. Jemal A, Ward E, Hao Y, Thun M. Trends in the leading causes of death in the United States, 1970–2002. JAMA 2006;295(4):393–394.

28. Lopez AD, Shibuya K, Rao C, et al. Chronic obstructive pulmonary disease: Current burden and future projections. Eur Respir J 2006;27:397–412.

29. Global Initiative for Chronic Obstructive Lung Disease (GOLD). Global Strategy for the Diagnosis, Management, and Prevention of Chronic Obstructive Pulmonary Disease (2007). http://www.goldcopd.com/Guidelineitem.asp?l1=2&l2=1&intId=989 (accessed December 2008).

30. Gorecka D, Gorzelak K, Sliwinski P, Tobiasz M, Zielinski J. Effect of long term oxygen therapy on survival in patients with chronic obstructive pulmonary disease with moderate hypoxaemia. Thorax 1997;52(8):674–679.

31. Poole PJ, Veale AG, Black PN. The effect of sustained-release morphine on breathlessness and quality of life in severe chronic obstructive pulmonary disease. Am J Respir Crit Care Med 1998;157:1877–1880.

32. Masood, AR, Reed, JW, Thomas SH. Lack of effect of inhaled morphine on exercise-induced breathlessness in chronic obstructive pulmonary disease. Thorax 1995;50:629–634.

33. Mitch WE. Chronic kidney disease. In: Goldman L, Ausiello D, eds. Goldman: Cecil Medicine (23rd ed). Philadelphia, PA: Saunders Elsevier; 2007: chap 131.

34. Cowie CC, Port FK, Wolfe RA, Savage PJ, Moll PP, Hawthorne VM. Disparities in incidence of diabetic end-stage renal disease according to race and type of diabetes. N Engl J Med 1989;321:1074–1079.

35. U.S. Renal Data System. USRDS 2008 Annual Data Report: Atlas of Chronic Kidney Disease and End-Stage Renal Disease in the United States. National Institutes of Health; National Institute of Diabetes and Digestive and Kidney Diseases 2008. Available from http://www.usrds.org/adr.htm.

36. Weisbord SD, Carmody SS, Bruns FJ, et al. Symptom burden, quality of life, advance care planning and the potential value of palliative care in severely ill hemodialysis patients. Nephrol Dial Transplant 2003;18(7):1345–1352.

37. Owens DA. Palliative and End Stage Renal Disease. J Hosp Palliat Nurs 2006;8(6):318–319.

38. CMS Pub 100–2. Medicare Benefit Policy Manual (2004). Chapter 9, Coverage of hospice services under hospital insurance, §10, 10/21, 40.19, 40.24; Chapter 11, End stage renal disease (ESRD), § 50.6.1.4.

39. Poppel DM, Cohen LM, Germain MJ. The renal palliative care initiative. J Palliat Med 2003;6:321–326.

40. Singer PA. Advance care planning in dialysis. Am J Kidney Dis 1999;33:688–693.

41. Cohen LM, Germain MJ, Poppel DM. Practical considerations in dialysis withdrawal: "To have that option is a blessing". JAMA 2003;289(16):2113–2119.

42. Davison SN, Rosielle DA. Withdrawal of dialysis: Decision-making. Fast Facts and Concepts. September 2008; 207. Available from http://www.eperc.mcw.edu/fastfact/ff_207.htm.

43. Cohen LM, Germain M. Poppel D, Woods A, Kjellstrand CM. Dialysis discontinuation and palliative care. Am J Kidney Dis 2000;36(1):140–144.

44. Davison SN. Pain in hemodialysis patients: Prevalence, cause and management. Am J Kidney Dis 2003;42:1239–1247.

45. Dean M. Opioids in renal failure and dialysis patients. J Pain Symptom Manage 2004;28(5):497–504.

46. Wolfson C, Wolfson DB, Asgharian M, et al. Clinical Progression of Dementia Study Group. A reevaluation of the duration of survival after the onset of dementia. N Engl J Med. 2001;344(15):1160–1161.

47. Samus QM, Rosenblatt A, Steele C, Baker A, Harper M, et al. The association of neuropsychiatric symptoms and environment with quality of life in assisted living residents with dementia. Gerontologist 2005;45(1):19–26.

48. Trinh N, Hoblyn J, Mohanty S, Yaffe K. Efficacy of cholinesterase inhibitors in the treatment of neuropsychiatric symptoms and functional impairment in Alzheimer's disease. JAMA 2003;289(2):210–216.

49. Kaduszkiewicz H, Wiese B, Van den Bussche H. Self-reported competence, attitude and approach of physicians towards patients with dementia in ambulatory care: Results of a postal survey. BMC Health Serv Res 2008;8:54.

50. FDA news. FDA Approves Memantine (Namenda) for Alzheimer's Disease; 2003. Available at http://www.fda.gov/bbs/topics/news/2003/new00961.html. (accessed December 19, 2008).

51. Weschules DJ, Maxwell TL, Shega JW. Acetylcholinesterase inhibitor and N-Methyl-D-aspartic acid receptor antagonist use among hospice enrollees with a primary diagnosis of dementia. J Palliat Med 2008;11(5):738–745.

52. Elici-Evcime Y, Breitbart W. An update on the use of antipsychotics in the treatment of delirium. Palliat Support Care 2008;6:177–182.

53. Schnieder L, Dagerman K, Insel P. Efficacy and adverse effects of atypical antyipsychotics for dementia: Meta-analysis of randomized, placebo-controlled trains. Am J Geriatr Psychiatry 2006;14(3):191–202.

54. Landes AM, Sperry SD, Strauss ME. Prevalence of apathy, dysphoria, and depression in relation to dementia severity in Alzheimer's Disease. J Neuropsychiatry Clin Neurosci 2005;17:343–349.

55. AGS Panel on Persistent Pain in Older Persons. The management of persistent pain in older persons. J Am Geriatr Soc 2002;50:1–20.

56. Bernabei R, Gambassi G, Lapane K, et al. Management of pain in elderly patients with cancer. JAMA 1998;279(23):1877–1882.

57. Herr K, Coyne PJ, Key T, et al. Pain assessment in the nonverbal patient: Position statement with clinical practice recommendations. Pain Manag Nurs 2006;7(2):44–52.

58. Lane P, Kuntupis M, MacDonald S, et al. A pain assessment tool for people with advanced Alzheimer's and other progressive dementias. Home Healthc Nurse 2003;21(1):32–37.

59. AGS Panel on Persistent Pain in Older Persons. The management of persistent pain in older persons. JAGS 2002;50:S205–S224.

60. Ersek M, Cherrier MM, Overman SS, Irving GA. The cognitive effects of opioids. Pain Manag Nurs 2004;5(2):75–93.

61. Li I. Feeding tubes in patients with severe dementia. Am Fam Physician 2002;65:1605–1610.

62. D'Agata E, Mitchell S. Patterns of antimicrobial use among nursing home residents with advanced dementia. Arch Intern Med 2008;168(4):357–362.

63. Mumm J, Hanson L, Zimmerman S, Sloane P, Mitchell CM. Is Hospice Associated with Improved End-of-Life Care in Nursing Homes and Assisted Living Facilities? J Am Geriatr Soc 2006;54:490–495.

64. Shega JW, Hougham GW, Stocking CB, Cox-Hayley D, Sachs GA. Patients dying with dementia: Experience at the end of life and impact of hospice care. J Pain Symptom Manage 2008;35(5):499–507.

65. Connor SR, Tecca M, LundPerson J, Teno J. Measuring hospice care: The National Hospice and Palliative Care Organization National Hospice Data Set. J Pain Symptom Manage 2004;28(4):316–328.

66. Stuart B. The NHO Medical Guidelines for Non-Cancer Disease and local medical review policy: Hospice access for patients with diseases other than cancer. Hosp J 1999;14(3–4):139–154.

67. Amyotrophic Lateral Sclerosis (ALS) Association. Who gets ALS. 2008 Sep 1(1):[1 screen] Available from http://www.alsa.org/als/who.cfm. (accessed December 30, 2008).

68. Mitsumoto H, Rabkin JG. Palliative care for patients with amyotrophic lateral sclerosis. JAMA 2007;298(2):207–216.

69. Corcia P, Meininger V. Management of amyotrophic lateral sclerosis. Drugs 2008;68(8)1037–1048.

70. Rowland LP, Shneider MA. Amyotrophic lateral sclerosis. N Eng J Med 2001;344(22):1688–1700.

71. De Simone GG, Eisenchlas JH, Junin M, Pereyra F, Brizuela R. Atropine drops for drooling: A randomized controlled trial. Palliat Med 2006;20(7):665–671.

72. Miller RG, Rosenberg JA, Gelinas DF, et al. Practice parameter: The care of the patient with amyotrophic lateral sclerosis (an evidence-based review). Neurology 1999;52(7):1311–1323.

73. Bach JR. Amyotrophic Lateral Sclerosis: Prolongation of life by noninvasive respiratory aids. Chest 2002;122(1):92–98.

74. Chen JJ, Trombetta DP, Fernandez HH. Palliative management of Parkinson's Disease: Focus on nonmotor, distressing symptoms. J Pharm Prac 2008;21:262–272.

75. Chen JJ, Swope DM. Pharmacotherapy for Parkinson's Disease. Pharmacotherapy 2007;27(12):162S–173S.

76. Weaver FM, Follett K, Stern M, et al. Bilateral deep brain stimulation vs best medical therapy for patients with advanced Parkinson disease. JAMA 2009;301(1):63–73.

77. Friedman JH, Fernandez HH. Atypical antipsychotics in Parkinson's sensitive populations. J Geriatr Psychiatry Neurol 2002;15:156–170.

78. Kurlan R, Cummings J, Raman R, Thal L. Quetiapine for agitation or psychosis in patients with dementia and parkinsonism. Neurology 2007;68:1356–1363.

# 37

*Polly Mazanec and Joan T. Panke*

# Cultural Considerations in Palliative Care

*Life is pleasant. Death is peaceful. It's the transition that's troublesome.—Isaac Asimov*

◆ **Key Points**

◆ *Quality palliative care requires attention to patient and family cultural values, practices, and beliefs.*

◆ *A multidimensional assessment of culture is essential to planning palliative care for patients and families.*

◆ *An individual's culture encompasses multiple components, including ethnicity, age, race, gender, and religion/spirituality.*

This chapter defines culture and the complexity of its components as they relate to palliative care. It emphasizes how recognizing one's own values, practices, and beliefs impact care. Finally, selected palliative care concepts and issues influenced by culture are discussed. This chapter is not intended to be a "cookbook" approach to describing behaviors and practices of different cultures as they relate to palliative care but, rather, a guide to raising awareness of the significance of cultural considerations in palliative care.

## Culture and Palliative Care Nursing

The essence of palliative nursing is to provide holistic supportive care for the patient and the family living with a life-limiting illness. Palliative nursing strives to meet the physical, emotional, social, and spiritual needs of the patient and family across the disease trajectory.[1] To meet these needs, nurses must recognize the vital role that culture has on one's experience of living and dying. The beliefs, norms, and practices of an individual's cultural heritage guide one's behavioral responses, decision-making, and actions.[2] Culture shapes how an individual makes meaning out of illness, suffering, and death.[2,3] Nurses, along with other members of the interdisciplinary team, partner with the patient and family to ensure that patient and family values, beliefs, and practices guide the plan of care. *The Clinical Practice Guidelines for Quality Palliative Care* recommend attention to cultural considerations for patients and families living with a life-limiting illness and facing the transition to end of life (Table 37–1).[4]

The following case illustrates the distress experienced by the patient, family, and health-care team when cultural implications of care are not considered.

**Table 37–1**
**Clinical Practice Guidelines for Quality Palliative Care—Cultural Aspects of Care**

**Guideline 6.1 The palliative care program assesses and attempts to meet the culture-specific needs of the patient and family.**
Criteria:
- The cultural background, concerns, and needs of the patient and their family are elicited and documented.
- Cultural needs identified by team and family are addressed in the interdisciplinary team care plan.
- Communication with patient and family is respectful of their cultural preferences regarding disclosure, truth-telling, and decision-making.
- The program aims to respect and accommodate the range of language, dietary, and ritual practices of patients and their families.
- When possible, the team has access to and utilizes appropriate interpreter services.
- Recruitment and hiring practices strive to reflect the cultural diversity of the community.

*Source*: www.nationalconsensusproject.org.

CASE STUDY
*Cultural Issues in a Man with Severe Head Injury*

Mr. B is a 54-year-old male who suffered severe head injury from a car accident. He was successfully resuscitated at the scene and intubated, and he is currently in the intensive care unit (ICU). Tests reveal minimal brain activity. It is unlikely that he will recover any brain function beyond primitive brain stem function. The primary team, along with consulting services, agrees that at best he will remain in a persistent vegetative state.

Mr. B is single and has no living relatives. His stepfather is his closest family relation and lives out of state. Information obtained from the stepfather includes that the patient's mother died after a long battle with cancer 6 months ago in an ICU and on a ventilator. He also relates that Mr. B is of the Jewish faith, and he and his stepfather were planning on spending the upcoming high holidays together. The stepfather, very distraught, states that Mr. B is all the family he has and asks that all efforts be attempted to save him. He plans to travel to the hospital within the week. Friends and coworkers have been visiting, but no one, including the stepfather, is aware of whether Mr. B had completed any advance directives. A family meeting is planned for the day after the stepfather arrives.

**Questions to Consider in This Case Are:**

1. What cultural issues might arise with this case?
2. What religious/spiritual issues might impact decision-making?

3. Who might the palliative team involve to assist in ascertaining religious or cultural aspects of care?
4. Who should be involved in the family meeting?

## Increasing Diversity in the United States Population

As the United States becomes increasingly diverse, the range of treasured beliefs, shared teachings, norms, customs, and languages challenge the nurse to understand and respond to a wide variety of perspectives. The population in the United States is predicted to exceed 28 million people by 2008.[5] Population statistics from the 2000 National Census illustrate that cultural diversity is increasing among the five most common panethnic groups, which are federally defined as American Indian/Alaskan native, Asian/Pacific Islander, African-American, Hispanic, and white.[6] The Hispanic population, a very heterogeneous group including Mexican-Americans and Latinos, is the largest and fastest growing minority group in the United States.[7] Census 2010 is gathering statistics and developing materials for specific ethnic groups earmarked in 2010 (Table 37–2). Trends suggest that by 2042, the combined minority groups, which currently make up one-third of the U.S. population, will become the majority.[5] Diversity among age groups is also changing as the population ages. In 2030, one in five citizens will be 65 years or older and the 85-year and older age group is expected to more than triple between 2008 and 2050. It is quite probable that intergroup diversity will also increase, adding to the complexity of culturally competent care and the potential for cultural clashes.

With the changes in cultural diversity in the U.S. population comes increasing diversity in the nursing workforce. Nurses must be aware of how one's own cultural beliefs and norms shape professional practice and differ from the beliefs and norms of patients and families for whom they care.

**Table 37–2**
**Ethnic Groups, Census 2010**

American Indian/Alaskan Native
Other Pacific Islanders
Hispanic
Asian
Eastern European
African-American
Haitian

*Source*: https://ask.census.gov/cgi/bin/askcensus (Accessed December 20, 2008).

## Culture Defined

Culture is the "learned, shared and transmitted values, beliefs, norms and life ways of a particular group that guide their thinking, decision, actions in patterned ways—a patterned behavioral response."[8] Culture is shaped over time in a dynamic system in which the beliefs, values, and lifestyle patterns pass from one generation to another.[9] Although culture is often mistakenly thought of as race and ethnicity, the definition of culture expands far beyond, encompassing such dimensions as gender, age, differing abilities, sexual orientation, religion, financial status, residency, employment, and educational level.[2] Each cultural component plays a role in shaping patient and family responses to life-threatening illness.

A broad definition of culture recognizes the various subcultures an individual may associate with that shape experiences and responses in any given situation. The nurse must be constantly aware that the culture of the health-care system and the culture of the nursing profession, as well as personal beliefs, shape how he or she responds to interactions with patients, families, and colleagues.

## Components of Culture

### Race

The commonly held misconception that "race" refers to biological and genetic differences and "ethnicity" refers to cultural variation is outmoded. Race exists not as a natural category but as a social construct.[10] Any discussion of race must include the harsh reality of racism issues and disparities that have plagued society and continue to exist even today. Recent studies have demonstrated the discrimination of persons of certain races regarding health-care practices, treatment options, and hospice utilization.[11–13] When viewed in relation to specific races, morbidity and mortality statistics point to serious gaps in access to quality care. Racial disparities are still evident, even after adjustments for socioeconomic status and other access-related factors are taken into account.[14]

There is often an underlying mistrust of the health-care system. Memories of the Tuskegee syphilis study and segregated hospitals remain with older African-Americans.[15] The combination of mistrust and numerous other complex variables influence palliative care issues such as medical decision-making and advance care planning.[16,17] Compounding the situation is the fact that health-care providers often do not recognize existing biases within systems or themselves.[14,18] These unknown biases may add to the perceived discrimination experienced.[14,18,19]

### Ethnicity

Ethnicity refers to "a group of people that share a common and distinctive racial, national, religious, linguistic, or cultural heritage."[19] The values, practices, and beliefs shared by members of the same ethnic group may influence behavior or response. Ethnicity has been identified as a significant predictor of end-of-life preferences and decision-making.[18] Currently, there are more than 100 ethnic groups and more than 500 American Indian Nations in the United States.[19]

It is important to note that although an individual may belong to a particular ethnic group, he or she may not identify strongly with that group.[8] For example, members of the same family from the same ethnic group may have very different ideas about what is acceptable practice concerning important palliative care concepts such as communication with health-care professionals, medical decision-making, and end-of-life rituals. The tendency to assume that an individual will respond in a certain way because he is a member of an ethnic group contributes to stereotyping. This can lead to inappropriate interventions and unnecessary distress. The nurse should assess each individual's beliefs and practices rather than assuming that he or she holds the beliefs of a particular group. Note that many studies have demonstrated that regardless of race or ethnicity, all persons share common needs at the end of life: being comfortable, being cared for, sustaining or healing relationships, having hope, and honoring spiritual beliefs.[18,20]

### Gender

Cultural norms dictate specific roles for men and women. The significance of gender is evident in areas such as decision-making, caregiving, and pain and symptom management. It is important to have an awareness of family dominance patterns and determine which family member or members hold that dominant role. In some families, decision-making may be the responsibility of the male head of the family or eldest son; in others, it may be the eldest female. For example, those of Asian ethnicity who follow strict Confucian teaching believe that men have absolute authority and are responsible for family decision-making.[21] Discussing prognosis and treatment with a female family member is likely to increase family burden and distress and may result in significant clashes with the health-care team.[22]

### Age

Age has its own identity and culture.[2] Age cohorts are characterized by consumer behaviors, leisure activities, religious activities, education, and labor force participation.[23] Each group has its own beliefs, attitudes and practices, which are influenced by their developmental stage and by the society in which they live. The impact of a life-limiting illness on persons of differing age groups is often influenced by the loss of developmental tasks associated with that age group.[24] As the U.S. population ages, the importance of addressing the unique needs of elders becomes more evident. Consider also the cultural impact of this aging population on caregiving issues, medical decision-making, and end-of-life choices.

## Differing Abilities

Individuals with physical disabilities or mental illness are at risk of receiving poorer quality healthcare. Those with differing abilities constitute a cultural group in themselves and often feel stigmatized. This discrimination is evident in cultures where the healthy are more valued than the physically, emotionally, or intellectually challenged.[2] If patients are unable to communicate their needs, then pain and symptom management and end-of-life wishes are not likely to be addressed. Additionally, this vulnerable population's losses may not be recognized or acknowledged, putting individuals at risk for complicated grief. Taking time to determine an individual's goals of care—regardless of differing abilities—and identifying resources and support to improve quality of life is essential.

## Sexual Orientation

Sexual orientation may carry a stigma when the patient is gay, lesbian, or transgendered. In palliative care, these patients have unique needs because of the legal and ethical issues of domestic partnerships, multiple losses that may have been experienced as a result of one's sexual orientation, and unresolved family issues. Domestic partnerships, which are sanctioned by many cities and states in the United States, grant some of the rights of traditional married couples to unmarried homosexual couples who share the traditional bond of the family.[2] However, many cities and states do not legally recognize the relationship. Durable Power of Attorney for Health Care must be completed. Without such documentation, decision-making follows state guidelines. If legal documents have not been drafted prior to death of a partner, then survivorship issues, financial concerns, and lack of acknowledgment of bereavement needs may cause additional distress and complicate grief.[2]

## Religion and Spirituality

Religion is the belief and practice of a faith tradition, a means of expressing spirituality. Spirituality, a much broader concept, is the life force that transcends our physical being and gives meaning and purpose.[24] Although religion and spirituality are complementary concepts, these terms are often mistakenly used interchangeably. It should be noted that an individual may be very spiritual but not practice a formal religion. In addition, those who identify themselves as belonging to a religion may not necessarily adhere to all the practices of that religion. As with ethnicity, it is important to determine how strongly the individual aligns with his or her identified faith and the significance of its practice rituals.

Religious beliefs can significantly influence a person's decisions regarding treatment and care. These beliefs can be at the cornerstone of decisions regarding continuation or discontinuation of life-prolonging therapies for some people.[25] Additionally, religious beliefs can strongly influence how patients and families understand illness and suffering.[25]

An example can be taken from the case presented at the beginning of this chapter. It was noted that the patient was Jewish, and it was important to him that his friends and family shared his faith. Consulting with a Rabbi and chaplain services will assist not only in supporting the family and friends of the patient during critical decisions but will also help to clarify specific religious beliefs and practices necessary for decisions regarding ongoing care of the patient. In this case, it was the Rabbi who helped clarify with which denomination of Judaism the patient was affiliated. The Rabbi worked closely with family, who described that the Jewish faith shaped the fabric of their lives, and thus the Rabbi was able to tap into important Jewish traditions for the patient and family, recite appropriate initial prayers, focus on forgiveness, and then complete the final prayers. The family spoke with the Rabbi about the meaning of suffering and finding meaning in the suddenness of this catastrophic trauma. Eventually, the ventilator was removed and the patient died peacefully.

Chaplains, clergy from a patient's or family member's religious group—ideally their own community clergy—are key members of the interdisciplinary palliative care team. Those who turn to their faith-based communities for support may find the emotional, spiritual, and other tangible support they need when dealing with a life-limiting illness.[16,26] Keep in mind, however, that some individuals who are struggling with misconceptions of the tenets of their own faith may experience spiritual distress and need spiritual intervention from caring chaplains or spiritual care counselors.

Spirituality is in the essence of every human being. It is what gives each person a sense of being, meaning, purpose, and direction.[27] It transcends the self to connect with others and with a higher power, independent of organized religion. One's sense of spirituality is often the force that helps transcend loss and suffering.[28,29] Spiritual distress can cause pain and suffering if not identified and addressed. Assessing spiritual well-being and attending to spiritual needs, which may be very diverse, is essential to quality of life for patients and families confronting end of life. A case example that emphasizes the importance of spirituality follows.

A 72-year-old woman with end-stage heart failure was nearing end of life. She had no formal religious practice but was a very spiritual person who found meaning and purpose in the nature surrounding her home. Every day of her life, she made a trip to the creek behind her house and spent time sitting with the water, rocks, and natural beauty. When she could no longer go to the creek, the palliative care team suggested that the family "bring the creek to her." For the remainder of her life, her grandson went to the creek daily and brought her a pail full of fresh water and rocks so that she could dip her hand in them and be one with nature again. She died peacefully at home, with her creek and rocks at her side.

## Socioeconomic Status

One's socioeconomic status, place of residence, workplace, and level of education are important components of one's cultural

**Table 37–3**
**Key Cultural Assessment Questions**

*Formal cultural assessments are available for the nurse to use (see resources Table 37–4). Remember that a checklist does not always instill trust. Below are some suggestions for ascertaining key cultural preferences from both patients and family caregivers.*

- Tell me a little bit about yourself (e.g., for families, your mother, father, siblings, etc.).
- Where were you born and raised? (If an immigrant, "How long have you lived in this country?")
- What language would you prefer to speak?
- Is it easier to write things down, or do you have difficulty with reading and writing?
- To whom do you go for support (family friends, community, or religious or community leaders)?
- Is there anyone we should contact to come be with you?
- I want to be sure I'm giving you all the information you need. What do you want to know about your condition? To whom should I speak about your care?
- Who do you want to know about your condition?
- How are decisions about healthcare made in your family? Should I speak directly with you, or is there someone else with whom I should be discussing decisions?
- (*Address to patient or designated decision maker*) Tell me about your understanding of what has been happening up to this point? What does the illness mean to you?
- We want to work with you to be sure you are getting the best care possible and that we are meeting all your needs. Is there anything we should know about any customs or practices that are important to include in your care?
- Many people have shared that it is very important to include spirituality or religion in their care. Is this something that is important for you? Our chaplain can help contact anyone that you would like to be involved with your care.
- We want to make sure we respect how you prefer to be addressed, including how we should act. Is there anything we should avoid? Is it appropriate for you to have male and female caregivers?
- Are there any foods you would like or that you should avoid?
- Do you have any concerns about how to pay for care, medications, or other services?

**Death rituals and practices**
- Is there anything we should know about care of the body, about rituals, practices, or ceremonies that should be performed?
- What is your belief about what happens after death?
- Is there a way for us to plan for anything you might need both at the time of death and afterward?
- Is there anything we should know about whether a man or a woman should be caring for the body after death?
- Should the family be involved in the care of the body?

identity and play a role in palliative care. For example, those who are socioeconomically disadvantaged face unique challenges when seeking healthcare and when receiving treatment. Financial costs, including pain medications, medical tests, treatments and drugs not covered by limited insurance plans, transportation and childcare, add additional burden.

However, regardless of financial status, an estimated 25% of families are financially devastated by a serious terminal illness.[2] Patients experiencing disease progression, or in whom treatment side effects preclude the ability to work, are forced to confront profound losses: loss of work and income, loss of identity, and loss of a network of colleagues. Those who are educationally disadvantaged struggle to navigate the healthcare system and to find information and support. Patients and families in a supportive community have increased access to resources at end of life compared to other, more vulnerable populations, such as those in prison and the homeless.[2]

## Conducting a Cultural Assessment

There are many tools available to help with cultural assessment. These tools include the components of culture discussed in this chapter. However, doing a cultural assessment involves questions that necessitate the development of a trusting relationship. When meeting the patient and family early in the disease trajectory, the palliative care nurse has the advantage of time to establish such a relationship. This luxury of time is not always available. Using the skill of presence and active listening is often more beneficial than using a standardized tool. Checklists do not necessarily build trust and can be burdensome. Simple inquiries into patient and family practices and beliefs can assist the nurse in understanding needs and goals. Asking the patient and/or the family member to tell you about him/herself or the family and then listening to those narratives is powerful. The patient and family often give clues that trigger important questions to ask to clarify patient and family needs and goals. Table 37–3 provides examples of trigger questions.

## Selected Palliative Care Issues Influenced by Culture

Culture impacts all aspects of palliative care. This section focuses on cultural considerations regarding selected palliative care issues and concepts.

## Communication

Communication is the foundation for all encounters between clinicians, patients, and family members. When the clinicians and the patient–family unit are from different ethnic or cultural backgrounds, relating news regarding a poor prognosis, or "bad news," can be challenging. Williams et al.[30] relate that for African-Americans it is the establishment of a relationship with the clinician, where the clinician seeks to understand individual concerns of the patient and family, that provides a foundation for all future communication and decision-making.

When a patient has a serious or life-threatening illness, the sharing of medical information will shape how decisions are made. Clinicians are challenged to build trusting relationships with patients and families by listening to their individual and group concerns, beliefs, and values. General communication principles should be utilized at all times. These include (1) adequate preparation for communicating medical facts; (2) selecting a setting that is private and free from distractions; (3) using appropriate nonverbal communication styles, sitting down, maintaining eye contact, and conveying that the clinician is not rushed; and (4) expressing empathy and responding to patient and family emotional responses.[31]

Other key factors to consider include being acutely aware of the words used to convey medical facts and recognizing that common phrases used among medical personnel may not be terms readily understood by patients and families. Additionally, it is important to clarify who the decision-maker in the family is and with whom information should be shared (patient, family, or both). The dominant language and dialect spoken and the literacy level of both patient and primary family caregiver(s) are also critical factors to establish.

The communication of poor prognosis directly to the patient may be avoided in some cultures to protect the patient from losing hope. Ideally, preferences for communication, including full disclosure of a terminal diagnosis and poor prognosis, are best discussed early in the clinician–patient relationship when the patient is relatively healthy. When this is not possible, clinicians should take time to reflect on their own bias, listen to patient and family concerns, determine individual and group norms, and engage in an ongoing dialogue about such preferences. Such measures will strengthen the relationship and show respect for the unique ways in which a family group functions.[31,32]

Awareness of verbal and nonverbal communication styles assists the nurse in establishing trusting relationships, showing respect for variations, and identifying potential communication barriers early to avoid potential conflicts. Communication is an interactive, multidimensional process, often dictated by cultural norms, and provides the mechanism for human interaction and connection. Given the complexities of communicating diagnosis, prognosis, and progression of a life-limiting disease, there is no "one size fits all" approach.[31]

If there is a language barrier, a professionally trained interpreter of the appropriate gender should be contacted. Although it has been suggested that family members should not be asked to serve as interpreters because this may force them into an uncomfortable role should sensitive issues arise, use of professional interpreters does not take the place of determining what is culturally appropriate to disclose. Adequate cultural assessment must be completed prior to discussions, whether or not family or medical interpreters are used to communicate medical information.[31] When using an interpreter, direct all verbal communication to the patient/family rather than the interpreter. Ongoing clarification that information is understood is critical.

Touch can be a powerful communication tool in palliative care; however, although intended to communicate reassurance and caring, touch may invade personal space and privacy, resulting in considerable distress.[31] Norms regarding appropriateness of touching members of the opposite sex are important to note. How close you should be to another, or the concept of personal space, is closely related to communication styles. Sitting too close to a patient may be considered intrusive or disrespectful. On the other hand, sitting or standing far away from the patient may communicate disinterest and lack of caring. Asking the individual for guidance on these issues will avoid a great deal of unintended discomfort and misunderstandings. Additionally, finding out if there are norms related to greetings (e.g., formal/informal; appropriateness of touch, handshake, smile) should also be considered. Attention to acceptable forms of nonverbal communication is as important as knowledge of verbal communication customs; for example, certain gestures, eye contact, and silence may be acceptable in some cultures yet unacceptable in others.

## Medical Decision-Making

Over the past 40 years in the United States, ethical and legal considerations of decision-making have focused on patient autonomy.[33] This focus replaced the more paternalistic approach of decision-making as solely the physician's responsibility, with an approach that emphasizes a model of shared responsibility with the patient's active involvement.[34] The Patient Self-Determination Act of 1991 sought to further clarify and to protect an individual's health-care preferences with advance directives.[35] The principle of respect for patient autonomy points to a patient's right to participate in decisions about the care he/she receives. Associated with this is the right to be informed of diagnosis, prognosis, and the risks and benefits of treatment to make informed decisions. Inherent in the movement for patient autonomy is the underlying assumption that all patients want control over their health-care decisions. Yet, in fact, for some individuals, patient autonomy may violate the very principles of dignity and integrity it proposes to uphold and may result in significant distress.[36]

This European-American model of patient autonomy has its origin in the dominant culture, a predominantly white, middle-class perspective that does not consider diverse cultural perspectives.[33] This shared decision-making model is not the norm in many cultures.[31,37] Emphasis on autonomy as the guiding principle assumes that the individual, rather than the family or other social group, is the appropriate decision-maker.[31,33] However, in many non-European-American cultures, the concept of interdependence among family and community members is more valued than individual autonomy.[33] Cultures that practice family-centered decision-making, such as the Korean-American and Mexican-American cultures, may prefer that the family, or perhaps a particular family member rather than the patient, receives and processes information.[38,39] For example, the traditional Chinese concept of "filial piety" requires that children, especially the eldest son, are obligated to respect, care for, and protect their parents.[21] Based on the values and beliefs of this culture, the son is obligated to protect the parent from the worry of a terminal prognosis.

Patient autonomy may not be seen as empowering but, rather, may seem burdensome for patients who are too sick to have to make difficult decisions.[32] The label of "truth-telling" itself is misleading.[36] Although full disclosure may not be appropriate, it is never appropriate to lie to the patient. If the patient does not wish to receive information and/or telling the patient violates the patient's and family's cultural norms, the health-care provider may not be respecting the patient's right to autonomously decide not to receive the information. Some cultures believe that telling the patient he has a terminal illness strips away any and all hope and causes needless suffering and may indeed hasten death.[40,41] The nurse must consider the harm that may occur when the health system or providers violate cultural beliefs and practices.[42] Assessing and clarifying the patient and family's perspectives, values, and practices may prevent a cultural conflict.[22] The nurse is in a key position to advocate these critical patient and family issues (see Table 37–3 for examples of questions to ask). By asking how decisions are made and whether the patient wishes to be involved in both being told information or participating in the decision-making process, patient autonomy is respected, and individual beliefs and values are honored.[32]

### Discontinuation of Life-Prolonging Therapies

Another issue with the potential for cultural conflict surrounds decision-making regarding the discontinuation or withholding of life-sustaining treatments. Inherent in the decision is that the patient will most likely die.[34] Attitude surveys evaluating initiating and terminating life-prolonging therapies have demonstrated differences among several ethnic groups. Research suggests that groups including African-Americans, Chinese-Americans, Filipino-Americans, Iranian-Americans, Korean-Americans, and Mexican-Americans were more likely to start and to continue such therapies than were European Americans when such measures were felt by the health-care team to be futile.[10,18,43] When making difficult decisions, family members often feel that by agreeing to withdrawal of life-prolonging therapies, they are in fact responsible for the death of their loved one. For families who believe that it is the duty of children to honor, respect, and care for their elders, they may feel obligated to continue futile life-sustaining interventions. Allowing a parent to die may violate the principles of "filial piety" and bring shame and disgrace on the family.[21]

Recognize also that the words used in these decisions, including "do not resuscitate" and "withdrawal of life support" all have negative connotations and involve the removing of something or the withholding of a particular intervention. The clinician is encouraged to be acutely aware of how information or questions are phrased. A suggestion is to use words that convey benefit versus burden of all therapies. Words and phrases that may seem clear to the health professional often get literally lost in translation regardless of whether the parties are speaking the same language.

Because many ethical conflicts arise from differences in patients', families', and providers' values, beliefs, and practices, it is critical that individual members of the health-care team be aware of their own cultural beliefs, understand their own reactions to the issue, and be knowledgeable about the patients' and families' beliefs to address the conflict.[22]

### Meaning of Food and Nutrition

Across cultures, there is agreement that food is essential for life to maintain body function and to produce energy.[44] Food serves another purpose in the building and maintaining of human relationships. It is used in rituals, celebrations, and rites of passage to establish and maintain social and cultural relationships with families, friends, and others. Because of food's importance for life and life events, a loss of desire for food and subsequent weight loss and wasting can cause suffering for both the patient and family. Culturally appropriate foods may be used to improve health by groups who have strong beliefs about particular foods and their relationship to health.

Families often need clear guidance and explanations when a patient is no longer able to enjoy favorite foods or family mealtime rituals because of declining physical ability. It is imperative that the health-care team understands the meaning attached to food in a palliative care setting, when decisions regarding the potential burden of providing artificial nutrition and hydration for an imminently dying patient are discussed. Exploring alternative ways in which the family can care for the patient through physical, spiritual, or emotional means of support will allow families to interact with the patient in ways that are meaningful to them and reflect individual beliefs, values, and preferences.

## Pain and Symptom Management

Pain is a highly personal and subjective experience. Pain is whatever the person says it is and exists whenever the person says it does.[45] Culture plays a role in the experience of pain, the meaning of pain, and the response to pain. A biocultural model of pain suggests that social learning from family and group membership can influence the psychological and physiological processing of pain, which then affects the perception and modulation of pain.[46] The meaning of pain varies among cultural groups. For some, pain is a positive response that demonstrates the body's ability to fight against disease or the dying process. For others, pain signifies punishment and its value lies in the patient's ability to withstand the suffering and work toward resolution and peace.[47]

Strong beliefs about expressing pain and expected pain behaviors exist in every culture.[48] Pain tolerance varies from person to person and is influenced by factors such as past experiences with pain, coping skills, motivation to endure pain, and energy level. Western society appears to value individuals that exhibit a high pain threshold. As a result, those with a lower threshold, who report pain often, may be labeled as "difficult patients."

Pain assessment should be culturally appropriate, using terms that describe pain intensity across most cultural groups. "Pain," "hurt," and "ache" are words commonly used across cultures. These words may reflect the severity of the pain, with "pain" being the most severe, "hurt" being moderate pain, and "ache" being the least severe.[2] The health-care team should focus on the words the patient uses to describe pain. To help facilitate an understanding of the severity of the pain experienced by someone who does not speak English, the providers should use pain-rating scales that have been translated into numerous languages.[45] Although it is important to base the assessment on the patient's self-report of pain intensity, it may be necessary to rely on nonverbal pain indicators such as facial expression, body movement, and vocalization to assess pain in the nonverbal, cognitively impaired patient, the older adult, or the infant, who are all at risk for inaccurate assessment and undertreatment of pain.[2,45]

Racial, ethnic, age, and gender biases in pain management have been identified and documented.[49–51] Studies of gender variations in pain response have identified differences in sensitivity and tolerance to pain as well as willingness to report pain.[50,52] Underidentification and undertreatment of pain is a well-recognized phenomenon in elder care.[53] Studies reveal that Hispanics, African-Americans, and females are less likely to be prescribed opioids for pain or may be unable to fill opioid prescriptions.[51,54]

Like pain, symptoms described by patients receiving palliative care may have meanings associated with them that reflect cultural values, beliefs, and practices. Assessment and management of symptoms such as fatigue, dyspnea, depression, nausea and vomiting, and anorexia/cachexia should be addressed within a cultural framework. For example, some cultural groups may be hesitant to disclose depression because it is considered a sign of weakness; instead it may be referred to as a "tired state." Using culturally appropriate language, the nurse will need to evaluate whether the symptom experienced is fatigue or depression.

Incorporating culturally appropriate nondrug therapies may improve the ability to alleviate pain and symptoms. Healing practices specific to cultures should be offered to the patient and family.[48] Herbal remedies, acupuncture, and folk medicines should be incorporated into the plan of care if desired. Keep in mind that certain nondrug approaches, such as hypnosis and massage, may be inappropriate in some cultures.[44]

## Death Rituals and Mourning Practices

The loss of a loved one brings sadness and upheaval in the family structure across all cultures.[48] Each culture responds to these losses through specific rituals that assist the dying and the bereaved through the final transition from life. It is important to note that rituals may begin before death and may last for months or even years after death. Respecting these rituals and customs will have tremendous impact on the healing process for family members following the death and leave a positive lasting memory of the loved one's end-of-life experience. The nurse should make sure that any required spiritual, religious, or cultural practices are performed and that there is appropriate care of the body after death.

For example, dying at home is especially important for Hmong-American elders who follow traditional beliefs.[55] The nurse in an acute care setting can be the advocate to ensure this tradition is honored. The family may consult a shaman to perform a ceremony to negotiate with the "God of the sky" to extend life. Additional ceremonies follow. Request for an autopsy or organ donation at the time of death is inappropriate because of the belief that altering the body will delay reincarnation. After the death, there is often much wailing and caressing of the body. The family prepares for an elaborate funeral with rituals to ensure that the loved one will "cross over" and continues with ceremonies for days following the funeral to make sure the soul joins its ancestors.[55]

The tasks of grieving are universal: to accept the reality of the loss, to experience pain of grief, to begin the adjustment to new social and family roles, and to withdraw emotional energy from the dead individual and turn it over to those who are alive.[56] The expressions of grief, however, may vary significantly among cultures. What is acceptable in one culture may seem unacceptable, or even maladaptive, in another. Recognizing normal grief behavior (vs. complicated grief) within a cultural context therefore demands knowledge about culturally acceptable expressions of grief.[48,56] It is important to note that rituals may begin before death and may last for months or even years after death. Some cultures may value being present at the time of death.

## Striving for Cultural Competence

Palliative care nurses value the importance of being culturally sensitive and striving for cultural competence. This sensitivity and competence is critical when working with patients with a life-limiting illness and their families.

Cultural competence refers to a dynamic, fluid, continuous process of awareness, knowledge, skill, interaction, and sensitivity.[57] The term remains controversial, as some question whether one care ever become "culturally competent."[58] However, cultural competence is an ongoing process, not an end-point. It is more comprehensive than cultural sensitivity, implying not only the ability to recognize and respect cultural differences but also to intervene appropriately and effectively. Five components essential in pursuing cultural competence are cultural awareness, cultural knowledge, cultural skill, cultural encounter, and cultural desire.[57]

Integrating cultural considerations into palliative care requires, first and foremost, that the nurse becomes aware of how one's own values, practices, and beliefs influence care. Cultural awareness begins with an examination of one's own heritage, family's practices, experiences, and religious or spiritual beliefs.[57] Because culture is a dynamic concept, it is important to re-assess one's own beliefs on a regular basis, reflecting on beliefs that may have changed with increasing knowledge and cultural encounters.

Each nurse brings his/her own cultural and philosophical views, education, religion, spirituality, and life experiences to the care of the patient and family. Cultural awareness challenges the nurse to look beyond his or her ethnocentric view of the world, asking the question "How are my values, beliefs, and practices different from the patient and family?" rather than "How is this patient and family different from me?" Exploring one's own beliefs will raise an awareness of differences that have the potential to foster prejudice and discrimination and limit the effectiveness of care.[2] Exploring answers to the same cultural assessment questions used for patients and families increases self-awareness (Table 37–3). Often this exploration identifies more similarities than differences. The universal aspects of life, family, trust, love, hope, understanding, and caring unite us all.

Acquiring knowledge about different cultural groups is the second component to gaining cultural competence, but knowledge alone is insufficient in providing culturally appropriate care. No one can expect to have in-depth knowledge of all cultural variations of health and illness beliefs, values, and norms. A suggested strategy is to identify the most common ethnic group/cultures living in the nurse's community and to integrate a basic understanding of norms and practices impacting issues likely to arise in palliative and end-of-life situations. To strengthen knowledge, one should seek out community members, organizations, faith communities, and leaders in a shared understanding of needs and concerns.

Knowledge gained of a particular group should serve only as a guide to understanding the unique cultural needs of the patient and family, which comes through individualized assessments. Other resources, such as cultural guides, literature, and web-based resources, are available to assist the nurse in acquiring knowledge about specific groups. Table 37–4

---

**Table 37–4**
**Web Resources for Acquiring Knowledge About Cultural Issues Affecting Healthcare**

**Cross Cultural Health Care Program (CCHPC): www.xculture.org**
CCHCP addresses broad cultural issues that impact the health of individuals and families in ethnic minority communities. Its mission is to serve as a bridge between communities and healthcare institutions

**Diversity Rx: http://DiversityRx.org**
This is a great networking website that models and practices policy, legal issues, and links to other resources.

**EthnoMed: http://ethnomed.org/**
The EthnoMed site contains information about cultural beliefs, medical issues, and other related issues pertinent to the healthcare of recent immigrants to the United States.

**Fast Fact & Concept #78; Cultural Aspects of Pain Management: www.eperc.mcw.edu/fastfact/ff_78.htm**
This website contains many "fast facts" regarding palliative care. Number 78 addresses important cultural considerations and provides assessment questions when working with patients in pain.

**Health Resources and Services Administration (HRSA): http://www.hrsa.gov/search**
When you search "culture" on this HRSA website, you will find information on health disparities including links to literacy and nutrition issues.

**Office of Minority Health: http://www.omhrc.gov**
This website has training tools for developing cultural competency.

**Transcultural Nursing Society: www.tcns.org**
The society (founded in 1974) serves as a forum to promote, advance, and disseminate transcultural nursing knowledge worldwide.

This list offers suggestions of several useful resources. The list is not intended to be exhaustive but serves as a starting point for gaining more information.

lists several useful web-based resources. It is important to remember that relying on culturally specific knowledge to guide practice, rather than individual assessment, is incongruent with culturally competent care.

Cultural skill is the third component of cultural competency. Skills in cultural assessment, cross-cultural communication, cultural interpretation, and appropriate intervention can be learned. Multiple tools are available to assess cultural behavior and beliefs. For the new nurse, key assessment questions, applicable in the palliative care setting, may be helpful in guiding the assessment (Table 37–3). However, nothing can replace sitting with the patient and family and asking them to tell the story of their heritage/family history and their cherished practices and beliefs.

The fourth component encompasses the concept of cultural encounters. Individuals with different ways of relating often misunderstand each others'cues. The more opportunities we have to engage with persons with differing values, practices, and beliefs, the more we learn about others and ourselves and the less likely we are to draw erroneous conclusions about each other. Active engagement with community leaders and use of learning tools such as case studies and role plays all help expose nurses to varied cultural experiences.[57,58] Increasing exposure to cultural encounters may also improve confidence in one's ability to meet the needs of diverse populations.[59]

The fifth and final component of cultural competence is cultural desire. This is the interest and openness with which the nurse strives to understand patients and families and the communities from which they come. Cultural desire is motivation to "want to" engage in the process of cultural competence as opposed to being "forced to" participate in the process. The desire is genuine and authentic and encourages the nurse to take advantage of cultural encounters and explore worlds beyond his/her own ethnocentric perspective. Such experiences lend opportunities for the nurse to grow both personally and professionally.[57]

## Summary

Given the changing population of the United States, we as nurses must advocate for the integration of cultural considerations in providing comprehensive palliative care. It is imperative that each of us moves beyond our own ethnocentric view of the world to appreciate and respect the similarities and differences in each other. We are challenged to embrace a better understanding of various perspectives. Becoming culturally competent first requires an awareness of how one's own cultural background impacts care. In addition, acquiring knowledge about cultures and developing skill in cultural assessment are essential to improving palliative care care to patients with life-limiting illnesses and their families.

This chapter encourages nurses to integrate cultural assessment and culturally appropriate interventions into palliative care. It is the hope of the authors that readers will enrich their practice by seeking new knowledge about different cultures through available resources and, most importantly, by using the most valuable resources on cultural considerations we have—our patients and their families.

REFERENCES

1. Coyle N. Introduction to palliative nursing care. In Ferrell BR, Coyle N, eds. Textbook of Palliative Nursing (2nd ed). New York, NY: Oxford University Press; 2006:5–11.
2. End-of-Life Nursing Education Consortium (ELNEC), http://www.aacn.nche.edu/elnec/ (accessed November 19, 2008).
3. Kagawa-Singer M, Blackhall L. Negotating cross-cultural issues at the end of life. JAMA 2001;286:2993–3001.
4. National Consensus Project for Quality Palliative Care. http://www.nationalconsensusproject.org (accessed December 8, 2008).
5. U. S. Bureau of the Census (2010). Current Population Reports, https://ask.census.gov/cgi/bin/askcensus (accessed December 20, 2008).
6. U.S. Bureau of the Census (2000). Current Population Reports, http://www.census.gov/ipc/www/usinterimproj (Internet release date March 18, 2004; accessed December 20, 2008).
7. Taxis JC. Mexican Americans and hospice care: Culture, control, and communication. J Hosp Palliat Nurs 2008;10:133–161.
8. Leininger M. Quality of life from a transcultural nursing perspective. Nurs Sci Quart 1994;7:22–28.
9. Giger JN, Davidhizar RE, Fordham, P. Multi-cultural and multi-ethnic considerations and advanced directives: Developing cultural competency. J Cult Divers 2006;13:3–9.
10. Crawley LM. Racial, cultural, and ethnic factors influencing end-of-life care. J Palliat Med 2005;8(Suppl.1):S-58–S-69.
11. McNeill J, Reynolds J, Ney M. Unequal quality of cancer pain management: Disparity in perceived control and propsed solutions. Oncol Nurs Forum 2007;34:1121–1139.
12. Ludke RL, Smucker DR. Racial differences in the willingness to use hospice services. J Palliat Med 2007;10:1329–1337.
13. Connor SR, Elwert F, Spence C. Christakis NA. Racial disparity in hospice use in the United States in 2002. Palliat Med 2008;22:205–213.
14. Smedley B, Stith A, Nelson A. Unequal treatment: confronting racial and ethnic disparities in health care (Report of the Institute of Medicine). Washington, D.C.: National Academy Press, 2003.
15. Brandon DT, Isaac LA, LaVeist TA. The legacy of Tuskegee and trust in medical care: is Tuskegee responsible for race differences in mistrust of medical care? J Natl Med Assoc 2005;97:951–956.
16. Bullock K. Promoting advanced directives among African Americans: A faith-based model. J Palliat Med 2006;9:183–195.
17. Kuczewski MG. Our cultures, our selves: toward an honest dialogue on race and end-of-life decisions. Am J Bioethics 2006;6:143–217.
18. Duffy SA, Jackson FC, Schim SM, Ronis DL, Fowler KE. Racial/ethnic preferences, esc preferences, and perceived discrimination related to end-of-life care. J Am Geriatr Soc 2006;54:150–157.
19. The Office of Minority Health: National Center on Minority Health and Health Disparities. http://www.ncmhd.nih.gov (accessed December 9, 2008).

20. Prince-Paul MJ. Relationships among communicative acts, social well-being, and spiritual well-being on the quality of life at the end of life in patients with cancer enrolled in hospice. J Palliat Med 2008;11:20–25.

21. Hsiung YY, Ferrans CE. Recognizing Chinese Americans' cultural needs in making end-of-life treatment decisions. J Hosp Palliat Nurs 2007;9:132–140.

22. Lapine A, Wang-Cheng R, Goldstein M, Nooney A, Lamb G, Derse A. When cultures clash: Physician, patient, and family wishes in truth disclosure for dying patients. J Palliat Care 2001;4:475–480.

23. Crawley L, Marshall P, Lo B, Koenig B. Strategies for culturally effective end-of-life care. Ann Inter Med 2002;136:673–679.

24. Sherman D. Cultural and spiritual backgrounds of older adults. In Matzo M, Sherman D, eds. Gerontologic Palliative Care Nursing. St. Louis, MO: Mosby; 2004:3–47.

25. Puchalski C, Heffner JE, Byock IR. Palliative and End-of-life Pearls. Philadelphia, PA: Hanley & Belfus, Inc., 2003.

26. Branch WT, Torke A, Brown-Haithco RC. The importance of spirituality in African- Americans' end-of-life experience. J Gen Intern Med 2006;21:1203–1205.

27. Highfield M. Providing spiritual care to patients with cancer. Clin J Oncol Nurs 2000;4:115–120.

28. Borneman T, Brown-Saltzman K. Meaning in illness. In Ferrell BR, Coyle N, eds. Textbook of Palliative Nursing (2nd ed). New York, NY: Oxford University Press; 2006:605–615

29. Ferrell B, Coyle N. The Nature of Suffering and the Goals of Nursing. New York, NY: Oxford University Press, 2008.

30. Williams SW, Hanson LC, Boyd C, et al. Communication, decision making, and cancer: What African Americans want physicians to know. J Palliat Med 2008;11:1221–1226.

31. Barclay JS, Blackhall LJ, Tulsky JA. Communication strategies and cultural issues in the delivery of bad news. J Palliat Med 2007;10:958–977.

32. Searight HR, Gafford J. Cultural diversity at the end of life: Issues and guidelines for family physicians. Am Fam Physician 2005;71:515–522.

33. Ersek M, Kagawa-Singer M, Barnes D, Blackhall L, Koenig B. Multicultural considerations in the use of advance directives. Oncol Nurs Forum 1998;25:1683–1701.

34. Scanlon C. Ethical concerns in end-of-life care. Am J Nurs 2003;103:48–55.

35. Federal patient self-determination act 19090, 42 U.S.C. 1395 cc(a).

36. Hancock K, Clayton JM, Parker SM, et al. Truth-telling in discusiing prognosis in advanced life-limiting illnesses: A systematic review. Palliat Med 2007;21:507–517.

37. Costantini M, Morasso G, Montella M, et al. Diagnosis and prognosis disclosure among cancer patients. Results from an Italian mortality follow-back survey. Ann Oncol 2006;17:853–859.

38. Kwak J, Salmon JR. Attitudes and preferences of Korean-American older adults and caregivers on end-of-life care. JAGS 2007;55:1967–1972.

39. Thomas R, Wilson DM, Justice C, Birch S, Sheps S. A literature review of preferences for end-of-life care in developed countries by individuals with different cultural affiliations and ethnicity. J Hosp Palliat Nurs 2008;10:142–161.

40. Blackhall L, Murphy S, Frank G, Michel V, Azen S. Ethnicity and attitudes toward patient autonomy. JAMA 1995;274:820–825.

41. Kraukauer EL, Crenner C, Fox K. Barriers to optimum end-of-life care for minority patients. JAGS 2002;50:182–190.

42. Fadiman A. The Spirit Catches You and You Fall Down. New York, NY: Farrar, Straus and Giroux, 1997.

43. Winter L, Dennis MR, Parker B. Religiosity and preferences for life-prolonging medical treatments in African-American and white elders:a mediation study. OMEGA 2007;56:273–288.

44. Chou F, Dodd M, Abrams D, Padilla G. Symptoms, self-care, and quality of life of Chinese American patients with cancer. Oncol Nurs Forum 2007;34:1162–1167.

45. McCaffery M, Pasero C. Pain: Clinical Manual (2nd ed). St. Louis, MO: Mosby, 1999.

46. Bates MS, Edwards WT, Anderson KO. Ethnocultural influences on variation in chronic pain perception. Pain 1993;52:101–112.

47. Meghani, SH. The meanings of and attitudes about cancer pain among African Americans. Oncol Nurs Forum 2007;34:1179–1186.

48. Spector R. Cultural Care: Guides to Heritage Assessment and Health Traditions (7th ed). Upper Saddle River, NJ: Pearson Education, 2009.

49. Anderson KO, Richman SP, Hurley J, et al. Cancer pain management among underserved minority out-patients: Perceived needs and barriers to optimal control. Cancer 2002;94:2295–2304.

50. Cleeland C. Undertreatment of cancer pain in elderly patients. JAMA 1998;279:1914–1915.

51. Morrison RS, Wallenstein S, Natale DK, Senzel RS, Huang LL. "We don't carry that"— failure of pharmacies in predominantly nonwhite neighborhoods to stock opioid analgesics. NEJM 2000;342:1023–1026.

52. Lasch K. Culture, pain, and culturally sensitive pain care. Pain Manage Nurs 2000;1(Suppl 3):16–22.

53. Reynolds KS, Hanson, LC, Henderson M, Steinhauser, KE. End-of-life care in nursing home settings: Do race or age matter? Palliat Support Care 2008;6:21–27.

54. Cohen LL. Racial/ethnic disparities in hospice care: A systematic review. J Palliat Med 2008;5:763–767.

55. Gerdner LA, Yang D, Tripp-Reimer T. The circle of life: end-of-life care and death rituals for Hmong-american elders. J Gerontol Nurs 2007;33:20–29.

56. Worden J. Grief Counseling and Grief Therapy (2nd ed). New York, NY: Springer, 1991.

57. Campinha-Bacote J. A model and instrument for addressing cultural competence in health care. J Nurs Educ 1999; 38:203–207.

58. Schimm SM, Doorenbos AZ, Boase NN. Enhancing cultural competence among hospice staff. Am J Hosp Palliat Med 2006;23:404–411.

59. Diver F, Molassiotis A, Weeks L. The palliative care needs of ethnic minority patients: Staff perspectives. Int J Palliat Nurs 2003;9:343–351.

# 38

*Susan Derby, Sean O'Mahony, and Roma Tickoo*

# Elderly Patients

*What a relief it is to find nurses and doctors who can see beyond the old woman in the bed and see the person who loved the smell of freshly baked bread, who could read for hours on end, and who loved and was loved........—An 80-year-old palliative care patient*

◆ **Key Points**
◆ *The majority of people who suffer from chronic disease are elderly.*
◆ *The trajectory of illness for the elderly is usually one of progressive loss of independence, with the development of multiple comorbid problems and symptoms.*
◆ *The last years of a frail elderly person's life are often spent at home in the care of family, with approximately 50% to 60% of the elderly dying in a hospital or long-term care facility.*
◆ *Evidence suggests that the end of life for many elderly is characterized by poor symptom control, inadequate advanced care planning, and increased burden on caregivers.*
◆ *Clinicians caring for the elderly often lack skills in providing palliative and end-of-life care.*
◆ *If we are committed to providing good end-of-life care to our population, clinicians must improve their care of elderly patients in all practice settings.*

Aging is a normal process of life, not a disease, and infirmity and frailty do not always have to accompany being old. It is expected that most of us will live well into our 70s or 80s, and the aging of the population is projected to continue well into the 21st century. Projected growth for the elderly population is staggering. During the next 20 years, the fastest-growing segment of the population will be in the group aged 85 years and older. During past decades, this increase in life expectancy has mainly resulted from improvements in sanitation and infectious disease control through vaccinations and antibiotics. Death from heart disease and atherosclerosis has decreased for all age groups in the elderly. Deaths for cancer in men over 65 years decreased in the 1990s after increasing for two decades. Hypertension decreased in white men but increased markedly in African-American men.[1]

Presently, the older population is growing older because of positive trends in the treatment of chronic diseases—cardiovascular and neurological, as well as cancer. This "swelling" of the older segment of the population reinforces the need for nurses, physicians, and all health-care professionals to understand the special palliative care needs of the elderly. In our society, the majority of people who have chronic disease are elderly. One of the major differences from younger groups in treating illness in the elderly population is the need for extensive family support and care during the last weeks and months of life. Older Americans at the end of life face 2 years or more of disability of sufficient severity to warrant assistance from someone else with their activities of daily living.[2,3]

## Comorbidity and Function

The elderly have many comorbid medical conditions that contribute an added symptom burden to this palliative care population. The presence of existing comorbidities and

**Table 38–1**
**Age-Specific Prevalence of Chronic Medical Conditions in Noninstitutionalized U.S. Adults (per 1000)**

|  | 18–44 Years | 45–64 Years | 65–74 Years | >75 Years |
|---|---|---|---|---|
| Arthritis | 52.1 | 268.5 | 459.3 | 494.7 |
| Hypertension | 64.1 | 258.9 | 426.8 | 394.6 |
| Heart disease | 40.1 | 129.0 | 276.8 | 349.1 |
| Hearing impairment | 49.8 | 159.0 | 261.9 | 346.9 |
| Deformity/orthopedic impairment | 125.3 | 160.6 | 167.9 | 175.5 |
| Chronic sinusitis | 164.4 | 184.8 | 151.2 | 160.0 |
| Visual impairment | 32.8 | 43.7 | 76.4 | 128.8 |
| Diabetes | 9.1 | 51.9 | 108.9 | 95.5 |
| Cerebrovascular disease | 1.9 | 17.9 | 54.0 | 72.6 |
| Emphysema | 1.6 | 15.2 | 50.0 | 38.9 |

*Source:* Seeman et al. (1989), reference 212.

disabilities renders them more susceptible to the complications of new illnesses and their treatments. The presence of chronic medical conditions is associated with disability and increased health-care use, including institutionalization and hospitalization in the elderly (Table 38–1). Forty percent of community-dwelling adults older than 65 years report impairment in their daily activities secondary to chronic medical conditions.[4] Sixteen percent of adults older than 65 years report impairment in walking, increasing to more than 32% in those older than 85 years. Comorbidity is highly prevalent in people over 65 years. In the United States, 49% of noninstitutionalized people over 60 years have two or more chronic conditions. Much higher percentages are seen in adults older than 65 years who are living in a nursing home or who are hospitalized.[4–11]

Between 1982 and 2004 there was a significant decline in the age-standardized prevalence of disability, which is largely attributed to a lower share of persons over 65 years living in institutions and a reduction in the the number of persons reporting some impairments in instrumental activities of daily living impairments (IADL), such as food shopping or using the telephone.[12] Between 1992 and 2004, the age-adjusted percentage of people aged 65 years and older with at least one functional limitation decreased from 34.7% to 29.2%.[13]

Between 1992 and 2003, prevalence rates for arthritis in persons over age 65 years increased from 55.2% to 58.6%, diabetes increased from 15.9% to 19.7%, hypertension increased from 51.1% to 59.2%, and obesity increased from 15% to 21.2%, whereas the reported prevalence of heart problems decreased slightly from 37.6% to 36.7%.[13]

Recent Organization for Economic Cooperation and Development (OECD) projections suggest that public expenditure on long-term care will increase from 1.1% of GDP in 2005 to 2.3% in 2050.[14] Regardless of the decline in disability in some countries, the aging of the population and the greater longevity of individuals can be expected to lead to increasing numbers of older people with severe disabilities and in need of long-term care.[14]

Three general stages of progression in chronic illness have been identified and include: early stage, diagnosis and initial management, middle stage, disease modification and adjustment to functional decline, late stage, and preparation for dying.[15]

An understanding of some of the very common geriatric syndromes should be thoroughly understood by the palliative care clinician and include dementia, delirium, urinary incontinence, and falls. These syndromes further complicate end of care planning, and end-of-life symptom management in this population.

## Sites of Residence and Place of Death

Sixty-six percent of older noninstitutionalized persons live in a family setting; this decreases with increasing age. Three of every five women older than 85 years live outside of a family arrangement. Rates of institutionalization are estimated to be 4% to 5% in the United States; this increases to 23% in the over-85-year-old population. The wide range of care settings for the elderly is reflected in the sites of death of the elderly.[8,16–19]

Over the past 100 years, the site of death has shifted from the home to institutions. Data from the National Institute on Aging's Survey of the Last Days of Life (SLDOL) indicate that 45% of the elderly who died spent the night prior to death in a hospital, 24% spent the night in a nursing home, and 30% died at home.[20] More recently, 43.2% of deaths for persons over 65 years were reported to have occurred in hospitals.[21] Nursing home deaths are increasingly common for the oldest old: approximately one-third of decedents aged 75 years and older died in skilled nursing facilities in 2001.[21] More than 90% of deaths at home, on hospice, or in nursing homes are now persons older than 65 years.[22]

In several studies, cancer and dementia are predictive of death at home rather than in institutions. Death in hospice appears to correlate with the local availability of hospice beds, as well as a diagnosis of cancer. For patients with a preference for death at home, the availability of home visits by physicians correlates with a higher rate of death at home. In patients expressing an initial wish to die at home, caregiver burnout and unrelieved symptoms are predictive of death in hospitals and hospice.[16-19] The available data suggest that with limited increase in the allocation of nursing support, dying patients' wishes to die at home can be met. Elderly women are more than twice as likely to be living alone than elderly men. More than half of women 75 years and older live alone.[16-19] Those living alone rely more heavily on the presence of social supports and assistance for the provision of healthcare.[16-19]

## Palliative Care in Nursing Homes

Today 1.6 million people reside in the 18,000 nursing homes in the United States. According to the 2000 census, 4.7% of those ages 75 to 84 years and 18.2% of those ages 84 years and older live in nursing homes nationwide. In 1999, 777,500 deaths occurred in nursing homes, which represented approximately 25% of all deaths in the United States. The average length of nursing home residence for those who died in these institutions was 2 years, compared with the 2.38-year average length of residence for all nursing home admissions.[23]

These figures clearly tell us that the vast majority of residents admitted to nursing homes are severely ill. Because of Medicare hospice regulations, those residents would largely not be certified as terminally ill (prognosis of 6 months or less) and would therefore be ineligible for hospice care for 75% of their stay in a facility. Although there has been a modest increase in the proportion of nursing home residents who are receiving hospice (from 1% to 2.5% of the total nursing home population), the vast majority continue not to receive hospice, and the duration of time that residents are on end-of-life care has remained at approximately 5 months. Other factors include time pressures and staff and leadership turnover.[24-28]

Other findings include the fact that few facilities have a "true" palliative care program; even in the model programs, 66.7% estimated that less than 15% of their patients were receiving palliative care.[29]

Pain management and end-of-life care in nursing homes represent management of the frailest individuals, often with minimal physician involvement. As many as 45% to 80% of nursing home residents have pain that contributes significantly to impaired quality of life.[30] Most mild pain in nursing homes is related to degenerative arthritis, low-back disorders, and diabetic and postherpetic neuropathy. Cancer pain accounts for the majority of severe pain.[31]

Barriers to palliative care in the nursing home include institutional, patient, and staff-related barriers (Table 38–2).

---

**Table 38–2**
**Barriers to Palliative Care in Nursing Homes**

**Institution-related**
Low priority given to palliative care management by administration
Limited physician involvement in care, weekly or monthly assessments
Limited pharmacy involvement, no on-site pharmacy
Limited RN involvement in care; inadequate nurse–patient staff ratios
Primary care being administered by nonprofessional nursing staff
Limited radiological and diagnostic services, which impairs determination of a pain diagnosis

**Patient-related**
Physiological changes of aging, which affects distribution, metabolism, and elimination of medications
Multiple chronic diseases
Polypharmacy
Impaired cognitive status and Alzheimer's-type dementia
Underreporting of pain because of fear of addiction, lack of knowledge, fear of being transferred
Sensory losses that impede assessment
Increased incidence of depression, which may mask reporting and assessment of pain

**Staff-related**
Lack of knowledge of symptom management at the end of life
Lack of knowledge in the assessment and management of chronic cancer pain
Lack of knowledge in use of opioid drugs, titration, and side-effect management
Fear of using opioids in elderly residents
Misconceptions about use of opioids in elderly patients (e.g., fear of addiction, "elderly feel less pain")
Lack of knowledge in use of nonpharmacological techniques
Lack of experience with other routes of administration including patient-controlled analgesia, transdermal, rectal, subcutaneous, and intravenous routes

*Source:* Adapted from Stein (1996), reference 213.

---

Current health policy and reimbursement structures discourage use of palliative care and hospice care for nursing home residents. Quality standards and reimbursement rules provide incentives for restorative care and technologically intensive treatments rather than labor-intensive palliative care. Reimbursement incentives and fears about adherence to state and federal regulations also limit its use. Data from nursing homes suggest that as many as 30% to 80% of nursing home residents receive inadequate pain management.[32-38]

In one study comparing analgesic management of dying patients in a nursing home who were enrolled or not enrolled in Medicare Hospice program, 15% percent of hospice residents and 23% of nonhospice residents who were in daily pain received no analgesics; 51% of hospice residents and 33% of nonhospice residents received regular treatment for pain. These findings suggest that for nursing home residents in pain, analgesic management is better for hospice patients, but for many residents, pain management is sporadic and often inconsistent with American Medical Directors Association Guidelines.[39]

Many other obstacles to palliative care have been identified, including lack of communication among decision-makers, lack of agreement on a course for end-of-life care, failure to implement a timely end-of-life care plan, and failure to recognize treatment futility.[40] Only about half of nursing home residents have do-not-resuscitate (DNR) orders, fewer than one in five have advance directives, and fewer (14%) have living wills and do-not-hospitalize directives (4%).[41,42] One of the most troublesome concerns expressed by staff who care for nursing home residents is the difficulty in assessing pain in the cognitively impaired elderly resident.

Approximately 90% of the 4 million Americans with dementia will be institutionalized before death.[43] One of the barriers to end-of-life care in this population is that advanced dementia is often not viewed as a terminal condition. Because of this, palliative care often is not initiated until the final stages of life. In one retrospective study using the data from the Minimum Data Set,[44,45] 1784 residents with advanced dementia and 918 residents with terminal cancer were compared. Residents with advanced dementia were older, lived longer, and had higher activity of living scores than the terminal cancer residents. Six months after admission to the nursing home, only 20% of the residents with advanced dementia were perceived as having a life expectancy of less than 6 months. At the last assessment before death, only 4.1% were recognized as having a prognosis under 6 months; 55% had a DNR order, compared with 86.1% of the cancer patients.[46] With respect to non-palliative interventions, residents dying with advanced dementia experienced more frequent uncomfortable or aggressive interventions at the end of life; 25% died with a feeding tube, 11% with restraints, and 10.1% with intravenous IV therapy. These findings suggest that palliative care for nursing home residents with advanced dementia is suboptimal and encourages use of educational strategies to promote palliative care to these patients.

## Ethical Issues in Providing Palliative Care in Nursing Homes

Although symptom management should be an integral part of the entire therapeutic continuum, intensive focus on palliation for elderly nursing home residents is typically an indication that the end of life is approaching. The issues that are raised and the decisions they require are some of the most difficult encountered in nursing homes. These decisions are often made by the older patient or, more often, the patient's family and the care team. Sometimes, however, the complex nature of such decisions and their profound consequences

create confusion or disagreement. Issues confronting staff include questions surrounding the patient's decisional capacity, how to best promote the patient's interests, and differences in goals and plan of care. When these clinical conflicts occur, a bioethics consultation can be especially helpful in gathering the key parties clarifying the issues, providing a forum for deliberation, helping to define the goals of care, and supporting the parties in resolving the conflict in ways that are mutually acceptable.[47,48]

Clinicians who work in nursing homes face increasing caseloads and often rely on decisions and opinions of caregivers that may ultimately not reflect the values or goals of the patient. Advance directives are often unavailable or lack sufficient specificity and clarity to impact decisions such as transfer to the acute care setting or the institution of life-prolonging treatments. The presence, stability, and willingness to discuss advance care planning (ACP) appears to depend on several factors, including communication issues, value differences, cultural issues, ethnicity, and mental capacity. Although much literature points toward the relationship between a patient's prior decision regarding future treatment choices, stability of nursing home residents' preferences for some life-prolonging therapies may vary over time. One study suggested that although a majority of residents consistently desired cardiopulmonary resuscitation over a 2-year period, fewer than half favored medical hydration and nutrition. However, as time progressed the proportion of residents willing to consider such interventions rose.[49,50] The majority of residents in nursing homes at the end of life are unable to make treatment decisions for themselves. This results in reliance on surrogates.[51]

The burden of decision-making about withdrawal of life-prolonging therapies may be lessened by affording the family the opportunity to explore goals of care with nursing home clinicians who have cared for their loved one over months or years, rather than being faced by unfamiliar hospital staff at critical times, in an emergent situation.

## Economic Considerations in Caring for the Elderly

The higher rates of disability and comorbidity in the elderly, which require the provision of long-term residential care as well as home care, result in considerable costs to health care.

Health Care Financing Administration data indicate that 6% to 8% of Medicare enrollees die annually and account for 27% to 30% of annual Medicare expenses.[52] However, spending on aggressive interventions is not a major component of the hospital costs incurred in the dying elderly. Only 3% of Medicare beneficiaries who die sustain high costs associated with aggressive interventions such as surgery, chemotherapy, or dialysis.

Although hospital costs in the last days of life are lower for the oldest old, the percentage of Medicare and Medicaid expenditure for nursing home care rises from 24% for the young-old (65–74 yr) to 62% for the oldest old (over 85 yr).[53,54] Most required residential care occurs in the last days of life. Many older adults with limited supplemental insurance may be unable to remain in their own homes.[55] Greater state support for home- and community-based services increases the likelihood of dying at home.

## Case Management and the Elderly: Providing Coordination of Care

Greater numbers of older adults living at home are managing multiple chronic conditions and disability. These patients often lack coordination of care. Their utilization of the health-care system may be episodic and unplanned, with the emergency department (ED) being an important source of medical care. The physician's evaluation in the ED, and acute care in general, is often time-limited. Their evaluation focuses on individual diseases as opposed to a function-based assessment and often does not give a complete picture of the older patient. Older patients with progressive illnesses may be at greater risk of polypharmacy, falls, functional decline, and institutionalization as a consequence of uncoordinated care.

Other consequences of chronic medical conditions such as pain and other untreated symptoms may also result in utilization of the ED.[56,57]

Case management is defined as a health care delivery process that provides quality healthcare, decreases fragmentation, enhances the client's quality of life, and contains costs. Case managers provide coordination of medical care and social services. Elders who receive case management services, including risk assessment and follow-up health education, experience fewer hospitalizations and have lower health-care costs.[58–60]

## Uncertainty of Prognosis and the Provision of Palliative Care

Providing palliative care to elderly patients is limited by the uncertain prognoses of many chronic illnesses in this population (congestive heart failure, chronic obstructive pulmonary disease [COPD], cerebrovascular disease, dementia). Because of the difficulty to accurately prognosticate and many other factors, most patients who have fatal illnesses do not use the Medicare hospice benefit until shortly before death.[61] Even the most complex prognostic scoring systems, such as the Acute Physiology Age Chronic Health Evaluation (APACHE), provide little information for the likelihood of an individual patient's death.[62]

The uncertain prognoses of chronic nonmalignant medical conditions can affect clinical decision-making. It may also lead to overuse of health-care resources in acute care settings, even when death is imminent. Routine use of screening measures such as the palliative performance scale in primary care, in the ED, and in long-term care settings may help distinguish between patients who are chronically ill and persons in whom death is likely in the following 12 months.[56]

## Advance Care Planning

Advance care planning is a *process* whereby a patient, in consultation with health-care providers, family members, and important others, makes decisions about his/her future healthcare. Grounded in the ethical principle of autonomy and the legal doctrine of consent, ACP helps to ensure that the norm of consent is respected should the patient become incapable of participating in treatment decisions. Health-care providers can play an important role by informing patients about ACP, directing them to appropriate resources, counseling them as they engage in ACP and helping them to tailor advance directives to their prognosis.[63]

Advance care planning assists individuals in preparing for a sudden unexpected illness from which they expect to recover, as well as the dying process and ultimately death. These conversations should begin when individuals are younger, healthy, and independent and should continue along the health/illness continuum, recognizing that goals of care and preferences may change as individuals develop chronic illness and functional decline, advancing disease, and frailty.[64] It is a not merely a document or an isolated event but dynamic planning that needs to be reviewed from time to time as the health status of a person changes.

The following steps must be taken prior to and when evoking advance care plans—both by the patient, their loved ones, and the health-care provider:

- Becoming educated about the topic, including understanding the documents, the process, and the benefits
- Exploring, clarifying, and documenting an individual's values, beliefs, goals of care, and expectations
- Understanding how to choose the best spokesperson (surrogate or agent) who is named in the state's legal document and who will work best with physicians and health-care providers to make decisions on the patient's behalf, then discussing wishes with the chosen spokesperson and alternate, family, physician, attorney, and spiritual advisor, as needed
- Understanding various life-sustaining treatments beyond cardiopulmonary resuscitation
- Recognizing practical issues related to maintaining document accessibility and the need to periodically review and update the documents.[65]

Having acquired the knowledge and education about the processes involved in ACP and via shared decision-making between patients, their caregivers, and the health-care providers, these wishes/plans can then be endorsed and ensured via the Advance Directives.

## Advance Directives

Advance Directives are written documents that may be an instruction directive, a proxy directive, or both. These extend the autonomy of competent patients to future situations in which the patient is incompetent. In effect they permit incompetent patients to exercise their autonomy rights through completing an instruction and/or proxy directive in advance of incompetency.[65]

### Instructive Directives

Instructive directives specify what life-sustaining treatments the person would or would not want in various health situations.[66] They often state the patient's wishes about life-sustaining treatment in various clinical situations. Patients with decision-making capacity have the right to refuse any treatment, and instructive directives extend that right when decision-making capacity is compromised. If an intervention is not legally available to any patient (e.g., euthanasia), then an instructive directive does not make that intervention available to a patient after they have lost decision-making capacity.

Directives can be difficult to complete, even for physicians. Most instructive directives are ambiguous and lack specific directions. Although directives often refer to "heroic life-prolonging measures," such measures are rarely defined. Generally, instructive directives fail to include direct references to when specific measures should be withheld or withdrawn in the context of incurable or terminal illness. Nevertheless, when people complete an instructive directive, they expect their wishes to be honored.[66]

Some states allow family members to execute a Natural Death Act Document after the patient loses decision-making capacity. This provides legal protection to physicians who withdraw life-prolonging interventions—protection that may encourage physicians to act in accordance with a patient's stated wishes.[66]

### Proxy Directives

A proxy directive is a document authorizing a specific person to make health-care decisions on behalf of a patient only after that person loses decision-making capacity.

When possible, ACP should take place soon after a diagnosis of a life-limiting or chronic disease is made, particularly one that is expected to cause declining mental and physical health. Alzheimer's disease is a good example of a chronic illness where an individual may lack or gradually lose the ability to think clearly. This change affects his/her ability to participate meaningfully in decision-making and also makes early legal and financial planning very important.[67] Although difficult questions often arise, ACP can help people with Alzheimer's disease and their families clarify their wishes and make well-informed decisions about healthcare and financial arrangements. When possible, ACP should take place soon after a diagnosis of early-stage Alzheimer's disease while the person can participate in discussions. People with early-stage Alzheimer's disease are often capable of understanding many aspects and consequences of legal decision-making. However, legal and medical experts say that many forms of planning can help the person and his family even if the person is diagnosed with later-stage Alzheimer's disease.[67]

In addition to the aforementioned advance directives, there are other medical and legal/financial planning documents that are coupled to ACP. Some such medical documents are:

- The *living will* describes and instructs how the person wants end-of-life healthcare managed.
- *Durable power of attorney for healthcare* gives a designated person the authority to make health-care decisions on behalf of the person with Alzheimer's disease.
- *The do not resuscitate (DNR) form* instructs healthcare professionals not to perform cardiopulmonary resuscitation in case of stopped heart or stopped breathing. A DNR order is signed by a doctor and put in a person's medical chart.[67]

### Legal/Financial Documents

- **Living will**: A living will indicates how a person's assets and estate will be distributed among beneficiaries after his/her death. It records a person's wishes for medical treatment near the end of life. It may specify the extent of life-sustaining treatment and major healthcare the person wants. It may also help a terminal patient die with dignity as well as protect the clinician or hospital from liability for carrying out the patient's instructions. These may also specify how much discretion the person gives to his/her proxy about end-of-life decisions.[67]
- **Durable Power of Attorney for Finances**: The Durable Power of Attorney for Finances gives a designated person the authority to make legal/financial decisions on behalf of the person.
- **Living Trust**: The living trust gives a designated person (trustee) the authority to hold and distribute property and funds for the individual.[67]

### The Importance of Advance Directives in Palliative Care

Advance directives are more relevant to palliative care than healthcare in general because of the high likelihood of deterioration and death among palliative patients. Generic advance directives fail to account for the different needs of people who might make use of them. The philosophy of palliative care probably predetermines many of the treatment choices usually offered in the instruction directives of advance directives. However, instruction directives do not necessarily need to be focused on the treatment choices. They can also be focused around patients' values, the goals of therapy, health states that patients consider to be worse than death, and symptoms such as pain. This approach to design instruction directives seems more appropriate to palliative care setting. It would help affirm goals of palliative care and facilitate discussion between patients and their families and the health-care providers. Moreover, the addition of a proxy directive can be very helpful in the palliative care context, particularly when there is dispute among family members regarding the appropriate direction of care.[65]

## Advance Directives and Decision-Making in the Elderly

Advance directives are especially important in elderly patients who are at high risk of morbidity and mortality. The presence, stability, and willingness to discuss ACP appears to depend on several factors, including communication issues, value differences, cultural issues, ethnicity, and mental capacity.[50,51] In one study of ACP among nursing home residents, two variables found to be associated with the reduced likelihood of having DNR and do-not-hospitalize orders or restricting feeding, medication, or other treatment were African-American ethnicity and less time in the facility.

Most studies support the notion that a patient's prior decision regarding treatment choices accurately reflects future choices.[68-71] However, some others show that patient preferences are subject to change and may be influenced by a number of factors as demonstrated by a 2-year prospective study conducted by McParland et al. to evaluate the durability over time of decisions made regarding terminal care of mentally intact nursing home patients and the influence of such factors as intervening illness, loss of significant others, and cognitive, emotional, and functional decline. Results of the study revealed that preferences regarding cardiopulmonary resuscitation and parenteral and enteral nutrition changed over both the 12- and 24-month study periods. Only degree of change in cognitive status proved to be predictive of changes in decision. Gender, presence or absence of depression, change in level of functional abilities and intercurrent illness or stressor did not influence change regarding life-sustaining therapy. This study suggests that periodic re-evaluation of advance directives should be performed and that ongoing discussions should be initiated with patients by health-care professionals.[72] Although this study focused on institutionalized patients but the principle of re-evaluation of goals of care should be practiced by health-care providers in all health-care settings. As per the philosophy of palliative care, these discussions should include the caregivers and the significant others in the patient's life as a means of providing holistic support via shared decision-making. It goes without saying that this would require time allocated toward having theses discussions by the health-care teams, which could pose a challenge and constraint on addressing ACPs.

It has also been brought to attention by a Hastings Center report that despite the hope that traditional advance directives would ensure that patient preferences are honored, numerous studies have found that only a minority (20%–30%) of American adults have an advance care directive and that these documents have limited effects on treatment decisions near the end of life.[73]

So, what is being done to promote the process of advance care planning?

## State Initiatives on Advance Care Planning

In 1991, Oregon state developed the "Physician Orders for Life-Sustaining Treatment" (POLST: www.polst.org), to honor end-of-life treatment preferences and to overcome some of the limitations of advance care directives.[74] The POLST paradigm is designed to improve end-of-life care by converting patients' treatment preferences into medical orders that are transferable throughout the health-care system. This paradigm is now implemented in multiple states, with many considering its use. It is designed to convert patient preferences for life-sustaining treatments into immediately actionable medical orders. The centerpiece of the program is a standardized, brightly colored form that provides specific treatment orders for cardiopulmonary resuscitation, medical interventions, artificial nutrition, and antibiotics. It is complemented based on conversations among health-care professionals with the patient and/or the appropriate proxy decisionmakers, in conjunction with any existing advance directive for incapacitated patients. The POLST form is recommended for persons who have advanced chronic progressive illness, who might die in the next year, or who wish to further define their preferences for treatment.[75]

As Oregon's program evolved, selected regulations rather than legislation were used to help with implementation. Other developing programs like West Virginia and New York sought legislation to facilitate POLST paradigm adoption. Each new program found that their approach needed to be thoughtfully tailored to state laws and regulations. An investigation by task force members, published in March 2008, underscores the need to understand state policies and rules in helping choose the best path for implementation.[75]

On July 7, 2008, in the state of New York, Governor David Paterson signed Chapter 197 of the Laws of 2008 allowing the use of an alternative DNR form, which is the Medical Orders for Life Sustaining Treatment (MOLST) form. MOLST is an alternative form and process for patients to provide their end-of-life care preferences to health-care providers across the spectrum of the health-care delivery system. MOLST may be honored by Emergency Medical Services (EMS), hospitals, nursing homes, adult homes, hospices, and other health-care facilities and their health-care provider staff. The MOLST form is a bright pink form that was piloted by the Rochester Health Commission under previous legislation for use by the EMS community in Onondaga and Monroe Counties.[76] MOLST has been reviewed annually since 2005 and has been adapted to meet clinical needs of the patients. The success of MOLST Pilot Project resulted in Governor Paterson signing a bill (PHL§2977(3)) that made MOLST a statewide law, thereby changing the scope of practice for EMS across New York State.[77]

The MOLST can be used in the community in lieu of the NYS Nonhospital DNR. In signing the legislation, Governor Paterson said, "People should be allowed as much say in their end-of-life care as they would have at any other time. This bill will allow many people who are critically ill to make enduring decisions on the care they will receive. These will be difficult decisions for every person to make, but they should have the freedom to make them."[78]

Addressing ACP can be complex and challenging and should be considered a dynamic process where the goals of care may need to be reset from time to time as the health status of the individuals and the resources available for their care change. Also, it would help to hold these discussions early and at the level of the community. To do so, the healthcare providers may need to incorporate these discussions in their practice as a standard of care. This may further require a motivation and commitment by educational institutions to train the future nurses, doctors, social-workers, and so forth on addressing advance care plans so that they are primed toward initiating and engaging in these discussions when they eventually are ready as individual health-care leaders or as part of the multidisciplinary health team.

To conclude, as commented by Murray and Jennings, we sometimes seem to act as though dying were solely the concern of the dying person. The fact is we die, as we live, in a web of vital and complex relationships. Culture needs time to catch up with end-of-life law. The next decades should be a time of education and soul-searching discussion in communities and at kitchen tables, as well as in health-care settings.[79]

## Family/Caregiver Issues

### Who are the Caregivers for the Elderly?

The term caregiver refers to anyone who provides assistance to someone else who needs it. "Informal caregiver" is a term used to refer to unpaid individuals, such as family members and friends, who provide care. These persons can be primary or secondary caregivers, full- or part-time, and can live with the person being cared for or live separately. "Formal caregivers" are volunteers or paid care providers associated with a service system. Estimates vary on the number of caregivers in the United States.

According to a National Long-Term Care Study (NLTCS), more than 7 million people are informal caregivers, defined here as spouses, adult children, other relatives, and friends who provide unpaid help to older people with at least one limitation in their activities of daily living. An estimated 15% of American adults are providing care for seriously ill or disabled adults.[80] Of these, an estimated 12.8 million Americans need assistance to perform activities such as eating, dressing, and bathing. About 57% are aged 65 years or older (7.3 million). Spouses accounted for about 62% of primary caregivers. Approximately 72% of caregivers are female.[81] The majority

of caregivers provide unpaid assistance for 1 to 4 years, and 20% provide care for 5 years or longer.[82] According to the 2000 National Hospice Care Survey (NHCS), 42% of patients enrolled in hospice programs were women and 33% were men. The majority (81%) were 65 years or older, and a significantly larger proportion of women than men were age 85 years or older. Men were more likely to have a spouse as their primary caregiver, whereas women were more likely to be cared for by a child or child-in-law. The most common diagnosis for most of the hospice care patients included neoplasm, heart disease, and COPD.[82]

## Involving Family in Caregiving for the Elderly

### What is the Burden on the Family?

The burden of caregiving has been well-documented in the literature and includes a greater number of depressive symptoms, anxiety, diminished physical health, financial problems, and disruption in work. The amount of concrete needs the patient has strongly relates to family and caregiver psychological distress and burden of care.[83] Elderly patients who are dying require varying levels of assistance with personal care, meal preparation, shopping, transportation, paying bills, and submitting forms related to health care. The level of physical care may be tremendous and includes bathing, turning and positioning, wound care, colostomy care, suctioning, medication administration, and managing incontinence. If the patient is confused or agitated, the strain is even greater, as 24-hour care may be necessary. In the palliative care setting, where the treatment goals are supportive and often include management of symptoms such as pain, respiratory distress, and delirium, the patient is frequently confined to home, with a greater burden placed on the live-in spouse or child.

In one study comparing the impact of caregiving in curative and palliative care settings, two study groups were evaluated: 267 patients received active, curative treatment, and 134 patients received palliative care through a local hospice. Patients in the palliative care group were more physically debilitated and had poorer performance status. The mean age was 59.7 years for the curative group and 57.9 years for the palliative care group. Caregiver quality-of-life measures demonstrated that family caregivers of patients receiving palliative care had lower quality-of-life scores and worse overall physical health than family caregivers of patients receiving curative care.[84] Families with low socioeconomic status and those with less education were more distressed by the patient's illness.

Transitions in spousal caregiving have been investigated in respect to the level/intensity of caregiving and its impact on the overall health of the caregiver. In 428 subjects who were assessed at four intervals over a 5-year period, those who transitioned to heavy caregiving had more depressive symptoms than those who transitioned into moderate caregiving. Heavy caregivers scored higher in the number of health-risk behaviors between the second and third observations, concluding that these outcomes become worse over time.[85] In another study of 231 caregivers of cancer patients who were at home, the goals were to evaluate family caregiver's quality of life, financial burden, and experience of managing cancer pain in the home.[86] Family caregivers scored worse in areas of coping with difficulty, anxiety, depression, happiness, and feeling in control. In areas of physical well-being, the greatest problems were sleep changes and fatigue. Other quality-of-life disruptions included interference with employment, lack of support from others, isolation, and financial burden. The estimated average time spent caregiving was more than 12 hours per day; the estimated time for pain management was more than 3 hours per day. Family caregivers reported worse outcomes than patients did in their perception of the pain intensity, pain distress to themselves, feeling able to control the pain, and family concern about pain in the future. Caregivers reported fear of future pain, fear of tolerance, and concern about addiction and harmful effects of analgesics. The authors concluded that educational programs in pain management are needed and that further educational efforts should also address the emotional aspects of managing cancer pain in the home. Interventions directed toward improving the quality of life of direct caregivers include educational programs, improvement in home care supports, psychoeducational programs, and improved access to healthcare professionals who provide symptom management and end-of-life care.

Family grief therapy during the palliative phase of illness has also improved the psychosocial quality of life of caregivers. Kissane and colleagues[87] used a screening tool to identify dysfunctional family members and relieve distress through a model of family grief therapy sessions. Smeenk and colleagues[88] demonstrated improved quality of life of direct caregivers after implementation of a transmural home care intervention program for terminal cancer patients. Macdonald[89] demonstrated that massage as a respite intervention for caregivers was successful in reducing physical and emotional stress, physical pain, and sleep difficulties. This nonpharmacological and noninvasive intervention is highly valued and accepted by caregivers because of its simplicity and beneficial effects.

## Pharmacological Considerations in Providing Symptom Management

Pharmacological intervention is the mainstay of treatment for symptom management in palliative care of the elderly patient. Knowledge of the parameters of geriatric pharmacology can prevent serious morbidity and mortality when multiple drugs are used to treat single or multiple symptoms or when, in the practice of chronic pain management, trials of sequential opioids (opioid rotation, or opioid switch) are used.

With normal aging there is a steady decline in physiological reserve capacity in most organ systems and dysregulation in others.[90] (These changes become apparent under stress and play an important role at the end of life when the goal is symptom control and comfort. Important physiological changes in the elderly patient will be outlined below.

### Pharmacokinetics

The four components of pharmacokinetics are absorption, distribution, metabolism, and excretion. In the absence of malabsorption problems and obstruction, oral medications are well-tolerated in the elderly population. With aging, there is some decrease in gastric secretion, absorptive surface area, and splanchnic blood flow. Most studies show no difference in oral bio-availability—the extent to which a drug reaches its site of action. There is little literature on the absorption of long-acting drugs in the elderly, including controlled or sustained-release opioids, and transdermal opioids commonly used in the treatment of chronic cancer pain in the elderly patient. Controlled-release dosage forms are generally more appropriate with drugs that have short half-lives (less than 4 hours) and include many of the shorter-acting opioids, including morphine and hydromorphone. Generally, it is safer to use opioids that have shorter half-lives in the elderly cancer patient.

Distribution refers to the distribution of drug to the interstitial and cellular fluids after it is absorbed or injected into the bloodstream. There are several significant physiological factors that may influence drug distribution in the elderly palliative care patient. An initial phase of distribution reflects cardiac output and regional blood flow. The heart, kidneys, liver, and brain receive most of the drug after absorption. Delivery to fat, muscle, most viscera, and skin is slower; it may take several hours before steady-state concentrations are reached. Although cardiac output does not change with age, chronic conditions, including congestive heart failure, may contribute to a decrease in cardiac output and regional blood flow.

This second phase of drug distribution to the tissues highly depends on body mass. Body weight generally decreases with age, but more importantly, body composition changes with age. Total body water and lean body mass decrease, whereas body fat increases in proportion to total body weight. The volume-of-distribution changes are mostly for highly lipophilic and hydrophilic drugs, and the elderly are most susceptible to drug toxicity from drugs that should be dosed on ideal body weight or lean body weight. Theoretically, highly lipid-bound drugs (e.g., long-acting benzodiazepines and transdermal fentanyl, both commonly prescribed to elderly patients) may have an increased volume of distribution and a prolonged effect if drug clearance is constant.[91] Water-soluble drugs (e.g., digoxin) may have a decreased volume of distribution and increased serum levels and toxicity if initial doses are not conservative. To avoid possible side effects in a frail elderly patient, it may be safe to start with one half the dose usually prescribed for a younger patient.

Another host factor that influences drug distribution is plasma protein concentrations.[92,93] Most drugs, including analgesics, are extensively bound to plasma proteins. The proportion of albumin among total plasma proteins decreases with frailty, catabolic states, and immobility, which is commonly seen in many elderly patients with chronic conditions. A decrease in serum albumin can increase the percentage of free (unbound) drug available for pharmacological effect and elimination. In this setting, standard doses of medications lead to higher levels of free (unbound) drug and possible toxicity.

The liver is the major site of drug metabolism. Hepatic metabolism of drugs depends on drug-metabolizing enzymes in the liver. The hepatic microenzymes are responsible for this biotransformation. With advanced age, there is a decrease in liver weight by 20% to 50% and liver volume decreases by approximately 25%.[94] Additionally, galactose clearance, a nondrug marker for hepatic functional mass, is decreased by 25% in advanced age. Associated with these changes in liver size and weight is a decrease in hepatic blood flow, normalized by liver volume. This corresponds to a decrease in liver perfusion of 10% to 15%. Drugs absorbed from the intestine may be subject to metabolism and the first-pass effect in the liver, accounting for decreased amounts of drug in the circulation after oral administration. The end result is decreased systemic bio-availability and plasma concentrations.[95] The process of biotransformation in the liver largely depends on the P-450 cytochrome. During biotransformation, the parent drug is converted to a more polar metabolite by oxidation, reduction, or hydrolysis. The resulting metabolite may be more active than the parent drug. The cytochrome P-450 has been shown to decline in efficiency with age. These altered mechanisms of drug metabolism should be considered when treating the elderly palliative care patient with opioids, long-acting benzodiazepines, and neuroleptics.

The effect of age on renal function is quite variable. Some studies show a linear decrease in renal function, amounting to decreased glomerular function; other studies indicate no change in creatinine clearance with advancing age.[95] Renal mass decreases 25% to 30% in advanced age, and renal blood flow decreases 1% per year after age 50.[95] There are also decreases in tubular function and reduced ability to concentrate and dilute the urine. Generally, the clearance of drugs that are secreted or filtered by the kidney is decreased in a predictable manner.

For example, delayed renal excretion of meperidine's metabolite, normeperidine, may result in delirium, central nervous system stimulation, myoclonus, and seizures. Meperidine is not recommended for chronic administration in any patient but is of special concern for elderly patients with borderline renal function. Other drugs that rely on renal excretion include nonsteroidal antiinflammatory agents, digoxin, aminoglycoside antibiotics, and contrast media.

## Medication Use in the Elderly: Problems with Polypharmacy

Older individuals use three times more medications than younger people do. They account for approximately 25% of physician visits and approximately 35% of drug expenditures.

Elderly patients are more likely to be prescribed inappropriate medications than younger patients.[95] Advancing age alone does not explain the risk of adverse drug reactions, and polypharmacy is a consistent predictor. As noted earlier, in the palliative care setting, elderly patients often have more than one comorbid medical condition, necessitating treatment with many medications, which places them at greater risk of adverse drug reactions. In addition, new medications not only place the elderly at risk of adverse drug reactions, they also increase the risk of significant drug interactions. For example, the addition of an antacid to an elderly patient already on corticosteroids for bone pain may significantly decrease the oral corticosteroid effect because of decreased absorption.

Understanding pharmacodynamics in relationship to age-related physiological changes can assist the clinician in evaluating the effectiveness and side-effect profile in the elderly palliative care patient (Table 38–3). When multiple drugs are used to treat symptoms, the side-effect profile may increase, potentially limiting the use of one or more drugs. For example, when using an opioid and a benzodiazepine in treating chronic pain and anxiety in the elderly patient, excessive sedation may occur, limiting the amount of opioid that can be administered. Table 38–4 outlines the components of a comprehensive medication assessment in the elderly palliative care patient.

---

**Table 38–3**

**Risk Factors for Medication Problems in the Elderly Palliative Care Patient**

1. Multiple health care prescribers (e.g., multiple physicians, nurse practitioners)
2. Multiple medications
3. Automatic refills
4. Age-related physiological pharmacokinetic changes
5. Age-related pharmacodynamic changes
6. Sensory losses: visual, hearing
7. Cognitive defects: delirium, dementia
8. Depression
9. Anxiety
10. Knowledge deficits related to indication, action, dosing schedule, and side effects of prescribed medication
11. Complex dosing schedule or route of administration
12. Comorbid medical conditions: frailty, cerebrovascular disease, cardiac disease, musculoskeletal disorders, advanced cancer
13. Self-medication with over-the-counter medications, herbal remedies
14. Lack of social support or lives alone
15. Alcoholism
16. Financial concerns
17. Illiteracy
18. Misconceptions about specific medications (e.g., addiction)
19. Language barrier

*Source*: Adapted from Walker et al. (1996), reference 214.

**Table 38–4**
**Medication Assessment in the Elderly Palliative Care Patient**

1. Identify prior problems with medications.
2. Identify other health care providers who prescribe medications.
3. Obtain a detailed history of present medication use at all patient contacts. Include over-the-counter and herbal remedies and dosage, frequency, expected effect, and side effects. When assessing efficacy of pain management, ask about PRN "rescue" doses.
4. Identify "high-risk" medications and assess for side effects or drug–drug interactions.
5. Evaluate the need for drug therapy by performing a comprehensive physical examination and symptom assessment, and obtain appropriate laboratory data.
6. Assess functional, cognitive, sensory, affective, and nutritional status.
7. Review patient's and family member's level of understanding about indications, dosing, and side effects.
8. Identify any concerns about medications (cost, fears, misconceptions).
9. Identify presence of caregiver or support person and include in all assessments.
10. Implement strategies to increase support if lacking (e.g., skilled or nonskilled home care nursing support, community groups, other family members, community-based day programs).

*Source:* Adapted from Walker et al. (1996), reference 214.

## Management During the Last Weeks of Life: Special Concerns During the Dying Process

Care during the last hours of life should be a fundamental component of every nurse and physician's training. Both patients and family members are in special need of assistance with decision-making about end-of-life care. Sykes has identified the need to make a diagnosis of dying, not only so that goals of care may be established and interventions tailored but also so that patients may be made aware, if they wish, so that end-of-life decisions can be made.[96]

Decisions about a place to die—either in hospital or at home—should be made, if possible, by the patient and their family. In a recent study in British Hospitals, only 45% of 2673 patients from 118 hospitals were informed by staff that they were dying.[97]

The concern about discussing death is the problem of prognostication. Physicians consistently overestimate patients' survival, and familiarity with the patients tends to decrease their ability to prognosticate.[98]

Predictors of death within days include the inability to take drinks larger than sips, semi-comatose state, inability to swallow pills, being bedridden, and, in some cases, death rattle. Other signs include mottled skin color in the extremities,

irregular breathing, and loss of the radial pulse. Difficulties in prognostication in the terminal stages of heart disease or dementia result from the lack of predictive prognostic factors, and thus hinder the provision of end-of-life care.[99]

Numerous studies have evaluated symptoms during the last weeks of life and indicate that patients experience a high degree of symptom distress and suffering. In one study by Seale and Cartwright,[100] there were age-related differences in the incidence of mental confusion, loss of bladder and bowel control, as well as seeing/hearing difficulties. There was no age-related difference in patients reporting pain (72%), trouble breathing (49%), loss of appetite (47%), drowsiness (44%), and other symptoms, including sleeplessness, constipation, depression, vomiting, and dry mouth.

In another study of 40 frail elderly patients admitted to the hospital, the most frequent diagnosis was chronic respiratory failure, loss of appetite, and weakness. Frail elderly patients were defined by age over 75 years, with the presence of numerous chronic diseases or geriatric syndrome (incontinence, falls, cognitive impairment, immobility, etc).[101]

The complex symptomatology experienced by elderly patients, especially those with cancer and multiple comorbidities, demands that an aggressive approach to symptom assessment and intervention be used. Geriatric patients differ from younger patients in all domains of care. At the end of life, the geriatric patient who is dying may also have a have a higher incidence of certain syndromes, including dementia, urinary incontinence, falls, hearing and visual problems, as well as limited family support.

Devising a palliative plan of care for the elderly patient who is highly symptomatic or who is actively dying requires ongoing communication with the patient and family; assessment of patient and family understanding of goals of care and religious, cultural, and spiritual beliefs; access to community agencies; psychological assessment; and patient and family preferences regarding advance directives.

Table 38–5 outlines dimensions of a palliative care plan for the elderly. The management of three prevalent and distressing symptoms experienced by the elderly at the end of life—dyspnea, pain, and delirium—is discussed below. Each of these symptoms is discussed in greater detail in other chapters.

## Dyspnea

Dyspnea may be one of the most frightening and difficult symptoms an elderly patient can experience. A subjective feeling of breathlessness or the sensation of labored or difficult breathing, dyspnea contributes to severe disability and impaired quality of life. Dyspnea and fear of dyspnea produce profound suffering for dying patients and their families. This section will outline the special needs for elderly patients, with a focus on physiological factors that increase the risk of dyspnea.

**Table 38–5**
**Dimensions of a Palliative Plan of Care for the Elderly Patient**

1. Assess extent of disease documented by imaging studies and laboratory data.
2. Assess symptoms, including prevalence, severity, and impact on function.
3. Identify coping strategies and psychological symptoms, including presence of anxiety, depression, and suicidal tendencies.
4. Evaluate religious and spiritual beliefs.
5. Assess overall quality of life and well-being. Does the patient feel secure that all that can be done for them is being done? Is the patient satisfied with the present level of symptom control?
6. Determine family burden. Is attention being paid to the caregiver so that burnout does not occur? If the spouse or caregiver is elderly, is he or she able to meet the physical demands of caring for the patient?
7. Determine level of care needed in the home if the patient is dying.
8. Assess financial burden on patient and caregiver. Is an inordinate amount of money being spent on the patient and will there be adequate provisions for the elderly caregiver when the patient dies?
9. Identify presence of advance care planning requests. Have the patient's wishes and preferences for resuscitation, artificial feeding, and hydration been discussed? Has the patient identified a surrogate decision-maker who knows their wishes? Is there documentation regarding advance directives?

*Source:* Adapted from "Improving care at the end of life" (1997), reference 215.

**Table 38–6**
**Risk Factors for Dyspnea in the Elderly Palliative Care Patient**

| Risk factor | Comment |
|---|---|
| **Structural factors** | |
| Increased chest wall stiffness | Increase in the work of breathing |
| Decrease in skeletal muscle, barrel chest, increase in anteroposterior diameter | Decrease in maximum volume expiration |
| Decrease in elasticity of alveoli | Decrease in vital capacity |
| **Other factors** | |
| Anemia | |
| Cachexia | |
| Dehydration | Drier mucous membrane, increase in mucous plugs |
| Ascites | |
| Atypical presentation of fever | Reduced febrile response, decreased WBC response |
| Heart failure | |
| Immobility | Increased risk of aspiration, DVT, PE |
| Obesity | |
| Recent abdominal, pelvic, or chest surgery | Increased risk of DVT, PE |
| Lung disease (COPD, lung cancer) | |

*Sources:* Adapted from Eliopoulos (1996), reference 216; Palange et al. (1995), reference 102.
COPD, chronic obstructive pulmonary disease; DVI, deep venous thrombosis; PE, pulmonary embolism; WBC, white blood cell.

## Physiological Correlates in the Elderly that Increase Risk of Dyspnea

The effects of aging produce a clinical picture in which respiratory problems can develop. With aging, the elastic recoil of the lungs during expiration is decreased because of less collagen and elastin. Alveoli are less elastic and develop fibrous tissue. The stooped posture and loss of skeletal muscle strength often found in the elderly contribute to reduction in the vital capacity and an increase in the residual volume of the lung. Table 38–6 outlines the pulmonary risk factors for the development of dyspnea in the elderly palliative care patient.

Respiratory muscle weakness may play a major role in some types of dyspnea. Palange and colleagues[102] found that malnutrition significantly affected exercise tolerance in patients with COPD by producing diaphragmatic fatigue. In patients with cachexia, the maximal inspiratory pressure, an indicator of diaphragmatic strength, is severely impaired. Cachexia and asthenia occur in 80% to 90% of patients with advanced cancer and are also prevalent in elderly patients with multiple comorbid psychiatric and medical conditions. These mechanisms may affect the development of dyspnea and fatigue in the elderly who have advanced nonmalignant and malignant disease. Ripamonti and Bruera[103] have suggested that in some patients, dyspnea may be a clinical presentation of overwhelming cachexia and asthenia.

The multiple etiologies of dyspnea in the dying elderly patient include both malignant (e.g., tumor infiltration, superior vena cava syndrome, pleural effusion), treatment-related (Adriamycin-induced cardiomyopathy, radiation-induced pneumonitis, pulmonary fibrosis), and nonmalignant causes (e.g., metabolic, structural).

Typically breathlessness may be episodic, but with rapid disease progression it often occurs at rest. Often dyspnea at the end of life occurs with other prominent end-of-life symptoms including cachexia, fatigue, and weakness, and decline in the cancer patient is more predictable and steadily downward.[104]

Two causes of dyspnea, deep vein thrombosis (DVT) and pulmonary embolism (PE), are prevalent in the elderly and are often unrecognized and undiagnosed. They may present as pleuritic chest pain with or without dyspnea and hemoptysis. The risk factors in the elderly include increased venous stasis in the legs, impaired fibrinolysis, coagulopathies, recent surgery, immobility, and congestive heart failure. Treatment depends on accurate diagnosis, and an estimate of risks versus benefits should be considered in deciding on a course of action. Ventilation-perfusion scans are the most reliable indicator of whether a PE has occurred, and the identification of a DVT as the source of the PE can be accomplished through noninvasive Doppler studies of the legs. Whether it is prudent or compassionate to perform these studies in the elderly patient who is dying should be considered. In the elderly patient who is not actively dying, diagnostic tests can be safely performed. Treatment with anticoagulants in addition to supportive symptom management will reduce the symptom burden and suffering.

## Treatment of Dyspnea

When possible, relief of dyspnea is aimed at treatment of the underlying disease process, whether malignant or nonmalignant in origin. Symptomatic interventions are used when the process is not reversible. Both pharmacological and nonpharmacological interventions should be employed. One patient may present with multiple etiologies; therefore, multiple interventions are indicated.

Therapeutic interventions are based on the etiology and include pharmacological (e.g., bronchodilators, steroids, diuretics, vasodilators, opioids, sedatives, antibiotics), procedural (e.g., thoracentesis, chest tube placement), nonpharmacological (e.g., relaxation, breathing exercises, music), radiation therapy, and oxygen. At the end of life, the pharmacological use of benzodiazepines, opioids, and corticosteroids remain the primary treatment.

Using opioids to manage dyspnea can relieve both the sensation of breathlessness as well as having other objective and subjective benefits including anxiety, pain cough, and cardiac pre-load and after-load.[105] The use of nebulized opioids has been evaluated and most of the studies conclude that they offer no greater benefit than systemic opioids.

The use of nebulized morphine has been reported as a treatment for dyspnea; systematic reviews have concluded that nebulized opioids are no more effective than nebulized placebo.[106]

A Cochrane Review, based on a meta-analysis with only three randomized controlled trials comparing nebulized morphine to placebo, concluded that there is no evidence to support the use of nebulized opioids for the treatment of breathlessness.[107] Another study indicated that both nebulized and subcutaneous morphine significantly reduced background dyspnea, although these results were not compared to a saline treatment arm.[108]

In another study comparing the effect on nebulized hydromorphone, systemic hydromorphone, and nebulized saline on relief of incident dyspnea in opioid-tolerant palliative care cancer patients found that each of the treatments resulted in statistically significant improvements in breathlessness, with no significant differences between treatments. The average age of the patient was 69 years, with a median of 40 days to death. The findings suggesting that systemic (oral or subcutaneous) breakthrough analgesic doses of hydromorphone provide rapid and significant relief for incident breathlessness are consistent with those reported for the effects of opioids on baseline intractable dyspnea.[109]

The results of this study are encouraging, suggesting the use of saline for the management of dyspnea in patients is a simple and easy intervention. The authors do not feel they could support clinical recommendations but suggested further trials.

The use of nebulized fursemide has been shown in several small, single-dose studies to result in bronchodilitation and reduction of breathlessness.[110,111] Fursosemide is a loop diuretic that when inhaled inhibit cough and protect against bronchoconstriction. In theory, aerosolized furosemide inhibits cough and prevents bronchospam and suppresses pulmonary C-fibers in bronchial epithelium.[112] The use of furosemide is largely free of side effects and may prove useful in patients at the end of life.

In conclusion, higher level clinical evidence consistently shows that aerosolized opioids are not effective in improving dyspnea or exercise tolerance in patients with chronic cardiopulmonary diseases including COPD and idiopathic pulmonary fibrosis.[113]

The physiological component of dyspnea may be relieved by supplemental oxygen, noninvasive positive pressure ventilation for hypercapneic adults, or blowing cool air on the face—measures that can used in the home or in the hospital. Nonpharmacological interventions should always be attempted, including relaxation therapy, acupuncture, music therapy, or massage.

A dyspnea scale should guide dose adjustments with the dual goal of providing dyspnea relief and minimizing the sedative effects. If the patient is unable to rate their dyspnea on a scale of 0 to 10, observational signs of dyspnea should be utilized.[114]

Often there is reluctance among staff to use opioids and sedatives in the elderly because of unfamiliarity with these medications, lack of experience in treating dyspnea in dying patients, low priority given to this symptom, or fear that these drugs may hasten death in the elderly. Table 38–7 outlines management guidelines based on presenting symptoms. Figure 38–1 reviews the overall assessment and management of dyspnea in the geriatric patient at the end of life.

CASE STUDY
*Management of Dyspnea in an Elderly Patient with Recurrent Head and Neck Cancer*

An 85-year-old man with recurrent squamous cell of the base of tongue presents to his palliative care team with increasing shortness of breath, which has grown progressively worse over the past week. The patient has been home with mild shortness of breath, which was

**Table 38-7**
**BREATHES Program for Management of Dyspnea in the Elderly Palliative Care Patient**

**B—bronchospasm.** Consider nebulized albuterol and/or steroids.

**R—rales/crackles.** If present, reduce fluid intake. If patient is receiving IV hydration, reduce fluid intake or discontinue. Consider gentle diuresis with Lasix 20–40 mg PO daily, ± spironolactone (Aldactone) 100 mg PO daily.

**E—effusion.** Determine on physical examination or chest x-ray. Consider thoracentesis or chest tube, if appropriate.

**A—airway obstruction.** If patient is at risk or has had aspiration from food, puree solid food, avoid thin liquids, and keep the patient upright during and after meals for at least 1 hour.

**T—tachypnea and breathlessness.** Opioids reduce respiratory rate and feelings of breathlessness as well as anxiety. Assess daily. If patient is opioid naïve, begin with morphine sulfate 5–10 mg PO q4h and titrate opioids 25%–50% daily/every other day as needed. Consider an anxiolytic such as lorazepam (be aware of potential for paradoxical response) 0.5–2 mg PO bid-tid. Use of a fan may reduce feelings of breathlessness.

**H—hemoglobin low.** Consider a blood transfusion if anemia is contributing to dyspnea.

**E—educate** and support the patient and family during this highly stressful period.

**S—secretions.** If secretions are copious, consider a trial of a scopalamine patch q72h, atropine 0.3–0.5 mg SC q4h PRN, glycopyrrolate (Robinul) 0.1–0.4 mg IM/SQ q4–12h PRN

*Sources:* Adapted from Storey and Knight (1996), reference 217; Ripamonti (1999), reference 218; Tobin (1990), reference 219; Kuebler (1996), reference 220.

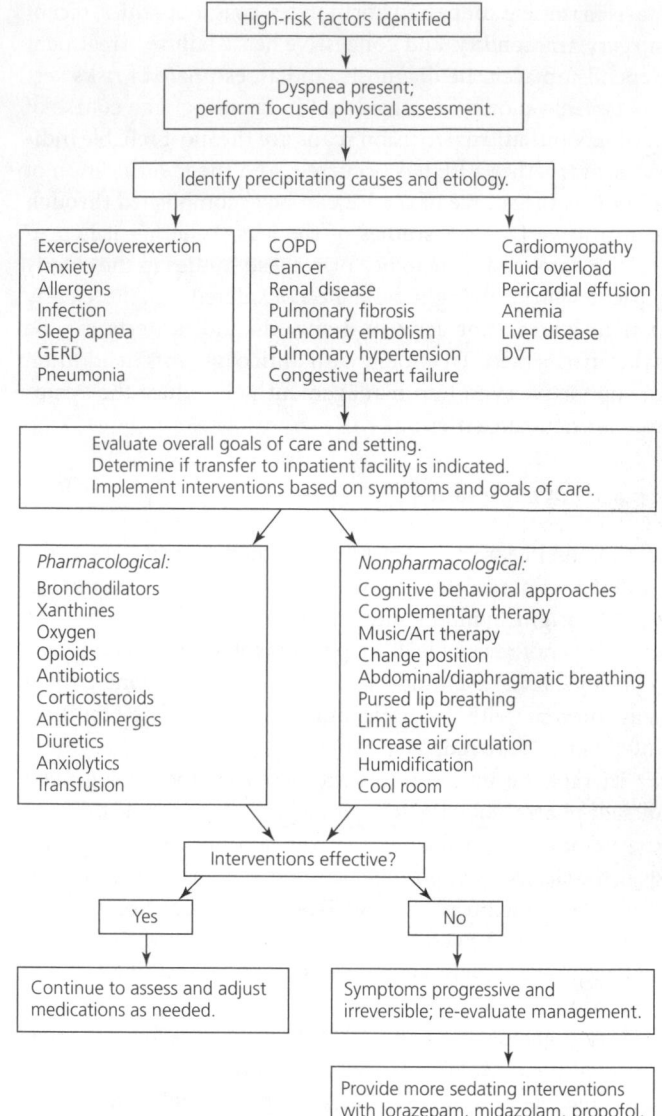

**FIGURE 38–1.** Dyspnea management in the geriatric patient at the end of life.

managed succesfully with 4 milligrams of intermittent hydromorphone every 4 hours prn. In the past he has received chemoradiation therapy to the tumor, and treatment concluded about 1 year ago. About 4 months ago he started experiencing pain in the lower right neck with some swelling, and imaging studies revealed recurrent disease. He has declined further radiation therapy because of the fear of mucositis and says he is ready to die. He is a very religious man and has put his "trust in God." A right pleural effusion was found 1 month ago, and he underwent two thoracentesis (the last one 5 days ago, when 1500 mL of pleuritic fluid was drained).

Past medications for dyspnea include 30 milligrams of morphine sulfate administered orally every 4 hours, which had produced sedation and delirium. He is also receiving 30 milligrams of prednisone orally two times daily for bronchospasm, and an albuterol inhaler (which he occasionally uses), senna, and a stool softener. Physical examination has revealed breath sounds decreased

bilaterally, an inspiratory stridor, and mild bilatoral wheezing. His respiratory rate is 26 per minute at rest, and he complains of feeling breathless and anxious. Pulse oximetry was 92% at rest, and he is using nasal oxygen (4 L/min). He is also very fatigued and cannot sleep at night. He is refusing further aggressive intervention and has signed a home DNR order.
❧

**At a Glance Assessment**

- Determine goals of care and clarify understanding between patient, family, and health-care providers.
- Management of dyspnea in the elderly patient at the end of life should be focused on the physical,

psychological, and spiritual domains of care. Relief of suffering should be a primary goal.

- Comprehensive management of dyspnea in the elderly patient at the end of life includes use of opioids, anxiolytics/sedatives, steroids and nonpharmacological interventions.

### Suggestions for Assessment and Intervention

1. Determine the etiology of the dyspnea in this patient. In this elderly cancer patient, dyspnea is multifactorial, including tumor progression in the upper airway as well as progression of pleural effusions. A chest X-ray has been done and has again revealed recurrent right pleural effusion. An X-ray of the neck has revealed progression of the tumor, compressing the trachea.

2. Review goals of care with the patient. It is clear to the staff that this patient is determined to not undergo further aggressive treatment, but he is willing to have X-rays or another thoracentesis if it would make him feel better. He wants to die at home, and his family is supportive of this decision.

3. He is given 10 milligrams of decadron every 6 hours in an attempt to reduce edema caused by the neck mass that is compressing his trachea. The members of the palliative care team feels that his life expectancy is very short, and their goal is to prevent the need for a tracheostomy.

4. Excessive fatigue is present in this patient, and a complete blood count has revealed a mild anemia, with no indication for a transfusion. A trial of a low-dose stimulant such as Ritalin administered 2.5 to 5 milligrams orally daily or twice a day is discussed but providers feel it should be used if the decadron fails to produce any stimulating effect on his fatigue.

5. The patient is receiving hydromorphone for dyspnea. The dose is increased by 50% to a dose of 6 milligrams orally every 4 hours to treat the tachypnea.

6. An anxiolytic– (0.5 mg of lorazepam) is prescribed orally every 4 to 6 hours with rescue doses if necessary.

7. Consider the benefit versus burden of additional interventions that are employed. The patient has agreed to medical interventions as well as another thoracentesis if necessary. The use of an intermittent draining pleural catheter has been discussed, and the patient has said he would consider it. The members of the palliative care team feel he can be evaluated in 3 days to determine if there is a need for a thoracentesis or indwelling pleural catheter.

8. Reduce the need for physical exertion. The patient has 24-hour home care, including family support, and an 8-hour daily home health aide. He has a hospital bed at home, is using a wheelchair, and has a bedside commode.

9. Address anxiety, providing support and reassurance. Reassure patient that symptoms can be controlled. The patient's son has asked what will happen if the patient becomes worse at home. The members of the palliative care team review the potential need for increasing sedating medications that would produce sedation at the end of life. The son feels greatly reassured.

10. Incorporate nonpharmacological interventions (e.g., progressive relaxation, guided imagery, and music therapy). The patient felt dyspnea relief from a fan, and used classical music to assist with his anxiety.

11. The patient is followed daily by a member of the palliative care team. Within 48 hours he feels better, his stridor has improved markedly, and he is able to drink some fluids. The steroids are keeping him up at night, so a small dose of a neuroleptic is added at bedtime, which is effective. He is still dyspneic after 5 days, and it is believed that an draining pleural catheter might further benefit him. A pigtail catheter is inserted and immediately drains 1000 milliliters. Over the next 2 weeks, the catheter drains approximately 300 milliliters daily, which allows him a great deal of symptomatic relief. The steroids are continued at the present dose, and the stridor is successfully treated. The patient dies 2 1/2 weeks later at home, in his bed.

## Treatment of Pain

The physiological changes accompanying advanced age have been discussed in this chapter; however, it is important to emphasize that the elderly are more sensitive to both the therapeutic and toxic effects of analgesics.

### Acetaminophen

Acetaminophen is one of the safest analgesics for long-term use in the older population and should be used for mild-to-moderate pain. It is particularly useful in the management of musculoskeletal pain and is often used in combination with opioids. In older patients with normal renal and liver function, it can be used safely and is highly effective for the treatment of osteoarthritis. In the setting of renal insufficiency, hepatic failure, or with patients who are drinking heavily or have a history of alcohol abuse, avoidance of acetaminophen is recommended.

### Nonsteroidal Antiinflammatory Drugs

Nonsteroidal antiinflammatory drugs (NSAIDs) are useful as initial therapy for mild-to-moderate pain and can be used as an additive with opioids and nonopioids. In particular, NSAIDs are useful in the treatment of nociceptive pain related to bone or joint disease. When used concurrently

**Table 38–8**
**Common Opioids and Their Metabolites**

| Opioid | Metabolite | Comment |
|---|---|---|
| Codeine | Codeine-6 glucuronide | May cause more nausea, vomiting, and constipation than other opioids. |
| Oxycodone | Noroxycodone, oxymorphone | |
| Dextropropoxyphene | Norpropoxyphene | Routine use is not advised because metabolites can accumulate with repetitive dosing. |
| Methadone | Metabolite inactive | Pharmacokinetics are variable. Renal excretion is pH dependent; fecal excretion accounts for the greatest part of clearance. |
| Hydromorphone | H3G, H6G | Eliminated by the kidney. |
| Fentanyl | Inactive and nontoxic metabolites | Highly lipophilic, which enables it to be absorbed through the skin. Less than 10% excreted in the urine. |
| Morphine | M3G, M6G | M6G accumulates in the blood and crosses the blood–brain barrier. |
| Meperidine | Normeperidine | Half as potent an analgesic as meperidine and 2 to 3 times more potent as a convulsant; toxicity is not reversed by naloxone; avoid chronic use because normerperidine accumulates with repeated dosing. |

with opioids, lower doses of opioids may be an additional benefit. NSAIDs are useful as initial therapy for mild-to-moderate pain and can be used as an additive with opioids and nonopioids. NSAIDs affect analgesia by reducing the biosynthesis of prostaglandins, thereby inhibiting the cascade of inflammatory events. They also have effects on pain receptors and nerve conduction and may have central effects.[115] The long-term use of traditional NSAIDs, such as aspirin and ibuprofen, are associated with gastrointestinal ulceration, renal dysfunction, and impaired platelet aggregration.[116,117] The cyclooxygenase-2 (COX-2) enzymatic pathway is induced by tissue injury or by other inflammation-inducing conditions.[118] There appears to be less risk of gastrointestinal bleeding with short-term use of the COX-2 selective NSAIDs.[119] In particular,[120–123] NSAIDs are useful in the treatment of nociceptive pain related to bone or joint disease. When used concurrently with opioids, lower doses of opioids may be an additional benefit.

Elderly patients with a history of ulcer disease are most vulnerable to the side effects of these drugs, which can cause renal insufficiency and nephrotoxicity. Cognitive dysfunction has been reported with the use of salicylates, indomethacin, naproxen, and ibuprofen. Also, NSAIDs are problematic in elderly patients with congestive heart failure, peripheral edema, or ascites. In the palliative setting, consideration should be given to the risks versus the benefits to the elderly patient. If, for example, the use of NSAIDs provides effective analgesia and the life expectancy of the patient is limited (days to weeks), then it is probably prudent to initiate this therapy.

## Opioids

In older patients with moderate-to-severe pain who have limited prior treatment with opioids, it is best to begin with a short-half-life agonist (morphine, hydromorphone,

oxycodone). Shorter half-life opioids are generally easier to titrate than longer half-life opioids such as levorphanol or methadone and may have fewer side effects in the elderly. Recent research has demonstrated the importance of both liver biotransformation of metabolites and renal clearance of these metabolites. Most opioids are converted to substances that may have a higher potency than the parent compound or produce more adverse effects with repeated dosing and accumulation.[124] Table 38–8 outlines the most commonly used opioids and their metabolites.

When prescribing opioids in the older population, it is be helpful to obtain baseline renal function studies. A normal serum creatinine does not indicate normal renal function; it is prudent to determine a 24-hour creatinine clearance to accurately determine renal function.

Morphine is the most commonly prescribed opioid because of its cost and ease of administration. Morphine can be administered as an immediate-release tablet or a liquid formulation in a controlled-release tablet administered every 8 to 12 hours (MS Contin) or every 24 hours (Avinza, Kadian). Plasma clearance of morphine decreases with age;[125] therefore, elderly patients should be carefully monitored for any signs of sedation or confusion. In the setting of impaired renal function, morphine should not be used in the elderly patient.

When administering morphine for long-term use, the metabolites of morphine—morphine-3 and -6 glucuronide—may accumulate with repeated dosing, especially in the setting of impaired renal or hepatic function.[125–127] If, after a few days of treatment with morphine, the elderly patient develops side effects that include sedation, confusion, or respiratory depression, it may mean that there is an accumulation of these metabolites, and the opioid should be changed.

Hydromorphone (Dilaudid) is available in oral tablets, liquids, and parenteral formulations and will soon be available in a long-acting preparation. The main metabolite of hydromorphone (H3G) may lead to myoclonus, hyperalgesia, and seizures, especially in the setting of renal failure.[128] Oxycodone is a synthetic opioid available in a long-acting formulation (OxyContin), as well as immediate-release tablets and a liquid preparation. In the oral formulation, it is one-third to one-half more potent than oral morphine. The cost of OxyContin may be prohibitive to some patients on limited incomes.

Fentanyl is a highly lipophilic soluble opioid, which can be administered spinally, transdermally, transmucosally, and intravenously. Transdermal fentanyl (Duragesic) is especially useful when patients cannot swallow, have difficulty adhering to an oral regimen, or have side effects to other opioids. There is some suggestion that transdermal fentanyl may produce less constipation when compared with long-acting morphine. Fever, cachexia, obesity, and ascites may have a significant effect on absorption, predictability of blood levels, and clinical effects.[129,130] The fentanyl patch can be used safely in the older patient, but patients should be monitored carefully. Prior to initiating therapy with the transdermal patch, one should begin with a short-acting opioid (5 mg of oxycodone every 4 hours) and to monitor the patient over 5 to 7 days. If this dose is tolerated, conversion to a 25-mcg fentanyl patch can be safely done. If, after initiation with the fentanyl patch, side effects develop, it is important to remember that they may persist for long periods (hours or even days) after the patch is removed. However, the frail elderly, who have experienced multiple side effects from other opioids, may not do well with this route of administration.

One way of providing for rescue dosing is the oral transmucosal route of administration. Fentanyl citrate may be attempted; it is composed of fentanyl on an applicator that the patient massages or rubs against the oral mucosa or a lozenger that is placed between the gum and the teeth. Absorption occurs rapidly, and many patients begin to have relief after 5 to 10 minutes. This formulation is especially useful in settings where rapid onset of analgesia is needed, such as with severe breakthrough pain or during a procedure or dressing change. This formulation is only to be used in opioid-tolerant patients who are already receiving an around-the-clock opioid to manage baseline pain. Adults should start with 200 mcg, and the dose should be titrated as needed.[131]

Methadone can be safely used in the older adult, provided they are carefully monitored. Methadone is a mu-receptor agonist with a long half-life (ranging from 8 to 90 hours) and allows for prolonged dosing intervals.[132] The long half-life increases the potential for drug accumulation and side effects before the development of steady state blood levels, thus placing the patient at risk for sedation and possible respiratory depression. Therefore, close monitoring of these patients should be done during the first 7 to 10 days of treatment. When initiating the drug, obtaining a baseline EKG is recommended because of the possibility of QT wave abnormalities.[133,134] and the development to a specific type of ventricular fibrillation called torsades de pointes.[133,134] Methadone may bind as an antagonist to the N-methyl-D-aspartate (NMDA) receptor, which may be useful in the management of neuropathic pain.[135] From a cost perspective, it is

one of the less costly opioids, making it appealing to some patients on limited incomes.

As in younger individuals, the use of meperidine for the management of chronic cancer pain is not recommended. The active metabolite of meperidine is normeperidine, which is a proconvulsant. The half-life of normeperidine is 12 to 16 hours. With repeated dosing, accumulation of normeperidine can result in central nervous system excitability, with possible tremors, myoclonus, and seizures. Table 38–9 outlines guidelines for opioid use in the elderly patient.

Parenteral routes of administration should be considered in elderly patients who require rapid onset of analgesia or require high doses of opioids that cannot be administered orally. They may be administered in a variety of ways, including the IV and subcutaneous route, using a patient-controlled analgesia (PCA) device. A careful evaluation of the skin in the elderly patient should be done before initiation of subcutaneous administration. If the patient has

**Table 38–9**
**Opioid Use in the Elderly Patient at the End of Life**

| Opioid | Comments |
| --- | --- |
| Morphine | Observe for side effects with repeated dosing; continuous or sustained release may not be tolerated even after a trial with immediate release |
| Hydromorphone (Dilaudid) | Short half-life; may be safer than morphine |
| Propoxyphene (Darvon, Darvocet) | Avoid use—metabolite causes CNS and cardiac toxicity |
| Codeine | May cause excessive constipation, nausea and vomiting |
| Methadone | Use cautiously, long half-life may produce excessive side effects; requires careful monitoring, especially during first 72 hours after initiation. If it is indicated, it may be safer to use a short-acting opioid as a rescue dose |
| Pentazocine (Talwin) | Opioid agonist/antagonist should not be used; may cause CNS side effects (delirium, agitation) |
| Transdermal fentanyl patch | Long half-life (12–24 hr) is used cautiously in the frail elderly or in elderly with multiple comorbid conditions; cannot titrate easily. If side effects develop, will last at least 12 to 24 hours after patch is removed |
| Meperidine | Avoid use in elderly because of CNS toxicity |
| Oxycodone | Useful for moderate to severe pain control |

*Source:* Adapted from McCaffery and Pasero (1999), reference 221.

---

**Table 38–10**
**Indications for a Subcutaneous or Intravenous PCA Pump**

- Oral route not tolerated—patient cannot swallow (postoperative nausea/vomiting)
- Oral absorption impaired or variable
- Bowel obstruction—partial or complete
- Escalating pain that needs to be managed quickly
- Severe breakthrough or incident-related pain
- Dose-limiting side effects with other routes of administration exist
- When managing pain and other symptoms at the end of life
- Suspected misuse/abuse of other opioids via other routes of administration

---

excessive edema, a very low platelet count, or skin changes related to chronic steroid use, then absorption may be impaired or subcutaneous tissue may not sustain repeated dosing, even with a permanent indwelling butterfly catheter. Infusion devices with the capability of patient-administered rescue dosing can be safely used in the elderly cancer patient provided that they have clear understanding on how to use the rescue button. It is important to remember that severe cognitive impairment should not deter the use of IV administration, especially in the elderly patient at the end of life. In patients who are cognitively impaired, the pca button should be removed. Choice of analgesics and routes of administration must be based on individual assessment of each patient. Table 38–10 outlines indications for a subcutaneous or IV PCA pump.

## Dose Titration

After initiation with an opioid, a stepwise escalation of the opioid dose should be performed until adequate analgesia or intolerable side effects develop. The increased sensitivity of the elderly to opioid side effects suggests that careful titration and escalation should be performed.[136] It is generally safe to begin with a dose that is 25% to 50% less than the dose for a younger adult, especially if the elderly patient is frail or has a history of side effects from prior opioid use. Generally, it is safe to titrate opioids 25% to 50% every 48 hours, although a less aggressive approach may be necessary in elderly patients.

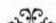

CASE STUDY
*A 90-Year-Old Woman with Metastatic Breast Cancer*

An 90-year-old woman with metastatic breast cancer and extensive bone disease is receiving 15 milligrams of morphine sulfate orally every 4 hours and is reporting inadequate pain relief, with a pain intensity of 7 out of 10. She is also is experiencing intermittent nausea and

vomiting. She was previously on tramadol (50 mg) every 6 hours but had worsening pain in the low back and ribs and was rotated to morphine about 3 days ago. Since starting on morphine, she has reported having bad dreams, confusion, and agitation, which has been corroborated by her family. She has been in bed most of the time. The family also reports constipation, with no bowel movement for 5 days. Today she was admitted to the local emergency room and was given lorazepam (1 mg IV) for agitation and morphine sulfate (2 mg IV) two times for pain. Her confusion and agitation worsene and she is admitted. The patient mentions that she had a DNR order several months ago when she had fallen at home and fractured a rib. The family wants an aggressive evaluation for the delirium, and a brain MRI is done and is normal except for some age-related changes.

Once on the unit, she becomes more agitated and complains of severe pain. An opioid infusion of morphine sulfate (1 mg/hr) is started but fails to produce anagesia and her agitation worsens. A psychiatry consult is called and the patient is started on ativan (1 mg every 6 hours) around the clock. By day 2 the patient is worse, with worsening agitation and delirium.

### At a Glance Assessment and Management

- A comprehensive assessment of the elderly patient with delirium should include a determination of the etiology of delirium, including common predisposing factors (fever, infection, tumor, altered metabolism of drugs, alcohol, comorbid conditions, urinary/bowel retention). Often the cause is multifactorial.
- A careful history of onset and duration of symptoms as well as severity of symptoms should be determined, and dementia should be ruled out. A Mini Mental Status Exam is done and is performed at intervals throughout the course of her delirium.
- When possible, the underlying cause should be identified and treated.
- In this patient, the goals of care are reviewed with the family members, who decide to aggressively try to reverse the delirium. The patient is already DNR.
- Pharmacological management should always include administration of a neuroleptic as a first line treatment.
- Incorporate nonpharmacological interventions when appropriate.

*Case Analysis.* What evaluation of this patient should be done and how should her delirium be managed?

1. The etiology of the confusion should be determined. A careful review of all medications should be done and all centrally acting medications discontinued. In

this patient, the only recent additional medication is morphine.

2. Appropriate laboratory data (electrolytes, renal and liver function) should be obtained to determine if there is any metabolic etiology for her confusion. Electrolytes and liver function studies are normal. BUN is 65 and serum creatinine is 2.3, which is doubled from 3 months ago.

3. A review of all medications is done, with careful attention to centrally acting medications. There does not seem to be any other etiology to the delirium other than the recent switch to morphine. In this patient a change in opioid is indicated, because morphine metabolites—namely morphine-6 glucuronide—may be accumulating in the setting of altered renal function, causing her delirium.

4. The lorazepam is stopped because it is felt to be contributing to her agitation, and the patient is started on a neuroleptic: haloperidol (1 mg every 6 hours) around the clock.

5. An evaluation for the etiology of the nausea and vomiting is done. A history of onset, duration, temporal characteristics, and exacerbating/relieving factors is obtained from her family. A thorough physical examination is performed, with special attention to the abdominal and rectal examination. The physical examination reveals that bowel sounds are present, and the rectal exam reveals retained feces in the rectal vault.

6. An abdominal X-ray is done and shows extensive retained feces but no bowel obstruction.

7. It has been determined that the etiology of the nausea and vomiting is related to severe constipation.

8. The severe constipation may also be contributing to the development of confusion.

9. The decision is made to switch the patient to another opioid. In selecting another opioid, factors to consider include half-life, duration of action, and route of administration. The decision is made to start the patient on a continuous infusion of fentanyl. The equianalgesic dose table should be used as a guide. Because of the existence of incomplete cross-tolerance between drugs, advanced age, and cognitive changes, the alternative opioid should be reduced by 50%.

10. Disimpaction is attempted but cannot be tolerated. A bowel regimen of an oil-retention enema followed by a Fleets enema is tolerated, and the patient has a large bowel movement. The plan is to start the patient on an oral regimen of Senokot (2 tabs orally twice a day) and Colace (300 mg orally daily) when the delirium clears.

11. Within 24 hours of discontinuance of the morphine and lorazepam, the patient's mental status begins to clear and her agitation calms significantly. By day 3 she is almost back to baseline and out of bed.

## The Use of Adjuvant Analgesics for Pain

Several nonopioid medications have been found to be analgesic. These drugs alter, attenuate, or modulate pain perception. They may be used alone or in combination with opioids or nonopioid analgesics to treat many different pain syndromes, including neuropathic pain. Included in this category are antidepressants, anticonvulsants, N-methyl-D-aspartate (NMDA) antagonists, corticosteroids, and local anesthetics. All of these medications have side-effect profiles that can be especially harmful to the older patient, and careful monitoring is required.

Tricyclic antidepressants (TCAs) have been the most widely studied class of adjuvant medications for neuropathic pain. The action of these drugs probably results from interruption of norepinephrine and serotonin-mediated mechanisms in the brain.[137] Side effects—namely the anticholinergic side effects—often limit the use of these medications. Dry mouth, urinary retention, constipation, blurred vision, tachycardia, and delirium are some of the more common side effects. Nortriptyline, a secondary amine, may be preferred in the older adult because it produces less orthostatic hypotension than amitriptyline, and desipramine may have lesser anticholinergic side effects than amitriptyline. TCAs are contra-indicated in patients with coronary artery disease, narrow-angle glaucoma, and significant prostatic hyperplasia. When initiating therapy, start the dose low, monitor patients, and titrate the dose slowly.

Anticonvulsants are used to control sharp, shooting, burning, electric, and stabbing pain, which are typical sensations found in patients with neuropathic pain. Their analgesic effect is believed to be related to the slowing of peripheral nerve conduction in primary afferent fibers.[138] Several different anticonvulsants are useful for neuropathic pain, including carbamazepine, gabapentin, phenytoin, and valproic acid. Carbamazepine should be used cautiously because of the side-effect profile—blood dyscrasias can occur.[139] Gabapentin is believed to have several different mechanisms of action, including NMDA antagonist activity. The most effective analgesic doses range from 900 milligrams to 3600 milligrams per day, in divided doses every 8 hours.[140,141] Evidence supports the efficacy of gabapentin in several painful disorders, including diabetic neuropathy,[141] postherpetic neuralgia,[142] thalamic pain, spinal cord injury,[142] and restless legs syndrome.[143] The starting dose in elderly patients can begin as low as 100 milligrams a day, titrated by 100 milligrams a day every 3 days, until the onset of analgesia. The most commonly reported side effects of gabapentin are somnolence, dizziness, ataxia, tremor, and fatigue. More recently, pregabalin, an analog of the neurotransmitter γ-aminobutyric acid (GABA), is being used to treat neuropathic pain, including postherpetic neuralgia and diabetic peripheral neuropathy.[144,145] Other anticonvulsants that have been used in the management of neuropathic pain include lamotrigine (Lamictal), topiramate (Topamax), zonisamide (Zonegran), and levetiracetam (Keppra). NMDA antagonists are believed to block the binding of excitatory amino acids, such as glutamate, in the spinal cord. Medications that inhibit this receptor interfere with the transmission of pain across the synaptic area. Methadone, ketamine, and dextromethorphan are all NMDA antagonists believed to have analgesic effects in the management of neuropathic pain.[146–148] Ketamine should be used with caution because of its psychomimetic effects, and routine use is not recommended. At the end of life, it has been used in the management of refractory neuropathic pain.[149] Corticosteroids have specific and nonspecific effects in managing pain, including treatment of painful nerve or spinal cord compression, reducing tissue edema and inflammation, and by lysis of some tumors. The mechanism of effect is by inhibition of prostaglandin synthesis and decreasing edema surrounding neural tissues.[150] Corticosteroids are the standard treatment for malignant spinal cord compression (dexamethasone 16–96 mg/day). They may be useful in the management of painful malignant lesions involving the brachial or lumbosacral plexus, hepatic enlargement, distension, and pain.[151,152] Corticosteroids are also helpful in the management of bone pain as well as in the treatment of bowel obstruction.[153,154] Corticosteroids may also be useful in the management of nausea and vomiting. In the older adult, corticosteroids should not be used concurrently with NSAIDs because of the potential increased risk of bleeding.

Local anesthetics have been shown to relieve pain when administered orally, topically, intravenously, and intraspinally. Mexiletine has been useful when anticonvulsants have failed.[155] Topical local anesthetic gels and topical Lidoderm patches have been useful in the management of postherpetic neuropathy[156] and other neuropathic pain syndromes, including peripheral neuropathy, postthoracotomy pain, stump neuroma, complex regional pain syndrome, radiculopathy, and postmastectomy pain.[157] Lidoderm patches (5%) should be applied 12 hours on–12 hours off, within a 24-hour period. They have an excellent safety profile; systemically active serum levels of lidocaine do not occur, and patients can cut the patches to fit small areas. In many older patients, the patches may provide an opioid-sparing effect—the patient may use less opioid analgesia within a 24-hour period. Intravenous lidocaine boluses at doses of 1 to 5 milligrams/kilogram (maximum 500 mg) administered over 1 hour, followed by a continuous infusion of 1 to 2 milligram/kilogram/hour have been reported to reduce intractable neuropathic pain in the palliative care and hospice setting.[158]

Bisphosphonates inhibit osteoclast-mediated bone resorption and alleviate pain from metastatic bone disease and multiple myeloma.[159,160] Analgesic effects can occur in 2 to 4 weeks and, therefore, might not be suitable for patients at the end of life. Pamidronate disodium and zoledronic acid are used in patients with metastatic lesions from breast and prostate cancer. Pamidronate sodium has been shown to reduce pathological fractures in patients with breast cancer.[161] Patients should be monitored with serum calcium levels because hypocalcemia can occur.

Calcitonin may be given subcutaneously or intranasally to relieve pain associated with osteoporotic fractures.[162] Usual doses are 100 to 200 IU/day and are usually well-tolerated. At the end of life, this is probably not a practical or helpful intervention.

Radiation therapy is extremely helpful in relieving painful bone lesions. In many instances, single-fraction external beam therapy can be used. Onset of relief can be fairly rapid, often within days of treatment, and may be a helpful intervention when patients are having side effects to opioid therapy. Unless a single fraction is considered, at the end of life it is not a practical intervention.

Radionuclide therapy is often helpful when there is widespread bony metastatic disease that cannot be easily targeted with localized radiotherapy.[163] Strontium (Metastron) is a radiopharmaceutical calcium analog taken up by the skeleton into active sites of bone remodeling and metastasis. A large clinical trial demonstrated that strontium was an effective adjuvant to local radiotherapy and that it reduced disease progression, decreased new sites of pain, and decreased systemic use.[164] The latency of response can be as long as 2 to 3 weeks, and patients should continue their opioid therapy. Because of this delayed onset of analgesia, patients who are actively dying are not candidates. Side effects associated with strontium use include thrombocytopenia and leucopenia. Samarium lexidronam (Quadramet) is a radiopharmaceutical that has an affinity for bone and concentrates in areas of bone turnover with hydroxyapatite, which is useful for metastatic bone pain. Patients should also be instructed that a transitory pain flare can occur, and analgesics may need to be titrated.

## Invasive Approaches for the Management of Pain

Anesthetic and neurosurgical approaches are indicated when conservative measures using opioids and adjuvant analgesics have failed to provide adequate analgesia or when the patient is experiencing intolerable side effects. The use of these approaches is not contra-indicated in the older adult. The clearest indication for these approaches is intolerable central nervous system toxicity. These procedures include regional analgesia (spinal, intraventricular, and intrapleural opioids), sympathetic blockade and neurolytic procedures (celiac plexus block, lumbar sympathetic block, cervicothoracic [stellate] ganglion block), or pathway ablation procedure (chemical or surgical rhizotomy, or cordotomy). At the end of life, these approaches may be useful in some older patients who have intractable pain that cannot be managed with systemic treatment.

## Nonpharmacological Approaches: Complementary Therapies

Physical and psychological interventions can be used as an adjunct with drugs and surgical approaches to manage pain in the older adult. These approaches carry few side effects and, when possible, should be tried along with other approaches. In selecting an approach in the dying patient, factors that should be considered include physical and psychological burden to the patient, efficacy, and practicality. If the patient has weeks to live, these strategies may allow for a reduction in systemic opioids and diminish adverse effects.

Cognitive-behavioral interventions include relaxation, guided imagery, massage, distraction, and music therapy. The major advantages of these techniques are that they are easy to learn, safe, and readily accepted by patients. Cognitive and behavioral interventions are helpful to reduce emotional distress, improve coping, and offer the patient and family a sense of control. Other physical interventions such as reflexology and massage therapy have been shown to relieve pain and produce relaxation.[164,165]

## End-of-Life Pain Management in the Nursing Home: A Special Challenge

Challenges in end-of-life care for nursing home residents are multiple, and for many the disease trojectory is complicated by multiple illnesses, limited family support, cognitive changes, and communication difficulties. Many patients do not have assigned health-care agents, and it is often the case that end-of-life discussions are not held until an emergency occurs. The complexity of needs for the elderly patient necessitates that the geriatric clinician have palliative care expertise.[166]

Conventional models of palliative care often focus on the cancer patient, and this may not meet the needs of elderly patients not suffering from cancer, who often have multiple comorbid illnesses and a different trajectory at the end of life.[167]

Cognitively impaired nursing home residents present a special barrier to pain assessment and management.[168-172] Residents of nursing homes exhibit very high rates of cognitive impairment.[173] Most studies of nursing home residents reveal that cognitively impaired nursing home residents are prescribed and administered significantly less analgesic medication—both in number and in dosage of pain drugs—than their more cognitively intact peers.[174]

Reasons for lack of attention to residents' pain include inadequate assessment tools and little formal staff education in pain management or palliative care. Studies suggest that persons enrolled in nursing home hospice programs, many of whom are dying or with dementia, are more likely to have better pain control and symptom management.[175]

Inadequate pain assessment and management in nursing homes is widespread, and for many patients at the end of life, unnecessary treatments and interventions are often employed.[176]

Assessment of pain in cognitively impaired elderly at the end of life remains a special challenge. Mild-to-moderate cognitive impairments seem to be associated with a decrease in propensity to report pain.[174] In severely cognitively impaired individuals, assessment is often difficult because these individuals frequently cannot verbalize their reports of pain. In their evaluation of 217 elderly patients with significant cognitive impairment, Ferrell and colleagues[177] found that 83% could complete at least one pain scale, with the McGill Present Pain Intensity Scale having the highest completion rate, and 32% were able to complete all of the scales presented.

The best way to assess pain is to ask the individual. In the cognitively impaired elderly, it is difficult to assess pain. The ability of caregivers, either family or staff, to assess pain in this population is crucial. In one study of caregiver perceptions of nonverbal patients with cerebral palsy, more than 80% of the caregivers used aspects of crying and moaning to alert them to a pain event.[177] In another study evaluating a measurement tool for discomfort in noncommunicative patients with advanced Alzheimer's disease, indicators of pain included noisy breathing, negative vocalizations, facial expression (content, sad, or frightened), frown, and body language (relaxed, tense, or fidgeting).[169]

There is some evidence that cognitively impaired elderly individuals' facial expressions of pain depend on the cause of the underlying cognitive disorder, including hemispheric dysfunction and type of dementia; however, facial expressions and body language can be very useful indicators of pain.

In one study evaluating the impact of a Palliative Care Educational Resource Team on nursing home staff, a comprehensive program was offered to 108 nursing staff and 61 certified nursing assistants. The program lasted 4 days. Results in pre- to postknowledge increased, and practice changes as evidenced by supervisor evaluations suggested improvement. The authors suggested alternative ways to deliver the content, including use of electronic and train-the-trainer programs.[178]

In other studies looking at cancer patients admitted to nursing homes, evidence suggests that regardless of the site of cancer, patients receiving hospice care appear to obtain better pain relief than those not enrolled.[179] Recommendations for improving end-of-life care to cancer patients in nursing homes include discussions of goals of care, implementation of clinical pathways for pain and nonpain cancer-related symptoms.[180]

## Cognitive Changes: The Challenges of a Diagnosis of Delirium or Dementia

Delirium may often be superimposed upon dementia in the elderly patient. In clinical practice, it is important to distinguish whether the delirious patient has an underlying dementia. When an elderly demented patient becomes delirious, it should be assumed that an organic precipitating factor—metabolic, drug-induced, acute illness—is the cause, and the patient should be evaluated for the etiology and treated. The distinction is not always apparent.

Both delirium and dementia feature global impairment in cognition. Obtaining a careful history from family members or caregivers to learn about the onset of symptoms is probably the most important factor in making the distinction. Generally, acute onset of cognitive and attention deficits and abnormalities, whose severity fluctuates during the day and tends to increase at night, is typical of a delirium. Delirium, in general, is a transient disorder that seldom lasts for more than a month, whereas dementia is a clinical state that lasts for months or years.[181] Dementia implies impairment in short- or long-term memory associated with impaired thinking and judgment, with other disturbances of higher cortical function or with personality change.[182]

Older adults with chronic illnesses are especially vulnerable to delirium as a result of inter- and intrahospital transfers, intensive care unit psychosis, and delirium associated with medication errors.

Alzheimer's Dementia is the most prevalent progressive neurodegenerative disease. It begins with minute memory impairment and ultimately leads to the loss of all mental and physical function. A person with Alzheimer's Dementia lives an average of 8 years from diagnosis and could live as many as 20 years. There is some evidence to suggest that rate of deterioration in activities of daily living correlate with the burden of neurofibrillary tangle count.[183] The prevalence of people with Alzheimer's Dementia in the United States is estimated to be more than 4 million.[184] Currently available therapies, such as the anticholinesterase inhibitors, may delay progression of Alzheimer's Dementia and defer requirement for institutionalization but have limited impact on memory; however, if uncovered by payers, they represent considerable expense to caregivers who are also required to pay for formal homecare in the absence of "skilled need" for homecare.[185]

The prediction of survival in end-stage dementia is particularly challenging for hospice providers who must make difficult decisions regarding eligibility for the Medicare hospice benefit when patients "outlive" the hospice benefit. Conversely to patients with terminal cancer, in which decline is typically a straight downward course, the disease trajectory for patients with end-stage dementia is marked by slow deteriorations in function over several years, with reduced levels of activities of daily living interspersed with periods of marked deterioration in parallel with urosepsis and pneumonia; this is in contrast to cancer, where death is usually heralded by a period of pronounced functional deterioration in the last 3 months of life.[186]

## Delirium in the Elderly Patient at the End of Life: Prevalence, Etiologic Factors and Treatment

### Prevalence

Delirium is a frequently occurring consequence of advanced cancer and is characterized by disturbances in arousal, perception, cognition, and psychomotor behavior.[187,188] In all settings, delirium is a common symptom in the elderly medically ill and cancer patient. The presence of delirium contributes significantly to increased morbidity and mortality. Estimates of the prevalence of delirium range from 25% to 40% in cancer patients at some point during their disease,

and in the terminal phases of disease, the incidence increases to 85%.[187–189] In elderly hospitalized patients, delirium prevalence ranges from 10% to 40% and up to 80% at the end of life. One of the major problems in the treatment of delirium in the elderly patient is lack of assessment by hospital staff, especially if the patient is quiet and noncommunicative.

Delirium can be categorized into three clinical subtypes, based on either motor or arousal disturbances: hypoactive, hyperactive, and mixed. The hypoactive type is characterized by psychomotor retardation, lethargy, sedation, and reduced awareness of surroundings.[190] The hyperactive subtype is more commonly characterized by restlessness, agitation, hypervigilence, hallucincations, and delusions.[191]

### Predisposing and Etiological Factors

The etiology of delirium in the medically compromised and dying elderly patient is often multifactorial and may be nonspecific. In an elderly patient, delirium is often a presenting feature of an acute physical illness or exacerbation of a chronic one or of intoxication with even therapeutic doses of commonly used drugs.[182] Numerous factors appear to make the elderly more susceptible to the development of delirium (Table 38–11).

Delirium can result from the direct effects of the disease on the central nervous system, metabolic reasons (including organ failure), electrolyte imbalance, infection, hematological disorders, nutritional deficiencies, paraneoplastic disorders, hypoxemia, chemotherapeutic agents, immunotherapy, vascular disorders, hypothermia, hyperthermia, uncontrolled pain, sensory deprivation, sleep deprivation, medications, alcohol or drug withdrawal, diarrhea, constipation, or urinary retention. Various drugs can produce delirium in the medically ill or elderly patient (Table 38–12). In the palliative care setting, multiple medications are generally required to control symptoms at the end of life. Prospective data suggest a prevalence of delirium in 28% to 42% of patients with advanced cancer on admission to a palliative care unit.[192] Given the projected increase in the numbers of elderly patients, health-care providers will encounter the need for management of delirium in the elderly more frequently.

Other risk factors for the development of delirium include advanced age, cancer, preexisting cognitive impairment, hip fractures, and severe illness.[193–195] In cancer patients, risk factors that have been identified include advanced age, cognitive impairment, low albumin level, bone metastases, and the presence of hematological malignancy. In one study that determined risk factors for delirium in oncology patients, specific etiological factors in the elderly were identified and included reduced cholinergic reserves of the brain, high prevalence of cognitive impairment and comorbid disease, visual and hearing loss, and impaired metabolism of drugs.[196,197]

The diagnosis of delirium in an elderly patient carries serious risks. Delirium produces distress for patients, families, and health-care providers. Depending on the severity of symptoms (fluctuating cognitive changes, hallucinations,

**Table 38–11**
**Factors Predisposing the Elderly to Delirium**

| Factor | Comments |
|---|---|
| Age-related changes in the brain | Atrophy of gray and white matter |
| | Senile plaques in hippocampus, amygdala, middle cerebral cortical layers |
| | Cell loss in frontal lobes, amygdala, putamen, thalamus, locus ceruleus |
| | Alzheimer's disease, cerebrovascular disease |
| **Brain damage** | |
| Reduced regulation and resistance to stress | Visual, hearing loss |
| Sensory changes | Prolonged immobility, Foley catheters |
| Infection | |
| Intravenous lines | Pulmonary and urinary tract infections |
| | Reduced ability to metabolize and eliminate drugs |
| Impaired pharmacokinetics | Vitamin deficiency as a result of prolonged illness |
| Malnutrition | Folate deficiency may directly cause delirium |
| Multiple comorbid diseases | Cancer and cardiovascular, pulmonary, renal, and hepatic disease |
| | Endocrine disorders, including hyperthyroidism and hypothyroidism |
| | Fluid and electrolyte abnormalities |
| Reduced thirst | Hypovolemia |
| Reduction of protein-binding of drugs | Enhanced effect of opioids, diuretics |
| Polypharmacy | Use of sedatives, hypnotics, major tranquilizers |

*Sources:* Adapted from Lipowski (1989), reference 181, and Inouye et al. (1996), reference 193.


**Table 38–12**
**Drugs Commonly Causing Delirium in the Elderly**

| Classification | Example |
|---|---|
| Antidepressants | Amitriptyline, doxepin |
| Antihistamines | Chlorpheniramine, diphenhydramine, hydroxyzine, promethazine |
| Diabetic agents | Chlorpropamide |
| Cardiac | Digoxin, dipyridamole |
| Antihypertensives | Propranolol, clonidine |
| Sedatives | Barbiturates, chlordiazepoxide, diazepam, flurazepam, meprobamate |
| Opioids | Meperidine, pentazocine, propoxyphene |
| Nonsteroidal antiinflammatory agents | Indomethacin, phenylbutazone |
| Anticholinergics | Atropine, scopolamine |
| Antiemetics | Trimethobenzamide, phenothiazine |
| Antispasmodics | Dilomine, hyoscyamine, propantheline, belladonna alkaloids |
| Antineoplastics | Methotrexate, mitomycin, procarbazine, Ara-C, carmustine, fluorouracil, interferon, Interleukin-2, L-asparaginase, prednisone |
| Corticosteroids | Prednisone, dexamethasone |
| $H_2$-receptor antagonists | Cimetidine |
| Lithium | |
| Acetaminophen | |
| Salicylates | Aspirin |
| Anticonvulsant agents | Carbamazepine, diphenylhydantoin, phenobarbital, sodium valproate |
| Antiparkinsonian agents | Amantadine, levodopa |
| Alcohol | |

*Source:* Adapted from Lipowski (1989), reference 181.

agitation, or emotional lability), patients often require one-to-one observation, chemical, and—rarely—physical restraints. Falls and pressure ulcers are associated with the hyperactive and hypoactive subtypes.[198] Delirium in terminally ill patients is a reliable predictor of approaching death within days to weeks, and hospital mortality rates among elderly patients with delirium range from 22% to 76%.[199]

Given the projected increase in the numbers of elderly patients, health-care providers will encounter management of delirium in the elderly more frequently. To reduce the risk of polypharmacologically induced delirium, it is prudent to add one medication at a time, evaluating its response, before adding another medication.

Delirium in the elderly patient is often undertreated for several reasons, including lack of assessment tools, inadequate knowledge of early signs of confusion, and inadequate time spent with the patient to determine cognitive function—all factors that lead to underdiagnosis. In addition, behavioral manifestations of delirium may include a variety of symptoms that may be interpreted as depression or dementia.

Inouye established a multifactorial model of delirium in the elderly, with baseline predisposing factors and the addition of various insults.[194] The factors that have been identified to be contributory to baseline vulnerability in the elderly include visual impairment, cognitive impairment, severe illness, and an elevated blood urea nitrogen/creatinine ratio of 18 or greater. Other factors that have been identified in the elderly include advanced age, depression, electrolyte imbalance, poor functional status, immobility, Foley catheter, malnutrition, dehydration, alcohol, and medications, including neuroleptics, opioids, and anticholinergic drugs. Finally, delirium in an elderly patient is often a precursor to death and should be viewed as a grave prognostic sign.[200]

Alcohol withdrawal may be a cause of delirium in the elderly. In one study, organic mental syndromes were diagnosed in more than 40% of elderly alcoholics admitted for alcohol abuse, and delirium was found in about 10% of these.[201] Illness, malnutrition, or concurrent use of a hepatotoxic drug or one that is metabolized by the liver may result in increased sensitivity of the elderly to alcohol. Alcohol, combined with other medications, especially centrally acting medications, can produce delirium in the elderly.

The diagnosis of delirium in an elderly patient carries with it serious risks. An agitated delirious patient may climb out of bed; pull out Foley catheters, IV lines, and sutures; and injure staff in an attempt to protect themselves from a perceived threat. Mental status questionnaires are relatively easy to administer, and an examination should be performed on all patients with mental status changes. The Mini-Mental State Exam, a 10-item test, is easy to administer to an elderly patient.[202] Other delirium screening and evaluation tools have been developed, including the Delirium Rating Scale-Revised,[203] Confusion Assessment Method,[204] Cognitive Test for Delirium,[205] and Memorial Delirium Assessment Scale.[206]

### Treatment of Delirium

Treatment of delirium includes an identification of the underlying cause, correction of the precipitating factors, and symptom management of the delirium. In the very ill or dying patient, however, the etiology may be multifactorial, and the cause is often irreversible.

Ensuring safety is critical, and specialized training is needed to monitor these patients; often these patients cannot be managed at home.[207] When caregivers are elderly, it may be necessary to advise hospitalization so that the elderly patient can be given the support and care they require.

If delirium is occurring in the dying elderly patient and the goal of care has been identified as the promotion of comfort and relief of suffering, diagnostic evaluations (imaging and laboratory studies) would not prove beneficial.

Interventions that may be helpful include restoration of fluid and electrolyte balance, environmental changes, and supportive techniques such as elimination of unnecessary stimuli, provision of a safe environment, and measures that reduce anxiety. In many cases, the etiology of delirium may be pharmacological, especially in the elderly patient. All nonessential and central nervous system-depressant drugs should be stopped. The use of Foley catheters, IV lines, and physical restraints should be minimized; consider the use of gentle massage or music to facilitate sleep hygiene. Figure 38–2 reviews the overall assessment and management of delirium in the geriatric patient at the end of life.

Pharmacological treatment includes the use of sedatives and neuroleptics. Breitbart and Jacobsen[208] demonstrated that the use of lorazepam alone in controlling symptoms of delirium was ineffective and contributed to worsening cognition. These authors advocate the use of a neuroleptic such as haloperidol, along with a benzodiazepine, in the control of an agitated delirium. Other neuroleptics, such as risperidone and olanzapine, have also been used to treat delirium in the elderly and may have fewer side effects. The oral route is preferred, although in cases of severe agitation and delirium, the parenteral route should be used. In one study by Breitbart, 79 cancer patients were treated for delirium with olanzapine and age over 70 years was found to be the most powerful predictor of poorer response to olanzapine treatment. Other factors included history of dementia, central nervous system spread of disease, and hypoxia as delirium etiologies.[209] A Cochrane Review of drug therapy for delirium in terminally ill patients concluded that, based on a single study,[210] haloperidol is the most suitable medication for treatment of patients with delirium near the end of life, with chlorpromazine as an acceptable alternative.[211]

❧

### Summary

Elderly patients who are dying should be able to receive skillful and expert palliative care. This means that clinicians must become knowledgable about the aging process—the

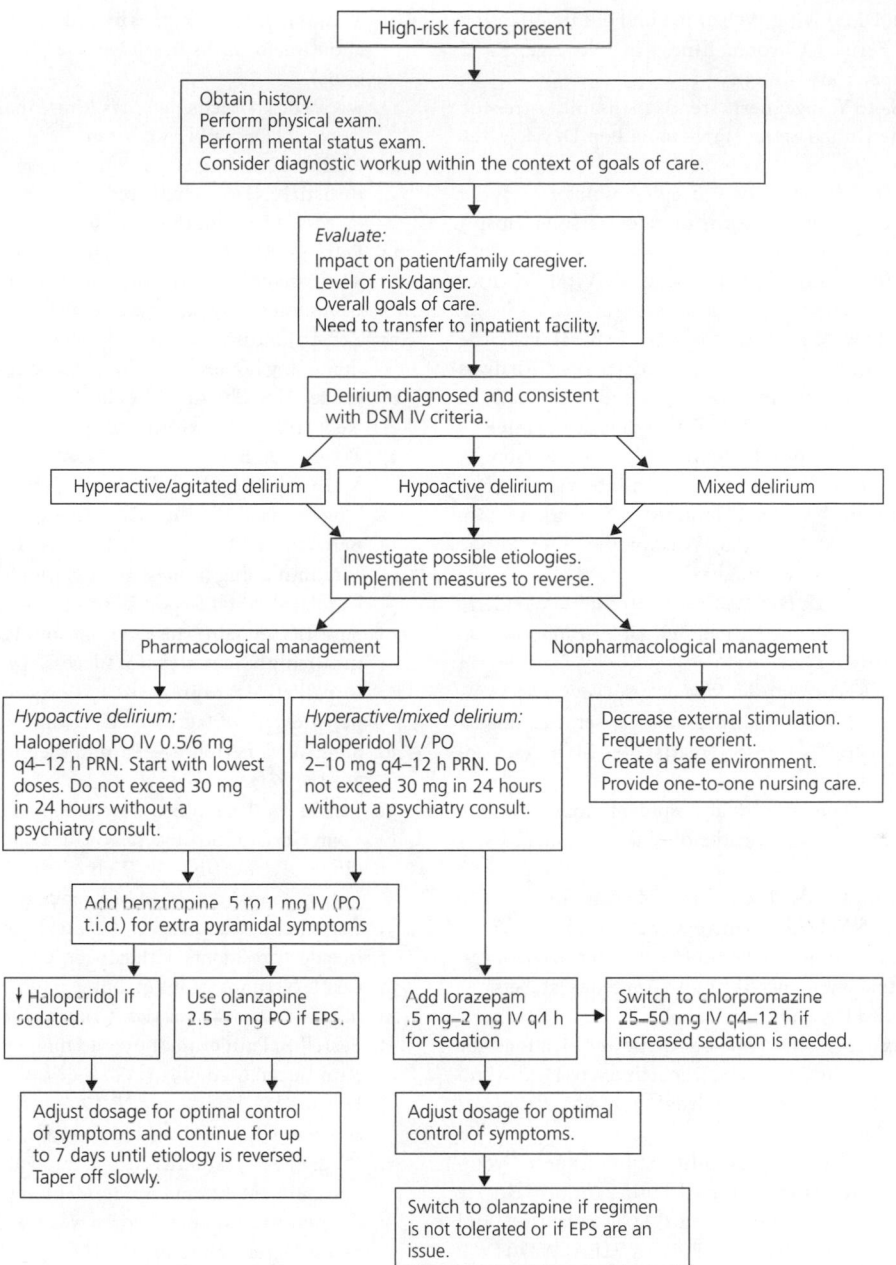

**FIGURE 38–2.** Delirium management in the geriatric patient at the end of life. *Source*: Adapted from Memorial Sloan-Kettering Cancer Center algorithm for pharmacologic management of delirium (August 14, 2001).

physiological changes that normally occur with aging and the impact of progressive disease on an already frail system. Management of symptoms at the end of life in the elderly patient is different from the younger age group because of their altered response to medications, their fear of taking medication, and the need to involve and educate informal and formal caregivers, who are often elderly themselves.

Pain, respiratory distress, and delirium are the three most common symptoms in the elderly patient who is dying. Relief of these symptoms is a basic priority for care of the dying elderly patient. Continued assessment of the patient will allow

for drug changes, dose adjustments, and relief of distressing symptoms. Providing relief from these symptoms will help facilitate a peaceful death, one that is remembered as such by family and friends.

REFERENCES

1. Trends in Causes of Death Among the Elderly Robinson K 2001 NCHS accessible at www.cdc.gov/nchs/data/ahcd/agingtrends/01death.pdf (accessed December 10, 2009).

2. Lynn J, Adamson DM. Living Well at the End of Life Adapting Health Care to Serious Chronic Illness in Old Age. Rand Health White Paper 2003 WP-137.

3. Crimmins EM, Saito Y, Ingegneri. Trends in disability-free life expectancy in the United States, 1970–1990. Pop Develop Rev 1997;23:555–572.

4. Foley D, Brock D. Demography and epidemiology of dying in the U.S. with emphasis on deaths of older persons. Hosp J 1998;13:49–60.

5. National Center for Health Statistics. Monthly Vital Statistics Report 1995;43.

6. Grulich A, Swerdlow A, Dos Santos Silva I, Beral V. Is the apparent rise in cancer mortality in the elderly real? Analysis of changes in certification and coding of cause of death in England and Wales, 1970–1990. Int J Cancer 1995;63:164–168.

7. National Center for Health Statistics, Moss A, Parson V. Current estimates from the National Health Interview Survey, United States 1985. In: Vital Health Statistics, ser. 10, no. 160. DHHS Pub. No. (PHS) 860–1588. Washington, DC: Public Health Service, 1986:13, 82–83, 106, 118.

8. Foley DJ, Miles TP, Brock DB, Phillips C. Recounts of elderly deaths: Endorsements for the Patient Self-Determination Act. Gerontologist 1995;35:119–121.

9. Seeman I. National Mortality Followback Survey: 1986 summary. United States. Vital Health Statistics, ser. 20, no. 19. DHHS Pub. No. (PHS) 92–1656. Hyattsville, MD: National Center for Health Statistics.

10. Foley D, Brock D. Demography and epidemiology of dying in the U.S. with emphasis on deaths of older persons. Hosp J 1998;13:49–60.

11. Wallace R, Woolson R, eds. The Epidemiological Study of the Elderly. New York, NY: Oxford University Press, 1992.

12. Duke Clinical Research Institute Limited Data Set. www. nltcs. aa.duke/index.htm2.www.cms.hhhsgov/Limited DataSets/11_ MCBS.asp (accessed December 10, 2009).

13. Changes in elderly disability rates and the implications for health care utilization and cost: US. Department of Health and Human Services http://aspe/hhs/gov/daltcp/reports/hcutlces/ htm (accessed December 31, 2008).

14. Lafortune G, Balestat G, the Disability Study Expert Group Members. OECD Trends in severe disability among elderly people: Assessing the evidence in 12 OECD countries and the future implications. OECD DELSA/HEA/WD/HWP 2007:2.

15. Kapo, J, Morrison L, Liao S. Palliative care for the old adult. J Pall Med 2007;10(1):185–209.

16. Fried T, Pollack D, Drickamer M, Tinetti M. Who dies at home? Determinants of site of death for community-based long-term care patients. J Am Geriatr Soc 1999;47:25–29.

17. Groth-Janucker A, McCusker J. Where do elderly patients prefer to die? Place of death and patient characteristics of 100 elderly patients under the care of a home healthcare team. J Am Geriatr Soc 1983;31:457–461.

18. McWhinney IR, Bass M, Orr V. Factors associated with location of death (home or hospital) of patients referred to a palliative care team. CMAJ 1995;152:361–367.

19. Townsend J, Frank A, Fermont D, et al. Terminal cancer and patients' preference for place of death: A prospective study. BMJ 1990;301:415–417.

20. Losonczy KG, White LR, Brock DB. Prevalence and correlates of dementia: Survey of the last days of life. Public Health Rep 1998;113:273–280.

21. Trends in nursing homes by bed size. http://www.cdc.gov.nchs/ about/major/nnhsd/trendsnurse.htm (accessed December 10, 2009).

22. www.cdc.gov/nchs/data/dvs.MortFinal2004_Wortable 309.pdf (accessed December 10, 2009).

23. National Nursing Home Survey 1999. www.cdc.gov/nchs/data/ nnhsd/NNHS599selectedchar_homes_beds_residents.pdf (accessed December 10, 2009).

24. Petrisek AC, Mor V. Hospice in nursing homes: A facility-level analysis of the distribution of hospice beneficiaries. Gerontologist 1999;39:3:279–290.

25. Zerzan J, Stearns S, Hanson L. Access to palliative care and hospice in nursing homes. J Am Med Assoc 2000:284(19):2489–2494.

26. Carter JM, Chichin E. Palliative Care in the Nursing Home. New York, NY: Oxford University Press, 2003.

27. Travis SS, Bernard M, Dixon S, McAuley WJ, Loving G, McLanahan L. Obstacles to palliation and end of life care in a long term care facility. Gerontologist 2002:42(3):342–349.

28. Bercovitz A, Decker FH, Jones A, Remsburg RE. End-of-life care in nursing homes: 2004 National Nursing Home Survey. Natl Health Stat Report 2008;8(9):1–23.

29. Susan Rosendahl-Masella S, Sansone P, Phillips M. Palliative care in nursing homes, steps for success: A guide to developing a quality palliative care program. P18. http://www.scherviercares.org/ pc_booklet.pdf (accessed December 11, 2009).

30. Stein WM, Ferrell BA. Pain in the nursing home. Clin Geriatr Med 1996;12:601–613.

31. Ferrell BA, Ferrell BR, Osterweil D. Pain in the nursing home. J Am Geriatr Soc 1990;38:409–414.

32. Singer P, Martin DK, Kelner M. Quality end-of-life care. Patient's perspective. JAMA 1999;281:163–198.

33. Bernabei R, Gambassi G, Lapane K, et al. Management of pain in elderly residents with cancer. JAMA 1998;279:1877–1882.

34. Castle N. Innovations in dying in the nursing home: The impact of market characteristics. Omega 1998;36:227–240.

35. Ferrell B. Pain evaluation and management in nursing homes. Ann Intern Med 1995;123:681–687.

36. Hanson LC, Henderson M. Care of the dying in long-term care settings. Clin Geriatr Med 2000;16:225–237.

37. Wagner AM, Goodwin M, Campbell B, et al. Pain prevalence and pain treatments for residents in Oregon nursing homes: Communication breakdown was associated with the failure to assess Geriatr Nurs 1997;18:268–272.

38. Teno J. Looking beyond the "form" to complex interventions needed to improve end-of-life care. J Am Geriatr Soc 1998;46:1170–1171.

39. Miller SC, Mor V, Wu N, Gozalo P, Lapane K. Does receipt of hospice care in nursing homes improve the management of pain at the end of life? J Am Geriatr Soc 2002;50:507–515.

40. Travis SS, Bernard M, Dixon S, McAuley WJ, Loving G, McClanahan L. Obstacles to palliation and end-of-life care in a long-term care facility. Gerontologist 2002;42:342–349.

41. Teno JM, Branco KJ, Mor V, et al. Changes in advance care planning in nursing homes before and after the Patient Self Determination Act: Report of a five state survey. J Amer Geriatr Soc 1997;45:939–944.

42. Castle N, Mor V. Advance care planning in nursing homes. Pre- and postpatient self-determination act. Health Serv Res 1998;33:101–124.

43. Smith GE, Kokmen E, O'Brien PC. Risk factors for nursing home placement in a population-based dementia cohort. J Am Geriatr Soc 2000;48:519–525.

44. Morris JN, Hawes C, Fries BE, et al. Designing the national resident assessment instrument for nursing homes. Gerontologist 1999;30:293–307.

45. Hawes C, Morris JN, Phillips CD, Mor V, Fries BE, Nonemaker S. Reliability estimates for the minimum data set for nursing home resident assessment and care screening (MDS). Gerontologist 1995;35:172–178.

46. Mitchell SL, Kiely DK, Lipsitz LA. The risk factors and impact on survival of feeding tube placement in nursing home residents with severe cognitive impairment. Arch Intern Med 1997;157:327–332.

47. Dubler NN, Liebman CB. Bioethics Mediation: A Guide to Shaping Shared Solutions. New York, NY: United Hospital Fund; 2004:1–19.

48. Back AL, Arnold RM. Dealing with conflict in caring for the seriously ill: "It was just out of the question." JAMA 2005;293(11):1374–1381.

49. Emanuel L, Madelyn I, Webster JR. Ethical aspects of geriatric palliative care. In: Morrison RS, Meier DE, eds. Geriatric Palliative Care. New York, NY: Oxford University Press; 2003:55–78.

50. Phipps E, True G, Harris D, et al. Approaching the end-of-life: Attitudes, preferences and behaviors of African-American and white patients and their family caregivers. J Clin Onc 2003;21(3):549–554.

51. Nolan DA, Larnette RM, Veira BL. Dying on an aged care ward—decision making and pain relief. Mature Med 2000;October–November:178–182.

52. Gornick M, McMillan A, Lubitz J. A longitudinal perspective on patterns of Medicare payments. Health Aff (Millwood) 1993;12:140–150.

53. Perls TT, Wood ER. Acute costs and the oldest old. Arch Intern Med 1996;156:759.

54. Riley G, Potosky A, Lubitz J, Kessler L. Medicare payments from diagnosis to death for elderly cancer patients. Med Care 1995;33:828–841.

55. O'Mahony S. Blank A, Persaud J, et al. Report of a palliative care and case management project for elderly patients in the emergency department in an urban medical center. J Urban Health 2008;85(3):443–451.

56. O'Mahony S. Cancer pain, prevalence and undertreatment. In: Portenoy RK, Breura E, eds. Cancer Pain. New York, NY: Cambridge University Press; 2003:38–47.

57. Adams WL, McIlvain HE, Lacy NL, et al. Primary care for the elderly people: Why do doctors find it so hard. Gerontologist 2002;42:835–842.

58. Zander K. Nursing case management: Strategic management of cost and quality outcomes. J Nurs Adm 1988;18(5):23–30.

59. Whitehall C. Emergency department case management. Developing strategies and outcomes. In: Cohen EL, Cesta TG, eds. Nursing Case Management: From Essentials To advanced Practice Applications. St. Louis, MO: Mosby; 2001; 16:173–184.

60. O'Mahony S, Martino-Starvuggi F. Palliative care and the elderly: Complex case management. In: Blank AE, O'Mahony S, Selwyn A, eds. Choices in Palliative Care: Issues in Health Care Delivery. New York, NY: Springer; 2007:169–183.

61. Riley G, Lubitz J, Prihoda R, Rabey E. The use and costs of Medicare services by cause of death. Inquiry 1987;24:233–244.

62. Knaus W, Wagner DP, Draper EA, et al. The APACHE prognostic system: Risk prediction of hospital mortality for critically ill hospitalized adults. Chest 1991;100:1619–1636.

63. Lavery JV, Dickens BM, Boyle JM, Singer PA. Bioethics for clinicians: (6) Advance care planning. CMAJ 1996;155: 1689–1692.

64. Bomba P. Advance care planning along the continuum. Case Manager 2005;6(2):68–72.

65. Singer PA. Advance directives in palliative care. J Pall Care 1994;10(3):111–116.

66. Ethical and legal dimensions of treating life-limiting illness in Hospice and Palliative Care Training for Physicians: A self study program, 2008: Third edition, UNIPAC six.

67. Alzheimer's Disease Fact Sheet. http://www.nia.nih.gov/NR/rdonlyres/B92E702C-AA10-4245-9E52-C8BE1C61601C/10446/508ADEARFactsheetLegal08AUG27.pdf (accessed December 10, 2009).

68. McAuley WJ, Travis SS. Advance care planning among residents in long-term care. Am J Hos Palliat Care 2003;20:529–530.

69. Danis M, Garrett J, Harris R, Patrick DL. Stability of choices about life-sustaining treatments. Ann Int Med 1994;120:567–573.

70. Emanuel LL, Emanuel EJ, Stoeckle JD, Hummel LR, Barry MJ. Advanced directives. Stability of patient's treatment choices. Arch Int Med 1994;154:209–217.

71. Rosenfeld KE, Wenger NS, Phillips RS, et al. Factors associated with change in resuscitation preference of seriously ill patients. The SUPPORT Investigators. Study to Understand Prognoses and Preferences for Outcomes and Risks of Treatment. Arch Intern Med 1996:156(14):1558–1564.

72. McParland E, Likourezos E, Chichin E, Castor, Paris BEC. Stability of preferences regarding life-sustaining treatment: A two-year prospective study of nursing home residents. Mount Sinai J Med 2003;70:85–92.

73. Hickman SE, Hammes BJ, Moss AH, Tolle SW. Hope for the future: Achieving the original intent of advance directives. Hastings Center Report 2005;356:S26–S30.

74. Hickman SE, Sabatino CP, Moss AH, Jessica WN. The POLST (Physician Orders for Life-Sustaining Treatment) Paradigm to Improve End-of-Life Care: Potential state legal barriers to implementation. J Law Med Ethics 2008;36(1):119–140.

75. History of the POLST paradigm initiative: http://www.ohsu.edu/ethics/polst/developing/history.htm (accessed January 2, 2009).

76. EMS Policy Document. http://www.health.state.ny.us/nysdoh/ems/pdf/08-07.pdf (accessed January 2, 2009).

77. http://www.compassionandsupport.org/pdfs/professionals/training/MOLST_Update_August_2008.pdf. (accessed January 2, 2009).

78. Medical Orders for Life-Sustaining Treatment (MOLST) Frequently Asked Questions (FAQs). December 2008: http://www.health.state.ny.us/professionals/patients/patient_rights/molst/frequently_asked_questions.htm (accessed December 10, 2009).

79. Murray TH, Jennings B, "The quest to reform end of life care: Rethinking assumptions and setting new directions." Improving end of life care: Why has it been so difficult? Hastings Center Report 2005:Spec No:S52–S57.

80. Otten A. About 15% of U.S. adults care for ill relatives. Wall Street Journal, April 22, 1991, B1.

81. Stone R, Cafferata GI, Sangl J. Caregivers of the frail elderly: A national profile. Gerontologist 1987;27:616–626.

82. National Center for Health Statistics. National home and hospice care data. Hyattsville, MD: U.S. Department of Health and Human Services, 2000.

83. Schott-Baer D, Fisher L, Gregory C. Dependent care, caregiver burden, hardiness, and self-care agency of caregivers. Cancer Nurs 1995;18:299–305.

84. Weitzner MA, McMillan S, Jacobson P. Family caregiver quality of life: Differences between curative and palliative cancer treatment settings. J Pain Sympt Manage 1999;17:418–428.

85. Burton LC, Zdaniuk B, Schulz R, Jackson S, Hirsch C. Transitions in spousal caregiving. Gerontologist 2003;43:230–241.

86. Ferrell BR, Grant M, Borneman T, Juarez G, Ter Veer A. Family caregiving in cancer pain management. J Palliat Med 1995;2:185–195.

87. Kissane DW, Block S, McKenzie M, McDowell AC, Nitzan R. Family grief therapy: A preliminary account of a new model to promote healthy family functioning during palliative care and bereavement. Psychooncology 1998;7:14–25.

88. Smeenk FW, de Witte LP, Van Haastregt JC, Schipper RM, Biezeman HP, Crebolder HF. Transmural care of terminal cancer patients. Nurs Res 1998;47:129–136.

89. Macdonald G. Massage as a respite intervention for primary caregivers. Am J Hosp Palliat Care 1998;15:43–47.

90. White K, Cohen HJ. The older cancer patient. Med Clin N Am 2006;90:967–982.

91. Greenblatt DJ, Harmatz JS, Shader RI. Clinical pharmacokinetics of anxiolytics and hypnotics in the elderly: Therapeutic considerations. Clin Pharmacokinet 1991;21:165–177, 262–273.

92. Vestal RE, Montamat SC, Nielson CP. Drugs in special patient groups: The elderly. In: Melmon KL, Morrelli HF, Hoffman BB, Nierenberg DW, eds. Clinical Pharmacology: Basic Principles in Therapeutics (3rd ed). New York, NY: McGraw-Hill; 1992:851–874.

93. Avorn J, Gurwitz HH. Principles of pharmacology. In: Cassel CK, Cohen HJ, Larson EB, et al. eds. Geriatric Medicine (3rd ed). New York, NY: Springer; 1997:55–70.

94. Vestal RE. Aging and pharmacology. Cancer 1997;89:1302–1310.

95. Aparasu RR, Sitzman SJ. Inappropriate prescribing for elderly outpatient. Am J Health Syst Pharm 1999;56:433–439.

96. Sykes N. End of life issues. Eur J Cancer 2008;44:1157–1162.

97. National Care of the Dying Audit—Hospitals (NCDAH). Royal College of Physicians: Summary Report, December 5, 2007.

98. Glare P, Virik K, Jones M, et al. A systematic review of physicians' survival predictions in terminally ill cancer patients. BMJ 2003;327:195–200.

99. Coventry PA, Grande GE, Richards DA, Todd CJ. Prediction of appropriate timing of palliative care for older adults with non-malignant life-threatening disease: A systematic review. Age Aging 2005;34:218–227.

100. Seale C, Cartwright A. The Year Before Death. Brookfield, VT: Ashgate Publishing Company: 1994.

101. Saavedra Munoz G, Martin Barreto Pilar Ma. Frail Elderly and Palliative Care. Psicothema 2008;20(4):571–576.

102. Palange P, Forte S, Felli A, Galassetti P, Serra P, Carlone S. Nutritional state and exercise tolerance in patients with COPD. Chest 1995;107:1206–1212.

103. Ripamonti C, Bruera E. Dyspnea: Pathophysiology and assessment. J Pain Symptom Manage 1997;13:220–232.

104. Booth S, Moosavi SH, Higginson IJ. The etiology and management of intractable breathlessness in patients with advanced cancer: A systematic review of pharmacological therapy. Nat Clin Pract Oncol 2008;5:2:90–100.

105. Cachia E, Ahmedzai SH. Breathlessness in cancer patients. Eur J Cancer 2008;44:1116–1123.

106. Joyce M, McSweeney M, Carrieri-Kohlman KL, Hawkins J. The use of nebulized opioids in the management of dyspnea: Evidence synthesis. Oncol Nurs Forum 2004;31:3:551–561.

107. Jennings AL, Davies AN, Higgins JPZT, Broadley K. Opioids for palliation of breathlessness in termimal illness. Cochrane Review. In The Cochrane Library, Issue 3. New York, NY: Oxford Update Software; 2003.

108. Bruera E, Sala R, Spruyt O, Palmer L, Zhang T, Willey J. Nebulized versus subcutaneous morphine for patients with cancer dyspnea: A preliminary study. J Pain Symptom Manage 2005;29(6):613–618.

109. Charles MA, Liz R, Fiona Israel M. Relief of incident dyspnea in palliative cancer patients: A pilot, randomized controlled trial comparing nebulized hydromorphone, systemic hydromorphone and nebulized saline. J Pain Sympt Manage 2008;36(1):29–38.

110. Kohara H, Ueoka H, Aoe K, et al. Effect of nebulized furosemide in terminally ill cancer patients with dyspnea. J Pain Symptom Manage 2003;26:962–967.

111. Moosavi SH, Binks PA, Lansing RW, Topulus GP, Banzett RB, Schwartzman RM. Effects of inhaled furosemide on air hunger induced in healthy humans. Respir Physiol Neurobiol 2007;156:1–8.

112. Ong K-C, Kor A-C, Chong W-F, Earnest A, Wang Y-T. Effects of inhaled furosemide on exertional dyspnea in chronic obstructive pulmonary disease. Am J Resp Crit Care Med 2004;169(9):1028–1033.

113. Kallet RH. The role of inhaled opioids and furosemide for the treatment of dyspnea. Resp Care 2007;52(7):900–910.

114. Lanken PN, Terry PB, DeLisser HM, et al. An official american thoracic society clinical policy statement: Palliative care for patients with respiratory diseases and critical illnesses. Am J Resp Crit Car Med 2008;177:912–927.

115. Vane JR, Botting RM. Anti-inflammatory drugs and their mechanism. Inflamm Res 1998;47(Suppl 2):S78–S87.

116. Mercandate S. The use of anti-inflammatory drugs in cancer pain. Cancer Treat Rev 2001;27:51–61.

117. Perez Gutthann S, Garcia Rodriguez LA, Raiford DS, Duque Oliart A, Ris Romeu J. Nonsteroidal anti-inflammatory drugs and the risk of hospitalization for acute renal failure (comment). Arch Intern Med 1996;156:2433–2439.

118. Cryer B, Feldman M. Cyclooxygenase-1 and cyclooxygenase-2 selectivity of widely used nonsteroidal anti-inflammatory drugs. Am J Med 1998;104:413–421.

119. Simon LS, Weaver Al, Graham DY, et al. Anti-inflammatory and upper gastrointestinal effects of celecoxib in rheumatoid arthritis: A randomized controlled trial. JAMA 1999;282:1921–1928.

120. Juni P, Rutjes AW, Dieppe PA. Are selective COX-2 inhibitors superior to traditional nonsteroidal anti-inflammatory drugs? BMJ 2002;324(7353):1538, erratum.

121. Juni P, Dieppe P, Egger M. Risk of myocardial infarction associated with selective COX-2 inhibitors: Questions remain. (comment). Arch Intern Med 2002;162:2639–2640, author reply 2640.

122. Wright JM. The double-edged sword of COX-2 selective NSAIDs. (comment) Can Med Assoc J 2002;167:1131–1137.

123. Peterson WL, Cryer B. COX-1-sparing NSAIDs—is the enthusiasm justified? (comment). JAMA 1999;282:1961–1963.

124. Mercadante S, Arcuri E. Opioids and renal function. J Pain 2004;5:2–19.

125. Kaiko RF, Wallenstein SL, Rogers AG, Grabinski PY, Houde RW. Narcotics in the elderly. Med Clin N Am 1982;66:1079–1089.

126. Anderson G, Jensen NH, Christup L, Hansen SH, Sjogren P. Pain, sedation and morphine metabolism in cancer patients during long-term treatment with sustained-release morphine. Palliat Med 2002;16:107–114.

127. Smith MT. Neuroexcitatory effects of morphine and hydromorphone: Evidence implicating the 3-glucuronide metabolites. Clin Exp Pharmacol Physiol 2000;27:524–528.

128. Wright AW, Mather LE, Smith MT. Hydromorphone-3-glucuronide: A more potent neuroexcitant than its structural analogue, morphine-3 glucuronide. Life Sci 2001;69:409–420.

129. Menten J, Desmedt M, Lossignol D, Mullie A. Longitudinal follow-up of TTS-fentanyl use in patients with cancer-related pain: Results of a compassionate–use study with special focus on elderly patients. Curr Med Res Opin 2002;18:488–498.

130. Radbruch L, Sabatowski R, Petzke F, Brunsch-Radbruch A, Grond S, Lehman KA. Transdermal fentanyl for the management of cancer pain: A survey of 1005 patients. Palliat Med 2001;15:309–321.

131. Coluzzi PH, Schwartzberg L, Conroy JD, et al. Breakthrough cancer pain: A randomized trial comparing oral transmucosal fentanyl citrate (OTFC) and morphine sulfate immediate release (MSIR). Pain 2001;91:123–130.

132. Shaiova, L, Berger A, Blinderman CD, et al. Consensus guideline on parenteral methadone use in pain and palliative care. Palliat Support Care 2008;6:165–176.

133. Kornick CA, Kilborn MJ, Santiago-Palma J, et al. QTC interval prolongation associated with intravenous methadone. Pain 2003;105:499–506.

134. Cruciani R. Methadone: To ECG or not to ECG…That is still the question. J Pain Sympt Manage 2008;36:5:545–552.

135. Morley JS, Bridson J, Nash TP, Miles JB, White S, Makin MK. Low-dose methadone has an analgesic effect in neuropathic pain: A double-blind randomized controlled crossover trial. Palliat Med 2003;9:73–83.

136. Popp B, Portenoy RK. Management of chronic pain in the elderly: Pharmacology of opioids and other analgesic drugs. In: Ferrell BR, Ferrell BA, eds. Pain in the Elderly. Seattle, WA: IASP Press; 1996:21–34.

137. Max MB. Antidepressants and analgesics. In: Fields HL, Liebeskind JC, eds. Progress in Pain Research and Management, Vol 1. Seattle, WA: IASP Press; 1994:229–246.

138. Leo RJ, Singh A. Pain management in the elder: Use of psychopharmacologic agents. Ann Long-Term Care 2002;10:37–45.

139. Lipman AG. Analgesic drugs for neuropathic and sympathetically maintained pain. Clin Geriatr Med 1996;12:501–515.

140. Wiffen PJ, McQuay HJ, Edwards JE, Moore RA. Gabapentin for acute and chronic pain. Cochrane Database Syst Rev 2005;3:CD005452.

141. Rowbotham M, Harden N, Stacey B, Bernstein P, Magnus-Miller L. Gabapentin for the treatment of postherpetic neuralgia: A randomized controlled trial. JAMA 1998;280:1837–1842.

142. Ahn SH, Park HW, Lee BS, et al. Gabapentin effect on neuropathic pain compared among patients with spinal cord injury and different durations of symptoms. Spine 2003;28:341–347.

143. Garcia-Borreguero D, Larrosa O, de la Llave Y, Verger K, Masramon X, Hernandez G. Treatment of restless legs syndrome with gabapentin: A double-blind, cross-over study. (comment). Neurology 2002;59:1573–1579.

144. Baron R, Brunnmuller U, Brasser Matthias, May Michael, Binder A. Efficacy and safety of pregabalin in patients with diabetic peripheral neuropathy or postherpetic neuralgia: Open-label, non-comparative, flexible-dose study. Eur J Pain 2008;2:850–858.

145. Lesser H, Sharma U, LaMoreaux L, Poole RM. Pregabalin relieves symptoms of painful diabetic neuropathy: A randomized controlled trial. Neurology 2004;63:2104–2110.

146. Portenoy RK, Prager G. Pain management: Pharmacological approaches. In: von Gunten CF, ed. Palliative Care and Rehabilitation of Cancer Patients. Boston, MA: Kluwer Academic Publishers; 1999:1–29.

147. Nelson KA, Park K, Robinovitz E, Tsigos C, Mas MB. High-dose oral dextromethorphan versus placebo in painful diabetic neuropathy and postherpetic neuralgia. Neurology 1997;48:1212–1218.

148. Visser E, Schug SA. The role of ketamine in pain management. Biomed Pharmacother 2006;6:341–348.

149. Coyle N, Layman-Goldstein M. Pain assessment and management in palliative care. In: Matzo M, Sherman D, eds. Palliative Care Nursing: Quality Care to the End of Life. New York, NY: Springer: 2001:422.

150. Watanabe S, Bruera E. Corticosteroids as adjuvant analgesics. J Pain Symptom Manage 1994;9:442–445.

151. Mercadante S, Fulfaro F, Casuccio A. The use of corticosteroids in home palliative care. Support Cancer Care 2001;9:386–389.

152. Woolridge JE, Anderson CM, Perry MC. Corticosteroids in advanced cancer. Oncology (Huntington) 2001;15:225–236.

153. Ettinger AB, Portenoy RK. The use of corticosteroids in the treatment of symptoms associated with cancer. J Pain Symptom Manage 1988;3:99–103.

154. Feuer DJ, Broadley KE. Corticosteroids for the resolution of malignant bowel obstruction in advanced gynaecological and gastrointestinal cancer. Cochrane Database Syst Rev 2000;(3):CD001219.

155. Sloan P, Basta M, Storey P, von Guten C. Mexiletine as an adjuvant analgesic for the management of neuropathic pain. Anesth Analg 1999;89:760–761.

156. Galer BS, Jensen MP, Ma T, Davis PS, Rowbotham MC. The lidocaine patch 5% effectively treats all neuropathic pain qualities: Results of a randomized, double-blind, vehicle-controlled, 3-week efficacy study with use of the neuropathic pain scale. Clin J Pain 2002;18:297–300.

157. Devers A, Galer BS. Topical lidocaine patch relieves a variety of neuropathic pain conditions: An open label study. Clin J Pain 2000;16:205–208.

158. Ferrini R, Paice JA. Infusional lidocaine for severe and/or neuropathic pain. J Support Oncol 2004;2:90–94.

159. Walker K, Medhurst SJ, Kidd BL, et al. Disease modifying and anti-nociceptive effects of the bisphosphonate, zoledronic acid in a model of bone cancer pain. Pain 2002;100:219–229.

160. Rizzoli R. Bisphosphonates and reduction of skeletal events in patients with bone metastatic breast cancer. Ann Oncol 2004;15:700–701.

161. Hortobagyi GN, Theriault RL, Porter L, et al. Efficacy of pamidronate in reducing skeletal complications in patients with breast cancer and lytic bone metastases. Protocol 19 Aredia Breast Cancer Study Group. N Engl J Med 1996;335:1785–1791.

162. Gennari C, Agnusdei D, Camporeale A. Use of calcitonin in the treatment of bone pain associated with osteoporosis. Calcif Tissue Int 1991;49(Suppl 2):s9–s13.

163. Giammarile F, Mognetti T, Resche I. Bone pain palliation with strontium-89 in cancer patients with bone metastases. Q J Nucl Med 2001;45:78–83.

164. Rhiner M, Ferrell BR, Ferrell BA, Grant MM. A structured nondrug intervention program for cancer pain. Cancer Pract 1993;1:137–143.

165. Weinrich SP, Weinrich MC. The effect of massage on pain in cancer patients. Appl Nurs Res 1990;3a:140–145.

166. Kristjanson, J Walton J, Toyce C. End of life challenges in residential aged care facilities: A case for a palliative approach to care. Int J Pall Nurs 2005;11(3):127–129.

167. Kristjanson LJ, Walton J, Toyce C. Palliative care for the aged community: An australian perspective. In: Morse C, ed. The Art of Ageing in a Global Community: Lessons from Three Nations. Baywood Publishers, New York; 2005.

168. Farrell MJ, Katz B, Helme RD. The impact of dementia on the pain experience. Pain 1996;67:7–15.

169. Hurley AC, Volicer BJ, Hanrahan PA, Houde S, Volicer L. Assessment of discomfort in advanced Alzheimer patients. Res Nurs Health 1992;15:369–377.

170. Porter FL, Malhotra KM, Wolf CM, Morris JC, Miller JP, Smith MC. Dementia and response to pain in the elderly. Pain 1996;68:413–421.

171. Sengstaken EA, King SA. The problem of pain and its detection among geriatric nursing home residents. J Am Geriatr Soc 1993;41:541–544.

172. Stein WM, Ferrell BA. Pain in the nursing home. Clin Geriatr Med 1996;12:601–613.

173. Kaasalainen S, Middleton J, Knezacek S, et al. Pain and cognitive status in the institutionalized elderly: Perceptions and interventions. J Gerontol Nurs 1998;24:24–31.

174. Parmelee A. Pain in cognitively impaired older persons. Clin Geriatr Med 1996;12:473–487.

175. Mumm J, Hanson L, Zimmerman S, Sloane P, Mitchell CM. Is hospice associated with improved end of life care in nursing homes and assisted living facilities? J Am Ger Soc 2006;54:490–495.

176. Teno JM, Mor V, DeSilva K, Kabumunto G, Mor V. use of feeding tubes in nursing home residents with severe cognitive impairment. JAMA 2002;287:3211–3212.

177. Ferrell BR, Grant M, Chan J, Ahn C, Ferrell BA. The impact of cancer pain education to family caregivers of elderly patients. Oncol Nurs Forum 1995;22:1211–1218.

178. Ersek M, Grant MM, Kraybill BM. Enhancing end-of-life care in nursing homes: Palliative care educational resourse team (PERT) program. J Pall Med 2005;8(3):556–566.

179. Hall P, Schroeder C, Weaver L. The last 48 hours of life in long term care. A focused chart audit. J Am Ger Soc 2002;50:501–506.

180. Rodin MB. Cancer patients admitted to nursing homes: What do we know? JAMA 2008;149:156.

181. Lipowski Z. Delirium in the elderly patient. N Engl J Med 1989;2:578–582.

182. Costa PT, William TF, Somerfield M, et al. Recognition and Initial Assessment of Alzheimer's Disease and Related Dementias. Clinical Practice Guideline No. 19. Pub. No. 97-0702. 1996. Rockville, MD: U.S. Department of Health and Human Services, Public Health Service, Agency for Health Care Policy and Research.

183. Marshal GA, Fairbanks LA, Tekin S, Vinters HV, Cummings JL. Neuropathological correlates of activities of daily living in Alzheimer's Disease. Alzheimer Dis Assoc Disord 2006;20(1):56–59.

184. Hebert LE, Scherr PA, Bienias JL, Bennett DA, Evans DA. Alzheimer disease in the US population: Prevalence estimates using the 2000 census. Arch Neurol 2003;60:1119–1122.

185. Cummings JL. Alzheimer 's Disease. N Engl J Med 2004;351:56–67.

186. Lunney JR, Lynn J, Foley DJ, Lipson S, Guralnik JM. Patterns of functional decline at the end of life. JAMA 2003;289(18):2387–2392.

187. Massie MJ, Holland J, Glass E. Delirium in terminally ill cancer patients. Am J Psychiatry 1983;140;1048–1050.

188. Foreman MD. Acute confusion in the elderly. Ann Rev Nurs Res 1993;11:3–30.

189. Breitbart W, Bruera E, Harvey C, Lynch M. Neuropsychiatric syndromes and psychological symptoms in patients with advanced cancer. J Pain Symptom Manage 1995;10:131–141.

190. Spiller JA, Keen JC. Hypoactive delirium: Assessing the extent of the problems for the inpatient specialist palliative care. Palliat Med 2006;20(1):17–23.

191. Stagno D, Gibson C, Breitbart W. The delirium subtypes: A review of prevalence, phenomenologyathophysiology, andtreatmentresponse. Palliat Support Care 2004;2(2):171–179.

192. Bruera E, Miller L, McCallion J, Macmillan K, Krefting L, Hanson J. Cognitive failure in patients with terminal cancer: A prospective study. J Pain Symptom Manage 1992;7:192–195.

193. Inouye S, Charpentier PA. Precipitating factors for delirium in hospitalized elderly persons: Predictive model and interrelationship with baseline vulnerability. JAMA 1996;275:852–857.

194. Francis J, Martin D, Kapoor WN. A prospective study of delirium in hospitalized elderly. JAMA 1990;267:827–831.

195. Rockwood K. Acute confusion in elderly medical patients. J Am Geriatric Soc 1989;37:150–154.

196. Schor JD, Levkogg SE, Lipsitz LA, et al. Risk factors for delirium in hospitalized elderly. JAMA 1992;267:827–831.

197. Ljubisavljevic V, Kelly B. Risk factors for development of delirium among oncology patients. Gen Hosp Psychiatry 2003;25:345–352.

198. O'Keefe ST, Lavan JN. Clinical significance of delirium subtypes in older people. Age Ageing 1999;28:115–119.

199. Maltoni M, Caraceni A, Brunelli C, et al.; Steering Committee of the European Association for Palliative Care. Prognostic factors in advanced cancer patients: Evidence-based clinical recommendations—a study by the Steering Committee of the European Association for Palliative Care. J Clin Oncol 2005;23(25):6240–6248.

200. Lawlor PG, Fainsinger RL, Bruera ED. Delirium at the end of life: Critical issues in clinical practice and research. JAMA 2000;284:2427–2429.

201. Maltoni M, Caraceni A, Brunelli C, et al.; Steering Committee of the European Association for Palliative Care. Prognostic factors in advanced cancer patients: Evidence-based clinical recommendations-a study by the Steering Committee of the European Association for Palliative Care. J Clin Oncol 2005;23(25):6240–6248.

202. Folstein MF, Folstein SE, McHugh PE. "Mini-Mental Status": A practical method for yielding the cognitive state of patients for clinicians. J Psych Res 1975;12:189–198.

203. Trzepacz PT. The Delirium Rating Scale: Its use in consultation-liaison research. Psychosomatics 1999;40(3):193–204.

204. Inouye K, Vandyck C, Alessi C, Balkin S, Siegal AP, Horwitz RI. Clarifying confusion: The confusion assessment method, a new method for the detection of delirium. Ann Intern Med 1990;113(12):941–948.

205. Hart RP, Levenson J, Sessler C, Best A, Schwartz S, Rutherford L. Validation of a cognitive test for delirium in medical ICU patients. Psychosomatics 1996;37(6):533–546.

206. Breitbart W, Rosenfeld B, Roth A, Smith MJ, Cohen K, Passik S. The Memorial Delirium Assessment Scale. J Pain Symptom Manage 1997;13(3):128–137.

207. Breitbart W, Alici Y. Agitation and delirium at the end of life. JAMA 2008;300(24):2898–2910.

208. Breitbart W, Jacobsen PB. Psychiatric symptom management in terminal care. Clin Geriatr Med 1996;12:329–347.

209. Breitbart W, Tremblay A, Gibson C. An open trial of olanzapin for the treatment of delirium in hospitalized cancer patients. Psychosomatics 2002;43:175–182.

210. Breitbart W, Marotta R, Platt M, et al. A double-blind trial of haloperidol, chlorpromazine, and lorazepam in the treatment of delirium in hospitalized AIDS patients. Am J Psychiatry 1996;153:2:231–237.

211. Jackson KC, Lipman AG. Drug therapy for delirium in terminally ill patients. Cochrane Database Syst Rev 2004;2:CD004770.

212. Seeman T, Guralnik J, Kaplan G, Knudsen L, Cohen R. The health consequence of multiple morbidity in the elderly. The Alameda County Study. J Aging Health 1989;1:5066.

213. Stein W. Barriers to effective pain management in the nursing home. In: Ferrell B, ed. Pain in the Nursing Home. Clinics in Geriatric Medicine Pain Management. Philadelphia, PA: W.B. Saunders; 1996:604.

214. Walker MK, Marquis DF; NICHE Faculty. Ensuring medication safety for older adults. In: Abraham I, Bottrell M, Fulmer T, Mezey MD, eds. Geriatric Nursing Protocols for Best Practice. New York, NY: Springer; 1996:131–144.

215. Field M, Cassel C; Committee on Care at the End of Life, Institute of Medicine. Approaching Death: Improving Care at the End of Life. Washington, DC: National Academy Press: 1977:50–86.

216. Eliopoulos C. Respiratory problems. In Gerontological Nursing (4th ed). Philadelphia, PA: J.B. Lippincott; 1996:277–290.

217. Storey P, Knight CF, Unipac Four. Management of Selected Nonpain Symptoms in the Terminally Ill. A Self-study Program. Gainesville, FL: American Academy of Hospice and Palliative Medicine; 1996:25–32.

218. Ripamonti C. Management of dyspnea in advanced cancer patients. Support Care Cancer 1999;7:233–243.

219. Tobin M. Dyspnea: Pathophysiologic basis, clinical presentation, and management. Arch Intern Med 1990;150:1604–1613.

220. Kuebler KK. Hospice and palliative care clinical practice protocol: Dyspnea. Hosp Nurs Assoc 1996:1–28.

221. McCaffery M, Pasero C. Pain: Clinical Manual. St. Louis, MO: Mosby; 1999:179–180.

# 39

*Anne Hughes*

# Poor, Homeless, and Underserved Populations

*Can you give me respect?...Respect me...If you got something to say, listen. Don't jump to conclusions...Treat me as I'm treating you. Give me respect; I give you respect. Don't play (with) my intelligence.—Bill, 41-year-old African-American with AIDS and paraplegia secondary to a gunshot injury*

◆ **Key Points**
◆ *Poor people are at risk for poor quality of life and poor-quality deaths.*
◆ *People whose lives have been filled with physical and emotional deprivation may be suspicious of attempts to engage them in "shared" decision-making to limit therapy, regardless of its likely benefits or burdens.*
◆ *Some poor people have medical comorbidities and other social characteristics that have marginalized them in society.*
◆ *Poor people's interactions with the health-care system are frequently marked by rejection, shame, and lack of continuity of care.*

Poverty is inextricably linked to increased morbidity, premature mortality, and limited access to both preventive healthcare and ongoing medical care. Beyond the medical outcomes of poverty, the personal and social costs are substantial and often invisible. People who are poor constitute a *vulnerable population*, a term used in community health to describe social groups at greater risk for adverse health outcomes. The root causes of this vulnerability typically are low socioeconomic status and a lack of access to resources.[1] The Institute of Medicine's report, which evaluated racial and ethnic disparities in healthcare, failed to address the role of poverty in disparities.[2] However, the role of poverty in contributing to inequalities, independent of race and ethnicity, is difficult to decipher because class and race are often closely intertwined.[3,4] Some believe poverty may be most responsible for disparities in healthcare.[4]

Although much has been written about end-of-life care in the United States,[5-8] with few exceptions, little has been said about those in our society who live at its margins, such as the urban poor.[9-12i] To be poor and to have a progressive, life-threatening illness presents more challenges than either one of these conditions alone. As Taipale elegantly notes, "Poverty means the opportunities and choices most basic to human development are denied [p. 54]."[13] Consider the following questions: What type of death would a person hope for who doesn't have a home or lives in a room without a phone, a toilet, or kitchen? What are the meanings of life-threatening illness and death when premature death is an all-too-common part of life? What matters at the end of life if most of your life has been spent trying to survive day to day? All of these questions, in part, introduce us to the worlds of the poor who are confronting a life-threatening illness. Physical, psychological, and spiritual deprivation aren't all that poor people contend with—deprivation also harms the moral self and the ability both to act and to live autonomously.[14]

The purpose of this chapter is to examine the characteristics of the poor as an underserved population that place them at risk when palliative care is indicated . In particular, this chapter looks at a subset of the poor who are homeless or marginally housed and how this affects both access to and quality of care at the end of life. The recent economic downturn affecting the United States and the world has increased the numbers of persons "doing without." However, this chapter focuses on persons whose "membership" in this group is more long term and not the result of an identifiable global economic crisis; similarly, this chapter does not address the experiences of persons living in extreme poverty in resource-limited countries around the world.

The experience of being poor is not singular or universal, as poor persons are as diverse a population as the nonpoor. Case studies are used to illustrate the concepts discussed and to demonstrate the need for the more research to guide practice. The cases described are composite and reflective of the author's clinical practice and dissertation research[12e] in a metropolitan area that is greatly impacted by HIV/AIDS and homelessness. Therefore, these cases are not generalizable to all the poor or even to all the homeless. Poverty is only one social determinant that affects health status and access to resources. Persons with many vulnerabilities (e.g., being poor AND a member of a minority community, elderly, or having other medical problems) are at the greatest risk for adverse outcomes at the end of life.[15]

| Table 39–1 | |
|---|---|
| **States Whose Poverty Rates Exceed National Average (12.5%) for 3-Year Average 2005–2007** | |
| **State** | **People in Poverty (%)** |
| Alabama | 15.2 |
| Arizona | 14.7 |
| Arkansas | 15.1 |
| California | 12.7 |
| District of Columbia | 19.2 |
| Georgia | 13.5 |
| Kentucky | 15.7 |
| Louisiana | 17.1 |
| Mississippi | 21.1 |
| Montana | 13.4 |
| New Mexico | 16.3 |
| New York | 14.4 |
| North Carolina | 14.1 |
| Oklahoma | 14.7 |
| South Carolina | 13.4 |
| Tennessee | 14.8 |
| Texas | 16.4 |
| West Virginia | 15.2 |

*Source:* U.S. Census, (http://www.census.gov/hhes/www/poverty/poverty07/stategrid.xls).

## Epidemiology of Poverty in the United States

More than 37 million Americans (approximately one in eight) are poor.[16] The poverty line established by the federal government is based on annual household income. In 2007, a single adult under age 65 years was considered poor if his/her income was less than $10,787, and a family of four (with one adult and three children under age 18 years) was considered poor if their annual income was less than $21,100.[16] Table 39–1 lists states in which the poverty level exceeds the national average of 12.5% for the period of 2005 through 2007. Most experts believe the federal definition of poverty underestimates the true prevalence of poverty in the United States. For example, the poverty line (annual household income) does not capture cost-of-living differences across the country nor out-of-pocket medical costs.

The faces of the poor in the United States disproportionately include persons of color, children, foreign-born individuals, and single-parent families.[16] African-Americans have the highest rates of poverty in the United States (24.5%), followed by Hispanics (21.5%), Asian/Pacific Islanders (10.2%), and whites (8.2%) according to the U.S. Census Bureau Report for 2007.[16] Children have greater rates of poverty than young and middle-aged adults and the elderly. Forty three percent of children under age 18 years in the United States and living in a female-headed household were poor compared with 8.5% of children living with two married parents.[16]

Although poverty is not confined to urban areas, as evident in Table 39–1 (which includes many states with large rural populations), 80% of the poor live in or near the more populous metropolitan areas, and 43% of all the poor live in inner (or principal) cities.[16] Most of the poor have access to some type of housing or shelter, even if the basic accommodations (telephone, cooking and refrigeration, heat, water, private toilet, and bathing facilities) are inadequate. However, for a small subset, housing is marginal or unavailable. This subset is the focus of the following discussion.

## Definition and Prevalence of Homelessness

Homelessness is defined in the Stewart McKinney Homeless Act as a condition under which persons "lack fixed, regular and adequate night-time residence" or reside in temporary housing such as shelters and welfare hotels.[17] Calculating the number of Americans homeless or marginally housed is extremely difficult. Most cross-sectional studies fail to capture persons transiently homeless—the hidden homeless, or those staying with family members, those living in cars or encampments, and others living in single-room occupancy hotels (SROs), sometimes known as welfare hotels. Many of the poor and, in particular, the chronically homeless avoid contact with social and health services.

According to the National Coalition for the Homeless, on any given night between 440,000 to 840,000 Americans are homeless; as many as 3.5 million Americans experience homelessness in a given year.[18] Persons who are homeless are not members of a homogenous group. Some are street people and chronically homeless, whereas others are homeless because of a financial crisis that put them out of stable housing (this number is expected to climb given the recent global economic crisis). Street people may be more reluctant to accept services and may have much higher rates of concurrent substance abuse and mental illness (i.e., dual diagnosed).[19] Homeless persons frequently are also persons of color, veterans, victims of domestic violence, the mentally ill, and substance abusers.[20] Although the rates of mental illness and substance abuse are higher in the homeless than persons who are stably housed, assuming that all the poor or, for that matter, that all homeless suffer from these problems only contributes to stereotypes that fail to see the person who is before us.[17] Domestic violence, mental illness, and substance abuse are not confined to the poor; therefore, poverty does not cause these problems, although it may well exacerbate them.

## Health Problems Associated with Homelessness and Poverty

Numerous health problems are associated with homelessness. Many of these problems are related to environmental factors such as exposure to weather conditions, poorly ventilated spaces, unsafe hotels and street conditions, and high-crime neighborhoods, where the poor tend to live.[21] These health problems (Table 39–2) include malnutrition, lack of access to shelter and bathing facilities, problems related to drug and alcohol use, chronic mental illness, and violence-related injuries. One-fifth of the homeless have a major psychiatric illness.[20] About one in three homeless persons abuse drugs and alcohol.[20] Drugs and alcohol are sometimes used to self-medicate distressing psychiatric symptoms (e.g., anxiety, depression).

A meta-analysis of the influence of income inequality and population health concluded that although the direct effects of poverty on population health were not evident, the individual effects of poverty on health status are irrefutable.[22] Consider the case of coronary artery disease (CAD): the link between onset of CAD and low socioeconomic status has been established and is believed to be related to lifestyle factors, such as dietary habits, smoking, and physical activity.[23] Poor cardiac outcomes among the poor may also be related to limited access to standard medical care.[23,24] Persons who are poor, on average, have shorter life expectancies than those whose incomes are higher.[25] Men in Harlem have life expectancy rates comparable to those living in developing countries, such as Bangladesh.[4]

In urban areas, health-care services for the poor are often provided by public health departments, teaching hospitals, faith communities, and non-governmental organizations. These services typically are overburdened and unable to meet the needs of the poor and the growing number of Americans who are uninsured who access them.[12f] For many of the poor, the Emergency Department (ED) has become the primary source of medical care.[10]

**Table 39–2**
**Health Problems Associated with Homelessness**

| Causes | Manifestations |
| --- | --- |
| Malnutrition | Dental problems, tuberculosis, wasting |
| Lack of shelter and access to bathing facilities | Skin infections, lice, cellulitis, podiatric problems, hypothermia, tuberculosis |
| Drug and alcohol use | Overdose, seizures, delirium, sexually transmitted infections (such as HIV, hepatitis B, hepatitis C), trauma, falls, cirrhosis, heroin nephropathy, esophageal varices |
| Chronic mental illness | Paranoid ideation, antisocial behaviors, psychosis, suicide |
| Violence-related injuries | Assaults, homicides, rape |

## Poverty, Life-Threatening Illness, and Quality of Life

Poor people endure a heavier burden of cancer according to a report from the American Cancer Society.[4] The key findings of the impact of poverty on cancer care—irrespective of race and ethnicity—are listed in Table 39–3. Generally, poor people encounter substantial barriers to obtaining quality cancer care, experience more pain and suffering, and are more fatalistic about cancer.

Understanding the role race and ethnicity play in the end-of-life experience of the urban poor is complex. Nevertheless, three studies examined the impact of economic resources on quality of life for persons with life-threatening illnesses.[26-28] Being poor (defined as having an annual income of less than $20,000) negatively affected the quality of life reported by mostly white (85%) men who were newly diagnosed with prostate cancer, although low income was not related to quality-of-life over time. However, the lack of health insurance did predict worse quality of life for men with prostate cancer over time but not at baseline.[27] In a qualitative study of heterosexual couples in which only one partner was HIV-positive, the investigators were surprised to learn the "benefits" of having AIDS in providing poor persons with access to subsidized housing, food, and other social services.[26] Indeed, these researchers noted that given policy changes in welfare programs, having an AIDS diagnosis was a commodity that brought with it benefits that the poor were otherwise ineligible to receive. In other words, for poor people, having AIDS improved their quality of life. In a cross-sectional study of 212 adults with heart failure who were predominantly female (68%) and Africa-American (53%), quality of life was not related to physiological measures of heart function but was correlated with greater income, social support, and positive health beliefs.[28] Economic resources were associated with improved quality of life.

| Table 39–3<br>Poverty and Cancer: Findings from an American Cancer Society Report |
| --- |
| • Poor people lacking access to quality healthcare are more likely to die of cancer than nonpoor.<br>• Poor people experience greater cancer-related pain and suffering.<br>• Poor people facing significant barriers to getting health insurance often do not seek necessary care if they are unable to pay for it.<br>• Poor people and their families make extraordinary sacrifices to obtain and pay for care.<br>• Cancer education and outreach efforts are insensitive and irrelevant to the lives of many poor people.<br>• Fatalism about cancer is common among the poor and often prevents them from accessing care. |
| *Source:* Adapted from Freeman (2004), reference 4. |

| Table 39–4<br>Insights About the Dying Poor |
| --- |
| • Poverty inflicts substantial harm throughout life.<br>• Poverty exacerbates indignity and suffering throughout dying.<br>• Patients/families are often mistrustful and angry about the care received.<br>• Patients, at the same time, are often grateful for the care received.<br>• Spirituality plays an important role in providing strength and resilience when dying.<br>• Social isolation increases suffering.<br>• Hidden and sometimes unexpected sources of support can emerge from family and community.<br>• The emergency room is the front door to healthcare.<br>• The organization of medical care is frequently fragmented and lacks continuity.<br>• Funerals are important rituals, and their cost creates enormous stress for survivors. |
| *Source*: Adapted from Moller (2004), reference 10. |

In the book, *Dancing with Broken Bones: Portraits of Death and Dying Among Inner City Poor*, Moller poignantly recounts and photographically documents the stories of poor patients followed by an oncology clinic in a midwest city. His insights about the suffering of the urban poor are exquisite: "…the dying poor are the quintessential violators of the American dream; they live in the shame of poverty and with the unpleasantness of dying [p. 10]."[10] Because much of a person's "worth" in American society is connected with social status indicators such as occupation and income, the poor represent those who haven't made it. Being poor becomes a matter of personal failure rather than a social problem.[29] From Moller's longitudinal qualitative study of poor inner-city patients, their families, and their health-care providers, the researcher drew a number of conclusions, which are listed in Table 39–4. His work can perhaps be summed up by saying that the indignities of being poor in America are only intensified when that person is also dying; this finding is corroborated by other researchers.[12e,12f,12h] Unlike persons who are not poor, dying is not always feared in the same way, because for some persons who are socially or economically disadvantaged, dying may represent freedom from the misery of living.[12f]

## Clinical Presentations of Advanced Disease in the Poor

Persons who are poor frequently present with advanced disease. In addition to the late-stage disease presentation, many have significant comorbidities that affect both the palliation of symptoms and the course and treatment of underlying illnesses. These clinical management issues usually occur within the context of complex psychosocial situations, as the following cases illustrate:

CASE STUDY
### A 49-Year-Old Man with AIDS

Bill, a charmingly personable 41-year-old African-American man with AIDS and spinal cord injury, has been living in an AIDS-dedicated nursing home for over 12 years off and on, mostly on for the last 5 years except when hospitalized. Bill is dependent in most ADLs including transfers but is able to feed himself, perform his own oral hygiene and grooming, and get around in a motorized wheelchair. He enjoys writing poetry and loves to ride around in his chair. Bill resists his nurses' efforts to reposition him in the wheelchair or back in bed to relieve pressure on his coccyx. Bill's mother lives out of state and he has no other close relatives or friends who are in contact with him regularly. From time to time when Bill can borrow a phone, he calls his mother. Bill's past attempts to return to the community were hampered by lack of support system and Bill's feeling like a "sitting duck" in the high-crime area where most of the wheelchair-accessible SROs were located. Bill's spinal cord injury and paraplegia secondary to a gunshot wound predate his diagnosis with advanced HIV disease ( his HIV diagnosis occurred more than 15 years ago). His other medical problems include liver disease secondary to Hepatitis C and alcohol abuse, chronic obstructive pulmonary disease (COPD), stage IV pressure ulcer on coccyx, history of crack cocaine and heroin use, depression, and occasional delusional thinking. Bill was a drug dealer who even tried selling drugs at the nursing home when he was first admitted. Periodically he has had positive urine toxicology screens for cocaine and occasionally was found to have alcohol on his breath.

After his spinal cord injury, Bill was hospitalized for a presumed suicidal drug overdose. Currently Bill is taking antiretrovirals, bronchodilators, antidepressant therapy, and opioids for pain, which are administered by the nursing staff at the home. Although the staff believe Bill has pain, they are aware of his drug use, and that he "cheeks" his prescribed opioid to sell to another patient.

Comorbidities, especially those related to drug use and violence, complicate symptom management and other medical management.[30] As Bill's case study illustrates, there are several competing factors that may influence his providers' willingness to aggressively manage his pain. Persons known to be chemically dependent are often denied treatment for pain because of providers' concerns of aberrant or drug-hoarding behaviors. Will Bill take the medication as ordered? What should the nurse say/do when Bill insists he does not need to be observed swallowing his medications or when he insists that he does not like the taste of the liquid opioid? Is he likely to try again to sell his opioids for cocaine? How does one manage the severe pain of a patient who has diverted opioids in the past and whose actions may have compromised the safety of other patients? Pain experts have noted that some providers question the use of opioids for any nonmalignant pain syndrome and ethical dilemmas arise when assessing and managing pain in these complex situations.[30a] Who then will prescribe opioid medications? If Bill is seen by a covering provider rather than his primary care provider will he need to negotiate the need for analgesia with the new doctor ? Does the pharmacy that provides medications to the nursing home carry them? Morrison and colleagues[31] reported that pharmacies in predominantly non-white neighborhoods in New York City were less likely to carry opioids for pain management than were pharmacies in neighborhoods serving predominantly white communities. Most health-care facilities and housing programs serving the poor are located in inner cities rather than in middle class or affluent communities, where more whites live. Poor social conditions, criminal activity, and the threat of violence are significant barriers to effective pain management for persons with life-threatening illnesses.[12] In the nursing home, Bill is carefully monitored but the nurses remain concerned that he is using drugs again when he is quite drowsy and insisting that his pain is not well-controlled. How can the nurse know for sure that he is in pain and not merely "drug seeking" for income or to self-medicate the suffering of his everyday existence? Some questions are philosophical and cannot simply be answered clinically.

In addition to these quandaries, for many persons who are poor and others lacking adequate health insurance, access to treatment is a significant factor that influences symptom management. For example, if an antiemetic prescribed to relieve the chronic nausea experienced by a poor person with pancreatic cancer is not covered on the Medicaid formulary, or the person is not eligible for any drug-assistance program, then the range of medications used to manage the nausea is severely limited.

High-tech methods to control symptoms are probably not an option for the person who lives in a tent encampment. Most poor persons are institutionalized to manage uncontrolled symptoms and to provide both chronic and terminal care that cannot be managed sufficiently on the street or in the shelter.[10]

The management of symptoms associated with progressive illness is further complicated by end-organ diseases, such as liver or renal disease, that may alter the pharmacokinetics of medications used to palliate symptoms. Clinically significant drug–drug and drug–nutrient interactions are common with antiretrovirals that Bill is taking. Determining whether a patient is experiencing an adverse drug reaction is not easy when the person has comorbidities, has rapidly progressive disease, is malnourished, or may be continuing to use alcohol or other substances.

Comorbidities also affect the health-care providers' ability to realistically estimate prognosis and the nature of symptoms or problems that might occur down the road. Bill has lived with AIDS for more than 15 years. Prior to the introduction of antiretroviral therapy and prophylaxis of opportunistic infections in the mid-1990s, in all probability he would not have survived this life-threatening condition. Now Bill is more likely to succumb to complications associated with his spinal cord injury or substance abuse.[31a] Charting the dying trajectory for the chronic progressive illness may be conceivable, but superimposing the acute illnesses and injuries that the very poor live with and manage creates jagged peaks and valleys in a downward course. How quickly the life-threatening illness will progress becomes a prognostication puzzle; some persons who have been living on the street truly seem to have had nine lives.

Because Bill is in a setting in which his medications and treatments are administered, treatment adherence is less a concern. If Bill were living in a less supervised setting, then this would be another issue about which health-care providers would likely be quite concerned—Despite the prevalence of substance abuse among the poor, lack of attention to self-care activities cannot be assumed in all drug users. Some homeless persons who use drugs manage complex HIV antiretroviral regimens that require scrupulous attention regarding when to eat, which other medications may or may not be taken at the same time, and the necessary several-times-a-day dosing.[32] Race, class, and housing status cannot be used as surrogate predictors of who abuses drugs and alcohol or who will adhere or not adhere to treatment demands.

## More Psychosocial Factors Influencing Palliative Care Available to the Poor and Homeless

Health-care professionals committed to supporting patients' right to a *good death* may be challenged when working with the poor and the homeless. The good death is described as: (1) free from avoidable distress and suffering; (2) in accord with the patient and family's wishes; and (3) consistent with clinical, cultural, and ethical standards.[5] Bad deaths, in contrast, are accompanied by neglect, violence, or unwanted and senseless medical interventions.[5] Persons who are poor or homeless are at risk for not-so-good deaths.[12a] Many persons have had episodic contact with the health-care system during acute illnesses or life-threatening trauma and may wind up receiving life-saving therapies such as mechanical ventilation, vasopressors, dialysis, and other therapies. All too often, the client does not have an advance directive or a surrogate decision-maker to articulate his/her wishes. Furthermore, in the absence of a competent patient or family directing otherwise, the technological imperative of hospitals and physicians in training may see saving a life at any cost of greater value.[5] Nevertheless, what constitutes a good or bad death is a question that can only be answered by an individual, if such a question is even relevant, and cannot be predicted based on group membership or economic resources.[33]

Basic survival needs (food, shelter, clothing, protection) are of primary concern to the poor—often of greater and more pressing importance than the existential crisis of facing one's own mortality. Seeing others die prematurely, often under violent or disturbing circumstances, or alone and forgotten, may be an all-too-common experience for this population.[34,12g] Table 39–5 lists challenges to providing a good death in this population. The lack of resources, both economic and human, limit the palliative options available to the person who is poor. In the movie *The Wizard of Oz*, Dorothy's refrain, "There's no place like home, there's no place like home," speaks of an almost faraway magical experience of which many who are poor and dying cannot even dream. Housing is so essential to health that for those of us who do not worry about having a roof over our heads at night, its importance is taken for granted. Many persons who are poor and don't have enough to get by are often trying to figure out how to find a place to stay. And for those with a place to live, the concerns may be keeping the utilities (lights, heat, water) on and having enough money for other needs.

In addition to basic survival needs of the poor that influence their end-of-life experiences are their relationships with the health-care professionals who care for them. Health-care professionals can and often do stigmatize patients for their appearance or lack of hygiene. Sometimes the presence of body odor leads to rejection. Historical events and power differential in patient–provider roles can also affect such relationships. For example, the African-American experience with the medical care system includes the Tuskegee experiment and other instances of abuse. Many African-Americans feel betrayed by the predominantly white medical care system and believe their trust in the system has been violated.[35]

Because many of the poor receive care in public health-care systems or indigent care settings that often serve as teaching hospitals, continuity of care is often an illusion.[10] Additionally, discussions about limiting therapy or do-not-resuscitate decisions may be regarded as an attempt by the dominant culture to withhold possibly life-sustaining therapy. Some individuals and communities fear being treated "like a guinea pig" and refuse to participate in clinical trials when offered. The sometimes-conflicted relationships

---

**Table 39–5**
**Psychosocial Challenges in Providing Palliative Care to the Poor**

- Patient is homeless or has unstable or unsafe housing, with inadequate basic facilities (phone, private bathroom, refrigerator, and cooking facilities).
- Getting to appointments is difficult without reliable transportation.
- Lack of money limits options and often contributes to chaotic lives.
- Patient has fragile or nonexistent support system (e.g., no primary caregiver, caregiver who is unable to provide necessary care, caregiver also sick, no surrogate or proxy decision-maker, estranged from family, history of family violence or abuse).
- Many poor people who have encountered rejection or shame when accessing healthcare services avoid contact and are slow to trust even well-meaning healthcare professionals.
- Poor people who obtain healthcare usually do so without benefit of a long-term relationship with a primary care provider or a case manager familiar with their history that can help them navigate a complex care-delivery system.
- Most healthcare or specialized palliative care services are geographically remote from where poor people live. Some service providers curtail services to the poorest communities because of concerns about staff safety.
- Behavioral problems (e.g., drug hoarding, selling prescriptions, hostility, psychiatric illness, substance abuse) can affect patient relationships with health-care providers.
- It is difficult to assess the decision-making capacity and goals of patients who are cognitively impaired, intoxicated, or brain-injured.
- Many patients, including the poor, are asked to make treatment decisions without sufficient information about the implications of the decisions, and in the context of a patient–provider relationship that has enormous power imbalances.
- There is little evidence available on which to base therapeutic interventions because this population is not included in clinical trials.

*Source:* Adapted from Moller (2004), reference 10.

---

that poor people have with health-care providers and systems related to care at the end of life is again powerfully captured by Moller:

> ...Perhaps even more poignant than the anger and disappointment of dissatisfied patients is the absence of resentment on the part of those who have every reason to be upset with the care they receive. It is fair to suggest that, for some, this lack of assertiveness and anger has its roots deep within the experience of poverty. Living every day with chaos, stress, and the indignity of inner-city poverty creates, for many, a level of tolerance that most of us would find intolerable. In this regard, it is not unusual for

patients to accept care with which they are unhappy because they have accepted a lifetime of economic and social indignities about which they are unhappy. In a strange sense, many patients often felt their suffering in the face of disease was just, "one more bad thing to endure." Thus despite many variations in form and meaning, disease and dying are often borne with a sense of equanimity that flows from constant adjustments required by a life lived in poverty [p. 1].[10]

## CASE STUDY
### A 35-Year-Old Man with Liver Cancer

Danny is a 53-year-old African-American man with liver cancer and end-stage heart disease (New York Heart Disease Class IV) and multiple other comorbidities, including a history of psychosis (controlled when he takes antipsychotic medications) and polysubstance abuse (his drug of choice is crack cocaine). Danny has been chronically homeless and spent some of his youth incarcerated in a penitenary in the South—in fact, Danny was born in jail. He is enrolled in the ED psychosocial case management program, in part to decrease his ED use (Danny had over 75 visits to the ED of a public hospital in 1 year). Danny's psychiatric social worker/case manager has worked over time to develop a relationship with him, to secure stable housing, and to help Danny receive the medications and medical appointments needed to manage his mental illness and heart disease and to palliate his liver cancer. Danny is the father of eight daughters and a son. One daughter was murdered by her husband. "What are you going to do, that's life," Danny commented when interviewed for a study exploring dignity among persons with advanced disease.[12e,12f] He is no longer in touch with his ex-wife or most of his children but periodically remains in contact with his 83-year-old mother. Danny's illness narrative is woven into his life (e.g., what he was doing at the time, following a psychiatric hospitalization and not the cancer or heart disease symptoms that resulted in his seeking healthcare). Danny believes he is going to live forever. According to his social worker, Danny has outlived most physicians' prognostications, which undoubtedly contributes to his beliefs. His outliving the doctors' prognosis made Danny question if doctors can always be believed.

Danny hates being "prejudged" by health-care providers because he is African-American and a drug user.[12e,12f] At times, these labels have contributed to his feeling of being spoken down to or ignored, which makes him angry and has resulted in his leaving clinics or hospitals against medical advice. Danny is annoyed that all the doctors keep telling him he is going to die. After all, "(he's) still here." He does not want to be asked about his end-of-life wishes, because he's still alive.

Heart disease and liver cancer are not the only chronic illnesses Danny and his family have been dealing with; Danny has a history of severe mental illness that have required previous hospitalization. Mental illness obviously is not confined to the poor. However, incorporating palliative care in the care of persons with mental illnesses is not easy regardless of their socioeconomic class. The literature to guide practice on palliative care and mental illness is sparse. In 2008, a literature review published by the Mental Health Foundation in England underscored the lack of evidence on which to base practice.[35a] The review noted that research and practice guidelines in palliative care typically address depression, anxiety, delirium, and cognitive impairment, which may be secondary to the lifethreatening condition.[35b] Few, if any, explored how persons with severe mental illnesses cope with life-threatening illness, although such patients may be a greater risk for presenting with advanced medical diseases.[35a]

Danny's story also raises a number of complex issues influenced by culture, historical discrimination, and the process of end-of-life decision-making. For some African-Americans, according to Crawley, death is seen as a struggle to overcome and, for others, a welcomed friend that precedes going home to heaven.[35] Danny is not ready to die, he does not regard death in his immediate future; perhaps dying, like living, is one more struggle to be overcome. Danny receives care in a public hospital from an oncology fellow whose different race, education, and occupation may contribute to different world views. Because Danny is living with two life-threatening conditions, his care is comanaged and poorly coordinated. When to introduce the option of hospice is difficult[35c]; it is even more difficult for communities who have felt marginalized or ignored by the dominant culture. For some patients, poor and nonpoor alike, hospice is equated with giving up, with not having hope. Given Danny's focus on living and his expressed desire not to think about or talk about dying, how can hospice be brought up without disregarding his expressed wishes? Is hospice likely to alter Danny's ED use when he has an urgent symptom or concern? Would hospice be able to provide services to his SRO and make visits at night to high-crime neighborhoods? Why must a person who has been receiving aggressive treatment to control disease shift to an approach whose goal is a peaceful and dignified death, when he has been struggling to live? These questions are not unique to the poor who are dying.

## CASE STUDY
### A 55-Year-Old Woman with Ovarian Cancer

Sally is a 55-year-old white woman with advanced ovarian cancer who lives in an SRO. She's had debulking surgery and many cycles of chemotherapy. Sally is a widow, without children, who has lived in the same 100-square-foot room for "many years." The bathroom she shares with the other tenants on her floor is around the corner and down the hall. She has no kitchen—only a hot plate and small refrigerator. Sally was raised in foster care and never had any contact with her biological family. Whenever asked about her support system Sally consistently replies, "I have no family." She completed eighth grade of her formal education but studies and frequently refers to the written cancer patient education materials she received from the American Cancer Society. Sally worked as a domestic, cleaning homes for rich families, until she was brutally raped, left critically ill, and hospitalized for an extended period more than 20 years ago. Sally's survival after that violent trauma was uncertain and almost miraculous. How horribly ironic that Sally would be diagnosed with ovarian cancer after surviving a brutal rape. When her tumor marker increases, Sally admits to being scared that the tumor may have extended to other organs, but she remarks "There's nothing you can do about it. Worrying don't do no good." Sally's faith is very important to her as a source of comfort and companionship. When asked about any worry she might have related to her cancer, Sally states, "No, because if I'm concerned, I pray to God and tell Him to show me the way so I get through it...I'm very close to God and if I have problems, I just pray to God." Listening to a TV televangelist and studying the Bible and other religious texts on CDs is how Sally spends most of her day in her room. She even takes her religious CDs and player to listen to while she is getting her chemotherapy at the outpatient infusion center. Sally's faith has helped her manage the worry of cancer and to find strength to cope with its demands. When interviewed for a study to understand the meaning and experience of dignity, Sally asks, "What does dignity mean? I got to know what it means before I can answer the questions [pp. 1114]."[12f]

Sally's story documents the difficult backgrounds and socially isolated experience of many of the poor.[12f] Sally's story also illuminates the enriching role that religion and spirituality can play in patients' lives. [10,12f,35d] Spiritual beliefs and practices help some to make sense of their world, to cope with adversity (whether serious illness or poverty), and to find meaning in suffering. Faith surely seems to play this role for Sally. The role that faith plays in the lives of the poor may not differ from the role faith plays in the lives of the nonpoor; although for the poor faith may be more a beacon of relief in a world that is hostile, rejecting, and marginalizing. Sally's question about dignity reminds us that some concepts central to palliative care, such as dignity, may not be understood to those for whom we care; however, the meaning of dignity at the end of life is hardly unambiguous and consensual.[12e,12h,35e] Sally's prophetic question may be the question researchers, clinicians, and policymakers also find themselves struggling to answer.

### Where and How Homeless People Die

Limited data are available regarding the socioeconomic factors, places of death, and immediate causes of death of the homeless.[36–38] Similar to those who are not poor, most poor people die in institutions. For those who are homeless, dying on the street or in jail is another fact of life.[39]

In 2003, 169 homeless persons died in San Francisco.[38] The profile of the homeless who died is the following: male (85%), average age of 42 years, and disproportionally more whites and African-Americans than live in San Francisco.[36] Drug and alcohol were directly associated with 60% of these deaths. Chronic alcohol abuse and acute alcohol intoxication were also listed as causes of death in the homeless in Georgia.[40] Hypothermia was also noted as a cause of death among the homeless in Chicago and in Georgia.[40,41] Accidental deaths resulting from fires, falls, and pedestrian–motor vehicle accidents, as well as drowning and violent deaths related to homicide and suicide were also reported in the homeless.[40]

Researchers in Boston studied the use of healthcare by the homeless for the year prior to their deaths.[37] Chart reviews were completed for all patients reported to the state death registry who had participated in a health-care program for the homeless. The actual circumstances of the death were not studied; however, the causes of death as listed on death certificates were noted. For the 5-year study period, 558 deaths were reported. Unlike the previous results, which examined coroner's cases, 81% of the deaths were attributed to natural causes (such as HIV/AIDS-related conditions, heart disease, cancer, and other unspecified causes), and only 19% resulted from external causes such as homicide, suicide, motor vehicle injuries, and drug overdoses.[37] Similar to the homeless who died in San Francisco, most were male (86%), between ages 25 and 44 years (56%), white (59%), and had a history of substance abuse (76% used alcohol). In addition, 28% were mentally ill.[37]

### Palliative Care Models for Working with the Poor

Several hospitals serving the urban poor have developed palliative care programs to address their specific needs.[42–44] The longest-running program (since 1986) is a nurse-directed program that serves critically ill patients who are unlikely to survive hospitalization in a trauma level I hospital in the Midwest. This supportive care team has documented decreased use of health-care resources and family satisfaction.[42] Another program, an interdisciplinary palliative care service based in a public hospital, follows patients and their families in the community and serves as a bridge when the patient is transferred to a nursing home or hospice for continuing care.[43] A third program, is an HIV/AIDS disease-specific palliative care consult service in New York City in a Bronx hospital serving the poor. The multidisciplinary team consults with both inpatient services and outpatient providers. The primary reasons for consultation included goals of care, pain, and psychsocial issues.[44]

## Strategies for Working with the Poor and Homeless Who Happen to be Dying

Working with the very poor can be challenging. Generations of internalized hopelessness, poor self-awareness, differing perceptions of time (everything seeming to take much longer), and difficulties navigating the many bureaucracies necessary to obtain services surely frustrate patients and caregivers alike.[45] Some have suggested modifying expectations to these realities and recognizing small successes as strategies to address these factors.[45]

On the other hand, for many persons who live on the street, survival skills are keenly developed. Knowing when a food bank opens, where to get clothing, when shelter-bed waiting lines begin to form, or how to get benefit checks without an address requires remarkable ingenuity and discipline. Needless to say, as with persons who are not poor, wide variations in abilities, resources, and relationships with health-care professionals exist.

Obviously, stable housing is critical to providing palliative care. Researchers noted the benefits of supportive housing to minority elders in East Harlem, including better psychological outcomes and increased use of informal supports.[46] In a qualitative study of nurses who care for persons who are disenfranchised, the researcher used the metaphor of a wall to describe the separation that nurses believed their clients experienced from society.[47] The disenfranchised in this study included the poor, mentally ill, immigrants, persons with substance abuse, and/or those with stigmatizing life-threatening illness. The nurses described three key themes in how they engaged their disenfranchised clients: (1) making a human connection with the client; (2) creating a community connection for their disconnected clients; and (3) making self-care possible.

In summary, developing therapeutic relationships with the poor and homeless requires (1) expecting the person's trust to be earned over time (sometimes a long time) and not be taken for granted; (2) respecting the person's humanity, no matter how they look, what they say, and what feelings in us they evoke; (3) appreciating the person's unique story as influencing his/her response to illness and death; and, finally, (4) recognizing and addressing maladaptive behaviors.[29,39,48] Table 39–6 includes a list of helpful suggestions to reach a difficult-to-engage client.

In addition to the interpersonal interventions to engage the client in a therapeutic interaction, nurses are often required to become knowledgeable about the availability of and the services provided by community agencies. Knowing which agencies or services are involved with a client and communicating with them assures consistency of approach and continuity of care. Advocacy is often required to access services such as pain management, substance abuse treatment, mental health services, and social services for housing and money management. To truly improve end-of-life care for the poor, nurses need to advocate for public policies that assure access to safe and stable housing, health insurance, and client-centered, community-based primary care.

| Table 39–6 |
| --- |
| **Helpful Suggestions When Engaging a Difficult-to-Engage Client** |

- Address anyone older than 40 years of age by the title of Mr. or Ms. Ask permission to be on a first-name basis.
- Do not hestitate to shake hands.
- Be prepared to meet people who are more intelligent, more perceptive, and more wounded than you expect.
- Be tolerant. How would you react if you were in that situation?
- Don't make promises you can't keep.
- Don't take it personally.
- Taking time out helps prevent burnout.
- Get to know the community.
- If you feel you have to save the human race, do it one person at a time.
- Providing material assistance (e.g., clean socks, food, hygiene kits) opens people up.
- Usually the most difficult clients are those most in need. Throw the word *noncompliant* out of your vocabulary.
- Make eye contact. If the person does not like eye contact or becomes agitated, avoid using it.
- Keep in mind that people who live intense lives may not particularly like unasked-for physical contact.
- Don't be afraid to ask "stupid" questions; patients' answers are better than your assumptions.
- Adjust your expectations and accept small victories with satisfaction.

*Source:* Patchell (1997), reference 48.

## Summary

Providing palliative care to the poor, especially the homeless, is extremely challenging. Comorbid illnesses, illnesses associated with poverty, and clarifying the etiology of presenting symptoms may seem almost impossible at times. Psychosocial risk factors and strained relationships with health-care providers sometimes result in the client receiving futile or unwanted medical interventions at an advanced stage of illness. Clarifying with a patient what constitutes a good death for him/her can be humbling when the patient tells you he or she wants simply to have shelter and to feel safe. Meeting the palliative care needs of this vulnerable population will require innovative practice and education models.

## Acknowledgments

The author gratefully acknowledges the research and educational grant support of the American Cancer Society Doctoral Scholarship in Nursing; National Institute of Nursing Research, Ruth L. Kirschstein National Research Service Award F31NR079923; Oncology Nursing Society (ONS) Foundation

Small Research Grant Award; ONS Doctoral Scholarship; UCSF Alpha Eta Research Award, Sigma Theta Tau Chapter and UCSF Graduate Student Research Award. She dedicates this chapter to the memory of Sally and Danny who while no longer in this world, their stories and others like them, continue to enlighten us.

## REFERENCES

1. Flaskerud JH, Winslow BJ. Conceptualizing vulnerable populations health-related research. Nurs Res 1998;47:69–78.
2. Smedley BD, Stith AY, Nelson AR. Unequal Treatment: Confronting Racial and Ethnic Disparities in Health Care. Washington, DC: National Academy Press, 2002.
3. Koenig BA, Gates-Williams J. Understanding cultural differences in caring for dying patients. West J Med 1995;163:244–249.
4. Freeman HP. Poverty, culture and social injustice: Determinants of cancer disparities. CA Cancer J Clin 2004;54:72–77.
5. Field MJ, Cassel CK. Approaching Death: Improving Care at the End of Life. Washington, DC: National Academy Press, 1997.
6. Foley KM, Gelband H. Improving Palliative Care for Cancer. Washington, DC: National Academy Press, 2001.
7. Krakauer EL, Crenner C, Fox K. Barriers to optimum end-of-life care for minority patients. J Am Geriatr Soc 2002;50:182–190.
8. SUPPORT. A controlled trial to improve care for seriously ill hospitalized patients: the study to understand prognoses and preferences for outcomes and risks of treatment (SUPPORT). JAMA 1995;274:1591–1598.
9. Gibson R. Palliative care for the poor and disenfranchised: A view from the Robert Wood Johnson Foundation. J R Soc Med 2001;94:486–489.
10. Moller DW. Dancing with Bones: Portraits of Death and Dying Among Inner-City Poor. New York, NY: Oxford University Press, 2004.
11. O'Neill JF, Romaguera R, Parham D, Marconi K. Practicing palliative care in resource-poor settings. J Pain Symptom Manage 2002;24:148–151.
12. Soares LGL. Poor social condition, criminality and urban violence: Unmentioned barriers for effective cancer pain control at the end of life. J Pain Symptom Manage 2003;26:693–695.
12a. Hughes A. Poverty and palliative care in the US: Issues facing the urban poor. Int J Pall Nurs 2005;11:6–13.
12b. Song J, Ratner ER, Bartels DM. (2005). Dying while homeless: Is it a concern when life itself is such a struggle? J Clin Ethics 2005;16(3):251–261.
12c. Norris WM, Nielsen EL, Engelberg RA, Curtis JR. Treatment preferences for resuscitation and critical care among homeless persons. Chest 2005;127(6):2180–2187.
12d. Kushel MB, Miaskowski C. End-of-life care for homeless patients: "She says she is there to help me in any situation." JAMA 2006;297(3):305.
12e. Hughes AM. (2007). "Can you give me respect?" Experiences of the Urban Poor with Advanced Disease. Unpublished Dissertation, University of California San Francisco.
12f. Hughes A, Gundmundsdottir M, Davies B. Everyday struggling to survive: Experiences of the urban poor living with advanced cancer. Oncol Nurs Forum 2007;34(6):1113–1118.
12g. Song J, Bartels DM, Ratner ER, Alderton L, Hudson B, Ahluwalia JS. Dying on the streets: Homeless persons' concerns and desires about end of life care. J Gen Intern Med 2007;22(4):435–441.
12h. Hughes A, Davies B, Gudmundsdottir M. "Can you give me respect?" Experiences of the urban poor on a dedicated AIDS nursing home unit. J Assoc Nurses AIDS Care 2008;19(5):342–356.
12i. Francoeur RB, Payne R, Raveis VH., Shim H. Palliative care in the inner city. Patient religious affiliation, underinsurance, and symptom attitude. Cancer 2007;109(2 Suppl):425–434.
13. Taipale V. Ethics and allocation of health resources: The influence of poverty on health. Acta Oncol 1999;38:51–55.
14. Blacksher E. On being poor and feeling poor: Low socio-economic status and the moral self. Theor Med Bioeth 2002;23:455–470.
15. Aday LA. At Risk in America: The Health and Health Care Needs of Vulnerable Populations (2nd ed). San Francisco, CA: Jossey-Bass, 2001.
16. DeNavas-Walt C, Proctor BD, Smith JC. 2008. Income, poverty and health insurance coverage in the United States: 2007. http://www.census.gov/prod/2008pubs/p60-235.pdf (accessed January, 2009)
16a. U.S. Census Bureau, http://www.census.gov/hhes/www/poverty/poverty07/tables07.html (accessed January, 2009).
17. National Coalition for the Homeless. 2008. Who is homeless? Fact Sheet #3 from http://www.nationalhomeless.org (retrieved January 9, 2009).
18. National Coalition for the Homeless. How many people experience homelessness? Fact sheet #2 http://www.nationalhomeless.org (accessed January 9, 2009).
19. Fellin P. The culture of homelessness. In: Manoleas P, ed. Cross-Cultural Practice of Clinical Case Management in Mental Health. New York, NY: Haworth Press; 1996:41–77.
20. National Coalition for the Homeless. 2002. Who is homeless fact sheet. Available at: http://www.nationalhomeless.org (accessed December 27, 2004).
21. Strechlow AJ, Amos-Jones T. The Homeless as a vulnerable population. Nurs Clin N Am 1999;34:261–274.
22. Lynch J, Davey Smith G, Harper S, Hillemeier M, Ross N, Kaplan GA, Wolfson M. Is income inequality a determination of population health? Part I. A systematic review. Millbank Q 2004;82:5–99.
23. Horne BD, Muhlestein JB, Lappe DL, et al. Less affluent area of residence and lesser-insured status predict an increased risk of death or myocardial infarction after angiographic diagnosis of coronary disease. Ann Epidemiol 2003;14:143–150.
24. Fang J, Alderman MH. Is geography destiny for patients in New York with myocardial infarction? Am J Med 2003;115:448–453.
25. Lynch J, Davey Smith G, Harper S, Hillemeier M. Is income inequality a determinant of population health? Part 2. U.S. national and regional trends in income inequality and age- and cause-specific mortality. Millbank Q 2004b;82:355–400.
26. Crane J, Quirk K, van der Straten A. "Come back when you're dying," the commodification of AIDS among California's urban poor. Soc Sci Med 2002;55:1115–1127.
27. Penson DF, Stoddard ML, Pasta DJ, Lubeck DP, Flanders SC, Litwin MS. The association between socioeconomic status, health insurance coverage, and quality of life in men with prostate cancer. J Clin Epidemiol 2001;54:350–358.

28. Clark DO, Tu W, Weiner M, Murray MD. Correlates of health-related quality of life among lower income, urban adults with congestive heart failure. Heart Lung 2003;32:391–401.

29. Kiefer CW. Health Work with the Poor: A Practical Guide. New Brunswick, NJ: Rutgers University Press, 2000.

30. O'Connor PG, Selwyn PA, Schottenfeld RS. Medical care for injection drug users with human immunodeficiency syndrome. N Engl J Med 1994;331:450–459.

30a. Sullivan M, Ferrell B. Ethical Challenges in the Management of Chronic Nonmalignant Pain: Negotiating Through the Cloud of Doubt. J Pain 2005;6(1):2–9.

31. Morrison RS, Wallenstein S, Natale DK, Senzel RS, Huang LL. "We don't carry that"—failure of pharmacies in predominantly nonwhite neighborhoods to stock opioid analgesics. N Engl J Med 2000;342:240–248.

31a. Sackoff JE, Hanna DB, Pfeiffer MR, Torian LV. Causes of death among persons with AIDS in the era of highly active antiretroviral therapy: New York City. Ann Intern Med 2006;145(6):397–406.

32. Bangsberg D, Tulsky JP, Hecht FM, Moss AR. Protease inhibitors in the homeless. JAMA 1997;278:63–65.

33. Tong E, McGraw SA, Dobihal E, Baggish R, Cherlin E, Bradley EH. What is a good death? Minority and non-minority perspectives. J Palliat Care 2003;19:168–175.

34. Kozol J. Amazing Grace: The Lives of Children and the Conscience of a Nation. New York, NY: Perennial Publishers, 1995.

35. Crawley L, Payne R, Bolden J, Payne T, Washington P, Williams S. Palliative and end-of-life care in the African American community. JAMA 2000;284:2518–2521.

35a. Ellison, N. 2008. Mental Health and Palliative Care Literature Review. http://www.mentalhealth.org.uk/publications/?entryid5=62815&char=M (accessed January, 2009).

.35b. National Consensus Project. 2004. Clinical Practice Guidelines for Quality Palliative Care. http://www.nationalconsensus-project.org/Guideline.pdf (accessed September 10, 2006).

35c. Casarett D, Quill TE. "I'm not ready for Hospice:" Strategies for timely and effective hospice discussions. Ann Intern Med 2007;146(6):443–449.

35d. Hughes A, Gudmundsdottir M, Davies B. Exploring Spirituality in the Urban Poor with Advanced Cancer (poster abstract). Oncol Nurs Forum. 2008;35:535.

35e. Street AF, Kissane DW. 2001. Constructions of dignity in end-of-life care. J Palliat Care 2001;17(2):93–101.

36. Bermudez R, von der Werth L, Brandon J, Aragon T. San Francisco Homeless Deaths Identified from Medical Examiner Records: December 1997–November 1998. San Francisco, CA: Department of Public Health, 1999.

37. Hwang SW, O'Connell JJ, Lebow JM, Bierer MF, Orav EJ, Brennan TA. Health Care Utilization Among Homeless Adults Prior to Death. J Health Care Poor Underserved 2001;12:50–58.

38. Dineen JK. Increase in homeless death rate on city's streets. San Francisco Examiner, August 28, 2003. http://www.examiner.com/article/index.cfm/i/082803n_homeless (accessed December 27, 2004).

39. Patchell T. Nowhere to run: portraits of life on the street. Turning Wheel J Soc Engag Buddhism 1996;Fall:14–21.

40. CDC. Deaths among the homeless—Atlanta, Georgia. Morbid Mortal Report 1987;36:297–299.

41. CDC. Hypothermia-related deaths—Cook County, Illnois. Morbid Mortal Report 1991;42:917–919.

42. Campbell ML, Frank RR. Experience with an end-of-life practice at a university hospital. Crit Care Med 1997;25:197–202.

43. Gramelspacher GP. 2001. End-of-life ethics. American Medical Association. http://www.ama-assn.org/ama/pub/category/5145.html (accessed December 27, 2004).

44. Selwyn PA, Rivard M, Kappell D, et al. 2002. Palliative care for AIDS at a large urban teaching hospital: Program description and preliminary outcomes. www.edc.org/lastacts/ (accessed January 11, 2009).

45. Kemp C. Terminal Illness: A Guide to Nursing Care (2nd ed). Philadelphia, PA: Lippincott Williams & Wilkins, 1999.

46. Cleak H, Howe JL. Social networks and use of social supports of minority elders in East Harlem. Social Work Health Care 2002;38:19–38.

47. Zerwekh JV. Caring on the ragged edge: Nursing persons who are disenfranchised. Adv Nurs Sci 2000;22:47–61.

48. Patchell T. Suggestions for Effective Outreach. San Francisco: San Francisco Department of Public Health, Homeless Death Prevention Project, 1997.

# 40

*Betty D. Morgan*

# End-of-Life Care for Patients with Mental Illness and Personality Disorders

*My mom, she was schizophrenic all her life, but when she was regulated on her medicines she was good, really good. She was a good mother when she was herself—that's what we would call it "being herself." She was like that at the end. I'm so glad we had that time. —A son whose mother died of breast cancer after long-term mental illness*

♦ **Key Points**

♦ *Enhanced communication skills with an emphasis on therapeutic communication are needed to work with patients with Serious Mental Illness (SMI) and Personality Disorders (PD)*

♦ *Capacity/Competency Issues may arise when working with people with SMI and PD, however, simply having a diagnosis of SMI or PD does not necessarily indicate lack of capacity or competency*

♦ *Redefinition of family may need to take place in order to include the patient's support system in their care*

♦ *Consultation/Collaboration is essential in caring for the population of people with SMI or PD to meet the needs of the patient and their support system*

Approximately 26.2% of Americans (about one in four) aged 18 years and older are diagnosed with a mental disorder in any given year. This translates to more than 57 million people in the United States. A smaller number of people, approximately 6% of Americans (1 in 17) suffer from a serious mental illness (SMI) such as schizophrenia, bipolar disease, and severe depression.[1] Comorbidity is common; almost half of the people who are diagnosed with a mental disorder meet criteria for a second mental disorder, with mood, anxiety, and addictive disorders being the most common comorbid illnesses.[1] The Global Burden of Disease study presented data revealing that mental illness, including suicide, makes up 15% of the burden of disease in the United States, more than the burden caused by all cancers combined.[2]

People with SMI reportedly die 20 to 25 years earlier than the general population worldwide.[3] The increase in mortality has been associated with both natural and "unnatural" causes of death, with unnatural causes defined as suicide, homicide, and accidental death.[4] Comorbid medical illnesses that are commonly observed in those with SMI include hypertension, cardiac disease, diabetes and other metabolic conditions, respiratory illnesses, obesity, renal disease, cerebrovascular disease, cancer and HIV/AIDS.[5] Additionally, an estimated one-third to one-half of the homeless people in the world have schizophrenia.[6,7]

This chapter examines what is known about palliative care and the mentally ill, including those with SMI and personality disorders (PDs). Special issues related to communication and treatment are presented as well as strategies for care for this population. Issues related to capacity and competency for decision-making as it relates to those with SMI and end-of-life care is also discussed. Collaboration and consultation between providers is essential in providing end-of-life care for those with SMI.

## Research Related to SMI and End-of-Life Care

Little research has been conducted in end-of-life issues with people with SMI, and those who have SMI have been under-served in terms of palliative care. Capacity of patients to make end-of-life decisions, provider concerns that end-of-life discussions would be upsetting, and lack of provider training and comfort in conducting discussions about end-of-life care have been cited as barriers to care and research.[7] Foti and colleagues demonstrated that a group of community-residing adults with SMI were able to designate treatment preferences for end-of life care in response to scenarios involving end-of-life situations.[8] Participants chose aggressive pain management in a scenario including pain and incurable cancer and were divided in their responses between waiting for a defined period before turning off life-support, terminating life support immediately, and keeping the person alive indefinitely for a patient with an irreversible coma. The researchers also provided follow-up with participants who were distressed by the research questions but found that none required crisis intervention or were so distressed that psychiatric decompensation was a risk.[9]

## Barriers to Care for Patients with Mental Illness

There are several barriers to consistent medical care for those with a mental illness; these barriers exist in primary care settings and apply to palliative care settings as well. Lack of preventive care or an ongoing relationship with a medical provider is a key issue for people with mental illness. People with SMI often seek care later in the course of the disease, resulting in costly services and complex care needs. Inadequate support systems that are common among those with SMI affect their ability to access medical care and navigate the complex health system. Adherence is a major problem in the treatment of people with SMI, and adherence to medical regimes for this population is compounded by mental health and addictive problems, homelessness, or lack of transportation to get to medical providers. Lack of financial resources may complicate the patient's ability to receive timely care or treatment. Finally, stigma affects communication about all aspects of care of the medical illness, including assessment, explanation of treatment options, adherence, and the development of a trusting relationship with the patient.[5]

## Serious Mental Illness

Psychotic symptoms may occur as a result of certain medical conditions, substance abuse, schizophrenia, schizoaffective disorder, mania, dementia, and depression. SMI includes illnesses such as schizophrenia and other psychotic disorders,

bipolar disease, and severe depression. A brief discussion of each of these illnesses will be presented; however, depression is described in detail in another chapter of the book. Treatment issues and special concerns in communication will be discussed as they relate to palliative care.

## Schizophrenia

Schizophrenia affects approximately 1% of U.S. population. However, it accounts for 40% of mental health facility beds and 9% of all hospital beds. It is a devastating illness to those who are affected by the illness—either the patient or the family of the patient. Several types of schizophrenia exist, including paranoid, catatonic, and undifferentiated schizophrenia. The symptoms of schizophrenia include what are referred to as positive symptoms (exaggerated or distorted function) and negative symptoms (diminution or loss of normal function). The positive symptoms include delusions, hallucinations, and disorganized and bizarre behavior and speech as well as deterioration of social behavior. The negative symptoms include flattened affect, decreased range and intensity of expression, anhedonia, restricted thought and speech, amotivation, apathy, and difficulty in mental focus and ability to sustain attention.[6,7] Other psychotic disorders, including schizoaffective disorder, delusional disorder, brief psychotic disorder, and shared psychotic disorder (folie au deux), share many of the same psychotic symptoms with schizophrenia.[6,7]

Some of the more limiting symptoms of psychotic disorders that are of particular concern in palliative care settings are the ability to participate in decision-making, perceptual difficulties that can affect sensory integration, concrete thought processes, and difficulty in attention and concentration. The effect of perceptual difficulties has been demonstrated in research related to pain sensation in people with schizophrenia. Patients with schizophrenia may have reduced sensitivity to pain, and this could lead to delays in care or treatment.[10]

## Treatment of Psychotic Disorders

Treatment is based on symptom management. Psychopharmacological and nonpsychopharmacological interventions are both utilized to treat psychotic disorders; however, nonpsychological interventions may not be effective unless interfering hallucinations or delusions are brought under some degree of control.

### Pharmacological Treatment

Table 40–1 lists first-generation or typical antipsychotics. These medications, developed in the 1950s and 1960s were very effective in the treatment of the positive symptoms, and some—but not all—of these medications had effect on negative symptoms. The negative side effect profiles of these medications, including extrapyramidal symptoms (EPS), tardive

**Table 40–1**
**Antipsychotic Medications**

| First Generation (Typicals) | Second Generation (Atypicals) |
|---|---|
| Chlorpromazine (Thorazine) | Clozapine (Clozaril) |
| Thioridizine (Mellaril) | Risperidone (Risperidol) |
| Perphenazine (Trilafon) | Olanzapine (Zyprexa) |
| Trifluoperazine (Stelazine) | Quetiapine (Seroquel) |
| Fluphenazine (Prolixin) | Ziprasidone (Geodon) |
| Thiothixene (Navane) | Aripiprazole (Abilify) |
| Haloperidon (Haldol) | |
| Loxapine (Loxitane) | |
| Molindone (Moban) | |
| Pimozide (Orap) | |

*Source*: Adapted from Bezchlibnyk-Butler, et al., reference 24; Moller, reference 7.

dyskinesia (TD), and anticholinergic effects, had a profound effect on quality of life and medication adherence.[11]

In the 1980s the second-generation or atypical antipsychotics were developed (Table 40–1). These medications reduced both the positive and negative symptoms associated with schizophrenia, improved cognition, and were useful in treatment for patients who were considered treatment-refractory. The side effect profile of the second-generation drugs showed lower rates of EPS and TD and fewer anticholinergic effects. However, the emergence of metabolic syndrome, including pronounced weight gain, diabetes, hyperlipidemia, and hypercholesterolemia, has resulted in the need for close monitoring of their use in treating psychotic disorders.[11] These medications result in cardiovascular problems and compound the existing higher prevalence of cardiovascular problems in people with schizophrenia.

Pharmacological treatment of psychotic symptoms in conjunction with palliative care treatment should be closely monitored by consultation with the psychiatric providers. Any change in mental status should be immediately evaluated. Screening for the presence of delirium, which can occur frequently at end of life should occur with any change in mental status. It should not be assumed that the psychiatric illness is the cause of a mental status change until a physical cause is ruled out. Several of the typical and atypical antipsychotic medications share common metabolic pathways with opioid analgesics. Inhibition or potentiation of the antipsychotic or the opioid medication is possible; therefore, close monitoring is essential.[11]

### Right to Refuse Medication

In the 1970s psychiatric patients filed lawsuits related to their rights to refuse medication treatment. Legal decisions in Massachusetts and New York, the states where the most prominent cases were filed, resulted in different approaches to the problem. The Massachusetts decision resulted in the *Rogers decision*, which decreed that a guardian needed to be appointed for incompetent patients to deal strictly with the psychiatric medication in question and that the final decision would be left to a judge. The concept of substituted judgment—that is, what the person would consent to if they were competent—is how the judge evaluated the question of whether to give the guardian the right to overrule the patient's right to refuse medication.[12] Other states have panels, independent consultants, or psychiatrists make the decision about right to refuse medication. It is important to know the state law about the right to refuse medication so that each nurse can practice within the rules and regulations under which he/she is governed.

### Nonpharmacological Treatments

Nonpharmacological interventions include psychotherapeutic strategies such as supportive psychotherapy, cognitive-behavioral therapy (CBT), group therapy, and complementary therapies. Collaborative care with psychiatric providers can include additional supportive therapy to assist patients facing a terminal illness. People with SMI face the same end-of-life concerns as patients without mental illness, such as dealing with pain and suffering, fear of what lies ahead, fear of becoming a burden, spiritual concerns, financial concerns, and difficulty "saying goodbye."[13] People with schizophrenia may need additional support and extra time to process medical information. This extra support is best provided by professionals who already have a relationship with the patient, and the psychiatric providers should be included in discussions of treatment options in the palliative care setting.

### Advanced Directives

Advanced directives, in terms of decisions about psychiatric care in a future emergency situation, have been a focus of concern over the last decade. Providing a patient with the opportunity to discuss their wishes, in advance, has assisted with the need to have a legal competency hearing to determine a course of treatment. Including a discussion of the patient's wishes for end-of-life care is an area that needs further exploration in psychiatric settings. Research has indicated a low rate of advanced directives for either psychiatric care or medical care in patients with SMI.[14]

### Capacity and Competency

The ability to make decisions about treatment is a cornerstone of good palliative care. Controversy can occur when a person loses the capacity to participate in informed decision-making, or a competent person refuses life-sustaining treatments.

A general rule is that all competent persons have the right to make their own decisions, even when decisions conflict with what a majority would decide under similar circumstances.[15] When the patient is a person who has schizophrenia or another psychiatric disorder, the ability to make decisions may be compromised by psychotic thought processes. However, having a diagnosis of a mental illness, even one with psychotic features, does not automatically mean that a person is incompetent.[15] When treatment decisions of the patient are questioned by providers and there is no advanced directive about treatment wishes, then a psychiatric evaluation must be requested.

Capacity indicates the ability to understand the problem and make decisions. A psychiatric provider makes a "clinical assessment of the patient's capacity to function in certain areas."[16] Competency is a legal term and is decided by a court of law based on the capacity assessment of a psychiatric provider. Competency is usually confined to a specific area or task, such as the ability to make a will, the ability to testify in court, decision-making capacity, or the right to refuse treatment.[15] Applebaum & Grisso outlined four criteria used to determine capacity to consent to treatment[17]:

- Patient expression of a preference
- Ability to understand the illness, the prognosis with and without treatment, and the risks and benefits of the treatment (factual understanding)
- An appreciation of the significance of the facts (significance of the facts)
- Ability to use the information in a rational way to reach a decision in a logical manner (rationality of the thought processes).

Intense pain, depression, delirium, dementia, and psychosis are the most common causes of incompetence.[15] However, the existence of one of these conditions does not necessarily mean that a person is incompetent. Careful assessment of each individual is necessary to determine capacity and competency. Competency is a legal term, but most courts do accept the evaluation of capacity provided by the psychiatric professional. A patient is not deemed competent or incompetent until a court of law rules.

## Aggression and Psychotic Disorders

Patients enter health-care systems in great distress, and palliative care settings are no exception. When the patient has a SMI the distress may be even greater than in the general population, because people with SMI may have inadequate coping resources and are in a crisis state when dealing with a life-threatening illness. Most often, people become aggressive when they feel threatened in some way. The aggressive behavior may be the result of perceptual problems, such as hallucinations or delusions, and the aggressive behavior often masks a lack of confidence in self. Aggressive behavior may be a way to enhance self-esteem by overpowering others.[18]

There are some important predictors of aggressive behavior, including impulsivity, hostility, family history of violent or abusive behavior, substance use, and irritability.[19] Prevention of aggressive behavior focuses on early recognition of escalating behaviors, such as pacing, nonverbal expressions, yelling, or an angry tone of voice. Allowing the person a chance to talk may defuse the situation. It is important for the nurse to use nonthreatening body language, and to communicate with a calm but firm voice while conveying respect for the patient and his/her feelings. Allowing the patient some choice about the situation is often a way to help the patient gain some control.[19]

## Communication Issues and Psychotic Disorders

The cornerstone of both palliative care and psychiatric care is the importance of communication and the establishment of a trusting, therapeutic relationship between the nurse and the patient. Traditionally, psychiatric providers are not comfortable with medically ill patients and medical providers are not comfortable with psychiatrically ill patients. Additionally, many people with mental illness are housed in nontraditional settings. Staff of any of these settings, including medical hospital units, palliative care units, or psychiatric units as well as the homeless shelters, prisons, and nursing homes may be ill-equipped to deal with psychiatric problems in the face of terminal illness. Education of all staff about mental illness and end-of-life care in these settings will result in better care for patients with SMI.[5]

There are additional communication issues and strategies involved when providing palliative care to those with psychotic illnesses. The role of stigma affects all aspects of care and communication. Patients may conceal or not report pain and other symptoms because of fear of the meaning of the symptom, self-blame, guilt, anger, or denial. As mentioned previously, mental status changes should be evaluated for a medical cause of delirium before assuming that altered perceptions or hallucinations are the result of psychotic disorder.

If the patient is delusional or hallucinating, then a safety assessment should be completed and arrangements made to keep the patient safe from self-harm. The content of the hallucinations or delusions can be very important. Any thoughts or hallucinations that the patient expresses concerning the need to die or presence of command hallucinations telling the person to die require immediate psychiatric consultation. Patient safety mechanisms, such as evaluation by emergency services (for outpatient settings) or use of sitters or frequent observation (for inpatient settings) should be instituted until the psychiatric assessment can occur.

Maintaining a calm presence and use of a quiet tone of voice, nonthreatening demeanor, and stance are important strategies when dealing with all patients who are psychotic. Decrease of environmental stimuli, such as turning off a radio or television, will decrease distractions and help the patient focus on the immediate medical care. Because the ability to concentrate or pay attention may be affected by the mental illness, detailed explanations may be needed, with additional time allowed for the patient to process the information. Conversations focused on understanding what the patient has processed about the information may need to take place over lengthened periods of time. Patients may also tend to focus on concrete parts of the information, and it can be helpful to provide alternative ways to view the situation if a patient appears to be stuck or focused on one particular aspect of the issue. Occasionally, people with psychotic disorders may become more focused and less psychotic in the face of a life-threatening illness.

Patients with SMI who are actively hallucinating or delusional, as well as those who may be delirious and experiencing altered perceptions, should receive explanations of all physical care to be delivered. Before touching the patient, it is important to let he/she knows what is to be done, as the patient might misinterpret the touch and react as if he/she is being assaulted. Patients with SMI may have a different sense of private space and may also react to violations of personal space.

## Redefinition of Family

For many people with SMI there are strained, distant, or nonexistent ties with family of origin. Some of this disconnection may result from years of strain, disappointment, financial burden, and fear caused by threatening behavior. For many people with SMI who are cared for by the state government, long-term relationships with psychiatric providers or staff of mental health housing programs have become a substitute for family. The inclusion of these staff into the palliative care team is essential to ensuring that the treatment will be properly performed and for providing the day-to-day intensive support that may be required for the patient. Similarly to family, staff will also have their own particular needs for support because most psychiatric providers do not have end-of-life care experience or education. Fellow patients with SMI are the other component of family that needs to be considered in palliative care of people with SMI. Occasionally, long-term relationships with other people with SMI are the most significant relationships in the person's life. Special needs for support should be considered for this group of people as well. Although palliative care staff may not be involved in delivering this support, the collaborative partnerships with psychiatric providers should be available for support for this group of people.

CASE STUDY
*A 54-Year-Old Woman with Schizophrenia*

Joan is a 54-year-old white woman who was diagnosed with schizophrenia at age 24 years. She has had multiple hospitalizations and is currently living in a group home. She sees a psychiatrist every 2 months and has visits at the group home by a psychiatric nurse who administers her Prolixin deconoate injection every month. Her caseworker at the group home reports to the nurse and psychiatrist that she is very concerned about the patient's physical health. It has been 3 years since Joan has seen a medical provider (she has refused to go to appointments that have been set up for her), and Joan has become fatigued and has lost 23 pounds in the last 9 to 10 months.

After much discussion between providers and the patient, arrangements are made for the caseworker to go with Joan to her medical appointment. The physician who examines Joan notes a large mass on her left breast and after completing diagnostic tests has confirmed a diagnosis of stage 4 breast cancer. Joan is reluctant to discuss the treatment options provided for her, and the psychiatric team is attempting to involve her family in care planning. Joan is estranged from her closest relative, an older sister who lives a half-hour from Joan's group home. Joan does not seem to be reacting to the diagnosis and cuts short attempts to discuss her care and the need for treatment. Her caseworker is successful in contacting the sister, who agrees to visit Joan and discuss treatment options.

At the first visit Joan is very pleased to see her sister. The caseworker meets with the two of them and discusses the cancer diagnosis and the treatment options. Joan's response to her sister is, "I don't want to be like Momma was…" The sister tells the caseworker that their mother had breast cancer and was treated with chemotherapy when she and Joan were ages 10 years and 12 years, respectively. Their mother was very sick with the treatment and unable to really participate in their lives and died during chemotherapy. She says that she believes that Joan would not want to go through that, given her poor prognosis. This is new information for the members of the psychiatric team, who had been encouraging Joan to participate in the treatment. The caseworker is especially opposed to stopping the effort to get Joan to accept treatment and feels that she is not getting the best advice from her sister. The sister is in support of comfort and compassionate care only for Joan and is happy that they have been able to reconnect before Joan dies.

This case illustrates several issues of importance:

- The importance of family and history
- The need for regular medical care of patients with SMI
- Need for expansion of definition of family—often residential treatment staff are the ones with daily contact and may best know the patient's wishes regarding care; they may also have their own grieving and bereavement process that should be accounted for

## Bipolar Disease

People with bipolar disorder have more co-occurring medical conditions—especially cardiovascular disease and other problems related to metabolic syndrome—than those with other chronic mental illnesses.[20] As with psychotic disorders like schizophrenia, the use of second-generation antipsychotic medications as mood stabilizers for those with bipolar disease has increased the risk of diabetes and subsequent cardiovascular disease among people with this diagnosis.[20]

Bipolar disease is included under the diagnostic category of mood disorders and includes major depressive disorder as well as bipolar disease, which is described as Bipolar I or Bipolar II.[6] Depression is discussed in detail in Chapter 20. Bipolar I is described with periods of depression and some periods of an elevated mood, either hypomania or mania. Symptoms of hypomania or mania include an inflated self-esteem, grandiosity, decreased need for sleep, pressured speech, flight of ideas, increase in activities, and excessive involvement in pleasurable activities that have a high potential for consequences.[6] Severe mania can present more with symptoms of agitation than euphoria and often includes psychotic episodes as well. Bipolar II is characterized by at least one depressive episode and at least one hypomanic episode but with a history of full mania.[6]

Treatment of bipolar disorder includes mood-stabilizing medications such as lithium and other drugs (Table 40–2). When patients are in a manic state or a severe depression, they may lack decision-making capacity but are then capable of making decisions when they become stable. A psychiatric provider should be a part of the palliative care team and

provide close follow-up for people with bipolar disorder. Any medications used in treatment of the underlying medical illness should be reviewed for their potential to induce a manic episode.[13] As with psychotic disorders, there are many psychotherapeutic interventions that are utilized in treatment of people with bipolar disorder, but patients frequently need to be stabilized with medications before these treatments are able to be utilized effectively.

## Communication Issues and Bipolar Disorder

Communicating with someone during a manic episode can be difficult because patients may be emotionally labile, very talkative (with pressured speech), may not be able to stop and listen or concentrate, and often reject help.[21] Patients can be quite charming and even entertaining during some stages of a manic episode. Staff members need to see these presentations as a part of the illness and not join in grandiose discussions or plans. Patients may need to be gently redirected so that they do not go off on tangents unrelated to the medical issue at hand. They may also need firm but caring limits set on behaviors that might affect others' care, such as wandering into other patients' rooms, becoming inappropriately involved in others' care, and intrusion in staff conversations with other patients. Assisting patients in calming behaviors such as sitting quietly with the patient or closing the door to the room to decrease external stimuli are strategies that may be helpful. Inclusion of the psychiatric provider in the team will allow for communication of information about the best approach to take with an individual suffering from [with] bipolar disorder.

Often, one of the first symptoms of a manic episode is the decreased need for sleep. Early reporting of change of sleep habits is important because it is easier to help someone regain stability early in the course of a manic episode. If the patient is beginning to exhibit signs of mania and/or psychosis, then assessment of safety issues and the potential for suicide must be considered. The importance of early intervention in escalating symptoms and good interteam communication cannot be emphasized enough when caring for someone with bipolar disorder.

CASE STUDY

*A 45-Year-Old Man Suffering from Bipolar Disease*

Jim is a 45-year-old white male suffering from bipolar disease. He has had a very difficult course of his disease, with multiple hospitalizations following suicide attempts. Additionally, he has HIV and Hepatitis C. His HIV is in good control, and he has been fairly consistent in taking his HIV medications for the last 9 months. For the last 2 years, he has been followed for supportive therapy by a Psychiatric Clinical Nurse Specialist.

His older brother is the only family member who has remained involved in his life and has had to act as his guardian for a number of years because of Jim's psychosis

---

**Table 40–2**
**Mood Stabilizers**

**Antimania medications**
- Lithium (Eskalith, Lithobid)
- Lithium citrate

**Benzodiazepines**
- Alprazalam (Xanax)
- Chlordiazepoxide (Librium)
- Clonazepam (Klonopin)
- Diazepam (Valium)
- Lorazepam (Ativan)
- Oxazepma (Serax)
- Prazepam (Centrax)

**Anticonvulsants**
- Valproic Acid (Depakene, Depakote)
- Lamotrigine (Lamictal)
- Carbamazepine (Tegretol)
- Gabapentin (Neurontin)
- Oxcarbazepine (Trileptal)
- Topiramate (Topamax)
- Tiagabine (Gabatril)

**Calcium channel blockers**
- Verapamil (Calan)
- Nifedipine (Adalat, Procardia)
- Nimodipine (Nimotop)

*Source*: Adapted from Bezchlibnyk-Butler, et al., reference 24.

during manic episodes as well as his severe depression. The brother was told years ago that Jim is likely to succeed in killing himself at some point because of the severity of his bipolar disease.

Jim was diagnosed with pancreatic cancer 4 months ago and has been given less than a year to live. The physician discusses his care with Jim and his brother and has primarily followed the brother's wishes for Jim's care. Shortly after this diagnosis, Jim stops taking all of his medications and is rehospitalized with severe depression and suicidal thoughts. He has recompensated and returned to his mental health halfway house. He now wants to live and is very meticulous in adhering to his medication regimen. Hospice and palliative care services were started about 1 month ago. The Psychiatric Clinical Nurse Specialist and hospice nurse convene a team meeting to coordinate care among providers.

His brother has been unable to accept the diagnosis and continues to want very aggressive treatment for Jim, whereas Jim's psychiatric caseworker believes that Jim is starting to focus on comfort care. His brother talks freely about how psychiatric staff expected him to die years ago from his bipolar disease and how he never gave up hope for a better life for his brother. The coordinated care team has set up a meeting with Jim and his brother to discuss continuing care.

This case highlights several factors that are important in the palliative care of patients with mental illness:

- Some patients with suicidal histories may put suicidal tendencies aside in the face of a terminal illness and fight to live, in a different way than their history would indicate, as long as their quality of life is satisfactory.
- Chronic severe mental illness may have depleted family coping resources.
- Family may be in a crisis as a result of unexpected medical illness in addition to mental illness.
- The fact that the brother has had to make decisions for psychiatric care in the past does not preclude the patient's right to make decisions about end-of-life care.
- If the patient is not currently suicidal or psychotic, then his right to make decisions about ending aggressive treatment should be discussed with both the patient and his brother at length to help determine the best course of action.

## Personality Disorders and Palliative Care

People with PDs can present major challenges for palliative care providers, partly because of the stigma associated with PDs. Personality traits are enduring patterns of perceiving, relating to, and thinking about the world and how one relates to the world.[6] The enduring patterns of response and behavior deviate from social norms and present in the areas of:

- Cognition (ways of perceiving self, others, events)
- Affectivity (range, intensity, lability, appropriateness)
- Interpersonal functioning
- Impulse control

There is a lack of flexibility and maladaptive behavior that can cause impairment in function and distress for the person.[6]

All humans have vulnerabilities that are accentuated when the person is under stress. Approaching personality traits as vulnerabilities that are accentuated by stress, and therefore result in the use of predictable coping mechanisms, can be a useful way to change stigmatized attitudes toward people with PDs. It is important to identify traits or vulnerabilities and move beyond labels so that treatment can be geared to preparing for the expected response, minimizing maladaptive coping mechanisms and replacing them with more functional coping mechanisms.

PDs are grouped into three clusters based on some descriptive similarities. Cluster A PDs include paranoid, schizoid, and schizotypal.

PDs and people with these disorders often appear odd, eccentric, or paranoid. People with paranoid PD have a pervasive distrust and suspiciousness of others. The person will be reluctant to trust or confide in anyone and may suspect that others are trying to cause him/her harm.[6] The person with schizoid PD has a pervasive pattern of detachment from relationships, even with family. This person prefers solitary activities, lacks close relationships, and may be emotionally detached or have a flat affect. People with schizotypal PD are uncomfortable with close relationships and have cognitive distortions, including ideas of reference, odd beliefs or magical thinking, unusual perceptions, odd thinking and speech, inappropriate affect, and social anxiety.[6]

Cluster B PDs include antisocial PD, borderline (BPD), histrionic PD, and narcissistic PD. People with this group of PDs often appear dramatic, emotional or erratic, and it is this cluster that often presents the biggest challenge to health care providers.[6] The person with antisocial PD has a pervasive disregard for, and violation of, the rights of others. They fail to conform to most social norms and can be impulsive, irritable, and aggressive at times. People with BPD have a lifelong pattern of instability of interpersonal relationships and self-image and either idealize or devalue others, or fluctuate between the two views of the same person. People with BPD are impulsive in ways that are damaging to themselves and frequently have recurrent suicidal behavior. They have a chronic feeling of emptiness and therefore constantly seek attention and contact with others to fill themselves.[6]

People with histrionic PD have a pattern of excessive emotionality and attention-seeking and can be inappropriately provocative or sexually seductive. People with these traits are easily influenced by others and often consider relationships to be more intimate than they actually are.

People with narcissistic PD need admiration, lack empathy for others, and have a sense of entitlement.[6]

Cluster C PDs include avoidant PD, dependent PD, and obsessive-compulsive PD. These disorders share anxiety and fear as their major characteristics.[6] The person with avoidant PD is hypersensitive to negative evaluation, has feelings of inadequacy and is severely restrained in relationships. This person is reluctant to take personal risks or engage in new activities.[6] Someone with dependent PD has an excessive need to be taken care of that exhibits itself by submissive and clinging behavior and fear of separation. People with this PD have difficulty making decisions and need a lot of advice and reassurance from others. They have difficulty expressing disagreement with others because of fear of loss of support.

Finally, obsessive-compulsive PD is evidenced by a preoccupation with orderliness, perfectionism, and control. The person with obsessive-compulsive PD shows perfectionism that interferes with completion of tasks, is inflexible and overly conscientious, may be unable to throw out useless objects, and is miserly toward spending for self and others. This person may be quite rigid and stubborn in thought and behavior.[6]

## Treatment of Personality Disorders

By description, PDs are enduring patterns and, therefore, are not likely to change rapidly. Current evidence does suggest that people with PDs can be treated, but realistic goals must be established for treatment. Symptom management and specific therapies such as CBT and dialectical behavioral therapy (DBT) have demonstrated effectiveness with specific PDs.[22] The relationship with a psychiatric provider is a primary tool in the treatment of people with PDs. Comorbid psychiatric conditions are common with PD, so symptom management of anxiety, depression, and other psychiatric symptoms is important to improve quality of life.

## Communication Issues and Personality Disorders

Some general principles related to communication with patients with PD can be identified. Clear information provided verbally and in writing with repeated discussions about the information can help with distortions and misinterpretation that are common in people with PDs. A calm and nonjudgmental approach is also the cornerstone of good communication in the process of developing a therapeutic relationship with patients. All discussion of suicidal ideation should be taken very seriously and a thorough psychiatric assessment should be performed, even when repeated threats of suicide occur. The therapeutic alliance may take a long time to develop, but nonetheless the development of this alliance is a goal for treatment. CBT techniques are helpful for people with PD to examine maladaptive ways of viewing their environment. Supportive therapy is useful in helping people with PD adjust to the issues that arise in palliative and end-of-life care.

Obstacles to therapeutic communication that occur with people suffering from [with] PD include issues such as resistance, transference, countertransference, and boundary violations.[23] Resistance is often unconscious and is usually employed to avoid anxiety. Transference also occurs when a patient unconsciously transfers feelings or attitudes from one person in their life onto the health-care provider.[23] Countertransference is the emotional reaction of the health-care provider toward the patient, stimulated by their own past feelings toward someone in their personal life. Boundary violations occur when the health-care provider goes beyond the standards of a therapeutic relationship and enters a more social relationship with a patient.

Communication issues with patients suffering from Cluster A disorders focus on the establishment of a therapeutic relationship, because distrust, suspiciousness, and withdrawal from interpersonal interactions are common. Engaging a nonthreatening approach and allowing the patient to engage with the provider at his/her own speed is very important. The intensity of a one-to-one conversation may be difficult for those with Cluster A PD; therefore, focusing conversation on an external issue or task may be a helpful way to lessen the intensity.

Communication with people with Cluster B disorders are often the most problematic for health-care providers. People with these disorders tend to have an increased risk of suicide, violence toward others, and self-mutilating behaviors as well as chronic low self-esteem, ineffective coping, and impaired social interactions.[22] Volatile changes in emotion as well as splitting behaviors are characteristic of BPD. Development of a consistent approach will minimize the patient's ability to split staff and minimize the heightened feelings that can arise in caring for this population.

Providers should be alert for their own countertransference reactions toward patients with PD, as this is a common issue. Patients with PD can evoke strong reactions from staff that may interfere with delivery of quality care. Staff support in working through these reactions so that care is not affected can be provided through consultative relationships with psychiatric providers. Many Psychiatric Clinical Nurse Specialists have experience with staff support groups to handle such issues.

Communication issues with people suffering from Cluster C diagnoses also focus on the development of a therapeutic relationship geared toward assisting patients in identifying their fears and anxiety as it relates to palliative care treatment and issues.[23] Helping people identify their anxiety, decrease the maladaptive response to the anxiety, and increase their supportive relationships with others are essential issues in dealing with people with in this cluster.

CASE STUDY
### A 39-Year-Old Woman with Colon Cancer

Eileen is a 39-year-old woman suffering from colon cancer. She has been hospitalized twice in the last 6 months and is now readmitted to the oncology unit. The staff is not pleased to hear about her readmission because she was a management problem on her last admission. She was frequently upset with the night shift nurses and called the patient advocate several times a week to complain about them. She also left the unit frequently and was not available at treatment times. She complained bitterly about one nurse and demanded someone else care for her when that nurse was assigned her care. This nurse is very upset and asks the nurse manager to assign Eileen's care to another nurse. The nurse manager calls the psychiatric consultation nurse and asks for help in developing a plan of care for the patient and requests a meeting with the nursing staff to discuss the plan and their feelings about the Eileen as a patient.

## Summary

Palliative care providers often feel poorly prepared to deal with people with SMI and/or PD. Conversely, psychiatric providers feel poorly prepared to deal with medical care and end-of-life care. Collaborative partnerships can enhance the care given to people with SMI who are in need of palliative care services. Care delivery sites need to be examined for the optimal situation to provide both palliative care and treatment in an environment that also is able to provide optimal support and treatment by psychiatric providers. If the patient has a preference for a place to receive end-of-life care, all attempts possible can be made to address this preference. If the person considers a halfway house or psychiatric unit to be their home, and they desire to die at home, attempts to provide end-of-life care in that setting should be discussed just as it would be with a person wanting to die in their more traditional home.

Nurses have often been instrumental in making this kind of care possible in a situation that has not previously involved this level of care. As strong advocates for their patients, nurses have found a way to push themselves into new arenas of care and have developed new collaborative partnerships for the ultimate benefit of their patients. Collaboration between psychiatric providers and palliative care providers is a new area in which nurses can lead the way to ultimately provide new skills for each other and meaningful end-of-life experiences for people with SMI as well as their families.

REFERENCES

1. http://www.nimh.nih.gov/health/topics/statistics/index.shml (accessed November 20, 2008).
2. Lopez AD, Mathers CD, Ezzati M, Jamison DT, Murray CJL. Global Burden of Disease and Risk Factors. New York, NY: The Oxford University Press, 2006.
3. Parks J, Svendsen D, Singer P, Foti M. 2006. Morbidity and mortality in people with serious mental illness. National Association of State Mental Health Program Directors (NASMHPD) Medical Directors Council. Alexandria, VA. 22314. http://www. nasmphd.org/generalFiles/publications/med_directors.pub (accessed on November 20, 2008).
4. Hiroeh U, Appleby L, Mortensen PB, Dunn G. Death by homicide, suicide and other unnatural causes in people with mental illness: A population-based study. Lancet 2001;358(9299): 2110–2112.
5. Baker, A. Palliative and end-of-life care in the serious and persistently mentally ill population. J Am Psych Nurses Assoc 2005;11(5):298–303.
6. American Psychiatric Association (APA). Diagnostic and Statistical Manual of Mental Disorders (4th ed, text rev) (DSM-IV-TR). Washington DC: APA, 2000.
7. Moller MD. Neurobiological responses and schizophrenia and psychotic disorders. In: Stuart GW, Laraia MT, eds. Principles and Practice of Psychiatric Nursing (8th ed). St. Louis, MO: Mosby, 2005.
8. Foti ME. "Do it your way": A demonstration project on end-of-life care for persons with serious mental illness. J Palliat Med 2003;6(4):661–669.
9. Foti ME, Bartels SJ, Van Citters AD, Merriman MP, Fletcher KE. End-of-Life treatment preferences of persons with serious mental illness. Psychiatr Serv 2005;56(5):585–591.
10. Kudoh A, Ishihara H, Matsuki A. Current perception thresholds and postoperative pain in schizophrenic patients. Reg Anesth Pain Med 2000;25(5):475–479.
11. Chan P. Psychopharmacology. In: Fortinash KM, Holoday Worret PA. Psychiatric Mental Health Nursing (4th ed). St. Louis, MO: Mosby, 2008.
12. Laben JK, Yorker BC. Legal issues in advanced practice psychiatric nursing. In: Burgess AW. Advanced Practice Psychiatric Nursing. Stamford, CT: Appleton & Lange, 1998.
13. Miovic M, Block S. Psychiatric disorders in advanced cancer. Cancer 2007;110(8):1665–1676.
14. Srebnick DS, La Fond JQ. Advance directives for mental health treatment. Psychiatr Serv 1999;50(7):919–925.
15. Schouten R, Brendel RW. Legal aspects of consultation. In: Stern TA, Fricchione GL, Cassem HNH, Jellinek MS, Rosenbaum JF, eds. Massachusetts General Hospital Handbook of General Hospital Psychiatry (5th ed). Philadelphia, PA: Mosby: 2004.
16. Schouten R, Brendel RW. Legal aspects of consultation. In: Stern TA, Fricchione GL, Cassem HNH, Jellinek MS, Rosenbaum JF, eds. Massachusetts General Hospital Handbook of General Hospital Psychiatry (5th ed). Philadelphia, PA: Mosby: 2004:356.
17. Applebaum PS, Grisso T. Assessing patient's capacities to consent to treatment. N Engl J Med. 1988;319:1635–1638.
18. Hamolia CD. Preventing and managing aggressive behavior. In: Stuart GW, Laraia MT. Principles and Practice of Psychiatric Nursing (8th ed). St. Louis, MO: Mosby, 2005.
19. American Psychiatric Nursing Association (APNA). Coping with aggressive behavior in patients with schizophrenia: A roundtable discussion. Counseling Points: Enhancing Patient Communication for the Psychiatric Nurse. September 2006. Ridgewood, New Jersey: Delaware Media Group.
20. Kilbourne AM, Post EP, Nossek A, Drill L, Cooley S, Bauer MS. Improving medical and psychiatric outcomes among individuals with Bipolar disorder: A randomized controlled trial. Psych Serv 2008;59(7):760–768.

21. McCasland LA. Providing hospice and palliative care to the seriously and persistently mentally ill. J Hosp Palliat Nurs 2007;9(6):305–313.

22. Marcus PE. Personality disorders. In: Fortinash KM, Holoday Worret PA. Psychiatric Mental Health Nursing (4th ed). St. Louis, MO: Mosby, 2008.

23. McDonald SF. Therapeutic communication. In: Fortinash KM, Holoday Worret PA. Psychiatric Mental Health Nursing (4th ed). St. Louis, MO: Mosby, 2008.

24. Bzchlibnyk-Butler KZ, Jeffries JJ. Clinical Handbook of Psychotropic Drugs (16th ed). Toronto, Canada: Hofgrefe & Huber Publishers, 2006.

# 41

*Deborah Witt Sherman and Carl A. Kirton*

# Patients with Acquired Immunodeficiency Syndrome

*I thank God that there are medications to treat AIDS, but there are serious side effects and they can make you feel quite sick. Yet, I want to live, and I will do everything possible to stay alive. Some people say AIDS is now a chronic disease. There are other medications to treat my symptoms, and there is my belief in God that lifts my spirit. My family helps me care for my kids, but it is hard on everyone. We all need support because we are all suffering one way or another.*
—Anonymous patient

◆ ***Key Points***
◆ *With HIV/AIDS, the severity, complexity, and unpredictability of the illness trajectory have blurred the distinction between curative and palliative care.*
◆ *The focus of AIDS care must be on improving quality of life by providing care for the management of pain and other symptoms, while addressing the emotional, social, and spiritual needs of patients and their families throughout the illness trajectory.*
◆ *With up-to-date knowledge regarding HIV disease, including changes in epidemiology, diagnostic testing, treatment options, and available resources, nurses can offer effective and compassionate care to patients and families at all stages of HIV disease.*

In 28 years, AIDS has escalated from a series of outbreaks in scattered communities in the United States and Europe to a global health crisis. Although the biomedical paradigm of highly active antiretroviral therapy (HAART) has significantly reduced the mortality from HIV in the developed world and has transformed AIDS into a manageable chronic illness, the reality in developing countries is that people are not "living with AIDS" but, rather, "dying from AIDS" because of a lack of access to medications and appropriate healthcare.[1] In the late stages of HIV, there is a false dichotomy created between disease-specific, curative therapies and symptom-specific palliative therapies.[2] Although little attention has been given in the past to palliative care as a component of AIDS care, it is now realized that the palliation of pain, symptoms, and suffering must occur throughout the course of a life-threatening disease, not just in the final stages near the end of life. AIDS has stimulated the need to evaluate clinical practice when curative and palliative care interface. No longer should there be an abrupt demarcation between palliative care and treating disease in individuals with life-threatening, progressive illnesses.[3] Both the public and health professionals have been troubled by the reality of over- and undertreatment of pain and symptoms in individuals with life-threatening illnesses who may suffer severe, unremitting pain in their final days.[4] Such concern extends to the care of patients with HIV and the resultant illness of AIDS because no cure has yet been found. Therefore, the focus of care must be on improving quality of life by providing palliative care for the management of pain and other physical symptoms while addressing the emotional, social, and spiritual needs of patients and their families throughout the illness trajectory. Although current therapies have increased the life expectancy of people with HIV/AIDS, the chance of experiencing symptoms related not only to the disease but to the effects of therapies also increases. Furthermore, palliative measures can be beneficial in ensuring tolerance of and adherence to difficult pharmacological regimens.[5]

Because patients are surviving longer in the latter stages of illness, an integrated model must be developed to provide comprehensive care for patients with advanced AIDS and their families.[2] This chapter provides an overview and update of the comprehensive care related to HIV/AIDS and addresses the palliative care needs of individuals and families living with and dying from this illness. With this information, nurses and other health-care professionals will gain the knowledge to provide effective and compassionate care, recognizing the need for both curative and aggressive care as well as supportive and palliative therapies to maximize the quality of life of patients and their family caregivers.

## Overview and Update: Incidence, Historical Background, Epidemiology, and Pathogenesis

### Incidence of HIV/AIDS

HIV/AIDS is a worldwide epidemic affecting more than 33 million people. An estimated 2.5 million acquired HIV in 2007, and an estimated 2.1 million people died from AIDS.[6] In 2008 the Centers for Disease Control and Prevention (CDC) reported that from the beginning of the epidemic through December 2006, there were more than 1,014,797 reported cases of AIDS in the United States. Of these cases, 783,786 cases were males, 189,566 were females, and an estimated 9,144 cases were children under age 13 years.[7] In the United States, the estimated number of deaths of persons with AIDS is 565,927, including 540,436 adults and adolescents, and 5,369 children under age 15 years.[7] Although HIV is no longer a leading cause of death in the United States, in populations and nations without access to antiretorviral therapy and treatments for opportunistic infections, AIDS remains a life-threatening and progressive illness that marks the final stage of a chronic viral illness.

### Historical Background of HIV/AIDS

In the early 1980s, cases were reported of previously healthy homosexual men who were diagnosed with *Pneumocystis carinii* (now known as *Pneumocystis jiroveci*) pneumonia and an extremely rare tumor known as Kaposi's sarcoma (KS). The number of cases doubled every 6 months, with further occurrence of unusual fungal, viral, and parasitic infections, and researchers realized that the immune systems of these individuals were being compromised. Over time, reports began to emerge of the appearance of similar unsual infections and immune system destruction beyond the homosexual community. This new disease was also seen among heterosexual partners, IV substance users, persons with hemophilia, individuals receiving infected blood products, and children born to women with the disease. These epidemiological changes alerted health professionals to the existence of an infectious agent transmitted via infected body fluids, particularly through sexual transmission and blood products.[8]

Origins of HIV can be traced through serum studies to 1959, when crossover mechanisms between humans and primates via animal bites or scratches in Africa led to HIV transmission. In 1981, the virus was identified and named lymphadenopathy-associated virus (LAV). By 1984, the term had been changed to human T-lymphocytic virus type III (HTLV-III) and in 1986 renamed the human immunodeficiency virus type 1 (HIV-1). HIV-1 accounts for nearly all the cases reported in the United States, whereas a second strain, HIV-2, accounts for nearly all the cases reported in West Africa. There have only been 79 cases of HIV-2 reported in the United States, the majority occurring in immigrants from Africa.

Globally, AIDS is characterized as a volatile, unstable, and dynamic epidemic that has spread to new countries around the world. It has become increasingly complex because of the viruses' ability to mutate and crosses all socioeconomic, cultural, political, and geographic borders.[9] To date, the following scientific progress has been made in combating the infection: (1) the virus has been identified; (2) improved methodologies for screening for HIV infection have been implemented; (3) vaccines have been tested; (4) biological and behavioral cofactors have been identified related to infection and disease progression; (5) prophylactic treatments are available to prevent opportunistic infections; (6) HIV RNA quantitative assays, which measure viral load (VL), have become essential to evaluate the response of the disease to treatment; and (7) the latest advances in treatment involve the use of combination antiretroviral therapies.[10] However, epidemiological evidence heightens concern regarding changes in the population affected and the morbidity and mortality still associated with the disease.

### HIV Pathogenesis and Classification

Like all viruses, the HIV virus survives by reproducing itself in a host cell, usurping the genetic machinery of that cell, and eventually destroying the cell. The HIV is a retrovirus whose life cycle consists of (1) attachment of the virus to the cell, which is affected by cofactors that influence the virus's ability to enter the host cell; (2) uncoating of the virus; (3) reverse transcription by an enzyme called reverse transcriptase, which converts two strands of viral RNA to DNA; (4) integration of newly synthesized proviral DNA into the cell nucleus, assisted by the viral enzyme integrase, which becomes the template for new viral components; (5) transcription of proviral DNA into messenger RNA; (6) movement of messenger RNA outside the cell nucleus, where it is translated into viral proteins and enzymes; and (7) assembly and release of mature virus particles out of the host cell.[10]

These newly formed viruses have an affinity for any cell that has the CD4 molecule on its surface, such as T lymphocytes and macrophages, which become major viral targets. Because CD4 cells are the master coordinators of the immune system response, chronic destruction of these cells severely compromises individuals' immune status, leaving the host susceptible to opportunistic infections and eventual progression to AIDS.

HIV and AIDS are not synonymous terms but, rather, refer to the natural history or progression of the infection, ranging from asymptomatic infection to life-threatening illness characterized by opportunistic infections and cancers. This continuum of illness is associated with a decrease in CD4 cell count and a rise in HIV-RNA VL.[11] However, in monitoring disease progression, it should be noted that although low CD4 cell counts are generally correlated with high VLs, some patients with low CD4 counts have low VLs and vice versa. Therefore, the most reliable current measurement of HIV activity is the VL, and the more consistent surrogate marker is the percentage of lymphocytes that are CD4 cells, rather than the absolute CD4 cell count.[12]

The natural history of HIV infection begins with primary or acute infection. This occurs when the virus enters the body and replicates in large numbers in the blood. This leads to an initial decrease in the number of T cells. Viral load climbs during the first 2 weeks of the infection. Within 5 to 30 days of infection, the individual experiences flu-like symptoms characteristic of a viremia such as fever, sore throat, skin rash, lymphadenopathy, and myalgia. Other manifestations of primary HIV infection include fatigue, splenomegaly, anorexia, nausea and vomiting, meningitis, retro-orbital pain, neuropathy, and mucocutaneous ulceration.[13] The production of HIV antibodies results in seroconversion, which generally occurs within 6 to 12 weeks of the initial infection. The amount of virus present after the initial viremia and the immune response is called the viral set-point.

Clinical latency refers to the chronic, clinically asymptomatic state in which there is a decreased VL and resolution of symptoms of the primary infection. It was previously believed that in this period, the virus lay dormant in the host cells. However, recent advances in the understanding of pathogenesis of the virus have revealed that there is continuous viral replication in the lymph nodes. Because more than 10 billion copies of the virus can be made every day during this period, early medical intervention with combination antiretroviral therapy is recommended. Al-Harthi et al. (2000) demonstrated that when antiretroviral therapy is used as an early intervention in non-acute HIV infection, it potentially reverses immune-mediated damage .[14]

Early symptomatic stage occurs after years of infection and is apparent by conditions indicative primarily of defects in cell-mediated immunity. Early symptomatic infection generally occurs when CD4 counts fall below 500 cells/mm³ and the HIV VL copy count increases above 10,000/mL up to 100,000/mL, which indicates a moderate risk of HIV progression and a median time to death of 6.8 years. There are frequently mucosal clues, ranging from oral candidiasis and hairy leukoplakia to ulcerative lesions. Gynecological infections are the most common reasons women have a medical examination. There are also dermatological manifestations, which include bacterial, fungal, viral, neoplastic, and other conditions such exacerbation of psoriasis, severe pruritus, or the development of recurrent pruritic papules.[13]

Late symptomatic stage begins when the CD4 count drops below 200 cells/mm³ and the VL generally increases above 100,000/mL. This CD4 level is recognized by the CDC as the case definition for AIDS. Opportunistic infections or cancers characterize this stage and result in multiple symptoms. In addition to such illnesses as KS, *Pneumocystis jiroveci* pneumonia, HIV encephalopathy, and HIV wasting, diseases such as pulmonary tuberculosis, recurrent bacterial infections, and invasive cervical cancer are sometimes seen.[6] Advanced HIV disease stage occurs when the CD4 cell count drops below 50 cells/mm³ and the immune system is so impaired that death is likely within 1 year. Common conditions are central nervous system (CNS) non-Hodgkin's lymphoma, KS, cytomegalovirus (CMV) retinitis, or *Mycobacterium avium* complex (MAC).[13] In the late stages of the disease, most individuals have health problems such as pneumonia, oral candidiasis, depression, dementia, skin problems, anxiety, incontinence, fatigue, isolation, bed dependency, wasting syndrome, and significant pain.[14] Research regarding AIDS patients experiencing advanced disease confirms the multitude of patient symptoms and factors that contribute to mortality. In a study of 83 hospitalized patients with AIDS, factors contributing to higher mortality included the type of opportunistic infections, serum albumin level, total lymphocyte count, weight, CD4 count, and neurological manifestations.[15] Of 363 patients with AIDS who were referred to community palliative care services, the most severe problems throughout care were patient and family anxiety and symptom control.[16] In the last month of life, a retrospective study of 50 men who died from AIDS indicated that the most distressing symptoms included pain, dyspnea, diarrhea, confusion, dementia, difficulty swallowing and eating, and loss of vision. Dehydration, malnutrition, and peripheral neuropathy were also important problems.[17]

## Palliative Care as a Natural Evolution in HIV/AIDS Care

From the earliest stages of HIV disease, symptom control becomes an important goal of medical and nursing care to maintain the patient's quality of life. Therefore, palliative care for patients with HIV/AIDS should be viewed not as an approach to care only in the advanced stage of the illness but as an aspect of care that begins in the early stage of illness and continues as the disease progresses.[18]

With the occurrence of opportunistic infections, specific cancers, and neurological manifestations, AIDS involves multiple symptoms not only from the disease processes but also from the side effects of medications and other therapies. Patients with AIDS present with complex care issues because they experience bouts of severe illness and debilitation alternating with periods of symptom stabilization.[19] In one model of care, AIDS palliation begins when active treatment ends. Although this model limits service overlap and is economical, it creates not only the ethical issue of when to shift from a curative to a palliative focus but also promotes discontinuity of care and possible discrimination. Conversely, a second model of AIDS care recognizes that AIDS treatment is primarily palliative, directed toward minimizing symptoms and maximizing the quality of life, and necessitates the use of antiretroviral drugs, treatment of infections and neoplasms, and provision of high levels of support to promote the patient's quality of life over many years of the illness.[20] Selwyn and Rivard[21] emphasize that although AIDS is no longer a uniformly fatal disease, it is an important cause of mortality, particularly for ethnically diverse populations with comorbidities such as hepatitis B and C, end-organ failure, and various malignancies. Further, Shen, Blank, and Selwyn (2005) conducted a study based on patients ($n$ = 230) in a large urban New York Medical Center who had been referred to the HIV palliative care team. They reported that close to half of all deaths for these patients were attributable to non-AIDS-specific causes, including cancer and end-organ failure. Further, age and markers of functional status were more predictive of mortality than traditional HIV prognostic variables, suggesting the need to reconsider the current value of prior prognostic variables.[22]

Although thousands of individuals continue to suffer and die from AIDS, the division between curative-aggressive care and supportive-palliative care is less well-defined and more variable than in other life-threatening illnesses such as cancer. With HIV/AIDS, the severity, complexity, and unpredictability of the illness trajectory have blurred the distinction between curative and palliative care. Other continuining challenges associated with HIV/AIDS are the societal stigmatization of the disease and, therefore, the greater emotional, social, and spiritual needs of those experiencing the illness, as well as their family and professional caregivers who experience their own grief and bereavement processes.

Resources aimed at prevention, health promotion and maintenance, and end-of-life care must be available through health-care policies and legislation.[23] Not only the treatment of chronic debilitating conditions but also the treatment of superimposed acute opportunistic infections and related symptoms is necessary to maintain quality of life. For example, IV therapy and blood transfusions, as well as health prevention measures such as ongoing IV therapies to prevent blindness from CMV retinitis, must be available to patients with AIDS to maintain their quality of life.

Palliative care is therefore a natural evolution in AIDS care. Core issues of comfort and function, which are fundamental to palliative care, must be addressed throughout the course of the illness and may be concurrent with restorative or curative therapies for persons with AIDS.[23] The management decisions for patients with advanced AIDS revolve around the ratio between benefits and burdens of the various diagnostic and treatment modalities and the patient's expectations and goals, as well as anticipated problems.[24] In the face of advanced HIV disease, health-care providers and patients must determine the balance between aggressive and supportive efforts, particularly when increasing debility,

wasting, and deteriorating cognitive function are evident. At this point, the complex needs of patients with HIV/AIDS and the needs of their families require the coordinated care of an interdisciplinary palliative care team, involving physicians, advanced practice nurses, staff nurses, social workers, dietitians, physiotherapists, and clergy.[25] Because in palliative care the unit of care is the patient and family, the palliative care team offers support not only for patients to live as fully as possible until death but also for the family to cope during the patient's illness and in their own bereavement.[26] Palliative care core precepts of respect for patient goals, preferences, and choices; comprehensive caring; and acknowledgment of caregivers' concerns support the holistic and comprehensive approach to care needed by individuals and families with HIV/AIDS. The components of high-quality HIV/AIDS palliative care, as identified by health-care providers, include competent, skilled practitioners; confidential, nondiscriminatory, culturally sensitive care; flexible and responsive care; collaborative and coordinated care; and fair access to care.[26]

Although the hospice and palliative care movement developed as a community response to those who were dying primarily of cancer, the advent of the AIDS epidemic made it necessary for hospices to begin admitting patients with AIDS. This meant applying the old model of cancer care to patients with a new infectious, progressive, and terminal disease.[27] Unlike the course of cancer, which is relatively predictable once the disease progresses beyond cure, AIDS patients experience a series of life-threatening opportunistic infections. It is not until wasting becomes apparent that the course of AIDS achieves the predictability of cancer.[28] Furthermore, although the underlying goal of AIDS care remains one of palliation, short-term aggressive therapies are still needed to treat opportunistic infections.[29] Additionally, unlike cancer palliation, AIDS palliation deals with a fatal infectious disease of primarily younger people, which requires ongoing infection control and the management of symptoms.[30]

## Barriers to Palliative Care

The neglect of the palliative care needs of patients with HIV also relates to certain barriers to care, such as reimbursement issues. Specifically, public and private third-party payers have reimbursed end-of-life care only when physicians have verified a life expectancy of less than 6 months to live.[30] Given the unpredictability of the illness trajectory, many patients with AIDS have been denied access to hospice care. Currently, these policies are under review, and the 6-month limitation is being extended so that patients with AIDS will be eligible for comprehensive care, with control of pain and other symptoms along with psychological and spiritual support offered by hospice/palliative care.

Until recently, a second barrier to access to hospice/palliative care for patients with AIDS has been the cost of continuing the administration of antiretroviral therapies and other medications to prevent opportunistic infections. The estimated cost of treatment for AIDS patients in hospices could amount to twice the cost of treating patients with cancer—particularly when the costs of medications are included—and cost remains an important issue for hospices. Financing of such therapies for patients with AIDS is now being addressed by hospice/palliative care organizations.

The third barrier to palliative care is the patients themselves, many of whom are young, clinging to the hope of a cure for AIDS, and unwilling to accept hospice care. However, the current emphasis on beginning palliative care at the time of diagnosis of a life-threatening illness may shift the perception of palliative care as only end-of-life care and help promote palliative care as an aggressive approach to care throughout the course of the illness to ensure their quality of life. Indeed, media and Internet coverage of government and private initiatives to improve the care of the seriously and terminally ill in the United States is informing patients, families, and nurses of the philosophy and precepts of palliative care, the availability of palliative care for life-defining illnesses, and the rights of patients to receive excellent end-of-life care, as well as the obligations of health professionals to provide such care across health-care settings.

A review of the evidence of barriers and inequality in HIV care by Harding et al. (2005) found that there is increased complexity in the balance of providing concurrent curative and palliative therapies given the prolongation of lifespan as a result of HAART therapy. Harding and colleagues believe that palliative care should not solely be associated with terminal care and propose four recommendations:

1. the need for multidimensional palliative care assessment for differing populations;
2. basic palliative care skills training for all clinical staff in standard assessments;
3. development of referral criteria and systems for patients with complex palliative care needs;
4. the availability of specialist consultation across all settings.[31]

Finally, Harding, Karus, and Easterbrook (2005) systematically reviewed the effects of models of palliative care on patient outcomes. Although they found that there is a lack of experimental and standardized methods, with most studies being descriptive, correlational studies, their review of the literature supports improvement in palliative care outcomes in home palliative and inpatient hospice care in measures of pain, symptom control, anxiety, insight, and spiritual well-being.[32]

### Criteria for Palliative Care

Grothe and Brody[27] suggest that four criteria be considered regarding the admission of AIDS patients to hospice: functional ability, statistical prognosis, CD4 count and VL, and history of opportunistic infections. These criteria give a better understanding of the patient's prognosis and needs. The complex needs of patients with advanced AIDS also indicate the need for an interdisciplinary approach to care offered by

hospice/palliative care. The continual review of hospice policies in accordance with the changes in the disease is encouraged. Indeed, developing different models of care, such as enhanced home care, hospice care, day care, or partnerships with community hospitals or agencies, and conducting cost-benefit analysis will be important in meeting the health-care needs of patients with AIDS and their families in the future.[14]

Important advances are currently being made in the field of palliative medicine and nursing, involving an active set of behaviors that continue throughout the caregiving process to manage the pain and suffering of individuals with HIV/AIDS. Health professionals have the responsibility to be knowledgable about the various treatment options and resources available for pain and symptom management. They must know about pharmacological agents' actions, side effects, and interactions, as well as alternative routes of medication administration. And they must be able to inform patients of their options for care—documenting their preferences, wishes, and choices; performing a complete history and physical assessment; and collaborating with other members of the interdisciplinary team to develop and implement a comprehensive plan of care.[26]

### Health Promotion and Maintenance in Promoting the Quality of Life of Persons with HIV/AIDS

As palliative care becomes an increasingly important component of AIDS care from diagnosis to death,[23] and given the definition of palliative care as the comprehensive management of the physical, psychological, social, spiritual, and existential needs of patients with incurable progressive illness,[26] palliative care must involve ongoing prevention, health promotion, and health maintenance to promote the patient's quality of life throughout the illness trajectory. With HIV/AIDS, health promotion and maintenance involves promoting behaviors that will prevent or decrease the occurrence of opportunistic infections and AIDS-indicator diseases, promoting prophylactic and therapeutic treatment of AIDS-indicator conditions and preventing behaviors that promote disease expression.[4]

With no current cure, the health management of patients with HIV/AIDS is directed toward controlling HIV disease and prolonging survival while maintaining quality of life.[33] Quality of life may be defined as the impact of sickness and healthcare on an ill person's daily activities and sense of well-being.[34,35] Furthermore, quality of life varies with disease progression from HIV to AIDS. To understand quality of life means to understand the patient's perceptions of his/her ability to control the physical, emotional, social, cognitive, and spiritual aspects of the illness.[45] Quality of life is therefore associated with health maintenance for individuals with HIV/AIDS, particularly as it relates to functioning in activities of daily living, social functioning, and physical and emotional symptoms.[36] In a study regarding the functional quality of life of 142 men and women with AIDS, Vosvick and colleagues[37] concluded that maladaptive coping strategies were associated with lower levels of energy and social functioning and that severe pain interfered with daily living tasks and was associated with lower levels of functional quality of life (physical functioning, energy/fatigue, social functioning, and role functioning). Therefore, health promotion interventions should be aimed at developing adaptive coping strategies and improving pain management.

Health promotion and maintenance for patients with HIV/AIDS must acknowledge patients' perceived health-care needs. Based on a study of 386 HIV-infected persons, it was determined that the health-care challenges perceived by patients with HIV/AIDS across hospital, outpatient, home, and long-term care settings included decreased endurance, physical mobility, and changes in sensory perception, as well as financial issues—specifically lack of income and resources to cover living and health-care expenses.[38] Furthermore, based on a sample of 162 hospitalized men and women with AIDS, Kemppainen reported that the strongest predictor of decreased quality of life was depression, which accounted for 23% of the variance, with other symptoms accounting for 9.75% and female gender accounting for an additional 8%.[39] Additionally, active involvement in the process of nursing care contributed 13.4% to the variance in quality of life. These results indicate the health-care challenges and physical, emotional, and interactional needs of patients with AIDS. In addition to managing pain and other symptoms, a comprehensive and compassionate approach to care is necessary as the illness progresses. Furthermore, enhancing immuno-competence is critical at all stages of illness, as is treating the symptoms brought on by the disease or related to prophylactic or treatment therapies. Palliation of physical, emotional, and spiritual symptoms—particularly as experienced in the late symptomatic and advanced stages of HIV disease—is considered the final stage of a health-and-disease-prevention approach and will be discussed later in this chapter.[9]

Through all stages of HIV, health can be promoted and maintained through diet, micronutrients, exercise, reduction of stress and negative emotions, symptom surveillance, and the use of prophylactic therapies to prevent opportunistic infections or AIDS-related complications.

## Diet

A health-promoting diet is essential for optimal function of the immune system. Deficiencies in calorie and protein intake impair cell-mediated immunity, phagocytic function, and antibody response. Therefore, an alteration in nutrition is associated with impaired immune system function, secondary infections, disease progression, psychological distress, and fatigue. In patients with AIDS, common nutritional problems are weight loss, vitamin and mineral deficiencies, loss of muscle mass, and loss or redistribution of fat mass. The redistribution of fat is characterized by increased abdominal girth,

loss of fat from the face, and a "buffalo hump" on the back of the neck, which may result from the administration of antiretroviral therapy.[40] Patients with HIV/AIDS often have reduced food or caloric intake, malabsorption, and altered metabolism. Reduced food or caloric intake frequently results from diseases of the mouth and oropharynx, such as oral candidiasis, anular cheilitis, gingivitis, herpes simplex, and hairy leukoplakia. Incidence of diseases of the gastrointestinal (GI) tract that can cause malabsorption (such as CMV, MAC, cryptosporidiosis, and KS) increases for individuals with CD4 counts of 50 or less and may adversely affect their nutritional status.[41] Metabolic alterations may result from HIV infection or secondary infections, as well as abnormalities in carbohydrate, fat, and protein metabolism.[37] Hussein[42] believes that a good diet is one of the simplest ways to delay HIV progression and will bolster immune system function and energy levels and help patients live longer and more productive lives. A diet with a variety of foods from the five basic food groups—including 55% of calories from carbohydrates, 15% to 20% of calories from proteins, and 30% of calories from fats—is important in supporting immune function.[43] It is recommended to have two or three servings daily from the protein and dairy groups, seven to 12 servings from the starch and grain group, two servings of fruits and vegetables rich in vitamin C, as well as three servings of other fruits and vegetables.[43]

## Micronutrients

Research has indicated that HIV-infected individuals have lower levels of magnesium, total carotenes, total choline, and vitamins A and $B_6$, yet higher levels of niacin than noninfected individuals.[44] A linkage has been reported between vitamin A (β-carotene) deficiency and elevated disease progression and mortality.[45] Correcting both vitamin A and $B_6$ deficiencies has been hypothesized to restore cell-mediated immunity, and vitamin-supplement trials are underway. Current research supports the increase in dietary intake of n-3 polyunsaturated fatty acids, arginine, and RNA to increase body weight and stave off wasting caused by malabsorption. Increase in concentrations of amino acids such as arginine has also been found to preserve lean muscle mass.[44]

## Exercise

A consistent outcome of the effects of exercise on immune function is the increase in natural killer-cell activity, although variable results have been reported on the effects of exercise on neutrophil, macrophage, and T- and B-cell function and proliferation.[46] In a review of exercise studies, LaPerriere and colleagues[47] reported a trend in CD4 cell count elevation in all but one study, with the greatest effect from aerobic exercise and weight training. The CDC[48] recommends a physical exercise program of 30 to 45 minutes four or more times a week as a health-promoting activity to increase lung capacity, endurance, energy, and flexibility and to improve circulation.

Massage has also been linked to natural killer-cell activity and overall immune regulation, as reported in a research study of 29 HIV-infected men who received daily massages for 1 month.[49] Patient reports of less anxiety and greater relaxation related to exercise and massage are regarded by both patients and practitioners as important laboratory markers.[44]

## Stress and Emotions

Stress and negative emotions have also been associated with immunosuppression and vulnerability to disease. In a study of 96 HIV-infected homosexual men without symptoms or antiretroviral medication use, Leserman and colleagues[50] reported that higher cumulative average stressful life events, higher anger scores, lower cumulative average social support, and depressive symptoms were all predictive of a faster progression to both the CDC AIDS classification and a clinical AIDS condition. Stress of living with HIV/AIDS is related to the uncertainty regarding illness progression and prognosis, stigmatization and discrimination, and financial concerns as disabilities increase with advancing disease. Persons with AIDS frequently cite the avoidance of stress as a way of maintaining a sense of well-being.[51] The use of exercise and massage and other relaxation techniques, such as imagery, meditation, and yoga, have been reported as valuable stress-management techniques.[52] Cognitive–behavioral interventions have also been shown to improve certain aspects of quality of life of women with AIDS ($n = 330$), specifically in terms of cognitive functioning, health distress, and overall health perceptions. However, no changes were observed in energy/fatigue, pain, or role or social functioning.[53]

Health promotion also involves health beliefs and coping strategies that support well-being despite protracted illness. A study of 53 patients diagnosed with AIDS demonstrated that long-term survivors used numerous strategies to support their health, such as having the will to live and positive attitudes, feeling in charge, maintaining a strong sense of self and a sense of humor, and expressing their needs. Other health-promotion strategies frequently used by these patients included remaining active, seeking medical information, talking to others, socializing and pursuing pleasurable activities, finding good medical care, and seeking counseling.[54] Cohen examined the relationship between the use of humor to cope with stress (coping humor) and perceived social support, depression, anxiety, self-esteem, and stress, based on a sample of 103 patients with HIV/AIDS.[55] The results indicated that patients who used more coping humor were less depressed, expressed higher self-esteem, and perceived greater support from friends. However, the use of coping humor did not buffer stress, anxiety, or immune-system functioning. Stress can also be associated with the financial issues experienced by patients with HIV/AIDS. Therefore, health promotion may involve financial planning, identification of financial resources available through the community, and public assistance offered through Medicaid.

It must also be recognized that additional physical and emotional stress is associated with the use of recreational drugs such as alcohol, chemical stimulants, tobacco, and marijuana because these agents have an immunosuppressant effect and may interfere with health-promoting behaviors.[56] The use of such substances may have a negative effect on interpersonal relationships and is associated with a relapse to unsafe sexual practices.[57] Interventions for health promotion include encouraging patients to participate in self-health groups and harm-reduction programs to deal with substance-abuse problems.

## Symptom Surveillance

Throughout the course of their illness, individuals with HIV require primary care services to identify early signs of opportunistic infections and to minimize related symptoms and complications. This includes a complete health history, physical examination, and laboratory data, including determination of immunological and viral status.

## Health History

In the care of patients with HIV/AIDS, the health history should include the following[12]:

- History of present illness, including a review of those factors that led to HIV testing
- Medical history, particularly those conditions that may be exacerbated by HIV or its treatments, such as diabetes mellitus, hypertriglyceridemia, or chronic or active Hepatitis B infection
- Childhood illnesses and vaccinations for preventing common infections such as polio, DPT, or measles
- Medication history, including the patient's knowledge of the types of medications, side effects, adverse reactions, drug interactions, and administration recommendations
- Sexual history, regarding sexual behaviors and preferences and history of sexually transmitted diseases, which can exacerbate HIV progression
- Lifestyle habits, such as the past and present use of recreational drugs, including alcohol, which may accelerate progression of disease, or cigarette smoking, which may suppress appetite or be associated with opportunistic infections such as oral candidiasis, hairy leukoplakia, and bacterial pneumonia
- Dietary habits, including risks related to food-borne illnesses such as Hepatitis A
- Travel history to countries in Asia, Africa, and South America, where the risk of opportunistic infections increase
- Complete systems review to provide indications of clinical manifestations of new opportunistic infections or cancers, as well as AIDS-related complications both from the disease and its treatments

## Physical Examination

A physical exam should begin with a general assessment of vital signs and height and weight, as well as overall appearance and mood. A complete head-to-toe assessment is important and may reveal various findings common to individuals with HIV/AIDS, including those mentioned below.[12]

- Oral cavity assessment may indicate candida, oral hairy leukoplakia, or KS.
- Funduscopic assessment may reveal visual changes associated with CMV retinitis; glaucoma screening annually is also recommended.
- Lymph node assessment may reveal adenopathy detected at any stage of disease.
- Dermatological assessment may indicate various cutaneous manifestations that occur throughout the course of the illness such as HIV exanthema, KS, or infectious complications such as dermatomycosis.
- Neuromuscular assessment may indicate various central, peripheral, or autonomic nervous systems disorders and signs and symptoms of conditions such as meningitis, encephalitis, dementia, or peripheral neuropathies.
- Cardiovascular assessment may reveal cardiomyopathy.
- GI assessment may indicate organomegaly—specifically splenomegaly or hepatomegaly—particularly in patients with a history of substance abuse, as well as signs related to parasitic intestinal infections; annual stool of guaiac and rectal examination, as well as sigmoidoscopy every 5 years, are also parts of health maintenance.
- Reproductive system assessment may reveal occult sexually transmitted diseases or malignancies as well vaginal candidiasis, cervical dysplasia, pelvic inflammatory disease, or rectal lesions in women with HIV/AIDS. They may also reveal urethral discharge and rectal lesions or malignancies in HIV-infected men. Health maintenance in individuals with HIV/AIDS also includes annual mammograms in women, as well as testicular exams in men and prostate-specific antigen annually.

## Laboratory Data

CD4 counts—both the absolute numbers and the CD4 percentages—should be evaluated to assist the health practitioner in therapeutic decision-making about treatments of opportunistic infections and antiretroviral therapy. It is the strongest predictor of disease progression and patient survival.[58] The quantitative RNA level or VL can be useful as a marker of disease progression but is primarily used as a measure of the effectiveness of antiretroviral therapy. The DHHS Panel on Clinical Practices for the Treatment of HIV recommends that the CD4 count and the VL be measured upon entry into care and every 3 to 6 months thereafter.[58] The patient's HIV-RNA (VL) should be measured immediately before a patient is started on HAART and again 2 to 8 weeks after treatment is initiated to determine the effectiveness of the therapy. With adherence to the medication schedule, it is expected that the HIV-RNA will decrease to undetectable levels (<50 copies/mL) after 16 to 24 weeks of the intitiation of therapy.[58] If a patient does not significantly respond to therapy, the clinician should evaluate adherence, repeat the test, perform a genotyping or phenotyping resistance assay, and rule out malabsorption or drug interactions.

The decision regarding laboratory testing is based on the stage of HIV, the medical processes warranting initial assessment or follow-up, and consideration of the patient-benefit-to-burden ratio. Complete blood counts are often measured with each VL determination or with a change of antiretroviral therapy, particularly with patients on drugs known to cause anemia. Chemistry profiles are done to assess liver function, lipid status, and glycemia every 3 to 6 months or with a change in therapy and are determined by the patient's antiretroviral therapy, baseline determinations, and co-infections. Abnormalities in these profiles may occur as a result of antiretroviral therapy. Increasing hepatic dysfunction is evident by elevations in the serum transaminases (AST, ALT, ALP, LDH). Blood work should also include Hepatitis C serology (antibody), Hepatitis B serology and *Toxoplasma* IgG serology.[59]

Urine analysis should be done annually unless the person is on antiretroviral therapy, which may require more frequent follow-up to check for toxicity. Annual Papanicolaou (Pap) smears are also indicated, with recommendations for Pap smears every 3 to 6 months in HIV-infected women who are symptomatic. Syphilis studies should be performed annually; however, patients with low positive titers should have follow-up testing at 3, 6, 9, 12, and 24 months. Gonorrhea and chlamydia tests are encouraged every 6 to 12 months if the patient is sexually active. In addition, HIV-infected persons should be tested for IgG antibody to *Toxoplasma* soon after the diagnosis of HIV infection to detect latent infection with *T. gondii*. *Toxoplasma*-seronegative persons who are not taking a PCP prophylactic regimen known to be active against Toxoplasma enecephalitis (TE) should be retested for IgG antibody to Toxoplasma when their CD4+ counts decline to less than 100 cells/μL to determine whether they have seroconverted and are therefore at risk of TE.[12]

All persons should be tested for latent tuberculosis infection (LTBI) at the time of their HIV diagnosis regardless of their TB risk category and then annually if negative. LTBI diagnosis can be achieved with the use of tuberculin skin test (TST) or by or interferon-γ release assay using the patient's serum.. A TST is considered positive in patients with induration of greater than or equal to 5 mm. An interferon-γ release assay is reported as positive or negative. Any positive test warrants chest radiograph for active disease and consideration of antituberculosis therapy based on history, laboratory, physical, and radiographic findings.

## Prophylaxis

The primary strategy to prevent the development of opportunistic infections is to avoid exposure to microorganisms in the environment. Second, the immune system can be supported and maintained through the administration of prophylactic and/or suppressive therapies, which decrease the frequency or severity of opportunistic infections.[12] Primary prophylaxis is the administration of a pharmacological agent to prevent initial infection, whereas secondary prophylaxis is the administration of a pharmacological agent to prevent future occurrences of infection.[12] However, because of the effectiveness of HAARTs, there has been a significant decrease in the incidence of opportunistic infections. Therefore, prophylaxis for life for HIV-related co-infections is no longer necessary in many cases.[59] If HAART restores immune system function as evident by a rise in CD4 counts, then clinicians may stop administering primary prophylaxis under defined conditions.[59] The advantages to ending preventive prophylaxis for opportunistic infections in selected patients is a decrease in drug interactions and toxicities, lower cost of care, and greater adherence to HAART regimens.[59] Table 41–1 describes the common opportunistic infections and recommended prophylactic and alternative regimens.[60] In the late symptomatic and advanced stages of HIV disease, when CD4 counts are low and VL may be high, prophylaxis remains important to protect against opportunistic infections. Therefore, throughout the illness trajectory, and even in hospice settings, patients may be taking prophylactic medications, thus requiring sophisticated planning and monitoring.

Additionally, HIV-infected individuals are at risk for severe diseases that are vaccine preventable, such as Hepatitis A and B, tetanus, influenza, pneumococcal and measles, rubella, and mumps. Table 41–2 presents vaccine-preventable illnesses and interventions. Von Gunten and colleagues suggest the continuation of prophylaxis in hospice and palliative care settings for patients with AIDS as long as patients are able to take oral medications.[61] This is because there is a high risk of reactivation and dissemination of diseases that can result in a high number of symptoms. Suppressive therapy for herpes infections is also continued to prevent painful lesions. Von Gunten and colleagues also recommend the following plan regarding prophylaxis and suppressive therapy in hospice/palliative care:[61]

1. If the patient is clinically stable and wants to continue prophylaxis, then continue drug therapy.
2. If side effects occur and the patient continues to be otherwise stable, then consider alternative regimens.
3. If the patient is intolerant of prophylaxis and/or the regimens are burdensome, then discontinue medications.

Although these recommendations were made in 1995, they are still applicable to patients with AIDS who are enrolled in hospice.

## Indications for Antiretroviral Therapy Across the Illness Trajectory

Without a cure for HIV, all treatments are essentially palliative in nature to slow disease progression and limit the occurrence of opportunistic infections, which adversely affect quality of life. The CD4 cell count and VL are used in conjunction to determine the initiation of antiretroviral therapy.

The goal of initiating HAART is to achieve maximum long-term suppression of HIV-RNA and to restore or preserve immune system function and thereby reduce morbidity and mortality and promote quality of life.[59] The potential risks versus benefits of early or delayed initiation of therapy for asymptomatic patients must be considered. The benefits of early therapy include earlier suppression of viral replication, preservation of the immune system functioning, prolongation of disease-free survival, and a decrease in the risk of HIV transmission.[59] However, the risks of early therapy initiation include lower quality of life caused by the adverse effects of therapy, problems with adherence to therapy, and subsequent drug resistance, with the potential limitation of future treatment options as a result of premature administration of available drugs. There is further concern regarding the risks of severe toxicities associated with certain antiretroviral medications, such as elevations in serum levels of triglycerides and cholesterol, alterations in fat distribution, or insulin resistance and diabetes mellitus.[58] Given the available data in terms of the relative risk for the progression to AIDS, the evidence supports the initiation of therapy for asymptomatic HIV-infected patients with a CD4 T-cell count of less than 350 cells/mm$^3$ or with an AIDS-defining history. Antiretroviral therapy should also be started regardless of CD4 in pregnant patients who have HIV-associated kidney disease and patients co-infected with Hepatitis B when treatment is indicated.[62] If a patient has a CD4 count greater than 350 cells/mm$^3$, arguments can be made for both conservative and aggressive approaches to therapy. However, the decision to start therapy for the asymptomatic patient in this range involves discussion with the patient regarding his/her willingness, ability, and readiness to begin therapy and the risk for disease progression given the VL as well as CD4 count. The aggressive approach to initiating therapy early is supported by studies that indicate suppression of plasma HIV-RNA is easier to maintain when CD4 counts are higher and VLs are lower.[58]

It is further recommended that all patients with symptomatic infection be treated with antiretrovirals regardless of CD4 count or plasma viral levels. If a patient is acutely ill with an opportunistic infection or other complication of HIV, then the timing of antiretroviral therapy initiation should be based on drug toxicity, ability to adhere to the treatment regimen, drug interactions, and laboratory abnormalities. However, maximally suppressive regimens should be used, and patients with advanced AIDS should not discontinue therapy during an acute opportunistic infection or malignancy unless there is drug toxicity, intolerance, or drug interactions.[58]

**Table 41–1**
**Opportunistic Infections and Treatments: Prophylaxis to Prevent First Episode of Opportunistic Disease in Adults and Adolescents Infected With HIV**

| Pathogen | Indication | First Choice | Alternative |
|---|---|---|---|
| *Pneumocystis jirovecii pneumonia (PCP)* | CD4+ count <200 cells/µL or oropharyngeal candidiasis<br><br>CD4+% <14% or history of AIDS-defining illness<br><br>CD4+count >200 but <250 cells/µL if CD4+ count monitoring every 1 to 3 months is not possible | Trimethoprim-sulfamethoxazole (TMP-SMX), 1 double strength (DS) by mouth (PO) daily; or 1 single strength (SS) daily | • TMP-SMX 1 DS PO three times weekly (TIW); or<br>• Dapsone 100 mg PO daily or 50 mg PO twice daily (BID); or<br>• Dapsone 50 mg PO daily + pyrimethamine 50 mg PO weekly + leucovorin 25 mg PO weekly; or<br>• Aerosolized pentamidine 300 mg via Respigard II™ nebulizer every month; or<br>• Atovaquone 1,500 mg PO daily; or<br>• (Atovaquone 1,500 mg + pyrimethamine 25 mg + leucovorin 10 mg) PO daily |
| *Toxoplasma gondii encephalitis* | Toxoplasma IgG positive patients with CD4+ count <100 cells/µL<br><br>Seronegative patients receiving PCP prophylaxis not active against toxoplasmosis, should have toxoplasma serology retested if CD4+ count decline to <100 cells/µL<br><br>Prophylaxis should be initiated if seroconversion occurred | TMP-SMX, 1 DS PO daily | • TMP-SMX 1 DS PO TIW; or<br>• TMP-SMX 1 SS PO daily;<br>• Dapsone 50 mg PO daily + pyrimethamine 50 mg PO weekly + leucovorin 25 mg PO weekly; or<br>• (Dapsone 200 mg + pyrimethamine 75 mg + leucovorin 25 mg) PO weekly;<br>• (Atovaquone 1,500 mg ± pyrimethamine 25 mg + leucovorin 10 mg) PO daily |
| *Mycobacterium tuberculosis infection*<br><br>(Treatment of latent TB infection or LTBI) | (+) diagnostic test for latent TB infection (LTBI), no evidence of active TB, and no prior history of treatment for active or latent TB;<br><br>(−) diagnostic test for LTBI, but close contact with a person with infectious pulmonary TB and no evidence of active TB;<br><br>A history of untreated or inadequately treated healed TB (i.e., old fibrotic lesions) regardless of diagnostic tests for LTBI, and no evidence of active TB | Isoniazid (INH) 300 mg PO daily or 900 mg PO BIW for 9 months—both plus pyridoxine 50 mg PO daily; or<br><br>For persons exposed to drug resistant TB, selection of drugs after consultation with public health authorities | • RIF 300 mg PO daily × 4 months; or<br>• RFB (dose adjusted based on concomitant ART) × 4 months |
| *Disseminated Mycobacterium avium complex (MAC) disease* | CD4+ count <50 cells/µL—after ruling out active MAC infection | Azithromycin 1,200 mg PO once weekly; or<br>Clarithromycin 500 mg PO BID; or<br>Azithromycin 600 mg PO twice weekly | • RFB 300 mg PO daily (dosage adjustment based on drug–drug interactions with ART)—rule out active TB before starting RFB |
| *Streptococcus pneumoniae infection* | CD4+ count >200 cells/µL and no receipt of pneumococcal vaccine in the past 5 years<br><br>CD4+ count <200 cells/µL—vaccination can be offered<br><br>In patients who received PPV when CD4+ count <200 cells/µL, but has increased to > 200 cells/µL in response to ART | 23-valent polysaccharide pneumococcal vaccine (PPV) 0.5 mL IM × 1<br><br>Revaccination every 5 years may be considered | |

| Disease | Indication | Prophylaxis/Vaccine |
|---|---|---|
| Influenza A and B virus infection | All HIV-infected patients | Inactivated influenza vaccine 0.5 mL IM annually |
| *Histoplasma capsulatum* infection | If CD4+ count ≤150 cells/μL and at high risk because of occupational exposure or live in a community with a hyperendemic rate of histoplasmosis (>10 cases/100 patient-years) | Itraconazole 200 mg PO daily |
| Coccidioidomycosis | Positive IgM or IgG serologic test in a patient from an endemic area; and CD4+ count <250 cells/μL | Fluconazole 400 mg PO daily / Itraconazole 200 mg PO BID |
| Varicella-zoster virus (VZV) infection | <u>Pre-exposure prevention:</u> Patients who have not been vaccinated, have no history of varicella or herpes zoster, or are seronegative for VZV & have CD4+ count ≥200 cells/μL<br><br>Note: routine VZV serologic testing in HIV infected adults is not recommended<br><br><u>Postexposure</u>—close contact with a person who has active varicella or herpes zoster: For susceptible patients (those who have no history of vaccination or of either condition, or are known to be VZV seronegative) | <u>Pre-exposure prevention:</u> Primary varicella vaccination (Varivax), 2 doses (0.5 mL SQ) administered 3 months apart<br><br>If vaccination results in disease due to vaccine virus, treatment with acyclovir is recommended<br><br><u>Postexposure therapy:</u> Varicella-zoster immune globulin (VariZIG) 125 IU per 10 kg (maximum of 625 IU) IM, administered within 96 hours after exposure to a person with active varicella or herpes zoster<br><br>Note: As of June 2007, VariZIG can be obtained only under a treatment IND (1–800-843-7477, FFF Enterprises)<br><br>• VZV-susceptible household contacts of susceptible HIV-infected persons should be vaccinated to prevent potential transmission of VZV to their HIV-infected contacts<br><br><u>Alternative postexposure therapy:</u><br>• Post exposure varicella vaccine (Varivax) 0.5 mL SQ × 2 doses, 3 months apart if CD4+ count >200 cells/μL; or<br>• Pre-emptive acyclovir 800 mg PO 5 times/day for 5 days<br>• These two alternatives have not been studied in the HIV population |
| Human Papilloma Virus (HPV) Infection | Women aged 15 to 26 | HPV quadravalent vaccine 0.5 mL IM months 0, 2, and 6 |
| Hepatitis A virus (HAV) infection | Patients with chronic liver disease, injection drug users, or men have sex with men Some experts might delay vaccination until CD4+ count >200 cells/μL | Hepatitis A vaccine 1 mL IM × 2 doses, at 0 and 6 to 12 months<br><br>IgG antibody response should be assessed one month after vaccination; non-responders should be revaccinated |
| Hepatitis B virus (HBV) Infection | All HIV patients without evidence of prior exposure to HBV should be immunized with HBV vaccine, including patients with CD4+ count <200 cells/μL<br><br>*Patients with isolated anti-HBc* (consider screen for HBV DNA prior to vaccination to rule out occult chronic HBV infection)<br><br><u>*Vaccine nonresponders:*</u> Defined as Anti-HBs <10 IU/mL 1 month after a vaccination series<br><br>For patients with low CD4+ count at the time of first vaccination series, some experts might delay revaccination until after a sustained increase in CD4+ count with ART. | Hepatitis B vaccine IM (Engerix-B 20 mcg/mL or Recombivax 10 mcg/mL) at 0, 1, and 6 months<br><br>Anti-HBs should be obtained one month after completion of the vaccine series<br><br>Revaccinate with a second vaccine series |
| Malaria | Travel to endemic area | Recommendations are the same for HIV-infected and -uninfected patients. One of the following 3 drugs is generally recommended depending on location: atovaquone/proguanil, doxycycline, or mefloquine. Please refer to the following website for the most recent recommendations based on region and drug susceptibility http://www.cdc.gov/malaria/ |

**Table 41–2**
**Vaccine Preventable Illnesses and Immunization Schedule for HIV-Infected Adults**

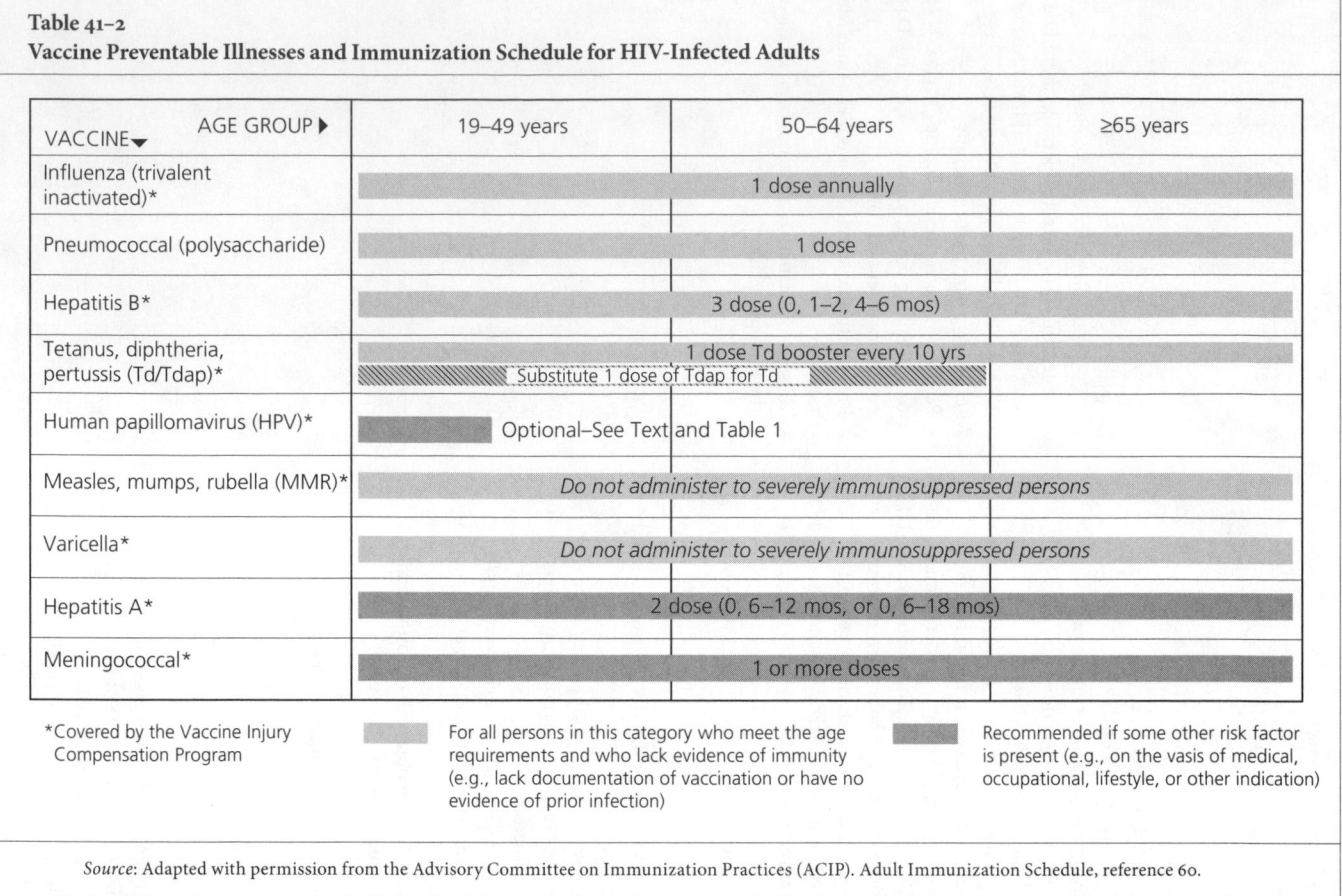

| VACCINE ▾    AGE GROUP ▶ | 19–49 years | 50–64 years | ≥65 years |
|---|---|---|---|
| Influenza (trivalent inactivated)* | 1 dose annually | | |
| Pneumococcal (polysaccharide) | 1 dose | | |
| Hepatitis B* | 3 dose (0, 1–2, 4–6 mos) | | |
| Tetanus, diphtheria, pertussis (Td/Tdap)* | 1 dose Td booster every 10 yrs | | |
| | Substitute 1 dose of Tdap for Td | | |
| Human papillomavirus (HPV)* | Optional–See Text and Table 1 | | |
| Measles, mumps, rubella (MMR)* | *Do not administer to severely immunosuppressed persons* | | |
| Varicella* | *Do not administer to severely immunosuppressed persons* | | |
| Hepatitis A* | 2 dose (0, 6–12 mos, or 0, 6–18 mos) | | |
| Meningococcal* | 1 or more doses | | |

*Covered by the Vaccine Injury Compensation Program

☐ For all persons in this category who meet the age requirements and who lack evidence of immunity (e.g., lack documentation of vaccination or have no evidence of prior infection)

☐ Recommended if some other risk factor is present (e.g., on the vasis of medical, occupational, lifestyle, or other indication)

*Source*: Adapted with permission from the Advisory Committee on Immunization Practices (ACIP). Adult Immunization Schedule, reference 60.

## Antiretroviral Therapy Used to Treat HIV Infection

Antiretroviral drugs are broadly classified by the phase of the retrovirus life-cycle that the drug inhibits.

- Nucleoside reverse transcriptase (NRTIs) interfere with the action of an HIV protein called reverse transcriptase, which the virus needs to make new copies of itself.
- Non-nucleoside reverse transcriptase inhibitors (nNRTIs) inhibit reverse transcriptase directly by binding to the enzyme and interfering with its function.
- Protease inhibitors (PIs) target viral assembly by inhibiting the activity of protease, an enzyme used by HIV to cleave nascent proteins for final assembly of new virons.
- Integrase inhibitors inhibit the enzyme integrase, which is responsible for integration of viral DNA into the DNA of the infected cell.
- Entry inhibitors (fusion inhibitors and CCR5 antagonist) interfere with binding, fusion and entry of HIV-1 to the host cell by blocking one of several targets. Maraviroc and enfuvirtide are the two available agents in this class.

## Recommended Antiretroviral Therapy for Patients Naïve to Antiretroviral Therapy

Patients naïve to antiretroviral therapy should be started on a combination regimen that consists of either:

- 1-NNRTI + 2 NRTI or
- PI (preferably boosted with ritonavir) + 2 NRTI

The preferred nNRTI is Efavirenz, and the preferred PI is either Atazanvir, Darunavir, Fosemprenavir, or Lopinavir. The prefered NRTIs to be used in combination with the aforementioned drug are tenofovir + emtricitabine. When alternatives to the preferred regimen are needed for treatment, the prescriber should consult the latest treatment recommendations.

## Reasons to Change a Regimen

A change in regimen may be necessary because of insufficient viral suppression evident by an increase in VL, inadequate increase in CD4 cell counts, or evidence of disease progression, as well as adverse clinical effects on the patient or compromised adherence caused by the inconvenience of difficult regimens. However, the decision to change therapy should account for whether other drug choices are available because another regimen may also be poorly tolerated or fail to result in better viral suppression, and such a change may limit future treatment options.[59] The criteria for considering changing a patient's antiretroviral regimen include:

- Incomplete Virologic Suppression: when the HIV VL is greater than 400 copies after 24 weeks or greater than 50 copies after 48 weeks of therapy or there is a virologic rebound after complete virologic supression
- Persistent decline in CD4 cell or failure to achieve an adequate CD4 response despite virologic supression
- The occurrence or recurence of HIV-related events after at least 3 months on an antiretrovral regimen

Clinicians should consult with HIV specialists when considering a change in regimen. Furthermore, the change in an antiretroviral regimen can be guided by drug-resistance tests, such as genotyping and phenotyping assays. Drug resistance is a major short-term risk associated with any level of viral replication.[39]

### Concern Regarding Drug Interactions

Considerations should also be given to possible drug interactions such as pharmacokinetic interactions, which occur when administration of one agent changes the plasma concentration of another agent, and pharmacodynamic interactions, which occur when a drug interacts with the biologically active sites and changes the pharmacological effect of the drug without altering the plasma concentration. For example, in palliative care, drug interactions have been reported for patients who are receiving methadone for pain management and who begin therapy with the nNRTI nevirapine. These individuals have reported symptoms of opioid withdrawal within 4 to 8 days of beginning nevirapine because of its effect on the cytochrome P-450 metabolic enzyme CYP3A4 and its induction of methadone metabolism.[62] See Table 41–3 on antiretroviral medications for dosages, common side effects, special instructions, and drug interactions.

### Use and Continuation of Antiretrovirals in the Hospice/ Palliative Care Setting and in Patients With Organ Failure

The current to aims of antiretroviral therapy are to prevent progression to AIDS, prevent the direct effects and symptoms of HIV disease (such as dementia, neuropathy, and diarrhea), and to prevent the complications of AIDS. According to Von Gunten and colleagues, the continuation of antiretroviral therapy in hospice or palliative settings is often contingent on the feelings of patients regarding the therapy.[61] Patients can be asked, "How do you feel when you take your antiretroviral medications?" Because medications may still symbolize hope, patients who enter hospice may have a greater acceptance of their mortality and wish to stop antiretrovirals because of the side effects. Other patients may wish to

continue antiretroviral therapy because of its symptom relief and the prevention of future symptoms related to opportunistic infections. Von Gunten and colleagues suggest the following plan: [61]

1. If the drug causes burdensome symptoms, then discontinue.
2. If the patient no longer wants the drug, then discontinue.
3. If the patient is asymptomatic and wants the drug, then continue with close clinical assessment.
4. Discontinue the measurement of VLs and CD4 counts and help the patient focus on relief of symptoms.

In the hospice and palliative care settings, it is important for clinicians to discuss with patients and families their goals of care to make important decisions regarding the appropriateness of curative, palliative, or both types of interventions. More specifically, examples of clinical decisions about palliative or disease-specific care include: [63]

- The use of blood transfusions, psychostimulants, or corticosteroids to treat fatigue in patients with late-stage AIDS
- Aggressive antiemetic therapy for PI-induced nausea and vomiting or discontinuation of such antiretroviral therapies, given severe side effects
- Continued suppressive therapy for CMV retinitis to prevent blindness, or use of amphotericin B for azole-resistant candidiasis for patients who wish to continue eating, or other prophylactic medications in dying patients
- Palliative treatment of disseminated MAC in patients with advanced disease who are unwilling to take anti-infectives or withdrawal of MAC or PCP prophylaxis in patients who are expected to die soon
- Use of HAART for short-term palliation of symptoms related to high VLs or withdrawal of HAART after evident treatment failure, with assessment of medical risk–benefit and emotional value of therapy
- Decisions to initiate HAART in newly diagnosed late-stage patients

Selwyn and Rivard suggest that decisions regarding these issues need to be based on the specific goals of care, such as quality of life or life prolongation, the use of palliative care interventions to relieve the side effects of other medications, and the use of certain diseasespecific therapies to enhance quality of life, as well as the decision to not prolong life when a certain threshold is met, such as progressive dementia.[63]

The use of antiretrovirals must also be seriously considered for patients who have organ dysfunction or failure, given changes in hepatic and renal function and the effects on drug elimination. For example, patients with renal impairment may be at greater risk for zidovudine-induced hematological toxicity resulting from lowered production of erythropoietin. In addition, because of the markedly decreased clearance of ZVD and increased drug half-life, it is recommended that

**Table 41-3a**
**Characteristics of Nucleoside (NRTIs) and Non-Nucleoside Reverse Transcriptase Inhibitors (Non-NRTIs)**

| Generic Name (abbreviation)/ Trade Name | Formulation | Dosing Recommendations | Food Effect | Oral Bioavailability | Serum Half-Life | Intracellular Half-Life | Elimination | Adverse Events |
|---|---|---|---|---|---|---|---|---|
| **NRTIs** | | | | | | | | |
| Abacavir (ABC) ZIAGEN TRIZIVIR— w/ZDV+3TC EPZICOM— w/3TC | ZIAGEN 300 mg tablets or 20 mg/mL oral solution TRIZIVIR ABC 300 mg + ZDV 300 mg + 3TC 150 mg EPZICOM ABC 600 mg + 3TC 300 mg | ZIAGEN 300 mg BID or 600 mg once daily TRIZIVIR 1 tablet BID EPZICOM 1 tablet once daily | Take without regard to meals; Alcohol increases abacavir levels 41%; abacavir has no effect on alcohol | 83% | 1.5 hours | 12–26 hours | Metabolized by alcohol dehydrogenase and glucurononyl transferase. Renal excretion of metabolites 82% TRIZIVIR & EPZICOM– not for patients with CrCl < 50 mL/min | • Hypersensitivity reaction that can be fatal, symptoms may include fever, rash, nausea, vomiting, malaise or fatigue, loss of appetite, respiratory symptoms such as sore throat, cough, shortness of breath • Lactic acidosis with hepatic steatosis (rare but potentially life-threatening toxicity with use of NNRTIs) |
| Didanosine (ddI) VIDEX EC, Generic didanosine enteric coated (dose same as VIDEX EC) | VIDEX EC 125-, 200-, 250-, 400-mg capsules Buffered tablets (non-EC) are no longer available. VIDEX 10 mg/mL oral solution | Body weight ≥ 60 kg: 400 mg once daily* with TDF: 250 mg once daily < 60 kg: 250 mg once daily* with TDF: 200 mg once daily *Preferred dosing with oral solution is twice daily (total daily dose divided into two doses) | Levels decrease 55%; Take 1/2 hour before or 2 hours after meal | 30–40% | 1.5 hours | >20 hours | Renal excretion 50% Dosage adjustment in renal insufficiency | • Pancreatitis • Peripheral neuropathy • Nausea • Lactic acidosis with hepatic steatosis is a rare but potentially life-threatening toxicity associated with use of NRTIs. |
| Emtricitabine (FTC) EMTRIVA ATRIPLA—w/ EFV+TDF TRUVADA—w/ TDF | EMTRIVA 200 mg hard gelatin capsule and 10 mg/mL oral solution ATRIPLA EFV 600 mg + FTC 200 mg + TDF 300 mg TRUVADA FTC 200 mg + TDF 300 mg | EMTRIVA 200 mg capsule once daily or 240 mg (24 mL) oral solution once daily ATRIPLA 1 tablet once daily TRUVADA 1 tablet once daily | Take without regard to meals | 93% | 10 hours | >20 hours | Renal excretion Dosage adjustment in renal insufficiency ATRIPLA—not for patients with CrCl <50 mL/min TRUVADA—not for patients with CrCl <30 mL/min | • Minimal toxicity • Lactic acidosis with hepatic steatosis (rare but potentially life-threatening toxicity with use of NRTIs.) • Hyper-pigmentation/ skin discoloration |

| Drug | Formulation | Dose | Food effect | Bioavailability | Serum half-life | Intracellular half-life | Elimination | Adverse effects |
|---|---|---|---|---|---|---|---|---|
| Lamivudine (3TC) EPIVIR COMBIVIR—w/ZDV EPZICOM—w/ABC TRIZIVIR—w/ZDV+ABC | EPIVIR 150 or 300 mg tablets or 10 mg/mL oral solution COMBIVIR 3TC 150 mg + ZDV 300 mg EPZICOM 3TC 300 mg + ABC 600 mg TRIZIVIR 3TC 150 mg + ZDV 300 mg + ABC 300 mg | EPIVIR 150 mg BID or 300 mg once daily COMBIVIR 1 tablet BID EPZICOM 1 tablet once daily TRIZIVIR 1 tablet BID | Take without regard to meals | 86% | 5–7 hours | 18–22 hours | Renal excretion Dosage adjustment in renal insufficiency COMBIVIR, TRIZIVIR & EPZICOM—not for patients with CrCl <50 mL/min | • Minimal toxicity<br>• Lactic acidosis with hepatic steatosis (rare but potentially life-threatening toxicity with use of NRTIs) |
| Stavudine (d4T) ZERIT | ZERIT 15, 20, 30, 40-mg capsules or 1 mg/mL oral solution | Body weight ≥60 kg: 40 mg BID Body weight <60 kg: 30 mg BID | Take without regard to meals | 86% | 1.0 hour | 7.5 hours | Renal excretion 50% Dosage adjustment in renal insufficiency | • Peripheral neuropathy<br>• Lipodystrophy<br>• Pancreatitis<br>• Lactic acidosis with hepatic steatosis—higher incidence than w/other NRTIs<br>• Hyperlipidemia<br>• Rapidly progressive ascending neuromuscular weakness (rare) |
| Tenofovir Disoproxil Fumarate (TDF) VIREAD ATRIPLA—w/ EFV+FTC TRUVADA—w/ FTC | VIREAD 300 mg tablet ATRIPLA EFV 600 mg + FTC 200 mg + TDF 300 mg TRUVADA TDF 300 mg + FTC 200 mg | VIREAD 1 tablet once daily ATRIPLA 1 tablet once daily TRUVADA 1 tablet once daily | Take without regard to meals | 25% in fasting state; 39% with high-fat meal | 17 hours | >60 hours | Renal excretion Dosage adjustment in renal insufficiency ATRIPLA—not for patients with CrCl <50 mL/min TRUVADA—not for patients with CrCl <30 mL/min | • Asthenia, headache, diarrhea, nausea, vomiting, and flatulence<br>• Renal insufficiency, Fanconi syndrome<br>• Potential for osteopenia<br>• Lactic acidosis with hepatic steatosis (rare but potentially life-threatening toxicity with use of NRTIs) |

(continued)

**Table 41-3a**
**Characteristics of Nucleoside (NRTIs) and Non-Nucleoside Reverse Transcriptase Inhibitors (Non-NRTIs)** (*continued*)

| Generic Name (abbreviation)/ Trade Name | Formulation | Dosing Recommendations | Food Effect | Oral Bioavailability | Serum Half-Life | Intracellular Half-Life | Elimination | Adverse Events |
|---|---|---|---|---|---|---|---|---|
| Zidovudine (AZT, ZDV) RETROVIR COMBIVIR— w/3TC TRIZIVIR— w/3TC+ABC | RETROVIR 100 mg capsules, 300 mg tablets, 10 mg/mL intravenous solution, 10 mg/mL oral solution COMBIVIR 3TC 150 mg + ZDV 300 mg TRIZIVIR 3TC 150 mg + ZDV 300 mg + ABC 300 mg | RETROVIR 300 mg BID or 200 mg TID COMBIVIR 1 tablet BID TRIZIVIR 1 tablet BID | Take without regard to meals | 60% | 1.1 hours | 7 hours | Metabolized to AZT glucuronide (GAZT). Renal excretion of GAZT. Dosage adjustment in renal insufficiency COMBIVIR & TRIZIVIR— not for patients with CrCl < 50 mL/min | • Bone marrow suppression: macrocytic anemia or neutropenia • Gastrointestinal intolerance, headache, insomnia, asthenia • Lactic acidosis with hepatic steatosis (rare but potentially life-threatening toxicity associated with use of NRTIs) |
| **Non-NRTIs** | | | | | | | | |
| Delavirdine (DLV)/ RESCRIPTOR | 100-mg tablets or 200-mg tablets | 400 mg 3 times/day; four 100 mg tablets can be dispersed in ≥3 oz. of water to produce slurry; 200 mg tablets should be taken as intact tablets; separate dose from antacids by 1 hour | Take without regard to meals | 85% | 5.8 hours | | Metabolized by cytochrome P450 (3A inhibitor); 51% excreted in urine (<5% unchanged); 44% in feces | • Rash* • Increased transaminase levels • Headaches |
| Efavirenz (EFV)/ SUSTIVA Also available as ATRIPLA— with FTC + TDF | 50-, 100-, 200-mg capsules or 600-mg tablets ATRIPLA EFV 600 mg + FTC 200 mg + TDF 300 mg | 600 mg daily on an empty stomach, at or before bedtime | High-fat/high-caloric meals increase peak plasma concentrations of capsules by 39% and tablets by 79% take on an empty stomach | Data not available | 40–55 hours | | Metabolized by cytochrome P450 (3A mixed inducer/ inhibitor); No dosage adjustment in renal insufficiency if EFV is used alone; ATRIPLA— not for patients with CrCl <50 mL/min | • Rash* • Central nervous system symptoms† • Increased transaminase levels • False-positive cannabinoid test • Teratogenic in monkeys‡ |

| Etravirine (ETR)/ INTELENCE | 100-mg tablets | 200 mg twice daily following a meal | Take following a meal. Fasting conditions reduce drug exposure by approximately 50% | Unknown | 41 ± 20 hours | Metabolized by cytochrome P450 (3A4, 2C9, and 2C19 substrate, 3A4 inducer, 2C9 and 2C19 inhibitor) | • Rash* • Nausea |
| Nevirapine (NVP)/ VIRAMUNE | 200-mg tablets or 50 mg/5 mL oral suspension | 200 mg daily for 14 days; thereafter, 200 mg by mouth twice daily | Take without regard to meals | >90% | 25-30 hours | Metabolized by cytochrome P450 (3A inducer); 80% excreted in urine (glucuronidated metabolites; <5% unchanged); 10% in feces. Not recommended in patients with moderate-to-severe hepatic impairment (Child Pugh B or C). Dosage adjustment in hepatic insufficiency recommended | • Rash including Stevens-Johnson syndrome* • Symptomatic hepatitis, including fatal hepatic necrosis, have been reported‡ |

*During clinical trials, NNRTI was discontinued because of rash among 7% of patients taking nevirapine, 4.3% of patients taking delavirdine, 1.7% of patients taking efavirenz, and 2% of patients taking etravirine. Rare cases of Stevens-Johnson syndrome have been reported with the use of all four NNRTIs, the highest incidence seen with nevirapine use.

†Adverse events can include dizziness, somnolence, insomnia, abnormal dreams, confusion, abnormal thinking, impaired concentration, amnesia, agitation, depersonalization, hallucinations, and euphoria. Overall frequency of any of these symptoms associated with use of efavirenz was 52%, as compared with 26% among controls subjects; 2.6% of those persons on efavirenz discontinued the drug because of these symptoms; symptoms usually subside spontaneously after 2–4 weeks.

‡Symptomatic, sometimes serious, and even fatal hepatic events (accompanied by rash in approximately 50% of cases) occur with significantly higher frequency in treatment-naive female patients with prenevirapine CD4 counts >250 cells/mm³ or in treatment-naive male patients with prenevirapine CD4 counts >400 cells/mm³. Nevirapine should not be initiated in these patients unless the benefit clearly outweighs the risk. This toxicity has not been observed when nevirapine is given as single doses to mothers or infants for prevention of mother-to-child HIV transmission.

**Table 41–3b**
**Characteristics of Protease Inhibitors (PIs)**

| Generic Name/ Trade Name | Formulation | Dosing Recommendations | Food Effect | Oral Bioavailability | Serum Half-Life | Route of Metabolism | Storage | Adverse Events |
|---|---|---|---|---|---|---|---|---|
| **Atazanavir (ATV)/ REYATAZ** | 100 mg, 150 mg, 200 mg, 300 mg capsules | 400 mg once daily (unboosted ARV only recommended for PI-naïve pts) <u>With efavirenz or tenofovir TDF, or for ARV-experienced pts:</u> (ATV 300 mg + RTV 100 mg) once daily <u>With EFV in treatment-naïve pts:</u> (ATV 400 mg + RTV 100 mg) once daily | Administration with food increases bioavailability. Take with food; avoid taking simultaneously with antacids | Not determined | 7 hours | Cytochrome P450 3A4 inhibitor and substrate Dosage adjustment in hepatic insufficiency recommended | Room temperature (up to 25°C or 77°F) | • Indirect hyperbilirubinemia<br>• Prolonged PR interval—1st degree symptomatic AV block in some pts<br>• Use with caution in pts with underlying conduction defects or on concomitant medications that can cause PR prolongation<br>• Hyperglycemia<br>• Fat maldistribution<br>• Possible increased bleeding episodes in pts with hemophilia<br>• Nephrolithiasis |
| **Darunavir (DRV)/ PREZISTA** | 300 mg, 400 mg, 600 mg tablets | <u>ARV-naïve pts:</u> (DRV 800 mg + RTV 100 mg) once daily <u>ARV-experienced pts:</u> (DRV 600 mg + RTV 100 mg) BID Unboosted DRV is **not** recommended | Food ↑ Cmax & AUC by 30%—should be administered with food | <u>Absolute bioavailability:</u> DRV alone—37%; w/RTV—82%; | 15 hours (when combined with RTV) | Cytochrome P450 3A4 inhibitor and substrate | Room temperature (up to 25°C or 77°F) | • Skin rash (7%)—DRV has a sulfonamide moiety, Stevens-Johnson syndrome & erythrema multiforme have been reported.<br>• Hepatotoxicity<br>• Diarrhea, nausea<br>• Headache<br>• Hyperlipidemia<br>• Transaminase elevation<br>• Hyperglycemia<br>• Fat maldistribution<br>• Possible increased bleeding episodes in pts with hemophilia |

| Drug | Formulation | Dosing | Effect of Food | Bioavailability | Serum Half-Life | Metabolism/Elimination | Storage | Adverse Events |
|---|---|---|---|---|---|---|---|---|
| **Fosamprenavir (FPV)/ LEXIVA** | 700 mg tablet or 50 mg/mL oral suspension | ARV-naïve pts: • FPV 1,400 mg BID or • (FPV 1,400 mg + RTV 100–200 mg) once daily or • (FPV 700 mg + RTV 100 mg) BID PI-experienced pts (once daily dosing not recommended): • (FPV 700 mg + RTV 100 mg) BID or With EFV (FPV boosted only): • (FPV 700 mg + RTV 100 mg) BID or • (FPV 1,400 mg + RTV 300 mg) once daily | No significant change in amprenavir pharmacokinetics in fed or fasting state | Not established | 77 hours (amprenavir) | Amprenavir is a cytochrome P450 3A4 inhibitor, inducer, and substrate Dosage adjustment in hepatic insufficiency recommended | Room temperature (up to 25°C or 77°F) | • Skin rash (19%) • Diarrhea, nausea, vomiting • Headache • Hyperlipidemia • Transaminase elevation • Hyperglycemia • Fat maldistribution • Possible increased bleeding episodes in patients with hemophilia |
| **Indinavir/ CRIXIVAN** | 200 mg, 333 mg, 400 mg capsules | 800 mg every 8 hours; With RTV: (IDV 800 mg + RTV 100–200 mg) BID | Unboosted IDV: Levels decrease by 77% Take 1 hour before or 2 hours after meals; may take with skim milk or low-fat meal RTV-boosted IDV: Take with or without food | 65% | 1.5–2 hours | Cytochrome P450 3A4 inhibitor (less than ritonavir) Dosage adjustment in hepatic insufficiency recommended | Room temperature 15°–30°C (59°–86°F), protect from moisture | • Nephrolithiasis • GI intolerance, nausea • Indirect hyperbilirubinemia • Hyperlipidemia • Headache, asthenia, blurred vision, dizziness, rash, metallic taste, thrombocytopenia, alopecia, and hemolytic anemia • Hyperglycemia • Fat maldistribution • Possible increased bleeding episodes in pts with hemophilia |
| **Lopinavir + Ritonavir (LPV/r)/ KALETRA** | Each tablet contains LPV 200 mg + RTV 50 mg Oral solution: Each 5 mL contains LPV 400 mg + RTV 100 mg Note: Oral solution contains 42% alcohol | LPV 400 mg + RTV 100 mg (2 tablets or 5 mL) BID or LPV 800 mg + RTV 200 mg (4 tablets or 10 mL) once daily (**Note:** once-daily dosing only recommended for treatment-naive pts; not for pregnant women or patients receiving EFV, NVP, FPV, or NFV) With EFV or NVP: For ARV-experienced pts: LPV 600 mg + RTV 150 mg (3 tablets) BID or LPV 533 mg + RTV 133 mg (6.7 mL oral solution) BID with food | Oral tablet—No food effect; take with or without food Oral solution— Moderately fatty meal ↑LPV AUC & Cmin by 80% & 54%, respectively; take with food | Not determined in humans | 5–6 hours | Cytochrome P450 (3A4 inhibitor and substrate) | Oral tablet is stable at room temperature Oral solution is stable at 2°–8°C until date on label; is stable when stored at room temperature (up to 25°C or 77°F) for 2 months | • GI intolerance, nausea, vomiting, diarrhea (higher incidence with once-daily than twice-daily dosing) • Asthenia • Hyperlipidemia (esp. hypertriglyceridemia) • Elevated serum transaminases • Hyperglycemia • Fat maldistribution • Possible increased bleeding episodes in patients with hemophilia |

(continued)

Table 41–3b
**Characteristics of Protease Inhibitors (PIs)** *(continued)*

| Generic Name/ Trade Name | Formulation | Dosing Recommendations | Food Effect | Oral Bioavailability | Serum Half-Life | Route of Metabolism | Storage | Adverse Events |
|---|---|---|---|---|---|---|---|---|
| Nelfinavir (NFV)/ VIRACEPT | 250 mg, 625 mg tablets<br>50 mg/g oral powder | 1,250 mg BID or 750 mg TID | Levels increase two- to threefold<br>Take with meal or snack | 20%–80% | 3.5–5 hours | Cytochrome P450 3A4 inhibitor and substrate | Room temperature 15°–30°C (59°–86°F) | • Diarrhea<br>• Hyperlipidemia<br>• Hyperglycemia<br>• Fat maldistribution<br>• Possible increased bleeding episodes among patients with hemophilia<br>• Serum transaminase elevation |
| Ritonavir (RTV)/ NORVIR | 100 mg capsules or 80 mg/mL oral solution | As pharmacokinetic booster for other PIs: 100 mg–400 mg per day in 1–2 divided doses (please refer to other PIs for specific dosing recommendations)<br>600 mg every 12 hours (when ritonavir is used as sole PI) | Levels increase 15%<br>Take with food if possible; this may improve tolerability | Not determined | 3–5 hours | Cytochrome P450 (3A4 > 2D6) substrate; Potent 3A4, 2D6 inhibitor | Refrigerate capsules<br>Capsules can be left at room temperature (up to 25°C or 77°F) for ≤30 days; Oral solution should NOT be refrigerated | • GI intolerance, nausea, vomiting, diarrhea<br>• Paresthesias—circumoral and extremities<br>• Hyperlipidemia, esp. hypertriglyceridemia<br>• Hepatitis<br>• Asthenia<br>• Taste perversion<br>• Hyperglycemia<br>• Fat maldistribution<br>• Possible increased bleeding episodes in patients with hemophilia |
| Saquinavir tablets and hard gel capsules (SQV)/ INVIRASE | 200 mg hard gel capsules, 500 mg tablets | (SQV 1,000 mg + RTV 100 mg) PO BID<br>Unboosted SQV is not recommended | Take within 2 hours of a meal | 4% erratic (when taken as sole PI) | 1–2 hours | Cytochrome P450 (3A4 inhibitor and substrate) | Room temperature 15°–30°C (59°–86°F) | • GI intolerance, nausea and diarrhea<br>• Headache<br>• Elevated transaminase enzymes<br>• Hyperlipidemia<br>• Hyperglycemia<br>• Fat maldistribution<br>• Possible increased bleeding episodes in patients with hemophilia |

| Tipranavir (TPV)/ APTIVUS | 250 mg capsules | (TPV 500 mg + RTV 200 mg) PO BID Unboosted TPV is **not** recommended | No clinically significant change in TPV pharmacokinetics in fed or fasting state | Not determined | 6 hours after single dose of TPV/ RTV | TPV— Cytochrome P450 (3A4 inducer and substrate) Net effect when combined with RTV—CYP 3A4 inhibitor and CYP 2D6 inhibitor | Refrigerated capsules are stable until date on label; if stored at room temperature (up to 25°C or 77°F)— must be used within 60 days | • Hepatotoxicity—clinical hepatitis including hepatic decompensation has been reported, monitor closely, esp. in patients with underlying liver diseases<br>• Skin rash—TPV has a sulfonamide moiety, use with caution in patients with known sulfonamide allergy<br>• Rare cases of fatal and nonfatal intracranial hemorrhages have been reported. Most patients had underlying comorbidity such as brain lesion, head trauma, recent neurosurgery, coagulopathy, hypertension, alcoholism, or on medication with increase risk for bleeding<br>• Hyperlipidemia (esp. hypertriglyceridemia)<br>• Hyperglycemia<br>• Fat maldistribution<br>• Possible increased bleeding episodes in patients with hemophilia |

*Dose escalation for Ritonavir when used as sole PI: Days 1 and 2: 300 mg two times; Days 3–5: 400 mg two times; Days 6–13: 500 mg two times; Day 14: 600 mg two times/day.

**Table 41-3c**
**Characteristics of Fusion Inhibitors**

| Generic Name (abbreviation)/ Trade Name | Formulation | Dosing Recommendations | Food Effect | Oral Bioavailability | Serum half-life | Route of Metabolism | Storage | Adverse Events |
|---|---|---|---|---|---|---|---|---|
| Enfuvirtide (T20)/ FUZEON | • Injectable—in lyophilized powder • Each vial contains 108 mg of enfuvirtide, reconstitute with 1.1 mL of Sterile Water for injection for delivery of approximately 90 mg/1 mL | 90 mg (1 mL) sub-cutaneously BID | Not appli-cable | Not applicable | 3.8 hours | Expected to undergo catabolism to its constituent amino acids, with subsequent recycling of the amino acids in the body pool | Store at room temperature (up to 25°C or 77°F) Reconstituted solution should be stored under refrigeration at 2°C–8°C (36°F–46F°) and used within 24 hours | • Local injection site reactions—almost 100% of patients (pain, erythema, induration, nodules and cysts, pruritus, ecchymosis) • Increased bacterial pneumonia • Hypersensitivity reaction (<1%)—symptoms may include rash, fever, nausea, vomiting, chills, rigors, hypotension, or elevated serum transaminases; rechallenge is not recommended |

**Table 41-3d**
**Characteristics of CCR5 Antagonists**

| Generic Name (abbreviation)/Trade Name | Formulation | Dosing Recommendations | Food Effect | Oral Bio-availability | Serum Half-Life | Route of Metabolism | Storage | Adverse Events |
|---|---|---|---|---|---|---|---|---|
| Maraviroc (MVC)/ SELZENTRY | 150-mg, 300-mg tablets | • **150 mg BID** when given with strong CYP3A inhibitors (with or without CYP3A inducers) including PIs (except tipranavir/ritonavir) • **300 mg BID** when given with NRTIs, enfuvirtide, tipranavir/ritonavir, nevirapine, and other drugs that are not strong CYP3A inhibitors • **600 mg BID** when given with CYP3A inducers, including efavirenz, rifampin, etc. (without a CYP3A inhibitor) | No food effect; take with or without food | 23% for 100-mg dose and 33% (predicted) for 300 mg | 14–18 hrs | Cytochrome P450 (CYP3A substrate) | Room temperature | Abdominal pain, cough, dizziness, musculoskeletal symptoms, pyrexia, rash, upper respiratory tract infections, hepatotoxicity, orthostatic hypotension. |

**Table 41-3e**
**Characteristics of Integrase Inhibitors**

| Generic Name (abbreviation)/Trade Name | Formulation | Dosing Recommendations | Food Effect | Oral Bioavailability | Serum Half-Life | Route of Metabolism | Storage | Adverse Events |
|---|---|---|---|---|---|---|---|---|
| Raltegravir (RAL)/ ISENTRESS | 400-mg tablets | 400 mg BID | Take with or without food | Not established | ≈ 9 hrs | UGT1A1-mediated glucuronidation | Room temperature | Nausea, headache, diarrhea, pyrexia, CPK elevation |

the daily dosage of ZVD be reduced by approximately 50% in patients with severe renal dysfunction (CrCL, 25 mL/min), for those receiving hemodialysis, and for those with hepatic dysfunction.[64] Additionally, because of reduced drug clearance, patients should be monitored for ZVD-related adverse effects.

As many of the antiretroviral agents are metabolized by the liver and excreted by the kidney, knowledge of pharmacokinetic properties of antiretroviral drugs is recommended to monitor drug therapy for efficacy and safety.[64] Table 41–4 presents the suggested dosing recommendations for antiretroviral agents in patients with organ dysfunction.

### Adherence to Therapy

Adherence, which is "the extent to which a person's behavior coincides with medical and health advice,"[65] is essential to health maintenance for patients with HIV/AIDS because nonadherence to antiretroviral therapy may lead to HIV drug resistance. Medication adherence is defined as the ratio of medication doses taken to those prescribed. The gold standard for medication adherence requires that more than 95% of the regimen be taken to achieve full supression, More recent adherence studies that utilized boosted PIs and nNRTIs suggest that boosted PIs and efavirenz may be more forgiving of lapses in adherence because of their longer half-lives.[66,67] Simplifying the patient's HAART regimen to decrease the number of medications taken and the number of times the patient has to take medications can improve adherence.[70] Assessment of adherence is most often done by self-report, with studies showing that it is a valid indicator of adherence.[68] Important aspects of assessment include asking patients to bring their medications to a health visit, to describe their pill-taking regimens, to review the number of doses taken in 24 hours, and to ask about problems taking the medications and effects of the medications.[69] Factors not predictive of adherence include age, sex, race, education, occupation, and socioeconomic status,[70] whereas factors predictive of adherence include the following:[71]

- Patient characteristics, such as physical and emotional health, material resources, cultural beliefs, self-efficacy, social support, personal skills, and HIV knowledge
- Clinician factors, including interpersonal style and availability, as well as assessment, communication, and clinical skills
- Medication regimen factors, such as frequency, number, and size of pills, taste of pills, storage, side effects, effectiveness, and cost
- Illness factors, including symptoms duration, severity, and stigma

Adherence to medication regimens can be improved through educational, behavioral, and social interventions, specific to the patient, clinician, and medication regimen (Table 41–5).[69] An established partnership and an open, trusting, and supportive relationship between patient and clinician remain key factors in promoting not only adherence to medication regimens but support of all health-promotion and management initiatives to delay disease progression and AIDS-related complications.

## AIDS-Related Opportunistic Infections and Malignancies

Opportunistic infections are the greatest cause of morbidity and mortality in individuals with HIV. Given the compromised immune system of HIV-infected individuals, there is a wide spectrum of pathogens that can produce primary, life-threatening infections, particularly when the CD4 cell counts fall below 200 cells/mm³. Given the weakened immune systems of HIV-infected persons, even previously acquired infections can be reactivated. Most of these opportunistic infections are incurable and can at best be palliated to control the acute stage of infection and prevent recurrence through long-term suppressive therapy. Additionally, patients with HIV/AIDS often experience concurrent or consecutive opportunistic infections that are severe and cause a great number of symptoms. Table 41–6 reviews the various categories of opportunistic infections and malignancies with regard to epidemiology/pathogenesis, presentation and assessment, diagnosis, and interventions.

### Pain and Symptom Management in HIV

Patients with HIV/AIDS require symptom management not only for chronic debilitating opportunistic infections and malignancies but also for the side effects of treatments and other therapies. There are five broad principles fundamental to successful symptom management: (1) taking the symptoms seriously, (2) assessment, (3) diagnosis, (4) treatment, and (5) ongoing evaluation.[72]

- *Taking the symptoms seriously* implies that symptoms often are not observable and measurable. Therefore, self-report of the patient should be taken seriously by the practitioner and acknowledged as a real experience of the patient. An important rule in symptom management is to anticipate the symptom and attempt to prevent it.[30] Assessment and diagnosis of signs and symptoms of disease and treatment side effects require a thorough history and physical examination. Questions regarding when the symptom began and its location, duration, severity, and quality, as well as factors that exacerbate or alleviate the symptom, are important. Patients can also be asked to rate the severity of a symptom by using a numerical scale from 0 to 10, with 0 being "no symptom" and 10 being

**Table 41–4**
**Antiretroviral Dosing Recommendations in Patients with Renal or Hepatic Insufficiency**

| Antiretrovirals | Daily Dose | Dosing in Renal Insufficiency | | | | Dosing in Hepatic Impairment |
|---|---|---|---|---|---|---|
| Nucleoside Reverse Transcriptase Inhibitors—Note: Use of fixed-dose combination NRTI (± NNRTI) of: ATRIPLA, COMBIVIR, TRIZIVIR, EPZICOM—not recommended in patients with CrCl <50 mL/min; use of TRUVADA—not recommended in patients with CrCl <30 mL/min | | | | | | |
| Abacavir* (ZIAGEN) | 300 mg PO BID | No need for dosage adjustment | | | | No dosage recommendation |
| Didanosine (VIDEX EC) | ≥60 kg 400 mg PO once daily | | | **Dose** | | No dosage recommendation |
| | | CrCl (mL/min) | >60 kg | <60 kg | | |
| | | 30–59 | 200 mg | 125 mg | | |
| | | 10–29 | 125 mg | 125 mg | | |
| | | <10 | 125 mg | not recommended* | | |
| | <60 kg 250 mg once daily | CAPD or HD patients >60 kg: use same dose as CrCl <10 mL/min | | | | |
| | | CAPD or HD patients <60 kg: not recommended* | | | | |
| | | *Use oral solution | | | | |
| Didanosine oral solution (VIDEX) | ≥60 kg 200 mg PO twice daily or 400 mg PO once daily | | **Dose (once daily)** | | | No dosage recommendation |
| | | CrCl (mL/min) | >60 kg | <60 kg | | |
| | <60 kg 250 mg once daily or 125 mg twice daily | 30–59 | 200 mg | 150 mg | | |
| | | 10–29 | 150 mg | 100 mg | | |
| | | <10 | 100 mg | 75 mg | | |
| | | CAPD or HD patients >60 kg: use same dose as CrCl <10 mL/min | | | | |
| Emtricitabine (EMTRIVA) | 200 mg oral capsule PO once daily or 240 mg (24 mL) oral solution PO once daily | CrCl | capsule | solution | | No dosage recommendation |
| | | 30–49 | 200 mg q48h | 120mg q24h | | |
| | | 15–29 | 200 mg q72h | 80 mg q24h | | |
| | | <15 | 200 mg q96h | 60 mg q24h | | |
| | | or HD* | | | | |
| | | CrCl (mL/min) | | **Dose** | | |
| | | 30–49 | | 150 mg q24h | | |
| | | 15–29 1 | | 50 mg × 1, then 100 mg q24h | | |
| | | 5–14 | | 150 mg × 1, then 50 mg q24h | | |
| | | <5 | | 50 mg × 1, then 25 mg q24h | | |
| | | or HD* | | | | |

| Drug | Dose | CrCl (mL/min) | Dose | | |
|---|---|---|---|---|---|

| Lamivudine* (EPIVIR) | 300 mg PO once daily or 150 mg PO BID | | | | No dosage recommendation |

**Stavudine (ZERIT)** — No dosage recommendation

| | | CrCl (mL/min) | Dose | |
|---|---|---|---|---|
| | | | **>60 kg** | **<60 kg** |
| | ≥60 kg: 40 mg PO BID | 26–50 | 20 mg q12h | 15 mg q12h |
| | <60 kg: 30 mg PO BID | 10–25 or HD* | 20 mg q24h | 15 mg q24h |

| Tenofovir (VIREAD) | 300 mg PO once daily | CrCl (mL/min) | Dose | | No dosage recommendation |
|---|---|---|---|---|---|
| | | 30–49 | 300 mg q48h | | |
| | | 10–29 | 300 mg twice weekly | | |
| | | ESRD or HD* | 300 mg q7d | | |

| Tenofovir + Emtricitabine (TRUVADA) | 1 tablet PO once daily | CrCl (mL/min) | Dose | | No dosage recommendation |
|---|---|---|---|---|---|
| | | 30–49 | tablet q48h | | |
| | | <30 | not recommended | | |

| Zidovudine* (RETROVIR) | 300 mg PO BID | "Severe" renal impairment (CrCl < 15 mL/min) or HD*: 100 mg TID or 300 mg once daily | | | No dosage recommendation |

**Non-Nucleoside Reverse Transcriptase Inhibitors**

| Delavirdine (RESCRIPTOR) | 400 mg PO TID | No dosage adjustment necessary | | | No recommendation; use with caution in patients with hepatic impairment |
|---|---|---|---|---|---|

| Efavirenz (SUSTIVA) | 600 mg PO once daily | No dosage adjustment necessary | | | No recommendation; use with caution in patients with hepatic impairment |
|---|---|---|---|---|---|
| Efavirenz/tenofovir/emtricitabine (ATRIPLA) | One tablet PO once daily | ATRIPLA™—not recommended if CrCl <50 mL/min | | | |

| Etravirine (INTELENCE) | 200 mg PO BID following a meal | No dosage adjustment necessary | | | No dosage adjustment for Child-Pugh Class A or B. Has not been evaluated in patients with Child-Pugh Class C |
|---|---|---|---|---|---|

| Nevirapine (VIRAMUNE) | 200 mg PO BID | No dosage adjustment necessary | | | Contraindicated in patients with Child-Pugh Class B or C |
|---|---|---|---|---|---|

(continued)

**Table 41-4**

**Antiretroviral Dosing Recommendations in Patients with Renal or Hepatic Insufficiency** (*continued*)

| Antiretrovirals | Daily Dose | Dosing in Renal Insufficiency | Dosing in Hepatic Impairment | |
|---|---|---|---|---|
| **Protease inhibitors** | | | | |
| Atazanavir (REYATAZ, ATV) | 400 mg PO once daily or (ATV 300 mg + RTV 100 mg) once daily | No dosage adjustment for patients with renal dysfunction not requiring hemodialysis  Treatment-naïve patients on hemodialysis: ATV 300 mg + RTV 100 mg once daily  Treatment-experienced patients on hemodialysis: ATV or RTV-boosted ATV not recommended | **Child-Pugh Score** | **Dose** |
| | | | 7–9 | 300 mg once daily |
| | | | >9 | not recommended |
| | | | RTV boosting is not recommended in patients with hepatic impairment | |
| Darunavir (PREZISTA, DRV) | (DRV 800 mg + RTV 100 mg) PO once daily (ARV-naïve pts) (DRV 600 mg + RTV 100 mg) PO BID | No dosage adjustment necessary | No dosage adjustment in patients with mild-to-moderate hepatic impairment. DRV is not recommended in patients with severe hepatic impairment. | |
| Fosamprenavir (LEXIVA, FPV) | 1,400 mg PO BID; or (FPV 1,400 mg + 100–200 mg RTV) PO once daily; or (FPV 700 mg + RTV 100 mg) PO BID | No dosage adjustment necessary | **Child-Pugh Score** | **Dose** |
| | | | 5–8 | 700 mg BID |
| | | | 9–12 | not recommended |
| | | | Ritonavir boosting should not be used in patients with hepatic impairment | |
| Indinavir (CRIXIVAN) | 800 mg PO q8h | No dosage adjustment necessary | Mild to moderate hepatic insufficiency because of cirrhosis: 600 mg q8h | |
| Lopinavir/ritonavir (KALETRA) | 400/100 mg PO BID or 800/200 mg PO once daily (only for treatment-naïve patients) | No dosage adjustment necessary | No dosage recommendation; use with caution in patients with hepatic impairment | |
| Nelfinavir (VIRACEPT) | 1,250 mg PO BID | No dosage adjustment necessary | No dosage recommendation; use with caution in patients with hepatic impairment | |
| Ritonavir (NORVIR) | 600 mg PO BID | No dosage adjustment necessary | No dosage adjustment in mild hepatic impairment; no data for moderate to severe impairment, use with caution | |
| Saquinavir (INVIRASE, SQV) | (SQV 1,000 mg + RTV 100 mg) PO BID | No dosage adjustment necessary | No dosage recommendation; use with caution in patients with hepatic impairment | |
| Tipranavir (APTIVUS) | (TPV 500 mg + RTV 200 mg) PO BID | No dosage adjustment necessary | No dosage recommendation; use with caution in Child-Pugh Class A; TPV/RTV is contraindicated in pts with moderate to severe (Child-Pugh Class B & C) hepatic insufficiency | |
| **Fusion inhibitors** | | | | |
| Enfuvirtide (FUZEON) | 90 mg SUB-Q q12h | No dosage adjustment necessary | No dosage recommendation | |
| **CCR5 antagonists** | | | | |
| Maraviroc (SELZENTRY) | The recommended dose differs based on concomitant medications because of drug interactions. See Table 41–3d for detailed dosing information. | No dosage recommendation; use with caution. Patients with CrCl <50 mL/min should receive MVC and CYP3A inhibitor only if potential benefits outweigh the risk. | No dosage recommendations. Concentrations will likely be increased in patients with hepatic impairment. | |

## Integrase inhibitors

| | | | |
|---|---|---|---|
| Raltegravir (ISENTRESS) | 400 mg twice daily | No dosage adjustment. | No dosage adjustment. |

**Creatinine Clearance calculation:**

$$\text{Male: } \frac{(140\text{-age in yr}) \times \text{weight (kg)}}{72 \times \text{S.Cr.}} \text{ ; Female: } \frac{(140\text{-age in yr}) \times \text{weight (kg)} \times 0.85}{72 \times \text{S.Cr.}}$$

## Child-Pugh Score

| Component | Score Given | | |
|---|---|---|---|
| | **1** | **2** | **3** |
| Encephalopathy* | None | Grade 1–2 | Grade 3–4 |
| Ascites | None | Mild or controlled by diuretics | Moderate or refractory despite diuretics |
| Albumin | >3.5 g/dL | 2.8–3.5 g/dL | <2.8 g/dL |
| Total Bilirubin OR | <2 mg/dL (<34 µmol/L) | 2–3 mg/dL (34 µmol/L to 50 µmol/L) | >3 mg/dL (>50 µmol/L) |
| Modified Total Bilirubin** | <4 mg/dL | 4–7 mg/dL | >7 mg/dL |
| Prothrombin time (sec prolonged) OR INR | <4 / <1.7 | 4–6 / 1.7–2.3 | >6 / >2.3 |

HD* = dose after dialysis on dialysis days, HD = hemodialysis, CAPD = chronic ambulatory peritoneal dialysis, ESRD = End Stage Renal Disease.

*NB: Encephalopathy Grades—Grade 1: Mild confusion, anxiety, restlessness, fine tremor, slowed coordination; Grade 2: Drowsiness, disorientation, asterixis; Grade 3: Somnolent but rousable, marked confusion, incomprehensible speech, incontinence, hyperventilation; Grade 4: Coma, decerebrate posturing, flaccidity

**Modified Total Bilirubin used to score patients who have Gilbert's syndrome or who are taking indinavir **Child-Pugh Classification**—Child-Pugh Class A = score 5–6; Class B = score 7–9; Class C = score >9.

**Table 41–5**
**Interventions to Improve Antiretroviral Medication Adherence**

| Type of Intervention | Specific Examples |
|---|---|
| **Interventions addressing the patient** | |
| Key patient education topics | Dynamics of HIV infection |
| | Purpose of antiretroviral therapy |
| | All names of medications |
| | Reasons for dose and administration requirements |
| | Potential side effects |
| | Techniques for managing side effects |
| Cues and reminders for patient | Detailed daily schedule |
| | Doses planned to coincide with daily habits (favorite TV program, morning news) |
| | Medication boxes and timers (available from some pharmaceutical companies) |
| | Prepoured medications |
| | Unit-of-use packaging |
| Patient involvement in therapeutic plan | Contributes to choice of antiretroviral combination |
| | Self-control of medications for side effects |
| | Anticipatory planning for weekends, vacations |
| Rewards and reinforcements | Positive feedback: falling HIV RNA level, rising CD4+ cell count, fewer clinic appointments |
| Social support for adherence | Involvement of significant others |
| | Support groups |
| | Peer counseling and buddy plans |
| | Treatment of concomitant conditions such as substance abuse, depression |
| | Case management and financial assistance |
| | Home visits and telephone follow-up |
| **Interventions addressing the clinician** | |
| Continuing education regarding | Importance of adherence |
| | Factors associated with adherence |
| | Techniques to increase adherence |
| | Teaching skills |
| | Communication skills |
| | Effective management of side effects |
| Cues and reminders for the clinician | User-friendly medication review forms |
| | Tables and checklists in the clinical chart |
| | Patient teaching tools |
| Social support | Involvement of colleagues |
| | Team approach |
| | Administrative approval for additional time spent with patient on adherence concerns |
| **Interventions addressing the regimen** | Once- or twice-a-day dosing regimens |
| | Use of fewer pills per day |
| | Use of smaller pills or capsules |
| | Improved taste |
| | Simpler storage requirements |
| | Fewer side effects |
| | Increased effectiveness |
| | Decreased cost |

*Source:* Williams (1999), reference 69. Copyright 1999 with permission from Elsevier.

**Table 41-6**
**Opportunistic Infections and Malignancies Associated with HIV/AIDS**

| Types of Infections and Malignancies | Epidemiology/Pathogenesis | Presentation and Assessment | Diagnosis | Interventions |
|---|---|---|---|---|
| **Fungal infections** | | | | |
| *Candida albicans* | Ubiquitous organism. Occurs with immunosuppression/alteration in mucous membranes or skin. Early manifestation of HIV. Predictor of disease progression. Human-to-human transmission possible. Oropharyngeal candidiasis common. | Oral *Candida* manifests as pseudomembranous white patches, easily removed, leaving erythematous or bleeding mucosa. Vaginal candidiasis manifests with pruritus and curdlike vaginal discharge. Esophageal candidiasis manifests with dysphagia. *Candida* leukoplakia cannot be removed. | Often presumptive by tissue inspection. Wet mount and/or potassium hydroxide (KOH) smear showing budding hyphae. Esophageal diagnosis by endoscopy with biopsy. Diagnosis by culture is unreliable. | Mucotaneous infection treated locally with clotrimazole troches, nystatin suspension, fluconazole, miconazole, or amphotericin B |
| *Coccidioides immitis* (Coccidioidomycosis) | Endemic to south western United States. Acquired by inhalation of spores. Occurs with CD4+ count <250 μL. | May be asymptomatic or with progressive signs of fever, malaise, weight loss, cough, fatigue. | Chest radiographs may show diffuse interstitial or nodular infiltrates. Definitive diagnosis by culture or direct visualization of the organism in sputum, urine, or CSF. | System amphotericin B, followed by lifelong suppressive therapy with oral fluconazole |
| *Cryptococcus neoformans* (Cryptococcosis) | Ubiquitous organism. Aerosolized and inhaled. Most common life-threatening infection in AIDS. *Cryptococcus* meningitis photophobia, has a high mortality rate. | Meningitis is most common clinical manifestation, with headache, fever, stiff neck, lethargy, and confusion. Symptoms develop over 2–4 wk. Cranial nerve palsies occur. Decreased vision; can lead to blindness. Cryptococcal pneumonia may present with cough, dyspnea. Infection may disseminate to bone marrow, kidney, liver, spleen, lymph nodes, heart, oral cavity, and prostate. | Serum cryptococcal antigen is 99% indicative. Examination of CSF. Infection of extrameningeal sites diagnosed with India ink and culture of tissues and specimens. MRI or CT scan can show cryptococcoma. Chest radiographs show diffuse or focal infiltrates with or without mediastinal adenopathy. | Acute therapy with amphotericin B with or without fluconazole, then lifelong suppression with fluconazole |
| *Histoplasma capsulatum* | Endemic to midwest and south central United States. Spores are inhaled. Occurs with CD4+ counts <100 μL. | Cough with fever. Often disseminated disease rather than pneumonitis. Signs and symptoms include fever, weight loss, night sweats, nausea, diarrhea, abdominal pain. | Chest radiographs show diffuse bilateral interstitial infiltrates. One third have normal chest radiograph; 5–10% have cutaneous lesions. | Amphotericin B for serious illness or itraconazole or fluconazole for mild disease. Lifelong therapy of itraconazole or fluconazole |
| **Mycobacterial infection** | | | | |
| *Mycobacterium tuberculosis* (TB) | Increase in infections attributable to the high incidence of HIV infection. HIV infection may lead to reactivation of latent TB infection. Outbreaks of multidrug-resistant TB. Caused by inhalation of infectious particles that are aerosolized. Can have latent infection with no symptoms of active TB. Extrapulmonary TB may occur in 70% of HIV-infected patients; TB decreases CD4+ count and increases viral load. | Fever, weight loss, night sweats, and fatigue are initial complaints. With pulmonary TB, dyspnea, hemoptysis, and chest pain may occur. Extrapulmonary sites such as lymph nodes, bones, bone marrow, joints liver, spleen, skin, and CSF may show TB. | Positive PPD is defined as >5 mm of induration at 48–72 h using Mantoux intradermal method. Check for anergy with use of mumps and *Candida*. Chest radiographs show apical or cavitary infiltrates, and may show intrathoracic adenopathy. Diagnosis confirmed by sputum for acid-fast bacilli (AFB) stain. Blood cultures for AFB should be obtained. | Four-drug regimen with isoniazid, rifampin, pyrazinamide, and either streptomycin or ethambutol. Prophylaxis with isoniazid or rifampin for individuals without current active TB. |

*(continued)*

**Table 41–6**
**Opportunistic Infections and Malignancies Associated with HIV/AIDS** (*continued*)

| Types of Infections and Malignancies | Epidemiology/Pathogenesis | Presentation and Assessment | Diagnosis | Interventions |
|---|---|---|---|---|
| *Mycobacterium avium intracellulare* (MAC) | Composed of *M. avium* and *M. intracellulare*, two related species. Exists in water, soil, and foodstuffs. Person-to-person transmission is not likely. Most common cause of systemic bacterial infection in AIDS. Disseminated disease frequently the cause of mortality in advanced HIV disease. | Respiratory symptoms uncommon. MAC bacteremia is the most common syndrome. Fever, fatigue, weight loss, anorexia, nausea and vomiting, night sweats, diarrhea, abdominal pain, hepatosplenomegaly, and lymphadenopathy are common symptoms. | Positive cultures from normally sterile sites (e.g., blood, bone marrow, lymph nodes). Confirmed by biopsy with AFB stain. Lab studies usually demonstrate anemia and elevated alkaline phosphatase. | Macrolide (clarithromycin or azithromycin) and rifabutin and ethambutol for acute treatment. Prophylaxis with rifabutin or clarithromycin or azithromycin |
| **Viral infections** | | | | |
| Cytomegalovirus (CMV) | Ubiquitous, human herpesvirus. Most common cause of serious opportunistic disease in AIDS. May have contracted primary infection in childhood or young adulthood. Occurs in >40% of patients with CD4+ count <50/μL. | CMV retinitis most common form; if untreated, can quickly lead to blindness. May be asymptomatic or with painless loss of visual acuity and symptoms of floaters or visual field defects, or conjunctivitis. GI tract is second most common site, with symptoms of dysphagia, abdominal pain, odynophagia, fever, bloody diarrhea, and colitis. | CMV retinitis on ophthalmoscopic exam shows creamy yellow-white exudate with retinal hemorrhage. GI CMV is demonstrated by endocscopy showing ulceration and tissue biopsy. | High doses of ganciclovir or foscarnet, followed by lifelong daily IV infusions, with maintenance doses of one of these two medications |
| Herpes simplex virus (HSV) | HSV-1 transmitted primarily by contact with mucous membranes and salivary secretions. HSV-2 spread by sexual transmission. Risk with CD4+ count <100/μL. | Cutaneous ulcerative, vesicular painful lesions on any part of the body, particularly face, genitals, or perianal area. May cause esophagitis with dysphagia and odynophagia. | Visual infection with confirmation by viral swab culture. If vesicle is present, it should be unroofed with 18-gauge needle and swabbed over the base of the ulcer. | Acyclovir is used in primary therapy. IV acyclovir for severe HIV infection or HSV encephalitis. Topical acyclovir ointment to relieve subjective symptoms. Maintenance therapy with acyclovir to prevent reactivation. |
| Varicella-zoster virus (VZV) (herpes zoster—shingles) | Herpesvirus; may be initial presentation of HIV infection. Recurrent or disseminated VZV is seen with advanced HIV disease. Primary VZV is chickenpox. | Radicular pain, a localized burning, followed by localized maculopapular rash along a dermatome progressing to fluid-filled continuous vesicles. Postherpatic neuralgia may persist for months after lesions have healed. Visceral dissemination to lung, liver, or CNS is life threatening. | Clinical appearance. Cutaneous scrapings stained with fluorescein-conjugated monoclonal antibodies to confirm presence of VZV antigens. | Acyclovir, famciclovir, ganciclovir, or foscarnet for acute treatment |
| Human papilloma virus (HPV) | Most prevalent STD. Occurs with increased frequency in immunocompromised patients | Genital and perianal warts in men and women. Internal warts may also occur. | Cytological dysplasia evident on smears. | Trichloroacetic acid 50% or podophyllin 25% or podofilox or 5-fluorouracil cream for acute treatment. Electrosurgery or surgical excision |

| | | | | |
|---|---|---|---|---|
| **Protozoal infections** | | | | |
| *Cryptosporidium parvum* | Transmitted through fecally contaminated water or food. May spread person-to-person in HIV-infected individuals. Oocyts can remain active outside the body for 2–6 mo. Major cause of diarrhea when $CD_{4+}$ count <200/μL. | Profuse watery diarrhea, severe crampy abdominal pain, nausea, flatulence, weight loss, electrolyte imbalance, dehydration. May lead to malabsorption and wasting syndrome. | Confirmed by modified acid-fast or fluorescent antibody stain of stool specimen or small bowel biopsy. | Restore immune system with HAART. No currently approved specific agent. Paromomycin or nitrazoxanide may be beneficial. |
| *Toxoplasma gondii* | Occurs worldwide in humans and domestic animals, particularly cats. Oocyts transmitted in infected meats, eggs, vegetables, and other food products. Major cause of neurological morbidity and mortality, especially in individuals with $CD_{4+}$ count <100 μL. | Toxoplasmosis encephalitis most common with headache, fever, altered mental status, focal neurological deficits, and seizures. | Laboratory studies nonspecific. CT scan with contrast or brain MRI shows multiple diffuse mass lesions with edema. Examination of CSF usually is not helpful. | Pyrimethamine and folinic acid as first-line treatment for acute infection. Second-line treatment with clindamycin or atovaqu-one-oneor clarithromycin or mycin. Lifelong prophylaxis with TMP-SMX for those with CD4+ count <100/μL. |
| *Isospora belli* | Distributed throughout the animal kingdom and endemic to parts of Africa, Chile, and Southeast Asia. Transmission through direct contact with infected animals, persons, or contaminated water. Shed in the stool of humans or host animals. Latino and foreign-born persons are at greater risk. | Profuse watery, diarrhea, with stool output averaging 8–10 bowel movements per day, steatorrhea, headache, fever, malaise, abdominal pain, vomiting, dehydration, and weight loss. | Identification of oocytes in the stool. Suggest minimum of four stool specimens taken for patients with AIDS. A rapid autofluorescence technique may help in making a more rapid and reliable diagnosis. | TMP-SMX or pyrimethamine for acute treatment. Maintenance treatment with either agent. |
| Microsporidia | Includes multiple species that are pathogenic to humans. Worldwide distribution. Occurs with CD4+ count <100 μL. Fecal–oral transmission by ingestion of spores. Can live outside body for for up to 4 months | Profuse watery diarrhea, with crampy abdominal pain, malabsorption, weight loss, and wasting. | Poor staining qualities. Detection requires endoscopy with small bowel biopsy. | HAART has led to the resolution of this infection. Albendazole and octreotide have proved beneficial. |
| **Bacterial infections** | | | | |
| *Streptococcus pneumoniae* and *Haemophilus influenzae* (community acquired) | Most common causes of bacterial pneumonia in HIV-infected individuals. Occurs five times more frequently with $CD_{4+}$ <200 μL. Reaches the lungs through inhalation, aspiration of secretions from mouth or oropharynx, or spread by blood from another site. | Abrupt onset with fever, cough with purulent sputum, and systemic toxic effects. | Chest radiograph shows dense segmental or lobar consolidation. Chest radiograph may show nodular patterns or diffuse interstitial infiltrates. | Clarithromycin or azithromycin used to treat or prevent infection. Low-dose TMP-SMX as secondary prophylaxis for sinopulmonary infections. Vaccination against *H. influenzae* in persons with HIV infection. |

(continued)

**Table 41–6**
**Opportunistic Infections and Malignancies Associated with HIV/AIDS** *(continued)*

| Types of Infections and Malignancies | Epidemiology/Pathogenesis | Presentation and Assessment | Diagnosis | Interventions |
|---|---|---|---|---|
| *Pseudomonas aeruginosa* | Important pathogen in late HIV disease. Isolated from soil, water, plants, and animals. Most frequently acquired nosocomial pulmonary or cutaneous infection. High rate of relapse in those who survive initial infection. | Fever, cough, dyspnea, chest pain, sinusitis. May have recurrent cellulitis. | Blood and sputum cultures. Focal chest radiograph similar to other bacterial pneumonias. | Optimize immunological status because PCP or MAC prophylaxis is not effective in prevention of *Pseudomonas*. Treatment requires two or more antipseudomonal agents. |
| *Salmonella* species | Gram-negative bacteria pathogenic in both animals and humans. *Salmonella typhi* causes typhoid fever. Nontyphoid *Salmonella* species cause infection in patients with AIDS. Transmitted person to person by oral–fecal route, and by infection in animals such as chickens. *Salmonella* gastroenteritis results from exposure to infected pets or animal-derived foodstuffs such as poultry or eggs. HIV-infected patients are at risk for *Salmonella* bacteremia with or without GI disease. | Bacteremia without signs of localizing infection and nonspecific signs of septicemia. GI presentation includes diarrhea or abdominal pain. | Bacterial culture of blood. *Salmonella* enteritis is diagnosed by positive stool cultures. Other localized disease is diagnosed by culture of CSF or aspirated fluid. | Ampicillin, fluoroquinolone, ciprofloxacin, cefotaxime, ceftriaxone, or TMP-SMX for acute treatment. TMP-SMX or amoxicillin for maintenance treatment. |
| **Pneumocystis infections** *Pneumocystis carinii* | One of most common opportunistic infections in HIV infection. Most common cause of pulmonary disease. Without prophylaxis, occurs with CD4+ count <200 μL. | Fever, dyspnea, a nonproductive cough; 2% of patients develop spontaneous pneumothorax. | Sputum induction, bronchoalveolar lavage. Arterial blood gases show hypoxia. LDH elevated. | TMP-SMX or dapsone as first-line treatment. Pentamidine or clindamycin as second-line therapy. TMP-SMX for prophylaxis. |
| **Malignancies** Non-Hodgkin's lymphoma (NHL) | Rate of NHL is 73 times higher in HIV-infected individuals than in the general population. Greater chance of NHL with $CD_{4+}$ count <50/μL and in older white men. Caused by uncontrolled proliferation of lymphatic tissue, usually arising in the lymph nodes, spleen, liver, and bone marrow. Brain is the most common site of involvement. In patients with HIV disease, 80%–90% of the NHL is extranodal, making lymph node–based tumors uncommon. | Nonspecific symptoms of unexplained fever, weight loss, and night sweats. Elevated serum LDH. Localizing symptoms depend on site of tumor. Neurological deficits if NHL of the brain. NHL of GI tract manifests with abdominal pain, weight loss, or GI bleeding. Small-bowel lymphoma may lead to obstructive jaundice and small-bowel intussusception. | Biopsy of specimens or cytological examination of tissue fluid. CT scan of brain or abdomen. | CNS lymphoma treated with radiation with poor survival (3 mo.). Disease outside CNS treated with chemotherapy. Assess and treat for neutropenia secondary to chemotherapy. Antiretroviral agents may enhance clinical response to chemotherapy. |

| | | | |
|---|---|---|---|
| Kaposi's sarcoma (KS) | Classic KS is a rare, unusual neoplasm that usually affects older men of Jewish and Mediterranean ancestry; it is different from KS of HIV infection, which is most frequently seen in HIV-infected men, who have sex with men, and is the most common HIV-associated malignancy. It is associated with specific sexual practices and geographic locations. | Seen in any tissue but most often found in GI tract, mucous membranes, lymph nodes, and skin. Identified as patch, plaque, and/or nodular lesions of any size, color or configuration on the trunk, arms, head, or neck. Lesions in GI tract may be associated with bleeding pain, weight loss, and diarrhea. GI lesions are visualized by barium studies and are best evaluated endoscopically. Histological examination of tissue biopsy to confirm the diagnosis. | Treatment based on immunological status and symptoms. KS lesions are highly sensitive to radiation therapy. Isolated KS lesions can be treated with cryotherapy or laser surgery. Interferon-alpha with antiretroviral agents may be beneficial, as may single agent or combination chemotherapy. |
| Cervical invasive cancer | HIV-infected women have a 7-to-10 greater chance of developing precancerous or cancerous cervical lesions and a higher rate of recurrence after cervical intraepithelial neoplasia (CIN) excisions. Progression of CIN (cervical dysplasia) to carcinoma of the cervix is slow in immunocompromised women. Incidence of AIDS-defining cervical cancer appears to be higher in women who are injecting substance users, are black, and live in the southern United States. | Early stages are asymptomatic and usually identified by PAP smear. Vaginal bleeding, usually postcoital, is most common symptom. Metrorrhagia and malodorous, blood-tinged vaginal discharge may be present. Advanced disease may cause pelvic, back or leg pain, hematuria, rectal bleeding, or bladder and bowel involvement. PAP smear to determine the presence of abnormal cells, visible lesions, or both. Recommended that HIV-infected women have a PAP smear twice in the first year after diagnosis. If both are negative then a yearly PAP smear is recommended. If PAP smear is abnormal than a colposcopy is recommended. | Treatment of CIN and cervical cancer is carbon dioxide laser therapy, conization, cryosurgery, or electrocautery. Treatment of invasive cancer depends on the stage of the disease and may include surgery, radiation, or chemotherapy. |

*Sources:* Murphy and Flaherty (2003), reference 59.

"extremely severe." Such scales can also be used to rate how much a symptom interferes with activities of daily life, with 0 meaning "no interference" and 10 meaning "extreme interference."

- Many patients seek medical care for a specific symptom, which requires a focused history, physical exam, and diagnostic testing. Throughout the continuum of HIV, CD4 counts and percentages, VLs, and blood counts and chemistries may provide useful information for the management of the disease and its symptoms. Assessment of current medications and complementary therapies, including vitamin therapy, past medical illness that may be exacerbated by HIV disease, and the administration regimen of chemotherapy and radiation therapy should also be ascertained to determine the effects of treatment, side effects, adverse effects, and drug interactions. However, when treatment is no longer effective, as in the case of extremely advanced disease, practitioners must reevaluate the benefits versus burden of diagnostic testing and treatments, particularly the need for daily blood draws or more invasive and uncomfortable procedures. When the decision of the practitioners, patient, and family is that all testing and aggressive treatments are futile, their discontinuation is warranted.

- Treatment of opportunistic infections and malignancies often requires support of the patient's immune system, antiretroviral therapy to decrease the VL and improve CD4 cell counts, and medications and therapies to cure the patient of opportunistic infections or merely palliate the associated symptoms. Indeed, the treatment of symptoms to improve quality of life plays an important role in the management of HIV throughout the course of the illness.[18] In the case of many infections, acute treatment is followed by the regular dosing or maintenance therapy to prevent symptom recurrence. To maximize the quality of life, each patient's treatment regimen and plan of care should be individualized, with documentation of the treatment response and ongoing evaluation.

- Ongoing evaluation is key to symptom management and to determining the effectiveness of traditional, experimental, and complementary therapies. Changes in therapies are often necessary because concurrent or sequential illness or conditions occur.[72]

In an article regarding the symptom experience of patients with HIV/AIDS, Holzemer[73] emphasizes a number of key tenets, specifically: (1) the patient is the gold standard for understanding the symptom experience; (2) patients should not be labeled "asymptomatic" early in the course of the infection because they often experience symptoms of anxiety, fear, and depression; (3) nurses are not necessarily good judges of patients' symptoms, as they frequently underestimate the frequency and intensity of HIV signs and symptoms; however, following assessment, they can answer specific questions about a symptom, such as location, intensity, duration, and so forth; (4) nonadherence to treatment regimens is associated with greater frequency and intensity of symptoms; (5) greater frequency and intensity of symptoms leads to lower quality of life; (6) symptoms may or may not correspond with physiological markers; and (7) patients use few self-care symptom management strategies other than medication.

Pain and symptom assessment and management have been related to quality of life in patients with HIV/AIDS. Using data from a nationally representative cohort of HIV patients ($n = 2267$), Lorenz et al. reported that symptoms were significantly related to health-related quality of life and that the functional status and well-being of patients with HIV was inextricably linked to their symptoms.[74]

### Pain Management

Pain management must become more integrated in the comprehensive care offered to patients with AIDS. In a study to identify the most common sites of pain in patients with advanced AIDS, Norval reported that lower limb pain was the most prevalent (66%), followed by mouth pain (51%), headache (42%), throat pain (40%), and chest pain (18%).[75] Of the respondents, 34% indicated that pain was the worst overall symptom, with the average number of pains experienced as three.[75] In a longtitudinal study based on 95 patients with AIDS, Frich and Borgbjerg reported the overall incidence of pain as 88%, with 69% suffering moderate-to-severe constant pain that interfered with daily living.[76] Pain conditions were associated with opportunistic infections, KS, and lymphoma as well as neuropathic pain conditions.[76] The most common locations of pain were extremities (32%), head (24%), upper GI tract (23%), and lower GI tract (22%).[76] The survival rate of patients without pain was significantly higher than in those who reported pain.[76] Shofferman and Brody reported that more than half of the patients with advanced AIDS who were cared for in hospice experienced pain.[77] In a study by Breitbart and colleagues, only 8% of patients who reported severe pain (score of 8–10 on a pain intensity scale) in an AIDS-patient cohort received a strong opioid, as recommended by the World Health Organization (WHO) pain-management guidelines.[78] Cleeland and colleagues also reported significant undermedication of pain in AIDS patients (85%), which far exceeds the published reports of undertreated pain in cancer populations.[79]

The inadequate assessment and treatment of pain often occurs because of societal, practitioner, and patient barriers and limitations. For example, with regard to pain management, society fears addiction to opioids and has not distinguished between the legitimate and illegal use of drugs. Practitioners may have inadequate knowledge and misconceptions about pain management, whereas patients often fear pain because it is suggestive of advanced disease, and they are reluctant to report pain because they desire to be perceived as "good" patients.

Pain syndromes in patients with AIDS are diverse in nature and etiology. For patients with AIDS, pain can occur in more than one site, such as pain in the legs (peripheral neuropathy reported in 40% of AIDS patients), which is often associated with antiretroviral therapy such as AZT, as well as pain in the abdomen, oral cavity, esophagus, skin, perirectal area, chest, joints, muscles, and head. Pain is also related to HIV/AIDS therapies such as antiretroviral therapies, antibacterials, chemotherapy (such as vincristine), radiation, surgery, and procedures.[74] Following a complete assessment, including a history and physical examination, an individualized pain management plan should be developed to treat the underlying cause of the pain, which often arise from underlying infections associated with HIV disease.[81]

The principles of pain management in the palliative care of patients with AIDS are the same as for patients with cancer and include regularity of dosing, individualization of dosing, and using combinations of medications. The three-step guidelines for pain management (as outlined by WHO) should be used for patients with HIV disease.[82] This approach advocates for the selection of analgesics based on the severity of pain. For mild-to-moderate pain, anti-inflammatory drugs such as non-steroidal anti-inflammatory drugs (NSAIDs) or acetaminophen are recommended. However, the use of NSAIDs in patients with AIDS requires awareness of toxicity and adverse reactions because they are highly protein-bound, and the free fraction available is increased in AIDS patients who are cachetic or wasted.[69] For moderate-to-severe pain that is persistent, opioids of increasing potency are recommended, beginning with opioids such as codeine, hydrocodone, or oxycodone (each available with or without aspirin or acetaminophen), and advancing to more potent opioids such as morphine, hydromorphone (Dilaudid), methadone (Dolophine), or fentanyl either intravenously or transdermally. In conjunction with NSAIDs and opioids, the following adjuvant therapies are recommended:[83]

- Tricyclic antidepressants, heterocyclic and noncyclic antidepressants, and serotonin reuptake inhibitors for neuropathic pain
- Psychostimulants to improve opioid analgesia and decrease sedation
- Phenothiazine to relieve anxiety or agitation
- Butyrophenones to relieve anxiety and delirium
- Antihistamines to improve opioid analgesia and relieve anxiety, insomnia, and nausea
- Corticosteroids to decrease pain associated with an inflammatory component or with bone pain
- Benzodiazepines for neuropathic pain, anxiety, and insomnia

Caution is noted, however, with use of PIs because they may interact with some analgesics. For example, Ritonavir has been associated with potentially lethal interactions with meperidine, propoxyphene, and piroxicam. PIs must also be used with caution in patients receiving codeine, tricyclic antidepressants, sulindac, and indomethacin to avoid toxicity.

Furthermore, for patients with HIV who have high fevers, the increase in body temperature may lead to increased absorption of transdermally administered fentanyl.

To ensure appropriate dosing when changing the route of administration of opioids or changing from one opioid to another, the use of an equianalgesic conversion chart is suggested. As with all patients, oral medications should be used, if possible, with round-the-clock dosing at regular intervals and the use of rescue doses for breakthrough pain. Often, controlled-release morphine or oxycodone are effective drugs for patients with chronic pain from HIV/AIDS. In the case of neuropathic pain, often experienced with HIV/AIDS, tricyclic antidepressants such as amitriptyline or anticonvulsants such as Neurontin can be very effective.[83] However, the use of neuroleptics must be weighed against an increased sensitivity of AIDS patients to the extrapyramidal side effects of these drugs.[83] If the cause of pain is increasing tumor size, radiation therapy can also be very effective in pain management by reducing tumor size, as well as the perception of pain. Tables 41–7 and 41–8 present the nonopiate analgesics for pain management in patients with AIDS and opioid analgesics for the management of mild-to-moderate pain and from moderate-to-severe pain in patients with AIDS, respectively.

### Tolerance, Dependence, and Addiction

Physiological tolerance refers to the shortened or diminished effect of a drug resulting from exposure to the drug and, therefore, the need for increasing doses to maintain effect. In the case of opioids, tolerance to analgesic properties of the drug appears to be uncommon in the clinical setting, whereas tolerance to adverse effects such as respiratory depression, somnolence, and nausea is common and favorable. Most patients can remain on stable doses of opioids for prolonged periods of time. If an increase in opioid dosage is needed, then it is usually because of disease progression. Another expected physiological response to opioids is physical dependence, which occurs after 3 to 4 weeks of opioid administration, as evidenced by withdrawal symptoms after abrupt discontinuation. If a drug is to be discontinued, halving the daily dose every 1 to 2 days until the dose is equivalent to 15 mg of morphine will reduce withdrawal symptoms.[83]

Tolerance to opioids does not imply addiction, as addiction is a compulsive craving for a drug for effects other than pain relief and is extremely uncommon in patients who are terminally ill. Furthermore, studies have demonstrated that although tolerance and physical dependence commonly occur, addiction (psychological dependence) is rare and almost never occurs in individuals who do not have histories of substance abuse.[83] However, it should be noted that a certain percentage of patients with HIV/AIDS will have a history of substance abuse, either past or current, that needs to be recognized so that their pain can be managed appropriately, as well as other symptoms for which they are self-medicating. Healthcare providers in palliative care are often concerned with the

**Table 41–7**
**Nonopioid Analgesics for Pain Management in Patients with AIDS**

| Analgesic Nonopiate | Starting Dose (mg/day) | Plasma Duration (hours) | Half-Life (hours) | Comments |
|---|---|---|---|---|
| Aspirin | 650 | 4–6 | 3–12 | The standard for comparison among nonopioids. GI toxicity. May not be as well tolerated as some newer analgesics. |
| Ibuprofen | 400–600 | 4–8 | 3–4 | Can inhibit platelet function. |
| Acetaminophen | 650 | 4–6 | 2–4 | Overdosage produces hepatic toxicity. Not antiinflammatory. Lack of GI and platelet toxicity. |
| Choline magnesium trisalicylate | 700–1500 | 12 | 8–12 | Believed to have less GI toxicity than other NSAIDs. No effect on platelet aggregation. |
| Naproxen | 250–500 | 8–12 | 13 | Lower incidence of side effects than other agents. |
| Indomethacin | 25–75 | 8–12 | 4–5 | Available in sustained release in the United States. |
| COX-2 inhibitor: Celecoxib | 100–200 mg q.d. or bid | 3–5 | 11 | Not used for patients <18 y. Maximum daily dose is 400 mg. Growing concern regarding cardiac toxicities, especially with long term use. |

*Source:* Portenoy (1997), reference 132.

administration of opioids to patients who have a history of substance abuse, who are in methadone maintenance programs, or who currently are abusing drugs. Therefore, these patients often receive ineffective pain management. Consistent use of a standard pain scale and regular monitoring of drug consumption by one nurse and one physician can be helpful in ongoing assessment and pain management because it limits potential abuse. Oral administration of medications also lowers abuse potential. Given that substance-abusing patients have greater tolerance to morphine derivatives and benzodiazepines because of previous exposure to these drugs, increased dosage may be necessary for effective pain management, or the interval between doses should be shortened. Furthermore, the dosages of medications should be carefully monitored to avoid overdosing, given the possibility of hepatic failure in substance-abusing patients. Simultaneous use of agonists and antagonists are avoided in all populations because they provoke withdrawal symptoms.

### Alleviating Opioid Side Effects

Although opioids are extremely effective in pain management for patients with HIV, their common side effects must be anticipated and minimized. In medically fragile populations, such side effects may also result from other comorbid conditions rather than from opioid analgesia itself; therefore, a complete assessment is warranted. Medications and treatments to alleviate opioid side effects include:

- Nausea and vomiting, treated with prochlorperazine (Compazine), metoclopramide (Reglan), haloperidol (Haldol), granisetron (Kytril), and ondansetron (Zofran); (a change in the opioid may also be necessary)

- Constipation, treated by increasing fiber in the diet, stimulating cathartic drugs such as bisacodyl or senna, or hyperosmotic agents such as sorbitol or lactulose
- Sedation, treated by reducing the opioid in each dose or decreasing the frequency, as well as the ingestion of caffeine, and administration of dextroamphetamine or methylphenidate (again, a change in the opioid may be warranted)
- Confusion, treated by lowering the opioid dose, changing to a different opioid or Haldol
- Myoclonus, treated with clonazepam (Klonopin), diazepam (Valium), and baclofen (Lioresal), or a change in the opioid
- Respiratory depression, prevented by starting at a low dose in opioid-naïve patients and being aware of relative potencies when changing opioids, as well as differences by routes of administration. Naloxone (Narcan) may be administered to reverse respiratory depression but should be used with caution in patients who are opioid-tolerant because of the risk of inducing a withdrawal state. Dilute one ampule of naloxone (0.4 mg) in 10 mL of normal saline and titrate to the patient's respirations.[83]

### Management of Other Symptoms Experienced With HIV

For patients with HIV/AIDS, suffering occurs from the many symptoms experienced at the various stages of the illness. Based on a sample of 1128 HIV-infected patients, Fantoni and colleagues reported that the most commonly experienced symptoms were fatigue (65%), anorexia (34%), cough

**Table 41–8**
**Opioid Analgesics for Mild to Moderate to Severe Pain in Patients with AIDS**

| | Recommended Dose (mg) | Peak Effect (hours) | Duration (hours) | Plasma Half-Life (hours) | Comments |
|---|---|---|---|---|---|
| **For mild to moderate pain** | | | | | |
| Codeine (with or without acetaminophen) <br> Tylenol #2 acetaminophen 300 mg + codeine 15 mg <br> Tylenol #3 acetaminophen 300 mg + codeine 30 mg <br> Tylenol #4 Acetaminophen 300 mg + codeine 60 mg | 30–60 PO | 1–2 | 3–4 | 2–3 | Metabolized to morphine; often used to suppress cough. When acetaminophen is added, there is a ceiling dose of 4 g/day. |
| Hydrocodone (with acetaminophen combinations in Lorcet, Lortab, Vicodin, others) | 30 PO | 1–2 | 3–6 | 2–4 | When acetaminophen is added, there is a ceiling dose of 4 g/day. |
| Oxycodone (with or without acetaminophen) <br> Roxicodone (a single-entity oxycodone) <br> Percoset (oxycodone 5 mg + acetaminophen 325 mg) <br> Roxicet (oxycodone 5 mg + acetaminophen 500 mg) | 20–30 PO | 1–2 | 3–6 | 2–3 | Toxicity is the same as morphine. Used with acetaminophen for moderate pain. Available as a single agent for severe pain. Equianalgesic to morphine when not combined with acetaminophen. |
| Oxycodone (sustained release)—oxycodone SR | 20–40 PO | 1 | 8–12 | 2–3 | — |
| Oxycodone (controlled release)—OxyContin | 20–30 PO | 3–4 | 8–12 | 2–3 | — |
| **For moderate to severe pain** | | | | | |
| Morphine (immediate release) | 20–60 PO 10 <br> IM, IV, SC | 1–2 <br> 0.5–1 | 3–6 <br> 3–4 | 2–3 <br> 2–3 | Standard of comparison for the opioid analgesics. Constipation, nausea, and sedation are common side effects. Respiratory depression is rare. |
| Morphine (controlled release)—MS Contin | 20–60 PO | 3–4 | 8–12 | 2–3 | — |
| Morphine (sustained release)—Kadian, Oramorph SR | 20–60 PO | 4–6 | 24 | 2–3 | Kadian is only QD dosing. |
| Hydromorphone (Dilaudid) | 7.5 PO | 1–2 | 3–6 | 2–3 | Short half-life. |
| Hydromorphone (sustained release)—Palladone | 1.5 IM, IV | 0.5–1 | 3–4 | 2–3 | Toxicities similar to other opioids. |
| Methadone (Dolophine) | 20 PO 10 IM | 1–2 <br> 0.5–1.5 | 4 -> 8 <br> 4 -> 8 | 12 > 150 <br> 12 > 150 | Requires close monitoring for toxicity due to long half-life and careful titration. |
| Levorphanol (Levo-Dromoran) | 4 PO <br> 2 IM | 1–2 <br> 0.5–1 | 3–6 <br> 3–6 | 12–15 <br> 12–15 | Long half-life requiring careful titration in the first week. |
| Fentanyl | — | — | — | 7–12 | Can be administered as a continuous IV or SC infusion; 100 mcg/h is roughly equianalgesic to morphine 4 mg/h. |
| Fentanyl transdermal (Duragesic) | — | — | 48–72 | 16–24 | 100 mcg transdermal system is approximately equianalgesic to morphine 4 mg/h. Not suitable for rapid titration. If patient has pain after 48 h, increase the dose or change the patch every 48 h. |
| Fentanyl transmucosal (Actiq) | 200 mcg (1–2 units) q3h PRN but no more than 4 units/day. The unit is to be sucked and not chewed. Recosing within a single pain episode can occur 15 min after the previous unit has been completed or 30 min after the start of the previous unit. | 0.5 | — | 7 | Unit is administered as a "lozenge" on a stick that is to be sucked. Used for breakthrough pain as a rescue dose for cancer patients. Not to be used with opioid-naïve patients due to life-threatening hypoventilation. Recent research findings suggest that the onset of effect is faster than oral morphine and the same as IV morphine. |

*Source:* Portenoy (1997), reference 127.

(32%), and fever (29%).[84] Based on a sample of 207 patients with AIDS, Holzemer and colleagues also found that 50% of the participants experienced shortness of breath, dry mouth, insomnia, weight loss, and headaches.[85] The records of 50 men who died of AIDS between 1988 and 1992 indicated the distressing symptoms of dyspnea, diarrhea, confusion, dementia, and difficulty eating and swallowing. Therefore, care in the last month of life is often directed at the palliation of symptoms.[17] Indeed, the last stage of HIV infection is often marked by increasing pain, GI discomfort, and depression.[9] Patients may be suffering from inflammatory or infiltrative processes and somatic and visceral pain. Neuropathic pain is commonly a result of the disease process or the side effect of medications.[86] Based on a sample of 92 HIV-positive men, Avis, Smith, and Mayer[87] also reported that quality of life was more related to symptoms as measured by the Whalen's HIV Symptom Index than CD4 counts or hemoglobin. Based on a longitudinal pilot study of patients with advanced AIDS ($n = 63$), Sherman et al. reported that the most prevalent symptoms for AIDS patients, based on the Memorial Symptom Assessment Scale (MSAS), were lack of energy (75%), pain (73%), worry (65%), dry mouth (64%), feeling sad (62%), shortness of breath (58%), difficulty sleeping (57%), cough (57%), and numbness/tingling (51%), which significantly affected quality of life.[88] With the myriad of symptoms experienced by patients with HIV across the illness trajectory, health-care practitioners need to understand the causes, presentations, and interventions of common symptoms, as presented in Table 41–9 to enhance the quality of life of patients.

## Nonpharmacological and Complementary Interventions for Pain and Symptom Management

Nonpharmacological interventions for pain and symptom management can also be effective in the care of patients with HIV. Bed rest, simple exercise, heat or cold packs to affected sites, massage, transcutaneous electrical stimulation, and acupuncture can be effective physical therapies with this patient population. Psychological interventions to reduce pain perception and interpretation include hypnosis, relaxation, imagery, biofeedback, distraction, and patient education. In cases of refractory pain, nerve blocks and cordotomy are available neurosurgical procedures for pain management. Increasingly, epidural analgesia is an additional option that provides continuous pain relief. Therapeutic massage and healing touch have been shown to effectively reduce short-term pain in cancer patients.[89]

The 10 most commonly used complementary therapies and activities reported by 1106 participants in the Alternative Medical Care Outcomes in AIDS study were aerobic exercise (64%), prayer (56%), massage (54%), needle acupuncture (48%), meditation (46%), support groups (42%), visualization and imagery (34%), breathing exercises (33%), spiritual activities (33%), and other exercise (33%).[89] Clearly, patients with HIV seek complementary therapies to treat symptoms, slow

the progression of the disease, and enhance their general well-being. Nurses' knowledge, evaluation, and recommendations regarding complementary therapies are important aspects of holistic care. Milan et al. found that more than 90% of inner-city, middle-aged, heterosexual women and men ($n = 93$) who were at risk for or who had HIV reported use of complementary and alternative medicine in the prior 6 months.[90]

## Psychosocial Issues for Patients With HIV/AIDS and Their Families

Uncertainty is a chronic and pervasive source of psychological distress for persons living with HIV, particularly as it relates to ambiguous symptom patterns, exacerbation and remissions of symptoms, selection of optimal treatment regimens, the complexity of treatments, and the fear of stigma and ostracism. Such uncertainty is linked to negative perceptions of quality of life and poor psychological adjustment.[91] However, many practitioners focus on patient's physical functioning and performance status as the main indicators of quality of life, rather than on the symptoms of psychological distress such as anxiety and depression.[92] Based on a sample of 203 patients with HIV/AIDS, Farber and colleagues reported that positive meaning of the illness was associated with a higher level of psychological well-being and lower depressed mood and contributed more than problem-focused coping and social support to predicting both psychological well-being and depressed mood.[93] During the late stages of AIDS, minority women ($n = 220$) expressed high levels of psychological disturbance on the Psychiatric Symptom Index, which were significantly related to their mothers' reports of having non-HIV-related medical conditions, spending time in bed during the past 2 weeks, having more activity restrictions, and having difficulty caring for children as a result of ill health.[94] In a study of the problems and needs of HIV/AIDS patients during the last weeks of life, Butters and colleagues used the Support Team Assessment Schedule (STAS) to determined that symptom control, patient and family anxiety, spiritual needs, and communication between patient and family were their greatest needs.[95] Furthermore, Friedland and colleagues identified the determinants of quality of life in a sample of 120 individuals with HIV/AIDS.[96] Income, emotional support, and problem-and perception-oriented coping were positively related to quality of life, whereas tangible support and emotion-focused coping were negatively related. Ragsdale and Morrow emphasized the importance of focusing on the psychosocial aspects of life in patients with HIV/AIDS because patients reported a repetitive cycle of emotional changes with slight physical changes.[34] Disfigurement, the symptoms associated with the disease and its treatment, and the contagious nature of the disease add to the psychological distress associated with HIV/AIDS.

Nurses must also be cognizant of issues such as the experience of multiple losses, complicated grieving, substance abuse, stigmatization, and homophobia, which contribute to

**Table 41–9**
**Selected Symptoms Associated with HIV/AIDS**

| Symptom | Cause | Presentation | Interventions |
|---|---|---|---|
| Fatigue (asthenia) | HIV infection<br>Opportunistic infections<br>AIDS medications<br>Prolonged immobility<br>Anemia<br>Sleep disorders<br>Hypothyroidism<br>Medications | Weakness<br>Lack of energy | Treat reversible causes.<br>Pace activities with rest periods/naps.<br>Ensure adequate nutrition.<br>Use relaxation exercises and meditation.<br>Take warm rather than hot showers or baths.<br>Use cool room temperatures.<br>Administer dextroamphetamine 10 mg/day PO. |
| Anorexia (loss of appetite and cachexia (wasting) | Metabolic alterations caused by cytokines and interleukin-1<br>Opportunistic infections<br>Nutrient malabsorption from intestines<br>Chronic diarrhea<br>Depression<br>Taste disorders | Diminished food intake<br>Profound weight loss | Treat reversible causes.<br>Consult with dietitian about choice of food.<br>Make food appealing by color and texture.<br>Avoid noxious smells at mealtime.<br>Avoid fatty, fried, and strong-smelling foods.<br>Offer small, frequent meals and nutritious snacks.<br>Encourage patients to eat whatever is appealing.<br>Provide high-energy, high-protein liquid supplements.<br>Use appetite stimulants such as megesterol acetate 800 mg/day PO or dronabinol 2.5 mg PO qd or bid.<br>Testosterone administered by 5 mg transdermal patch to increase weight gain and muscle mass. |
| Fever (elevated body temperature) | Bacterial toxins<br>Viruses<br>Yeast<br>Antigen–antibody reactions<br>Drugs<br>Tumor products Exogenous pyrogens | Body temperature >99.5°F (oral), 100.5°F (rectal), or 98.5°F (axillary)<br>Chills, rigor<br>Sweating, night sweats<br>Delerium<br>Dizziness<br>Dehydration | Treat reversible causes.<br>Maintain fluid intake.<br>Use loose clothing and sheets, with frequent changing.<br>Avoid plastic bed coverings.<br>Exceptionally high temperature may require ice packs or cooling blankets.<br>Administer around-the-clock antipyretics such as acetaminophen or ASA, 325–650 mg PO q6–8 h. |
| Dyspnea (short-ness of breath) and cough | Bronkospasm<br>Embolism<br>Effusions<br>Pulmonary edema<br>Pneumothorax<br>Kaposi's sarcoma<br>Obstruction<br>Opportunistic infections<br>Anxiety<br>Allergy<br>Mechanical or chemical irritants<br>Anemia | Productive or nonproduc-tive cough<br>Crackles<br>Stridor<br>Hemoptysis<br>Inability to clear secretions<br>Wheezing<br>Tachypnea<br>Gagging<br>Intercostal retractions<br>Areas of pulmonary dullness<br>Anxiety | Treat reversible causes.<br>Elevate bed to Fowler's or high Fowler's position.<br>Provide abdominal splints.<br>Administer humidified oxygen therapy to treat dyspnea.<br>Use fans or open windows to keep air moving for dyspnea.<br>Remove irritants or allergens such as smoke.<br>Teach pursed-lips breathing for patients with obstructive disease.<br>Use frequent mouth care to decrease discomfort from dry mouth.<br>Treat bronchospasm.<br>Suppress cough with dextromethorphan hydrobromide 15–45 mg PO q4 h PRN, or opioids such as codeine 15–60 mg PO q4 h even if taking other opioids for pain, or hydrocodone 5–10 mg PO q4–6 h PRN, or morphine 5–20 mg PO q4 h PRN (may be increased) to relieve dyspnea, cough, and asso-ciated anxiety.<br>For hyperactive gag reflex use nebulized lidocaine 5 mL of 2% solution (100 mg) q3–4 h PRN. |

(continued)

**Table 41–9**
**Selected Symptoms Associated with HIV/AIDS** *(continued)*

| Symptom | Cause | Presentation | Interventions |
|---|---|---|---|
| Diarrhea | Idiopathic HIV enteropathy | Flatulence | Treat reversible causes. |
| | Diet | Multiple bowel movements/day | Maintain adequate hydration. |
| | Bowel infections (bacteria, parasites, protozoa) | Cramps/colic | Replace electrolytes by giving Gatorade or Pedialyte. |
| | Chronic bowel inflammation | Hemorrhoids | Give rice, bananas, or apple juice to reduce diarrhea. |
| | Medications | | Increase protein and calories. |
| | Obstruction with overflow incontinence | | Avoid dairy products, alcohol, caffeine, extremely hot or cold foods, spicy or fatty foods. |
| | Stress | | Maintain dignity while toileting. |
| | Malabsorption | | Provide ready access to bathroom or commode. |
| | | | Maintain good perianal care. |
| | | | Administer medications such as Lomotil 2.5–5.0 mg q4–6 h; Kapectolin 60–120 mL q4–6 h (max 20 mg/day); Imodium 2–4 mg q6 h (max 16 mg/day); or aregoric (tincture of opium) 5–10 mL q4–6 h. |
| Insomnia (inability to fall asleep or stay asleep) | Anxiety | Early morning awakening | Treat reversible causes. |
| | Depression | Nighttime restlessness | Establish a bedtime routine. |
| | Pain | Fear | Reduce daytime napping. |
| | Medications | Nightmares | Avoid caffeinated beverages and alcohol. |
| | Delirium | | Take a warm bath 2 h before bedtime. |
| | Sleep disorders such as sleep apnea | | Use relaxation techniques. |
| | Excess alcohol intake | | Provide an environment conducive to sleep (dark, quiet, comfortable temperature). |
| | Caffeine | | Administer anxiolytics such as benzodiazapines (use for <2 wk because of dependency), antidepressants (helpful over long term), or other sedatives such as Benadryl. |
| Headache | Infections such as encephalitis, herpes zoster, meningitis, toxoplasmosis | Pain in one or more areas of the head or over sinuses | Treat reversible causes. |
| | Sinusitis | | Suggest chiropractic manipulation. |
| | | | Provide message therapy. |
| | | | Use relaxation therapy. |
| | | | Apply TENS. |
| | | | Use stepwise analgesia. |
| | | | Administer corticosteroids to reduce swellings around space-occupying lesions. |

*Sources:* Coyne et al. (2002), reference 128.

patients' sense of alienation, isolation, hopelessness, loneliness, and depression. Such emotional distress often extends to the patient's family caregivers as they attempt to provide support and lessen the patient's suffering yet are often suffering from HIV themselves. Reciprocal suffering is experienced by family caregivers as well as patients, and there is the need to improve their quality of life through palliative care.[97]

### Psychosocial Assessment of Patients With HIV

Psychosocial assessment of patients with HIV is important throughout the illness trajectory, particularly as the disease progresses and there is increased vulnerability to psychological distress. Psychosocial assessment includes the following:

- Social, behavioral, and psychiatric history, which includes the history of interpersonal relationships, education, job stability, career plans, substance use, preexisting mental illness, and individual identity
- Crisis points related to the course of the disease as anxiety, fear, and depression intensify, creating a risk of suicide
- Life-cycle phase of individuals and families, which influences goals, financial resources, skills, social roles, and the ability to confront personal mortality
- Influence of culture and ethnicity, including knowledge and beliefs associated with health, illness, dying, and death, as well as attitudes and values toward sexual behaviors, substance use, health promotion and maintenance, and health-care decision-making
- Past and present patterns of coping, including problem-focused and/or emotion-focused coping
- Social support, including sources of support, types of supports perceived as needed by the patient/family, and perceived benefits and burdens of support
- Financial resources, including health-care benefits, disability allowances, and the eligibility for Medicaid/ Medicare

### Depression and Anxiety in Patients With HIV

Because AIDS is a life-threatening, chronic, debilitating illness, patients are at risk for such psychological disorders as depression and anxiety. Among persons living with HIV/ AIDS, the prevalence of depression has been estimated at 10% to 25%[98] and is characterized by depressed mood, low energy, sleep disturbance, anhedonia, inability to concentrate, loss of libido, weight changes, and possible menstrual irregularities.[99] It is also important to assess whether depressed patients are using alcohol, drugs, and opioids.

Patients with HIV who are diagnosed with depression should be treated with antidepressants to control their symptoms.[100] Selective serotonin reuptake inhibitors (SSRIs) are as effective as tricyclic antidepressants but are better tolerated because of their more benign side effect profile. Further, SSRIs may interact with such antiretroviral medications as

protease inhibitors and nNRTIs; therefore, initial SSRI dosage should be lowered with careful upward titration and close monitoring for toxic reactions.[100] Serotonin and norepinephrine reuptake inhibitors such as venlafaxine and duloxetine are newer antidepressants that also are useful in treating chronic pain. Tricyclic antidepressants are indicated for treating depression only in patients who do not respond to newer medications.[100] It is noted that monoamine oxidase inhibitors may interact with multiple medications used to treat HIV and should therefore be avoided. Medication interaction and liver function profiles should be considered before antidepressant therapy is initiated.

Because depression is a common symptom in patients with HIV/AIDS, research studies have also focused on other factors that relate to depression in this patient population. Schrimshaw examined whether the source of unsupportive social interactions had differential main and interactive relations with depressive symptoms among ethnically diverse women with HIV/AIDS ($n = 146$).[101] After controlling for demographic variables, Schrimshaw found that unsupportive social interactions with family had a major effect in predicting more depressive symptoms and that there was a significant interaction between unsupportive interactions from a lover/ spouse and friends, which predicted high levels of depressive symptoms. Arrindell examined differential coping strategies, anxiety, depression, and symptomatology among African-American women with HIV/AIDS ($n = 30$).[102] The results indicated that the majority of women used emotion-focused coping; however, there were no main effects for coping strategies on psychological distress and no significant difference between symptomatology and coping strategies. An inverse relationship was reported between psychological distress and social support, with less distress reported when women had financial assistance from their families and friends. There was a relationship reported between symptomatology and anxiety, with those who were asymptomatic reporting no anxiety.

Anxiety is often associated with the stresses of HIV or may result from the medications used to treat HIV disease, such as anticonvulsants, sulfonamides, NSAIDs, and corticosteroids.[102] Generalized anxiety disorder is manifested as worry, trouble falling asleep, impaired concentration, psychomotor agitation, hypersensitivity, hyperarousal, and fatigue.[103]

The treatment for patients with anxiety is based on the nature and severity of the symptoms and the coexistence of other mood disorders or substance abuse. Short-acting anxiolytics such as lorazepam (Ativan), and alprazolam (Xanax) are beneficial for intermittent symptoms, whereas buspirone (BuSpar) and clonazepam (Klonopin) are beneficial for chronic anxiety.[100]

For many patients experiencing psychological distress associated with HIV, participation in therapeutic interventions such as skill-building, support groups, individual counseling, and group interventions using meditation techniques can provide a sense of psychological growth and a meaningful way of living with the disease.[104,105] Such interventions are particularly helpful for patients with HIV/AIDS who may not have disclosed their sexual orientation or substance-abusing history to their families. Often, significant stress is associated with sharing such information, particularly when such disclosures occur during the stage of advanced disease. However, the need for therapeutic communication and support from all health professionals caring for the patient and their family exists throughout the illness continuum. Furthermore, fear of disclosure of the AIDS diagnosis and stigmatization in the community often raises concern in the family about the diagnosis stated on death certificates. Practitioners may therefore write a nonspecific diagnosis on the main death certificate and sign section B on the reverse side to signify to the registrar general that further information will be provided at a later date.

Often many members of a single family are infected and die because of the transmission of the disease from sexual partners and through childbirth. In the homosexual community and substance-abusing community, multiple deaths have also resulted in complicated mourning. The anxiety, depression, sadness, and loneliness associated with these multiple deaths and unending experiences of loss must be recognized and support must be offered. Community resources and referrals to HIV/AIDS support groups and bereavement groups are important in emotional adjustment to these profound losses.

## Spiritual Issues in AIDS

The spiritual care of the patient and the ability of the community to support patients with HIV/AIDS may be unique opportunities for both personal and societal growth and transcendence. Mellors and colleagues examined the relationship of self-transcendence and quality of life in a sample of 46 individuals with HIV/AIDS.[106] The results demonstrated that overall self-transcendence for this sample was relatively high. Quality of life was higher than reported in previous research, yet those with disease progression, evident by the diagnosis of AIDS, had lower quality of life than those who were asymptomatic or symptomatic with CD4 counts greater than 200 cells/mm[3]. There was no significant difference in self-transcendence between groups, but those with AIDS were more inclined to accept death and refrained from dwelling on the past or unmet dreams. There was a moderate positive correlation between self-transcendence and quality of life.[116–118]

As health professionals, assessment of the patient's spiritual needs is an important aspect of holistic care. Learning about patients' spiritual values, needs, and religious perspectives is important in understanding their perspectives regarding their illnesses and their perceptions and meaning of life and its purpose, suffering, and eventual death. According to Elkins and colleagues, spirituality is a way of being or experiencing that comes about through an awareness of a transcendent dimension and identifiable life values with regard to self,

others, nature, and God.[107] An understanding of the patient's relationship with self, others, nature, and God can inform interventions that promote spiritual well-being and the possibility of a "good death" from the patient's perspective.

Patients living with and dying from HIV have the spiritual needs of meaning, value, hope, purpose, love, acceptance, reconciliation, ritual, and affirmation of a relationship with a higher being.[108] Assisting patients to find meaning and value in their lives, despite adversity, often involves a recognition of past successes and their internal strengths. Respectful behavior toward patients demonstrates love and acceptance of the patient as a person. Encouraging open communication between the patient and family is important to work toward reconciliation and the completion of unfinished business.

### CASE STUDY
### *Will Stillers, a Patient With MAC*

Will Stillers, a 28-year-old homosexual male, was admitted to the inpatient palliative care unit for fever, fatigue, anorexia, nausea and vomiting, and weight loss. He had 20 episodes of liquid diarrhea each day. As a differential diagnosis, he was tested for HIV. Findings indicated a CD4 count of 45 cells/mm[3] and a VL of 142,000 mL, indicative of the advanced stage of HIV. His laboratory work indicated anemia and an elevated alkaline phosphatase. MAC was confirmed by biopsy with AFB stain. Physical examination revealed hepatosplenomegaly and inguinal lymphadenopathy.

Will was started on azithromycin and rifabutin to treat MAC, as well as a HAART regimen of one potent PI and two NRTIs—specifically atazanavir + ritonavir (PI)—and emtricitabine and tenofovir disoproxil fumarate (Truvada) to treat his advanced stage of AIDS. Will had been estranged from his mother and sister, who lived on the West Coast. However, he had a very close friend, Carl, who viewed himself as Will's guardian given that he had known Will for many years, and his mother was friends with Will's mother when she lived in New York. Will lived with Carl and was considered a family member. After Will's infection improved, he returned to Carl's 4th-story walk-up. Will still had difficulty "holding down" food but ate small frequent meals, which he prepared for Carl and himself. Will's only interest was in cooking because he was trained as a chef. He was very weak but enjoyed cooking as his creative outlet and viewed it as an opportunity to contribute to the household.

The diarrhea improved with medications, but Will was still too insecure to leave the house because he was more comfortable having immediate access to a toilet. He still felt very weak and was also concerned about his ability to climb stairs. Within the month, Will became more depressed and isolated. Although a home health aide visited for a few hours each day, there was minimal verbal interaction between them. Will began to stay in bed for long periods of time during the day. He wondered if he was ever going to recover but hoped some day to get his own apartment and be well enough to work. Will was treated with an antidepressant, and within weeks his mood improved. His appetite increased and his physician was encouraged by his response to the HAART therapy. His physician discussed advance directives, and Will asked Carl to be his health care proxy, as Carl knew Will's wishes and preferences.

Over the next 2 months, Will's quality of life improved because he was free of opportunistic infections, and although unemployed, he kept busy with household activities. Carl and Will had a wide circle of friends, but unfortunately many were also living with HIV/AIDS. Over the next 3 months, three of their friends died. Will understood the fragility of his condition and was adherent to his medication regimen. However, night sweats, fever, and diarrhea returned, and he was readmitted to the hospital within 6 months of his initial hospitalization with an exacerbation of MAC and severe dehydration. The palliative care team was asked for a consultation by the AIDS specialist. The advanced practice nurse developed a very supportive relationship with Will and Carl. She listened attentively to Will's fears and concerns and provided a caring presence that helped him to relax. They discussed his relationship with his mother and sister, and he asked the nurse to call his sister and tell her about his hospitalization. Will was coming to terms with his diagnosis and was ready to move beyond old hurts in his relationship with his family. Although he did not have a strong religious faith, Will asked for the chaplain to visit because he was trying to come to terms with his own suffering and the death of his friends.

Over the next few weeks, Will's infection began to resolve, and the advanced practice nurse promised him that when he felt better, she would bring him a meal from his favorite "soul food" restaurant where he once worked. Will's sister and mother asked to come to see him. On the day they arrived, Will's condition took an unexpected turn for the worse. With Carl and his family at his side, Will's fever began to rise and he became delirious. Several tests were conducted to identify other potential sources of the infection, and other possible reasons for the delirium. His symptoms were treated with Haldol and antipyretics. However, within the next day, Will slipped into a coma and died. In a letter found at his bedside, Will thanked his physicians and the members of the palliative team for their care. He said that without their support, he never would have reconciled with his mother and sister. He knew that his illness was advanced and did not expect to regain his health. He thanked Carl for his unconditional friendship and care. He said, "I feel that you are my older brother whom I could always count on–no matter what." Members of the palliative care team were surprised at his sudden death but also understood the uncertainty of living with advanced AIDS. In a celebration of his life, the palliative care team brought Will's favorite foods from the restaurant where he worked, and asked Will's family to join them to celebrate his loving spirit and his life. In remembrance, tears were shed because of the tragic death of this promising young man who had touched their hearts, yet the importance of unconditional love, caring presence, and the joys of everyday life, such as sharing a meal, were reinforced by the message he left.

As with many life-threatening illnesses, patients with AIDS may express anger with God. Some may view their illness as a punishment or are angry that God is not answering their prayers. Expression of feelings can be a source of spiritual healing. Clergy can also serve as valuable members of the palliative care team in offering spiritual support and alleviating spiritual distress. The use of meditation, music, imagery, poetry, and drawing may offer outlets for spiritual expression and promote a sense of harmony and peace.

In a grounded-theory study of hope in patients with HIV/AIDS, Kylma and colleagues found that patients had an alternating balance between hope, despair, and hopelessness based on the possibilities of daily life.[108] They experienced losses such as loss of joy, carefree time, safety, self-respect, potential parenthood, privacy, and trust in self, others, systems, and God. However, there was hope as they received strength by seeing their life from a new perspective as well as an acceptance of the uncertainty of life and the value of life. Hope was described as a basic resource in life and meant the belief that life is worth living at the present and in the future, with good things still to come. Despair meant losing grip, unable to take hold of anything, whereas hopelessness implied giving up in the face of an assumably nonexistent future, which was the opposite of hope.

For all patients with chronic, life-threatening illness, hope often shifts from hope that a cure will soon be found to hope for a peaceful death with dignity, including the alleviation of pain and suffering, determining one's own choices, being in the company of family and significant others, and knowing that their end-of-life wishes will be honored. Often, the greatest spiritual comfort offered by caregivers or family for patients comes from active listening and meaningful presence by sitting and holding their hands and showing them that they are not abandoned and alone.

Spiritual healing may also come from life review, as patients are offered an opportunity to reminisce about their lives, reflect on their accomplishments, reflect on their misgivings, and forgive themselves and others for their imperfections. Indeed, such spiritual care conveys that even in the shadow of death, there can be discovery, insight, the completion of relationships, the experience of love of self and others, and the transcendence of emotional and spiritual pain. Often, patients with AIDS, by their example, teach nurses, family, and others how to transcend suffering and how to die with grace and dignity.

### Advanced Care Planning

Advanced planning is another important issue related to end-of-life care for patients with HIV/AIDS. Most patients with AIDS have not discussed with their physicians the kind of care they want at the end of life, although more homosexual men have executed an advance directive than injection-drug users or women.[109] Nonwhite patients with AIDS report that they do not like to talk about the care they would want if they were very sick and are more likely to feel that if they talk about death, it will bring death closer. Conversely, white patients were more likely to believe that their doctor was an HIV/AIDS expert and good at talking about end-of-life care and to recognize they have been very sick in the past and that such discussions are important.[102] According to Ferris and colleagues,[110] health-care providers can assist patients and families by (1) discussing the benefits of healthcare and social support programs, unemployment insurance, worker's compensation, pension plans, insurance, and union or association benefits; (2) emphasizing the importance of organizing information and documents so that they are easily located and accessible; (3) suggesting that financial matters be in order, such as power of attorney or bank accounts, credit cards, property, legal claims, and income tax preparation; (4) discussing advance directives or power of attorney for care and treatment, as well as decisions related to the chosen setting for dying; and (5) discussing the patient's wishes regarding their death—Whom does the patient want at the bedside? What rituals are important to the dying patient? Does the patient wish an autopsy? What arrangements does the patient want regarding the funeral services and burial? Where should donations in remembrance be sent? It is important to realize that these issues should be discussed at relevant stages in the person's illness, in a manner that is both respectful to the patient's wishes and strengths and that promotes the patient's sense of control over his/her life and death.

Health-care providers must also understand the concept of capacity, a "state in which the person is capable of taking legal acts, consenting or refusing treatment, writing a will or power of attorney."[110] In assessing the patient's competency, the health provider must question whether the decision-maker knows the nature and effect of the decision to be made and understands the consequences of his/her actions and determine if the decision is consistent with an individual's life history, lifestyle, previous actions, and best interests.[110]

When an individual is competent, and in anticipation of the future loss of capacity, he/she may initiate advance directives such as a living will and/or the designation of a health-care proxy who will carry out the patient's health-care wishes or make health-care decisions in the event that the patient becomes incompetent. The patient may also give an individual the power of attorney regarding financial matters and care or treatment issues. Advance directives include the patient's decisions regarding such life-sustaining treatments as cardiopulmonary resuscitation, use of vasoactive drips to sustain blood pressure and heart rate, dialysis, artificial nutrition and hydration, and the initiation or withdrawal of ventilatory support. The signing of advance directives must be witnessed by two individuals who are not related to the patient or involved in the patient's treatment. Individuals who are mentally competent can revoke their advance directives at any time. If a patient is deemed mentally incompetent, state statutes may allow the court to designate a surrogate decision-maker for the patient.

## Palliative Care Through the Dying Trajectory

Death from AIDS usually results from multiple causes, including chronic infections, malignancies, neurological disease, malnutrition, and multisystem failure.[111] However, even for patients with HIV/AIDS for whom death appears to be imminent, spontaneous recovery with survival of several more weeks or months is possible. The terminal stage is often marked by periods of increasing weight loss and deteriorating physical and cognitive functioning. The general rule related to mortality is that the greater the cumulative number of opportunistic infections, illnesses, complications, and/or deviance of serological or immunological markers in terms of norms, the less the survival time. Survival time is also decreased by psychosocial factors such as a decrease in physical and emotional support as demands increase for the caregivers, feelings of hopelessness by the patient, and older age (>39 years).[112] In the terminal stage of HIV, decisions related to prevention, diagnosis, and treatment pose ethical and clinical issues for both patients and their health-care providers because they must decide on the value and frequency of laboratory monitoring, use of invasive procedures, use of antiretroviral and prophylactic measures, and patients' participation in clinical trails.

The dying process for patients with advanced AIDS is commonly marked by increasingly severe physical deterioration, leaving the patient bedbound and experiencing wasting, dyspnea at rest, and pressure ulcers. Ultimately, patients become dependent on others for care. Febrile states and changes in mental status often occur as death becomes more imminent. Maintaining the comfort and dignity of the patients becomes a nursing priority. Symptomatic treatments, including pain management, should be continued throughout the dying process, as even obtunded patients may feel pain and other symptoms.

The end of life is an important time for individuals to accept their own shortcomings and limitations and differences with significant others so that death may be accepted without physical, psychosocial, and spiritual anguish. At the end of life, patients with AIDS may have a desire for hastened death. Based on a sample of 128 terminally ill patients with AIDS who were receiving palliative care, Pessin[113] found that there was a significant association between desire for a hastened death and cognitive impairment, with memory impairment providing an independent and unique contribution to desire for hastened death. Curtis and colleagues[114] also examined the desire of AIDS patients for less life-sustaining treatment as associated with the medical futility rationale. It was reported that 61% (n = 35) of patients with advanced AIDS accepted the medical futility rationale as it applied to their medical care at the end of life, including the use of mechanical ventilation. However, because 26% (n = 15) thought the medical futility rationale was probably acceptable and 10% ($n = 5$) said it was definitely not acceptable, clinicians invoking the medical futility rationale should consider the diversity of these patient attitudes toward care at the end of life. Through an interdisciplinary approach to care, health professionals can assist patients with the following: reducing their internal conflicts, such as fears about the loss of control, which can be related to a desire for hastened death; making end-of-life decisions regarding medical treatments that are consistent with their values, wishes, and preferences; promoting the patient's sense of identity; supporting the patient in maintaining important interpersonal relationships; and encouraging patients to identify and attempt to reach meaningful but limited goals.

Because palliative care also addresses the needs of family, it is important to consider the vulnerability of family members to patients' health problems at the end of life. In a study of the health status of informal caregivers ($n = 76$) of persons with HIV/AIDS, Flaskerud and Lee[115] found that caregiver distress regarding a patient's symptoms, anxiety, and education was related to depressive symptoms and that depressive symptoms, anger, and functional status of patients with AIDS were related to poorer physical health of informal caregivers. Therefore, members of the palliative care team can provide much-needed assistance not only to patients but their families.

In a 2-year longitudinal pilot study regarding quality of life for patients with advanced cancer and AIDS, Sherman et al. found that although patients with advanced AIDS ($n = 63$) reported a total lower quality of life compared to patients with advanced cancer ($n = 38$), AIDS caregivers ($n = 43$) reported greater overall quality of life, psychological well-being, and spiritual well-being than cancer caregivers ($n = 38$).[128] Sherman and colleagues have posed that even as death approaches, health professionals can identify changes in quality of life and appropriate interventions to improve quality of life outcomes for HIV/AIDS patients.[116]

As illness progresses and death approaches, health professionals can encourage patients and family members to express their fears and end-of-life wishes. Encouraging patients and families to express such feelings as "I love you," "I forgive you," "Forgive me—I am sorry," "Thank you," and "Good-bye" is important to the completion of relationships.[117] Peaceful death can also occur when families give the patient permission to die and assure them that they will be remembered.

### Loss, Grief, and Bereavement for Persons With HIV/AIDS and Their Survivors

Throughout the illness trajectory, patients with HIV disease experience many losses: a sense of loss of identity as they assume the identity of a patient with AIDS; loss of control over health and function; loss of roles as the illness progresses; loss of body image because of skin lesions, changes in weight, and wasting; loss of sexual freedom because of the need to change sexual behaviors to maintain health and prevent transmission

to others; loss of financial security through possible discrimination and increasing physical disability; and loss of relationships through possible abandonment, self-induced isolation, and the multiple deaths of others from the disease.[119] In a study of AIDS-related grief and coping with loss among HIV-positive men and women ($n = 268$), Sikkema and colleagues[119] reported that the severity of grief reaction to AIDS-related losses was associated with escape-avoidance and self-controlling coping strategies, the type of loss, depressive symptoms, and history of injection drug use. For health-care professionals, each occurrence of illness may pose new losses and heighten the patient's awareness of his or her mortality. Therefore, each illness experience is an opportunity for health professionals to respond to cues of the patients in addressing their concerns and approaching the subject of loss, dying, and death. Given that grief is the emotional response to loss, patients dying from AIDS may also manifest the signs of grief, which include feelings of sadness, anger, self-reproach, anxiety, loneliness, fatigue, shock, yearning, relief, and numbness; physical sensations such as hollowness in the stomach, tightness in the chest, oversensitivity to noise, dry mouth, muscle weakness, and loss of coordination; cognitions of disbelief or confusion; and behavior disturbances in appetite, sleep, social withdrawal, loss of interest in activities, and restless overactivity.[120]

Upon the death of the patient, the patient's family and significant others enter a state of bereavement, or a state of having suffered a loss, which is often a long-term process of adapting to life without the deceased.[120] Family and significant others may experience signs of grief, including a sense of presence of the deceased, paranormal experiences or hallucinations, dreams of the deceased, and a desire to have cherished objects of the deceased and to visit places frequented by the deceased. The work of grief is a dynamic process that is not time-limited nor predictable.[121] It may be that those left behind never "get over" the loss but, rather, find a place for it in their life and create through memory a new relationship with their loved one.

Families and partners of patients with AIDS may experience disenfranchised grief, defined as the grief that persons experience when they incur a loss that is not openly acknowledged, publicly mourned, or socially supported.[122] Support is not only important in assisting families in the tasks of grieving but is also important for nurses who have established valued relationships with their patients. Indeed, disenfranchised grief may also be experienced by nurses who do not allow themselves to acknowledge their patient's death as a personal loss or who are not acknowledged by others, such as the patient's family or even professional colleagues, for having suffered a loss.

For all individuals who have experienced a loss, Worden[123] has identified the tasks of grieving as (1) accepting the reality of the death; (2) experiencing the pain of grief; (3) adjusting to a changed physical, emotional, and social environment in which the deceased is missing; and (4) finding an appropriate emotional place for the person who died in the emotional life of the bereaved.

To facilitate each of Worden's tasks, Mallinson[121] recommends the following nursing interventions:

- Accept the reality of death by speaking of the loss and facilitating emotional expression.
- Work through the pain of grief by exploring the meaning of the grief experience.
- Adjust to the environment without the deceased by acknowledging anniversaries and the experience of loss during holidays and birthdays; help the bereaved to problem solve and recognize their own abilities to conduct their daily lives.
- Emotionally relocate the deceased and move on with life by encouraging socialization through formal and informal avenues.

The complications of AIDS-related grief often come from the secrecy and social stigma associated with the disease.[124] Reluctance to contact family and friends can restrict the normal support systems available for the bereaved.

In addition to a possible lack of social support, the death of patients with AIDS may result in complicated grief for the bereaved, given that death occurs after lengthy illness, and the relationships may have been ambivalent. Through truthful and culturally sensitive communication, health professionals can offer families support in their grief and promote trust that their needs are understood and validated.

## Summary

The care of patients with HIV/AIDS requires both active treatment and palliative care throughout the disease trajectory to relieve the suffering associated with opportunistic infections and malignancies. With up-to-date knowledge regarding HIV, including changes in epidemiology, diagnostic testing, treatment options, and available resources, nurses can offer effective and compassionate care to patients, alleviating physical, emotional, social, and spiritual suffering at all stages of HIV. Patients can maintain a sense of control and dignity until death by establishing a partnership with their health-care professionals in planning and implementing their healthcare, as well as through advanced care planning to insure that their end-of-life preferences and wishes are honored. The control of pain and symptoms associated with HIV/AIDS enables the patient and family to expend their energies on spiritual and emotional healing and the possibility for personal growth and transcendence, even as death approaches. Palliative care offers a comprehensive approach to address the physical, emotional, social, and spiritual needs of individuals with incurable progressive illness throughout the illness trajectory until death. Therefore, palliative care preserves patients' quality of life by protecting their self-integrity, reducing a perceived helplessness, and lessening the threat of exhaustion of coping resources.[125-131] Through effective and compassionate nursing care, patients with AIDS can achieve a sense of inner well-being even at death, with the potential to make the transition from life as profound, intimate, and precious an experience as their birth.[117]

REFERENCES

1. Watt G, Burnouf T. AIDS—past and future. N Engl J Med 2002;346:710–711.
2. Selwyn P, Forstein M. Overcoming the false dichotomy of curative vs palliative care for late-stage HIV/AIDS: "Let me live the way I want to live, until I can't." JAMA 2003;90:806–814.
3. O'Neill JF, Marconi K, Surapruik A, Blum N. Improving HIV/AIDS services through palliative care: A HRSA perspective. J Urban Health 2000;77:244–254.
4. Bolin J. Pernicious encroachment into end-of-life decision making: Federal intervention in palliative pain treatment. Am J Bioeth 2006;6:34–36.
5. O'Neill J, Alexander C. Palliative medicine and HIV/AIDS. HIV/AIDS Management in Office Practice 1997;24:607–615.
6. UNAIDS/WHO (2007) AIDS epidemic update: December 2007. UNAIDS. Geneva 2007.
7. Centers for Disease Control and Prevention. National Center for HIV, STD, and TB prevention: HIV/AIDS Surveillance report. 2008. http://www.cdc.gov/hiv/topics/surveillance/resources/reports/2006report/default.htm (accessed November 22, 2008).
8. Sherman DW, Ouellette S. Moving beyond fear: Lessons learned through a longitudinal review of the literature regarding health care providers and the care of people with HIV/AIDS. In: Sherman DW, ed. HIV/AIDS Update Nursing Clinics of North America. Philadelphia, PA: W.B. Saunders; 1999:1–48.
9. Flaskerud JH, Ungvarski P. 1999. HIV/AIDS: A guide to primary care management. Philadelphia, PA: W.B. Saunders, 1999.
10. Andrews L. The pathogenesis of HIV infection. In: Ropka ME, Williams, AB, eds. HIV Nursing and Symptom Management. Sudbury, MA: Jones & Bartlett Publishers; 1998:3–35.
11. Melroe NH, Stawarz KE, Simpson J. HIV RNA quantitation: Marker of HIV infection. J Assoc Nurses AIDS Care 1997;8:31–38.
12. Guidelines for Prevention and Treatment of Opportunistic Infections in HIV-Infected Adults and Adolescents. 2008, http://aidsinfo.nih.gov/contentfiles/Adult_OI.pdf (accessed December 15, 2008).
13. Orenstein R. Presenting syndromes of human immunodeficiency virus. Mayo Clin Proc 2002;77:1097–1102.
14. Al-Harthi L, Siegel J, Spritzler J, Pottage J, Agnoli M, Landay A. Maximum suppression of HIV replication leads to the restoration of HIV-specific responses in early HIV disease. AIDS 2000;14:761–770.
15. Gerard L, Flandre P, Raguin G, Le Gall JR, Vilde JL, Leport C. Life expectancy in hospitalized patients with AIDS: Prognostic factors on admission. J Palliat Care 1996;12:26–30.
16. Butters E, Webb D, Hearn J, Higginson I. Prospective audit of eight HIV/AIDS community palliative care services. Int Conf AIDS 11(2):223.
17. Malcolm J, Dobson P. Palliative care of AIDS: The last month of life. Annual Conf Aust Soc HIV Med 1994;6:266.
18. Barnes R, Barrett C, Weintraub S, Holowacz G. Hospital response to psycho-social needs of AIDS inpatients. J Palliat Care 1993;9:22–28.
19. Bloomer S. Palliative care. J Assoc Nurses AIDS Care 1998;9:45–47.
20. Malcolm JA. What is the best model for AIDS palliative care? Annual Conf Aust Soc HIV Med 1993;5:60.

21. Selwyn P, Rivard M. Palliative care for AIDS: Challenges and opportunities in the era of highly active anti-retroviral therapy. J Palliat Med 2003;6:475–487.

22. Shen JM, Blank A, Selwyn PA. Predictors of mortality for patients with advanced disease in an HIV palliative care program. J Acquir Immune Defic Syndr 2005;40:445–447.

23. Higginson I. Palliative care: A review of past changes and future trends. J Public Health Med 1993;15:3–8.

24. Sherman DW. Palliative care. In: Kirton C, Talotta D, Zwolski K, eds. Handbook of HIV/AIDS Nursing. Philadelphia: W.B. Saunders; 2001:173–194.

25. Post L, Dubler N. Palliative care: A bioethical definition, principles, and clinical guidelines. Bioethics Forum 1997;13:17–24.

26. National Consensus Project for Quality Palliative Care. Clinical practice guidelines for quality palliative care. 2004. http://www.nationalconsensusproject.org (accessed February 11, 2009).

27. Grothe TM, Brody RV. Palliative care for HIV disease. J Palliat Care 1995;11:48–49.

28. Fraser J. Sharing the challenge: The integration of cancer and AIDS. J Palliat Care 1995;11:23–25.

29. Malcolm JA, Sutherland DC. AIDS palliative care demands a new model. Med J Aust 1992;157:572–573.

30. Walsh TD. An overview of palliative care in cancer and AIDS. Oncology 1991;6:7–11.

31. Harding R, Easterbrook P, Higginson IJ, Karus D, Raveis VH, Marconi K. Access and equity in HIV/AIDS palliative care: A review of the evidence and responses. Palliat Med 2005;19:251–258.

32. Harding R, Karus D, Easterbrook P, Raveis VH, Higginson IJ, Marconi K. Does palliative care improve outcomes for patients with HIV/AIDS? A systematic review of the evidence. Sex Transm Infec 2005;81:5–14.

33. Burgoyne RW, Tan DH. Prolongation and quality of life for HIV-infected adults treated with highly active antiretroviral therapy (HAART): A balancing act. J Antimicrob Chemother 2008;61:69–473.

34. Ragsdale D, Morrow J. Quality of life as a function of HIV classification. Nurs Res 1992;39:355–359.

35. Ragsdale K, Kortarba J, Morrow J. Quality of life of hospitalized persons with AIDS. Image 1992;24:259–265.

36. Nichel J, Salsberry P, Caswell R, Keller M, Long T, O'Connell M. Quality of life in nurse case management of persons with AIDS receiving home care. Res Nurs Health 1996;19:91–99.

37. Vosvick M, Koopman C, Gore-Felton C, Thoresen C, Krumboltz J, Spiegal D. Relationship of functional quality of life to strategies for coping with the stress of living with HIV/AIDS. Psychosomatics 2003;44:51–58.

38. Baigis-Smith J, Gordon D, McGuire DB, Nanda J. Healthcare needs of HIV-infected persons in hospital, outpatient, home, and long-term care settings. J Assoc Nurses AIDS Care 1995;6:21–33.

39. Kemppainen J. Predictors of quality of life in AIDS patients. J Assoc Nurses AIDS Care 2001;12:61–70.

40. Keithley J, Swanson B, Murphy M, Levin D. HIV/AIDS and nutrition implications for disease management. Nurs Case Manag 2000;5:52–62.

41. Rene E, Roze C. Diagnosis and treatment of gastrointestinal infections in AIDS. In: Kotler D, ed. Gastrointestinal and Nutritional Manifestations of AIDS. New York, NY: Raven Press; 1991:65–92.

42. Hussein R. Current issues and forthcoming events. J Advan Nurs 2003;44:235–237.

43. Aron J. Optimization of nutritional support in HIV disease. In: Watson RR, ed. Nutrition and AIDS. Boca Raton, FL: CRC Press; 1994:215–233.

44. Freeman EM, MacIntyre RC. Evaluating alternative treatments for HIV infection. Nurs Clin North Am 1999;34(1):147–162.

45. Semba R, Graham P, Caiaffa J. Maternal vitamin A deficiency and mother-to-child transmission of HIV-1. Lancet 1994;343:1593–1597.

46. Nieman D. Exercise immunology: Practical applications. Int J Sports Med 1996;18:91–100.

47. LaPerriere A, Klimas N, Fletcher M, et al. Change in CD4 cell enumeration following aerobic exercise training in HIV-1 disease: Possible mechanisms and practical applications. Int J Sports Med 1997;18:56–61.

48. Centers for Disease Control and Prevention. Physical activity and health: A report of the surgeon general. Morb Mortal Wkly Rep 1996;45:591–592.

49. Ironson G, Field T, Scafidi F, et al. Massage therapy is associated with enhancement of the immune system's cytotoxic capacity. Int J Neurosci 1996;84:205–217.

50. Leserman J, Petitto J, Gaynes B, et al. Progression to AIDS, a clinical AIDS condition and mortality: Psychosocial and physiological predictors. Psychol Med 2002;32:1059–1073.

51. Sherman DW, Kirton C. Hazardous terrain and over the edge: The survival of HIV-positive heterosexual minority men. J Assoc Nurses AIDS Care 1998;9:23–34.

52. Eller LS. Effects of two cognitive-behavioral interventions on immunity and symptoms in persons with HIV. Ann Behav Med 1995;17:339–344.

53. Lechner S, Antoni M, Lydston D, et al. Cognitive-behavioral interventions improve quality of life in women with AIDS. J Psychosom Res 2003;54:252–261.

54. Remien RH, Rabkin JG, Williams JBW. Coping strategies and health beliefs of AIDS longterm survivors. Psychol Health 1992;6:335–345.

55. Cohen M. The use of coping humor in an HIV/AIDS population. Dissertation Abs Int 2001;61:4976.

56. Casey K. Malnutrition associated with HIV/AIDS. Part one: Definition and scope, epidemiology, and pathophysiology. J Assoc Nurses AIDS Care 1997;8:24–34.

57. Sherman DW, Kirton CA. Relapse to unsafe sex among HIV-positive heterosexual men. Appl Nurs Res 1999;12:91–100.

58. U.S. Department of Health and Human Services. Guidelines for using antiretroviral agents among HIV-infected adults and adolescents. 2008. http://aidsinfo.nih.gov/contentfiles/AdultandAdolescentGL.pdf (accessed December 15, 2008).

59. Murphy R, Flaherty J. Contemporary Diagnosis and Management of HIV/AIDS Infections. Newtown, PA: Handbooks in Health Care, 2003.

60. Adult Prevention and Treatment of Opportunistic Infections Guidelines Working Group. Guidelines for Prevention and Treatment of Opportunistic Infections in HIV-Infected Adults and Adolescents [DRAFT]. 2008:1–289. http://aidsinfo.nih.gov/contentfiles/Adult_OI.pdf (accessed December 15, 2008).

61. Von Gunten CF, Martinez J, Neely KJ, Von Roenn JH. AIDS and palliative medicine: Medical treatment issues. J Palliat Care 1995;11:5–9.

62. Panel on Antiretroviral Guidelines for Adult and Adolescents. Guidelines for the use of antiretroviral agents in HIV-1-infected

adults and adolescents. Department of Health and Human Services. 2008:1–139. http://www.aidsinfo.nih.gov/ContentFiles/AdultandAdolescentGL.pdf (accessed December 15, 2008).

63. Selwyn P, Rivard M. Palliative care for AIDS: Challenges and opportunities in the era of highly active anti-retroviral therapy. J Palliat Med 2003;6:475–487.

64. Hilts AE, Fish DN. Antiretroviral dosing in patients with organ dysfunction. AIDS Reader 1998;8:179–184.

65. Haynes RB, Taylor DW, and Sackett DL. Compliance in Health Care. Baltimore, MD: Johns Hopkins University Press, 1979.

66. Bangsberg DR. Less than 95% adherence to nonnucleoside reverse-transcriptase inhibitor therapy can lead to viral suppression. Clin Infect Dis 2006;43(7):939–941.

67. Raffa JD, Tossonian HK, Grebely J, et al. Intermediate highly active antiretroviral therapy adherence thresholds and empirical models for the development of drug resistance mutations. J Acquir Immune Defic Syndr 2008;47(3):397–399.

68. Chesney, M. Adherence to HIV/AIDS treatment. In Program of Adherence to New HIV Therapies: A Research Conference. Office of AIDS Research, Washington, DC: National Institutes of Health, 1997.

69. Williams AB. Adherence to highly active antiretroviral therapy. Nurs Clin North Am 1999;34:113–127.

70. Meichenbaum D, Turk C. Facilitating Treatment Adherence: Practitioner's Guidebook. New York, NY: Plenum, 1987.

71. Haynes RB, McKibbon KA, Kanani R. Systematic review of randomized trials of interventions to assist patients to follow prescriptions for medications. Lancet 1996;348:383–389.

72. Newshan G, Sherman DW. Palliative care: Pain and symptom management in persons with HIV/AIDS. Nurs Clin North Am 1999;34(1):131–145.

73. Holzemer W. HIV/AIDS: The symptom experience: What cell counts and viral loads won't tell you. Am J Nurs 2002;102:48–52.

74. Lorenz KA, Cunningham WE, Spritzer LK, Hays RD. Changes in symptoms and health-related quality of life in a nationally representative sample of adults in treatment for HIV. Quality Life Res 2006;15:951–958.

75. Norval DA. Symptoms and sites of pain experienced by AIDS patients. South African Med J 2004;94:450–454.

76. Frich LM, Borgbjerg FM. Pain and pain treatment in AIDS patients: A longitudinal study. J Pain Symptom Manage 2000;19:339–347.

77. Shofferman J, Brody R. Pain in far advanced AIDS. In: Foley KM, Bonica JJ, Ventafriddaet V, eds. Advances in Pain Research and Therapy, vol. 16. New York, NY: Raven Press; 1990:379–386.

78. Breitbart W, Passik S, Rosenfeld B, McDonald M, Thaler H, Portenoy H. Undertreatment of pain in AIDS. (abstract) American Pain Society, 13th Annual Meeting, November 10–14, 1994.

79. Cleeland CS, Gonin R, Hatfield AK, et al. Pain and its treatment in outpatients with metastatic cancer: The eastern co-operative group's cooperative study. N Engl J Med 1994;300:592–596.

80. Coyle N, Layman-Goldstein M. Pain assessment and pharmacological interventions. In: Matzo M, Sherman D, eds. Pallitaive Care Nursing: Quality Care to the End of Life (2nd ed). New York, NY: Springer Publishers; 2006:345–405.

81. American Pain Society. Principles of Analgesic Use in the Treatment of Acute Pain and Cancer Pain (3rd ed). Skokie, IL: American Pain Society, 1992.

82. Jacox A, Carr D, Payne R, Berde CB, Breitbart W. Clinical Practice Guideline Number 9: Management of Cancer Pain. Washington, DC: U.S. Department of Health and Human Services, Public Health Service, Agency for Health Care Policy and Research (Pub. No. 94–0592), 1994:139–141.

83. Trescot AM, Standiford H, Hansen H, Benyamin R, et al. Opiods in the management of chronic non-cancer pain: An update of American Society of the Interventional Pain Physicians' (ASIPP) Guidelines. Pain Physician 2008;11:S5–S62.

84. Fantoni M, Ricci F, Del Borgo C, et al. Multicentre study on the prevalence of symptoms and somatic treatment in HIV infection. Central Italy PRESINT Group. J Palliat Care 1997;13:9–13.

85. Holzemer W, Henry S, Reilly C. Assessing and managing pain in AIDS care: the patient perspective. J Assoc Nurses AIDS Care 1998;9:22–30.

86. Reiter G, Kudler N. Palliative care and HIV. Part II: Systemic manifestations and late stage illness. AIDS Clin Care 1996; 8:27–30.

87. Avis N, Smith K, Mayer K. The relationship among CD4, hemoglobin, symptoms, and quality of life domains in a cohort of HIV-positive men. Int Conf AIDS 1996;11:116 (abstract).

88. Sherman DW, Ye XY, McSherry CB, Parkas V, Calabrese M, Gatto M. Symptom assessment of patients with advanced cancer and AIDS and their family caregivers: The results of a quality-of-life pilot study. Am J Hosp Palliat Care 2007; 24(5):350–365.

89. Post-White J, Kinney ME, Savik K, Gau JB, Wilcox C, Lerner I. Therapeutic massage and healing touch improve symptoms in cancer. Integr Cancer Ther 2003;2:332–344.

90. Milan FB, Arnsten JH, Klein RS, et al. Use of complementary and alternative medicine (CAM) in inner-city persons with or at risk for HIV infection. AIDS Patient Care STDS. 2008;22:811–816.

91. Brashers DE, Neidig JL, Reynolds NR, Haas SM. Uncertainty in illness across the HIV/AIDS trajectory. J Assoc Nurses AIDS Care 1998;9:66–77.

92. Grassi L, Sighinolfi L. Psychosocial correlates of quality of life in patients with HIV infection. AIDS Patient Care STDS 1996;10:296–299.

93. Farber E, Mirsalimi H, Williams K, McDaniel J. Meaning of illness and psychological adjustment to HIV/AIDS. Psychosomatics 2003;44:485–491.

94. Silver E, Bauman L, Camacho S, Hudis J. Factors associated with psychological distress in urban mothers with late-stage HIV/AIDS. AIDS Behav 2003;7:421–431.

95. Butters E, Higginson I, George R. Palliative care needs of patients referred to two HIV/AIDS community teams. Int Conf AIDS 1993;9(1):522.

96. Friedland J, Renwick R, McColl M. Coping and social support as determinants of quality of life in HIV/AIDS. AIDS Care 1996;8:15–31.

97. Sherman DW. Reciprocal suffering: The need to improve family caregiver's quality of life through palliative care. J Palliat Med 1998;1:357–366.

98. Atkinson JH, Grant I. Natural history of neuropsychiatric manifestations of HIV disease. Psychiatr Clin North Am 1994;17:33.

99. McEnany GW, Hughes AM, Lee KA. Depression and HIV. Nurs Clin North Am 1996;31:57–80.

100. Repetto MJ, Petitto JM. Psychopharmacology in HIV-infected patients. Psychosom Med 2008;70:585–592.

101. Schrimshaw R. Relationship-specific unsupportive social interactions and depressive symptoms among women living with HIV/AIDS: Direct and moderating effects. J Behav Med 2003;26:297–313.

102. Arriendel J. Differential coping strategies, anxiety, depression, and symptomatology among African-American women with HIV/AIDS. Dissertation Abs Int. Section B: The Sciences & Engineering. 2003;64:1481. US: Univ MicroFilms International.

103. Capaldini L. HIV disease: psychosocial issues and psychiatric complications. In: Sande MS, Volberding PA, eds. The Medical Management of AIDS. Philadelphia, PA: W.B. Saunders; 1997:217–238.

104. Chesney MA, Folkman S, Chambers D. Coping Effectiveness training decreases distress in men living with HIV/AIDS. Int Conf AIDS 1996;11:50.

105. Kinara, M. Transcendental meditation: A coping mechanism for HIV-positive people. Int Conf AIDS 1996;11:421.

106. Mellors M, Riley T, Erlen J. HIV, self-transcendence and quality of life. J Assoc Nurses AIDS Care 1997;8:59–69.

107. Elkins D, Hedstrom LJ, Hughes L, Leaf JA, Saunders C. Towards a humanistic-phenomenological spirituality. J Humanistic Psychol 1998;28:5–18.

108. Kylma J, Vehvilainen-Julkunen K, Lahdevirta J. Hope, despair and hopelessness in living with HIV/AIDS: A grounded theory study. J Adv Nurs 2001;33:764–775.

109. Curtis R, Patrick D, Caldwell E, Collier A. Why don't patients and physicians talk about end of life care?: Barriers to communication for patients with acquired immunodeficiency syndrome and their primary care clinicians. Arch Intern Med 2000;160:1690–1696.

110. Ferris F, Flannery J, McNeal H, Morissette M, Cameron R, Bally G. Palliative care: A comprehensive guide for the care of persons with HIV disease. Toronto, ON: Mount Sinai Hospital/Casey House Hospice, 1995.

111. Wood C, Whittet S, Bradbeer C. ABC of palliative care. BMJ 1997;315:1433–1436.

112. Goldstone I, Kuhl D, Johnson A, Le Clerc, McCleod A. Patterns of care in advanced HIV disease in a tertiary treatment centre. AIDS Care 1995;7:47–56.

113. Pessin H. The influence of cognitive impairment on desire for hastened death among terminally ill AIDS patients. Dissertation Abs Int 2001;62:2963.

114. Curtis R, Patrick D, Caldwell E, Collier A. The attitudes of patients with advanced AIDS toward use of the medical futility rationale in decisions to forgo mechanical ventilation. Arch Intern Med 2000;160:1597–1601.

115. Flaskerud J, Lee P. Vulnerability to health problems in female informal caregivers of persons with HIV/AIDS and age-related dementias. J Adv Nurs 2001;33:60–68.

116. Sherman DW, Ye XY, McSherry C, Parkas, V, Calabrese M, Gatto M. Quality of life of patients with advanced cancer and acquired immune deficiency syndrome and their family caregivers. J Palliat Med 2006;9:948–963.

117. Byock I. Dying Well: The Prospect for Growth at the End of Life. New York, NY: Riverhead Books, 1997.

118. Welsby P, Richardson A, Brettle R. AIDS: Aspects in adults. In: Doyle D, Hanks G, MacDonald N, eds. Oxford Textbook of Palliative Medicine (2nd ed). New York, NY: Oxford University Press: 1998:1121–1148.

119. Sikkema K, Kochman A, DiFranceisco W, Kelly J, Hoffman R. AIDS-related grief and coping with loss among HIV-positive men and women. J Behav Med 2003;26:165–181.

120. Rando T. Grief, Dying, and Death: Clinical Interventions for Caregivers. Champaign, IL: Research Press, 1984.

121. Mallinson RK. Grief work of HIV-positive persons and their survivors. In: Sherman DW, ed. HIV/AIDS Update. Nurs Clin North Am. Philadelphia, PA: W.B. Saunders; 1999:163–177.

122. Doka K. Disenfranchised Grief: Recognizing the Hidden Sorrow. Lexington, MA: Lexington Books, 1989.

123. Worden J. Grief Counseling and Grief Therapy: A Handbook for the Mental Health Practitioner. New York, NY: Springer Publications, 1991.

124. Maxwell N. Responses to loss and bereavement in HIV. Prof Nurse 1996;12:21–24.

125. Centers for Disease Control and Prevention Guidelines for the Prevention of Opportunistic Infections in Persons with Human Immunodeficiency Virus. Morbid Mortal Week Rep 1999;48(RR-10):40–43.

126. Centers for Disease Control and Prevention. Recommendations of the Advisory Committee on Immunization Practices (ACIP): Use of vaccines and immune globulins in persons with altered immunocompetence. Morbid Mortal Week Rep 1993;42 (RR-5):5.

127. Portenoy RK. Contemporary Diagnosis and Management of Pain in Oncologic and AIDS Patients. Newtown, PA: Handbooks in Health Care, 1997.

128. Coyne P, Lyne M, Watson AC. Symptom management in people with AIDS. Am J Nurs 2002;102:48–57.

129. McNaghten AD, Hanson DL, Jones, JL, Dworkin MS, Ward JW, Adult/Adolescent Spectrum of Disease Group. Effects of antiretroviral therapy and opportunistic illness primary chemoprophylaxis on survival after AIDS diagnosis. AIDS 1999;13:1687–1695.

130. U.S. Department of Health and Human Services. USPHS/IDSA Guidelines for the Prevention of Opportunistic Infections in Persons Infected with Human Immunodeficiency Virus. 2001. http://aidsinfo.nih.gov/guidelines/ (accessed March 24, 2005).

131. Bayes R. A way to screen for suffering in palliative care. J Palliat Care 1997;13:22–26.

# 42

Kenneth L. Kirsh, Peggy Compton, and Steven D. Passik

# Caring for the Drug-Addicted Patient at the End of Life

*You've stuck with me and helped me through a lot when other docs would have given up on me.*
*— Patient with metastatic breast cancer who also had a frank addiction problem and was found to be selling and trading medications for cocaine; her eventual management is described later in the chapter*

♦ **Key Points**

♦ *With the changing face of cancer and other advanced diseases progressing, patients are living for longer periods of time, which creates new challenges in treating pain and potential addiction issues on a longer term basis.*

♦ *Identifying addiction in patients with advanced disease is not an easy task, and old conceptions of addiction such as tolerance and dependence need to be re-examined.*

♦ *Patients with advanced disease and comorbid addiction are difficult to manage but can be successfully treated with careful documentation and planning.*

♦ *Remember that the patient with advanced disease and comorbid addiction has two diseases that need treatment: one of drug addiction and one of chronic pain.*

Substance use disorders are a consistent phenomenon in the United States, with estimated base rates of 6% and 15%.[1-4] This prevalence of drug abuse certainly touches medically ill patients and can negatively influence how pain is treated. Because of these issues and despite the fact that national guidelines exist for the treatment of pain disorders such as cancer, pain continues to be undertreated, even at the end of life.[5-7] In cancer, approximately 40% to 50% of patients with metastatic disease and 90% of patients with terminal cancer or other advanced diseases are reported to experience unrelieved pain.[5-7] Furthermore, inadequate treatment of cancer pain is an even greater possibility if the patient is a member of an ethnic minority, female, elderly, a child, or a substance abuser.[8] Therefore, for multicultural patients, we sometimes have conflicting multiple biases in pain treatment that can lead to poor management, mutual suspicion and alienation, and suffering unless these biases are adequately addressed. Finally, although we must consider the potential of abuse, misuse, and diversion with palliative patients, we must never let this worry generate fear on the part of the practitioner which could ultimately lead to further undertreatment of pain as discussed above. The following case is an extreme example of when this fear can lead to poor patient care.

## CASE STUDY

### A 65-Year-Old Man With Newly Diagnosed, Stage IV Pancreatic Cancer

The father of one of the authors was a 65-year-old man who presented to a major midwestern medical center with extreme jaundice. During the work-up in hospital, he was diagnosed with very late-stage pancreatic cancer. Despite no history of drug abuse, alcoholism, or any other potential warning signs, the physicians decided to discharge the patient because there were no feasible curative treatment options. The family members present asked for help and clarification but were told the patient should get his affairs in order and "go home to die." The physicians involved initially offered no prescriptions for pain management upon discharge, stating that they were not comfortable with writing for "narcotics" [as a side note, "narcotics" refers to the legal side of these substances when a crime is involved, whereas "opioids" is the term appropriate for medical use of them]. Eventually, the patient was sent home with a prescription for a total of 20 oxycodone/acetaminophen 5/325 mg. The author quickly intervened, helped the patient to switch hospital systems, and ultimately saw that the patient got appropriate care.

## Incidence of Substance Use Disorders in Patients With Advanced Disease

Although few studies have been conducted to evaluate the epidemiology of substance abuse in patients with advanced illness, substance use disorders appear to be relatively rare within the tertiary-care population with cancer and other advanced diseases. Findings from a consultations review performed by the Psychiatry Services at Memorial Sloan-Kettering Cancer Center revealed that requests for management of issues related to substance abuse consisted of only 3% of the consultations.[9,10]

While the incidence of substance use disorders is much lower in patients with advanced disease than in society at large, in community-based medical populations, and emergency medical departments, this may not represent the true prevalence in the advanced illness spectrum overall. Institutional biases or a tendency for patients' underreporting in tertiary care hospitals may be reflective of the relatively low prevalence of substance abuse among advanced patients. Social forces may also inhibit patients' reporting of drug use behavior. Many drug abusers are of lower socioeconomic standing and feel alienated from the health-care system and, therefore, may not seek care in tertiary care centers. Furthermore, those who are treated in these centers may not acknowledge drug abuse for fear of stigmatization.[9–11] Additionally, minority patients are treated in such settings more often than are Caucasians.

## Issues in Defining Abuse and Addiction in the Medically Ill

It is difficult to define substance abuse and addiction in patients with advanced illness, as the definitions of both terms have been adopted from addicted populations without medical illness. Furthermore, the pharmacological phenomena of tolerance and physical dependence are commonly confused with abuse and addiction. The use of these terms is so strongly influenced by sociocultural considerations that it

may lead to confusion in the clinical setting. Therefore, the clarification of this terminology is necessary to improve the diagnosis and management of substance abuse when treating patients with advanced disease.[10]

Substance abuse concentrates on the psychosocial, physical, and vocational harm that occurs from drug-taking, which makes identifying drug-taking behaviors more difficult in patients with advanced illness who are receiving potentially abusable drugs for legitimate medical purposes. In contrast, substance dependence emphasizes chronicity and includes the dimensions of tolerance and physical dependence. Because of the possibility that patients may develop these effects as a result of therapeutic drug use, it is inapplicable to use this terminology in the medically ill. Not only does the existing nomenclature complicate the effort to distinguish the drug-taking behaviors of patients with advanced disease that are appropriately treated with potentially abusable drugs, it also impedes the communication that is fundamental for proper pain management and medical care.[9,10]

## Theoretical Problems in the Diagnosis of Substance Use Disorders

Because substance abuse is increasingly widespread in the population at large, patients with advanced disease who have used illicit drugs are more frequently encountered in medical settings. Illicit drug use, actual or suspected misuse of prescribed medication, or actual substance use disorders create the most serious difficulties in the clinical setting, complicating the treatment of pain management. However, the management of substance abuse is fundamental to adherence to medical therapy and safety during treatment. Also, adverse interactions between illicit drugs and medications prescribed as part of the patient's treatment can be dangerous. Continuous substance abuse may alienate or weaken an already tenuous social support network that is crucial for alleviating the chronic stressors associated with advanced disease and its treatment. Therefore, a history of substance abuse can impede treatment and pain management and increase the risk of hastening morbidity and mortality among advanced patients, which can only be alleviated by a therapeutic approach that addresses drug-taking behavior while expediting the treatment of the malignancy and distressing symptoms, as well as addiction.[11]

When assessing drug-taking behaviors in the patient with advanced disease, issues exist that increase the difficulty in arriving at a diagnosis of abuse or addiction. These issues include the problem of undertreatment of pain, sociocultural influences on the definition of aberrancy in drug-taking, and the importance of cancer-related variables.[9,10]

### Pseudoaddiction

Various studies have provided compelling evidence that pain is undertreated in populations with advanced disease.[5–7]

Clinical experience indicates that the inadequate management of symptoms and related pain may be the motivation for aberrant drug-taking behaviors. Pseudoaddiction, coined by Weissman and Haddox, is the term used to depict the distress and drug-seeking that can occur in the context of unrelieved pain, such as similar behaviors in addicts.[12] The main factor of this syndrome is that sufficient pain relief eliminates aberrant behaviors.

The original paper on pseudoaddiction was a four-page, single case study of a 17-year-old man presenting with leukemia and complaining of chest wall pain. The case was made that undertreated pain created behavioral changes that looked much like iatrogenic addiction in the patient and resulted in a crisis regarding the clinical interactions between the healthcare team and patient. Clinically, pseudoaddiction is not uncommonly seen in outpatients, those with and those without histories of chemical dependency. Interestingly, patients with chemical dependency are often set up for pseudoaddiction. Their unique pharmacological needs, combined with the ambivalence clinicians feel about their treatment, render them a likely to be underdosed. With regard to the range of behaviors to which the term has been applied, it is important to note that the original patient's behaviors as described in the paper were relatively tame. In pain lectures and case discussions, it would not be uncommon to hear the use of illicit drugs and alcohol described as evidence of pseudoaddiction. That they might be desperate attempts to improve analgesia is not categorically impossible, but the degree of conviction that clinicians express about it as a possibility has clearly changed.

The potential for pseudoaddiction creates a challenge for the assessment of a known substance abuser with an advanced illness. Clinical evidence indicates that aberrant behaviors impelled by unrelieved pain can become so dramatic in this population that some patients appear to return to illicit drug use as a means of self-medication. Others use more covert patterns of behavior, which may also cause concerns regarding the possibility of true addiction. Although it may not be obvious that drug-related behaviors are aberrant, the meaning of these behaviors may be difficult to discern in the context of unrelieved symptoms.[9,10]

### Distinguishing Aberrant Drug-Taking Behaviors

Whereas abuse is defined as the use of an illicit drug or a prescription drug without medical indication, addiction refers to the continued use of either type of drug in a compulsive manner regardless of harm to the user or others. However, when a drug is prescribed for a medically diagnosed purpose, less assuredness exists as to the behaviors that could be deemed aberrant, thereby increasing the potential for a diagnosis of drug abuse or addiction. Although it is difficult to disagree with the aberrancy of certain behaviors, such as intravenous injection of oral formulations, various other behaviors are less blatant, such as a patient experiencing unrelieved pain who is taking an extra dose of prescribed opioids.[9,10]

The ability to categorize these questionable behaviors as apart from social or cultural norms is also based on the assumption that certain parameters of normative behavior exist. Although it is useful to consider the degree of aberrancy of a given behavior, it is important to recognize that these behaviors exist along a continuum, with certain behaviors being less aberrant (such as aggressively requesting medication) and other behaviors more aberrant (such as injection of oral formulations). Empirical data defining these parameters do not exist regarding prescription drug use (Table 42–1). If a large portion of patients were found to engage in a certain behavior, it may be normative, and judgments regarding aberrancy should be influenced accordingly.[9,10]

We know more scientifically about aberrant behaviors, their prevalence and meaning today than we did in the mid-1990s. We know that many patients will have at least a few aberrant behaviors in a 6-month period.[12a] We also know that once a patient has demonstrated four behaviors in their lifetime, they have an 85% likelihood of meeting DSM-IV criteria for substance use disorder.[12b] But there is still much to be learned, confirmed, replicated, and studied.

The importance of social and cultural norms also raises the possibility of bias in the determination of aberrancy. A clinician's willingness to classify a questionable drug-related behavior as aberrant when performed by a member of a certain social or ethnic group may be influenced by bias against that group. Based on clinical observation, this type of prejudice has been found to be common in the assessment of drug-related behaviors of patients with substance abuse histories. Regardless of whether the drug-abuse history is in the past or present, questionable behaviors by these patients may immediately be labeled as abuse or addiction. The possibility of

Table 42–1
**Sample Behaviors More or Less Likely To Indicate Aberrancy**

| Less Indicative of Aberrancy | More Indicative of Aberrancy |
| --- | --- |
| Drug hoarding during periods of reduced symptoms | Prescription forgery |
| Acquisition of similar drugs from other medical sources | Concurrent abuse of related illicit drugs |
| Aggressive complaining about the need for higher doses | Recurrent prescription losses |
| Unapproved use of the drug to treat another symptom | Selling prescription drugs |
| Unsanctioned dose escalation one or two times | Multiple unsanctioned dose escalations |
| Reporting psychic effects not intended by the clinician | Stealing or borrowing another patient's drugs |
| Requesting specific drugs | Obtaining prescription drugs from nonmedical sources |

bias in the assessment of drug-related behaviors also exists for patients who are members of racial or ethnic minority groups different from that of the clinician.[9,10] The following case study illustrates the point that aberrant behaviors do not have a universal interpretation (including the illegal and obviously worrisome ones) and must be understood in the context of the patient's care.

CASE STUDY
*A 54-Year-Old Man With Pancreatic Cancer*

A 54-year-old man was introduced to our practice. He had just been released from a prison sentence and shortly thereafter was diagnosed with end-stage pancreatic cancer. He was significant for a history of drug use and robbery. Given his poor prognosis, the patient was placed in hospice care, but the staff became increasingly worried that the patient appeared overly sedated most days but was complaining of increasing pain and was running out of medications early. This increased until he was a candidate to be discharged from hospice because of the growing suspicions. Working together with hospice, the staff were able to gain his confidence and learned that the patient's son was stealing his pain medications and overdosing the patient on promethazine to keep him quiet. When asked why he did not tell the staff sooner, the patient responded: "I just got out of prison and am dying. I don't want my last act to be sending my son to jail." The home situation was altered and the patient was able to stay in hospice and achieve adequate pain care and ultimately a good death.

## Disease-Related Variables

Changes caused by progressive diseases, such as cancer, also challenge the principal concepts used to define addiction. Alterations in physical and psychosocial functioning caused by advanced illness and its treatment may be difficult to distinguish from the morbidity associated with drug abuse. In particular, alterations in functioning may complicate the ability to evaluate a concept that is vital to the diagnosis of addiction: "use despite harm." For example, discerning the questionable behaviors can be difficult in a patient who develops social withdrawal or cognitive changes after brain irradiation for metastases. Even if diminished cognition is clearly related to pain medication used in treatment, this effect might only reflect a narrow therapeutic window rather than the patient's use of analgesic to acquire these psychic effects.[9,10]

To accurately assess drug-related behaviors in patients with advanced disease, explicit information is usually required regarding the role of the drug in the patient's life. Therefore, the presence of mild mental clouding or the time spent out of bed may have less meaning than other outcomes, such as noncompliance with primary therapy related to drug use or

behaviors that threaten relationships with physicians, other health-care professionals, and family members.[9,10]

## Appropriate Definitions of Abuse and Addiction for Advanced Illness

A more appropriate definition of addiction would exemplify that it is a chronic disorder characterized by "the compulsive use of a substance resulting in physical, psychological, or social harm to the user and continued use despite the harm."[13] Although this definition is not without fault, it emphasizes that addiction is essentially a psychological and behavioral syndrome.[9,10]

A differential diagnosis should also be considered if questionable behaviors occur during pain treatment. A true addiction (substance dependence) is only one of many possible interpretations. A diagnosis of pseudoaddiction should also be taken into account if the patient is reporting distress associated with unrelieved symptoms. Impulsive drug use may also be indicative of another psychiatric disorder, the diagnosis of which may have therapeutic implications. On occasion, aberrant drug-related behaviors appear to be causally remotely related to a mild encephalopathy, with perplexity concerning the appropriate therapeutic regimen. On rare occasions, questionable behaviors imply criminal intent. These diagnoses are not mutually exclusive.[9,10]

Varied and repeated observations over a period of time may be necessary to categorize questionable behaviors properly. Perceptive psychiatric assessment is crucial and may require evaluation by consultants who can elucidate the complex interactions among personality factors and psychiatric illness. Some patients may be self-medicating symptoms of anxiety, depression, insomnia, or problems of adjustment (such as boredom caused by decreased ability to engage in usual activities and hobbies). Yet others may have character pathology that may be the more prominent determinant of drug-taking behavior. Patients with borderline personality disorders, for example, may impulsively use prescription medications that regulate inner tension or improve chronic emptiness or boredom and express anger at physicians, friends, or family. Psychiatric assessment is vitally important for both the population without a prior history of substance abuse and the population of known substance abusers who have a high incidence of psychiatric comorbidity.[14]

## Cultural Issues in the Treatment of Substance Use Disorders

As noted earlier, cancer pain continues to be grossly undertreated despite the availability of guidelines for its clinical management, with patients who are members of an ethnic minority or substance abusers having a greater risk of inadequate treatment of cancer pain.[5-7] In fact, various studies have documented that minority patients receive insufficient pain treatment compared to nonminority patients when being treated for pain caused by a variety of sources.[15-17] Because minority patients with advanced illness are undertreated for pain, they may be at greater risk of being misdiagnosed if exhibiting behaviors of pseudoaddiction.

Recently, more attention has been given to the significant influence that age, gender, and ethnicity have on the issues and treatment of substance abuse. Certain issues must be considered when implementing substance abuse treatment with the minority patient who is suspected of having a substance use disorder.[18]

First and foremost, it must be recognized that immense diversity exists within the different sociocultural groups themselves. Any given minority patient may possess beliefs, values, or drug-taking behaviors that greatly differ from the majority of the sociocultural group of which the patient is a member. In addition to ethnic orientation, attention must also focus on other sociocultural factors such as age, gender, sexual orientation, income, education, geographic location, and level of acculturation.[18] Ascribing certain cultural characteristics to all patients of a particular minority group may lead to stereotyping, alienating patients, and compromising treatment effectiveness.[19] Although the perfect scenario would be to accurately understand all of the possible cultural issues that influence the patient within the context of his/her life circumstances, this is difficult and may be impractical.[1,18] Therefore, it is particularly important to respond to cultural needs in the treatment of substance abuse, because sociocultural factors greatly effect the manifestation of the disease. Consequently, clinicians must often acclimate their therapeutic approaches to accommodate the patient's sociocultural orientation.[18]

## Risks in Patients With Current or Remote Histories of Drug Abuse

There is a lack of information regarding the risk of abuse or addiction during or subsequent to the therapeutic administration of potentially abusable drugs to medically ill patients with a current or remote history of abuse or addiction.[9] The possibility of successful long-term opioid therapy in patients with cancer or chronic nonmalignant pain has been indicated by anecdotal reports, particularly if the abuse or addiction is remote.[20-22]

Because it is commonly accepted that the likelihood of aberrant drug-related behavior occurring during treatment for medical illness will be greater for those with a remote or current history of substance abuse, it is reasonable to consider the possibility of abuse behaviors occurring when using different therapies. For example, although no clinical evidence exists to support that the use of short-acting drugs or the

---

**Table 42–2**
**Basic Principles for Prescribing Controlled Substances to Patients With Advanced Illness and Issues of Addiction**

Choose an opioid based on around-the-clock dosing.
Choose long-acting agents when possible.
As much as possible, limit or eliminate the use of short-acting or "breakthrough" doses.
Use nonopioid adjuvants when possible, and monitor for compliance with those medications.
Use nondrug adjuvants whenever possible (e.g., relaxation techniques, distraction, biofeedback, TNS, communication about thoughts and feelings of pain).
If necessary, limit the amount of medication given at any one time (i.e., write prescriptions for a few days' worth or a week's worth of medication at a time).
Use pill counts and urine toxicology screens as necessary.
If compliance is suspect or poor, refer to an addictions specialist.

---

parenteral route is more likely to cause questionable drug-related behaviors than other therapeutic strategies, it may be prudent to avoid such therapies in patients with histories of drug abuse.[9] Table 42–2 presents a basic set of principles pertaining to prescribing controlled substances to this patient population.

## Summary of Issues

Clinicians should understand that essentially any drug that acts upon the central nervous system or any route of administration has the potential to be abused. Therefore, a more comprehensive approach that recognizes the biological, chemical, social, and psychiatric aspects is necessary to effectively manage patients with substance abuse histories. Using this strategy extends beyond merely avoiding certain drugs or routes of administration—it also affords practical means to manage risk during cancer treatment.[9]

## Clinical Management of Advanced-Disease Patients With Substance Use Histories

The most challenging issues in caring for patients with advanced disease typically arise from patients who are actively abusing alcohol or other drugs. This is because patients who are actively abusing drugs experience more difficulty in managing pain.[23] Patients may become caught in a cycle where pain functions as a barrier to seeking treatment for addiction with another addiction, possibly complicating treatment for chronic pain.[24] Also, because pain is undertreated, the risk of binging with prescription medications and/or other substances increases for drug-abusing patients.[23]

## General Guidelines

The following guidelines can be beneficial, whether the patient is actively abusing drugs or has a history of substance abuse. The principles outlined assist clinicians in establishing structure, control, and monitoring of addiction-related behaviors, which may be helpful and necessary at times in all pain treatment.[25]

Recommendations for the long-term administration of potentially abusable drugs, such as opioids, to patients with a history of substance abuse are based exclusively on clinical experience. Research is needed to ascertain the most effective strategies and to empirically identify patient subgroups who may be most responsive to different approaches. The following guidelines broadly reflect the types of interventions that might be considered in this clinical context.[10,25]

## Multidisciplinary Approach

Pain and symptom management is often complicated by various medical, psychosocial, and administrative issues in the population of advanced patients with a substance use disorder. The most effective team may include a physician with expertise in pain/palliative care, nurses, social workers, and, when possible, a mental health-care provider with expertise in the area of addiction medicine.[10,25]

## Assessment of Substance Use History

In an effort to not offend, threaten, or anger patients, many times clinicians avoid asking patients about drug abuse. There is also often the expectation that patients will not answer truthfully. However, obtaining a detailed history of duration, frequency, and desired effect of drug use is vital. Adopting a nonjudgmental position and communicating in an empathetic and truthful manner is the best strategy when taking patients' substance abuse histories.[11,25]

In anticipating defensiveness on the part of the patient, it can be helpful for clinicians to mention that patients often misrepresent their drug use for logical reasons, such as stigmatization, mistrust of the interviewer, or concerns regarding fears of undertreatment. It is also wise for clinicians to explain that in an effort to keep the patient as comfortable as possible, by preventing withdrawal states and prescribing sufficient medication for pain and symptom control, an accurate account of drug use is necessary.[11,25]

The use of a careful, graduated-style interview can be beneficial in slowly introducing the assessment of drug abuse. This approach begins with broad and general inquiries regarding the role of drugs in the patient's life, such as caffeine and nicotine and gradually proceeds to more specific questions regarding illicit drugs. This interview style can also assist in discerning any coexisting psychiatric disorders, which can significantly contribute to aberrant drug-taking behavior.

Once identified, treatment of comorbid psychiatric disorders can greatly enhance management strategies and decrease the risk of relapse.[11,25]

## Use of Risk Assessment Tools

As stated above, potential opioid use must be accompanied by risk stratification and management. Given time constraints, a full psychiatric interview may not be feasible and thus time sensitive measures are clearly needed to help in this endeavor. However, until very recently, there were nearly no validated screening tools for the prediction of aberrant behaviors in pain patients. This need has been acknowledged and there has been a substantial increase in addiction-related screening tools.[25a] Many screening tools contain items on personal and family history of addiction as well as other history-related risk factors, such as pre-adolescent sexual abuse, age, and psychological disease. Some of the tools are particular to pain management, whereas others are simply risk factors for addiction in general. The rather sudden and large volume of tools available is both a blessing (in that we have choices) and a curse (in that it is sometimes difficult to determine which is most applicable to a particular practice). As a final note, it must be remembered that these are tools for clinical decision-making and should not be viewed as necessarily diagnostically accurate. Whatever tool the clinician chooses, it is advised that the screening process be presented to the patient with the assurance that no answers will negatively influence effective pain management.

## Setting Realistic Goals for Therapy

The rate of recurrence for drug abuse and addiction is high. The stress associated with advanced illness and the easy availability of centrally acting drugs increases this risk. Therefore, total prevention of relapse may be impossible in this type of setting. Gaining an understanding that compliance and abstinence are not realistic goals may decrease conflicts with staff members in terms of management goals. Instead, the goals might be perceived as the creation of a structure for therapy that includes ample social/emotional support and limit-setting to control the harm done by relapse.[11,25]

There may be some subgroups of patients who are unable to comply with the requirements of therapy because of severe substance use disorders and comorbid psychiatric diagnoses. In these instances, clinicians must modify limits on various occasions and endeavor to develop a greater variety and intensity of supports. This may necessitate frequent team meetings and consultations with other clinicians. However, pertinent expectations must be clarified, and therapy that is not successful should be modified.[11,25]

## Evaluation and Treatment of Comorbid Psychiatric Disorders

Extremely high comorbidity of personality disorders, depression, and anxiety disorders exist in alcoholics and other patients with substance abuse histories.[14] The treatment of depression and anxiety can increase patient comfort and decrease the risk of relapse or aberrant drug-taking.[11,25]

### Preventing or Minimizing Withdrawal Symptoms

Because many patients with drug abuse histories use multiple drugs, it is necessary to conduct a complete drug-use history to prepare for the possibility of withdrawal. Delayed abstinence syndromes, such as those that may occur after abuse of some benzodiazepine drugs, may be particularly diagnostically challenging.[11,25]

### Considering the Therapeutic Impact of Tolerance

Patients who are active substance abusers may be tolerant to drugs administered for therapy, which will make pain management more difficult. The magnitude of this tolerance is never known. Therefore, it is best to begin with a conservative dose of therapeutic drug and then rapidly titrate the dose, with frequent reassessments until the patient is comfortable.[9,22] Also, it must be remembered that opioids, pharmacologically speaking, still have no ceiling.[25b] Cancer patients and those with progressive disease can still be treated with gradually increasing doses, and opioids can still be titrated to effect or toxicity with no arbitrary number of milligrams constituting a limit.

### Applying Pharmacological Principles to Treating Pain

Widely accepted guidelines for cancer pain management must be used to optimize long-term opioid therapy.[26,27] These guidelines stress the importance of patient self-report as the base for dosing, individualization of therapy to identify a favorable equilibrium between efficacy and side effects, and the value of monitoring over time.[25] They also are strongly indicative of the concurrent treatment of side effects as the basis for enhancing the balance between both analgesia and adverse effects.[28]

Individualization of the dose without regard to the size, which is the most important guideline for long-term opioid therapy, can be difficult in populations with substance abuse histories.[25] Although it may be appropriate to use care in prescribing potentially abusable drugs to these populations, deciding to forego the guideline of dose individualization without regard to absolute dose may increase the risk of undertreatment.[29] Aberrant drug-related behaviors may develop in response to unrelieved pain. Although these behaviors might be best understood as pseudoaddiction, the incidence of such behaviors serves to verify clinicians' fears and encourages greater prudence in prescribing.[25]

Another common misconception is the use of methadone. Clinicians who manage patients with substance abuse histories must comprehend the pharmacology of methadone because of its dual role as a treatment for opioid addiction and as an analgesic.[30,31] Methadone impedes withdrawal for significantly longer periods than it relieves pain. That is, abstinence can be prevented and opioid cravings lessened with a single dose, whereas most patients appear to require a minimum of three doses daily to obtain sustained analgesia. Although patients who are receiving methadone maintenance for treatment for opioid addiction can be administered methadone as an analgesic beyond the guidelines of the addiction treatment program, this usually necessitates a substantial modification in therapy, including dose escalation and multiple daily doses.[11,25]

From a pharmacological stance, the management of such a change does not pose difficult issues. It can, however, create substantial stress for the patient and clinicians involved in the treatment of the addiction disorder. Because the drug has been classified as addiction therapy, as opposed to pain therapy, some patients express disbelief in the analgesic efficacy of methadone. Others wish to continue the morning dose for addiction even if treatment throughout the remainder of the day uses the same drug at an equivalent or higher dose. Some clinicians who work at methadone clinics are willing to continue to be involved and prescribe opioids outside the program, and others wish to relinquish care.[25]

### Selecting Appropriate Drugs and Route of Administration for the Symptom and Setting

The use of long-acting analgesics in sufficient amounts may help to minimize the number of rescue doses needed, lessen cravings, and decrease the risk of abuse of prescribed medications, given the possible difficulty of using short-acting formulations in patients with substance abuse histories. Rather than being overly concerned regarding the choice of drug or route of administration, the prescription of opioids and other potentially abusable drugs should be carried out with limits and guidelines.[11,25]

Many clinicians now respond to particularly high doses with rotation to another opioid. This practice is based on capitalizing on incomplete cross-tolerance, or the unique pharmacology of methadone in particular, to bring doses down while maintaining or improving efficacy and changing the balance of efficacy to toxicity.[32,33] Some clinicians set arbitrary dose limits for the various opioids. Others stopped using certain opioids they perceived as of higher risk or street value. Still others became so disillusioned as to stop using opioids altogether.

### Recognizing Specific Drug Abuse Behaviors

In an effort to monitor the development of aberrant drug-taking behaviors, all patients who are prescribed potentially abusable drugs must be evaluated over time. This is particularly true for those patients with a remote or current history of drug abuse, including alcohol abuse. Should a high level of concern exist regarding such behaviors, frequent visits and regular assessments of significant others who can contribute information regarding the patient's drug use may be required. To promote early recognition of aberrant drug-related behaviors, it may also be necessary to have patients who have been actively abusing drugs in the recent past submit urine specimens for regular screening of illicit, or licit but unprescribed, drugs. When informing the patient of this approach, explain that it is a method of monitoring that can reassure the clinician and provide a foundation for aggressive symptom-oriented treatment, thus enhancing the therapeutic alliance with the patient.[11,25]

## Using Nondrug Approaches as Appropriate

Many non-drug approaches can be used to assist patients in coping with chronic pain in advanced illness. Such educational interventions may include relaxation techniques, ways of thinking of and describing the experience of pain, and methods of communicating physical and emotional distress to staff members (see Table 42–2). Although non-drug interventions may be helpful adjuvants to management, they should not be perceived as substitutes for drugs targeted at treating pain or other physical or psychological symptoms.[11,25]

## Inpatient Management Plan

In designing the inpatient management of an actively abusing patient with advanced illness, it is helpful to use structured treatment guidelines. Although the applicability of these guidelines may vary from setting to setting, they provide a set of strategies that can ensure the safety of the patient and staff, control the patient's manipulative behaviors, allow for supervision of illicit drug use, enhance appropriate use of medications for pain and symptom control, and communicate an understanding of pain and substance abuse management.[11,25]

Under certain circumstances, such as actively abusing patients who are scheduled for surgery, patients should be admitted several days in advance, when possible, to allow for the stabilization of the drug regimen. This time can also be used to avoid withdrawal and to provide an opportunity to assess whether modifications to the established plan are necessary.[11,25]

Once established, the structured treatment plan for the management of active abuse must proceed conscientiously. In an effort to assess and manage symptoms, frequent visits are usually necessary. It is also important to avoid drug withdrawal, and to the extent possible, prescribed drugs for symptom control should be administered on a regularly scheduled basis (see Table 42–2). This helps to eliminate repetitive encounters with staff that center on the desire to obtain drugs.[11,25]

Treatment management plans must be designed to represent the clinician's assessment of the severity of drug abuse. Open and honest communication between clinician and patient to stress that the guidelines were established in the best interest of the patient is often helpful. However, in cases where patients are unable to follow these guidelines despite repeated interventions from the staff, discharge should be considered. Clinicians should discuss this decision for patient discharge with the staff and administration, while considering the ethical and legal ramifications of this action.[11,25]

## Outpatient Management Plan

Alternative guidelines may be used in the management of the actively abusing patient with advanced illness who is being treated on an outpatient basis. In some instances, the treatment plan can be coordinated with referral to a drug rehabilitation program. However, patients who are facing end-of-life issues may have difficulty participating in such programs. Using the following approaches may be helpful for managing the complex and more difficult-to-control aspects of care.

## Using Written Agreements

Using written agreements that clearly state the roles of the team members and the rules and expectations for the patient is helpful when structuring outpatient treatment. Basing the level of restrictions on the patient's behaviors, graded agreements should be enforced that clearly state the consequences of aberrant drug use.[11,25] Figure 42–1 provides a sample contract for the initiation of opioid therapy. This template can be modified and structured to fit individual practices and clinics, but it is a good general indication of the responsibilities of the patient as well as the provider.

## Guidelines for Prescribing

Patients who are actively abusing must be seen weekly to build a good rapport with staff and afford evaluation of symptom control and addiction-related concerns. Frequent visits allow the opportunity to prescribe small quantities of drugs, which may decrease the temptation to divert and provide a motive for not missing appointments[11,25] (see Table 42–2).

Procedures for prescription loss or replacement should be explicitly explained to the patient, with the stipulation that no renewals will be given if appointments are missed. The patient should also be informed that any dose changes require prior communication with the clinician. Additionally, clinicians who are covering for the primary care provider must be advised of the guidelines that have been established for each patient with a substance abuse history to avoid conflict and disruption of the treatment plan.[11,25]

## Using 12-Step Programs

The clinician should consider referring the patient to a 12-step program with the stipulation that attendance be documented for ongoing prescription purposes. The clinician may wish to contact the patient's sponsor in an effort to disclose the patient's illness and that medication is required in the treatment of the illness. This contact will also help to decrease the risk of stigmatizing the patient as being noncompliant with the ideals of the 12-step program.[11,25]

# Opioid Medication Consent Form

PATIENT NAME: _____     SSN: _____

The purpose of this Agreement is to clarify expectations and prevent misunderstandings about certain medicines I will be taking for pain management. This is to help both my doctor and I comply with the law regarding controlled prescription drugs. I understand that this Agreement is essential to the trust and confidence necessary in a doctor/patient relationship and that my doctor will treat me based on this Agreement.

I understand that if I break this Agreement, my doctor may decide to stop prescribing these pain-control medicines. In this case, my doctor may taper off the medicine (i.e., slowly decrease) over a period of several days, as necessary to avoid withdrawal symptoms. Also, a drug-dependence treatment program may be recommended.

### GOALS OF OPIOID TRIAL/TREATMENT
The purpose of this medication is to increase your ability to function at work and at home. Success will be measured by your activity level, not your report of pain.

### RISKS OF OPIOID TRIAL/TREATMENT
This medication has the potential to cause an addiction. Physical tolerance and dependence occurs with regular use of a narcotic, but this is different from addiction. For a person's health, safety and protection, this medication may be stopped if there is a concern about addiction.

### ADDICTION BEHAVIOR
- a lot of time & energy focused on obtaining medication
- continuing to take medications despite being told to stop
- decline in family and/or work functioning
- loss of interest in other life activities (e.g., hobbies, social activities)
- consistent misuse of medications (see below)

### MISUSE OR ABUSE OF MEDICATION
- taking more medication than prescribed
- use of pain medications that have not been prescribed by this program
- use of alcohol to manage pain
- high number of emergency room visits seeking medication
- failing to use other recommended pain management techniques (e.g., physical therapy, relaxation techniques, TNS unit)
- getting medication from more than one doctor
- using someone else's opioid medication
- reports of lost or stolen medication
- asking only for medications with a high street value

### GUIDELINES FOR OPIOID PRESCRIPTIONS

*Our Responsibility*
- Medication will only be prescribed by a SINGLE PROVIDER.
- Medication will be prescribed on a "by-the-clock" schedule.
- Lost or stolen prescriptions or medications will not be replaced.
- OPIOID MEDICATIONS WILL NOT TYPICALLY BE FILLED OVER THE PHONE.
- If an opioid taper is unsuccessful, medical care will be provided. Referral to facilities specializing in medication detoxification may be necessary.

**Figure 42–1.** Pain management guidelines: opioid medication consent form.

**Opioid Medication Consent Form (Continued)**

*Your Responsibility*
- A person is responsible for his or her medications, and needs to make sure that prescriptions are filled correctly. Therefore, they need to make certain that the pharmacy gives them the correct number prescribed.
- No increases in medication doses will be made without the approval of the prescribing physician.
- If a person takes more medication than is prescribed, he or she will run out of medication before being given more.
- Narcotic medication use questions should be made during normal business hours, Monday through Friday, 8:00 A.M. to 4 P.M.
- Patients are expected to be on time for all appointments including those not related to refills medications. You will be asked to come in before a medication is to be refilled at times.

*Informed Consent*
- I will communicate fully with my doctor about the character and intensity of my pain, the effect of the pain on my daily life, side effects, and how well the medicine is helping to relieve the pain.
- I may be asked to bring unused medications to clinic with me for a "pill count" to ensure that I am using the medication as prescribed.
- I consent to submit to a blood or urine test if requested by my doctor to determine my compliance with my program of pain control medicine.
- I will not use any illegal controlled substances, including marijuana, cocaine, etc., as these will interact poorly with my pain medications.
- I will not share, sell, or trade my medication with anyone as these are dangerous to use when not under a doctor's care.
- I will not attempt to obtain any pain medicines, including opioid pain medicines, stimulants, or anti-anxiety medicines from any other doctor.
- I authorize the doctor and my pharmacy to cooperate fully with any city, state or federal law enforcement agency, including this state's Board of Pharmacy, in the investigation of any possible misuse, sale, or other diversion of my pain medicine. I authorize my doctor to provide a copy of this Agreement to my pharmacy. I agree to waive any applicable or right of privacy or confidentiality with respect to these authorizations.

If these guidelines are not met, you may be discharged from the program.

I, the undersigned, agree that the above guidelines have been explained to me, and that my questions and concerns regarding this treatment have been adequately answered. I agree to comply with the above guidelines. I have a copy of this document.

Signed: _____ Date: _____

Physician/Clinician: _____ Date: _____

Witness: _____ Date:_____

**Figure 42–1.** (*continued*)

## Urine Toxicology Screens

Periodic urine toxicology screens should be performed for most patients to encourage compliance and detect the concurrent use of illicit substances. This practice, as well as how positive screens will be managed, should be clearly explained to the patient at the beginning of outpatient therapy. A response to a positive screen generally involves increasing the guidelines for continued treatment, such as more frequent visits and smaller quantities of prescribed drugs.[11,25]

## Family Sessions and Meetings

The clinician, in an effort to increase support and function, should involve family members and friends in the treatment plan. These meetings will allow the clinician and other team members to become familiar with the family and additionally assist the team to identify family members who are using illicit drugs. Offering referral of these identified family members to drug treatment can be portrayed as a method of gathering support for the patient. The patient should also be prepared to cope with family members or friends who may attempt to buy or sell the patient's medications. These meetings will also assist the team in identifying dependable individuals who can serve as a source of strength and support for the patient during treatment.[11,25] A final case study illustrates how a highly complicated patient with advanced cancer was managed in cooperation with hospice nurses to treat her pain and control aberrant behavior.

CASE STUDY
### A 37-Year-Old Woman With Breast Cancer

A 37-year-old woman was diagnosed with stage IV breast cancer with metastases to bone upon initial diagnosis. The patient was found to be a polysubstance abuser who was often dealing her medications to purchase cocaine. In addition, she would also overuse her medications and showed a pattern of increased use when dealing with emotional issues. Further, she was diagnosed with borderline personality disorder and had significant marital issues, including periods of physical violence. The patient was admitted to rehabilitation programs on several occasions and had periods of successful control followed by frequent relapse. The patient survived for a total of 11 years and eventually died when her cancer spread to the central nervous system, and home hospice had to be engaged. The challenge with treating the patient centered on the chronic nature of her condition and need to keep a coherent plan of care together over a number of years across a multitude of professionals. Remembering that addiction is a cyclical disease with periods of recovery followed by relapse is important, especially with concerns over not being overly punitive on relapses and the issue of diversion.

## Summary

Treating patients who are experiencing chronic pain from advanced illness and a substance use disorder is both complicated and challenging, because each can significantly complicate the other. Patients are living longer with advanced disease and pain concerns. We are no longer able to justify high-dose opioid therapy in a vacuum without trying to assess and manage addiction and abuse behaviors. In addition, the management of an advanced patient who is actively abusing drugs and is a member of an ethnic minority is more perplexing because of cultural differences that may exist. Using a treatment plan that involves a team approach that recognizes and responds to these complex needs is the optimum strategy to facilitate treatment. Although pain management may continue to be challenging even when all treatment plan procedures are implemented, the health-care team's goal should be providing the highest level of pain management for all patients with substance use disorders.

REFERENCES

1. Substance Abuse and Mental Health Data Archive. Treatment episode data set, 2005. Substance Abuse and Mental Health Data Archive. Available at: http://webapp.icpsr.umich.edu/cocoon/SAMHDA-SERIES/00056.xml?token=2 (accessed December 2008).
2. Groerer J, Brodsky M. The incidence of illicit drug use in the United States 1962–1989. Br J Addiction 1992;87:1345–1351.
3. Paulson M 3rd, Dekker AH. Healthcare disparities in pain management. J Am Osteopath Assoc 2005;105(6 Suppl 3):S14–S17.
4. Regier DA, Myers JK, Kramer M, Robins LN, Blazer DG, Hough RL, Eaton WW, Locke BZ. The NIMH epidemiology catchment area program. Arch Gen Psychiatry 1984;41:934–941.
5. Ramer L, Richardson JL, Cohen MZ, Bedney C, Danley KL, Judge EA. Multimeasure pain assessment in an ethnically diverse group of patients with cancer. J Transcultural Nurs 1999;10:94–101.
6. Glajchen M, Fitzmartin RD, Blum D, Swanton R. Psychosocial barriers to cancer pain relief. Cancer Pract 1995;3:76–82.
7. Ward SE, Goldberg N, Miller-McCauley V, Mueller C, Nolan A, Pawlik-Plank D, Robbins A, Stormoen D, Weissman DE. Patient-related barriers to management of cancer pain. Pain 1993;52:319–324.
8. Rupp T, Delaney KA. Inadequate analgesia in emergency medicine. Ann Emerg Med 2004;43(4):494–503.
9. Passik SD, Portenoy RK. Substance abuse issues in palliative care. In Berger A, Portenoy R, Weissman D, eds. Principles and Practice of Supportive Oncology. Philadelphia, PA: Lippincott Williams & Wilkins; 1998:513–524.
10. Passik SD, Portenoy RK, Ricketts PL. Substance abuse issues in cancer patients, part 1: Prevalence and diagnosis. Oncology 1998;12:517–521.
11. Passik SD, Portenoy RK. Substance abuse disorders. In Holland JC, ed. Psycho-oncology. New York, NY: Oxford University Press; 1998:576–586.
12. Weissman DE, Haddox JD. Opioid pseudoaddiction—an iatrogenic syndrome. Pain 1989;36:363–366.

12a. Passik SD, Kirsh KL, Whitcomb LA, Schein JR, Kaplan M, Dodd S, Kleinman L, Katz NP, Portenoy RK. Monitoring outcomes during long-term opioid therapy for non-cancer pain: Results with the pain assessment and documentation tool. J Opioid Manage 2005;1(5):257–266.

12b. Fleming MF, Balousek SL, Klessig CL, Mundt MP, Brown DD. Substance use disorders in a primary care sample receiving daily opioid therapy. J Pain 2007;8(7):573–582. Epub May 11, 2007.

13. Rinaldi RC, Steindler EM, Wilford BB. Clarification and standardization of substance abuse terminology. JAMA 1988; 259:555–557.

14. Sullivan MD, Edlund MJ, Steffick D, Unutzer J. Regular use of prescribed opioids: Association with common psychiatric disorders. Pain 2005;119(1–3):95–103. Epub November 17, 2005.

15. Anderson KO, Mendoza TR, Valero V, Richman SP, Russell C, Hurley J, DeLeon C, Washington P, Palos G, Payne R, Cleeland CS. Minority cancer patients and their providers. Cancer 2000;88:1929–1938.

16. Reynolds KS, Hanson LC, Henderson M, Steinhauser KE. End-of-life care in nursing home settings: Do race or age matter? Palliat Support Care 2008;6(1):21–27.

17. Burgess DJ, Crowley-Matoka M, Phelan S, Dovidio JF, Kerns R, Roth C, Saha S, van Ryn M. Patient race and physicians' decisions to prescribe opioids for chronic low back pain. Soc Sci Med 2008;67(11):1852–1860. Epub October 15, 2008.

18. Seale JP, Muramoto ML. Substance abuse among minority populations. Subst Abus 1993;20:167–180.

19. Finn P. Addressing the needs of cultural minorities in drug treatment. J Subst Abuse Treat 1994;11(4):325–337.

20. Dunbar SA, Katz NP. Chronic opioid therapy for nonmalignant pain in patients with a history of substance abuse: Report of 20 cases. J Pain Symptom Manage 1996;11:163–171.

21. Gonzales GR, Coyle N. Treatment of cancer pain in a former opioid abuser: Fears of the patient and staff and their influences on care. J Pain Symptom Manage 1992;7:246–249.

22. Burton-MacLeod S, Fainsinger RL. Cancer pain control in the setting of substance use: Establishing goals of care. J Palliat Care 2008;24(2):122–125.

23. Kemp C. Managing chronic pain in patients with advanced disease and substance related disorders. Home Healthc Nurse 1996;14:255–261.

24. Savage SR, Kirsh KL, Passik SD. Challenges in using opioids to treat pain in persons with substance use disorders. Addict Sci Clin Pract 2008;4(2):4–25. Available at: http://www.drugabuse.gov/PDF/ascp/vol4no2/Challenges.pdf (accessed December 10, 2009).

25. Passik SD, Portenoy RK, Ricketts PL. Substance abuse issues in cancer patients, part 2: Evaluation and treatment. Oncology 1998;12:729–734.

25a. Passik SD, Kirsh KL, Casper D. Addiction-related assessment tools and pain management: Instruments for screening, treatment planning, and monitoring compliance. Pain Med 2008;9(S2):S145–S166.

25b. Coluzzi F, Pappagallo M; National Initiative on Pain Control. Opioid therapy for chronic noncancer pain: Practice guidelines for initiation and maintenance of therapy. Minerva Anestesiol 2005;71(7–8):425–433.

26. Christo PJ, Mazloomdoost D. Cancer pain and analgesia. Ann N Y Acad Sci 2008;1138:278–298.

27. American Pain Society. Principles of Analgesic Use in the Treatment of Acute Pain and Cancer Pain (5th ed). Glenview, IL: Author, 2003.

28. Dy SM, Asch SM, Naeim A, Sanati H, Walling A, Lorenz KA. Evidence-based standards for cancer pain management. J Clin Oncol 2008;26(23):3879–3885.

29. Breitbart W, Rosenfeld BD, Passik SD, McDonald MV, Thaler H, Portenoy RK. The undertreatment of pain in ambulatory AIDS patients. Pain 1996;65:243–249.

30. Fainsinger R, Schoeller T, Bruera E. Methadone in the management of cancer pain: A review. Pain 1993;52:137–147.

31. Smith HS, Kreek MJ, Johnson C, Kirsh KL. Methadone and methadone issues. In Smith HS, Passik SD, eds. Pain and Chemical Dependency. New York, NY: Oxford University Press; 2008:113–122.

32. Wirz S, Wartenberg HC, Elsen C, Wittmann M, Diederichs M, Nadstawek J. Managing cancer pain and symptoms of outpatients by rotation to sustained-release hydromorphone: A prospective clinical trial. Clin J Pain 2006;22(9):770–775.

33. Zimmermann C, Seccareccia D, Booth CM, Cottrell W. Rotation to methadone after opioid dose escalation: How should individualization of dosing occur? J Pain Palliat Care Pharmacother 2005;19(2):25–31.

# 43   Palliative Care of Cancer Survivors

*Mary S. McCabe and Nancy G. Houlihan*

*The goal is to bring quality to the lives we fought so hard to keep. We want lives that are rich; we want children; and we want to be well and happy.—Cancer Survivor*

*It isn't accomplished by knowing every curve in the road ahead. Instead, the headlights shine a light on what's immediately in front of us—that's all. And that's what's necessary—shining a light on the few feet ahead, and then the next few feet, and on and on…and before we know it we have traveled the whole trip in the dark.—Cancer Survivor*

- ◆ **Key Points**
- ◆ *There are approximately 12 million cancer survivors in the United States.*
- ◆ *Being told you are cancer-free does not mean you are free of the consequences of the disease.*
- ◆ *Seventy-two percent of cancer survivors are over age 60 years and have coexisting medical conditions that complicate posttreatment recovery to maximum health.*
- ◆ *Childhood cancer survivors carry a heavy burden of medical and psychological problems resulting from their experience with cancer.*
- ◆ *Improvements are needed in the coordination of care for cancer survivors to assure optimal quality of life.*
- ◆ *Cancer diagnosis and treatment affects the family as well as the patient.*

Just as palliative care has faced many challenges in reaching its full potential as a specialty within the health-care continuum, so it is with survivorship care. Until recently, the primary focus in oncology was on the diagnostic and treatment phases of care. It wasn't until the 2006 publication of the seminal report by the Institute of Medicine (IOM), *From Cancer Patient to Cancer Survivor: Lost in Transition*, that national attention has been given to the specific health issues and resulting care needs of cancer survivors[1] (see Figure 43–1). Fortunately, there is a growing body of knowledge about the lingering and late consequences of cancer and its treatment, greater understanding about the interventions needed to address these problems, a focus on developing models for optimal care delivery, and an awareness of the key role nurses play in the delivery of survivorship care.[2–4]

## The Intersection of Palliative Care and Cancer Survivorship

The essentials of palliative care—attention to physical pain and suffering, including existential distress; the inclusion of the family as a unit of care; and interdisciplinary care—are all relevant to and needed by the cancer survivor.[5] Although many survivors recover quickly and completely from the toxicities of cancer treatment, the words of one survivor—"being free of the cancer is not being free of its consequences"—ring true for many others. Survival after a cancer diagnosis can come at a price in terms of medical, psychosocial, and existential problems. For example, chronic pain may be the result of surgery and radiation in a young adult treated for a rare head and neck tumor; fatigue may last for years in a survivor treated for Hodgkin's disease; severe anxiety may prevent the social reintegration of a patient treated for leukemia with a stem cell transplant; and lymphedema of the leg may impede

**The Cancer Control Continuum**

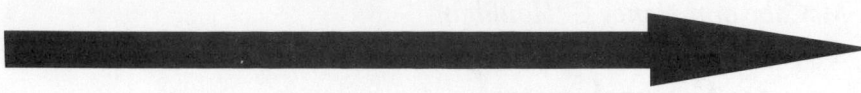

| Prevention | Early Detection | Diagnosis | Treatment | Survivorship | End-of-Life Care |
|---|---|---|---|---|---|
| —Tobacco Control | —Cancer Screening | —Oncology consultations | —Chemotherapy | —Long-term follow-up/surveillance | —Palliation |
| —Diet | | —Tumor staging | —Surgery | —Late-effects Management | —Spiritual issues |
| —Physical activity | —Awareness of cancer signs and symptoms | | —Radiation therapy | | —Hospice |
| —Sun exposure | | —Patient counseling and decision making | —Adjuvant therapy | —Rehabilitation | |
| —Virus exposure | | | —Symptom management | —Coping | |
| —Alcohol use | | | —Phychosocial care | —Health promotion | |
| —Chemoprevention | | | | | |

**Figure 43–1.** The Cancer Control Continuum. *Source*: With permission, Hewitt and Stovall (2006), reference 1.

the function of a person treated for a sarcoma. In each of these cases, the application of palliative care strategies can reduce and/or eliminate the problems.

## Challenges of Survivorship

In discussing the palliative care needs of cancer survivors, it is important to first understand who is considered a cancer survivor and what cancer survivorship means. As reported by the President's Cancer Panel, the time at which a person diagnosed with cancer becomes a survivor has a variety of interpretations depending on the focus of the group doing the defining.[6] A widely embraced definition states that a person is a survivor from the moment of diagnosis and that family members are included in the survivorship experience throughout the trajectory. Both the National Coalition for Cancer Survivorship and the National Cancer Institute's Office of Cancer Survivorship have adopted this definition:[1]

> *An individual is considered a cancer survivor from the time of diagnosis, through the balance of his or her life. Family members, friends and caregivers are also impacted by the survivorship experience and are therefore included in this definition.*

For the purposes of highlighting a set of often neglected issues requiring the palliative care interventions, this chapter focuses, as did the IOM report, on the survivorship experience following first diagnosis and treatment and prior to the development of a recurrence of the initial cancer. This phase of care has been given relatively little attention until recently, often because the care ends abruptly once treatment is completed or because the follow-up care becomes episodic and focuses on disease recurrence and not on a comprehensive approach to posttreatment needs.

The acute toxicities associated with cancer treatment (chemotherapy, radiation, and surgery) are well-characterized, and considerable research has appropriately focused on their amelioration. Professional medical and nursing societies have made the education about these interventions a central focus. Now, with the rapidly growing number of cancer survivors, it is time to do the same for the long-term and late effects of cancer treatment. The long-term effects are those that begin during treatment and become chronic, continuing well beyond the end of treatment. As defined by Aziz, the late effects of treatment are those that occur after treatment has ended but "manifest later with the unmasking of hitherto unseen injury to immature organs by developmental processes or as a result of failure of compensatory mechanisms because of the passage of time or organ senescence."[7]

Because cancer is a disease of the elderly, with the overwhelming majority of survivors being over age 60 years, these long-term and late effects add significant morbidity to the lives of elderly cancer survivors, and if not identified and treated, they may not only add to the burden of illness but significantly impact quality of life (QoL) and even survival itself.[8]

The negative consequences of cancer treatment are not restricted to physical domains. There is a known set of important psychosocial concerns as well.[9,10] In addition, although the diagnosis and treatment phases are widely recognized as being psychologically challenging for all patients and their families, there are a subset of survivors who experience long-term psychological distress or problems later in their survivorship. Studies have identified risk factors for developing these problems, including anxiety, depression, poor adjustment—all of which influence posttreatment recovery, health, and overall well-being.[11,12]

## Special At-Risk Groups

### Pediatric Survivors

One of the most important successes in oncology has been in pediatrics, where over 80% of children and adolescents treated for cancer become long-term survivors.[13] There are an estimated 270,000 pediatric cancer survivors in the United States—1 in every 640 adults between the ages of 20 and 39 years.[14] However, as these young people grow into adulthood, they face (often serious) health consequences of their cancer treatment that may not become evident for many years.[15] Both the organ system damage and psychological impact of having been treated at such a young age creates a need for ongoing care focused on prevention, surveillance, early detection, and management of late treatment effects.

Numerous seminal survivorship studies have been conducted with participants who are in the Childhood Cancer Survivor Study (CCSS; a multi-institutional cohort of long-term cancer survivors diagnosed with a pediatric malignancy from 1970–1986) to determine the prevalence, incidence, and severity of chronic health conditions in adult survivors of pediatric cancers; the risk of chronic conditions compared with their siblings; and the subpopulations of survivors at highest risk for severe, debilitating, or life-threatening health conditions.[15,16] A 2006 study of more than 10,000 survivors showed that risk of chronic health conditions was high—particularly for second cancers, cardiovascular disease, renal dysfunction, musculoskeletal problems, and endocrinopathies—and that the incidence of these conditions and others increases over time.[15] Survivors were eight times as likely as their siblings to have severe or life-threatening conditions, and there were particular treatment combinations, especially those including chest, abdominal, or pelvic radiation, which were associated with a tenfold increase in risk for severe or life-threatening conditions. Overall, in patients treated 30 years ago, almost three-fourths have a chronic health condition; one-third have multiple conditions; and more than 40% experience severe, life-threatening, disabling, or fatal conditions, such as heart attacks or second cancers.[15]

The important future challenge in survivorship care is the identification and treatment of these conditions to assure the long-term health and well-being of this unique group of survivors. One well-established effort exists at academic medical centers, where long-term follow-up clinics for pediatric cancer survivors provide the specialized care required for their complex problems. Unfortunately, it has been reported that less than 20% of adult survivors of childhood cancers are followed at a cancer center or by a knowledgeable professional such as an oncologist.[17] This leaves much work to be done in educating the survivor and other health-care providers about needed surveillance, symptom identification, and proper management. Fortunately, an important resource for assuring quality care for this group of survivors that can be made widely available for use by any provider of survivorship care are the Long-Term Follow-Up Guidelines for Survivors of Childhood, Adolescent, and Young Adult Cancers developed by The Children's Oncology Group. The guidelines are available at (http://www.survivorshipguidelines.org/) and represent an important guide to the management of survivors of pediatric cancers.[18] The dissemination of this resource to both survivors of pediatric cancers and the health-care community involved in their care is a critical next step in which nurses can play a crucial role when caring for these individuals.

### Bone Marrow Transplant/Hematopoietic Stem Cell Transplantation Survivors

Bone marrow transplant, or the more current term *hematopoietic stem cell transplantation* (HSCT), is a curative treatment for many patients with cancer, including those with relapsed and/or high-risk acute and chronic leukemia and subsets of patients with lymphoma and multiple myeloma.[19] Advances in therapeutic approaches over the last decade, including the use of diverse sources of stem cells, reduced-intensity conditioning regimens, and improvements in supportive care, have decreased the morbidity and mortality rates for most HSCT recipients and increased the number of eligible patients, including the elderly and those without suitably matched donors.[20] As a result, there are increasing numbers of transplants performed annually and greater expectations for long-term survival. A recent study of patients who are disease-free at 2 years after allogeneic HSCT indicated a 90% probability of surviving 5 years and an 80% probability of surviving 15 years after transplant.[21]

Despite these advances in toxicity reduction, the physical late effects of transplant continue to include the risk of secondary malignancies, pulmonary complications, cataracts, sterility, and graft-versus-host disease (GVHD).[22] A comprehensive analysis of disease and treatment-related factors associated with late mortality in a large cohort of allogeneic HSCT recipients demonstrated mortality rates twice as high as that of the general population and that survivors face challenges affecting their overall health and well-being.[21] As the number of survivors increase, the long-term effects on the QoL of patients and families becomes more important. Although many transplant recipients report normal QoL, the majority indicate a poorer QoL relative to pre-morbid status and when compared to healthy peers, including low energy levels and sleep difficulties, low self-esteem, sexual difficulties, psychological distress, and impaired social relationships.[22,23] Functional well-being is reported as lower in transplant recipients in comparison to siblings, as measured by decreased likeliness to be married, greater likeliness to have difficulty holding a job because of a health problem, lower household income, and more difficulty obtaining health and life insurance.[21] Measures of emotional well-being after transplant reveal that those undergoing transplant in childhood or young adulthood score higher in coping abilities than older transplant recipients and tend to have a less passive, more positive, and mature style of coping than their peers.[23] A study of the presence of posttraumatic stress disorder in HSCT recipients revealed that patients at risk were those with a pretransplant measurement of poor social support combined with avoidance coping.[24]

Chronic graft-versus-host disease (cGVHD) remains the most significant complication affecting QoL and overall outcomes in long-term survivors after transplant.[19] It is the chief cause of nonrelapse-related death.[21] Incidence of cGVHD has increased along with the number of allogeneic HSCTs performed, affecting an estimated 50% of long-term survivors.[21] cGVHD can involve almost any organ but most commonly affects the skin, mouth, mucosa, liver, eyes, and lungs in addition to the hematopoietic and lymphoid organs. Clinical manifestations can vary in both severity and clinical course.[20] Traditionally, treatment requires immunosuppression with corticosteroids (prednisone) along with calcineurin inhibitors (cyclosporin or tacrolimus) as the primary therapy. Newer agents and techniques are under study for prevention, primary treatment, and treatment of steroid refractory or dependent disease.[25] Balancing the treatment of symptoms while maintaining sufficient immune function to protect against opportunistic pathogens is the greatest challenge because infections that occur as a result of lymphopenia are the major cause of death in cGVHD.[20]

A multidisciplinary approach to the supportive care of patients with cGVHD is essential. Potential side effects of treatment include infections, osteoporosis, hypertension, hyperglycemia, renal insufficiency, and hyperlipidemia as well as reduced QoL and psychosocial disturbances.[25] Care includes antimicrobial and antifungal prophylaxis as well as nutritional support and physical therapy. The National Institutes of Health Consensus Development Project for Clinical Trials in Chronic Graft Versus Host Disease published recommendations for standardized monitoring and treatment with an emphasis on supportive care.[26] Identification of patients at greatest risk for posttransplant difficulties—whether physical, psychological, or functional—and implementing appropriate interventions for prevention and management is an important step in achieving a better QoL for this ever-growing number of long-term survivors.

## Elderly Survivors

Of the estimated 12 million cancer survivors in the United States, 60% (6.5 million) are age 65 years and older.[13] By 2030 there will be 71 million Americans age 65 years and older, accounting for 20% of the population.[13] If current trends continue, then the increase in survival rates coupled with the aging population present a major challenge to our healthcare system charged with the posttreatment care of this rapidly growing number of Americans.

The posttreatment health of older cancer survivors is influenced by multiple factors, including toxicity of treatment, presence of symptoms and/or late effects, coexisting comorbid health conditions, social resources, and normative ageing.[27] Physical and social functioning are the most common health domains adversely affected. A recent review of the research literature found that older cancer survivors reported higher rates of comorbid health problems compared to older adults without a cancer history.[27] Although it is unclear whether these conditions are late treatment effects, it appears that the coexistence of comorbid health conditions (whatever their cause) can exacerbate the effects of cancer and treatment on the posttreatment health of older adults.[13] With respect to mental health, cancer in older adults may occur in the context of other losses, isolation, and constraint on social resources, thus putting strain on coping mechanisms.[28]

Care for the projected numbers of older cancer survivors presents new challenges with predictions of shortages in the number of oncologists and geriatricians. The role of nurses, particularly geriatric nurse practitioners, will grow in importance as the complexities of posttreatment and comorbid conditions of aging converge. There is much to be studied in elderly cancer survivors so that appropriate guidelines for surveillance and follow-up interventions can be developed. Research on physiological and psychological effects of therapy; QoL and physical function; risk of coexistence of comorbid conditions and disability; and control and prevention of late effects have all been identified as important to the provision of care to this expanding population.[29]

## Socioeconomically Disadvantaged Survivors

Cancer patients who are socioeconomically disadvantaged face greater challenges compared to patients who have adequate resources.[30,31] The stress of a cancer diagnosis adds enormous burden to the physical, psychological, and financial deprivation already experienced by the poor. With limited health-care choices already, the complexity and expense of therapies can become overwhelming for disadvantaged cancer patients.[32] Often, essentials such as food and shelter remain the first priority. Cancer survivors who live in poverty remain vulnerable even after the acute treatment period has ended. They have limited access to ongoing medical care and may not be aware of the importance of ongoing follow-up. Therefore, they are less likely to receive treatment for comorbidities and are less likely to receive psychosocial services. Follow-up care for needed services of long-term and late effects are most often not attainable. Palliative care services needed by the survivor, in particular, may be overlooked because access to healthcare may abruptly end once cancer treatment is completed. Sadly, these barriers faced by the socioeconomically underserved survivor mirror the problems faced by the poor in general and are outlined in an American Cancer Society report: poor people experience more cancer related pain; poor people often do not seek necessary care if they are unable to pay for it; and cancer education and outreach efforts are often insensitive and irrelevant to the lives of many poor people, and fatalism about cancer is common among the poor and often prevents them from accessing care.[30]

The challenges to improving the care of the disadvantaged cancer survivor are tied to the important issue of assuring access to quality care for the poor in general. It requires community-based approaches that incorporate health-care access into a broader plan for housing, social services, and job training.

꧁꧂

## Selected Symptoms of Importance in Survivor Care

### Fatigue

Fatigue is the most common symptom associated with cancer and its treatment.[33] Cancer-related fatigue is defined as a "distressing, persistent, subjective sense of tiredness or exhaustion related to cancer or cancer treatment that is not proportional to recent activity and interferes with usual functioning."[34] Prevalence and severity depend on the disease stage, treatment type, and treatment phase. It occurs most frequently among patients receiving chemotherapy with or without radiation therapy. Fatigue is multidimensional and reported by patients in terms of perceived energy, mental capacity, and psychological status.[35] Fatigue can interfere with normal functioning and lead to negative effects on QoL.[36,37] Although the study of fatigue generally is focused on the active treatment period, fatigue may persist for a significant time afterward. A national survey of cancer patients more than 1 year posttreatment using consensus-based diagnostic criteria for cancer-related fatigue (CRF) showed a prevalence of CRF of 17% with 64% of survivors reporting some fatigue-related problem.[38]

Fatigue has been well-documented in specific survivor populations. Minton and Stone conducted a literature review to characterize and quantify the phenomenon of posttreatment fatigue (PTF) in breast cancer survivors that is distinguishable from fatigue related to aging and comorbidities seen in the general population.[39] In studies of women less than 2 years after treatment completion, PTF have been as high as 20% to 30%, with a significant difference between treated women and controls. Longer term studies, longer than 2 years posttreatment, have shown significant disturbances compared to the general population up to 5 years after treatment, most notably in respect to physical functioning and mental fatigue. Data suggest that in affected women, any improvement is seen only after 2 years and that fatigue may continue up to 5 years. Longitudinal studies suggest the existence of ongoing PTF but with improvement in fatigue symptoms over time. A significant minority of women still experience PTF up to 5 years, with a wide variation in prevalence. The authors conclude that fatigue is not a phenomenon that occurs solely during breast cancer treatment and should not be dismissed without palliative care interventions.

Prevalence of chronic fatigue (CF), defined as elevated fatigue levels lasting longer than 6 months, is 2.5 to 3 times higher in Hodgkin's Lymphoma (HL) survivors than in the general population.[40] Most studies attribute excess fatigue to the late effects of treatment. However, prospective data suggest that fatigue is a significant problem at diagnosis and does not remit with effective treatment.[41] Fatigue in HL survivors may be multifactorial and could relate to ongoing disruption of pro-inflammatory cytokines that are part of the underlying disease as well as endocrine, respiratory, and circulatory alterations as well as comorbid conditions.[40,41] Survivors of HL do report a reduced QoL related to fatigue, persistent after resolution of treatment effects.[40] Further research is needed to understand the etiology of this long-term complication of HL so that effective assessment and interventions can be employed.

Evaluation of CRF is difficult because of the subjectivity of measurement and is complicated by a wide range of symptoms consistent with psychological impairment, low physical performance, pain, and depression.[37] Surveys of patients, caregivers, and oncologists have revealed that fatigue is rarely discussed and that few recommendations for treatment are offered, particularly with survivors.[37] Assessment of fatigue at follow-up visits is important to determine the impact on the patient's adjustment after treatment. Identification of physiological conditions (such as persistent anemia) or psychological factors (such as depression) can help in initiating appropriate management. Educating patients and caregivers about pharmacological and nonpharmacological strategies to reduce symptoms is essential. The National Comprehensive Cancer Network (NCCN) incorporated specific interventions for fatigue monitoring and management for cancer survivors into the latest version of their Cancer-Related Fatigue guidelines. The guidelines Cancer Related Fatigue: Interventions for Patients on Long Term Follow-up are available on the NCCN website http:/www.nccn.org/professionals/physician_gls/PDF/fatigue.pdf.[34]

### Chronic Pain

Chronic pain in cancer survivors is an underappreciated and underreported symptom that can result from chemotherapy, radiation surgery, or a combination of any of the three modalities. Until recently, there was limited focus by the health-care team on pain as an important consequence of treatment, and patients were often reluctant to discuss this symptom for fear it was a poor prognostic sign about their survival.[42,43] The types of pain experienced by survivors are complex, are difficult to diagnose, and may begin during treatment (e.g., taxane neuropathy) or occur many years later (e.g., radiation-induced plexopathy). Chronic pain caused by cancer therapy may be further complicated by preexisting pain in the elderly and further intensified by untreated anxiety and depression.

### Chemotherapy

Painful peripheral neuropathies caused by the chemotherapy agents vincristine, platinum, taxanes, thalidomide, and borteximib have been well-described, and although this pain most often resolves over time without intervention, it can remain intensely painful in a small group of survivors.[44,45] Its severity may be increased by preexisting neuropathy caused by diabetes or alcoholism. Treatment includes antineuropathic pain medications, and physical therapy is an important component of a plan of care focused on maximum functioning.

Corticosteroids are an integral part of treatment regimens for some cancers, such as leukemia and myeloma, and are known to cause osteonecrosis or avascular necrosis. Usually occurring within 3 years of steroid treatment, osteonecrosis primarily affects the bones of the weight-bearing joints, leading to limited range of motion and pain. In one study of adult patients treated for lymphoblastic disease, 55% of adult patients developed avascular necrosis.[46] Unfortunately, there is often limited awareness of this significant problem and no consistent diagnostic standards exist. Because adolescents may be more susceptible to the development of osteonecrosis as a result of maturing bones, particular attention should be paid to joint pain symptoms in young adults who have received steroids as part of cancer treatment.[47]

## Radiation

The late effects of radiation include connective tissue fibrosis and nerve damage and, when present, put women treated for breast cancer at risk for chronic pain in the breast and arm. Additionally, radiation-induced brachial plexopathy can occur in breast cancer survivors as well. The initial presentation of this painful syndrome varies in time to initiation and types of symptoms. The incidence of painful, disabling brachial plexopathy ranges from 1% to 5% depending on the radiation dose, technique, and concurrent chemotherapies, and 9% of women have at least a mild plexopathy.[46]

Individuals who have received pelvic radiation are another group at risk for chronic pain. Studies have identified that pelvic pain in survivors treated for cervical and prostate cancers may result from pelvic insufficiency fractures, enteritis, visceral dysfunction, or nerve damage.[48] In each of these patient groups, the presentation of new onset pain requires a careful assessment that includes a review of prior cancer treatment because the chronic pain syndrome resulting from radiotherapy has a delayed onset of many years. This is one of the key reasons for ongoing careful assessment of the cancer survivor and for health-care providers to be knowledgeable about the survivor's prior cancer therapy.

## Surgery

Chronic pain syndromes resulting from cancer surgery are most common in survivors who have undergone an amputation and who have been treated for thoracic and breast cancers. Although nearly all amputees experience phantom sensations, only a subset has reported phantom limb pain.[49] The predisposing factors for phantom limb pain include pre-amputation pain, severe postoperative pain, and a more proximal amputation.[50] The interplay between chronic pain and physical disability in amputees is a complex one, and researchers have found that ongoing functional impairment is most closely correlated with severe stump pain, the level of the amputation, and significant phantom sensation.[49] This information provides an important guide for the focus of combined pain and rehabilitation interventions.

Numerous studies have evaluated the incidence of chronic postthoracotomy pain in patients with lung cancer. Although there is usually gradual improvement over time, 60% of patients continue to report pain significant enough for analgesic use at 1 year, and prolonged chronic pain may have an incidence of as high as 50%, with half of these individuals reporting moderate-to-severe pain.[51,52] This intensity and chronicity of pain then leads to functional limitations that become an impediment to the survivor's recovery and may also affect psychological domains.

Chronic pain after breast cancer surgery is seen in as many as 50% of mastectomy patients and is characterized into specific types: phantom breast pain, intercostobrachial neuralgia, neuroma pain, and other nerve injury pain.[53] Studies have identified that the pain can be present in the arm, neck, shoulder, axilla, chest, or breast, and it is influenced by the type of surgical procedure.[54] Although it was hoped that the newer breast-conserving surgical procedures would reduce the incidence of chronic pain, this has not been demonstrated as true. In fact, in one survey, women undergoing a breast-sparing surgery with axially node dissection had a higher incidence of chronic pain.[55] Tasmuth et al. have shown that the best predictor of chronic pain in breast cancer survivors is the severity of acute postoperative pain.[54] This acute pain may be related to anxiety and depression and postoperative complications—all issues that require palliative care interventions.

## Sleep Disorders

Although sleep disorders are known to be associated with various medical conditions, only limited attention has been paid to the impact of sleep quality in cancer patients—particularly in cancer survivors. Insomnia has been reported in adult cancer patients beginning during treatment with a prevalence of 30% to 50% and remaining as high as 23% to 44% following treatment.[56] In a unique study of survivors of pediatric cancers, the prevalence was much lower (16.7%) but varied greatly by diagnosis, with 50% of survivors of pediatric leukemia reporting sleep difficulties.[57] Not only are sleep difficulties common in cancer patients, they are also of major concern as a source of emotional and physical distress in these individuals.[58,59]

There are numerous important factors that contribute to the experience of sleep disorders. In particular, fatigue, physical pain, and depression all are known to impact sleep in adults and are specifically known to increase the likelihood of insomnia.[60] Unfortunately, far less is known about these symptoms in the cancer population. Servaes et al. have shown that fatigue is a distressing and common symptom estimated to be as high as 70% to 96% in recently treated adult cancer patients across diagnoses, but it also has been found to be present years after completion of cancer therapy.[61] Chronic pain in cancer survivors is also an understudied and underreported problem and contributes significantly to sleep disorders when unrelieved. Although many surveys have identified the relationship between depressive feelings and insomnia, studies in cancer patients have been rare. In a recent study of cancer patients, Davidson et al. found that individuals who experienced "ups and downs" of mood were prone to insomnia, thus suggesting that mood variability is associated with insomnia.[60]

While continuing to describe the prevalence and type of sleep disorders and their relationship to other cancer-related symptoms and treatment exposures, it is critical that studies be conducted focusing on the formal assessment of sleep quality in cancer patients along with adaptive interventions that can be evaluated and made part of a palliative care plan. For example, Hoyt et al. have proposed that an avoidance-oriented coping style may negatively impact mood and sleep, thus having implications for psychological interventions in this group.[62] In addition, given the complex nature of sleep disorders in survivors, treatments focused on reducing cognitive arousal and pain would be useful palliative care strategies. Mendelson has offered that short-term pharmacological interventions may be useful as well.[63] Most importantly, because of the immensely negative impact of sleep disturbance on the QoL of cancer survivors, palliative care interventions targeted to the array of related and contributory symptoms are essential for recovery.

## Cognitive Dysfunction

Increasingly, research is focused on the identification and understanding of the cognitive changes associated with cancer and its treatment.[64] Although it is known that cancers involving the central nervous system (CNS) and treatments involving cranial surgery and radiation cause cognitive impairment, most research to date has focused on non-CNS cancers.

Breast cancer has been the focus of the greatest number of studies in response to the anecdotal reporting of changes in memory and concentration, termed "chemo brain," in breast cancer survivors that received adjuvant chemotherapy and hormonal therapy.[65] Although most breast cancer patients report some cognitive changes during active treatment, the symptoms resolve over time. However, in a subset of patients, cognitive changes associated with chemotherapy, hormonal therapy, and biological response modifiers may be longlasting or permanent.[66] Recent prospective studies have demonstrated that some degree of cognitive dysfunction exists prior to breast cancer treatment, suggesting the disease rather than the treatment as a cause.[67] Multiple factors have been found to influence, and possibly increase, risk for cognitive changes, either independently or in interaction with chemotherapy. These include older age at treatment, lesser intelligence and

education, anxiety and depression, fatigue, menopause, and prior hormonal therapy.[66] Overall, the symptoms of cognitive dysfunction are often subtle and complex. They are related to memory, concentration, and executive functioning.[64] Such impairment can impact a survivor's ability to function normally, impeding the attainment of personal, professional, and general QoL goals.[33]

Various interventions are being evaluated to reduce or prevent chemotherapy-induced cognitive decline. Pharmacological interventions (including psychostimulants, cholinesterase inhibitors, and gingko biloba) and cognitive rehabilitation may improve memory and concentration.[68] To guide the development of future interventions of this distressing symptom, the results of longitudinal studies are needed to provide greater understanding of the extent of cognitive deficits created by cancer and chemotherapy, the number of patients affected, and the factors that contribute.[69] The use of functional MRI may add a new dimension to pre- and posttreatment assessment in understanding the patterns of regional brain activation, and greater understanding of genetic factors may identify targets for agents that could prevent or reduce cognitive effects.[9,70] Future research hopefully will provide answers to the many questions about this phenomenon in cancer therapy.

## Psychological Effects

Nearly all cancer patients experience some level of psychological distress, including depression, sadness, anxiety, fear, worry, anger, or panic.[9] For most individuals, distress remits during the first 24 months after diagnosis, and individuals evidence few late or long-term psychological effects.[10] For some, however, the cancer experience triggers a psychological response that has a lasting impact, leading to poor adjustment and functional limitations extending across the survivorship trajectory.[71]

## Depression

Estimates of the prevalence of depression in cancer survivors vary from 0% to 38% for major depression and 0% to 58% for depression spectrum syndromes.[72] Variability is attributable to multiple factors, including variations in cancer site, cancer treatment, age, disease, stage at diagnosis, and time from diagnosis and completion of treatment.[73] It is likely that many people affected by subclinical depression go undetected. Depression symptoms are more common in those with cancers of the head and neck, pancreas, lung, and breast and are less common in colon and gynecological cancers and lymphoma.[74] Depression and posttraumatic stress disorder (PTSD) are reported in older adults who continue to experience cancer-related illness symptoms.[75]

PTSD can be a debilitating effect of cancer.[71] Although some studies report a prevalence as high as 32%, the majority of studies suggest a prevalence of PTSD in the range of 5% to 15%, which exceeds the prevalence in the general population.[76] Symptoms include cognitive avoidance, emotional reactivity, hypervigilance, sleep disruption, difficulty concentrating, intrusive thoughts related to cancer and treatment, fear of recurrence, and physical reactions such as heart palpitations or nausea.[77] Risk factors for the development and severity of depression and PTSD are reported as persistent physical problems; poor psychosocial or familial adjustment to cancer; avoidant coping style; lower socioeconomic status, educational, or financial resource level; younger age at diagnosis; female gender; poor premorbid physical and mental health; prior traumas or a current or prior negative stressful event; inadequate social support; cancer stage and type; and treatment severity.[74] Although many patients do not meet the full criteria for cancer-related depression and PTSD, subclinical syndromes are not uncommon.[77] One study of PTSD following bone marrow transplant strongly supported the view that high-avoidance coping and low social support played a causal role in the development of PTSD symptomatology and were interactive in severity.[24] Because both depression and PTSD are treatable problems, it is critical to assess individuals with symptoms and those who are at risk as part of routine survivorship care.

## Anxiety

Similarly to other psychological effects of cancer, anxiety is not disabling in the majority of cancer survivors. The prevalence of anxiety disorders has been estimated to be 6% to 23%, with variations based on similar factors to depression.[78] Anxiety in an individual with cancer is often associated with the meaning and interpretation of specific events that occur as part of the illness.[78] Most cancer survivors experience anxiety over the possibility of a cancer recurrence. Anxiety related to posttreatment surveillance visits and testing is commonly reported. Although fear of recurrence is normal after cancer treatment, fear that is severe and persistent can significantly impact QoL and diminish everyday functioning.[72] Anxious individuals experience and report more symptoms related to their cancer than others. They monitor their bodies for symptoms of relapse and may use maladaptive patterns of reassurance-seeking as a coping mechanism, which can perpetuate anxiety.[78] Anxiety is often a component of depression, and evidence of one should lead to assessment of the other.[72]

Psychological response to cancer is a function of two classes of variables: the stress and burden posed by the cancer experience and the resources available to cope with the stress and burden. The balance of these variables determines the psychological health of the cancer survivor in the short and long term.[71] Overall, certain factors can predict poor adjustment and functional limitations over time. These include such factors as receipt of chemotherapy, social isolation or conflict, expectancies for low level of control and negative outcomes, and avoidance of thoughts and feelings about cancer.[10] Protective factors that can be incorporated into interventions to treat anxiety include counseling survivors about having emotionally supportive relationships, using active coping strategies such as problem solving, positive reappraisal, and emotional expression.[10] It is important to note that many individuals extract positive meaning and benefit from their experience with cancer such as enhanced personal relationships, deepened appreciation for life, increased personal strength, greater spirituality, valued change in life priorities and goals, and greater attention to health-promoting behaviors.[79] Survivors also report that the positive and negative sequelae of cancer coexist.[77]

Assessment of long-term psychological effects in cancer survivors at follow-up visits is essential for implementation of effective interventions. Research shows that survivors who receive an intervention designed to improve function or well-being do better than those who do not.[74] The majority of interventions studied include the use of support groups, which have been shown to reduce distress, not only in patients but families. Physical activity can have positive effects on psychosocial measures, including depression, anxiety, self-esteem, and QoL.[80] Despite the evidence, relatively few survivors avail themselves of mental health services in general, or support group interventions specifically. Lack of insurance coverage is a likely factor and should be addressed locally for the individual and nationally as part of health-care reform.[81]

CASE STUDY

*Surviving is Not Survivorship: The Future Contribution of Palliative Care*

John is a 23-year-old who was diagnosed with Hodgkin's Disease when he was a junior in college. Because of the intensity of the treatment, John dropped out of college and returned home to live with his parents. Eventually, he was able to graduate from college, but he has lost touch with most of his classmates.

Because of the radiation and chemotherapy he received, John has chronic fatigue, as well as pain and decreased range of motion in his shoulder. He was also treated for depression in the first year after therapy was completed.

John receives physical therapy for the muscle atrophy in his neck and shoulder but has not found anyone who can help him with his chronic pain. He is reticent to apply for a promotion at work because he is concerned that his fatigue may limit his success in a new position. His employer doesn't know about his cancer history. John is in a serious relationship with a young woman, and he is quite anxious about discussing his cancer history, especially because he doesn't know if the treatment has affected his fertility.

As one can see from this case study, the challenges for cancer survivors as they become a greater and larger force in the American population are many. First is the education of health-care providers—particularly nurses—about the medical, psychological, social, and spiritual problems facing cancer survivors. Second is the development of communication tools to be shared between the survivor and health-care professionals outlining these potential problems, along with plans for follow-up care. Third, greater professional education and training about how to conduct a careful assessment to identify these long-term and late effects of treatment. Fourth, survivors should receive aggressive palliative care interventions for their symptoms. Finally, there should be greater public discussion and debate about how best to employ and provide insurance reimbursement for the comprehensive approach used by palliative care experts to individuals living with and beyond their cancer.

REFERENCES

1. Hewitt M, Greenfield S, Stovall E. From Cancer Patient to Cancer Survivor: Lost in Transition. Washington, DC: Institute of Medicine and National Research Council of the National Academies, 2006.
2. McCabe MS, Jacobs L. Survivorship care: Models and programs. Semin Oncol Nurs 2008;24:202–207.
3. Oeffinger KC, McCabe MS. Models for delivering survivorship care. J Clin Oncol 2006;24:5117–5124.
4. Rowland JH, Hewitt M, Ganz PA. Cancer survivorship: A new challenge in delivering quality cancer care. J Clin Oncol 2006;24:5101–5104.
5. Ferrell BR, Coyle N. For every nurse–a palliative care nurse. In Ferrell BR, Coyle N, eds. Textbook of Palliative Nursing. New York: Oxford University Press; 2006:IX.
6. President's Cancer Panel: Living Beyond Cancer: Finding a New Balance. Bethesda, MD: National Cancer Institute, 2004.
7. Azis NM, Rowland JH. Trends and advances in cancer survivorship research: Challenge and opportunity. Semin Radiat Oncol 2003;13:248–266.
8. Rowland JH. Cancer survivorship: Rethinking the cancer control continuum. Semin Oncol Nurs 2008;24:145–152.
9. Andrykowski MA, Lykins E, Floyd A. Psychological health in cancer survivors. Semin Oncol Nurs 2008;24:193–201.
10. Stanton AL. Psychological concerns and interventions for cancer survivors. J Clin Oncol 2006;24:5132–5137.
11. Stanton AL, Revenson TA, Tennen H. Health psychology: Psychosocial adjustment to chronic disease. Ann Rev Psychol 2007;58:565–592.
12. Meyerowitz BE, Oh S. Psychosocial response to cancer diagnosis and treatment. In Miller SM, Bowen DJ, Croyle RT, eds. Handbook of Behavioral Science and Cancer. Washington, DC: American Psychological Association, 2008;110–128.
13. Reis LAG, Melbert D, Krapcho M, et al. SEER Cancer Statistics Review, 1975–2004. Bethesda, MD: National Cancer Institute, 2006.
14. Hewitt M, Wiener SL, Simone JV. Childhood Cancer Survivorship: Improving Care and Quality of Life. Washington, DC: The National Academies Press, 2003.
15. Oeffinger KC, Mertens A, Sklar CA, et al. Chronic Health Conditions in Adult Survivors of Childhood Cancer. N Engl J Med 2006;355:1572–1582.
16. Mertens AC, Yasui Y, Neglia JP, et al. Late mortality experience in five-year survivors of childhood and adolescent cancer: The Childhood Cancer Study Group. J Clin Oncol 2001;19:3163–3172.
17. Oeffinger KC, Mertens AC, Hudson MM, et al. Health care of young adult survivors of childhood cancer: A report from the Childhood Cancer Survivor Study. Ann Fam Med 2004;2:61–70.
18. Children's Oncology Group Long-Term Follow-Up Guidelines for Survivors of Childhood, Adolescent, and Young Adult Cancers. Available at: http://www.survivorshipguidelines.org/ (accessed February 18, 2009).
19. Appelbaum FR. Hematopoietic-cell transplantation at 50. N Engl J Med 2007;357:1472–1475.
20. Joseph RW, Couriel DR, Komanduri KV. Chronic graft-versus-host disease after allogeneic stem cell transplantation: Challenges in prevention, science, and supportive care. J Support Oncol 2008;6:361–372.
21. Bhatia S, Francisco S, Carter A, et al. Late mortality after allogeneic hematopoietic cell transplantation and functional status of long-term survivors: Report from the Bone Marrow Transplant Survivor Study. Blood 2007;110:3784–3792.
22. Andrykowski MA, Greiner CB, Altmaier EM, Burish TG, Antin JH, Gingrich R, McGarigle C, Henslee-Downey PJ. Quality of life following bone marrow transplantation: Findings from a multicentre study. Br J Cancer 1995;71:1322–1329.
23. Helder DI, Bakker B, de Heer P, van der Veen F, Vossen JMJJ, Wit JM, Kaptein AA. Quality of life in adults following bone marrow transplantation during childhood. Bone Marrow Transplant 2004;33:329–336.
24. Jacobsen PB, Sadler IJ, Booth-Jones M, Soety E, Weitzner MA, Fields KK. Predictors of posttraumatic stress disorder symptomatology following bone marrow transplantation for cancer. J Consult Clin Psychol 2002;70:235–240.
25. Reddy P, Arora M, Gulmond M, Mackall CL, Weisdorf D. GVHD: A continuing barrier to the safety of allogeneic transplantation. Biol Blood Marrow Transplant 2008;15(1 Suppl):162–168.
26. Couriel D, Carpenter PA, Cutler C, et al. Ancillary therapy and supportive care of chronic graft-versus-host disease: National institutes of health consensus development project on criteria for clinical trials in chronic graft-versus-host disease: V. Ancillary therapy and Supportive Care Working Group Report. Biol Blood Marrow Transplant 2006;12:376–396.
27. Bellizi KM, Rowland JH. Role of comorbidity, symptoms and age in the health of older survivors following treatment for cancer. Ageing Health 2007;3:625–635.
28. Bellizi KM. Expressions of generativity and posttraumatic growth in adult cancer survivors. Int J Aging Hum Dev 2004; 58:247–267.
29. Rao AV, Demark-Wahnefried W. The older cancer survivor. Crit Rev Oncol Hematol 2006;60:131–143.
30. Freeman HP. Poverty, culture and social injustice: Determinants of cancer disparities. Cancer J Clin 2004;54:72–77.
31. Foley KM, Gelband H. Improving Palliative Care for Cancer. Washington, DC: National Academy Press, 2001.
32. Penson DF, Stoddard ML, Pasta DJ, Lubeck DP, Flanders SC, Litwin MS. The association between socioeconomic status, health insurance coverage, and quality of life in men with prostate cancer. J Clin Epidemiol 2001;54:350–358.
33. Portenoy RK, Thaler HT, Kornblith AB, et al. Symptom prevalence, characteristics, and distress in a cancer population. Qual Life Res 1994;3:183–189.
34. Cancer-Related Fatigue: Interventions for Patients on Long-Term Follow-Up. V.2.2009 National Comprehensive Cancer Network, Practice Guidelines in Oncology. Available at: http://www.nccn.org/professionals/physician_gls/PDF/fatigue.pdf (accessed February 16, 2009).

35. Cella D, Peterman A, Passik S, et al. Progress toward guidelines for the management of fatigue. Oncology 1998;12:369–377.

36. Irvine D, Vincent L, Graydon JE, et al. The prevalence and correlates of fatigue in patients receiving treatment with chemotherapy and radiotherapy: A comparison with the fatigue experienced by healthy individuals. Cancer Nurs 1994;17:367–378.

37. Curt GA, Breitbart W, Cella D, et al. Impact of cancer–related fatigue on the lives of patients: New findings from the fatigue coalition. Oncologist 2000;5:353–360.

38. Cella D, Davis K, Breitbart W, Curt G. The fatigue coalition cancer-related fatigue: Prevalence of proposed diagnostic criteria in a United States sample of cancer survivors. J Clin Oncol 2001;19:3385–3391.

39. Minton O, Stone P. How common is fatigue in disease-free breast cancer survivors? A systematic review of the literature. Breast Cancer Res Treat 2008;112:5–13.

40. Hjermstad MJ, Oldervoll L, Fossa SD, Holte H, Jacobsen AB, Loge JH. Quality of life in long term Hodgkin's disease survivors with chronic fatigue. Eur J Cancer 2006;42:327–333.

41. Ganz PA, Naipour CM, Pauler DK, et al. Health status and quality of life in patients with early-stage Hodgkin's disease treated on southwest oncology group study 9133. J Clin Oncol 2003;21:3512–3519.

42. Sun V, Borneman T, Piper B, Koczywas M, Ferrell B. Barriers to pain assessment and management in cancer survivorship. J Cancer Surviv 2008;2:65–71.

43. Burton AW, Fanciullo GJ, Beasley RD, Fisch MJ. Chronic pain in the cancer survivor: A new frontier. Pain 2007;8:189–198.

44. Chaudhry V, Rowinsky EK, Sartorius SE, Donehower RC, Cornblath DR. Peripheral neuropathy from taxol and cisplatin combination chemotherapy: Clinical and electrophysiological studies. Ann Neurol 1994;35:304–311.

45. Andre T, Boni C, Mounedji – Boudiaf L, et al. Oxaliplatin, fluorouracil and leucovorin as adjuvant treatment for colon cancer. N Engl J Med 2004;350:2343–2351.

46. Chan-Lam D, Prentice AG, Copplestone JA, Weston M, Williams M, Hutton CW. Avascular necrosis of bone following intensified steroid therapy for acute lymphoblastic leukemia and high-grade malignant lymphoma. Br J Haematol 1994;86:227–230.

47. Mattano LA, Sather HN, Trigg ME, Nachman JB. Osteonecrosis as a complication of treating acute lymphoblastic leukemia in children: A report from the Children's Oncology Group. J Clin Oncol 2000;18:3262–3272.

48. Ogino I, Okamoto N, Ono Y, Kitamura T, Nakayama H. Pelvic insufficiency fractures in postmenopausal women with advanced cervical cancer treated with radiotherapy. Radiother Oncol 2003;68:61–67.

49. Borsje S, Bosmans JC, van der Schans CP, Geertzen JHB, Dijkstra PU. Phantom pain: A sensitivity analysis. Disabil Rehabil 2004;26:905–910.

50. Smith J, Thompson JM. Phantom limb pain and chemotherapy in pediatric amputees. Mayo Clin Proc 1995;70:357–364.

51. Perttunen K, Tasmuth T, Kalso E. Chronic pain after thoracic surgery: A follow-up study. Acta Anaesthesiol Scand 1999;43:463–467.

52. Kalso E, Perttunen K, Kaasinen S. Pain after thoracic surgery. Acta Anaesthesiol Scand 1992;36:96–100.

53. Jung BF, Ahrendt GM, Oaklander AL, Dworkin RH. Neuropathic pain following breast cancer surgery: Proposed classification and research update. Pain 2003;104:1–13.

54. Tasmuth T, Kataja M, Blomqvist C, von Smitten K, Kalso E. Treatment related factors predisposing to chronic pain in patients with breast cancer—a multivariate approach. Acta Oncol 1997;36:625–630.

55. Wallace MS, Wallace AM, Lee J. Pain after breast surgery; a survey of 282 women. Pain 1996;66:195–205.

56. Savard J, Morin CM, Insomnia in the context of cancer: A review of a neglected problem. J Clin Oncol 2001;19:895–908.

57. Mulrooney DA, Ness KK, Neglia JP, et al. Fatigue and sleep disturbance in adult survivors of childhood cancer: A report from the Childhood Cancer Survivor Study (CCSS). Sleep 2008;31:271–281.

58. Ginsburg ML, Quirt C, Ginsburg AD, MacKillop WJ. Psychiatric illness and psychosocial concerns in patients with newly diagnosed lung cancer. Can Med Assoc J 1995;152:701–708.

59. Whelan TJ, Mohide EA, Willan AR, et al. The supportive care needs of newly diagnosed cancer patients attending a regional cancer center. Cancer 1997;80:1518–1524.

60. Davidson JR, MacLean AW, Brundage MD, Schulze K. Sleep disturbance in cancer patients. Soc Sci Med 2002;54:1309–1321.

61. Servaes P, van der Werf S, Prins J, Verhagen S, Bleijenberg G. Fatigue in disease-free cancer patients compared with fatigue in patients with chronic fatigue syndrome. Support Care Cancer 2001;9:11–17.

62. Hoyt MA, Thomas KS, Epstein DR, Dirksen SR. Coping style and sleep quality in men with cancer. Ann Behav Med 2009;37(1):88–93.

63. Mendelson WB. Pharmacotherapy of insomnia. Psychiatr Clin N Am 1987;10(4):555–563.

64. Vardy J, Wefel JS, Ahles T, Tannock IF, Schagen SB. Cancer and cancer-therapy related cognitive dysfunction: An international perspective from the Venice cognitive workshop. Ann Oncol 2007;19:623–629.

65. Ganz PA. Cognitive dysfunction following adjuvant treatment of breast cancer: A new dose-limiting toxic effect? J Natl Cancer Inst 1998;90:182–183.

66. Ahles TA, Saykin AJ. Breast cancer chemotherapy-related cognitive dysfunction. Clin Breast Cancer 2002;3(Suppl 3):S84–S90.

67. Wefel JS, Witgert ME, Meyers CA. Neuropsychological sequelae of non-central nervous system cancer and cancer therapy. Neuropsychol Rev 2008;18:121–131.

68. Ferguson RJ, Ahles TA, Saykkins AJ, McDonalds BC, Furstenberg CT. Cognitive-behavioral management of chemotherapy related cognitive changes. Psychooncology 2007;16:772–777.

69. Ahles TA, Saykin AJ. Candidate mechanisms for chemotherapy-induced cognitive changes. Nat Rev Cancer 2007;7:192–201.

70. Correa DD, Ahles TA. Cognitive adverse effects of chemotherapy in breast cancer patients. Curr Opin Support Palliat Care 2007;1(1):157–162.

71. Stein KD, Syrjala KL, Andrykowski MA. Physical and psychological long-term and late effects of cancer. Cancer 2008;112 (Suppl):2577–2590.

72. Massie MJ. Prevalence of depression in patients with cancer. J Natl Cancer Inst Monogr 2004;32:57–71.

73. Pasquini M, Biondi M. Depression in cancer patients: A critical review. Clin Pract Epidemiol Ment Health 2007;3:2.

74. Alfano CM, Rowland JH. Recovery issues in cancer survivorship: A new challenge for supportive care. Cancer J 2006;12: 432–443.

75. Deimling GT, Kahana B, Bowman KF, Schaefer ML. Cancer survivorship and psychological distress later in life. Psychooncology 2002;11:479–494.

76. Kangas M, Henry JL, Bryant RA. Posttraumatic stress disorder following cancer: A conceptual and empirical review. Clin Psychol Rev 2002;22:499–524.

77. Cordova MJ, Andrykowski MA. Responses to cancer diagnosis and treatment: Post-traumatic stress and posttraumatic growth. Semin Clin Neuropsychiatry 2003;8:286–296.

78. Stark DPH, House A. Anxiety in cancer patients. Br J Cancer 2000;83:1261–1267.

79. Stanton AL, Bower JE, Low CA. Posttraumatic growth after cancer. In Calhoun LG, Tedeschi RG, eds. Handbook of Posttraumatic Growth: Research and Practice. Mahwah, NJ: Lawrence Erlbaum; 2006:138–175.

80. Schwartz AL. Physical activity after a cancer diagnosis: Psychosocial outcomes. Cancer Invest 2004;22:82–92.

81. Hewitt M, Rowland JH. Mental health service use among adult cancer survivors: Analysis of the National Health Interview Survey. J Clin Oncol 2002;20:4581–4590.

# VI

# End-of-Life Care Across Settings

# 44 Marilyn Bookbinder

# Improving the Quality of Care
# Across All Settings

*Never doubt that a small group of thoughtful, committed citizens can change the world. Indeed, that's the only thing that ever has.—Margaret Mead*

♦ **Key Points**

♦ *Quality palliative care is a result of intelligent systematic efforts to raise standards of care.*

♦ *Tools are available to assist in the monitoring and measurement of structure, process, and competency in the delivery of palliative care.*

♦ *Outcome measures are needed to evaluate the impact of innovative change on patient and family quality of life, health-care systems, and professional practice.*

One system for addressing health and end-of-life (EOL) care is the inclusion of quality methodologies designed to improve education, streamline health-care bureaucracies, help measure costs, and even address how people feel about their jobs. Whether or not your organization is accredited by the Joint Commission on Accreditation of Health Care Organizations (JCAHO) or mandated to use a quality improvement (QI) methodology, a planned-change approach is needed to achieve positive outcomes and to cultivate an infrastructure that maintains optimal standards of care for those at the end of life.

This chapter provides perspectives on QI-based initiatives in U.S. health-care organizations across settings and populations and discusses their impact on patient, professional, and system outcomes in palliative care. Principles of QI and structural, process, and outcome approaches to conducting QI studies are introduced. A case study is presented of a care-path for end of life that the author and colleagues pilot-tested. It is used to establish the linkages between QI principles and practice to improve EOL care. The chapter closes by showcasing nurses within interdisciplinary teams who are providing leadership in the field of quality and palliative care.

## The Terminology Turmoil

Quality improvement is increasingly commonplace in the lexicon of industry and government health-care systems in the United States. Typically, QI is used to describe a process for improving things. Although the terms vary, distinct vocabulary, tools, and techniques used to conduct QI studies are the same. Other labels include continuous quality improvement (CQI), total quality management (TQM), total quality systems (TQS), quality systems improvement (QSI), total quality (TQ), and performance improvement.[1]

Because consensus regarding these terms is unlikely, it is recommended that each organization define a methodology and terms that apply across the board and be consistent in their use. This will encourage users of QI to read beyond labels and to examine the meaning behind concepts and the value of teamwork in achieving goals. For the purposes of this chapter, QI is defined generically as the label for the philosophy driving a systematic approach to improving clinical practice, systems, issues, education, and research.

## Quality Improvement in Healthcare

### What Is Quality Improvement?

As a philosophy, QI is broadly defined as "a commitment and approach used to continuously improve every process in every part of an organization, with the intent to exceed customer expectations and outcomes." As a management approach, QI is a way of doing business—a way to stimulate employees to become part of the solution by improving the ways care is delivered, identifying the root causes of problems in systems, designing innovative products and services, and evaluating and continuously improving.[2]

The concepts of QI go back to the 1920s, with pioneers in the field such as Deming, Shewhart, Juran, and Ishikawa. W. Edwards Deming, an American engineer and statistician most widely known for his efforts to assist Japan in its quest for quality after World War II, was all but unknown in his own country (United States) until the 1980s. In fact, the Deming prize, Japan's highest award for industrial productivity and quality, was first awarded to an American company, Florida Electric and Light Company, in 1989. To date, no health-care organizations have received the Deming prize. Joseph Juran, also involved in the Japanese quality transition in the 1940s and 1950s, added the concepts of planning and control to the quality process and addressed the "costs" of poor quality, which includes wasted effort, extra expense, and defects. Readers wanting more detail about the rationale and statistical methods behind QI philosophy and methods are referred to the writings of Deming and others.[2]

Although Deming's quality method has been used extensively in industry with much success, it has only been adapted to education and healthcare since the early 1990s. The U.S. Health Care Reform Act of 1992[3] fueled the need for QI methods and better control over inconsistencies in services. Effects of the reform include: (1) increased managed-care contracts in health systems and reductions in reimbursement; (2) reorganization and downsizing of hospitals and staff; (3) cross-training and the development of multipurpose personnel; (4) shorter hospital stays for patients; and (5) a shift in the provision of services from hospital care to ambulatory and home care.

The most recognized symbol of quality in healthcare remains the JCAHO. JCAHO accredits and certifies more than 15,000 health-care organizations and programs in the United States to meeting certain performance standards.

The urgent need for health-care reform in the United States has propelled private and professional organizations to form coalitions to assist the United States in making Healthy People 2010 become a reality (i.e., improve quality and years of *healthy* living). In the last decade, organizations such as the Institute for Healthcare Improvement spurred by the Rand Corporation and Don Berwick, leader in Quality Improvement, have provided leadership for health-care professionals striving to improve quality and costs in their organizations. With the help of web-based learning systems, virtual teams of professionals can join national and regional collaborative efforts around specific content areas, offering mentorship and resources.

## Introducing the Beth Israel Medical Center Case to Improve End-of-life Care

Table 44–1 describes six key principles of QI, based on the doctrines of W. Edwards Deming. These principles were applied to a QI project to improve EOL care at Continuum's Beth Israel Medical Center (BIMC) in New York City in early 2001 and are still applicable today.[4] At BIMC, chart reviews of inpatient deaths and other sources of data provided evidence that EOL care could be improved. The purpose of the 1-year pilot study, funded by a New York State Quality Measurement grant, was to create a benchmark for the care of the imminently dying inpatient.

The QI process begins and ends with customers, determining their needs and creating products that meet or exceed their expectations. To achieve the necessary improvement, multidisciplinary teams are to break down barriers between disciplines and departments, promote collaboration and mutual respect among health-care workers, and encourage "buy-in" from front-line staff. In the BIMC pilot study, to determine the causes of variation in EOL care, a 28-member team was formed to involve staff integral to the EOL process on five pilot units: oncology, geriatrics, hospice, medical intensive care, and step-down unit. Early in the study, QI techniques of brainstorming and flowcharting were used to identify health system barriers and to identify possible strategies for dealing with them.

Quality improvement teams use a systematic, scientific approach and statistical methods to study problems and make decisions. This paradigm encourages an environment of life-long learning and promotes a team approach to identifying and developing the "best practices." The BIMC project identified a critical need for multidisciplinary education and teambuilding. For example, monthly QI meetings included a segment of the American Medical Association's (AMA's) Education for Physicians on End-of-Life Care[5] training program. Discussions, led by Russell K. Portenoy, M.D., a co-investigator for the AMA project and co-chair of the Palliative Care for Advanced Disease (PCAD) QI team, and leader in palliative care, provided team members fundamental

**Table 44–1**
**Principles of Quality and Application for Improving End-of-Life Care**

| Principle | Discussion | Application |
|---|---|---|
| 1. Customer-driven | The focus is on customers, both internal and external, and understanding them. Teams strive to achieve products/services to better meet needs and exceed expectations of customers. | Chart reviews of patient deaths reveal areas to improve: Documentation regarding advance directive discussions, symptom management effectiveness, spiritual and psychosocial care, treatment decisions in last 48 hours of life. Focus groups with caregivers reveal need for better communication with health professionals about patient's progress. |
| 2. System optimization and alignment | Organizations/teams are systems of interdependent parts, with the same mission and goals for customers. Optimizing performance of the entire system means aligning the processes, technology, people, values, and policies to support team efforts to continually improve. | Hospital-wide multidisciplinary CQI team is formed to reduce variation in EOL care with three standardized tools that provide guidelines for care (carepath), documentation, and physician orders. Ongoing resources from Pain and Palliative Care available to pilot unit staff (one advanced practice nurse). |
| 3. Continual improvement and innovation | Focus shifts to processes of care and using a systematic and scientific approach. Methods seek to reduce and control unnecessary process variation and improve outcomes. | Flowcharting and brainstorming techniques help identify current activities and unit norms for EOL care regarding establishing goals of care, advance directives, respecting patient and family preferences, and barriers to implementing goals of project. |
| 4. Continual learning | Resources are available to develop a culture in which people seek to learn from each other and access new sources of evidence. Feedback mechanisms support the use of evidence to drive improvements. | Extensive literature searches and team expertise guide development of clinical tools and educational materials. Team members receive education regarding issues in EOL care, viewing of Education in Palliative and End-of-Life Care (EPEC). Adult learning principles guide sequencing and content of educational sessions for unit staff (e.g., physiology of dying). |
| 5. Management through knowledge | Decision-making is based on knowledge, confirmed with facts about what is "best practice," and guided by statistical thinking. | Team uses FOCUS-PDSA methodology to structure study processes. Content experts in EOL, measurement, outcomes, and QI guide sampling, selected outcome measures, and graphic display of data. |
| 6. Collaboration and mutual respect | Organizations/teams engage everyone in the process of improvement and in the discovery of new knowledge and innovations. Mutual respect for the dignity, knowledge, and potential, contributions of others is valued by members. | Team forms subcommittees to develop materials in four areas based on expertise and interest: Carepath development, flow sheet, physicians' orders. Implementation (timeline for phases of planning, launching, rollout, evaluation, dissemination, and decisions to adopt practice changes). Education (staff, patient, and family) Outcomes (patient, family, staff knowledge, process audit of new tools). |

information about the components of good EOL care, as well as opportunities to voice their own ideas and concerns.

The QI team worked in four subcommittees over a 5-month period to reach the implementation schedule of the project. One subcommittee developed the PCAD pathway, which has three parts: a multidisciplinary care path, a flow sheet for daily documentation of care, and a physician's order sheet that includes suggested medications for treating 15 of the most prevalent symptoms at EOL. The other three subcommittees addressed (1) education of nurses, physicians, other staff, patients, and families; (2) a timeline and detailed plan

for implementation, education, and evaluation of PCAD; and (3) tools and methods for evaluating patient, family, staff, and system outcomes of the project.

## The Effectiveness of Quality Improvement

Those wanting to improve quality by using best evidence quickly learn the value of the Cochrane Collaboration, an international not-for-profit organization, providing up-to-date high-quality, and timely research evidence about the effects of healthcare. Readers are encouraged to search the Cochrane Library for the results of an interventional protocol reviewing continuous quality improvement and its effects on professional practice and patient outcomes. One of the principle objectives of the review will be to determine the relative effectiveness of continuous QI approaches compared with standard health-care practices, the sustainability of the outcomes, and the associated costs. The review includes the effects of modifying information flows (e.g., paper or electronic records), material flows (e.g., a blood sample sent to a laboratory), patient flows (e.g., patients through outpatient department), or combinations of these (e.g., annual review of specific patient groups). Strategies used for implementing the approach will also be included, such as educational materials, educational meetings, educational outreach, or opinion leaders/product champions, marketing, or use of other media.[6]

The Joint Commission's Journal on Quality and Patient Safety annually publishes profiles of the Joint Commission Ernest Amory Codman Award recipients. One 2008 award recipient, Mission Hospital, of Mission Viejo, California, illustrates the positive outcomes that teams can achieve and the effectiveness of quality efforts on outcomes. This hospital improved care for seriously ill patients in the emergency department or on medical-surgical floors rather than the intensive care unit (ICU). The program used a specialized nurse-driven rapid response team with the goal of reducing deaths associated with non-ICU cardiac/respiratory arrests by bringing to the necessary staff to the bedside to help the patient. Mission Hospital's program reduced cardiac or respiratory arrests outside the ICU from 36 to 16 during a 1-year period, and the associated mortality rate for floor code patients decreased from 62% to 23% during the same timeframe. Unanticipated transfers of patients from the noncritical care units to the ICU also dropped significantly—from 8% of all transfers per hospital discharge to 5%—by intervening before their conditions deteriorated. This is just one example of how positive changes in outcomes are occurring through quality initiatives.[7]

Given the emphasis in healthcare on using QI to achieve high quality at reduced costs, nurses can expect to see increases in accountability in the following areas: performance monitoring, participation in multidisciplinary team meetings, education in quality improvement, implementation of process improvement approaches, use of flowcharts and other tools and techniques for data gathering, restructuring of workflow patterns and removal of barriers to patient care, development and use of quality indicators, and focus on patient and caregiver outcomes.

## The Need for Quality Improvement in Palliative Care

The World Health Organization defines palliative care as the "the active total care of patients whose disease is not responsive to curative treatment…when control of pain, of other symptoms and of psychological, social and spiritual problems is paramount."[8] Palliative care is often referred to as supportive care or comfort care that seeks to prevent, relieve, alleviate, lessen, or soothe the symptoms of disease without effecting a cure.

The Institute of Medicine's (IOM's), landmark report, *Approaching Death: Improving Care at End of Life*[9] published by a 12-member medical nursing expert committee summarized four areas needing improvement: the state-of-the-knowledge in EOL care, evaluation methods for measuring outcomes, factors impeding high-quality care, and steps toward agreement on what constitutes "appropriate care" at end of life. These major findings suggested starting points for QI work in America:

- *Patient care*: Too many people suffer needlessly at the end of life, both from errors of omission (when caregivers fail to provide palliative and supportive care known to be effective) and from errors of commission (when caregivers do what is known to be ineffective and even harmful).
- *Organizations*: Legal, organizational, and economical obstacles conspire to obstruct reliably excellent care at the end of life.
- *Education*: The education and training of physicians and other health-care professionals fail to provide them with knowledge, skills, and attitudes required to care well for the dying patient.
- *Research*: Current knowledge and understanding are inadequate to guide and support consistent practice of evidence-based medicine at the end of life.

The IOM report includes results from the national SUPPORT study, which produced over 104 publications supporting the deficiencies in care and citing the frequency of aggressive medical treatment at end of life (deaths occurring in the ICU) and the lack of adequate symptom management (conscious patients with moderate to severe pain).[10]

The need to identify quality care at EOL for oncology patients has also been a priority. Through its Evidence-Based Practice Centers (EPCs), the AHRQ sponsored the development of a Technical Evidence Report (TEP) on "Cancer Care Quality Measures: Symptoms and End-of-Life Care."[11] The TEP identified evidence-based quality measures to support quality assessment and improvement in the palliative care of cancer patients in the areas of pain, dispend, depression, and advance care planning. Of the 537 articles that met the TEP criteria for review, only 25 contained quality measures: 21 on advance care planning, 4 on depression, 2 on dyspnea, and 12 on pain, of which only a few had been specifically tested in a cancer population. These findings suggest that little progress has been made in standardizing the assessment of the quality of care delivered and are key research areas in which nurse researchers can make a difference.

The next segment of this chapter highlights approaches to improving quality palliative care in the IOM's four areas of identified need: patient care, organizations, education, and research. Donabedian's classic framework for defining and improving quality will be used: structure, process, and outcome components.[12]

## Improving Structure, Process, and Outcomes in Palliative Care

### Structure

Quality improvement models can provide structure to an EOL care program. In addition to explaining the interrelationship of program parts, a systematic approach guides the activities of people performing QI as well as assuring the validity and relevance of a study. QI experts agree that "quality is never an accident" and that it is "always the result of intelligent effort, intent, and vigilance to make a superior thing." To achieve this, QI teams need a systematic methodology to follow. Although various models have evolved, all of them support the notion of QI as an unceasing, organization-wide effort that focuses people and systems on improving the processes of work. They are not intended for policing or blaming people for errors after the fact.

The oldest and most frequently used methodology designed to support "intelligent effort" is the FOCUS-PDCA cycle, which illustrates the BIMC team's application of each step in the cycle (see Appendix 44–1). The details and application of the FOCUS-PDCA cycle and tools and techniques for conducting QI studies have been described more fully elsewhere.[11–14] The PDCA (plan–do–check–act) portion of the cycle, will be called by its more commonly used name today, the PDSA (plan–do–study–act). The FOCUS-PDSA methodology is briefly described below using the BIMC example. Its first five steps are aimed at team-building, clarifying the nature and scope of the improvement needed, and gathering information about the culture and setting in which the study will be done.

### FOCUS

- *Find a process to improve.* The focus for the BIMC study was care of imminently dying inpatients on the five hospital units known to have the highest volume of patient deaths. Chart reviews of patient deaths investigated 2 years earlier identified the need for the study.
- *Organize to improve a process.* A 28-member QI team spanned departments and disciplines to address EOL issues, such as ethics, social work, chaplains, pharmacists, nurses, and physicians. Experts in the Department of Pain and Palliative Care and EOL took the lead.
- *Clarify what is known.* Flowcharts were created to map the ideal process of care and increase dialogue among

the team's disciplines about "why" the care varied. Based on the results, the team regrouped into four concurrent subcommittees: (1) care path development; (2) implementation; (3) education; and (4) evaluation, including searches of internal and external sources of evidence and rationale in EOL care.
- *Understand variation.* Brainstorming techniques helped the team elicit reasons for variations in the care process and identify potential barriers. An Ishikawa diagram (to display cause and effect) was used to show the barriers; materials, methods, people, and equipment categories were used. Subcommittees considered the barriers when planning and implementing the program.
- Select a process improvement. The four subcommittees developed evidence-based interventions, including the three-part PCAD care path, educational materials, a timeline for the work of implementation, and appropriate tools to measure professional, patient and family, and system outcomes. The FOCUS step prepares the team for the PDSA cycle.

### The PDSA Cycle: Plan–Do–Study–Act

Also known as the Shewhart Cycle,[2] the PDSA constitutes the evaluation aspect of the study. It is an iterative problem-solving process, with staff involvement, and uses measurement to monitor progress toward defined goals as changes are applied. The implementation of these steps during the BIMC pilot follows. The PDSA cycle used by the education subcommittee is highlighted.

- *Plan.* In this step, a timeline of activities for the 1-year pilot prepared administration, team members, and others with direction, goals, and resources. The sample timeline in Appendix 44–1 illustrates the various phases involved in launching the pilot project: the planning phase, roll-out or introduction phase, implementation, evaluation, and dissemination and reporting phases. Then the study design is crafted. This includes determination of sample size and selection, what data will be collected and by whom, what tools will be used and when they will be applied, what training will be conducted and by whom, and who will perform data analysis. Table 44–2 outlines principles for assuring the quality of data.
- *Do.* The interventions are implemented and data collection begins. In the BIMC study, several pre-measures were obtained, including baseline knowledge, using the Palliative Care Quiz for Nurses,[15] chart reviews, and focus groups with staff to obtain baseline data.
- *Check.* The results of data collection are analyzed by the team and the next steps formulated. For example,

**Table 44–2**
**Principles for Assuring the Quality of Data**

| Principle | Key Point |
|---|---|
| Validity/reliability | There is accuracy and consistency in data collection. |
| Completeness | Measurement system includes a policy for missing data and timeliness of collection. |
| Sampling method | Sample size is determined by power analysis to ensure representativeness of population. |
| Outlier cases | Measurement systems make efforts to validate or correct outliers. |
| Data specification | There are standardized definitions and terminology for transmission/use of data across departments. |
| Internal standards | Prespecified data-quality standards are tailored for individual performance measures. |
| External standards | There is a commitment to implementing data sets, codes, methodologies developed by accrediting bodies (e.g., government, professional organizations) for data use across health care systems. |
| Auditability | Data are traceable to the individual case level. |
| Monitoring process | Ongoing data-measurement process in place is based on prespecified standards. |
| Documentation | Data standards and findings are recorded and available for review. |
| Feedback | Performance systems regularly provide summary reports on data quality to organization leadership. |
| Education | Performance systems provide support through education, on-site visits, and guidelines to ensure quality data. |
| Accountability | Measurement systems are responsible for data quality and dissemination to participating members. |

## Measures and Repeated Use of the Cycle

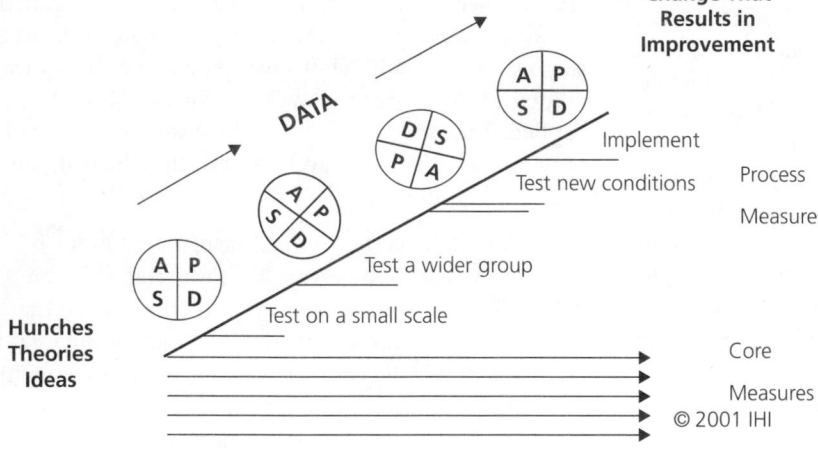

**Figure 44–1.** General approach to sequential PDSA cycles. *Source:* Copyright IHI.

the BIMC group used the findings from the knowledge pretest to identify areas for continuing education. Through consensus, members agreed that knowledge items answered incorrectly by 15% of staff would be targeted for continued education.

- *Act.* Action plans are developed. The BIMC team gave monthly feedback to the QI team, pilot units, and the hospital QI department in a quarterly report. Knowledge scores on pilot units were lowest on items about the dying process. The pretest scores and staff requested education in "the physiology of dying." To address an educational need at the BIMC team level, videos from the End of Life Care for Physicians Education Consortium were shown at monthly

meetings. Discussions were led by the department's palliative care experts.

The PDSA rapid cycle process has been used successfully by many QI teams in national Improvement for Healthcare Initiative (IHI) collaboratives to improve EOL care.[16] In this model, teams are formed, including senior leadership, acknowledging buy-in, and support for the effort from the start. During a year's time, members are coached by IHI faculty with additional three 1-day educational sessions, online discussions groups, on-site visits by faculty, and telephone conference calls of frequently discussed topics, such as advance directives, pain and symptom management, and bereavement care. Figure 44–1 shows the general approach to sequential PDSA cycles. Teams are encouraged to make small changes rapidly and, once met, to repeat the PDSA cycle with the next phase of the process or move to another process. This rapid cycle method has helped many achieve positive results within weeks to months. Encouraging teams to reach their targeted goals quickly reinforces team-building and motivates the teams to examine other processes. More detailed readings on the rapid cycle approach and the results of studies can be found in *Improving Care for the End-of-Life: A Sourcebook for Healthcare Managers and Clinicians.*[17]

## Standards of Care Provide Structure

Quality in clinical settings begins with well-defined standards of care that are accepted as authoritative by professionals. Such standards represent acknowledged conditions against which comparisons can be made and levels of excellence are judged. They serve to establish consistency, expectations, and patterns for practice. They articulate what health-care professionals do and whom they serve, and they define what clinical services and resources are needed. Standards also provide a framework against which quality of care can be measured and constantly improved.

In QI, the term benchmark is used to refer to "the search for the best practices that consistently produce best-in-the-world results"[18]—the gold standard. Nurses leading QI teams are increasingly joining benchmarking associations such as the Association for Benchmarking Health Care™[18] (http://www.abhc.org/) and the Six Sigma Health Care Benchmarking Association™ (http://www.sixsigmabenchmarking.com/6shcba.html)[19] that offer mentorship, education, newsletters, and participation in benchmarking studies relevant to their health-care needs. Standards of care,[20] guidelines,[21,22] and principles of professional practice from national associations[23] position papers from professional associations[23 26] and research models for EOL care[27–29] are further examples of structures available to clinicians seeking to make improvements in the appropriateness, effectiveness, and cost-effectiveness of care.

If explicit, guidelines can describe appropriate management of specific symptoms and at provide a basis for assessment, treatment, and possible outcomes. However, if the evidence is weak, as is the case for much of EOL care, guidelines or standards need to be supported with recommendations made through consensus.

In 2004, two documents containing standards for palliative care clinicians were released. The first, published by the Center to Advance Palliative Care, was the "Crosswalk of JCAHO Standards and Palliative Care—with PC Policies, Procedures and Assessment Tools."[30] This document provides hospitals with the policy and administrative foundation for delivering palliative care services that are consistent with JCAHO standards. Its intent is to assist programs in implementing quality palliative care in accordance with JCAHO Standards. The document can be accessed at www.capc.org.

One example of a standard from the crosswalk relative to palliative care is within the provision of care standards (PC.5.50). It states that care, treatment, and services are provided in an interdisciplinary, collaborative manner. To implement this standard, a palliative care team would provide documentation of assessments, planning, and treatments from physicians, nurses, social work, and perhaps a chaplain. The team has policies and procedures that address the standard, including the timing and scope of performing initial assessments and reassessments, patient care planning and guidelines for staff about patient and family conferences, and assessment and treatment of pain and symptoms. The document suggests tools to implement the standards and document how they've been met, such as a consultation report, progress notes, spiritual care assessment, social work consultation note, initial assessment, plan of care, patient and family care conference record, and a palliative care intervention form.

The second key document published was the National Consensus Project for Quality Palliative Care.[31] This project produced guidelines for quality palliative care programs that represent a consensus opinion of the major palliative care organizations and leaders in the United States and that are based both on the available scientific evidence and expert professional opinion. These clinical practice guidelines have become the accepted means of promoting consistency, comprehensiveness, and quality across eight domains of healthcare. Fundamental processes that cross all domains include assessment, information sharing, decision-making, care planning, and care delivery at EOL. Adoption of these guidelines in the United States will help to promote high-quality care to persons living with life-threatening and debilitating chronic illness.

## Process

Answering the question "What are the processes for giving care to a dying patient?" can generate many ideas for QI work. Process refers to the series of linked steps (but not necessarily sequential), which by design deliver a set of results. Quality improvement operates on the principle that people do their best but are constrained by faulty health-care processes that need to be addressed. Nurses' routine process for assessment, diagnosis, reassessment, treatment, documentation, and evaluation of patient care are critical to producing positive patient and family outcomes. Specifically, assessment and reassessment of pain, dyspnea, agitation, delirium, nausea, diarrhea, and constipation are important symptoms leading to nursing interventions that can reduce the suffering of dying patients.

As clinicians have been challenged to deliver high-quality care at lower cost, there has been an explosion of tools designed to reduce variability in the processes of care. Algorithms and clinical pathways are two such tools that offer streamlined strategies for multidisciplinary teams to monitor and manage the processes of patient care. These tools define desired patient outcomes for specific medical conditions and delineate the optimal sequence and timing of interventions to be performed by health-care professionals.

## Algorithms and Standardized Orders Streamline Processes

Algorithms are step-by-step guides used by busy clinicians in their day-to-day work. The Providence Hospice in Yakima, Washington is a model program of QI thinking applied in daily practice and service. Their pocket-size handbook of standing orders and algorithms, "Symptom Management Algorithms for Palliative Care,"[32] is one of the most widely used by clinicians. The symptom-management algorithms allow for a team approach involving the referring physician, medical director, nurse, pharmacist, patient, and family caregivers. Quality improvement results have been positive thus far at Yakima. In one study, use of an algorithm reduced the turnaround time of medication delivery to home hospice patients from 24 to 48 hours to less than 2 hours. Other topics in the handbook include algorithms for pain and other distressing symptoms, such as mucositis, anxiety, and terminal agitation and dyspnea. Figure 44–2 shows an example of an algorithm to improve the management of dyspnea developed at Dartmouth-Hitchcock Medical center (Lebanon, New Hampshire).[33] The approach offers clinicians a methodology for assessing and directing treatment options and includes pharmacological and nonpharmacological interventions. Others are available at http://www.intelli-card.com/photos/Dyspnea.pdf.[34]

## Clinical Pathways Reduce Variation in Processes of Care

The term pathway refers to clinical trails that form a structured, multidisciplinary action plan. It defines the key events, activities, and expected outcomes of care for each discipline during each day of care. Pathways are evidence-driven, reflect best practices, and delineate the optimal sequence and timing of interventions. The goal of using a pathway is to "reduce variation" in services and practices, thus reducing costs and negative patient outcomes."[35,36] Table 44–3 shows a six-step process for developing pathways. Table 44–4 lists commonly used elements of care and interventions. Reducing variation in any process (clinical decision-making or care delivery) takes three steps. The first step is to study the process as it currently operates (usually done through flowcharting) to identify potential sources of variation and to gather data about which activities are likely to achieve the desirable outcomes. The second step is to stabilize the process by getting everyone to use the same procedures, equipment, materials, and so forth. This is usually done by giving timely feedback to users, educating about procedures, and involving them in tweaking the process. The third step is to measure again and repeat the process until control within agreed-upon limits is reached.

The BIMC QI team's pilot test of a clinical pathway is described in the next section. The Palliative Care for Advanced Disease pilot was on three units—oncology, geriatrics, and the hospice units—and two medical units served as control units.

## Pilot-Test of a Pathway to Improve End-of-Life Care

The BIMC QI team's Carepath subcommittee designed an evidenced-based PCAD pathway consisting of three parts: (1) a Care Path—the interdisciplinary plan of care; (2) a Daily Patient Care Flow Sheet for documentation of assessments and interventions (including automatic referrals to social work and chaplaincy); and (3) a standardized Physician Order Sheet, with suggestions for medical management of 15 symptoms prevalent at the EOL (see Appendix 44–1 or go to http://www.StopPain.org/professional).[37] This three-part pathway was designed to guide interdisciplinary management of the imminently dying inpatient once the patient's primary physician had ordered PCAD (Table 44–5).

Implementation of PCAD in daily care on the three pilot units confirmed the enormous complexity of "implementation" and predicting the timing of a patient's death.[34] Although "imminently dying" was defined for the study as "hours to two weeks until death," nurses and physicians reported discomfort about making this decision. Each patient was assessed for eligibility during daily morning report or at weekly discharge planning rounds by answering the question "Whose death would not surprise you this admission?" Designated nurse leaders on each unit served as the liaisons between staff and primary physicians to request a patient's enrollment into PCAD. During the 3-month start-up period, multidisciplinary teams reported that their greatest challenge was identifying patients who were imminently dying. As patients were identified by nurses as candidates, barriers to implementing PCAD began to surface: patients and families wanted "everything done" to continue curative treatment; a physician evaluated a patient as "fragile" and unable to hear "bad news"; a patient's physical status changed dramatically in 24 hours, from dying to "rallying" and preparing for discharge; or a house staff physician felt that he was already prescribing PCAD and could not see the benefit of enrollment.

There were several positive outcomes of the PCAD pilot. Results included: (1) a heightened awareness by staff of the disease trajectory (such as initial diagnosis, curative treatment, life-prolonging treatment, palliative care, symptomatic palliative care, and care of the imminently dying) and the importance of knowing patient wishes for this admission; (2) increased discussions about the goals of care and the rationale for treatment orders; (3) increased symptom assessments and interventions; and (4) increased awareness of the need to identify patients requiring referral to hospice and pain medicine and palliative care for symptom management and family support following discharge.

Debriefing was included in the implementation of the care path. Sessions held with staff after a patient died became an important aspect of the PCAD process. Staff were encouraged to discuss their satisfaction or dissatisfaction with the experience of the PCAD pathway. Such questions as "Were the patient's wishes honored?," "Were unnecessary tests/procedures performed?," "Did the patient have a peaceful death?," "Were symptoms controlled?," and "What is the

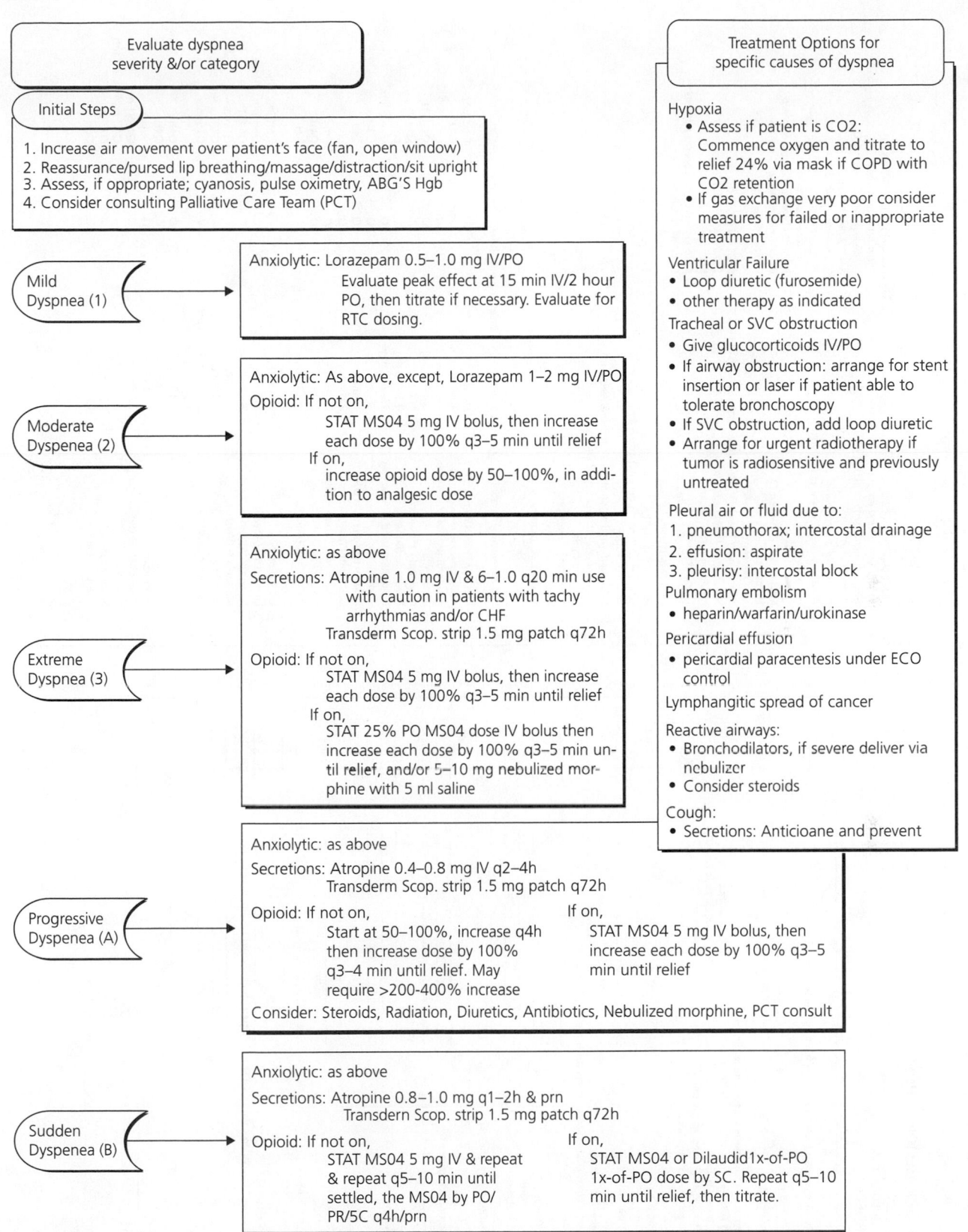

**Figure 44–2.** Algorithm designed to improve the management of dyspnea. *Source*: Developed at Dartmouth-Hitchcock Medical Center, Lebanon, NH, 198, used with permission.

## MARY HITCHCOCK MEMORIAL HOSPITAL
Lebanon, NH
Last Breaths (Resource #)
DOCTOR'S ORDERs
DATE/TIME:

Draft

**1. Evaluate severity of dyspnea:** (see reverse side for scale description)

| 0 | 1 | 2 | 3 | 4 | 5 | 6 | 7 | 8 | 9 | 10 |
|---|---|---|---|---|---|---|---|---|---|---|
| no dyspnea | | mild dyspnea | | | moderate dyspnea | | | | extreme dyspnea | |

**2. Useful nonpharmacological methods to reduce dyspnea**
- ☐ Positioning (sit, lean forward, elevate head)
- ☐ Direct fan toward patient
- ☐ Breathing strategies (Pursed lip breathing)
- ☐ Guided imagery, desensitization

- ☐ Reassurance
- ☐ Nasal cannula (c̄ O2 ___)
- ☐ Mask (c̄ O2 ___)

**3. Medication Categories**

| | Dose | Route | Frequency |
|---|---|---|---|
| EXPECTORANTS | | | |
| ☐ Glycerol Buaļacolate | | | |
| MUCOLYTIC AGENTS | | | |
| ☐ Acetylcysteine (Mucomyst) | | | |
| OPIOIDS (BE SURE TO FOLLOW-UP WITH BOWEL ORDERS WHEN PRESCRIBING OPIOIDS) | | | |
| ☐ Morphine Sulfate | | | |
| SEDATIVES/ANXIOLYTICS | | | |
| ☐ Diazepam (Valium) | | | |
| ☐ Lorazepam (Ativan) | | | |
| ☐ Midazolam (Versed) | | | |
| ☐ Promethazine (Phenergan) | | | |
| ☐ Chlorpromazine (Thorazine) | | | |
| STEROIDS | | | |
| ☐ Prednisone | | | |
| ☐ Dexamethasone (Decadron) | | | |
| ANTIMUSCARINICS | | | |
| ☐ Atropine | | | |
| ☐ Scopalamine patch | | | |
| ☐ Levsin | | | |
| DIURETICS | | | |
| ☐ Furosemide (Lasix) | | | |
| ☐ Bumelanide (Bumex) | | | |
| COUGH SUPPRESSANTS | | | |
| ☐ Benzonate (Tessalon) | | | |
| ☐ Codeine | | | |
| NEUROLEPTICS | | | |
| ☐ Haloperidol (Haldol) | | | |
| INHALED MEDS (nebulizer for patients with COPD and hypercapnia should be air and not oxygen) | | | |
| ☐ Morphine | | | |
| ☐ Lidocaine | | | |
| ☐ Saline | | | |
| BRONCHODILATORS | | | |
| ☐ Albuterol | | | |

Physician Signature _____ / RN Signature _____ / Secretary Signature

Print Physician Name: _____  Beeper Number: _____

---

## DYSPNEA SCALE

**MILD DYSPNEA (1–3)**
Usually can sit and lie quietly
May be intermittent or persistent
Worsens with exertion
No or mild anxiety during SOB
Breathing not observed as laboured
No cyanosis

**MODERATE DYSPNEA (4–7)**
Usually persistent
May be new or chronic
SOB worsens if walk or exert; settles partially with rest
Pause while talking q30 sec
Breathing mildly laboured
Cyanosis usual

**EXTREME DYSPNEA (8–10)**
Agonizing air hunger
Talk only 2–3 words between gasps for air
Very frightened
Exhausted—tries to sit and lean forward, falls back
Total concentration on breathing
Cyanosis usual
+/– resp. congestion
+/– confusion
Maybe cold, clammy

**PROGRESSIVE DYSPNEA (A)**
Often acute on chronic
Worsening over few days/wks
Anxiety present
Often awaken suddenly with SOB.
+/– cyanosis
+/– onset confusion
Laboured breathing awake & asleep
Pause while talking q15 sec
Cough often present

**SUDDEN DYSPNEA (B)**
Sudden onset (min. to few hrs.)
High anxiety & fear
Agitation with very laboured respirations
Pause while talking
+/– resp. congestion
~+/– acute chest pain
+/– diaphoresis
+/– confusion

Use incremental titration until, when asked, "Is your breathing easy now?" the patient replies, "Yes."

| MEDICATION CATEGORIES | DOSE | ROUTE | FREQUENCY |
|---|---|---|---|
| Acetylcysteine (Mucomyst) | 10% 2–20 ml | nebulizer | QID |
| Albuterol (Proventil, ventolin) | 1–2 puffs | MDI | QID |
| Atropine | 0.4–1.0 mg | PO/SC | Q4-12H |
| Benzonate (Tessalon) | 100 mg | PO | Q4-6H |
| Butemide (Bumex) | 0.5–2.0 mg | IV | prm |
| Chlorpromazine (Thorazine) | 25–100 mg | PO | Q4-6H/prn |
| Codeine | 30 mg | PO | Q3-4H |
| Dexamethasone (Decadron) | 1–4mg | PO | QID |
| Diazepam (Valium) | 2–10 mg | PO | prm |
| Furosemide (Lasix) | 20–80 mg | FO | prm |
| Glycerol guaiacolate | 5 ml | IV | Q4H |
| Haloperidol (Haldol) | .5–30 mg | PO | Q4H |
| Levsin | | IV | I6H |
| Lidocaine 2% | 2.5–5 ml | nebulizer | Q6H prm |
| Lorazepam (Ativan) | 1–2 mg | PO | Q8H/prm |
| Metaproterenol (Alupent) | 20 mg | PO | Q6-8H |
| Midazolam (Versed) | 1–10 mg | IV | Q10min |
| Morphine | 5–10 mg | nebulizer | Q4H or 4 hourly prm |
| Morphine Sulfate | 5–10 mg (initial bolus) | 1V | Q15 min |
| | 2.5–5 mg/hr (infusion), or | | |
| | 5–10 mg, or | PO | Q4H |
| | 2–5 mg | SC | Q4H |
| Prednisone | 10–15 mg | PO | ~ TID |
| Promethazine (Phenergan) | 25–50 mg | nebulizer | Q4-6H/prm |
| Saline | 5 ml | patch | Q4H or 4 hourly prm |
| Scopalamine | 1.5 mg | | Q72H |
| Theophylline | 100 200 mg | PO | Q6H |

**Figure 44–2.** (continued).

**Table 44–3**
**The Six-Step Process for Developing a Care Path**

1. Identify high-volume, high-priority case types, review medical records, review and evaluate current literature to characterize the specific problems, average length of stay, critical events, and practical outcomes.
2. Write the critical path, defining the sequence and timing of functions to be performed by physicians, nurses, and other staff.
3. Have nurses, physicians, and other disciplines involved in the process review the plan of care.
4. Revise the pathway until consensus on care components is reached.
5. Pilot-test the pathway and revise as needed.
6. Incorporate pathway patient management into quality-improvement programs, which include monitoring and evaluating patient care outcomes.

**Table 44–4**
**Routine Elements of Care Paths**

- Physical elements
- Medications
- Nutrition and dietary
- Vital signs, intake and output, weight
- Comfort assessment
- Safety and activity
- Diagnostic lab work
- Intravenous use
- Transfusions
- Diagnostic tests
- Psychosocial and spiritual needs
- Referrals and consultations
- Patient and family counseling and education

**Table 44–5**
**Goals of the Palliative Care for Advanced Disease Pathway**

- Respect patient autonomy, values, and decisions.
- Continually clarify goals of care.
- Minimize symptom distress at end of life.
- Optimize appropriate supportive interventions and consultations.
- Reduce unnecessary interventions.
- Support families by coordinating services.
- Eliminate unnecessary regulations.
- Provide bereavement services for families and staff.
- Facilitate the transition to alternate care settings, such as hospice, when appropriate.

family's likelihood for complicated grieving and the need for follow-up?" generated much dialogue and opportunities for teaching and grief resolution. Overall, staff expressed appreciation for the opportunity to talk about experiences of patient care and the personal involvement in caring for a patient and family whom they may have known over several admissions. Another positive outcome for unit nurses was using the PCAD Daily Flow Sheet. Hospice nurses reported that the pathway got all disciplines on the same page in terms of goals of care. They said it provided them with an easy and comprehensive system for documenting the assessment and intervention of key elements in EOL care: comfort; physical, psychosocial, and spiritual care as well as patient and family support.

Quality improvement team members also identified several areas that the hospital needed improvement during the pilot period: (1) clearer definition and measure of the concept of "comfort care"; (2) the need for a forum for educating voluntary physician staff, who have less unit/hospital involvement than staff physicians; (3) documentation of spiritual care and issues; (4) systematic identification of families at risk for complicated grieving; and (5) resources about local bereavement services and education for families.

At the organizational level, results of the pilot suggested that PCAD is a means for: (1) increasing multidisciplinary team discussions of patients' goals of care during hospitalization; (2) reducing the variation in the documentation of care of imminently dying patients, placing emphasis on comfort, patient and family wishes, and closure for caregivers; (3) increasing staff awareness of patients who are imminently dying or in need of palliative care services, long-term care, hospice, and bereavement care; (4) improving symptom assessment and the use of evidence-based interventions, and (5) identifying areas in EOL care for continual improvement in BIMC's organizational, education, practice, and evaluation systems.[35–37]

The PCAD pathway, education, and evaluation tools have been dissseminated widely. As of January 2009, nearly 25,000 clinicians, from all settings, have downloaded the pathway and materials from http:/www.stopPain.org. A replication study of the PCAD project was conducted by the Veterans Administration of Brooklyn, New York.[38] The VA team has translated PCAD for the electronic medical record and reported similar positive results such as increased documentation of goals of care, decreased length of stay in ICU, and fewer interventions in the last days of life.

## Outcomes

Outcomes refer to results of actions or nonaction to structures, processes, patients and caregrivers, professionals, and systems within the organizaton. Reduced symptom distress, improved family satisfaction with and reduced costs of EOL care, and improved perceived support of families with physicians are all examples of outcomes relevant to quality EOL care.

Clinicians will need to become competent at measuring outcomes of their care. Federal and state governments, private purchasers, physicians, nurses, insurers, labor unions, health plans, hospitals, and accreditation organizations, among others, have placed pressure on organizations to address some of the significant quality problems in U.S. health-care systems (http://www.ahcpr.gov/qual).[39] The Centers of Medicare and Medicaid Services recently implemented a set of pay-for-performance initiative to support better quality care of Medicare beneficiaries. About 100 such initiatives are in progress across the country. The general intent is to reward doctors for providing better care. We will need to improve our ability to measure and report the quality of care being delivered. Such reporting prompts a closer look at provider and health-care practices, both as feedback for clinicians and as publicly available scorecards for consumer evaluation. This movement is not new. In fact, with just a click of a mouse, consumers can instantly access free performance data that allow them to compare the standards of care provided by hospitals, home health agencies, nursing homes and HMOs, and emergency rooms (http://consumers.ipro.org/index/compare-hosp).[40]

Two approaches are described for measuring outcomes in palliative care at the unit level. Teams can use use a single indicator of a quality of service or multiple measures.

## Quality Improvement Indicators: Measures of Organizational Performance

A clinical indicator is typically defined as a quantitative measure that evaluates the quality of important patient care and support-service activities. Indicators that directly affect quality services typically include such factors as timeliness, efficiency, appropriateness, accessibility, continuity, privacy and confidentiality, participation of patients and families, and safety and supportiveness of the care environment. Although they are not direct measures of quality, indicators serve as "screens" or "flags" that direct attention to specific performance areas that should be targets for ongoing investigation within an organization.

Institutions that have had a JCAHO survey recently have experienced the shift in focus of performance from competence and skills ("Is the organization able to provide quality services?") to productivity and outcomes ("To what extent does the organization provide quality services?"). For example, rather than requesting a review of the institution's policy and procedure manual for a pain management program, surveyors might evaluate whether pain standards have been implemented and to what extent they have had an effect on patients' satisfaction with care or patient understanding of side effects associated with specific analgesics. Surveyors are now using a tracer methodology, whereby the surveyor interviews the nurse caring for the patient, and if more information seems needed, the surveyor may interview the patient and/or family member about their satisfaction.

Nurses will need to be knowledgeable in systems of care as the accreditation process promises to get more rigorous in areas affecting our largest and most costly group of citizens: the ill elderly.

Indicators can reflect a performance measure such as competence or safety. Competence means that individuals or the organization have the ability (e.g., education, behavioral skills) to provide quality services; safety means that those abilities are translated into actions that achieve quality outcomes. Results of indicators can reveal deviations from the norm and may warn of impending problems. Indicators may require a single-item measure, multiple items, or multiple tools. Indicators are typically expressed as an event or ratio (percentage).

Examples of structure, process, and outcome indicators that are clinical (patient care), professional (competence), and administrative (satisfaction) are described here.

1. *Structural indicators* are derived from standards of care and need to be aligned with the mission, philosophy, goals, and policies of a hospital, department, or unit. Structure standards measure whether the authorized norms are being followed. For example, a standard and its accompanying policy may read that all (100%) patients admitted to the hospital require discussion and documentation about advanced directives within 48 hours of admission. The percentage obtained would indicate the extent to which adherence to the 100% goal is being met. A structural indicator on an oncology unit might read:

   Number of records with documentation of discussion of advanced directives/Total number of patients who were admitted to the oncology unit (determined period)

Another structural indicator relates to staff competence. This indicator may reflect a standard and policy that requires all staff working on a geriatrics unit pass a competency in EOL care. The competency might consist of written exam (cognitive) and demonstration of skill (behavioral) in the use of an EOL pathway (see Appendix 44–1 for sample knowledge quiz in palliative care). For this indicator, a threshold is determined for successful completion, such as 90% on the written exam plus three return demonstrations in the use of the pathway. Low results on this indicator might suggest the need to send key nurses to an EOL care training for nurses (ELNEC). Readers can visit http://www.aacn.nche.edu/ELNEC/ to read more about ELNEC's national effort and courses available.[41]

2. *Process indicators* measure a specific aspect of nursing practice that is related to flow of work: flow of information, materials, or patient care. Examples of process indicators might include pain screening, assessments, implementation of an intervention, reassessment, prompt management of

complications, and documentation. These indicators describe "how care is to be delivered and recorded." Sometimes it may be difficult to separate process indicators from outcome indicators. For example, if an improvement study is directed toward reducing discomfort related to dyspnea in dying patients, then the indicator might involve the process of assessment of respirations, obtaining an order, and giving appropriate medication within a designated time period. The indicator might read that 100% of patients with severe dyspnea will be asssessed and treated with appropriate medications within a 2-hour period. Another segment of the same process may produce an indicator that reads that 100% of patients treated for severe dyspnea will achieve relief (reduction to mild dyspnea) within 8 hours. The indicator would read: Time severe dyspnea treated to time of relief (mild dyspnea) (in minutes)/ Each patient reaching mild reflief within 8 hrs is scored a yes.

Number of patients with severe dyspnea reaching mild dyspnea within 8 hrs/The total number of patients experiencing severe dyspnea (designated period)

Low results on this indicator might prompt a special QI team to investigate the barriers to nonadherence. The team may learn that the dyspnea measure is too difficult to administer, too time-consuming, or too confusing to assess mild, moderate, and severe dyspnea. Is the computer screen's field for documenting care not easy to use? Were physician's orders not appropriate for treating severe dyspnea? Were calls made to providers with delays in answering? Any of these pieces of the process could trigger a new look at the process of reaching mild relief of this symptom, including testing the use of a dyspnea algortihm.

3. *Outcome indicators* measure what does or does not happen after something is or is not done. Many organizations have shifted their focus from examining the documentation of processes of care to measuring outcomes of care and learning which treatment works best, under what conditions, by which individuals, and at what cost. Examples of outcome indicators for quality EOL care include family satisfaction with care (family), symptom control (patient), respect for patient preferences, family support and communication, and referral for ethics consultation if no health-care agent is identified. The goal of implementing a multidisciplinary pathway to improve care of dying patients might be to achieve a family satisfaction with care rating of 90% very satisfied, using a 0 to 5 scale (0 = very dissatisfied to 5 = very satisfied). A standard for the oncology unit might read that designated family members will be contacted at 3 to 4 months following the patient's death for an interview about

satisfaction with care. The indicator would read: 90% of families will report being very satisfied with care when asked about overall satisfaction with the patient's care in the last days of life. In this example, the response rate from families should ideally be over 50% so that findings are used with confidence and not viewed as biased.

## Number of Families Scoring Very Satisfied With Overall Care/Number of Persons Completing Satisfaction Survey Following the Death of a Family Member (Designated Period)

Although few tested methods currently exist to adequately measure the quality of care at EOL, Twaddle et al. reported one of the first attempts at benchmarking the quality of palliative care services in 35 academic hospitals.[42] The research team used a multicenter, cross-sectional, retrospective design, and reviewed 1596 patient records against 11 key performance measures (KPMs; Table 44–6) derived from evidence-based practice standards. Results suggested wide variability in adherence among hospitals, ranging from 0% to 100% (with 0 meaning no adherence and 100% meaning complete adherence). Greater improvement in KPMs indicated greater improvement in quality outcomes, cost, and length of stay. Institutions that benchmarked above 90% did so by incorporating KPMs into care processes and using systematized triggers, forms, and default pathways. Results of this study suggest that a "palliative care bundle" (i.e., selected KPMs) leads to improvement in areas of deficiency when all components of care are given to patients. For example, patients who had pain and other symptoms and who were assessed within 48 hours of admission were more likely to report relief of the symptom within the same timeframe than those patients who were not assessed.

---

**Table 44–6**
**Areas for Improving Quality Care at the End of Life**

1. Physical and emotional symptoms
2. Support of function and autonomy
3. Advance planning
4. Aggressive care near death, including preferences about site of death, CPR, and hospitalization
5. Patient and family satisfaction
6. Global quality of life
7. Family burden
8. Survival time
9. Provider continuity and skill
10. Bereavement

*Source:* American Geriatrics Society (1996), reference 29.

## Building Evidence in Quality Palliative Care

A synthesis of the evidence in key elements of palliative care was recently published by palliative care experts and the British Journal Publishing Group. The review addressed the control of common symptoms such as pain, dyspnea, and fatigue; communication and goal setting; and effective efficient transition management. Readers are encouraged to consult *"Putting Evidence Into Practice: Palliative Care"* as a resource when searching for best practices.[43] In terms of coordination of care, the review found moderate-quality evidence that specialized palliative care services improved family satisfaction but evidence on patient satisfaction, quality of life, and symptoms control was less clear-cut. A systematic review of specialized palliative care found 22 randomized controlled trials. Problems with study implementation or analysis were common. Insufficient power, including high withdrawal rates, typically limited the potential for finding a positive effect. The best evidence of effectiveness was family satisfaction, with 7 of 10 studies indicating a positive effect. The review identified no good evidence that specialist care improved symptoms. Indications that usual care was not sufficient included indicators such as patient and/or family distress and symptoms not responding to usual management.[44]

A new area of study for researchers interested in improving quality patient care is implementation, the work of putting the evidence into practice (i.e., evidence-based practice) on a routine basis. The science of nursing implementation, according to Achterberg, Shoonhovern, and Grol[44] requires an analytical deliberate process of identifying the determinants of implementation and choosing the appropriate strategies to achieve successful behavior change. They describe common determinants of success to include factors such as knowledge, cognitions, attitudes, routines, social influence, the organization, and its resources. The author's review of the literature showed that strategies such as reminders, decision support, and use of information and communication technology, records, and combined strategies are often effective in encouraging implementation of innovations. The authors recommend using relevant theories to go from identification of determinants to selection of strategies. For example, if a team is interested in improving knowledge deficits in advance care planning, active learning strategies derived from social cognitive theory (such as role modeling or observing an ethics committee at work) might prove more beneficial than traditional lectures. The authors also recommend the need to pilot an innovation and conduct evaluations to assure that the intended changes are delivered as planned. Without this check, a lack of effect may be attributed to inadequate implementation of the strategy.

Joan Teno, M.D., of the Center for Gerontology and Health Care Research at Brown University, together with faculty and staff at the Center to Improve Care of the Dying, has assembled a comprehensive annotated bibliography

---

### Table 44–7
#### Executive Summary of the Toolkit of Instruments to Measure End-of-Life Care

Chart review instrument, surrogate questionnaires, patient questionnaires
Measuring quality of life
Examining advance care planning
Instruments to assess pain and other symptoms
Instruments to assess depression and other emotional symptoms
Instruments to assess functional status
Instruments to assess survival time and aggressiveness of care
Instruments to assess continuity of care
Instruments to assess spirituality
Bibliography of instruments to assess grief
Bibliography of instruments to assess caregiver and family experience
Instruments to assess patient and family member satisfaction with the quality of care

*Source:* Teno (1998), reference 45.

---

of instruments to measure the quality of care at EOL. The Toolkit of Instruments to Measure End-of-Life Care includes a Patient Evaluation, After-Death Chart Review, and After-Death Caregiver Interview.[45] A recent addition to the toolkit is the mortality follow-back survey of family members or other knowledgable informants representing 1,578 decedents' perceptions of the last place of care.[46] Teno's current research project, Data Analysis and Reports for Toolkit Instruments, refines the toolkit and measures for users. Table 44–7 shows additional outcome measures suggested for improving EOL care. A review of the current literature related to each tool in the kit can be found at http://www.chcr.brown.edu/pcoc/toolkit.htm.[45]

Donabedian stated that "achieving and producing health and satisfaction, as defined for its individual members, is the ultimate validator of the quality of care." There has been limited research in examining satisfaction among terminally ill patients and families. However, for most dying patients, satisfaction may be the most important outcome variable for themselves and their families. Professor Irene J. Higginson, Ph.D., an international leading researcher for more than two decades, has been using the audit cycle, a feedback process similar to QI methods, to improve outcomes in palliative care. Currently at King's College School of Medicine and Dentistry and St. Christopher's Hospice in London, England, she notes the difficulties in obtaining outcome information, such as quality of life, from the weakest group of patients.[47] She supports the need to test the use of proxies to obtain this important information. One tool currently available for clinicians that is used to measure the quality of life for patients with terminal illness is the Missoula-VITAS quality of life

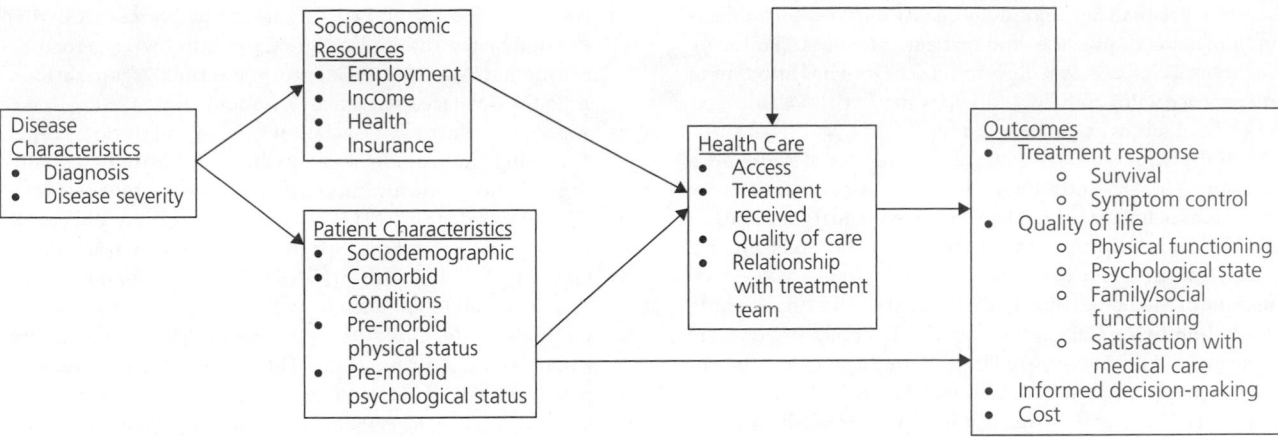

**Figure 44–3.** Model of outcomes research in the medically ill. *Source*: Kornblith (1999), reference 51, with permission.

index.[48] Readers seeking measures and indicators to be used in clincial audits are referred to *"Clinical and Organizational Audit in Palliative Medicine."*

Measures of family satisfaction in palliative care such as the FAMCARE scale[49] are also available. FAMCARE is based on qualitative research that asks family members to list indicators of quality of palliative care from the patient's perspective and their own. A similar instrument, the National Hospice Organization Family Satisfaction Survey,[50] is an 11-item survey that asks about satisfaction with aspects of hospice care.

Figure 44–3 presents a model used by the BIMC Department of Pain Medicine and Palliative Care for outcomes research in the medically ill. The model illustrates the feedback loop between outcomes and healthcare. Outcomes research requires ongoing data collection and analysis that feeds into the modification of guidelines for clinical practice, resulting in improved patient, caregiver, professional, and systems outcomes, including costs.[51] Appendix 44–1 presents an early BIMC Palliative Care Initial Consultation Tool located at http://www.stoppain.org. The tool can be used to screen patients for key components of palliative care and resources needed from an interdisciplinary team. The symptom assessment portion of the form is a validated instrument, the Memorial Symptom Assessment Scale-Condensed.[52] This data can be used to evaluate changes in symptoms within individuals and among groups of patients.

## Summary

Nurses are poised to have pivotal roles in improving the quality of care of the dying in the decade ahead. As nurses, we need to continue to learn what works and what does not work for patients and families in our practice settings and to stay active in developing and testing QI models, tools, and interventions toward better EOL care. Nurses are providing leadership in areas of clinical practice,[53–55] education,[41,56,57] and

research.[58–63] Nurses need to continue to test interventions for improved symptom management, developing models for assuring "best practices" using research,[64] and integrating QI methods into palliative care practices[65–69] and curricula in nurses' education.[70] Nurses will need to strengthen their involvement in national and international efforts that educate professionals and consumers and influence health-care policy in EOL care issues.

To survive, health-care systems must be able to change and improve rapidly. Healthcare, as with any other service operation, requires systematic innovation efforts to remain competitive, cost-efficient, and up-to-date. If the quality of EOL care is to improve, nurses will need to have expert knowledge about making change: how to encourage it and how to manage and to evaluate it within and across organizations and settings. This knowledge needs to be coupled with the methods and know-how to produce change. Clinical audits and feedback are a means to encourage dialogue among all ranks of staff, disciplines, and services. Nurses with expertise in QI methods and tools can provide necessary leadership in designing and testing strategies to improve EOL care.

REFERENCES

1. Kelly D. Applying quality management in healthcare: A sysytems Approach (2nd ed). Chicago, IL: Washington DC: Health Administration Press, AUPHA Press, 2007.

2. Deming WE. Out of the Crisis. Massachusetts Institute of Technology Center for Advanced Engineering Study. Cambridge: MIT Press, 1986.

3. Coile RC, Jr. Health care: Top 10 trends for the "era of health reform." Hosp Strategy Rep 1993;5:3–8.

4. Bookbinder MB, Blank AE, Arney E, et al. Improving end-of-life-care: Development and pilot-test of a clinical pathway. J Pain Symptom Manage 2005;29(6):529–543.

5. American Medical Association. Education for Physician's on End-of-Life Care (EPEC). www.epec.net (accessed January 2, 2009).

6. Rogers S, Brennan S. Continuous quality improvement: Effects on professional practice and patient outcomes (Protocol). Cochrane Database Syst Rev 2001;(4):CD003319. http://mrw.interscience.wiley.com/cochrane/clsysrev/articles/CD003319/frame.html (accessed January 1, 2009).

7. JCAHO National Health Care Award for Performance Measurement. http://www.jointcommissioncodman.org/pressrelease/christianacare.aspx (accessed January 1, 2009).

8. World Health Organization. Cancer Pain Relief and Palliative Care. Geneva: WHO, 1989.

9. Institute of Medicine. In: Field MJ, Cassel C, eds. Approaching Death: Improving Care at the End of Life. Committee on Care at the End of Life, Division of Health Care Services, Institute of Medicine. Washington, DC: National Academy Press, 1997.

10. SUPPORT Principal Investigators. A controlled trial to improve care for seriously ill hospitalized patients: The Study to Understand Prognoses and Preferences for Outcomes and Risks of Treatments (SUPPORT). JAMA 1995;274:1591–1598.

11. Lorenz K, Lynn K, Dy S, et al. 2006. Cancer care quality measures: Symptoms and end-of-life care. Evidence Report/Technology Assessment No. 137. (Prepared by the Southern California Evidence-Based Practice Center under Contract No. 290–02-003.) AHRQ Publication No. 06-E001. Rockville, MD: Agency for Healthcare Research and Quality. http://www.ahrq.gov/downloads/pub/evidence/pdf/eolcanqm/eolcanqm.pdf (accessed May 24, 2007).

12. Donabedian A. Evaluating the quality of medical care. Milbank Q 1996;44:166–203.

13. American Hospital Corporation. FOCUS-PDCA Methodology. Sponsored by Medical Risk Management Associates Consulting and Software Development Specialists. http://www.sentinel-event.com/focus-pdca_index.php (accessed January 21, 2009).

14. Bookbinder M, Kiss M, Coyle N, Brown M, Gianella A, Thaler H. Improving pain management practices. In: McGuire D, Yarbro C, Ferrell B, eds. Cancer Pain Management (2nd ed). Boston, MA: Jones and Bartlett; 1995:321–361.

15. Ross M, McDonald B, McGuinness J. The palliative care quiz for nurses. J Adv Nurs 1996;23:128–137.

16. Institute for Healthcare Improvement. Boston, MA. http://www.ihi.org/ihi (accessed January 10, 2009).

17. Lynn J, Schuster JL, Wilkinson A. Simon LN. Improving Care for the End of Life: A Sourcebook for Health Care Managers and Clinicians. New York, NY: Oxford University Press, 2007.

18. Association for Benchmarking Health Care™. http://www.abhc.org/ (accessed January 2, 2009).

19. Six Sigma Health Care Benchmarking Association™. http://www.sixsigmabenchmarking.com/6shcba.html (accessed January 2, 2009).

20. National Hospice Organization, National Council for Hospice and Specialists in Palliative Care Services. Making palliative care better: Quality improvement, multi professional audit and standards. Arlington, VA: Author, 1997.

21. American Association of Colleges of Nursing (AACN). Peaceful death: Recommended competencies and curricular guidelines for end-of-life nursing care. Washington DC: Author, 2002.

22. National Hospice Organization, Working Party on Clinical Guidelines in End-of-Life Care. Changing gears: Guidelines for managing care in the last days of life in adults. Arlington, VA: Author, 1997.

23. American Medical Association: Council on Scientific Affairs. Good care of the dying patient. JAMA 1996;275:474–478.

24. American Society of Pain Management Nurses (ASPMN). Position Statement: End-of-Life Care. http://www.geronurse-online.net/MainMenuCategory/PartnerOrganizations/ASPMN.aspx (accessed January 3, 2009).

25. American Nurses Association (ANA). Position Paper: Foregoing nutrition and hydration. http://www.nursingworld.org/MainMenuCategories/ANAMarketplace/ANAPeriodicals/OJIN/TableofContents/Vol31998/No3Dec1998/References.aspx (accessed January 3, 2009).

26. Oncology Nursing Society (ONS). Oncology Nursing Society and Association of Oncology Social Work Joint Position on End-of-Life Care. Revised 7/2007. http://www.ons.org/Publications/positions/EndOfLifeCare.shtmlpublications/positions/EndOfLifeCare.shtml (accessed January 3, 2009).

27. Cassel CK, Foley K. Principles for care of patients at the end-of-life: An emerging consensus among the specialties of medicine. Milbank Memorial Fund: NY, 1999. http://www.milbank.org/endoflife/ (accessed January 3, 2009).

28. Canadian Palliative Care Association. Palliative Care: Towards a Consensus in Standardized Principles of Practice. 1995. http://www.library.vcu.edu/tml/bibs/nursing.html (accessed January 21, 2005).

29. American Geriatrics Society (AGS). American Geriatrics Society (AGS) Position Statement: The Care of Dying Patients. AGS Ethics Committee. 1996. http://www.american geriatrics.org/products/positionpapers/careofd.shtml (accessed January 21, 2006).

30. Crosswalk of JCAHO Standards and Palliative Care—with PC Policies, Procedures and Assessment Tools. http://www.capc.org (accessed January 21, 2009).

31. The National Consensus Project for Quality Palliative Care (NCP). http://www.nationalconsensusproject.org/ (accessed January 21, 2009).

32. Wrede-Seaman L. Symptom Management Algorithms: A Handbook for Palliative Care (3rd ed). Yakima, WA: Intellicard, 2005. http://www.Intelli-card.com (accessed January 2, 2009).

33. Dartmouth-Hitchcock Medical Center: Hematology/Oncology Group. A dyspnea algorithm. Lebanon, NH: Author, 1998.

34. Dyspnea Treatment Algorithm. http://www.intelli-card.com/photos/Dyspnea.pdf (accessed January 2, 2009).

35. Ellershaw J. Care of the dying: Clinical pathways—an innovation to disseminate clinical excellence. Innovations in End-of-Life Care 2001;3(4). http://www2.edc.org/lastacts/ (accessed January 21, 2005).

36. National Hospice Organization. A Pathway for Patients and Families Facing Terminal Illness. Arlington, VA: Author, 1997.

37. Continuum Health Partners, Inc., Beth Israel Medical Center, Department of Pain Medicine and Palliative Care. Palliative Care for Advanced Disease (PCAD) Care Path. (CQI Team on End-of-Life Care), NY. http://www.stoppain.org (accessed January 1, 2009).

38. Luhrs CA, Meghani S, Homel P, et al. Pilot of a pathway to improve the care of imminently dying oncology inpatients in a Veterans Affairs (VA) Medical Center. J Pain Symptom Manage 2005;29(6):544–551.

39. Quality and Patient Safety. Agency for Healthcare Research and Quality (AHRQ). http://www.ahcpr.gov/qual/ (accessed January 10, 2009).

40. Compare Hospitals, Nursing Homes, Home Health Agencies, HMOs. http://consumers.ipro.org/index/compare-hosp (accessed January 10, 2009).

41. American Association of Colleges of Nursing (AACN) and City of Hope, CA. The End-of-Life Nursing Education Consortium (ELNEC) project. http://www.aacn.nche.edu/elnec/ (accessed January 1, 2009).

42. Twaddle ML, Maxwell TL, Cassel JB, et al. Palliative care benchmarks from academic medical centers. J Pall Med 2007;10:86–98.

43. Brunnhuber K, Nash S, Meier DE, Weissman DE, Woodcock J. Putting Evidence into Practice: Palliative Care. London, England: BMJ Publishing Group, 2008.

44. Achterberg TV, Schoonhoven L, Grol R. Nursing implementation science: How evidence-based nursing requires evidence-based implementation. J Nurs Scholar 2008;40:302–310.

45. Teno J. Center to Improve Care of the Dying. Toolkit of instruments to measure end-of-life. 1998. http://www.chcr.brown.edu/pcoc/toolkit.htm (accessed January 10, 2009).

46. Teno JM, Clarridge BR, Casey V, et al. Family perspectives on end-of-life care at the last place of care. JAMA 2004;291:88–93.

47. Higginson, IJ, Clinical and organizational audit in palliative medicine. In: Doyle D, Hanks G, Cherny N, Calman K, eds. Oxford Textbook of Palliative Medicine (3rd ed). Oxford, England: Oxford University Press; 2004:184–196.

48. Byock IR. Merriman MP. Measuring quality of life for patients with terminal illness: The Missoula-VITA quality of life index. Palliative Med 1998;12:231–244.

49. Kristjanson LJ. Validity and reliability testing of the FAMCARE scale: Measuring family satisfaction with advanced cancer care. Soc Sci Med 1993;36:693–701.

50. National Hospice Organization. Family Satisfaction Survey. Arlington, VA: Author, 1996.

51. Kornblith A. Outcomes research in palliative care. Newsletter: Department of Pain Medicine and Palliative Care, Beth Israel Medical Center, New York, NY, 1999;2:1–2.

52. Chang VT, Hwang SS, Kasimis B, Thaler HT. Shorter symptom assessment instruments: The Condensed Memorial Symptom Assessment Scale (CMSAS). Cancer Invest 2004;22(4):526–536.

53. McCaffery M, Pasero C. Pain: Clinical Manual (2nd ed). St. Louis, MO: Mosby, 1999.

54. Duggleby WD, Degner L, Williams A, et al. Living with hope: Initial evaluation of a psychosocial hope intervention for older palliative home care patients. J Pain Symptom Manage 2007;33:247–257.

55. Hughes, RG, O'Mara A, *Kovner CT*. Palliative wound care at the end of life. *Home Health Care Manag Pract* 2005;17(3):196–202.

56. Matzo M, Sherman D, eds. Palliative Care Nursing: Quality Care to the End of Life (2nd ed). New York, NY: Springer Publishing, 2006.

57. Core Curriculum for the advanced practice hospice and palliative nurse. 2007. http://www.hpna.org/Publications_APNCC.aspx (accessed January 3, 2009).

58. Steeves R, Kahn D. Understanding a good death: James's story. In: Ferrell BR, Coyle N, eds. Textbook of palliative nursing (2nd ed). Oxford, England: Oxford University Press; 2006:1209–1216.

59. Coyle N. The hard work of living in the face of death. J Pain Symptom Manage 2006;32:266–274.

60. Ferrell BR, Grant M. Nursing research. In: Ferrell BR, Coyle N, eds. Textbook of palliative nursing (2nd ed). Oxford, England: Oxford University Press; 2006:1094.

61. Gordon DR, Dahl JL, Miaskowski C, et al. American Pain Society Recommendations for Improving the Quality of Acute and Cancer Pain Management American Pain Society Quality of Care Task Force. Arch Intern Med. 2005;165: 1574–1580.

62. Campbell ML, Happ MB, Hultman T, et al. The HPNA Research Agenda for 2009–2012. J Hosp Palliat Nurs 2009;11(1):10–18.

63. Johnson VMP, Teno JM, Bourbonniere M, Mor V. Palliative Care Needs of Cancer Patients in U.S. Nursing Homes. J Pall Med 2005,8(2):273–279.

64. Wysocki A, Bookbinder M. Implementing clinical practice changes: A practical approach. Home Health Care Manag Pract 2005;17(3):164–174.

65. Strassels SA, Blough DK, Hazlet TK, et al. Pain, demographics, and clinical characteristics in persons who received hospice care in the United States. J Pain Symptom Manage 2006; 32(6):519–531.

66. Johnson VMP, Teno JM, Bourbonniere M, et al. Palliative care needs of cancer patients in US nursing homes. J Palliat Med 2005;2(8): 273–279.

67. Brechtl JR, Murshed S, Homel P, Bookbinder M. Monitoring symptoms in patients with advanced illness in long-term care: A pilot study. J Pain Symptom Manage 2006,32(2): 168–174.

68. Jones KR, Fink RM, Clark L, Hutt E, Vojir CP, Mellis BK. Nursing home resident barriers to effective pain management: Why nursing home residents may not seek pain medication. J Am Med Dir Assoc 2005;6(1):10–17.

69. Hanson LC, Reynolds KS, Henderson M, Pickard CG. A quality improvement intervention to increase palliative care in nursing homes. J Palliat Med 2005;8(3):576–584.

70. Buhr GT, White HK. Quality improvement initiative for chronic pain assessment and management in the nursing home: A pilot study. J Am Med Dir Assoc 2006;7(4): 246–253.

**Sample CQI study proposal to improve end-of-life care**
**using FOCUS-PDCA**

*F*ind a process to improve.

Set the boundaries by defining the beginning and end points of the process.

**Opportunity statement**

An opportunity exists to improve <u>EOL care for the imminently dying inpatient,</u>
*(Name the process.)*
beginning with <u>a physicians' order for the Palliative Care for Advanced Disease care path</u>
ending with <u>death or discharge to homecare, hospice, or residential facility.</u>
*(Set boundaries.)*
This effort should improve <u>patient comfort and family satisfaction with EOL care</u>
*(Name outcome measure)*
for <u>hospitalized oncology, geriatric, hospice, and intensive care unit patients.</u>
*(Name the customers.)*

The process is important to work on now because <u>good EOL care is an institutional priority, no</u>
<u>benchmarks are currently available in the US, and no standard approach is used at BIMC* to</u>
<u>assess and treat patients who are imminently dying.</u>
*(State significance.)*

*O*rganize to improve the process.

Form a multidisciplinary CQI team; establish roles, rules, and meeting times.

**Multidisciplinary Team (22 members)**
Department of Pain Medicine and Palliative Care
MDs, nurses, social workers, psychologist, chaplain
Hospital departments
Ethics
Pediatrics
Nutrition
Quality improvement
Pharmacy
Outcomes measurement (research grants and contracts)
Pilot units (Oncology, Geriatrics, Intensive Care, Hospice)
Nurse managers, case managers, clinical nurse specialists

---

* BIMC: Beth Israel Medical Center

*C*larify what is known.

**FLOWCHART OF PALLIATIVE CARE FOR
ADVANCED DISEASE (PCAD) CARE PATH**

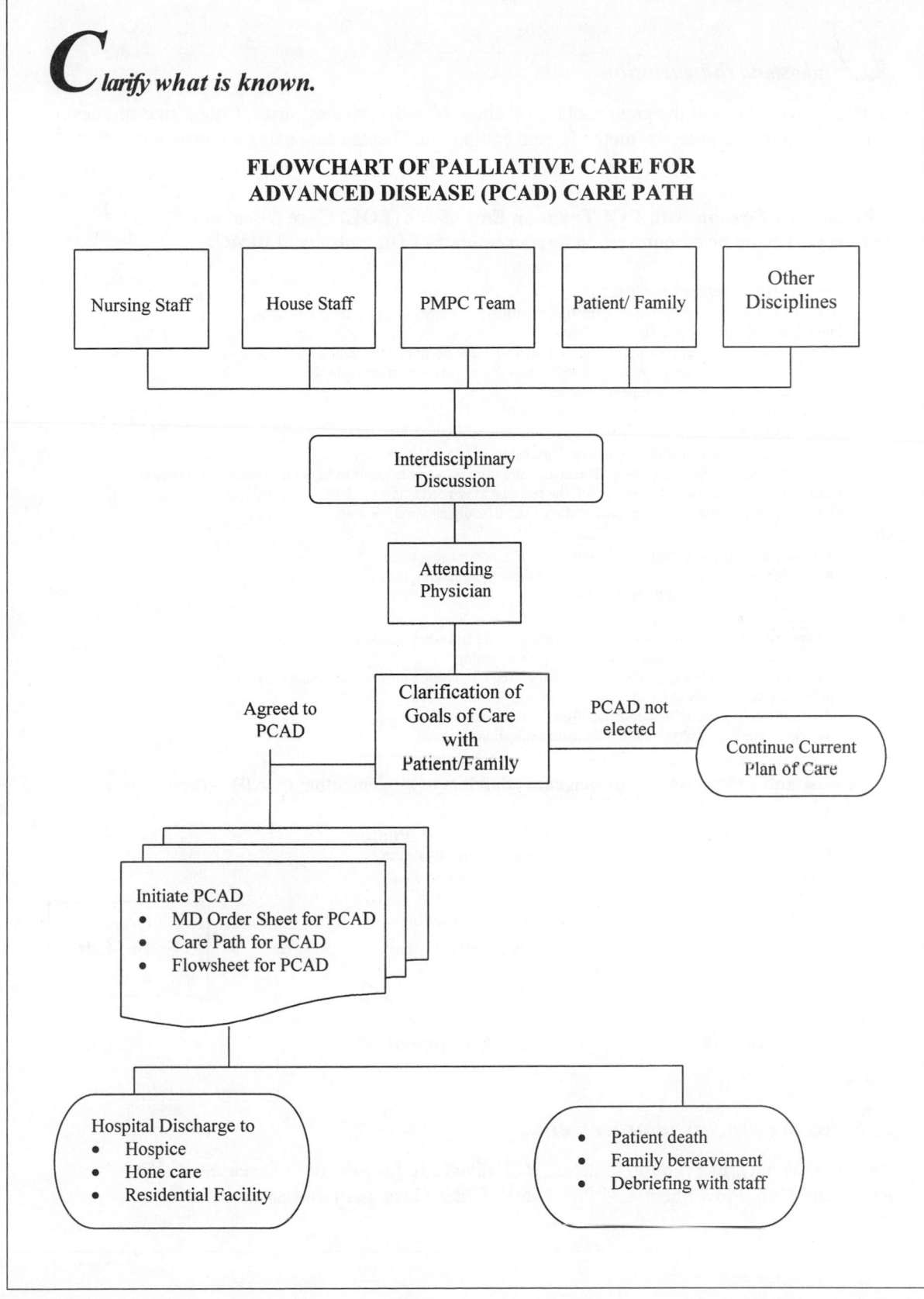

Nursing Staff

House Staff

PMPC Team

Patient/ Family

Other Disciplines

Interdisciplinary Discussion

Attending Physician

Clarification of Goals of Care with Patient/Family

Agreed to PCAD

PCAD not elected

Continue Current Plan of Care

Initiate PCAD
- MD Order Sheet for PCAD
- Care Path for PCAD
- Flowsheet for PCAD

Hospital Discharge to
- Hospice
- Hone care
- Residential Facility

- Patient death
- Family bereavement
- Debriefing with staff

# *U*nderstand the variation

Brainstorm with those at the grass roots level about why the process varies. Categorize sources of variation by people, materials, methods, and equipment. Display data using a cause-and-effect diagram.

**Brainstorming Session with CQI Team on End-of-life (EOL) Care Question:**
**What barriers could be encountered in implementing an EOL Pathway at BIMC?**

*EOL awareness/ discomfort/readiness*:
> What is "end-of-life care?" When is treatment palliative vs. life ending? How do we choose?
> Patient, family, readiness/awareness of dying
> Physician, family, patient willingness to acknowledge that death is imminent
> Issues of truth telling: family may not know status of patient prior to the pathway
> Physician discomfort with stopping treatment
> Medical uncertainty about when to stop treatment

*Team communication*:
> Physician and nurse discomfort in discussing change in treatment strategy
> Is it the physician's decision alone? The heath care team as a whole needs to be acknowledged in decision.
> Definition of terms. Need to define who the team is. May need a new model.
> Nurses' comfort—may be put in the middle of team/family attending and decisions.

*Unit resistance*:
> Resistance of unit teams. May see this project as "another thing to do."
> Large-scale resistance. Some may not see that there is something to "fix."
> Organizational pressure to discharge quickly.

*Knowledge deficit*:
> Assumptions about pastoral care (patient, family, staff) and what the experience will be.
> Knowledge deficit about medical and nursing interventions
> How to implement the care path and encourage people to speak up front rather than later
> Large cultural diversity at BIMC
> Education needed about biomedical analysis and ethical problems
> Physician/patient and physician/family communication skills

**Cause and Effect (Ishikawa) Diagram (Barriers to implementing PCAD)**—Themes above

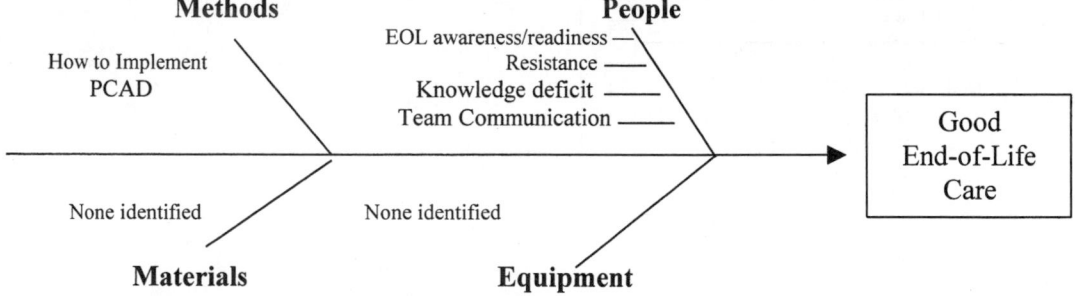

# *S*elect the process improvement.

Describe the new intervention in detail. Palliative Care for Advanced Disease (PCAD) Care Path: Care Path, Flow Sheet, and Physicians' Order Sheet **(see following pages)**

**BETH ISRAEL HEALTH CARE SYSTEM** ☐ **PETRIE DIVISION** ☐ **NORTH DIVISION** ☐ **KINGS HWY DIVISION**

**Care Path:** *PALLIATIVE CARE for ADVANCED DISEASE*

| PRE-ADMISSION CONSIDERATION/ ADMISSION CRITERIA | DISCHARGE OUTCOMES | |
|---|---|---|
| ☐ Disease at Advanced Stage – limited life expectancy _____ | ☐ Discharge to Community: Hospice _ Home Care _ Alternative Care Facility _ Home _ or | STAMP ADDRESSOGRAPH NAME OF SERVICE/ATTENDING/ HOUSE MD |
| ☐ HCP: Agent _____ ☐ DNR ☐ Primary Caregiver _____ ☐ Next of Kin | ☐ Patient expired/Bereavement resources provided to family | |

| **PLAN:** | **START DATE:** | **ONGOING DAYS:** |
|---|---|---|
| TREATMENTS/ INTERVENTIONS/ ASSESSMENTS | 1) CLARIFY GOALS OF PALLIATIVE CARE FOR ADVANCED DISEASE (PCAD) WITH PATIENT AND/OR FAMILY <br> 2) FACILITATE DISCUSSION & DOCUMENTATION OF ADVANCE DIRECTIVES: <br> Identify designated individuals & roles in decision-making: <br> 1) Health Care Agent    3) Primary Caregiver <br> 2) Durable Power of Attorney    4) Next-of-kin <br> Identify patient/family preferences regarding: <br> • Health Care Proxy    • Resuscitation Status/DNR <br> • Living Will <br> 3) INITIATE PHYSICIAN ORDER SHEET/REVIEW DAILY <br> 4) COMFORT ASSESSMENT to include <br> • Pain and symptom management needs <br> • Psychosocial coping, anticipatory grieving, and social/cultural needs <br> • Spiritual issues and distress <br> 5) VS – None unless useful in promoting pt/family comfort <br> 6) ASSESS FOR AND PROVIDE ENVIRONMENT CONDUCIVE TO MEET PATIENT & FAMILY NEEDS | REPEAT CARE PATH DAILY <br><br> DOCUMENT IN: <br> DAILY PATIENT CARE FLOW SHEET <br> PROGRESS NOTES |
| PAIN MANAGEMENT | 1) ASSESS PAIN Q 4 HR and evaluate within 1 hr post intervention. Complete pain assessment scale. Anticipate pain needs. | |
| TESTS/PROCEDURES | 1) USUALLY UNNECESSARY for patient/family comfort <br> (All lab work and diagnostic work is discouraged) | |
| MEDICATIONS | 1) Medication regimen focus is the RELIEF OF DISTRESSING SYMPTOMS. | |
| FLUIDS/NUTRITION | 1) DIET: Selective diet with no restrictions <br> • Nutrition to be guided by patient's choice of time, place, quantities and type of food desired. Family may provide food. <br> • Educate family in nutritional needs of dying patient <br> 2) IVs for symptom management only <br> 3) TRANSFUSIONS for symptom relief only <br> 4) INTAKE AND OUTPUT – consider goals of care relative to patient comfort <br> 5) WEIGHTS – consider risks/benefits relative to patient comfort | |

**REPEAT CARE PATH DAILY**

**DOCUMENT IN:**
DAILY PATIENT CARE FLOW SHEET
PROGRESS NOTES

**ACTIVITY**

1) ACTIVITY DETERMINED BY PATIENT'S PREFERENCES AND ABILITY. Patient determines participation in ADLs, i.e., turning and positioning, bathing, transfers

**CONSULTS**

1) INITIATE referrals to institutional specialists to optimize comfort and enhance quality of life (QOL) only.

**PSYCHOSOCIAL NEEDS**

1) PSYCHOSOCIAL COMFORT ASSESSMENT of:
   - Patient
   - Primary caregiver
   - Grieving process of patient & family

2) PSYCHOSOCIAL SUPPORT: Referral to Social Work
   - Offer emotional support
   - Support verbalization and anticipatory grieving
   - Encourage family caring activities as appropriate/individualized to family situation and culture
   - Facilitate verbal and tactile communication
   - Assist family with nutrition, transportation, child care, financial, funeral issues
   - Assess bereavement needs

**SPIRITUAL NEEDS**

1) SPIRITUAL COMFORT ASSESSMENT
   - Spiritual supports
   - Spiritual needs and/or distress

2) SPIRITUAL SUPPORT: Referral to Chaplain
   - Provide opportunity for expression of beliefs, fears, and hopes
   - Provide access to religious resources
   - Facilitate religious practices

**PATIENT/FAMILY EDUCATION**

1) ASSESS NEEDS AND PROVIDE EDUCATION REGARDING:
   - Goals of Palliative Care for Advanced Disease
   - Physical and psychosocial needs during the dying process
   - Coping techniques/Relaxation techniques
   - Bereavement process and resources

**DISCHARGE PLANNING**

1) FOR DISCHARGE TO COMMUNITY: Referral to Pain Medicine & Palliative Care/ Hospice/Home Care/Social Work as needed.

2) AT TIME OF DEATH:
   - Post Mortem care observing cultural and religious practices and preferences
   - Provide for care of patient's possessions as per family wishes
   - Bereavement support for family and staff

©Continuum Health Partners, Inc., Department of Pain Medicine & Palliative Care 1999

*This document is to be used as a guideline only. Each case should be evaluated and treated individually based upon clinical findings.*

# Beth Israel Health Care System
Carepath: Palliative Care for Advanced Disease
**DAILY PATIENT CARE FLOW SHEET**

ADDRESSOGRAPH

**DATE:**

| □ DNR | □ NO DNR | □ HCP | □ NO HCP | HCP AGENT: | | CAREGIVER: |
|---|---|---|---|---|---|---|

**COMFORT ASSESSMENT:** Comfort Level  Patient states or appears to be
1. Always comfortable   2. Usually comfortable   3. Sometimes comfortable   4. Seldom comfortable   5. Never comfortable

| TIME (per MD order) | | | | | | | | |
|---|---|---|---|---|---|---|---|---|
| PATIENT Comfort Level (Indicate number) | | | | | | | | |

| VITAL SIGNS ONLY AS ORDERED | T | | | | | | | | |
|---|---|---|---|---|---|---|---|---|---|
| | P | | | | | | | | |
| | R | | | | | | | | |
| | BP | | | | | | | | |

| | | | | | | | | | | PAIN/RELIEF SCALE KEY | | | SEDATION SCALE |
|---|---|---|---|---|---|---|---|---|---|---|---|---|---|

**P AI N**

| TIME | | | | | | | |
|---|---|---|---|---|---|---|---|
| LOCATION | | | | | | | |
| PAIN RATING | | | | | | | |
| RELIEF/SEDATION | | | | | | | |

PAIN/RELIEF SCALE KEY
NONE ← 0 1 2 3 4 5 6 7 8 9 10 → WORST
COMPLETE RELIEF        NO RELIEF

SEDATION SCALE
0 Alert
1 Awake but drowsy
2 Drowsy/Easily awakened
3 Sleeping/Easily awakened
4 Sleeping/Difficult to awaken
5 Unarousable

\* See Progress Note     A = Assessment     I = Intervention     Check mark = present or done     \* Needs MD Order

| | | Time | | | | | | Time | | | | | | | Time | | | |
|---|---|---|---|---|---|---|---|---|---|---|---|---|---|---|---|---|---|---|
| **E Y E S** | A | Moist/Clear | | | | **B R E A T H I N G** | A | Rate: Normal | | | | **N U T R I T I O N** | A | Full meal | | | |
| | | Inflamed | | | | | | Rapid | | | | | | > 50% | | | |
| | | Dry/Crusted | | | | | | Slow | | | | | | < 50% | | | |
| | | | | | | | | Rhythm: Reg | | | | | | Refused | | | |
| | | | | | | | | Irregular | | | | | | Nausea/vomiting | | | |
| | I | Routine Care | | | | | | Depth: Normal | | | | | | NPO | | | |
| | | _Artificial Tears | | | | | | Shallow | | | | | | Dysphagia | | | |
| | | _Oint/Lubricant | | | | | | Labored | | | | | | | | | |
| | | | | | | | | Secretions: None | | | | | | | | | |
| | | | | | | | | Mild | | | | | I | Diet as tolerated | | | |
| **L I P S** | A | Smooth/moist | | | | | | Copious | | | | | | NG/G tube | | | |
| | | Dry/Cracked | | | | | | Breath sounds: | | | | | | Enteral feeding | | | |
| | | Ulcerated | | | | | | Clear | | | | | | Feeding set changed | | | |
| | | | | | | | | Diminished | | | | | | Residual vol-cc's | | | |
| | | | | | | | | Absent | | | | | | Placement check | | | |
| | I | Routine Care | | | | | | Crackles | | | | | | Meds as ordered | | | |
| | | Topical Lubricant | | | | | | Wheeze | | | | | | | | | |
| | | | | | | | | Dyspnea | | | | **I V** | A | IV site | | | |
| | | | | | | | | | | | | | | No S&S infil/phleb | | | |
| **M O U T H** | A | Moist | | | | | | | | | | **L I N E S** | | Dry & intact | | | |
| | | Dry | | | | | I | None | | | | | | | | | |
| | | Coated | | | | | | Reposition | | | | | | IV Dsg change | | | |
| | | Stomatitis | | | | | | _O2 via_ _@_ _lpm | | | | | I | IV Tubing change | | | |
| | | | | | | | | Suctioning q ___ | | | | | | See progress note | | | |
| | I | Routine Care | | | | | | Trach Care | | | | | | Cap Change | | | |
| | | *Artificial Saliva | | | | | | Elevate HOB | | | | | | Huber needle change | | | |
| | | _Magic Wash | | | | | | Fan | | | | | | | | | |
| | | Meds as ordered | | | | | | Meds as ordered | | | | | | | | | |

| **Time** | | | | | | **Time** | | | | | | **Time** | | | |
|---|---|---|---|---|---|---|---|---|---|---|---|---|---|---|---|
| **M** | **A** | Bedbound | | | | **S** | **A** | Normal | | | | **F** | **A** | Engaged w pt | | |
| **O** | | OOB Chair | | | | **L** | | Interrupted Cycle | | | | **A** | | Coping w loss | | |
| **B** | | Amb w Assist | | | | **E** | | Insomnia | | | | **M** | | Distressed | | |
| **I** | | OOB ad lib | | | | **E** | | | | | | **I** | | | | |
| **L** | | BR Privileges | | | | **P** | **I** | Modify Environment | | | | **L** | | | | |
| **I** | **I** | T&P per pt comfort | | | | | | Relaxation | | | | **Y** | **I** | Goals of care reviewed | | |
| **T** | | ROM q___ | | | | | | Meds as order | | | | | | Encourage verbal | | |
| **Y** | | Assistive Device | | | | | | | | | | | | & non-verbal | | |
| | | ___Ted Stocking(s) | | | | **P** | **A** | Awake/alert | | | | | | communication w pt | | |
| | | Side Rails Up | | | | **S** | | Responds to voice | | | | | | Family Meeting | | |
| **E** | **A** | Voiding qs | | | | **Y** | | Resp to tactile stim | | | | | | Bereavement | | |
| **L** | | Anuria | | | | **C** | | Unresponsive | | | | | | support | | |
| **I** | | Incontinent Urine | | | | **H** | | Oriented | | | | | | | | |
| **M** | | Bowel Movement | | | | **O** | | Confused | | | | | | | | |
| **I** | | Incontinent Feces | | | | **S** | | Hallucinating | | | | | | | | |
| **N** | | Diarrhea | | | | **O** | | Calm | | | | | | | | |
| **A** | | Constipation | | | | **C** | | Anxiety | | | | **M** | | AM Care | | |
| **T** | | | | | | **I** | | Agitated | | | | **I** | | PM Care | | |
| **I** | **I** | ___Foley Catheter | | | | **A** | | Depression | | | | **S** | | PresUlcer Prev Plan | | |
| **O** | | Texas Catheter | | | | **L** | | Spiritual distress | | | | **C** | | Fall Prev Plan | | |
| **N** | | Inc't Pads | | | | | | | | | | **E** | | Precautions: | | |
| | | ___Enema | | | | | **I** | Emotional support | | | | **L** | | Isolation: | | |
| | | Meds as ordered | | | | | | Verbal/tactile | | | | **L** | | Siderails Up | | |
| | | | | | | | | stimulation | | | | **A** | | ID Bracelet | | |
| | | | | | | | | **Social Worker visit** | | | | **N** | | Allergy Bracelet | | |
| **S** | **A** | Normal/Intact | | | | | | **Chaplain visit** | | | | **E** | | DNR Bracelet | | |
| **K** | | Feverish | | | | | | | | | | **O** | | Post Mortem care | | |
| **I** | | Diaphoretic | | | | | | | | | | **U** | | | | |
| **N** | | Pressure Ulcer Stg___ | | | | | | | | | | **S** | | | | |
| | | Ostomy site D/I | | | | **Comments/Progress Notes** | | | | | | | | | | |
| | | Edema | | | | | | | | | | | | | | |
| | | Pruritis | | | | | | | | | | | | | | |
| | | Cool/Mottled | | | | | | | | | | | | | | |
| **W** | **I** | Site | | | | | | | | | | | | | | |
| **O** | | Dressing___ | | | | | | | | | | | | | | |
| **U** | | Dry & Intact | | | | | | | | | | | | | | |
| **N** | | Drain___ | | | | | | | | | | | | | | |
| **D** | | Drainage | | | | | | | | | | | | | | |
| | | Odor | | | | | | | | | | | | | | |
| **C** | | Ostomy site care | | | | | | | | | | | | | | |
| **A** | | Tube site care | | | | | | | | | | | | | | |
| **R** | | | | | | | | | | | | | | | | |
| **E** | | | | | | | | | | | | | | | | |

**PATIENT/FAMILY EDUCATION:**     **See IPFER**

**PCAD Care Path:**     **Initiated**     **Reviewed/Continue With Plan Of Care**     ☐ **Revised (See Progress Note)**

**OTHER NURSING DOCUMENTATION:**
  ☐ **I & O SHEET**     ☐ **RESTRAINT FLOW SHEET**     ☐ **NEURO-ASSESSMENT**     ☐ **OTHER_____**

| SIGNATURE/TITLE | DATE | SHIFT | INITIALS | SIGNATURE/TITLE | DATE | SHIFT | INITIALS |
|---|---|---|---|---|---|---|---|
| 1. | | | | 6. | | | |
| 2. | | | | 7. | | | |
| 3. | | | | 8. | | | |
| 4. | | | | 9. | | | |
| 5. | | | | 10. | | | |

## Beth Israel Health Care System
**DOCTOR'S ORDER SHEET**
**PALLIATIVE CARE FOR ADVANCED DISEASE**

ADMISSION HT_____ ADMISSION WEIGHT_____

ADDRESSOGRAPH AREA

| ORDERS OTHER THAN MEDICATION/INFUSION | MEDICATION/INFUSION (Specify route & directions) |
|---|---|

**ORDERS OTHER THAN MEDICATION/INFUSION**

1  Primary Diagnosis:

2  Activate PCAD Care Path

3  Anticipated time on PCAD Care Path:
   ___ hours  ___days  ___weeks  ___unknown

4  Allergies:

5  Diet: ☐ No restrictions (food may be provided by caregiver)
   ☐ NPO   ☐ Other:

6  Activity: ☐ OOB as tolerated   ☐ OOB with assistance

7  Vital Signs: ☐ Discontinue
   ☐ Daily   ☐ q shift   ☐ q ___hours

8  Comfort Assessment: ☐q __ hr ☐q 2 hr ☐q 4 hr ☐q shift

9  Weight:   ☐ None   ☐ q _____ day(s)

10 I & O:   ☐ None   q _____

11 Visiting: ☐ Open visiting, nurse-restrictions apply
   ☐ Per routine policy
   ☐ Other:

12 DNR:   ☐ Yes   ☐ No

13 PCAD Care Path will include (specify if otherwise):
   Psychosocial Care – Social Work Referral
   Spiritual Care – Chaplaincy Referral

14 Consults:
   ☐ Pain Medicine & Palliative Care Consult
   ☐ Ethics Consult
   ☐ Hospice Consult
   ☐ Other:

15 Labs: ☐ Discontinue all previous standing orders
   ☐ Continue previous lab orders
   ☐ Other labs:

16 Oxygen Therapy: _____L/min via_____

17 Other orders:

**MEDICATION/INFUSION (Specify route & directions)**

1. Assess patient for the following symptoms:
   Anxiety & Insomnia        Hiccups
   Confusion/Agitation       Nausea/Vomiting
   Constipation              Pain
   Depressed Mood            Pruritis
   Diarrhea                  Stomatitis
   Dyspnea                   Terminal Secretions
   Fever                     (Noisy Respirations)
   *See reverse side for suggestions for pain management and symptom control*

2. DISCONTINUE ALL PREVIOUS MED ORDERS

3. ORDERS:

| CLERK | DATE | TIME | NURSE'S SIGNATURE | PRESCRIBER'S SIGNATURE | ID# | DATE | TIME |
|---|---|---|---|---|---|---|---|
| | | | | | | | |

©Continuum Health Partners, Inc., Department of Pain Medicine & Palliative Care 1999

*The following are medications for consideration in treating pain and symptoms of patients on PCAD:*

## PAIN MANAGEMENT
**For Opioid-Naïve Patient:**
Morphine Sulfate 15 mg po or 5 mg SQ/IV.
Repeat q 1 hr until pain relief is adequate. Begin Morphine Sulfate 30 mg po or 10 mg SQ/IV q 4 hr ATC or begin IV Morphine Sulfate basal infusion at 2 mg per hour and 2 mg SQ/IV q 1 hr prn.

**For Opioid-Treated Patient:**
If pain uncontrolled, increase fixed schedule dose by 50%.

Many non-opioid analgesics are available and should be considered after opioid therapy has been optimized. If pain remains uncontrolled, consider consult to Department of Pain Medicine and Palliative Care (Beeper #6702).

## ANXIETY & INSOMNIA
Lorazepam 0.5mg po/SQ/IV BID-TID q HS for anxiety.
Temazepam 15 – 30 mg po q HS for anxiety/ insomnia.
Clonazepam 0.5 – 2 mg po BID-TID for anxiety/myoclonus.

## CONFUSION/AGITATION
Haloperidol 0.5 mg po/SQ/IV. Repeat q 30 minutes until symptom intensity declines.
Haloperidol 0.5 – 5 mg po/SQ/IV q 4 hr prn.

## CONSTIPATION
Lactulose 30 ml po q 2 hr prn until constipation relieved.
When symptom improves, begin Lactulose 30 ml po q 12 hr.
Warm Fleets Enema TIW prn

To prevent constipation:
Senokot 1 – 2 tabs po BID and
Colace 1 – 2 tabs po BID.

## SYMPTOMS OF DEPRESSION
**If anticipated survival is in weeks:**
Begin SSRI, e.g., Paroxetine 20 mg po daily, and titrate to effect.

**If anticipated survival is in days:**
Methylphenidate 2.5 mg po q morning and at noon and escalate daily to 5 – 10 mg po q morning and at noon or Pemoline 18.75 mg po q morning and at noon and escalate daily to 37.5 mg po q morning and at noon.
Higher doses may be needed.

*Consider Liaison Psychiatry consultation*

## DIARRHEA
Loperamide 4 mg po q 4 hr prn

## DYSPNEA
**For Opioid-Naïve Patient:**
Morphine Sulfate 5 – 15 mg po or 2 – 5 mg SQ/IV. Repeat q 1 hr, if needed. When symptom is improved, begin Morphine Sulfate 30 mg po or 10 mg SQ/IV q 4 hr ATC; or begin Morphine Sulfate basal infusion at 2 mg per hour and 2 mg SQ/IV q 1 hr prn.

**For Opioid-Treated Patient:**
If dyspnea uncontrolled, increase fixed schedule dose by 50%.
*If breathlessness continues*, add Lorazepam 0.5mg po or SQ/IV prn. Repeat q 60 minutes if needed until symptom intensity declines, then begin 1 mg po/SQ/IV q 3 hr.

Additional therapies may include:
Dexamethasone 16 mg po/IV, followed by 4 mg po/IV q 6 hr
Albuterol 2.5 mg via nebulization q 4 hr prn if wheezing present

## FEVER
Acetaminophen 650 mg po/PR q 4 hr prn, and/or
Dexamethasone 1.0 mg po/SQ/IV q 12 hr prn

## HICCUPS
Chlorpromazine 10 – 25 mg po/IM TID prn
Haloperidol 0.5 – 2 mg po/SQ/IV TID – QID

## INTRACTABLE SYMPTOMS, MANAGEMENT OF
*Consider referral to Department of Pain Medicine & Palliative Care (Beeper # 6702).*

## IV HYDRATION
Consider decreasing IV rate to 0.5 – 1 liter/24 hr

## NAUSEA/VOMITING
Metoclopromide 10 mg po/IV q 4 hr prn, or
Prochlorperazine 10 mg po/IV q 4 hr or 25 mg PR q 8 hr prn with or without Dexamethasone 4 mg po/IVPB q 6 hr

## PRURITIS
Diphenhydramine 25 – 50 mg po/IV q 12 hr
Hydrocortisone 1 % cream to affected areas q 6 hr
Dexamethasone 1.0 mg po daily alone or in combination with above

## STOMATITIS
Viscous lidocaine 2 % to painful areas prn
Clotrimazole 10 mg troche 5 times daily
Nystatin S & S q 6 hr prn
Magic Mouthwash prn

## TERMINAL SECRETIONS (NOISY RESPIRATIONS)
Scopolamine patches 1.5 – 3 mg 72 hr, or
Scopolamine 0.4 mg SQ q 4 – 6 hr

## PLAN—DO—CHECK—ACT (the Shewhart cycle)

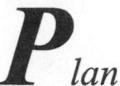*lan*

Create a timeline of resources, activities, training, and target dates. Develop a data collection plan, the tools for measuring outcomes, and thresholds for determining when targets have been met.

### Timeline for One-Year Pilot CQI EOL Project

#### Phase 0 – Planning

| | |
|---|---|
| Jan – June | Formalize CQI Team for the development of a clinical pathway. Clarify knowledge of processes: review literature and existing data sources, conduct brainstorming, flowcharting with pilot units. Evaluate and synthesize literature, tools, other data gathered. Identify content for Care Path. Develop and pilot audit tool for chart reviews. Create database, codebook, and scoring guidelines for data entry. Identify patient outcome assessment tools. Identify family outcome assessment tools. Identify staff assessment tools. Refine study tools/procedures. Develop staff education. Develop caregiver educational materials. |
| June 21 | Medical Records review |
| Aug 2 | Tools Committee review |
| July 3 | Committee on Scientific OSA Application and Approval |

#### Phase I – Launching the Project

| | |
|---|---|
| August 2 | Meet with hospital leadership—Introduction to Palliative Care for Advanced Disease Care Path<br>• PCAD Care Path, MD Orders, and Flow sheet<br>• Timeline for Education/Evaluation |
| August 11 | Introduction of PCAD Care Path to medical staff |

## Phase II – Unit Implementation and Education of PCAD Care Path

|  | Cohort 1 | Cohort 2 | | Cohort 3 |
|---|---|---|---|---|
| • Meet with unit leaders of pilot units | June 21 | September 15 | July 21 | October 11 |
| • Pre-test | August 23–25 | September 27 | September 14 | TBS |
| • Unit leadership team meeting | TBS | October 5 | October 12 | TBS |
| • Introduction of PCAD Care Path to unit staff | August 31–September 1 | September 27–September 30 | October 22 | TBS |
| • In-service of unit staff | September 1 September 2 September 3 | October 4–October 6 | October 25–October 26 | TBS TBS TBS |
| • Rollout of Care Path | September 6 | October 11 | November 1 | TBS |
| • Brainstorming—educational needs | October 11 | November 8 | December 13 | December 6 |
| • Educational series | September–February | October– March | November–April | November–April |
| • Focus groups | October & January | November & February | December & March | December & March |
| • Feedback / closure / continuation | March | April | May | May |
| • Post-test | March | April | May | May |

## Phase III – Evaluation

Chart Reviews using Chart Audit Tool (CAT) (Total =330)

| | | |
|---|---|---|
| June–Aug | • 20 retrospective audits for 5 pilot units | (Total = 100) |
| Sep 1999–Mar 2002 | • 20 retrospective audits for 2 control units | (Total = 40) |
| | • 10 during implementation audits for 5 pilot units | (Total = 50) |
| | • 20 post implementation audits for 5 pilot units | (Total = 100) |
| | • 20 post implementation audits for 2 control units | (Total = 40) |

Each patient on PCAD Care Path as admitted.

| | |
|---|---|
| Sep 1999–Mar 2002 | Tool: Teno's After Death (interview or mailed survey) |
| Dates TBD | Staff survey post-tests (4 mo post-initiation of PCAD) Tool: Palliative Care Quiz |
| Sep 1999–Mar 2002 | Process Audits (PAT) Ongoing throughout time patient on PCAD Care Path |
| Sep 1999–Mar 2002 | Brainstorming sessions and focus groups with staff to identify education 1–2 mo after each unit begins PCAD |

## Phase IV – Reporting

| | |
|---|---|
| April 15, 2002 | Report to grant agency, hospital, and unit staff |

# *D*<sub>o</sub>

Collect data and monitor the intervention until fully implemented.

## Palliative Care Quiz for Nurses (PCQN)

Name: _____

**Background Information:**

Department/ Service

| | |
|---|---|
| 1. Nursing | 2. Social work |
| 3. Medicine | 4. Pharmacy |
| 5. Surgery | 6. Chaplaincy |
| 7. Critical care | 8. Other (describe) |

Unit: _____

Age: _____

Sex:
1. Male
2. Female

Years of experience in discipline:
1. 0–5
2. 6–10
3. >10

Educational preparation:
1. HS diploma
2. Associate degree
3. Baccalaureate degree
4. Masters' degree
5. Postgraduate degree

Previous education/ training in palliative care:
1. No
2. Yes (describe) _____

_____

_____

_____

_____

_____

*The 20-item survey that follows is used with permission.  Ross, M. M.,  McDonald,B., & McGuinness, J. (1996).  The palliative care quiz for nurses (PCQN): the development of an instrument to measure nurses' knowledge of palliative care. Journal of Advanced Nursing, 23:125-137.*

Please circle your response to the items below using the following key:

**T = True**          **F = False**          **DK = Don't Know**

1. Palliative care is appropriate only in situations where there is evidence of a downhill trajectory or deterioration.   T    F    DK

2. Morphine is the standard used to compare the analgesic effect of other opioids.   T    F    DK

3. The extent of the disease determines the method of pain treatment.   T    F    DK

4. Adjuvant therapies are important in managing pain.   T    F    DK

5. It is crucial for family members to remain at the bedside until death occurs.   T    F    DK

6. During the last days of life, the drowsiness associated with electrolyte imbalance may decrease the need for sedation.   T    F    DK

7. Drug addiction is a major problem when morphine is used on a long-term basis for the management of pain.   T    F    DK

8. Individuals who are taking opioids should follow a bowel regime.   T    F    DK

9. The provision of palliative care requires emotional detachment.   T    F    DK

10. During the terminal stages of an illness, drugs that can cause respiratory depression are appropriate for the treatment of severe dyspnea.   T    F    DK

11. Men generally reconcile their grief more quickly than woman.   T    F    DK

12. The philosophy of palliative care is compatible with that of aggressive treatment.   T    F    DK

13. The use of placebos is appropriate in the treatment of some types of cancer pain.   T    F    DK

14. In high doses, codeine causes more nausea and vomiting than morphine.   T    F    DK

15. Suffering and physical pain are synonymous.   T    F    DK

16. Demerol is not an effective analgesic in the control of chronic pain.   T    F    DK

17. The accumulation of losses renders burnout inevitable for those who seek work in palliative care.   T    F    DK

18. Manifestations of chronic pain are different from those of acute pain.   T    F    DK

19. The loss of a distant or problematic relationship is easier to resolve than the loss of one that is close or intimate.   T    F    DK

20. The pain threshold is lowered by anxiety or fatigue.   T    F    DK

# $C_{heck}$

Analyze findings, graph results, and evaluate reasons for variations. If targets are reached, set a date to stop or decrease the frequency of monitoring. Summarize what was learned.

**Sample: Results of Palliative Care Knowledge Quiz, Preimplementation of PCAD**

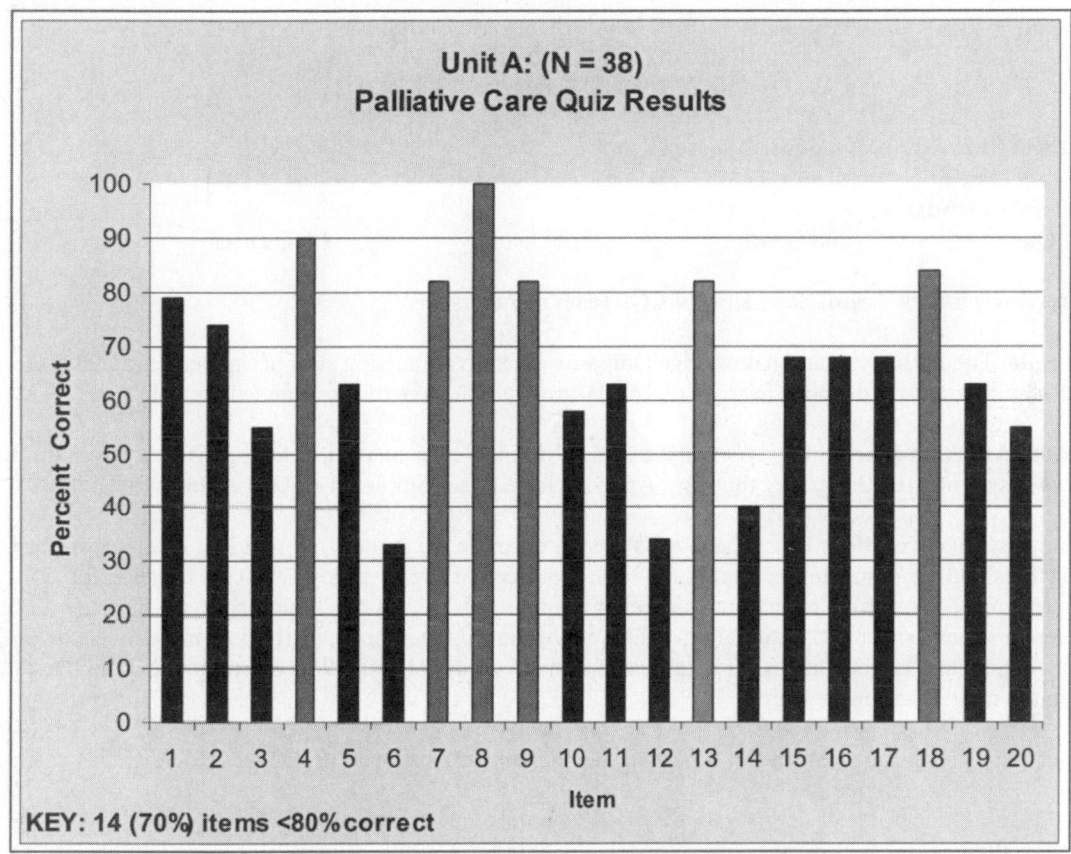

Unit A: (N = 38)
Palliative Care Quiz Results

KEY: 14 (70%) items <80% correct

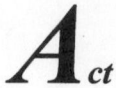*ct*

Act on what is learned and determine the next steps. If successful, act to hold the gain achieved and work at making the intervention a part of standard operating procedure.. If not successful, analyze the sources of failure, design new solutions, and repeat the PDCA cycle.

**Sample: Quarterly Reporting Form**

BETH ISRAEL MEDICAL CENTER
PAIN MEDICINE AND PALLIATIVE CARE
QUALITY IMPROVEMENT STUDY REPORT

**Title of Study**: Improving End-of-Life Care

**Date(s) of study**:
1st Quarter ✓          2nd Quarter__          3rd Quarter__          4th Quarter __

**Interdisciplinary Team**: See listing of CQI Team members.

**Sample**: The Palliative Care Knowledge Quiz was given to all nursing staff preimplementation of the Palliative Care for Advanced Disease (PCAD) Care Path on three of five planned units thus far.

**Findings:** In this quarter, we report on the results of knowledge surveys. A total of 90 staff from three units has completed the survey thus far.  Analyses have been completed on Unit A described below.

**Analysis/interpretation**: Unit A, above, is used to describe the process of providing feedback to staff. The threshold for competency was set for 80%. Fourteen of twenty items (70%) are targeted for improvement. No formal education has been given thus far. This data will be used to (a) measure change pre and post an educational series and use of the PCAD in practice, (b) determine levels of competency and targeted areas for continued education, and (c) to stimulate discussion and dialogue with the multidisciplinary team.

**Conclusion**: Continued education is needed to integrate palliative care principles into the mainstream of daily clinical practice.

**Action Plan / Step 1:** In-services are scheduled in Quarter 2, 2000.  All survey answers will be shared. The Pain Medicine and Palliative Care team will lead a discussion, supported by research results, about the 14 items for which staff answered <80% correctly.  Three content areas were identified: end-of-life issues, pain treatment and side effects, and philosophy of palliative care.
**Step 2:** Based on the dialogue and discussion, subsequent in-services using case-based teaching, will be scheduled. A post-test survey is planned following 6 months of implementation PCAD on each unit.

**Follow-up plan:**  We will report progress at monthly CQI Team meetings. Next report will include chart audit results.

Beth Israel Medical Center-Department of Pain Medicine and Palliative Care

## PALLIATIVE CARE CONSULTATION FORM

Patient's Name: _____    Date Completed: _____/_____/_____

Admission Date: _____/_____/_____    Chart # _____    Date of Follow-up: ____/_____/_____

Days from Admission: _____    Insurance: _____    Completed by: _____

I. BACKGROUND
1. Gender: [1] Male    [2] Female

2. Age: _____    Date of Birth: _____/_____/_____

3. Race/Ethnicity:[1] White-Non-Hispanic   [2] Black-Non-Hispanic   [3] Hispanic-White   [4] Hispanic-Black
            [5] Asian                [6] Other

4. Marital Status: [1] Single (*never married*) [2] Married (*living with partner*) [3] Separated [4] Divorced [5] Widowed

5. Household [*circle all that apply*]: [1] Lives Alone [2] Spouse/Partner [3] Children [4] Parents [5] Other Relative

6. Religion:  [1] Catholic  [2] Protestant  [3] Jewish  [4] Muslim  [5] Hindu  [6] Other _____  [7] None

7. Language: [1] English as primary language [2] Other: _____, but can speak & understand English
   [3] Non-English speaking

8. Primary Medical Diagnosis: [1] _____
                              [2] _____
                              [3] _____

9. Where seen:    [1] Inpatient-hospital   [2] Inpatient-nursing home   [3] Outpatient-office/clinic   [4] Home

10. Reason for consult: [1] Pain   [2] Other symptoms   [3] Management of imminent death   [4] Other _____

SECTIONS II – VII  TO BE COMPLETED BY A MEDICAL HEALTH PROFESSIONAL MD/PA/RN

## II. COGNITIVE STATUS

11. COGNITIVE IMPAIRMENT
    [1] Normal
    [2] Mild Impairment; some memory loss or cognitive disability, but does not interfere with functioning; some confusion or
        disorientation, but brief and resolves quickly
    [3] Moderate impairment; memory loss, confusion or disorientation interfering with functioning, but *no* interference with
        activities with daily living (ADL)
    [4] Severe impairment; confusion, delirium, memory loss interfering with ADL; frank mental retardation.
    [5] Comatose; vegetative state; not conscious

12. DECISIONAL CAPACITY
    [1] Normal – Has decisional capacity
    [2] Cognitively impaired, but has decisional capacity
    [3] Global incompetence, lacks decisional capacity

## III. PATIENT SELF-DETERMINATION/ADVANCE DIRECTIVES
13. Circle all treatment preferences/advance directives, with supporting documents
    [1] Living will                                    [4] Court appointed guardian
    [2] Do not resuscitate (DNR)                       [5] Patient chooses not to discuss
    [3] Health care proxy, durable power of attorney   [6] Don't know

    A. If no Health Care Proxy; Who would you like to speak for you if you were not able to speak for yourself?
       Name: _____ Phone #: _____

Beth Israel Medical Center-Department of Pain Medicine and Palliative Care

## IV. COMMUNICATION

14. METHOD OF COMMUNICATION
    [1] Speaking [2] Language Barrier [3] Sign Language (*for hearing impaired*) [4] Writing Only [5] None

15. DEGREE OF INDEPENDENCE IN COMMUNICATING
    [1] Functional; independent with all aspects of communication (speaking, hearing, sight), with or without glasses, hearing aids, or communication devices
    [2] Moderate assist; communicates ź 50% of the time
    [3] Dependent; unable to communicate with others

## V. PHYSICAL/ACTIVITY STATUS

16. PRESSURE ULCERS
    [1] None
    [2] Mild [Stage I/II]: Injury to skin, Partial loss of skin layers
    [3] Severe [Stage III/IV]: Deep craters in skin that extends down to but not through underlying fascia; breaks in skin exposing muscle or bone; extensive destruction, tissue necrosis, or damage to muscle, bone or supporting structures (e.g., tendons)

17. BOWEL AND BLADDER FUNCTION
    [1] Independent in bowel and bladder function, with full self-care, including ostomy/catheter, if present
    [2] *Not* incontinent, but some assistance needed in managing bathroom or bedpan or ostomy/catheter, if present
    [3] Rarely incontinent; requiring substantial assistance in managing bathroom or bedpan or ostomy/catheter, if present
    [4] Occasionally incontinent; requires full assistance in managing bathroom or bedpan or ostomy/catheter, if present
    [5] Fully incontinent or unable to assist in management of ostomy/catheter, if present
    [6] Don't know

18. PERFORMACE STATUS
    [0] Normal activity
    [1] Capable of all self-care, is ambulatory, but restricted in physicallythan 50% of waking hours strenuous activity, able to carry out work of a light or sedentary
    [2] Ambulatory, capable of all self-care activities, but unable to carry out any work activities; up and about more than 50% of waking hours
    [3] Capable of only limited self-care; confined to bed greater
    [4] Completely disabled; cannot carry on any self-care; nature (e.g., light housework, office work) totally confined to bed/chair

19. NUTRITIONAL INTAKE
    [1] Normal
    [2] Modified Independent; intake limited, need for modification unknown
    [3] Requires diet modification to swallow solid foods and liquids (puree, thickened fluids)
    [4] Combined oral and tube feeding
    [5] Tube feeding only
    [6] No oral intake (NPO) and no tube feeding

20. PRACTICAL SUPPORT WITH ESSENTIAL TASKS (e.g., cooking, cleaning, shopping)
    [1] Needs assistance in essential tasks which is not available
    [2] Needs assistance in essential tasks which is often unreliable or incomplete
    [3] Needs assistance in essential tasks which is sometimes inadequate or available only for less critical tasks such as banking
    [4] Needs assistance in essential tasks is usually available; assistance in less critical tasks is incomplete and unreliable; other responsibilities limit helper availability
    [5] Assistance is available and adequate for any need

## VI. SOCIAL SUPPORT

21. The emotional support I have had from my family and friends has been:
    [1] As much as I wanted    [2] Very adequate   [3] Adequate        [4] Inadequate        [5] Very Inadequate

Beth Israel Medical Center-Department of Pain Medicine and Palliative Care

**VII.  SPIRITUALITY** (*Skip if Patient is Globally Incompetent*)

22.  How important is your religion or spiritual beliefs in your everyday life?
    [1] Not at all important    [2] A little    [3] Somewhat    [4] Important    [5] Very important

23.  During your current illness, how much comfort and strength are you finding from your religion or spiritual beliefs?
    [1] None  [2] A little  [3] Some  [4] A lot  [5] Great strength/comfort  [6] Not religious

NOTES:

_____

_____

_____

_____

_____

_____

_____

SECTIONS VIII - IX TO BE COMPLETED BY PATIENT/FAMILY MEMBER OR HEALTH PROFESSIONAL

**VIII. SYMPTOMS** (*CMSAS-Condensed* Memorial Symptom Assessment Scale)
    If the patient has any of the following symptoms, how severe and distressing are they now?
    <u>Specify who is responding</u>:   [1]  Patient   [2]  Family member, friend, other   [3]  Health Care Professional

How much did this symptom bother or distress you in the past 7 days?

| Symptom | Present | Not at all | A little Bit | Some what | Quite a bit | Very much |
|---|---|---|---|---|---|---|
| Lack of energy | Y  N | 0 | 1 | 2 | 3 | 4 |
| Lack of appetite | Y  N | 0 | 1 | 2 | 3 | 4 |
| Pain | Y  N | 0 | 1 | 2 | 3 | 4 |
| Dry mouth | Y  N | 0 | 1 | 2 | 3 | 4 |
| Weight Loss | Y  N | 0 | 1 | 2 | 3 | 4 |
| Feeling drowsy | Y  N | 0 | 1 | 2 | 3 | 4 |
| Shortness of breath | Y  N | 0 | 1 | 2 | 3 | 4 |
| Constipation | Y  N | 0 | 1 | 2 | 3 | 4 |
| Difficulty sleeping | Y  N | 0 | 1 | 2 | 3 | 4 |
| Difficulty concentrating | Y  N | 0 | 1 | 2 | 3 | 4 |
| Nausea | Y  N | 0 | 1 | 2 | 3 | 4 |

**How frequently did these symptoms occur during the last week?**

| Symptom | Present | Rarely | Occasionally | Frequently | Almost constantly |
|---|---|---|---|---|---|
| Worrying | Y  N | 1 | 2 | 3 | 4 |
| Feeling sad | Y  N | 1 | 2 | 3 | 4 |
| Feeling nervous | Y  N | 1 | 2 | 3 | 4 |

References:
Kaasa, T, Loomis, J, Gillis, K Bruera, E, & Hanson, J. (1997) The Edmonton Functional Assessment Tool: preliminary Development and
    Evaluation for Use in Palliative Care. JPSM 13(1):10-19.
Coyle, N, Goldstein, M, Passik, S, Fishman, B & Portenoy, R. (1996). Development and  validation of a patient needs assessment tool
    (PNAT) for oncology clinicians. Cancer Nursing. 19(2):81-92.
Oken, M.M, Creech, RH, Tormey, DC, Horton, J, Davis, TE, McFadden, & ET, Carbone, PP. (1982). Toxicity and Response Criteria Of the
    Eastern cooperative Oncology Group (ECOG). Am J Clin Oncol 5:649-655.
Chang, VT, Hwang, SS, Kasimis, B & Thaler, H. (2004). Shorter symptom assessment instruments: the Condensed Memorial Symptom
    Assessment Scale (CMSAS). Cancer Invest  22(4):526-36.
National Pressure Ulcer Advisory Panel Report. 1996. Pressure ulcer staging. Wound Ostomy and Continence Society. 4(3).

# 45

*Sarah A. Wilson*

# Long-Term Care

*My father's nurse suggested we think about hospice care for him. He was 93 and living in a long term care facility. His care was excellent, and I could not really imagine how it might need to change. Since he was declining and I trusted the nurse's assessment, I agreed. His decline became more rapid. As each new problem appeared, the hospice nurses worked with the staff to assure his comfort and ours. I cherish those final days and am so thankful for the expertise of the nurses who accompanied us in the journey.—Daughter, talking about her father*

◆ **Key Points**
◆ *The older people are, the more likely they are to die in a nursing home.*
◆ *Elderly residents in long-term care settings often have multiple chronic illnesses and are among the most frail Americans.*
◆ *Unlicensed personnel provide a substantial proportion of long-term care and should be included in palliative care education efforts.*

Quality end-of-life (EOL) care in nursing homes is becoming more important as the number of older adults increases, and managed care continues to minimize hospital stays. Nursing home residents are sicker today and have different care needs. Although nursing homes were not established as sites for terminal care, they are becoming the place where many people die. Statistics on the place of death tell us little about the environment where someone lived and died. This chapter addresses nursing homes, the environment of nursing homes, the staff, the care of dying residents, and model programs to support dying residents.

The terms *institutional care* and *long-term care* have been used interchangeably in reference to nursing home care, although neither is synonymous with *nursing home care*. *Long-term care* refers to a continuum of services addressing the health, personal care, and social service needs for persons who need help with activities of daily living as a result of some functional impairment.[1] Services may be provided in the home, the community, or a nursing home.

## History of Nursing Homes

Before the late 1970s, nursing homes were the primary source of care that could not be provided by families for persons needing long-term care. Nursing homes have been described as the offspring of the almshouse and boarding house and the stepchild of the hospital.[2] In the mid-19th century, older people who were poor, sick, or disabled and without family support had few options other than the almshouse.[3] Private homes for the aged emerged as an alternative to public almshouses after the passage of the Social Security Act in the 1930s. Women who were caring for their ill family members at home took in other patients to help pay the bills. From these small homes, proprietary nursing homes evolved.

## Growth of Nursing Homes

The growth of nursing homes from the 1930s to the 1960s was related to six key factors[2]: (1) Old Age Assistance allowed a portion of the elderly to directly purchase services; (2) payments were made directly to facilities for the care of older adults, easing the state's financial obligations and creating a source of payment for care; (3) construction loans and loan guarantees were available through the federal Hill–Burton Act, the Small Business Administration, and the Federal Housing Authority; (4) the Kerr–Mills Program extended financial participation to medically indigent older adults; (5) the American Association of Nursing Homes became a strong lobby for those with interests in the new industry; and (6) in a limited way the federal government began to develop some standards for nursing homes. The growth of nursing homes occurred largely by chance; however, with the passage of Medicare and Medicaid in 1965, nursing homes became an industry.

The number of certified nursing homes decreased from 19,100 in 1985 to 16,100 in 2004.[4] Nursing homes cared for about 1.46 million residents in 2005.[5] These numbers are low given the growing elderly population. The majority of nursing homes are proprietary or profit-making. Nursing homes are licensed or certified to designate the level of care provided and method of reimbursement. Approximately 82% of nursing homes are certified by Medicare and Medicaid. Skilled nursing facilities (SNFs) are also certified for Medicare funding. Medicare provides for up to 100 days of skilled care in a nursing home following a 3-day hospitalization. However, reimbursement for nursing home care by Medicare is restricted by narrowly defining what "skilled" is and by limiting the duration of the "skilled" benefit. The yearly cost of nursing home care in 2006 was $75,000 for a private room and $66,795 for a semiprivate room.[4] Medicaid is the primary payor for most nursing facilites; approximately 65% of nursing home residents have Medicaid.[5] Most elderly who need nursing home care for more than a few weeks spend or liquidate all their resources to qualify for Medicaid.

## Population Demographics and Nursing Homes

The population of the United States continues to increase. One of the most significant developments is the growth of the older population. The large number of people who were born between 1946 and 1964, commonly referred to as "Baby Boomers," contributes to the "graying of America." Statistics from the 2000 Census reflect the influence of Baby Boomers. Thirty million people are over age 65 years and account for 12.4% of the population.[6] This number is expected to double in the next 20 years. By 2030, one in five Americans will be 65 years or older.[7] "The fastest growing segment of our population is centenarians, the number has doubled every decade since 1970."[7] The second fastest growing age group consists of persons 85 years and over. The number of the elderly age 85 years and older population is expected to more than triple between 2008 and 2050, from 5.4 million to 19 million.[8]

Nineteen percent of the people aged 65 years and older are members of minority groups.[5] The growing diversity in the older adult popualtion has implications for healthcare. Disaparities continue to exist among the white and non-white populations. Health-care providers need to become culturally competent and representative of the diverse cultural groups they care for.

Demographic changes in the older adult population will have a major impact on healthcare in terms of services needed, delivery of healthcare, and education of health-care providers. Older persons have more health problems, use more health services, and are hospitalized more often for longer stays than younger persons.

Five percent is most often cited as the proportion of older adults living in nursing homes. However, this is misleading because the use of nursing homes increases with age. The characteristics and needs of nursing home residents have changed with the implementation of the prospective payment system for Medicare. Nursing homes are experiencing changes in the reasons for admission and discharges. The intensity of care has increased as more people enter nursing homes as a result of early hospital discharge. Some people are entering nursing homes for a relatively short stay and rehabilitation, others are being discharged home, and still others are being transferred to hospitals in the final stages of life and ultimately die there.

Death occurs more frequently among older adults in institutions than at home among family and friends. A widespread belief is that the majority of older people die in hospitals. In fact, the older people are, the more likely they are to die in nursing homes.[9] It is estimated that by the year 2040 40% to 50% of all deaths will occur in long-term care settings.[9] Although nursing homes were not established as places for terminal care, they are increasingly becoming such facilities.

## Regulation of Nursing Homes

Nursing homes are highly regulated. The number of rules and regulations have led some to compare the regulations to those of nuclear power plants. The nursing home population is viewed as a population of vulnerable adults who need protection, which, in combination with the history of patient abuse by some providers, has led to a strong tradition of regulation by federal and state governments. Most of the effort in quality assessment has been directed toward detecting problems; less has been devoted to assessing and acknowledging good care.[10]

Almost two decades ago, concern with the quality of care in nursing homes led Congress to commission the Institute of Medicine (IOM) to study nursing homes. The recommendations of the IOM Committee on Nursing Home Regulation, as well as many consumer advocacy groups, led Congress to enact major reforms in nursing home regulations as part of the Omnibus Budget Reconciliation Act of 1987 (OBRA 87).[11]

The intent of OBRA 87 was to improve the quality of care by establishing a single set of certification conditions for all nursing homes.[12] In addition, these regulations addressed residents' care, rights, and quality of life. A key aspect of OBRA 87 was that residents have the right to be free of physical and chemical restraints. The emphasis of regulations shifted toward addressing outcomes of care.

Some improvements have been noted in nursing homes since OBRA 87 was implemented.[12] The focus on residents' rights and the empowerment of residents in care decisions have been identified as one of the most significant accomplishments of OBRA 87.[12] Perhaps most significant regulation was the overall reduction in the use of both physical and chemical restraints. No provisions were made for improving reimbursement to increase staffing. The emphasis of OBRA 87 was rehabilitation, restoration, and improvement in function rather than the provision of quality EOL care.[13]

### Accreditation

Nursing homes may apply for voluntary accreditation by the Joint Commission on Accreditation of Healthcare Organizations (JCAHO), an organization created for the accreditation of hospitals that has expanded to include home health agencies and nursing homes, among other health-care institutions. The facility pays a fee for the inspection to determine if JCAHO standards are being followed. Some nursing homes that seek JCAHO accreditation believe that it adds to a facility's credibility and makes it more marketable to the consumer.

In summary, growth in nursing homes has been proportionate with the increasing elderly population, and the need for long-term care services will continue to increase as the population ages. Palliative care is an important component of nursing home care. Along with understanding the structure of nursing homes, it is important to consider the sociocultural environment of these institutions.

## Sociocultural Environment of Nursing Homes

The sociocultural environment of nursing homes differs from other health-care institutions: the average length of stay is longer, physician visits are less frequent, the majority of primary care providers are nursing assistants, and registered nurses (RNs) constitute a small portion of the home's full-time equivalent (FTE) employees.

### Length of Stay

The length of stay in nursing homes is either short term or long term. In most nursing homes, the length of stay varies, although there is greater movement of residents into and out of nursing homes as a result of early hospital discharges. The short-term resident is usually someone under age 75 years who stays in the nursing home for 4 to 6 weeks for rehabilitation after an acute illness, such as a stroke or hip replacement. The long-term resident is usually older than age 75 years and has numerous chronic diseases and functional and cognitive impairments. The average length of stay in a skilled nursing facility is 892 days from admission to discharge.[14] Almost half (47.7%) of all nursing home residents have some form of dementia.[15] The 1999 National Nursing Home Study indicated that the typical resident is a female, age 85 years and older, and needs assistance with one or more activities of daily living and instrumental activities of daily living.[16] Older people who die in a nursing home have dying trajectory of fragility, with 60% having a diagnosis of a stroke or a hip fracture.[17] Between 50% and 60% of all deaths in SNFs are residents with a diagnosis of dementia.[17]

## Studies of Death and Dying in Nursing Homes

Early studies of death and dying focused on hospitals as the place of death. The attitudes of hospital staff toward dying patients, the stresses encountered by nurses in caring for dying patients and families, and communication with dying patients and families were described in these studies.[18–21] More recent studies of death and dying have focused on other settings, including nursing homes. The setting of care has a direct influence on the older adult's quality of life at the EOL.[22,23] A "good death" is not assured in nursing homes. Studies of death and dying in nursing homes have examined family perceptions of nursing homes, physician involvement in care, nursing home staff, symptom management, referrals to hospice, and barriers to quality EOL care.

### Family Perceptions of Nursing Homes

The public and families of nursing home residents may have unrealistic expectations of nursing homes. It is a difficult decision for families to decide on nursing placement. Families expect the same type of care to be provided in the nursing home that was provided in the hospital. For example, families may believe a physician will visit every day instead of once a month. The media reinforces negative images of nursing homes. Cases of abuse and poor management receive more attention in the media than positive images of nursing homes.

Teno[23] conducted the first large national study to examine family perspectives on the quality of EOL care in institutional settings and home. Family members were surveyed to determine if the adequacy or quality of EOL care differed in hospitals, nursing homes, and home. A mortality follow-up survey was used, and 1,578 decedents were represented. Nearly one-fourth of all respondents reported the patient did not receive adequate treatment for pain and dyspnea. Family members of persons whose last place of care was a nursing home or a home with home health nursing services had higher rates of reported unmet needs for pain compared with persons who had home hospice services. One-fourth of the families reported problems with physician communication.

Nursing home residents were less likely to have been treated with respect at the EOL. The family members of decedents who received home hospice care were more likely to report a favorable dying expereince.[23]

Cartwright[13] reviewed nursing research in nursing homes and assisted-living facilities as places of care for the dying. She noted a large discrepancy between family and staff perceptions of the quality of EOL care in nursing homes.

### Physician Involvement

Physician visits to residents in nursing homes are often limited to once every 30 days. Federal regulations require physicians to make at least one visit every 60 days to nursing home residents, in contrast to the acute care environment, where physicians usually see patients every day. The nurse in the nursing home is responsible for communicating any changes in a resident's condition to the physician. If the physician does not respond in a timely manner, then the medical director intervenes. As noted earlier, physician involvement in nursing homes is limited. Families expect more frequent physican visits, as the severity of the resident's illness increase and the resident becomes more frail.[24] Shield et al. conducted in-depth interviews with 54 family members or others who were close to the decedents.[24] The participants were asked how they communicated with healthcare providers with an emphasis on physicians. Physicians were described as "missing in action" in nursing homes.[24] Some families never met the physician, and others had difficulty getting information about their family member from the physician. Comments about "missing physicians" often occurred in the context of inadequate staffing. Nursing homes present some barriers to physician involvement, such as low payments and complex regulations for reimbursement.

### Nursing Home Staff

Nursing homes and hospitals differ in the type of staff employed and in staffing patterns. The acute care hospital has a higher ratio of professional staff to patients than the nursing home. Nursing assistants, the primary caregivers in nursing homes, spend the most time with residents and constitute more than 32% of a nursing home's FTE employees. In comparison, RNs constitute only 7.6% of the FTE employees.[16,17] Licensed practical nurses (LPNs) constitute 10.6% of the nursing home's FTE employees.[16,17] Approximately 50% of SNFs do not have an RN on duty 24 hours a day. Proprietary nursing homes have fewer RNs (6.8%) per 100 beds than nonprofit or government nursing homes (9.1%).[16,17]

The educational level and preparation of staff in the two types of institutions also differ. The LPN program may be completed in 12 to 24 months and has a limited amount of educational content devoted to geriatrics, palliative care, and death and dying. Most nursing assistants have not completed high school, work for low pay, and receive few benefits. The work assigned to nursing assistants is often difficult and stressful, with little recognition of their contribution to resident care.

Increasing staff in nursing homes is often perceived as a way to improve quality of care. However adding more staff may not be associated with better outcomes. The use of "head counts" does not address the quality of care.[25] In a study of over 6,000 nursing homes, Castle and Engberg reported that resident care was influenced not only by staffing but also by the consistency of care, care coordination, and care practices.[25]

Nurses' lack of ability to supervise unlicensed personnel influences the quality of care.[26] Preparing nurses for a supervisory role varies from classes and workshops to no programs. Nurses' workloads and staffing also affect the ability of nurses to supervise unlicensed personnel. A limitation of this study was a small sample size in one geographic area.[26] Further studies should include a larger sample size in diverse geographic areas.

### Symptom Management

One of the major themes reported in the IOM study of care at the EOL was that too many people suffer from pain that could be prevented or relieved with the use of existing knowledge and therapies.[11] Several studies have documented the poor control of pain in nursing home residents.[11,23,27] Instruments to assess pain in residents with cognitive impairment are inadequate. Staff often lack knowledge of the assessment and management of pain.[27,28] Palliative care educational programs have been effective in increasing staff knowledge of pain management in nursing homes. A comprehensive discussion of pain assessment and management are found in Chapters 6 and 7.

### Referrals to Hospice

Nurses are in a key position to influence referrals to hospice based on their assessment of changes in the residents' condition.[29] The benefits of hospice care include better pain management, fewer hospitalizations, greater satisfaction with care, and decreased costs. Late referrals to hospice allows little time to control symptoms and provide support to residents and families.In a study of nursing home referrals to hospice and the timing of referrals, Welch et al.[29] reported that nurses' ability to recognize signs of terminal decline and beliefs about hospice care were significant factors in determining whether residents were referred to hospice. The nursing homes in this study did not have any procedures for assessing terminal status or eligibility for hospice care.[29] Beliefs about hospice included: nursing home could provide better care than hospice because they know the residents better; hospice does not provide value to EOL care; and hospice care is for the "very end." Nurses need education to address misconceptions of hospice and how to assess signs of terminal decline.

### Barriers to Quality End-of-Life Care

The nursing home environment has some barriers to quality EOL care. Nursing home residents are a vulnerable population with complex chronic health problems. The number of nursing home residents is expected to increase. Nursing home staff need to be provided with the skill set to care for these residents. Educational programs are needed to address pain and symptom management, assessment of terminal decline, and how to support to dying residents and families.

Pain management is an area of concern. Physicians depend on nurses to assess and report pain and may be unaware of measures that can be used to control pain in nursing homes. For example, some physicians are unaware that morphine can be given intravenously in many nursing homes. In addition, LPNs receive little education in pain management. Nursing homes are extremely concerned about state and federal regulations and have few protocols for pain management. Pain management is further complicated by the large number of cognitively impaired residents who are unable to communicate if they are in pain.

There is a lack of evidence-based research in the delivery of model programs for quality EOL care in nursing homes. Many nursing homes are apprehensive about participating in research studies because of the costs involved, both in monetary terms as well as staff time required. Studies are needed to address issues of protection of study subjects, because many elderly persons in nursing homes are unable to give informed consent. It is important that the researchers clearly explain the purpose(s) of the research and its objectives, the potential benefits to the nursing home, the time and costs involved, and the amount of staff involvement necessary. Researchers should meet with nursing home administration and staff during the course of the study to discuss the study progress and identify any problems. They should also meet with family members to explain the research project. Once the study is complete, the researchers should provide feedback to the nursing home.

In summary, studies of death and dying in nursing homes have described family perceptions of care, physician involvement in nursing homes, nursing home staff, symptom management, referrals to hospice and barriers to providing EOL care in nursing homes. Further study needs to be done to learn more about the experience of dying in long-term care facilities. Institutional policies and practices need to change to achieve better outcomes in the management of pain. Finally, reimbursement mechanisms need to change to provide quality EOL care in nursing homes.

## Caring for Dying Residents

This section explores issues related to the care of dying residents in nursing homes, including advance directives, ethical issues, spiritual support, provision of hospice services, support for dying residents and their families, and recognition of the impact of loss on staff.

### Advance Directives

Nursing home residents have the right to participate in decisions about their care, including EOL care. The passage of the federal Patient Self-Determination Act (PSDA) in 1990 required all health-care agencies that receive federal funding to recognize advance directives. The purpose of the PSDA was to encourage greater awareness and use of advance directives. OBRA 87 regulations emphasized that residents have the right to self-determination, including the right to participate in care planning and the right to refuse treatments. Residents are usually informed of their rights, including the right to advance directives at the time of admission to the nursing home, which is a stressful time for both resident and family members. Families report making these decisions in the context of guilt and overwhelming burden related to nursing home admission. Nursing home residents with dementia are less likely to have advance directives or a family member to make decisions on their behalf.[30]

Resnick, Schurr, and Stone[31] examined data from the 2004 National Nursing Home Survey to determine the most recent prevalence of advance directives in nursing home residents. The prevalence of advance directives increased from 53% in 1996 to 69.6% in 2004.[32] Non-white residents were less likely to have completed advance directives. This may have been associated with cultural differences and a lack of trust in health-care providers. Teno et al.[32] used a mortality follow-back survey, to study the relationship between advance directives and quality EOL care. There was some improvement in communicating with families regarding what to expect when a family member was dying. However, concerns still remain how we treat dying residents with dignity and respect. Completing an advance directives does not assure quality EOL care.[32]

### Ethical Issues

Autonomy is based on the assumption that an individual is the best judge of what is in his/her best interest. Nursing homes have been criticized as dehumanizing and promoting dependence. Autonomy gives meaning to one's life, and with regard to nursing homes, it means being able to direct and influence others in decisions regarding daily living situations.[33] The routines, regulations, and restricted opportunities in nursing homes have been described as enemies of autonomy, and the regimentation contributes to a "loss of control." Most nursing homes were designed based on a hospital or medical model of care, which focuses on routines and tasks. The medical model tends to foster a paternalistic approach of "we know what is best." The physical environment of the nursing home also limits autonomy. Space is limited, with most residents sharing a room and toilet facilities that restrict privacy and space for personal possessions. Residents may also wander in and out of others' rooms. The environment could be more individualized by using personal furnishings and creating a homelike common area, such as a dining room.

One of the most difficult and sometimes controversial ethical issues involves decisions regarding food and hydration. Food in all societies is part of the ongoing cycle of daily interaction and activity around which much of family life is organized and that is symbolic of life and caring. Families may continue to try to feed their relatives when they are no longer able to eat. Nursing home staff can assist families by explaining that it is normal to lose appetite at the EOL and that the body only takes in what it needs. Trying to force someone to eat may cause more harm than good. Families should understand that there is a risk of aspiration as a person gets weaker. Nursing staff may encourage families to offer small amounts of liquids, ice chips, or popsicles.

The following case study illustrates some of the ethical issues at the EOL in nursing homes.

CASE STUDY
*Jim's Dilemma*

Jim is 78 years old and lives at Shorehaven Nursing Home. He has two adult children, Lisa and Jim Jr. Jim lived with his wife in a small apartment until she died 2 years ago. Since then it has become increasingly difficult for Jim to cook meals and manage the apartment. He stopped driving 8 months ago because his vision was poor. Lisa and Jim Jr. were concerned about their father being safe at home. They discussed Shorehaven Nursing Home with their dad and were surprised when he agreed to be admitted to the facility. Jim has adjusted well to Shorehaven and has made new friends. He enjoys playing cards with his new friends. Jim sits with his friends for meals; this is a social time for him, and he loves to eat.

Jim notices he has some blood with his stools. At first he ignores it, but when it persists he becomes concerned and asks to see his physican. It has been over 6 years since Jim had a colonoscopy, so the physican recommends another. Jim agrees, because his last colonoscopy went well he isn't concerned. The results of the colonoscopy reveal that Jim has colon cancer and needs to have part of his colon removed. He is hospitalized and has a colon resection. Jim's prognosis is poor. He returns to Shorehaven and does well for 4 months, then he becomes progressively weaker and has problems eating. When Jim tries to eat, he has difficulty swallowing. Jim is concerned about becoming weaker and having difficulty eating. He discusses this with his children. Jim wants to know what will happen if he can't eat. Can he get food by some other means? Jim believes he will starve to death and have a painful death. Jim and his family decide to talk to the nurse about this.

What are the issues in this case? What decisions need to be made? Who will be most affected by the decision? Would a family conference be helpful to discuss artificial food and hydration? What options does Jim have? What are some possible benefits and consequences of Jim's decision? Would the Hospice and Palliative Care Nurses Association position on artificial nutrition and hydration be helpful in this situation? Would the American Nurses Association (ANA) Code of Ethics be useful in making a decision? The ANA Code of Ethics address the person's rights to

self-determination and primacy of the patient's interests. How do these principals apply in this case? What is the nurse's role in the family conference? How can he/she be helpful to Jim and his family? Should anyone else be involved in the conference? What can be learned from this case?

To answer the above questions, consider the following: Is the primary issue whether Jim should have artificial nutrition and hydration if he is no longer able to eat? What are Jim's goals for his care? What are Jim's values? Does Jim understand how artificial food and hydration can be provided? The risks and benefits? How would you address Jim's comments about starving and experiencing painful death? Does current research on artificial food and hydration address this? Is the Hospice and Palliative Care Nurses Association position on artificial nutrition of any help in planning how to respond to Jim and his family? Does this case illustrate the importance of advance directives and the need to discuss the goals of care?

## Providing Support to Dying Residents and Their Families

Nursing home staff may provide support to dying residents and their families in coping with the eventual loss of the family member. It is important that nurses communicate openly with families, explain changes in the patient's/resident's condition, and answer questions honestly. Listening is an important communicative skill. Active listening is usually more helpful than judging or giving advice. Effective active listening skills include being able to convey that you want to listen, that you want to be helpful, and that you accept the other's feelings. When communication is a concern for staff, it may be helpful to role-play some representative situations. For example, role-playing can teach what to say on the telephone when informing a family member that their relative is dying and how to help families decide about options.

Families have identified a number of caring behaviors of nursing staff that helped them cope with the eventual loss of their relative.[34] It was important to families for staff to take the time to come to residents' rooms and ask how they were doing. Families also identified that listening to the family's concerns and getting answers to their questions were helpful. Staff also demonstrated concern for families in other ways, such as asking if they would like a cup of coffee or getting a comfortable chair for a family member. Families appreciated the fact that the staff respected their privacy and seemed to know when they wanted to be left alone.

It is important for families to understand the dying process. Staff may explain signs and symptoms of approaching death to families and keep them informed of what is changing and why. If the family is not present, they should be kept informed by telephone. Family decisions, such as being present at the time of death or not being present, should be respected. Every effort should be made to notify families early enough that they may be present at the time of death, if that is their wish. Families may be encouraged to reminisce together. They may participate in providing care by holding a hand or giving a backrub. Staff should remind families that although the family member cannot respond, the sound of familiar voices may be a source of comfort.

There are some barriers to providing support for dying residents and families in the nursing home environment. The lack of privacy in most nursing homes is a problem, and it is often difficult to find a private area to talk to families and residents. One social worker commented that "dying is almost a public spectacle in the nursing home." Another barrier is the lack of staff time to spend with dying residents and families, as the staffing patterns of most nursing homes do not account for labor-intensive care at the end of life.

## Providing Spiritual Support

An important component of palliative care is spiritual support. Spirituality is often associated with religion, but the two are not identical. Religion is a means of expressing spirituality and refers to feelings, beliefs, and behaviors associated with a faith community. Spirituality is broader than religion and relates to "meaning-making," to have meaning and purpose in life.[35] Spirituality influences a resident's needs, decision-making, coping, and understanding of illness.[36] Spirituality is common to all people; however, how people understand and practice spirituality varies from person to person. Spiritual support is an integral part of supportive care. The search for meaning or spiritual comfort at the EOL is often guided by religious or philosophical beliefs. Spiritual well-being in relation to the EOL has been described as "meaningful existence, ability to find meaning in daily experience, ability to transcend physical discomfort, and readiness for death."[36] Families and residents may fear the future and have questions about life in general. Residents are usually asked about their religious affiliation and the name of their clergy at the time of admission to most nursing homes, but, unfortunately, this may be the only time spirituality is mentioned. Spiritual needs vary and can change at the EOL.

Private, religiously affiliated nursing homes usually have pastoral care available, and most have a room that is designated as a chapel. Many nursing homes have funeral and memorial services for residents. Nonprivate nursing homes usually attempt to make arrangements for pastoral care through volunteer clergy in the community. Some have been successful with these arrangements, but some nursing home staff have stated that it is difficult to find clergy when needed.

Meeting the spiritual needs of dying residents and their families has been identified as an educational need of nursing home staff. Staff often are aware of spiritual needs but are unsure of what to do or say and what would be considered acceptable to their facilities in meeting spiritual needs. Listening and presence are important interventions that help to establish a connection between the caregiver and the resident.[35] Listening allows the resident the opportunity to express

feeling such as grief or happiness. Presence is *being* with the dying person. Staff may use a number of interventions to provide spiritual care, including praying with the resident and family, reading the Bible or other religious works, journaling, singing hymns, and providing time for solitude, all of which may help decrease the loneliness and separation persons are experiencing. Staff should avoid imposing their beliefs on residents and families and if the resident is not interested in spirituality it should not be pursued.

With proper staff education and training, most barriers to providing spiritual support in nursing homes can be eliminated. Continuing education programs need to be developed to address staff needs for education on spirituality. Staff need to know the facility's policies regarding spiritual care. Many nursing homes do not have a space designated as a meditation room or chapel. It is important for families and residents to have a private, quiet area where they can meditate. If pastoral care is not available in the nursing home, it may be arranged by contacting local clergy or layleaders in the community.

## Providing Support for Staff

Nursing staff form an attachment to residents that may be defined as a strong emotional bond and connectedness that develops between residents and staff over time.[37] Attachment is fostered by staff efforts to treat residents as "family." The nursing home is "home" for many residents, as some live there for years, so that staff often experience feelings of loss and sadness when a resident dies.

Staff members need to be able to talk about their feelings of loss when a resident dies. It is necessary for nursing homes to develop programs to assist staff in coping with the loss of a resident. Allowing staff time to talk about a resident at staff meetings, sharing memories of a resident, and planning a memorial for residents who have died may be helpful. Other staff members should acknowledge that the loss must be difficult when they know a particular staff member was close to a certain resident.

The loss of a resident may also be stressful for other nursing home residents. Residents develop friendships with other residents over time; they may have shared a room with the resident or sat next to the resident for meals. The death may remind residents of their own mortality. Residents may want to attend the funeral of the deceased resident, or the nursing home may have a memorial service or time of remembrance. Staff should acknowledge the loss and what it means to other residents.

In summary, the nursing home environment influences the care of residents at the end of life. Nursing home staff need to be comfortable talking with residents and families about death and dying. The staff's assessment of a resident's terminal status and beliefs about hospice influence the timing and referral to hospice.[30] Knowledge of pain management is as important in nursing homes as it is in other settings. Families should be included in the care of dying residents, and their need for privacy should be respected. Model programs have been developed to enhance the quality EOL care in nursing homes, as described in the following section.

## Model Programs for Quality End-of-Life Care in Nursing Homes

The place for EOL care influences the experience of dying.[22] Nursing homes are unique settings and experience challenges providing quality EOL care. Educational programs have been developed to address specific needs in nursing homes. The majority of these programs are designed primarily for nurses. Few programs addresss the needs of nursing assistants and other unlicensed staff in nursing homes. This section describes two exemplary programs to address the educational needs of nurses and unlicensed staff in nursing homes.

### Palliative Care Educational Resource Team

The Palliative Care Educational Resource Team (PERT) is a comprehensive curriculum designed for nurses and nursing assistants in nursing homes.[27] The purpose of PERT was to enhance the quality of EOL in nursing homes by providing staff with the knowledge, skills, and confidence needed to care for dying residents.[27] The course content for nurses and nursing assistants was offered as a 4-day-long monthly class. Nurses and nursing assistants attended the majority of classes together. This helped to acknowlege the contributions of both licensed and unlicensed staff. Participants were given a copy of the course syllabus, class notes, and reference materials. In addition, a user-friendly PERT website (www. swedishmedical.org/pert) was developed, which contained course content, extensive bibliographies, and links to other resources. Sixty-one nursing assistants and 108 licensed staff from 44 facilities participated in PERT. Participants completed evaluations prior to and 6 months after the program. The participant's immediate supervisor evaluated the participant's performance prior to the program and 6 months after completion. The PERT program was effective in enhancing the expertise of nursing home staff; there were significant increases in the participant's knowledge, skills, and confidence in providing EOL care.[27]

A PERT train-the-trainer program format was developed to increase staff and facility participation and reach a wider geographic area.[28] This format allowed educators to attend the program and conduct in-services in their facilities. All participants received a copy of the curriculum as well as a CD with an electronic copy of the curriculum. Curriculum materials included PowerPoint presentations, slides in a Adobe Portable Document Format (PDF), module outlines, resource materials, and quizzes. Participants rated the course as comprehensive, current, and appropriate for long-term care facilities. Confidence in teaching EOL content increased significantly after completing the course. Six months after completion of the course, 87% of the participants had conducted one in-service program.[28]

### End of Life Nursing Education Consortium

The End of Life Nursing Education Consortium (ELNEC) was initiated in response to the need to improve palliative care education for nurses and to provide quality EOL care for dying persons and their families. The American Asssociation of Colleges of Nursing and City of Hope Medical Center colloborated to develop a national palliative care education program for nurses. Nationally recognized experts in palliative care contributed to the curriculum with input from an advisory board and reviewers. ELNEC was developed in a train-the-trainer format. The first ELNEC program was offered in January 2001; since then, five additional curricula have been developed for diverse speciality areas. Nurses who complete ELNEC courses are provided with a hard copy of the course syllabus, a CD of the syllabus, numerous references, PowerPoint slides, a palliative care textbook, assessment tools, and other resources. ELNEC is nationally known for excellence in EOL care education. Nurses who complete ELNEC training are empowered to become palliative care educators and leaders. Information about ELNEC is available at http://www.aacn.nche.edu/elnec.[38]

### End of Life Nursing Education Consortium-Geriatric Training Program

The ELNEC Geriatric Training Program was developed to address the unique needs of nurses in long-term care facilities and hospices that serve those facilities.[38] Nurses who work with geriatric populations in other settings may also benefit from the program. Applicants to the ELNEC Geriatric Training Program are competitively selected. Part of the application process includes participating in a precourse survey, providing a statement of goals for attending and agreeing to particpate in follow-up surveys.[38] Funding for the ELNEC-Geriatric Training curriculum and pilot course was initially provided by the California HealthCare Foundation[38] and has been sustained by the Archstone Foundation.

The curricula for the ELNEC Geriatric Training Program includes teaching modules for nursing assistants and other unlicensed staff.[38] As previously mentioned, nursing assistants provide the majority of care in long-term care facilities, including nursing homes. The ELNEC teaching modules were modified to include geriatric content, and sessions were added to address the educational needs of nursing assistants and other unlicensed staff.[38] For example, the module "Pain Assessment and Management" includes assessment of pain in olders adults, additional content on pain assessment for nonverbal patients or those with dementia, and a session for education of nursing assistants.[38] Another example is the module "Loss, Grief and Bereavement." This module includes grief in LTC residents, nurses, and nursing assistants with an additional session for education of nursing assistants. Participants evaluate the program at 1 month, 4 months, and 12 months following completion of the program. The results of the evaluations indicate the ELNEC Geriatric Program is an effective model for educating geriatric nurses and nursing assistants in EOL care. Examples of program implementation include the following.

- A hospice taught a session on Grief, Loss, and Bereavement for licensed and unlicsensed staff and videotaped it to make it availabe for all three shifts. The staff "loved it." The session validated everyone's concern and allowed them to express their grief as well as support each other.
- A hospice completed a needs assessment and formed a pain management committee.
- One organization started palliative care teams in seven of eight facilities. Education programs have been started at every facility to increase awareness of how the EOL experience can be individualized, they refer to this as "Sacred Journey." "Sacred Journey" kits are provided for each facility and can be customized to fit the needs of their residents.
- A facility is collaborating with nursing faculty to have clinical students receive ELNEC training.
- One facility created the first staff retreat with the theme of self-care and caregiver fatigue. The "Loss & Grief" module was helpful in planning the retreat. The retreat was so successful that it will become an annual event.
- One facility developed a presentation on pain management for volunteers.
- One organization offers multiple formats for relief on pain. For example, pet therapists, journaling, fresh air, comfort foods, a glass of wine or beer, and hugs and hand-holding.
- A long-term care facility initiated a palliative care screening tool for all admissions.
- A facility has initiated one topic on EOL issues for monthly family council meeting. Family particpation has been very good, and they are interested in talking about these issues.

## Recommendations for Change

The quality of end-of-life care in nursing homes can be improved. The following are some recommendations for change: (1) reimbursement for nursing home care needs to be increased; (2) nursing home staff should include more professional staff, and the ratio of staff to residents should be increased; (3) nurses and nursing assistants need education on palliative care; (4) environmental modifications should be made to improve quality of life and human dignity; and (5) hospice and palliative care concepts should be incorporated in nursing homes.

## Reimbursement

Reimbursement and regulations in nursing homes are often impediments to quality EOL care. Policymakers and the public need to be educated about the cost of nursing home care. Reimbursement should change from an emphasis on procedures to a focus on continuing comfort measures and palliation. Nursing homes receive most of their revenue from private-pay residents and Medicaid. Medicaid rates need to be increased to reflect the labor-intensive nature of long-term care. The IOM[11] recommends that additional research projects on the use of financial and other resources to improve quality of care and outcomes in nursing homes be funded. An issue closely related to reimbursement is the number and type of staff in nursing homes.

## Nursing Home Staff

The relationship between the ratio of RNs to residents and quality of care has been clearly established in nursing homes.[11,17,22] Considering the projected growth in the elderly population, the need for RNs in nursing homes is expected to increase. In addition, nursing home residents will be sicker as a result of shorter hospital stays. A major barrier to increased staffing in nursing homes is the fiscal limits of government support. Registered nurses' salaries are lower in nursing homes than in hospitals, and vacancy rates are higher.[11] Nursing homes are starting to use advance practice nurses to deal with the complex needs of older adults. Advance practice nurses, geriatric nurse practitioners, and clinical specialists in geriatrics can improve outcomes and contribute to the quality of care. Nurses and nursing assistants need education on providing palliative care in long-term care facilities. The ELNEC program provides evidence that education on palliative care does make a difference in quality EOL.

Nursing assistants provide the most direct care for residents and have the least amount of training. Their work is often difficult, with few rewards—salaries are low and there are few benefits. The care provided by nursing assistants is important to residents' quality of life, yet they are often paid little more than minimum wage. Interaction with professional staff is limited because of the demands of the nursing assistants' work. Nursing assistants should be provided with training for their jobs, and salaries should be increased. Efforts need to be made to include nursing assistants as part of the team.

## Environmental Modifications

The environment of nursing homes needs to be changed to promote resident autonomy and quality of life. Residents should be consulted about the type of living arrangement they prefer. For example, some residents may prefer a single room with space for personal belongings, whereas others may appreciate sharing the room with someone for companionship. Nursing homes should be designed to accommodate residents' preferences. Common areas, such as the dining room and lounge, need to be more homelike, with separate conversational areas. Space should be designated for a meditation room to allow residents and families a quiet place. The elderly in nursing homes are often deprived of natural light. Some simple environmental modifications may improve the older adults' visual abilities—for example, using colors to enhance contrast, using curtains to control glare, and placing chairs in positions to enhance illumination. Biological changes occur within the brain in response to different levels of bright-light exposure, and these changes may affect hormones and neurotransmitters responsible for regulating mood, energy, sleep, and appetite. The change of seasons and light and dark affect mood and energy level. In the fall and winter months, when it's dark and cool, people may be more prone to depression and lethargy. Most people feel better on days when the sun is shining. The nursing home environment may be modified to make better use of light by using broad-spectrum fluorescent and daylight-simulating lights.

## Incorporation of Hospice and Palliative Care Concepts

Palliative care concepts should be an integral part of nursing home care. The emphasis of care should be directed toward the quality of life at the EOL. Both the resident and family should participate in care planning. The nursing home environment should be a therapeutic milieu that addresses the physical, psychological, social, and spiritual needs of all residents. Research by nurses is needed to improve EOL care in nursing homes. Nurses can make a difference in the quality of EOL care in nursing homes. It is hoped that the reader will incorporate some of the suggestions discussed in this chapter to make a difference in the delivery of EOL care for nursing home residents.

REFERENCES

1. Miller CA. Nursing for Wellness in Older Adults. Philadelphia, PA: Lippincott Williams & Wilkins, 2008.
2. Kane RL. The evolution of the American nursing home. In Binstock RH, Cluff LE, Von Mering O, eds. The Future of Long-Term Care: Social and Policy Issues. Baltimore, MD: Johns Hopkins University Press; 1996:145–168.
3. Holstein M, Cole TR. The evolution of long-term care in America. In: Binstock RH, Cluff LE, Von Mering O, eds. The Future of Long-Term Care: Social and Policy Issues. Baltimore, MD: Johns Hopkins University Press; 1996:19–48.
4. Houser AN. A Nursing Home Research Report. 2007. AARP Public Policy Institute. Available at: http://www.aarp.org/research/longtermcare/nursinghomes/fs10r_homes.html#FOOT2 (accessed Novemeber 20, 2008).
5. Houser AN, Fox-Grange W, Gibson MJ. Across the States: Profiles of Long-Term Care and Independent Living. 2006. AARP Public Policy Institute. Available at: http://assets.aarp.org/rgcenter/health/d18763_2006_ats.pdf (accessed December 2, 2008).
6. U.S. Bureau of the Census: Statistical Abstracts of the United States: 2002. Washington, DC: U.S. Government Printing Office.
7. Touhy T. Gerontological nursing and an aging society. In Ebersole P, Hess P, Touhy T, Jett K, Luggen AS, eds. Toward Healthy Aging: Human Needs and Nursing Response (7th ed). St. Louis, MO: Mosby Elsevier; 2008:15.
8. U.S. Census Bureau. Press Release: An Older and More Diverse Nation by Midcentury. Released August 14, 2008. Available at: http://www.census.gov/Press-Release/www/releases/archives/population/012496.html (accessed December 4, 2008).
9. Matzo ML, Sherman DW. Gerontological Palliative Care Nursing. St. Louis, MO: C.V. Mobsy Press, 2004.
10. Kane RA. Long-term care and a good quality of life: Bringing them closer together. Gerontologist 2001;42:314–320.
11. Institute of Medicine (IOM). Improving the Quality of Care in Nursing Homes. Washington, DC: National Academy Press, 1986.
12. Marek KD, Rantz MJ, Fagin CM, Krejci JW. OBRA '87 has it resulted in better quality care? J Gerontol Nurs 1996;122:28–36.
13. Cartwright JC. Nursing homes and assisted living facilites as places for dying. Annu Rev Nurs Res 2002;20:231–266.
14. Jones A. The National Nursing Home Survey: 1999 summary. National Center for Health Statistics. Vital Health Stat 2002;13(152):1–125.
15. Magaziner J, German P, Zimmerman SI, et al. The prevalence of dementia in a statewide sample of new nursing home admissions aged 65 and older: Diagnosis by expert panel. Epidemiology of dementia in nursing homes research group. Gerontologist 2000;40:663–672.
16. National Center for Health Statistics. Health United States, 2003. DHHS Publication No. 2003–1232. Hyattsville, MD: U.S. Department of Health and Human Services, 2003.
17. Lunney JR, Lynn J, Hogan C. Profile of older Medicare decedents. J Am Geriatr Soc 2002;50:1108–1112.
18. Mass M, Buckwalter K, Specht J. Nursing staff and quality of care in nursing homes. In Institute of Medicine. Nursing Staff in Hospitals and Nursing Homes: Is It Adequate? Washington, DC: Academy Press; 1986:361–425.
19. Germain C. Cancer Unit: An Ethnography. Wakefield, MA: Nursing Resources, 1979.
20. Glaser BG, Strauss AL. A Time for Dying. Chicago, IL: Aldine Publishing Company, 1968.
21. Mumma CM, Benoliel JQ. Care, cure, and hospital dying trajectories. Omega 1984;85:275–288.
22. Mezey M, Dubler NN, Mitty E, Brody AA. What impact do setting and transitions have on the quality of life at the end of life and the quality of the dying process? Gerontologist 2002;42:54–67.
23. Teno JM, Clarridge BR, Casey V, et al. Family perspective on end of life care in the last place of care. JAMA 2002;291:88–93.
24. Shield R, Wetle T, Teno J, Miller S, Welch L. Physicians "missing in action": Family perspectives on physician and staffing problems in end-of-life care in the nursing home. J Am Geriatr Soc 2005;53:1651–1657.
25. Castle NG, Engberg J. Further examination of the influence of caregiver staffing levels on nursing home quality. Gerontologist 2008;48:464–476.

26. Siegel E, Young H, Mitchell P, Shannon S. Nurse preparation and organizational support for supervision of unlicensed assistive personnel in nursing homes: A qualitative exploration. Gerontologist 2008;48:453–463.

27. Ersek M, Grant M, Kraybill B. Enhancing end-of-life care in nursing homes: Palliative Care Educational Resource Team (PERT) Program. J Palliat Med 2005;8:556–566.

28. Ersek M, Miller Kraybill B, Hansen NR. Evaluation of a train-the-trainer program to enhance hospice and palliative care in nursing homes. J Hosp Palliat Nurs 2006;8:42–49.

29. Welch LC, Miller SC, Martin EW, Nanda A. Referral and timing of referral to hospice care in nursing homes: The significant role of staff members. Gerontologist 2008;48: 477–484.

30. Mitchell SL, Kiely DK, Hamel MB. Dying with advance dementia in a nursing home. J Palliat Med 2004;7:808–816.

31. Resnick HE, Schuur JD, Heineman J, Stone R, Weissman JS. Advance directives in nursing home residents aged ≥65 Years: United States 2004. Am J Hosp Palliat Care 2009;25(6): 476–482.

32. Teno J, Gruneir A, Schwartz Z, Nanda A, Wetle T. Association between advance directives and quality of end of life care: A national study. J Am Geriatr Soc 2007;55:189–194.

33. Semradek J, Gammoth L. Prologue to the future. In Gammoth LM, Semradek J, Tomquist EM, eds. Enchancing Autonomy in Long-term Care: Concepts and Strategies. New York, NY: Springer; 1997:207–218.

34. Wilson SA, Daley BJ. Family perspectives of dying in long term care. J Gerontol Nurs 1999;25(11):19–25.

35. Puchalski DM, ed. A Time for Listening and Caring: Spirituality and the Care of the Chronically Ill and Dying. New York, NY: Oxford University Press, 2006.

36. Ferrell BR, Coyle N, eds. Textbook of Palliative Nursing (2nd ed). New York, NY: Oxford University Press, 2006.

37. .Wilson SA, Daley BJ. Attachment/detachment: Forces influencing care of the dying in long term care. J Palliat Med 1998;1:21–34.

38. Kelly K, Ersek M, Virani R, Mallory P, Ferrell BJ. End-of-life nursing education consortium geriatric training program improving palliative care in community geriatric care settings. J Gerontol Nurs 2008;34(5):29–35.

# 46

*Paula Milone-Nuzzo, Ruth McCorkle, and Elizabeth Ercolano*

## Home Care

*My wife's diagnosis came out of the blue. Even though she had stage 4 ovarian cancer, the doctors started treating her with chemotherapy right after surgery. I thought I could take care of her myself, but when she came home from the hospital we both were unprepared. Several days later she was readmitted and almost died. I knew I had to have help the next time she came home and the home care nurses taught me to help with her care. I don't know why we did not get the help the first time.—Husband of a woman with ovarian cancer*

♦ **Key Points**

♦ Home care for terminal patients can be used to improve their quality of life. Often, home care interventions can be provided on a short-term basis when clients experience a crisis that requires focused interventions.

♦ Nurses are the leaders and essential members of the home care team. Advanced practice nurses can have an impact on the cost, access to, and quality of care provided to terminally ill patients.

♦ Patients with complex problems need family caregivers who are taught to provide care in the home. Caregiving can be extremely stressful for family members and may adversely affect the health of the caregiver. Home care providers should assist family caregivers to maintain their health.

♦ Palliative home care should be provided by a team of providers, including physicians, mental health workers, therapists, nurses, and paraprofessionals.

Originally, palliative care in home care nursing was associated with patients who were clearly near the end of life. The contemporary philosophy of palliative care had its beginnings in England in 1967, when Dame Cicely Saunders founded St. Christopher's Hospice. Home and respite care continue to be a major component of that program. Palliative care, by definition, focuses on the multidimensional aspects of patients and families, including physical, psychological, social, spiritual, and interpersonal components of care. These components of care need to be instituted throughout all phases of the illness trajectory and not only at the point when patients qualify for hospice services. Palliative care also needs to be given across a variety of settings and not be limited to inpatient units.

The primary purpose of palliative care is to enhance the quality and meaning of life and death for both patients and loved ones. To date, health professionals have not used the potential of palliative care to maximize the quality of life of patients in their homes. In this chapter, we discuss home care as an environment that provides unique opportunities to promote palliative care for patients and families throughout their illnesses. The chapter gives background information on what home care is, its historical roots, the types of providers available to give services, the regulatory policies controlling its use, examples of models of palliative home care programs, and recommendations to professionals for facilitating the use of home care in palliative care, concluding with a case study illustrating key elements of palliative care provision in the home.

## Historical Perspective on Home Care Nursing

The period spanning the middle of the 20th century, during which patients were routinely cared for in acute care hospitals, may turn out to have been but a brief period in medical history. Before that time, patients were cared for primarily at home by their families. Today social and economic forces are interacting to avoid hospitalization, if possible, and to return patients home quickly if hospitalized. Although at face value these changes seem positive, they have highlighted gaps and deficiencies in the current health-care delivery system.

Scientific advances have allowed us to keep patients with diseases such as cancer alive increasingly longer despite complex and chronic health problems. The burden of their care usually falls on families, who often are not adequately prepared to handle the physically and emotionally demanding needs for care that are inherent in chronic and progressive illnesses. In addition, family members often become primary care providers within the context of other demands, such as employment outside the home and competing family roles. The necessity among most of the nation's family members to assume employment outside the home and to alter those arrangements when faced with a sick relative has created an immeasurable strain on physical, emotional, and financial resources. The increasing responsibilities of the family in providing care in the face of limited external support and the consequences of that caregiving for patient and family raise important challenges for clinicians.[1]

The origins of home care are found in the practice of visiting nursing, which had its beginnings in the United States in the late 1800s. In 1859, William Rathbone of Liverpool, England, established the modern concept of providing nursing care in the home. Rathbone, a wealthy businessman and philanthropist, set up a system of visiting nursing after a personal experience, when nurses cared for his wife at home before her death. In 1859, with the help of Florence Nightingale, he started a school to train visiting nurses at the Liverpool Infirmary, the graduates of which focused on helping the "sick poor" in their homes.[2]

As in England, caring for the ill in their homes in the United States focused, from its inception, on the poor. Compared to the upper and middle class who received frequent visits from the family physician, either in their homes or in the hospital pay wards, treatment of the sick poor seemed careless at best. Visiting nurse associations (VNAs) in the United States were established by groups of people who wanted to assist the poor to improve their health. In 1885 and 1886, visiting nurse services developed in Buffalo, New York, Boston, and Philadelphia that focused on caring for the middle-class sick as well as the sick poor.[2]

During World War II, as physicians made fewer home visits and focused instead on patients who came to their offices and were admitted to hospitals, the home care movement grew, with nurses providing most of the health and illness care in the home. Up until the mid-1960s, not-for-profit VNAs developed in major cities, small towns, and counties throughout the United States. Under their auspices, nurses focused on providing health services to women and infants and illness care to the poor in their homes, whereas most acute care was provided to patients in hospitals.[2]

The face of home care in the United States changed dramatically with the passage of an amendment to the Social Security Act that enacted Medicare in 1965. Home care changed from almost exclusively care for well mothers and children and the sick poor to a program that focused on care of the sick elderly in their homes. In 1967, there were 1753 home care agencies, a large percentage of which were not-for-profit VNAs. Almost 50 years later, in 2006, there were 8838 home care agencies, with the largest percentage of agencies represented by the proprietary sector.[3] Not only did the types of agencies change, the acuity of patients increased and the development of technology allowed for the delivery of highly complex care in the home setting. The structural changes in the health-care delivery system associated with the passage of the Medicare legislation in 1965 provided the foundation for the contemporary practice of home care nursing in the United States.

The 1990s brought a new challenge, managed care, to healthcare in general and home care specifically in the United States. The most significant impact of managed care on home care was a decrease in the number of visits allowed per patient per episode of illness. The result was a decline in the amount of home care patients received, causing a stabilization of the rapid growth in the home care delivery system. The American Balanced Budget Act of 1997 (PL 105–33) mandated the implementation of a prospective payment system for home care for Medicare beneficiaries. In this system, home care agencies receive a designated dollar amount per episode of illness to provide care for a Medicare patient based on the patient's admitting diagnosis and other factors related to physical and functional status. Just as the Diagnostic Related Group (DRG) system caused a significant decline in the number of hospital beds in the 1980s, the prospective payment system (PPS) for home care has resulted in significant shrinkage of the home health-care industry as a result of patients receiving fewer visits per episode of illness. Between 1998 and 2000, Medicare Home care spending fell from $14 billion to $9.2 billion. One of the major initiatives of PPS was the requirement that all Medicare patients be assessed on admission, every 60 days and at discharge using a standardized assessment tool called Outcomes and Assessment Information Set (OASIS ). This tool is used to determine the patient's case mix weight, which partially defines reimbursement to the home care.[4] As home care agencies have become adept at working within the PPS, utilization of home care service has begun to rebound. Between 2000 and 2006, utilization of home care increased by 26%.[3]

## Definition of Home Care Nursing

Home care, home healthcare, and home care nursing can be confusing terms to both providers and consumers, because they are often used interchangeably. Numerous definitions of home care have been provided by the many professional and trade associations that address home care issues (National Association for Home Care, Consumer's Union, American Hospital Association, American Medical Association, Center for Medicare and Medicaid Services, etc.). Common to all the definitions is the recognition that home care is care of the sick and well in the home by professionals and paraprofessionals, with the goal to improve health, enhance comfort, and improve the quality of life of clients. Home care nursing is defined here as "...the provision of nursing care to acutely ill, chronically ill, terminally ill and well patients of all ages in their residences. Home care nursing focuses on health promotion and care of the sick while integrating environmental, psychosocial, economic, cultural, and personal health factors affecting an individual's and family's health status."[5]

## Home Care Use in the United States

Home care is a diverse industry that provides a broad scope of care to patients of all ages. In 2000, it was estimated that slightly less than 8 million people received home care services for acute illness, long-term health conditions, permanent disability, and terminal illness.[3] Although home care is provided to a large number of people, it still represents a very small percentage of national health-care expenditures. Home care represented only 3% of the total national health expenditure in 2006, whereas hospital care consumed 37% and physician services 25%,[6] demonstrating the cost-efficient nature of home care practice.

The majority of patients (67.5%) who received home care were discharged primarily to urban home care agencies.[7] As the reimbursement for home care visits has decreased and the cost of home visiting in rural areas has increased because of increased travel time, many rural home care agencies have been forced to close, limiting access to home care for the population in the region. The federal government has been inconsistent in its payment of additional dollars to home care agencies that provide care in rural settings.

The demographic picture of home health-care recipients shows a predominately female (63.8%) and white (90.3%) population. The majority (86.1%) of home care patients are age 65 years and older, although home care is provided to patients of all ages, from birth to death. The most common primary diagnosis for home care patients is diseases of the circulatory system, including heart disease. Other common primary diagnoses of patients receiving home care are diseases of the musculoskeletal system and connective tissue, diabetes mellitus, diseases of the respiratory system, endocrine, nutritional, and metabolic diseases and immunity disorders.[3] A primary diagnosis of malignant neoplasm represents only 3.1% of home health-care patients,[3] whereas it accounts for 52% of all patients in hospice.[7] Clearly, non-hospice home care has not been used adequately as an integral part of care for cancer patients and families as they have endured the physical and emotional demands of complex cancer treatments and move across the acute, chronic, and terminal phases of their disease. This is an ideal context in which the need for palliative care should drive an increased use of home care services.

## Types of Home Care Providers

Home care providers are traditionally characterized as either formal or informal caregivers. Informal caregivers are those family members and friends who provide care in the home and are unpaid. It is estimated that almost three-quarters of the elderly with multiple comorbidities and severe disabilities who receive home care rely on family members or other sources of unpaid assistance. The majority of those providing informal home care are female, older than 46 years of age, and are providing assistance approximately 20 hours per week.[1] The type of care provided by informal caregivers ranges from routine custodial care, such as bathing, to sophisticated skilled care, including tracheostomy care and intravenous medication administration. Informal caregivers assume a considerable physiological, psychological, and economic burden in the care of their significant other in the home. When layered on top of existing responsibilities, caregiver tasks compete for time, energy, and attention. As a result, caregivers frequently describe themselves as financially impacted and emotionally and physically drained.[1] In a qualitative study of 15 family caregivers, Strang and Koop[8] found that several factors facilitated or interfered with caregiver coping. One factor that interfered with caregiver coping was the competence of the formal caregiver. When formal caregivers were less than competent, caregiving burden was intensified. The economic cost of providing informal care in the home also places a significant burden on caregivers. With the shift toward community-based care, numerous costs have shifted to the patient and caregiver. Out-of-pocket financial expenditures include medications, transportation, home medical equipment, supplies, and respite services, all of which increase in utilization as the patient's condition worsens.[9] These costs are non-reimbursable and often invisible but are very real to families who are trying to provide care on a fixed income.

Formal caregivers are those professionals and paraprofessionals who are compensated for the in-home care they provide. In 2007, an estimated 867,100 persons were employed in home health agencies. In home care, nurses represent 21% of the formal caregivers providing care to patients in Medicare-certified home care agencies. Home health aides also represent a large proportion of the formal caregivers in home care and are expected to increase in number in upcoming years.[10] Table 46–1 describes the professionals and paraprofessionals who represent the range of home care providers in home health agencies.

## Reimbursement Mechanisms

Home health services are reimbursed by both commercial and government third-party payers as well as by private individuals. Government third-party payers include Medicare,

**Table 46–1**
**Types of Providers in Home Care**

| Type of Provider | Roles and Responsibilities |
|---|---|
| **Nurses** | |
| Registered nurses (RNs) | Deliver skilled care to patients in the home. Considered to be the coordinator of care. |
| Licensed practical nurses (LPNs) | Deliver routine care to patients under the direction of a registered nurse. |
| Advanced practice nurses (APNs) | Coordinate total patient care to complex patients, supervise other nurses in difficult cases related to their specialty, develop special programs, and negotiate for reimbursement of services. Teach patients and caregivers special skills and knowledge. |
| **Therapists** | |
| Physical therapists | Deliver skilled care that includes assessment for assistive devices in the home. Perform therapy procedures with the patient, and teach the patient and family to assist in treatment. Assist patient to improve mobility. Can also serve as coordinator of care for certain patients. |
| Occupational therapists | Focus on improving physical, mental, and social functioning. Rehabilitation of the upper body and improvement of fine motor ability. |
| Speech therapists | Rehabilitation of patients with speech and swallowing problems. |
| Respiratory therapists | Provide support to patients using respiratory home medical equipment such as ventilators. Perform professional respiratory therapy treatments. |
| **Other clinical staff** | |
| Social workers | Help patients and families identify needs and refer to community agencies. Assist with applications for community-based services and provide financial assistance information. |
| Dietitians | Provide diet counseling to patients with special nutritional needs. |
| **Paraprofessionals** | |
| Home health aides | Perform personal care, basic nursing tasks (as opposed to skilled), and incidental homemaking. |
| Homemakers | Homemakers perform housekeeping and chores to ensure a safe and healthy home care environment. |

Medicaid, Tricare, and the Veterans Administration system. These government programs have specific requirements that must be met for the coverage of services. Commercial third-party payers include insurance companies, health maintenance organizations (HMOs), preferred provider organizations (PPOs), and case management programs. Commercial insurers often allow for more flexibility in their requirements than Medicare. For example, the home care nurse may negotiate with an insurance company to obtain needed services for the patient on the basis of the cost-effectiveness of the home care plan, although that service may not be routinely covered.

## Medicare

Medicare is a federal insurance program for the elderly (65 years and older), the permanently disabled, and persons with end-stage renal disease in the United States and is the single largest payer for home health services. To be eligible for this program, an individual or spouse must have paid into Social Security. Medicare is a federal program and, as such, the benefits are the same from state to state. The Centers of Medicare and Medicaid Services (CMS), a department in the federal government, regulates payments for services under

Medicare. The Centers of Medicare and Medicaid Services contracts with insurance companies called fiscal intermediaries to process Medicare claims that are submitted from home care agencies.

Since agencies are now reimbursed using a prospective payment methodology, home care has gained increased flexibility for the services provided under Medicare. In the former fee-for-service model, designated and specific home care providers were paid for each visit made. Today, home care agencies are responsible for assuring that the patients achieve their health outcomes in the most efficient manner. If a home care agency suggests the most effective plan of care would be to integrate alternative and complementary therapies or mental health therapy into a patient's plan of care, it will not reduce or increase the amount of payment received from the government.

There are five criteria (summarized in Table 46–2) that a patient must meet for home care services to be reimbursed by Medicare.

Medicare is the main payer of hospice services in the United States under the Medicare Hospice Benefit, which Congress first enacted as part of Medicare Part A in 1982 under the Tax Equity and Fiscal Responsibility Act (TEFRA;

**Table 46–2**
**Criteria for Home Care Reimbursement Under Medicare**

| Criterion | Description |
|---|---|
| Homebound | A patient is considered homebound if absences from the home are rare and short of duration and attributable to the need to receive medical treatments. |
| Completed plan of care | A plan of care for home care services must be completed in Centers for Medicare and Medicaid services (CMS) forms 485 and 487. The plan of care must be signed by a physician. |
| Skilled service | Medicare defines skilled service as one provided by a registered nurse, physical therapist, or speech therapist. Skilled nursing services include skilled observation and assessment, teaching, direct care and management, and evaluation of the plan of care. |
| Intermittent and part-time | Part-time means that skilled care and home health aide services combined may not exceed 8 hours per day or 28 hours per week. Intermittent means that skilled care is provided or needed on fewer than 7 days per week or less than 8 hours of each day for periods of 21 days or less, with extensions for exceptional circumstances. |
| Reasonable and necessary | The services provided must be reasonable for the patient given the diagnosis and necessary to assist the patient to achieve the expected outcomes. |

P.L. 97-248). The law was in effect from 1983 until 1986, when Congress made hospice a permanent part of the Medicare program.[11] The impetus behind Medicare's hospice benefit came from the recognition that the regulations and restrictions for traditional Medicare were not well-suited to meet the needs of terminally ill patients.

Medicare hospice was designed primarily as a home care benefit that included an array of services to assist care providers in the clinical management of the terminally ill in the home.[12] However, the regulations for hospice care also require home care providers to have in-patient hospice beds available for terminally ill patients who are unable to remain in their homes. Recognizing that hospice is a philosophy of care rather than a place for care, it seems appropriate that hospice care is given in a variety of settings.

For a patient to elect the Hospice Medicare benefit, the patient must waive the traditional Medicare benefit. By electing the Hospice Medicare benefit, the patient is acknowledging the terminal nature of the illness and opting no longer to have curative treatment.

## Medicaid

Medicaid is an assistance program for the poor, some disabled persons, and children. Unlike Medicare, Medicaid is jointly sponsored by the federal government and the individual states. Therefore, Medicaid coverage varies from state to state. These differences can often be dramatic and in some cases dependent on the state's financial solvency. Eligibility for Medicaid is based on income and assets and is not contingent on any previous payments to the federal or state governments.

Unlike the requirements of the Medicare program, Medicaid covers both skilled and unskilled care in the home and usually does not require that the recipient be homebound. To qualify for the home care benefits under Medicaid,

patients must meet income eligibility requirements and have a plan of care signed by a physician, and the plan of care must be reviewed by a physician every 60 days.

## Commercial Insurance

Many commercial insurance companies are involved in health insurance for individuals or groups. These local or national companies often write policies that include a home care benefit. Commercial insurers often cover the same services covered by Medicare in addition to preventive, private duty, and supportive services, such as a home health aide or homemaker. Commercial insurance companies cover patients of all ages, including Medicare patients with supplemental insurance policies that cover health-care expenditures not reimbursed by Medicare.

Supplemental insurance policies are a source of confusion and anxiety among home care patients, often when families are under increased stress because of the complexity of the health situation for one of its members. Nurses should encourage families to carefully review the specifics of the supplemental insurance policy, including copays, annual review of benefits, anticipated out-of-pocket costs, and pharmacy costs. Families should recognize that when changing a supplemental insurance carrier, you may also have to change the home care provider, because some supplemental policies state which home care provider will be reimbursed for services.

Commercial insurance often includes a maximum lifetime benefit as part of the policy. The high cost of high-technology care forces a growing number of patients to reach this maximum rather quickly and face the loss of coverage. This has resulted in the development of case-management programs administered by insurance companies. The case manager projects the long-term needs and costs of care for the patient and develops a plan with the patient to meet those needs in a cost-efficient manner. Consideration is given to the life expectancy of the patient in relationship to the maximum lifetime benefit.

Unlike the Medicare program, in which negotiation for services is not an option, it may be important for home care nurses to identify the needed services for a patient with a commercial insurance plan and intervene to obtain funding for those services. When working with an insurance case manager, the home care nurse must be specific about the services the patient will need, the overall cost of those services, and the expected outcome related to the services requested. The more precisely the home care nurse can portray the impact of the care plan on the patient outcomes with objective data, the more inclined the case manager will be to authorize services. Insurance companies are very concerned with the satisfaction of their enrollees. Patients and families should be empowered to make their voices heard about the services they need to remain safe in the home. If out-of-network services or special pricing is negotiated with the insurance case manager, written documentation of the agreement should be included in the patient's record. Ideally, the patient should be given a copy of this agreement in the event that any disputes over payment occur.

## The Home Health–Hospice Connection

For a patient to receive the full array of hospice services under Medicare, the care must be provided by a certified hospice provider. To be reimbursed, home care agencies that are not certified hospice providers must refer their terminally ill patients to an agency that carries the certification. This regulation affects clinical care in several ways. Home care nurses have a long history of developing strong and intimate bonds with patients and families. As patients progress toward the terminal phase of their illnesses, it is emotionally difficult for home care nurses to refer their patients to hospice providers. At times, it is equally as difficult for a family to accept the referral, knowing that they will have to give up "their nurse." The home care nurse and the family may believe that the relationship that has developed among the patient, the family, and the home care nurse is more important than any additional benefits the hospice might bring.

Although families may feel that they are getting sufficient home care in the terminal phases of the patient's life from their traditional home care agency, they are not able to take advantage of the prescription drug components of the hospice benefit, which may result in significant financial burden. They also usually do not receive supportive services such as pastoral care and bereavement follow-up, which are integral to the hospice program. Because the emotional impact of the patient's death is unknown at the time the patient makes the decision to forego a hospice referral, it is impossible to predict the significance of a service such as bereavement follow-up. In addition, hospice nurses are skilled in pain management in the terminal phases of life. This is one of the areas in which hospice care can be most effective for patients and their families. The non-hospice home health agency and the hospice provider offer important services, especially nursing care to patients at the end of life; strengthening mechanisms that facilitate transitions between these two types of services is essential. See Chapter 2 for a comprehensive discussion of the hospice admission criteria, including the certification by the physician of a terminal diagnosis and the six-month rule.

## Cancer as a Prototype for Home Care Use in Palliative Care

Over the years cancer has shifted from a terminal illness to a chronic disease. Patients with advanced disease and guarded prognoses initially may be treated as if their disease is curable rather than progressive and terminal. Although the philosophical underpinnings and goals of curative and palliative treatments are quite different, an individual who has advanced disease is often treated first with a curative approach.[13] During this time, it is important that there is frequent communication among the patient, family, and health-care team as the disease, its stage, and the patient's response to treatment is understood.[14,15] The course of the patient's disease depends on the type of cancer and its biology. Some courses are faster than others and some patients often experience disease-free intervals and multiple treatments before the cancer becomes terminal.[16] The experience of living with progressive disease and effects of the treatment can have physical, social, and emotional consequences that ultimately affect the patient's quality of life. Characteristics of advanced cancer that require coordinated palliative care include multiple physical needs, intense emotional distress manifested by anxiety and depression, and complex patient and caregiver needs. The goals of palliative care are best achieved if care is initiated early, and one of the most efficient ways of monitoring patients' needs is to coordinate the overall plan of management with home nursing care during times of crisis to decrease fragmentation and promote continuity.

## Needs of Patients With Cancer and Their Caregivers

Because of the continued trend to discharge hospitalized patients as soon as possible, the increasing use of ambulatory care services, and the increasing use of complex therapies, the needs for ongoing monitoring and teaching of patients and families has never been greater. Family members, often without the assistance of any formal home care services, are assuming primary responsibility for the care of patients at home.[17] This demand on families is not new, although the caregiver role has changed dramatically from promoting convalescence to providing high-technology care and psychological support in the home. Members of a patient's family are of vital importance in meeting the patient's physical and psychological needs and accomplishing treatment goals.[18] Cancer family caregivers represent a sizable and diverse segment of the population who are making major contributions to their families, communities, and the health-care system, often at the expense of their own health and well-being.[19]

Research to identify patient-defined home care needs began in the 1980s and has increased steadily since the 1990s. An early study identified pain, sleep, and elimination management as major patient needs.[20] Wellisch and colleagues[21] investigated the types and frequency of problems experienced by two separate groups of seriously ill cancer patients and their families in their homes in the Los Angeles area and explored the types of interventions that helped to reduce the problems. The five most frequent problem categories identified included somatic side effects, including pain; patient mood disturbance; equipment/technology problems; family relationship impairment; and patient cognitive impairment. Interventions reported to be effective included reinforcement to the patient and family, counseling, and emotional support. They noted that patients with cognitive deficits had special needs, and their family members were at high risk for ongoing problems. Although these two studies were accomplished more than 25 years ago, the findings remain relevant today. There have been numerous review articles that have documented these needs across the disease and treatment courses.[22,23] Evidence suggests that both patients and their families benefit from home care services directed at their needs, including physical and psychological distress.[24,25]

Similarly, numerous review articles have summarized the needs of family members who provide care to patients with cancer.[26-30] Generally, researchers have found that a significant number of cancer caregivers exhibit psychological distress and physical symptoms throughout the palliative phase of care. Predictors of caregiver distress included a number of patient-related variables, including more advanced stages of cancer, younger age, disability, and complex care needs.[31,32] In addition, there have been a number of individual studies to document the specific needs of caregivers. For example, Carter[33] described sleep and depressive symptoms in 47 caregivers of patients with advanced cancer and found severe fluctuations in sleep patterns. Caregivers reported they suffered progressive sleep deprivation that affected their emotions and ability to continue as caregivers. Others have shown that the patient's physical status and severity of their symptoms affected caregiver's activity restriction, financial loss, and levels of intimacy[34] as well as psychological status, including both depression [35-37] and anxiety.[38-40] There is no question that patients have a better quality of life when they have an informed and competent caregiver at home; however, the financial burden of caregiving may prevent many family members from assisting. In 2001, the annual cost associated with family caregiving to individuals with cancer was conservatively estimated at $1 billion dollars.[41] This cost evaluation is based on survey data from the Asset and Health Dynamic Study (AHEAD; $n = 7443$), accounting solely for direct patient care hours and valuing those hours at $8.17/hour. The cost of family caregiving far exceeds $1 billion dollars when one considers the health and social consequences incurred by the caregiver. Cancer family caregivers are a valuable and indispensable resource whose needs should be accurately identified so that interventions to support their caregiving can be efficiently tested and supplied.

Patients and caregivers consistently report the need for information.[42,43] Their search for information can be extensive, as they use many sources for obtaining information, including the Internet. Caregivers may be more active than patients in seeking information, and often initiate a search for information to supplement the information provided by health professionals. Caregivers need information about specific treatments, what to expect, the ways to manage symptoms, and available community resources. Caregivers also need information on the emotional aspects of the illness and patients' expected course of recovery, both physically and emotionally.[44] Table 46–3 summarizes the patient and caregiver's needs for information over the course of illness and can vary from one phase to another.[45]

In general, the literature on the needs of cancer patients and caregivers of cancer patients highlights: (1) that patients are increasingly being treated in ambulatory clinics and have ongoing, unmet complex care needs with little or no use of home or palliative care referrals; (2) that caregivers are assuming more and more responsibility for monitoring patients' status and providing direct care in the home with little instruction or opportunities for respite; (3) that as patients' physical status changes, caregivers have a high proportion of unmet needs themselves; (4) that the caregiving experience encompasses both positive and negative elements[46]; and (5) that the conceptualization of caregiver burden is linked to negative reactions to caregiving.[47]

## Models of the Delivery of Palliative Care

Although the field of palliative care is still a relatively new discipline, there have been major advances in the establishment of programs—primarily hospital-based programs with recent expansion to outpatient clinics.[48,49] Many of these programs have demonstrated significant improvements in symptom management and satisfaction with care. There has been little research specifically testing the effects of home care interventions on patient outcomes in palliative care.[50] For palliative care to flourish in home care, there must be systems that can facilitate it and clinicians who are knowledgeable about the state of the science. A growing body of evidence suggests that input from specialists in palliative care can improve the quality of patient care and reduce costs.[51,52] Kuebler and Bruera recommend a collaborative consultative Internet relationship to support clinicians in providing comprehensive palliative

**Table 46–3**
**Information Needs of Patients and Caregivers Throughout Palliative Care**

| Diagnostic Phase | Hospital Phase | Treatment Phase | Survivorship Phase | Recurrent Phase |
|---|---|---|---|---|
| • Type and purpose of diagnostic procedures that will be performed<br>• When test results can be expected<br>• The person who is coordinating the care<br>• Common emotions that develop while awaiting diagnosis (e.g., anxiety, uncertainty)<br>• How to talk to people about the diagnosis<br>• Making treatment decisions, pros/cons of options | • Type of surgery planned<br>• When pathology report will be available<br>• Expected length of hospitalization and time to recover<br>• Role limitations to anticipate when patient is discharged<br>• The effects of illness on other family members<br>• Concerns about pain and other common symptoms | • Type and length of treatments planned<br>• Anticipated side effects and when they may occur<br>• Ways to reduce side effects<br>• Likelihood of temporary role changes<br>• Availability of education, support groups, and community resources<br>• How and who to talk with about the patient's or caregiver's unresolved concerns | • When follow-up exams or tests are necessary<br>• Common concerns during this phase (e.g., fear of recurrence)<br>• Importance of balancing needs of patient and family<br>• Availability of education, support groups, and community resources<br>• Adjusting to a new self-image<br>• Working after cancer treatment, financial issues | • Type of treatment planned<br>• Anticipated side effects, when they may occur, and ways to manage them<br>• Common feelings during this phase (e.g., uncertainty, sadness, fear, growth)<br>• Ways to maintain hope regardless of recurrence<br>• Availability of support groups and community resources |

interventions for patients in a timely manner. They tested the model between a rural palliative care nurse practitioner and an urban medical research physician. Preliminary results show promise, and its potential success could enhance care of the persons living within underserved or remote areas around the world.[53] Many countries, other than the United States, provide healthcare with government support and realize the potential cost savings.[54,55] These countries have delivered palliative care in the patient's home successfully for a number of years, including Great Britain, Canada, Sweden, Italy and Australia. Also, France has instituted three levels of home care, with the most recent including specialized home care for cancer patients with the assistance of pharmacists.[56]

## Patient and Caregiver Palliative Care Interventions

Nurse counseling or care management is the most frequently studied approach to delivering information and support to cancer patients and their caregivers. Earlier meta-analyses of randomized trials of nursing interventions suggest that many are effective in reducing symptoms of cancer or its treatment[57] as well as symptoms of anxiety, depression, and psychological distress.[58] However, because of the mixture of different intervention components, these meta-analyses are of limited help in identifying the intervention elements that contribute to their effectiveness. Randomized trials conducted by McCorkle[59] and others[60–62] have demonstrated that nursing interventions directed at improving patient and family self-management skills have reduced symptoms, improved function, reduced re-hospitalizations, improved mood and mental

health status, reduced psychological distress, and improved survival among patients during cancer treatment. Cognitive behavioral interventions with an emphasis on problem-solving delivered by trained oncology nurses have been shown to reduce symptoms.[60] To illustrate, Given and colleagues[62] tested a cognitive behavioral intervention among solid tumor patients undergoing chemotherapy that began with collaborative problem identification by patient and nurse. The nurse would then propose interventions that would be collaboratively evaluated, and an action plan would be developed. These were supported by classes focused on self-management, problem-solving, and communication with providers. Those receiving the experimental intervention reported significantly less severe symptoms at 10- and 20-week follow-ups. Efforts to give patients with cancer and their families the information, skills, and confidence needed to manage the physical, psychosocial, and communication challenges associated with cancer and its care seem warranted by the literature. Progress in this area could be accelerated by the systematic use by home care nurses through the Internet[63]; access to the researchers' symptom management toolkit is readily on the Web for both clinicians and patients.[64]

There have also been several literature reviews of interventions conducted with caregivers of patients with cancer.[65,66] Northouse and McCorkle categorized the interventions described in these studies into four broad intervention areas: (1) supportive-educative, (2) caregiving skills/symptom management, (3) coping skills, and (4) relationship-focused interventions.[67–71] These are not necessarily discrete categories because some interventions address more than one area. The reviews indicate that positive results related to improvement in caregivers' coping skills and knowledge. Studies that focused on education for palliative and hospice care had a tendency to show decreases in caregiver stress.[72] In addition, there have been a number of programs developed to teach caregivers direct care responsibilities for patients in the home that have had positive outcomes on patients and caregivers.[73,74] Unfortunately the majority of this evidenced-based research rarely is adopted into clinical practice.

## Recommendations for Facilitating the Use of Home Care Nursing in Palliative Care

Home care nursing is an ideal mechanism to deliver effective palliative care; however, for a number of reasons, it has been underutilized. Patients who need palliative care have complex and often challenging physical and psychological problems. Palliative care for specific types of diseases requires knowledgeable and competent clinicians. It is common for professional staff nurses in home care agencies to lack the knowledge and expertise to manage patients' symptoms and to teach caregivers the skills they need to manage the day-to-day problems they encounter in caregiving. And yet repeatedly, home care nurses are placed in the position of being responsible for patients who have palliative care needs. One potential solution is to teach the staff to use evidence-based research to remain current in the advances in palliative care. The rationale for promoting evidence-based palliative care is straightforward, but there are major challenges to achieving the goal of translating palliative care research into everyday clinical practice. Maybe the most difficult challenge is persuading the staff to change how they deliver care.[75] Schumacher and colleagues used standard pain management strategies to teach the staff to change their practice in the home.[76] Another successful strategy has been the use of medication kits containing prescription medications to treat pain and dyspnea to use with dying patients as they approach death.[77] In addition, for palliative care to be successful in the home, physicians and other experts must work collaboratively with nurses and be available to solve problems as they arise. It is often easier for physicians to admit patients to the hospital than to work with home care nurses to keep patients at home.

The state of the science in home care was reviewed for this chapter. Results from these studies have not been systematically incorporated into clinical practice where services are reimbursed. However, we identified critical factors in these studies that, if adopted, could become the basis of successful home care palliative nursing. These include the following:

1. *Staff nurses who are responsible for direct patient care in the home must have contact with experts who have specialized knowledge and skills related to the disease-specific needs of patients.*

   Experts can include any member of a palliative care program, but usually include an advanced practice nurse (APN) or palliative care physician. The term "advanced

practice nurse" used here is defined as a professional nurse, including clinical nurse specialists and nurse practitioners, who has graduated from a master's program in a specialty field such as an oncology advanced practice program. To assist the staff nurse in dealing with the complexity of palliative care, either a palliative care physician or an APN should serve as a supervisor/consultant to the team and be directly involved in clinical decisions. There may be fewer than needed opportunities for APNs working directly in home care agencies because of the perception that they are too costly to employ. As agencies move to prospective payment and greater efficiency, the role of the APN may factor more prominently in home care agencies. Advanced practice nurses may also work independently and provide care to a group of patients, such as case managers from an ambulatory clinic. As a result of the Balanced Budget Act of 1997 (PL 105-55), APNs—specifically clinical nurse specialists and nurse practitioners—practicing in any setting can be directly reimbursed at 85% of the physician fee schedule for services provided to Medicare beneficiaries. In home care, this change has the potential to facilitate access to care for patients who do not have access to a home care agency or other primary care provider, specifically those in rural and underserved areas.

2. *Because of the barriers to entering hospice care, home care nurses must become knowledgeable and highly skilled in providing palliative care to patients.*

   This will require not only the development of skills in a new area of clinical expertise but also a paradigm shift in the way home care nurses view the episode of care for patients in the home. Home care has traditionally been viewed as a component of the long-term care delivery system. Although the number of home visits per episode of illness has decreased significantly, home visits tend to be spread out over a greater period of time, usually a 60-day certification period. For patients requiring palliation, home care may need to be very intensive over a relatively short period of time (2–4 weeks). In this model, the home care nurse can assist the patient and family in methods of managing symptoms and coping with the caregiving role. In the long term, as the patient's disease progresses, the patient and caregivers will need "booster" visits, but the majority of visits and care may be given in short periods of time, when the patient and caregivers are most in need. Telephone visits to provide care have been shown to be an effective strategy for chronic illnesses in which the needs are for support and education. Home care can also be used for short durations in crisis situations. By providing intensive home care for short durations, patients can be helped to address current issues in the most effective way. These short but intensive interventions can improve quality of life and may also impact survival outcomes for some patients.

3. *Patients are usually hospitalized when symptoms get out of control and their disease is unstable. When patients are hospitalized, comprehensive discharge planning and follow-up by nurses skilled in palliative care is needed to ensure that the plan is implemented, evaluated, and modified as needed.*

Patients with complex problems including distressing symptoms need assistance to make a smooth transition from the hospital to their homes, and caregivers need access to information, skills training, and resources to help with providing essential assistance. A referral to a home care agency may also be necessary for successful outcomes. The complexity of symptom management following hospitalization may require the advanced skills of an APN or other expert in palliative care to provide consultation to the home care nurse or to implement a plan of care with a patient and family. Access to these nurses may be based in a variety of settings, such as hospital-based clinics, private offices, and home care agencies. The multidisciplinary care provided by nurses, physicians, paraprofessionals, social workers, chaplains, and pharmacists is essential to the development of positive outcomes. As members of the multidisciplinary team, physicians must work in collaboration with other professionals across settings to provide comprehensive care to patients and families. Collaboratively, the team determines the amount of care needed, the most appropriate setting for care, and the type of interventions required to improve the patient's quality of life.

4. *Patients who have complex problems and receive home care nursing need family caregivers who are willing and able to learn the skills to provide care.*

Standardized educational programs to teach family caregivers skills to provide care are needed and should be a part of routine home nursing care.

In the event these caregivers are ill themselves, additional or complementary services need to be provided to help with the patients' care. Nurses providing home care for ill patients should conduct ongoing assessments of family caregivers, including their health and demands made upon them.

5. *The use of innovative models must be considered as a strategy for providing care to patients and families.*

Telephone visits have been shown to be an effective strategy to help families cope with the caregiver role. Traditionally, specific criteria have been used to define the requirements for home care services. These criteria need to be re-examined in light of our increased understanding of disease patterns, treatment effects, and patient responses to illness. In the future, we need to consider alternative ways of delivering services to patients and family caregivers. Telephone contacts have been shown to be an effective strategy to help families cope with the

caregiver role. Under prospective payment for home care, home care providers are no longer constrained by the per-visit method of reimbursement, and telephone visits can be integrated into the plan of care. The use of alternative and complementary therapy, nutritional counseling or mental health therapies has been made financially reasonable as a result of the move to prospective payment. Telehealth programs have also been used effectively with patient populations at home.[78] Other technology interventions could include the use of the Internet or E-mail.[79] As the technology becomes less expensive, increased opportunity to implement these strategies will occur.

A growing number of cancer patients are being discharged from the hospital following surgery or other cancer treatments to be cared for at home by family caregivers who have chronic illnesses themselves, as described by the following case study.

CASE STUDY
## Mrs. W, a Woman with Stage IV Ovarian Cancer

Ms. W was a 66-year-old semi-retired nurse behavioral therapist with stage 4 ovarian cancer treated by total abdominal hysterectomy and additional surgery because of metastases in the abdominal cavity. Because of the advanced stage of her cancer, she was treated with one course of carboplatin and paclitaxol during her hospital stay. Ms. W's other medical history included diverticulosis and depression. She lived with her husband Richard, a 68-year-old psychotherapist. Their three adult children lived out-of-state and were not available to assist her postsurgery.

Ms. W was discharged home within 6 days of her surgery without home care services. Within 2 days, she noted redness and swelling around her incision site, and her temperature was elevated to 101 degrees. She also was experiencing diminished appetite, diarrhea, loss of stamina, sleep disturbance, and forgetfulness and remained bed-bound, with occasional trips to the bathroom. She required assistance with bathing and dressing. Concerned about changes in the appearance of her incision and elevated temperature, she visited the gynecological–oncology APN before her scheduled postoperative visit. During the office visit, Ms. W's husband expressed his concern about his wife's appetite problems and loss of independence. He also identified himself as a willing caregiver but expressed feeling overwhelmed trying to balance his work and home demands.

The APN assessed an unstable situation at home, ordered skilled home nursing visits twice a day to manage the wound, and requested home health aide care to assist Ms. W with her activities of daily living. She counseled the couple to arrange for homemaker services to assist with meal preparation and housekeeping. Because of the unstable course of Ms. W's illness and the potential for her to decline further from ongoing, rigorous chemotherapy approximately every 3 weeks, her oncology APN contacted

Ms. W by phone twice a week between office visits. The APN used the phone conversations to assess symptoms, alter plans of care around any troubling symptoms, and assess progress toward independence in activities of daily living. The APN relied on the home care nurses to provide information about the status of her wound and whether the home resources were effective. Within a month, Ms. W had made substantial progress; her wound had healed and she was able to function independently, although fatigue interfered with her quality of life and her capacity to resume her full prediagnosis schedule. Because of Ms. W's positive physical health outcomes, her home care nurses discontinued their services after a month of care. However, during an office with her APN, Ms. W expressed feeling distressed about her persistent sleep disturbance and a generalized feeling of anxiety. The APN approached Ms. W about contacting a psychotherapist for an evaluation of her symptoms. Ms. W agreed and entered into psychotherapy with medication management. The APN also counseled Ms. W about strategies to self-manage those chronic features of her illness, including fatigue, anxiety, and minor neuropathy in her fingers. They also outlined self-management strategies to promote her general health.

Upon completion of her course of chemotherapy nearly 6 months after her surgery, Ms. W was able to resume work on a part-time basis and traveled out-of-state with her husband to visit their children. She acknowledged feeling confident about her ability to live in a quality way with the chronic aspects of her disease. Her husband reported a relief from his earlier distress.

Ms. W's cancer remained in remission for another 6 months. When the disease progressed, chemotherapy was initiated again. Complications of this progression were abdominal ascites, constipation, difficulty breathing, weakness, loss of appetite, and generalized pain. She became increasingly sedentary and relied more and more on her husband. Ms. W and her husband wanted to continue chemotherapy, and she wanted to remain in her home, a decision that her husband endorsed. The APN instituted palliative care services in the home, consisting of skilled nursing visits, home health aide support, and counseling by palliative care social worker and pastoral staff. Ms. W's plan of care included pain management, nutritional and bowel management, support with activities of daily living, and psychological and spiritual counseling. Ms. W's psychotherapist agreed to phone conversations to deal with Ms. W's feelings around her physical decline. The APN worked closely with the palliative care social worker, who periodically visited Ms. W and her husband. The social worker spent time with her husband, helping him to prepare for the inevitable outcome. Ms. W received weekly chemotherapy directed toward controlling the spread of the cancer to bring symptom relief. Despite the resources in her home, Ms. W fell, requiring hospitalization. During her inpatient stay, she developed a delirium that was resistant to treatment. She became less able to engage in her care and relate to others. The inpatient social worker, acting on direction from Ms. W's APN and gynecological-oncologist, presented the option of inpatient hospice care to her husband. Although grief-stricken, he agreed, and Ms. W died at the inpatient hospice 1 week later with her husband by her side. The APN visited Mr. W 2 weeks after his wife's death. They reviewed the care Ms. W had received, and the nurse reinforced what a good job he did with helping her stay at home for as long as she did. Mr. W's grief gradually lessened; he was contacted several times by the nurse and social worker to assess how he was adjusting.

## Summary

For palliative care to be a viable component of the service provided by home care agencies, changes are needed in both the structure of home care and the mechanisms for reimbursement. The regulations for the provision of home care under Medicare must be substantively modified to allow increased access to palliative care. Under the current regulations in the United States, the physician is the only provider who has the ability to order and to supervise a home plan of care through home care agencies. The literature is consistent in its description of the positive role APNs play in supporting both the patient and family caregivers in the home, yet APNs are not given the authority to direct patient care through home care agencies for patients who need palliative care. Exceptions do exist through hospital-based programs. For example, Memorial Sloan Kettering Cancer Center (New York) has a successful hospital-based supportive care program that provides palliative care in the home for patients. This program is directed by an APN, and services are billed through the outpatient service. Regulations that support the critical role APNs play in the clinical management of patients at home who require palliative care and that legitimize the APN's ability to order and to supervise the plan of care are essential. The few successful models in hospital-based and ambulatory clinics could be implemented in home care agencies.

Additionally, the historical structure of Medicare reimbursement was a disincentive for the use of APNs in home care agencies. Because of the regulatory changes in reimbursement to prospective payment, APNs could play an increasingly important role in the delivery of effective home care. As the demographics of the home care population change and the complexity of clinical problems increase, agencies can ill afford to be without expert clinical providers or, at the very least, access to consultative services.

The earlier case study had a successful outcome, although the current home care delivery system is fragmented; however, the care in this case was effective because it was under the coordination of a palliative care team based in a cancer comprehensive center. The need for palliative care to be integrated into both home care as well as hospice care is essential for the provision of a continuum of care to patients at the end of life. For these changes to be integrated into the care delivery system, regulations need to be changed to allow home care nurses to provide end-of-life care in situations in which hospice care is unavailable, or at the request of the patient or family. Creative strategies are needed to translate effective evidence-based interventions into standard clinical care, such as access to resources through the Internet.

In summary, home care is an important component of palliative care. Clinical and regulatory barriers have forced palliative care in the home to be provided by certified hospices at the end of life. Structural changes in home care are needed to fully integrate palliative care into the home care delivery system and at different times of crisis throughout the illness course. Additionally, the role of APNs must be fully acknowledged and reimbursement mechanisms established to integrate palliative care into home care for both patients and family caregivers.

REFERENCES

1. American Association for Retired People, Valuing the Invaluable; The Economic Value of Family Caregiving, 2008 Update. Available at: http://www.aarp.org/research/housing-mobility/caregiving/i13_caregiving.html (accessed November 25, 2008).
2. Clement-Stone S, Eigsti D, McGuire S. Comprehensive Health Nursing (4th ed). St. Louis, MO: Mosby, 1995.
3. National Association for Home Care. Basic Statistics about Home Care, updated 2008. Available at: http://www.nahc.org/facts/08HC_Stats.pdf (accessed December 1, 2008).
4. Centers for Medicare and Medicaid Services, OASIS Background. Available at: http://www.cms.hhs.gov/OASIS/02_Background.asp#TopOfPage (accessed December 6, 2008).
5. American Nurses Association. HomeHealth Nursing: Scope and Standards of Practice. Silver Springs, MA: American Nurses Association, 2008.
6. Keehan S, Sisako A, Truffler C, Smith S, Sisko A, Cowan C. Health spending projections through 2017 the baby boom generation is coming to medicare. Health Aff 2008;27(2):w145–w155.
7. National Center for Health Statistics, Health, United States 2005 with Chartbook on Trends of the Health of Americans. Hyattsville, MD, 2005.
8. Strang V, Koop PM. Factors which influence coping: Home-based family caregiving of persons with advanced cancer. J Palliat Care 2003;19:107.
9. Zhu CW, Scarmeas N, Torgan R, et al. Clinical characteristics and longitudinal changes of informal cost of Alzheimer's disease in the community. J Am Geriatr Soc 2006;10:1596–1602.
10. U. S. Department of Labor, Bureau of Labor Statistics. National Industry-Occupation Employment Matrix: Data for 2006. Washington, DC: 2006. Available at: http://data.bls.gov/oep/servlet/oep.nioem.servlet.ActionServlet (accessed December 15, 2008).
11. U. S. House of Representatives. Committee on Ways and Means, 1998 Green Book. Washington, DC: 105th Congress, 2nd session, 1998.
12. National Association for Home Care, Hospice Facts and Stats, updated 2008. Available at: http://www.nahc.org/facts/HospiceStats08.pdf (accessed December 5, 2008).

13. Harrington S, Smith T. The role of chemotherapy at the end-of-life: "When is enough, enough?" JAMA 2008;299:2667–2678.
14. Kirk P, Kirk I, Kristjanson L. What do patients receiving palliative care for cancer and their families want to be told? A Canadian and Australian qualitative study. BMJ 2004;328:1343–1347.
15. Schfield P, Carey M, Love A, Nehill C, Wein S. Would you like to talk about your future treatment option? Discussing the transition from curative cancer treatment to palliative care. Palliat Med 2006;20:397–406.
16. Murray S, Kendall M, Boyd K, Sheikh A. Illness trajectories and palliative care. BMJ 2002;330:611–612.
17. Given BA, Given CW, Kozachik S. Family support in advanced cancer. CA Cancer J Clin 2001;51:213–231.
18. Hudson P, Aranda S, Kristjanson L. Meeting the supportive needs of family caregivers in palliative care: Challenges for health professionals. J Palliat Med 2004;7:19–25.
19. Haley WE, LaMonde LA, Han B, Narramore S, Schonwetter R. Family caregiving in hospice: Effects on psychological and health functioning among spousal caregivers of hospice patients with lung cancer or dementia. Hospice J 2001;15:1–18.
20. Googe MC, Varricchio CG. A pilot investigation of home health care needs of cancer patients and their families. Oncol Nurs Forum 1981;8:24–28.
21. Wellisch D, Fawzy F, Landsverk J, Pasnau R, Wocott D. Evaluation of psychosocial problems of the home-bound patient: The relationship of disease and sociodemographic variables of patients to family problems. J Psychosoc Oncol 1983;1:1–15.
22. Teunissen S, Wesker W, Kruitwagen C, et al. Symptom prevalence in patients with incurable cancer: A systematic review. J Pain Symptom Manage 2007;34:94–104.
23. Whitmer K, Pruemer J, Nahleh Z, et al. Symptom management needs of oncology outpatients. J Palliat Med 2006;9:628–630.
24. Peters L, Sellick K. Quality of life of cancer patients receiving inpatient and home based palliative care. J Adv Nurs 2006;53(5):524–533.
25. McCorkle R, Dowd M, Ercolano E, et al. Effects of a nursing intervention on quality of life outcomes in post-surgical women with gynecological cancers. Psychooncology 2009;18(1):62–70.
26. Finlay J, Higginson I, Goodwin D, et al. Palliative care in hospital, hospice, at home: Results from a systematic review. Ann Oncol 2002;13(Suppl):257–264.
27. Northouse LL. The impact of cancer on family: Overview of the literature. Int J Psychiatry Med 1984;14(3):87–113.
28. Lewis FM. The impact of cancer on the family: A critical review of the literature. Patient Educ Couns 1986;8:269–289.
29. Laizner A, Shedga L, Barg F, McCorkle R. Needs of family caregivers of persons with cancer: A review. Semin Oncol Nurs 1993;9:114–120.
30. Kristjanson JL, Norby PA. The family's cancer journey: A literature review. Cancer Nurs 1994;17:1–17.
31. Sales E, Schultz R, Biegel D. Predictors of strain in families of cancer patients review of the literature. J Psychosoc Oncol 1990;10:1–26.
32. Goldstein NE, Concato J, Fried TR, Kasl SV, Johnson-Hurzeler R, Bradley EH. Factors associated with caregiver burden among caregivers of terminally ill patients with cancer. J Palliat Care 2004;20:38–43.
33. Carter PA. Caregivers' descriptions of sleep changes and depressive symptoms. Oncol Nurs Forum 2002;29:1277–1283.

34. Williamson G, Shaffer, D, Schultz, R. Activity restriction and prior relationship history as contributors to mental health outcomes among middle-aged and older spousal caregivers. Health Psychol 1998;17:152–162.

35. Given B, Wyatt G, Given C, et al. Burden and depression among caregivers of patients with cancer at the end of life. Oncol Nurs Forum 2004;31(6):1105–1115.

36. Bradley EH, Prigerson H, Carlson MD, Cherlin E, Johnson-Hurzeler R, Kasl SV. Depression among surviving caregivers: Does length of hospice enrollment matter? Am J Psychiatry 2004;161:2257–2262.

37. Harding R, Higginson IJ, Donaldson N. The relationship between patient characteristics and career psychological status in home palliative cancer care. Support Care Cancer 2003;11:638–643.

38. Andrews SC. Caregiver burden and symptom distress in people with cancer receiving hospice care. Oncol Nurs Forum 2001;28:1469–1474.

39. Cameron J, Franche R, Cheung A, Stewart D. Lifestyle interference and emotional distress in family caregivers of advanced cancer patients. Cancer 2002;94:521–527.

40. Sherif T, Jehani T, Saadani M, Andejani A. Adult oncology and chronically ill patients: Comparison of depression, anxiety and caregivers' quality of life. East Mediterr Health J 2001;7:502–509.

41. Hayman JA, Langa KM, Kabeto MU, et al. Estimating the cost of informal caregiving for elderly patients with cancer. J Clin Oncol. 2001;19:3219–3225.

42. National Alliance of Caregiving and AARP, Caregiving in the U.S. 2004.

43. Echlin KN, Rees CE. Information needs and information-seeking behaviors of men with prostate cancer and their partners: A review of literature. Cancer Nurs 2002;25:35–41.

44. Northouse LL, Peters-Golden H. Cancer and the family: Strategies to assist spouses. Semin Oncol Nurs 1993;9(2):74–82.

45. Northouse L, McCorkle R. Spouse caregivers of cancer patients in psycho oncology. In Holland J, Jacobsen P, Loscalzo M, McCorkle R, eds. Psycho-oncology. New York: Oxford Press; 2010:1907–1978, Chapter 72.

46. Milberg A, Strang P. Meaningfulness in palliative home care: An interview study of dying cancer patients' next of kin. Palliat Support Care 2003;1:171–180.

47. Proot I, Aby-Saad H, Crebolder H, Goldstein M, Luker K, Widdershoven G. Vulnerability of family caregivers between burden and capacity. Scand J Caring Sci 2003;17:113–121.

48. Byock I, Twohig J, Merriman M, Collins K. Promoting excellence in end-of-life care: A report on innovative models of palliative care. J Palliat Med 2006;9:137–151.

49. Follwell M, Burman D, Le L, et al. Phase II study of an outpatient palliative care intervention in patients with metastatic cancer. J Clin Oncol 2009;27(2):206–213.

50. Hughes S, Weaver F, Giobbie-Hurder A, et al. Effectiveness of team-managed home-based primary care: A randomized multicentertrial. JAMA 2000;284:2877–2885.

51. Kralik, D, Anderson, B. Differences in home-based palliative care service utilization of people with cancer and non-cancer conditions. J Nurs Healthcare Chronic Illness 2008;17(11):429–435.

52. Griffin J, Koch K, Nelson J, Cooley M. Palliative care consultation, quality-of-life measurements, and bereavement for end-of-life care in patients with lung cancer. Chest 2007;132:404S–422S.

53. Kuebler K, Bruera E. Interactive collaborative consultation model in end-of-life care. J Pain Symptom Manage 2000;20:202–209.

54. Corner J, Hallisday D, Haviland J, et al. Exploring nursing outcomes for patients with advanced cancer following intervention by Macmillan specialist palliative care nurses. J Adv Nurs 2003;4:561–574.

55. Bostrom B, Hinic H, Lundberg D, Fridlund B. Pain and health-related quality of life among cancer patients in final stage of life: A comparison between two palliative care teams. J Nurs Manage 2003;11:189–190.

56. Charles B. Home health care in France. Pharm World Sci 1990;12:23.

57. Meyer TJ, Mark MM. Effects of psychosocial interventions with adult cancer patients: A meta-analysis of randomized experiments. Health Psychol 1995;14(2):101–108.

58. Sheard T, Maguire P. The effect of psychological interventions on anxiety and depression in cancer patients: Results of two meta-analyses. Br J Cancer 1999;80(11):1770–1780.

59. McCorkle R. A program of research on patient and family caregiver outcomes: Three phases of evolution. Oncol Nurs Forum 2006;33(1):25–31.

60. Given BA, Given CW, Sikorskii A, Jeon S, Sherwood P, Rahbar M. The impact of providing symptom management assistance on caregiver reaction: Results of a randomized trial. J Pain Symptom Manage 2006;32:433–443.

61. Miaskowski C, Dodd M, West C, Schumacher K, Paul SM, Tripathy D, Koo P. Randomized clinical trial of the effectiveness of a self-care intervention to improve cancer pain management. J Clin Oncol 2004;22(9):1713–1720.

62. Given C, Given B, Rahbar M, et al. The effect of a cognitive behavioral intervention on reducing symptom severity during chemotherapy. J Clin Oncol 2004;22(3):507–516.

63. Strecher VJ. Internet methods for delivering behavioral and health-related interventions (eHealth). Ann Rev Clin Psychol 2007;3:53–76.

64. Family Care Research Program. Michigan State University. Family Education Issues: Symptom Management, 2009. Available at: http://www.cancercare.msu/edu (accessed October 22, 2009).

65. 65.Harding R, Higginson I. What is the best way to help caregivers in cancer and palliative care? A systematic literature review of interventions and their effectiveness. Palliat Med 2003;17:63–74.

66. Pasacreta JV, McCorkle R. Cancer care: Impact of interventions on caregiver outcomes. Annu Rev Nurs Res 2000;18:127–148.

67. Budin WC, Hoskins CN, Haber J, et al. Breast cancer: Education, counseling, and adjustment among patients and partners: A randomized clinical trial. Nurs Res 2008;57:199–213.

68. Lewis FM, Cochrane BB, Fletcher KA, et al. Helping her heal: A pilot study of an educational counseling intervention for spouses of women with breast cancer. Psychooncology 2008;17:131–137.

69. Northouse LL, Mood DW, Schafenacker A, et al. Randomized clinical trial of a family intervention for prostate cancer patients and their spouses. Cancer 2007;110:2809–2818.

70. Hudson P, Aranda S, Hayman-White K. A psycho-educational intervention for family caregivers of patients receiving palliative care: A randomized controlled trial. J Pain Symptom Manage 2005;30:329–341.

71. Manne S, Babb J, Pinover W, Horwitz E, Ebbert J. Psycho-educational group intervention for wives of men with prostate cancer. Psychooncology 2004;13:37–46.

72. McMillan SC, Small BJ, Weitzner M, et al. Impact of coping skills intervention with family caregivers of hospice patients with cancer. Cancer 2006;106:214–222.

73. Northouse L, Kershaw T, Mood D, Schafenacker A. Effects of a family intervention on the quality of life of women with recurrent breast cancer and their family caregivers. Psychooncology 2005;14:478–491.

74. Ferrell B, Hudson P, Aranda S, Hayman-White K. A psycho-educational intervention for family caregivers of patients receiving palliative care: A randomized controlled trial. J Pain Symptom Manage 2005;30:329–341.

75. Jacobosen P. Promoting evidence-based psychosocial care for cancer patients. Psychooncology 2009;18(1):6–13.

76. Schumacher KL, Koresawa S, West C, et al. Putting cancer pain management regimens into practice at home. J Pain Symptom Manage 2002;23:369–382.

77. Bishop M, Stephens L, Goodrich M, Byock I. Medication kits for managing symptomatic emergencies in the home: A survey of common hospice practice. J Palliat Med 2009;12:37–43.

78. Van den Brink JL, Moorman PW, de Boer MF, et al. Impact on quality of life of a telemedicine system supporting head and neck cancer patients: A controlled trial during the postoperative period at home. J Am Med Inform Assoc 2007;14(2):198–205.

79. Bowles K, Baigh A. Applying research evidence to optimize telehomecare. J Cardiovasc Nurs 2007;22(1):5–15.

# 47

*Jennifer McAdam and Kathleen Puntillo*

# The Intensive Care Unit

*This is the thing that is keeping me going, is thinking that she is comfortable. Everybody has been encouraging me to come when I get ready. I can walk in, I can turn the music on. I can ask them to suction her. They give her the mouth hygiene or whatever. And I'm sure that is for me, it makes me feel better. I told her, 'Oh, they are washing your face, cleaning your eyes out, this is going to make you feel better', and I pat her a little and change her music tapes…I think that my concern now is that she is comfortable, that she is not in any undue distress, but anything that can be done to make her comfortable…—Mother of a 43-year-old woman who died in the intensive care unit[1]*

♦ **Key Points**

♦ *Although an intensive care unit (ICU) is rarely the place where patients would choose to die, transition from aggressive to end-of-life care is a frequent occurrence.*

♦ *Optimal transitional care in ICUs requires clear communication among patients, family members, and care providers from multiple disciplines.*

♦ *At the end of life, the appropriateness of procedures should be assessed, unnecessary procedures eliminated, and the pain associated with necessary procedures treated appropriately.*

♦ *Analgesics should be administered to dying patients in the amounts necessary to decrease pain and symptoms without concern about the milligram dose required.*

♦ *Pain and symptom assessment and management, although challenging in an ICU setting, are primary roles and contributions of the ICU nurse.*

♦ *Decisions to forgo life-sustaining therapies are made when the burden of aggressive treatment clearly outweighs the benefits. There are two methods of withdrawing ventilator therapy: immediate extubation and terminal weaning. Guidelines exist for each of these methods of withdrawal.*

♦ *Optimal family care occurs at any point along the patient's dying trajectory by providing access, information, support, and involvement in caregiving activities.*

An ICU is, by tradition, the setting in which the most aggressive care is rendered to hospitalized patients. Patients are admitted to an ICU so that health professionals can perform minute-to-minute titration of care. The primary goals of this aggressive care are patient resuscitation, stabilization, and recovery from the acute phase of an illness or injury. However, many patients die in ICUs. It is estimated that 540,000 people die in the United States each year after admission to ICUs.[2] Stated otherwise, almost one in five Americans receives ICU services before death. Intensive care unit deaths account for 59% of all hospital deaths and 80% of all terminal inpatient costs.[2] In one study, the rate of ICU admissions at the end of life increased significantly with advanced age and multiple comorbidities, with one-third of all ICU deaths resulting from pnuemonia and sepsis.[3] Therefore, it is clear that management of the process of dying is common in ICUs.[4]

In the high-technology environment of an ICU, it may be difficult for health professionals and families of dying patients to acknowledge that there are limits to the effectiveness of medical care. However, it is important to focus on providing the type of care that is appropriate for the individual patient and the patient's family, be it aggressive life-saving care or palliative end-of-life care. This chapter discusses the provision of palliative care in ICUs. Specifically, challenges and barriers to providing such care in ICUs are described, and recommendations are offered for the provision of symptom assessment and management. Current issues related to withholding and withdrawing life-sustaining therapies are covered. Recommendations are offered for attending to the needs of families as well as health-care providers who care for ICU patients at the end of life. Finally, an international agenda for improving end-of-life care in ICUs is presented.

## The Limitations of End-of-Life Care in Intensive Care Units

Although many deaths occur in ICUs, an ICU is rarely the place that one would choose to die.[5] Health professionals in ICUs, frequently uncertain about whether a patient will live or die, are caught between the opposing goals of preserving life and preparing the patient and family for death. It is important for professionals to realize that a patient's death is not necessarily an indication of ineffective care. Yet, there are serious limitations to the care provided to seriously ill and dying patients and their families. Communication between physicians and patients may be poor;[6] physicians often may not implement patients' refusals of interventions;[7] patients may be overly optimistic about the outcomes of cardiopulmonary resuscitation (CPR) and other technological treatments;[8] and many hospitalized patients die in moderate-to-severe pain and with other troubling symptoms.[9,10]

In a landmark study, more than 5,000 seriously ill hospitalized patients or their family members were asked questions about the patients' pain (SUPPORT).[11] Almost one-half of these patients had pain during the previous 3 days, and almost 15% had pain that was moderately or extremely severe and occurred at least half of the time. Of those with pain, 15% were dissatisfied with its control. In another study measuring the real-time symptom experiences of 50 chronically critically ill ICU patients, over 90% of the sample were symptomatic, with 45% reporting moderate-to-severe levels of pain and a significant majority reporting other distressing symptoms, such as thirst, fatigue, dyspnea, confusion, fright, and sadness.[10] These findings stress the importance of attending to the assessment and management of pain and other symptoms in all ICU patients.

## Planning Palliative Care for Intensive Care Unit Patients

Providing comfort to patients should accompany all ICU care, even during aggressive attempts to prolong life. However, if a patient is not expected to survive, the focus shifts to an emphasis on palliative care. It is often extremely difficult in an ICU to determine the appropriate time for a change of focus in care. A transition period occurs during which the health professionals, the patient's family, and sometimes the patient recognize the appropriateness of withdrawing and/or withholding treatments and begin to make preparations for death. The transition period (i.e., the time from decision to death) may be a matter of minutes or hours, as in the case of a patient who has sustained massive motor vehicle injuries, or it may be a matter of weeks, as in the case of a patient who has undergone bone marrow transplantation and has multiple negative sequelae while in the ICU. Clearly, this time difference must be recognized as a factor that can influence

the experience of a patient's family members. When patients rapidly approach death, their family members may not have time to overcome the shock of the trauma and adjust to the possibility of death. On the other hand, when death is prolonged, family frustration and fatigue may be part of their experience. Health professionals who are sensitive to these different experiences can individualize their approaches and interventions for family members.

The death trajectory in the ICU usually follows one of the following patterns: a patient in good health that suffers a catastrophic event such as an intracranial bleed; a patient with several comorbities that presents with a new acute problem; a patient with an exacerbation of their chronic condition; or an elderly patient progressively declining with a life-threatening illness.[12] However, the transition from aggressive care to death preparation has not been well-operationalized. The transition period is clearly uncomfortable for many health-care professionals because clinically useful prediction models recognizing which patietnts have the highest risk of death in the ICU remain elusive.[12] Scenarios concerning end-of-life decision-making in the absence of patient or family input are especially challenging. Although some guidelines exist to assist ICU professionals through the processes of maintaining, limiting, or stopping life-sustaining treatments,[13] there are no well-tested standards to assist in the decision-making process. Therefore, it is important for ICU professionals to consider the following steps when caring for patients at risk for not surviving their ICU course:

1. Identify and communicate the goals of care for the patient at least once a day. Ascertain whether the patient has developed an advance directive, whether a family member has durable power of attorney, and whether the patient has communicated a preference about CPR. In a retrospective review of 50 charts of patients who had life support withdrawn in the ICU, 32% had no documentation of an advance directive and 16% had no documentation of resuscitation status.[14]

2. Outline the steps that need to be taken to accomplish the goals of care and evaluate their effectiveness. Technology should not drive the goals of care. Instead, technology should be used, when necessary, to accomplish the goals, and its use should be minimized when the primary goal is achievement of a peaceful death.

3. Use a multidisciplinary team approach to decision-making regarding transition to end-of-life care. All team members, including the patient's family, should reach a consensus—sometimes through negotiation—that the withdrawal of life support and a peaceful death are the appropriate patient outcomes.[4,15,16]

4. In a situation where the patient lacks decision-making capacity and surrogate representation it is recommended that a court appoints a guardian on behalf of the patient or to have safeguards put in place to protect the patient's interests such as mandatory ethics committee review. It

is generally not recommended that the physician makes the decision in isolation.[8,13]

5. Develop and communicate the palliative care plan to professionals and family, and identify the best persons for implementing the various actions in the plan.

6. Developing a plan of care may include enlisting the assistance of in-hospital palliative care staff and/or hospice services. The major goals in any palliative care plan are to provide optimal symptom management, provide psychosocial and spiritual support, provide patient- and family-centered care, coordinate care across settings, and provide staff support.[17]

## Symptom Assessment and Management: Essential Components of Palliative Care

### Pain Assessment

Health-care professionals have an ethical mandate to provide comfort to patients entrusted in their care.[18] However, in spite of advances in pain assessment and management techniques, hospitalized patients continue to receive inadequate pain management.[19] Pain research focusing on dying ICU patients remains scarce, but advances that have been made in the assessment of pain in other critically ill patient populations can be applied to dying patients.[20–22] The patient's report of pain is still considered to be the most valid source, and seeking this information from the patient should be attempted whenever possible. Some ICU patients, even if they are being mechanically ventilated, may be able to use simple numeric or word rating scales, word quality scales, and body outline diagrams if they are provided. However, many critically ill patients are unable to self-report because of their disease process, technological treatment interventions (e.g., mechanical ventilation), or the effects of medications (e.g., opioids, benzodiazepines [BZDs]). The use of BZD infusions may make patients too sedated to respond to pain, although pain may still be present. On the other hand, the use of the anesthetic agent propofol or of neuromuscular blocking agents (NMBAs) such as vecuronium may limit or entirely mask the patient's ability to express or show any behavioral signs of pain. It is essential that clinicians understand that propofol and NMBAs have no analgesic properties, although visible signs of pain disappear during their use. If these agents are used, they must be accompanied by infusions of analgesics, sedatives, or both. In these situations, the nurse may enlist the assistance of family members or friends in their evaluation of the patient's discomfort. The nurse can ask them about any chronic pain experienced by the patient or methods used by the patient at home to decrease pain or stress. This information can then be incorporated into the patient's care plan. In a recent study, the ICU patients' reports on a 0 to 10 numeric rating scale and their nurses' estimation of the patients' pain on a similar scale were within one numeric level of each other 73% of the time.[23] Thus, there is early support that the ICU nurse might be a valid proxy reporter of patient pain.

When patients are too ill to communicate their pain through self-report, clinicians can conduct systematic observations of behaviors that might be indicative of pain. Recently Li and colleagues published a systematic review of objective pain measures that can be used in critically ill patients.[24] These measures include the Behavioral Pain Scale that was developed to quantify pain in sedated, mechanically ventilated patients.[21] Items on this scale include facial expressions, upper limb movements, and compliance with mechanical ventilation. Since its development, the Behavioral Pain Scale's validity and reliability have advanced through testing in other ICU patient groups.[20,22]

A second behavior observation scale that can be considered is the Critical-Care Pain Observation Tool.[25] It, too, prompts the assessor to view the patient's facial expressions, movements, ventilator compliance, and, additionally, muscle tension. Its psychometric properties have been evaluated in several studies.[25–27] The use of scales helps clinicians assess specific pain behaviors in patients who are unable to self-report. However, behavioral measures are only proxies for the patient's subjective reports, although they are frequently the only measures available. As another proxy measure, nurses can use their imaginations to identify possible sources of pain by asking the question, "If I were this patient and had intact sensations, what might be making me uncomfortable?" Even if patients are not exhibiting behavioral or physiological signs of pain, it does not mean that they are pain free.

### Procedural Pain

Before and during the transition from aggressive care to end-of-life care, critically ill patients undergo many diagnostic and treatment procedures. Many of these, such as central, arterial, and peripheral line placements, nasogastric tube placements,[28] chest tube removal,[29,30] and endotracheal suctioning,[30] are quite painful and may be the primary cause of suffering at the end of life. Turning, one of the most ubiquitous procedures performed in acute and critical care settings, was shown to be the most painful of six commonly performed procedures.[31] Other procedures that may be unnecessary, painful, and unpleasant include central line insertions,[21] wound débridement, frequent dressing changes,[31] and the use of sequential compression devices.[21] Paice and colleagues[32] demonstrated through a chart review that 71% to 100% of 57 patients in a medical ICU had numerous procedures during their last 48 hours of life. These procedures included IV medications and fluids, urinary catheters, antibiotics, X-ray studies, enteral feeding tubes, and ventilators. In spite of this knowledge, routine and frequently conducted procedures continue to cause pain in ICU patients.[33] Nurses can act as "gatekeepers" by evaluating the appropriateness of procedures being planned for patients, especially after a decision has been made to end life support, and they can advocate for their omission. Helping patients avoid iatrogenic suffering is a fundamental part of palliative care. Practice guidelines should include recommendations that anticipating and treating pain be part of procedural instructions.[33] The most important procedures for patients to experience at the end of life are those that promote comfort. Yet, when necessary procedures must be performed, the nurse can facilitate pain management before, during, and after procedures.

### Pharmacological Management of Pain

Numerous categories of analgesics and types of modalities exist for administration to critically ill patients.[34] As in all situations, the selection of analgesics should depend on the specific pain mechanism, and the route and modality should be matched to their predictability of effectiveness. Although no comprehensive survey of pain management techniques used for dying ICU patients has been reported, the most common analgesic intervention is use of IV opioids. Choosing the best opioid and method of delivery will depend on factors such as the patient's body composition (e.g., amount of adipose tissue), development of tolerance, and the adverse effect profiles of the various opioids.[34] Use of a continuous infusion of an opioid allows for titration of the drug to a level of analgesic effectiveness and for maintenance of steady plasma levels within a therapeutic range. Table 47–1 presents basic principles in using opioids in critically ill patients.[34] Additionally, health-care professionals may consider the administration of intermittent opioid boluses for breakthrough pain. (See Table 47–2 for information on opioids commonly used in the ICU setting.)

Clearly, concerns about patients becoming tolerant of or dependent on opioids are misplaced during terminal care. What is important is that professionals recognize the development of tolerance, which is the need for larger doses of opioid analgesics to achieve the original effect,[35] and increase the dosage as necessary. There is no ceiling effect from opioids; the dose can be increased until the desired effect is reached or intolerable side effects develop. If it is the family's wish to have the opioid infusion decreased in a sedated patient to assess that the patient is able to participate in end-of-life decision-making, this must be done slowly and carefully. Opioid-dependent patients are at high risk of developing withdrawal symptoms,[35] which would seriously increase their discomfort. In this situation, physical dependence can be addressed by gradually lowering the opioid dose while carefully assessing for signs of pain or withdrawal.

Titration of analgesics to achieve the desired effect is one of the most challenging and important contributions that ICU nurses can make to the comfort care of dying patients. The desired effect can often be described as use of the least amount of medication necessary to achieve the greatest comfort along with the optimum level of tranquil awareness. In ICU settings, concern may arise that administration of analgesics in the amounts necessary to provide comfort could

---

**Table 47–1**
**Basic Tenets of Pain Management for Critically Ill Patients**

All health-care professionals should be considered patient advocates for effective pain control and this advocacy may require intervention on the patient's behalf regardless of perceived or actual hierarchal roles.

Most (if not all) critically ill patients will likely experience pain at some point during their ICU stay.

The clinician should err on the side of presuming pain is present when patient input for pain assessment is not possible, objective measures of pain are conflicting, or when pain is difficult to distinguish from other problems.

It is easier to prevent the escalation of pain through early recognition and control rather than manage the pain effectively after it is out of control.

Analgesics should be started prior to or concomitantly with sedative agents possessing little or no analgesic effects if there is any suspicion of pain.

*Source:* With permission, Erstad et al. (2009), reference 34.

---

"cause" death. It is essential that ICU health professionals understand the "double-effect" principle. In brief, the double-effect principle states that administration of analgesics to dying patients in the amounts necessary to decrease pain and suffering—although possibly causing unintentional hastening of death—is a good, ethically sound way to treat a dying patient.[36] This principle, framed in ethics, provides support to such an action when the clinician's moral intent is directed primarily at alleviating suffering rather than intending to kill. In fact, critical care investigators have found no relationship between the terminal patient's duration of survival and use of opioids.[37,38] When the ICU patient is approaching death, the most important aim of care should be to make the patient's dying as comfortable as possible. Effective symptom control may be one of the last interventions offered to dying patients and their families.[39]

### Nonpharmacological Management of Pain

Nonpharmacological interventions for pain management complement, but do not substitute for, the use of pharmacological interventions. Numerous therapies may be used by critical care nurses to augment the administration of medications to promote patient comfort. They include the use of distraction (e.g., music, humor), relaxation techniques (e.g., visual imagery, rhythmic breathing), and massage.[40] Complementary therapies are low-cost, easy to provide, and safe, and many clinicians can implement them with little difficulty or resources. There is research evidence that ICU nurses do use these types of therapies in their practice.[39] A group of 22 ICU nurses caring for 24 patients were asked about their use of nonpharmacological therapies for patients' symptoms. Nurses reported the use of nonpharmacologic interventions such as music, distraction, touch, and talk. However, they did

**Table 47–2**
**Characteristics of Opioids Commonly Used in the ICU Setting**

| Opioid | t ½β (h) | Cl (mL/kg/min) | Vc/Vdss (L) | logP | Cost | Metabolism | Unique Concerns[a] |
|---|---|---|---|---|---|---|---|
| Morphine | 1.5–5 | 14 | 25/225 | 1.2 | $ | Demethylation[c] | Bradycardia/hypotension; bronchospasm; active metabolite |
| Hydro-morphone | 3 | 20 | 25/300 | 1.2 | $ | Demethylation[c] | Dosing errors related to high potency versus morphine |
| Fentanyl | 1.3–3 | 13 | 15/325 | 4.1 | $ | Demethylation | Muscle rigidity |
| Remifentanil | 0.05[b] | 50 | 10/30 | 1.8 | $$$ | Esterases | Bradycardia/hypotension |

t ½β = half-life of beta-elimination phase, Cl = clearance, Vc/Vdss = volumes of distribution of the central compartment and at steady state, logP = log of octanol/water partition coefficient.

[a]These are particular concerns with individual agents; common adverse effects associated with all opioids, such as respiratory and central nervous system depression are not listed.

[b]Degraded by plasma esterases so this is a context sensitive half-time.

[c]3-Glucuronide metabolite accumulation with morphine or hydromorphone may result in neuroexcitatory toxicity; the 6-glucuronide metabolite of morphine has analgesic and sedative properties similar to the parent compound; both metabolites may accumulate with high doses or renal dysfunction.

*Source*: With permission, Erstad et al. (2009), reference 34.

not immediately recognize them as such. Family members can be encouraged to assist with the provision of comfort measures and may welcome this way of participating in care and decreasing their sense of helplessness. Family involvement is discussed in further detail in a later section of this chapter.

## Anxiety, Agitation, and Sedation

An important part of palliative care in the ICU is assessment and treatment of anxiety and agitation. In one study of 171 ICU patients with a high risk of dying, 58% reported feeling anxious and rated this symptom at a moderate level of intensity.[9] There are many reasons for a dying patient to be anxious, agitated, or both. Assessment of anxiety and agitation provides the practitioner with information that can guide the use of specific interventions. It is imperative to assess for these symptoms because they have been associated with nosocomial infections, unplanned extubations,[41] shortness of breath, increase in blood pressure and heart rate, and combative behavior.[42]

### Assessment of Anxiety and Agitation

Simple numeric rating scales for anxiety can be used if the patient can self-report to identify how much the patient is psychologically bothered. Critical care clinicians and patients are familiar with the use of the 0 to 10 numeric rating scales for pain. "Anxiety" word anchors can be substituted for pain word anchors so that the numeric rating scales also can be used to quantify the degree of distress.

Common behavioral or physiological signs of anxiety include trembling, restlessness, sweating, tachycardia, tachypnea, difficulty sleeping, and irritability. Several agitation/sedation assessment scales are available (e.g., Sessler, Grap & Ramsay 2008).[43] These scales can be printed on the patient flowsheet or on a separate form and used as a bedside assessment tool. Nurses can plan periodic and simultaneous assessments of pain and agitation using pain rating scales and agitation scales. The frequency with which the scales are used depends on the patient's condition and the schedule for evaluating treatment interventions.

### Pharmacological Management to Promote Sedation in Anxious or Agitated Patients

Along with opioids, other categories of sedating drugs are frequently used in the ICU, especially for patients who are mechanically ventilated. Several guidelines,[44] algorithms,[45] and review articles[43,46,47] exist regarding the use of analgesics and sedatives. Often, the goal of combined analgesic-sedative therapy is to promote physical and psychological comfort. Practice decisions include choosing the right type and combination of medications; determining whether to use interrupted sedative infusions (which provide opportunities for patient assessment) or continuous infusions[47]; determining appropriate clinical endpoints for pharmacological interventions; and evaluating the effectiveness of sedation protocols on practices and outcomes.[48]

The appropriate pharmacological agent to control agitation and anxiety is selected according to the desired effect. For example, uncomplicated anxiety is best treated with BZDs, whereas paranoia, panic, and fear accompanied by delusions and hallucinations may require the addition of antipsychotic agents. BZDs are excellent agents for anxiolysis, but they possess no analgesic or psychological properties. Concomitant use of BZDs, opioids, and certain neuroleptic agents may relieve anxiety-provoking symptoms through a synergistic action.[49,50] When used together, these drugs can be administered in lower doses less frequently, have fewer side effects, and can decrease or delay development of tolerance or dependence through the use of smaller doses of each drug. At lower doses, BZDs reduce anxiety without causing central nervous system sedation or a decrease in cognitive or motor function. With increasing dosages, inhibition of motor and cognitive functions as well as central nervous system depression does occur. Sufficiently high doses can induce hypnosis and coma.[49]

The most frequently used BZDs in critical care are midazolam and lorazepam. When midazolam is used as a continuous infusion, the dose can be 1 to 2 milligrams/hour for mild sedation or as high as 20 milligrams/hour for severe agitation if the patient is mechanically ventilated (see Table 47–3). If the degree of sedation is not adequate, then the serum level of midazolam can be raised by one to three small bolus IV injections while simultaneously increasing the infusion rate.[47]

Lorazepam gives effective sedation and anxiety relief over a longer period than midazolam. Cardiovascular and respiratory effects occur less frequently with this drug than with other BZDs. It may also act synergistically with haloperidol, a neuroleptic agent discussed later in this chapter. Lorazepam can be administered intravenously, intramuscularly, or orally. Intravenous doses may be 2 to 6 milligrams every 4 to 6 hours. In the critical care setting, it can also be administered as an infusion at 1 to 10 milligrams/hour and titrated to clinical effect.[47,51] As with opioids, tolerance to BZD effects can develop in critically ill patients, especially those receiving midazolam infusions. Midazolam should be also used in caution with patients with renal insufficiency.[47,52] Additionally, BZD dependence can occur, evidenced by symptoms such as dysphoria, tremor, sweating, anxiety, agitation, muscle cramps, myoclonus, and seizures on abrupt medication withdrawal, and BZDs such as lorazepam have been associated with ICU delirium.[51]

Propofol is a highly lipophilic IV sedative/hypnotic agent that has a very rapid onset of action and short duration. It is indicated for use in the ICU to control agitation and the stress response in patients who are mechanically ventilated and those who require deep sedation for procedures.[44,53] However, propofol has no analgesic properties and must always be used in conjunction with analgesics whenever the patient might experience pain. During initial use of propofol, a drop in systolic blood pressure, mean arterial blood pressure, and heart rate may occur in patients with fluid deficits and in those receiving opioids. The rapid loss of clinical effect of propofol renders it a valuable sedative agent in the critical care environment. Continuous infusion doses may range from 5 to 150 micrograms/kilogram/minute (see Table 47–3).[47] The short effective half-life of propofol allows rapid clinical evaluation of the patient's level of consciousness and determination of the minimum dose required for effective sedation. This may make it a useful drug during situations in which intermittent interaction with professionals and family members is desired.[49]

It is important that patients in ICUs be routinely assessed for the presence of delirium using available and reliable tools such as The Delirium Screening Checklist or the CAM-ICU.[54] Haloperidol is a frequently used neuroleptic for critically ill patients with delirium. A loading dose of 2 milligrams can be administered, followed by twice that dose repeated every 15 to 20 minutes while agitation persists. Doses as high as 400 milligrams have been reported, but adverse effects may occur with these high doses.[44] This drug has few cardiovascular effects unless given rapidly, in which case vasodilation and hypotension may occur. Haloperidol does not depress respirations; rather, it has a calming effect on agitated, disoriented patients, making them more manageable without causing excessive sedation. However, haloperidol has some significant adverse effects, such as reduction of the seizure threshold, precipitation of extrapyramidal reactions, and prolongation of the QT interval leading to torsades de pointes.[54] Once a haloperidol drug dosage has been established, it should not be necessary to increase the dose to obtain the same effect over time, because tolerance should not occur. Clinicians may try other atypical antipsychotic medications (e.g., olanzapine, quetiapine, and ziprasidone) in treating delirium with fewer side effects than Haldol.[55]

## Nonpharmacological Interventions for Anxiety and Agitation

Numerous interventions exist that may promote tranquility and sedation in a critical care environment. These include control of environmental noise and the use of clocks, calendars, and personal articles such as pictures from home. Music therapy can be used to decrease anxiety and pain as well as promote sleep. As noted earlier, imagery and relaxation techniques also provide a means of distraction for patients and help to alleviate anxiety.[56]

The act of physically caring for a patient and providing gentle touch is a major source of comfort for patients in critical care. Taking the time to provide simple measures such as back rubs and massages, repositioning the patient, smoothing bed linen wrinkles, removing foreign objects from the bed, providing mouth and eye care, and taping tubes to maintain patency and inhibit pulling effectively promotes comfort and decreases anxiety. Family member participation in caregiving activities, such as bathing, massages, and back rubs, can have a powerful calming effect on patients and promote sleep and psychological integrity.

For alert patients, increasing opportunities for control is a strategy that can reduce the sense of helplessness that often accompanies patients who are critically ill. This sense of control can be promoted by allowing alert patients to make decisions about the timing of interventions. Facilitating contact and communication with clergy, psychologists, or psychiatrists, if appropriate, can help to alleviate the distress experienced by both patients and families.

**Table 47–3**
**Pharmacological Symptom Management**

| Symptom | Drug Type Most Frequently Used | Method of Administration | Usual Dose* |
|---|---|---|---|
| Pain | Opioids (e.g., morphine, fentanyl, hydrocodone, methadone) | Continuous IV infusions with use of intermittent boluses for procedure-related pain or during treatment withdrawal | Continuous infusion: 1–10 mg/h morphine equivalents<br>Bolus: 1–5 mg IV morphine equivalent slow push; titrate to effect |
| Anxiety/ Agitation | Benzodiazepines (e.g., lorazepam, midazolam) | Same as for opioids | Continuous midazolam infusion: 1–20 mg/h<br>Bolus midazolam: 2–5 mg IV<br>Continuous lorazepam infusion: 1–10 mg/h<br>Bolus lorazepam: 2–6 mg IV every 4–6 hours |
|  | Haldol | IV boluses | Bolus: 0.5–20 IV |
|  | Propofol | Continuous IV infusion | Continuous: 50–150 mcg/kg/min |
| Dyspnea | Oxygen | Multiple methods (e.g., nasal cannula, mask, ventilator) | Concentration as needed |
|  | Opioids (e.g., morphine) | Continuous IV infusion and/or IV bolus; or per nebulizer | See above for IV doses<br>Per nebulizer: 2.5 mg in 3 mL saline (preservative free) or sterile water q4h |
|  | Benzodiazepines | See above | See above |
|  | Bronchodilators (e.g., Alupent) | Per nebulizer | Alupent: 2.5 mL 0.4–0.6% solution |
|  | Diuretics (e.g., Lasix) | IV bolus, slow push | Bolus Lasix: 20–40 mg IV |
|  | Anticholinergics (e.g., atropine) | Per nebulizer | Atropine: 0.025 mg/kg diluted with 3–5 mL saline three or four times daily; doses not to exceed 2.5 mg |

*Drug doses are general recommendations. Dosing should be individualized to a particular patient. Under usual circumstances, start with low doses, wait for effect, and titrate to desired effect.

Sources: Jacobi et al. (2002), reference 44; Kompanje et al. (2008), reference 78; Kuebler (2002), Treece et al. (2004), reference 82; reference 136; Mularski (2004), reference 135; Truog et al. (2001), reference 134.

## Other Distressing Symptoms

Scant research has been conducted on symptoms experienced by ICU patients who are at high risk of dying. A notable exception was the study by Puntillo and colleagues.[9] These investigators specifically focused on the self-reported symptom experiences of ICU patients who were at high risk of dying. Investigators used a 10-item symptom checklist measuring both intensity (scale 0–3) and distress (scale of 0–3) of symptoms such as pain, fatigue, shortness of breath, restlessness, anxiety, sadness, hunger, fear, thirst, and confusion. Their sample consisted of 171 patients (mean age: 58 years; 64% male), and 34% were mechanically ventilated, and 19% died during their ICU stay. The most prevalent symptoms included fatigue (75%), thirst (71%), and anxiety (56%). Symptoms lower in prevalence but reported to be moderately distressful by patients included: shortness of breath, pain, confusion, fear, and sadness. This study demonstrated that a significant proportion of patients at high risk of dying in ICUs experience substantial emotional amd physical symptoms.

ICU nurses play a major role in alleviating distressing symptoms such as thirst, sleeplessness, and general discomfort experienced by patients at the end of life. Because nurses are the health-care providers who are constantly at the bedside, they can assess the presence of these symptoms, advocate for effective pharmacological therapy, use additional nursing comfort measures, and provide for continuity of therapy. Symptom management is a special contribution that ICU nurses can make to their patients at the end of life.

## End-of-Life Practice Issues: Withholding and Withdrawing Life-Sustaining Therapies

Limiting life-sustaining therapies in an ICU is becoming more common. It is estimated that withholding or withdrawing of life support precedes up to 75% of deaths in ICUs.[57–59] Generally, life-sustaining treatment is withdrawn when death is believed to be inevitable despite aggressive interventions.

The President's Commission for the Study of Ethical Problems in Medicine and Biomedical and Behavioral Research[60] supported the right of a competent patient to refuse life-sustaining and life-prolonging therapy. The Commission also noted that there is no moral difference between withholding and withdrawing therapy. Numerous critical care-related professional organizations have published position papers in support of the patient's autonomy regarding withholding and withdrawal decisions.[8,61,62]

If patients are unable to make treatment decisions, then these decisions must be made on the patient's behalf by surrogates or by the health-care team.[6] Optimally, patients' living wills or advance directives can provide the direction for decisions related to treatment withholding or withdrawal. However, only 10% to 20% of patients complete them.[63,64] When surrogates are asked to participate in decision-making, it is recommended that a family centered decision-making approach be used.[16,65] This type of decision-making is recommended for major decisions involving limiting life-sustaining treatments when survival is unlikely but possible or when survival may come with significant impairment.[16]

Promoting a family-centered decision-making philosophy includes incorporating the dimensions of shared decision-making and by improving communication using the VALUE technique. Both are briefly described here:

Shared decision-making removes the burden from any one person, whether that be a family member or a physician. It includes the following broadly defined dimensions:

1. Assess the patient's prognosis and provide complete and consistent medical information to the family.
2. Elicit the patient's preferences, goals, and values.
3. Assess the family's preference for their role in decision-making (this can range from letting the physician decide to the family member assuming all responsiblity for the decision).[66]

The VALUE communication technique improves the quality of the communication process between ICU clinicians and family members during end-of-life care conferences.[65,67] This approach incorporates the following steps:

Value family statements
Acknowledge family emotions
Listen to the the family
Understand the patient as a person through the family
Elicit family questions

This commication strategy was tested on family members of 126 patients dying in French ICUs in a randomized controlled trial. The family members received either standard care or the intervention (VALUE technique) during their end-of-life care conference. Those family members who received the intervention had significantly lower symptom prevalence of posttraumatic stress disorder (PTSD), anxiety, and depression.[65]

Other suggestions that ICU clinicians can incorporate in their practice to improve the quality of care during this challenging time include:

- Conducting a patient and family care conference within 72 hours of an admission to an ICU[68]
- Ensuring the care conference occurs in a private setting[69]

- Ensuring that the care conference is multidiscplinary (including nurses, physicians, respiratory therapists, and other clinicians)[69]
- Encouraging ICU clinicians to spend more time listening and less time talking with family members[70]
- Educating ICU clinicians to use empathetic statements[71]
- Assuring the family that the patient will not suffer[72]
- Emphasizing that the health-care team will not abandon the patient or family during this time no matter the outcome of the conference.[16,73]

Family members often struggle with concern that they are doing the right thing. Providing clear, consistent infomration about the patient's prognosis (albeit in the face of prognostic uncertainty) provides support for families in their decision-making.

When a decision to forgo life-saving therapy is made in an acute care setting, there should be a concerted effort to evaluate all therapies all therapies, including blood products, hemodialysis, vasopressors, mechanical ventilation, total parenteral nutrition, antibiotics, IV fluids, and tube feedings, to assess whether these treatments could make a positive contribution to the patient's comfort.[8,74] Withdrawal of therapies should be preceded by chart notations of DNR orders and a note documenting the rationale for comfort care and removal of life support.[75] There should be a clear plan of action and provision of information and support to the family. Adequate documentation of patient assessments, withdrawal decisions and plans, therapy withdrawal orders, and patient and family responses during and after withdrawal is essential.[7,8,16,76] There is considerable variability regarding physician documentation of discussions with families regarding withdrawal of life support.[74,76] This lack of documentation may infer—rightly or wrongly—lack of interactions with families about treatment decisions.[14]

## Withdrawal of Ventilator Therapy With Consideration of Analgesic and Sedative Needs

It is important to understand the methods by which mechanical ventilation may be removed. The primary goal during this process should be to ensure that patients and family members are as comfortable as possible, both psychologically and physically. Two primary methods of mechanical ventilation removal exist: immediate extubation and terminal weaning (Table 47-4). Debates continue as to which of these methods is optimal for the patient, and often the method is determined according to the physician's, patient's, or family members' comfort levels.[57,76,78] However in one study, Gerstel and colleagues reported a significant increase in family satisfaction with immediate extubation before death of their loved one in the ICU.[74]

Although there is considerable variability regarding the preferred approach to withdrawal,[7,12,79] recommendations regarding

**Table 47–4**
**Methods of Mechanical Ventilation Withdrawal**

| Immediate Extubation | Terminal Weaning |
| --- | --- |
| **Description** | |
| Abrupt removal of the patient from ventilator assistance by extubation after suctioning (if necessary). Humidified air or oxygen is administered to prevent airway drying. | Physicians or other members of the ICU team (e.g., respiratory therapists, nurses) gradually withdraw ventilator assistance. This is done by decreasing the amount of inspired oxygen, decreasing the ventilator rate and mode, removal of positive end-expiratory ressure (PEEP), or a combination of these maneuvers. Usual time from ventilator to T-piece or extubation: 15–60 min. |
| **Positive aspects** | |
| Patient free of technology; dying process less likely to be prolonged; intentions of the method are clear. | Allows titration of drugs to control symptoms; maintains airway for suctioning if necessary; patient does not develop upper airway obstruction; longer time between ventilator withdrawal and death; moral burden on family may be less because method appears less active. |
| **Negative aspects** | |
| Noisy breathing, dyspnea may be distressful to patient/family. | May prolong dying; patient unable to communicate; machine between patient and family. |
| **Time course to death** | |
| Unpredictable. Usually shorter than with terminal weaning. | Unpredictable. |

*Sources:* Truog et al. (2008), reference 8; Szalados et al.(2007), reference 57; Campbell (2007), reference 76.

specific procedures for withdrawal are available.[4,8,78,80] Table 47–5 presents a protocol for withdrawal of mechanical ventilation for the clinician's consideration that includes specific recommendations regarding use of analgesics and sedatives (see Curtis article).[82] Consensus guidelines on the provision of analgesia and sedation for dying ICU patients support the titration of analgesics and sedatives based on the patient's requests or observable signs indicative of pain or distress.[8,81] The guidelines emphasize that no maximum dose of opioids or sedatives exists, especially considering that many ICU patients receive high doses of these drugs over their ICU time-course. Anticipatory dosing, as opposed to reactive dosing, is recommended by some to avoid patient discomfort and distress.[7,8,57,76,78] A group of researchers surveyed 143 nurses and 61 physicians to assess the usefulness of using a standardized order form for the withdrawal of life support. The majority of nurses (84%) reported the form was helpful and were mostly satisfied with the sedation and mechanical ventilation sections. Almost all of the physicians (95%) reported that the form was helpful and were mostly satsified with the sedation, mechanical ventilation, and death preparation sections.[82]

It is important to provide comfort to dying patients, who could experience pain and distress. Several investigators studying patients receiving morphine or morphine equivalents and benezodiapines prior to mechanical ventilation withdrawal reported no difference in time to death according to opioid dose.[37,83] Therefore, clinicans should strive for symptom control at the end of life. Attention must also be paid to involvement of the family in decision-making, providing support to the family, and good documentation of decisions and treatments. However, documentation has been found to be lacking for patients who die after ventilator withdrawal.[14] Without proper documentation, evaluation of competent and compassionate care is limited.

Patients should be withdrawn from NMBAs before withdrawal from life support. The use of NMBAs (such as vecuronium) makes it almost impossible to assess patient comfort; although the patient appears comfortable, he/she may be experiencing pain, respiratory distress, or severe anxiety. The use of NMBAs prevents the struggling and gasping that may be associated with dying but not the patient's suffering.[8,78] The horror of such a death can only be imagined. The withdrawal of these agents may take considerable time for patients who have been receiving them chronically, and patients continue to have effects from lingering active metabolites.[57]

As mentioned earlier, research to guide the practice of ventilator withdrawal and factors associated with withdrawal is scant. One group of researchers assessed the process of withdrawal of life support in 155 ICU patients. They reported that 62.6% died after extubation, and 58% of those died with an airway in place.[83] Wunsch and colleagues reveiwed the charts of patients who had life-support treatments withdrawn to identify factors associated with this process. They found wide variablity in practice; however, overall, forgoing active life-supporting treatment decisions were associated with older patient age, severe pre-existing medical conditions, emergency surgery, and CPR in the 24 hours prior to admission.[77] Finally, other investigators reported that most ICU clinicians used a stuttering withdrawal process (removing one treatment at a time) and that on average removal of life-support treatment was prolonged (lasting longer than 1 day). In this study, they found that factors such as younger patient age,

**Table 47–5**
**A Protocol for the Withdrawal of Mechanical Ventilation**

I. Anticipate and prevent distress
  A. Review process in advance with patient (if awake), nurse, and family. Identify family goals during withdrawal (e.g., ability to communicate versus sedation). Arrange a time that allows the family to be present, if they wish.
  B. Provide for special needs (e.g., clergy, bereavement counselor). Assess respiratory pattern on current level of respiratory support.
  C. Use opioids and/or benzodiazepines* to control respiratory distress (i.e., respiratory rate >24 breaths per minute, use of accessory muscles, nasal flaring, >20% increase in heart rate or blood pressure, grimacing, clutching). In patients already receiving these agents, dosing should be guided by the current dose.
  D. In the absence of distress, reduce intermittent mandatory ventilation (IMV) rate to less than 10 and reassess sedation.
  E. Discontinue therapies not directed toward patient comfort:
    1. Stop neuromuscular blockade after opioids and/or benzodiazepines have been started or increased.[†]
    2. Discontinue laboratory tests, radiographs, vital signs.
    3. Remove unnecessary tubes and restraints.
    4. Silence alarms and disconnect monitors.

II. Optimize existing function
  A. Administer breathing treatment, if indicated.
  B. Suction out the mouth and hypopharynx. Endotracheal suctioning before withdrawal may or may not be advisable depending on patient distress and family perception. Consider atropine (1–2.5 mg by inhalation q6h), scopolomine (0.3–0.65 mg IV q4–6h), or glycopyrrolate (1–2 mg by inhalation q2–4h) for excessive secretions.
  C. Place the patient at least 30 degrees upright, if possible.

III. Withdraw assisted ventilation[‡]
  A. In general, changes should be made in the following order[§]:
    1. Eliminate positive end-expiratory pressure (PEEP).
    2. Reduce the fractional oxygen content of inspired air ($FIO_2$).
    3. Reduce or eliminate mandatory breaths.
    4. Reduce pressure support level.
    5. Place to flow-by or T-piece.
    6. Extubate to humidified air or oxygen.
  B. Constant reevaluation for distress is mandatory. Treat distress with additional bolus doses of opioids and/or benzodiazepines equal to hourly drip rate and increase drip by 25–50%.
  C. Observe for postwithdrawal distress, a medical emergency. A physician and nurse should be present during and immediately after extubation to assess the patient and to titrate medications. Morphine (5–10 mg IV q10 min) or fentanyl (100–250 μg IV q3–5 min) and/or midazolam (2–5 mg IV q7–10 min) or diazepam (5–10 mg IV q3–5 min) should be administered.

*Drug doses are difficult to specify because of the enormous variability in body weight and composition, previous exposure, and tolerance. In opioid-naïve patients, 2–20 mg morphine or 25–250 μg fentanyl, followed by an opioid infusion of one-half of the loading dose per hour, is a reasonable initial dose.

†Usually the effects of neuromuscular blocking agents (NMBAs) can be reversed within a short period, but it may take days to weeks if patients have been receiving NMBAs chronically for management of ventilatory failure.61 Neuromuscular blockade masks signs of discomfort. Therefore, clinicians should feel that the patient has regained sufficient motor activity to demonstrate discomfort.

‡There is no one sequence applicable to all patients because their clinical situations are so variable. The pace of changes depends on patient comfort and may proceed as quickly as 5–15 min or, in an awake patient to be extubated, over several hours.

§Patients who require high levels of ventilatory support may die after small adjustments such as reduction or elimination of PEEP or decrease in $FIO_2$ to 21%. In such patients, the physician should be present during and immediately after the change in therapy to assess the patient.

*Sources:* Kompanje et al. (2008), reference 78; Szalados et al. (2007), reference 57; Treece et al. (2006), reference 125; https://depts.washington.edu/eolcare/instruments/wls-orders2.pdf.

longer ICU stay, more life-sustaining interventions, and more decision-makers involved led to prolonged withdrawal.[74]

Regardless of the methods, factors, or processes used to withdraw life-sustaining therapies, the critical care nurse plays a major role during the decision and implementation of withdrawal of patients from mechanical ventilation. Increased nursing involvement can help provide optimal care to these patients. Specifically, the nurse can ensure that a rationale for, and all elements of, the plan have been adequately discussed among the team, patient, and family. The nurse can ensure that adequate time is given to families and their support persons, such as clergy, to reach as good a resolution as possible. The family needs reassurance that they and the patient will not be left alone and that the patient will be kept comfortable with the use of medications and other measures. As discussed earlier, opioids, alone or in combination with BZDs, are used during withdrawal to ensure that patients are provided the optimal degree of comfort.

## Care for the Family of the Dying Intensive Care Unit Patient

Although the focus of care in many critical care areas is on the critically ill patient, nurses and other clinicians with family care skills realize that comprehensive patient care includes care of the patient's family. A family-centered approach to care is strongly supported by a consensus guideline[84] and acknowledges a reciprocal and all-important relationship between the family and the critically ill family member.[85-87] A change in one affects the other, and vice versa. Current research describes that an ICU experience for family members can be stressful (especially when their loved one dies in the ICU) and has been associated with symptoms of PTSD, anxiety, depression, and complicated grief.[88-91] Therefore, no discussion of palliative care in the ICU is complete without also discussing care of the dying patient's family. Family is defined here as any significant other who participates in the care and well-being of the patient.

The clinical course of any given critically ill, dying patient can vary tremendously, ranging from a rapid unfolding over several hours to a gradual unfolding over several days, weeks, and even months. Of course, the manner in which a family copes is also highly variable. Caring for families at any point along the dying trajectory, however, encompasses major aspects of access, information and support, and involvement in caregiving activities.

### Access

A crucial aspect of family care is ensuring that the family can be with their critically ill loved one. Historically, critical care settings have severely restricted family access and discouraged lengthy family visitation. Commonly cited rationales to limit family access include concerns regarding space limitations, patient stability, infection, rest, and privacy; the negative effect of visitation on the family; and clinicians' performance abilities. Some of these concerns have merit, whereas others, such as adverse patient-related issues and a negative effect on the family, have not been borne out in the research literature.

Many ICUs around the world routinely limit visitors to two at any one time.[92,93] Space limitations in critical care areas can be profound, because most ICUs were designed for efficient use of life-saving machinery and staff and were not intended for end-of-life vigils by large, extended families. Ensuring that all interested family members have access to their loved one's bedside can present challenges to the often already narrow confines of the ICU. However, family members of dying loved ones should be allowed more liberal access (both in visiting time and in number of visitors allowed).[84,87] Patients are confronting what may be the most difficult of life passages, and therefore, they may need support from their family members. In a current study of 209 patients, 149 family members, and 43 ICU workers, researchers assessed their perceptions of unrestricted visiting hours in the ICU. They reported that family members were more satisfied with this practice; however, ICU nurses and physicians stated moderate interruptions to patient care. Nurses reported a slight delay in organizing nursing care, and physicians reported greater unease when they were assessing the patient and perceived greater family stress, but they also perceived greater family trust.[93]

There is a growing body of literature that supports family access to patients during invasive procedures and resuscitation. Facilitating family access during such times has come to be known as facilitating family presence, a practice supported by the Emergency Nurses Association[94] and the Society of Critical Care Medicine.[84] Several authors have reviewed the impact of family presence on patients and have found that family members thought their presence benefitted their loved ones by being present to comfort and support them.[95-97] Studies examining family satisfaction with family presence have yielded similar results, and several studies have demonstrated no adverse psychological effects on the part of family members after the witnessed resuscitation.[95,98]

Because children as young as 5 years have been reported to have an accurate concept of death,[88] their visitation needs should also be considered when a family member is dying. There is support for letting children visit the patient and become familiar with the care the patient is receiving. Visitation has the potential to help the child cope and gives the child a chance to say goodbye. If ICU clinicians account for the child's developmental status and properly prepare the child, then children can visit a critically ill family member in the ICU without ill effects.[84,99]

Finally, caring for the critically ill, dying patient and his/her family can call forth feelings of failure for clinicians bent on finding a cure and force health-care providers to reflect on their own mortality.[100] Perhaps this helps to explain why so many health-care providers believe that family presence is stressful and disruptive to the health-care team caring for the critically ill patient.[95,101] Although research does not support these findings, this topic remains controversial. Currently it has been recommended that hospitals establish formal programs that allow immediate family members to be present during resuscitation. This program should include trained staff to support the family, assess the family for distress, educate the family regarding the process, and debrief after the process.[102] The emotional burden for health-care providers when providing palliative care is discussed later in this chapter.

### Information and Support

Information has been identified as a crucial component in family coping and satisfaction in critical care settings.[103,104] Support, in the form of clinicians' caring behaviors and interactions, is enormously influential in shaping the critical care experience for both patients and their families.[103,104] In the context of caring for a critically ill, dying patient, however, nurses and physicians alike have reported high stress related to "death-telling," or notifying family members of the patient's death or terminal prognosis.[100,105,106] These same studies and articles point to the fact that few health-care providers feel they have the skills and knowledge necessary to counsel families effectively during this emotionally charged time. The ethical principle of honesty and truth-telling collides with the limits of knowing the truth precisely when there is clinical ambiguity and also collides with the suffering imposed on a family having to face the hard truth. Compassionate truth-telling requires dialogue and relationship, timing, and attunement,[107] all of which are relational aspects that are frequently overlooked in the hectic pace of the ICU. Add patient, family, and health-care provider culture to the equation, and one can readily understand why communication between involved parties is a less-than-perfect science.[7] The educational implications for clinicians are addressed later in this chapter.

Overall satisfaction with end-of-life care has been shown to be significantly associated with completeness of information received by the family member, support and care shown to the patient and family, consistency in staff, and satisfaction with the amount or level of healthcare received.[84,87,108] Family conferences have been used extensively as a means to improve communication between health-care providers and family members, and the few studies that have investigated best practices in relation to the timing, content, and participants necessary for optimal communication during a family conference have shown improved satisfaction and lower emotional distress for family members.[65,67]

Some hospitals have created interdisciplinary teams of helping professionals to work with hopelessly ill patients and their families in an effort to meet patients' and families' physical, informational, and psychosocial needs.[15,17,103,109] Such teams usually include a nurse, physician, chaplain, and social worker. Working in concert with the nurses and physicians at the bedside, these interdisciplinary teams can more fully concentrate on end-of-life issues so that, theoretically, no patient or family needs go unmet during this time.

Finally, because feelings of grief in surviving family members are still commonly unresolved 1 year after a loved one's death, many critical care units across the lifespan have organized bereavement follow-up programs.[65,110] These programs typically involve contacting the surviving family (by telephone or mail) monthly for some period of time and at the 1-year anniversary of their loved one's death. In addition to remembering and supporting the family, these programs have also been shown to help health-care providers cope with the loss as well. Another suggestion that may be helpful to family members is that the ICU staff can hold memorial services twice a year for family/friends of the patient to reconnect with the critical care staff. During this service, names of those who have died in the past 6 months are read. A reception is held afterward that gives everyone, especially the staff, an opportunity to reflect on their work and to honor the people they have served.[111]

## Involvement in Caregiving Activities

Few interventional studies have examined the effect of family involvement on critically ill patients and their families, yet families should have the opportunity to be helpful.[112] One study qualitatively assessed the roles family members assume when their loved one is at high risk of dying in the ICU.[113] Families in this study discussed their roles as patient protector, facilitator, historian, coach, voluntary caregiver, and actively present person. These roles were extremely important to family members and gave them a sense of purpose. Acknowledging the contributions of family members and involving them in caregiving activities can be beneficial. These activities can range from minor activities (such as assisting with oral care or rubbing the dying patient's feet) to major activities (assisting with postmortem care). This involvement may be helpful for family members in working through their grief by demonstrating their love in caring and comforting ways. Being involved in meaningful caregiving activities can make a family member feel useful rather than useless and helpful rather than helpless.[112–114]

Although physical death occurs in the dying patient, the social death is felt in the patient's surviving family. Because the perception of death lingers at the family level long after the physical death has occurred, involving family members who are interested in participating in their loved one's care may go far to provide closure, comfort, and connection. Nurses' facilitation of family involvement in their dying loved one's care is a practical family intervention that should be more widely employed if humane and comprehensive palliative care is desired.[113]

## Care for the Caregiver of the Dying Intensive Care Unit Patient

*It's only human to hurt, to cry, to grieve, when a person who's influenced you in some way has died. Please cry with your patients and their families; it's okay for you to grieve too.[115]*

Numerous studies have described the tension between the cure-oriented critical care setting and palliative care.[116–119] The bedside health-care provider, typically a nurse, often feels caught between differing perceptions held by physicians and family members concerning patient progress and treatment goals. Facilitating and coordinating dialogue and consensus between these groups as well as caring for the dying patient and family can be physically and emotionally exhausting. If the dying process is prolonged, the nurse can become frustrated and fatigued. Although health-care providers often cope with this stress by emotionally disengaging themselves from the charged atmosphere, emotional distancing has been shown to hamper skill acquisition and the development of involvement skills.[120,121] Involvement skills are defined here as the cluster of interpersonal skills that enable a nurse and the patient and family to establish a relational connection. This section discusses two strategies to help health-care providers sustain their caring practices and extend their involvement skills—namely, sharing narratives and death education.

### Sharing Narratives

Debriefing, either formally or informally, has been used effectively in many settings to discuss and process critical incidents; analyze health-care providers' performance in terms of skill, knowledge, and efficiency; and learn, both personally and institutionally, from mistakes and system breakdown.[109,122,123] Sharing stories or narratives of practice can be used to achieve the same goals, but telling stories from practice also enables clinicians to (1) increase their skill in recognizing patient and family concerns; (2) learn to communicate more effectively with patients, families, and other health-care providers; (3) reflect on ethical comportment and engaged clinical reasoning; and (4) articulate clinical knowledge development.[122,123]

Creating the interpersonal and institutional space in which to both tell and actively listen to stories from practice also enables health-care providers to share skills of involvement and sustaining strategies. These understandings can provide clinicians with guidance—and, in some cases, corrective action—to intervene in ways that are true to the patient's condition and to the patient's and family's best interests.[105,122,123] Through reflection and dialogue with others, nurses and other health-care providers can pool their collective wisdom and extend their care of dying patients and their families.

### Death Education

Closely coupled with sharing clinical narratives is the use of seminars and other reflective exercises aimed at preparing nurses and other health-care providers for the care of dying patients and their families. Death education often consists of didactic and experiential classes. Participants in these classes are encouraged to reflect on and share their own perceptions and anxieties about death, as well as their attitudes toward care of the dying patient and his/her family. This approach has been used with varying degrees of success with nurses, nursing students, and physicians.[105,122,124] Because many health-care providers feel uneasy and ill-prepared to effectively care for terminally ill patients and their families, this is a promising strategy that deserves more implementation and research.

Additionally, integrating palliative care into the ICU requires preparation and education of ICU clinicians. The main components include:

- Educating critical care staff about palliative care (e.g., prinicples of shared decision-making, communication techniques, symptom management, and practices of withdrawal of life support). This step can be accomplished through lectures, pamphlets, teaching videos, and poster boards.[67,125]
- Training local ICU champions who can serve as role models and facilitate behavior change. This can

be completed through half-day or full-day training sessions.[67,125]
- Collecting feedback on quality improvement data (e.g., family member s' satsifaction with care or family member s' ratings of the quality of death and dying).[67,125]
- Finally utilizing system supports and hospital resources to develop family informational pamphlets, (e.g., "get to know me" posters for patients rooms and developing withdrawal of life support forms).[67,111,126]

## An International Agenda to Improve Care of Dying Intensive Care Unit Patients

Considerable emphasis has been placed on improving care at the end of life for ICU patients. Several books that comprehensively and specifically address ICU end-of-life care have been published[127,128] and another is forthcoming.[129] A Robert Wood Johnson-sponsored national ICU Peer Workgroup on end-of-life care conducted several education and research initiatives related to this topic. One of these initiatives was the development of quality indicators for end-of-life care in ICUs.[109] These quality indicators can provide a framework for interventions to improve care of the dying in ICUs. The Society of Critical Care Medicine held a symposium in 2006 entirely devoted to improving the quality of end-of-life care through interventions that work.[130] An international consensus statement and a task force guideline have been published to provide evidence on end-of-life care in ICUs and to make recommendations for research and practice improvements.[8,84] The Robert Wood Johnson Foundation funded demonstration projects in four ICUs in the United States. These demonstration projects developed palliative care models for ICUs and assessed the impact on the quality of care for patients and their families.[131] It is anticipated that findings from these demonstration projects will guide national and international practice improvements.

## Summary

As noted by Todres and colleagues,[132] "There is not one best way to die." However, the authors believe that provision of a pain-free, ethically intact, and dignified death is the right of all ICU patients. Research has offered little guidance for managing the issues that surround ICU patient deaths. However, Chapple[133] presented important goals to consider during an ICU patient's dying process: (1) honor the patient's life; (2) ensure that the patient and the family are not abandoned; (3) provide a sense of moral stability; and (4) ensure the patient's safety and comfort. Intensive care unit nurses can feel privileged to strive toward the accomplishment of those goals.

CASE STUDY
*Positive End-of-Life Care in the Intensive Care Unit*

Submitted by Cathy Schuster, RN, from the University of California, San Francisco Moffitt-Long Hospital Adult Medical-Surgical ICU.

Mrs. F was an active woman in her early 50s. She had been experiencing some health issues, and after a visit to her family physician she was diagnosed with stage 3 lung cancer with metastasis and scleroderma. She decided that she wanted everything done. Her goal was to return to her favorite activity, which was hiking in the mountains. The plan was for Mrs. F and her friends to talk to the surgeon the following day about her options, including the possibility of a lung transplant.

Unfortunately, Mrs. F became very ill the next afternoon, experiencing respiratory distress, altered mental status, and hypotension. She required intubation and mechanical ventilation and was subsequently transferred to the ICU. Intravenous fluids were given, and a vasopressor was started for her hypotension. Her son, who was listed as Mrs. F's Durable Power of Attorney for Healthcare, was notified and stated he was on his way to the ICU.

At 11:00 the following morning, the patient's son, his wife, and the patient's sister met with the physicians, Mrs. F's primary nurse, and a social worker. The health-care team answered all of the family's questions and concerns about Mrs. F's condition. The health-care team updated the family on her current condition and prognosis. Unfortunately, Mrs. F had not regained consciousness since entering the ICU.

The medical and nursing staff continued to pursue aggressive treatment, but the family expressed concern about her comfort. The health-care team assured the family that the Mrs. F would be made comfortable. Mrs. F's condition did not improve, and it was then decided by the health-care team and the family to withhold chest compressions and defibrillation. A "Do Not Resuscitate" order was completed.

Her family and friends kept constant vigil at her bedside, talking to her and reading to her. The primary nurses and physicians kept the family informed about the many changes in her condition and the treatments they were administering. Unfortunately, Mrs. F's situation worsened over the next 7 days. Her hypotension did not respond to maximum doses of three vasopressors, fluids, and antibiotics. Her mechanical ventilatory support required higher levels of oxygen, positive end expiratory pressure, and respiratory rate to maintain her oxygenation and ventilation. She was suffering from severe septic shock and adult respiratory distress syndrome.

Another family meeting was held. The family was told that Mrs. F's prognosis was grave and that she was not expected to survive. The decision was made to withdraw life support. All family and friends arrived at the hospital from distant cities in time. The son wanted to proceed with the withdrawal of support after the conference. The health-care team used a preprinted "Withdrawal of Life Support" order set and a new "Do Not Resuscitate" order was written to stipulate the withholding of all resuscitative efforts.

After the family conference, Suzanne, Mrs. F's primary nurse, prepared the room for the family. The monitor alarms and the overhead lights were turned off, and the door was closed. The nurse played soft music and a low light was positioned in the corner to provide a chapel-like setting. The primary nurse placed a blue butterfly sign, which read "Please Honor Family Private Time," outside Mrs. F's door to request a respectful quiet outside the room. This sign also informed all staff that a patient was actively dying and that a special visiting policy had been initiated. Visiting was then unlimited for Mrs. F's family. All family and friends could come and go as they wished throughout the day and night. The primary nurse also ordered a comfort care food basket for the family from the hospital kitchen containing a variety of drinks, fruits, and chips. The primary nurse paged the chaplain from the Spiritual Care Services Department to provide support and care to the patient and her family during this challenging time.

When the family returned to the bedside, they wanted to know more details, such as the various steps of withdrawal and what to expect ("Will she move?" and "Will she gasp for breath?"). Suzanne, the primary nurse, addressed each of their concerns and instructed them regarding what to expect, such as the bradyarrthymias that would appear on the cardiac monitor and the changes in breathing patterns. Suzanne spoke about the medications that she would be giving Mrs. F while she closely monitored for any signs of distress or discomfort by assessing the heart rate, blood pressure, respiratory rate, and observing for agitation or diaphoresis.

Per the "Withdrawal of Life-Support" orders, Suzanne initiated a continuous morphine infusion to ensure that Mrs. F was free of discomfort and pain. An infusion of an anxiolytic, Midazolam, was started to provide relief of anxiety and fear. Suzanne continuously assessed Mrs. F for signs and symptoms of discomfort. The "Withdrawal of Life-Support" orders include a reference guide to inform and guide staff on the various aspects of providing caring for an actively dying patient. As Mrs. F was hypotensive because of her sepsis, Suzanne also looked at her respiratory effort and facial expression and for any restlessness to indicate that Mrs. F was in distress. After Suzanne was assured that Mrs. F was free of pain and anxiety, she stopped the three vasopressors that were supporting her blood pressure. Suzanne noted that there was a hint of a frown on her forehead and administered a bolus of morphine and Midazolam to assure that Mrs. F was comfortable. At the family conference, it had been decided that Mrs. F would not be extubated. This would serve to save the family from hearing the distressing noise caused by oral secretions collecting in the back in her throat. Susanne continued giving oral and endotracheal suctioning to Mrs. F only as needed.

Mrs. F was gradually weaned from her mechanical ventilator support per the "Withdrawal of Life-Support" orders for terminal weaning. She was removed from the ventilator and placed on T-piece with room air. Throughout the process, Suzanne watched for any sign that Mrs. F was uncomfortable or in distress and administered medication as necessary.

After 4 minutes on T-piece, Mrs. F stopped breathing. The withdrawal of her life support lasted 1 hour. During this time, Suzanne encouraged the family to touch and talk to Mrs. F. Some friends combed her hair, while others massaged her feet and hands. During this hour some of her friends chanted in the room. They told Suzanne that the purpose of the chanting was to ease Mrs. F's soul into the next world.

After Mrs. F's family and friends said their last goodbyes, Mrs. F's son and wife each gave Suzanne a tearful hug and thanked Suzanne for the special care she gave to their mother. In parting, Suzanne provided them several pamphlets to provide referrals for grief counseling, guidelines for decedent paperwork, and a hospital contact number for further assistance.

A short time later, a butterfly bereavement card was sent from the staff of the ICU to Mrs. F's son to express their sorrow and sympathy over his loss. This card was signed by her primary care nurses and the other staff members who cared for her in the ICU.

## REFERENCES

1. Puntillo K. Unpublished data, 2003.

2. Angus DC, Barnato AE, Linde-Zwirble WT, et al. Use of intensive care at the end of life in the United States: An epidemiologic study. Crit Care Med 2004;32(3):638–643.

3. Seferian EG, Afessa B. Adult intensive care unit use at the end of life: A population-based study. Mayo Clin Proc 2006;81(7):896–901.

4. Curtis JR. Caring for patients with critical illness and their families: The value of the integrated clinical team. Respir Care April 2008;53(4):480–487.

5. Ryder-Lewis M. Going home from ICU to die: A celebration of life. Nurs Crit Care 2005;10(3):116–121.

6. Luce JM, White DB. The pressure to withhold or withdraw life-sustaining therapy from critically ill patients in the United States. Am J Respir Crit Care Med 2007;175(11):1104–1108.

7. Reynolds S, Cooper AB, McKneally M. Withdrawing life-sustaining treatment: Ethical considerations. Surg Clin North Am 2007;87(4):919–936, viii.

8. Truog RD, Campbell ML, Curtis JR, et al. Recommendations for end-of-life care in the intensive care unit: A consensus statement by the American College [corrected] of Critical Care Medicine. Crit Care Med 2008;36(3):953–963.

9. Puntillo K, Arai S, Gropper M, Cohen H. The Prevalence, Intensity and Distress of Symptoms in High-Risk ICU Patients. 2008 (abstract). Annual Meeting of the American Association of Critical Care Nurses.

10. Nelson J, Meier DE, Litke A, Natale DA, Siegel RE, Morrison SR. The symptom burden of chronic illness. Crit Care Med 2004;32(7):1527–1534.

11. The SUPPORT Principal Investigators. A controlled trial to improve care for seriously ill hospitalized patients: The study to understand prognoses and preferences for outcomes and risks of treatments (SUPPORT). JAMA 1995; 274(20):1591–1598.

12. Cook D, Rocker G, Giacomini M, Sinuff T, Heyland D. Understanding and changing attitudes toward withdrawal and withholding of life support in the intensive care unit. Crit Care Med 2006;34(11 Suppl):S317–S323.

13. White DB, Curtis JR, Lo B, Luce JM. Decisions to limit life-sustaining treatment for critically ill patients who lack both decision-making capacity and surrogate decision-makers. Crit Care Med 2006;34(8):2053–2059.

14. Kirchhoff KT, Anumandla PR, Foth KT, Lues SN, Gilbertson-White SH. Documentation on withdrawal of life support in adult patients in the intensive care unit. Am J Crit Care 2004;13(4):328–334.

15. Puntillo KA, McAdam JL. Communication between physicians and nurses as a target for improving end-of-life care in the intensive care unit: Challenges and opportunities for moving forward. Crit Care Med 2006;34(11 Suppl):S332–S340.

16. Curtis JR, White DB. Practical guidance for evidence-based ICU family conferences. Chest 2008;134(4):835–843.

17. Billings JA, Keeley A, Bauman J, et al. Merging cultures: Palliative care specialists in the medical intensive care unit. Crit Care Med 2006;34(11 Suppl):S388–S393.

18. Herr K, Coyne PJ, Key T, et al. Pain assessment in the nonverbal patient: Position statement with clinical practice recommendations. Pain Manag Nurs 2006;7(2):44–52.

19. Teno JM, Clarridge BR, Casey V, et al. Family perspectives on end-of-life care at the last place of care. JAMA 2004;291(1):88–93.

20. Young J, Siffleet J, Nikoletti S, Shaw T. Use of a Behavioural Pain Scale to assess pain in ventilated, unconscious and/or sedated patients. Intensive Crit Care Nurs 2006;22(1):32–39.

21. Payen JF, Bru O, Bosson JL, et al. Assessing pain in critically ill sedated patients by using a behavioral pain scale. Crit Care Med 2001;29(12):2258–2263.

22. Aissaoui Y, Zeggwagh AA, Zekraoui A, Abidi K, Abouqal R. Validation of a behavioral pain scale in critically ill, sedated, and mechanically ventilated patients. Anesth Analg 2005;101(5):1470–1476.

23. Ahlers SJ, van Gulik L, van der Veen AM, et al. Comparison of different pain scoring systems in critically ill patients in a general ICU. Crit Care 2008;12(1):R15.

24. Li D, Puntillo K, Miaskowski C. A review of objective pain measures for use with critical care adult patients unable to self-report. J Pain 2008;9(1):2–10.

25. Gelinas C, Fillion L, Puntillo KA, Viens C, Fortier M. Validation of the critical-care pain observation tool in adult patients. Am J Crit Care 2006;15(4):420–427.

26. Gelinas C, Johnston C. Pain assessment in the critically ill ventilated adult: Validation of the Critical-Care Pain Observation Tool and physiologic indicators. Clin J Pain 2007;23(6):497–505.

27. Gelinas C, Fillion L, Puntillo KA. Item selection and content validity of the Critical-Care Pain Observation Tool for nonverbal adults. J Adv Nurs 2008;65(1):203–126.

28. Morrison RS, Ahronheim JC, Morrison GR, et al. Pain and discomfort associated with common hospital procedures and experiences. J Pain Symptom Manage 1998;15(2):91–101.

29. Puntillo KA. Dimensions of procedural pain and its analgesic management in critically ill surgical patients. Am J Crit Care 1994;3(2):116–122.

30. Puntillo K, Ley SJ. Appropriately timed analgesics control pain due to chest tube removal. Am J Crit Care 2004;13(4):292–301; discussion 302; quiz 303–294.

31. Puntillo KA, White C, Morris AB, et al. Patients' perceptions and responses to procedural pain: Results from Thunder Project II. Am J Crit Care 2001;10(4):238–251.

32. Paice JA, Muir JC, Shott S. Palliative care at the end of life: Comparing quality in diverse settings. Am J Hosp Palliat Care 2004;21(1):19–27.

33. Siffleet J, Young J, Nikoletti S, Shaw T. Patients' self-report of procedural pain in the intensive care unit. J Clin Nurs 2007;16(11):2142–2148.

34. Erstad B, Puntillo K, Gilbert H, Grap M, Li D, Medina J. General pain management principles in the critically ill. Chest 2009;135(4):1075–1086.

35. Society AP. Principles of Analgesic Use in the Treatment of Acute Pain and Cancer Pain (5th ed). Glenview, IL: American Pain Society, 2003.

36. Campbell ML. Treating distress at the end of life: The principle of double effect. AACN Adv Crit Care 2008;19(3):340–344.

37. Chan JD, Treece PD, Engelberg RA, et al. Narcotic and benzodiazepine use after withdrawal of life support: Association with time to death? Chest 2004;126(1):286–293.

38. Campbell ML, Bizek KS, Thill M. Patient responses during rapid terminal weaning from mechanical ventilation: A prospective study. Crit Care Med 1999;27(1):73–77.

39. Puntillo KA, Smith D, Arai S, Stotts N. Critical care nurses provide their perspectives of patients' symptoms in intensive care units. Heart Lung 2008;37(6):466–475.

40. Titler MG, Rakel BA. Nonpharmacologic treatment of pain. Crit Care Nurs Clin North Am 2001;13(2):221–232.

41. Jaber S, Chanques G, Altairac C, et al. A prospective study of agitation in a medical-surgical ICU: Incidence, risk factors, and outcomes. Chest 2005;128(4):2749–2757.

42. Pun BT, Dunn J. The sedation of critically ill adults: Part 1: Assessment. The first in a two-part series focuses on assessing sedated patients in the ICU. Am J Nurs 2007;107(7):40–48; quiz 49.

43. Sessler CN, Jo Grap M, Ramsay MA. Evaluating and monitoring analgesia and sedation in the intensive care unit. Crit Care 2008;12(Suppl 3):S2.

44. Jacobi J, Fraser GL, Coursin DB, et al. Clinical practice guidelines for the sustained use of sedatives and analgesics in the critically ill adult. Crit Care Med 2002;30(1):119–141.

45. Schweickert WD, Kress JP. Strategies to optimize analgesia and sedation. Crit Care 2008;12(Suppl 3):S6.

46. Sessler CN, Wilhelm W. Analgesia and sedation in the intensive care unit: An overview of the issues. Crit Care 2008; 12(Suppl 3):S1.

47. Sessler CN, Varney K. Patient-focused sedation and analgesia in the ICU. Chest 2008;133(2):552–565.

48. Robinson BR, Mueller EW, Henson K, Branson RD, Barsoum S, Tsuei BJ. An analgesia-delirium-sedation protocol for critically ill trauma patients reduces ventilator days and hospital length of stay. J Trauma 2008;65(3):517–526.

49. Gommers D, Bakker J. Medications for analgesia and sedation in the intensive care unit: An overview. Crit Care 2008; 12(Suppl 3):S4.

50. Fraser GL, Riker RR. Sedation and analgesia in the critically ill adult. Curr Opin Anaesthesiol 2007;20(2):119–123.

51. Pandharipande P, Shintani A, Peterson J, et al. Lorazepam is an independent risk factor for transitioning to delirium in intensive care unit patients. Anesthesiology 2006;104(1):21–26.

52. Liu LL, Gropper MA. Postoperative analgesia and sedation in the adult intensive care unit: A guide to drug selection. Drugs 2003;63(8):755–767.

53. Carson SS, Kress JP, Rodgers JE, et al. A randomized trial of intermittent lorazepam versus propofol with daily interruption in mechanically ventilated patients. Crit Care Med 2006;34(5):1326–1332.

54. Pun BT, Ely EW. The importance of diagnosing and managing ICU delirium. Chest 2007;132(2):624–636.

55. Skrobik YK, Bergeron N, Dumont M, Gottfried SB. Olanzapine vs haloperidol: Treating delirium in a critical care setting. Intensive Care Med 2004;30(3):444–449.

56. Pun BT, Dunn J. The sedation of critically ill adults: Part 2: Management. Am J Nurs 2007;107(8):40–49; quiz 50.

57. Szalados JE. Discontinuation of mechanical ventilation at end-of-life: The ethical and legal boundaries of physician conduct in termination of life support. Crit Care Clin 2007;23(2):317–337, xi.

58. Prendergast TJ, Claessens MT, Luce JM. A national survey of end-of-life care for critically ill patients. Am J Respir Crit Care Med 1998;158(4):1163–1167.

59. McLean RF, Tarshis J, Mazer CD, Szalai JP. Death in two Canadian intensive care units: Institutional difference and changes over time. Crit Care Med 2000;28(1):100–103.

60. President's Commission for the Study of Ethical Problems in Medicine and Biomedical and Behavioral Research. Deciding to Forgo Life-Sustaining Treatment: A Report on Ethical, Medical and Legal Issues in Treatment Decisions. Washington DC: U.S. Government Printing Office, 1983.

61. Thompson BT, Cox PN, Antonelli M, et al. Challenges in end-of-life care in the ICU: Statement of the 5th International Consensus Conference in Critical Care: Brussels, Belgium, April 2003: Executive summary. Crit Care Med 2004;32(8):1781–1784.

62. American Association of Critical Care Nurses. Position Statement: Withholding and/or Withdrawing Life-Sustaining Treatment. Newport Beach, CA: AACN, 1999.

63. Whetstine LM. Advanced directives and treatment decisions in the intensive care unit. Crit Care 2007;11(4):150.

64. Tillyard AR. Ethics review: 'Living wills' and intensive care—an overview of the American experience. Crit Care 2007;11(4):219.

65. Lautrette A, Darmon M, Megarbane B, et al. A communication strategy and brochure for relatives of patients dying in the ICU. N Engl J Med 2007;356(5):469–478.

66. White DB, Curtis JR. Establishing an evidence base for physician-family communication and shared decision making in the intensive care unit. Crit Care Med 2006;34(9):2500–2501.

67. Curtis JR, Treece PD, Nielsen EL, et al. Integrating palliative and critical care: Evaluation of a quality-improvement intervention. Am J Respir Crit Care Med 2008;178(3):269–275.

68. Glavan BJ, Engelberg RA, Downey L, Curtis JR. Using the medical record to evaluate the quality of end-of-life care in the intensive care unit. Crit Care Med 2008;36(4):1138–1146.

69. Pochard F, Azoulay E, Chevret S, et al. Symptoms of anxiety and depression in family members of intensive care unit patients: Ethical hypothesis regarding decision-making capacity. Crit Care Med 2001;29(10):1893–1897.

70. McDonagh JR, Elliott TB, Engelberg RA, et al. Family satisfaction with family conferences about end-of-life care in the intensive care unit: Increased proportion of family speech is associated with increased satisfaction. Crit Care Med 2004;32(7):1484–1488.

71. Selph RB, Shiang J, Engelberg R, Curtis JR, White DB. Empathy and life support decisions in intensive care units. J Gen Intern Med 2008;23(9):1311–1317.

72. Stapleton RD, Engelberg RA, Wenrich MD, Goss CH, Curtis JR. Clinician statements and family satisfaction with family conferences in the intensive care unit. Crit Care Med 2006;34(6):1679–1685.

73. West HF, Engelberg RA, Wenrich MD, Curtis JR. Expressions of nonabandonment during the intensive care unit family conference. J Palliat Med 2005;8(4):797–807.

74. Gerstel E, Engelberg RA, Koepsell T, Curtis JR. Duration of withdrawal of life support in the intensive care unit and association with family satisfaction. Am J Respir Crit Care Med 2008;178(8):798–804.

75. O'Mahony S, McHugh M, Zallman L, Selwyn P. Ventilator withdrawal: Procedures and outcomes. Report of a collaboration between a critical care division and a palliative care service. J Pain Symptom Manage 2003;26(4):954–961.

76. Campbell ML. How to withdraw mechanical ventilation: A systematic review of the literature. AACN Adv Crit Care 2007;18(4):397–403; quiz 344–395.

77. Wunsch H, Harrison DA, Harvey S, Rowan K. End-of-life decisions: A cohort study of the withdrawal of all active treatment in intensive care units in the United Kingdom. Intensive Care Med 2005;31(6):823 831.

78. Kompanje EJ, van der Hoven B, Bakker J. Anticipation of distress after discontinuation of mechanical ventilation in the ICU at the end of life. Intensive Care Med 2008;34(9):1593–1599.

79. Willms DC, Brewer JA. Survey of respiratory therapists' attitudes and concerns regarding terminal extubation. Respir Care 2005;50(8):1046–1049.

80. End-of-Life Care Research Program. Integrating palliative and critical care (video). 2008. Available at: http://depts.washington.edu/eolcare/instruments/index.html (accessed December 24, 2008).

81. Hawryluck LA, Harvey WR, Lemieux-Charles L, Singer PA. Consensus guidelines on analgesia and sedation in dying intensive care unit patients. BMC Med Ethics 2002;3:E3.

82. Treece PD, Engelberg RA, Crowley L, et al. Evaluation of a standardized order form for the withdrawal of life support in the intensive care unit. Crit Care Med 2004;32(5):1141–1148.

83. Rocker GM, Heyland DK, Cook DJ, Dodek PM, Kutsogiannis DJ, O'Callaghan CJ. Most critically ill patients are perceived to die in comfort during withdrawal of life support: A Canadian multicentre study. Can J Anaesth 2004;51(6):623–630.

84. Davidson JE, Powers K, Hedayat KM, et al. Clinical practice guidelines for support of the family in the patient-centered intensive care unit: American College of Critical Care Medicine Task Force 2004–2005. Crit Care Med 2007;35(2):605–622.

85. Kirchhoff KT, Walker L, Hutton A, Spuhler V, Cole BV, Clemmer T. The vortex: Families' experiences with death in the intensive care unit. Am J Crit Care 2002;11(3):200–209.

86. Kirchhoff KT, Song MK, Kehl K. Caring for the family of the critically ill patient. Crit Care Clin 2004;20(3):453–466, ix–x.

87. Kirchhoff KT, Faas AI. Family support at end of life. AACN Adv Crit Care 2007;18(4):426–435.

88. Siegel MD, Hayes E, Vanderwerker LC, Loseth DB, Prigerson HG. Psychiatric illness in the next of kin of patients who die in the intensive care unit. Crit Care Med 2008;36(6):1722–1728.

89. Pochard F, Darmon M, Fassier T, et al. Symptoms of anxiety and depression in family members of intensive care unit patients before discharge or death. A prospective multicenter study. J Crit Care 2005;20(1):90–96.

90. Azoulay E, Pochard F, Kentish-Barnes N, et al. Risk of posttraumatic stress symptoms in family members of intensive care unit patients. Am J Respir Crit Care Med 2005;171(9):987–994.

91. Anderson WG, Arnold RM, Angus DC, Bryce CL. Posttraumatic stress and complicated grief in family members of patients in the intensive care unit. J Gen Intern Med 2008;23(11):1871–1876.

92. Lee MD, Friedenberg AS, Mukpo DH, Conray K, Palmisciano A, Levy MM. Visiting hours policies in New England intensive care units: Strategies for improvement. Crit Care Med 2007;35(2):497–501.

93. Garrouste-Orgeas M, Philippart F, Timsit JF, et al. Perceptions of a 24-hour visiting policy in the intensive care unit. Crit Care Med 2008;36(1):30–35.

94. Emergency Nurses Association. Presenting the Option for Family Presence (2nd ed). Park Ridge, IL: ENA, 2001.

95. Mangurten JA, Scott SH, Guzzetta CE, et al. Family presence: Making room. Am J Nurs 2005;105(5):40–48; quiz 49.

96. Harteveldt R. Benefits and pitfalls of family presence during resuscitation. Nurs Times 2005;101(36):24–25.

97. Eichhorn DJ, Meyers TA, Guzzetta CE, et al. During invasive procedures and resuscitation: Hearing the voice of the patient. Am J Nurs 2001;101(5):48–55.

98. Booth MG, Woolrich L, Kinsella J. Family witnessed resuscitation in UK emergency departments: A survey of practice. Eur J Anaesthesiol 2004;21(9):725–728.

99. Ihlenfeld JT. Should we allow children to visit ill parents in intensive care units? Dimens Crit Care Nurs 2006;25(6):269–271.

100. McMillen RE. End of life decisions: Nurses perceptions, feelings and experiences. Intensive Crit Care Nurs 2008;24(4):251–259.

101. Grice AS, Picton P, Deakin CD. Study examining attitudes of staff, patients and relatives to witnessed resuscitation in adult intensive care units. Br J Anaesth 2003;91(6):820–824.

102. Critchell CD, Marik PE. Should family members be present during cardiopulmonary resuscitation? A review of the literature. Am J Hosp Palliat Care 2007;24(4):311–317.

103. Wall RJ, Curtis JR, Cooke CR, Engelberg RA. Family satisfaction in the ICU: Differences between families of survivors and nonsurvivors. Chest 2007;132(5):1425–1433.

104. Gries CJ, Curtis JR, Wall RJ, Engelberg RA. Family member satisfaction with end-of-life decision making in the ICU. Chest 2008;133(3):704–712.

105. Moores TS, Castle KL, Shaw KL, Stockton MR, Bennett MI. 'Memorable patient deaths': Reactions of hospital doctors and their need for support. Med Educ 2007;41(10):942–946.

106. Hough CL, Hudson LD, Salud A, Lahey T, Curtis JR. Death rounds: End-of-life discussions among medical residents in the intensive care unit. J Crit Care 2005;20(1):20–25.

107. Benner P. A dialogue between virtue ethics and care ethics. Theor Med 1997;18(1–2):47–61.

108. Mularski RA, Heine CE, Osborne ML, Ganzini L, Curtis JR. Quality of dying in the ICU: Ratings by family members. Chest 2005;128(1):280–287.

109. Mularski RA, Curtis JR, Billings JA, et al. Proposed quality measures for palliative care in the critically ill: A consensus from the Robert Wood Johnson Foundation Critical Care Workgroup. Crit Care Med 2006;34(11 Suppl):S404–S411.

110. Valks K, Mitchell ML, Inglis-Simons C, Limpus A. Dealing with death: An audit of family bereavement programs in Australian intensive care units. Aust Crit Care 2005;18(4):146,148–151.

111. The End-of-Life Nursing Educational Consortium. End-of-Life Educational Modules. 2008. Available at: http://www.aacn.nche.edu/ELNEC/ (accessed December 29, 2008).

112. Williams CM. The identification of family members' contribution to patients' care in the intensive care unit: A naturalistic inquiry. Nurs Crit Care 2005;10(1):6–14.

113. McAdam JL, Arai S, Puntillo KA. Unrecognized contributions of families in the intensive care unit. Intensive Care Med 2008;34(6):1097–1101.

114. Engstrom A, Soderberg S. The experiences of partners of critically ill persons in an intensive care unit. Intensive Crit Care Nurs 2004;20(5):299–308; quiz 309–210.

115. Reese CD. Please cry with me: Six ways to grieve. Nursing (Lond) 1996;26(8):56.

116. Hamric AB, Blackhall LJ. Nurse-physician perspectives on the care of dying patients in intensive care units: Collaboration, moral distress, and ethical climate. Crit Care Med 2007;35(2):422–429.

117. Embriaco N, Papazian L, Kentish-Barnes N, Pochard F, Azoulay E. Burnout syndrome among critical care healthcare workers. Curr Opin Crit Care 2007;13(5):482–488.

118. Brosche TA. A grief team within a healthcare system. Dimens Crit Care Nurs 2007;26(1):21–28.

119. Badger JM. Factors that enable or complicate end-of-life transitions in critical care. Am J Crit Care 2005;14(6):513–521.

120. Brunelli T. A concept analysis: The grieving process for nurses. Nurs Forum 2005;40(4):123–128.

121. Benner P, Tanner CA, Chesla CA. Expertise in Nursing Practice: Caring, Clinical Judgment, and Ethics. New York, NY: Springer, 1996.

122. Rushton CH, Reder E, Hall B, Comello K, Sellers DE, Hutton N. Interdisciplinary interventions to improve pediatric palliative care and reduce health care professional suffering. J Palliat Med 2006;9(4):922–933.

123. Ihlenfeld JT. Applying personal reflective critical incident reviews in critical care. Dimens Crit Care Nurs 2004;23(1):1–3.

124. Ferrell B. End-of-life education for nurses. Topics Adv Pract Nurs eJ 2007;7(2).

125. Treece PD, Engelberg RA, Shannon SE, et al. Integrating palliative and critical care: Description of an intervention. Crit Care Med 2006;34(11 Suppl):S380–S387.

126. Available at: http://nursing.ucsfmedicalcenter.org/docshares/ComfortCareOrders.pdf (accessed October 18, 2009).

127. Medina J, Puntillo K. Palliative and end-of-life care issues in critical care. In: AACN Protocols for Practice. Sudbury, MA: Jones & Bartlett Publishers International, 2006.

128. Curtis JR, Rubenfeld GD. The Transition from Cure to Comfort. New York, NY: Oxford University Press, 2001.

129. Rocker G, Puntillo K, Azoulay E, Nelson J. End-of-Life in the Intensive Care Unit. London: Oxford Publishing, in press.

130. Lexy, M, Curtis JR. Improving end of life care in the intensive care unit. Crit Care Med. 2006;34 (11):s301.

131. Promoting Excellence in End-of-Life Care. Grantees: Promoting Palliative Care Excellence in Intensive Care. Available at: http://www.aacn.org/WD/Palliative/Content/grantees.pcms?menu=Practice (accessed December 29, 2008).

132. Todres ID, Armsrong A, Lally P, Cassem EH. Negotiating end-of-life issues. New Horiz 1998;6:374–382.

133. Chapple HS. Changing the game in the intensive care unit: Letting nature take its course. Crit Care Nurse 1999;19(3):25–34.

134. Truog RD, Cist AF, Brackett SE, et al. Recommendations for end-of-life care in the intensive care unit: The Ethics Committee of the Society of Critical Care Medicine. Crit Care Med 2001;29(12):2332–2348.

135. Mularski RA. Pain management in the intensive care unit. Crit Care Clin 2004;20(3):381–401; viii.

136. Kuebler K. Dyspnea. In: Kuebler K, Berry P, Heidrich D, eds. End of Life Care: Clinical Practice Guidelines. Philadelphia, PA: W.B. Saunders Company; 2002:301–315.

# 48

*Jeanne Robison and Anna R. Du Pen*

# The Outpatient Setting

*The doctors, nurses and staff at the clinic are like family . . . .they have supported us through it all, from the day last year that we were told the prognosis, through the treatments, the ups and downs. . . . So we decided to come by the clinic after her funeral today for a few more hugs and to thank them for all they have done.—Elaine, family member*

♦ ***Key Points***
♦ *Twenty-four-hour accessibility to health-care providers is critical to providing palliative care to outpatients.*
♦ *Evaluation and management of physical, emotional, and spiritual distress at each office visit are primary components of outpatient palliative care.*
♦ *Active listening in the office and at telephone triage contributes greatly to individualizing the plan of care.*
♦ *Providing a sense of control for patients and their families is an integral part of palliative care.*

Dramatic changes over the last two decades have resulted in shorter and shorter hospital stays, longer survival with chronic debilitating disease, and smaller, fractured families—all of which have contributed greatly to increased use of outpatient services. Outpatient care is delivered in private practice offices, free-standing clinics, and hospital-based outpatient settings. Individuals with chronic and terminal illnesses receive care over time in the outpatient clinic or office setting. In these settings, significant long-term relationships develop among providers, patients, and families. As patients move toward the end of life, visits to the clinic provide an excellent opportunity to assess the patient's and family's needs, desires, struggles, and fears.

The months or years spent providing and receiving care in an outpatient setting are fundamental to establishing trust between the care team and the patient. This trusting relationship is vital both early in the disease continuum and at the end of life. Building this relationship is a critical component of the palliative nursing role.[1,2]

Unlike in an acute care setting, patients and families have time scheduled with physicians and staff to address their needs. This allows families to avoid the frustration of waiting in a hospital room trying to connect with a physician or nurse to raise issues or ask questions. The patient's and family's questions are answered and processed at one visit, and further clarifying questions and detailed responses can ensue at the next office visit.

In most cases, an outpatient setting is more intimate and less crisis-driven than a hospital setting. On the other hand, patients may experience excessive time in the waiting room and may be in very different stages of disease than others surrounding them. In the best situation, patients and families meet and support each other, and facilities use waiting room space to make educational materials readily available.

The new frontier of delivering palliative care is the establishment of outpatient palliative care clinics.[3] Early palliative care programs were primarily hospital-based.

In this tertiary model, the inpatient palliative care team was called to assist patients and their families in addressing acute palliative care needs. Historically palliative care and hospice services have been offered very late in the disease trajectory. A recently published review of over 60,000 patient deaths from cancer over a 10-year period from New Jersey and Pennsylvania indicated that over two-thirds of patients never received hospice and for those who did, greater than 25% were admitted to hospice less than 3 days prior to death.[4] Underutilization of palliative care services at the end of life for patients with advanced heart failure and chronic obstructive pulmonary disease (COPD) have also been reported.[5,6] Today, palliative principles of care are being integrated "upstream" of the active dying phase into traditional oncology, cardiology, or internal medicine outpatient care delivery or are accessed within separate specialty outpatient palliative care clinics.

## Outpatient Palliative Care Models

In many ways the structure of the traditional outpatient clinic visit lends itself to the integration of palliative care. In addition to taking a history, performing a physical examination, and reviewing medication history, the clinician can effectively integrate a discussion about advance directives into the routine. Treatment plans can be discussed and negotiated with the patient. An assessment of pain and symptoms can be done at the time vital signs are taken or during telephone triage. The pain management standards for outpatient care from the Joint Commission on Accreditation of Healthcare Organizations (JCAHO)[7] can be used to help incorporate pain and symptom management into the routine documentation of outpatient care.

Studies have shown that patients treated in the outpatient setting by dedicated palliative care teams have improvement physical, psychological, and spiritual health outcomes and evidence of earlier advanced care planning.[8,9] Individuals also make fewer visits to emergency rooms or urgent care centers, and the number of hospitalizations declines.[8] The quality of end-of-life care is enhanced when treatment of the disease comes into balance with identification and management of evolving palliative care needs in the outpatient setting. Table 48–1 outlines the benefits of outpatient palliative care.

Many hospital-based palliative care services began as inpatient consultation services and have evolved into more comprehensive inpatient and outpatient programs.[3] These clinics have the advantage of providing continuity of care to patients after discharge and of insuring the plan of care established in the hospital is working when the patient returns home. These programs generally start with a half-day clinic every week, often "borrowing" space from an established clinic, and gradually increase their patient base through hospital follow-ups and, eventually, outpatient referrals.

---

**Table 48–1**
**Advantages of Outpatient Palliative Care**

- Meets the palliative care needs of patients living in the community
- Facilitates earlier referral for palliative care among specialty practices and raises awareness of this focus
- Provides follow-up and improved continuity of discharged patients
- Provides patients with a sense of confidence that they have support in community
- Improves ability for coordination of the palliative care visit with other sub-specialist or primary care visits
- Enhances overall disease management
- Allows more time for patient and family support and education
- Improves communication between palliative care team, patient and primary care providers
- Gives opportunity for palliative care staff to work with patients earlier in the disease trajectory
- Provides an opportunity for palliative care teams to target special populations in need that may not require frequent hospitalizations, such as patients with chronic neuromuscular disease
- Targets another setting for education, training and research in the arena of palliative care
- Offers an economical way to manage care and reduce hospital stays and readmissions

*Source:* Adapted from Meier (2008), reference 3.

---

Another model involves the outpatient-based palliative care clinics. Many of these evolved out of traditional "pain clinics" into more comprehensive palliative care outpatient clinics. These clinics are generally staffed by palliative care physicians, nurses, social workers, and volunteers. The challenges in operating these clinics include adequate facilities, logistical support, reimbursement, and establishing referral relationships with primary care providers. Despite these difficulties, palliative care clinics are experiencing significant growth. The palliative care clinic at Dartmouth grew from 283 outpatient visits in 2001 to 1233 visits in 2007.[3] The palliative clinic load at the Princess Margaret Hospital in Toronto increased from 1 half-day clinic per week in 2002 to 5 full days per week in 2006.[10]

Despite the growth of specialty palliative care clinics, the most common approach to palliative care delivery is one that integrates palliative care principles into primary care. In this model, clinicians caring for patients with incurable or terminal illnesses incorporate palliative care initiatives within their practices without "contracting this service out" to another provider. Biases exist, and some outpatient clinics prefer to deliver this care themselves for fear of fragmenting care or "losing" patients. Strategies to providing this integrated palliative care while managing complex diseases include investing in additional staff, such as registered nurses, social workers, financial counselors, nutritionists, and advanced practice nurses (APN) who can help the primary physician meet the needs of this population without referral to another care provider.

## The Advanced Practice Nurse Role

Advanced practice nurses have played a major role in the development of palliative care programs in the United States.[11,12] Master's degree nursing programs, focusing on palliative care, were launched in the late 1990s. Today, certification in palliative care for APNs is available, although licensing and certification for APNs differs from state to state. This is a growing specialty among APNs both in the inpatient and outpatient setting, with a trend for the majority of palliative care APNs to be licensed nurse practitioners. Nurse practitioners working in palliative care clinics serve to provide consultative services to patients with diseases such as COPD, congestive heart failure, multiple sclerosis, or cancer. The role of these consultative clinics is to assist the primary care provider with specific recommendations and to comanage the patients if requested. Advanced practice nurses in these roles may staff symptom management clinics or conduct hospital or home consultations.

With a growing number of outpatient palliative care programs, the need for APNs with this training and focus will intensify. A constant variable in providing outpatient palliative care is the need for adequate reimbursement. Palliative care providers also need experience and expertise in recommending and/or prescribing pain and symptom management medications. Nurse practitioners will continue to be highly desired members of outpatient palliative care teams as they help meet both of these challenges.

In the outpatient setting, the primary role of the APN is to provide clinical consultation regarding the palliative needs of the patient with a serious illness. This role may be as a member of an outpatient palliative care team or within a specialty practice whose population requires frequent palliative care attention. For example, oncology APNs often have dual roles in the outpatient cancer center, providing antitumor therapy for some patients while treating symptoms in other patients who have elected to follow a palliative course. Nurse practitioners managing advanced cardiac patients prescribe therapy for heart arrhythmias and manage electrolyte imbalances in one exam room while educating a patient and family in the next room about completing a Physicians Orders for Life Sustaining Treatment (POLST) form. These practitioners move back and forth several times a day, caring for patients undergoing active treatment while consulting with other patients with primarily palliative care needs. The challenge for these practitioners is to incorporate discussions about advanced care planning and symptom management education earlier rather than later in the course of care.

The broad educational focus of nurses with a master's degree or higher arms them with other abilities that are critical for building and maintaining effective palliative care programs. These nurses bring with them the ability to not only contribute clinically but to serve as educators, researchers, and administrative leaders within palliative care programs.

## Strategies for Integrating Palliative Care into the Outpatient Setting

A combination of philosophical mission, strategic planning, and bottom-line pragmatism is necessary to integrate palliative care successfully into the current outpatient medical model (Figure 48–1). The philosophical mission must come from the institution, and the strategic planning from administration, but practical, day-to-day implementation occurs in the clinical practice at the hands of nurses and physicians. Integration of palliative care must begin at the initial visit and continue through the ongoing evaluation and management process.

### Assessment

Assessment of the patient's and family's goals and preferences begins during the initial meeting. In most outpatient settings, a baseline history, a physical examination, and a review of radiographic and laboratory tests accompany a review of preventive, general, or specialty health-care needs during the first few office visits. An evaluation of current health needs and preventive health issues can be followed by a routine review of end-of-life care preferences. If such a discussion is delayed and occurs during a later or exacerbated illness, then the patient and family are much more likely to fear that death is imminent or that the doctor is "holding something back." This makes it much more difficult for all involved to reach clarity concerning the patient's goals. Table 48–2 shows a sample clinic conversation.

If the patient already has a life-threatening diagnosis, it is appropriate to establish a routine for assessing pain, fatigue, nausea, and other physical, psychological, and functional parameters early in treatment. It is critically important to establish a standard approach to assessing the palliative care

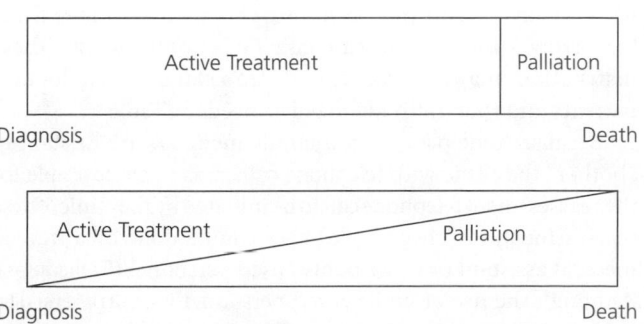

**Figure 48–1.** Active treatment versus palliative care depicted in a mutually exclusive "old" model and an integrated "new" model.

Table 48–2
**Sample Dialogue for Opening Advanced Directive Discussion**

**Nurse:** Mrs. Jones I notice in your chart here we do not have a copy of your living will.

**Mrs. Jones:** Well the doctor has told me I am doing ok.

**Mr. Jones:** We like to think positive.

**Nurse:** Of course, and your tests today are very positive. However, part of taking care of you and your family is for us to understand your wishes from day one. I will have our social worker bring in some materials for you to review at home. I will sit down with you next week when you are back for treatment.

needs of the patient and family in the outpatient setting. To save time and obtain preliminary information, patients may be given a standard form to fill out before the examination (Figure 48–2). This can also help narrow the priority issues for the visit. In one study, the use of a "question prompt list" decreased unmet informational needs about "what to expect in the future" among patients and caregivers ($p = 0.003$).[13] Electronic forms are increasingly being used; they may be accessed through a waiting room kiosk or even over the internet from the patient's home.

Patients and their families should be educated early about the importance of symptom assessment and reporting as well as about evaluation of treatment efficacy and side effects. Establishing the patient and family as part of the team improves outcomes. As always, the patient's goals of care become the central focus for facilitating optimized palliative care. Table 48–3 shows a sample dialogue.

Reassessment of pain and symptoms should occur with new or continuing problems and with a reasonable frequency and method. For example, if a patient with pain level of 7 on a scale of 10 is seen in the office for opioid titration, an explicit follow-up assessment plan should be established before the patient leaves the clinic. A clinic nurse should telephone the patient in a day or two, or alternatively, the patient or a family member should call the office nurse if the pain level does not drop below 4 within a day or two. Patient instructions should be specific, such as, "Call the clinic if you go 3 days or longer without having a normal bowel movement," or "Call the clinic tomorrow if the antinausea medicine is not working." These instructions may be incorporated into a standard handout for patients and then individualized as needed (Table 48–4).

Because some patients and family members are hesitant to "bother" the clinic with telephone calls, it is often desirable for the reassessment telephone call to be initiated by the clinic. These reassessment, or "check-back," calls can be done by a trained medical assistant or other nonlicensed personnel (Table 48–5). Although the use of nonlicensed personnel is controversial, it is increasingly accepted as part of the priorities for containing spiraling costs. Training in the triage of critical symptom problems is the key to optimal use of nonlicensed staff.

An organized reminder system for callbacks should be instituted. With newer electronic medical records (EMR), charts can be "flagged" to remind the provider or assistant to follow up with a patient at a later date. The electronic note can then be built on to show the chain of communication and intervention. This is a benefit of the EMR and improves documenation and communication in the outpatient setting. As with telephone triage, the caller must be given clear criteria for what to do with the information obtained (e.g., document resolved problems, report unresolved problems to the provider). Criteria for further follow-up can be established so that unresolved symptoms identified by the office nurse or medical assistant at telephone triage lead to notification of the physician and further revision of the treatment plan. For example, any new problems should be triaged by a registered nurse or physician. Table 48–6 shows a sample of the electronic medical record document.

Patients who have a knowledge deficit about their medications or treatment regimen require one or more follow-up calls from a registered nurse or pharmacist. It is extremely helpful to provide the patient with written descriptions of medication changes or significant changes in the plan of care.

New or escalating symptoms require timely response by the outpatient team. A reasonable time-frame should be set for follow-up of new problems. Ideally, the patient should be seen within 12 hours after the onset of new symptoms—essentially the same day, if possible. This is particularly true for patients with significant symptom management issues, for whom trips to the emergency room or urgent care center would be extremely tiring and would result in the patient's being evaluated without all pertinent data available. Any patient with significant new or escalating symptoms who is seen in an emergency room should be seen again in the outpatient setting within 24 to 48 hours. If the patient receives home care or is involved with a hospice, an initial evaluation can be performed at home with telephone contact with the clinic. If home care or hospice care is not in place, an escalation of symptom management problems often is a very good indication that these resources should be initiated immediately.

Palliative care goals should be identified and evaluated by the clinic staff on an ongoing basis. Assessment of the palliative needs of the patient should begin within the first few office visits, become a standard part of routine interactions, and should increase in scope and frequency as the patient's disease process progresses.

### Evaluation and Management

The focus in the outpatient setting is evaluation and management of acute and chronic conditions. The evaluation and management codes drive reimbursement and consequently dictate documentation requirements. The "evaluate and treat" construct is deeply entrenched in the traditional medical model. However, neither the reimbursement-driven evaluation and management process nor the traditional medical model lends itself to the inclusion of palliative care. In

**Pain and Symptom Management
Waiting Room Checklist**

Patient Name:_____

Date:              _____

Since you saw your doctor last have you had any "new" pain or symptoms?

(circle one)

Yes   No

The level of pain is described on a 0 to 10 scale where 0 is no pain and 10 is the worst pain you can imagine. Please circle the number that best indicates the level of pain you have had over the last 24 hours:

| 0 | 1 | 2 | 3 | 4 | 5 | 6 | 7 | 8 | 9 | 10 |
|---|---|---|---|---|---|---|---|---|---|----|
| No Pain | | Mild | | Discomforting | | Distressing | | Horrible | | Excruciating |

Check the box beside all of the below words that describe your pain

☐ aching     ☐ burning     ☐ shooting     ☐ throbbing

☐ tender     ☐ sharp       ☐ stabbing     ☐ cramping

**Please indicate which symptoms you are currently experiencing:**

| | No | Yes | If yes, is the symptom | | | If yes, how long has it been |
|---|---|---|---|---|---|---|
| | | | ✓ Mild | ✓ Moderate | ✓ Severe | |
| Nausea | | | | | | |
| Hard/infrequent bowel movements | | | | | | |
| Drowsiness | | | | | | |
| Shortness of Breath | | | | | | |
| Dry Mouth | | | | | | |
| Feeling Very Tired | | | | | | |
| Stomach ache after my pills | | | | | | |
| Muscle jerking/twitching | | | | | | |
| Bad dreams or "seeing things" that are not there | | | | | | |

(circle one)

Are you having any problems with your medications?

Yes   No

Is there <u>anything</u> that you feel is a priority to discuss at today's clinic appointment? (if yes, please indicate what)

_____

_____

_____

**Figure 48–2.** Patient waiting room checklist for pain and symptom assessment. The questions relate to pain and any side effects of analgesics—information that can facilitate discussion of symptom management.

fact, one of the most persistent problems in palliative care is the "hospice as last resort" assumption of some providers, which causes referrals from the hospital or outpatient setting to a hospice agency within the last days of life. The concept of incorporating palliative care prior to suspension of active treatment has historically not been covered by insurance as a separate service and therefore has been slow to develop in most programs. In addition, the "hospice" versus "palliative care" versus "pain specialist" verbage has confused some primary care providers, leading them to ask "Where does the palliative component of our role intersect with the palliative care specialist role?"

Some providers historically have worried that hospice would "take over" the patient. In some cases, this concern has resulted in an "us-or-them" mentality. Integration of palliative care principles into primary practice at all levels along

**Table 48–3**
**Sample Dialogue for Goal-Oriented Pain Assessment**

**Nurse:** Mr. Edwards, in addition to treating your disease, we also want to be successful at relieving your symptoms. What's your pain level today on the 0 to 10 scale?

**Mr. Edwards:** Oh, don't worry about my pain—its only a 6 today.

**Nurse:** You mentioned that your pain is 6 out of 10, but I see that you haven't been taking as much pain medicine as the doctor ordered for you. What level of pain relief would be your goal?

**Mr. Edwards:** Well, it would be nice to be down around a 4, but the medicine is so darn expensive that I try not to use it unless it gets pretty bad.

**Nurse:** I see…your goal would be to get the pain down to a 4, or so if the cost factor wasn't there…is that right? Well, let's ask Dr. Jones if there is a less expensive drug that would work for you. We could also check to see if the drug company has a program to help out with the cost of the medication. I'll have the financial counselor make some calls.

---

**Table 48–4**
**Handout Reminder List for Patients**

Your comfort is important to us. This is a reminder to call us if you are having any of the problems listed below:
☐ Any new pain
☐ Pain that is constantly above a 5 on 0–10 scale, even with your pain medicine
☐ Severe episodes of pain, even with your pain medicine
☐ Stools that are hard and difficult to pass, or if you are moving your bowels only every 2nd or 3rd day.
☐ Feeling very drowsy after taking your medicine
☐ Having bad dreams or "seeing things"
☐ Nausea, vomiting, or stomach pain after taking your medicine
☐ Muscle twitching or jerking
☐ Other

**Other Issue Important to Discuss with the Doctor or Nurse**

1) Call the clinic tomorrow if the nausea medicine is not working
2) Call the clinic tomorrow if the pain is still > 4/10
3) Call the clinic if you are not getting enough instructions or how to take your medicines
4) Not being able to afford your medicines
5) Worries about taking pain medicine

---

**Table 48–5**
**Sample Dialogue for "Check-Back" Calls**

Mr. Edwards this is Jesse from Dr. Jones' office. I'm calling to check back on Mr. Edwards' constipation since we increased his stool softeners. Has he had a normal bowel movement today?

Mr. Smith, this is Jesse from Dr. Jones' office. I'm calling to check back on your nausea. Is that antinausea medicine working for you?

---

**Table 48–6**
**Sample Documentation from Electronic Medical Record**

*2/10/09: 15:30*
Susan please call Mr. Thomas tomorrow to see if nausea is better. If he has had no improvement please route this to the triage RN and have her call him. **J. Smith, ARNP**

*2/11/09: 10: 00*
Mr. Jones called today and he had a rough night. Pain is an 8/10 and he is still nauseated. He was told triage nurse would be calling within the next twenty minutes. **S. White, MA**

*2/11/09 10:05*
Mary, can you please call and triage issues with Mr. Jones. He needs urgent call back for new pain. **S. White, MA**

*2/11/09: 10:15*
Call back to Mr. Jones. He has new pain in lower back and weakness in his right leg. Patient was advised to come in for immediate evaluation. Discussed with J. Smith, ARNP. Urgent appointment made with oncology nurse practitioner for 11:00 AM today. MRI notified we may require work in for MRI. **M. Roberts, RN**

---

diagnosis with active treatment and then abruptly, shortly before death, switching to a purely palliative model. The "new" model depicts the health-care system using active and palliative care concurrently, with a primarily active treatment focus at diagnosis, integration along the trajectory, and a primarily palliative focus at death (see Figure 48–1).

A good example is the patient with heart failure described in the case study that follows.

CASE STUDY
*Mr. T, a 54-Year-Old Male with a History of MI*

Over the course of many years of treatment Mr. T develops a close relationship with the providers in his cardiology office. At age 54 Mr. T had his first myocardial infarction and was referred to a cardiologist. He and his family felt this was a "call to action" and listened attentively as the cardiologist and his nurse recommended a variety of lifestyle changes including diet and exercise, as well as blood pressure monitoring and cholesterol lowering medications. He sees the physicians, nurse practitioners, and nurses in the

---

with further development of the palliative care discipline as a consulting service are key to resolution of these issues.

Many clinicians reject the stark line drawn between active treatment and palliative care and successfully merge these concepts in outpatient care. Conceptually, this model was described by the World Health Organization.[14] The "old" model depicts health-care system involvement starting from

cardiology office every 6 to 12 months for the next ten years developing confidence and trust in their management of his cardiac care. At age 65 he has acute shortness of breath and atrial fibrillation and is rushed to the hospital where he is found to be having ischemic changes. In the ICU Mr. T and his family are greatly comforted by the presence of the familiar face of his cardiologist. He recommends coronary bypass surgery, indicates that he is referring Mr. T to the heart surgeon that he feels is the best, and reassures them that he will continue to watch over him during and after the procedure. Mr. T recovers from surgery and makes regular visits to the cardiology practice every six months. Years go by and the trust and confidence that has built up between Mr. T and the providers in the practice grows into genuine affection, frequently underscored with jokes about how they are all growing grey together. In his late 70s Mr. T has recurrent atrial fibrillation, increasing aortic stenosis, and signs of heart failure. During this time, education regarding palliative strategies for preventing sequelae of the disease (such as dypnea on exertion and easy fatigability, or chest pain) are discussed alongside aggressive measures (possible valve replacement) during many outpatient encounters. As the disease progresses, discussions in the exam room have less emphasis on "cure" and more emphasis on "control." At age 79 Mr. T has increasing shortness of breath at rest and elects to go forward with aortic valve replacement. Once again, the cardiologist and cardiac nurse practitioner follow him closely during and after surgery alongside the cardiac surgery team. Although the surgeon is in charge of his care, Mr. T and his family look to the cardiology team as their primary medical experts and source of support. Mr. T rallies after surgery and is able to make some trips back east to visit family, spend time with his grandchildren, and remain active in his church. He visits the cardiology practice now every 3 to 6 months where the primary focus now is monitoring and managing his heart failure. Late in the process, much more time is spent on quality-of-life issues, such as energy conservation techniques, assistive devices, and home oxygen. At age 82 Mr. T and his wife move into assisted living. He often uses a wheelchair to go to meals in the dining room as ambulating causes too much fatigue. He finds it more difficult to travel to office visits and many of his contacts with the practice are now by phone and are almost exclusively about control of his dyspnea. During his last visit to the practice the familiar faces of the doctors and nurses bring a smile to Mr. T's face. They again reminisce about their long journey together. The nurse practitioner indicates that the heart failure is progressing and the treatment to control it is no longer working. She recommends hospice and assures them that there are strategies that can be used to control symptoms as the heart continues to fail. There is not a dry eye in the room. All the staff give Mr. T hugs with many reassurances that they will keep in touch through the hospice team. Mr. T no longer travels to the clinic but is often in the thoughts of those providers.

Another example is an elderly gentleman with metastatic prostate cancer who has decided not to pursue any more aggressive care but has developed severe pain, rated as 9 on a scale of 0 to 10, that radiates from his back down his legs. His opioid therapy has been increased aggressively over the past week, and he is now somnolent between periods of extreme pain. His wife also notices he needs more help getting out of bed because his legs "won't hold him up." The patient and his wife explain that their goals are to keep his pain under control and to keep him as functional as possible. If metastatic spinal compression is suspected, then palliative radiation may be the best strategy to meet the patient's and family's goals. In such situations, a very clear understanding of the patient's and family's goals of care—well-defined and known to both outpatient providers and palliative care providers—facilitates the best possible outcomes.

Treatment algorithms or protocols can promote efficiency in the clinic and enhance outcomes. These tools can be successfully put into place and implemented by both clinic nurses and home care or hospice nurses. One such algorithm was used in outpatient oncology and resulted in improved pain management.[15] The Cancer Pain Algorithm is a decision tree model for pain treatment that was developed as a practical interpretation of the Agency for Health Care Policy and Research Guidelines for Cancer Pain Management. The algorithm consists of a bulleted set of analgesic "guiding principles" for use with opioids, nonsteroidal anti-inflammatory drugs, tricyclic antidepressants, and anticonvulsants and addresses drug side effects. For example, the statement "Titrate to efficacy or side effects" is an underlying principle throughout the algorithm. Drug choice decisions depend on pain assessment data. The flow chart directs the oncology nurse or oncologist to side effect protocols, equianalgesic conversion charts, and a primer for intractable pain.

Figure 48–3 represents the high-level algorithm decision-making flow chart. Etiology and location correlate the pain with its known tumor or treatment-related source or indicate the need for further diagnostic work-up. Pain intensity is based on self-report on a scale from 0 to 10, where 0 is no pain and 10 is the worst pain imaginable. Pain character is divided into nociceptive versus neuropathic components; the character of the pain is the primary variable to direct the choice of nonopioid or coanalgesic therapies. The frequency and method of reassessment are outlined for the practitioner based on the results of the last pain assessment contact. An algorithm reference tool contains drug-specific content (e.g., titration parameters, side-effect protocols) and a number of highly specific flow charts. The algorithm process is intended as a team effort, relying on the network of physician, clinic nurse, home care nurse, and family caregiver as a cohesive outpatient unit, all applying the principles of the algorithm as they relate to the individual patient.

Another concept now used in outpatient care is that of the care coordinator. In cancer centers, these nurses are

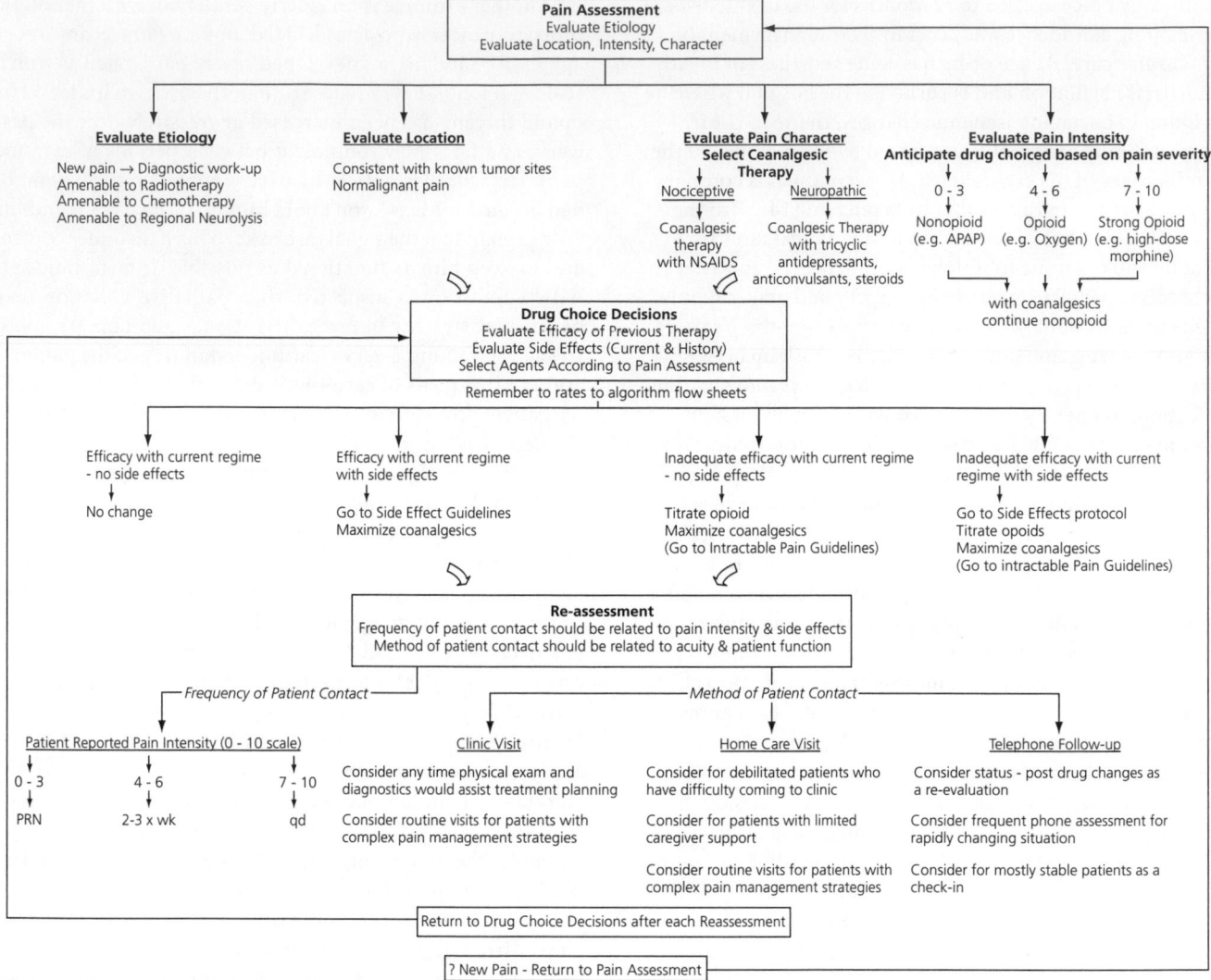

**Figure 48–3.** Du Pen Cancer Pain Algorithm. An algorithm designed to aid decision making in outpatient management of cancer pain.

sometimes referred to as "nurse navigators." Regardless of their title, care coordinators in a variety of outpatient settings help to guide the patient and the family through the myriad of services. The nurse coordinator utilizes critical pathways, or algorithms of her specialty, to plan the patient's course and provides feedback to the physician weekly. A treatment plan becomes a "road atlas," and the nurse steers the patient's care to the key stops along the way. These stops may be time for educational sessions, follow-up diagnostic studies, interdisciplinary consultations, meetings with social workers or financial counselor, home health and hospice referrals, or a variety of other patient-specific services. This model works well for outpatient services that generally are disconnected from one another and that might be overlooked under strained resources. Nurses who work as care coordinators in these settings require orientation and continuing education in palliative care to effectively incorporate a palliative focus into the care pathway.

## Critical Building Blocks for Outpatient Palliative Care

The two major benefits of the outpatient setting are a more intimate, structured environment and more time to develop long-term relationships. Numerous critical elements provide an excellent framework for integrating basic palliative care concepts into almost any outpatient setting. Improving provider accessibility to patients and caregivers, promoting active listening by all staff, providing a sense of control over decision-making, and continuously assessing psychological and spiritual distress of patients and their families are the building blocks to successful outpatient palliative care.[8,9,16,17]

### Accessibility

In the outpatient setting, accessibility is critical to the palliative care of patients. Having 24-hour support available to patients and their caregivers helps reduce anxiety and, when necessary, facilitates identification of after-hours problems that require immediate attention, such as escalating pain or shortness of breath. The clerk or other nonlicensed personnel who answer the telephone should receive very clear instructions on how to distinguish problems that require immediate attention. For example, billing questions and insurance issues receive callbacks, whereas pain, shortness of breath, and changes in level of consciousness require a nurse or physician to take the call. These criteria should be agreed upon by all and followed consistently. Calls that require high-level triage should be handled by trained nurses armed with protocols and standing orders that have been approved by the patient's physician. The triage system should include procedures for bringing patients into the clinic for same-day evaluation or for admission to the hospital. Such a system has three main benefits: (1) the patient sees the nurse as a qualified member of the team who is available and ready to assist; (2) the patient and family caregivers become more confident in making adjustments to medications for pain or symptom management; and (3) telephoning allows the nurse to reassess, reassure, and reinforce the teaching that has taken place. Table 48–7 shows an example of palliative care management via an outpatient phone triage system.

Advanced practice nurses improve accessibility for patients undergoing palliative care management. Many nurse practitioners share on-call responsibilities with physicians, thereby alleviating some of the workload that 24-hour accessibility requires. Flexible scheduling of APNs can allow for "same-day work-ins," nursing home visits, or home visits, as circumstances require.

Oncology nurses are often comfortable opening a dialogue with patients about pain, fatigue, weight loss, and appetite but are less comfortable handling conversations about death and dying or loss.[18] Cardiovascular clinic nurses are skilled at assessing for fluid overload and evaluating for home oxygen eligibility for the end-stage heart failure patient but less comfortable handling conversations about intubation and feeding tubes. If a formerly hopeful patient with a "fighter" attitude responds with "I don't think I can do this anymore," the active listener understands that a transition is occurring. Time must be set aside for this patient, either immediately or with a plan for a follow-up telephone call or family conference. Time spent proactively facilitating these transitions almost always saves crisis-induced time spent later in the patient's course.

Another critical component of active listening involves identifying barriers to effective palliative care. The classic example of a barrier to care is the fear of opioid addiction. A clinic nurse often first identifies the patient's or family member's concern about taking opioids. It is important to discuss this attitudinal barrier early and frequently. Another barrier to pain management at the end of life is the belief that using pain medications hastens death. Because of this belief, family members may resist optimizing opioids and adjuvants at the end of life. In addition to verbal instructions at the time of the clinic visits, written materials on the rationale and role of

| Table 48–7 |
|---|
| **Triage Phone Note** |

Incoming call: 8:00

**Call from:** Machintosh, J.P. (MR # 800005469)

**Call taken by:** Janet Smith, MA

**Details for reason:** Called at 8:00 am having more constipation since increasing morphine dosage.

**Summary of call:** Patient reports better pain control but also reports constipation. No fever, no abdominal pain or nausea. Recommended patient initiate stool softener and laxative per protocol. I will alert triage nurse to check back with him tomorrow. Patient given list of symptoms to call back within next 12 hours.

**Action taken:** Phone call completed, constipation protocol initiated, sent to Triage Nurse for follow up

**Follow-up for phone call**

**Details for follow-up action taken:** Have checked back with patient today. Current bowel regimen is working well. He feels pain control is adequate. Reinforced need to call us if symptoms return.

**Follow-up action taken:** Phone call completed, Provider notified

**Follow-up by:** Susan Jones, RN

symptom management in end-of-life care can be extremely helpful.

Another issue that is frequently present and often requires active facilitation by clinic staff is the social context of care. The cost of care is an increasing concern and is an area that patients and families are frequently uncomfortable discussing. This often results in conflicts that are identified only late in the course of care. Distressing issues may arise concerning long-term care—particularly the distribution of financial support and caregiving responsibilities among family members. Whenever possible, prompt initiation of family conferences or referrals to social workers or financial counselors are advisable.

## Providing a Sense of Control

Helping chronically and terminally ill patients regain a sense of control is a key element in managing the helplessness many patients experience. Interventions that can promote a sense of control in the outpatient setting include allowing patients to remain dressed during most office calls, at least until an examination is required; reducing the clinical, white-coat formality; and providing a safe, nonthreatening, private place for meetings with patients and their families. These accommodations return a sense of control and dignity to the patient. Another critical component of providing a sense of control is having an active patient education component. Giving patients and families the knowledge that they need to make decisions is a great empowerment. Practical information regarding how to "negotiate the system," how to get help after hours, and how to communicate with health-care professionals in a way that gets them the information they need are all important components of patient education.

## Tuning in to Distress

Psychological and spiritual health are often profoundly affected by life-threatening illness. In a recent study conducted at Duke University, cancer patients were audiotaped during outpatient encounters with their oncologists. Patients expressed anxiety (46%), fear (25%), depression (12%), and anger (9%). Issues that brought up these emotions included symptoms and functional concerns (66%), medical diagnoses and treatment (54%), social issues (14%), and the health-care system (9%).[19] Identifying distress early in the palliative care continuum allows for early intervention, prevention of comorbid psychological problems, and improved quality of life.

Easy-to-use, inexpensive, brief, noninvasive, and generally well-accepted self-reporting questionnaires can be used in the outpatient setting. Two good examples are the Hospital Anxiety and Depression Scale (HAD)[20] and the Distress Thermometer.[21] The HAD consists of 14 questions to which the client answers "yes" or "no." This tool omits somatic complaints and focuses on questions that can help differentiate anxiety and depression. Despite its title, it has also been successfully used in the outpatient setting.[22] The Distress Thermometer has been tested in men with prostate cancer. It consists of a visual analog scale made to look like a thermometer, with the bottom of the thermometer reading 1, or no distress, 5 being moderate distress, and 10 (at the top of the thermometer) being extreme distress. Distress is defined in a generic sense of unpleasant stress. This is a simple scale that can be used at the beginning of each office visit or on a regular basis (e.g., quarterly). Responses can be used to open discussions of the symptoms of distress experienced by a client in the outpatient setting. For example, the clinician may say, "I see that you're feeling a moderate amount of distress. Can we talk about what you're feeling?"

Spiritual distress can be equally devastating to the patient and family. Hearing "What did I do to deserve this?" or "How could God let this happen to my husband?" from a patient or family member is a cue that spiritual support is needed. Some health-care systems have chaplains available in the outpatient setting. Many churches and synagogues provide outreach ministries to the gravely ill. Other nontraditional means of spiritual support include meditation and rituals to explore the meaning of events. Whenever possible, the clinic should be given a list of community resources for spiritual support.

## The Three C's of Outpatient Palliative Care: Cooperation, Communication, and Closure

At the heart of palliative care in the outpatient setting are the three concepts of cooperation, communication, and closure. The outpatient setting is the site of cooperation among patient, family, and outpatient staff. This cooperation expands to the agencies within the community that are caring for the patient. This may include home health-care nurses, long-term care staff, local pharmacists, neighbors and friends of the client, and the local church. The physician and APNs cooperate to provide easy access to care. The specialist and primary care physician, who both often monitor the patient in the outpatient setting, cooperate to provide the most comprehensive care. Care in the outpatient setting is not provided in isolation, but by a well-coordinated and dedicated community team.

Central to this cooperation is good communication. Communication begins with active listening, fostered in the outpatient setting. Efficient and accurate documentation of patient teaching, telephone calls, and interventions is the key to continuity of care. Various tools have been developed for use in the outpatient setting to improve this communication.

Not yet addressed, but also important in the outpatient setting, is closure. Bereavement is an issue for nurses, physicians, and staff in the outpatient setting.[23] As patients become sicker and eventually homebound, the outpatient staff is no longer able to see the patients, despite being in close contact with family and home care staff over the telephone. In many cases, this early separation from the patient complicates the ability of the outpatient staff to come to closure with what often has been a long-term relationship with the patient. This abrupt loss of connection can be a significant source of bereavement for staff.

Outpatient nurses may have had years to assess the families or caregivers' previous experiences with death, the support available, and the coping resources of those who have suffered the loss. This familiarity with the family or caregiver helps the nurse in the outpatient setting provide better support to grieving loved ones.

Often, family members or caregivers are drawn back to the outpatient setting to say final goodbyes or give gifts of thanks to staff members who may have become as close as family to the patient and caregivers. Staff should prepare for this visit by being informed of the patient's death. Work should stop for a moment to embrace the returning family members and give them time to tell the story of the death and share feelings of grief and joyful memories of the deceased. Gifts or pictures brought by the family should be accepted graciously. Many offices take time out each month to send cards to families of patients who have died.

Staff of the outpatient clinic, the front desk receptionist, the medical assistant, the nurse, and the physician may experience grief after the loss of a patient. Often, staff require support through the deaths of patients dear to them. It is important to allow for special opportunities to celebrate the lives and mourn the deaths of these patients. Attending funerals, keeping scrapbooks, and having occasional symbolic tributes to patients can help staff through the grieving process. Occasionally, it may be helpful to provide professional counseling or to send staff members on a retreat, where feelings regarding death and loss can be shared. Caregivers, as well as family and friends, need closure when death comes. In the outpatient setting, this affords all who have experienced the loss support on the journey toward healing.

## Summary

The outpatient setting has both advantages and disadvantages. As more and more patients with end-stage disease choose to remain in their homes, the outpatient clinic has become the main point of contact for care and coordination of resources. Relationships are developed over many years, creating a sense of trust that fosters the comprehensive care that is at the heart of palliative medicine.

Strategies for providing palliative care in this setting apply to all diseases. The concepts of active listening, promoting patient control, assessing for distress, and promoting access to care all improve the delivery of palliative care in the outpatient clinic. The use of nurse-staffed telephone triage systems, nurse practitioners, and tools for assessing palliative care needs benefits both the terminally ill patient and the patient with advanced chronic disease. Care algorithms and critical pathways assist staff in implementing research-based interventions to prevent suffering and promote quality of life. Finally, the three C's of outpatient palliative care emphasize the necessity of coordination, communication, and closure.

There is perhaps a fourth quality needed when caring for chronically or terminally ill clients in the outpatient setting; commitment. Through a commitment to alleviate suffering and promote quality of life, caregivers in the outpatient setting assist patients in finding physical, psychological, and spiritual wellness, even at the end of the disease trajectory.

REFERENCES

1. Fitch MI, Mings D. Cancer Nursing in Ontario: Defining nursing roles. Can Oncol Nurs J 2003;13:28–44.
2. Mok E, Chiu PC. Nurse–patient relationships in palliative care. J Adv Nurs 2004;48:475–483.
3. Meier DE, Beresford L. Outpatient clinics are a new frontier for palliative care. J Palliat Med 2008;11:823–828.
4. Setoguchi S, Earle CC, Glynn R, et al. Comparison of prospective and retrospective indicators of the quality of end of life cancer care. J Clin Oncol 2008;26:5671–5678.
5. Daley A, Matthews C, Williams A. Heart failure and palliative care services working in partnership: Report of a new model of care. J Palliat Med 2006;20:593–601.
6. Au DH, Udris EM, Fihn SD, McDonell MB, Curtis R. Differences in health care utilization at the end of life among patients with chronic obstructive pulmonary disease and patients with lung cancer. Arch Intern Med 2006;13:326–331.
7. Prepublication 2010 Standards. http://www.jointcommission.org/Standards/ (accessed November 10, 2009).
8. Rabow MW, Dibble SL, Pantilat SZ, McPhee SJ. The comprehensive care team: A controlled trial of outpatient palliative medicine consultation. Arch Intern Med 2004;164:83–91.
9. Strasser F, Sweeney C, Willey J, Benisch-Tolley S, Palmer JL, Bruera E. Impact of a half-day multidisciplinary symptom control and palliative care outpatient clinic in a comprehensive cancer center on recommendations, symptom intensity, and patient satisfaction: A retrospective descriptive study. J Pain Symptom Manage 2004;27:481–491.
10. Zimmerman C, Seccareccia D, Clarke A, Warr D, Rodin G. Bringing palliative care to a Canadian Cancer Center: The palliative care program at Princess Margaret Hospital. Support Care Cancer 2006;14:982–987.
11. Coyne P. The evolution of the advanced practice nurse within palliatie care. J Palliat Med 2003;6:769–770.
12. Meier D, Beresford L. Advanced practice nurse in paliative care: A pivotal role and perspective. J Palliat Med 2006;9:624–627.
13. Clayton JM, Butow PN, Tattersall MHN, et al. Randomized controlled trial of a prompt list to help advanced cancer patients and their caregivers to ask questions about prognosis and end of life care. J Clin Oncol 2007;25:715–723.
14. World Health Organization. Cancer Contol—Knowledge into Action: Palliative Care. Geneva: World Health Organization, 2007.
15. Du Pen A, Du Pen S, Hansberry J, et al. An educational implementation of a cancer pain algorithm for ambulatory care. Pain Manag Nurs 2000;1:116–128.
16. Back AL, Arnold RM, Baile WF, Tulsky JA, Fryer-Edwards K. Approaching difficult communication tasks in oncology. CA Cancer J Clin 2005;55:164–177.
17. Walling A, Lorenz KA, Dy SM, et al. Evidence-based recommendations for information and care planning in cancer care. J Clin Oncol 2008;26:3896–3902.
18. Sivesind D, Parker PA, Cohen L, et al. Communicating with patients in cancer care: What areas do nurses find most challenging? J Cancer Educ 2003;18:202–209.
19. Anderson WG, Alexander SC, Rodriquez KL, et al. "What concerns me is…" Expression of emotion by advanced cancer patients during outpatient visits. Support Care Cancer 2008;16:803–811.
20. Moorey S, Greer S, Watson M, et al. The factor structure and factor stability of the Hospital Anxiety and Depression Scale in patients with cancer. Br J Psychiatry 1991;158:255–259.
21. Roth AJ, Kornblith AB, Batel-Copel L, Peabody E, Scher HI, Holland JC. Rapid screening for psychologic distress in men with prostate carcinoma: A pilot study. Cancer 1998;82:1904–1908.
22. Zigmond AS, Snaith RP. The hospital anxiety and depression scale. Acta Psychiatr Scand 1983;67:361–370.
23. Valentino RL. Recognizing and responding to grief: Concepts to guide daily practice. Adv Nurse Pract 2001;9:52–55.

# 49 Rehabilitation and Palliative Care

*Donna J. Wilson and Kathleen Michael*

*Long after lung surgery, my fatigue was so debilitating the marathon walks I thrived on seemed a distant memory, Several months of exercise during my many rounds of chemotherapy treatments, my energy improved enough so I could enjoy my family and friends as long as I am living.*
*—A patient*

◆ **Key Points**
◆ *Rehabilitation principles are applicable to palliative care to enhance quality of life.*
◆ *Interdisciplinary care is a key concept in rehabilitation.*
◆ *Rehabilitation in palliative care can prevent disability and complications.*
◆ *Mobility and self-care are the critical components of physical functioning in palliative care.*

CASE STUDY
*A 64-Year-Old Female with Lung Cancer*

AD, age 58 years, was in her usual state of good health as a homemaker, enjoyed traveling with husband on business trips, playing cards, and organizing parties. She was slim and exercised four times a week, although exercise was not her favorite activity. She was loved by all, always giving of herself to others. AD went for her yearly routine physical. A chest X-ray showed an abnormality; therefore, it was repeated, and the second X-ray showed a right upper lobe mass. A CT scan confirmed the mass and a fine needle aspiration biopsy was positive for adenocarcinoma non-small cell lung cancer (NSCLC). She was completely asymptomatic and specifically had no cough, hemoptysis, dyspnea, wheezing, fever, or weight loss. AD did smoke occasionally in high school and was not exposed to secondhand smoke. At the time of thoracotomy, disease was discovered in four mediastinial lymph nodes. Chemotherapy was soon instituted after surgical recovery and then radiotherapy. During her chemotherapy, she continued to exercise five times a week. Her exercises included breathing exercises, treadmill walking for 20 minutes, squats, upper body lightweight training, and stretching. She enjoyed doing the breathing exercises because she felt her lateral chest expand and felt the relaxation from the deep breathing. The breathing was performed slowly, rhythmical, and under control. Her breathing pattern was coordinated each exercise. When bending forward to do a stretch, she would blow out through her lips, bend forward, and then breathe slowly to hold the stretch. Most importantly, AD was reminded not to hold her breath with each exercise. She would commonly complain that her exercise workout was more painful than the chemotherapy but it maintained her strength so she could enjoy dinner with family and friends each night. In her usual fashion, she continued her work as a party organizer. After chemotherapy and radiation, her chest X-ray was clear, only to find another lung lesion a year later. A surgical resection was performed, and her postoperative course was uneventful. AD did admit the exercise might be keeping her strong but continued to express she did not like exercising. Her family and friends were her great support and were always there to push, encourage, and love her. In fact her friends would call when she was on the treadmill. She would put the phone on speaker and chat for 20 minutes and the time went fast.

For several years, AD's life was normal without cancer and she maintained a 15-minute exercise program and treadmill walking. Then one evening, she had a seizure. She was diagnosed with recurrent lung cancer metastatic to the brain. AD had a resection of the right occipital brain metastasis. She completed whole-brain radiotherapy as well as chemotherapy and continued her exercise program. The exercises were modified, but she wanted to be strong physically to enjoy dinners with her family. Maintaining strength of the large muscle groups is most important—for example, doing chair squats with minimal assistance and walking outside with support. Her family and the rehabilitation team adapted her activities of daily living to maintain her function as much as possible to prevent feeling of helplessness and hopelessness. She demonstrated good muscle tone and strength of her arms and legs, with the exception of her big toes, which were numb from peripheral neuropathy. Reflexology was started with some relief. AD was alert and oriented but experienced difficulty with short-term memory loss. To reduce the stress from memory loss she would do things she enjoyed, such as look at family pictures, listen to music for relaxation, or talk to her closest friends. She had a Karnofsky performance scale of 80%. Over the next several months, she was stable until the cancer was metastatic to her spine. This created increased pain and muscle weakness but she continued to walk with the use of a walker and continued to have dinner with family and friends. The rehabilitation team and family members adapted her exercises to maintain the activities she requested, such as going to the bathroom and family gatherings each evening. Many of the exercises were performed in bed and chair. Breathing exercises were performed three to four times a day with instruction, and a family member or the home health aide would provide gentle pressure to her lateral chest wall as she breathe out to lengthen her exhalation. This was intended to increase a larger volume of air removed from the lung so she could take a larger breath in with ease. As she lost more control and ambulation was more difficult, her family and the rehabilitation team were meticulous about her safety. The rehabilitation team provided support for her family and friends, discussing role changes and coping with loss of someone special. This is a case where exercise maintained independence and self-care that suited the patient's abilities and lifestyle.

Her husband said, "No matter the stage of her illness there was always some level of physical activity you could do to maintain her independence. The exercises rebuilt her muscular strength and endurance, reduced fatigue, regained range of motion and flexibility, and relieved anxiety, anger, and stress while restoring her energy level and hope each day we shared together. Thank you."

Even when it is not reasonable to expect cure or reversal of disease processes or to restore a previous level of functioning and independence, a rehabilitative approach to nursing care adds quality to the experience of life's completion. Grounded in respect for each unique patient, rehabilitation nurses address palliative and end-of-life care with concern for restoring the patient's physical and emotional balance. This will enhance feelings of self-confidence, independence, preserving hope, human dignity, and autonomy. They involve social, spiritual, and functional support systems. Rehabilitation nursing interventions are designed to help patients and families make the most out of each day in the context of the disease trajectory. The language of rehabilitation nursing is a language shared with those who practice palliative care.

Rehabilitation nurses work with the concepts of independence and interdependence, self-care, coping, access, and quality of life, skillfully weaving them into the assessment, planning, implementation, and evaluation of nursing care.[1,2] Although the focus is on physical function, fundamental to this practice is the acceptance of varieties of life experiences, including those at life's end. The true challenge in a rehabilitation program is to change or maintain the patient's exercise program so they can be mobile and not become a burden for their caretakers in view of their poor prognosis.

This chapter applies concepts of rehabilitation to palliative care across settings. The case study presented above demonstrates the application of rehabilitative nursing care with a life-threatening illness. A review of the literature demonstrating the effects of physical exercise in the palliative care patient follows. Finally, numerous strategies are discussed for use of rehabilitation techniques to prevent disability and complications in advanced disease.

## Rehabilitation Nursing

Rehabilitation nursing in any context concerns itself with adaptation. As life proceeds to its end, adaptation to a new state allows beings to remain whole: to interact with their environments, to experience human relationships, and to achieve personally meaningful goals. Rehabilitation nurses find themselves at work in every phase of growth, development, and dying, as individuals strive to adapt across the continuum of life.

Rehabilitation nurses care for persons with incurable progressive disease states in a variety of settings. Whether care is patient-, provider-, or facility-centered, the merging of rehabilitation and palliative nursing approaches is evident. Both services are symptom control-oriented, solving functional physical or psychological problems to improve the patient's quality of life.

Research had demonstrated that exercise is the nonpharmacological therapy for managing fatigue, mobility, and self-care. A mild-to-moderate intensity exercise program for patients and family can be designed in an acute, subcute, long-term or hospice care setting. Chair aerobics is an exercise program including breathing exercises, stretching, arm and leg movements for flexibility, lightweight training, and chair squats. As documented in the literature, chair exercises slow the decline of fatigue and physical well-being in patients with advanced breast cancer.[50] The beneficial effects of physical fitness are physiological, such as enhanced rest, improved muscular strength, improved delivery of oxygen-rich blood to the brain and tissues, reduced fatigue, and better sleep patterns, flexibility, and range of motion. The psychological effects are important to enhance one's quality of life, such as coping ability, reduced stress, regaining self-confidence, mood elevation, sharpening mental functioning, and decreased depression. The benefits may be small, but engaging the patient and family together decreases everyone's feelings of helplessness by maintaining some muscle strength and physical activity.

Another approach to maintain quadriceps muscle function is neuromuscular electrical stimulation.[51] This study is a controlled pilot study of a home-based program with lung cancer patients.[52]

A pilot study by Oldervoll and colleagues provided an outpatient hospital-based structured exercise program for 1 hour twice a week for 6 weeks.[53] This exercise program focused on strength-promoting activities such as aerobic exercises using large muscle groups in a standing or sitting position, bicycling, upper and lower body strength exercises, chair squats, balance, and optional abdominal exercises. At the end of the 6 weeks, the patients fatigue level was less, their ability to do self-care activities was improved and the response to physical activity played a role in maintaining independence.

A physical function assessment tool for the palliative care patient has received little attention until now. Helbostad and colleagues reviewed the literature for all existing instruments that had physical function items to assess this patient population's physical performance.[54] This study describes the first steps for the development of a new instrument to measure the physical function of cancer patients receiving palliative care. The goal of this instrument will describe specific types of exercise and explain the complementary roles of structured exercise and daily activity. The rehabilitation professional can then design an exercise program that suits a patient's ability.

*Acute comprehensive inpatient rehabilitation units* are set up in such a way that complex medical-surgical issues may be managed concurrently with the functional processes of comprehensive rehabilitation.[3] For example, patients with metastatic cancer affecting their bones may have significant care needs related to mobility and activities of daily living, well-addressed in an inpatient rehabilitation setting.

For many patients with terminal illness, the transition to an acute rehabilitation unit represents a crucial point in their health-care experience. It is a time when the future comes into focus, and goals are defined based on the likely disease progression. Sometimes a short stay on an inpatient rehabilitation unit makes it possible for patients to return to a home setting, because of the gains in independent function that may be realized. Patients and family members may begin to face limited prognoses, decline in abilities, and changes in roles. Through an interdisciplinary therapeutic process, care needs are clarified, and skills and adaptation strategies are taught to patients and those who will care for them outside of the hospital.

*Subacute rehabilitation facilities* provide additional therapy activities, such as physical, occupational, or speech therapy, based on patient need, endurance, and tolerance. The pacing and amount of therapy are gaged according to individualized goals. As in comprehensive inpatient rehabilitation units, the aim is to facilitate improved physical function and as much independence as possible, even as the disease process moves the patient toward death. For example, patients with advanced disease who are too frail to participate in a full acute rehabilitation program may benefit from the slower-paced rehabilitation of a subacute setting.

*Long-term care settings*, such as skilled nursing facilities, are often places where lives are completed. Specialized *geriatric facilities* focus on the care needs of aging persons, often requiring specialized rehabilitation interventions. In both of these settings, rehabilitation nurses may plan and direct care delivery and make sure that patient and family concerns are kept in the forefront. Attention is paid to optimizing function and self-care, as well as addressing physical care issues.

*Hospice settings* may also provide a venue for a rehabilitative approach to end-of-life care. Careful planning of care to account for limitations, yet promote function and autonomy, is a key factor in smoothing the transition to an inevitable death. Rehabilitative techniques and strategies make it easier for caregivers to manage increasing deficits, thereby protecting patient comfort and dignity through the dying process.

*Pediatric rehabilitation* is focused on guiding the development of children to minimize disability and handicap that may result from physical or cognitive impairment. There are situations in pediatric rehabilitation in which palliative care comes into play, and efforts are directed toward enhancing the normal function of both patient and family through the course of disease. For example, the family members of a child with progressive neuromuscular disease may learn how to use adaptive devices to position the child in a wheelchair for comfort and social interaction as well as for physiological function.

In the *insurance industry* and *managed care systems*, rehabilitation nurses have the opportunity to advocate for the needs of persons with disease or disability and to reduce barriers to their access to care and resources. Near the end of a terminal disease course, planning and resource management are essential to ensure optimal care without undue economic and emotional burdens to families. *Case management* is an expanding practice area for rehabilitation nurses, usually with multidisciplinary relationships. Because palliative care needs are unique to individuals and require coordination of the care across disciplines, usual or episodic patterns of delivery and resource use may prove inadequate. The implementation of care pathways in palliative care requires careful and compassionate guidance and evaluation, tailored to meet individual strengths, abilities, needs, and preferences.[3,4]

Finally, care of dying patients frequently occurs at *home*. Successful end-of-life care at home is the preference of many patients and families. Such care depends on skill, concern, keen assessment, and creative problem-solving. For the reasons shown in each setting, rehabilitation and palliation are compatible. The critical importance of the nurse is to identify a safe exercise program to achieve sufficient autonomy, with mobility and activities of daily living decreasing everyone's feelings of helplessness.

## Rehabilitation Nursing and Palliative Care

Rehabilitation nursing adds value in the arena of palliative care. As future health-care services center on needs, preferences, and informed consent of patients and families in our society, there is less emphasis on cure, illness, paternalism, and prescription. More attention is directed to self-care and client participation, holistic wellness, primary care and prevention, and the quality attributes of care as defined by the consumer.[1]

Patient/family-centered care is clearly appropriate for the unique experience of dying. Enabling a kind of wellness to exist even at the point of death, such as the experience of a "good death," fits with the rehabilitation philosophy. Many rehabilitation nursing actions center on supporting physiological function and preventing complications, goals that are still appropriate at the end of life. Finally, rehabilitation has long been concerned with understanding and measuring quality of life, whether related to physical, psychosocial, or spiritual domains.

The real value of a rehabilitative approach to the nursing care of persons with declining health lies in the foundations of rehabilitation nursing practice. As defined by the Association of Rehabilitation Nurses and the Oncology Nursing Society in 2005, it is imperative that ongoing research and education in rehabililitation be funded to find ways to improve care.[4a] Rehabilitation nurses:

- attend to the full range of human experiences and responses to health and illness;
- deal with families coping with lifelong issues;
- provide a holistic approach to care;
- facilitate team dynamics and integration;
- educate patients and their families to help them control and manage a wide range of challenges associated with chronic illness or disability;
- form partnerships with patients and other health-care providers to attain the best possible outcomes.

The hallmark of rehabilitation is interdisciplinary collaboration. The synergy of collaboration enhances the value of rehabilitation nursing interventions and ensures that patient needs are addressed from a variety of perspectives.[5–9] Typically, the rehabilitation team consists of physicians with specialized training in Physical Medicine and Rehabilitation; rehabilitation nurses; physical, occupational, speech, respiratory, and recreation therapists; exercise physiologists; dietitians; social workers; and others as required to address particular needs (Table 49–1). Effective teamwork requires mutual understanding and synchrony of the roles and responsibilities of each member. When the rehabilitation team works in synergy, it serves patients and families across the continuum of life.

---

**Table 49–1**
**Role of Interdisciplinary Rehabilitation Team Members**

**Physiatrists:** Direct the rehabilitation team in providing comprehensive, integrated, patient-centered care.

**Rehabilitation nurses:** Address physical care needs, such as mobility, daily living skills, bowel and bladder care, skin care, medications, and pain management, and coordinate the overall rehabilitation process.

**Physical therapists:** Address strength, endurance, mobility, activity level, equipment needs, range of motion, balance and stability, and education about ongoing exercise programs to facilitate independent function.

**Occupational therapists:** Address energy conservation needs, upper-extremity strength and function, self-care and home management skills, need for assistive devices, perceptual evaluation and guidance, and education for adaptation needs.

**Speech/language pathologists:** Address expressive and receptive communication needs as well as eating and swallowing issues.

**Social workers:** Address home care and extended care needs; provide patient and family with counseling and resources.

**Rehabilitation psychologists:** Address complex emotional and psychological needs of patients and families, guide the team in psychosocial care, and provide comprehensive psychological testing.

**Vocational counselors:** Address concerns and options related to school or work.

**Recreation therapists:** Address adaptation of leisure skills, recreational activities, socialization, stress management, establishment of therapeutic environment, and enhancement of normalization.

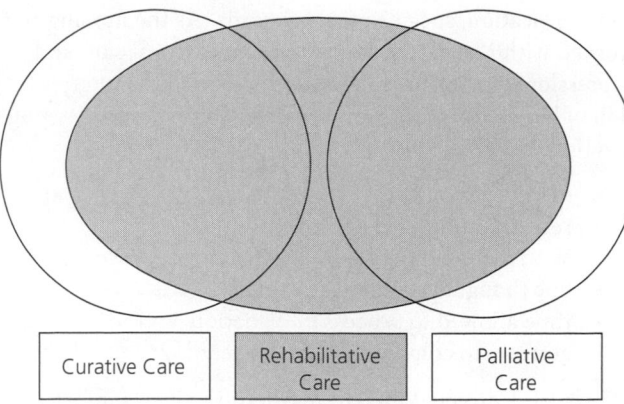

**Figure 49–1.** A conceptual framework for curative, palliative, and rehabilitative care.

## Conceptual Framework

It is a common view that rehabilitation has a place somewhere between curative and palliative care.[10] Rehabilitation does not really seem to fit with curative processes, where care issues resolve with specific treatments, and patients' levels of function and independence ultimately return to normal. Nor does rehabilitation seem in keeping with the irrevocable progress toward death, because rehabilitation implies a return to a previous way of living through adaptation. However, rehabilitation has concerns at each point of the continuum from wellness to death. In wellness, the concern is to prevent health problems and reduce factors that might lead to illness and disability. At the end of life, the concern is to promote autonomy and dignity by enhancing function, independence, and self-care as much as possible.

To conceptualize how rehabilitation nursing fits with care at the end of life, it is helpful to consider a diagrammatic representation (Figure 49–1). In this diagram, curative and palliative care are pictured as two discrete spheres. Rehabilitation overlaps both substantially. In each sphere there is a place for rehabilitation. At the junction between curative and palliative care, rehabilitation may find its greatest impact.

## Rehabilitation Principles Applied to Palliative Care

The rehabilitation of patients with palliative care needs should begin as early as possible. As soon as functional deficits are observed or anticipated, appropriate consultation with members of the rehabilitation team should be initiated. Certain diagnoses, such as progressive neuromuscular diseases; malignancies affecting the brain, spinal cord, or skeletal system; organ failure; and many other conditions that result in functional impairments, should trigger mobilization of the rehabilitation team.

The goals of rehabilitation are to prevent secondary disability, to enhance the functions of both affected and unaffected systems, and to help patients adapt to their physical and social environments by means of physical restoration and adaptive devices.[6]

Rehabilitation nursing strategies focus on:

- Caring for whole persons in their social and physical environments
- Preventing secondary disability
- Enhancing function of both affected and unaffected systems
- Facilitating use of adaptive strategies
- Promoting quality of life.

To illustrate the rehabilitation strategies as they may be applied in actual palliative nursing care situations, some case studies are offered here. The stories serve to illuminate the role of rehabilitation nursing in palliative care and represent common issues with many rehabilitation patients.

## Caring for Whole Persons in Their Social and Physical Environments

Appreciating each person as a unique individual is extremely important to the rehabilitation process. Whereas it may be evident to rehabilitation professionals that certain goals and interventions would suit the patient's needs, it is even more important to find congruence with the patient's own perceived and stated goals and values.

CASE STUDY
*Edna W, A 60-Year-Old Woman with a Lung Transplant*

With a history of rapidly worsening chronic obstructive pulmonary disease, 60-year-old Edna W was faced with few options. As every breath became a struggle, she wondered how she could go on with her life and whether it was worth continuing the fight. She had already lost so much of what was important to her: mobility, independence, and social relationships. Now she found herself homebound, exhausted, and unable to carry on even a telephone conversation with friends and family she so cherished.

After much consultation and deliberation, she agreed that lung transplantation was the only course of treatment that would afford her the function and independence she believed made her life worthwhile. She received the transplanted lungs after a relatively short wait. But her expectations of returning to wellness were not to be fulfilled. Ms. W began an extraordinarily complicated postoperative course and a journey that would lead her to a life's end on which she had not planned.

Initially, Ms. W required prolonged ventilatory support. She struggled with infection and rejection of her new lungs.

She experienced shock, sepsis, and distress; her records thickened with stories of heroics and near misses, of technology, of miracles, and of persistent argument with fate. She had established with her family that she would want everything possible done to preserve her life, and thus the critical balancing act went on for months. Just as her condition seemed to be stabilizing, she had a massive stroke, resulting in dense hemiplegia and loss of speech/language function.

She was admitted to the inpatient rehabilitation medicine service to focus on mobility, self-care, and speech functions to help her to return home with her family. She progressed very slowly, with numerous complications related to her pulmonary status, immunosuppression, and cardiovascular deterioration.

A second stroke left her with even more-limited language and cognitive function. She required maximum assistance for all activities of daily living, and she ceased to make progress toward her rehabilitation goals. Her pulmonary function declined. Her family recognized that they would not be able to meet her care needs at home. Further evaluation of her lungs revealed that she had developed a lymphoma, for which, in her case, no treatment could be offered. Her prognosis plummeted, with the likelihood of death in a matter of weeks.

The focus of her rehabilitation care shifted. No longer would it be reasonable to expect her to reach the level of independence she would need to return home. A rigorous exercise program was not going to change the trajectory of her disease and might, in fact, sap her energies and contribute to more frustration and discomfort.

By talking with family and friends, the rehabilitation team learned that Ms. W was strong-willed, stubborn, and difficult but deeply loved. She was seen as the matriarch of the family. For most of her adult life, she had balanced her responsibilities as a single parent with her work as a postal clerk. She was characterized as determined and cantankerous, impatient, critical, and quick to frustrate. Her family was close and extremely important to her. She had a wide circle of friends. Her four sons took turns visiting her in the hospital and sincerely wanted to get her back home again.

With these facts in mind, the rehabilitation team designed communications and interventions that took into account the personal traits and values that were particular to Ms. W. They knew that she would have difficulty tolerating frustration. They knew that she would need to feel in control as much as possible. They also knew that involvement of her family and friends would be essential. They anticipated the effects of prolonged stress on the family unit and recognized the profound loss the family would sustain as her life concluded.

Rehabilitation nursing actions focused first on communication. Because of her dense aphasia, she was unable to verbalize her thoughts or feelings. Instead, she perseverated on one word, growing increasingly agitated when people were unable to understand her. A speech therapist was involved in setting up nonverbal methods of communication, such as picture boards. As the nursing staff worked with Ms. W, they tuned into behavioral cues and expressions. Family members also helped in the interpretation of her attempts to communicate. Strategies for communication included:

- direct eye contact;
- relaxed, unhurried approach;
- slow, distinct phrases in normal tone of voice;
- one thought presented at a time;
- time allowed to process information; and
- gestures to convey and clarify meaning;

Efforts were directed toward maintaining her comfort and dignity. Whenever possible, she was supported in making her own choices. Occupational and physical therapies concentrated on interventions that would promote her autonomy. Functional activities, such as dressing, grooming, and eating, allowed her opportunities to exercise her independence. Access to her physical environment was accomplished through the use of adaptive devices and wheelchair mobility skills. As her condition deteriorated, it was more difficult to ascertain her desires. Inclusion of family members became more important, both for carrying out her wishes as they knew them and for giving the family the active role in her care that they wanted.

Throughout the course of Ms. W's final illness, spiritual and psychosocial support were priorities. With her ability to communicate so severely impaired, her needs for support might have been misunderstood or overlooked. She was suddenly unable to serve as the source of stability and strength for her family, and roles and expectations were greatly changed. The rehabilitation nurses, the psychologist, the social worker, and the chaplain worked together to counsel and care for both patient and family.

When death came, the family described a mixture of feelings of relief, sorrow, and satisfaction. Through their sadness, they recognized the efforts of the rehabilitation team to preserve Ms. W's uniqueness and integrity as a human being. Thus, they would remember her.

❦

❦

## Preventing Secondary Disability

Whatever the disease process, persons in declining states of health are at risk for development of unnecessary complications. Even at the end of life, complications can be prevented, thereby enhancing a person's comfort, function, independence, and dignity. Treatment of one body system must not compromise another. For example, patients who are bedbound are at risk for development of muscular, vascular, integumentary, and neurological compromise, which could result in secondary disability.

CASE STUDY
*JB, A Man with Amyotrophic Lateral Sclerosis*

JB knew his days were numbered, irrevocably ticking away with the advance of his amyotrophic lateral sclerosis. Bit by bit, his body functions eroded. Weakness began in his lower extremities, then spread to his trunk and upper extremities. He was troubled with spasticity, which soon made ambulation almost impossible. He depended on his wife to help him with all of his daily living activities but continued to get out each day in his electric wheelchair, to work with the city government on disability policies. When he went on the ventilator to support his breathing, he likened his health to driving an old truck down a mountain road: no way to stop, no way to turn around, nothing to do but drive on home.

As JB's disease progressed, he was at risk for the development of secondary disabilities. Concerns included the potential development of edema, contractures, and skin breakdown. JB lacked the normal muscular activity that would promote vascular return, and he developed significant edema in his extremities. Knowing that "edema is glue" when it comes to function, rehabilitation nursing actions included range-of-motion exercises and management of dependent edema with compression and elevation.[1]

Spasticity complicated positioning of JB's limbs. It was important to avoid shortened positions that favored the flexors, because that would allow contractures to occur. Contractures would further limit his mobility and function, so he and his wife were taught a stretching program as well as the use of positioning devices and splints to maintain joints in neutral alignment.

Because of his impaired mobility, JB was at risk for skin breakdown. He enjoyed spending a lot of time in his wheelchair. Although his sensation was basically intact, he was not able to react to the message of skin pressure and change his position. JB learned how to shift his weight in the wheelchair, by either side-to-side shifts or tilt-backs. A small timer helped remind him of pressure releases every 15 minutes when he was up in his chair. In addition, a special wheelchair cushion protected bony prominences with gel pads.

## Enhancing Function of Both Affected and Unaffected Systems

A chief concern in rehabilitative care is enhancing function of both affected and unaffected body systems, thereby helping patients to be as healthy and independent as possible. In palliative care, many care issues involve the interconnections of body systems and the need to enlist one function to serve for another.

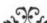

CASE STUDY
*Mr. O'Neill, A Man with Metastatic Prostate Cancer*

Paul O'Neill had been a successful attorney for 30 years. A burly, loud-spoken Irishman, he prided himself in bringing life and laughter everywhere he went. Although diagnosed and treated for prostate cancer, he never slowed the hectic pace of his law practice or his busy social calendar. In fact, he had little time to pay attention to the ominous symptoms that were developing that indicated the advance of his disease.

When he sought medical attention at last, the cancer had metastasized to his spine, resulting in partial paralysis and bowel and bladder impairment. Orthopedic spine surgeons attempted to relieve pressure on his spinal cord with the hope of restoring motor and sensory function. However, when they performed the surgery, they found that the cancer had spread extensively, and they were unable to significantly improve his spinal cord function. Radiation followed, but it had little effect on the spreading cancer.

Mr. O'Neill was stunned. He could not believe the turn his life had taken. Suddenly, nothing seemed to work. He had to depend on others for the first time in his life. He felt like "some kind of freak," unable to move his legs or even manage normal bodily functions. His bulky frame became a heavy burden as he tried to relearn life from a wheelchair. He wrestled with the unfairness of the situation, finally promising himself that he would "go out in style." He wanted to get home as soon as possible, so as not to waste his precious remaining time.

Mr. O'Neill spent 12 days on the inpatient rehabilitation unit, then transitioned to home with continued therapies and nursing care. He died 2 months later, at home with his family present.

In Mr. O'Neill's case, several body systems were at risk for complications, although not all were directly affected by the disease process. Mobility was a critical concern. Bowel and bladder management also presented challenges. His neurological deficits and rapidly progressing disease, combined with his size and the need to learn new skills from a wheelchair level, placed him at risk for development of contractures, skin breakdown, and deep vein thrombosis. Problems with bowel and bladder function put him at risk for constipation, distention, and infection. He experienced severe demoralization. In keeping with his wishes, the rehabilitation nursing staff designed a plan for Mr. O'Neill and his family to follow at home.

Priority rehabilitation nursing issues included the following:

- Managing fatigue related to advancing disease
- Pain control
- Promoting mobility and independence
- Managing neurogenic bowel and bladder

- Alleviating social isolation related to the effects of terminal illness
- Anticipatory grieving and spiritual care.

## Managing Fatigue Related to Advancing Disease

The rehabilitation team planned Mr. O'Neill's care to protect his periods of rest throughout the day. They knew that his therapy would be more effective and his ability to carry over new learning of functional activities would be better if he were in a rested state. His sleep–wake cycle was restored as quickly as possible. Occupational therapists taught him strategies for energy conservation in his activities of daily living, including the use of adaptive devices, planning, and pacing.

## Pain Control

Mr. O'Neill initially described his pain as always with him, dull and relentless, wearing him down. Rehabilitation nurses evaluated his responses in relation to different medications and dosage schedules, as well as nondrug pain control interventions such as positioning and relaxation. The most effective method of pain control for Mr. O'Neill was scheduled doses of long-acting morphine, coupled with short-acting doses for breakthrough or procedural pain. This method of pain management is frequently used in rehabilitation settings, because it does not allow pain to become established, and the patient does not have to experience a certain level of pain and then wait for relief. It also minimizes sedative effects. With his pain under better control, Mr. O'Neill was able to actively participate in his own care and make deliberate decisions about his goals.

## Promoting Mobility and Independence

### Bed Positioning

Positioning and supporting of the body in such a way that function is preserved and complications are prevented is an important consideration in mobility. As Mr. O'Neill's disease progressed and he experienced increasing weakness and fatigue, he spent more and more time in bed. Teaching of patient and family focused on the techniques of bed mobility and specific precautions to prevent complications.

Supine lying was minimized because of Mr. O'Neill's high risk for sacral skin breakdown. Even with a pressure-reducing mattress, back-lying time needed to be restricted. To reduce shearing forces, the bed was placed in reverse Trendelenburg position to raise the head, rather than cranking up just the head of the bed. Draw sheets were used to move Mr. O'Neill, again to prevent shearing. Shearing is a force generated when the skin does not move as one with the structures beneath it. Stretching and breakage of capillaries

and subcutaneous tissues contributes to the potential for deep skin breakdown.

Positioning of the lower extremities is important to prevent complications such as foot drop, skin breakdown, contractures, and deep vein thrombosis. When the patient is supine, care should be taken to support the feet in neutral position. This can be accomplished by using a footboard or box at the end of the bed or by the application of splints. Derotational splints were placed on Mr. O'Neill's lower legs to keep his hips in alignment, to prevent foot-drop contractures, and to reduce the risk of heel breakdown. Range-of-motion exercises were done at least twice daily.

When Mr. O'Neill was side-lying, pillows were employed to cushion bony prominences and maintain neutral joint position. His uppermost leg was brought forward, and the lower leg was straightened to minimize hip flexion contractures. Frequently overlooked as a positioning choice, prone lying offers advantages not only of skin pressure relief and reduction in hip flexion contractures, but also in promoting greater oxygen exchange.[7] Mr. O'Neill's bed position was alternated between back, both sides, and prone at least every 2 hours.

### Sitting

There are many physiological benefits of upright posture. Blood pressure, digestive and bowel functions, oxygenation, and perception are geared toward being upright. Weight-bearing helps to avert skeletal muscle atrophy. Sitting, standing, and walking provide for changes in scenery and enhance the ability to socialize. This was an important consideration for Mr. O'Neill, who experienced emotional distress at the social isolation his illness imposed.

It is important to choose seating that supports the patient, avoiding surfaces that place pressure on bony prominences. A seat that is angled back slightly helps keep the patient from sliding forward. Placing the feet on footrests or a small box or stool may add comfort, as may supporting the arms on pillows or on a table in front of the patient. Sitting time should be limited, based on patient comfort, endurance, and skin tolerance. Mr. O'Neill followed a sitting schedule that increased by 15 minutes a day until he was able to tolerate about 2 hours of upright time. That was enough time to carry out many of his personal activities, yet not so much as to overly tire him.

Planning for Mr. O'Neill's return home involved careful assessment of his equipment needs. Physical and occupational therapists conducted a home evaluation to determine how he would manage mobility and self-care activities and what equipment would be appropriate. Family members practiced using equipment and devices under the guidance of the rehabilitation team. The objective was to simplify the care as much as possible, while supporting Mr. O'Neill's active participation in his daily activities.

Examples of home care equipment often include commodes, wheelchairs, sliding boards, Hoyer lifts, adaptive devices such as reachers, dressing sticks, long-handled sponges, tub/shower benches, hospital beds, and pressure-relieving mattresses. Examples of home modifications include affixing handrails and grab bars, widening doors, using raised toilet seats, and installing stair lifts and ramps.

### Management of Neurogenic Bowel and Bladder

For Mr. O'Neill, the loss of bowel and bladder function was especially distressing. It placed him in a position of dependence and impinged on his privacy. It reinforced his feelings of isolation and being different. The focus of rehabilitation nursing interventions was to mimic the normal physiological rhythms of bowel and bladder elimination. By helping Mr. O'Neill gain control of his body functions, nursing staff hoped to promote his confidence, dignity, and feelings of self-worth.

Bowel regulation and continence were achieved by implementing a classic bowel program routine. Mr. O'Neill was especially prone to constipation caused by immobility and the effects of pain medications. The first intervention was to modify his diet to include more fiber and fluids. He also took stool softener medication twice daily. His bowel program occurred after breakfast each morning, to take advantage of the gastrocolic reflex. He was assisted to sit upright on a commode chair. A rectal suppository was inserted, with digital stimulation at 15-minute intervals to accomplish bowel evacuation. The patient and his wife were taught how to manage this program at home. Although reluctant at first, Mr. O'Neill became resigned to the necessity of this bowel program and worked it into his morning routine. His wife, eager to help in any way she could, also learned the techniques. Once a regular pattern of elimination was established, Mr. O'Neill no longer experienced incontinence.

For bladder management, nursing staff implemented a program of void trials and intermittent catheterization. The patient learned to manage his own fluid intake and to catheterize himself at 4-hour intervals, thereby preventing overdistension or incontinence. However, as his disease progressed, he opted for an indwelling urinary catheter because it was easier for him to manage. There is a continuous need to evaluate and individualize rehabilitation goals and to alter goals as patients experience more advanced disease.

### Alleviating Social Isolation Related to the Effects of Terminal Illness

With a history of active social involvement, Mr. O'Neill had great difficulty with the limitations his disease imposed on his energy level and his ability to remain functional. He did not want others to see him as incapacitated in any way. He did not want to be embarrassed by his failing body. The rehabilitation team concentrated on solving the physical problems that could be solved. A recreation therapist assessed his leisure and avocational interests and prescribed therapeutic activities that would build his confidence in social situations. Together, the team helped him learn to navigate around architectural barriers and helped him to practice new skills successfully from a wheelchair level.

### Anticipatory Grieving and Spiritual Care

Mr. O'Neill concentrated on making plans and settling financial matters in preparation for his death. He continued to set goals for himself and to maintain hope, but the nature of his goals shifted. Initially, he was concerned with not becoming a burden to his family and focused on his physical functioning. As his mobility and endurance flagged and he had to rely more on others for assistance with basic care needs, he began to change his goals. Some of his stoicism fell away. He revealed his feelings more readily and described the evolution of his emotions. Now the focus became his relationships: an upcoming wedding anniversary, a son's graduation from law school. Rehabilitation nurses, home care nurses, the psychologist, and the social worker supported the patient and his family as they began to grieve the past that would never return and the future that was not to be. Pastoral care was a significant part of the process, as Mr. O'Neill struggled with spiritual questions and sought a peaceful understanding of what was happening to him. The rehabilitation team endeavored to help the patient live all the days of his life, by helping body and soul continue to function.

### Facilitating Use of Adaptive Strategies

The ability of patients to continue to participate actively in living their lives has much to do with successful adaptation to changes in function. Even at the end of life, a patient's capacity to adapt remains. Everyday activities may become very difficult to perform with advancing disease. However, rehabilitation nursing actions that promote communication, the use of appropriate tools and equipment, family participation, and modifications to the environment all enhance the process of adaptation.

### Communication

Opening the doors to communication is the most important rehabilitation nursing intervention. By removing functional barriers to speech, by teaching and supporting compensatory strategies, and by allowing safe opportunities for patients and families to discuss difficult issues around death and dying, rehabilitation nurses perform a critical function in the adaptation process.

### Tools and Equipment

Many adaptive devices are available to patients and families that enhance functional ability and independence. Rehabilitation offers the chance to analyze tasks with new eyes and solve problems with creativity and individuality. Examples of useful tools to assist patients in being as independent as possible include reachers, dressing aids such as sock-starters, elastic shoelaces, and dressing sticks. For some patients, adapted eating utensils increase independence with the activity of eating and thereby support nutritional intake. Modifications to clothing may permit more efficient toileting and hygiene, conserving both energy and dignity.

### Family Participation

As illustrated in the previous case studies, the involvement of family and friends has multifaceted benefits. Because of the social nature of humankind, presence and involvement of family and friends has great importance at the end of life. Family members may seek involvement in the caring activities as an expression of feelings of closeness and love. They may try to find understanding, resolution, or closure of past issues. For the person at the end of life, the presence of family, friends, and even pets may be a powerful affirmation of the continuity of life.

### Modifications to Environment

Rehabilitation professionals are keenly aware of the effect of the environment of care on function, independence, and well-being. The physical arrangement of furnishings can be instrumental, not only in promoting patient access to the environment, but also in the ease with which others care for the patient. The environment can be made into a powerful tool for orientation, for spatial perception, and for preserving a territorial sense of self.

Light has a strong effect not only on visual perception but also on mood and feelings of well-being. Light can be a helpful tool in maintaining day–night rhythms and orienting patients to time and place.[8] Sound is also an important environmental variable. For example, music has been implicated as a therapeutic intervention in both rehabilitation and palliative care.[9]

## Promoting Quality at the End of Life

The concept of quality of life is linked to function and independence. Patients often describe their satisfaction with life in terms of what they are able to do. Important determinants of quality of life include (1) the patient's own state, including physical and cognitive functioning, psychological state, and physical condition; (2) quality of palliative care; (3) physical environment; (4) relationships; and (5) outlook.[10] Rehabilitation zeroes in on the essential components of mobility, self-care, cognition, and social interaction, which define what people can do.

CASE STUDY
*LN, A 42-Year-Old Woman With a Malignant Brain Tumor*

LN, age 42 years, had just started her own consulting business when she began to experience headaches and visual

disturbances. At first, she attributed her symptoms to the long hours and stress related to building her business. But when she experienced weakness of her left side, she knew that something more serious was happening.

She had a glioblastoma multiforme growing deep in her brain. Surgery was performed to debulk the tumor, but in a matter of weeks it was clear that the mass was growing rapidly. A course of radiation was completed to no avail. Her function continued to decline, and it seemed that every body system was affected by the advancing malignancy. Now her left side was densely paralyzed, she had difficulty swallowing and speaking, and her thinking processes became muddled.

Her family was in turmoil. On one hand, they resented the disruption her sudden illness imposed on their previously ordered lives. On the other hand, they wanted to care for her and make sure that her remaining time was the best that it could be. As they watched her decline day by day, ambiguities in their relationships surfaced, and conflicts about what would define quality of life emerged.

Rehabilitation's part in promoting quality of life at the end of life is several-fold. Rehabilitation is a goal-directed process. Realistic, attainable goals based on the patient's own definition of quality of life drive the actions of the team. In the area of physical care, rehabilitation strategies support energy conservation, sequencing and pacing, maintaining normal routines, and accessing the environment. Beyond that, rehabilitation nurses facilitate effective communication and problem-solving with patients and families. They offer acceptance and support through difficult decision-making and help mobilize concrete resources.

When rehabilitation nurses approach care, it is with the goal of enhancing function and independence. In LN's case, the brain tumor created deficits in mobility, cognition, and perception. Also, more subtle issues greatly influenced the quality of her remaining time. It was important to understand how the patient would define the quality of her own life and to direct actions toward protecting those elements.

### Promoting Dignity, Self-Image, and Participation

LN's concept of quality of life was evident in how she participated in her care and the decisions that she made about her course of treatment. The rehabilitation team learned that LN's mother had died several years earlier of a similar brain tumor. Caring for her mother had solidified her beliefs about not wishing to burden others. Part of LN's definition of quality of life was that she would not be dependent on others.

LN prided herself on being industrious and self-sufficient. To her, the ability to take care of herself was a sign of success. Rehabilitation nurses and therapists focused on helping to manage symptoms of advancing disease so that she would be able to do as much for herself as possible. This included adaptive techniques for daily living skills, pain management, eating, dressing, grooming, and bowel and bladder management. Even with her physical and cognitive decline, retaining her normal routines helped to allay some feelings of helplessness and to promote a positive self-image.

### Control, Hope, and Reality

As her illness progressed, LN felt she was losing control. It became difficult for her to remember things, and expressing herself became more laborious and frustrating. She slept frequently and seemed disconnected from external events. Her family understood her usual desire for control and made many attempts to include her in conversations and to support her in making choices.

At first, her concept of hope was tied to the idea of cure. Radiation therapy represented the chance of cure. When that was completed without appreciable change in her tumor, some of her feelings of hopefulness slipped away. She sank into a depression. Her family was alarmed: LN's psychological well-being was a critical component in her own definition of quality of life. Treating her depression became a priority issue for the rehabilitation team. Through a combination of rehabilitation psychological counseling and antidepressant medications, her dark mood slowly lifted. Hope seemed to return in a different form, less connected to an event of cure and more a part of her interactions with her daughter and sister.

### Family Support

Another significant area that related to quality of life for LN had to do with social well-being. She struggled with the idea of becoming a burden to her family and realized that she was losing control over what was happening to her. Her relationships with others in her life were complex, and now they were challenged even further. At the same time, her family members wrestled with memories of the mother's death and feared the responsibilities for care that might be thrust upon them.

The rehabilitation team tried to help the patient and her family work through their thoughts, feelings, and fears and helped them to find ways to express them. The team arranged several family conferences to discuss not only the care issues but also the changes in roles and family structure. Whenever possible, the team found answers to the family's questions and made great effort to keep communications open. Creating safe opportunities for the family to express their ambivalence and conflict helped move them toward acceptance. The family was able to prepare in concrete ways for the outcome they both welcomed and dreaded.

### Understanding Outcomes

In rehabilitation, there is a strong emphasis on the measurement of patient outcomes. Since the 1950s, many functional

| Table 49–2 |
| --- |
| **Measures of Functional Outcomes** |
| Barthel Index[15] (Mahoney 1958) |
| Dartmouth COOP Functional Health Assessment Charts[16] |
| Edmonton Functional Assessment Tool[17] |
| Functional Activities Questionnaire[18,19] |
| Functional Independence Measure[13,14] |
| Functional Status Index[20,21] |
| Index of Independence in Activities of Daily Living (ADL)[22] |
| Kenny Self-Care Evaluation[23] |
| Lambeth Disability Screening Questionnaire[24] |
| Medical Outcomes Study Physical Functioning Measure[25] |
| Physical Self-Maintenance Scale[26] |
| PULSES Profile[27] |
| Rapid Disability Rating Scale[11] |
| Self-Evaluation of Life Function Scale[28] |
| Stanford Health Assessment Questionnaire[29] |

assessment instruments have been developed and used to help quantify the changes that occur in patients as a result of care and recovery. Some instruments to measure functional and physical outcomes are applicable to the assessment of patients within the last month of life.

There are more than a dozen functional outcome measurement tools in common use in rehabilitation settings in the United States and Canada (Table 49–2). Measurement of self-care and mobility are central to rehabilitation, but the functions and behaviors required to lead a meaningful life are much broader. They may include cognitive, emotional, perceptual, social, and vocational function measurements as well.

For measuring function in the last 30 days of life, three scales may be particularly useful. The Rapid Disability Rating Scale (RDRS-2)[11] has a broad scope to include items related to activities of daily living, mental capacity, dietary changes, continence, medications, and confinement to bed. The Health Assessment Questionnaire (HAQ)[12] is a widely used instrument that summarizes the patients' areas of major difficulty. The Functional Independence Measure (FIM) is an ordinal scale that quantifies 18 areas of physical and cognitive function in terms of burden of care.[13,14] These scales are appropriate to palliative care because they focus on specific aspects of function that relate to patients' independence. The scales may be used to determine whether interventions at the end of life serve to foster independence and function for as long as possible.

There is also strong interest in the field of rehabilitation in measuring patients' perceptions of quality of life. When the measured domains are considered, the connection between rehabilitation and end-of-life care becomes evident. Most of the measurements of quality of life have to do with physical, cognitive, social, and spiritual function, the chief concerns of the rehabilitation practitioner (Table 49–3).

Outcome measurements matter because they can reveal a lot about the quality of life experienced by persons near the

**Table 49–3**
**Examples of Quality-of-Life Measure**

| Name of Instrument | Domains Measured |
| --- | --- |
| CARES-SF[30] | Rehabilitation and quality of life for patients with cancer |
| Chronic Respiratory Disease Questionnaire[31] | Measuring outcomes of clinical trials for patients with chronic obstructive pulmonary disease |
| City of Hope Quality of Life, Cancer Patient Version[32] | Physical well-being, psychological well being, and spiritual well-being |
| COOP Charts[16] | Screen patients in an outpatient setting |
| Daily Diary Card-QOL[33] | Changes in quality of life related to symptoms induced by chemotherapy |
| EORTC QOL-30[34] | Physical function, role function, cognitive function, emotional function, social function, symptoms, and financial impact |
| FACT-G[35] | Patients undergoing cancer treatment |
| Ferrans and Powers Quality of Life Index[36] | Satisfaction with and importance of multiple domains |
| FLIC[37] | Physical/occupational function, psychological state, sociability, and somatic discomfort |
| HIV Overview of Problems Evaluation Systems (HOPES)[38] | Rehabilitation and quality of life for patients with HIV |
| Hospice Quality of Life Index—Revised[39] | Physical, psychological, spiritual, social, and financial well-being |
| McGill Quality of Life Questionnaire[40] | Quality of life at the end of life |
| Medical Outcomes Study, Short Form | Physical functioning, role limitations, bodily pain, social functioning, mental health, |
| Health Survey[25] | vitality, and general health perceptions |
| National Hospice Study Quality of Life Scale[41] | Quality of life at end of life |
| Nottingham Health Profile[42] | Physical, social, and emotional health problems and their impact on functioning |
| Quality of Life Index[43] | General physical condition, important human activities, and general quality of life |
| Quality of Life for Respiratory Illness Questionnaire[44] | Chronic nonspecific lung disease |
| Quality of Well-Being Scale[45] | Mobility, physical activity, social activity, and 27 symptoms |
| Sickness Impact Profile[46] | How an illness affects a person's behavior |
| Southwest Oncology Group Quality of Life Questionnaire[47] | Function, symptoms, and global quality of life measures |
| Spitzer QL-Index[48] | Activity level, social support, and mental well-being |
| VITAS Quality of Life Index[49] | Symptoms, function, interpersonal domains, well-being, and transcendence |

end of life. For example, by assessing at intervals, it is possible to determine how much function patients retain as they approach death. By identifying and measuring differences in this experience, it is possible to determine the essential interventions and care activities that contribute to the highest levels of functional independence up to the end of life.

Further research is needed to:

- Establish norms and indications for the application of rehabilitation in palliative care
- Determine cost-effectiveness of rehabilitation interventions
- Determine optimal time frames for providing rehabilitation services after the onset of disease
- Define variables having the greatest impact on patient outcomes

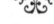

## Summary

Rehabilitation nursing approaches have value in palliative care. Regardless of the disease trajectory, nurses can do something more to preserve function and independence and positively affect perceptions of quality of life, even at its end. Rehabilitation nurses facilitate holistic care of persons in their social and physical environments. They direct actions toward preventing secondary disability and enhancing both affected and unaffected body systems. They foster the use of adaptive strategies and techniques to optimize autonomy. The deliberate focus of rehabilitation nurses on function, independence, dignity, and the preservation of hope makes a fitting contribution to care at the end of life.

REFERENCES

1. Hoeman S. Rehabilitation Nursing: Process and Application (3rd ed). St. Louis, MO: Mosby, 2002.

2. American Nurses' Association. Rehabilitation Nursing—Scope of Practice: Process and Outcome Criteria for Selected Diagnoses. Kansas City, MO: American Nurses' Association, 1988.

3. Doloresco L. CARF: Symbol of rehabilitation excellence. Sci Nurs 2001;18:165,172.

4. Maloof M. The 1989 CARF nursing standards: Guidelines for implementation. Commission of Accreditation of Rehabilitation Facilities. Rehabil Nurs 1989;14:134–136.

4a. Association of Rehabilitation Nurses Position Statements. Available at: http://rehabnurse.org/profresources/pappropr.html (accessed March 7, 2005).

5. Fox E. Predominance of the curative model of medical care: A residual problem. JAMA 1997;278:761–763.

6. Hansen S, Swiontkowski MF. Orthopedic Trauma Protocols. New York, NY: Raven Press, 1993.

7. Ciesla ND. Chest physical therapy for patients in the intensive care unit. Phys Ther 1996;76:609–625.

8. Stewart K, Hayes BC, Eastman CI. Light treatment for NASA shift workers. Chronobiol Int 1995;12:141–151.

9. Halstead MT, Roscoe ST. Restoring the spirit at the end of life: Music as an intervention for oncology nurses. Clin J Oncol Nurs 2002;6:332–336.

10. Cohen SR, Leis A. What determines the quality of life of terminally ill cancer patients from their own perspective? J Palliat Care 2002;18:48–58.

11. Linn M, Linn BS. The Rapid Disability Rating Scale-2. J Am Geriatr Soc 1982;30:378–382.

12. Steen V, Medsger TA. The value of the Health Assessment Questionnaire and special patient-generated scales to demonstrate change in systemic sclerosis patients over time. Arthritis Rheum 1997;40:1984–1991.

13. Stineman M, Shea JA, Jette A, et al. The Functional Independence Measure: Tests of scaling assumptions, structure, and reliability across 20 divers impairment categories. Arch Phys Med Rehabil 1996;77:1101–1108.

14. Granger C, Brownscheidle CM. Outcome measurement in medical rehabilitation. Int J Technol Assess Health Care 1995;11:262–268.

15. Mahoney FI, Barthel DW. Functional evaluation: The Barthel Index. Md State Med J 1965;14:61–65.

16. Nelson EC, Landgraf JM, Hays RD, Wasson JH, Kirk JW. The functional status of patients: How can it be measured in physicians' offices? Med Care 1990;28:1111–1126.

17. Kaasa T, Loomis J, Gillis K, Bruera E, Hanson J. The Edmonton Functional Assessment Tool: Preliminary development and evaluation for use in palliative care. J Pain Sympt Manage 1997;13:10–19.

18. Pfeffer R, Kurosaki TT, Harrah CH, Chance JM, Filos S. Measurement of functional activities in older adults in the community. J Gerontol 1982;37:323–329.

19. Pfeffer R, Kurosaki TT, Chance JM, Filos S, Bates D. Use of the mental function index in older adults: Reliability, validity, and measurement of change over time. Am J Epidemiol 1984; 120:922–935.

20. Jette A, Deniston OL. Inter-observer reliability of a functional status assessment instrument. J Chronic Dis 1978;31:573–580.

21. Jette A. Functional capacity evaluation: An empirical approach. Arch Phys Med Rehabil 1980;61:85–89.

22. Katz S, Ford AB, Moskowitz RW, Jackson BA, Jaffe MW. Studies of illness in the aged. The Index of ADL: A standardized measure of biological and psychosocial function. JAMA 1963;185:914–919.

23. Schoening H, Anderegg L, Bergstrom D, Fonda M, Steinke N, Ulrich P. Numerical scoring of self-care status of patients. Arch Phys Med Rehabil 1965;46:689–697.

24. Patrick DL, Darby SC, Green S, Horton G, Locker D, Wiggins RD. Screening for disability in the inner city. J Epidemiol Community Health 1981;35:65–70.

25. Stewart A, Hays RD, Ware JE. The MOS Short Form general health survey: Reliability and validity in a patient population. Med Care 1988;26:724–735.

26. Lawton M, Brody EM. Assessment of older people: Self-maintaining and instrumental activities of daily living. Gerontologist 1969;9:179–186.

27. Moskowitz E. PULSES profile in retrospect. Arch Phys Med Rehabil 1985;66:647–648.

28. Linn M, Linn BS. Self-Evaluation of Life Function (SELF) scale: A short, comprehensive self-report of health for elderly adults. J Gerontol 1984;39:603–612.

29. Fries J, Spitz PW, Young DY. The dimensions of health outcomes: The health assessment questionnaire, disability and pain scales. J Rheumatol 1982;9:789–793.

30. Schag C, Ganz PA, Heinrich RL. Cancer Rehabilitation Evaluation System–Short Form (CARES-sf): A cancer specific rehabilitation and quality of life instrument. Cancer 1991;68:1406–1413.

31. Guyatt G, Berman LB, Townsend M, Pugsley SO, Chambers LW. A measure of quality of life for clinical trials in chronic lung disease. Thorax 1987;42:773–780.

32. Ferrell B, Dow KH, Grant M. Measurement of quality of life in cancer survivors. Qual Life Res 1995;4:523–531.

33. Gower N, Rudd RM, Ruiz De Elvira MC, et al. Assessment of quality of life using a daily diary card in a randomised trial of chemotherapy in small-cell lung cancer. Ann Oncol 1995;6:575–580.

34. Aaronson NK, Ahmedzai S, Bergman B, et al. The European Organization for Research and Treatment of Cancer QLQ-C30: A quality of life instrument for use in international clinical trials in oncology. J Natl Cancer Inst 1993;85: 365–376.

35. Cella D, Tulsky DS, Gray G, et al. The Functional Assessment of Cancer Therapy scale: Development and validation of the general measure. J Clin Oncol 1993;11:570–579.

36. Ferrans C, Powers MJ. Quality of life index: Development and psychometric properties. ANS Adv Nurs Sci 1985;8:15–24.

37. Finkelstein D, Cassileth BR, Bonomi PD, Rucksdeschel JC, Ezdinli EZ, Wolter JM. A pilot study of the Functional Living Index–Cancer (FLIC) scale for the assessment of quality of life fore metastatic lung cancer patients. Am J Clin Oncol 1988;11:630–633.

38. Schag CA, Ganz PA, Kahn B, Petersen L. Assessing the needs and quality of life of patients with HIV infection: Development of the HIV Overview of Problems–Evaluation System (HOPES). Qual Life Res 1992;1:397–413.

39. McMillan SC, Mahon M. Measuring quality of life in hospice patients using a newly developed Hospice Quality of Life Index. Qual Life Res 1994;3:437–447.

40. Cohen S, Mount BM, Strobel MG, Bui F. The McGill Quality of Life Questionnaire: A measure of quality of life appropriate for people with advanced disease. Palliat Med 1995;9:207–219.

41. Greer D, Mor V. An overview of National Hospice Study findings. J Chronic Dis 1986;39:5–7.

42. Hunt SM, McKenna SP, McEwen J, Backett EM, Williams J, Papp E. A quantitative approach to perceived health status: A validation study. J Epidemiol Community Health 1980;34:281–286.

43. Padilla G, Presant C, Grant MM, Metter G, Lipsett J, Heide F. Quality of life index for patients with cancer. Res Nurs Health 1983;6:117–126.

44. Maille A, Koning CJ, Zwinderman AH, Willems LN, Dijkman JH, Kaptein AA. The development of the Quality of Life for Respiratory Illness Questionnaire (QOL-RIQ): A disease-specific quality of life questionnaire for patients with mild to moderate chronic non-specific lung disease. Respir Med 1997;91:297–309.

45. Kaplan RM, Atkins CJ, Timms R. Validity of a quality of well-being scale as an outcome measure in chronic obstructive pulmonary disease. J Chronic Dis 1984;37:85–95.

46. Bergner M, Bobbitt RA, Pollard WE, Martin DP, Gilson BS. The Sickness Impact Profile: Validation of a health status measure. Med Care 1976:14:57–67.

47. Moinpour C, Hayden KA, Thompson IM, Feigle P, Metch B. Quality of life assessment in Southwest Oncology Group Trials. Oncology (Huntingt) 1990;4:79–84,89,104.

48. Spitzer W, Dobson AJ, Hall J, et al. Measuring quality of life of cancer patients: A concise QL index for use by physicians. J Chronic Dis 1981;34:585–597.

49. Byock I, Merriman MP. Measuring quality of life for patients with terminal illness: The Missoula-VITAS quality of life index. Palliat Med 1998;12:231–244.

50. Headley JA, Ownby KK, John LD. The effect of seated exercise on fatigue and quality of life in women with advanced breast cancer. Oncol Nurs Forum 2004;31:997–983.

51. Maddocks M, Mockett S, Wilcock A. Re: The effect of a physical exercise program in palliative care: A phase ll study. J Pain Symptom Manage 2006;32:513–515.

52. Maddocks M, Lewis M, Chauhan A, Manderso C, Hocknell J, Wilcock A. Randomized controlled pilot study of neuromuscular electrical stimulation of the quadriceps in patients with non-small cell lung cancer. J Pain Symptom Manage (in press).

53. Oldervoll LM, Loge JH, Paltiel H, et al. The effect of a physical exercise program in palliative care: A Phase ll Study. J Pain Symptom Manage 2006;31:421–430.

54. Helbostad JL, Holen JC, Jordhoy MS, Ringdal GI, Oldervoll L, Kaasa MD. A first step in the development of an international self-report instrument for physical functioning in palliative cancer care: A systematic literature review and an expert opinion evaluation study. J Pain Symptom Manage 2009;37:196–205.

## SUGGESTED READINGS

Association of Rehabilitation Nurses. Rehabilitation Nursing (journal published bimonthly). Glenview, IL.

Association of Rehabilitation Nurses. Position statements [online], 2004. Available at: http://www.rehabnurse.org/profresources/index.html#positions (accessed February 4, 2005).

Davis MC. The rehabilitation nurse's role in spiritual care. Rehabil Nurs 1994;19:298–301.

Edelman CL, Mandle CL. Health Promotion Throughout the Lifespan (3rd ed). St. Louis, MO: Mosby–Year Book, 1994.

Field MJ, Cassel CK, eds. Approaching Death: Improving Care at the End of Life. Washington, DC: National Academy Press, 1997.

Frank C, Hobbs N, Stewart G. Rehabilitation on palliative care units. J Palliat Care 1998;14:50–53.

Glick OJ. Interventions related to activity and movement. Nurs Clin North Am 1992;27:541–568.

Granger CV, Gresham GE, eds. Functional Assessment in Rehabilitation Medicine. Baltimore, MD: Williams & Wilkins; 1984:99–121.

Hoeman SP. Pediatric rehabilitation nursing. In Molnar G, ed. Pediatric Rehabilitation (2nd ed). Baltimore, MD: Williams & Wilkins; 1992.

Kottke SJ, Stillwell GK, Lehman JS. Krusen's Handbook of Physical Medicine and Rehabilitation (4th ed). Philadelphia, PA: WB Saunders, 1990.

O'Brien T, Welsh J, Dunn F. ABC of palliative care: Non-malignant conditions. BMJ 1998;316:286–289.

O'Neill B, Fallon M. ABC of palliative care: Principles of palliative care and pain control. BMJ 1997;315:801–804.

O'Neill B, Rodway A. ABC of palliative care: Care in the community. BMJ 1998;316:373–377.

Rehabilitation Nursing Foundation. Rehabilitation Nursing—Concepts and Practice: A Core Curriculum (3rd ed). Glenview, IL: Author, 1993.

Rehabilitation Nursing Foundation. Application of Rehabilitation Concepts to Nursing Practice [independent study program]. Glenview, IL: Author, 1995.

Rehabilitation Nursing Foundation. Advanced Practice Nursing in Rehabilitation: A Core Curriculum. Glenview, IL: Author, 1997.

Wood C, Whittet S, Bradbeer C. ABC of palliative care: HIV infection and AIDS. BMJ 1997;315:1433–1436.

## RESOURCES

American Academy of Physical Medicine and Rehabilitation (AAPM&R)
One IBM Plaza, Suite 2500, Chicago, IL 60611
http://www.aapmr.org

American Congress of Rehabilitation Medicine (ACRM)
4700 W. Lake Avenue, Glenview, IL 60025
http://www.acrm.org

Association of Rehabilitation Nurses (ARN)
4700 W. Lake Avenue, Glenview, IL 60025-1485
http://www.rehabnurse.org

Commission for the Accreditation of Rehabilitation Facilities (CARF)
4891 E. Grant Road, Tucson, AZ 85712
http://www.carf.org

Rehabilitation Foundation, Inc.
600 S. Washington St. Suite 301A, Naperville, IL 60540
http://www.rfi.org

# 50

*Garrett K. Chan, Margaret L. Campbell, and Robert Zalenski*

# The Emergency Department

*"We were trained to rescue patients in the ED—I can't just stand by and let someone die."*
—Emergency physician and former residency director

◆ **Key Points**

◆ *Palliative care can be provided to all patients who present to the emergency department (ED).*

◆ *Each seriously ill or injured person triaged in an ED presents in a crisis that has physical, emotional, social, and spiritual components.*

◆ *The growing number of patients presenting to the ED at the end of life means an increase in the proportion of patients for whom the default resuscitation approach is less applicable.*

◆ *Rapid identification of treatment goals with the terminally ill patient or surrogate prevents unwanted resuscitation and application of burdensome life-prolonging therapies.*

◆ *The most prevalent distressing symptoms that require immediate attention for the patient who is dying in the ED are pain and dyspnea.*

◆ *Unrestricted access of the family to the dying patient can be successfully implemented in the ED.*

◆ *An unexpected death in the ED requires a different approach to preparing the body for viewing that consists of minimizing delays, judicious draping, and information about next steps to help the survivors with bereavement.*

Each year, there approximately 119 million visits to the ED and approximately 561,000 patients who die in the ED or hospital.[1] The ED is a fast-paced and high-stress environment where decisions are made quickly and, at times, with suboptimal levels of information.[2] Although the ED may be chaotic and relationships among providers, patients, and families are hastily forged, emergency clinicians play a crucial role in influencing the trajectory of the patient's care and matching helpful interventions with the goals and expectations of the patient and family. Palliative care is central to good emergency nursing and medical care.

This chapter on palliative care in the ED is designed to assist in recognizing and addressing the needs of ill and injured patients and their families. Once emergency clinicians recognize that all patients who present to the ED are eligible to receive palliative care, nurses and physicians can tailor the plan of care from a broader range of interventions to help patients and families in crisis. From this perspective, the key questions to be added to the basic ED assessment include the following: Is the patient/family aware of the stage of illness and the likelihood of cure? What are their preferences for care, and how rapidly can we establish treatment goals? What can be done to relieve distressing symptoms? What can be done to ease the family's distress and meet their needs?

The workload in the ED is such that for most patients, the "greet, treat, and street" approach must necessarily prevail to prevent crowding.[3] All patients can benefit from palliative care principles such as appropriate symptom management, emotional/psychological care, social care, spiritual/existential care, advanced care planning, or bereavement care for survivors. For a smaller number of patients who present with severe uncontrolled symptoms and organ failure that is not curable, recommendations made to lessen suffering and respect preferences for care can provide a rewarding sense of satisfaction for provider, patient, and family. There are a growing number of elderly persons in this country, and care teams are likely to face an increased incidence of terminally ill patients presenting to the ED who can be guided into the positive outcomes that palliative care can provide.[4,5]

Emergency nurses and physicians traditionally view themselves as foot soldiers in the trenches fighting against the enemy, dying, and death. The criterion of success is whether the patient was admitted to the hospital or discharged to the community alive. Death is regarded as failure; it may be blamed on the disease or the patient's response but must not be blamed on a clinician's lack of willingness to "do everything" to keep the ED patient alive. In this view, every ED case can be dichotomized into success or failure based on whether the patient left the ED with return of spontaneous circulation.

Smith and colleagues conducted a qualitative study investigating the attitudes, experiences, and beliefs of emergency providers about palliative care in the ED.[6] They conducted focus groups of nurses, social workers, ED technicians, and attending and resident physicians. Six distinct themes emerged: (1) participants equated palliative care with end-of-life care; (2) participants disagreed about the feasibility and desirability of providing palliative care in the ED; (3) patients for whom a palliative approach has been established often visit the ED because family members are distressed by end-of-life symptoms; (4) lack of communication between outpatient and ED providers leads to undesirable outcomes (e.g., resuscitation of patients with a do-not-resuscitate [DNR] order); (5) conflict around withholding life-prolonging treatment is common); and (6) training in pain management is inadequate. Obstacles to palliative care in the ED included attitudinal and structural barriers. Attitudinal barriers included concepts such as "palliative care is not a major focus of ED providers"; "situations are emotionally challenging for providers"; and not being able to 'act' is frustrating. Structural barriers described stated that the environment was not appropriate; ED providers do not know patients as well as outpatient providers; patients with palliative care needs and families sometimes are considered lower priority; and long ED wait times are particularly burdensome for patients with palliative care needs.

These findings illustrate the urgent need for emergency and palliative care clinicians to educate other emergency clinicians, conduct research projects, and design programs that improve the delivery of palliative care to ED patients.

~~~

## Recognizing Poor Prognoses

Experienced emergency nurses and physicians are able to recognize the gravely and terminally ill, who arrive with severe distressing symptoms, altered mental status, or imminent death. Examples are an 80-year-old with advanced dementia, decubiti, severe cachexia, and aspiration pneumonia; a 60-year-old with marked cachexia, dyspnea, and metastatic non-small-cell lung cancer who has received surgery, radiation, and two courses of chemotherapy; a 50-year-old man

with cardiac arrest, in pulseless electromechanical dissociation despite 20 minutes of three rounds of resuscitative therapy; or a 60-year-old with severe diabetes and poorly controlled hypertension who has declined dialysis and is now in pulmonary edema with distressing dyspnea.

To help clarify thinking about patients who die, researchers have conceptualized them by placing them in one of five "dying trajectories": (1) terminal illness, such as cancer; (2) sudden death, if younger than age 80 years and previously healthy; (3) organ failure, such as congestive heart failure (CHF) and chronic obstructive pulmonary disease (COPD); (4) frailty, such as with dementia, bed-bound, or with multiple recurrent hospitalizations; and (5) other. Data from Medicare decedents shows that 47% were considered to have died of frailty, 22% were on a cancer-like trajectory, 16% had organ failure, 7% had sudden death, and 8% were in the "other" category.[7]

Within each trajectory, death can be considered expected or unexpected by the provider or patient/family. If death is expected or known by the provider only, this is termed closed awareness; if known by provider and patient, it is called open awareness. Other possibilities are that neither the provider nor the patient is aware that the patient is dying (no awareness) or that the patient is aware but the provider is not, which can be termed "hidden awareness."[8] Assessment here has great implications, because the type of awareness of death (open vs. closed vs. no) often determines the ability of the provider to render optimal care.

Each trajectory has implications for a palliative approach to the patient. Sometimes such discussions take place in the ED, as they should if the ED clinicians recognize that the reflex curative/restorative ED procedure is in fact the "wrong" thing for the patient and family. More commonly, such decisions are "turfed" to the admitting team by default, although prudence would dictate that ED providers not hand off such discussions on nights or weekends, when the patient might die before others have had a chance to establish or review goals of care.

*Patients with terminal illness* who present with advanced disease and distressing symptoms should be assessed for their awareness of their prognosis. One approach is to say to the patient, "Tell me what you understand about your cancer." Patients (or surrogates) with open awareness are good candidates to begin a palliative care approach in the ED, rather than resuscitation and admission to the intensive care unit (ICU). Palliative-directed intervention in the ED can help avoid the worst-case scenario: uncomfortable interventions in unrecognized terminal illness that result in a moribund patient who is unprepared for death and unable to make choices to forgo further nonbeneficial interventions.

*Patients who die suddenly* present a number of challenges to ED clinicians. In general terms, they often leave behind loving family members who are not yet aware of their death. Patients who die unexpectedly of acute renal, respiratory, or heart failure are ideal candidates for the default ED approach and are amenable to all aggressive resuscitative efforts—unless there is an advance directive to withhold them. When death occurs in the ED after an attempt at resuscitation, the surviving families are ill-equipped to cope with the news and require intensive interventions directed at bereavement care. Studies have revealed that families want to be informed of the death in a compassionate and unhurried manner; to be reassured that the patient's belongings will be properly handled; to be told what to do next (e.g., how to contact a funeral home); and to have the opportunity for follow-up with the hospital to answer unresolved questions.[9-11] Development and implementation of ED-focused bereavement guidelines enhance the quality of care provided to the family after an unexpected loss.[12-14]

*Patients with organ failure*—notably those with CHF or COPD—are usually resuscitated or pronounced dead in the ED. Because the chance of pulling a patient through one more episode is relatively high, this course of action, conforming to the default ED approach, is often the road of least resistance and the most appropriate course. Inquiring about treatment preferences for resuscitative therapy is important if the patient is still alert or the family is available. Patients who arrive in extremis with clear expressions of their wishes, such as documented and confirmed forgoing of resuscitation, and hospice patients seeking comfort care that outstrips the home's resources should continue to have their preferences honored by the ED team.

*Patients dying on the frailty trajectory* should have had ample time for their or their surrogate's preferences to be established before the ED visit. As with patients with organ failure, they should have these preferences assessed and their awareness of dying probed. Admission for a palliative care approach rather than ICU admission could be considered.

The fact that growing numbers of patients are presenting to the ED at the end of life means an increase in the proportion of patients for whom the "default" ED approach is less applicable. This calls for a growing sensitivity of ED clinicians for greater skills in palliative care. Emergency department staff must become comfortable with the decisions that patients or their surrogates make regarding forgoing resuscitative interventions and accepting natural death.[15] Emergency department staff are highly trained to rescue and, as with other specialty areas in the hospital, can provide the requisite palliative care interventions to patients and their families who may be dying in the ED.

CASE STUDY
*ES, 34-Year-Old Man with Cystic Fibrosis[16]*

ES was a 34-year-old man who has been fighting cystic fibrosis since birth. ES was sitting on the ambulance gurney, cross-legged with his elbows on his knees and his head down. In his lap, he brought with him to the hospital an Oregon form for advance directives called Physician's Orders for Life Sustaining Treatment (POLST), indicating he had a DNR order and would only want limited interventions, not intubation because he had "terminal cystic fibrosis." The emergency staff were able to contact ES's primary care provider who confirmed that ES wanted comfort measures only and knew that ES was dying.

ES rapidly became unresponsive, and his oxygen saturation dropped precipitously. When his breathing became more labored, he was given small doses of lorazepam and morphine to ease his symptoms. The ED staff spoke with his foster mother via phone, who was unable to accompany him because she was caring for another person with cystic fibrosis at home. The mother lived 2 hours away and would come as soon as she could. She understood that ES might die before she could get to the hospital. The ED nurses and physician took turns sitting by ES's side, talking with him, holding his hand, not wanting him to be alone. ES died quietly in the ED about 3 hours later.

## Establishing Treatment Goals

When the seriously ill patient presents to the ED, rapid identification of treatment goals with the patient or the surrogate of an incapable patient is indicated and may prevent unwanted resuscitation and the application of other potentially burdensome life-sustaining therapies. Likewise, if palliative care treatment goals are established rapidly after an attempt at resuscitation, the patient and family can be afforded a quick transition from resuscitation to comfort by a skilled, compassionate ED intervention to withdraw unwanted life support. Establishment of palliative care treatment goals in the ED can be inhibited by lack of prognostic information, the lack of any prior relationship with the patient or surrogate, a need for rapid action, and the fear of liability if life is not extended.[17,18] Hopefully, clinicians in EDs will begin to see themselves as ideally positioned to identify and treat palliative care emergencies—such as pain crises—and adopt the goals of prevention of suffering and enabling of a "good death." This development will expand the ED concept of success.

Most physicians (78%) responding to a survey study about cardiopulmonary resuscitation (CPR) indicated that they would honor legal advance directives about resuscitation.[17] However, despite more than a decade of experience with the Patient Self-Determination Act,[19] there continues to be a paucity of persons who have completed an advance directive. In the general U.S. population, only 15% of Americans have an advance directive,[18] but among frail, elderly nursing home residents the prevalence of advance directive completion increases to 45% to 60%.[20-22]

Even if the advance directive accompanies the patient to the ED, it may have limited usefulness in guiding emergency management. One study found that, although 44% of nursing home residents seen in the ED had advance directives, the advance directives frequently addressed only CPR and did not address other life-supporting strategies (e.g., intubation) with the same frequency.[21] Yet, even a limited advance directive provides the ED clinician with a starting point for a conversation about treatment preferences. The ED clinician can open the discussion with a request for clarification of the preferences expressed in the directive, and the conversation about contemporaneous diagnosis and treatment recommendations and preferences will flow. After ascertaining the patient's or surrogate's understanding about the illness, the clinician might ask, "I see you already have wishes about CPR; will you tell me more about your preferences for treatment?"

In the absence of an advance directive, or if the advance directive is ambiguous, the ED staff are obliged to engage in a decision-making process at the earliest opportunity after identifying or inferring the patient's terminal prognosis. This conversation may occur before or after an attempt at resuscitation. A discussion with the patient who has retained decision-making capacity about diagnosis, prognosis, and relevant treatment options is a challenging process in the ED, because the patient may have no prior relationship with the ED staff and may be lacking bonds of trust and rapport. Furthermore, this type of clinician–patient conversation is ideally held in privacy and quiet, and the ED environment is not always a conducive setting. A creative approach to finding a quiet room or screening area around the patient is needed.

Cognitive impairment is highly prevalent in terminally ill patients—particularly those whose death is imminent—and it may preclude them from having the capacity to make decisions about treatment.[23,24] Reliance on a valid surrogate decision-maker, usually a family member or close friend, becomes necessary. Surrogates appointed by the patient through an advance directive have pre-eminence in decision-making. In the absence of a patient-appointed proxy, many states have enacted surrogacy statutes, often relying on a next-of-kin hierarchy, to direct clinicians. Clinicians need to know the provisions of their own state when seeking a surrogate decision about treatment. Table 50–1 details the core components of a discussion about end-of-life treatment options.

### CASE STUDY
#### HR, An 88-Year-Old Woman with Dementia

HR is an 88-year-old woman brought to the ED from her nursing home. She is in the terminal stage of dementia by physical examination and report from the nursing home, yet treatment goals have never been established with her only surviving family member, a niece. HR is curled into a fetal position and has stage III and IV sacral, trochanter, and heel decubiti. She is febrile, she has leukocytosis, and her chest radiograph is consistent with aspiration pneumonia. Her respiratory pattern and blood gas analysis predict imminent respiratory failure. The ED staff are in consensus that this patient would benefit from a palliative care approach rather than intubation and admission to the ICU.

The ED social worker calls the patient's niece and asks her to come to the hospital as soon as possible. On her

---

| Table 50–1 |
| --- |
| **Core Components of a Discussion about End-of-Life Treatment Goals** |

Prepare in advance.

- Identify the diagnosis/prognosis.
- Determine what the patient or surrogate already knows.
- Seek assistance from support personnel (e.g., chaplain, social worker, patient advocate).

Establish a therapeutic milieu.

- Identify a private and quiet place in the emergency department where everyone can sit and be seen and heard.
- Minimize interruptions.

Seek patient and surrogate knowledge about diagnosis and prognosis.

- Correct inaccuracies and misconceptions.
- Provide additional information.

Communicate effectively.

- Avoid jargon, slang, and acronyms.
- Demonstrate empathy.
- Be honest and direct.

Make a palliative care treatment recommendation.

- Provide rationale for recommendations.
- Answer questions.

Seek patient or surrogate agreement with recommendation.

*Source:* Reference 53.

---

arrival, an ED physician, nurse, and the social worker sit with the niece, discuss the patient's diagnoses and prognosis, and make a recommendation about comfort care. The niece agrees, thanks the team, and reports that no one has ever raised this option with her in the past. She believes that her aunt has "suffered enough" and should "pass naturally and peacefully." The hospital's palliative care service is consulted by the ED for admission, rather than the ICU.

After the goals of treatment have been determined with the patient or surrogate, the relevant interventions can be identified. A focus on palliation rather than resuscitation indicates that reduction of symptom distress and attention to patient and family grief are the priorities of patient and family care.

## Symptom Management: Pain and Dyspnea

The most prevalent symptoms that produce distress in the patient with advanced illness and require immediate attention are pain and dyspnea.[24] The nursing process (i.e., assessment, planning, intervention, and evaluation) guides effective symptom management in the ED.

The gold standard for pain assessment is the patient's self-report. When the patient is able to self-report, his/her appraisal of pain intensity, location, quality, and possible causes should be sought. A documented trend using a numeric rating or visual analog scale is standard and permits continuous assessment and re-evaluation over time and across caregivers. Pain occurs as result of trauma, somatic disorders, and common ED procedures.[25,26]

Critically ill patients and those with cognitive impairments may not be able to provide a self-report; in such cases, a combination of measures is used to validate the assessment. Behaviors such as facial grimacing, restlessness, moaning, muscle tension, tachycardia, tachypnea, clenched fists, closed eyes, and diaphoresis may be cues to unrelieved pain.[26,27]

Analgesics are the standard agents for managing pain in the terminally ill patient. Nonsteroidal anti-inflammatory drugs have a limited role for treatment of mild-to-moderate pain and bone pain, and conservative use is recommended in the geriatric patient. Opioids, with the exception of meperidine, are the drugs of choice for moderate-to-severe pain, and antidepressants or anticonvulsants are used for neuropathic pain.[28]

The route is chosen according to patient characteristics and goals of analgesia, including the desired rapidity of response. Intravenous or subcutaneous administration affords the most rapid onset of action. Oral, sublingual, or buccal administration causes the least patient burden when there is an intact oral cavity. Transdermal medication is useful for long-acting, chronic analgesia; it should not be used as the first-line strategy, because of the long delay in onset of action, and/or if the therapeutic dose has not been determined, as may be the case with an ED patient. The intramuscular route is discouraged because of poor absorption and patient discomfort.[27,28]

Analgesics are titrated according to the patient's responses; therefore, frequent reassessment to evaluate effectiveness is indicated. Although an individual patient may experience toxicity, there are no dose ceilings when using opioids, and titration to therapeutic effect may require high doses in patients with opioid tolerance or severe pain. Equianalgesia tables and consultation with pain specialists may be used to guide appropriate dosing.[27,28]

Similarly to pain, dyspnea and any associated respiratory distress must be assessed frequently in high-risk patients, because many pulmonary, cardiac, and neuromuscular terminal illnesses produce breathing distress. The gold standard for this subjective experience is the patient's self-report, using either a numeric or a visual analog scale. Behavioral cues are useful if the patient is unable to self-report and include tachypnea, tachycardia, accessory muscle use, a paradoxical breathing pattern, restlessness, nasal flaring, and a fearful facial expression.[29,30]

Treatment of dyspnea or respiratory distress can be organized into three categories: prevention, treatment of the underlying cause, and palliation of symptom distress. Prevention of dyspnea in the dying ED patient warrants maximizing treatments that have proven beneficial to the patient, including enhancing ventilator synchrony if the patient is going to remain ventilated, avoiding volume overload, and continuing oxygen and nebulized bronchodilators. Measures to correct metabolic acidosis may also be useful to decrease the work of breathing and thereby decrease respiratory distress.[31,32]

Treating underlying causes of dyspnea may be useful, particularly if the benefit of the treatment is not in disproportion to the burden. If death is not imminent, the patient may benefit from antibiotics, corticosteroids, paracentesis, pleurodesis, or bronchoscopy.

Numerous strategies have demonstrated effectiveness for palliation of terminal dyspnea, including optimal positioning, oxygen, and sitting in front of a fan. Upright positioning that affords the patient an optimal lung capacity is useful, especially for patients with COPD.[33] Oxygen has been shown to be more effective than air in hypoxemic cancer patients and in patients with advanced COPD. However, other investigators reported no difference in cancer patients' respiratory comfort in response to oxygen compared with air, and increased ambient air flow, fans, and cold air have also been found to be therapeutic.[33] Oxygen can be more burdensome than beneficial in the patient who is near death, particularly if a face masks is employed, because the mask produces a feeling of suffocation. The individual patient's report or behavior in response to oxygen determines its usefulness. The comatose patient does not require oxygen while dying.

Opioids are the mainstay of pharmacological management of terminal dyspnea, and their effectiveness has been demonstrated in clinical trials. A meta-analysis of 18 double-blind, randomized, placebo-controlled trials of opioids in the treatment of dyspnea from any cause revealed a statistically positive effect on the sensation of breathlessness ($P = 0.0008$). Meta-regression indicated a greater effect in studies using oral or parenteral opioids than in studies using nebulized opioids. In subgroup analysis, the COPD studies had essentially the same results as the cancer studies.[34] In the ED, parenteral access is almost universal, obviating the need for other routes of administration except in special or unusual circumstances. Doses for treating dyspnea are patient-specific, and as with opioid use in the management of pain, no ceiling should be placed on dosage. The dose should be rapidly titrated until the patient reports or displays respiratory comfort. Frequent bedside evaluation to assess the efficacy of the medication is essential.

Fear and anxiety may be components of the respiratory distress experienced by the dying ED patient. The addition of a benzodiazepine to the opioid regimen has demonstrated success in patients with cancer and with advanced COPD.[35] As with opioids, these agents should be titrated to effect. Care of the attendant family to reduce their fear, anxiety, and grief warrants as much effort as that directed to the patient's needs.

## Family Presence

Studies have consistently demonstrated that families want to be close to their terminally ill loved ones.[36,37] Family access promotes cohesion, affords the opportunity for closure, and may soothe the patient. Unrestricted access of the family to the dying patient is a standard of care in hospitals and nursing homes. The family of the patient who is dying in the ED should be afforded this same benefit. There is growing evidence and support for the successful implementation of families at the side of loved ones during resuscitation and invasive procedures in the ED.[38-40] Although additional "outcomes" research is still needed. It follows that if families and patients can be accommodated with open access to one another in the ED during procedures, then unrestricted visiting for the dying patient and grieving family is possible. Emergency departments may consider first implementing a family presence program in children or adults with nontraumatic cardiac arrest, and then extending successful practices to traumatic cardiac arrest. The latter involves special challenges, especially when gang violence is suspected.

Ideally, the patient and family should be separated from the harried milieu of the ED while dying or waiting for a hospital bed yet should remain visible and accessible for close monitoring and care. Movement to a quieter area in the ED, such as the observation care unit or an isolation room, may serve this purpose, particularly if there is space for a few chairs and the attendant family. Limiting visitors to only two at a time has no rationale if the patient is dying and there is a large, loving family.

## Death Notification and Requests for Organ/Tissue Donation

Delivery of adverse diagnoses and death notification entails all of the communicative skills of the ED staff. A framework for communicating bad news is helpful. There are four temporally ordered segments in the approach to breaking bad news: the preparation, the content, the survivor's response, and the close.

Key elements of the *preparation phase* include a private setting, with determination of what the family already knows about the illness or accident. Important elements of the *content phase* include a "warning shot." For example, the physician might say, "There has been a factory accident, and I am sorry to say that I have bad news." The news should then be stated clearly: "Your husband died in the accident." Drawn-out deliveries may be more comfortable for the staff, but they are not helpful to the anxious family member.[40]

To cast death notification in an easily learned format, similarly to the way other procedures are taught, a procedural competency model has been developed.[41] Table 50–2 summarizes the steps.

Deaths that are out of cycle (e.g., death at a young age), out of context (e.g., death was not expected because oncologist overestimated length of life remaining), or sudden are the hardest for families to bear. Ideally, contact information for bereavement counselors or for support groups in the community should be given to the family.

| Table 50–2 |
| --- |
| **Elements of an Empathic Death Disclosure** |

Introduce self/role.
- Sit down.
- Assume comfortable communication distance.
- Tone/rate of speech acceptable.
- Make eye contact.
- Maintain open posture.

Give advance warning of bad news.
- "I'm afraid I have bad news."

Deliver news of death clearly.
- Use direct terms such as "dead" or "died."
- Use no medical jargon.
- Use language that is clear and easily understood.

Tolerate survivor's reaction.
Explain medical attempts to "save" patient.
Offer viewing of deceased.
Offer to be available to survivor.
Conclude appropriately.
- Offer condolences and leave.

*Source:* Quest et al. (2002), reference 41. Copyright 2002, with permission from The Society for Academic Emergency Medicine.

Federal law (Public Law 99-5-9; Section 9318) and Medicare regulations mandate that hospitals give surviving family members the chance to authorize donation of their family member's organs and tissues. Most families are receptive to requests for donation, and many take consolation in helping others despite their own tragic loss. Studies have shown that it is essential to approach relatives for this purpose only after death notification is completed, allowing a temporal separation between death notification and the request for organs. Also, a higher response rate is obtained if the requesting personnel have received specific training for this purpose.[42,43]

One of the most difficult tasks caregivers must complete is to witness the acute grief reaction of the family after they have received the news of unexpected death. The newly bereaved is literally broken from the world in which he/she formerly lived. There is often an unreal feeling of disbelief or suspension in time and insulation from place. The bereaved can feel hopeless, frustrated, and often very angry. It is important for the caregiver to "stay with" the bereaved during this initial grief reaction, which can be brief or last for several minutes. If duties prevent staying put, then the caregiver should most definitely return after the bereaved's initial emotions have subsided. It is only then that the bereaved family member is able to re-engage in rational thought, and at that point he/she needs answers to the when, where, what, and how questions about the death. Reassurances about the patient's not having suffered, if based in reality, may prove helpful to the bereaved.[44]

A fine tradition from the U.S. military mandates that an officer and aid (a team) stay with the bereaved family until they are released. Although this may be harder to achieve in the ED, the same sense of solemn duty could be embraced by staff members performing death notification. The tone of voice, words, bearing, and demeanor of the individual performing death notification will be seared into the mind and hearts of the bereaved forever. Death notification is an immense responsibility and must be done well. Family witness to resuscitation efforts is an alternative method of death disclosure. The bad outcome and the intensity of life-saving efforts are communicated over a period of 20 minutes, rather than 2 minutes.

## Care of the Body and Bereavement Care for the Survivors

It is commonly accepted that long-term outcomes are better for those who are able to see the deceased body of a loved one. Viewing the body helps those who are grieving acknowledge and begin to come to terms with the death.[45] If the death is expected, the body should be bathed and laid out neatly on the stretcher with the eyes closed, and the preparation should be completed before the family arrives. Families who are present at the time of death may want to participate in body preparation. In some cultures, rituals at the time of death require family involvement and should be accommodated within reason in the ED. For example, in some Moslem traditions, the body is turned to face east, and persons of the same gender and religion as the deceased perform the *post mortem* care. Some families may want private time with the body of the deceased, but others may want a supportive person from the hospital staff, such as a nurse, aide, or chaplain, to remain in attendance.[46]

If the death is unexpected, such as from an accident or sudden illness, the family members who are arriving at the ED need a different approach to viewing the body. After learning of the death, the family may demonstrate an urgency to see the body, and delays for cleaning and laying out may produce more distress; similarly, not seeing the body because of disfigurement or mutilation causes distress to the bereaved. Seeing the deceased and the evidence of the injury or accident, along with the accoutrements of the attempts at resuscitation, gives a subliminal message to the family that the ED staff did all they could. The ED nurse should allow the family access to the deceased at the earliest possible opportunity and should use judicious draping to cover the most severe disfigurements.

Bereavement care for the survivors can come in many forms. One helpful strategy is to have an information packet of commonly asked questions and who to contact at the hospital for information; a list of funeral homes; medical examiner and autopsy fact sheets; and a list of resources for grief and for specific populations or situations, such as victims of violence, sudden infant death syndrome, or loss after a miscarriage. Other strategies for providing bereavement care is

to acknowledge the loss and being present with survivors immediately after delivering the bad news.

CASE STUDY
### HP, A Victim of a Motorcycle Accident

While riding his motorcycle, HP was hit by a truck and dragged. He sustained a closed head injury, a severe scalp laceration, comminuted fractures of both femurs and of the left humerus, rib fractures bilaterally, and a ruptured spleen. He died in the ED during trauma resuscitation.

The frantic family members arrived at the hospital shortly after death was pronounced and screamed to see the patient. The resuscitation room looked like a tornado had touched down, with empty supply wrappers, intravenous fluid bags, and soiled dressings on the counters and floor. The deceased was bloody, with his torn clothing partially removed or cut off, and bone was protruding from his left arm and both legs. He had bilateral chest tubes, a Foley catheter, three large-bore angiocaths, and an endotracheal tube that had to remain in place for the medical examiner.

The nurse recognized the family's need to see the body as quickly as possible. She enlisted a nurse's aide to rapidly reduce the amount of debris on and around the stretcher. She draped the body to cover the worst injuries, including the exposed bones, and washed the deceased's face and hands. A handtowel covered the scalp wound without covering the face. Within 5 minutes the nurse had prepared the body and room for the family.

The nurse escorted the weeping family to see the body and remained unobtrusively nearby in case anyone fainted. She also answered questions about the injuries and the magnitude of the efforts to resuscitate. Later, after the family was more composed, the nurse explained the procedures for referral to the county medical examiner and the need to identify a funeral home. She also gave the family the business card of a trauma counselor who specialized in bereavement counseling. The nurse found a quiet, private place for the family to wait until they reached an emotional calm that would allow them to drive home safely.

The use of cadavers to practice procedures such as endotracheal intubation in the ED has been commonplace as an integral part of resident training.[46-49] Current ethical norms do not permit this practice without contemporaneous consent from the surviving family or evidence from a patient's advance directives that this would be acceptable. Consent is standard elsewhere in healthcare, and respect for the newly dead and for the survivors warrants this same standard. Recent legal cases have held that families have property rights to the bodies of their loved ones, and the use of cadavers without consent poses a liability risk. Studies have shown that most patients or families are willing to have procedures performed after death if permission is obtained in advance. An empathetic expression of condolences, followed by a sensitive request to permit procedures, may yield the teaching–learning opportunity while demonstrating respect for the deceased and their family.

❧

❧

## Novel Approaches to Increase Palliative Care in the Emergency Department

With the recognition that palliative care should be provided concurrently with curative care or by itself when curative therapies have failed, new innovations to increase the awareness and incorporation of palliative care principles have been created.

### End-of-Life Nursing Education Consortium-Critical Care

The End-of-Life Nursing Education Consortium-Critical Care (ELNEC-CC) curriculum is a joint collaboration between the City of Hope National Medical Center and the American Association of Colleges of Nursing and is designed to train emergency and critical care nurses in palliative and end-of-life care.[50] ELNEC-CC is a comprehensive training program that covers content areas of symptom management, communication strategies, care at the end of life, ethics, cultural issues, and loss and bereavement. The goal is to assist nurses in expanding their holistic care of the patients and families. Extensive support materials such as a CD, binder of printed materials, case studies, textbooks, and other educational materials are provided to participants to educate colleagues about palliative and end-of-life care in critical care settings.

### Education in Palliative and End-of-Life Care-Emergency Medicine

The Education in Palliative and End-of-life Care-Emergency Medicine (EPEC-EM) is another educational curriculum designed to teach emergency clinicians about palliative and end-of-life care so that clinicians can incorporate these skills and interventions into their daily practices.[51] EPEC-EM provides core clinical competencies in palliative and end-of-life care for emergency clinicians through teaching modalities that incorporate interactive lecture, case vignettes, and role-play among others. Palliative and end-of-life topics are presented, such as trajectories of approaching death, prognoses of illnesses, rapid palliative care assessment, establishing goals of care, ethical and legal issues, withholding and withdrawing treatment, family-witnessed resuscitation, and pain and symptom management.

### A Palliative Care and Case Management Team in the Emergency Department

O'Mahony and colleagues established a pilot project at Montefiore Medical Center to investigate the effect of advanced practice palliative care nurses based in the ED on the disposition of chronically ill geriatric patients, linkage with hospital-based palliative care services, and patient and family satisfaction with symptom control.[52] The advanced practice nurses (APNs) rounded with the emergency team to identify patients that may be appropriate for palliative care services and conducted a clinical consultation, if agreed upon by the emergency team and the patient. Education was provided to the emergency staff on topics such as indications for referral to palliative care, hospice eligibility, and how to access additional palliative care services.

Over a 14-month period, the APNs screened charts of more than 950 patients and conducted 894 consultations. Ninety percent of patients were admitted to the medical center. Two hundred sixty-three patients were referred to home care organizations, 83 received homecare services, and of the 287 patients who were referred to hospice, 91 received hospice services. Linkage to hospital-based palliative care services decreased to a median of 3 days, and the number of admissions to the palliative care unit from the ED increased to between 10 and 15 patients per month. Patient and family satisfaction with the pilot project after discharge from the ED increased, especially in the areas of physical symptom management and communication with people close to them on the Missoula Vitas Quality of Life Index. However, patients also described a "loss of ability to do many of the things that I like" and a general sense of loss of life's value.

This pilot program illustrates the benefits of collaborating with the palliative care team in determining goals of care, deciding on appropriate disposition, providing appropriate symptom management, linking patients with additional palliative care resources, and increasing patient and family satisfaction. A palliative care team presence in the ED has been reported to increase the amount of palliative care being delivered and can assist emergency clinicians immediately in a chaotic environment.[6]

❧

## Summary

Dying care in the ED can be complicated by the milieu and by the usual "resuscitative" expectations of this environment. A default view of ED success is whether the patient left the ED with return of spontaneous circulation. The fact that a growing number of patients are presenting to the ED at the end of life demands palliative care competency by ED staff. In most EDs, there are clinicians who are willing to guide terminally ill patients or their surrogates toward a palliative care approach, in which success is redefined as preventing suffering and enabling a good death.

The paucity of patients with written advance directives or advance planning for the terminal illness necessitates rapid establishment of treatment goals with the dying patient or surrogate in the ED. This is accomplished through compassionate communication about diagnosis and prognosis and recommendations for a palliative care treatment focus.

An abundance of evidence about managing pain and dyspnea is available to guide the ED staff in reducing symptom distress. Similarly, optimal caring for the grieving family has been informed by research and includes effective communication about prognosis or death notification and timely access to the patient before or after death.

Personal and professional satisfaction with comprehensive dying care in the ED can be achieved by ED staff. Compassionate recommendations made to decrease suffering and ensure respect for the dying patient afford the survivors a positive experience, even in the face of loss.

## REFERENCES

1. Pitts SR, Niska RW, Xu J, Burt CW. National hospital ambulatory medical care survey: 2006 emergency department summary. National health statistics reports; no. 7. Hayattsville, MD: National Center for Health Statistics, 2008.

2. Chan GK. End-of-Life models and emergency department care. Acad Emerg Med 2004;11(1):79–86.

3. Karpiel M. Improving emergency department flow: Eliminating ED inefficiencies reduces patient wait times. Healthcare Exec 2004;19(1):40–41.

4. Lawson BJ, Burge FI, McIntyre P, Field S, Maxwell D. Palliative care patients in the emergency department. J Palliat Care 2008;24(4):247–255.

5. Smith AK, Fisher J, Schonberg MA, et al. Am I doing the right thing? Provider perspectives on improving palliative care in the emergency department. Ann Emerg Med 2009;54(1):86–93.

6. Meir D, Berensford L. Fast response is key to partnering with the emergency department. J Palliat Med 2007; 10(3):641–645.

7. Lunney JR, Lynn J, Hogan C. Profiles of older Medicare decedents. J Am Geriatr Soc 2002;50:1108–1112.

8. Seale CL, Addington-Hall J, McCarthy M. Awareness of dying: Prevalence, causes, and consequences. Soc Sci Med 1997;45:477–485.

9. Fanslow J. Needs of grieving spouses in sudden death situations: A pilot study. J Emerg Nurs 1983;9:213–216.

10. Parrish GA, Holdren KS, Skiendzielewski J, Lumpkin OA. Emergency department experience with sudden death: A survey of survivors. Ann Emerg Med 1987;16:792–796.

11. Walters DT, Tupin JP. Family grief in the emergency department. Emerg Med Clin North Am 1991;9:189–206.

12. Adamowski K, Dickinson G, Weitzman B, Roessler C, Carter-Snell C. Sudden unexpected death in the emergency department: Caring for the survivors. CMAJ 1993;149:1445–1451.

13. Lipton H, Coleman M. Bereavement practice guidelines for health care professionals in the emergency department. Int J Emerg Ment Health 2000;2:19–31.

14. Williams AG, O'Brien DL, Laughton KJ, Jelinek GA. Improving services to bereaved relatives in the emergency department: Making healthcare more humane. Med J Aust 2000;173:480–483.

15. Schears RM. Emergency physicians' role in end-of-life care. Emerg Med Clin North Am 1999;17:539–559.

16. Schmidt, TA. Futility-futilis-the leaky vessel. Ann Emerg Med 2000;35:614–617.

17. Marco CA, Bessman ES, Schoenfeld CN, Kelen GD. Ethical issues of cardiopulmonary resuscitation: Current practice among emergency physicians. Acad Emerg Med 1997;4:898–904.

18. Marco CA, Larkin GL, Moskop JC, Derse AR. Determination of "futility" in emergency medicine. Ann Emerg Med 2000;35:604–612.

19. Patient Self Determination Act 1990, incorporated into the Omnibus Budget Reconciliation Act 1990, 42 U.S.C. 1395 cc (a).

20. Lynn J, Schuster JL, Kabcenell A. Improving Care for the End of Life. New York, NY: Oxford University Press, 2000.

21. Lahn M, Friedman B, Bijur P, Haughey M, Gallagher EJ. Advance directives in skilled nursing facility residents transferred to emergency departments. Acad Emerg Med 2001;8:1158–1162.

22. McCauley WJ, Travis SS. Advance care planning among residents in long-term care. Am J Hosp Palliat Care 2003;20:353–359.

23. Cassell EJ, Leon AC, Kaufman SG. Preliminary evidence of impaired thinking sick patients. Ann Intern Med 2001;134(12):1120–1123.

24. Solano JP, Gomes B, Higginson IJ. A comparison of symptom prevalence in far advanced cancer, AIDS, heart disease, chronic obstructive pulmonary disease and renal disease. J Pain Symptom Manage 2006;31(1):58–69.

25. Morrison RS, Ahronheim JC, Morrison GR, et al. Pain and discomfort associated with common hospital procedures and experiences. J Pain Symptom Manage 1998;15:91–101.

26. Puntillo KA, Morris AB, Thompson CL, Stanik-Hutt J, White CA, Wild LR. Pain behaviors observed during six common procedures: Results from Thunder Project II. Crit Care Med 2004;32(2):421–427.

27. Herr, K, Bjoro K, Decker S. Tools for assessment of pain in nonverbal older adults with dementia: A state-of-the-science review. J Pain Symptom Manage 2006;31(2):170–192.

28. American Pain Society. Principles of Analgesic Use in the Treatment of Acute Pain and Cancer Pain (5th ed). Glenview, IL: American Pain Society, 2003.

29. Truog RD, Campbell ML, Curtis JR, et al. Recommendations for end-of-life care in the Intensive care unit: A consensus statement by the American College [corrected] of Critical Care Medicine. Crit Care Med March 2008;36(3):953–963.

30. Campbell ML. Respiratory distress: A model of responses and behaviors to an asphyxial threat for patients who are unable to self-report. Heart Lung 2008;37(1):54–60.

31. Campbell ML. Nurse to Nurse Palliative Care. New York, NY: McGraw-Hill Publishing Company, 2009.

32. Navigante AH, Cerchietti LC, Castro MA, Lutteral MA, Cabalar ME. Midazolam as adjiunct therapy to morphine in the alleviation of severe dyspnea perception in patients with advanced cancer. J Pain Symptom Manage 2006;31(1):38–47.

33. Campbell ML. Terminal dyspnea and respiratory distress. Criti Care Clin North Am 2004;30:403–417.

34. Jennings AL, Davies AN, Higgins JP, Gibbs JS, Broadley KE. A systematic review of the use of opioids in the management of dyspnoea. Thorax 2002;57:922–923.

35. Light RW, Stansbury DW, Webster JS. Effect of 30 mg of morphine alone or with promethazine or prochlorperazine on the exercise capacity of patients with COPD. Chest 1996;109:975–981.

36. Hampe SO. Needs of the grieving spouse in a hospital setting. Nurs Res 1975;24:113–120.

37. Steinhauser KE, Christakis NA, Clipp EC, MdNeilly M, McIntyre L, Tulsky JA. Factors considered important at the end of life by patients, family, physicians, and other care providers. JAMA 2000;284:2476–2482.

38. Duran CR, Oman KS, Abel JJ, Koziel VM, Szymanski D. Attitudes toward and beliefs about family presence: A survey of healthcare providers, patients' families, and patients. Am J Crit Care 2007;16(3):270–279.

39. Swinburn CR, Mould H, Stone TN, Corris PA, Gibson GJ. Symptomatic benefit of supplemental oxygen in hypoxemic patients with chronic lung disease. Am Rev Respir Dis 1991;143:913–915.

40. Booth S, Kelly MJ, Cox NP, Adams L, Guz A. Does oxygen help dyspnea in patients with cancer? Am J Respir Crit Care Med 1996;153:1515–1518.

41. Quest TE, Otsuki JA, Banja J, Ratcliff JJ, Heron SL, Kaslow NJ. The use of standardized patients within a protocol competency model to teach death disclosure. Acad Emerg Med 2002;9:1326–1333.

42. DeJong W, Franz HG, Wolfe SM, et al. Requesting organ donation: An interview study of donor and nondonor families. Am J Crit Care 1997;7:13–23.

43. Garrison RN, Bentley FR, Rague GH, et al. There is an answer to the shortage of donor organs. Surg Gynecol Obstet 1991;173:391–396.

44. Fraser S, Atkins J. Survivors' recollections of helpful and unhelpful emergency nurse activities surrounding sudden death of a loved one. J Emerg Nurs 1990;16:13–16.

45. Haas F. Bereavement care: Seeing the body. Nurs Stand 2003;17(28):33–37.

46. Fourre MW. The performance of procedures on the recently deceased. Acad Emerg Med 2002;9:595–598.

47. Berger JT, Rosner F, Cassell EJ. Ethics of practicing medical procedures on newly dead and nearly dead patients. J Gen Intern Med 2002;17:774–778.

48. Moore GP. Ethics seminars: The practice of medical procedures on newly dead patients—is consent warranted? Acad Emerg Med 2001;8:389–392.

49. Alden AW, Ward KLM, Moore GP. Should post-mortem procedures be practiced on recently deceased patients? A survey of relatives' attitudes. Acad Emerg Med 1999;6:749–751.

50. Ferrell BR, Dahlin C, Campbell ML, Paice JA, Malloy P, Virani R. End-of-life nursing education consortium (ELNEC) training program: Improving palliative care in critical care. Crit Care Nurs Q 2007;30:206–212.

51. Emanuel LL, Quest T, eds. The Education in Palliative and End-of-Life Care for Emergency Medicine (EPEC-EM) Curriculum. The EPEC Project. Chicago, IL: Author, 2007.

52. O'Mahoney S, Blank A, Simpson J, et al. Preliminary report of a palliative care and case management project in an emergency department for chronically ill elderly patients. J Urban Health: Bull NY Acad Med 2008;85(3):443–451.

53. Campbell ML. Communicating a poor prognosis and making decisions. In: Foregoing Life-Sustaining Therapy: How to Care for the Patient Who Is Near Death. Aliso Veijo, CA: American Association of Critical-Care Nurses, 1998:19–41.

# 51

*Betty R. Ferrell, Gloria Juarez, and Tami Borneman*

# The Role of Nursing in Caring for Patients Undergoing Surgery for Advanced Disease

*My doctor told me that I need surgery, but the surgery will not cure my cancer. To have to go through all this just to make sure I don't get obstruction in my colon, makes you wonder if its worth it at all. What if I go through the procedure and still end up getting obstructed?—A patient*

♦ **Key Points**

♦ *Patients and their family caregivers facing surgery for advanced disease have complex physical and psychosocial needs.*

♦ *Patients and family members require support as they make decisions regarding the benefits and burdens of treatments for advanced disease.*

♦ *Palliative surgeries affect physical, psychological, social, and spiritual well-being as well as additional health system outcomes.*

---

CASE STUDY
### Marcella Gutierrez, A 42-Year-Old Woman with Gastric Cancer

Marcella Gutierrez was a 42-year-old Hispanic woman who immigrated from Mexico 8 years ago and lived in Southern California. She and her husband, Jose, had four children, and the youngest was 11 years old. About 4 months prior, Mrs. Gutierrez began to notice gastrointestinal symptoms such as pain, early satiety, and excessive indigestion. After attempting to treat the symptoms using over-the-counter medications and herbal treatments without success, she was evaluated at a community clinic and was found to have gastric cancer. The family sought care at a large University Cancer Center and placed great confidence in the fact that Marcella's cancer would be cured because one of her cousins was treated successfully there 5 years before. At the surgical consult, the oncology surgeon explained the seriousness of her cancer as well as results from diagnostic imaging, which showed widespread metastases to the lung. When the surgeon discussed treatment options with the family, Marcella and Jose and their extended family voiced their desire for aggressive treatment. Marcella voiced her desire to "try anything" to treat the cancer, and she repeated her confidence in the abilities of the surgeon and his team to save her life. The surgeon attempted to explain to Marcella, her husband, and their extended family that the planned surgical procedure was not curative and that the procedure was primarily offered for symptom control. Both Marcella and Jose stated that they had faith in God as well as the skills of the surgeon and again voiced their confidence that Marcella's cancer would be cured. Later that evening (the day before the planned surgery), the evening nurse approached Marcella for discussion of surgical consent. Marcella voiced that she had no questions and was eager to sign off on any surgical consent needed, because

959

the sooner she had the surgery, the sooner her cancer would be cured.

This case illustrates the numerous complexities of caring for patients with advanced disease for whom surgical treatment may be an option. The nurse is faced with caring for a patient with advanced cancer and a poor prognosis, yet both the patient and family are expecting a "miracle." There are many complex cultural and social factors affecting her decisions for care as well. The nurse is challenged to work with the patient, her family, the physician, and other interdisciplinary colleagues to provide the best information and support for this family while also anticipating the many immediate postoperative needs as well as the longer term symptom management and disease issues. This case is only one example of the incredibly complex and challenging needs of patients undergoing surgery for advanced disease.

## Decision-Making in Palliative Surgery

Patients facing advanced disease are often in the position of making difficult choices regarding treatments. Patients often face a critical juncture of determining when they should continue disease-focused treatments such as chemotherapy, radiation, or surgery and when it is time to stop such treatments. Even amid the recognition of advanced disease, patients frequently seek aggressive treatment with the hope of prolonging their survival, even if only for a matter of months—or of possibly enhancing their quality of life (QOL) through the relief of symptoms.[1-3]

Figure 51–1 is derived from research in the area of palliative surgery conducted at the City of Hope National Medical Center.[4] The model demonstrates that the process of making decisions about palliative surgery involves influences from the patient, the family, and the health-care team. Patients and families must weigh the potential benefit versus the harm of the surgery proposed, whereas the health-care team considers factors such as the difficulty of the procedure, the duration of hospitalization, recovery time, chance of achieving the goal, anticipated durability of the intervention, and anticipated disease progression.[5-7] It becomes evident in reviewing these factors that much of the decision-making involves great individual variation, so that it is difficult to estimate who might benefit most from more aggressive intervention. For example, the patient with a poor prognosis resulting from an extremely advanced gastrointestinal tumor, who subsequently lives

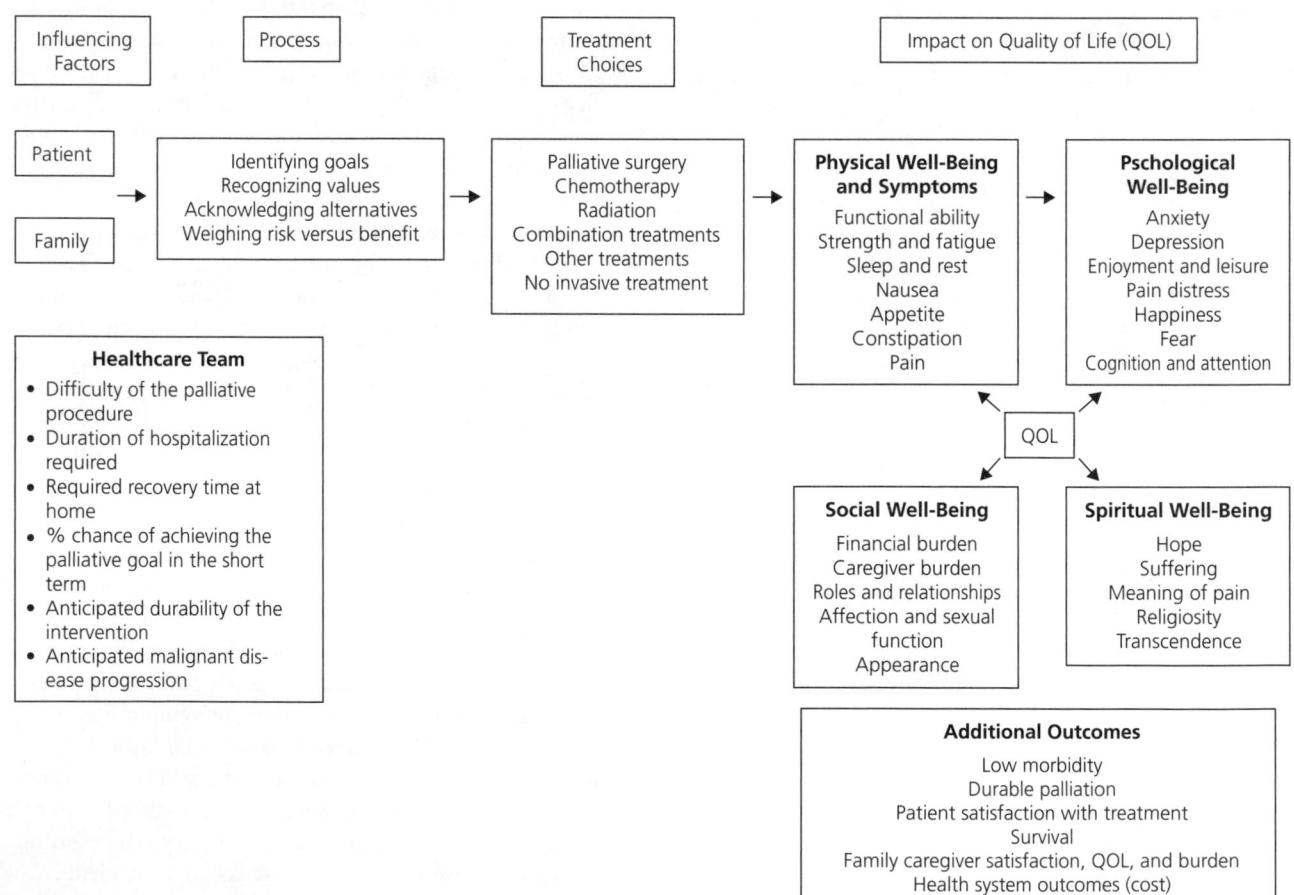

**Figure 51–1.** Clinical decision-making in palliative surgery. *Source:* Ferrell et al. (2003), reference 4.

twice the original duration anticipated, may well have been the patient who could have benefited from surgery to relieve obstruction for abdominal pressure causing severe nausea, vomiting, or bowel problems.

The process of making decisions involves a focus on goals of care, recognizing the values of the patient, acknowledging alternatives, and always weighing the risks versus benefits.[8] As surgeries have become more advanced in technique, it is often possible to do very extensive surgery on an outpatient basis or with very short hospitalization time. This reduced "burden" makes it more likely that patients may opt for surgical procedures. Given the many symptoms or problems resulting from advanced disease, patients consider a variety of treatment choices, including surgery, chemotherapy, radiotherapy, or a combination of treatments.

The outcomes of this process of decision-making are depicted in Figure 51–1 as affecting all dimensions of QOL. Physical well-being and symptoms, as well as function, are almost always affected by treatment choices.[9] Psychological well-being, including anxiety and depression as well as fears, is also influenced by treatment choices.[10] Patients and families have often reflected that, although a particular treatment may have not prolonged survival, it gave them a tremendous sense of assurance that everything possible was being done to treat the illness. In the realm of social well-being, the choices of treatments have very significant impacts on the patient's roles and relationships as well as the burden on caregivers.[11–13]

Although invasive, "high-tech" treatments may be thought of as adding to the caregiver burden; in advanced disease, the failure to aggressively treat problems commonly results in heightened burden. For example, a patient who declines surgery relatively early in the course of an advanced gastrointestinal tumor may then experience much worse nausea, vomiting, diarrhea, and subsequent complications that could result in a more intense caregiver burden than would have been required after earlier surgery.

Finally, spiritual well-being is greatly influenced by decisions regarding palliative surgery, because patients rely on their faith and religion in making treatment choices.[1,2] One of the strongest themes throughout palliative care research at the COH has been the concept of hope.[2] This concept is covered in greater detail in Chapter 29, but it certainly applies closely to the topic of palliative surgery. Patients may perceive that surgery, even if presented as only palliative in nature, is still potentially curative or life-prolonging, and therefore may opt for surgery with unfounded hope for a cure.[14]

The model in Figure 51–1 illustrates how important it is for nurses to provide education, counseling, and support as patients and families wrestle with treatment choices. It also is not uncommon for patients and families to have different perspectives and conflicting opinions. For example, a patient with advanced disease may opt for no further invasive treatments and instead focus on measures of comfort. At the same time, family members may press for the patient to endure continued procedures for even the smallest possibility of prolonged survival.

## Research in Palliative Surgery

There has been limited research in the field of palliative care and even far more limited focus on the area of palliative surgery. Recent studies have begun to document both the lack of research in the field and the limitations of existing research.[15–17] Leaders in the field of palliative surgery have documented that few studies evaluating these procedures have included measures of patient QOL, symptom management, or psychosocial concerns.[18]

Research in the area of palliative surgery was initiated at the COH in 2000, and since that time a series of studies has been conducted involving collaboration between the Division of Nursing Research and the Department of Surgery. Table 51–1 summarizes phases of this research to date. The studies included a review of surgical cases to determine the extent of palliative surgery use at a cancer center, which was followed by a prospective review of cases that led to research evaluating decision-making by patients and family members.[19] To broaden understanding of palliative surgery beyond one cancer center, phase III involved a survey of 419 surgeon members of the Society of Surgical Oncology.[20,21] A very important finding of this research was the identification of ethical dilemmas faced by surgeons, such as providing patients with honest information without destroying hope and preserving patient choices.

These early studies have led to clinical investigations exploring symptom management and QOL outcomes, as well as longitudinal measures, in an effort to capture the effects of palliative surgery and its potential impact on symptoms and QOL.[22] These studies have also provided an opportunity to incorporate qualitative methods for exploration of patient and family caregiver experiences.[1,2]

## Patient Perspectives

The research at COH has explored patient perspectives of surgery through in-depth individual interviews conducted preoperatively and postoperatively, as well as assessment of symptoms and QOL. Table 51–2 includes some representative comments from patients' perspectives of QOL after surgery. As this study demonstrated, patients may believe that surgery is their only option to avoid progression and eventual death from their disease. The presence of physical symptoms has been found to be a key motivator for seeking surgical intervention. Even those patients who recognize that surgery is not curative may aggressively seek surgical approaches to relieve distressing physical symptoms such as pain, gastrointestinal symptoms, bleeding, odors, and other problems. These studies

**Table 51–1**
**Description of Program of Research**

### Phase I

Surgical Palliation at a Cancer Center (Krouse et al. [2001], reference 26)

**Design:** Retrospective review of surgical cases ($n$ = 1915) during a 1-year period with a 1-year survival follow-up. This descriptive study began exploration of the extent of palliative surgery and identification of patient outcomes.

**Key findings:** Palliative surgeries (PS) comprised 240 (12.5%) of 1915 surgical procedures. There were 170 major and 70 minor procedures. Neurosurgical (46.0%), orthopedic (31.3%), and thoracic (21.5%) surgical procedures were frequently PS. The most common primary diagnoses were lung, colorectal, breast, and prostate cancers. Length of hospital stay was 12.4 days (range, 0–99 days). Mortality was 21.9% for surgical procedures classified as major and 10.0% for those classified as minor. The investigators concluded that in significant numbers of PS mortality was high; however, a significant number of patients had short hospital stays and low morbidity. PS should remain an important part of end-of-life care. Patients and their families must be aware of the high risks and understand the clear objectives of these procedures.

### Phase II

Advancing the Evaluation of Palliative Surgery for Cancer Patients (Krouse et al. [2002], reference 19)

**Design:** Prospective review of PS ($n$ = 50). Pilot testing of interview guide for use with patients/family caregivers and surgeons to explore decision-making and goals.

**Key findings:** Prospective design allowed expansion of outcomes to include quality of life (QOL) and exploration of the involvement of family caregivers.

### Phase III

Indications and Use of Palliative Surgery—Results of Society of Surgical Oncology (SSO) Survey (McCahill [2002a and 2002b], references 20 and 21)

**Design:** Mailed survey (110 items) of members of the SSO ($n$ = 419 responses). This phase was intended to provide a national perspective on the topic of PS and to expand knowledge of surgeons' decision-making.

**Key findings:** Surgeons estimated 21% of their cancer surgeries as PS in nature; 43% of respondents believed PS was best defined based on preoperative intent, 27% based on postoperative factors, and 30% on patient prognosis. Only 43% considered estimated patient survival time an important factor in defining PS, and 22% considered 5-year survival rate important. Patient symptom relief and pain relief were identified as the two most important goals in PS, with increased survival the least important. On a scale of 1 (uncommon problem) to 7 (common problem), surgeons reported that the most common ethical dilemmas in PS were providing patients with honest information without destroying hope and preserving patient choice. On a scale of 1 (not a barrier) to 7 (severe barrier), surgeons rated the most severe barriers to optimum use of PS as limitations of managed care and referral to surgery by other specialists. The least severe barriers were surgeon avoidance of dying patients and surgery department reluctance to perform PS.

### Phase IV

A Prospective Evaluation of Palliative Outcomes for Surgery of Advanced Malignancies (McCahill [2003], reference 22)

**Design:** Prospective evaluation of patients undergoing PS ($n$ = 59) with longitudinal measures for 1 year. Outcomes were expanded to provide more detailed evaluation of symptom management and QOL. Qualitative evaluation included in-depth interviews of patients, family caregivers, and surgeons before and after surgery to further describe decisions and outcomes related to surgery.

**Key findings:** Preoperatively, surgeons identified 22 operations (37%) as PS, 37 (63%) as curative. Thirty-three patients (56%) were symptomatic preoperatively, and symptom resolution was documented in 79% surviving >30 d. Good to excellent palliation, defined as "more than 70% symptom-free non-hospitalized days relative to postoperative days of life," was achieved in 53% of PS patients. Among patients with postoperative survival <6 mo, 63% had good to excellent palliation. The majority of symptomatic patients undergoing major surgery for advanced malignancies attained good to excellent symptom relief. The researchers concluded that outcome measurements other than survival are feasible and are likely to play an important role in defining surgery as an important component of multimodality palliative care.

### Phase V

A Comparison of Resource Consumption in Curative and Palliative Surgery (Cullinane et al. [2003], reference 18)

**Design:** Prospective evaluations of all surgeries performed over a 3-month period ($n$ = 302) with 6-month follow-up. The investigators extended the outcomes of surgery to be evaluated based on Phases I–IV.

**Key findings:** Over a 4-month period, the outcome and service needs of 302 consecutive patients with malignancy undergoing surgeon-defined PS or curative surgery were evaluated. Previous treatment history, comorbidities, symptoms, procedures, outcome, and use of supportive services were collected. Patients were monitored for 6 months after the surgical procedures performed for cure (breast or prostate cancer) or for palliation (breast, lung, and bone/soft tissue tumors). There were 3 (1%) curative and 4 (6%) palliative deaths during the surgical admission. Mean hospital stay was 5.1 days (range, 0–58 days) for curative surgery patients and 1.9 day (range, 0–34 days) for PS patients. After discharge, a total of 4690 encounters with the cancer center occurred, including 1676 encounters with surgery, 1595 encounters with medical oncology, 1006 encounters with radiation oncology, 226 visits to medical specialists, and 187 visits with supportive services. Mean number of encounters for curative and PS patients were 15 and 17, respectively, ($P$ = 0.41). Curative patients were more likely to have visits with therapeutic intent, including chemotherapy ($P$ = 0.01) and radiation ($P$ = 0.003). Readmission occurred in 82 (34%) of curative and 28 (48%) PS patients during the 6-month period ($P$ = 0.04). PS patients were more likely to be admitted for symptom management ($P$ = 0.0001), whereas curative surgery patients were more likely to be admitted for repeat procedures ($P$ = 0.006).

*(Continued)*

---

**Table 51–1**
**Description of Program of Research** (*contiued*)

**Phase VI**

Concerns of Family Caregivers of Cancer patients Facing Surgery for Advanced Malignancies (Borneman et al. [2003], reference 1)

**Design:** Family caregivers were assessed before planned PS and at 2 weeks and 6 weeks after surgery. Quantitative assessment of caregiver QOL occurred at each time point. A subset of nine caregivers also participated in a structured interview before surgery and at 2 weeks after surgery.

**Key findings:** The study findings indicate important family caregiver QOL concerns and needs for support at the time surrounding surgery for advanced disease. Psychological issues were most pronounced with common needs of uncertainty, fears regarding the future, and loss. Family caregivers voiced concerns about surgical risks and care after surgery and experienced recognition of the patient's declining status. The investigators concluded that surgery is an important component of palliative care and is an area requiring further research and clinical attention.

---

**Table 51–2**
**Patient Perspectives on Quality of Life and Surgery**

**Surgery-only option**

"Because this is one of the slower—slower growing cancers, radiation and chemo wouldn't have helped at all. So there was—there was no option other than—other than the surgery—there was no option."

**Gastrointestinal symptoms**

"I used to always, I had the constant urge that I was going to have a bowel movement. Well, I did not have a bowel movement, but, and this urge is so strong I, I'd go in and sit on the toilet. And then, of course, I would pass some mucus and stuff. Um, there for a while before the surgery, oh, it was just terrible. And a lot of it would be quite bloody. And, ah, you know, I had a good day yesterday. I had a good night last night and the night before that I had a good night."

**Psychological well-being**

"But now I feel even the surgery's not complete. I still have my tumor in my kidney. But that is not operable based on what [the doctor] told me. Just, just a few alternatives. You know, it's a surgery, remove the whole kidney? Or do the gene therapy? Or do the freezing or burn technique, you know. So there's still a chance."

**Postsurgery quality of life**

"Yeah. Every time my friend, or whoever, has cancer, I told them don't give up. Find an alternative. If you're rejected by this doctor, don't just give up. Keep on trying whatever possible, whatever you have to go through. So, that's the only way. A lot of my friends are cancer patients. When they come to the end of the tunnel, they don't know how to do and they are so depressed, I say don't worry. We already have the problem. You got to face it. Your worry doesn't help. You know, you got to ask God to give you a day. Use the medical technology available …Somebody may save you. You know, a miracle. This could happen to you, too. It happened to me many times."

*Source:* Ferrell et al. (2003), reference 4.

---

also demonstrated that tremendous psychological stress and anxiety are induced by the need to make decisions about surgical options. Having surgery in advanced disease seems to be a stark reality given the extent of the disease. Also, it is not uncommon to find evidence of far more advanced disease during the surgery than was originally known.

The COH investigators also investigated differences in resource utilization of surgical patients following curative or palliative procedures. Results showed that the number of resources utilized was similar in both groups but that the nature of interactions were different.[18] This suggests that resource needs are different for the two treatment intents. In a separate analysis of advanced gastrointestinal cases, Podnos and colleagues described the effect of palliative surgical procedures on symptoms and overall QOL. The most common symptoms reported were pain and obstruction.[23] The frequency of primary symptoms improved postoperatively, but overall QOL decreased over time.[7]

## Family Caregivers

The palliative surgery research at the COH has also described the concerns of family caregivers of patients undergoing palliative surgeries for advanced malignancies. Family caregivers ($n = 45$) were assessed before planned palliative surgery and at 2 weeks and 6 weeks after surgery.[8] Quantitative assessment of caregiver QOL occurred at each interval. A subset of nine caregivers also participated in structured interviews before surgery and 2 weeks after surgery. Caregiver concerns, QOL, and decision-making were evaluated. Findings of the study indicated that family caregivers have important QOL concerns and needs for support before and after surgery for advanced disease. Psychological issues were most pronounced, and common concerns included uncertainty, fears regarding the future, and loss. Further analysis suggested that family caregivers also experienced disruptions in overall QOL that were similar to those experienced by patients.[24] Caregivers' distress levels were high prior to surgery, and overall distress continued to worsen over time and after the surgery. Financial burden for caregivers included transportation, medications, and other services that were not covered by insurance. In a path analysis of variables influencing caregiver burden in palliative care, Grov and colleagues found a direct significant association between caregiver depression and caregiver burden.[25] The effects of other variables, such as patient's symptom status, social support, and caregiver overall QOL, on caregiver burden were all mediated by caregiver depression.[25]

Family caregivers had concerns about surgical risks and patient care needs after surgery and voiced recognition of the declining status of patients. The needs of family caregivers are multiple and complex, requiring ongoing assessment to provide interventions that help them cope and ultimately improve their QOL. This important topic requires further research and clinical attention.

Table 51–3 includes examples of family caregivers' perspectives provided both preoperatively and postoperatively. Families articulated their concerns about the surgery and its risks and were more concerned than patients about potential negative consequences of surgery.[8] Family members often

discussed the benefits of surgery, with a strong sense from both patients and family caregivers that surgery is always a good option because "to take it out" must increase one's chance for survival. For family members, however, the postoperative period was most often one of incredible stress as they faced the reality that the patient's prognosis was not likely to have changed and that surgery may in fact have revealed more evidence of advanced disease. For many patients, the surgical experience became a "roller coaster," in which they grasped for hope for a cure from surgery, even if intended as palliative, but the hope was balanced by recognition of the patient's decline in status.

## Nursing Care of Patients Undergoing Palliative Surgery

The care of patients undergoing palliative surgery is often focused more on the medical aspects, yet nursing care is essential throughout all phases of preoperative, intraoperative, immediate postoperative, and postoperative recovery and discharge. This is a critical time, with numerous

---

**Table 51–3**
**Family Caregivers' Perspectives**

**Preoperative**
*Concerns about surgery and risks*
"I'm scared. I worry about just him getting through it ... for the first few days, I'll still be worried, and I'll just be glad when he comes home. I'll be glad to do anything, you know, just to have him come home again. I know it's good to know the truth, and I'm glad that [the doctor] was so up front with us. But it's just so hard to deal with. Surgery's very scary. The chemotherapy and radiation was not scary. I knew he would get sick, but I knew that there was no chance of him dying from it. This is a whole different animal."

*Benefits of surgery*
"I think it's a good thing. Because, you know, your immune system concentrates on, like, if you have a tumor, they concentrate all over the body. By taking this out, this is a big thing that, you know, it has cancer in it. By taking that out I feel like maybe her body can concentrate on other parts a little bit better than with, you know, with this in her. And then they're going to take the one out of her hip and I, I think it's a good thing. I'm glad that she's having the surgery."

**Postoperative**
*No change in prognosis*
"It was more of a quality-of-life thing. They'd like to get her eating, like to get her home. Like to get her spending her time in a way that she finds, you know, enjoyable. But, um, they're not planning on curing her or anything like that, I think she is aware of the prognosis. But, you know, like she said, she wants to still be in the treatment category more than, she doesn't want hospice at this point. So, although she knows that, she's not ready to just say that's it and prepare to die. She's wanting to do whatever she can to keep going."

*Uncertain survival*
"The last day, of course, he was sleeping. I couldn't stand to even see him because his eyes were all swollen and his face was all swollen. But he never woke up on that second day anyway. That very morning, [the doctor] told me that it would be a long, slow recovery, but he was going to do okay and he had a 50–50 chance that morning. And that was at about 9 o'clock in the morning. And at 7 o'clock that night, [the doctor] told me he wasn't going to make it through the night. Do you know how that can throw a person emotionally? Do you? You have no idea what kind of an emotional roller coaster I was on for those 13 days. One day, everything's looking better. The next day everything was just horrible. I'm surprised I didn't end up having a heart attack myself or a nervous breakdown."

*Source:* Borneman et al. (2003), reference 1.

transitions between care settings, and nurses can play a vital role in ensuring continuity across settings such as the operating room, intensive care unit (ICU), postoperative surgical unit, and home care. A prime example is the role of nursing in ensuring pain management by assessing a patient's chronic pain problem at the time of admission to plan adequate analgesia as the patient is admitted for surgery. The nurse then works collaboratively with the physician and the pharmacist to plan the analgesic orders for the transition from the oral analgesics used preoperatively to an appropriate regimen after surgery. Additional monitoring is needed because the patient's pain may escalate after major surgery and also to ensure the appropriate changes as the patient goes from chronic oral medications at home to parental administration in the postoperative period and in the ICU. Maintaining adequate analgesia after discharge from the ICU to the postoperative unit and then to home care is essential for the patient's timely discharge to home and remains a requirement during recovery. This simple example of just one aspect of care, pain management, illustrates the vital role of nursing during this very acute phase of treatment.

Patients with advanced disease often undergo surgery with the goal of palliation to achieve a longer survival, even when cure is not a realistic goal. The following case illustrates this point.

CASE STUDY
*Robert Newsom, A 62-Year-Old Man with Rectal Cancer*

Robert Newsom was a 62-year-old African-American man with stage IIIa rectal cancer who underwent neoadjuvant chemoradiation followed by anterior resection of his rectum. After a prolonged postoperative course and extensive recovery phase, Mr. Newsom was able to return to work as a security guard for a local bank. About 4 months after his initial surgery, Mr. Newsom was admitted to the hospital with abdominal pain, dehydration, and nausea and vomiting that was refractory to antiemetics. The final diagnosis was malignant bowel obstruction, secondary to recurrence of his rectal cancer as well as chronic adhesions, a complication from his previous surgical procedure. The surgical team met with Mr. Newsom and his wife to explain the status of his recurrence and treatment options for the malignant bowel obstruction. Because of the extent and location of the recurrence, it was suggested that a nonsurgical approach be taken to manage the obstruction with the use of octreotide. Other options, such as surgical removal of a portion of the recurrent tumor as well as the site of adhesion, were also discussed. The surgeon also wanted to discuss the fact that the recurrence meant that any procedure would only be palliative and not curative and that Mr. Newsom's prognosis was likely to worsen. Mr. Newsom and his wife voiced their strong faith and belief that God would guide the surgeon in helping him with removal of all his remaining cancer.

Mr. Newsom and his wife also voiced an important goal for them: to make sure, at all costs, that Mr. Newsom would live to see their son's college graduation in 6 months. This was a particularly significant event, because Mr. Newsom's son would be the first in their family ever to receive an undergraduate degree.

This case illustrates the role of palliative surgery and the benefit of extending patient survival to achieve life goals even if a cure is not possible. Nurses would play a vital role in Mr. Newsom's care, including aggressive management of his existing symptoms and additional psychosocial support required at that critical time in his illness, as he and his family confronted the reality of his worsening disease. Continued attention would also be needed after surgery to monitor Mr. Newsom's progress. For example, if his disease progressed more rapidly or if he developed postoperative complications that could have lead to shorter survival, it might have been necessary to work with the family to realize what choices they could have made if he had not lived to see the graduation. Supporting Mr. Newsom's faith and the spiritual crisis that might have developed if he believed that God had failed him was essential. This case also illustrates the vital role of nurses in monitoring patients after surgery to assist with transitions to home care/hospice or palliative care programs.

## The Goal of Symptom Relief

The following case study illustrates the goal of symptom relief in palliative surgery.

CASE STUDY
*Beatrice Anderson, An 80-Year-Old Woman with Breast Cancer*

Beatrice Anderson is an 80-year-old Native American woman who was diagnosed with advanced breast cancer approximately 8 months prior. Ms. Anderson had discovered a fungating lesion on her right breast and had been experiencing severe pain as the lesion continued to grow but did not seek medical care. Instead, she relied on traditional Native American healers and treatments, believing that her pain and the lesion would become smaller with the traditional treatments. When the lesion continued to grow and bleed and the pain became unbearable, Ms. Anderson was evaluated and informed of her diagnosis. She opted for supportive care only and initially was not interested in the possibility of surgery or chemotherapy; however, she did voice her desire for aggressive symptom management with the goal of reducing her pain and maintaining her function and independence "as long as possible." Ms. Anderson moved from her rural tribal community into the home of her daughter in an urban metropolitan area. Ms. Anderson was evaluated by the pain specialist at a local hospital. She was started on a pain regimen, but the regimen alone was unsuccessful in achieving significant pain relief as the lesion on her breast continued to grow. At this point, Ms. Anderson was referred to a surgeon and was presented with the option of lumpectomy to remove the fungating lesion. At first her daughter was hesitant in having her mother undergo such an extensive surgery at age 80 years. However, Ms. Anderson insisted on having the surgery if it would help with achieving some pain relief. The nurse practitioner in the surgical clinic met with the patient and family, as well as the surgeon, to describe the procedure and the expected postoperative course. Ms. Anderson underwent surgery and recovered without any major complications, with the exception of an infection acquired during her postoperative stay at the hospital. Her pain significantly improved, although she remained on pain medications on an as-needed basis. She continued to be monitored by the pain specialist at the hospital.

This case illustrates the role of surgery in relieving severe symptoms that have been unresponsive to less aggressive means. It also illustrates the importance of evaluating the patient's goals of care and circumstances as well as the fact that quite often surgical intervention, although considered to be invasive or aggressive, may be the best option even in the face of advanced disease.

## Psychosocial Issues Affecting Palliative Surgery

Patients facing advanced disease and critical associated decisions related to treatment options also present with complex psychosocial and spiritual needs. The following case illustrates complex issues in patients who are torn between the desire to survive and weariness and readiness for life's end.

CASE STUDY

*Katherine Kowolski, A 59-Year-Old Woman with Esophageal Cancer*

Mrs. Kowolski was a 59-year-old Russian immigrant who came to the United States 20 years ago with her husband. They owned a small janitorial service business. The Kowlaskis had three children who had all completed college and were doing well. The family prospered as successful small business oweners. Three years ago, Mr. Kowolski passed away suddenly from cardiac arrest. Since then, Mrs. Kowolski battled chronic depresssion, and the family's small business suffered from her devastating loss. Approximately 2 years after

her husband's death, Mrs. Kowolski was diagnosed with esophageal cancer and underwent neoadjuvant chemoradiation plus surgery to remove the primary tumor. Her postoperative course was complicated by numerous problems, including a chronic problem with digestion, swallowing, and pain. She experienced a fairly sharp decline in status 6 months later.

Mrs. Kowolski made her wishes very clear: she did not want life-sustaining treatment and did not want to be treated any further. She felt that she had become a burden for her three children. Over the past month, Mrs. Kowolski developed worsening dysphagia and was found to have recurrent disease. The surgeon recommended a surgical procedure to remove some of the recurrent tumor but stated that it might not be possible to remove all of the tumor given its location. Mrs. Kowolski hesitantly agreed to the surgery. She mentioned to the nursing staff that she had hoped that it wouldn't come to this, stating, "I think I'm dying from the inside out." The surgical resident came to obtain her consent for the surgical procedure. Mrs. Kowolski became extremely angry and hostile when the resident informed her that her "do-not-resuscitate" order would have to be rescinded for her to have surgery, because it was the hospital's policy that all patients entering surgery were at full code status. Mrs. Kowolski told the resident that she and her deceased husband would haunt him for the rest of his career if he should "rob her the opportunity to die" if God deemed it should be so during surgery. After the resident left, a nurse came to the bedside to talk with Mrs. Kowolski. While in tears, Mrs. Kowolski stated that she still wanted the surgery, but she couldn't imagine that the surgeons would want to resuscitate her if the need should arise during surgery. After she became much calmer, Mrs. Kowolski admitted to the nurse, "On the other hand, I wish that maybe my heart would stop during surgery so that it would be easier for everyone if I could die quickly."

The case of Mrs. Kowolski illustrates the complexities of dealing with patients with advanced disease. Cultural, spiritual, and psychosocial issues are important influences. This case also illustrates the importance of nursing leadership in creating policies and procedures that support the goals of palliative care. Many institutions have eliminated their requirement for full code status on patients undergoing surgery and now honor the request to avoid resuscitation even if its need should occur during surgery. Mrs. Kowolski's clinical signs of depression are also important to evaluate in considering her overall plan of care. A patient's wish for death should never be dismissed, and such information should be shared with the surgical staff. Instances such as this are also primary examples for incorporating psychiatry or psychology: evaluation of her depression is essential, and attention to her emotions would be needed before the surgery as well as in the follow-up period. Nurses play a critical role in attending to the communication around this issue and in acting as the patient's advocate in all stages of care and across settings.

## Summary

Palliative nursing care extends across all treatment modalities, and patients undergoing surgery require intensive support and care. Nurses play a critical role in patient and family communication, establishing goals of care and expert management of symptoms. There is a need for continued research to address this area of palliative care and for continued advancements of clinical nursing expertise to best serve these patients and families.[26,27]

REFERENCES

1. Borneman T, Chu DZJ, Wagman L, et al. Concerns of family caregivers of patients with cancer facing palliative surgery for advanced malignancies. Oncol Nurs Forum 2003;30: 997–1005.

2. Borneman T, Stahl C, Ferrell BR, Smith D. The concept of hope in family caregivers of patients with cancer at home. J Hosp Palliat Nurs 2002;4:21–23.

3. Angelos P. Palliative philosophy: The ethical underpinning. Surg Oncol Clin North Am 2001;10:31–38.

4. Ferrell BR, Chu DZJ, Wagman L, et al. Patient and surgeon decision making regarding surgery regarding advanced cancer. Oncol Nurs Forum 2003;30:E106–E114.

5. Bradley CJ, Clement JP, Lin C. Absence of cancer diagnosis and treatment in elderly Medicaid-insured nursing home residents. J Natl Cancer I 2008;100(1):21–31.

6. Hofmann B, Haheim LL, Soreide JA. Ethics of palliative surgery in patients with cancer. Br J Surg 2005;92(7):802–809.

7. Podnos YD, Juarez G, Pameijer C, Choi K, Ferrell BR, Wagman LD. Impact of surgical palliation on quality of life in patients with advanced malignancy: Results of the decisions and outcomes in palliative surgery (DOPS) trial. Ann Surg Oncol 2007;14(2):922–928.

8. Miner TJ, Jaques JP, Shriver CD. A prospective evaluation of patients undergoing surgery for the palliation of an advanced malignancy. Ann Surg Oncol 2002;9:696–703.

9. Burke CC. Surgical treatment. In: Miakowski C, Buchsel P, eds. Oncology Nursing: Assessment and Clinical Care. St. Louis, MO: Mosby; 1999:29–58.

10. Milch RA, Dunn GP. Communication: Part of a surgical armamentiarium. J Am Coll Surg 2001;193:449–451.

11. Andrews SC. Caregiver burden and symptom distress in people with cancer receiving hospice care. Oncol Nurs Forum 2001;28:1469–1474.

12. Given BA, Gicen CW, Kozachik S. Family support in advanced cancer. CA: A Cancer J Clin 2001;51:213–231.

13. Langenhoff BS, Krabbe PF, Wobbes T, Ruers TJ. Quality of life as an outcome measure in surgical oncology. Br J Surg 2001;88:643–652.

14. Bruera E, Sweeney C, Calder K, Palmer L, Benisch-Tolley S. When the treatment goal is not cure: Are cancer patients equipped to make informed decisions? J Clin Oncol 2001;20:503–513.

15. Velovich V. The quality of quality of life studies in general surgical journals. J Am Col Surg 2001;193:288–296.

16. Dunn GP. The surgeon and palliative care. Surg Oncol Clin North Am 2001;10:7–24.

17. Easson AM, Crosby JA, Librach SL. Discussion of death and dying in surgical textbooks. Am J Surg 2001;182:34–39.

18. Cullinane CA, Borneman T, Smith DD, Chu DZ, Ferrell BR, Wagman LD. The surgical treatment of cancer: A comparison of resource utilization following procedures performed with a curative and palliative intent. Cancer 2003;98(10):2266–2273.

19. Krouse R, Ferrell BR, Nelson RA, Juarez G, Wagman LC, Chu D. Advancing the Evaluation of Palliative Surgery for Cancer Patients. Unpublished manuscript, 2002.

20. McCahill LE, Krouse R, Chu DZJ, et al. Indications and use of palliative surgery: Results of Society of Surgical Oncology survey. Ann Surg Oncol 2002;9:104–112.

21. McCahill LE, Krouse RS, Chu DZJ, et al. Decision making in palliative surgery. J Am Coll Surg 2002;195:411–423.

22. McCahill LE, Smith D, Borneman T, et al. A prospective evaluation of palliative outcomes for surgery of advanced malignancies. Ann Surg Oncol 2003;10:654–663.

23. Podnos YD, Juarez G, Pameijer C, Uman G, Ferrell BR, Wagman LD. Surgical palliation of advanced gastrointestinal tumors. J Palliat Med 2007;10(4):871–876.

24. Juarez G, Ferrell B, Uman G, Podnos Y, Wagman LD. Distress and quality of life concerns of family caregivers of patients undergoing palliative surgery. Cancer Nurs 2008;31(1):2–10.

25. Grov EK, Fossa SD, Sorebo O, Dahl AA. Primary caregivers of cancer patients in the palliative phase: A path analysis of variables influencing their burden. Soc Sci Med 2006; 63(9):2429–2439.

26. Krouse RS, Nelson RA, Ferrell BR, et al. Surgical palliation at a cancer center: Incidence and outcomes. Arch Surg 2001;136:773–778.

27. Krouse RS, Ferrell BR, Nelson RA, Juarez G, Wagman LC, Chu D. Advancing the evaluation of palliative surgery for cancer patients. Unpublished manuscript, 2002.

# 52 Virginia Sun

# Palliative Chemotherapy and Clinical Trials in Advanced Cancer: The Nurse's Role

*I decided to enroll in a clinical trial and see what it does for me. I have been told that the chances of the new drug doing anything to my cancer is small, but I'm willing to take even a 1% chance that it might actually shrink it. What have I got to lose at this point?—A patient*

♦ ***Key Points***
♦ *Patients with advanced cancer are often caught between the dichotomy of continuing aggressive treatment and the focus on quality supportive and palliative care.*
♦ *Faced with difficult decisions, patients and families become especially vulnerable and may experience heightened physical, psychological, social, and spiritual distress.*
♦ *Palliative chemotherapy uses systemic antineoplastic agents to treat symptoms of incurable malignancies and maintain quality of life.*
♦ *Nurses can help alleviate suffering by supporting patients and families through changes in treatment intent, the decision-making process, and supportive care needs during palliative chemotherapy.*

Nurses have always been in the forefront of managing treatment-related symptoms. In an ever-changing and complex health-care setting, optimal care requires a transdisciplinary approach. This approach is especially valued in an oncology setting, where patients frequently present with complex disease- and treatment-related symptoms. These often debilitating symptoms negatively affect the quality of life (QoL) of patients and their extended families.[1] For patients with advanced cancer, treatment options are often limited. It is usually at this stage of the cancer continuum that discussion of palliative modalities of treatment occurs. These palliative modalities often include—but are not limited to—radiation, surgery, and chemotherapy. It is also during this stage of the continuum that physicians discuss the use of investigational therapeutic agents as an attempt to control the disease. However, it is not uncommon for patients and families to be faced with difficult decisions. Patients with advanced cancer are often caught between the dichotomy of continuing aggressive treatment and the focus on quality supportive and palliative care.[2] The debate of treatment futility often comes into play at this stage of the cancer continuum, because patients and families are faced with a shorter life expectancy and all standard therapeutic regimens have failed to control the spread and proliferation of the tumor itself. Faced with these difficult decisions, patients and families become especially vulnerable and may experience heightened physical, psychological, social, and spiritual distress.[3]

In advanced malignancies, the choice between palliative chemotherapy, clinical trial, or best supportive care may be difficult. This chapter describes the use of chemotherapy and cancer investigational agents as a palliative treatment for patients with advanced cancer. Emphasis is placed particularly on the role of palliative chemotherapy and the dichotomy between clinical trials of cancer investigational therapeutic agents and palliative care. Finally, an in-depth analysis of the role of nurses in supporting patients and families receiving palliative chemotherapy or investigational agents through clinical trials is discussed.

## Definitions

Palliative chemotherapy, in its broadest sense, is the use of systemic antineoplastic agents to treat an incurable malignancy.[4] In most medical literature, the efficacy of palliative chemotherapy is reported through data regarding tumor response rate, duration of response, and survival benefit.[5] However, the purpose of these studies usually is not the investigation of these agents for palliation of symptoms, although most subjects accrued in these clinical trials are deemed incurable.[6] It is only in recent years that symptom palliation has become an important aspect in the design and evaluation of cancer clinical trials. The majority of the symptom palliation research incorporated into therapeutic clinical trials focuses on QoL as a prognostic factor for better patient outcomes.[7] Other, more specific definitions used to describe palliative chemotherapy include the relief of cancer-induced symptoms.[4,8] This refers to the use of antineoplastic agents with the expectation of prolonged survival and improved QoL, which includes the relief and prevention of adverse symptoms that are indicative of advanced malignancies.[4,8]

## Curative versus Palliative Chemotherapy

As a primary therapy, chemotherapy may be potentially beneficial in the prolongation of survival in the advanced stages of cancer. However, the majority of malignancies in adults are incurable with chemotherapy. Although the development of adjuvant chemotherapy has resulted in a decrease in recurrence rates, the data show that there is no significant difference in disease-free survival.[4] Therefore, the majority of patients living with cancer will experience recurrence of disease, and it is this population that may also receive palliative chemotherapy.

Trends in the aggressiveness of cancer care at the end of life have been explored in the literature. Earle and colleagues identified several indicators of aggressive care, including intensive use of chemotherapy, low rates of hospice use, emergency room visits, hospitalization, and intensive care unit (ICU) admissions.[9] In a subsequent study to characterize end of life treatment aggressiveness in older adults on Medicare, the investigators found that rates of palliative chemotherapy treatment increased from 27.9% to 29.5% between 1993 and 1996.[10] For patients who received palliative chemotherapy, 15.7% received treatments up to 2 weeks before death.[10] An increasing proportion of patients used hospice services, but the services were primarily initiated within the last 3 days of life.[10] An updated analysis published in 2008 showed that the aggressiveness of care continued to increase, with more patients being referred to hospice within 3 days of death.[11] In both sets of analysis, elderly, female, non-white, and unmarried patients were less likely to receive aggressive care.[10–12] Other studies reported similar trends in treatment aggressiveness at the end of life for advanced lung cancer and ovarian cancer.[12,13] Studies have also found that many palliative chemotherapy treatments are initiated within 30 days of death.[14] In a retrospective cohort analysis of Medicare beneficiaries at the end of life, Emanuel and colleagues found that palliative care chemotherapy use was similar for patients with breast, colon, and ovarian cancer compared to those with less chemosensitive cancers, such as pancreatic, hepatocellular, or melanoma.[16]

When the disease has metastasized to other organ systems, the primary goal of using chemotherapy in advanced disease is to control the patient's symptoms and maintain QoL.[8] The rationale for palliating direct or indirect symptoms of cancer is multifaceted, but it is important for practitioners to remember that not all patients are suitable for palliative chemotherapy. Standard chemotherapy should not be offered to all patients with metastatic malignancies. A predicted toxicity of treatment should preclude any consideration for the use of palliative chemotherapy.[4,8] The benefit-to-toxicity ratio of treatment should be seriously considered. Subtherapeutic doses of chemotherapy should never be given to maintain hope in a patient's prognosis.[8] Such a false sense of hope may prove to be even more distressing and may induce tremendous suffering for patients and families.

Several prognostic factors have been used in chemotherapeutic treatments of cancer to determine palliative treatment modality. One of the most important prognostic factors is performance status.[4] A severely debilitated patient with a restricted performance status is more likely to sustain excessive chemotherapy toxicity. The site of metastasis outside the primary tumor can also be prognostic of patient response to symptoms related to treatment.[8] These tumor-specific prognostic factors are crucial because they can assist nurses in defining an incurable disease.

The decision to treat or not to treat is based not only on clinical indicators but also on the patient's perspective. Chemotherapy involves a commitment on the part of the patient and family to travel to the treating institution on a scheduled basis. Repeated hospitalizations, venipunctures, cannulations, investigations, and assessments over and beyond the actual administration of chemotherapy are inevitable routines of cancer treatment. These factors need to be addressed with patients and families in an effort to facilitate the decision-making process.

## Quality of Life Concerns in Palliative Chemotherapy

The assessment of QoL has increasingly become a key measure in cancer clinical trials, in conjunction with other measures such as tumor response, disease-free survival, and overall survival.[17] Some of the parameters commonly included in QoL measurement tools are factors that affect the quality of a patient's physical, psychological, social, and spiritual well-being.[4] Quality of Life should be used clinically to weigh the benefit-to-toxicity ratio of palliative chemotherapy. Aside from assessing antitumor effects and the toxicity of chemotherapy, the overall positive or negative impact of the treatment on QoL must also be addressed.[18] An ideal situation in which palliative chemotherapy might be beneficial is one in which the treatment does not alter survival duration but does positively affect QoL.[8]

Very few prospective studies have investigated the QoL benefits of supportive care versus a combination of palliative chemotherapy plus supportive care for the management of advanced, incurable malignancies. The average prolongation of survival with chemotherapy compared with best supportive care has not been fully described in literature. An increasing number of studies has reported the potential palliative benefits of chemotherapy.[19–25] Shanafelt and colleagues[25] performed a systematic analysis of 25 randomized, controlled clinical trials comparing cytotoxic chemotherapy with best supportive care. Sixteen of the clinical trials involved patients with non-small-cell lung cancer. The results indicated that there is a modest relationship between response rate and both median and 1-year survival rate for patients with non-small-cell lung cancer treated with cytotoxic chemotherapy.[25]

A meta-analysis of randomized clinical trials of best supportive care versus chemotherapy for unresectable non-small-cell lung cancer was performed to allow for better determination of the actual statistical significance of the treatment effect.[26] There was a survival benefit in the range of 6 to 10 weeks for those patients treated with palliative chemotherapy. However, this benefit was seen only in patients who had an adequate performance status. Patients with Eastern Cooperative Oncology Group (ECOG) performance status of 3 or 4 had no benefit from chemotherapy.[26] In summary, it appears that palliative chemotherapy is effective only for a select group of patients in the lung cancer population. A strong predictor of positive treatment benefit is related to the patient's performance status.[26]

In a study of patients with unresectable metastatic or locally advanced non-small-cell lung cancer, subjects were randomly assigned to receive either best supportive care or two different chemotherapy regimens ($n = 150$).[27] Survival was 8 to 15 weeks longer for the chemotherapy + supportive care arm, but improved survival was observed only in patients who had a high ECOG performance status (0 or 1) and a weight loss of less than 5 kilograms. Moreover, about 40% of subjects were judged to have sustained severe, life-threatening, or lethal toxicities.[27] Very few patients showed improvement in performance status or gained weight during chemotherapy treatment.[27] Finally, in a meta-analysis that sought to determine the benefits and harms of palliative chemotherapy in patients with locally advanced or metastatic colorectal cancer, results from the analysis of 13 randomized, controlled trials found an improvement of 16% with median survival of 3.7 months.[28] However, the investigators found that the overall quality of evidence for palliative chemotherapy in relation to treatment toxicity, symptom control, and QoL was poor.[28]

The QoL of family caregivers was addressed in a study to compare the impact of cancer caregiving in curative and palliative settings.[29] Family caregivers of patients receiving palliative care had significantly lower QoL scores and lower overall physical health scores.[29] There was no additional significant variability in caregiver QoL scores after adjustments for patient performance status and treatment status. These results suggest that patients' poor performance status is a predictor of low QoL in the palliative care setting that also affects caregivers' QoL.[29] The data reinforce the importance of supporting families as well as the impact on their QoL and on the patient's well-being when the treatment intent is palliative.

## When and How Long to Treat?

Multiple factors need to direct the decision-making process when considering palliative chemotherapy for patients with advanced cancer. The goal at this juncture in the cancer continuum is to relieve or prevent tumor-induced symptoms, with the potential of prolonging survival.[8] Patients who are symptomatic from malignancy, and those who are expected to be symptomatic soon, are typically considered for treatment initiation within a few days or weeks.[4] This indication for palliative chemotherapy, although proven to be somewhat beneficial for effective palliation in oncologic emergencies, is appropriate for only selected patients.[4] Local treatments with palliative radiation or surgery are also common treatment modalities in advanced malignancies.

A more difficult scenario of whether to delay or begin palliative chemotherapy occurs with patients who are asymptomatic from malignancy. In these circumstances, especially with tumor types that are less responsive to chemotherapy, the general consensus is that the benefit-to-toxicity ratio may be more heavily weighted toward the toxicity side.[4] In such situations, treatment may be withheld and the patient closely monitored until symptomatic progression is evident.

CASE STUDY
### Mr. S, A Patient with Pancreatic Cancer

Mr. S is a 46-year-old business man who was diagnosed with metastatic pancreatic cancer 3 months ago. At the time of diagnosis, he had widespread disease in his liver. Mr. S has been experiencing abdominal pain that is escalating. He is also losing weight and utilizes the wheelchair on a regular basis because of his decreasing energy level. His wife has been his primary caregiver. Mr. S has decided to continue treatment because of his 2-year-old daughter. He is started on single agent Gemcitabine as a palliative chemotherapy regimen in an attempt to control his pain and symptoms. After one cycle (3 weeks) of treatment, there are some improvements to his pain. However, after the second cycle, Mr. S's condition deteriorates, with dropping blood counts, increasing fatigue, and worsening of pain. At this point,

Mr. S relies completely on a wheelchair for ambulation. His pain is also not controlled by standard pain medications. Mr. S's medical oncologist refers him to a pain specialist for a nerve block to manage his pain, with very little success. Throughout this time, Mr. S insists on continuing with palliative chemotherapy treatment with dose reductions and schedule changes. He is finally referred to hospice, and passes away 1 week after referral

In this case, a focus on watchful waiting or aggressive supportive care was indicated. In general, at later stages of disease, pancreatic cancer is not very chemosensitive. Mr. S's performance status was gradually declining; therefore, he could be anticipated to experience more difficulties with treatment side effects if palliative chemotherapy was given. The chemotherapy did not have a long-term effect on Mr. S's pain. Aggressive supportive care involving experts such as pain specialists would have been beneficial for symptom management and QoL for this patient immediately following diagnosis. In such cases, the health-care team should also provide Mr. S's family with adequate information regarding the pros and cons of palliative chemotherapy at this stage of the cancer trajectory. Another important aspect of caring for Mr. S was to support his family. Because Mr. S's decision to receive palliative chemotherapy was for his children, supportive care experts who specialize in working with young families or children should have been included to aid Mr. S in treatment decision-making.

### Decision-Making: Accept, Reject, or Continue

After the initial shock of receiving a cancer diagnosis, patients and families must battle anxiety-provoking concerns such as dying from the disease, financial burdens, disease-related pain, and treatment-related toxicities. The general public often perceives chemotherapy as an extremely toxic.[30] These concerns are very much related to patient and family decision-making processes, especially when the intent to treat is to palliate symptoms. There are also concerns about whether patients are equipped with enough information to help make informed decisions. The current evidence suggests that patients with advanced, incurable cancers are not given clear information about the survival gain of palliative chemotherapy.[31] Other evidence suggests that patients perceive themselves to be well-informed, but information about prognosis and alternatives to palliative chemotherapy are still lacking.[32,33] There is also evidence that suggests that patients with advanced cancer perceive much benefit from cancer treatments in general.[34] Patients in general are willing to be treated for as little as 1 month of extra survival.[35] Slevin and associates investigated the differences between patients' attitudes to either mild or intensive cancer chemotherapy and the attitudes of health-care providers, such as physicians and nurses.[36] Cancer patients were more likely to accept intensive treatment with debilitating toxicities in exchange for an extremely small probability of cure, prolongation of life, and symptom relief.[37-44] Medical oncologists were more likely to accept aggressive treatment than were general practitioners. Oncology nurses, not surprisingly, were more divided on the aggressiveness of treatment. The nurses' perceptions fell between aggressive treatment and wanting more information on the benefit-to-toxicity ratio.[37]

Silvestri and coworkers conducted a study to determine how patients with advanced non-small-cell lung cancer valued the tradeoff between the survival benefit of chemotherapy and its toxicities.[44] Data were qualitatively collected through the use of three scripted scenarios. Patients' willingness to accept chemotherapy varied widely ($n = 81$). Many would choose chemotherapy for a likely survival benefit of 3 months only if the treatment positively affected QoL as well.[44] The investigators found that the conflict between patients' preferences and the actual care they received greatly affected their decision-making. It appears that some patients did not receive the treatment they would have chosen had they been fully informed in their previous choice of treatment.[44]

Koedoot and colleagues investigated patient treatment preferences and decision-making processes in regard to palliative chemotherapy or best supportive care.[45] The actual treatment decision was the main outcome of the study. At baseline, the majority of subjects preferred to undergo chemotherapy rather than watchful waiting.[45] The majority of subjects also eventually chose treatment with chemotherapy. Treatment preference and a deferring style of decision-making were predictors of actual treatment choice. Treatment preference is positively explained by striving for length of life and negatively explained by striving for QoL.[45] The results indicated that it is still questionable whether the purpose of palliative chemotherapy is made clear to patients.[46] This emphasizes the need for health-care providers to attach further attention to the process of information-giving and shared decision-making in patients with advanced cancer.[45]

### The Role of Nurses in Palliative Chemotherapy

Through randomized clinical trials and meta-analyses, the incorporation of chemotherapy into the palliative care setting has been shown to have survival benefits for patients with advanced cancer whose disease is incurable. However, these benefits are seen only in patients with higher baseline performance status and in those who are asymptomatic from their metastatic malignancies. Hence, it is evident that palliative chemotherapy, although effective in palliating certain disease-related symptoms, has limited benefits for all advanced cancer patients. Therefore, it is important for nurses, as integral team members in the transdisciplinary approach of oncology palliative care, to support patients and families through the difficult path of answering the quintessential question: to treat or not to treat? Nurses can help alleviate further anguish and suffering for patients with advanced cancer and their families in three crucial areas related to palliative chemotherapy: change in treatment intent, decision-making, and supportive care through treatment choice.

## Change in Treatment Intent

When curative intent of treatment becomes impossible, practitioners should begin to address the intent to treat as palliation of disease-related symptoms. This initial communication is traditionally the domain of the treating physician. However, with more and more collaborative practices emerging among nurses, advanced practice nurses (APNs), and physicians, it is becoming apparent that a transdisciplinary approach offers the best support for patients and families during this difficult and vulnerable time.[1] Communication of difficult news should best be conducted in a prearranged consultation session in which the treating physician, nurse, and social worker together deliver the information to the patient, the family, and other individuals who are integral to the decision-making process. Nurses can foster this transdisciplinary approach of delivering difficult news through collaboration and communication with experts across disciplines. Nurses are often the first to recognize the need for dialogue between the health-care team and the patient/family regarding treatment intent and prognosis.[47] Therefore, nurses can advocate for patients by recommending and organizing these important communication sessions to alleviate unnecessary suffering for patients and families.

CASE STUDY
### Mrs. J, A Patient with Metastatic Rectal Cancer

Mrs. J, a 56-year-old Hispanic female who emigrated from Mexico to the United States 20 years ago, has metastatic rectal cancer to the peritoneum. She has been treated with chemoradiation, followed by more palliative chemotherapy. She wants to be aggressive with treatment despite her poor prognosis. Functionally, Mrs. J has been doing well, and her symptoms, such as pain, are well-controlled. Mrs. J maintains maintains a positive outlook on life for the sake of her family and wants to remain functional as long as possible. During a routine computed tomographic scan to assess disease status, it is revealed that she has progressive disease despite the palliative chemotherapy. Mrs. J speaks some English and is accompanied by her husband, who speaks no English, and her daughter, who speaks fluent English, to talk with the health-care team about the treatment options.

In this case, a consultation session is warranted. The objective of the session is threefold: (1) to present the difficult news of further disease progression and failure of treatment; (2) to re-evaluate treatment intent; and (3) to make recommendations for treatment. An interpreter should be onhand during the session to ensure that the patient and the family understand the situation. Before divulging the difficult news, it is important to assess for cultural needs in terms of communicating bad news. The health-care team should understand how much information patients want to know and how much they already know. This assessment guides the consultation session. If supportive care experts such as a psychologist or chaplain are not available to be present during the session, then it is vital that they be accessible to intervene during this very difficult and sensitive time of the cancer trajectory.

## Decision-Making

Once the change in treatment intent has been discussed, the next step is to guide patients and families through an informed decision-making process to either continue on aggressive treatment or focus on symptom relief. Again, this information should be delivered in a setting where all practitioners involved in the care of the patient and family are present. If this scenario is not possible, it is imperative for members of the health-care team to communicate and follow-up with each other regarding details of the information disclosed to the patient and family. In presenting this information, it is important to avoid the use of medical jargon and to use resources such as information leaflets and diagrams to assist the patient and family in informed decision-making.[8] Nurses, having expertise in educating patients and families, can facilitate the availability of these visual resources and present them to patients and families.

Some patients might find it helpful to meet other similar patients or to access supportive care services such as psychology or chaplaincy. Nurses can encourage and facilitate these desires by initiating referrals to these services. A compassionate and ethical approach to review the medical situation with the patient and family is essential to providing them with an informed assessment of possible treatment choices.[4] It is important to include in the treatment choices the use of hospice services and nonchemotherapy palliative care, depending on the patient's individual situation. Another important aspect to consider is the awareness of specific cultural needs and differences. Patient and family desires for open communication and participation in decision-making are greatly influenced by both ethnicity and religion, so it is important to assess these needs and ensure cultural sensitivity before presenting the information.[4]

When discussing the possibility of palliative chemotherapy as a treatment choice, it is essential, before presenting statistical evidence, to learn about other specific factors that may affect the decision-making process. Nurses can facilitate and perform the assessment to obtain this vital information. Questions should focus on the following factors: (1) questions and decisions that need to be addressed in the patient's or family's lives; (2) a special upcoming event or specific unfinished business that must be completed; and (3) fears about dying or spiritual issues that need interventions from other supportive care services.[4] Nurses can play a particularly important role in facilitating information-gathering on the third factor: fear of dying and spiritual needs. Fear of dying and spirituality represent a much-ignored area in the general medical literature but have been shown to have significant impact on the QoL of cancer patients, especially when disease is incurable.[48] Nurses can facilitate the patient's and family's search for spiritual understanding of their situation and alleviate existential suffering by first acknowledging patient's fears and distress. Facilitation of open communication regarding existential suffering can help alleviate fears of dying.[48] Nurses must be compassionate listeners and allow patients and families a forum to discuss their deepest fears concerning the seemingly impending and inevitable terminality of their disease.

### Supportive Care through Treatment Choice

If palliative chemotherapy is the treatment choice, support for patients and families through treatment becomes the most important objective for nurses. Education regarding the common and expected side effects of the specific chemotherapy regimens can foster a sense of control over symptom management and prevent unnecessary anxiety-provoking episodes related to poorly managed side effects. The use of written materials that list and explain common side effects can be helpful in facilitating the learning process for patients and families. Most importantly, nurses can assist in the continuous assessment of patient and family needs, focusing not only on the physical but also on the psychological, social, and spiritual domains.[49] Communication during this difficult and vulnerable phase of the disease trajectory is key to the success of quality cancer care. Nurses can serve as a bridge of communication by fostering continued dialogue on the goals of treatment between patients/families and the health-care team. This bridge of communication, although often difficult to sustain, is essential in a truly transdisciplinary model of care. Open and clear communication among health-care team members can guide the assessment of patient and family needs but can also alleviate suffering by maintaining consistency in the amount and types of information provided. Inconsistencies in vital communication factors in palliative chemotherapy, such as treatment intent, often create false hopes and distress for patients and families.[4]

If palliative chemotherapy is not the chosen plan of treatment, patients and families frequently experience a profound sense of abandonment.[4] This sense of abandonment is most often directed toward health-care providers. Patients and families, after living through the initial treatment phase of the cancer trajectory wherein follow-up with physicians and nurses is routine, suddenly lose the security of being assessed on a regular basis. Nurses can assist in alleviating this sense of abandonment through reassurance that follow-up care will remain in place. If referral to hospice is warranted, then nurses can act as a liaison to attending physicians and hospice services to foster a smooth transition between care settings and to maintain continuity of care.

## Clinical Trials and Advanced Cancer

Several reports published or commissioned by government advisory boards such as the National Cancer Policy Board and the Institute of Medicine noted that the quality of end-of-life care in the United States is seriously deficient.[6] Many oncology professional organizations assert that hospice is the best-developed model of end-of-life care in the U.S. healthcare delivery system.[6] Hospice offers quality palliative care using a transdisciplinary approach. With the rising interest in palliative care for terminally ill patients, there has also been a dramatic increase in interest regarding palliative care specifically for advanced cancer patients.

Patients with advanced cancer are often offered the opportunity to enroll in a phase I clinical trial. Although research on new therapeutic agents is crucial to the oncology specialty, it is not uncommon that patients who enroll in phase I trials are forced to forgo the use of services such as hospice and palliative care. This dichotomy is primarily a result of U.S. federal policy. Medicare and insurance policies deny hospice coverage to patients with terminal cancer who enroll as participants in phase I studies. However, it is precisely this population of cancer patients who would benefit from comprehensive palliative care. It is important to note that phase I studies are designed to determine the toxicity and maximum tolerated dose of potential treatments, mostly for currently incurable cancers. These studies are not designed, and do not have the intended purpose, to have a therapeutic effect. In fact, studies have shown that therapeutic effects from cancer investigational therapeutic agents occur in only 2% to 4% of subjects enrolled in a phase I clinical trial.[50,51] It is also ironic that the entry criteria for phase I trials is similar to the disease state criteria for admission into hospice—but it is precisely this dichotomy that renders a patient ineligible for the quality palliative care services that hospice provides.[6]

Patients who enter investigational cancer trials participate, in part, because of protocol eligibility such as disease and functional criteria. Many advanced-stage cancer patients who make decisions to participate in cancer clinical trials are also characterized by a highly motivated personality.[52] They feel that active treatment is best for them.[53] Other factors identified with enrollment may include altruism and the influence of the physician.[54] Patient expectations include a response to therapy, a reduction in symptoms, and improved and increased communication with their physicians.[55-57] Preliminary findings also have suggested that patients who choose to enroll in experimental trials are slightly more spiritual than other patients with advanced cancer who choose not to participate.[58] Therapeutic efforts are often equated with superior QoL and are measured against no other options. By contrast, patients and families believe palliative care is a passive choice, the equivalent of "no care."

When faced with decision-making regarding their plan of care, the current evidence suggests that there is controversy about whether patients with advanced incurable cancers fully understand the choices that are available to them. Studies have found that patients are aware of other alternatives at the end of life, but their overwhelming need to fight their cancer at any cost prevents them from seriously considering the other alternatives.[59,60] Patients who would qualify for hospice services as regulated by Medicare have very little understanding of admission criteria and services rendered.[61] It is unlikely that patients who are potential study participants understand fully that to enroll in a clinical trial means that they must temporarily forgo the opportunity of receiving comprehensive palliative care.[6] Furthermore, there are no informed consent documents that disclose the risk of losing hospice benefits when enrolled in a clinical trial. Within the informed consent documents for cancer investigational therapeutic agents, there are no descriptions in the benefits and risks section that address the risk of temporarily losing hospice eligibility.[62] This loss of eligibility is not permanent; rather, patients and families can enroll and disenroll from hospice benefits whenever they choose.

## Tensions Between Palliative Care and Clinical Research

Despite significant progress in research and treatments, the diagnosis of cancer creates fear and turmoil in the lives of every cancer patient and the family. Cancer disrupts all components of social integration—family, work, finances, and friendships—as well as the patient's psychological status. Over the extended course of the illness, physical changes and deterioration create multiple and complex demands on the patient and family. These demands, in conjunction with significant financial assaults, generate a negative synergy, which is often ignored in the care of patients with advanced disease.

Patients with advanced, incurable cancers are especially vulnerable and therefore have many unique needs in coping with their disease.[63] Hence, it is helpful to tailor treatment to the specific needs of each individual and family to fulfill personal goals and maintain QoL. This is precisely what a comprehensive palliative care program can provide. At the same time, many patients faced with the terminality of their disease want and seek new innovative therapies. In the absence of further evidence-based and effective standard therapy, clinical trials offer a sense of hope for a potential cure.[63] But for patients who choose to participate in a clinical trial, there are often no guarantees of benefit, and there is the added possibility of harm and discomfort in the form of physical and psychological distress.

The impact of clinical trial participation on physical symptoms related to advanced cancer is complex, and there is a paucity of data regarding the extent of these symptoms.[63] Similarly to standard treatment agents, experimental agentscause side effects. The difference in the side effect profile of a well-established agent versus an experimental agent

lies in the anticipation of symptoms. Well-established agents have well-documented side effect profiles that can be anticipated and predicted and therefore better controlled or even prevented in certain situations. The novelty of experimental agents, however, renders their side effects unpredictable. There is a tremendous amount of uncertainty about what effects an experimental agent might have on a particular patient.

Palliative care stands in contrast to disease-directed therapy at most cancer centers in the United States. The rift between them creates a dissonance for development of clinical research protocols and for recruitment of some groups of patients into cancer clinical trials. Only one-third of all cancer patients receive formal palliative care through hospice, and often this occurs only in the final days of life.[64] Although advanced cancer should be a time of refocusing and resolution, the hospice referral process often occurs during crisis situations. As disease advances, a positive relationship exists between increased physiological symptom severity and the patient's level of emotional distress and overall QoL. An inability to complete end-of-life tasks may lead to patient dissatisfaction as well as complicated family/caregiver stress and grief after the death.[64–66]

## Quality of Life Concerns for Clinical Trial Participants

Although the structure and requirement of a clinical trial protocol mandates the inclusion of a plan of action for unexpected physical symptoms, these plans often are focused on pharmacological interventions only. For example, if nausea and vomiting is an anticipated or expected side effect, a protocol of which antiemetic agents to use is written into the clinical trial protocol itself. However, the psychological and social distress from this side effect is not included in the plan. A clinical trial protocol generally does not include plans that specifically state the need for referrals to other allied health professionals, such as palliative care specialists and psychologists.[6]

The psychological and cognitive symptoms of patients participating in research studies vary.[63] Some patients may be distressed to be told that they are not eligible for inclusion into clinical trials. Research subjects may also have difficulty when an experimental treatment fails, which often mandates the withdrawal of subjects from the treatment protocol. One potential advantage of enrollment in clinical trials is that several members of the research team care for these patients. There are regularly scheduled visits, and that attention may affect the patient's psychological well-being. This added attention might lead to early detection of psychological symptoms that are indicative of depression, sadness, anxiety, or irritability.[63] Subtle changes in psychological effects might be readily detected by research personnel, and nurses are an integral part of this team. However, for this added attention to be beneficial to patients and families, it is important for research teams to work collaboratively with allied health professionals and palliative care specialists to address concerns in all areas of patient and family well-being.

Economic demands and caregiving needs may also be affected by clinical trial participation. Financial burdens may be increased for clinical trial participants even if the experimental agents are provided free of charge. The usual intensive monitoring and testing that can sharply increase with participation in clinical trials may not be covered by either the trial budget itself or the patient's insurance. The frequent visits for treatment, physician assessment, and various other procedures that are often mandated in clinical trial protocols may incur further economic burdens in terms of expenses for travel and room and board.[63]

The needs of caregivers and families may also change with clinical trial participation. Families experience tremendous physical, psychological, social, and spiritual concerns that are related to the patient's well-being. Physical symptoms such as fatigue can plague caregivers and families who are faced with the complex care of patients with advanced cancer.[30] The complexity of navigating through the health-care and insurance systems can place tremendous burdens on both patients and caregivers. Social exposure may be diminished for caregivers, because much of their days are spent caring for their loved ones.[30] Finally, the agony of being a witness to a loved one's suffering and the prospect of grief and bereavement in terminal illness may present caregivers with spiritual and existential distress.

Attending to the spiritual and existential needs of patients with advanced cancer is an important factor in the overall experience of patients and families facing the inevitability of terminal illness. It is often at this point in the cancer trajectory that patients experience the needs of altruism.[63] Patients and families who recognize the diminishing hope of survival may find comfort and solace in the possibility of contributing to the advancement of science through participation in clinical trials.[63] Others may choose to focus on using precious time to concentrate on more personal goals, such as unfinished business and QoL.

CASE STUDY
*Mrs. W, A Patient with Metastatic Colon Cancer*

Mrs. W is a 52-year-old African-American female with metastatic colorectal cancer to the liver. She lives with her husband and primary caregiver, Mr. W, and they have been married only for 6 months. Palliative chemotherapy was able to control disease progression and symptoms for 3 months, but the effect was not long-term. Following first-line palliative chemotherapy, Mrs. W was also treated with second- and third-line regimens, but efficacy for all was short-term. Mrs. W is worried about Mr. W, and she feels guilty about getting sick so early in their marriage. A decision is made to enroll in a clinical trial after failure of the third-line chemotherapy. Unfortunately, her disease

continues to worsen 2 months after initiation of the clinical trial treatment. Lately, Mr. W has become increasingly tearful when accompanying Mrs. W during her clinic visits.

In this case, it is clear that the caregiver is suffering tremendously. After surviving through several bouts of chemotherapy without much effect on the tumor, the impact of repeated discouragement weighs heavily on the patient's and caregiver's hearts. Mr. W has probably witnessed and supported Mrs. W through the agonies of treatment and continued progression of disease. One can anticipate that they will experience tremendous difficulties with regard to grief and bereavement. It is important, therefore, to recommend or establish support for the family. In this case, referral to supportive care experts might be warranted. The family should be provided with information on other types of support, such as support groups. It might be helpful to connect them with other caregivers, and to exchange experiences on caring for a terminally ill loved one.

## Perspectives Toward Clinical Trials

### Patient versus Nurses

The conduct of clinical trials involving human subjects raises ethical concerns for health-care professionals. In the process of decision-making in a clinical trial setting for patients with advanced cancer, the impact of nurses presents an additional element.[67] Nurses are involved in clinical trials both as clinical investigators and as caregivers for patients and families undergoing experimental treatments. In the clinical setting, nurses facilitate practitioner–patient communication and also serve as advocates.[67] Nurses often spend a considerable amount of time with patients and their families, and they are acutely aware of attitudes, needs, and concerns regarding participation.

Burnett and coworkers conducted a study to identify nurses' attitudes and beliefs toward cancer clinical trials and their perceptions of the factors influencing patients' participation.[67] A 59-item questionnaire was administered to nurses working in NCI-designated comprehensive cancer centers. Of the 417 nurses who responded, 96% reported that participation is important to improving standards of care, but only 56% believed that patients should be encouraged to participate in these clinical trials.[67] As a group, research nurses were more likely to have favorable views toward clinical trials and also about patient understanding regarding treatment plans and goals. On the other hand, nurses working in intensive care units and bone marrow transplant settings had more concerns regarding patient understanding and patient–physician communication. Ninety-two percent of nurses reported that patients entered a clinical trial with the belief that it would cure their cancer.[67] Sixty-eight percent of nurses reported the belief that patients participate in clinical trials because they hope to receive better medical care. Nurses also indicated their perception that nurses, as professionals, are more likely to respect patients' wishes and less likely to apply pressure on patients regarding clinical trial participation.[67] These results indicate the concerns that nurses working in oncology settings have toward the informed consent process of clinical trial participation and strongly suggest the need to develop nursing interventions to better support this process.

Aaronson and associates conducted a study to test the efficacy of a telephone-based nursing intervention on improving the effectiveness of the informed consent process in cancer clinical trials.[68] This randomized study compared the effectiveness of this nursing intervention in patients who were randomly assigned to either a standard informed consent procedure based on verbal explanation and written information or the standard informed consent process plus the supplementary telephone intervention (intervention group). Results showed that the intervention group was significantly better informed about the following: (1) the risks and side effects of treatment; (2) the clinical trial context of the treatment; (3) the objectives of the clinical trial; (4) the use of randomization in allocating treatment (if relevant); (5) the availability of alternative treatments; (6) the voluntary nature of the participation; and (7) the right to withdraw from the clinical trial. The intervention did not have any significant effect on patients' anxiety levels or on the rate of clinical trial accrual.[68]

Cox conducted a qualitative study to identify the psychosocial impact of participation in clinical trials, as experienced by the patients themselves.[69] The study sought to interpret patients' ways of coping with their individual situations and also to identify the consequences of trial involvement. Of the 55 patients involved in the study, the offer of a trial treatment was seen as a turning point for patients. Thirty patients (54%) described the offer of participation as being "the light at the end of a tunnel" because they perceived that hope was offered.[69] On the other hand, 58% of subjects described how the trial generated uncertainty, whereas 54% felt special, privileged, pleased, lucky, and honored to have been offered participation.[69] The majority of patients interpreted the offer of trial participation as being the right plan of action because their physicians offered it. Reasons for patients to accept trial participation included the desire to be in expert hands (54%) and the desire to help others (52%).[69]

As clinical trial initiation began and patients progressed through treatment, an overwhelming sense of being burdened by trial involvement was noted in all cases. These burdens focused on side effects and additional demands, such as blood tests and scans.[69] It was evident that these trial burdens were not fully anticipated by patients at the beginning of trial involvement. Nevertheless, most of the patients desired to persevere through treatment rather than withdraw.

At the conclusion of participation, patients expressed disappointment that the trial drug was not successful. An overwhelming sense of abandonment was a feature in all patients. Subjects were also eager to receive feedback on the trial in which they had participated.[69] Trial withdrawal resulting from disease progression or toxicity was a common feature for subjects in this study. Trial withdrawal and conclusion was a deeply distressing and stressful time for all patients. In addition to having to confront the realities of having a terminal illness and the lack of response to their last hope for "cure," patients also experienced a dramatic decrease in contact from health-care providers, which inevitably led to an overwhelming sense of abandonment.[69] These findings suggest that patients and families need support during and beyond the trial to deal with the major disruption that clinical trial participation might have on the overall dying trajectory. The investigators suggested that one way to overcome these issues is to consider early clinical trials in the context of a continuing palliative care program, in which the duty of care extends beyond trial involvement and in which death and dying concerns can be addressed.[69]

## The Role of Nurses in Caring for Clinical Trial Patients

Clinical trials of new investigational cancer therapeutics are a necessary component to the process of translating scientific discoveries into standard practice of care.[70] Oncology nurses have many different roles in the conduct of cancer clinical trials. First and foremost, the process of obtaining true informed consent is a critical factor, not only in improving patient accrual into clinical trials but also in the overall well-being of patients and their families. The informed consent process is an opportunity to provide accurate information regarding important factors that affect the patient's and family's decision-making process in advanced cancer. These factors include trial procedures and potential risks and benefits.[71] The initial informed consent process is also a time to correct any misconceptions and allay unfounded fears and to provide sufficient time for patients and families to thoughtfully consider clinical trial participation.[70] A predecisional support process provided by oncology nurses may influence the soundness of patients' decisions to enroll in clinical trials.[70] Nursing interventions that would assist in well-considered decisions include helping patients gather additional relevant sources of information, describing patients' roles and rights in studies, encouraging patients to define their own reasons for participating in clinical trials, and supporting patients in making decisions that correspond with their personal values and wishes.[72]

Nurses can also assist in educating not only clinical trial patients but also the extended community. Interventions aimed at increasing community awareness can foster better understanding of clinical trials and their importance in the advancement of treatment options and strategies for oncology patients.[70] The formation of clinical trial support groups for patients and families considering enrollment in research is another strategy that may provide necessary education and social support.[70] Strategies such as follow-up phone calls or E-mail messages while patients are considering clinical trial participation can have a positive effect on the decision-making process.[70]

Nurses are in an ideal position to promote awareness of the importance of clinical trials and subsequent improvements in patient care. The three key roles of nurses caring for clinical trial patients and their families are educator, patient advocate, and study coordinator.[73] As patient and family educators, nurses can have a tremendous impact on a patient's experience with clinical trial participation. Nurses are clinical interpreters who provide patients and families with explanations of highly complex and intricate protocols without using medical jargon.[73] Education about the specific protocol process, expectations at each stage, management of side effects, and the importance of communicating changes in health status to practitioners is integral to the oncology research setting.

As patient advocates, nurses play an important role in the critical gateway to clinical trial participation—the informed consent process.[73] Nurses bring to this role a patient-centered, holistic method of support. The nursing perspective is important in that it provides a framework within which patients and families are treated with dignity and respect. Clarification of reasons behind decisions to participate—whether physical, psychological, social, or spiritual—should be encouraged.

Advanced practice nurses such as clinical nurse specialists and nurse practitioners, can be an important factor in the conduct of clinical trials. Expertise in symptom management and clinical problem-solving is a key asset for APNs in the research setting. For example, nurse practitioners working in a clinical trial setting have an expanded scope of practice that allows them to perform routine follow-up physical examinations as well as diagnose and manage treatment complications.[26] This level of participation in patient and family care may enhance patient satisfaction, compliance, and retention.

### Summary

Of all the topics to which oncology health-care providers, palliative care specialists, and ethicists have devoted their attention, few raise as much heated debate as the dichotomy between active treatment and palliative care. The use of palliative chemotherapy and clinical trial participation as a treatment option for patients with advanced cancer has been at the heart of this debate for decades. There is a growing movement in the United States to integrate palliative care into clinical trials. However, there is still much work to be done. Frustration lies in the assumption that subjects who are actively treated for symptom palliation, whether through palliative chemotherapy or experimental agents, must forgo

a coordinated plan of care that involves quality palliative care.[74] It has become increasingly evident that this dichotomy should not exist—that is, patients and families can simultaneously receive therapy for palliation of symptoms and have access to quality palliative care. It is also increasingly evident that this quality care can be provided only through a transdisciplinary model of care. Nurses can help alleviate the tension between palliative care and disease-directed therapies through education, advocacy, and coordination of care. It is only by removing this dichotomy that patients with advanced cancer and their families can be provided with the highest quality of information to facilitate their decision-making process.

### REFERENCES

1. Joshi TG, Ehrenberger HE. Cancer clinical trials in the new millennium: Novel challenges and opportunities for oncology nursing. Clin J Oncol Nurs 2001;5:147–152.
2. Casarett DJ, Karlawish J, Henry MI, Hirschman KB. Must patients with advanced cancer choose between a phase I trial and hospice? Cancer 2002;95:1601–1604.
3. Ellison NM, Chevlen EM. Palliative chemotherapy. In: Berger AM, Portenoy RK, Weissman DE, eds. Principles and Practices of Palliative Care and Supportive Oncology. Philadelphia PA: Lippincott Williams & Wilkins; 2002:698–709.
4. Peppercorn JM, Weeks JC, Cook EF, Joffe S. Comparison of outcomes in cancer patients treated within and outside clinical trials: Conceptual framework and structured review. Lancet 2004;363:263–270.
5. Byock I, Miles SH. Hospice benefits and phase I cancer trials. Ann Intern Med 2003;138:335–337.
6. Osoba D. Lessons learned from measuring health-related quality of life in oncology. J Clin Oncol 1994;12:608–616.
7. McIllmurray M. Palliative medicine and the treatment of cancer. In: Doyle D, Hanks G, Cherny N, Calman K, eds. Oxford Textbook of Palliative Medicine. Oxford, England: Oxford University Press; 2004:229–239.
8. Earle CC, Park ER, Lai B, Weeks JC, Ayanian JZ, Block S. Identifying potential indicators of the quality of end-of-life cancer care from administrative data. J Clin Oncol 2003; 21(6):1133–1138.
9. Earle CC, Neville BA, Landrum MB, Ayanian JZ, Block SD, Weeks JC. Trends in the aggressiveness of cancer care near the end of life. J Clin Oncol 2004;22(2):315–321.
10. Earle CC, Landrum MB, Souza JM, Neville BA, Weeks JC, Ayanian JZ. Aggressiveness of cancer care near the end of life: Is it a quality-of-care issue? J Clin Oncol 2008;26(23):3860–3866.
11. Rose JH, O'Toole EE, Dawson NV, et al. Perspectives, preferences, care practices, and outcomes among older and middle-aged patients with late-stage cancer. J Clin Oncol 2004;22(24):4907–4917.
12. Temel JS, McCannon J, Greer JA, et al. Aggressiveness of care in a prospective cohort of patients with advanced NSCLC. Cancer 2008;113(4):826–833.
13. von Gruenigen V, Daly B, Gibbons H, Hutchins J, Green A. Indicators of survival duration in ovarian cancer and implications for aggressiveness of care. Cancer 2008;112(10):2221–2227.

14. Braga S, Miranda A, Fonseca R, et al. The aggressiveness of cancer care in the last three months of life: A retrospective single centre analysis. Psychooncology 2007;16(9):863–868.

15. Emanuel EJ, Young-Xu Y, Levinsky NG, Gazelle G, Saynina O, Ash AS. Chemotherapy use among Medicare beneficiaries at the end of life. Ann Intern Med 2003;138(8):639–643.

16. Sloan JA, Cella D, Frost MH, Guyatt G, Osoba D. Clinical Significance Consensus Meeting Group. Quality of life III: Translating the science of quality-of-life assessment into clinical practice—an example-driven approach for practicing clinicians and clinical researchers. Clin Ther 2003;25(Suppl):D1–D5.

17. Osoba D, Slamon DJ, Burchmore M, Murphy M. Effects on quality of life of combined trastuzumab and chemotherapy in women with metastatic breast cancer. J Clin Oncol 2002; 20:3106–3113.

18. Cullen MH, Billingham LJ, Woodroffe CM, et al. Mitromycin, ifosfamide, and cisplatin in unresectable non-small-cell lung cancer: Effects on survival and quality of life. J Clin Oncol 1999;17:3188–3194.

19. Glimelius B, Ekstrom K, Hoffman K, et al. Randomized comparison between chemotherapy plus best supportive care with best supportive care in advanced gastric cancer. Ann Oncol 1995;71:587–591.

20. Simmonds PC. Palliative chemotherapy for advanced colorectal cancer: Systematic review and meta-analysis. Colorectal Cancer Collaborative Group. BMJ 2000;321:531–535.

21. Doyle C, Crump M, Pintilie M, Oza AM. Does palliative chemotherapy palliate? Evaluation of expectations, outcomes, and costs in women receiving chemotherapy for advanced ovarian cancer. J Clin Oncol 2001;19:1266–1274.

22. Ellis PA, Smith IE, Hardy JR, Nicolson MC, Talbot DC, Ashley SE, Priest K. Symptom relief from MVP (mitomycin C, vinblastine and cisplatin) chemotherapy in advanced non-small-cell lung cancer. Br J Cancer 1995;71:366–370.

23. Burris HA 3rd, Moore MJ, Andersen J, et al. Improvements in survival and clinical benefit with gemcitabine as first-line therapy for patients with advanced pancreas cancer: A randomized trial. J Clin Oncol 1997;15:2403–2413.

24. Cunningham D, Pyrhonen S, James RD, et al. Randomized trial of irinotecan plus supportive care versus supportive care alone after fluorouracil failure for patients with metastatic colorectal cancer. Lancet 1998;352:1413–1418.

25. Shanafelt TD, Loprinzi C, Marks R, Novotny P, Sloan J. Are chemotherapy response rates related to treatment-induced survival prolongations in patients with advanced cancer? J Clin Oncol 2004;22:1966–1974.

26. Rapp E, Pater JL, Willan A, Cormier Y, Murray N, Evans WK. Chemotherapy can prolong survival in patients with advanced non small cell lung cancer: Report of a Canadian multicenter randomized trial. J Clin Oncol 1988;6:633–643.

27. Souquet PJ, Chauvin F, Boisel JP, et al. Polychemotherapy in advanced non-small-cell lung cancer A metaanalysis. Lancet 1993;342:19–30.

28. NSCLC Meta Analysis Collaborative Group. Chemotherapy in addition to supportive care improves survival in advanced non-small-cell lung cancer: A systematic review of meta-analysis of individual patient data from 16 randomized controlled trials. J Clin Oncol 2008;26:4617–4625.

29. Weitzner MA, McMillan SC, Jacobsen PB. Family caregiver quality of life: Differences between curative and palliative cancer treatment settings. J Pain Symptom Manage 1999;17:418–428.

30. Comis RL, Miller JD, Aldige CR, Krebs L, Stoval E. Public attitudes toward participation in cancer clinical trials. J Clin Oncol 2003;21:830–835.

31. Audrey S, Abel J, Blazeby JM, Falk S, Campbell R. What oncologists tell patients about survival benefits of palliative chemotherapy and implications for informed consent: Qualitative study. BMJ (Clinical research ed) 2008;337:a752.

32. Gattellari M, Voigt KJ, Butow PN, Tattersall MH. When the treatment goal is not cure: Are cancer patients equipped to make informed decisions? J Clin Oncol 2002;20(2):503–513.

33. Tattersall MH, Gattellari M, Voigt K, Butow PN. When the treatment goal is not cure: Are patients informed adequately? Support Care Cancer 2002;10(4):314–321.

34. Stiggelbout AM, de Haes JC. Patient preference for cancer therapy: An overview of measurement approaches. J Clin Oncol 2001;19(1):220–230.

35. de Haes H, Koedoot N. Patient centered decision making in palliative cancer treatment: A world of paradoxes. Patient Educ Couns 2003;50(1):43–49.

36. Slevin ML, Stubbs L, Plant HJ, Wlson P, Gregory WM, Armes PJ, Downer SM. Attitudes towards chemotherapy: Comparing view of patients with those of doctors, nurses, and general public. BMJ 1990;300:1458–1467.

37. Balmer CE, Thomas P, Osborne RJ. Who wants second-line, palliative chemotherapy? Psychooncology 2001;10(5):410–418.

38. Browner I, Carducci MA. Palliative chemotherapy: Historical perspective, applications, and controversies. Semin Oncol 2005;32(2):145–155.

39. Grunfeld EA, Maher EJ, Browne S, et al. Advanced breast cancer patients' perceptions of decision making for palliative chemotherapy. J Clin Oncol 2006;24(7):1090–1098.

40. Harrington SE, Smith TJ. The role of chemotherapy at the end of life: "When is enough, enough?" JAMA 2008;299(22):2667–2678.

41. Maltoni M, Amadori D. Palliative medicine and medical oncology. Ann Oncol 2001;12(4):443–450.

42. Markman M. Does palliative chemotherapy palliate? Support Oncol 2003;1(1):65–67.

43. Matsuyama R, Reddy S, Smith TJ. Why do patients choose chemotherapy near the end of life? A review of the perspective of those facing death from cancer. J Clin Oncol 2006;24(21):3490–3496.

44. Silvestri G, Pritchard R, Welch HG. Preferences for chemotherapy in patients with advanced non-small cell lung cancer: Descriptive study based on scripted interviews. BMJ 1998;317:771–775.

45. Koedoot CG, de Haan RJ, Stiggelbout AM, Stalmeier PF, de Graeff A, Bakker PJ, de Haes JC. Palliative chemotherapy or best supportive care? A prospective study explaining patients' treatment preference and choice. Br J Cancer 2003;89:19–26.

46. Koedoot CG, Oort FJ, de Haan RJ, Bakker PJ, de Graeff A, de Haes JC. The content and amount of information given by medical oncologists when telling patients with advanced cancer what their treatment options are: Palliative chemotherapy and watchful-waiting. Eur J Cancer 2004;40(2):225–235.

47. Aiken JL. Nursing roles in clinical trials. In: Klimaszewski D, Aiken JL, Bacon MA, DiStasio SA, Ehrenberger HE, Ford BA, eds. Manual for Clinical Trial Nursing. Pittsburgh, PA: Oncology Nursing Press; 2001:273–276.

48. Karigan M. Psychosocial considerations. In: Klimaszewski D, Aiken JL, Bacon MA, DiStasio SA, Ehrenberger HE, Ford BA, eds. Manual for Clinical Trial Nursing. Pittsburgh, PA: Oncology Nursing Press; 2001:173–176.

49. Decoster G, Stein G, Holdner E. Responses and toxic deaths in phase I clinical trials. Ann Clin Oncol 1990;1:175–181.

50. Estey E, Hoth D, Simon R, Marsoni S, Leyland-Jones B, Wittes R. Therapeutic response in phase I trials of antineoplastic agents. Cancer Treat Rep 1986;70:1105–1115.

51. Schutta KM, Burnett CB. Factors that influence a patient's decision to participate in a phase I cancer clinical trial. Oncol Nurs Forum 2000;27(9):1435–1438.

52. Daugherty CK. Impact of therapeutic research on informed consent and the ethics of clinical trials: A medical oncology perspective. J Clin Oncol 1999;17:1601–1617.

53. Daugherty C, Ratain MJ, Grochowski E, Stocking C, Kodish E, Mick R, Siegler M. Perceptions of cancer patients and their physicians involved in phase I trials. J Clin Oncol 1995;13:1062–1072.

54. Jenkins V, Fallowfield L. Reasons for accepting or declining to participate in randomized clinical trials for cancer therapy. Br J Cancer 2000;82:1783–1788.

55. Yoder LH, O'Rourke TJ, Etnye A, Spears DT, Brown TD. Expectations and experiences of patients with cancer participating in phase I clinical trials. Oncol Nurs Forum 1997;24:891–896.

56. Wendler D, Krohmal B, Emanuel EJ, Grady C. Why patients continue to participate in clinical research. Arch Intern Med 2008;168(12):1294–1299.

57. Daugherty CK, Fitchett G, Murphy PE, et al. Trusting God and medicine: Spirituality in advanced cancer patients volunteering for clinical trials of experimental agents. Psychooncology 2005;14(2):135–146.

58. Agrawal M, Emanuel EJ. Ethics of phase 1 oncology studies: Reexamining the arguments and data. JAMA 2003; 290(8):1075–1082.

59. Agrawal M, Grady C, Fairclough DL, Meropol NJ, Maynard K, Emanuel EJ. Patients' decision-making process regarding participation in phase I oncology research. J Clin Oncol 2006;24(27):4479–4484.

60. Oliverio R, Fraulo B. SUPPORT revisited: The nurse clinician's perspective. Study to understand prognoses and preferences for outcomes and risks of treatment. Holistic Nurs Pract 1998;13:1–7.

61. Horng S, Emanuel EJ, Wilfond B, Rackoff J, Martz K, Grady C. Descriptions of benefits and risks in consent forms for phase I oncology trials. N Engl J Med 2002;347:2134–2140.

62. Agrawal M, Danis M. End-of-life care for terminally ill participants in clinical research. J Palliat Med 2002;5:729–737.

63. Ferrell BR, Grant MM, Rhiner M, Padilla GV. Home care: Maintaining quality of life for patient and family. Oncology 1992;6(2 Suppl):136–140.

64. BrintzenhofeSzoc KM, Smith ED, Zabora JR. Screening to predict complicated grief in spouses of cancer patients. Cancer Pract 1999;7:233–239.

65. Schulz R, Beach SR. Caregiving as a risk factor for mortality: The Caregiver Health Effects Study. JAMA 1999;282: 2215–2219.

66. Burnett CB, Koczwara B, Pixley L, Blumenson LE, Hwang YT, Meropol NJ. Nurses' attitudes toward clinical trials at a comprehensive cancer center. Oncol Nurs Forum 2002; 28:1187–1192.

67. Aaronson NK, Visser-Pol E, Leenhouts G, et al. Telephone-based nursing intervention improves the effectiveness of the informed consent process in cancer clinical trials. J Clin Oncol 1996;14:984–996.

68. Cox K. Enhancing cancer clinical trial management: Recommendations from a qualitative study of trial participants' experiences. Psychooncology 2002;9:314–322.

69. Barrett R. A nurse's primer on recruiting participants for clinical trials. Oncol Nurs Forum 2002;29:1091–1098.

70. Rosse PA, Krebs LU. The nurse's role in the informed consent process. Semin Oncol Nurs 1999;15(2):116–123.

71. Sadler GR, Lantz JM, Fullerton JT, Dault Y. Nurses' unique role in randomized clinical trials. J Prof Nurs 1999;15:106–115.

72. Ocker BM, Plank DM. The research nurse role in a clinic-based oncology research setting. Cancer Nurs 2000;23:286–292.

73. Kapo J, Casarett D. Palliative care in phase I trials: An ethical obligation or undue inducement? J Palliat Med 2002;5:661–665.

# VII
# Pediatric Palliative Care

# 53

*Melody Brown Hellsten and Glen Medellin*

# Symptom Management in Pediatric Palliative Care

*What kind of God could do this to a child?—Mother of a symptomatic pediatric patient with advanced cancer*

◆ **Key Points**
◆ *Children are living longer with complex chronic medical conditions.*
◆ *This life prolongation may be accompanied by multiple acute and chronic health crises and challenges for the child and family.*
◆ *Symptom management for these children presents a unique challenge to care providers.*
◆ *Skilled and compassionate management of symptoms, with a family-centered approach, is an integral part of the care of a chronically ill child.*

Complex chronic conditions of childhood (Table 53–1) are defined as "any medical condition that can be reasonably expected to last at least 12 months, involves either multiple organs or one organ system severely enough to require specialty pediatric care, and some probability of hospitalization at a tertiary care center."[1,2] Using currently available demographic and epidemiological data, the estimated number of children currently living with complex chronic conditions of childhood could range from 2.2 to 3.7 million.[3–6]

In the past two decades, child mortality trends have shown a decrease in numbers of deaths from complex chronic conditions in middle childhood years, with stable to increased numbers of deaths in late adolescence and early adulthood.[6] This trend most likely reflects the ability of advancing medical science to provide life-prolonging management of children with complex chronic conditions. However, this life prolongation often comes at the cost of multiple acute and chronic health crises and challenges for the child and family, as well as increasing debilitation as the child's condition progresses, thereby increasing the possibility of suffering for the child and family. It is, therefore, imperative that care providers face the challenge of recognizing and attending to suffering as a concurrent obligation to providing scientifically based curative and life-prolonging treatment.[7] Unfortunately, fragmentation of healthcare, limited acknowledgment of terminal care needs of children, and a paucity of research on the impact of symptoms on quality of life and interventions aimed at managing distressing symptoms all create challenges in alleviating suffering for children with complex chronic conditions.[8]

This chapter focuses on issues related to the assessment and management of common non-pain symptoms in children and adolescents with complex medical conditions in the advanced and terminal stages. The unique issues related to children dying in pediatric and neonatal intensive care units are addressed in Chapters 55 and 57, respectively.

**Table 53–1**
**Categories of Complex Chronic Conditions of Childhood**

**Neurological conditions**
Congenital malformations of the brain
   Anencephaly
   Lissencephaly
   Holoprosencephaly
Cerebral palsy/Mental retardation
Neurodegenerative disorders
   Muscular dystrophies
   Spinal muscular atrophy
   Adrenoleukodystrophy
Epilepsy

**Cardiovascular conditions**
Malformations of the heart/great vessels
Cardiomyopathies
Conduction disorders/dysrhythmias

**Respiratory conditions**
Cystic fibrosis
Chronic respiratory disease
Respiratory malformations

**Renal conditions**
Chronic renal failure

**Gastrointestinal conditions**
Congenital anomalies
Chronic liver disease/cirrhosis
Inflammatory bowel disease

**Hematology/immunodeficiency**
Sickle cell disease
Hereditary anemias
Hereditary immunodeficiency
HIV/AIDS

**Metabolic conditions**
Amino acid metabolism
Carbohydrate metabolism
Mucopolysaccaridosis
Storage disorders

**Genetic conditions**
Trisomy 18
Chromosome 22 deletions
Other congenital disorders

**Malignancy**
Leukemias/lymphomas
Brain tumors
Sarcomas
Neuroblastoma

## Assessing Sources of Suffering in Advanced Childhood Illness

### Family-Centered Care

Family-centered care is based on the understanding that the family is the child's primary source of strength and support and that the perspectives and information provided by families, children, and young adults are important in clinical decision-making.[8–14] In considering symptom management within the context of family-centered care, it is necessary to assess the family system as a whole, as well as its individual members, to identify all sources of suffering that may require intervention. Interdisciplinary collaboration with chaplains, social workers, psychologists, and child-life therapists will contribute to the overall assessment of the ill child, parents, and siblings.

The focus of family-centered care is to develop a process of shared decision-making over the course of the child's and family's illness experience that is based in the interpersonal relationship between the child and family and their health-care providers. The physician and healthcare team must come to know the child and family as individuals and provide diagnostic, prognostic, and treatment information in a manner sensitive to the particular child's and family's experiences, values, beliefs, and available social and spiritual support.[15] Parents and children should be respected as the experts in their illness experience and management, and value must be given to their contribution to the plan of care. The child's and family's illness experience and goals of care, as well as the impact of a particular symptom on suffering and its effect on the child's function and quality of life, will influence the types of interventions considered as symptoms occur.

Illness Experience and Sources of Suffering Research exploring the experiences of families of children with complex chronic conditions provides a glimpse into their world. Uncertainty prevails as the parents move from the initial suspicion that something is wrong with their child to the confirmation that this is indeed the case.[16–19] Parents struggle to cope with the diagnosis and learn skills necessary to provide technical care and negotiate the care system for needed services and information.[20–23] Over time, as treatment continues, parents must live with ongoing uncertainty regarding the unpredictability of the illness, the ultimate outcome of their child's treatment, the challenges of parenting a seriously ill child, and the possibility of death.[24–28] The child may experience disability, physical pain, and other distressing symptoms as a result of the disease and treatments, severe alterations in their social world, and disruption of their developmental process.[29–34] Siblings may experience feelings of anger, guilt, anxiety, depression, and social isolation.[34–38]

Although the above picture gives an impression of tremendous struggle and individual distress in the family, there is also research that suggests there are aspects of family functioning that facilitate coping with this new family reality. Parents' adaptation and adjustment to their child's illness is facilitated by several factors, including gaining information regarding the disease, its treatment, and prognosis; good spousal communication, similar coping styles, and means of emotional expression; and sufficient social support.[34,39–41] Factors associated with adaptation of the ill child and siblings include having open communication and emotional support from parents during times of stress, having a wide range of coping skills, seeking information about the disease, and clarifying fears.[34,42–44]

Assessing and understanding the child's and family's unique experiences during the illness trajectory provides the care team with insight into what symptoms may contribute to the family's suffering. This assessment involves hearing the child's and family members' "story" as they have lived it during the course of the disease. It is important to elicit care that has been helpful in past experiences with the illness as well as care that was not helpful. Insight into what the family values regarding the role of spirituality or faith in God, the meaning they give to their experience of illness, and what activities or interactions the child and family identify as contributing to quality of life provide a context for identifying and managing symptoms that contribute to suffering for the child and family.

## Expectations and Goals of Care

Children with complex chronic conditions are a highly diverse population, with various illness trajectories that are often characterized by prognostic uncertainty, including sudden unexpected death, death from potentially curable disease, death from lethal congenital anomaly, and death from progressive conditions with intermittent health crises. The unpredictability and uncertainty of many of these disease trajectories often result in ongoing medical treatments aimed at cure or aggressive life-prolongation, with little attention to the suffering of the child or family.[8]

Generally, goals of care for children with serious, life-threatening, or limiting illness as they progress through their illness trajectory include interventions aimed at cure, life-prolongation with or without aggressive life-sustaining therapies, and care focused solely on interventions aimed at treating discomfort from symptoms as the disease moves into its terminal phase. Ideally, these goals would shift as the child, family, and primary health-care team discussed changes in quality of life, symptoms, and prognosis over the disease trajectory. It is very important that interventions aimed at maintaining maximal comfort and quality of life occur throughout the disease trajectory as well as through the terminal stages. Unfortunately, for many families, the presence of a do not resuscitate (DNR) order often leads to care professionals dismissing treatable illnesses or symptoms as "part of the dying process," thereby contributing to suffering for both the child and family.

The most difficult decision a parent must face is to change the focus of care from cure or aggressive life prolongation to focusing on comfort and terminal care. Wolfe and colleagues[45] reported on disparity between parents and care providers regarding the realization that a child with progressive cancer had no realistic chance for cure. Parents who came to that realization earlier were more likely to discuss hospice care, to establish a DNR order, and to change the focus of care from cancer-directed therapies to treatments focused on controlling discomfort; therefore, these parents experienced greater quality of home care.

Parents have reported that decisions to forgo further aggressive medical treatments and instead pursue care focused on comfort and quality of life occurred only after realizing that ongoing aggressive treatment would not bring about cure or further life prolongation, and they recognized the physical deterioration and suffering of their child. Once this realization is reached, parents report that the child's wishes and quality of life are major determinants of treatment decision-making.[45-49]

The first step to managing symptoms of children with advanced and terminal illness is a thorough assessment of the child's and family's expectations and goals of care. Interventions aimed at controlling symptoms must be compatible with the family's understanding of where their child is in the disease trajectory and their expectations of care, as well as the child's overall functional status and quality of life. For example, an adolescent with advanced muscular dystrophy may be attending school and participating in a religious community despite significant physical limitations. This level of function and quality of life may lead the child and family to desire aggressive ventilatory support for life prolongation in the event of an acute respiratory infection, with the hope that the child will be cured of the infection and resume his previous level of functioning. However, if the adolescent were home-bound and seriously debilitated as a result of progressive respiratory failure, he and his family may choose to pursue home management of respiratory discomfort without the use of ventilatory support to reduce suffering associated with intensive hospital-based interventions. In determining the expectations and goals of care with the child and family, it is important to discuss the balance between relieving and contributing to the child's suffering. The prevailing decision-making framework should not be based on whether an intervention is consistent with a palliative care focus but, rather, whether the intervention under consideration would provide relief from or contribute to the child's and family's suffering.

## Physical Symptoms and Suffering

Children dying as the result of complex chronic conditions experience numerous symptoms throughout their illness trajectory that can contribute to suffering and decreased quality of life (Table 53–2).

Managing these symptoms requires that health-care providers remain attentive in their assessment of the child's physical and emotional symptoms. Assessment should include the child's report of symptoms and how distressing he/she finds them, information based on parent observation of their child's condition, and health-care provider's knowledge of the pathophysiology of the underlying disease. Diagnostic tests should be considered carefully for the potential discomfort they may cause. Tests should be ordered only if they will help determine an intervention. A test should be questioned for its appropriateness if the results will not change management (e.g., MRI to document growth of known terminal tumor).

As mentioned earlier, symptoms experienced by children with advanced and terminal chronic illnesses are often interrelated. If a child reports a distressing symptom, it is

| Table 53–2 |
| --- |
| **Symptoms Contributing to Suffering in Advanced and Terminal Disease** |
| **General symptoms** |
| Fatigue |
| Anorexia |
| **Psychological/Emotional symptoms** |
| Anxiety/depression |
| **Neurological symptoms** |
| Seizures |
| Somnolence |
| **Respiratory symptoms** |
| Dyspnea |
| **Gastrointestinal symptoms** |
| Nausea/vomiting |
| Constipation |
| Diarrhea |

| Table 53–3 |
| --- |
| **Factors Contributing to Fatigue in Children with Advanced Disease** |
| **Disease/treatment** |
| Pain |
| Unresolved symptoms |
| Anemia |
| Malnutrition |
| Infection |
| Fever |
| Sleep disturbance |
| Debilitation |
| **Psychological factors** |
| Depression |
| Anxiety |
| Spiritual distress |

necessary to obtain a thorough assessment regarding the symptom's onset, severity, and effect on function and quality of life. The health-care provider must consider the likely cause of the symptom and determine the best course of intervention. For example, pain with urination may be related to an infection and amenable to treatment with antibiotics to cure the infection. Shortness of breath in a child with cystic fibrosis may be related to infection and amenable to treatment with antibiotics, with resolution of the symptom. However, it may also be related to progressive respiratory failure or disease progression. Oxygen therapy, opioids, ventilation and/or energy-conservation techniques may assist in relieving the severity of the symptom but will not eliminate the underlying cause. This distinction is important to discuss with the child and parent with regard to the goal of treatment and expectation of care in relation to the child's overall condition and quality of life.

Control of present symptoms as well as anticipation of distressing symptoms as disease progresses is imperative in attending to the suffering of children with advanced disease and their families. Following is a discussion of the most common symptoms associated with distress and suffering experienced by children with advanced illness. It is by no means an exhaustive presentation of all symptoms that children with complex chronic conditions may experience. Each symptom is discussed with regard to its general issues, causes, assessment, and pharmacological and nonpharmacological management. As discussed earlier, there is little evidence-based data on the management of non-pain symptoms in children with advanced disease. Much symptom management in pediatric palliative care is based on empirical approaches and extrapolation from adult hospice and palliative care literature.

An inherent difficulty in pharmacological management in pediatric palliative care is a lack of pharmacological dosing and side-effect information on infants, toddlers, and early school-aged children for many medications. Starting dosages of medications will vary depending on the age, weight, and clinical circumstances of the child. It is incumbent on physicians and nurses to consult with experienced pediatricians and pediatric hospice and palliative care providers for medication choices, appropriate doses, and titration for difficult cases of symptom management. For more information on pediatric pain management, see Chapter 59.

## Management of Symptoms During Disease Progression and End of Life

### General Systemic Symptoms

### Fatigue

The most comprehensive research in fatigue experienced by children with complex chronic illnesses has been in the area of childhood cancer. Fatigue has been described by young children with cancer as a "profound sense of being physically tired, or having difficulty with body movements such as moving legs or opening their eyes"; and as a "changing state of exhaustion that includes physical, mental, and emotional tiredness" by adolescents with cancer.[52–55] Fatigue, lethargy, lack of energy, and drowsiness have been reported in more than 50% of children with cancer, and has been described as moderately to severely distressing.[45,52,56] There is no clear incidence or prevalence of fatigue or its relation to distress or suffering in children with noncancer advanced illnesses.

Fatigue is a multidimensional symptom that can be related to disease, treatment, or emotional factors (Table 53–3). Assessment requires a multidimensional approach, which includes subjective and objective data to determine the degree of distress and potential causes of the child's fatigue. Subjective

**Table 53–4**
**Management of Fatigue in Children with Advanced Disease**

| Intervention | Dose | Comments |
|---|---|---|
| **Pharmacological management** | | |
| Blood transfusion | 10–15 mL/kg IV over 4 h | Premedicate with diphenhydramine (1 mg/kg/IV/PO, max dose 50 mg), acetaminophen (10–15 mg/kg PO) and hydrocortisone (2 mg/kg IV, max dose 100 mg) prior to transfusion if history of reaction. |
| Psychostimulants | | |
| • Methylphenidate | 0.3 mg/kg/dose PO bid | Dosage information for ≥6 y. Give doses in AM and early afternoon. May titrate by 0.1 mg/kg/dose to max of 2 mg/kg/day, gauge by child's desired activity level. May decrease appetite. |
| • Dextroamphetamine | 6–12 y 5 mg/day. May titrate in 5-mg increments weekly, 12 y 10 mg/day. May titrate in 10-mg increments weekly | Titrate according to child's desired level of activity. Will suppress appetite. |
| Sleep agents | | |
| • Chloral hydrate | 20–40 mg/kg/dose PO/PR | Tolerance to hypnotic effect occurs. Maximum of 50 mg/kg/24 h. Not recommended for use >2 weeks or 1 g/dose or 2 g/24 h. Taper dose in situations of prolonged use to avoid withdrawal. Syrup has unpleasant taste, chill or ask pharmacist to mix in flavored syrup. |
| • Diphenhydramine | 1 mg/kg IV/PO. Max dose 50 mg/dose | May cause paradoxical excitement, euphoria, or confusion. May use in children as young as 2 y. |
| • Lorazepam | 0.03–0.1 mg IV/PO. Max 2 mg/dose | Can cause retrograde amnesia. Taper dose with prolonged use. May use in infants and young children. |
| • Zolpidem | 10 mg PO qh | Use for adolescents, young adults. No dosing information in young children. |
| **Nonpharmacological management** | | |
| Nutritional supplementation (e.g., Boost®, Pediasure®, etc.) | | |
| Frequent rest, energy conservation | | |
| Physical/occupational therapies | | |
| Play therapy | | |
| Exploring fears/anxiety that may interfere with sleep | | |

*Source:* Ullrich et al. (2007), reference 52.

assessment involves asking children about their feelings of tiredness or lack of energy, how long they feel tired, when they feel most tired, and how it affected their ability to play or go to school. Objective assessment should include vital signs, presence of other symptoms such as dyspnea or vomiting, evaluation of hydration status, and muscle strength. Laboratory data may include parameters such as oxygen saturation, CBC/differential, and thyroid studies. Management of fatigue will vary depending on the underlying cause and may include both pharmacological and nonpharmacological interventions (Table 53–4). For more information on fatigue, see Chapter 8.

### Anorexia/Cachexia

Loss of appetite occurs in nearly all children with terminal illness. Anorexia involves the loss of desire to eat or a loss of appetite, with associated decrease in food intake. Cachexia is a general lack of nutrition that occurs over the course of a chronic progressive disease. Anorexia and cachexia are multidimensional in nature and are influenced by disease, treatment, and emotional factors[57,58] (Table 53–5). These symptoms are particularly distressing to parents of children with illness because they cause concern that the child is "starving to death." Food and meals have a social association with "caring" and are significant in family culture, activities, and ritual. In most instances, children will request favorite foods as a means of comfort and familiarity. It is important to assist parents in understanding their child's changing eating habits and nutritional needs as well as ways to redirect energies toward other caregiving activities. Table 53–6 provides additional suggestions for management of anorexia and cachexia.

Parents and health-care providers often struggle with personal and ethical dilemmas regarding fluid and nutrition management for children with terminal illness. The act of withholding medically provided fluids and nutrition (enteral feeds, total parenteral nutrition) is legally and ethically permissible for children with irreversible, progressive medical conditions when it is agreed upon by the health-care providers and family that such medically provided nutrition will increase the suffering and discomfort of the child and would not alter the progression of the disease or the outcome of death.[59–63] Such decisions are highly individual to the family and influenced by culture, religious tradition, and personal values.

Providing aggressive nutritional support does not usually improve the condition and, in fact, may add additional symptom burden for the child. Unfortunately, there is no clear data to guide the discussion of the risks/benefits of providing aggressive fluid and nutrition in terminally ill children. When medically provided nutritional interventions are chosen by a family, the challenge is balancing fluid and nutritional supplementation as appetite and metabolic needs decrease with advancing disease. Ideally, as the child's condition progresses, parenteral or enteral supplements can be

slowly weaned to promote comfort and decrease symptoms of increased congestion or secretions. For more information on anorexia and cachexia, see Chapter 8.

## Psychological/Emotional Symptoms

### Anxiety

Children with chronic illness may experience numerous anxiety-provoking events throughout their illness. Episodes of serious illness, hospitalizations, painful procedures, changes in independence and physical abilities, uncontrolled pain and other symptoms, and an uncertain future all can contribute to fear and anxiety.[64–67] The distinction between childhood fears and anxiety is crucial—childhood fears are specific and developmentally based (e.g., fear of the dark, fear of separation, fear of death), whereas anxiety is a generalized feeling of uneasiness without a known source.[68] Anxiety and depression may be comorbid conditions.

Anxiety in terminal illness is an expected reaction and should be assessed frequently. Toddlers and young children will generally have anxiety reactions that are an extension of the stress and anxiety levels of parents and other family members around them. These reactions may include irritability, clinginess, temper tantrums, and inconsolability. School-aged children and adolescents who can cognitively comprehend their illness and impending death may experience more adult-like symptoms, such as chronic apprehension, worry, difficulty concentrating, and sleep disturbance. Chaplains, child-life workers, and social workers are helpful in assessing children's fears, worries, and dreams. Children and adolescents under stress may regress behaviorally and emotionally; therefore, health-care professionals should be alert to changes in the child's coping or personality.

---

**Table 53–5**
**Factors Contributing to Anorexia/Cachexia in Advanced Disease**

**Physiological factors**
Uncontrolled pain or other symptoms
Feeding/swallowing problems
Poor oral hygiene and infections
Mouth sores
Nausea/vomiting
Constipation
Delayed gastric emptying
Changes in taste
**Psychological factors**
Depression
Anger
Stress

---

**Table 53–6**
**Management of Anorexia/Cachexia**

| Intervention | Dose | Comments |
|---|---|---|
| **Pharmacological management** | | |
| Megestrol | 10 mg/kg/dose PO bid | May cause headache, rash, hypertension |
| Dronabinol | 2.5 mg/kg/dose 3–4 times/day | Provides triple effect of antiemetic, appetite stimulant, mood elevation. May be used in young children. |
| Multivitamins | Infant drops 1 mL PO qd | Anecdotal evidence |
| Children's chewables | 1 tab qd | Suggests B vitamins increase appetite |
| **Nonpharmacological Management** | | |
| Prepare small portions of favorite foods. | | |
| Allow child to eat "comfort" foods, don't stress "balanced diet." | | |
| Use thickened liquids or soft foods. | | |
| Offer shakes, smoothies, and other high-calorie foods. | | |
| Provide nutritional drinks as tolerated. | | |
| Assist family in limiting stress over child's eating. | | |

*Source:* Santucci et al. (2007), reference 57.

## Depression

Little is known about the incidence or prevalence of clinical depression in children and adolescents living with chronic illness. Depression can be described as a broad spectrum of responses that range from "expected, transient, nonclinical sadness, to extremes of major clinical depressive disorders and suicidality."[64–67] Children are unique in their coping abilities, which are influenced by their age and developmental level. Often, during the course of terminal illness, most children remain focused on future hopes and continue to plan activities, even in the final days of life. This does not represent denial or being uninformed of their circumstance, rather a protective developmental function and should be gently supported by family and care providers.

Risk factors for depression in chronically ill children include frequent disruptions in important relationships, uncontrolled pain, and presence of multiple physical disabilities.[68] Existential factors related to impending death, concern for parents and other family members, and a personal or family history of preexisting psychological problems can also increase the risk for depression in chronically ill children. Suicidal thoughts or wishes are not common in terminally ill children and adolescents, but health-care providers should be alert to comments about wishing to die and use social workers or child-life therapists to assist in further assessment and management.

Assessment of depressive symptoms must account for the child's developmental level. Pediatric social workers and child-life therapists are good resources for assessing a child's emotional status. Somatic complaints such as lack of appetite, insomnia, agitation, and loss of energy may be the result of disease and cannot be considered hallmark signs of depression in ill children. More appropriate signs would include a persistent sad face and demeanor, tearfulness, irritability, and withdrawal from previously enjoyed activities and relationships. Siblings may exhibit persistent and significant decrease in school performance, hypersomnolence, changes in appetite or weight, and nonspecific complaints of not feeling well.[66] Parents should be assessed for depressed appearance, fearfulness, withdrawal, a sense of punishment, and mood that cannot be improved with good news and should be referred for further evaluation as needed.[50]

Pharmacological management of anxiety and depression should be considered if symptoms of anxiety and depression are debilitating. Consultation with appropriate psychiatric specialists for further evaluation and choice of agents is appropriate. Generally, management of anxiety and depression related to terminal illness in children involves nonpharmacological interventions aimed at addressing the underlying issues that are contributing to the symptoms. Both unconditional acceptance of the child's feelings and reassurance are powerful interventions for anxiety and depression. Facilitating open communication between children and their parents may also be helpful. Creative arts therapies, play, relaxation, storytelling, music, and games may assist in helping children begin to talk about their feelings. It is important to recognize that a certain level of anxiety and sadness is normal when facing death. Health-care providers must take caution to not be overly "cheerful" or insistent that a child discuss his/her feelings. Calm presence, active listening, and sitting quietly with a child will help to build trust. Adolescents in particular are very private about their thoughts and feelings, and if they choose to share them with a caregiver, confidentiality is an important factor in continuing a trusting relationship with the adolescent. For more information on depression, see Chapter 20.

## Neurological Symptoms

### Restlessness/Agitation

Restlessness is a state of hyperarousal in which there is the sensation of not being able to rest or remain in a relaxed position. Agitation in children may present as irritability, combativeness, or refusal of attention or participation. Causes of restlessness and agitation in children with advanced disease can include a variety of physical and psychological causes (Table 53–7).

Assessment should include observing for such behaviors as frequent position changes, twitching, inability to concentrate on activities, inconsolability, disturbed sleep–wake cycles, and moaning. Spiritual distress, disturbing dreams or nightmares, fears, and comorbid anxiety or depression should also be assessed. Treatment for agitation and restlessness should use both age-appropriate pharmacological and nonpharmacological techniques (Table 53–8). Benzodiazepines may be helpful in reducing mild-to-moderate agitation and increasing effectiveness of nonpharmacological interventions.[67,68]

In rare circumstances, children may experience such distressing restlessness or agitation as the result of unrelenting pain or other symptoms that the need for sedation may be considered. Sedation is generally indicated when distress cannot be controlled by any other means either because of limited time-frame or risk of excessive morbidity. Health-care professionals must determine what are truly uncontrollable pain or

---

**Table 53–7**
**Causes of Agitation/Restlessness in Children**

**Disease/Treatment-related Causes**
Uncontrolled pain or other symptoms
Metabolic disturbances
Infections
Hypoxemia
Constipation
Sleep disturbance

**Emotional causes**
Depression/anxiety
Fear
Change in family routine
Reaction to stress of other family members
Withholding of open information or open discussion
   with child

**Table 53-8**
**Management of Agitation/Restlessness**

| Intervention | Dose | Comments |
|---|---|---|
| **Pharmacological management** | | |
| Lorazepam | 0.03–0.1 mg IV/PO q4–6h, may titrate to max 2 mg/dose | Indicated for generalized anxiety<br>May increase sedation in combination with opioids<br>May use in infants and young children |
| Midazolam | 0.025–0.05 mg/kg/dose IV/SQ<br>0.3–1 mg/kg (max 20 mg) PR | Titrate to effect<br>Indicated for myoclonus related to prolonged opioid use, mild sedation<br>Short-acting, quickly reversed if overly sedated |
| Haloperidol | 0.05–0.15 mg/kg/day PO, IV, SQ divided 2–3 times per d | Indicated for agitation not responsive to benzodiazepines<br>Monitor for extra-pyramidal symptoms, treat with diphenhydramine as needed |
| **Nonpharmacological management** | | |
| Maximize pain and other symptom assessment and management. | | |
| Decrease environmental stress or stimulation. | | |
| Encourage open communication between child and family. | | |
| Provide relaxation/guided imagery. | | |
| Provide favorite books, videos, or music. | | |
| Encourage cuddling or holding by parents and other significant family members. | | |

*Source:* Wusthoff et al. (2007), reference 69.

symptoms versus undertreated pain and/or symptoms. Before considering sedation, it is important that all efforts have been made to achieve pain and symptom control. The goal of sedation is to relieve obvious suffering of the child by adding medications to induce sleep, but it is not intended to hasten death.

Presenting the option of sedation to a child and family requires a caring, open relationship between the treating health-care professionals and the family. If the child and family are opposed to sedation, they should be reassured that all efforts to relieve distress will continue. If the child and family choose sedation, there are a number of pharmacological agents available to produce the desired level of relief. Consultation with a hospice physician would be appropriate to determine the clinical appropriateness and best agents to use to achieve the desired comfort goals of the child and family.[69–72]

## Seizures

The risk for seizures in advanced and terminal disease is related to the nature of the underlying disease. Children with congenital malformations of the brain such as lissencephaly and congenital hydrocephaly, as well as other neurodegenerative diseases, often have seizures throughout their disease process. Children with malignancies of the central nervous system may experience seizures as an initial presentation of their illness or during disease progression. Children with advanced illnesses may also have seizure activity as a result of metabolic abnormalities, hypoxia, and neurotoxicity from medications. Seizure activity in children can present in a number of ways (Table 53–9). No matter what the cause, uncontrolled seizure is often one of the most distressing symptoms for parents. If a child has any risk for seizure

**Table 53-9**
**Seizure Patterns in Children**

**Infants and neonates**
Deviation of eyes
Pedaling or stepping movements of legs
Rowing movements of arms
Eye blinking or fluttering
Sucking or smacking lips
Drooling
Apnea
Tonic/clonic movements

**Older children**
Staring spells and deviated gaze
Unilateral or bilateral twitching, tremors
Generalized tonic/clonic movements

activity at the end of life, emergency medications such as diazepam suppositories should be available in the home. Management involves correcting the underlying cause when possible and adding appropriate prophylactic pharmacological agents such as phenobarbital, clonazepam, or lorazepam (Table 53–10).[67,68]

## Respiratory Symptoms

### Dyspnea

The experience of dyspnea is one of the most common nonpain symptoms reported by children and parents.[45,52,56] Dyspnea is the unpleasant sensation of breathlessness and

**Table 53–10**
**Management of Seizures at End of Life**

| Intervention | Dose | Comments |
|---|---|---|
| Phenobarbitol | *Loading dose*: Children 10–20 mg/kg IV, may titrate by 5 mg/kg increments q15–30 min until seizure controlled or to max of 40 mg/kg/dose | Generalized tonic-clonic seizures |
| | *Maintenance dose*: Infants/children 5–8 mg/kg/day in 1–2 divided doses. Therapeutic serum levels 1–50 µg/mL | Status epilepticus |
| Carbamazepine | <6 y *initial*: 5 mg/kg/day PO, titrate based on serum levels q5–7 d to dose of 10 mg/kg/day, then 20 mg/kg/day if necessary, give in 2–4 divided doses | Partial or complete seizures, generalized tonic-clonic, mixed seizure patterns |
| | 6–12 y *initial*: 100 mg/day or 10 mg/kg/day PO in 2 divided doses, increase by 200 mg/day in weekly intervals until therapeutic serum levels reached | |
| | >12 y–*Adult initial*: 200 mg PO bid, increase by 200 mg/day in weekly intervals until therapeutic serum levels reached | |
| Phenytoin | *Loading dose*: Infants/children 15–20 mg/kg IV | Generalized tonic-clonic seizures |
| | *Maintenance dose*: 6 mo–3 y: 8–10 mg/kg/day in divided doses; 4 y–6 y: 7.5–9 mg/kg/day in divided doses; 7 y–9 y: 7–8 mg/kg/day in divided doses; 10 y–16 y: 6–7 mg/kg/day in divided doses. Therapeutic levels 8–15 µg/mL for neonates, 10–20 µg/mL for children | Status epilepticus |
| Diazapam | 2–5 y: 0.5 mg/kg PR 6–11 y: 0.3 mg/kg PR >11 y: 0.2 mg/kg PR May repeat 0.25 mg/kg in 10 min PRN | Status epilepticus |

*Source:* Faulkner et al. (2006), reference 70.

can be particularly frightening for children. Diseases of childhood most associated with dyspnea include cystic fibrosis and other interstitial lung diseases, muscular dystrophy, spinal muscular atrophy, end-stage organ failure, and metastatic cancer. In each of these diseases, there can be a number of underlying causes (Table 53–11) that may be amenable to treatment.

The sensation of dyspnea is a subjective experience, and assessment should include the following: its effect on the child's functional status, factors that worsen or improve dyspnea, assessment of lung sounds, presence of pain with breathing, and oxygenation status. Extent of disease, respiratory rate, and oxygenation status may not always correlate with the degree of breathlessness experienced; therefore, patient report is the best indicator of the degree of distress. There is no validated tool to measure dyspnea; however, using a rating similar to a pain scale has proven anecdotally to provide some measure of distress and response to interventions.

Managing dyspnea depends on the suspected underlying cause of the symptom. Early in the terminal process, interventions for respiratory discomfort are aimed at improving respiratory effort. Antibiotics, oxygen, chemotherapy, or radiation to decrease tumor burden and noninvasive ventilation for children with muscular degenerative disease may be appropriate to treat the underlying cause. As the child becomes increasingly debilitated, the focus shifts to

**Table 53–11**
**Causes of Dyspnea**

**Physiological causes**
Tumor infiltration/compression
Aspiration
Pleural effusion, pulmonary edema, pneumothorax
Pneumonia
Thick secretions/mucous plugs
Bronchospasm
Impaired diaphragmatic excursion due to ascites, large abdominal tumors
Congestive heart failure
Respiratory muscle weakness due to progressive neurodegenerative disease
Metabolical disturbances

**Psychological causes**
Anxiety
Panic disorder

alleviating anxiety associated with respiratory changes and shortness of breath. There are a number of pharmacological choices for managing respiratory symptoms (Table 53–12). Opioids are the treatment of choice for managing dyspnea, as well as in treating a persistent cough. Anticholinergic medications assist in minimizing secretions. Bronchodilators

**Table 53–12**
**Management of Respiratory Symptoms**

| Agent | Dose | Comments |
|---|---|---|
| Morphine | 0.1–0.2 mg/kg/dose IV/SQ | Indicated for dyspnea, cough |
| | 0.2–0.5 mg/kg/dose PO | May need to titrate to comfort |
| Hydromorphone | 15 µg/kg IV q4–6h | |
| | 0.03–0.08 mg/kg/dose PO q4–6h | |
| Glycopyrrolate | 40–100 mg/kg/dose PO 3–4 times/day | Indicated for secretions, congestion |
| | 4–10 µg/kg/dose IV/SQ q3–4h | May give in conjuction with hyoscymine |
| Hyoscyamine | Infant drops (<2 y) | |
| | • 2.3 kg: 3 gtts q4 h; max: 18 gtt/day | |
| | • 3.4 kg: 4 gtt q4h; 24 gtt/day | |
| | • 5 kg: 5 gtt q4h; max: 30 gtt/day | |
| | • 7 kg: 6 gtt q4h; max: 36 gtt/day | |
| | • 10 kg: 8 gtt q4h; 48 gtt/day | |
| | • 15 kg: 10 gtt q4h; 66 gtt/day | |
| | 2–12 y: 0.0625–0.125 mg PO q4h; | |
| | max: 0.75 mg/day | |
| | >12 y: 0.125–0.25 mg PO q4h; | |
| | max: 1.5 mg/day | |
| Hydromet (solution combination of hydrocodone and homatropine) | 0.6 mg/kg/day divided 3–4 doses/day | |
| Albuterol | Oral: 2–6 y: 0.1–0.2 mg/kg/dose tid; max: 4 mg tid | Indicated for wheezing, pulmonary congestion |
| | 6–12 y: 2 mg/dose 3–4 times/day; max: 24 mg/day | Side effects include increased heart rate, anxiety |
| | >12 y: 2–4 mg/dose 3–4 times/day; max: 8 mg qid | |
| | *Nebulized:* 0.01–0.5 mL/kg of 0.5% solution q4–6h | |

*Source:* Lieben et al. (2006), reference 75.

promote increased air exchange in the lungs and can be helpful alone or in conjunction with opioids. Anxiolytic drugs can help reduce anxiety related to the feeling of shortness of breath and improve respiratory comfort.[52,73] As in other discussions of symptom management, it is important to determine with the child and family the level of intervention that is consistent with their perceptions of the child's suffering and quality of life. For more information on dyspnea, see Chapter 14.

### Terminal Respirations

In the final days to hours of life, respiratory patterns often change, initially becoming more rapid and shallow, then progressing to deep, slow respirations with periods of apnea, typically know as Cheyne-Stokes breathing. As the body weakens, pooling of secretions in the throat can lead to noisy respirations, sometimes referred to as "death rattle." Often at this point in disease progression, children are somnolent most of the time and do not report distress. However, these symptoms are particularly agonizing for parents and other family members to experience. Assessment should include monitoring changes in heart rate and respiratory rate, observing for distress, stridor, wheezing, and rales/rhonchi. Management

should focus on managing family distress by explaining the nature of the dying process, reassuring the family that the child is not suffering, administering appropriate anticholinergic medications to decrease secretions, and decreasing or discontinuing any fluids or enteral feedings that may exacerbate the development of secretions or fluid overload.

### Gastrointestinal Symptoms

#### Nausea/Vomiting

The pathophysiology of nausea and vomiting is often multifactorial; can be acute, anticipatory, or delayed; and requires careful assessment to determine underlying causes. Nausea and vomiting can cause extreme exhaustion and dehydration if not well-controlled. Underlying causes of nausea and vomiting may include decreased gastric motility, constipation, obstruction, metabolic disturbances, medication side effects or toxicity, and increased intracranial pressure.

A detailed assessment of the onset and duration, as well as the presence of concomitant symptoms (e.g., headache, visual disturbances) must be obtained. Medical management of nausea and vomiting is based on the suspected underlying cause (Table 53–13).

**Table 53-13**
**Management of Nausea/Vomiting**

| Agent | Dose | Comments |
|---|---|---|
| Ondansetron | 0.15 mg/kg/dose IV or 0.2 mg/kg dose PO q4h; max: 8 mg/dose | Indicated for opioid-induced nausea/vomiting |
| Metoclopromide | 1–2 mg/kg/dose IV q2–4h; max: 50 mg/dose | Indicated for nausea/vomiting related to anorexia, gastroesophageal reflux<br>Can cause dystonia |
| Promethazine | 0.5 mg/kg IV/PO q4–6h; max: 25 mg/dose | Indicated for nausea/vomiting related to obstruction, opioids<br>May increase sedation |
| Dexamethasone | 1–2 mg/kg IV/PO initially, then 1–1.5 mg/kg/day divided q6h; max: 16 mg/day | Indicated for nausea/vomiting related to bowel obstruction, intracranial pressure, medications<br>Side effects include weight gain, edema, and gastrointestinal irritation |

*Sources:* Santucci et al. (2007), reference 57; Karwacki et al. (2006), reference 76.

Corticosteroids may be helpful in reducing an intestinal obstruction. Antiemetic medications combined with medications to reduce secretions (e.g., glycopyrrolate) can be helpful in relieving nausea and vomiting related to intestinal obstruction. In cases of severe nausea and vomiting related to obstruction, placement of a nasogastric tube can decompress the stomach and provide comfort. Medications that promote gastric emptying (e.g., metoclopramide) or motility should not be used if obstruction is suspected. Steroids can provide relief from vomiting caused by increased intracranial pressure. Nausea and vomiting related to medications or anorexia may be managed by a number of antiemetic medications.[57,74] Relaxation techniques, deep breathing, distraction, and art therapies may assist in reducing anticipatory nausea. For more information on nausea and vomiting, see Chapter 10.

## Constipation

Constipation is a frequent symptom experienced by children with advanced and terminal illness and can occur even in children with limited oral intake.[57,74] Children and adolescents, in particular, become embarrassed if asked about bowel habits and will deny problems, leading to a severe problem. It is important to educate the child and family about the potential distress caused by constipation and determine with the child how to discuss this issue. Constipation occurs as a result of inactivity, dehydration, electrolyte imbalance, bowel compression or invasion by tumor, nerve involvement, and/or medications. Symptoms include anorexia, nausea, vomiting, colicky abdominal pain, bloating, and fecal impaction. Physical exam may reveal abdominal distension, right lower-quadrant tenderness, and fecal masses. A rectal exam should be done; however, it is important to gain the child's or adolescent's trust before such an invasive assessment. Ask the child which parent he or she would prefer to be present and have that parent sit near the child and provide reassurance and comfort. Assess the rectum for presence of hard impacted feces, an empty dilated rectum, or extrinsic compression of the rectum by a tumor, hemorrhoids, fissures, tears, or fistulas. Caution should be used in children with cancer who are neutropenic, and a digital exam should not be done unless absolutely necessary.

Management is aimed at preventing constipation from occurring, but if constipation has occurred, it should be treated immediately to avoid debilitating effects (Table 53–14).

Stool softeners should be given for any child at risk of constipation caused by opioid pain management or decreased activity. Softeners are most effective when children are well-hydrated, so the health-care provider should encourage the child to drink water as tolerated. Stimulant laxatives should be used if a child has not had a bowel movement for more than 3 days past that child's usual pattern. If these measures are not successful, stronger cathartic laxatives (e.g., magnesium citrate) or an enema may be used. If there is stool in the rectum and the child is unable to pass it, digital disimpaction may be necessary. The child should be prepared for the procedure and premedicated with pain and anti-anxiety medications. For more information on constipation, see Chapter 12.

## Diarrhea

Although diarrhea is far less common than constipation in children with terminal illnesses, it still may occur and contribute to a diminished quality of life.[57,74] Diarrhea may be caused by intermittent bowel obstruction, fecal impaction, medications, malabsorption, infections, history of abdominal or pelvic radiation, chemotherapy, inflammatory bowel disease, and foods with sorbitol and fructose (found frequently in juices, gum, and candy). Diseases related to increased risk of diarrhea include HIV/AIDS resulting from infections, cystic fibrosis related to malabsorption, and malignancies related to disease progression and treatment history.

---

**Table 53–14**
**Management of Constipation**

**Senna**
Children <12 y: 1–2 tablets PO qhs
2–4 y: Syrup: 1/4–1/2 tsp PO qhs
4–6 y: Syrup: 1/2–1 tsp PO qhs
6–10 y: Syrup: 1 tsp PO qhs

**Ducosate sodium**
Children < 3 y: 10–40 mg/day PO in 1–4 divided doses
3–6 y: 20–60 mg/day PO in 1–4 divided doses
6–12 y: 50–150 mg/day PO in 1–4 divided doses
Older than 12 y: 50–100 mg/day PO in 1–4 divided doses

---

**Table 53–15**
**Management of Diarrhea**

**Loperamide**
Initial doses: 2–5 y: 1 mg PO tid; 6–8 y: 2 mg PO bid; 8–12 y: 2 mg PO tid; after initial dose, 0.1-mg/kg doses after each loose stool (not to exceed the initial dose); >12 y: 4 mg PO × 1 dose; then 2 mg PO after each loose stool (maximum dose: 16 mg/day)

**Diphenoxylate and atropine**
2–5 y: 2 mg PO tid (not to exceed 6 mg/day)
5–8 y: 2 mg PO qid (not to exceed 8 mg/day)
8–12 y: 2 mg PO 5 times/day (not to exceed 10 mg/day)
>12 y: 2.5–5 mg PO 2–4 times/day (not to exceed 20 mg/day)

---

Assessment should include onset, suddenness, duration, and frequency of loose stools; incontinence; character of the stools (color, odor, consistency, presence of mucus or blood), bowel sounds, presence of palpable masses or feces, abdominal tenderness, and examination of the rectal area. Assessment of dehydration includes observation of mucous membranes for dryness, cracking, poor skin turgor, and generalized fatigue. Diet and medication history should be reviewed for potential causes of diarrhea.

Treatment is aimed at managing the underlying causes and the results of persistent diarrhea (Table 53–15). Dietary intervention should involve continued feeding of the child's regular diet as tolerated, as well as oral rehydration with electrolyte solutions as tolerated.[51] For debilitated children using incontinence garments, attention to skin condition and prevention of breakdown is imperative. For more information on diarrhea, see Chapter 12.

## Summary

Symptom management for children with advanced and terminal diseases presents a challenge to health-care providers. Suffering from uncontrolled symptoms can be prevented by knowledge of the child's underlying disease process, thorough assessment of the child and family for sources of suffering, advocacy for child and family needs, and the use of an interdisciplinary approach to management that includes appropriate pharmacological and nonpharmacological interventions.

REFERENCES

1. Feudtner C, DiGiuseppe DL, Neff JM. Hospital care for children and young adults in the last year of life: A population based study. BMC Med 2003;1:1–9.
2. Feudtner C, Feinstein JA, Satchell M, Zhao H, Kang TI. Shifting place of death among children with complex chronic conditions in the United States, 1989–2003. JAMA 2007;297(24):2725—2732.
3. US Census 2000. http://www.census.gov/main/www/cen2000. html (accessed October 22, 2009).
4. Bethell CD, Read D, Blumberg SJ, Newacheck PW. What is the prevalence of children with special health care needs? Toward an understanding of variations in findings and methods across three national surveys. Matern Child Health J 2008;12(1):1–14.
5. Bramlett MD, Read D, Bethell C, Blumberg C. Differentiating subgroups of children with special health care needs by health status and complexity of health care needs. Matern Child Health J 2009;13(2):151–163.
6. Feudtner C, Hays RM, Haynes G, Geyer JR, Neff JM, Koepsell TD. Deaths attributed to pediatric complex conditions: National trends and implications for supportive care services. Pediatrics 2001;107:e99.
7. Kane JR, Brown Hellsten M, Coldsmith A. Human suffering: The need for relationship-based research in pediatric end-of-life care. J Pediatr Oncol Nurs 2004;21:180–185.
8. Field MJ, Behrman RR. When children die: Improving palliative and end-of-life care for children and their families. Washington DC: National Academies Press, 2003.
9. Corlett J, Twycross A. Negotiation of parental roles within family-centred care: A review of the research. J Clin Nurs 2006;15(10):1308–1316.
10. Dokken D, Ahmann E. The many roles of family members in "family-centered care"—part I. Pediatr Nurs 2006;32(6):562–565.
11. Simms R, Cole FS. The many roles of family members in "family-centered care"—part II. Interview by Deborah Dokken. Pediatr Nurs 2007;33(1):51,52,70.
12. Williams L. The many roles of families in family-centered care—part III. Pediatr Nurs 2007;33(2):144–146.
13. Landis M. The many roles of families in "family-centered care"—part IV. Pediatr Nurs 2007;33(3):263–265.
14. Moretz JG, Black J. The many roles of families in family-centered care—part V. Interview by Deborah Dokken. Pediatr Nurs 2007;33(4):356–358.
15. Meltzer LJ, Steinmiller E, Simms S, Grossman M. The COMPLEX CARE Consultation Team, Li Y. Staff engagement during complex pediatric medical care: The role of patient, family, and treatment variables. Patient Educ Couns 2009;74(1):77–83.
16. Swallow VM, Jacoby A. Mothers' evolving relationship with doctors and nurses during the chronic childhood illness trajectory. J Adv Nurs 2001;36:755–764.

17. Stewart JL, Mishel MH. Uncertainty in childhood illness: A synthesis of the parent and child literature. Sch Inq Nurs Pract 2000;14:299–326.

18. Cohen MH. The stages of the prediagnostic period in chronic, life-threatening childhood illness: A process analysis. Res Nurs Health 1995;18:39–48.

19. Cohen MH. The unknown and the unknowable—managing sustained uncertainty. West J Nurs Res 2003;15:77–96.

20. Perrin EC, Lewkowicz C, Young MH. Shared vision: Concordance among fathers, mothers, and pediatricians about unmet needs of children with chronic health conditions. Pediatrics 2000;105:277–285.

21. Satterwhite BB. Impact of chronic illness on child and family: An overview based on five surveys with implications for management. Int J Rehabil Res 1978;1:7–17.

22. Mu PF. Transition experience of parents caring of children with epilepsy: A phenomenological study. Int J Nurs Stud 2008;45(4):543–551.

23. Sen E, Yurtsever S. Difficulties experienced by families with disabled children. J Spec Pediatr Nurs 2007;12(4):238–252.

24. Chen JY, Clark MJ. Family function in families of children with Duchenne muscular dystrophy. Fam Community Health 2007;30(4):296–304.

25. Steele R, Davies B. Impact on parents when a child has a progressive, life-threatening illness. Int J Palliat Nurs 2006;12(12):576–585.

26. Jantien Vrijmoet-Wiersma CM, van Klink JM, Kolk AM, Koopman HM, Ball LM, Maarten Egeler R. Assessment of parental psychological stress in pediatric cancer: A review. J Pediatr Psychol 2008;33(7):694–706.

27. Ware J, Raval H. A qualitative investigation of fathers' experiences of looking after a child with a life-limiting illness, in process and in retrospect. Clin Child Psychol Psychiatry 2007;12(4):549–565.

28. Farnsworth MM, Fosyth D, Haglund C, Ackerman MJ. When I go in to wake them … I wonder: Parental perceptions about congenital long QT syndrome. J Am Acad Nurse Pract 2006;18(6):284–290.

29. Angström-Brännström C, Norberg A, Jansson L. Narratives of children with chronic illness about being comforted. J Pediatr Nurs 2008;23(4):310–316.

30. Taylor RM, Gibson F, Franck LS. A concept analysis of health-related quality of life in young people with chronic illness. J Clin Nurs 2008;17(14):1823–1833.

31. Turkel S, Pao M. Late consequences of chronic pediatric illness. Psychiatr Clin North Am 2007;30(4):819–835.

32. Stewart JL. Children living with chronic illness: An examination of their stressors, coping responses, and health outcomes. Ann Rev Nurs Res 2003;21:203–243.

33. Sourkes BM. Armfuls of Time: The Psychological Experience of the Child with a Life-Threatening Illness. Pittsburgh, PA: University of Pittsburgh Press, 1995.

34. McSherry M, Kehoe K, Carroll JM, Kang TI, Rourke MT. Psychosocial and spiritual needs of children living with a life-limiting illness. Pediatr Clin North Am 2007;54(5):609–629.

35. Gursky B. The effect of educational interventions with siblings of hospitalized children. J Dev Behav Pediatr 2007;28(5):392–398.

36. Houtzager BA, Grootenhuis MA, Caron HN, Last BF. Sibling self-report, parental proxies, and quality of life: The importance of multiple informants for siblings of a critically ill child. Pediatr Hematol Oncol 2005;22(1):25–40.

37. Van Riper M. The sibling experience of living with childhood chronic illness and disability. Ann Rev Nurs Res 2003;21:279–302.

38. Sharpe D, Rossiter L. Siblings of children with a chronic illness: A meta-analysis. J Pediatr Psychol 2002;27:869–710.

39. Hopia H, Paavilainen E, Astedt-Kurki P. The diversity of family health: Constituent systems and resources. Scand J Caring Sci 2005;19(3):186–195.

40. Rolland JS, Walsh F. Facilitating family resilience with childhood illness and disability. Curr Opin Pediatr 2006;18(5):527–538.

41. Hendricks-Ferguson VL. Crisis intervention strategies when caring for families of children with cancer. J Pediatr Oncol Nurs 2000;17:3–11.

42. LeBlanc LA, Goldsmith T, Patel DR. Behavioral aspects of chronic illness in children and adolescents. Pediatr Clin North Am 2003;50:859–878.

43. Meijer SA, Sinnema G, Bijstra JO, Mellenbergh GJ, Wolters WH. Coping styles and locus of control as predictors for psychological adjustment of adolescents with a chronic illness. Soc Sci Med 2002;54:1453–1461.

44. Sloper P. Experiences and support needs of siblings of children with cancer. Health Social Care Commun 2000;8:298–306.

45. Wolfe J, Grier HE, Klar N, et al. Symptoms and suffering at the end of life in children with cancer. N Engl J Med 2000;342(5):326–333.

46. Hinds PS, Oakes L, Furman W, et al. End-of-life decision making by adolescents, parents, and healthcare providers in pediatric oncology: Research to evidence-based practice guidelines. Cancer Nurs 2001;24:122–134.

47. Vickers JL, Carlisle C. Choices and control: Parental experiences in pediatric terminal home care. J Pediatr Oncol Nurs 2000;17:12–21.

48. Friedman S, Gilmore D. Factors that impact resuscitation preferences for young people with severe developmental disabilities. Intellect Dev Disabil 2007;45(2):90–97.

49. Hammes BJ, Klevan J, Kempf M, Williams MS. Pediatric advance care planning. J Palliat Med 2005;8(4):766–773.

50. Whitney SN, Ethier AM, Frugé E, Berg S, McCullough LB, Hockenberry M. Decision making in pediatric oncology: Who should take the lead? The decisional priority in pediatric oncology model. J Clin Oncol 2006;24(1):160–165.

51. Kirschbaum MS. Life support decisions for children: What do parents value? Adv Nurs Sci 1996;19:51–71.

52. Ullrich CK, Mayer OH. Assessment and management of fatigue and dyspnea in pediatric palliative care. Pediatr Clin North Am 2007;54(5):735–756.

53. Hinds PS, Hockenberry M, Tong X, et al. Validity and reliability of a new instrument to measure cancer-related fatigue in adolescents. J Pain Symptom Manage 2007;34(6):607–618.

54. Hinds PS, Hockenberry M, Rai SN, et al. Nocturnal awakenings, sleep environment interruptions, and fatigue in hospitalized children with cancer. Oncol Nurs Forum 2007;34(2):393–402.

55. Hockenberry-Eaton M, Hinds P, O'Neill J. Developing a conceptual model for fatigue in children. Eur J Oncol Nurs 1999;3:5–11.

56. Collins JJ, Devine TD, Dick GS, et al. The measurement of symptoms in young children with cancer: The validation of the Memorial Symptom Assessment Scale in children aged 7–12. J Pain Symptom Manage 2002;23:10–16.

57. Santucci G, Mack JW. Common gastrointestinal symptoms in pediatric palliative care: Nausea, vomiting, constipation, anorexia, cachexia. Pediatr Clin North Am 2007;54(5):673–689.

58. Thompson A, McDonald A, Holden C. Feeding in palliative care. In: Goldman A, Hain R, Liben S, eds. Oxford Textbook of Palliative Care for Children. London and New York: Oxford University Press; 2006.

59. van der Riet P, Good P, Higgins I, Sneesby L. Palliative care professionals' perceptions of nutrition and hydration at the end of life. Int J Palliat Nurs 2008;14(3):145–151.

60. Jones BJ. Nutritional support at the end of life: The relevant ethical issues. Eur J Gastroenterol Hepatol 2007;19(5):383–388.

61. Porta N, Frader J. Withholding hydration and nutrition in newborns. Theor Med Bioeth 2007;28(5):443–451.

62. Carter BS, Leuthner SR. The ethics of withholding/withdrawing nutrition in the newborn. Semin Perinatol 2003;27:480–487.

63. Nelson LJ, Rushton CH, Cranford RE, Nelson RM, Glover JJ, Truog RD. Forgoing medically provided nutrition and hydration in pediatric patients. J Law Med Ethics 1995;23:33–46.

64. Kersun LS, Shemesh E. Depression and anxiety in children at the end of life. Pediatr Clin North Am 2007;54(5):691–708.

65. Mc Culloch, R, Hammell, J. Depression, anxiety, anger and delirium. In: Goldman A, Hain R, Liben S, eds. Oxford Textbook of Palliative Care for Children. London and New York: Oxford University Press; 2006.

66. Sourkes B. Psychological impact of life limiting illness on the child. In: Goldman A, Hain R, Liben S, eds. Oxford Textbook of Palliative Care for Children. London and New York: Oxford University Press; 2006.

67. Louis M, Prescott H. Impact of life limiting illness on the family. In: Goldman A, Hain R, Liben S, eds. Oxford Textbook of Palliative Care for Children. London and New York: Oxford University Press; 2006.

68. Hockenberry M, Wilson D, Winkelstein M, Kline N. Wong's Nursing Care of Infants and Children (8th ed). St. Louis, MO: Mosby, 2006.

69. Wusthoff CJ, Shellhaas RA, Licht DJ. Management of common neurologic symptoms in pediatric palliative care: Seizures, agitation, and spasticity. Pediatr Clin North Am 2007;54(5):709–733.

70. Faulkner KW, Thayer PB, Coulter DL. Neurological and neuromuscular symptoms. In: Goldman A, Hain R, Liben S, eds. Oxford Textbook of Palliative Care for Children. London and New York: Oxford University Press; 2006.

71. Claessens P, Menten J, Schotsmans P, Broeckaert B. Palliative sedation: A review of the research literature. J Pain Symptom Manage 2008;36(3):310–333.

72. Rietjens JA, Hauser J, van der Heide A, Emanuel L. Having a difficult time leaving: Experiences and attitudes of nurses with palliative sedation. Palliat Med 2007;21(7):643–649.

73. Postovsky S, Moaed B, Krivoy E, Ofir R, Ben Arush MW. Practice of palliative sedation in children with brain tumors and sarcomas at the end of life. Pediatr Hematol Oncol 2007;24(6):409–415.

74. de Graeff A, Dean M. Palliative sedation therapy in the last weeks of life: A literature review and recommendations for standards. J Palliat Med 2007;10(1):67–85.

75. Lieben S, Hain R, Goldman A. Respiratory symptoms. In: Goldman A, Hain R, Liben S, eds. Oxford Textbook of Palliative Care for Children. London and New York: Oxford University Press; 2006.

76. Karwacki MW. Gastrointestinal Symptoms. In: Goldman A, Hain R, Liben S, eds. Oxford Textbook of Palliative Care for Children. London and New York: Oxford University Press; 2006.

# 54 ❧❧ Lizabeth H. Sumner

# Pediatric Hospice and Palliative Care

*While we cannot relieve all suffering, we can help prepare these children and families for what comes. It is hard to imagine a situation that has a greater human imperative but far too often today it is not provided…Integrating palliative care from the time of a life-threatening condition is diagnosed should improve care for those children who will survive as well as for those who die and should help the families of both.—Richard E Berhman, MD, JD[1]*

- ◆ *Key Points*
- ◆ *Nursing responsibilities for the seriously ill child are multifaceted, both personally and professionally.*
- ◆ *Initial and ongoing education is essential in addressing the complex physical, emotional, spiritual, and practical needs and concerns of children and their families.*
- ◆ *A family-centered approach to caring for infants, children, and teens must view child and family members as a dynamic web of interconnected lives and relationships.*
- ◆ *Relieving suffering and improving quality of life, for even a brief life, can benefit not only the young patient but all those affected by the illness or death of the child, including siblings, parents, grandparents, other relatives, teachers, school friends, faith community, and neighbors, as well as the health-care professionals involved in their care.*
- ◆ *Nurses who care for dying infants and children and their families need a significant support system and opportunities for renewal and finding meaning for themselves.*

The death of an infant or a child is a special sorrow, leaving a devastating and enduring impact that demands of all of us the very best we can offer to prevent and relieve suffering—for the child as well as the family. Pediatric end-of-life care is very different from adult palliative care and hospice and thus requires specialized knowledge, training, and sensitivity to the unique needs of these families. Our American society promotes the fundamental value that children are our future. They represent our dreams, the promise of accomplishments yet to be fulfilled. With this is mind, why is it then that when these same children experience life-threatening conditions, they often find themselves adrift in a turbulent sea of fragments, care systems, and providers who are often unprepared personally and/or professionally to meet the full range of their intense needs?

❧❧

## Progress and Challenges

The advancement of palliative care as a model for care and for professional development in the United States has reached unprecedented levels in many types of settings. Following that surge is now a robust effort to develop and integrate programs and services for those facing a life-threatening diagnosis from a prenatal diagnosis of a lethal condition to young adults on the brink of adulthood. Since the last edition, growth has been evidenced on many fronts: legislative action, research, hospital-based palliative care, community-based hospice teams/programs, specialty areas of palliative care such as neonatal intensive care unit (NICU), and Emergency Department Oncology. Despite this growth in programs and education, the reality remains that parents and providers will typically choose the path of aggressively extending treatment until the very end of life. The pervasive stigma of what hospice means to the general public and health-care professionals remains a major obstacle for accessing pediatric hospice programs. National engagement is increasingly necessary to undo the misinformation of what hospice is and is not. Undoing the perceptions such as "hospice = no more hope, hospice = giving up; hospice = there's nothing more to do for the child; or death must be near," is a long-term and ongoing goal.

The ongoing painful dilemmas and struggles for families with infants and children who are facing end of life remain hidden from society's view, yet the demands and challenges of caring for a dying child are continually being addressed within hospitals and homes on a daily basis. Individuals, institutions, universities, and community organizations committed to infants and children with life-threatening illnesses and a growing number of hospice programs preparing to care for children are making a difference in addressing the needs of these children in their communities. The tragic irony for pediatric caregivers is that "end-of-life care" is often necessary at the beginning of young lives. Nurses are instrumental in incorporating this contradiction of beginnings and endings into a realistic and compassionate framework for the care of children and families dealing with terminal illnesses. The landmark report from the Institute of Medicine, *When Children Die: Improving Palliative and End-of-Life Care of Children and Their Families*, set forward the challenge and a "call to action" to improve all aspects of end-of-life care for children and families, including improved quality and access to pediatric hospice.[1] It became the catalyst for a cascade of national initiatives, research, funding, and heightened awareness that remains potent today. More specifics are addressed later in this chapter. In addition, The National Consensus Project Guidelines for Quality Palliative Care, published in 2004, also provide direction endorsed by many nationally respected entities for pediatric care within the overall perspective of care for all those—adults or children—facing life-threatening illness.[2]

The ultimate goal is not only to promote excellent palliative care from diagnosis through end-of-life care for these children but also to achieve success in heightening awareness in health-care professionals and the general public. Improving quality of life for even a brief life can benefit the patient and all those affected by the death of a young child.

Such a powerful wave goes beyond those most obviously affected—the parents and siblings. The rippling effect extends to grandparents, other relatives, teachers, school friends, family friends, and neighbors, as well as the many health-care professionals involved in their care and treatment. Each of these may also be deeply influenced by the child's illness and subsequent death. The extensive constellation of those impacted by this illness and death is exponentially greater than one might imagine (Figure 54–1). Compared to a terminally ill elderly adult, the comparatively larger number of people affected by a child's illness or impending death is significant. Few, if any, have had any previous experience with the death of a child. Typically, multiple physicians, care providers, suppliers, school professionals, and a variety of family members are involved with these children. Each has unique needs and roles in the child's experience. In addition, knowledge and skills regarding both palliative and curative care are essential to guide families through this transition in the focus of care. To establish a framework specific to this population the advisory council for the Children's Hospice and Palliative Care Coalition in California developed a definition to guide the state's efforts to radically change how care is provided and funded.

## Definition of Pediatric Palliative Care

*Developed by Children's Hospice & Palliative Care Coalition's Professional Advisory Committee, 2007*

> *Pediatric Palliative Care is both a philosophy of care and an organized, structured system of delivering care to children living with life threatening conditions and their families. The goal of Pediatric Palliative Care is to prevent and relieve suffering and to maximize quality of life for children of all ages, and their family members/ support systems.*

This family centered approach to care is provided by an interdisciplinary team of professionals including medicine, nursing, social work, chaplaincy, nutrition, pharmacy, therapists and other health care professionals. Pediatric Palliative Care offers expert pain and symptom prevention and management. Honest discussion around the child's medical condition serves as the foundation for collaborative decision-making regarding goals of care. This patient-focused, family centered, holistic health care incorporates the physical, emotional, social and spiritual needs of the child and family to enhance their capacity to cope with a life threatening condition.

Pediatric Palliative Care can be delivered concurrently with life-prolonging care or as the main focus of care and is treatment that should be started early in the trajectory of the condition. It preserves the integrity of the family during the condition progression, addressing anticipatory grief and bereavement support following the death."[3]

National Hospice and Palliative Care Organization (NHPCO) 2005 membership findings revealed 20% of hospice programs reported they actively provide or are developing

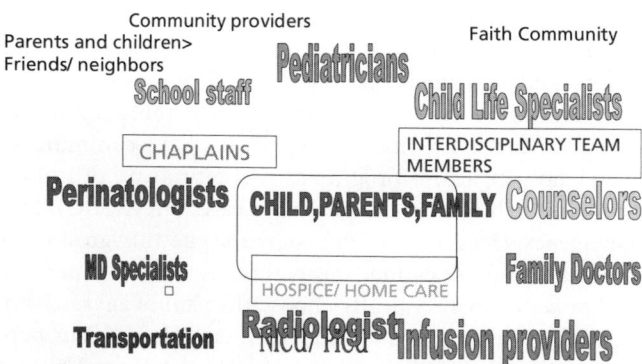

**Figure 54–1.** OTPN. Target group for pediatric palliative care.

pediatric palliative care programs. Over 64% of providers note that this care is provided outside of their traditional hospice program. In the same report, less than 1% of all patients served by member organizations are pediatric patients.[4] Since these findings were published, the NHPCO has made great strides to assist programs in caring for pediatric patients and has advocated for more training in adult hospice programs. They have made pediatric content more prominent and accessible at conferences, on websites, and in newsletter communication with their extensive membership.

How and where these services emerge varies widely, but there are some general models that apply across the country. They include: (1) community hospice-based program (may or may not include home health); (2) children's hospital-based palliative care program (which may or may not have a relationship to home-based services by home health or hospice); (3) freestanding hospice residence and related services; and (4) any combination of the previous components.

Intrinsic to the adaptation to palliative care for infants and children is that care (physical, emotional, spiritual, and social support) is firmly anchored in developmental standards and pertinent modifications to care based on the individual child's cognitive, emotional, physical, and spiritual development. In 2008 the NHPCO launched an effort to create pediatric-specific standards to guide programs and direct how care is rendered.[5] Input was gathered from many diverse stakeholders as well as opportunity to review and comment on the draft standards before they were finalized. Additionally, state hospice associations are supporting more localized efforts to advance the science and art of caring for children in their organizations by cosponsoring educational efforts with other entities such as the well-established and respected ELNEC curriculum created by the AACN and City of Hope. The Pediatric End of Life Nursing Education Consortium is designed to educate nurses as competent trainers when they return to their varied clinical practice settings in palliative care of infants and children facing end of life, as well as their loved ones. This curriculum has been recently revised to better reflect the maturing needs of pediatric palliative care and the emerging expansion of subspecialities of Perinatal and Neonatal approaches to palliative care. Children's hospitals with emerging palliative care programs are now offering more palliative care seminars and conferences to make offerings for education and professional development, creating their own community standard of care.

Palliative care for children has been integrated into recent national nursing professional practice guidelines and standards, such as Society of Pediatric Nursing, 2008.[6] Children's Hospice International *Standards of Hospice Care*. However, the standards are infrequently incorporated into organizational values and standards in predominantly adult patient organizations (Table 54–1).[7] An ongoing struggle remains for professional staff in pediatric care and for families, both of whom are dealing with end-of-life issues and are unprepared for the journey they are embarking on together. Requests on listservs and phone calls to programs for consultation are frequent from health-care professionals seeking peer consultation on the varied and complex issues faced in caring for this population. In the process, a "virtual professional community" has emerged across many specialty areas and across many miles and diverse expertise to respond to the very decentralized pediatric pallaitive care network. Advocacy for pediatric end-of-life and palliative care has evolved from both levels—from the bedside where nurses have advocated for their young patients for symptom management or on behalf of parents who need more information to make the difficult decisions about care and treaments. From the bedside setting, nurses attempt to influence their environment where children are critically ill or dying: identifying the "culture" of decision making, the expression of respect and dignity for each patient and level of respect for each other. It is vitally important for the health care team to establish an effective network for support and open communication within the unit or team; how to respond to each death; identify strategies for ameliorating the stress of a long and difficult shift. Bedside advocacy for good palliative care for the young patient and family can then influence other immediate settings. Next the sphere of influence can move to a larger area of impact—multiple units, across teams, between departments—to gather interest and commitment to make small but impactful changes. Success in reducing suffering, preserving quality of life, and reduced prifessional suffering can then be valued by increasing number of personnel. Leadership and administration is influenced by these growing changes and diverse perespectives that began at the bedside. They can move in multiple directions. State and national involvement can be as simple as writing letters and making calls or inviting a representative to a focus group or a community meeting or making a visit to their office. Regardless of where the seed takes root and sprouts, it usually begins with *an individual* making their voice heard. Change happens when someone takes that first step (see Figure 54–2; integrated approach to advocacy).

## Identifying the Children That Could Benefit From Hospice and Palliative Care

The trajectory toward end of life is widely varied among infants and children through adolescence. There are typically four generally recognized pathways of these conditions ending in death. In brief, they are sudden deaths, deaths from a potentially curable disease, death from a congenital anomaly that is lethal, deaths from a progressive condition that is rapidly growing, which results in a challenging group of patients (often referred to as the complex chronically ill child; IOM 2003). By age group, this same report highlights highest rate of death as between birth and age 1 year, with a high proportion occurring in first month of life.

For the sudden deaths (such as SIDS), the death is discovered after the fact or from an injury. These are particularly difficult because they often eliminate opportunity to say goodbye. Grief is intense and complicated.

**Table 54–1**
**Children's Hospice International Standards of Hospice Care of Children**

**Access to care**

**Principle**

Children with life-threatening, terminal illnesses and their families have special needs. Hospice services for children and their families offer developmentally appropriate palliative and supportive care to any child with a life-threatening condition in an appropriate setting. Children are admitted to hospice services without regard for diagnosis, gender, race, creed, handicap, age or ability to pay.

**Standards**

A.C.1. Hospice care services are accessible to children and their families in a setting that is desired and/or appropriate for their needs.

A.C.2. The hospice team is available to provide continuity of care to children and their families in the home and/or in an institutional setting.

A.C.3. The hospice program has eligibility admission criteria for the children and families they serve. Care plans are developed which take into consideration the child's prognosis, and the child and family's needs and desires for hospice services. Admission to the hospice care services does not preclude the child and family from treatment choices or hopeful, supportive therapies.

A.C.4. The hospice program provides information to the community and referral sources about the services that are offered, who qualifies, and how services may be obtained and reimbursed.

**Child and family as a unit of care**

**Principle**

Hospice programs provide family-centered care to enhance the quality of life for the child and family as defined by each child-and-family unit. It includes the child and family in the decision making process about services and treatment choices to the fullest degree that is possible and desired.

**Standards**

C.F.U.1. The unit of care is the child and family. Hospice provides family-centered care. The family is defined as the relatives and/or other significant persons who provide physical, psychological, social and/or spiritual support for the child.

C.F.U.2. The hospice program recognizes the unique, personal values and beliefs of all children and families. The hospice respects and maintains, as possible, the wishes and dignity of every child and his or her family.

C.F.U.3. The hospice program encourages that children and their families participate in decisions regarding care, including discontinuation of hospice care at any time, and maintains documentation related to consent, advance directives, treatments, and alternative choices of care.

C.F.U.4. The hospice program provides care that considers each child's growth, development and stage of family life cycle. Children's interests and needs are solicited and considered, but are not limited to those related to their illness and disability.

C.F.U.5. The hospice team seeks to assist each child and family to enjoy life as they are able, and to continue in their customary life-style, functioning and roles as much as possible, especially helping the child to live as normal a life as is possible.

**Policies and procedures**

**Principle**

The hospice program offers services that are accountable to and appropriate for the children and families it serves.

**Standards**

P.P.1. The hospice program establishes and maintains accurate and adequate policies and procedures to assure that the hospice is accountable to children, their families, and the communities they serve.

P.P.2. The hospice agency is in compliance with all local, state and federal laws and regulations which govern the appropriate delivery of hospice care services.

P.P.3. The hospice program provides a clear and accessible grievance procedure to families outlining how to voice complaints or concerns about services and care without jeopardizing services.

**Interdisciplinary team services**

**Principle**

Seriously ill children with life-threatening conditions and/or facing terminal stages of an illness and their families have a variety of needs that require a collaborative and cooperative effort from practitioners of many disciplines, working together as an interdisciplinary team of qualified professionals and volunteers.

**Standards**

I.T.1. The hospice program provides care to the child and family by utilizing a core interdisciplinary team which may include: the child, the family and/or significant others, physicians, nurses, social workers, clergy and volunteers.

I.T.2. Representatives of other appropriate disciplines are involved in the team as needed, i.e., physical therapy, occupational therapy, speech therapy, nutritional consultation, art therapy, music therapy. The team might also include psychologists, child life specialists, teachers, recreation therapists, play therapists, home health aides, nursing assistants, and other specialists or services as needed.

I.T.3. The hospice core team meets on a regular basis and an integrated plan of care is developed, implemented and maintained for every child and family.

*Source*: Children's Hospice International, http://www.chionline.org. Copyright 1993 Children's Hospice International. Reprinted with permission.

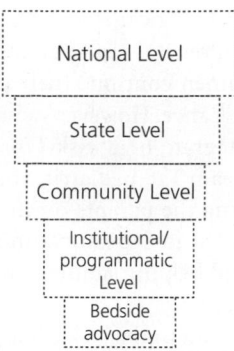

**Figure 54–2.** Integrative approach to advocacy for pediatric palliative care.

The next category of potentially curable disease usually evolves from initial response to treatment, return of disease, and then poor to no response to treatments. Preoccupation with therapies, labs, tests, or therapies may overshadow any discussion about possibility of dying, focusing on the tasks, and managing the medical aspects. Maximizing opportunities for comfort may be passed or delayed in the intensive search for cure and life-extending alternatives.

Sometimes the infants with congenital anomalies survive time of delivery; they usually survive only briefly,but they may live long enough to benefit from the comfort of palliative care, and maximum emotional and spiritual support can be offered to family while under the care of hospital/medical team before transitioning them to the reliable support in community for bereavement follow-up and ongoing support.

Finally, those children with the very extended and variable pathway through illness, those referred to as complex chronically ill children who are sick over a long period, have multiple peaks and valleys and extensive needs as time goes on for the family and child. Life can become consumed by the constant focus on appointments, therapy, transportation, shift care, special needs and ongoing obstacles to overcome in accessing adequate, or comprehensive, care.

Another widely used and well-established model for categorizing life-limiting conditions for the eligible children for palliative care approach is from the Association for Children's Palliative Care (ACT). They identify four groups.

> *Group 1*: Life-threatening conditions for which curative treatment may be feasible but can fail. Palliative care may be necessary during periods of prognostic uncertainty and when treatment fails (e.g., cancer, irreversible organ failures of heart or liver).
> *Group 2*: Conditions where premature death is inevitable, where there may be long periods of intensive treatment aimed at prolonging life and allowing participation in normal childhood activities (e.g. , cystic fibrosis and muscular dystrophy).
> *Group 3*: Progresive conditions without curative treatment options, where treatment is exclusively palliative and may commonly extend over several years (e.g., Batten's disease, mucopolysaccharidosis).

> *Group 4*: Conditions involving severe neurological disability that may cause weakness and susceptability to health complications and may deteriorate unpredictably but are not considered progressive (e.g., cerebral palsy).[8]

Becoming more "traditional" in palliative care are the hard to categorize but pertinent patients, including children discontinued from life-sustaining medical treatment following a motor vehicle accident or in the perinatal period who are not expected to survive and drowning accident victims who have not died immediately. The "entry" into these pathways varies greatly but subsequently, accessing palliative-oriented care is still challenging for all the emotional reasons one might imagine when it is a child's life at stake. Perhaps the best analogy is to emphasize the "titration" of care gradually in the direction of comprehensive symptom management and caring for the body, mind, and spirit of both child and family—titrating slowly from one sole focus of preserving life to adding/titrating up the measures to relieve suffering in tandem with the life-extending efforts. Nurses have an extraordinary role in gently and persuasively guiding families through this emotionally laden course, along with others in the care team. Nurses are present for the highest ratio of time with the child and family to create an impact and influence how care is perceived and how to interpret medical information upon which decisions are made.

## Perinatal Palliative Care

As the "umbrella" of palliative care for children is growing and becoming more defined, the emergence of a new population to be well-served by this approach has become well-established. *Perinatal* palliative care model has become well-known and is being replicated in many ways around the country and even internationally. When a parent receives a prenatal diagnosis that their unborn baby may not live to or perhaps much beyond delivery, the best practice of hospice (preventing and relieving suffering through an interdisciplinary team approach) is introduced *during pregnancy*. This has pushed the model for palliative care upstream into an arena of professionals and settings much less exposed to hospice or to palliative strategies to care.

"Perinatal hospice or palliative care is an innovative and compassionate model of support that can be offered to parents who find out during pregnancy that their baby has a fatal condition. As prenatal testing continues to advance, more families are finding themselves in this heartbreaking situation. Perinatal (perinatal means around the time of birth) hospice incorporates the philosophy and expertise of hospice into the care of this new population of patients. For parents who receive a terminal prenatal diagnosis and wish to continue their pregnancies, perinatal hospice helps them embrace whatever life their baby might have, before and after birth. Perinatal hospice support begins at the time of diagnosis, not just after the baby is born. It can be thought of as 'hospice in the womb' (including birth planning and preliminary medical decision-making before the baby is born) as well as more traditional hospice care after birth (if the baby lives longer than a few minutes or hours). This approach supports families through the rest of the pregnancy, through decision-making before and after birth, and through their grief. Perinatal palliative care also enables families to make meaningful plans for the baby's life, birth, and death, honoring the baby as well as the baby's family. Perinatal hospice is not a place. Ideally, it is a comprehensive team approach that includes obstetricians, perinatologists, labor & delivery nurses, neonatologists, NICU staff, chaplains/pastors and social workers (Calhoun & Hoeldtke 2000), as well as genetic counselors, therapists, and traditional hospice professionals. Perinatal hospice is a beautiful and practical response to one of the most heartbreaking challenges of prenatal testing."[9] Some programs emerge from a hospital setting, labor and delivery, NICU, and maternal child areas. Other times it arises from the community side in response to accessing hospice expertise and extending it into the prenatal period of care. However, it is often confused with bereavement support, as in perinatal loss following an infant death, pregnancy loss, or the spectrum of "birth-related tragedies." What distinguishes the perinatal palliatrive care approach is that the care and support begins before death, during pregnancy, and continues throughout pregnancy, through time of delivery and beyond, depending on how long the baby lives. It naturally creates a seamless continuum of care across settings (office to institution to home) across providers—traditional pregnancy care providers in collaboration with those focused on palliative care, advanced decisionmaking via a "birth plan" (see Table 54–2 and Figure 54–3.

At the beginning of this movement of perinatal hospice, mothers and parents were coming directly to hospices for help out of desperation, facing a prenatal diagnosis of a devastating nature for their unborn baby. These parents had decided to continue the pregnancy and treasure their child's life for as long as they could, yet they lacked any ongoing support. Their message was clear: "Finally, someone will just accept our decision and help our family deal with this experience. We don't want to just sit back and wait for our baby's death." Hospice professionals are trained to use an individualized approach to assist patients and families in dealing with life-threatening illnesses and their decisions concerning that experience. This unique group of parents faces the daunting challenge of anticipating and preparing for the birth *and* the possibility of death of their baby simultaneously. With the help of this unique program, they are given the opportunity to feel some level of control by making plans based on their individual needs for supporting themselves, their other children, the grandparents, and friends.[10,11]

The parents' goals and plans are discussed in collaboration with their physician. The physician is kept up to date regarding their psychological state and the development of their birthing plan. Prenatal nursing care is not a part of this program. These women continue their prenatal care under their physician's guidance. However some programs are hospital based and integrate high risk OB offices, NICU staff etc. into the care team. The pediatric hospice nurse may be involved in educating the parents on the diagnosis, helping them understand what to expect, planning for the possibility of home care, and helping siblings understand the baby's condition.

Perhaps as a reaction to the lack of responsiveness toward perinatal loss by the health-care system and society in general, these parents find ways to support each other. They experience truly disenfranchised grief, one not recognized as equal to the grief experienced with other types of death. The internet is rich with amazing and profoundly intimate resources and ideas, sharing of common experiences, practical help, opportunities to gain support, and even memorials to lost children. These parents discover help from within their isolation from others like themselves. Hospice (and hospital) professionals can gain valuable insight from their perspectives and excellent ideas on ways to improve support for these parents.

Initial feedback from the hospice bereavement counselors who work with these parents has highlighted the potential and anticipated impact of the perinatal hospice service. The bereaved parents who received help through perinatal palliative care demonstrated the following: they were more emotionally and spiritually prepared for their infant's death; they experienced less intense despair/sadness; they had better marital relationship communication and support; and they felt fewer "raw" intense emotions such as anger, rage, and uncertainty regarding the cause of death. The parents without hospice care during pregnancy and after birth seemed to demonstrate a more intense grieving experience, whereas the others expressed a sense of gratitude and peace surrounding the brief life of their child. Parents have told us that they are able to be fully present for their baby when he/she is born because of the planning and guidance beforehand. It also allowed them to maximize the limited time to truly celebrate and to welcome the baby before they had to say goodbye—an essential ingredient to their healing process.

Over time, the keepsakes accumulated during the pregnancy and birth—photographs and other objects—can assist young siblings and parents to integrate the loss of the child into their family experience. Before delivery, a family picture can be taken with the family gathered closely around the mother, all hands placed gently on her abdomen. Because the baby may die *in utero* or at birth, this earlier image may be helpful in recording and preserving his/her presence in their lives. The team provides paint, posterboard, and a memory box and then assists in obtaining handprints of the baby as well as of the entire family at the hospital to create another "family portrait." Because almost all NICUs and labor/delivery areas have developed procedures and activities for the experience of infant death, the hospice team works with the inpatient staff

**Table 54–2**
**Birthing Plan**

Dear staff at _____:

We have received the devastating news that our baby _____ has been diagnosed with _____. However imperfect his/her little body is, he/she is still our baby who we love and therefore chose to continue his/her life. Your kindness, compassion, and understanding during this difficult time are greatly appreciated. We believe that precious time with _____ is the only thing that will soothe the pain of those who love him/her.

We understand that decisions may need to be made after the birth, which were not anticipated. We ask only that you keep us informed so we can make the decisions together for what is best for _____. We ask that no interventions than those stated below be taken without approval from us and consideration be given to the precious nature of our brief time as a family.

Each of you can assist during this time by understanding and respecting our following wishes:

1. Please call our baby by his/her name _____. This is very comforting for us to hear.
2. In an effort to facilitate relaxation during labor and delivery, we would like_____ (selected music, shower, massage, etc.).
3. We prefer the same room for labor, delivery, and recovery.
4. In regards to fetal monitoring, we request ____external _____internal _____none.
   • We may desire to hear heartbeat initially before labor progresses.
5. If there is a loss of heartbeat prior to delivery, we do/do not wish to be informed.
6. We desire the following people in attendance _____ And that the birth is videotaped.
7. Any drugs used during labor should be given to _____ in the smallest dose that will be effective, to provide maximum pain relief and comfort while still allowing _____ to remain alert. Our other preferences in regards to pain management include _____.
8. We ask that _____ be able to cut the umbilical cord.
9. We request that oral/nasal suctioning only be used for comfort and no intubation without permission of the parents.
10. After our baby is born, we ask that _____ be quickly wiped, suctioned, wrapped in a blanket and handed to _____.
11. Following delivery, we wish to hold our baby immediately and that vital signs, weighing of baby, medications, and labs are postponed if possible.
12. We understand that our baby may be born with more or fewer problems than anticipated. If this is the case, we ask that our options be discussed with us and, if necessary, further diagnostic testing may be needed.
13. Other than the basic care needed after delivery, my husband and I would like to be left alone without interruption to have private time with our baby. (You may prefer for staff to check on you occasionally.)
14. We request that a liaison (i.e., nurse, social worker, chaplain) periodically give updates to the waiting family.
15. Additional family and friends that are special to us may be joining us as we celebrate our child's life.
16. If our baby cannot suck and or breastfeed, we wish to provide oral comfort with drops of expressed breast milk or formula.
17. We request that a ceremony be performed in accordance with our religious beliefs by _____ (baptismal, blessing).
18. If our child is to be placed in NICU, we request that we be provided with a private space for us to care for our child in private. Help us create a *sacred space* to share his/her brief life.
19. Please discuss any medications given to our baby to relieve pain and suffering with us prior to giving.
20. We wish to hold our baby as he/she is dying or after he/she has died.
21. We would like to bathe and touch our baby's precious little body as long as possible.
22. We would like to keep the following items as keepsakes: cord clamp, lock of hair, ID band, tape measure, crib card, baptismal certificate, weight card, hat/blanket/clothes, fetal monitor, tape, bulb syringe, footprints/handprints, thermometer, handprints of baby alone and with family, photographs-color and b/w. Anything with our baby's scent.
23. Upon discharge, please give us information on milk suppression and physical comfort measures for _____ (the mother).
24. Please allow my husband _____ or other designated person to spend the night in my room if possible.
   We understand that every birthing experience is unique and offer this only as a guideline to assist you and your family to decide what feels right for you.

*Source*: Liz Sumner (2009). Center for Compassionate Care. The Elizabeth Hospice.

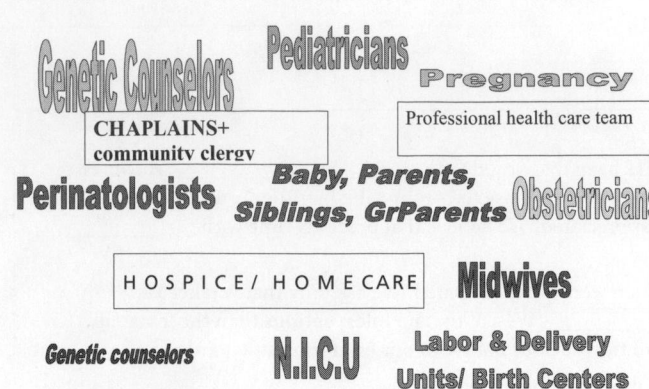

**Figure 54–3.** Constellation of support and providers. Perinatal palliative care.

as a bridge of continuity in the parents' experience. Planning the "who, what, when, and where" for the delivery and beyond is important. If this information is not shared with the hospital staff, time may be lost and opportunities missed forever for some critical experiences for the family.

Making both the pregnancy and the death more real helps reduce denial of the loss. Mourning the dead child is facilitated by visual reminders over which families can grieve.

## General Considerations For Pediatric Palliative and Hospice Care

See Table 54-3.

## Essential Elements In PPC
### (see Figure 54–4).

See Figure 54-5, "Needs of a child with a life threatening illness." The essential elements of palliative care for infants and children are similar in concept to those of all ages of patients, but the *practical elements* are truly a significant variable in the lives of younger families dealing with a serious and life-threatening condition. How we assist families to thrive—and yes, survive—this life journey is paramount. It needs to be woven into every aspect of nursing care—how does this affect their daily life, the life of the child, and the life of the family? Is this realistic care to teach them? Will their lives be totally focused on these tasks? Can we be flexible to make sure normalcy is still highly valued and considered in planning the care and treatment? The family must find ways to adjust daily and over time and still find time for work, other childrens' needs, family, and

some outlet for relief (school, church etc.). Table 54-4 shows some of the ways in which practical needs and issues can be addressed for families to be aware of resources, things to consider, how to ask for help, and so forth. *When a child is dying: The Supportive Care Handbook* lists many categories of who can help and how, from health-care professionals to friends.[12] Nurses can help ease fears and frustrations of the child along with normalizing the full range of normal feelings that may wax and wane over time. Painting a realistic picture for parents and family regarding what to expect as a child's condition changes, side effects to anticipate from medications, treatments, and therapies is empowering and fosters an environment of trust and respect at same time.

Core values of the approach to palliative care and hospice for children include:

- an individualized and family-centered approach that guides *how* team and nurses, in particular, approach the care provided;
- respect for the dignity and uniqueness of each infant, child, adolescent, or teen, regardless of the length of life or duration of illness and limitations imposed by the illness;
- goals and preferences elicited from and identified by the child and family and respected and implemented by the nurse and other team members;
- hope preserved and expressed in a variety of ways to sustain families and their beliefs through life and death of the child;
- enhancement and promotion of quality of life *and* quality of living for child and family;
- priority and value placed on sustaining relationships between child/parents/family and primary care/treatment team (timely response and solutions included); and
- coordination of care for an important and seamless continuum of care—among providers, between settings of care, and over time to *insure* adequate support.

### "Promise to Tell if it Will Hurt"

The author of the passage below is 7 years old and spent over 2 months in a hospital in the east with a rare and life-threatening auto-immune disease. Although grateful for her care, she summarized her "commandments" for other kids to benefit from and let people know how it felt being a child in the hospital.[13]

1. **Don't surprise me.** Tell me what you are going to do before you do it. Please let me know what you are doing way before you touch me.
2. **Always think of a less painful way of doing things and be organized.** Please bunch the tests together, it's not easy to get stuck no matter what they say. *(Anticipate and promote)*
3. **Be honest!** It upsets me more if they say something isn't going to hurt and then it does. Tell me the truth. *(Trust and respect)*

**Table 54-3**
**The Illness Experience: The Child and Adolescent**

| | Infant | Toddler | Preschooler | School-Age Child | Adolescent |
|---|---|---|---|---|---|
| Developmental task | Achievement of awareness of being separate from significant others | Invitation of autonomy | Creation of sense of initiative | Development of sense of industry | Achievement of a sense of identity |
| Impact of illness | Potential distortion of differentiation of self from parent/significant others | Interference with loss of developing sense of control, independence | Interference/loss of accomplishments such as walking, talking, controlling basic bodily functions. | Potential feelings of inadequacy/inferiority if autonomy and independences are compromised. | Potential alteration/relinquishment of newly acquired roles and responsibilities. |
| Cognitive age/stage | Sensorimotor (birth through 2 years) | Preoperational thought (2–7 years: egocentric, magical, little concept of bodily integrity | Preoperational thought: egocentric, magical tendency to use and repeat words they don't understand, providing own explanations and definitions. Literal translation of words. Inability to abstract. | Concrete operation thought (7–10+ years): beginning of logical thought but tendency to be literal. | Formal operational thought (11+ years): beginning of ability to think abstractly. Existence of some magical thinking (e.g., feeling guilty for illness) and egocentrism. |
| Major fears | Separation, strangers | Separation, Loss of control | Bodily injury and mutilation; loss of control; the unknown; the dark; being left alone. | Loss of control; bodily injury and mutilation; failure to live up to expectation of important others; death. | Loss of control; altered body image; separation from peer group. |
| Concept of illness | N/A | Phenomenism (2–7 years): Perceives external, unrelated, concrete phenomenon as cause of illness, e.g., "being sick because you don't feel well." Contagion: Perceives cause of illness as proximity between two events that occurs by "magic", e.g., "getting a cold because you are near someone who has a cold." | Phenomenism; contagion. | Contamination: Perceives cause as a person, object or action external to the child that is "bad" or "harmful" to the body, e.g., getting a cold because you didn't wear a hat. Internalization: Perceives illness a having an external cause but being located inside the body; e.g., "getting a cold by breathing in air and bacteria." | Physiologic: Perceives cause as a malfunctioning on nonfunctioning organ or process; can explain illness in sequence of events. Psychophysiologic: Realizes that psychologic actions and attitudes affect health and illness. |

(continued)

**Table 54–3**
**The Illness Experience: The Child and Adolescent** (*continued*)

| | Infant | Toddler | Preschooler | School-Age Child | Adolescent |
|---|---|---|---|---|---|
| Interventions | Provide consistent caretakers. Minimize separation from parents/ significant others. Decrease parental anxiety, which is projected to infant. Maintain crib/nursery as "safe place" in which not invasive procedures are performed. | Minimize separation from parents/ significant others. Keep security objects at hand. Provide simple, brief explanations. Explain and maintain consistent limits. Encourage participation in daily care, etc. Provide opportunities for play and play therapy. | Provide simple concrete explanations. Advance preparation is important: days for major events, hours for minor events. Verbal explanations are usually insufficient, so use pictures, models, actual equipment, medical play. | Provide choices whenever possible to increase the child's sense of control. Stress contact with peer group. Use diagrams, pictures and models for explanations, because thinking is concrete. Emphasize the "normal" things the child can do, because the child does not want to be seen as different. Reassure child he/she has done nothing wrong; hospitalization, etc., is not "punishment." | Allow adolescent to be an integral part of decision-making regarding care. Give information sensitively, since this age group reacts to content of information as well as the manner in which it is delivered. Allow as many choices and as much control as possible. Be honest about treatment and consequences. Stress what the adolescent can do for him or herself and the importance of cooperation and compliance. Assist in maintaining contact with peer group. |

*Source:* Armstrong-Dailey, A., & Zarboca, S. (2001). Hospice care for children (2$^{nd}$ ed., pp. 51–53). New York, NY: Oxford University Press. Reprinted with permission.

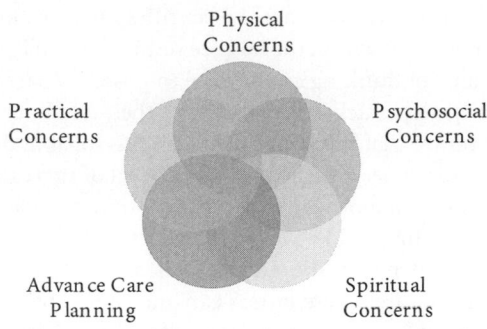

**Figure 54–4.** Essential elements in pediatric palliative care.

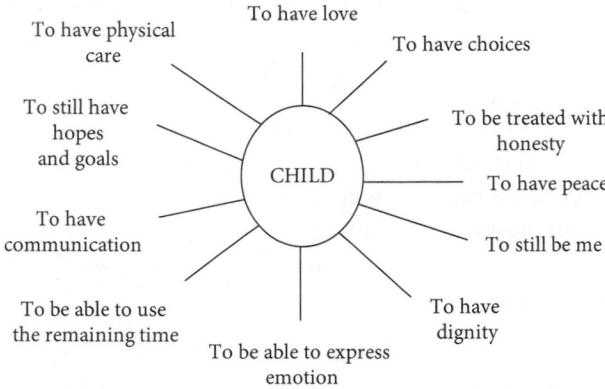

**Figure 54–5.** Needs of a child with life-threatening illness.
*Source*: Used with permission, Ann Goldman (1994).

4. **Ask permission before you put any part of your body on mine.** I often feel like a teddy bear with people squeezing and pushing my body parts. Wake me before you start doing something. Sometimes it should be okay for me to say no because I may not feel like being touched.

5. **Get down on my level.** If I am in bed, sit down. Don't stand over me, because it scares me. "Oh no, what is he going to say to me?" They look really big from where I am. When the doctor knelt down by my bed I wasn't scared any more.

6. **Try to keep the doctors and nurses who come in the room the same.** It is scary to wake up and see a whole group of new faces standing around my bed. Having the same nurse was nice; she learned the kind of things I like to do and helped me feel better about new things. *(Continuity)*

7. **Try not to wake me so many times!** Why do you have to wake me so many times during the night? *(Anticipate needs)*

8. **Dress normal.** Don't wear that white coat coming into my room; it always made me think something bad was going to happen or I was getting bad news. *(Trust and respect)*

9. **Get cable!** If this place is for kids, you need to have more children's programs for us, especially during the day.

---

**Table 54–4**
**Practical Needs and Concerns of Child and Family**

- **How do I get the help I need to keep us all afloat with so much to juggle?** No one wants to ask for help and no one knows HOW and when to help so….Solution: Help parents connect the helper with the "helpee"—refer to resources to learn how to mobilize friends, family, work friends, neighbors to establish a sustainable network of volunteers, friends and others through: SHARE THE CARE (WWW.SHARETHECARE.ORG) or LOTSA HELPING HANDS (Lotsahelpinghands.org).

- **Do I need to tell my child's school?** (The sick one or the well ones). Solution: Discuss the benefits of having someone from care team talk to school counselor/nurse/teacher to establish a safety net for child while at school as well as anticipate needs down the road (returning to school after illness or death, etc.).

- **How can I balance hope with the reality we face?** Solution: Nurses can offer time to reflect and share along the way and help parents see they both exist simultaneously. Hope allows for parents to move through each day. Help family identify realistic short-term goals like mini-wishes of what they hope for, allowing them to find success in accomplishing smaller milestones. As child condition declines they are holding on with one hand and having to let go with the other. The duality will remain while child is alive and after they are gone. Anticipation of what might come next by nurses can help prevent unnecessary suffering, worries, and fear.

- **Who do I call for what? When? How will I know what to do?** Solution: Prepare parents for range of things that may unfold as they are ready to take it in and then have a plan for which they can follow to take action. For example, for fear of sudden pain increase have stronger pain medicine on hand for crisis until they get in contact. Provide family with list of who their providers are, showing point person for each provider and numbers to call. Explain how on-call works for home setting or how to contact MD after hours, and so forth. Explain what to expect and which information to have ready.

- **What do I do if my child dies at home?** Solution: Nurses can provide written information that is gentle but clear on what this process will look like from a systems perspective—circulation, eating, elimination, awareness, temperature, physical appearance, and so forth. Offer them suggestions on how to comfort the child during these changes. This should be offered in both home setting with some preparation for hospital setting as well. The information needs to be communicated to those on alternate shifts to be consistent.

10. **Stop saying "It's no big deal."** I didn't like it when nurses said that when they took blood. It is a big deal to me. It is a big deal because you are taking something that's supposed to be in my body. It might not be a big deal because it is not happening to you.

Asking for feedback on the day-to-day care from children and families will always help us to gain insight into the other perspective from the bed.

### Barriers to Accessing Hospice Care

Barriers to accessing hospice or palliative care programs for pediatric patients differ from those for adult patients. Society's belief that "children shouldn't die," along with denial of the process, make end-of-life care for this population a distant and mysterious concept. Within the health-care profession, a profound silence of discomfort and denial exists regarding babies and children dying. In many cases, health-care professionals attitudes and denial become the greatest barrier to their patients'/families' ability to access additional options for expert palliative care and support services. In effect, this denies families the possibility of making an informed decision regarding the range of choices available during a child's illness. Excellence in advanced illness or end-of-life care as part of the continuum of clinical expertise should be readily available for families who may transition or alternate their focus of care from a strictly curative mode to one of comfort and quality of life.

The original hospice demonstration project in the 1980s was designed as a Medicare program for older adults with cancer as the "typical" disease process. The constantly changing continuum of needs in the pediatric population, from birth through 21-plus years (including diagnoses, variable prognoses, developmental issues and needs, and varying family situations), continues to make it difficult to "fit into" the adult-oriented guidelines for admission and standards of care. These only increase the barriers to access to appropriate care for the dying child and his/her support system. In addition, the eligibility for home health care is restricted enough to make that a barrier to care for those "more well" than children who meet eligibility criteria for hospice enrollment.

### Personal Issues and Biases

Nurses may experience emotional turmoil over their young patients' declining conditions and poor prognoses. The professional role of the nurse may quickly give way to the perspective of a parent, mother, or father toward the child. Expressions of transference may emerge and become problematic to the parents, the child, the nurse, or other team members. In programs where nurses are not clinically trained or emotionally prepared to manage pediatric patients, many issues can emerge as a result of their anguish. Previous losses of a similar nature, unresolved grief issues, conflicting beliefs regarding "supportive care-only" interventions, and insecurities and self-doubt are all common, even within the hospice setting. The "if it were my child" frame of thinking can even be imposed on parents who are already desperately struggling with their child's condition and the future that lies ahead for them. Personal and ethical dilemmas can emerge regarding withdrawal of aggressive care or nutritional support. Interdisciplinary ethics consultations can bring an invaluable contribution to the decision-making process and often raise the option of a hospice consult or referral to hospice care. These nurses can and should be mentored on an ongoing basis as they are exposed to the pediatric patient and family experience.It is not enough to just provide written material or a webinar; they need ongoing mentoring, opportunity to process and get feedback on the outcome of visits, interventions, communication, and real-time direction from experienced palliative care nurses and others. There are many excellent resources available to help even when time is limited before admission to a service, but that is not adequate. There needs to be commitment to avoid any unnecessary, avoidable distress to child/family as a result of the professional angst or lack of preparedness. *It is not about us,* it is about doing what is best for the patient and family.

### Professional Issues

Nurses working in predominantly adult-oriented care settings may lack pediatric physical assessment and symptom-management skills, as well as knowledge of the diverse disease processes and developmental stages and related needs essential to care for neonatal, pediatric, or adolescent patients. Those with a background in aggressive and curative care may find it difficult to support a family in transition to a palliative focus of care. A struggle for control may erupt between the family, the staff, and the child. By continually asking, "Whose need is this meeting?" one can maintain focus on the patient's care.

### Uncertainty in Determining the Child's Prognosis

State and federal regulations and standards governing hospice care and the clinical guidelines for ongoing appropriateness (Medicare and Medicaid) did not address pediatric patients when they were developed. Determining the required 6-months-or-less prognosis is extremely difficult for pediatric physicians because of the wide variability of prognoses in children, often varying from days to weeks or from months to years. Referral to hospice care by physicians also may represent them "giving up" on their young patients. The requirement to certify that the child will die within 6 months is often perceived as a direct assault on the practice of physicians. Parents may still wish to continue active treatment, which may, in fact, prolong their child's life to some extent, but they typically are not ready to "give up everything." Parents should not be forced to give up all treatment to avail themselves of help and guidance to actually make the transition to comfort care.

In addition, there is wide variability as to what—if any—treatments might be acceptable under hospice admission guidelines. Programs vary on whether blood products, antibiotics, infusions, lab tests, and so forth may be conisdered "too aggressive" an approach to care, expecting parents to surrender all means of therapies before enrollment in hospice. This threshold is simply too high for parents when they are seeking any way to achieve a longer life, buying time of weeks or months. The reality is that these interventions may in fact be specifically goal-oriented to relieve a symptom or to arrive at a near future goal or life milestone relationship or, at the least, to preserve quality of life for even a bit longer for family to be together. They usually are *not* considered curative, and thus the regulatory requirement of *foregoing curative treatments* is NOT a conflict. However, these interventions can become a great financial burden or unfeasible for many programs without substantial foundational support. Most hospice programs do not have the financial allowance to provide these more liberal interpretations. Although many treatments would indeed be considered "palliative" in nature versus curative, they would not be covered at too great a cost for typical programs. However, if one looks at this from an *access* perspective, it would be wise to try case-by-case individual considerations and to pursue additional funds to compliment the unreimbursed care rather than to expect all younger patients to accept hospice and to forfeit all treatments and therapies on which they have long been dependent. A gradual de-escalation in the intensity of care will arrive at the same result, and families could benefit from the earlier support of a palliative care team.

These families are not just "waiting longer for death" but are intentionally trying to maximize the "living time" they have left. The resiliency of children is often astounding in the face of information that says they should have only hours or days to live. Adult programs are penalized for patients who do not die fast enough by Medicare criteria, and the pediatric population is even more difficult to predict. Frequent case review and discussions with parents, physicians, the hospice or palliative care team, and, if possible, the child, ensure that everyone has the same goals and perceptions of the child's condition and appropriateness of care.

## Reimbursement Issues

The cost of caring for this population is often a barrier to pursuing pediatrics within a hospice program. Pediatric hospice or palliative care typically requires longer, more frequent home visits; longer time for family meetings and decision-making; more coordination of care with multiple physicians, other providers, and insurance companies; visits to schools by members of the team on behalf of the sick child or siblings; and hiring or access to pediatric experienced nurses, social workers, and child life specialists and aides. Ongoing therapies for palliation of distressing symptoms, including blood transfusions, antibiotics, chemotherapy, and enteral and gavage feedings, typically continues longer for children than adults. The cost and responsibility for covering these therapies may be an additional factor to home-based providers in deciding whether to serve children. Even inpatient settings face some challenges of the additional time and personnel needed for the pediatric palliative care family.

Many states have initiated Medicaid waiver programs that provide a concurrent model of both disease management and palliative care resources to address the whole picture of need for these families.

## Respecting What Parents Want and Need From Their Health-Care Providers

Nurses can support parents and families by identifying their concerns and fears regarding care at home, life outside the security of the hospital, what to expect at home, how they will know when to call for help, how to handle emergencies, and so forth. Nurses have an important role in creating the plans for how they can respond, to anticipate what may happen and have medications, resources, and contacts in place when the time comes. Imagine parents in the home as "first responders," and as such they need to have adequate access to what they need to respond to their child's issue when it arises to the best of their ability. For example, having an "emergency kit" of a few basic medications in one to two doses for common crisis situations can prevent needless fear and suffering with a timely response until help can arrive from a home care nurse. Educating parents as thoroughly as possible for transitions in care and settings will reduce anxiety and unneccesary problems faced at home. Imagine being suddenly thrust into the role of running and owning a new business, being totally responsible for its management and oversight; directing all the people involved 24/7 without any prior knowledge of this business. Imagine you have no preparation or previous experience in this business for assuming this role, yet you face immediate and serious consequences in stepping into that role. That is how parents feel when their child receives diagnosis of a serious illness. A foreign language is spoken all around you and no one translates for you. Our goal is to help parents and children feel confident as well as competent at home and in the hospital setting; to feel cared for and connected to their care team; to be respected in how their cultural and religious or spiritual beliefs influence decision-making and provision of care; and to preserve hope. Parents also desire to retain the responsibility and the right to be parent to their child or infant for whatever time they may have as well as to have control over time, routines, and ritualizing care to make their child feel safe and comfortable. Reducing powerlessness comes from offering elements of control and autonomy as they are each able to assume it. They want to have their child recognized as unique and special and have some semblance of "normalcy" and intimacy allowed in the framework of their existence, whether at home or in a facility. Discussing role and impact on sibling(s) and/or others at home is necessary on an ongoing basis. Assuming a posture of humble curiosity is welcomed by individuals of other cultures when one does not know the culture in-depth to reverse the power structure of who is "teacher" or "mentor." The communication between professional and parents and a child at the end of life must be grounded in caring and compassionate relationships. The work places special demands, not the least of which is an obligation to nurture relationships that can hold both vulnerability and suffering within their embrace: that which is experienced by our child patients and their families, and that which we experience within ourselves.[14] Moving back and forth fluidly between the experts and curious and respectful human beings needs to happen in context of a reciprocal view, not a unidirectional one such as "Delivering Bad News."

## Transitions: Between Settings and Caregivers to Minimize Disruption

Care taken at these critical junctures of change can be well-planned for and will minimize the feelings of surprise and lack of continuity and avoid fragmented communication. The bottom line is preparation and communication. Accountability for these must be a value in the clinical setting so everyone knows their role in insuring notification of who needs to know what and when. Plan ahead for supplies, medications, equipment, and resource people. Know who you are referring to for next caregivers—who can accept pediatric patients at home—identify who is the contact person for the inpatient setting for hand-off of report and updates over time. Because many of these relationships last for long periods of time, it is worth discussing who is best point person for passing on communication in a given setting and then revisiting this periodcially to insure things are working efficiently. Families most certainly feel the successful result or failure of this system for communication. If a child is leaving the facility, suggest a joint meeting with new providers and familiar ones to assist in transfer of trust and support, as well as the instructional aspect of insuring a smooth hand-off from one care team to another. Doing so can give parents confidence in the new nursing staff that will be assisting them in the next setting, whether it is from home to hospital or hospital to community-based nursing care. Clarify expectations on both sides (parents and nursing) and review what changes in the next setting and who to call. Making the effort up front will relieve parents of the uncertainties and insecurities of this "hand-off."

## When the Time Comes: Care at the Time of Death

Nothing can truly prepare a family for the actual death and final goodbyes at the time of dying, but there is much that can be done. In any setting, parents should be prepared for what is likely to occur—within a range of possibilities—and when, what it will look like, feel like, sound like, smell like, and so forth. Consider all the senses for both the adults and any other children who will be present. Parents often appreciate written handouts in language that is not too clinical or frightening so that when they feel they need or want to know, they have it to review. It gives them ways to talk about it as a family and prepare other children and relatives. Fears associated with dying process can include fears about what dramatic events can unfold, fear of being alone at time of death, and an unexpected emergency (realistic or not). Understanding the physical progression as death nears and the nearing death awareness that is common among children and adolescents may be reassuring. Now is the time to review goals for the desired setting for last days or hours of living, and, if possible and important for the family or the patient, nurses can try to facilitate this personal wish if local resources allow for safe and reliable care at home. It may be they desire a private space or room to themselves as a family. Several children's hospital's allocate a room as a "transitional care" room for caring for child as death approaches. Typically, changing locations close to end of life is not desired; however, for some it may be very important—we just need to be sure to inquire what is important to *the family*. Meeting family as soon as they arrive home is the ideal to assist them to settle in and get questions answered with supervision of initial care setting. At this time, families often begin the time of "nesting or cocooning," which reveals an almost reverse of birthing preparation for the next step. This becomes the *heart* of the home. Even the inpatient setting can become the gravitational force for loved ones to gather around the bedside. The tenderness and intimacy of these moments is beyond description and a very precious privilege for those at hand as nurses and other team members. Parents may have concerns about giving a final dose of pain medication, so reassuring them of need to continue comfort care is necessary. When the child has died, check to verify if presence at bedside is desired/needed or if they prefer to be alone. Offer a visit at home, even if just to assist in phone calls or help with some tasks or answer questions as family gathers. In hospital, the family may also just wish to be alone and tend to the child and each other in privacy because of the intimacy and anguish of the event. "Success" can also be measured when family feels confident enough because of the previous mentoring to do this part on their own or asks to be left alone in the hospital setting. Cultural and religious practices may guide what happens at time of death and immediately following, but generally time is allowed for bathing, dressing, holding or rocking child, offering prayers, obtaining handprints (if not obtained before), cutting a lock of hair, and gathering the clothing items that may have the child's scent on them (to be preserved in a timely manner in a zipper bag). Sibling and parents or others can send along a little something with the child's body as symbolic way to remain connected while apart (see Table 54–5).

## Creating a Sacred Space

When a baby or child is dying, the very space becomes a sacred space and following the death inspires something to be done to "hold" that space in dignity for a brief period of time to honor the fact that something very profound happened.

**Table 54–5**
**When the Time Comes: How to Help When a Child Dies in the Home—by Sumner**

*When the call comes in that a baby or child has died in the home, it may be a challenge and even a bit overwhelming to think of what you will do to be of help and comfort to the grieving family. Below are some guidelines that may help you approach the situation a bit more prepared and thus more capable of making the process a little less painful for the parents and family.*

1. Most parents may not directly ask for a home visit, but usually appreciate and often—benefit from a visit at the time of the child's death. Just having someone there to help orchestrate the process when they may be feeling overwhelmed and paralyzed by their grief will be helpful. If they refuse, then there are still things to do over the phone that will be helpful for them. It is most likely that they will not need the nurse or other team members to stay for the entire time until the child is taken from the home.

2. The family should be allowed to have as much time as they need with their baby or child before the mortuary comes to take their child's body. It may seem unusual to you that they would want to keep the body for many hours, but it is a very final step to have their child taken from the home. The mortuary can be notified with the appropriate information required at time of death but informed that the family will contact them directly when they are ready.

3. Try to suggest to the parents/caregivers to take some private time alone with their child, without all the family around. This is a very intimate and personal time for them and may help to facilitate the process of "letting go" and saying goodbye. Others in the family may also wish to have some private time with the child to say a personal goodbye.

4. Encourage the parents/adults present to give any other children in the home or family the choice to go in and say goodbye. Children of most any age are able to decide for themselves if they want to see the child who has died. By just offering the child the choice, it has given the child a sense of control during an unfamiliar and unsettling experience. They will remember that someone thought enough of them and their relationship with the person who died to give them the chance to say goodbye. The child should be prepared in simple language for what the child will look and feel like, that they will not move, and so forth. It's a good idea to remove any tubing from infusions, oxygen tubing, catheters, and so forth to normalize the appearance at the bedside as much as possible. Someone he/she feels safe with should accompany the child. If the family plans on cremation, this may be the last opportunity for them to see their sibling, thus there may not be a second chance if not now. The child may wish to go in for just a "peek" or they may be curious and want to stay around. Whatever length of time the child chooses to stay is okay and should be up to them.

5. Allow parents to have the time they need to perform any private rituals or activities, which may include bathing the little one, redressing the child into something special, rocking, a blessing or time for prayer around the bedside. They may wish to have their priest, minister, or chaplain come to the home.

6. Offer the parents the suggestion of saving a lock of hair if they have not already done so. They may not feel comfortable doing this themselves and may wish for the staff person to do this. The nape of the neck or the back of the head is the best places to obtain a swatch of hair. It can be tied with a piece of yarn, thread or ribbon. The hair can be placed in an envelope and sealed. Explain that they may not wish to look at it or have it now but that some day they may be glad they had this small remembrance, something tangible that connects them to their loved one, their precious child. A comfortable way to present these suggestions to the family is to say that these are some ideas and suggestions that other parents/families have found to be comforting. They may choose to do all or none of these activities, the point is to make it meaningful for themselves as a family.

7. There are instances when the family may want to take pictures of the child after death. They may wish to keep them for relatives who live away or for cultural reasons. A family may ask for your assistance to do so, or they may obtain them at the mortuary.

8. If the primary team has not already done so, it may be important to offer the suggestion of taking handprints and/or footprints of the infant or child. Someone could go out to purchase an inkpad, poster paints or tempera paints if nothing is available in the home with which to improvise. These supplies are available to the staff in the resource area. Keep a soapy washcloth or alcohol handy to quickly remove the coloring from the extremity. It's best to try to do the prints as soon as possible before any stiffening of the body sets in. Again, if there are other children in the home it will be significant to obtain at least one print for the sibling to have for later on. Other family members can add their handprints also, creating a "family portrait" of hands.

9. When contacting the mortuary, emphasize that it was a child that died so that they will be sensitive to the situation they will face. When they arrive at the home, the family may need to say a last goodbye. Rather than have the child taken from the home by the mortuary attendants, we have found that is much less painful if one of the adults/parents carries the child out to the vehicle and surrenders over their child to the arms of the attendants. Parents have told us it felt less traumatic than if they stood back and the baby was taken out by "strangers." Occasionally this process becomes an informal processional to accompany the child out of the home for the last time.

10. If at all possible when the child is ready to be carried out of the home, ask the attendant to keep the child's face and head uncovered and not enclosed completely. The use of the body bag is very distressing and offensive to most parents/family. Perhaps the child can be wrapped in special blanket and/or a sheet. Sometimes the driver is willing to take the little one partially covered like this until away from the home, and then secure the child's body after leaving the area. Siblings can add a special keepsake to accompany the child's body (e.g., a note, flower, drawing, or stuffed toy).

11. Remind the family of the local bereavement support resources available to them (community or your own organization) and how/when the primary team will be following up. Request that arrangements for funeral/memorial service be communicated to the child's care team unless it is private, family-only. If visits are made after hours, notify primary team, including MDs, of how the family is coping and report on events surrounding the child's death. The primary team can follow-up with their sick child's or sibling's school with permission from the parents.

This also allows for a breathing space between assignments or use of that space. Some programs place a rose on the bed, a special sign on the door, or an image of a dove, butterfly, nightlight, or leaf to subtly designate this sacred space. Honoring and respecting the space also models to staff that it is not just "business as usual," for a brief time at least. At home, the sleeping area can be tidied up but not stripped for a time. Same signage or symbolism might be comforting. Again handling the transitions with care makes these painful circumstances a bit more bearable. Allowing the father to carry the child out to the vehicle that will transport to mortuary (if permissable by local regulations) can be a powerful and loving tribute, like an honor guard, and this is a task the father can assume as a final loving act of care. Siblings can tuck a note or picture or flower in with child as a symbol of their connectedness.

Following the time of death, the nursing staff benefits from the support of supervision to allow for a brief respite, break, or time away from setting. In some instances, they are given lighter caseload or, if necessary, have time to debrief with another colleague, chaplain, or other designee. The moral and spiritual distress comes from accompanying the family through such emotional territory; even when death comes gently and peacefully, it takes an emotionally resilient person to adjust and switch to the next task at and. Preserving the meaning and satisfaction from this demanding work requires self-discipline and intentionality to tend to one's own spirituality and whatever it takes for renewal and reflection on outside time or in even a few minutes a nurse finds in the day. Great wisdom can be gained, burdens lessened, and insights gained in a staff support encounter or a more clinical debrief session, sharing what strategies worked and how to improve keeps the care and approaches in continual development and growth.

Participating in community-based programs, coalitions regarding children's health-care issues, collaborations on grief and loss of children, and presenting cases at grand rounds and professional meetings are all excellent ways to connect with other providers and develop vital linkages for a thriving pediatric palliative care program. Trust is transferred between inpatient and home care/hospice staff as a result of seeing, hearing, and experiencing what the other has to offer. The patients and families become more confident if they sense the confidence in those who make the referral. Once trust and accountability have been established, they can form a strong and lasting foundation that can be passed on to new members as they join the team. The need for ongoing, honest, and open communication between the two groups is critical.

Agencies and institutions are challenged with the moral responsibility to make the right decision for the dying child and his/her family, informing them of all relevant options to best meet the needs of the child. It may be in the child's best interest for a home care agency to refer the child to another, more appropriately qualified provider, such as a hospice program, if the program is better equipped to provide end-of-life care for the child. The multidimensional experience of a terminal illness requires attention to all aspects of the child's, parents', and siblings' needs, including spiritual, physical, emotional, and psychosocial needs. An individual nurse may feel overwhelmed by the enormous burden of trying to meet all those needs alone or may experience intense frustration and helplessness in not being able to do so at all within the limitations of traditional home health care. Difficulties can also arise when a referral to hospice care is offered but refused by families based on unfamiliarity and perhaps dependency on the home health care nurse.

Possible solutions to this situation might be a joint case conference to discuss the family's issues and concerns or making a few joint, overlapping visits to transfer trust and to ease the often well-established relationships to the hospice team. These may be nonreimbursed visits, but they may create an openness between the two programs and increase referrals. These visits may require discussions with the parents regarding their fears and concerns and how their needs might be met.

## Transitioning Between Adult and Pediatric Patients: Staffing Issues

Many hospices are not staffed with nurses who are comfortable dealing with babies, young children, and adolescents who are dying or with the unique issues of the parents and/or extended family. Because the family's outlook is greatly influenced by the personalities and reactions of the staff, a special degree of confidence and caring is required.[15] After-hours staffing poses a particular challenge, and sometimes a hardship, on the agency and its staff. Adult care staff may be unwilling or incapable of caring for pediatric patients. The most serious outcome would be added stress and uncertainty imposed by the very experts from whom families are seeking refuge and comfort. Partnering with pediatric staff to train other staff as well as thorough reporting to the after-hours staff are helpful actions. Anticipation of needs and problems with a plan for appropriate treatment can minimize and even prevent symptom crises. Implementing a curriculum-based training on caring for the seriously ill or dying child can be done in a variety of ways. Interdisciplinary case discussions, 1-hour lunch-and-learn sessions to cover key care issues, scheduled over several weeks can result in a commitment from nursing and other staff to then form a committee or a special task force. Small funding can even help to support a training program in palliative care strategies for symptom management, communication, addressing culture and spirituality, bereavement, ethics and decision-making in the neonatal and pediatric end-of-life milieu. As mentioned previously, the curriculum available currently include the Pediatric ELNEC curriculum of 10 modules with cases, key references, supplemental teaching tools and resources, current practice highlights, and models of excellence. The Initiative for Pediatric Palliative Care (IPPC) sponsored by the Educational Development Center (EDC) is an interdisicplinary model of case-based experiential training, usually held in a retreat-style event for 3 days; small group and plenary structure and accompanying films as instructional medium as well as the curriclum is available at www.ippcweb.org.[16] A distinguishing feature is the emphasis on including parents in the role as faculty and peer in the training. With proper preparation and clear expectations, hearing from parents—the firsthand experts—can be an invaluable asset to the learning experience. The National Hospice and Palliative Care Organization (NHPCO) has a pediatric curriculum that is currently being revised to address the ongoing demand for training for adult hospice programs to be prepared to care for children as well as to address the pediatric palliative care issues for a larger audience, interdisciplinary in focus. In a related special focus, Association of Women's Health and Neonatal Nursing has a well-respected established curriculum on Perinatal Loss, which was revised in 2008–2009 to incorporate the elements of perinatal palliative care in its curriculum; this curriculum is utilized in hospitals around the country to meet competency goals in this area.

## Cultural Issues

Various cultures approach the child with a terminal illness differently. This involves decision-making, communication, openness with the patient, the role of the parents in protecting the child from the truth about his/her condition, the role that religion or faith plays in health-care issues, and determination of who can translate for the family respectfully. Language barriers and lack of translation options can create great obstacles to providing adequate care. For example, parents may direct staff not to address the dying process with the child so as not to discourage the child. They may believe that in saying "it" aloud, it will cause "it" to come to pass. Or simply speaking of death may be too direct within the context of their culture. Hope is often intertwined in cultural issues and in the expression of that culture within the experience of serious illness. For some families, this may necessitate frequent and ongoing reteaching and subsequent validation that a plan for collaborative care has been respected. These issues of decision-making are of particular relevance to adolescents, as they play a more active role in decision-making regarding illness and end-of-life care.[17]

## Crossing Over into the Adult World

Pediatric palliative care professionals can be an outstanding resource to the colleagues who care for adult patients who have children impacted by their illness. Focus on the children in adult patient families is not typically as extensive as with siblings in a pediatric case. They may not be seen by the medical team, invisible in the complex network of settings and providers, or may be shielded from the experience and not well-identified. However, they do exist and they do need support and attention from early in the illness through bereavment after the parent or grandparent

has died. Typically, a wide variety of bereavement support is available in many communities that address the grieving child who has had a death but do not address the needs and concerns or including of children *prior* to the death. It is here that the nurse or other team member in palliative care for children can be a wealth of knowledge, guidance, and expertise for those caring for the adult patient with children in family. This one area of intersection between the world of adult and pediatric palliative and hospice care gives hope to the author that indeed all children will have their emotional needs met as the family faces a serious illness and end of life—that children will have their grief honored, have the choice and blessing to be part of the journey with their parent or other family member, and be prepared and supported in age-appropriate care. Once the person dies, there is no going back to obtain detailed remembrances, keepsakes, letters, and intimate moments and conversations. This is also a strategy to justify the expert pediatric trained staff when they can be utilized in both areas or they enhance the care for families at the other end of the spectrum of care. Their interventions include opportunities for play and art activities; rituals and keepsake activities for themselves or the family; therapeutic games; and storybooks on coping with feelings and illness, grief and loss, death and dying, the life cycle of nature, funerals, and so forth. The place to begin is helping them with understanding the illness itself, then how to understand the emotional and behavioral changes they are experiencing in the family and especially changes in their loved one who is sick. Nurses can help them know how to ask for information so they can better understand what's going on aorund them. They benefit from help in how to express their feelings in a healthy and safe way. Children benefit from having this type of guidance *before* the parent has died. These children are often considered invisible in the care setting if they are not physically present and yet have much at stake for decades of adjustment ahead of them. Like siblings in pediatric hospice care, they deserve special attention and individual support when a parent or other loved one is nearing end of life.

The family-centered care team extends the circle of care to involve the child's or childrens' school in its web of support for the family (whether sick child or parent). Typically (with parental permission), the staff will confer or even meet with the teacher, school counselor, or nurse to include them in the plan of care. The aim is to facilitate more involvement of the child in the illness experience before the death occurs, maximizing their support systems as well as their ability to cope with the death when it does occur. A great deal can be done to better prepare children for the death and loss of a loved one by early intervention. Besides anticipatory grieving, many practical issues, fears, and concerns emerge for the children and their caregivers. In addition, the team provides adult caregivers with strategies and education regarding children's needs during the loved one's illness and in bereavement. The expertise of those familiar with developmental issues and needs of children can be an invaluable resource to adult palliative and hospice care programs to achieve a truly family centered and holistic approach. Children take the grief and loss from the death a parent or sibling along with them into the years ahead. We must do what we can before the death to provide them with the understanding, tools, insights and inner resources that will help them navigate the path that lies ahead for them in the years to come.

Families are never fully prepared for a child to be gone from their lives. The palliative care nurse can take steps to assist them down the long road of bereavement by helping them create tangible reminders of and treasures from their child's life, no matter how short or long it was. Families might create a memory box with the child using special things that remind the child of favorite activities, trips, people, accomplishments—anything that helps to celebrate the child's life. Letters and journals can also be created by parents, the sick child, and siblings and friends. The most popular activity with families is doing handprints. This is done by making handprints of the baby or child, along *with* those of the parents, siblings, and others, using tempera or poster paint to create a unique family portrait. Ear prints can be taken of a baby with anomalies of the extremities and as another way of preserving something physical of the child. An "All About Me" booklet can be created over time through regular visits of a volunteer or family member, capturing the child's identity before and after the illness and his/her role as part of a family. Schoolmates can send notebooks or letters back and forth to stay connected, and later these can become lovely remembrances of friendships.

The possibilities are endless, and these tangible keepsakes may help siblings and parents stay better connected to memories and significant events as they pass through developmental milestones over the years. These physical tokens may help relatives find their way back to special memories and events concerning their loved one. These treasures may help them to survive their experience a bit more whole, having a "toolbox" to help them integrate this tremendous loss into their being and may help them to create a sense of meaning about the experience over time. The author refers to them as "Landmarks for Memories." The definition of these two words makes a concrete image of why they are so important.

- *Landmark*: A fixed marker, as a concrete block indicating a boundary line. An event marking an important phase of development or decisive moment in history. Building or site that has historical and often aesthetic importance.
- *Memory*: The mental faculty of retaining and recalling past experiences; the act of an instance of remembrance: recollection; something remembered; the fact of being remembered.

Through the physical connection or experience with concrete objects and items of personal significance, family and friends can literally find their way back to a connection or trigger a connection to a memory of the deceased child through connecting with these tangible keepsakes. Examples include ordinary and special clothing, toys, favorite food items, photos, scented items, things to remember scents they loved, and favorite activity symbols. Then over years to come, when they need it, the loved one can reconnect through these boxes containing "treasures."

## Overview of Nursing Care Issues for Pediatric Palliative Care

Nursing responsibilities when caring for a dying infant or child are extensive. An awareness of "total suffering" requires that the nurse understand the interconnectedness of these four aspects of the experience of illness and suffering: physical, emotional/psychological, spiritual, and social. Each component greatly affects the others. In the words of Attig, "Suffering is the experience of brokenness. Illness unravels the pattern that belongs uniquely to each child, interrupting the ongoing stories of children's lives."[18] Nurses must assess for imbalances and indications of suffering in each of these areas to appropriately intervene. Without physical comfort, a child has little energy to be "present" to those around him/her and engage in meaningful exchanges. Management of symptoms in infants, children, and adolesecents requires the same degree of diligence and aggressive intervention as that used for adult patients.

Symptoms in children are generally similar to those in adults. However, discomfort/seizure management, pain in nonverbal patients, and feeding issues are more common. The age and developmental level of the child directly influence the selection of pain assessment tools, intervention strategies, route of medication, and type of medication. Many excellent resources are available to nurses for gaining competence in pain and symptom management for children. In addition, families require practical help, information, explanations, and support. Attention must be paid to the practical issues of preparing for pediatric-appropriate supplies, medications, formulas, feeding tubes, medical equipment, documentation, and teaching tools for parents and children. A gently written, parent-friendly handout on the signs and symptoms of approaching death is an invaluable tool.

## Interaction with School

To provide education, support, and resources to classmates, teachers, and other parents, the team goes to the school of the sick child. The bridge developed between the hospice and palliative care professionals and schools has become a standard element of pediatric palliative care, another characteristic distinguishing it from adult palliative care. The unit of care becomes: child + family + school. The onsite support may vary depending on resources available, but printed materials, phone consultation with faculty and administration, or case meetings at school can make good use of time and disseminate helpful approaches and resources and identify who to call for help.

## Support for Siblings

Two unique areas of concern when dealing with a pediatric population are the issues of the parents and those of the siblings. Siblings require explanations along the way and opportunities to be included, not excluded, from these experiences that affect the entire family. Siblings relish the chance to be helpers to nurses and parents as a way to feel important and contribute to the tasks at hand. Helping serves to validate their relationship with the sick child, can diminish their feelings of helplessness, and may well affect how they integrate the loss over time.

As mentioned earlier, similarly to the children of adult patients, the goal for siblings of terminally ill children is to enhance their feelings of involvement to the greatest degree possible while the sibling is alive to facilitate a healthy grieving process. The attempt to assist in achieving "effective coping with and grieving for" the sibling must begin when the sick child is diagnosed, because the family is changed profoundly from that moment.

Strategies for including siblings in care may be as simple as the nurse including the siblings in his/her visit or bedside check in the hospital, asking to see their rooms or favorite toys, or reading a story together. Joint visits with a social worker are highly effective in spreading the attention and interventions among the sick child, siblings, and parents. It is important to repeatedly evaluate the well child's level of understanding about the sibling's condition. Family meetings are also a good setting in which to discuss how everyone is doing (including the patient), how they each perceive the situation, how their needs are (or are not) being met, and how their fears and concerns can be addressed. With parents' permission, an occasional small treat for the sibling is a simple gesture that may help make the well children feel special and included. Hospice and hospital volunteers make an excellent addition to the team for the specific role of being available to the sibling for a picnic, playing outside, reading, or a specific project or memory-making activity. A really simple, inexpensive and memorable activity is handprinting with the whole family. The sick baby or child is handprinted with poster board and tempera or poster paint and the rest of the family's handprints are placed around the child's. The activity lifts the family from focusing on the tasks of the illness to a playful yet reverent level. Subsequently, the print becomes a treasure for the family. The same activity can be done with children of a dying adult as a keepsake for the children. Siblings may wish to have their own set of prints as well. Parents and children are also given "memory boxes" to store treasures in. The best example for this is using photo storage boxes as inexpensive durable containers that can be decorated with photos on lid, stickers, or the handprint of child (adult patients can use these activities for their children as well).

## Support for Parents

To counterbalance the overwhelming sense of powerlessness and helplessness parents frequently feel, nurses can help to identify ways in which they can feel more in control. For example, with ongoing preparation for anticipated changes in the child's condition, a nurse can have medications in the home or instructions written for whom and when to call for assistance.[19]

Typically, parents of dying children have two overriding concerns: a fear of a sudden or acute increase in pain that they will be unable to manage, especially as death approaches, and fear of a crisis situation or unexpected change in condition, including how and when death may occur. It is critical to address these issues on an ongoing basis.

The need to feel a sense of control is also relevant to the sick child, who may be fearful from experiencing so many physical and emotional changes. Nurses can assist parents with methods to help their child gain control over aspects of his/her experience, retain choices regarding care, and feel comfortable with a daily routine, all of which have great affirmational value. Managing medication regimens and symptoms is a daunting task for parents, having enormous impact on the family.[20] Nurses should consider the overall responsibilities of parents for managing care as well as maintaining family routines when planning medication and treatment regimens with the physician. "Partnership for Parents" now fills a void for parents facing a child's diagnosis through a Web-based resource—available to anyone, anywhere—starting from time of diagnosis, through treatment phase, and as disease progresses, facing possibility of end of life and time surrounding dying process, and finally into bereavement following the death of their baby or child. The Children's Hospice and Palliative Care Coalition in CA has established this unprecedented and evolving presence when parents need it most. It was created with extensive parent review, writing, and overall involvement along with many professionals who are experts in the field. It has created a source for comfort, support, validation, and tender reassurance for parents to access at any time, day or night, when the concerns are on their minds, and they have place to turn now for help and information.[21]

## Preserving Hope and Questioning God in the Midst of Serious Illness

A common characteristic of pediatric patients and their families is a prevailing and powerful experience of hope, evidenced in their language and decision-making. It is important to preserve and nurture hope during all stages of the child's life-threatening illness. No matter how grim the situation, one should always strive to deal with matters in a positive, yet realistic, manner. The focus of hope inevitably must change over time—for example, from hope for cure, to hope for a longer remission than previously, to hope that the child can continue to be cared for at home, or to hope that the child will die without pain. Hope has a powerful and practical place within these families. With the presence of hope, parents speak of being able to continue their caregiving responsibilities, having the strength to put one foot in front of the other, and being able to carry on in their day-to-day existence. Without hope, the burden of the child's impending death would be utterly paralyzing. Hope offers opportunities for growth for the child and family. Examples of a child's hopes are a wish to return to school once more, to celebrate an important birthday, or to reach a significant milestone or rite of passage. Other expressions of hope include planning for a visit from grandparents, having friends gathered together, or even gaining the understanding that their loved ones will, indeed, survive after they die.

Addressing spiritual needs of children and families is an area with great need for improvement.[22] Views on life and living are seriously challenged, if not shattered, at least temporarily when a child has a life-threatening illness. Reactions are visceral, distressing, and visual in how parents describe the impact of the diagnosis. Most people have some kind of belief system—a way of looking at their lives, the meaning of their existence, and a connection to something outside of themselves. This view can be a lifeline to "survival" for families as they work through the many challenges to their changed world. "Why is this happening to me? Why me? Why our child?" Despite the gravity of the future, there are somehow times of profound joy and tenderness, and even celebration, that are beyond common description. Their deepest fears and dark moments may be lifted to some degree by seeking the insight and comfort that one's beliefs may offer. Parents and children need to be encouraged to hold onto them and allow support from friends, family, community, clergy, hospital/palliative care team, and even nature to wrap them in care and comfort.

## Hospice and Palliative Care for Infants

When a dying child is an infant, the need for hope is similar, but time constraints are severe. Parents may need support and encouragement to consider going home with their baby to have the opportunity to "welcome baby home." They may be offered a selection of "keepsake" activities to consider to preserve the presence of their little one's life and record the connectedness they had for such a brief period. For them, it may be a simultaneous greeting and farewell. Strengthening this experience may help diminish long-term psychological implications for parents and siblings. Palliative care in neonatal intensive care and other settings of infant care has evolved in many levels.[23]

CASE STUDY
*Baby Michael*

Baby Michael was born with a hypoplastic left ventricle and was not expected to survive more than a few days. His parents were determined to take him home with them for whatever time they could manage and were eager to plan and fulfill this hope. The team worked quickly with the NICU team to arrange for his discharge and to be met at home by a pediatric hospice nurse and social worker. At

home, they were admitted to the hospice program and settled in as family gathered to be with Michael. Together, they created the opportunity to welcome Michael into the family and into their home. Michael kept them awake a lot with typical new baby needs. He died quietly in the early morning hours of the following day. Although to many it seemed tragic, his parents were grateful that they had been able to truly be parents for 1 day. In those hours, they were able to etch some precious yet ordinary memories that other parents have and experience the normal stresses as well as provide the comfort all babies need.

The implications for staff in caring for dying infants and children are enormous. Some are more suited for this field than others. Key personal attributes of those identified as successful in this role include a high tolerance for ambiguity and flexibility; an appreciation for individual differences; good external support networks; a realistic awareness of personal limits; a joy for life in general; a sense of humor; an open communication style; a tendency to value self-awareness as an asset; empathy; and a willingness to learn continually. Being able to function in a self-directed mode facilitates using one's own resourcefulness to meet the challenges of an ever-fluctuating schedule.

Perhaps the most basic necessary characteristic is a comfort with death. Only by coming to terms with one's own thoughts and feelings about death is it possible to adapt philosophically to working with children who will die. Swanson-Kauffman developed a model of caring for nurses dealing with perinatal loss. She stated that fundamental to caring is understanding the personal meanings of the loss; resonating emotionally with the mother's feelings; offering realistic support, nurture, and protection; facilitating the expression of grief; and helping maintain her faith in her capacity to come through her loss as a functioning, whole person.[24] These also apply to the baby's father.

Even a brief life is mourned for a very long time. Seeds for more effective grieving may be planted for the long journey ahead to recovery and healing.

## The Future Unfolding for Pediatric Palliative Care

Ongoing efforts for change and reform are still needed for addressing the ethical issues related to removing life-sustaining therapies when the prognosis is bleak and de-escalating extremely aggressive care with a dying child and the needs of medically fragile children who have a slowly deteriorating condition to the needs of children who die in the emergency department or in the ICU on intensive support. Prospective hospice, home health, and intensive care nurses need to be acclimated to the reality that infants and children tragically do die, and it will take many more trained and competent professional nurses to make the best care both possible and available to all those who so need and deserve it. Infants, children, adolescents, and young parents are part of the continuum of palliative care.

There is much to be done to support these families and advance the quality of end-of-life care for infants and children. Each step toward increasing awareness regarding these issues is a step forward on behalf of the children who are dying without access to all the resources available to them and their loved ones.

Nurses who choose to care for dying infants and children and their families need a significant support system themselves to maintain the difficult and delicate task of balancing perspectives. However, in doing so, nurses receive a spiritual treasure that only comes from experience with these children, parents, siblings, and others around them—heightened awareness of how very precious life is. Families share their wisdom from their tragedy, urging others to make the most of each moment in their own lives with their own loved ones. The courage and strength observed in families on this pilgrimage is humbling and strengthening at once. Those who stand "close to the fire" cherish and are grateful for the opportunity to be eyewitnesses to one of life's most intimate and powerful experiences.

*I did not know how it would impact me. No patient young or old will ever feel the same after caring for this child.—A hospice nurse*

Through collaborative efforts among leaders in pediatric palliative and hospice care, children's healthcare, and various branches of government, plans are moving forward for appropriations and site applications for various demonstration projects. Pediatric palliative care aims to raise the consciousness of our society, which claims to value children as a treasured resource. If this is so, then we must treasure them and honor them in sickness and in health, in living and dying, until death do they part from us.

REFERENCES

1. Field MJ, Behrman RE. When Children Die: Improving Palliative and End-of-Life Care for Children and Their Families (Report of the Institute of Medicine Task Force). Washington, DC: National Academy Press, 2003.
2. National Consensus Project Guidelines for Quality Palliative Care. 2004. http://www.nationalconsensusproject.org (accessed February 7, 2005).
3. Children's Hospice Coalition. 2007. www.childrenshospice.org (accessed October 2009).
4. NHPCO. November 2006. NEWSLINE.
5. Pediatric Palliative Care Standards, Alexandria, VA: National Hospice and Palliative Care Organization, 2009.
6. Society of Pediatric Nursing. Scope and standards of Practice. July 2008.
7. Children's Hospice International. 1993. http://www.chionline.org (accessed October 2009).
8. Association for children with life-threatening or terminal conditions and their families (ACT). Royal College of Paediatrics and Child Health A Guide to the Development of Children's Palliative Care Services (2nd ed). ACT, Bristol, 2003.
9. Perinatal Hospice: A gift of time. www.perinatallhospice.org. (accessed October 2009).
10. Taking palliative care into pregnancy and perinatal loss: qa model for community collaboration. Washington, DC: National Association of Perinatal Social Workers. October 2003.
11. Sumner L, Kavanaugh K, Moro T. Extending palliative care into pregnancy and the immediate newborn period: The state of the practice of perinatal palliative care. J Perinat Neonatal Nurs 2006;20(1):113–116.
12. Seyda B, Fitzsimons A, Rothman E. When a Child Is Dying: The Supportive Care Handbook. Chapel Hill: Compassionate Passages, Inc. 2002.
13. Walter Vincent Brooks. Washington post 9/1,2002. Monique Olivia McIntyre.
14. Browning D. To show our humanness-relational and communicative competence in pediatric palliative care. Bioethics Forum 2003;18(3/4):23–28.
15. Stevens M. Psychological adaptation of the dying child. In: Doyle D, Hanks GWC, Cherny N, Calman K, eds. Oxford Textbook of Palliative Medicine (3rd ed). Oxford: Oxford University Press; 2004:798–806.
16. Initiative for Pediatric Palliative Care: www.pediatricpalliativecare.org or www.ippcweb.org (accessed October 2009).
17. Edwards J. A model of palliative care for the adolescent with cancer. Int J Palliative Nurs 2001;7:485–488.
18. Attig T. Beyond pain: The existential of children. J Palliat Care 1996;12:20–23.
19. Laasko H, Paunonen-Illonen M. Mothers' experience of social support following the death of a child. J Clin Nurs 2002;11:176–185.
20. Ferrell BR, Rhiner M, Shapiro B, et al. The Family experience of cancer and pain management in children. Cancer Pract 1994;2:441–446.
21. Partnerhsip for Parents: A Support Network for Parents of Children with Serious Illnesses. www.partnershipforparents.org (accessed October 2009).
22. Davies B, Brenner P, Orloff S, Sumner L, Worden W. Addressing spirituality in pediatric hospice and palliative care. J Palliat Care 2002;18:59–67.
23. Catlin A, Carter B. Creation of a neonatal end-of-life palliative care protocol. J Perinatol 2002;22:184–195.
24. Swanson-Kauffman K. Caring in the instance of unexpected early pregnancy loss. Top Clin Nurs 1986;8:37–46.

# 55

*Marcia Levetown, Melody Brown Hellsten, and Barbara Jones*

# Pediatric Care: Transitioning Goals of Care in the Emergency Department, Intensive Care Unit, and In Between

*Every word that was said the day Becky died is indelibly etched in my mind. I have replayed the words in my mind a million times. It's a never-ending tape.—Pam Borchart[1]*

♦ **Key Points**

♦ *Most children who die experience acute, unexpected death.*

♦ *Attention to the grieving family and organized bereavement programs can improve the outcome of emergency department (ED) deaths.*

♦ *Chronically ill children also often die in the intensive care unit (ICU); effective advance care planning, often beginning in the ICU and involving the child when possible, can prevent this.*

♦ *Compassionate, respectful, effective, consistent, bidirectional communication is a high priority for families of children who die in the ICU.*

♦ *Parents need to maintain a parenting role when their child is ill, even during invasive procedures and CPR.*

♦ *Parents need ackowledgment of their love and efforts and assistance with their spiritual needs.*

♦ *Clarity of facts and ethical principles among family and staff enables good medical decision-making and prevents regrets.*

♦ *The vast majority of children die after forgoing ICU interventions; this event can be transformed into a celebration of life.*

♦ *Grief and bereavement of family and staff must be addressed; clear evidence about effective interventions is lacking.*

♦ *Autopsies and post-death conferences can be very reassuring to parents.*

Palliative care is comprehensive, transdisciplinary care focused on promoting the maximal quality of life for patients living with a life-threatening illness and their families.[2–5] It can and should occur from the earliest recognition of a life-threatening condition and can be concurrent with efforts to prolong life.[3–7] Palliative care is as applicable in the emergency department (ED)[8–10] and in the intensive care unit (ICU) setting[11–16] as it is in the home;[3–5] this is a critically important issue for children who die, since the vast majority of childhood deaths occur in an ICU setting.[17–23] In fact, Wanzer and colleagues[24] state:

> *As sickness progresses toward death, measures to minimize suffering should be intensified. Dying patients may require palliative care of an intensity that rivals that of curative efforts. Even though aggressive curative techniques are no longer indicated, profe ssionals and families are still called on to use intensive measures— extreme responsibility, extraordinary sensitivity, and heroic compassion.*

Scrupulous attention to communication, symptom control, social support for the family and patient, and grief management have not been a traditional focus of health-care delivery or training for emergency and critical care personnel.[25–31] Working together in effective interdisciplinary teams, learning new ways of communicating, using protocols where appropriate, and new tools for patient and family assessment, we can meet these patients' and their families' needs for a peaceful, family-centered death.[32–36] Specific suggestions for family-centered and palliative care in the ED and ICU have recently been published.[8–14,37–40] Nurses can and should play a key role in effecting this philosophy of care. Although individuals and families differ in the details and nuances of their conception of a good death, common themes emerge[11,27,41–47] (see Table 55–1).

---

**Table 55–1**
**Elements Enabling a Good Death**

- Clear, honest, and easily accessible information provided throughout the illness
- Anticipatory guidance to limit suffering
- Compassion
- Symptom control
- Social support
- Support for parents to maintain a significant parenting role
- Unfettered access to the ill child
- Spiritual support
- Adequate space and means for self-care
- Sibling needs assessment and assistance
- Bereavement care and contact by healthcare providers

---

Given that few children ill enough to be in the ICU can participate in the discussion, research has centered primarily on the needs of their families.

## Epidemiology of Pediatric Death

Approximately 53,000 children die annually in the United States. Infants (children under age 1 year), who account for more than 50% of childhood deaths, die primarily of congenital defects and prematurity; however, sudden infant death syndrome (SIDS) and trauma (including unintentional injury and homicide) account for 12% of infant deaths. For children age 1 year to 24 years, 61% of deaths are the result of trauma, while the remaining 39% are the result of cancer, congenital anomalies, and metabolic defects.[48] Traumatic injury and unexpected overwhelming illness occurring in previously healthy children usually call for initial resuscitative measures provided in ED and ICU settings; many of these children will unavoidably die there, too.[10,16,18–20,22,37,49] In fact, 20% of childhood deaths are declared in the emergency department each year,[8] whereas 4.6% of pediatric ICU and 10% to 20% of trauma ICU admissions end in death, together accounting for 40–90% of childhood deaths.[15,17] Consideration of palliative care issues must therefore be a part of the care plan for critically ill or injured children at admission to the ED and the PICU, as well as at discharge if the child survives.[8–10,12–14,16, 18,20,45,50] Bereavement care for families, including siblings, is a critical but often neglected need when pediatric death occurs in acute care settings.[8–10,12–14,16,20,27,38,47,50–59]

Regardless of the etiology, anticipated or unanticipated illness or injury, the care of a critically ill or injured child should be family-focused, while conveying fundamental respect and a culturally appropriate commitment to shared decision-making with the parent(s). All dying children and their families require appropriate (1) facilities, (2) information, (3) support, and (4) involvement in care and decision-making.[8–14,28,47,51–53,60–61]

## Palliative Care Considerations in the Emergency Department: Acute Unexpected Illness or Injury

Children experiencing a life-threatening event can present to the ED either having been transported by emergency medical system (EMS) providers after a potentially dramatic "on site" resuscitation effort or by frantic parents. The initial scene in the ED is often one of controlled chaos, with all personnel attending to the assessment and stabilization of the child. Some of these children are trauma victims, benefiting from a thorough assessment, rapid intervention, and pain control before a prognosis can be determined. For the child arriving in full arrest, the overwhelmingly likely outcome is death, whether in the ED or in the ICU a few days later.[62–73] In the absence of severe trauma, intoxication or congenital heart disease, primary cardiac causes of arrest among children are exceedingly rare. Thus, if cardiac arrest has occurred, either the child is irreversibly dying of multiorgan failure or has sustained prolonged hypoxemia; neither of these underlying causes of arrest is amenable to resuscitation with intact survival. Misperceptions of a high likelihood of good outcomes following resuscitation from cardiac arrest have been documented and must be addressed in the care of these children and their families.[74–78]

### Needs of Parents of Suddenly Ill/Injured Children in the ED

Assigning a professional to guide the parents from the moment of their arrival can facilitate communication, even given the severe time pressures of the ED.[9] This professional should greet the parents by name, introduce himself/herself and provide a card with his or her name and contact information. The family should be apprised of the child's situation, and the child should be referred to by name.[79,80] This guide should also address parents' practical needs, such as offering a blanket or water and assist to gather the family's supporters.[55] An interpreter should be summoned immediately, if needed.[8]

Especially in the ED, parents of acutely injured children prefer to be given timely, accurate, and consistent information that is easy to understand.[8–10] Information provided should be responsive to family members' questions and concerns. In addition, important issues of which the family may not be aware should be raised as needed. Extended family members or friends can often help the parents sort through the information and help them know what to ask. Although "information" emphasizes content, the nuances of "communication," or the process by which information is exchanged demands attention as well.[54,81] All family members of critically ill or dying children need to feel respected and valued. Grief under these extraordinarily stressful circumstances can be totally debilitating and incapacitating. This is the context in which parents are often asked to make decisions which, when worded poorly, imply choices between life and death; it may

**Table 55–2**
**Consensus Recommendations for Family Presence (FP) During Invasive Procedures and CPR**

1. Consider FP as an option for all families during pediatric procedures and CPR
2. Offer FP as an option when the child's care will not be interrupted and after an assessment of the parents for:
   Combative and threatening behavior
   Extreme emotional volatility
   Behaviors consistent with intoxication or altered mental status
   Disagreement among family members
   Threat to the safety of the health care team
3. If family is not provided with the option for FP, document the reasons why FP was not offered
4. Consider the safety of the health care team at all times
5. In-hospital transport and transfer settings should have written policies and procedures for FP; these should include but not be limited to:
   Definition of a facilitator
   Definition of family member, legal guardian, etc
   Definition of procedure
   Preparation of the family, including explanations, descriptions, and role of the family
   Process of escorting the family in and out of the treatment room
   Handling disagreements
   Providing support for the staff
6. Health care policies regarding FP should undergo legal review
7. Educate all health care providers
   Include education in FP in all core curricula for health care providers at all levels
   Include this education also in health care settings as part of hospital orientation

*Source:* Henderson and Knapp, J Emerg Nurs (2006), reference 83, used with permission.

also be also the context of their experience of the last hours with their child. Communication should ideally empower and strengthen parents' roles rather than marginalize them or imply they are outsiders in the circle of care for their child. In addition to frequent updates, nonverbal cues including eye contact and body language are the tangible means by which the values of family-centered are often expressed.[10]

Parents need to be given the opportunity to be with their child even when he or she is undergoing cardiopulmonary resuscitation or other invasive procedures.[8,41] Recent studies validate that parents can be present without disrupting the care process (see Table 55–2 for guidelines) and that their bereavement outcomes are enhanced when given this opportunity;[9,82–85] written policies and staff education are needed to translate the capacity for family presence during procedures into a reality.[86]

Gradual disclosure of the child's condition enables the parents to better absorb the information that the child is likely to or has died.[80] Although it is generally recommended that the attending physician should be responsible for the disclosure of death,[37] a study of parent preference found that parents preferred someone who is knowledgeable and compassionate and that they were unconcerned about the individual's title.[87] The child's usual care providers should be notified of the death as well, particularly the primary care pediatrician, who should be alerted to closely monitor the well-being of siblings in the aftermath of death.[8,9]

Emergency physicians typically have little to no training in the disclosure of death to a child's parents, and, not surprisingly, they find this activity to be one of the most stressful aspects of their jobs.[88] The stakes are high; every word said that day will linger in the parents' memories for the remainder of their lives, profoundly impacting their adaptation to the death. It is for this reason that the American Trauma Society has developed a program called "Second Trauma," providing interdisciplinary training on compassionate death disclosure (www.amtrauma.org). In addition, many first responder courses now incorporate teaching about managing death and grief.[8]

When a child dies in the ED, his/her parents generally prefer to be invited to be with their child's body in a private setting for as long as they need to stay;[37,55,89] they often wish to bathe and rock or hold the child's body. This may be difficult to accommodate in the ED, but has a tremendously beneficial effect on the family's recovery.[8] Ideally, the body will be cleaned up and fresh linens will be placed around it, with any disfiguring or gaping wounds covered, prior to inviting the parents to hold the child. Having the opportunity to speak with a chaplain and social worker at this time is often greatly appreciated. Even more importantly, parents need to understand the sequence of events, have their questions answered, and have friends bear witness to the death.[79] Parents often want a physical memento of their child, such as a lock of hair, a mold of the child's hand, or thei child's hospital bracelet and clothing.[8,9] Some programs have developed kits to ensure these items are available to families.[90] Some families appreciate being assured that the child's body will not be left alone until the funeral director or coroner comes to retrieve it.

Sudden, unexpected deaths are generally coroner's cases. In some instances, there may be a criminal investigation. This circumstance may prevent the removal of medical equipment from the child's body. It is important to explain these facts to the parents and to explain the necessity and potential benefits of autopsy.[8] Autopsy is further discussed later in this chapter.

If there is the potential that the child died from neglect or abuse, this must be investigated. Sometimes death is the result of intentional abuse by the parents or caregivers. Sometimes parents do not intend to harm their child, but are ignorant of how easy is it to severely injure a child, or they may have have poor impulse control. Most of the time, even if they caused the child's death, the parents did not intend to do so. They are hurting too, and their grief is all the more complex because of these factors. It may be difficult for nurses and other health-care professionals to reach out to parents who are suspected of having contributed to the child's death. Nonjudgmental support from the health-care team may help them begin to heal.

Sudden, unexpected death produces a high risk of complicated bereavement, regardless of the cause of death.[40,51,91] Parental grief commonly results in difficulty returning to work, severe anxiety and depression.[8,41,56] It is therefore important to provide a structured bereavement program for such families, including the opportunity to review the events of that day and to understand the autopsy results, which are generally available several weeks after the death.[8,55,92] Short- and long-term interventions are called for and should address the needs of siblings as a priority.[90] Suggestions for programs can be found in Oliver,[92] Cox,[90] and Foresman-Capuzzi.[79] At a minimum, a condolence card and a list of local grief resources should be provided. Bereaved parents appreciate a phone call from direct care providers as well.[38,51,59,93]

## Children with Chronic Life-threatening Conditions and the ICU

Unfortunately, even children with chronic illnesses and anticipated deaths most often die in the ICU.[18,19,21–23,94–96] This is less often a result of the circumstances of the death than to the lack of effective anticipatory guidance and advance care planning,[44,98–101] largely related to perceptions of an uncertain prognosis (Figure 55–1).[30,31]

Ideally, the patient and family facing a chronic, progressive, and ultimately fatal illness would be provided information gradually and recurrently, in an outpatient setting, tailored to the child's particular condition and the family's value system, orchestrated by a long-standing primary care physician.[6,7,102–106] Families need to understand the anticipated trajectory of the child's chronic condition and its associated symptoms; the interventions available for life-extension, their likely outcomes, benefits and burdens; the likely causes of death; the fact that symptoms can and will be controlled, regardless of the goals of care; and, most importantly, that that they will not be abandoned.[100] Pre-emptive discussions when the child is stable and can contribute to the discussion can aid in developing the family's preferences for care at the end of life and an associated coordinated plan of care, facilitating improved outcomes for these children and their families.[6,7,41,45] Parents state the opportunity for advance care planning provides them with comfort and assurance that their child received proper care.[103,104] Unfortunately, these conversations occur infrequently, leaving the burden to ICU personnel who have just met this chronically and now critically ill child. Crises are not the ideal time to ensure thoughtful decisions based on long-held values; nevertheless, patience and compassion can frequently lead to good outcomes.[13,15,33,105,107] Nurses often play a leading role in initiating such discussions. Ideally, the patient's medical home should be contacted to facilitate the most appropriate care plan.[9,106]

In approaching parents and children about considering limitations of medical intervention now or at a future date, it is important to understand that parents need to feel that they have done everything that is "appropriate," that they have been good, brave, and loving parents, and that the child has "been a fighter." Their efforts and their concern must be acknowledged overtly.[108]

> *It was terribly important for us to do exactly what was right and necessary to help our daughter Our nurse and social worker made us feel that we Were, in fact, doing everything in our power to take care of our daughter.*
> —Kathleen and James Bula, parents[1]

Table 55–3 provides suggestions regarding how to begin this discussion in the setting of a stable period of a life-threatening condition. Additional advice is found in Mack and Wolfe, 2006.[6]

## Continuity and Coordination of Care Needs

Parents need to know what care venues are available to them in the community and how to access them to avoid recurrent, no-longer-beneficial ICU admissions in the setting of a chronic, life-limiting condition.[100,103,104] Children with terminal conditions and their families often want spiritual consultation and guidance, since it is very hard to understand why so tragic a thing as a child's death has to occur.[60,109,110] Above all, children and their families want to feel valued as individuals, with the awesomeness of the impending death duly noted and the opportunity for healing and growth at the end of life to be realized to the greatest extent possible. If end-of-life care is properly provided, fewer children with chronic, life-threatening conditions will die in the ICU, but instead

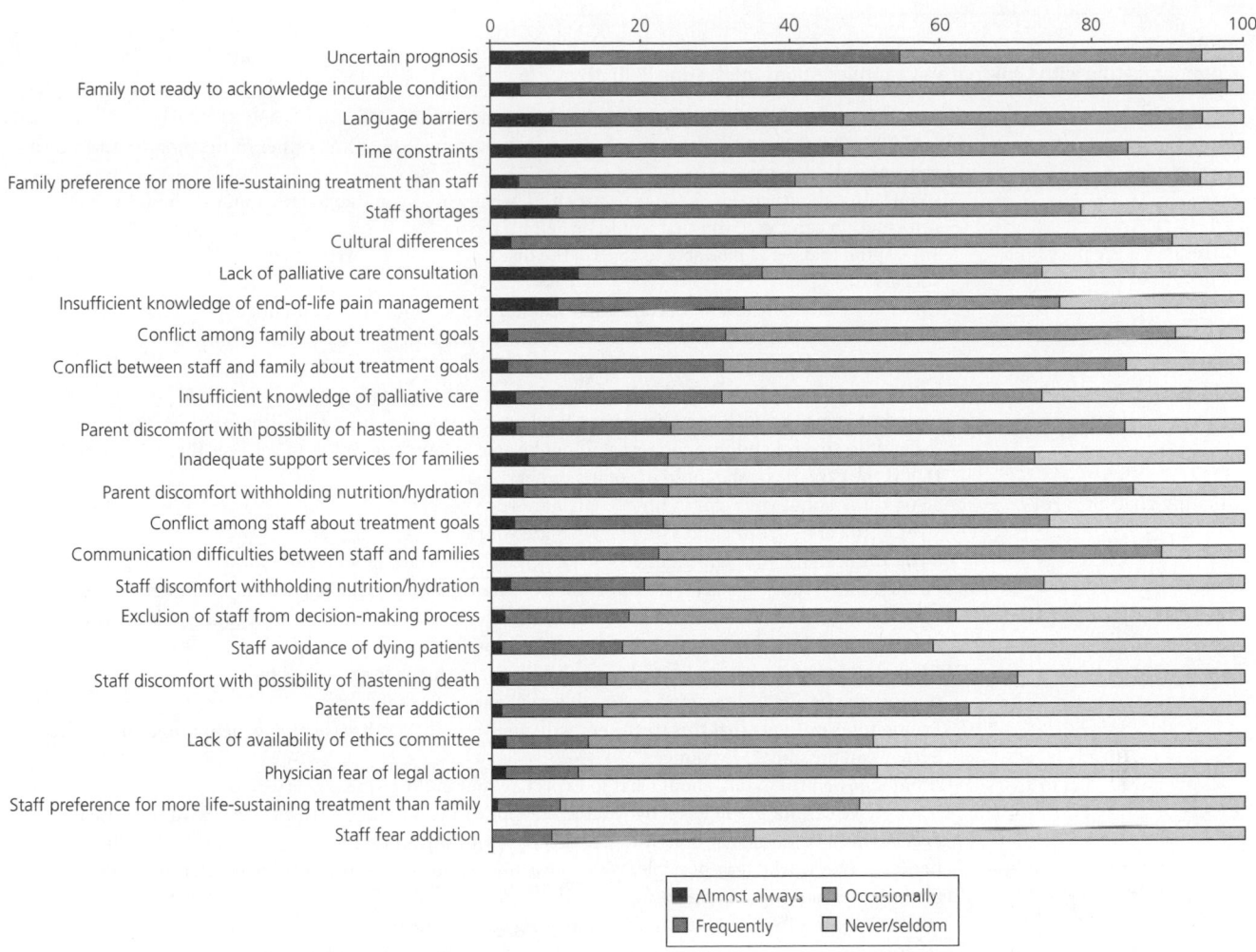

**Figure 55–1.** Barriers to pediatric palliative care. *Source*: Copyright ©2008 American Academy of Pediatrics, used with permission.

will die in a setting that they or their family prefer.[44,99,101] Accurate information increases the likelihood of a decision to forgo CPR.[75,76] Avoidable ICU deaths are taxing to the patient and family as well as the ICU personnel, who often begin to ask, "Are we doing this *to* the child or *for* the child?"[35,111]

Therapies that are not consistent with the child's and family's goals or that will not work given the child's condition should not be offered to children who have experienced chronic, progressive illness. In addition, misperceptions about the effectiveness of CPR in life-threatening conditions must be proactively addressed.[74,78] Proposals to forgo medical interventions should be presented with justifications and as a recommendation, not a choice for the family to make alone. Importantly, when suggesting what should no longer be done, describe what will be added or maintained to enhance the child's and family's quality of life. Most important are the promises to care;[51,100,112,113] to aggressively control symptoms; to be available; to assist (as a transdisciplinary team) in the arrangement of visits of family and friends; to facilitate the observation of important rituals; to provide spiritual guidance or affirmation (when desired); and to transfer

to alternate care settings (according to the patient's condition and the child's and family's wishes).[53] One suggested phrase that captures the essence of intensified caring with new goals is: "We will help your child live to his fullest to the very last moment, regardless of when that is. His comfort and yours are our top priority."

### Child Participation in Decision-Making

Most state advance directive laws do not specifically mention children. Although there is no legal mandate to address the issues of prognosis or potential future medical interventions and their expected benefits and burdens with chronically ill children, the intent of advance directives applies equally to children with decision-making capacity as it does to adults. Developing advance directives for children ensures that the wrenching decision-making process is well-considered and that the resulting care plan is enacted when the child's inevitable deterioration occurs, preventing an unwelcome

---

**Table 55–3**
**Communicating with Children and Families About Integrating Palliative Care**

| | |
|---|---|
| Beginning the conversation | "What is your understanding of what is ahead for your child?" |
| | "Would it be helpful to talk about how his or her disease may affect him or her in the months and years ahead?" |
| | "As you think about what is ahead for your child, what would you like to talk about with me? What information can I give you that would be helpful to you?" |
| Introducing the possibility of death | "I am hoping that we will be able to control the disease, but I am worried that this time we may not be successful." |
| | "Although we do not know for certain what will happen for your child, I do not expect that your child will live a long and healthy life, most children with this disease eventually die because of the disease." |
| | "I have been noticing that your child seems to be sick more and more often. I have been hoping that we would be able to make him or her better, but I am worried that his or her illness has become more difficult to control and that soon we will not be able to help him or her to get over these illnesses. If that is the case, he or she could die of his or her disease." |
| Eliciting goals of care | "As you think about your child's illness, what are your hopes?" |
| | "As you think about your child's illness, what are your worries?" |
| | "As you think about your child's illness, what is most important to you right now?" |
| | "You mentioned that what is most important to you is that your child be cured of his or her disease. I am hoping for that too. But I would also like to know more about your hopes and goals for your child's care if the time comes when a cure is not possible." |
| Introducing palliation | "Although I hope that we can control your child's disease for as long as possible, at the same time I am hoping that he/she feels as good as possible each day." |
| | "Although it is unlikely that this treatment will cure your child's disease, it may help him or her to feel better, and possibly to live longer." |
| Talking about what to expect | "Would it be helpful to talk about what to expect as your child's illness gets worse?" |
| | "Although we cannot predict exactly what will happen to your child, most children with this disease eventually have [difficulty breathing]. If that happens to your child, our goal will be to help him or her feel as comfortable as possible. We can use medications to help control his or her discomfort." |
| Talking to children | "What are you looking forward to most of all?" |
| | "Is there anything that is worrying you or making you feel afraid?" |
| | "Is there anything about how you are feeling that is making you feel worried or afraid?" |

*Source:* Mack and Wolfe (2006), reference 6.

---

ICU admission.[107] Families state that advance care planning for their children provides them peace and hope,[44,61,103–104] enabling them to decide based on the children's best interests and to include the child's perspective where possible.[61] It is recommended that the discussion be a longitudinal process, initiated early after the onset or discovery of life-threatening illness, maintained throughout the course of a child's illness and documented in written form.[6,7,104] Kreicbergs[101] found that parents who did not talk with their child about their impending deaths experienced bereavement complicated by regret, while parents who were open with their children uniformly had no regrets.

Advance care planning can prevent ED and ICU deaths for children who prefer to die at home. In a nationwide study, children who were informed about their prognoses and allowed to express a preference died at home four times more often than those who did not have that opportunity.[99] For this reason, whenever possible, the knowing child (who may be as young as 3 years if he or she has been chronically ill)

should have a voice in the discussion of the goals of medical intervention.[61,115–123] A father illustrates the importance of the child's voice well: "I think it makes it a little bit easier if they understand. In [my child's] case, he fully understands what's taking place, what's going on in his life, what's happening with his heart, and he knows that it's failing. My son says 'if I can't be me, then let me go'"(ref. 61, p 515). His wife advised that all chronically ill children be involved in their own life-and-death decisions, suggesting that small amounts of information along the way facilitated good decision-making. When the child cannot be involved, the impact of parental guilt ("I can't let my child go—it would mean I failed as a parent.") and family suffering on the decision-making process should be frankly discussed.[61] Reminding parents of their obligation to decide in their child's best interests and reassuring them that letting go is a loving decision can be helpful.

In states with out-of-hospital DNR laws, assuring these forms are appropriately executed (if the family chooses this option), the medical home physician[106] and local EMS are involved or at least notified and that hospice care is arranged can be very helpful to families. These activities increase the likelihood that the child will die at home, where most children and adults would prefer to die.[44,99,125]

In the ICU or ED, when the chronically ill child is not responding to stabilization or resuscitative efforts, the parents are often asked "Do you want us to do 'everything'?" This question does not fully encompass the possible benefits and burdens and probable outcomes of potential interventions. From the parent's perspective, there is no reasonable answer to this question but "Yes!" However, for informed consent to occur, the goals and the understanding of likely outcomes must be discussed and aligned before proceeding. To the physician, "everything" too often means everything to prolong survival, regardless of the quality of life.[111,126] For parents, other goals generally take precedence.[27,44,47,60,61,127,178] If the child's condition is stabilized and symptoms are aggressively controlled, more rational decision-making can take place. The terms used to discuss end-of-life planning and decisions are often ambiguous and do not enable informed consent.[128] The family could, for example, choose mechanical ventilation for respiratory distress or may prefer comfort management outside the ICU if extended survival is unlikely or is unduly burdensome for the child. Common medical colloquialisms are often misinterpreted by families. Table 55–4 provides suggested phraseology to ensure clear communication and to prevent perceptions of abandonment.

## Death Related to Chronic, Progressive Illness: Issues Relevant to ED and ICU Personnel

Although communicating news regarding the terminal phase of chronic disease is difficult and stressful for everyone, being uninformed of the severity of the situation is even more stressful for patients and families. One of the most common complaints of patients and families is the lack of accurate and clearly communicated information.[12,27,45,47,51,52,60,108,130–132,136] Done well, disclosure of the prognosis associated with a chronic condition often provides confirmation for families of what was already suspected, frequently resulting in relief and reduction of anxiety.[11,13,47,129–132]

Suggestions for discussing a poor prognosis in a way that is sensitive to the needs of the child and family, as well as the medical caregivers, are found in Table 55–5.

Unfortunately, even when advance directives have been thoughtfully crafted and executed, there are rarely mechanisms in place to honor these decisions. In addition, without reinforcement, parents may feel emotionally unprepared to follow through with their decisions to limit medical intervention. All too often, when the child begins to have the predicted deterioration, symptoms are inadequately controlled because no palliative care plan is in place and the patient appears in the emergency room *in extremis*.

## Patient and Family Needs in the Intensive Care Unit

Entering an ICU or ED is a frightening experience for both the child and family regardless of the presenting problem, prognosis, or treatment plan. The environment of care significantly impacts the ability of families to cope, particularly if the child dies.[11,12,47,53,133,134,136] Emergency department and critical care providers must strive to remember that the experience is new and often terrifying for children and families. Interventions to alleviate this type of suffering can improve the immediate experience of the child and the long-term outcomes for the parent.[8,9,135,136] Meert et al.[53] described several environmental needs of parents (see Table 55–6).

High levels of post traumatic stress disorder have been demonstrated among family members of ICU patients;[56,137,138] providing even the minimal information regarding how an ICU works, identifying the personnel involved and their functions, and teaching families how to access information has a dramatically beneficial effect. A simple explanatory brochure can lower ICU family PTSD rates by 50%.[135] In addition, support and honest communication is an important intervention. Compared with physicians, nurses are significantly less likely to agree that families are well informed and that ethical issues are well-discussed when assessing actual practice in their intensive care unit.[18,28,35] More collaborative education and regular case review on bioethical issues are needed as part of standard practice in the intensive care unit.[18,35,111,139]

### Needs of the Child in the Intensive Care Unit

In addition to being included in advance care planning and having meticulous symptom control, ill children also benefit from having a member of the care team attend specifically to his or her emotional needs. Ideally, the critical care unit has a social worker or child-life specialist who is immediately accessible and able to provide critical assessment, support, distraction and intervention for children who are alert and can participate. The benefits of this type of intervention can be seen in the following case example:

CASE STUDY
*A 10-Year-Old Girl with Leukemia*

Josephine, a 10-year-old African-American girl with recurrent acute myelogenouss leukemia, was transferred to the pediatric ICU for a bone marrow biopsy. Because Josephine was familiar with the procedure, she was frightened. The physicians and nurses determined that it would be better to allow her time to voice her concerns before beginning the procedure. The social worker encouraged her to draw a picture of her body and indicate what she was feeling. Josephine interpreted "feelings" to

**Table 55–4**
**Methods of Communicating Sensitive Healthcare Information and Perceptions of Communication**

| Usual Method of Communicating Message | How the Usual Communication May Be Perceived | Alternative Method of Communicating Message |
|---|---|---|
| "Do you want us to do CPR?" | "CPR would work if you would allow us to do it" | "Tell me what you know about" CPR. "CPR is most helpful for patients who are relatively healthy, and even then, only 1 of 3 patients survive. Many of Lisa's organs are not working. As you know, she is getting dialysis to clean her blood like her kidneys would have, a breathing machine for her lungs, and medicine to keep her blood pressure up. If her heart were to stop, it would not be because there is a problem with her heart (it is fine), but it would be because she is dying. All of our hearts stop when we die. So pumping on her heart, or "doing CPR" will not make her better. On the other hand, while I would recommend not doing CPR, I am not recommending stopping any other treatment she is receiving at this time. There is still a chance that she may get better. Let's hope for the best, but also plan for the worst. We will need to keep a close watch on her and keep you up to date on how she is doing. Do you have any questions?" "Let's talk again later today so I can update you. Is there anyone else I need to talk to?" |
| "Let's stop heroic treatment" | "We will provide less than optimal care" (What is heroic about performing invasive, painful, costly, nonbeneficial care?) | "At this time, I think the most heroic thing we can do is to understand how sick Jamal is and stop treatments that are not working for him. I think we should do all we can to ensure his comfort and yours, make sure there are no missed opportunities, and ensure we properly celebrate his life. I will follow your lead on this. Some ideas that have helped other families include getting him home with help for you if you wish, or you may choose to have his friends and your family come here instead and have a party; you can bring his clothes so that he will look like himself, bring in his music or a photo album and relive some of your best memories of him, make a mold of his hand so that you will always have his hand to hold, or anything else that would be a proper celebration of his life." |
| "Let's stop aggressive treatment" | "We will not be attentive to his needs, including symptom distress and need for comfort" | "We will do all we can to ensure he is as comfortable as possible." |
| "Aeisha has failed the treatment" | "The patient is the cause of the problem" | "We have tried all the proven treatments and even some experimental ones for Aiesha. Unfortunately, we did not get the results we had hoped for. I wish it were different!" |
| "We are recommending withdrawal of care for Marisa" | "We are going to abandon her and you" | "Marisa is too ill to get better. We need to refocus our efforts on making the most of the time she has left." |
| "There is nothing more we can do for Adam" | "We will allow him to suffer, we do not care about him, we only care about fighting the disease" | "We need to change the goals of our care for Adam. At this point we clearly cannot cure him, but that does not mean we can't help him and your family." |

| | |
|---|---|
| "Johnny is not strong enough to keep going" | "Johnny is a strong boy and he has fought hard with us to beat his disease. Unfortunately, as much as we wish we could, we cannot cure Johnny. At this point, we are hurting him rather than helping, giving him side effects, and keeping him from being at home or taking a trip, or whatever he really wants to do with the time he has left." |
| "We will make it so Thuy does not suffer" | "We will do everything we can to make Thuy comfortable." |
| "We need to stop active treatment for Dwayne" | "The goal of curing Dwayne's disease, despite the best efforts of a lot of smart and hard-working people, is no longer possible. We are so sorry and wish that that were different! I have cared for many children who are as sick as your son. It is very hard on all of us, especially you, his parents and family when the treatments do not work as we had hoped. Many parents like you have agreed to stop efforts to cure when they are not working, as difficult as that is. Would you like me to put you in touch with some of the other parents who have been through this too?" |
| "You are the final arbiter of your child's death" | "Bobby is lucky to have such excellent, loving and selfless parents. I know this is hard; we will get through it together. I am glad you agree with our recommendations to change the goals of care to better meet Bobby's needs. I will let my team know what we have decided." |
| "You are signing his death warrant" | |
| "Do you want us to stop Bobby's treatment?" | |
| "I am glad you agree. Will you sign Juan's do-not-resuscitate order?" | "There is no surgery, no medicine, and all the love you clearly feel for Juan will not make him better, he is just too sick. I wish it were different." (Silence) "I will change his orders to make sure he only gets tests and treatments that can help him now." |

CPR indicates cardiopulmonary resuscitation.
*Source:* Levetown (2008), reference 108. Used with permission obtained.

---

**Table 55–5**
**Breaking the Bad News**

---

1. Provide a "warning shot" or an introductory sentence before presenting the distressing information: "I am sorry that I have some bad news to tell you."

2. Provide an opportunity for supportive friends or family to be present when the information is shared: "Would you like to call someone to be with you when we talk?"

3. Tell the news in a private setting, with the physician, nurse, and social worker present. Bring the family (generally parents without the child first, depending on relationships and preferences) to a private conference room rather than speaking to them in the waiting room or the hall. Bring tissues. If appropriate and desired by the family, assist them in telling their children (patient and siblings) afterwards.

4. Sit down near the family, not across a table. Do not stand. Children and families want to be on an even plane with their caregivers. Look the family members in the eye to engender trust unless this is culturally undesirable. Ask them to tell you about their child and about any consistent values of the child and about the things that give him or her pleasure. Ask how much they want to know about his or her medical condition and prognosis. Ask them what they understand is happening. Clarify misconceptions, particularly about the cause of the problem, and attempt to assuage any guilt that may derive from having an inherited or developmental problem ("You did not wish for your child to have this") or from trauma or other causes. Then, let them know this news is difficult for you as well. Nurses can help guide the physician to present the truth in a jargon-free manner that is consistent with the family's educational level, sophistication, and stated desire for knowledge. Ask the family to explain what they understood was said. Clarify misconceptions. Then, solicit additional questions.

5. Be unhurried. If there is only a limited time available for the physician, let the family know: "I'm sorry the doctor only has 15 minutes now, but I will stay with you and answer any questions I can, and the doctor will be back later this afternoon to answer anything I can't and to update you." Don't look at your watch. Have the charge nurse or another nurse care for your patients while you sit with the family. Remind the other team members to give their beepers to someone else during the family meeting, when possible; otherwise, switch the beepers to vibrate mode.

6. Ideally, members of the multidisciplinary team participate as full members during the family conference.[48] The bedside nurse, chaplain, and social worker benefit from hearing the physician–family interaction. They can solicit questions, clarify misconceptions during the meeting and after the physician leaves, and address other facets of the patient's situation that the conversation with the physician evokes. Team members can also give the physician feedback regarding his or her communication with the patient and family, such as words they did not understand, and can help the physician address any unresolved issues at the next meeting. This technique requires interdisciplinary respect and cooperation, which are essential to successful, comprehensive end-of-life care; it prevents divisive misunderstandings between disciplines regarding suspected coercion or other undesirable communication.

7. Bring trainees to the family meeting. This allows the assigned nursing or medical student and resident to learn from directly observing the interdisciplinary critical care team, as well as the patient and family responses. It keeps trainees informed so that unnecessary and often damaging miscommunications do not occur. Trainees often get lost in the minutiae of the patient's laboratory values and vital signs and may unwittingly provide contradictory information to the family. However, do not overwhelm the family with white coats—have trainees take turns attending family meetings.

8. Be specific. The physician should present the options, include a description of life-sustaining treatments, the child's current status, the chance of survival, the probability of full recovery (and the probability of significant disability), and the possible effects of the child's long-term survival on the family.

---

represent both physical and emotional reactions, describing pain in her legs and stomach, feeling sad in her mind and confused in her intestines. She also noted that her eyes could not see. On probing, she said she could not see what her future would hold. As a result of this discussion, the medical staff understood the need to describe in more detail why the biopsy was necessary, how it would likely alleviate some of her pain and discussed her overall prognosis with her. Josephine began to feel calmer, feeling some control over what was happening to her. Respect for her concerns helped her trust her caregivers, enabling Josephine to receive the care she needed with less anxiety.

Although it is not always possible to delay a medical procedure in critical care, allowing time for the child to express feelings and have questions answered will reduce the natural anxiety associated with frightening or painful procedures, resulting in better outcomes.

## Compassionate, Effective, Consistent Bidirectional Communication with the Family and the Patient is Critical to Providing Care and to the Prevention of Suffering

Bartel[41] and Shudy[136] reviewed the needs and priorities of families whose child died in the ICU. Their findings again focused on effective and compassionate communication as a primary priority. Parents need to retain the role of caregiver and protector of their child and to function within the context of the family unit, regardless of circumstance. Nurses can be facilitators of this goal through policies and professional activities, including (see Table 55–7).

Truog et al.[13] reviewed the literature to determine evidence-based practice that will improve EOL care in the PICU. The six critical domains revealed were:

1. support of the family unit;
2. communication with the child and family about treatment goals and plans;
3. ethics and shared decision-making;
4. relief of pain and other symptoms;
5. continuity of care; and
6. grief and bereavement support.

Meyer[47] provided concrete examples of some of these domains of parents' preferences and priorities (see Table 55–8).

Families want bidirectional communication that is timely, complete, compassionate and consistent. Honest and accurate information is reassuring, even if it is bad news.[11,12,18,27,45,47,52,61,108,129] As quoted in Meert,[129] one bereaved parent stated:

*Things are just so unsettling that I think if you have an answer it's easier to deal with than not knowing.*

Information should be clearly and empathetically communicated from the earliest meeting to the family and followed by regular updates as the prognosis changes, even if the pace of change is very fast.[15,18,41,45,47,52,105,129] Parents want physicians to be accessible and to display a caring affect, to use lay language, and to speak at a pace in accordance with their ability to comprehend. Withholding prognostic information from parents can lead to false hopes and feelings of anger, betrayal, and distrust.[45,47,51,52,60,127,129]

## Strategies for Improving Team Communication

Nurses are often key professionals when it comes to communication with families in the ICU.[18,30,41] Being at the bedside, nurses often get to know the families and their concerns, values and priorities well and can enable the correct approach to best meet the needs of each family. Participation of the bedside nurse in daily rounds and in family meetings improves continuity of care and consistency of information and communication. The information that nurses gather

---

**Table 55–6**
**Environmental Needs of Parents Whose Child is Critically Ill**

1. Privacy and sufficient space
2. Easy access to the child, including during invasive procedures and CPR
3. Amenities enabling continuous access to the child:
   Nearby sleeping and bathing accommodations
   Vending machines or other food services
   A room to gather supporters in large numbers
   Comfortable seating in the child's room
4. Access to a phone when cell phones are not allowed
5. A clean, secure environment of care for their child and themselves
6. Secure storage
7. Need for assurance that everything that can be done to help is being done
8. Information resources, such as information on how to tell others your child has died

---

**Table 55–7**
**Nursing Faciliation of Parental Role Maintenance**

Providing clear information
Teaching the family about the child's condition and its management
Enabling and encouraging parent participation in the direct care of the child
Acknowledging the parents' concerns for the child and addressing them timely
Enabling parental presence 24 hours a day, particularly during procedures, including CPR.[47, 53, 133–134]
Preventing procedural pain

---

**Table 55–8**
**Parents' Priorities for Pediatric Palliative Care**

| | |
|---|---|
| Honest and complete information | "What we cannot handle is not knowing what is going on." |
| Ready access to staff | "Set a regular time for office hours at the bedside." |
| Communication and care coordination | "There were too many doctors explaining things." |
| Emotional expression and support by staff | "People need to feel that people really care, not that it's just a job." |
| Preservation of the integrity of the parent-child relationship | "Show more sincere compassion for the parents' and child's needs." |
| Faith | "Prayer and the services of my rabbi." |

*Source*: Meyer et al. (2006). 117(3): 649, Table 2, used with permission.

from patients and parents at the bedside is critically important to the entire team in understanding what the patient and family already know, what questions they have, and what further explanations or discussions are needed.[41] In addition, there is a need for excellent communication between nurses at shift change about what the family has been told and what they seem to understand. Parents often call at night to check on their children and get confused by conflicting messages. Strategies, such as primary nursing assignments and tools such as communication logs or a "goals of care" worksheet can improve overall communication and quality of care.[140]

Communication needs differ among families based on their education, personality, culture, experience and expectations. The recommended way to ensure communication meets the needs of these families is to ask about their communication preferences—do you prefer one main communication director; do you prefer to hear everyone's opinion, even if there is disagreement; do you want to know any time there is a change; do you want to participate in rounds; do you prefer to have a translator present; do you want detailed information or the bigger conceptual picture?

Creative means to accommodate family communication needs may include appointments for communication, a bedside journal allowing asynchronous communication, web-based technology including encrypted messaging and web-based cameras, email, interdisciplinary family meetings, and short discussions in person or by phone when a change occurs. Regardless of their individual preferences or the means of communication, parents need compassion and acknowledgement. In fact, compassion has both short- and long-term benefits for families, significantly impacting the likelihood of their successful adaptation to bereavement.[51,93]

### Effective Communication with Families

In complex environments like the ED and ICU, it is critical that members of the health-care team also communicate effectively with each other, in order to avoid confusion and resulting distress.[34,111,141] Communicating in highly technical and emotional circumstances can be difficult. Factors such as the family's willingness to acknowledge or accept a potential prognosis, physician bias regarding the goals of care, the management of and tolerance for uncertainty, and the emotions of the health-care professional and/or family all can create obstacles to open, honest communication regarding the child's condition and prognosis.[30,142,143] Positive communication styles are associated with being receptive to cues from patients and families, demonstrating genuine concern, moral responsibility, a caring presence and dedication.[144,145] Many clinicians try to "shield" parents from bad news, as they are reluctant to "take away hope." However, Mack's research has demonstrated that what parents define as hope differs from caregivers' perceptions. Parents hope for honest information that allows them to make the best decisions for and with their child and to have the capacity to ready themselves

for the inevitable with the support of their loved ones[61,127] (for more information on Communication Techniques, see Chapter 5).

### End-of-Life Family Conferences

End-of-life family conferences are formal, structured meetings between physicians, staff and family members. Guidelines for organizing these conferences take into account the specific needs of families, including reassurance that the patient's symptoms will be adequately managed; honest clear information about the patient's condition and treatment; a willingness on the part of physicians to listen and respond to family members and to address their emotions; attention to patient preferences; clear explanations about surrogate decision-making; and continuous, compassionate, and technically proficient attention to the patient's needs until death occurs. Means of improving end-of-life care have been identified in epidemiologic and interventional studies.[141,146,147] End-of-life family conferences constitute the keystone around which excellent end-of-life care can be built. Ideally all members of the interdisciplinary pediatric team will participate in the family conference.[30,34] Lautrette and colleagues provide excellent suggestions for conducting family meetings in their 2006 review of the evidence.[146]

### Medical Decision-Making: Clarity of Facts and Ethical Principles Among Family and Staff Enables Good Medical Decision-Making

Despite the benefits of formal family meetings, communication is a process, not an event. It works best if respect is demonstrated and trust is built. This can be accomplished by encouraging patients and families to talk, then listening without interruption (in fact, it has been demonstrated that families are more satisfied with communication the less the health-care providers speak[148]); acknowledging family and patient concerns and conflicts with other health-care professionals without indicting these colleagues; acknowledging errors and providing follow-up regarding the resolution for the patient and future patients; and by allowing families to arrive at decisions in a timeframe that is comfortable for them. Nonverbal cues such as eye contact, humility, and respect go a long way to building trust as well.

Effective communication enables solicitation of families' concerns, emotional reactions and values. Acknowledgement and validation of strong emotion is greatly appreciated by families, but is rarely offered.[105] These ingredients allow rational decisions to be made based on the facts as well as the values of the child and his or her family, preventing regret and significant parental morbidity.[20,45,60,61,99,103,104] Unfortunately, opportunities to communicate in this manner are often missed, particularly when strong emotions are present.[147] Meert and colleagues[52] found the following elements of communication are valued by parents whose children are nearing death:

- Comprehensive and complete information
- Clarity of information, use of clear language
- Ease of access to caregivers and their explanations throughout the course of care
- Pacing of information. Soliciting of parents' emotional responses and addressing their questions
- Consistency of information
- Honesty, lack of false hope
- Empathy as demonstrated by verbal, nonverbal and affective communication
- Summary statements and next steps

Azoulay et al.[137] investigated the risk of post-traumatic stress symptoms in families of ICU patients, finding a very high proportion with full-blown PTSD. The risk was increased among families who felt that insufficient time was available for receiving information; information was incomplete or difficult to understand; the family participated in end-of-life decision-making and when the patient died during the hospitalization.

### Time-Limited Trials

Throughout the time that the child is in the ICU receiving care, it is helpful to review the patient's progress continuously, monitoring the "big picture" of whether the patient is progressing along the hoped-for trajectory of improvement or whether he or she is deteriorating despite the best medical management. Daily or more frequent patient (when possible and appropriate) and the family updates of this information can facilitate reasonable decision-making, thereby avoiding burdensome and unhelpful care and diminishing the shock should death occur.[12,14,15,61] Letting the parents know when the child should reasonably be expected to show a response to treatment, anticipating outcomes and associated choices in advance and agreeing to meet again after the interval has passed (time-limited trails) to discuss progress provides the family time to adapt and to gather their supporters to hear the news with them, whether good or bad.

Recommendations for the next clinical step should be presented based on the team's experience with similar patients, the goals and values of the patient and family, and the observations of patient and family members during the meeting and the hospitalization overall. The benefits and burdens (including prolongation of suffering) of each potential care plan, the potential reversibility or irreversibility of the conditions being treated, the time frame for reevaluation, the projected future quality of life, and the comfort measures available if the ICU interventions are curtailed or discontinued must be explained to the family in a manner they can understand (Table 55–9).

When discussing the choice to forgo no-longer-beneficial medical interventions, the topic of current burdens of therapy as well as the probability of the hoped-for benefits must be clearly explained. Reassure the family that if ICU interventions are discontinued, the child will continue to receive attentive care for the relief of symptoms; describe the procedures to be undertaken, including the opportunities to observe important customs and rituals and the visitation allowances.[115]

The benefits of stopping ED or ICU treatments can be presented as limiting the harm to and the suffering of the child, and enabling the loving presence of the family rather than being surrounded by the health-care team engaged in non-beneficial resuscitative activities. When the option is inaccurately presented as "stopping care," it is not surprisingly usually rejected. This shorthand phraseology is perceived as cruel and callous; patients and families fear abandonment above all else.[100,112,113,149] Word choice is critical, as is a clear appreciation of the moral distinctions between killing and letting die from the underlying condition. Stating a child died "from" the discontinuation of "life support" creates confusion for families and professionals alike. Ongoing ignorance of the bioethical tenets supporting the discontinuation of ICU interventions among even senior pediatric clinicians was recently documented.[35,111] The goals of care and the principles underlying them must be clear in everyone's mind before proceeding, lest the tragedy of inaccurate perceptions of wrongdoing plague critical care providers[150] and family survivors.[151]

### End-of-Life Decision-Making

In most clinical situations, the justification to forgo disease-directed medical intervention in ICUs is physician assessment of poor prognosis for survival rather than quality-of-life considerations.[8,20,30,126,152–155] Parents, however, make their decisions based on the child's quality of life, degree of pain and suffering, likelihood of improvement, and physician's recommendations, as well as the child's "will to live," knowledge of

---

**Table 55–9**
**Evaluating Treatment Options**

- How realistic is it that the intervention will cure the disease?
- If not able to cure the disease, will the intervention prevent progression of the disease?
- Will the intervention improve the way the child feels?
- Could the intervention make the child feel worse? If so, for how long?
- What will it be like for this child to go through this treatment?
- What is likely to happen without the intervention?
- Will the intervention change the outcome for the child?
- What is the likely impact of this decision on the family?

*Source:* Levetown (1996), reference 157.

other deaths, and perceptions of the child's best interests.[47,61] Reassessing the goals of treatment only when the child is dying deprives the patient and family of earlier choices to limit suffering rather than extend the duration of life.[156,157] Children who cannot be cured and their families often have preferences regarding the value of medical interventions. Their opinions are not knowable by the medical team *a priori*; they must be actively solicited.[5,16,20,61,158–162] In addition, the child's perceptions of discomfort relative to various medical interventions may be very different than the medical caregivers' perceptions.[159,160,163,164] In fact, regardless of the presence of a terminal prognosis, patients and their surrogates have the right to forgo any medical intervention.[111,165–167]

### Consideration of Suffering and Future Quality of Life

Surrogates' (or parents') duties are to act on the child's wishes and in his or her best interests.[61,111,160–163,168–172] This role is sometimes not clear and therefore requires explanation. Surrogates more often request prolongation of a child's dying process rather than request discontinuation of ICU interventions too prematurely.[111] Thus, overriding any requests to terminate ICU interventions must be done with significant forethought and analysis. In addition, the motivation for requests to continue ICU interventions in the face of an extremely small likelihood of survival or a significantly poor quality of life must be explored fully. Guilt, fear and loss issues in particular should be examined:

- "What do you think caused his problems? You were away at work when the accident happened?"
- "Tell me about what has happened to your family as a result of your child's condition?"
- "It sounds like you've been through a lot. I wish I could make your child healthy and make it all okay again but unfortunately, there are limits to what medicine can do. The best we can reasonably hope for, medically, is…Does that change your perspective on treatment options? Our recommendation, based on all you've told us and our assessment of your child's condition is…."

Eliciting and demonstrating respect for the family's and child's (where applicable) values can be helpful in resolving decisional dilemmas.

A child's[114,119,159,163,169–171] or surrogates' requests to stop ICU interventions must be taken seriously in order to determine current sources of suffering, eliminating them where possible, reducing them, or changing the goals of care as needed; the request may indeed signal it is time to focus on maximizing comfort, regardless of impact on life expectancy.[12,45,47,61,163,164] Patient suffering must play a much more prominent role in the decision-making process if "good deaths" are to be attained for a higher proportion of patients.[6,30,31,44,99] ICU physicians and nurses must be educated on ethical principles in medical practice, particularly on autonomy, beneficence, nonmaleficence, and the construct of benefits vs.

burdens in making and guiding decisions; there remains substantial ignorance on these issues among even senior clinicians.[26,35,36,114,150,157,162] Personal biases regarding quality of life, fears of litigation and economic motivations for the withdrawal of ICU interventions should not play any role in the decision to forgo treatment.[152,158,172]

Within practical limitations, the patient's comfort should be the primary determinant of the process of end-of-life care. In several studies, vasopressors were withheld first, oxygen next, and mechanical ventilation next. However, oxygen supplementation and extubation may be preferred and more comfortable, potentially providing the opportunity for a last goodbye. In addition, withholding antibiotics and allowing the peaceful death associated with sepsis, without a trip to the ICU, may be the most humane option available for some children. In other cases, forgoing nutrition may ease nausea, and forgoing hydration may decrease the discomfort of renal failure or congestive heart failure.[168,173,174] Obviously, much depends on the child's symptoms, the clinical situation, and the child's and family's values and preferences. Effecting a philosophical change among medical decision-makers to proactively solicit children's and families' perspectives may be accomplished by educational intervention, although it is likely that cultural changes within institutions and protocol-driven practice may have more promise.[36,175]

### Forgoing No-Longer-Beneficial ICU Interventions: Review of the Patient Care Plan

After it has been determined that the child and family's primary goal is no longer simply the prolongation of life, because either the child's suffering is too great or the child will die no matter what more is done, the care plan must be reviewed in detail. The likely mechanisms of death must be determined; likely symptoms can then be anticipated and a care plan can then be created to address them proactively.[115,176] For example, if the child is likely to have seizures but cannot swallow, rectal or parenteral rapid-onset anticonvulsants should be written as a PRN order. It is not uncommon for the child to have several potential mechanisms for death; often, one route can be anticipated to be the most comfortable, such as dying from hyperkalemia or sepsis as opposed to hypoxemia. In this case, Kayexalate or dialysis as well as antibiotics should be discontinued, whereas oxygen supplementation should be continued. Developmentally-appropriate explanations about the possible course of events should be given to the child and family unless they refuse this information. It is unwise to predict an exact time of death, but approximations (with significant margin for error—e.g., minutes to hours, hours to days, days to weeks) are helpful for the family to arrange for the child's other loved ones and friends to visit before or be present at death.[12,14,51–53,108,177]

All interventions that either interfere with comfort or that do not enhance it should be discontinued.[12,14] For example, laboratory tests are not designed to enhance comfort. Sometimes in clinical practice, laboratory parameters, such as platelet counts, are monitored to "prevent" symptoms (such as bleeding) from arising. However, it is less intrusive to monitor the patient for clinical bleeding and treat if and when it arises, as desired. Medications that do not enhance comfort, often including antibiotics, should be considered for discontinuation. Even feeding and IV fluids may interfere with comfort if the child has pulmonary edema, heart failure, or renal failure; a decrease in or cessation of these therapies may enhance the child's comfort.[14,173,174] Removal of no longer needed devices, including monitoring equipment, should also be considered.

## Forgoing No-Longer-Beneficial Critical Care Interventions

Forgoing mechanical ventilation precedes most ICU deaths, allowing patients to die more peacefully from their underlying conditions.[12,14] Though a common phenomenon, it remains uncomfortable for many critical care practitioners. Initiating a meeting of those involved in the care of the patient to review the choice and hear concerns, as well as to guide the care, is very helpful in minimizing distrust and maintaining cohesion among the staff.[33,34,146,181] The use of protocols that outline the ethical principles underlying such choices have been found to be helpful in guiding decision-making and management of the extubuation by critical care physicians and nurses.[36]

Monitors, such as pulse oximeters, cardiorespiratory monitors, and the like should be removed in most cases.[12,150] They create physical barriers to being close, distract the family from attending to the child with their color displays and flashing lights, and emit distressing alarms that all have agreed not to respond to. They also create an excuse for caregivers to not enter the room. However, some families become so attached that removing these devices seems to them to be a form of abandonment and in these few cases, removal should not be carried out. When a family elects to forgo treatments in anticipation of death, visitation restrictions and many of the usual rules should be reconsidered.[11,47,53,134,136] Maximization of opportunities to hold the child or even invitations to family members to climb in bed with the child should be facilitated. Letting the family bathe the child and dress him or her in clothing of the child's or family's choice is often helpful. Other special requests should be honored if at all possible.

Engaging in family-centered rituals prior to forgoing critical care interventions is important, allowing unhurried family time while the child is still alive. As the family is approaching readiness for extubation, they should be reminded about what changes are likely in the child after extubation, making this difficult time easier. ("He may turn blue; we will treat this with morphine and oxygen if he looks uncomfortable. He may not breathe at all or may breathe comfortably for some time. His breathing may be noisy because his brain is not controlling the soft tissues in his throat. I do not know how long he will live, but I expect it will be on the order of (minutes, hours, days). I will stay with you until he is comfortable.") Positive thoughts about extubation are important to share as well. ("This will be the first time you see your daughter's beautiful face without tape and a tube interfering"; "I am giving you back your son as a child, not as a patient"; "You may be able to hear his voice for the first time in a while," depending on the age and circumstances of the child.)

### Extubation Technique

There is no single correct way to discontinue mechanical ventilation.[12,14,18,23,25,182] Although adult care practitioners most often wean the patient's ventilator settings and leave a "T tube" in place, there is some evidence that this is not what families prefer.[178]

Pediatric practitioners more often remove the tracheal tube.[18,180] Although some practitioners pre-medicate prior to changing ventilator settings,[182] others wait to see how the patient responds. In a study of the concerns of parents whose child had cancer regarding the last week of life, Pritchard[179] found that changes in consciousness were particularly disturbing. In another study, decision-making by parents of children in critical care settings was partially based on the parents' perceptions of the child's degree of suffering and will to live.[61] The desire to say a final goodbye is also very strong among some parents.[136] Therefore, it may be best practice to understand the parents' hopes for the final minutes to hours of their child's life, to educate them about the potential likelihood of achieving them, and then make every attempt to honor their wishes. The goal of preventing any discomfort at all calls for pre-emptive sedation, conflicting with a goal of a final goodbye, These considerations should be discussed in advance. Munson[182] recommends pre-bolusing in the care of neonates and having very clear mutual expectations among the staff about what signs indicate the need for treatment.

### Transfer to Alternative Care Settings

When children are acknowledged to be dying, it is common for extended family and loved ones to gather to support each other. Sometimes they may desire to perform rituals that are difficult to accommodate in the ICU setting. Thus, consideration of transfering to an alternate care setting may be helpful, even if it is only for a few hours.

If the child is anticipated to live for a few days once critical care interventions are discontinued, referral to hospice in the home care setting may be an option. Usually a 1- to 2-day stay in the hospital to ensure "stability" and to provide family and hospice caregiver teaching is needed. Alternatively, if the child will have significant distress in his or her final days, or the child and/or family prefer to stay in the hospital, admission to the floor, or preferably a palliative care unit, may be the best plan. As large a room as is needed to accommodate the child and his or her loved ones should be provided, if possible.[1,51,53,60] However, an agreement to transfer out of the

ICU must usually be predicated by an agreement to terminate the ventilator within hours of transfer.

## Aggressive Symptom Management in the Emergency Department and Intensive Care Unit

For more in-depth explanations of the management of these symptoms, see Part II, Symptom Assessment and Management. However, a few overarching principles deserve further mention.

Aggressive symptom control is a high priority for parents of children who die.[1,13,47,136,179] When critical care technologies are forgone, the most common symptom-distress risks are dyspnea, pain, and seizures.[12,14,180–182] Thus, meticulous care at the time of ventilator withdrawal, including the continuous presence of the physician and/or nurse, and protocols for symptom management are key to the effective prevention or immediate management of symptom distress.[12,14,36] When attended to by a skilled interdisciplinary team that focuses on these issues as primary concerns, symptoms are usually successfully prevented or rapidly mitigated. It is helpful to most families to affirm their decision and to explain the possible events in advance of their occurrence. For example:

*You are a brave and loving family. You have recognized that Brandon will not survive, regardless of further treatments and have opted not to prolong his dying process, but, rather, enable a proper goodbye, surrounded by love, friends, and family. This is probably the hardest thing you have ever done. Brandon is lucky you love him enough to do this for him. Do you have any concerns or questions I can address? (PAUSE) If not, let me go over the procedure for tomorrow. In order to keep Brandon comfortable, we will discontinue his IV fluids tonight so that he will breathe more comfortably. We will move him to the larger room in the morning. After your family and friends celebrate Brandon's life, when you and your family are ready, we will suction Brandon's breathing tube and then remove it from his windpipe. We will also stop the blood pressure medication. Brandon may breathe in a funny pattern—sometimes shallow and quick, sometimes like a yawn or hiccup, and sometimes not at all. He may also change color—he may become pale, red or even blue. We will stay with you; if he looks uncomfortable, we will give him medications every 5 minutes until he looks more comfortable according to you and to me. I will not leave your side until he is looking as comfortable as possible.*

### Pain

*We told them she didn't do well on morphine. We saw the pain she was in. For 48 hours we kept telling them it wasn't helping. No matter how much morphine they'd give her, she was flopping around on the bed. So we stood there the whole time…she was moaning in pain. [Crying] Those are the images that are the most painful, that she had to suffer. We were helpless. I'm sure they thought what they were doing would work; I'm sure for most kids it works. But for her, it didn't. At that time, we felt we weren't being taken seriously. It's still the image we wake up thinking about. (Excerpted from Contro[27])*

Pain in the ED is can be acute because of trauma, acute exacerbations of chronic pain for children with complex medical illnesses presenting with an emergent complication of the disease, and/or procedural pain. Age-appropriate assessment tools and evidence-based pain management approaches should be employed to minimize the pain experience of children in EDs.

Assessment and management of pain in the ICU setting is confounded by the likelihood of sedative and paralytic agents if the child is intubated. A number of scales are validated for the pediatric ICU patient, including the Premature Infant Pain Profile (PIPP), children's pain checklist, FLACC (Face, Legs, Activities, Cry, and Consolability) and COMFORT scales.[183–186] The Individualized Numeric Rating Scale was recently developed for children with severe cognitive impairment.[187] Primary nursing assignments facilitate symptom assessment and parents or usual caregivers are crucial resources for pain assessment.

The severity of reported or assessed pain dictates the category of analgesics or other interventions needed to relieve the pain, irrespective of etiology.[188] For example, according to the World Health Organization (WHO) pain management guidelines for children, severe pain, regardless of etiology, demands prompt treatment with a "strong opioid," such as morphine, hydromorphone (Dilaudid), fentanyl, or methadone.[189] In the vast majority of cases, pain can be rapidly controlled.[190] In the ICU and ED settings, parenteral administration of medications is most often indicated.

The occurrence of pain is not well-documented in the terminally ill pediatric ICU patient, but suspicion of pain must remain high, and presumptive treatment should occur if indications of pain are present. Where possible, each pain needs to be categorized not only by severity, but also by character (burning, gnawing, throbbing, sharp, crampy), location and radiation, duration, continuous or intermittent nature, and precipitating and relieving factors. The quality and timing of the pain suggest the etiology of the pain and dictate the most efficacious treatment. This ideal is very difficult to achieve in young or developmentally disabled children and in sedated or intubated patients. An empirical judgment of the etiology and physiology of the pain often dictates the choice of intervention in the ICU setting.

Burning pain in a patient who received neurotoxic chemotherapy or some anti-retroviral agents is a sign of neuropathic pain related to nerve injury. This pain is best treated with "adjuvant pain relievers" (medications most often used for other purposes, but which are effective in the relief of certain types of pain), such as tricyclic antidepressants and anticonvulsants along with "traditional" pain-relieving agents. It is crucial to stop the offending agent if it is still in use. Unfortunately, in the ICU setting, some adjuvants may not be of benefit because they must be given for at least 1 week to achieve effectiveness, or they are only available as oral preparations. Thus, depending on the patient's circumstance, the best pain management may be the use of nonpharmacological techniques, surgical, and anesthetic techniques where indicated,[191] and aggressive use of traditional pain relievers, including opioids and topical agents, such as topical lidocaine patches. Among opioids, methadone, which is available as a parenteral preparation, is most efficacious for neuropathic pain owing to its activity at numerous receptors, including the N-methyl-D-aspartate (NMDA) receptor.[192]

Concerns about addiction, a psychological phenomenon of craving a drug despite self-harm, are inappropriate in the ICU. Around-the-clock (ATC) analgesics should be provided, particularly in the setting of surgery, multiple trauma, and recurrent procedures.[193] Medications should be titrated to pain control using acetaminophen or nonsteroidal anti-inflammatory ATC pain relief (unless contraindicated) in addition to opioids for more severe pain, opioids and local anesthetics for procedure-related pain, and "adjuvant" analgesics for neuropathic pain. "As needed" or PRN opioid doses should be ordered for the alleviation of severe breakthrough pain and medications should also be available for the expected side effects of opioids, such as nausea, pruritus, urinary retention, and somnolence (when it is undesirable). Changing the specific opioid used[194] may also be considered for the management of refractory opioid-induced side effects when the child's expected survival is longer. Alternative routes of pain relief, such as epidurals for children who are excessively somnolent or who become delirious with systemically administered opioids may be of benefit in some cases.[188]

Respiratory depression in the face of pain is an uncommon occurrence even in children, despite aggressive use of opioids for pain relief.[195,196] Irregular breathing caused by pain can often be smoothed and regulated to promote optimal gas exchange when pain is relieved.

## Constipation

Constipation is very common in the ICU. Risk factors for constipation in the ICU include immobility, dehydration, and use of opioid, sedative and paralytic medications.[197] Nurses should consistently document bowel movement (BM) patterns and report lack of BMs greater than 2 days. Adjuvant stool softeners and laxatives should be initiated for any non-ambulatory, sedated or intubated patients. This is less of an issue for a child who is expected to die within 24 hours, as do most ICU patients undergoing the withdrawal or withholding of ICU interventions.[20,22,23] For more information on management of constipation see Chapter 53 in this text (symptom management).

## Dyspnea

*His breathing. It was a very shocking symptom. It was a scary symptom for us to see, and it hurt us as parents to watch because we knew how hard it was … he could hardly breathe. And every breath, we thought, that might be it. We kept holding our breath and thinking, 'That's it. He's not coming back,' and it was hard to see that, because it was so painful. It looked so painful to us. We're not sure if he was conscious enough for it to be painful for him. But as parents, it was very hard for us to watch that.[179]*

When the choice is to discontinue or to not initiate mechanical ventilation, scrupulous attention to the assessment and management of dyspnea must be explained and promised to the child (if capable of participating) and the family, and the promise must be realized. The idea that there may be a trade-off between relief of dyspnea and sedation, or even a slightly earlier death, must also be broached, concerns addressed and preferences elicited. In the few studies reviewing duration of survival related to the administration of morphine during withdrawal of mechanical ventilation, however, patients of all ages actually survive longer when liberal doses of morphine are used to ease the dyspnea.[12,14,35,182,195] Most families opt for enhanced comfort even in the face of a potentially foreshortened survival. However, patients occasionally are much less distressed than anticipated and are able to enjoy a few hours or even days with carefully titrated opioids, as needed.[198,199]

Dyspnea is a symptom that is even more distressing than pain to experience or witness. Behavioral correlates of the sensation of dyspnea observed in ICU patients are (in decreasing order): tachypnea and tachycardia, a fearful facial expression, use of accessory breathing muscles, paradoxical (diaphragmatic) breathing and nasal alar flaring.[200] Dyspnea can be difficult to control and requires intensive hands-on management and reassessment.[195] Several nonpharmacological approaches can be helpful,[201] such as limiting fluid intake, sitting the child upright, having a parent or other close family member or friend present, saying soothing words, and touching the child. In addition, having a small fan blow air across the child's face has been helpful in the hospice setting.

There are no published data on the treatment of dyspnea in children; clinical experience and the few small controlled studies done in adult patients support the use of opioids as the pharmacological agents of choice in the management of dyspnea.[202] Various recommendations for the pharmacological management of dyspnea exist.[12,14,34,182,195,203–205] Regardless of the protocol used, it is imperative that the child be continuously observed; the dose should be rapidly and aggressively escalated until relief is achieved.[206] The "correct" dose is established by titration to clinical effect; there is no maximal dose. Documentation should reflect dosing in response to distress and, optimally, will also note its resolution in response to treatment.

The expected response to opioids is gradual slowing of rapid respirations to a more normal level; respirations do not suddenly cease unexpectedly. Reversal with naloxone or other opioid antagonists should rarely, if ever, be undertaken in palliative care. Other pharmacologic aids in the management of dyspnea in the ICU include benzodiazepines to alleviate anxiety associated with, but not the sensation of, dyspnea; diuretics for children with pulmonary edema; and bronchodilators if there is an element of reactive airways disease. Withholding IV fluids or enteral feedings and adding anticholinergic agents will decrease excess secretions. Thorough suctioning of endotracheal tubes before extubation of mechanically ventilated children is helpful in preventing dyspnea and "death rattle." For more information on dyspnea, the reader is referred to Chapter 14.

## Palliative Sedation

Occasionally, a technique known as palliative (or sometimes "total") sedation is necessary to control refractory symptoms, most often pain, dyspnea, and intractable seizures. Within the palliative care community, palliative sedation has become a generally accepted option for refractory symptom management in adults. There are published articles for its use in children as well.[196] Although considered an "acceptable and justifiable form of euthanasia or physician-assisted suicide" (PAS) by some,[207-209] others see palliative sedation as the extension of the tenet that, above all, the health-care provider's duty is to relieve suffering. The intention is not to bring about the demise of the child (as in the case of PAS and euthanasia),[210,211] but rather to control the symptom, even at risk of death (principle of double effect).[180]

Regardless of the philosophical underpinnings that lead to the practice, palliative sedation is widely regarded in palliative care circles as the only humane solution to an otherwise uncontrollable and severely distressing problem. It is only undertaken after all other attempts at symptom control by an expert have failed to bring comfort. Full agreement of the child (when possible and usually accomplished in advance care planning discussions) and the family is required.[196] Explanations of the inability to reverse the underlying disease process must precede this decision. Some practitioners use barbiturates, which are particularly helpful in relieving agonal respirations, to decrease the patient's perception of terminal dyspnea and pain.[205]

Unfortunately, significant discomfort and uncertainty on the part of many critical care practitioners impede the availability of these therapeutic strategies.[111,181] Clinicians fear being perceived as the proximate cause of death resulting from the administration of opioids,[199] despite numerous well-known ethical opinions that the relief of symptoms is the primary obligation to the dying patient. Critical care nurses giving opioids to terminally ill patients withdrawn from mechanical ventilation reported that they believed they were engaging in euthanasia.[150] On the other hand, the administration of neuromuscular blocking agents, impeding the ability to assess dyspnea, can constitute euthanasia and should be avoided whenever possible.[212,213]

## Transforming Dying into a Celebration of Life

Most communication about forgoing "life support" concentrates on what will be stopped and not what will be enhanced or added.[61] Although we cannot help the child live longer, we can help parents properly celebrate the wonder of this child, his relationships, his value, and the impact he has had on the world.[11,13,60,90,109,110] Suggestions for accomplishing this celebration of life include:

- Inviting friends and extended family to visit with the family and child
- Bringing the child's own clothing and dressing him or her in it after a bath (the parent may choose to do this or ask to have the nurse do this)
- Removing no longer needed medical devices ("To make him your child again, and not a patient")
- Making a 3D plaster hand mold ("so you will always have your child's hand to hold")
- Bringing in photo albums to remember the good times that were had
- Bringing a camera or video to commemorate the celebration
- Offering families the opportunity to invite members of the family's congregation or others to provide spiritual support and guidance
- Bringing the child's favorite music, toys, videos, or other means of demonstrating the child's uniqueness
- Performing cultural, religious or family rituals as appropriate

Families have unique, individualized ways of acknowledging their child. One family may bring balloons and a sheet cake; another may choose to apply a teen's make-up and favorite cologne; a third might play videos of the teen's victorious football game. Easy access to a rocking chair or couch for the parent to hold the child (no matter how large) is helpful. Offer unlimited coffee, water, juice and soft drinks.

## The Butterfly Room

At the University of Texas Medical Branch at Galveston, an alternative care unit for children with life-threatening conditions called the Butterfly Room was created in 1995.[214] It is a homelike setting distinctly different from any other room in the hospital, with carpeting, wallpaper with butterflies, a kitchenette, TV, video game player and DVD player, pull-out sofa beds and chairs, padded window seats overlooking the Gulf of Mexico, and locked storage, as well as a place for the child to sleep (ohio warmer, crib, youth bed) with oxygen and suction at the head of the bed. It is as large as two semi-private rooms and is designed to accommodate the entire family. Meert's work supports such an environment of care as meeting the majority of families' needs near the time of death.[53]

One use of the room is for ICU patients who are expected to die within minutes to days following extubation, and who are thus generally not candidates for transfer home. After consultation with the family, reviewing the prognosis and goals of care, it is our practice to review the medical orders and discontinue all laboratory tests, all invasive equipment (extra IV sites, nasogastric tubes, urinary catheters, etc.), all monitors (including the recording of vital signs, fluid balance, and weights), and all medications other than those contributing to the comfort of the patient. Orders not to attempt resuscitation (DNAR) are written with the family's agreement. The child, who is still being mechanically ventilated, with vasopressors infusing as needed, is then moved from the ICU to the Butterfly Room, one floor and 150 feet away. Resuscitative medications, such as atropine and epinephrine, are brought in the elevator for unstable patients to ensure that the family will have a chance for final togetherness, but these medications have never been used. Cardiopulmonary resuscitation beyond these medications would not be done, however.

In the Butterfly Room, the child's loved ones are invited to sit in a rocking chair, or, in the case of an older child, they are invited to sit on a couch and hold the child. Even young siblings participate in this activity. Usually, each family member in turn will whisper loving thoughts and memories to the dying child. Numerous photographs are taken in most cases. The family is offered the opportunity to bathe the child, make handprints, footprints, or handmolds and dress the child in clothing of their choice. Other rituals specific to the family or their heritage may be undertaken. Once these events have taken place, with the family's acknowledgment of readiness, the respiratory therapist disables the alarms on the ventilator and the child is extubated by the physician. Opioids, benzodiazepines, and blow-by oxygen are immediately available. The interdisciplinary hospice team, including a spiritual leader of the family's choosing, if desired, a social worker, a child-life therapist for siblings, and the nurse and physician remain either in the room or close by, often mingling among the distressed relatives and listening to their concerns, providing explanations and empathy while attending to the patient's symptoms. Often, the child will seem to be dead for a few minutes, only to heave a sigh and turn pink for a few minutes. This may happen several times. When declaring death, it is critical to listen to the heart and to be certain of the death—waiting a little too long is better than being premature in this instance. A gentle acknowledgement ("He's gone") is often accompanied by an increase in the demonstration of grief. Depending on the relationships, a hug may be appreciated at the time.

### Notification of Death in the ED or ICU When Parents are not Present

Unless there are extremely extenuating circumstances, even if the death is expected, most experts strongly encourage that the notification of death be done in person. ("Mrs. Smith, I am afraid I have some bad news. Could you come in to discuss it?") Empathy can be more easily expressed in person by sitting close to the parents and siblings at the time of the discussion, perhaps even giving the bereaved a hug, or shedding a genuine tear.[8–14,27,37–41,48,51,54,55,57–61,79,87,89,90,93,105] These small tokens of warmth and understanding help the family to know that the medical team cared about the child as a person. Additionally, insistence that the family come in allows them to see the dead child's body, facilitating the acceptance of the death and allowing the family to participate in important rituals, such as bathing the child's body, sometimes assisting in the removal of equipment, or sitting vigil as some cultures require. These activities result in improved bereavement outcomes for the parents as well as the siblings. [52,88,92]

### Autopsy and Organ Donation

One of the most common complaints of bereaved families is that they still, even years later, do not understand the cause of their child's death.[8,37,52,129] Most of the time this is because of shock preventing integration of the information or based on poor or nonexistent communication. However, sometimes the cause of death was not known to the health-care providers; in still other cases, the physician is incorrect in his or her assessment. In fact, major unexpected findings related to death occurred in 28% of the autopsies in a recent pediatric study. Among 100 consecutive autopsies, these investigators found new information that had the potential to further clarify the cause(s) of a child's death (53% of cases); inform the future reproductive choices of either the parents (10%) or siblings (8%); affect siblings' future healthcare (6%); or contribute to patient care quality control (36%) or publishable knowledge (7%).[215] For these reasons, autopsy should be encouraged. Once the body is buried or cremated, the opportunity for this helpful information is gone forever.

Autopsies can be tailored to the needs of the family. Even the coroner's cases are not total body autopsies—they are limited to determining the cause of death. Most often, there is minimal disfigurement and an open-casket ceremony can still be performed, if desired. Moreover, in elective autopsies, parents can choose to limit the autopsy to the organ of interest. It is possible to take needle biopsies rather than to remove whole organs, if preferred, and a request can also be made to replace all organs back in their natural locations after the autopsy is performed. Many locales do not charge the family for the autopsy. There is generally no more than a 24-hour delay in removing the body to the funeral home if an autopsy is performed.

Many health-care providers believe that organ donation assists families of brain dead children to feel something good came of the death. Although this is true for some families, Bellali et al.[216] found that the bereavement outcomes for donor and nondonor families were more dependent on the families' perceptions of the meaning of the death, the way they were treated by the hospital personnel, the way the organ donation request was broached, and their own intrinsic world-view than by the fact of organ donation. Vane found that donation consent was more common if the family was approached by an attending physician, after time to absorb the fact of the death, and after time to gather supporters. A delay of eight hours enabled a donation rate increase from 23% to 86%.[217] In another study, families of brain dead patients report the need for privacy, acknowledgement, physical space, and bereavement follow-up.[218] Many of the parents of organ donors wanted follow-up information on the organ recipients' well-being.[219]

## Post-Death Conference

One of the most frequently recommended ways to provide needed bereavement support for families of patients who died in the ICU or ED is the post-death conference.[8–10,12–13,92,129] Especially in sudden, unanticipated deaths, families cannot absorb new information about how and why the child died. It takes several weeks to begin to think more clearly; at that point, feelings of despair arise as the questions pour in. Parents often erroneously feel they were told nothing and can become angry about not understanding what happened. In addition, if an autopsy was performed, families need a face-to-face appointment with the treating physician to explain the autopsy findings in understandable terms.[92,129,220,221] This explanation can provide the bereaved family with a profound sense of peace by affirming the cause of death, affirming the irreversibility of the problems, or determining a cause of death that was unknown antemortem.

Meert et al. studied ICU families' desires for a post-death meeting.[129] The majority preferred to meet with the ICU attending. The reasons noted for desiring such a meeting were:

- To review the sequence of events leading to the child's death, review the autopsy results in plain English
- To understand the risk to their existing or future children and any ways to prevent the same fate
- To get complete and honest information
- To be able to explain what happened to their familes and friends
- To get help, reassurance, and bereavement support
- To be able to help others
- To be able to express complaints and gratitude regarding their ICU experience.

The post-death conference has even been found to improve adaptation to loss. It enables monitoring of the family's grieving process and provides the opportunity for referral to counseling, if needed, for pathological grief reactions. In the absence of a face-to-face session, families consenting to an autopsy often complain that they had no follow-up and express anger and suspicion about the motivations for the autopsy. This post-death conference is also helpful for families who did not consent to autopsy, to answer their inevitable questions. Referrals can be made for families needing counseling or other assistance.

## Bereavement Care

Family-centered care is an essential approach to providing care to children and families during their stay in the PICU or ED; it does not end at the child's death.[1,8,9,11–14,47,93,222] Particularly after a sudden and traumatic event, the death of a child can lead to prolonged and often complicated grief for the parents, siblings and other family members.[56,91,51] Meert and colleagues[51] found that even those parents with strong coping skills suffered prolonged and intense grief reactions after the death of a child in the PICU. Acute death predicted longer and more complicated grief as compared with death from a chronic condition.[51] In this study, the strongest predictor of coping was the parents' level of physical health and wellness at the time of the death. Compassionate care from the PICU staff also seemed to predict better outcomes for the parents.[51] Meyer and colleagues[46] found that the majority of parents do not participate in bereavement support groups after the death of their child. For parents who do attend a support group, about half report that the experience was helpful.[46]

Oliver and Fallat found that parental grief was further complicated by unanswered questions and confusion about the medical decisions in that impacted their child.[56] Parents in this study also expressed delayed regret for not having had the opportunity to participate in organ donation. For parents whose child died a violent death, attendance at a support group and maintenance of religious connection can enable better adaptation in the long term.[223]

The following factors in the PICU were reported by parents as being beneficial to their adaptation to grief: parental presence at the time of death, adequate and timely information, and kindness and empathy from staff.[51] Unfortunately, because of a lack of rigorous study of interventions for bereaved parents and siblings following the death of a child in a PICU or ED, it is difficult to suggest evidence-based guidelines for care. A recent review of the literature concluded that more study is needed of replicable interventions in controlled trials.[224] However, there seems to be universal agreement that PICU and ED staff can positively impact the bereavement outcomes of parents by engaging in a thorough discussion of choices, provision of honest and timely information, and offering compassionate care.[51]

Studies have repeatedly shown an increased mortality rate of surviving spouses in the year following death.[225–227] A recent study of bereaved parents in Denmark showed a marked increase in mortality from natural (maternal) and unnatural causes (maternal and paternal),[228] though no similar study of siblings has been undertaken. The divorce rate among parents the first year after a child's death is higher than the national average (over the long term, however, the proportion returns to the national average of 50%). Parents have intense spiritual needs at the time of child's death in the PICU and during bereavement.[60,109,110] In the PICU, parents report drawing on spiritual guidance to assist them in end-of-life decision-making, to support them emotionally and to eventually make meaning out of their loss.[110]

A simple strategy of routinely sending a bereavement card 2 weeks following the death of a hospitalized adult patient was investigated. One year later, the bereaved survivors could consistently and without warning retrieve the card, indicating the importance to them of such a gesture. Remarks of survivors of patients who had died in the ED included, "At least I know my husband died among caring people."[229] Attending the deceased's funeral is an even more powerful demonstration of caring and may provide relief for the health-care provider as well.[60] When asked, bereaved parents remark that a simple card or call would have helped tremendously.[37,93,109]

### Memorial Services

A memorial service may also be offered.[230,231] This may take several forms; two are particularly suggested for the ICU. Families whose children have either come to the ICU recurrently, or those who have particularly bonded with the staff because of a child's prolonged stay or for other reasons, may be invited back to the unit with the families of a few other children who have died within the last month or 6 weeks for a ceremony of sharing. The family may bring a picture of the child, and the family and staff can exchange memories of the child. Songs may be sung, poems may be read, and prayers may be shared. Gratitude and admiration may be exchanged. In addition, all families bereaved of children could be invited to a group memorial service conducted on an annual or more frequent basis. One study of the bereavement care of families grieving a child's traumatic death included family contact at the hospital after discharge from the ED, attendance at the funeral home, a home visit, a meeting at a restaurant with the parents and 15 parental supporters 2 months following the death, for the purpose of educating parental supporters about the course of grief and the need for longer-term support and a parental interview approximately a year after the death.[92] Substantial improvement in parental outcome as measured by anxiety, depression, functional outcome and PTSD scales were demonstrated compared to historic controls.

### Grief of Health-Care Providers

Not only do children suffer and families and loved ones grieve, but we as health-care providers grieve for our patients, their families, and ourselves. We are exposed to pain and grief both vicariously and in empathy and are forced to confront the certainty of our own and our fellow humans' mortality on a daily basis. In caring for dying children, we are threatened by the reality that our own children, too, could die. The ability to share these feelings in a supportive environment, without sanction, and the ability to take leave to attend funerals can assist in increased job satisfaction and retention of highly-skilled emergency and critical care personnel. It can

also help to reinforce the humanity that makes us the health-care providers we can be.

Rushton and colleagues[212] found that health-care professionals suffer from grief and moral distress as well as from the stress of inadequate communication within the health-care team itself. Health-care providers do not always feel sufficiently supported to provide the type of compassionate and open communication that they want to offer to families. Health-care professionals from PICU, NICU and pediatric oncology units identify the following key factors which result in increased professional comfort and knowledge when caring for children who die:[212]

- Having a palliative care network
- Attending palliative care rounds
- Having access to patient care conferences and
- Bereavement debriefing sessions

These interventions increase the staff's ability to deal with their own grief, facilitate effective communication with staff and families, and increase knowledge of coping strategies.[212] In a study of the comfort and confidence levels of pediatric intensive care staff, Jones and colleagues[128] discovered that having 8 or more years of experience increased the confidence of staff, but not their comfort level. In this same study, physicians and nurses reported higher levels of confidence and comfort in providing medical and practical aspects of care than in the psychosocial aspects of care, for which they continue to have little formal training. Parker et al.[232] found that physicians report facing a number of dialectical tensions in compassionately communicating the death of a child in the emergency room. The internal tensions included clarity and compassion, trust and blame, empathy and professionalism, intimacy and nonintimacy, and certainty and uncertainty. All of these studies point to the increased need for training and support for health-care professionals in the PICU and ED in providing compassionate care while simultaneously addressing their own tensions, grief and moral distress. Clearly, standard preparatory medical and nursing education and years of experience are insufficient to mitigate the emotional challenges faced by providers in pediatric critical care. There are ongoing needs for support, debriefing, and self-compassion. In fact, the American Academy of Critical Care Medicine's (AACCM) consensus statement on end-of-life care in the ICU concluded that the unresolved grief of health-care professionals can impact the patient care provided and called for steps to be taken to alleviate caregivers' grief and moral distress.[12]

A variety of coping strategies have been described to help professionals manage the stress of caring for seriously ill children who eventually die.[31] Some coping strategies are personal and beneficial in the short term (e.g., engaging in self-care activities such as exercise, meditation, or journal-writing) or in the long term (e.g., developing a personal philosophy of care, engaging in self-reflection and self-awareness, committing to taking care of oneself). Other coping strategies are work-related, the most important being the development of supportive professional relationships that promote debriefing and enhance mutual support.[233-235] Health professionals seem to rely more on their colleagues than family and friends for support. The nature of this support differs, and includes the exchange of information (informational support); the clinical collaboration to meet patient needs (clinical or instrumental support); the sharing of personal feelings and experiences (emotional support); and the reflection and attribution of meaning to one's work experiences (meaning-making support). Opportunities for formal support (e.g., participation in support groups, stress-debriefing sessions, or supervision meetings) and informal support (e.g., time-out for discussions) are encouraged in different work settings, depending on the philosophy and goals of care, as well as on rules and regulations with regard to the team's functioning in the face of their patients' death.[234]

## Summary and Recommendations For Implementation

Improved end-of-life care begins with more highly-focused attention on the individual child and his or her preferences and values. Pediatric and neonatal ICU and ED practitioners are the caregivers for the vast majority of children who die; thus, they must have expertise in palliative care. Infants die primarily of congenital defects, prematurity, and SIDS. Children older than 1 year of age die primarily from trauma, thus predisposing them to die in the ED or ICU settings. The principles of palliative care must be applied to all children, even those whose fate is to die in the ED or ICU. Our challenge, as practitioners of pediatric emergency and critical care medicine, is to provide each of these children a "good death" and their families a more peaceful bereavement. This can be achieved by intensive attention to the child's and family's perspectives and goals, communication within the team and with the child and his or her loved ones, dedication to the meticulous prevention and management of symptoms, particularly during procedures—the most common source of discomfort in ill children—and effective bereavement follow-up.

### Recommendations to Enhance End-of-Life Care in the ICU and ED Setting

- Admission procedures should include a values history; solicitation of any advance directives for older, chronically ill children; and discussion of expressed preferences in light of the child's current situation. This should not be reserved only for imminently dying children. Waiting until that time only increases the chances that the child's preferences will never be known and the family's guilt will be unnecessarily increased in the event they are later called on to consent to the withdrawal of no-longer-beneficial medical interventions. Good coordination with primary care providers and specialists who have cared for the chronically ill child can be enormously helpful.

- Attention to pain and the relief of other symptoms, both during procedures and more generally, must become a priority for all children. This can be accomplished only with training and appropriate policies and documentation procedures, as well as emphasis by supervisors and attending physicians.

- Improved communication techniques must be employed that allow children or their surrogates to understand their options in a supportive and unbiased way. Guilt, missed opportunities, love, and existential and spiritual issues should be included in these discussions. Again, training must be developed and carried out. The importance of truly informed consent must be emphasized, demonstrated, and reflected in the practices of the opinion leaders within the unit.

- Cooperation, respect, and regular interdisciplinary rounds among the disciplines of nursing, medicine, social work, pastoral care, and, possibly, palliative care (and others as indicated, such as pharmacy, occupational therapy, physical therapy, child-life) will enhance the larger understanding of the child and his or her needs and facilitate the team's ability to assist the child with the accomplishment of his or her goals.

- Development of a celebration of life or similar protocol can transform the death of the child from a vigil to a recognition of the value of the individual while supporting the family.

- Establishment of a bereavement follow-up program, including the mailing of bereavement cards, autopsy debriefing or post-death sessions, "sharing sessions," and memorial services will improve the bereavement outcome for surviving loved ones and ED or ICU staff.

- Excused, paid absences for funeral attendance, formalized staff mentoring programs and facilitation of self-care will prevent burnout and turnover and allow the retention of the ideals and values that brought each staff member to the healing professions.

CASE STUDY
*FL, A Near-Drowning Victim*

FL, a 14-year-old Pakistani boy, suffered a near-drowning episode that compromised his central respiratory drive mechanism and left him neurologically devastated. His family was informed that he would not ever regain consciousness, nor would he be able to breathe on his own. They agreed to move him to the Butterfly Room to achieve a family-centered death. Orders not to attempt resuscitation were written in a clear and detailed manner. All laboratory analyses were discontinued and all monitors were removed.

Medications were reviewed and all were discontinued. Morphine and lorazepam were added for the management of dyspnea, IV fluids were discontinued, and scopolamine was administered for terminal secretions. One IV catheter was left intact, but all other invasive monitors, such as nasogastric tubes, urinary and arterial catheters, etc., were removed. During his transfer from the ICU to the Butterfly Room, FL remained mechanically ventilated.

Although FL had a small family, he belonged to a close-knit community. Thirty people of all ages came to be with him on his final day of life. They encircled the boy's bed, chanting but not touching him. After approximately 30 minutes, they approached the team and announced their readiness for the discontinuation of mechanical ventilation. One caregiver stated that she was unfamiliar with Pakistani traditions and customs, but had not observed anyone touching FL. She suggested that if touching was allowable and desirable for them, they were welcome to do so. The whole spirit of the group changed, with the circle drawing nearer the bed and men openly grieving and weeping, holding the boy and their wives, as well as each other. People stroked FL's face and body. After an hour, they again informed the team that they were now ready to have the mechanical ventilation discontinued.

FL's endotracheal tube (ETT) was suctioned; after extubation, he needed little pharmacological intervention. His loved ones chanted from the moment the ETT was removed. Each visitor, in turn, put small amounts of holy water in his mouth. Although the water bubbled out of his nose, a caregiver wiped it away, giving "permission" for the next person to engage in the ritual. After 27 minutes of nonstop chanting, FL died. A peaceful hush fell over the room, and all eyes turned to the same window leading to the outside.

### CASE STUDY
### *LF, A Newborn with Hypoplastic Left Heart Syndrome*

LF, a newborn girl, was diagnosed with hypoplastic left heart syndrome. After a full explanation of the surgical options, the family opted for palliative care. The mother preferred never to see LF again, because she feared bonding with her daughter. The baby was in the ICU but, because of her parents' decision, was not receiving ICU interventions. The parents were approached about the Butterfly Program, providing surrogate parents, and moving the baby to the Butterfly Room; they agreed. They decided to visit LF the next day. She was wearing normal baby clothes, being cared for and appearing like any other baby. When they saw that their daughter did not need highly-skilled care, the parents felt that they could care for her themselves at home with the help of the Butterfly Program. The next day, her parents took LF home; she lived well there and visited many churches for blessings, went to

numerous restaurants, had house guests, received several hospice visits, and was asymptomatic until two weeks of age, when she began to vomit and become intermittently cyanotic. The Butterfly Team (nurse, social worker, and physician) was summoned to the home. Further explanations of what was happening and assurances of the child's comfort were provided. The baby received one dose of morphine, but the family assessed that she did not need more. She died in her mother's arms 8 hours after the first cyanotic episode.

### CASE STUDY
### *Cameron, An Infant with a Mitochondrial Disorder*

"Cameron" was a 4-month-old boy born with a mitochondrial disorder, associated with a severe cardiomyopathy. His mother had brittle type 1 diabetes, resulting in pregnancy complications of a diabetic coma and quadriplegia. Traumatized by the situation, Cameron's father withdrew from the family. The maternal grandmother relocated from another state to care for her daughter and grandson until they could move home with her. Cameron was referred for hospice admission by the NICU attending, who had spent many hours with Cameron's mother and grandmother discussing the condition, prognosis and options for care. The family elected home hospice and an out of hospital DNR, doing well the first month. His mother suffered from severe depression, but enjoyed having him placed in bed with her. At each visit, the family discussed their wishes for moving to the grandmother's home. In the week prior to their move, Cameron began to show signs of a viral illness. The Hospice RN noted Cameron was mottled, febrile, tachypneic and tachycardic with poor perfusion, assessing he was likely to die from this episode. After notifying the neonatologist, the nurse told the mother and grandmother of the gravity of the child's condition and offered continuous care nursing support. After discussion, they requested transport to an ED. The Hospice RN honored the family's wishes, remaining with the family. Upon arrival, the ED attending physician conferred with the Hospice RN, then gently spoke with the grandmother while the ER staff rapidly assessed Cameron and began resuscitative measures, including bag-mask ventilation and chest compressions. On further discussion with the physician and the hospice nurse, the grandmother determined that the resuscitation would not benefit Cameron. She was brought to the bedside and the infant was placed in her arms and allowed to die comfortably. Cameron's father arrived with his mother within a few minutes of the death. His parents were placed in a quiet, secluded room and his grandmother brought the baby to them. ER nursing staff and the hospice nurse attended to the family until they felt comfortable releasing his body to a funeral home. Hospice provided bereavement services to the mother, father and the grandmother.

CASE STUDY
*Faith, An Adolescent with Recurrent Cancer*

"Faith" was a 14-year-old girl diagnosed with acute lymphocytic leukemia. Following induction chemotherapy, she had consolidation treatment and a bone marrow transplant from a matched sibling donor. Despite complications during the transplant, she recovered enough to be discharged home. A month later she developed respiratory distress leading to ICU admission. Her mother requested the presence of a trusted clinic nurse as Faith was notably anxious from the dyspnea and the impending intubation. The nurse calmed Faith with stories about a recent trip to a children's cancer camp and offered to sing a camp song for her. As the nurse began to sing a familiar camp song, Faith's mother and the ICU nurses and physician joined in. Faith was able to smile and relax while the group continued to sing as she was intubated. Thereafter, diagnostic tests confirmed the recurrence of Faith's leukemia, leading to her current complications. The transplant physician spoke at length with Faith's family over the next two days regarding her condition and her limited chance of recovery. The family felt that Faith would not want to remain intubated and unconscious and consented to the withdrawal of no-longer-beneficial treatments, including ventilation. They were provided time to contact family and friends and arrange for blessings from their congregation. They also brought in a CD player and played Faith's favorite song. When the ICU team began to withdraw the pressors and mechanical ventilation, the group sang along to the Everly Brother's "Dream" as Faith died peacefully, surrounded by family and friends.

REFERENCES

1. Maruyama N. Cited by: Field MJ and Behrman RE. Your child is dead. Am Coll Emerg Med News October 18, 1997. (Ref. 1, p. 113).

2. Billings JA. What is palliative care? J Palliat Med 1998;1:73–81.

3. Field MJ, Behrman RE, eds. When Children Die: Improving Palliative and End-of-Life Care for Children and Their Families. Washington, DC: National Academy Press, 2002.

4. American Academy of Pediatrics Committee on Bioethics and Committee on Hospital Care. Pediatric palliative care. Pediatrics 2000;106:351–357.

5. Himelstein BP. Palliative care for infants, children, adolescents, and their families. J Palliat Med 2006;9(1):163–181.

6. Mack JW, Wolfe J. Early integration of pediatric palliative care: For some children, palliative care starts at diagnosis. Curr Opin Pediatr 2008;18:10–14.

7. Baker JN, Hinds PS, Spunt SL, et al. Integration of palliative care practices into the ongoing care of children with cancer: Individualized care planning and coordination. Pediatr Clin North Am 2008;55:223–250.

8. O'Malley PJ, Brown K, Krug SE, the Committee on Pediatric Emergency Medicine Patient- and Family-Centered Care of Children in the Emergency Department. Pediatrics 2008;122:e511–e521.

9. Knapp J, Mulligan-Smith D, the Committee on Pediatric Emergency Medicine. Death of a child in the emergency department. Pediatrics 2005;115:1432–1437.

10. Wright JL, Johns CMS, Joseph JG. End of life care in emergency medical services for children. In: Fields M, Behrman RD, eds. When Children Die. Washington, DC: Institute of Medicine, National Academies Press; 2003:580–598, Appendix F.

11. Davidson JE, Powers K, Hedayat KM, et al. Clinical practice guidelines for support of the family in the patient-centered intensive care unit: American College of Critical Care Medicine Task Force 2004–2005. Crit Care Med 2007;35:605–622.

12. Truog RD, Campbell ML, Curtis JR, et al. Recommendations for end-of-life care in the intensive care unit: A consensus statement by the American Academy of Critical Care Medicine. Crit Care Med 2008;36:953–963.

13. Truog RD, Meyer EC, Burns JP. Toward interventions to improve end-of-life care in the pediatric intensive care unit. Crit Care Med 2006;34(11 Suppl):S373–S379.

14. Lanken PN, Terry PB, Delisser HM, et al. An official American Thoracic Society clinical policy statement: Palliative care for patients with respiratory diseases and critical illnesses. Am J Respir Crit Care Med 2008;177(8):912–927.

15. Mosenthal AC, Murphy PA, Barker LK, Lavery R, Retano A, Livingston DH. Changing the culture around end-of-life care in the trauma intensive care unit. J Trauma 2008;64(6):1587–1593.

16. Carter BS, Hubble C, Weise KL. Palliative medicine in neonatal and pediatric intensive care. Child Adolesc Psychiatr Clin N Am 2006;15(3):759–777.

17. Angus DC, Barnato AE, Linde-Zwirble WT, et al. Use of intensive care at the end of life in the United States: An epidemiologic study. Crit Care Med 2004;32(3):638–643.

18. Copnell B. Death in the pediatric ICU: Caring for children and families at the end of life. Crit Care Nurs Clin North Am 2005;17:349–360.

19. Brandon D, Docherty SL, Thorpe J. Infant and child deaths in acute care settings: Implications for palliative care. J Palliat Med 2007;10(4):910–918.

20. Garros D, Rosychuk RJ, Cox PN. Circumstances surrounding end of life in a pediatric intensive care unit. Pediatrics 2003;112:e371.

21. Carter BS, Howenstein M, Gilmer MJ, Throop P, France D, Whitlock JA. Circumstances surrounding the deaths of hospitalized children: Opportunities for pediatric palliative care. Pediatrics 2004;114:e361–e366.

22. Vats TS, Reynolds PD. Pediatric hospital dying trajectories: What we learned and what we can share. Pediatr Nurs 2006;32:386–392.

23. Zawistowski CA, DeVita MA. A descriptive study of children dying in the pediatric intensive care unit after withdrawal of life-sustaining treatment. Pediatr Crit Care Med 2004;5(3):216–223.

24. Wanzer SH, Federman DD, Adelstein SJ, et al. The physician's responsibility toward hopelessly ill patients: A second look. N Engl J Med 1989;320:844–849.

25. Sullivan AM, Lakoma MD, Block SD. The status of medical education in end-of-life care: A national report. J Gen Intern Med 2003;18:685–695.

26. Hilden JM. Emanuel EJ, Fairclough DL, et al. Attitudes and practices among pediatric oncologists regarding end of life care: Results of the 1998 American Society of Clinical Oncology survey. J Clin Oncol 2001;19:205–212.

27. Contro N, Larson J, Scofield S, Sourkes B, Cohen H. Family perspectives on the quality of pediatric palliative care. Arch Pediatr Adolesc Med 2002;156:14–19.

28. Contro NA, Larson JL, Scofield S, Sourkes B, Cohen HJ. Hospital staff and family perspecitives regarding quality of pediatric palliative care. Pediatrics 2004;114:1248–1252.

29. Kolarik RC, Walker G, Arnold RM. Pediatric resident education in palliative care: A needs assessment. Pediatrics 2006;117(6):1949–1954.

30. Davies B, Sehring SA, Partridge JC, et al. Barriers to palliative care for children: Perceptions of pediatric health care providers. Pediatrics 2008;121(2):282–288.

31. Liben S, Papadatou D, Wolfe J. Pediatric palliative care: Challenges and emerging ideas. Lancet 2008;371:852–864.

32. Mosenthal A, Murphy PA. Trauma care and palliative care: Time to integrate the two. J Am Coll Surg 2003;197:509–516.

33. Feudtner C. Collaborative communication in pediatric palliative care; a foundation for problem-solving and decision-making. Pediatr Clin North Am 2007;54:583–608.

34. Curtis JR. Caring for patients with critical illness and their families: The value of the integrated clinical team. Respir Care 2008;53(4):480–487.

35. Burns JP, Mitchell C, Griffith JL, Truog RD. End-of-life care in the pediatric intensive care unit: Attitudes and practices of pediatric critical care physicians and nurses. Crit Care Med 2001;29:658–664.

36. Treece PD, Engelberg RA, Crowley L, et al. Evaluation of a standardized order form for the withdrawal of life support in the intensive care unit. Crit Care Med 2004;32(5):1141–1148.

37. Ahrens W, Hart R, Maruyama N. Pediatric death: Managing the aftermath in the emergency department. J Emerg Med 1997;15:601–603.

38. Cook P, White DK, Ross-Russell RI. Bereavement support following sudden and unexpected death: Guidelines for care. Arch Dis Child 2002;87:36–38.

39. Levetown M. Breaking bad news in the emergency department: When seconds count. Top Emerg Med 2004;26:35–43.

40. Truog RD, Christ G, Browning DM, Meyer EC. Sudden traumatic death in children: We did everything, but your child did not survive. JAMA 2006;295:2646–2654.

41. Bartel DA, Engler AJ, Natale JE, Misra V, Lewin AB, Joseph JG. Working with families of suddenly and critically ill children: Physician experiences. Arch Pediatr Adolesc Med 2000;154:1127–1133.

42. Hinds PS, Gattuso JS, Fletcher A, et al. Quality of life as conveyed by pediatric patients with cancer. Qual Life Res 2004;13(4):761–772.

43. Hinds PS, Schum L, Baker JN, Wolfe J. Key Factors affecting dying children and their families. J Palliat Med 2005;8(Suppl 1):S-70–S-78.

44. Dussel V, Kreicbergs U, Hilden JM, et al. Looking beyond where children die: Determinants and effects of planning a child's location of death. J Pain Symptom Manage 2009; 37(1):33–43.

45. Meert KL, Thurston CS, Sarnaik AP. End-of-life decision-making and satisfaction with care: Parental perspectives. Pediatr Crit Care Med 2000;1(2):179–185.

46. Meyer EC, Burns JP, Griffith JL, Truog RD. Parental perspectives on end-of-life care in the pediatric intensive care unit. Crit Care Med 2002;30:226–231.

47. Meyer EC, Ritholz MD, Burns JP, Truog RD. Improving the quality of end-of-life care in the pediatric intensive care unit: Parents' priorities and recommendations. Pediatrics 2006;117:649–665.

48. Martin JA, Kung H-C, Mathews TJ, et al. Annual summary of vital statistics: 2006. Pediatrics 2008;121:788–801.

49. McCallum DE, Byrne P, Bruera E. How children die in hospital. J Pain Symptom Manage 2000;20:417–423.

50. Adamowski K, Dickinson G, Weitzman B, Roessler C, Carter-Snell C. Sudden unexpected death in the emergency department: Caring for the survivors. CMAJ 1993;149(10):1445–1451.

51. Meert KL, Thurston CS, Thomas R. Parental coping and bereavement outcome after the death of a child in the pediatric intensive care unit. Pediatr Crit Care Med 2001;2(4):324–328.

52. Meert KL, Eggly S, Pollack MM, et al. Parents' perspectives regarding a physician-parent conference after their child's death in the pediatric intensive care unit. J Pediatr 2007;151(1):50–55.e2.

53. Meert KL, Briller SH, Schim SM, Thurston CS. Exploring parents' environmental needs at the time of a child's death in the pediatric intensive care unit. Pediatr Crit Care Med 2008;9(6):623–628.

54. Dubin WR, Sarnoff JR. Sudden unexpected death: Intervention with the survivors. Ann Emerg Med 1986;15:54–57.

55. Fraser S, Atkins J. Survivors' recollections of helpful and unhelpful emergency nurse activities surrounding sudden death of a loved one. J Emerg Nurs 1990;16(1):13–16.

56. Oliver RC, Fallat ME, Traumatic childhood death; how well do parents cope? J Trauma 1995;39:303–308.

57. Edwardsen EA, Chiumento S, Davis E. Family perspective of medical care and grief support after field termination by emergency services personnel—a preliminary report. Prehosp Emerg Care 2002;6:440–444.

58. Merlevede E, Spooren D, Henderick H, et al. Perceptions, needs and mourning reactions of bereaved relatives confronted with a sudden unexpected death. Resuscitation 2004;61:341–348.

59. Wisten A, Zingmark K. Supportive needs of parents confronted with sudden cardiac death—a qualitative study. Resuscitation 2007;74:68–74.

60. Meert KL, Thurston CS, Briller SH. The spiritual needs of parents at the time of their child's death in the pediatric intensive care unit and during bereavement: A qualitative study. Pediatr Crit Care Med 2005;6(4):420–427.

61. Sharman M, Meert KL, Sarniak AP. What influences parents; decisions to limit or withdraw life support? Pediatr Crit Care Med 2005;6:513–518.

62. Slonim AD. Cardiopulmonary resuscitation outcomes in children. Crit Care Med 2000;28:3364–3366.

63. Sichting K, Berens R. Outcomes following resuscitations at Children's Hospital of Wisconsin. Crit Care Med 1997;25:A61.

64. Lantos JD, Miles SH, Silverstein MD, Stocking CB. Survival after cardiopulmonary resuscitation in babies of very low birth weight. N Engl J Med 1998;318:91–95.

65. Torres A, Pickert CB, Firestone J, Walter WM, Fiser DH. Long-term functional outcome of in-patient pediatric cardiopulmonary resuscitation. Pediatr Emerg Care 1997;13:369–373.

66. Schindler MB, Bohn D, Cox PN, et al. Outcome of out-of-hospital cardiac or respiratory arrest in children. N Engl J Med 1996;335:1473–1479.

67. American Heart Association. AHA guidelines for cardiopulmonary resuscitation and emergency cardiovascular are of pediatric and neonatal patients; Pediatric basic life support. Pediatrics 2006;117:e989–e1004.

68. Donoghue AJ, Nadkarni V, Berg RA, et al. Out-of-hospital pediatric cardiac arrest: An epidemiologic review and assessment of current knowledge. Ann Emerg Med 2005;46:512–522.

69. Gerein RB, Osmond MH, Stiell IG, Nesbitt LP, Burns S, OPALS Study Group. What are the etiology and epidemiology of out-of-hospital pediatric cardiac arrests in Ontario, Canada? Acad Emerg Med 2006;13:653–658.

70. Pitetti R, Glustein JZ, Bhende MS. Prehospital care and outcome of pediatric out-of-hospital cardiac arrest. Prehosp Emerg Care 2002;6:283–290.

71. Rodriguez-Nunez A, Lopez-Herce J, Garcia C, et al. Pediatric defibrillation after cardiac arrest: Initial response and outcome. Crit Care 2006;10:R113–R120.

72. Topjian AA, Berg, RA, Nadkarni VM. Pediatric cardiopulmonary resuscitation: Advances in science, techniques and outcomes. Pediatrics 2008;122:1086–1098.

73. Young KD, Gausche-Hill M, McClung CD, Lewis RJ. A prospective, population-based study of the epidemiology and outcome of out-of-hospital pediatric cardiopulmonary arrest. Pediatrics 2004;114:157–164.

74. Diem SJ, Lantos JD, Tulsky JA. Cardiopulmonary resuscitation on television: Miracles and misinformation. N Engl J Med 1996;334:1604–1605.

75. Murphy DJ, Burrows D, Santilli S, et al. The influence of the probability of survival on patients' preferences regarding cardiopulmonary resuscitation. N Engl J Med 1994;330:545–549.

76. O'Donnell H, Phillips RS, Wenger N, Teno J, Davis RB, Hamel MB. Preferences for cardiopulmonary resuscitation among patients 80 years or older: The views of patients and their physicians. J Am Med Dir Assoc 2003;4:139–144.

77. Ford D, Zapka JG, Gebregziabher M, Hennessy W, Yang C. Investigating critically ill patients' and families' perceptions of likelihood of survival. J Palliat Med 2009;12(1):45–52.

78. Marco CA, Larkin GL. Public education regarding resuscitation: Effects of a multi-media intervention. Ann Emerg Med 2003;42:256–60.

79. Foresman-Capuzzi J. Grief-telling: Death of a child in the emergency department. J Emerg Nurs 2007;33:505–508.

80. Wells PJ. Preparing for sudden death; social work in the emergency room. Social Work 1993;38:339–342.

81. Dear S. Breaking bad news: Caring for the family. Nurs Stand 1995;10:31–33.

82. Dingeman RS, Mitchell EA, Meyer EC, Curley MA. Parent presence during complex invasive procedures and cardiopulmonary resuscitation: A systematic review of the literature. Pediatrics 2007;120(4):842–854.

83. Henderson DP, Knapp JF. Report of the national consensus conference on family presence during pediatric cardiopulmonary resuscitation and procedures. J Emerg Nurs 2006;32:23–29.

84. Madden E, Condon C. Emergency nurses' current practices and understanding of family presence during CPR. J Emerg Nurs 2007;33(5):433–440.

85. Tinsley C, Hill JB, Shah J, et al. Experience of families during cardiopulmonary resuscitation in a pediatric intensive care unit. Pediatrics 2008;122(4):e799–e804.

86. Emergency Nurses' Association. Position statement on family presence at the bedside during invasive procedures and cardiopulmonary resuscitation. Rev 2005. Available at: http://www.ena.org/about/position/position/Family_Presence_-_ENA_PS.pdf (accessed February 2, 2009).

87. Jurkovich GJ, Pierce B, Pananen L, Rivara FP. Giving bad news: The family perspective. J Trauma 2000;48:865–873.

88. Ahrens WR, Hart RG. Emergency physicians' experience with pediatric death. Am J Emerg Med 1997;15:642–643.

89. Davies R. Mothers' stories of loss: Their need to be with their dying child and their child's body after death. J Child Health Care 2005;9(4):288–300.

90. Cox SA. Pediatric bereavement: Supporting the family and each other. J Trauma Nurs 2004;11:117–121.

91. Rando T. Treatment of Complicated Mourning. Champaign, IL: Research Press, 1993.

92. Oliver RC, Sturtevant JP, Scheetz JP, Fallat ME. Beneficial effects of a hospital bereavement intervention program after traumatic childhood death. J Trauma 2001;50:440–448.

93. Macdonald ME, Liben S, Carnevale FA, et al. Parental perspectives on hospital staff members' acts of kindness and commemoration after a child's death. Pediatrics 2005;116(4):884–890.

94. Feudtner C, Christakis DA, Zimmerman FJ, Muldoon JH, Neff JM, Koepsell TD. Characteristics of deaths occurring in children's hospitals: Implications for supportive care services. Pediatrics 2002;109(5):887–893.

95. Feudtner C, Feinstein JA, Satchell M, Zhao H, Kang TI. Shifting place of death among children with complex chronic conditions in the United States, 1989–2003. JAMA 2007;297(24):2725–2732.

96. Leuthner SR, Boldt AM, Kirby RS. Where infants die: Examination of place of death and home/hospice health care options in the state of Wisconsin. J Palliat Med 2004;7:269–277.

97. Serwint JR, Nellis ME. Deaths of Pediatric Patients: Relevance to their medical home, a urban primary care clinic. Pediatrics 2005;115:57–63.

98. Surkan PJ, Dickman PW, Steineck G, Onelöv E, Kreicbergs U. Home care of a child dying of a malignancy and parental awareness of a child's impending death. Palliat Med 2006;20(3):161–169.

99. Steele RG. Trajectory of certain death at an unknown time: Children with neurodegenerative life-threatening illnesses. Can J Nurs Res 2000;32(3):49–67.

100. Kreicbergs U, Valdimarsdóttir U, Onelöv E, Henter JI, Steineck G. Talking about death with children who have severe malignant disease. N Engl J Med 2004;351(12):1175–1186.

101. Spinetta JJ, Masera G, Eden T, et al. Refusal, non-compliance, and abandonment of treatment in children and adolescents with cancer: A report of the SIOP Working Committee on Psychosocial Issues in Pediatric Oncology. Med Pediatr Oncol 2002;38:114–117.

102. Hammes BJ, Klevan J, Kempf M, Williams MS. Pediatric advance care planning. J Palliat Med 2005;8:766–773.

103. Wharton RH, Levine KR, Buka S, Emanuel L. Advance care planning for children with special healthcare needs: A survey of parental attitudes. Pediatrics 1996;97:682–687.

104. Tulsky JA. Beyond advance directives: Importance of communication skills at the end of life. JAMA 2005;294:359–365.

105. AAP Committee on Children with Disabilities. Care coordination in the medical home: Integrating health and related systems of care for children with special health care needs. Pediatrics 2005;116:1238–1244.

106. Walsh-Kelly CM, Lang KR, Chevako J, et al. Advance directives in a pediatric emergency department. Pediatrics 1999;103;826–830.

107. Levetown M, AAP Committee on Bioethics. Communicating with children and families: From everyday interactions to skill in conveying distressing information Pediatrics 2008;121:e1441–e1460.

108. Feudtner C, Haney J, Dimmers MA. Spiritual care needs of hospitalized children and their families: A national survey of pastoral care providers' perceptions. Pediatrics 2003; 111(1):e67–e72.

109. Robinson MR, Thiel MM, Backus MM, Meyer EC. Matters of spirituality at the end of life in the pediatric intensive care unit. Pediatrics 2006;118(3):e719–e729.

110. Solomon MZ, Sellers DE, Heller KS, et al. New and lingering controversies in pediatric end-of-life care. Pediatrics 2005;116:872–883.

111. Quill TE. Nonabandonment: A central obligation for physicians. Ann Intern Med 1995;122:368–374.

112. Pellegrino ED. Nonabandonment: An old obligation revisited. N Engl J Med 1995;122:377–378.

113. Committee on Bioethics, American Academy of Pediatrics. Informed consent, parental permission and assent in pediatric practice. Pediatrics 1995;95:314–317.

114. Levetown M. Ethical aspects of pediatric palliative care. J Palliat Care 1996;12:35–39.

115. Wier R. Affirming the decisions adolescents make about life and death. Hastings Cent Rep 1997;27:29–40.

116. Doig C, Burgess E. Withholding life-sustaining treatment: Are adolescents competent to make these decisions? CMAJ 2000;162:1585–1588.

117. Nitschke R, Humphrey GB, Sexauer CL, Catron B, Wunder S, Jay S. Therapeutic choices made by patients with end-stage cancer. J Pediatr 1982;101:471–476.

118. Dreyer DR. Care of the dying adolescent: Special considerations. Pediatrics 2004;113:381–388.

119. Rushforth H. Practitioner review: Communicating with hospitalised children: Review and application of research pertaining to children's understanding of health and illness. J Child Psychol Psychiatr 1999;40:683–691.

120. McCabe MA. Involving children and adolescents in medical decision-making: Developmental and clinical considerations. J Pediatri Psychol 1996;21:505–516.

121. Attig T. Beyond suffering: The existential suffering of children. J Palliat Care 1996;12:20–23.

122. The George H. Gallup International Institute. Spiritual Beliefs and the Dying Process: Key Findings from a National Survey Conducted for the Nathan Cummings Foundation and the Fetzer Institute. Life at Risk, December 1997.

123. Levetown M, Pollack MM, Cuerdon TT, Ruttimann UE, Glover JJ. Limitations and withdrawals of medical intervention in pediatric critical care. JAMA 1994;272:1271–1275.

124. Mack JW, Wolfe J, Cook EF, Grier HE, Cleary PD, Weeks JC. Hope and prognostic disclosure. J Clin Oncol 2007;25(35):5636–5642.

125. Jones B, Sampson M, Greathouse J, Legett S, Higgerson R, Christie L. Comfort and confidence levels of health care professionals providing pediatric palliative care in the intensive care unit. J Soc Work End Life Palliat Care 2007;3(3):39–58.

126. Meert KL, Eggly S, Pollack M, et al. Parents' perspectives on physician-parent communication near the time of a child's death in the pediatric intensive care unit. Pediatr Crit Care Med 2008;9(1):2–7.

127. Field MJ, Behrman RE. Communication, goal setting and care planning. In: Field MJ, Behrman RE, eds. When Children Die: Improving Palliative and End-of-Life Care for Children and Their Families. Washington, DC: National Academy Press; 2002:104–140.

128. Levi RB, Marsick R, Drotar D, Kodish ED. Diagnosis, disclosure, and informed consent: Learning from parents of children with cancer. Int J Pediatr Hematol Oncol 2000;22:3–12.

129. Levinson W. Doctor-patient communication and medical malpractice: Implications for pediatricians. Pediatr Ann 1997;26:186–193.

130. Smith AB, Helfley GC, Anand KJS. Parent bed spaces in the PICU: Effect on parental stress. Pediatr Nurs 2007;33:215–221.

131. Sims JM, Miracle VA. A look at critical care visitation: The case for flexible visitation. Dimens Crit Care Nurs 2006;25(4):175–180.

132. Lautrette A, Darmon M, Megarbane B, et al. A communication strategy and brochure for relatives of patients dying in the ICU. N Engl J Med 2007;356(5):469–478. Erratum in: N Engl J Med 2007;357(2):203.

133. Shudy M, de Almeida ML, Ly S, et al. Impact of pediatric critical illness and injury on families: A systematic literature review. Pediatrics 2006;118(Suppl 3):S203–S218.

134. Azoulay E, Pochard F, Kentish-Barnes N, et al. Risk of post-traumatic stress symptoms in family members of intensive care unit patients. Am J Resp Crit Care Med 2005;171:987–994.

135. Peebles-Kleiger MJ. Pediatric and neonatal intensive care hospitalization as traumatic stressor: Implications for intervention. Bull Menninger Clin 2000;64:257–280.

136. Rushton CH, Reder E, Hall B, Comello K, Sellers DE, Hutton N. Interdisciplinary interventions to improve pediatric palliative care and reduce health care professional suffering. J Palliat Med 2006;9:922–932.

137. Narasimhan M, Eisen LA, Mahoney CD, Acerra FL, Rosen MJ. Improving nurse-physician communication and satisfaction in the intensive care unit with a daily goals worksheet. Am J Crit Care 2006;15(2):217–222.

138. Curtis JR, Patrick DL, Shannon SE, Treece PD, Engelberg RA, Rubenfeld GD. The family conference to improve communication about end-of-life care in the intensive care unit: Opportunities for improvement. Crit Care Med 2001;29(Suppl):N26–N33.

139. Sheldon LK, Barrett R, Ellington L. Difficult communication in nursing. J Nurs Scholarsh 2006;38(2):141–147.

140. Schulman-Green D, McCorkle R, Cherlin E, Johnson-Hurzeler R, Bradley EH. Nurses' communication of prognosis and implications for hospice referral: A study of nurses caring for terminally ill hospitalized patients. Am J Crit Care 2005;14(1):64–70.

141. Uitterhoeve R, de Leeuw J, Bensing J, et al. Cue-responding behaviours of oncology nurses in video-simulated interviews. J Adv Nurs 2008;61(1):71–80. Epub November 22, 2007.

142. Uitterhoeve R, Bensing J, Dilven E, Donders R, Demulder P, van Achterberg T. Nurse-patient communication in cancer care: Does responding to patient's cues predict patient satisfaction with communication. Psychooncology 2009;10:1060–1068.

143. Lautrette A, Ciroldi M, Ksibi H, Azoulay E. End-of-life family conferences: Rooted in the evidence. Crit Care Med 2006;34(11 Suppl):S364–S372.

144. Curtis JR, Engelberg RA, Wenrich MD, Shannon SE, Treece PD, Rubenfeld GD. Missed opportunities during family conferences about end-of-life care in the intensive care unit. Am J Resp Crit Care Med 2005;171:844–849.

145. McDonagh R, Ellott TB, Engelberg RA, et al. Family satisfaction with family conferences about end of life care in the intensive care unit: Increased proportion of family speech is associated with increased satisfactions. Crit Care Med 2001;29(2 Suppl):N26–N33.

146. West HF, Engelberg RA, Wenrich MD, Curtis JR. Expressions of nonabandonment during the intensive care unit family conference. J Palliat Med 2005;8(4):797–807.

147. Asch DA. The role of critical care nurses in euthanasia and assisted suicide. N Engl J Med 1996;334:1374–1379.

148. Campi CW. When dying is as hard as birth. New York Times, January 5, 1998.

149. Randolph AG, Zollo MB, Wigton RS, Yeh TS. Factors explaining variability among caregivers in the intent to restrict life-support interventions in a pediatric intensive care unit. Crit Care Med 1997;25:435–439.

150. Randolph AG, Zollo MB, Egger MJ, Guyatt GH, Nelson RM, Stidham GL. Variability in physician opinion on limiting pediatric life support. Pediatrics 1999;103(4):e46.

151. Tan GH, Totapally BR, Torbati D, Wolfsdorf J. End-of-life decisions and palliative care in a children's hospital. J Palliat Med 2006;9(2):332–342.

152. Asch DA, Hansen-Flaschen J, Lanken PN. Decisions to limit or continue life-sustaining treatment by critical care physicians in the United States: Conflicts between physicians' practices and patients' wishes. Am J Respir Crit Care Med 1995;151:288–292.

153. Hardart GE, Truog RD. Attitudes and preferences of intensivists regarding the role of family interests in medical decision-making for incompetent patients. Crit Care Med 2003;31:1895–1900.

154. Freyer DR. Children with cancer: Special considerations in the discontinuation of life-sustaining treatment. Med Pediatr Oncol 1992;20:136–142.

155. Doyal L, Henning P. Stopping treatment for end-stage renal failure: The rights of children and adolescents. Pediatr Nephrol 1994;8:768–791.

156. Committee on Bioethics, American Academy of Pediatrics. Guidelines on forgoing life-sustaining medical treatment. Pediatrics 1994;93:532–536.

157. Traugott I, Alpers A. In their own hands: Adolescents' refusals of medical treatment. Arch Pediatr Adolesc Med 1997;151:922–927.

158. President's Commission for the Study of Ethical Problems in Medicine and Biomedical and Behavioral Research. Deciding to Forgo Life-Sustaining Treatment: Ethical, Medical and Legal Issues in Treatment Decisions. Washington, DC: US Government Printing Office, 1983.

159. The Hastings Center. Guidelines on the Termination of Life-Sustaining Treatment and the Care of the Dying. Bloomington, IN: Indiana University Press, 1987.

160. American Medical Association. Withholding or withdrawing life-prolonging medical treatment. In: Code of Medical Ethics of the American Medical Association, 2008–2009 edition. Chicago, IL: American Medical Association; 1992.

161. Levetown M, Carter MA. Child-centred care in terminal illness: An ethical framework. In: Doyle D, Hanks GWC, MacDonald N, eds. Oxford Textbook of Palliative Medicine (2nd ed). Oxford: Oxford University Press; 1998: 1107–1119.

162. Leikin S. The role of adolescents in decisions concerning their cancer therapy. Cancer 1993;71:3342–3346.

163. King NMP, Cross AW. Children as decision-makers: Guidelinesw for pediatricians. J Pediatr 1989;115:10–16.

164. Leikin S. A proposal concerning decisions to forgo life-sustaining treatment for young people. J Pediatr 1989;115:17–22.

165. Alpert HR, Emanuel L. Comparing utilization of life-sustaining treatment with patient and public preferences. J Gen Intern Med 1998;13:175–181.

166. Nelson LJ, Rushton CH, Cranford RE, Nelson RM, Glover JJ, Truog RD. Forgoing medically provided nutrition and hydration in pediatric patients. J Law Med Ethics 1995;23:33–46.

167. Porto N, Frader J. Withholding hydration and nutrition in newborns. Theor Med Bioeth 2007;28:443–451.

168. Solomon MZ. The enormity of the task: SUPPORT and changing practice. Hastings Cent Rep Special Suppl 1995;25:S28–S32.

169. Horsburgh CR, Jr. Healing by design. N Engl J Med 1995;333:735–740.

170. Back AL, Arnold RM, Quill TE. Hope for the best, and prepare for the worst. Ann Intern Med 2003;138(5):439–443.

171. Gerstel E, Engelberg RA, Koepsell T, Curtis JR. Duration of withdrawal of life support in the intensive care unit and association with family satisfaction. Am J Respir Crit Care Med 2008;178:798–804.

172. Pritchard M, Burghen E, Srivastava DK, et al. Cancer-related symptoms most concerning to parents during the last week and last day of their child's life. Pediatrics 2008;121(5):e1301–e1309.

173. Burns JP, Mitchell C, Outwater KM, et al. End-of-life care in the pediatric intensive care unit after the forgoing of life-sustaining treatment. Crit Care Med 2000;28(8):3060–3066.

174. Curtis JR. Interventions to improve care during withdrawal of life-sustaining treatments. J Palliat Med 2005;8(suppl 1):S116–S131.

175. Munson D. Withdrawal of mechanical ventilation in pediatric and neonatal intensive care units. Pediatr Clin North Am 2007;54:773–785.

176. Stevens B, Johnston C, Petryshen P, Taddio A. Premature infant pain profile: Development and initial validation. Clin J Pain 1996;12:13–22.

177. Breau LM, Finley GA, McGrath PJ, Camfield CS. Validation of the non-communicating Children's Pain Checklist—postoperative version. Anesthesiology 2002;96:528–535.

178. Voepel-Lewis T, Merkel S, Tait AR, Trzcinka A, Malviya S. The reliability and validity of the Face, Legs, Activity, Cry, Consolability observational tool as a measure of pain in children with cognitive impairment. Anesth Analg 2002; 95:1224–1229.

179. van Dijk M, de Boer JB, Koot HM, Tibboel D, Passchier J, Duivenvoorden HJ. The reliability and validity of the COMFORT scale as a postoperative pain instrument in 0- to 3-year-old infants. Pain 2000;84:367–377.

180. Solodiuk J, Curley MA. Pain assessment in nonverbal children with severe cognitive impairments: The individualized numeric rating scale. J Pediatr Nurs 2003;18:295–299.

181. Friedrichsdorf SJ, Kang TI. The management of pain in children with life-limiting illnesses. Pediatr Clin North Am 2007;54:645–672.

182. World Health Organization and International Association for the Study of Pain. Cancer Pain Relief and Palliative Care in Children. Geneva: World Health Organization 1998.

183. Berde C, Sethna NF. Analgesics for the treatment of pain in children. N Engl J Med 2002;347:1094–1103.

184. Collins JJ. Intractable cancer pain in children. Child Adolesc Psych Clin N Am 1997;6:879–888.

185. Callahan RJ, Au JD, Paul M, Liu C, Yost CS. Functional inhibition by methadone of N-methyl, d-aspartate receptors expressed in Xenopus oocytes: Stereospecific and subunit effects. Anesth Analg 2004;98:653–659.

186. Zempsky WT. Optimizing the management of peripheral venous access pain in children: Evidence, impact and implementation. Pediatrics 2008;122(Suppl 3):S121–S170.

187. de Stouz ND, Bruera E, Suarez-Almazor M. Opioid rotation for toxicity reduction in terminal cancer patients. J Pain Symptom Manage 1995;10:378–384.

188. Partridge JC, Wall SN. Analgesia for dying infants whose life support is withdrawn or withheld. Pediatrics 1997;99:76–79.

189. Kenny NP, Frager G. Refractory symptoms and terminal sedation of children: Ethical and practical management. J Palliat Care 1996;12:40–45.

190. Santucci G, Mack JW. Common gastrointestinal symptoms in pediatric palliative care: Nausea, vomiting, constipation, anorexia and cachexia. Pediatr Clin North Am 2007;53:673–689.

191. Campbell ML. Terminal dyspnea and respiratory distress. Crit Care Clin 2004;20:403–407.

192. Daly BJ, Thomas D, Dyer MA. Procedures used in withdrawal of mechanical ventilation. Am J Crit Care 1996;5:331–338.

193. Campbell ML. Fear and pulmonary stress behaviors to an asphyxial threat across cognitive states. Res Nurs Health 2007;30:572–583.

194. Ullrich CK, Mayer OH. Assessment and management of fatigue and dyspnea in pediatric palliative care. Pedi Clin North Am 2007;54:735–756.

195. Bruera E, Macmillan K, Pither J, et al. Effects of morphine on the dyspnea of terminal cancer patients. J Pain Symptom Manage 1990;5:341–344.

196. Campbell ML. Managing terminal dyspnea: Caring for the patient who refuses intubation or ventilation. Dimens Crit Care Nurs 1996;15:4–11.

197. Cohen MH, Anderson AJ, Krasnow SH, et al. Continuous intravenous infusion of morphine for severe dyspnea. South Med J 1991;84:229–234.

198. Truog RD, Berde CB, Mitchell C, Grier HE. Barbiturates in the care of the terminally ill. N Engl J Med 1992;327:1678–1682.

199. Houlahan KE, Branowicki PA, Mack JW, Dinning C, McCabe M. Can end of life care for the pediatric patient suffering with escalating and intractable symptoms be improved? J Pediatr Oncol Nurs 2006;23(1):45–51.

200. Billings JA, Block SD. Slow euthanasia. J Palliat Care 1996;2:21–30.

201. Quill TE, Lo B, Brock DW. Palliative care options of last resort: A comparison of voluntarily stopping eating and drinking, terminal sedation, PAS, and voluntary, active euthanasia. JAMA 1997;78:2099–2104.

202. Quill TE, Dresser R, Brock DW. The rule of double effect—a critique of its role in end-of-life decision making. N Engl J Med 1997;37:1768–1771.

203. Mount B. Morphine drips, terminal sedation and slow euthanasia: Definitions and facts, not anecdotes. J Palliat Care 1996;2:31–37.

204. Roy DJ. On the ethics of euthanasia. J Palliat Care 1996;12:3–5.

205. Rushton CH, Terry PB. Neuromuscular blockade and ventilator withdrawal: Ethical controversies. Am J Crit Care 1995;4:112–115.

206. Truog RD, Burns JP, Mitchell C, Johnson J, Robinson W. Pharmacologic paralysis and withdrawal of mechanical ventilation at the end of life. N Engl J Med 2000;342(7):508–11.

207. Levetown M. Different and needing to be more available. Hosp Mag 1995;Winter:15–36.

208. Feinstein JA, Ernst LM, Ganesh J, Feudtner C. What new information pediatric autopsies can provide: A retrospective evaluation of 100 consecutive autopsies using family-centered criteria. Arch Pediatr Adolesc Med 2007;161(12):1190–1196.

209. Bellali T, Papadatou D. Parental grief following the brain death of a child: Does consent or refusal to organ donation affect their grief? Death Stud 2006;30(10):883–917.

210. Vane DW, Sartorelli KH, Reese J. Emotional considerations and attending involvement ameliorates organ donation in brain dead pediatric trauma victims. J Trauma 2001;51(2):329–331.

211. Lloyd-Williams M, Morton J, Peters S. The end of life experiences of relatives of brain dead intensive care patients. J Pain Symptom Manage 2009;37(4):659–664.

212. Bellali T, Papazoglou I, Papadatou D. Empirically based recommendations to support parents facing the dilemma of paediatric cadaver organ donation. Intensive Crit Care Nurs 2007;23(4):216–225.

213. McHaffie HE, Laing IA, Lloyd DJ. Follow up care of bereaved parents after treatment withdrawal from newborns. Arch Dis Child Fetal Neonatal Ed 2001;84:F125–F128.

214. Rankin J, Wright C, Lind T. Cross-sectional survey of parents' experience and views of the postmortem examination. BMJ 2002;324:816–818.

215. Heller KS, Solomon MZ; for the Initiative for Pediatric Palliative Care (IPPC) Investigator Team. Continuity of care and caring: What matters to parents of children with life-threatening conditions. J Pediatr Nurs 2005;20(5):335–346.

216. Murphy SA, Johnson LC. Finding meaning in a child's violent death: A five-year prospective analysis of parents' personal narratives and empirical data. Death Stud 2003;27:381–404.

217. Forte, AL, Hill,M, Pazder R, Feudtner C. Bereavement care interventions: A systematic review. BMC Palliat Care 2004;3:3 doi:10.1186/1472–684X-3–3. Available at: http://www.biomedcentral.com/1472–684X/3/3 (accessed January 26, 2009).

218. Helsing KJ, Szklo M. Mortality after bereavement. Am J Epidemiol 1981;114:41–52.

219. Clayton PJ. Mortality and morbidity in the first year of widowhood. Arch Gen Psychiatr 1974;30:747–750.

220. Parkes CM, Brown RJ. Health after bereavement: A controlled study of young Boston widows and widowers. Psychosom Med 1972;34:449–461.

221. Li J, Precht DH, Mortensen PB, Olsen J. Mortality in parents after death of a child in Denmark: A nationwide follow-up study. Lancet 2003;361:363–367.

222. Tolle SW, Bascom PB, Hickam DH, et al. Communication between physicians and surviving spouses following patient deaths. J Gen Intern Med 1986;1:309–314.

223. Platt J. The planning, organizing and delivery of a memorial service in critical care. Nurs Crit Care 2004;9:222–229.

224. Clark MA. A ritual for the closure of life when life is artificially supported, when the quality of life has gone. J Pastoral Care 1999;53:489–491.

225. Parker-Raley J, Jones B, Maxson T. Communicating the death of a child in the emergency department: The negotiation of dialectical tensions. J Healthc Qual 2008;30(5):20–31.

226. Brosche TA. A grief team within a healthcare system. Dimens Crit Care Nurs 2007;26:21–28.

227. Papadatou D, Papazoglou I, Petraki D, Bellali T. Mutual support among nurses who provide care to dying children. Illness Crisis Loss 1999;7:37–48.

228. Maytum JC, Heiman MB, Garwick AW. Compassion fatigue and burnout in nurses who work with children with chronic conditions and their families. J Pediatr Health Care July–August 2004;18(4):171–179.

# 56

*Pamela S. Hinds, Linda L. Oakes, and Wayne L. Furman*

# End-of-Life Decision-Making in Pediatric Oncology

*The diagnosis that the cancer came back and that there was nothing that could be done was understandable given the condition her body was in. It is more likely now that she will pass on from the infection than the cancer because the infection is in her bloodstream. It is a hard decision because you want your child to be with you. You have to think about your child and what is better for her. She already has two uncles and two baby sisters there (in heaven). She told us not to worry, that if she does die, she would go there and take care of them and she'd be OK. I just don't want her to suffer anymore. Twelve and a half years is long enough. It makes it a littler easier to put her in the hands of the Jesus and one day I'll see her again.—Mother who had made a "do not resuscitate" decision 48 hours previously on behalf of her 12-year-old daughter, who was dying of cancer*

♦ **Key Points**

♦ *Decision-making for parents facing the terminal illness of a child is, in most cases, extraordinarily difficult.*

♦ *Health-care providers can influence the extent to which patients and parents participate in end-of-life decision-making by communication style and timing of the discussion.*

♦ *Children and adolescents may need assistance making decisions based on their cognitive development, and each patient should be assessed as an individual to determine his or her competence.*

♦ *Preferences for treatment should be balanced between the child or adolescent patient and the caregiver or surrogate.*

♦ *Nurses have a professional responsibility to facilitate informed patient decisions at the end of life.*

Deciding to end a child's life, and involving a child in the decision to end his/her life, are startling concepts, but we in pediatric oncology participate in those considerations with parents, patients, and other members of the health-care team as a part of providing the highest-quality care for the child or adolescent with incurable cancer. Participating in end-of-life decisions is life-altering for the child or adolescent and for the family, but it can also be life-altering for the health-care provider. Clinical reports indicate that the way in which patients, family members, and health-care providers participate in end-of-life discussions and decision-making, and convey respect for the decision made can color all of their preceding treatment-related interactions, and may influence how well parents emotionally survive the dying and death of their child.[1,2] The manner in which end-of-life decision-making processes are completed may also contribute to the survival of health-care providers as compassionate and fully competent professionals.[3]

Despite the significant immediate and longer-term impact of participating in end-of-life decision-making for a child or adolescent with incurable cancer, guidelines for making or for facilitating such decisions have only recently become available.[4] Preparation for participating in end-of-life decision-making, though rare, is increasingly included in formal academic curricula[5,6] and other forms of clinician education[7] including online materials (e.g., www.ippceweb.org/; www.nhpco.org/). There is clearly a great need for more information that can be used to develop, test, refine and apply such guidelines into care of families whose child will not survive. The purposes of this chapter are (1) to offer a review of the current literature (both clinical and research-based) on end-of-life decision-making in pediatrics, with a special emphasis on pediatric oncology, and (2) to offer guidelines for the use of health-care professionals in assisting children, adolescents, their parents, and other health-care professionals in making such decisions. Table 56–1 defines key terms used in this chapter.

**Table 56–1**
**Key Terms Used in This Chapter**

*Decision*—The final choice between two or more treatment-related options.

*Phase I study*—The initial stage of human testing of a drug, in which the maximum tolerated dose is established; in oncology, the subjects are usually patients who have refractory disease.

*Do not resuscitate*—An order written in the medical record directing that no cardiopulmonary resuscitation is to be performed in the case of an acute event such as cardiac, respiratory, or neurological decompensation.

*Withdrawal of life-support*—Stopping a life-sustaining medical treatment such as mechanical ventilator therapy, pharmacological support of blood pressure, or dialysis, and vasoactive infusions.

*Life-sustaining medical treatment*—Interventions that may not control the patient's disease but may prolong the patient's life; these may include not only ventilator support, dialysis, and vasoactive infusions, but also antibiotics, insulin, chemotherapy, and nutrition and hydration provided by tubes and IV lines.

*Supportive care*—Comfort measures that exclude curative efforts but could include symptom management (such as pain relief and hydration) or symptom prevention (such as limited blood product support).

## Background

Advances in pediatric oncology have significantly increased the survival rates of patients during the past decade. The disease once thought to be universally fatal for children and adolescents is now viewed as a life-threatening, chronic illness that is potentially curable for many.[8–10] However, cancer remains the leading disease-related cause of death in children and adolescents, as ultimately 25% to 33% will die of their disease.[8,11–13] Indeed, approximately 2,200 children and adolescents die of cancer in the United States on an annual basis.[8,13,14] With treatment advances come more treatment options and more treatment-related decisions for patients, their parents, and their health-care providers.[15] Only a limited number of experiences with treatment decision-making occur for parents whose child is being treated for cancer as the majority of these children will be treated on a therapeutic protocol and according to which the child's treatment is directed. Most commonly, the parents' and most certainly the patients' first experience with treatment decision-making will be at the time when the disease becomes incurable. Parents and health-care providers report that the most challenging decision-making in pediatric oncology occurs when efforts to cure the cancer have failed.[16] A few parents report that end-of-life decision-making was not complicated for them because they had already decided what they would do if their child's cancer did not respond to treatment. However,

the majority of parents and health-care providers involved in the decision process describe this time as extraordinarily difficult. They attribute the difficulty to multiple and complex factors that must be considered, including the differing preferences of those involved in the actual decision-making or affected by it, and to intense emotions at a time when the parents' energy is depleted.

## Neonatal and Other Pediatric Specialties

End-of-life decision-making in pediatric oncology has been influenced by clinical and research reports from neonatal and other pediatric specialties and organizations. The growing commitment by professional associations to include pediatric patients and parents in end-of-life decisions marks a notable shift in care philosophy. Expectations that patients and their parents should be involved in these decisions have been formalized in policy statements of organizations such as the American Academy of Pediatrics,[17] the American Nurses Association,[18] the American Association of Critical Care Nurses,[19] the United Hospital Fund in its report on end-of-life care in New York,[20] the International Society of Pediatric Oncology (SIOP),[21] the collaborative precepts statements issued by the National Association of Neonatal Nurses, the Associaion of Pediatric Oncology Nurses and Last Acts (www.lastacts.org/palliativecare), and most recently from the Institute of Medicine.[14] In these published statements, the recommended patient and parental involvement is described as participative and mutual with health-care providers. Legislative rulings and legal decisions in some states and Canadian provinces support the participation of adolescents or mature minors in medical decision-making and in creating advance directives.[22–26] Regulatory bodies such as the JCAHO and health policy influencing groups such as the National Quality Forum are now becoming involved in directing or evaluating end-of-life care,[27,28] including patient and parental involvement in end-of-life decision-making. It is also likely that such involvement will be considered an indicator of the quality of end-of-life care and be linked to reimbursement for such care as is now being proposed for adult cancer patients.[29]

The actual extent to which patients and parents participate in end-of-life decision-making varies and can be influenced by the personal and professional preferences of the health-care provider.[30,31] For example, the way the health-care provider frames or words information about treatment options may influence the way a patient and family perceive the available alternatives.[32,33] Some advocate that the physician should assume the final responsibility for the decision,[34–36] whereas others believe that the parents should be the primary decision-makers.[37–39] Yet another view, espoused by few individuals, is that the adolescent patient should be the primary decision-maker, with his/her parents serving as consultants.[40] Even fewer sources advocate that children should be the primary decision-makers, but several advocate that children as young as 6[35,36,41,42] or 7 years old[23] should be involved in the decision-making.

The available reports on end-of-life decision-making that involve parents and health-care providers are predominantly from neonatal settings. End-of-life decisions in these settings often reflect the presenting condition of the infant. The number of immature and critically-ill neonates being admitted to neonatal intensive care units over the past 20 years has increased significantly as have the corresponding recommendations from health-care teams for end-of-life care.[43] The end-of-life decisions primarily considered include (1) limiting care, (2) withdrawing life-support, or (3) withholding life-support for infants who are extremely premature or have severe congenital abnormalities.[44-49] Most reports describe the decision-making as having been initiated when the intensivist determined that the infant had no chance for survival or no chance for quality of life. In most cases, parents agreed with the recommendations of the intensivist or the infant's attending physician. These descriptive reports are based on review of medical records. No information was obtained from parents about the factors they considered when making an end-of-life decision on behalf of their infant.

Two notable exceptions exist. In the first, Able-Boone and colleagues[50] interviewed parents and health-care providers of seriously ill infants regarding medical decision-making and the provision of health-care information. The parents emphasized their need and desire to be honestly informed of their child's health status. They expressed special appreciation of health-care professionals who drew pictures to convey technical information rather than relying only on words. Parents also expressed a strong need for information that is coordinated by the health-care team so that it is not confusing or contradictory.

The second study that recorded the values of parents in end-of-life decisions is the grounded-theory study in which Rushton[51] interviewed 31 parents of 20 hospitalized neonates with life-threatening congenital disorders about their decisions for or against implementing or continuing life-sustaining measures for their infants. Rushton concluded that the parents made these decisions based on their understanding of what it means to be a "good parent" for a neonate with a life-threatening congenital disorder. According to these parents, the characteristics of good parents for such neonates include putting the needs of the neonate first, not giving up, not taking the "easy" way out despite the self-sacrifice involved, and courage to pursue a "good" outcome for the child.

Reviews of the medical records of patients who have died in pediatric intensive care units (PICUs) show that withdrawal of life-support was chosen in 0% to 54% of cases,[52-56] and that limitation of supportive care (described as not escalating care efforts but providing hydration and pain comfort measures) was chosen in 26% to 46% of cases.[52,55] The wide range of these percentages may reflect cultural, ethnic, or religious differences: the lowest rate of withdrawal of life-support reported was from India and the highest rates were from PICUs in Europe, the United States, and the United Kingdom. Even within a single PICU setting, decision-making can reflect cultural differences. For example, the report from a Malaysian setting noted that Muslim parents declined end-of-life options at significantly higher rates than did non-Muslim parents.[53] Reports may also reflect the research method used. For example, Meyer and colleagues[57] relied upon surveys completed by parents to assess parental perceptions of pain control, decision-making, and social supports during their child's dying in a PICU. Parents reported that in most cases (n = 56; 90%), the physician initiated the end-of-life discussion, but in approximately half of those cases, parents had been privately considering an end-of-life decision. Factors identified by parents as influencing their decision-making included concerns about their child's quality of life, their child's chance of getting better, their child's pain or discomfort, advice of hospital staff, attitudes of hospital staff, and advice of friends or family members. Several medical record reviews of end-of-life characteristics of children dying of cancer have recently been completed. In general, the majority of these children and adolescents die of progressive disease with a medical order not to resuscitate (DNR). These characteristics indicate the child's likely death had been discussed with parents or family members. However, despite parental involvement in decision-making, the factors that influenced the decision-making and how the end-of-life discussions were initiated or facilitated were not included in the published reports. Recently published figures indicate that the majority (65% to 80%) of pediatric deaths are preceded by an end-of-life decision.[48,58,59] These figures suggest that pediatric health-care providers can correctly anticipate the likelihood of being involved in end-of-life decision-making and need to be competent in assisting families with such decision-making.

❦

## Participation of Children and Adolescents

Children and adolescents are not routinely involved in making end-of-life decisions on their own behalf, largely because of doubt on the part of parents and health-care providers that the child or adolescent has sufficient understanding of the clinical situation.[60-63] This doubt is based in part on adults' belief that children and adolescents are unable to appraise their well-being and are unaware of their life goals and values.[37] Buchanan and Brock[60] described children who are 9 years or older as competent to make certain decisions, but they did not study children's competence in end-of-life decision-making. The same authors also indicated that children of that age may be competent to make some decisions but not others, and that competence thus depends on the specific decision. According to Ariff and Groh,[64] a child's competence to make medical decisions is an ongoing developmental process that parallels other cognitive, moral, and emotional processes and is influenced by environment and by physical and mental illness. The capacity to make an end-of-life decision cannot be determined, then, on the basis of the child's or adolescent's competence in a different situation or decision. Instead, competence must be determined for each specific decision at a defined time point and under specific circumstances.[22] Recent cognitive studies on adolescent decision-making indicate that although adolescents are able to make decisions, they may be unaware of all possible options or may be unable to identify all possible consequences of those options.[65] Therefore, adolescents may need assistance in identifying, considering, and selecting end-of-life options.

Experiencing a life-threatening illness such as cancer and seeing others suffer and die from it may help a child to understand death and his or her own end-of-life circumstances.[26,66,67] Although they acknowledged that the competence to participate in decision-making differs with age and cognitive abilities, Burns and Truog[68] recommended that children and adolescents be involved early in the process of medical decision-making, including end-of-life decisions. In fact, Burns and Truog warned that if a child or adolescent is not involved early in the decision-making process, his or her ability to express an opinion may be lost before it can be exercised. Leikin[69] theorized that adolescents who have been treated for cancer have a clearer idea of the burdens and benefits of treatment options that are most acceptable to them. The ethical perspective is that adolescents have a conception of what is good for themselves. The treatment experience itself contributes to the adolescents' abilities to participate in end-of-life decision-making. A similar conclusion was reported by Hinds et al.[70] after analyzing data from interviews with 10- to 21-year-olds about their own end-of-life decision-making. These pediatric oncology patients were able to describe the decision they had made, the factors that influenced their decision-making, and their awareness of both likely short-term and long-term outcomes of their decision, including the effects the decision could have on others. These abilities comprise competence in participating in end-of-life decision-making on their own behalf. Impressively, the primary factor considered in their end-of-life decision-making was relationships with others and concern for them.

Our combined clinical and research experiences have convinced us that, as a general rule, seriously ill patients age 10 years and older are able to understand that they are participating in decisions about their cancer-related treatment and their lives, and are able to understand the options and the likely outcomes. Of course, some younger patients may also understand these issues and be competent to participate in end-of-life decisions, whereas some older patients may be less competent. Because of these very possible differences in understanding, each child needs to be individually assessed for his or her competence to participate. An assumption that a child is or is not competent to participate made without the assessment is not in the child's best interest.

Others have provided compelling support for the involvement of younger children in end-of-life decision-making. Nitschke and colleagues[41,42] reported that patients as young as age 6 years participated in end-of-life discussions in their pediatric oncology treatment setting. They described care conferences held with 43 families over a 6-year period in which children and adolescents with end-stage cancer, and their families, participated in discussions of therapeutic options, disease progression, lack of effective therapies, improbability of cure, and imminent death. The patients (who were ages 6–20 years) and their parents were offered the choice of Phase II investigational drugs or supportive care. According to this report, it was the patients who most frequently made the final decision. Fourteen chose further chemotherapy, 28 chose supportive care only, and 1 made no decision. Nitschke and colleagues also noted that patients younger than age 9 years understood that they were going to die soon of their disease. The authors concluded that children with cancer do have an advanced understanding of death and recommended that children as young as age 5 years have the capacity to make decisions about whether to continue therapy. This team did not investigate the specific factors considered by the patients, parents, and health-care providers and did not describe ways in which providers may have attempted to facilitate patient and parent decision-making.

A health-care team member who has established a relationship of trust with the child or adolescent and who has observed the child or adolescent in various challenging clinical situations is likely to be the best judge of competence in end-of-life decision-making. However, before initiating this assessment, the health-care team should discuss the purpose and process of the assessment, first as a group and then with the patient's parent or parents, and identify any areas of actual or potential disagreement between the team and the parents. Disagreements should be openly discussed, and participants should be allowed sufficient time to weigh the issues—another reason for initiating the end-of-life discussions in a timely manner. After the team and the parents agree on the intent and timing of the competence assessment, the team member, parent(s), and child or adolescent choose the location for the discussion. Most children younger than age 11 years prefer to have their parents present for this discussion.

Determining the child's or adolescent's competence requires establishing whether he/she understands the seriousness of the medical condition and understands that a decision point is at hand. If asked to explain the seriousness of the situation, the child or adolescent will use words or describe events that have personal, symbolic, or literal meaning. The health-care team can then use these same words to communicate with the patient about decision-making. Throughout the assessment, the child or adolescent will need reassurance from the health-care team member that the serious situation is not the fault of the child or adolescent.[71] The child or adolescent must also be able to indicate an understanding of the choices, including the potential consequences of each. In addition, the child or adolescent must show an understanding of how each choice made now could change future options. As McCabe and colleagues[25] emphasized, the health-care team member conducting the assessment must ensure that the child or adolescent does not feel coerced to make a certain choice. The team member should also ensure that the child or adolescent has access to the information needed to make a competent decision.[72] The team member needs to allow repeated opportunities for the child or adolescent to review the options and discuss concerns and to do so in a manner that is not rushed, and to provide different mechanisms (verbal, written, drawing) to facilitate expression of concerns or preferences.[73] It is especially important that the team member assess to what extent the child or adolescent wants to be included in the decision-making. That preference should be honored regardless of the personal preferences of team members.

Our experience is that children (some as young as age 7 years) have definite preferences regarding whether to participate in a Phase I clinical trial. Preferences most commonly reflect a desire to be home, to live a little bit longer, to play with a sibling or a friend, or to not feel sickly. Preferences regarding DNR status, although quite firmly expressed by some adolescents, tend to require more patient contemplation time. By the time this type of end-of-life decision-making needs to be considered, the members of the health-care team are very familiar with the child and the family and already have established a style of interacting. However, it is generally useful to preface the assessment of patient preference with a statement that conveys the important nature of what is about to be said, such as, "May I ask you to be quite serious with me for a few moments? I want to tell you something important about your [insert here the term used by the child when referring to the illness]. And I want you to tell me something, too." If the child conveys an inability to be serious at that moment, the team member needs to clarify whether that means the child only wants the "serious and important" topics to be discussed with the child's family, or if it means the child wants to try to be serious at a later time. Clinicians are encouraged to allow repeated opportunities for the child or adolescent to review the care options or concerns, to provide a variety of mechanisms to facilitate the child's expressions (such as using words, drawing, or writing), and to do so in a manner that is not rushed.

## Competence of Surrogates

Concern about patients' competence to participate in end-of-life decisions, although valid, may sometimes be exaggerated. As Levetown and Carter[72] wrote, it is relatively easy to usurp the autonomy of children and adolescents in end-of-life decision-making. This threat lends special importance to the use of guidelines for making end-of-life decisions. Guidelines could serve as formal reminders to health-care professionals to consider the preferences of children and adolescents to the extent that is possible or advisable. Of equal or greater concern is the competence of parents and health-care providers to make such decisions on behalf of the child or adolescent.

Making these decisions competently requires an understanding of their own values, the patient's values and goals, the treatment options, the likely outcome of each option, and the nature of the life-threatening illness. This imposes a short-term and a longer-term burden of unknown proportions on the parents and the health-care providers. A recent report indicates that parents and pediatric oncology patients have overlapping factors in their individual end-of-life decision-making on behalf of the ill patient.[70]

There are a limited number of empirically-based or theoretically-based guidelines for involving children, adolescents, or their parents in end-of-life decisions, but in clinical care stituations, the general assumption is that children younger than age 10 years are not competent to participate in such decision-making and that their parents are both competent and attentive to the best interests of their child.[25,37,68] This assumption is crucial because it tends to ensure that end-of-life decisions are made for seriously ill children and adolescents by their parents and health-care professionals. Legal rulings and common health-care practices support the role of parents as surrogates in this circumstance; it is rarely challenged, and health-care providers or others replace parental authority only in exceptional circumstances.[68] To feel competent, to be competent, and to be satisfied with their performance as surrogate decision-makers, parents and health-care providers need opportunities to exchange information about the child's preferences, the family's preferences, the child's chances of survival, the progression of the disease, and the intensity and intrusiveness of life-extending interventions and the likelihood of their effectiveness (including length of time gained). They also need to reflect on previous efforts to achieve cure and to question previous decisions. Competence of surrogates may also be affected by their realization of the likelihood of their child not surviving cancer. In one retrospective, descriptive study that included parent interviews and review of medical records, it was identified that physicians knew up to a year before the parents that the child would not survive.[74] Participating in end-of-life care planning is unlikely if the reality of the child's death is not yet in the parents' or surrogates' awareness. Competence of surrogate participation is also influenced by the challenges faced by health-care providers when trying to accurately predict timing of the dying.[75] However, only in a limited number of cases is the child's dying unexpected. Because of that, some degree of planning for preferred model of end-of-life care (home, home with hospice, hospital, hospital with hospice) is possible.[76,77] Matching the surrogates' preferences for end-of-life care might contribute to decreasing the morbidity of bereaved survivors.

## Participation of Patients and Parents

Previous studies indicate that the more informed parents become about their seriously-ill child's condition, the more they are able to participate in making decisions and advocating for their child.[78,79] Parents report that information is most helpful when it is provided gradually and repeatedly,[80] and respectfully in words that are easy to understand.[43] Including information about the prognosis, likely outcomes, a commitment not to allow suffering, and to respect religious beliefs have also been identified by parents as quite helpful at the time of end-of-life decision-making.[43,81,82] In addition, seeing the health-care team members treat the very ill neonate or child with respect and offer estimates of the appropriateness of the possible care as compared to its burdensome nature were both veiwed as helpful with end-of-life decision-making.[83] Stevens[84] recommends that parents be allowed to make tape recordings or bring friends or family members to the treatment-related discussions to help them later recall the details of the discussion. Other investigators suggest that parents differ in how much detailed information they desire[85] and in how much they want to participate in the actual decision-making[86,87] during periods of crisis in their child's illness. However, parental preferences about participation in end-of-life decision-making have not been well-studied.

In an international feasibility study, parents from pediatric oncology settings in Australia, Hong Kong, and the United States were interviewed about their decision-making on behalf of their ill child. There were clear differences among the countries in parental preference for involvement in decision-making. Mothers in Hong Kong were reluctant to participate in end-of-life decisions because of either their gender ("Women cannot make these decisions.") or their lack of expert knowledge ("I am only the mother. The doctor is the expert and he should decide.").[88] It remains unknown whether these parental preferences change between diagnosis and end of life. Regardless of their preference, all parents need reassurance from the health-care team that their child's condition is not their fault.[84]

The factors that parents consider at decision points in the treatment of their seriously ill child have only recently been studied. Using a phenomenological approach, Kirschbaum[89] interviewed 20 parents of children who had died in the previous 6 to 12 months. The parents had all made life-support decisions on behalf of their ill child. Various diagnoses were represented, including trauma, cancer, septic shock, liver failure, and congestive heart disease. Nine factors were identified as having influenced the parental decisions: (1) wanting life as the principal good for their child, (2) avoiding suffering and pain, (3) considering current and future quality of life, (4) respecting the individuality of the child, (5) defining and redefining the family, (6) having spiritual beliefs and explanations, (7) believing in natural or biological explanations, (8) considering the child's unique personality, and (9) having a favorable view of technology in health care.

In a retrospective study that conducted telephone interviews with 39 parents of 37 pediatric oncology patients who had died in the previous 6 to 24 months, Hinds and colleagues[16] were able to identify the factors most frequently considered by parents in end-of-life decision-making. The end-of-life decisions that were reported most frequently by these parents were choosing between a Phase I drug study and no further treatment ($n = 14$), maintaining or withdrawing life support ($n = 11$), and giving more chemotherapy or ending treatment ($n = 8$). The factor most considered in the parents' decision-making was "information received from health-care professionals." This information included facts, explanations, and opinions about their child's disease status, likelihood of survival, and complexities of continued care. Other factors parents frequently reported were "feeling supported by and trusting of the staff," which reflected the parents' sense that the health-care team listened and responded to their or their child's concerns and respected the parents' decisions, and "making decisions together with my child." This factor reflected the parents' comfort in having known and respected their child's wishes.

The parents also completed a 15-item questionnaire about the importance of each factor considered in their decision-making. The parents rated eight items as "very important" at least 50% of the time. The highest-rated factors included "recommendations received from health-care professionals," "things my child had said about continuing or not continuing treatment," "information received from health-care professionals," "my child's breathing problems," and "sensing that my child was no longer himself [herself]." These findings clearly indicate that information and recommendations received from health-care professionals are very important to parents who are making end-of-life decisions on behalf of their child, as is feeling certain of their child's desires about treatment.

The same research team has prospectively studied end-of-life decision-making by conducting interviews of parents, physicians, and when possible, the children or adolescents with incurable disease who had participated in making an end-of-life decision within the past week. The same factors noted in the retrospective study—related to trust, support, information, and advice—were also identified in the prospective study. In addition, parents cited these factors: wishing for the child's survival, reassuring themselves of the correctness of their decisions, questioning certain statements or behaviors of health-care professionals, and making decisions that would allow them to maintain communication with their dying child for as long as possible (Table 56–2).

CASE STUDY

*A Decision Agreement between Parents and the Health-Care Team*

A 12-month-old infant girl has been treated for an aggressive form of leukemia. It was clear that the disease was not responding to chemotherapy. The patient was transferred to the PICU when she began to experience respiratory distress. Initially, oxygen was administered by simple mask, but her breathing difficulties persisted and became more

**Table 56–2**
**Guidelines for the Health-Care Team to Use in Assisting Parents with End-of-Life Decision-Making**

1. At the time of diagnosis and throughout treatment, actively seek opportunities to provide information to the parent about treatment and the patient's response to treatment.
2. At the time of diagnosis and throughout treatment, involve the parent in treatment-related discussions and decision-making. Be available to discuss and rediscuss decisions and related concerns.
3. Encourage parents to talk with parents of other pediatric oncology patients.
4. Verbally and nonverbally reassure the parents that they are "good" parents who are committed to the well-being of their child.
5. Give assurances that everything that can be done to help the patient is being done and being done well.
6. As the child's disease progresses, provide clear verbal (and written, if desired by the parent) explanations of the child's status.
7. Inform parents of treatment options as they become available in the treating institution or elsewhere.
8. Include more than one health-care team member in end-of-life discussions with the parents.
9. When discussing end-of-life options with parents,
    a. Strongly emphasize the team's commitment to the patient's comfort and to providing expert care at all times.
    b. Offer professional recommendations.
    c. Describe how their child is likely to respond to each option (the child's physical appearance, ability to communicate, etc.).
    d. Give information about other support resources (ethics committees, social services, other health-care professionals, etc.).
10. When discussing end-of-life options with parents, anticipate
    a. Parents' vacillation between certainty and uncertainty about the decision.
    b. Parents' need for clarification and additional information to resolve their uncertainties.
    c. Parent's need for practical information about ways to explain the end-of-life decision to other family members.
    d. Being asked to give personal advice.
11. Allow parents private time to consider the options.
12. Maintain sensitivity to any specific ethnic, cultural, or religious preferences during the terminal stage.
13. Convey respect for the parents' right to change decisions, when clinically feasible.
14. Demonstrate commitment to maintaining the child's comfort and dignity, and to affirming the parents' role.
15. Do not question the parents' decision after it has been made.

evident within a few hours. The possibility of endotracheal intubation was first discussed among the health-care team members and then with the parents. During the meeting with the parents, the current symptoms of the little girl were discussed, the current disease status and its unresponsiveness to treatment were reviewed, and options of intubating or not intubating were considered. The parents then discussed the options privately with each other and in less than 30 minutes reached the decision that ventilatory support not be a part of their daughter's medical care. The parents said that knowing that their daughter was not going to be cured of the leukemia and understanding that the ventilator would help reduce their daughter's respiratory distress but not the leukemia were both factors that assisted them in making the decision. They credited their discussions with the doctors as key: "From the discussion we had with the doctors, we felt if it came to that point, the only reason for using a ventilator would be just to keep her breathing." An additional factor identified by the parents as influencing their decision-making was support from the health-care team. "Chaplain X and Dr. Y were real patient with us and understood the situation that we were in and did not seem to put pressure one way or another, or seem to think that we were making the wrong decision one way or another.... they told us the decision was actually ours. They let us know that, but they were supportive and also gave us their opinions."

CASE STUDY
*Disagreement between Parents*

A 1-year-old male infant with relapsed acute lymphoblastic leukemia was admitted for fever with persistent neutropenia following chemotherapy. Despite careful fluid management, he developed fluid overload and an enlarging abdomen from hepatomegaly secondary to leukemic infiltrates. His clinical status became more fragile with pleural and pericardial effusions and an increasing need for oxygen, administered first by nasal cannula and later by face mask. As his abdomen further enlarged, his pain increased prompting his primary team to initiate a fentanyl infusion with frequent nurse-administered boluses. Both parents participated in discussions with their son's care team to determine if the goal should continue to be for cure of his leukemia. When their son's primary physician informed them that a new type of chemotherapy might be helpful, the infant's father decided to do "whatever it takes to continue the fight for a cure for my son." The infant's mother wanted the focus of her son's care to be on comfort and advocated to have him at home for his final days surrounded by his family without all the sounds and interruptions that come from being in the hospital. However, her husband had always been the primary decision-maker in their family, and she ultimately chose to rely on him to make the decisions regarding their son's care, even when she disagreed with him. She stated that her husband needed more time and information to realize that cure "is not going to happen" and that by waiting for him to see that "everything was done" would help her husband after their son died. Relying on her own faith to "get us through this time," she believed that God would take care of them, including her son. However, the father revealed he wanted to believe God would help his son fight, and felt that God was punishing him in some way for not believing in Him fully all of his life. In the last 48 hours of their son's life, the laboratory findings indicated their son's peripheral blast count had increased to 70%. His mother noted that she found some comfort with the efforts to control her son's worsening abdominal pain with the rapidly enlarging abdomen. Gradually, the father accepted the support of the health-care team, including the primary physician, and recognized that his son was suffering and that he "[had] lost the fight" and "it [was] not fair to put him through any more treatment." With his son facing imminent transfer to the intensive care unit for ventilatory support, the father accepted the team's recommendation for the goal of care to shift to comfort. Many friends and family members arrived at the hospital to offer the young parents support. The infant son died in his mother's arms hours after the father's decision not to pursue more disease-directed therapy.

### CASE STUDY
#### Reluctant Agreement between Adolescent, Parents, and Health-Care Team

A 15-year-old male adolescent and former star pitcher for his high school baseball team had been aggressively treated for Ewing's sarcoma for 13 months. The primary site was his upper right arm, his pitching arm. A limb-sparing procedure had been successfully completed, but his disease had recurred and rapidly progressed. His pain was exceedingly difficult to manage and he openly spoke of his readiness to die. His mother continued to press for treatment options. They were advised of an open Phase I trial and were made aware of the experimental agent in the trial, and the toxicity-finding purpose of the trial, but were also advised by the treating team to consider only symptom management care efforts. The mother strongly urged her son to enroll in the Phase I trial. In a private meeting with one of his nurses, the adolescent confided that his personal preference was to go home to die but that he had not told his mother about that because he knew she was not ready yet for his death. The nurse asked for his permission to advocate on his behalf with his mother, but he thoughtfully declined, stating that enrolling in the trial was his final gift to his mother, a gift that he wanted very much to give her. With personal regret, the nurse accepted his choice without discussion with his mother and the adolescent enrolled in the trial and completed three courses before his

disease progressed. Although he continued to experience pain during those three courses, he remained certain of the importance of his decision because of its benefit for his mother.

### CASE STUDY
#### Adolescent and Parent Tension over End-of-life Treatment Decision-Making

A 15-year-old male with progressive large B-cell lymphoma recently began a new chemotherapy and was admitted for fever and symptom control (pain, nausea, fatigue, and pruritus). He and his parents were from a non-Western country and are in the United States for treatment without any other family support. He understood and spoke English, but his parents had a very limited understanding of English. Family members who remained in the home country of this patient were opposed to having the patient treated for his cancer by Western doctors. Before coming to the United States for treatment, the patient had lived away from his parents to attend a boarding school and while there made the majority of his own life decisions. His health-care team had arranged for his acupuncture treatments, which this adolescent regarded as beneficial for promoting his sleep. With his symptoms well-controlled, he was able to concentrate and play games on his laptop computer, an activity he enjoyed. The initial treatment goal for this patient had been a cure for his lymphoma with chemotherapy and an autologous bone marrow transplant. Both the patient and his parents realized that the likelihood of cure was low and that the greater likelihood was that the adolescent would not survive his disease. As treatment progressed, his parents were making treatment decisions including interventions for pain control. This led to conflict with his parents. Increasing metastatic disease in the mediastinal space led to episodes of painful coughing. His father urged his son "to fight the pain" and not ask for as many analgesics which the father thought led to itching and sedation; the patient cried and said, "Easy for you to say" resulting in his father feeling guilty for asking his son to avoid pain medicine because he feared that the narcotics were causing his son serious problems. The team learned that the parents' perceptions of pain interventions meant their son was worsening and dying. Over the last few days his life his respiratory effort increased and discussions were held with the adolescent and his parents regarding the option of discharging him with hospice support; however, the patient continued to say "I feel safer in the hospital." He had been reluctant to complete his My Wishes document, which would communicate his wishes if his disease continued to progress since he did not like to think about his dying. He wanted instead to proceed with more treatment for the lymphoma, stating "I would rather die from the chemotherapy than the cancer." He also stated "I do not like to be reminded I am sick and please talk to my parents about what is happening to me outside of my room. I just want to relax and do what I can do for fun such as play with my computer games rather than focus on my illness." Although suffering was reduced, evidenced by the patient's minimal ratings of pain, cough, pruritus, and nausea, tension between the patient and the staff with his parents existed due to their concern that their son was becoming addicted to medications. Interdisciplinary meetings were held to assure that the health-care team was honoring the patient's preferences, controlling his pain, maintaining trust, preventing suffering, and providing emotional support for this adolescent and his family.

Twenty patients participated in individual interviews about the end-of-life decision they had made. The factors most frequently considered in their decisions included "Being influenced by relationships with others," "Information from my doctor or my parents," "Wanting to be done with treatment," and "Worrying about my family."[71] These factors convey the interconnectedness between children or adolescents with incurable diseases and their families and health-care providers. All are affected by the decision-making process and the outcomes of the decision. This interconnectedness among the seriously ill child or adolescent, the family, and the health-care providers contributes to more agreements on end-of-life decisions than disagreements. Although rare, disagreements between the patient and parent, or between parents and health-care providers, do occur and are especially difficult for all involved. Disagreeing with a health-care professional who is deemed essential for their child's well-being and with whom a care alliance is desired is at best troubling for parents, but at worst disruptive to relationships and problem solving. When circumstances exist that allow a delay in the contested decision-making, a consultation with an ethicist or ethics board can facilitate decision-making. Involving the family, the patient who is deemed competent to participate in end-of-life decision-making, and the health-care team in the same meeting with the ethicist or ethics board is particularly helpful, as all perspectives can be considered. When a family and a health-care team do not have agreement, special measures must be initiated by the team leaders to support team members in their efforts to continue to deliver excellent care to the patient and family. Measures can include brief meetings with an esteemed institutional leader who openly acknowledges the sizable difficulty that the team is facing, having information-sharing or cathartic sessions with the ethicist, and developing strategies for handling similar future difficulties. Likewise, similar support measures need to be implemented for the family. In addition, regular opportunities to interact with the health-care team (such as care conferences) need to be established so that trust between the family and team can be fostered.

CASE STUDY

*Involving an Ethicist to Assist a Team in Anticipation of, During, or After an End-of-Life Decision*

A 7-year-old boy had a second recurrence of acute lymphoblastic leukemia. His leukemia was first diagnosed when he was 19 months old. The first recurrence occurred less than a year after completing the 3-year treatment protocol, and the second recurrence occurred 8 months after completing the treatment for relapsed leukemia. As his mother pointed out to the treating team, her son had had very few months in his life of feeling healthy. She conveyed reluctance to continue any curative efforts, preferring instead to have her son discharged from the inpatient unit so that she could take him home. The attending physician, an internationally recognized expert in the treatment of leukemia, strongly disagreed with the mother's stated preference and offered her information on the likelihood of cure (admittedly low) and emphasized his desire to continue curative efforts. When the mother firmly declined the option of further treatment, the physician told the mother that he considered the discharge to be "against medical orders" and noted that in the medical record. A nurse on the team later approached the physician and proposed a meeting with the team and an ethicist to discuss the decision. The physician agreed and the full team met a week later with an ethicist. The physician honestly acknowledged his sadness about the child's incurable disease, his liking of the child, and his concern that because the mother disagreed with his recommendation of further treatment, the health-care team might think less of him as a physician. The team and the ethicist reacted with surprise at the last admission and conveyed instead their strong respect for him and his efforts to be a good doctor and for the mother's efforts to be a good parent. The physician offered to write a letter to the mother expressing the team's support of her and her child and that the child would always have complete access to all of the care setting's resources. The mother telephoned the physician after receiving the letter to express her relief. Three weeks later, the mother brought her son to the hospital to die.

## Factors Considered by Health-Care Providers

The factors considered by health-care professionals in end-of-life decision-making on behalf of children and adolescents reveal important similarities and differences between nurses and physicians. Current reports indicate that nurses are more likely to reflect on the moral balance of the decision, that is, the goodness or lack thereof of extending a child's life if doing so also extends or increases the child's suffering,[90] whereas physicians first consider whether the child's life can be saved.[16] This difference can create tension within the health-care team and merits discussion by the team members. Nurses and physicians also identified a factor they both consider frequently in end-of-life decision-making for pediatric oncology patients: "respecting the patient's and family's preferences." This factor reflected the health-care professionals' efforts to inform the patient and family of all options and then to respect the choice they made. In a survey completed by 21 health-care professionals in pediatric oncology (16 physicians, 3 nurses, and 2 chaplains) regarding end-of-life decisions for patients with incurable cancer, the factors rated as most important included "discussions with the family of the patient," "thinking the patient would never get any better," "the belief that nothing else could help the patient," and "things the patient had said about continuing or not continuing treatment." Most of the participating health-care professionals also indicated that they did not make end-of-life decisions alone but sought the input of other team members.[16]

### Strategies for Facilitating Child, Adolescent, and Parent Involvement

End-of-life decision-making is a process that very likely begins at the time of diagnosis, when the patient and the parents are exposed to the seriousness of the illness, the possible risks of treatment, and the uncertainty of short-term and long-term treatment outcomes. When faced with the actual decision-making, a few parents and patients express a preference seemingly without hesitation or anguish. They are likely to have gained an earlier understanding of the situation; often, patients and parents who observe others undergoing end-of-life experiences begin to reflect on their own life values. More often, however, patients and parents require time to

think after becoming aware of the impending decision point and treatment options.[35] In both the briefer and longer contemplation periods, the decision-making capability evolves as treatment continues and understanding of the patient's situation increases. As noted in the American Academy of Pediatrics guidelines on forgoing life-sustaining treatment,[91] end-of-life decision-making is not a single event or one well-defined point in time.

It is essential that health-care providers realize that the end-of-life decision-making process begins early in treatment and evolves with each interaction between the provider, the patient, and the parent, and with each observation of or encounter with other seriously ill patients and their parents (Figure 56–1). Each interaction provides an opportunity for the health-care provider to build the patient's and family's trust in him or her as a source of information and support and as a care expert who can be relied on to do what is best for the patient.[16] Each interaction is also an opportunity for the provider to facilitate parents' efforts to function fully as parents—a role that becomes increasingly uncertain as parents deal with unfamiliar decisions. Feeling competent in their parenthood is especially crucial to parents who face end-of-life decisions on behalf of their child. Believing that they have acted as "good parents" in such a situation is likely to be very important to their emotional recovery from the dying and death of their child.

Decision-making by patients and parents is influenced not only by their interactions with the health-care team but also by the impressions they form through observations of and encounters with other patients and families in the care setting. As patients and parents learn about the treatment experiences and the positive or negative outcomes of other patients, they contemplate what it would be like to experience those situations themselves. A second type of personal experience that prompts this kind of reflection is an unexpected negative response to treatment, such as an adverse reaction

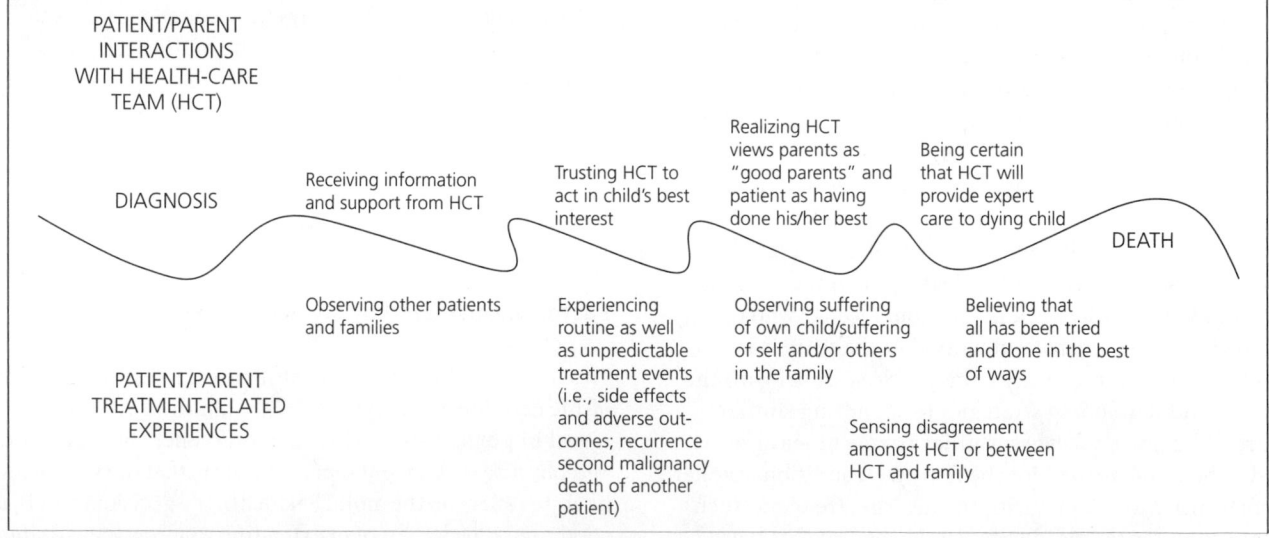

**Figure 56–1.** The interaction and experiences of pediatric oncology patients, their parents, and the members of their health-care team (HCT) from the point of diagnosis forward that influences end-of-life decision-making.

or even disease progression, after positive responses. When patients and parents feel well-informed by health-care team members about disease response to treatment and are routinely involved in treatment discussions and other decisions, they are being prepared for end-of-life decision-making, should it become necessary.

A third experience that prepares the patient and parents for end-of-life decision-making is the patient's experience of suffering and the parent's experience of witnessing that suffering and being unable to adequately relieve it. In our research with parents of children and adolescents who are experiencing a first or second recurrence of cancer, parents and guardians are more likely to contemplate ending curative efforts when they see their child in pain, unable to enjoy favorite activities, places, and people, or unable to find comfort.[85,87] Parents may react to the same experiences in different—even opposite—ways. The mother of a child treated for acute lymphocytic leukemia wrote in her guide for parents, friends, and health-care providers that an end-of-life decision is an "intensely personal decision."[92] Some parents seek to exhaust all possible treatments, whereas others hope only for sufficient time to prepare themselves and their child for the dying and death. A study by Hollen and Brickle[93] suggested that the socioeconomic status of parents of well adolescents helps to predict the quality of the parents' decision-making about their teenage children. However, no similar data are available that identify relationships between characteristics of parents whose child is seriously ill and their end-of-life decisions on behalf of their child.

## The Nurse's Role

The American Nurses Association's Position Statement on Nursing and the Patient Self-Determination Act[18] asserts that nurses have a professional responsibility to facilitate informed decision-making by patients about end-of-life options. The statement does not specify patient age, but other wording, such as that describing the nurse's responsibility for knowing state laws about advance directives, suggests that the statement is oriented toward adult patients. The document also asserts that the nurse is responsible for ensuring that advance directives are current and reflect the patient's choices. The ANA makes equally explicit assertions about the nurse's role in its position statement "Nursing Care and Do-Not-Resuscitate Decisions."[18] That position statement urges nurses to assume principal responsibility for ensuring that competent patients' preferences regarding resuscitation are honored, even if those preferences conflict with those of other health-care professionals and family members. Nurses are further urged to facilitate explicit discussions of the resuscitation order with the patient, family members, and health-care team, and to document the decisions clearly.

Several general studies about how nurses, physicians, and other health-care team members perceive end-of-life decision-making have revealed differences in role responsibilities and interpretations of care priorities.[47,94–98] These differences contribute to tension among team members. It is important that team members be aware of official statements

---

**Table 56–3**
**Guidelines for the Health-Care Team to Use in Assisting Each Other with End-of-Life Decision-Making**

1. Know the guidelines offered by specific disciplines regarding roles in end-of-life decision-making (i.e., the American Nurses Association's official statements on what the nurse is expected to do to help parents and patients make decisions), because it is possible that the guidelines differ from expectations held by others outside the discipline.

2. Before initiating end-of-life discussions with patients* and parents, all members of the health-care team should discuss and agree on
   a. The need for such a discussion.
   b. Which options are appropriate and available.
   c. Whether outside consultants, such as an ethics committee or external oncology expert, are needed to identify which options are in the best interest of the patient.
   d. Which other team members will participate in the discussion with the parents and patient.
   e. The time of the discussion and specific staff members who will participate.
   f. Which staff member will document the discussions in the medical record.
   g. Availability of the appropriate staff time and resources to address any questions parents and patients may have.
      Communicate to the team members who were not present at the patient-and-parent discussion what specific language was used to provide support to the parents and patient in making this decision.

3. Be available to team members and to the patient and parents to discuss and rediscuss decisions and related concerns.

4. Explore with the team all appropriate options to ensure that all that can be done is being done and being done well.

5. Inform other team members if feedback from or assessment of the patient, parents, or both indicates that any decision needs clarification or reconsideration.

* When considering whether the patient should be present during such discussions, evaluate the developmental stage of the patient and the severity of illness and symptoms at the time of the discussion.

issued by each discipline's professional association about role expectations. For example, the *Guidelines on Forgoing Life-Sustaining Medical Treatment* issued by the American Academy of Pediatrics[17] indicates that physicians are expected to provide adequate information to patients, parents, and "other appropriate decision-makers" about therapeutic options and their risks, discomforts, adverse effects, projected financial costs, potential benefits, and likelihood of success. In addition, physicians are expected to offer advice about which option to choose and to elicit questions from the patients and parents. Nurses should openly discuss expectations and team functions with other team members (Table 56–3) to prevent misunderstanding or disappointment about their perceived roles.

## Guidelines for End-of-Life Decision-Making in Pediatrics

End-of-life decision-making for children and adolescents who have been seriously and chronically ill necessitates consistent and careful attention to their most meaningful relationships.[99] The relationships of obvious importance are the relationship of child or adolescent with self and with family. Less obvious but also meaningful relationships are those between the patient and the health-care professionals, and between the family and health-care professionals (those who provide care for the child or adolescent or for the family). Because of the importance of these relationships

---

**Table 56–4**
**Guidelines for the Health-Care Team to Use in Assisting Pediatric Patients with End-of-Life Decision-Making**

1. Seek input of parents as to the timing and extent of information that should be offered to the patient about diagnosis, treatment options, and the likely response to treatment.
2. At the time of diagnosis and throughout treatment, actively seek opportunities to provide information to the child or adolescent that is appropriate to his or her developmental stage.
   a. For a child, assure parental presence during such discussions.
   b. For an adolescent, assure a discussion that includes the parents but offer to discuss with the patient alone as well.
3. Be available to discuss and rediscuss decisions and related concerns in a manner appropriate to the developmental stage of the patient.
4. With parental agreement, encourage the patient to interact with other pediatric oncology patients.
5. Convey verbally and nonverbally the recognition that the patient is trying his or her best and that the health-care team is committed to the patient's well-being.
6. Give assurances that everything that can be done to help the patient is being done and being done well.
7. As a patient's disease progresses, provide clear verbal (and written, if desired by the patient) explanations of the patient's status.
8. With parental agreement, inform the patient of treatment options as they become available in the treating institution or elsewhere.
9. Assess patient suffering and the need to change interventions to relieve such suffering.
10. When end-of-life options should be discussed with the patient, consult parents about the appropriate depth and timing of such discussions.
11. After receiving input from the parents and exploring the patient's readiness for information, discuss the end-of-life options, with
    a. A strong emphasis on the team's commitment to the patient's comfort and to providing expert care at all times.
    b. Professional recommendations.
    c. Descriptions about how the patient is likely to respond to each option (physical appearance, ability to communicate, etc.).
    d. Information about other support resources such as chaplains and ethicists.
12. Include more than one health-care team member in end-of-life discussions with the patient.
13. Allow the patient private time to consider the options with his or her parents.
14. Reassess the appropriateness of the chosen end-of-life options on an ongoing basis, remaining aware that patients will
    a. Vacillate between certainty and uncertainty about the decision.
    b. Need clarification and additional information to resolve uncertainties.
15. Convey respect for the patient's right to change decisions, when such changes are clinically feasible.
16. Maintain sensitivity to any specific ethnic, cultural, or religious preferences during the terminal stage.
17. Demonstrate continued commitment to providing symptom management, support of quality of life, and assurance of the parents' well-being.

in end-of-life decision-making, separate (although overlapping) guidelines are provided addressing how members of the health-care team can assist parents, patients (Table 56-4), and each other in making end-of-life decisions. The overlap in the guidelines reflects the parallel, and at times interacting, decision-making processes experienced by children, adolescents, and their parents. Health-care professionals will be most effective in implementing these guidelines if they first reflect on their feelings and concerns about the dying and death of children and adolescents and about participating in end-of-life decision-making. Research findings to date consistently indicate that when the child or adolescent participates as fully as possible in end-of-life decision-making, parents and health-care providers are more certain and more comfortable about the decision that is made.[15,88] Their belief that the decision reflects the child's or adolescent's preferences helps parents and health-care providers to make the decision and to recover emotionally from this painful experience.

## Acknowledgments

The authors express sincere appreciation to Linda Watts Parker for her careful formatting of this chapter, and to Sharon Naron for her thoughtful editing.

REFERENCES

1. Surkan P, Kreicbergs U, Valdimarsdottir U, et al. Perceptions of inadequate health care and feelings of guilt in parents after the death of a child to a malignancy: A population-based long-term follow-up. J Palliat Med 2006;9:317–331.

2. Kreichbergs U, Valdimarsdottir U, Onelov E, et al. Care-related distress: A nationwide survey of parents having lost their child to cancer. J Clin Oncol 2005;23:9162–9171.

3. Olson M, Hinds P, Euell K, et al. Peak and nadir experiences and their consequences described by pediatric oncology nurses. J Pediatr Oncol Nurs 1998;15:13–24.

4. Hinds P, Oakes L, Furman W, et al. End-of-life decision making by adolescents, parents, and healthcare providers in pediatric oncology. Cancer Nurs 2001;24:122–136.

5. Rothman M, Gugliucci M. End-of-life care curricula in undergraduate medical education: A comparison of allopathic and osteopathic medical schools. J Hosp Palliat Med 2008;25:354–360.

6. Wallace M, Grossman S, Campbell S, et al. Integration of end-of-life care content in undergraduate nursing curricula: Student knowledge and perceptions. J Prof Nurs 2009;25:50–56.

7. Baughcum A, Gerhradt C, Young-Saleme T, et al. Evaluation of a pediatric palliative care educational workshop for oncology fellows. Pediatr Blood Cancer 2007;49:154–159.

8. Ries L, Smith M, Gurney J, et al.Cancer Incidence and Survival Among Children and Adolescents: United States SEER Program 1975–1995, National Cancer Institute, SEER Program. NI Pub. No. 99-4649, Bethesda, MD, 1999.

9. Karian VE, Jankowski SM, Beal JA. Exploring the lived-experience of childhood cancer survivors. J Pediatr Oncol Nurs 1998;15:153–162.

10. Kazak AE. Psychological research in pediatric oncology (editorial). J Pediatr Psychol 1993;18:313–318.

11. Wolfe J, Grier ME. Care of the dying child. In: Pizzo P, Poplack D, eds. Principles and Practice of Pediatric Oncology (4th ed). Philadelphia, PA: Lippincott Williams & Wilkins; 2002:1477–1493.

12. Klopfenstein K, Hutchinson C, Clark C, et al. Variables influencing end-of-life care in children and adolescents. Pediatr Hematol Oncol 2001;23:481–486.

13. Wolfe J, Grier H, Klar N, et al. Symptoms and suffering at the end of life in children with cancer. N Engl J Med 2000;342:326–333.

14. Institute of Medicine. When Children Die: Improving Palliative and End-of-Life Care for Children and Their Families. Washington DC: National Academy Press, 2003.

15. Hinds P, Oakes L, Quaragnenti A, et al. Challenges and issues in conducting descriptive decision-making studies in pediatric oncology: A tale of two studies. J Pediatr Oncol Nurs 1998;15:10–17.

16. Hinds P, Oakes L, Furman W, et al. Decision making by parents and health care professionals for pediatric patients with cancer. Oncol Nurs Forum 1997;24:1523–1528.

17. American Academy of Pediatrics, Committee on Bioethics. Guidelines on foregoing life-sustaining medical treatment. Pediatrics 1994;93:532–536.

18. American Nurses Association, Task Force on the Nurse's Role in End-of-Life Decisions. Compendium of Position Statements on the Nurse's Role in End-of-Life Decisions. Washington, DC: American Nurses Association; 1991:1–14.

19. Lindquist R, Banasik J, Barnsteiner J, et al. Determining AACN's research priorities for the 90's. Am J Crit Care 1993;2:110–117.

20. Zuckerman C, Mackinnon A. The Challenge of Caring for Patients Near the End of Life: Findings from the Hospital Palliative Care Initiative. New York, NY: United Hospital Fund of New York; 1998.

21. Masera G, Spinetta JJ, Jankovic M, et al. Guidelines for assistance to terminally ill children with cancer: A report of the SIOP working committee on psychosocial issues in pediatric oncology. Med Pediatr Oncol 1999;32:44–48.

22. Awong L. Ethical dilemmas: When an adolescent wants to forgo therapy. Am J Nurs 1988;98:67–68.

23. Kluge EH. Informed consent by children: The new reality. CMAJ 1995;152:1495–1497.

24. Mayo TW. Withholding and withdrawing life-sustaining care: Legal issues. In: Levin D, Morriss F, eds. Essentials of Pediatric Intensive Care (Vol. 1). New York, NY: Churchill Livingstone; 1997:1091–1103.

25. McCabe MA, Rushton CH, Glover J, Murray MG, Leikin S. Implications of the Patient Self-Determination Act: Guidelines for involving adolescents in medical decision making. J Adolesc Health 1996;19:319–324.

26. Weir RF, Peters C. Affirming the decisions adolescents make about life and death. Hastings Center Rep 1997;27:29–34.

27. Joint Commission on the Accreditation of Healthcare Organizations. Shared Vision-New Pathways Resources. Available at: http://www.jcaho.org/accredited+organizations/svnp/index.htm (accessed December 23, 2009).

28. National Quality Forum (NQF). A National Framework and Preferred Practices for Palliative and Hospice Care Quality: A Consensus Report.Washington, DC: National Quality Forum; 2006.

29. Earle C, Park E, Lai B, et al. Identifying potential indicators or the quality of end-of-life cancer care from administrative data. J Clin Oncol 2003;21:1133–1138.

30. Edwardson SR. The choice between hospital and home care for terminally ill children. Nurs Res 1983;32:29–34.

31. Kollef MH. Private attending physician status and the withdrawal of life-sustaining interventions in a medical intensive care unit population. Crit Care Med 1996;24:968–975.

32. Miller DK, Coe RM, Hyers TM. Achieving consensus on withdrawing or withholding care for critically ill patients. J Gen Intern Med 1992;7:475–480.

33. Overbay JD. Parental participants in treatment decisions for pediatric oncology ICU patients. Dimens Crit Care Nurs 1996;15:16–24.

34. Campbell A, McHaffie H. Prolonging life and allowing death: Infants. J Med Ethics 1995;21:339–344.

35. Nelson L, Nelson R. Ethics and provision of futile, harmful, or burdensome treatment to children. Crit Care Med 1992;20:427–433.

36. Raffin TA. Withdrawing life support: How is the decision made? JAMA 1995;273:738–739.

37. Rushton C, Glover J Involving parents in decisions to forego life-sustaining treatment for critically ill infants and children. AACN clinical issues. Crit Care Nurs 1990;1:206–214.

38. Rushton C, Lynch M. Dealing with advance directives for critically ill adolescents. Crit Care Nurs 1992;12:31–37.

39. Zaner RM, Bliton MJ. Decisions in the NICU: The moral authority of parents. Child Health Center 1991;20:19–25.

40. Ross LF. Health care decision making by children: Is it in their best interest? Hastings Center Rep 1997;27:41–45.

41. Nitschke R, Humphrey G, Sexauer C, Catron B, Wunder S, Jay S. Therapeutic choices made by patients with end-stage cancer. J Pediatr 1982;10:471–476.

42. Nitschke R, Meyer W, Sexauer C, Parkhurst JB, Foster P, Huszh H. Care of terminally ill children with cancer. Med Pediatr Oncol 2000;34:268–270.

43. Williams C, Cairnie J, Fines V, et al. Construction of a parent-derived questionnaire to measure end-of-life care after withdrawal of life-sustaining treatment in the neonatal intensive care unit. Pediatrics 2009;123:e87–e95.

44. Cook LA, Watchko JF. Decision making for the critically ill neonate near the end of life. J Perinatol 1996;16:133–136.

45. De Leeuw R, Beaufort AJ, de Kleine MJ, van Harrewijn K, Kollee LA. Foregoing intensive care treatment in newborn infants with extremely poor prognoses. J Pediatr 1996;129:661–666.

46. Ragatz SC, Ellison PH. Decisions to withdraw life support in the neonatal intensive care unit. Clin Pediatr 1983;22:729–736.

47. Van der Heide A, van der Maas PJ, van der Wal G, et al. Medical end-of-life decisions made for neonates and infants in the Netherlands. Lancet 1997;350:251–255.

48. Wall SN, Partridge JC. Death in the intensive care nursery: Physician practice of withdrawing and withholding life support. Pediatrics 1997;99:64–70.

49. Whitelaw A. Death as an option in neonatal intensive care. Lancet 1986;2:328–331.

50. Able-Boone H, Dokecki PR, Smith MS. Parent and health care provider communication and decision making in the intensive care nursery. Child Health Care 1989;18:133–141.

51. Rushton C. Moral Decision Making by Parents of Infants Who Have Life-Threatening Congenital Disorders. Washington, DC: School of Nursing, Catholic University of America, 1994. PhD dissertation.

52. Guglani L, Lodha R. Attitudes towards end-of-life issues amongst pediatricians in a tertiary hospital in a developing country. J Tropical Pediatr 2008;54:261–264.

53. Goh AY, Lum LC, Chan PW, Bakar F, Chong BO. Withdrawal and limitation of life support in pediatric intensive care. Arch Disabled Child 1999;80:424–428.

54. Lantos JD, Berger AC, Zucker AR. Do-not-resuscitate orders in a children's hospital. Crit Care Med 1991;21:52–55.

55. Vernon DD, Dean JM, Timmons OD, Banner W, Allen-Webb EM. Modes of death in the pediatric intensive care unit: Withdrawal and limitation of supportive care. Crit Care Med 1993;21:1798–1802.

56. Burns J, Mitchell C, Outwater K, et al. End-of-life care in the pediatric intensive care unit after the forgoing of life-sustaining treatment. Crit Care Med 2000;28:3060–3066.

57. Meyer E, Burns J, Griffith J, et al. Parental perspectives on end-of-life care in the pediatric intensive care unit. Crit Care Med 2002;30:226–231.

58. Zawistowski C, DeVita M. A descriptive study of children dying in the pediatric intensive care unit after withdrawal of life-sustaining treatment. Pediatr Crit Care Med 2004;5:216–223.

59. Moore P, Kerridge I, Gillis J. Withdrawal and limitation of life-sustaining treatments in a paediatric intensive care unit and review of the literature. J Paediatr Child Health 2008; 44:404–408.

60. Buchanan A, Brock D. Deciding for Others: The Ethics of Surrogate Decision-Making. Cambridge, MA: Cambridge University Press, 1989.

61. Foley M. Children with cancer: Ethical dilemmas. Semin Oncol Nurs 1989;5:109–113.

62. Weithorn L, Campbell S. The competency of children and adolescents to make informed treatment decisions. Child Dev 1982;53:1589.

63. President's Commission for the Study of Ethical Problems in Medicine and Biomedical and Behavioral Research. Deciding to Forego Life-Sustaining Treatment: A Report on the Ethical, Medical and Legal Issues in Treatment Decisions. Washington, DC: U.S. Government Printing Office; 1983: 160–170, 197–220.

64. Ariff JL, Groh DH. In the best interests of the child: Ethical issues. In: Curley M, Smith J, Moloney-Harmon P, eds. Critical Care Nursing of Infants and Children. Philadelphia, PA: W.B. Saunders; 1996:126–141.

65. Beyth-Marom R, Fischhoff B. Adolescents' decisions about risks: A cognitive perspective. In: Schulenberg J, Maggs J, Hurrelmann K, eds. Health Risks and Developmental Transitions During Adolescence. Cambridge, MA: Cambridge University Press; 1997:110–135.

66. Hinds P, Martin J. Hopefulness and the self-sustaining process in adolescents with cancer. Nurs Res 1988;37:336–340.

67. Hinds P. Quality of life in children and adolescents experiencing cancer. Semin Oncol Nurs 1990;6:285–291.

68. Burns J, Truog R. Ethical controversies in pediatric critical care. New Horizons 1997;5:72–84.

69. Leikin S. The role of adolescents in decisions concerning their cancer therapy. Cancer 1993;71(Suppl):3342–3346.

70. Hinds P, Oakes L, Drew D. et al. Adolescents' end-of-life care preferences. J Clin Oncol 2005;23(36):9146–9154.

71. Goldman A. Life threatening illnesses and symptom control in children. In: Doyle D, Hanks G, MacDonald N, eds. Oxford Textbook of Palliative Medicine (2nd ed). New York, NY: Oxford University Press; 1998:1033–1043.

72. Levetown M, Carter M. Child-centered care in terminal illness: An ethical framework. In: Doyle D, Hanks G, MacDonald N, eds. Oxford Textbook of Palliative Medicine (2nd ed). New York, NY: Oxford University Press; 1998: 1107–1117.

73. Gowan D. End-of-life issues of children. Pediatr Transplant 2003;7(Suppl 3):40–43.

74. Wolfe J, Klar N, Grier H, et al. Understanding of prognosis among parents of children who died of cancer: Impact on treatment goals and integration of palliative care. JAMA 2000;284:2469–2475.

75. Schmidt L. Pediatric end-of-life care: Coming of age? Caring 2003;22:20–22.

76. Rowa-Dewar N. Do interventions make a difference to bereaved parents? A systematic review of controlled studies. Int J Palliat Nurs 2002;8:456–457.

77. Contro N, Larson J, Scofield S, et al. Family perspectives on the quality of pediatric palliative care. Arch Pediatr Adolesc Med 2002;156:14–19.

78. James LS, Johnson B. The needs of pediatric oncology patients during the palliative care phase. J Pediatr Oncol Nurs 1996;14:85–95.

79. Martinson IM, Cohen MH. Themes from a longitudinal study of family reactions to childhood cancer. J Psychosoc Oncol 1988;6:81–98.

80. Chesler MA, Barbarin OA. Difficulties of providing help in a crisis: Relationships between parents and children with cancer and their friends. J Soc Issues 1984;40:113–134.

81. Robinson M, Thiel M, Backus M, et al. Matters of spirituality at the end of life in the pediatric intensive care unit. Pediatrics 2006;118:e719–e729.

82. Meyer E, Ritholz M, Burns J, et al. Improving the quality of end-of-life care in the pediatric intensive care unit: Parents' priorities and recommendations. Pediatrics 2006;117:649–657.

83. Giannini A, Messeri A, Aprile A, et al. End-of-life decisions in pediatric intensive care. Recommendations of the Italian Society of Neonatal and Pediatric Anesthesia and Intensive Care (SARNePI). Pediatr Anesth 2008;18:1089–1095.

84. Stevens MM. Care of the dying child and adolescent: Family adjustment and support. In: Doyle D, Hanks G, MacDonald N, eds. Oxford Textbook of Palliative Medicine (2nd ed). New York, NY: Oxford University Press; 1998: 1057–1075.

85. Hinds PS, Birenbaum L, Clarke-Steffen L, et al. Coming to terms: Parents response to a first cancer recurrence. Nurs Res 1996;45:148–153.

86. Pyke-Grimm KA, Degner L, Small A, Mueller B. Preferences for participation in treatment decision making and information needs of parents of children with cancer: A pilot study. J Pediatr Oncol Nurs 1999;16:13–24.

87. Hinds P, Birenbaum L, Pedrosa A, Pedrosa F. Guidelines for the recurrence of pediatric cancer. Semin Oncol Nurs 2002; 18:50–59.

88. Hinds PS, Oakes L, Quargnenti A, et al. An international feasibility study on parental decision making in pediatric oncology. Oncol Nurs Forum 2000;27:1233–1243.

89. Kirschbaum MS. Life support decisions for children: What do parents value? Adv Nurs Sci 1996;19:51–71.

90. Davies B, Deveau E, deVeber B, et al. Experiences of mothers in five countries whose child died of cancer. Cancer Nurs 1998;21:301–311.

91. American Academy of Pediatrics, Committee on Bioethics. Informed consent, parental permission, and assent in pediatric practice. Pediatrics 1995;95:314–317.

92. Keene N. Childhood Leukemia: A Guide for Families, Friends and Caregivers. Sebastopol, CA: O'Reilly & Associates,1997.

93. Hollen PJ, Brickle BB. Quality parental decision making and distress. J Pediatr Nurs 1998;13:140–150.

94. Phillips RS, Rempusheski VF, Puopolo AL, Naccarato M, Mallatratt L. Decision making in SUPPORT: The role of the nurse. J Clin Epidemiol 1990;43(Suppl):55S–58S.

95. Randolph AG, Zollo MB, Wigton RS, Yeh TS. Factors explaining variability among caregivers in the intent to restrict life-support interventions in a pediatric intensive care unit. Crit Care Med 1997;25:435–439.

96. Randolph AG, Zollo MB, Egger MJ, Guyatt GH, Nelson RM, Stidham GL. Variability in physician opinion on limiting pediatric life support. Pediatrics 1999;103:S43.

97. Solomon MZ, O'Donnell L, Jennings MA, et al. Decisions near the end-of-life: Professional views on life-sustaining treatments. Am J Public Health 1993;83:14–23.

98. Walter SD, Cook DJ, Guyatt GH, et al. Confidence in life-support decisions in the intensive care unit: A survey of healthcare workers. Crit Care Med 1998;26:44–49.

99. Hume M. Improving care at the end of life. Qual Lett Healthc Lead 1998;10:2–10.

# 57 ❧ Palliative Care in the Neonatal Intensive Care Unit

*Carole Kenner and Marina Boykova*

*Why no miracle for my little one, so innocent, so small? Why so much suffering in such a short life? Should I have fought for her or spared her and let her go? The answers to my questions I will never know...until we meet again.—Kathleen Petzold, mother*

♦ **Key Points**
♦ *Palliative care in the neonatal intensive care unit (NICU) is as much a part of family-centered care and patient-focused care as any other aspect of care. Palliative care gives nurses the opportunity to do what nurses do best: nurture and care for the whole infant and family unit at a time of tremendous stress. It is the most intimate time that one can share with a family.*
♦ *Palliative care incorporates symptom management for the infant, and emotional, psychosocial, and spiritual support for the infant and family members. Family is defined by the parents and may include other children as well as grandparents and other close family members. The support is always provided in a cultural and developmental manner appropriate for each person. Palliative care is provided when a condition is life-threatening and may or may not result in death.*
♦ *Palliative care is the antithesis of what most professionals and families think about within the context of infant care. The primary focus of infant care is and should be life-prolonging care. Yet palliative and end-of-life (EOL) care are a part of neonatal nursing. In 2001 there were 27,568 infant deaths in the United States, with an infant mortality rate of 6.8 per 1,000 live births.[1] In 2008 this rate had risen to 28,000 infant deaths, placing the United States in 34th place globally.[2] Neonatal mortality accounts for about 60% of these infant deaths.[3] Thus it is obvious that the death of a newborn can be a part of the nurse's sphere of practice and requires that the nurse develops competencies in providing supportive palliative care, which may lead to a peaceful death.*

American society does not have a word for a parent who has lost a child—another challenge for the nurse. For example, the term "widow" is used for the surviving female spouse, but what do we call the surviving parent? There is no term, but the loss in many cases is more profound than a spousal loss, only because western culture no longer expects children to die before their parents. In fact, the role of parent is often viewed as gone when a baby dies. One nurse, prepared in palliative care, responded to a grieving mother whose baby was not likely to survive to term, "You are a mother now, and you will always be a mother, regardless of whether or not your baby survives. You have a baby and that makes you a mother." Although this was comforting to the mother, it points out the lack of good alternative language to describe a parent who has lost a child.

Other cultures may have words or strategies to support parents who have lost an infant, but American culture labels the person a bereaved parent and talks about another child in the parent's future or another child the parent may have.

This chapter presents the core values of palliative care within the context of providing culturally-appropriate, individualized, family-centered developmental care (IFCDC) and patient-focused care for infants receiving care in the NICU environment. The following case study will act as an exemplar of neonatal/pediatric palliative care.

To illustrate use of palliative care with the neonatal population, the following case study was supplied by team members from the Footprints Program (Continuity of Care Palliative Care Program), SSM Cardinal Glennon Children's Hospital, St. Louis, MO (used with permission).

❧

CASE STUDY
*Christian, A Newborn Patient with Holoprosencephaly*

March 8, 2001: We arrived at the hospital about 7 A.M. Within an hour we were told, "You're going to have a baby today!" During the next 6 hours, everything went spiraling downward. My doctor discovered I had hemolysis, elevated liver enzyme levels, low platelet count (HELLP) syndrome (my blood wasn't clotting and my liver and kidneys were shutting down). I was prepped for an emergency cesarean section and wheeled into the operating room. My husband, Matt, waited anxiously in the hallway for news of our new baby and my health. I can only imagine the fear he felt as a group of nurses carrying a small bundle rushed out of the operating room. I awoke in the recovery room and asked to see my husband and child. About 30 minutes later, Matt came into the room and bravely told me about our little boy and his problems. Christian was being transferred to SSM Cardinal Glennon Children's Hospital in St. Louis where he could be better evaluated. "Can I see him before he goes?" was all I could ask.

The transport team brought in a tiny 5-pound, 3-ounce, 17-inch baby boy with IVs, an oxygen mask, and monitors. Christian was handed to me, and I cradled my son in my arms. Matt said this was the proudest moment of his life. We had our first family photo and handed Christian back to the team after so few minutes. We were supposed to be celebrating the birth of our child but instead were overcome with worry, grief, and fear.

Over the next few days, we talked with many specialists in the NICU at Cardinal Glennon. Christian was diagnosed with holoprosencephaly, a condition in which the brain does not separate into two hemispheres. Christian also had cleft palate, cleft lip, and blindness, and was in constant seizure. We were told he would most likely not live beyond 2 weeks to 2 months, or, if we were lucky, 2 years.

After discussion, we determined we wanted Christian to experience every moment he could while he was alive. First and foremost, we wanted to take him home. Our NICU staff identified a program in the hospital that could help us make that desire a reality. They referred us to the Footprints Program (SSM Cardinal Glennon Hospital, St. Louis, MO); which cares for children with life-threatening and terminal illnesses. The Footprints staff identified a continuity physician who would direct Christian's care and gathered a team of our physicians, nurses, and chaplains to meet with Matt and me and our family members to make plans for Christian's eventual homecoming. Together, we identified our goals and our fears and, with help from the team, developed a plan of care for our son that would give him the best quality of life. While the NICU staff taught us how to care for Christian's basic physical needs, the Footprints staff contacted all of the care providers who would be involved in his care once he was home.... home health/hospice providers and the emergency medical services (EMS) community in our town. Because we expressed fear at what others might think if Christian died at home so soon after birth, the staff also contacted our local police department to let them know that Christian was seriously ill and not expected to live. A plan was in place! But we had yet to learn that Christian was the strongest person we had ever met!

Christian came home after 13 days in the NICU, and although scary, each day became easier. We focused on Christian, and with encouragement from the NICU and Footprints teams, made memories that would last forever. We took him outside to experience the wind in his hair, the sun on his face, and cold water on his feet. The next few months brought many changes. We needed to replace the feeding tube with a g-tube. We heard him cry for the first time, and although sad, it also made us smile. We visited the neurologist, and the doctor stated Christian was a "completely different baby than in the NICU." Christian was responding to his surroundings. He became a hospice dropout at the age of 6 months!

The Footprints team stayed very connected with follow-up phone conversations on a regular basis, encouraging us as Christian changed to redefine our goals and our hopes. We knew they were available to answer our questions at any time and always felt supported. We continued to give our son all of life's experiences—trick-or-treating (we ate the candy), snow on his face, and time in church. We were allowed to be Christian's parents and to leave some of the other more technical details to our care team. At a year, we met with the Footprints team and our physicians to reevaluate Christian's care plan, still focusing on the best quality of life we could give him, while keeping him with us as long as possible. We were also more prepared at that time to discuss arrangements for the time of Christian's death. Once again, we had a plan and all caregivers were notified of the revisions and new additions.

Despite several serious cases of pneumonia, Christian celebrated his second birthday, and he became a big brother. He lived to be 2 years, 8 months, and 2 days. We were able to hold him in our arms as his little body just wore out. His last moments were as we had wished, peaceful and at home with us. We are so glad we had a care plan in place. There were no arguments or questions. Arrangements basically fell into place. Our care plans focused on Christian's quality of life and helped us to focus on dignity at the time of his death. We were able to celebrate the life of our son each step of the way. The Footprints team continues to support us with phone calls and visits and is always available to help with any questions or issues we might still have.

Christian taught us about strength and hope, and what was truly important in life—love. Our lives are better—we are better—because Christian is a part of our family.
—Jennifer Anderson, Christian's Mom

## Case Summary

### We Wanted Christian to Experience Every Moment He Could While He Was Alive

Stated by Christian's mother, this goal is the essence of the best in neonatal palliative care. No one could predict the

**Table 57-1**
**Core Principles for Care of Patients (Newborns and Infants)**

- Respect the dignity of both child and caregiver.
- Be sensitive to and respectful of the family's wishes.
- Use the most appropriate measures that are consistent with the family's choices.
- Encompass alleviation of pain and other physical symptoms.
- Assess and manage psychological, social, and spiritual/religious problems.
- Ensure continuity of care—the child should be able to continue to be cared for, if so desired, by his/her primary care and specialist providers.
- Provide access to any therapy that may be realistically expected to improve the child's quality of life, including alternative or nontraditional treatments.
- Provide access to palliative care and hospice care.
- Respect the right to refuse treatment that may prolong suffering.
- Respect the physician's professional responsibility to discontinue some treatments when appropriate, with consideration for both child and family's preferences.
- Promote clinical evidence-based research on providing care at the end of life.

*Source*: Adapted from Cassel and Foley (1999), reference 4.

length of his short life; and this is often the case with newborn babies at NICU. For this family, his life was much longer than the predicted 2 weeks to 2 months. Thus, his life illustrates that neonatal palliative care must be planned in such a way as to meet the needs of the patient and family for whatever period of life the neonate has, in whatever environment that life is lived. The principles are the same regardless of the length or location of that life. Plan for death (the most peaceful and comfortable), support the parents, provide the best possible symptom relief for the neonate, honor the parents wishes, and at all times honor the life—while at the same time not denying that death is likely to occur prior to a usual lifetime of 70-plus years. With neonatal palliative care, perhaps even more so than adult palliative care, the critical element is for the health-care team and family to know the goals for the brief life and not just about advance care-planning choices. And as his mother described—to create memories of a life lived.

Excellence in palliative care can provide a positive outcome for the family and neonate even though the neonate cannot be cured. Health-care professionals can do much to make a difference. Let it never be said that "there is nothing we can do."

Palliative and EOL care is the antithesis of what most of us expect to provide to newborns. Yet this is a vital part of our professional skills. We have to start end-of-life care in the beginning of life. It is a privilege to be a part of birth and death, but it takes a professional who is adept at communicating, anticipating, and nurturing a family under tremendous grief to participate. It also requires acceptance that grief work extends to the health professional, and we must care for ourselves as we care for others.

## Core Principles and Philosophy of Care

As this case study points out, a shared interdisciplinary team approach, including the parents as part of the team, can make all the difference in how the end of life is experienced. As with any plan, there must be a shared understanding of how care is to be provided. Just as businesses and other enterprises have moved toward having a mission, vision, and core values or principles, so has palliative care. The mission, for example, of this text is to advance the knowledge of health professionals about palliative and EOL care. The vision of this book is that every individual and family will receive optimal palliative and EOL care. These core principles are the drivers of palliative care. Cassel and Foley[4] present the core principles for care of patients (newborns and infants) that are applicable to the NICU (Table 57-1).

Guiding principles only outline the key features of palliative care. Beyond that the nurse must understand the philosophy of care before employing these guidelines. Americans for Better Care of the Dying formulated seven promises they felt exemplified key aspects of palliative care.[5] These aspects were designed to constitute a contract between the health professional and the patient and family. These promises were adapted for use by the neonatal nurses. They are as follows:

1. *Good Medical Treatment*
   - Your baby will have the best of medical treatment and nursing care, aiming to prevent illness or disease progression, to promote survival, to encourage growth and development, to prevent known potential complications, and to ensure comfort.
   - Your baby will be offered proven diagnoses and treatment strategies that inhibit disease progression, enhance quality of life, and promote living fully although a condition is life-threatening.
   - We will use medical and nursing interventions that are in accord with best available standards of care and practice and consistent with your wishes and values.

2. *Never Overwhelmed by Symptoms*
   - Your baby will never have to endure overwhelming pain, severe breathing distress, or other overwhelming symptoms.
   - We will anticipate and prevent symptoms when possible. When symptoms occur, we will evaluate and address symptoms promptly.
   - We will treat severe symptoms, such as breathing difficulty, as emergencies.
   - We will use sedation when necessary to relieve symptoms that cannot be relieved in other ways near the end of life.

3. *Continuity, Coordination, and Comprehensiveness*
   - Your baby's care will be continuous, comprehensive, and coordinated.
   - We will be sure knowledgeable, caring, health-care professionals care for your baby.
   - We will make sure your baby and your family can count on an appropriate and timely response to needs.
   - We will make sure you can count on access to health-care professionals to answer questions.
   - We will try to minimize transitions among services, settings, and personnel; and when transitions are necessary, we will make sure they go smoothly.

4. *Well-Prepared, No Surprises*
   - You and your family will be prepared for everything that is likely to happen in the course of your baby's illness.
   - We will let you know what to expect if the illness worsens—and what we expect of you.
   - We will provide you with training and access to the supplies needed to handle your baby's predictable care needs.

5. *Customize Care, Reflecting Your Preferences*
   - Your wishes will be sought and respected and followed whenever possible.
   - We will tell you about the alternatives for care and services for your baby, and support you in making choices that matter to you.
   - If you wish, we will help your child to live out the end of life at home.

6. *Consideration for Patient and Family Resources (Financial, Emotional, and Practical)*
   - We will help you to consider your family's personal and financial resources, and we will respect your choices about their use.
   - We will inform families about services available in the community and the costs of those services.
   - We will discuss and address the concerns of family caregivers. When appropriate, we will make respite, volunteer, and home-aide care part of the care plan.
   - We will support families before, during, and after a loved one's death.

7. *Make the Best of Every Day*
   - We will do all we can to see that your baby and your family will have the opportunity to make the best of every day.
   - We will treat your baby as a person, not as a disease. What is important to the baby and family is important to the care team.
   - We will respond to the physical, psychological, social, and spiritual needs of your baby and family members.
   - We will support you before, during, and after your baby's death.

Using the mission, vision, core principles, and philosophy of palliative care as a backdrop, the neonatal and pediatric nursing community felt that the final step in formalizing a structure of care would be to construct precepts for the care. The Association of Pediatric Oncology Nurses (APON), National Association of Neonatal Nurses (NANN), and the Society of Pediatric Nurses (SPN) worked together to adapt the *Precepts of Palliative Care*, developed by the Last Acts Palliative Care Task Force, December, 1997. These precepts were originally written for the adult population and disseminated by the Last Acts Organization. The above organizations felt that newborns, infants, children, and their families represented a unique cohort of care where death was not expected or easily welcomed as a phase of the life cycle. The premise, however, is the same—that palliative care is comprehensive, holistic, and supportive, and it affirms life and regards dying as a profoundly personal process.[6]

So what does this mean for the neonatal nurse confronting a dying newborn or infant? It means that the nurse has to be present at the most difficult time for the family, to be fully attentive to the child and family, to separate his/her values regarding birth, life, and death from those of the family, and to clearly ask what it is that they need from their perspective. Of course, it means that the nurse must be ready to break the rules and turn over some control to the family, which is not something that most nurses feel comfortable doing. Nurses must adapt and individualize the care so that there is as much support for the positive development as possible for the infant and family. An IFCDC approach provides the context in which to render palliative and EOL care. This approach reminds the nurse that the families are parents first, and that they want to support their infant's development and preserve their role as parents. It is only after that role is solidified that parents can become the caregiver to a child that may or will die. For culturally competent care to reflect the complexity of care that is much broader than ethnicity, the nurse must be sensitive to cultural, ethnic, and religious values. A nurse must be appropriately prepared for this aspect of care. The main obstacles to good palliative care are the inability to appropriately communicate with brieving parents and a lack of knowledge about evidence-based pain management. The Institute of Medicine (IOM) *"Quality Chasm"* series puts forth a major competency of the 21st Century as patient focused care.[7,8] This competency aligns with IFCDC well as the definition is to place the patient as the center of care delivery while taking accounting for cultural values, believes, and wishes. In the case of a neonate, this definition includes the family unit. Why this is so important is that the IOM charges that quality care and patient safety are enhanced whent the patient and family becomes the central focus.

## Cultural Influences on Care

Cultural values and beliefs, both religious and ethnic, influence the family's view of pain, suffering, and end of life (Table 57–2). The neonatal nurse must incorporate these values and beliefs into the plan of care if it is to be effective and benefit the patient and family. Wong and colleagues[9] and the Texas Children's Cancer Center-Texas Children's Hospital[10] address cultural influence on care by outlining key aspects of health beliefs and practices that must be considered when providing any type of care. (For further information, *see* refs. 9 and 10).

For example, when working with a Native American family, the nurse must consider that they may want to combine healing ceremonies from their tribal rituals with western medicine to alleviate suffering. In this instance, ethnic and religious beliefs are intertwined. But in other instances, religious versus ethnic values must be incorporated into care.

It must be remembered that not every family that identifies themselves as Methodist, for example, strictly adheres to all principles of that faith. The nurse must determine what role religion plays with each family.[11] Additionally, we need to realize that for some cultures there is a biological birth and a social one. Social birth may not occur until it is clear that the infant will survive or until the infant has been given a name. How the family responds to the impending or possible death of the child will differ if the child is not considered a person until after a social birth.[12]

One example of religious belief affecting neonatal palliative care is that of an American Caucasian family strongly tied to the Catholic church. As their infant girl took a turn for the worst, the family was called. They immediately asked that she be baptized. The priest on call was unavailable and the family's priest was 2 hours away. Rather than take the chance that no priest would come before the infant's death, the nurse, a non-Catholic, baptized the baby. When the family arrived, they were reassured that yes, indeed, Angela had been baptized. The infant died peacefully in her parents' arms long before either priest arrived. The family expressed comfort in knowing she was held within the religious arms of the church's beliefs.

Rebagliato and colleagues[13] found that if this issue is examined at a global level, in addition to culture, in general the country context for the physician drives the type of palliative care rendered. Another obstacle is the lack of agreement among health professionals as to what constitues palliative

care.[14] Although some health professionals support children dying in their homes, the reality is that few pediatric hospice groups exist and even fewer for the neonate and family.[14,15] Catlin[16] studied 684 infants with life-threatening or chronic illnesses. She found that many infants stay six months or longer in the hospital with 20% of the NICU infants transferred to new and strange environment of the Pediatric Intensive Care Unit (PICU) to die even when care will most likely be futile. So despite having a palliative care protocol[17] supported at a national level, dissemination to individual institutions or units had not occurred. For the nurses, moral distress was noted as they were required to render futile and sometimes painful care.[16] As Anand suggests, health-care professionals must also understand current pharmacological treatment of pain and use the most effective methods tailored to the individual infant to eleviate distress.[18]

## Rights of Newborns and Their Families

In today's complex health-care delivery system, many families feel they have no rights. The American Hospital Association (AHA) took this to heart and in 1973 developed *A Patient's Bill of Rights*.[19] Keeping this tradition in the adult community, neonatal nurses have long recognized that even the most premature infant has rights, as does the family (Table 57–3). The rights presented here need to be considered whenever neonatal palliative care is being rendered.

Why is it so important to adapt rights to neonates and their families? Most neonatal health professionals recognize the unique needs of this population—their rights and their care needs. An infant has no history—as one family said, the infant does not know what the future possibilities are; there is no frame of reference. For the family, there are no memories of a past except prenatally, so palliative care is building a lifetime of memories. There are other aspects that are different as well. Table 57–4 summarizes these differences.

## Palliative Care Plan

Catlin and Carter[17] developed a palliative care protocol that has been disseminated widely since 2002 (see Appendix 57–1). Based on their research in neonatal palliative care, it is one of the only evidence-based plans available. It incorporates all of the elements previously discussed in this chapter. This protocol exemplifies the care that was provided in the chapter's opening exemplar—Christian's story. Their respect for the family wishes and alleviation of the pain and suffering were addressed. A team-integrated approach to care was used. Since its 2002 creation this protocol has formed the basis of many other dimensions of neonatal palliative care. For example, the National Association of Neonatal Nurses (NANN) in 2007 published a position statement on *"NICU Nurse Involvement*

**Table 57–2**
**Religious Influences**

| Religious Sect | Birth | Death | Organ Donation/Transplantation | Beliefs regarding Medical Care |
|---|---|---|---|---|
| Baptist | Infant baptism is not practiced. However, many churches present the baby and the parents to the congregation when they attend services for the first time after the birth. | It isn't mandatory that clergy be present at death, but families often desire visits from clergy. Scripture reading and prayer are important. | There is no formal statement regarding this issue. It is considered a matter of personal conscience. It is commonly regarded as positive (an act of love). | Some may regard their illness as punishment resulting from past sins. Those who believe in predestination may not seek aggressive treatment. Fundamentalist and conservative groups see the Bible as the infallible word of God to be taken literally. |
| Buddhist | Do not practice infant baptism. | Buddhist priest is often involved before and after death. Rituals are observed during and after death. If the family doesn't have a priest, they may request that one be contacted. | There is no formal statement regarding organ donation/transplantation. This is seen as a matter of individual conscience. | Believe that illness can be used as a tool to aid in the development of the soul. May see illness as a result of karmic causes. May avoid treatments or procedures on holy days. Cleanliness is important. |
| Church of Jesus Christ of Latter-day Saints (Mormon) | Infant baptism is not performed. Children are given a name and a priesthood blessing sometime after the birth, from a week or 2 to several months. In the event of a critically ill newborn, this might be done in the hospital at the discretion of the parents. Baptism is performed after the child is 8 years old. Church of Jesus Christ of Latter-day Saints feel that a child is not accountable for sins before 8 years of age. | There are no religious rituals performed related to death. | There is no official statement regarding this issue. Organ donation/ transplantation is left up to the individual or parents. | Administration to the sick involves anointing with consecrated oil and performing a blessing by members of the priesthood. While the individual or a member of the family usually requests this if the individual is unconscious and there is no one to represent him or her, it would be appropriate for anyone to contact the church so that the ordinance may be performed. Refusal of medical treatments would be left up to the individual. There are no restrictions relative to "holy" days. |
| Episcopal | Infant baptism is practiced. In emergency situations, request for infant baptism should be given high priority and could be performed by any baptized person, clergy or lay. Often in situations of stillbirths or aborted fetuses, special prayers of commendation may be offered. | Pastoral care of the sick may include prayers, laying on of hands, anointing, and/ or Holy Communion. At the time of death, various litanies and special prayers may be offered. | Both are permitted. | Respect for the dignity of the whole person is important. These needs include physical, emotional, and spiritual. |

| | | | |
|---|---|---|---|
| Society of Friends (Quakers) | Do not practice infant baptism. | Each person has a divine nature but an encounter and relationship with Jesus Christ is essential. | No formal statement, but generally both are permitted. | No special rites or restrictions. Leaders and elders from the church may visit and offer support and encouragement. Quakers believe in plain speech. |
| Islam (Muslim/Moslem) | At birth, the first words said to the infant in his/her right ear are "Allah-o-Akbar" (Allah is great), and the remainder of the Call for Prayer is recited. An Aqeeqa (party) to celebrate the birth of the child is arranged by the parents. Circumcision of the male child is practiced. | In Islam, life is meant to be a test for the preparation for everlasting life in the hereafter. Therefore, according to Islam, death is simply a transition. Islam teaches that God has prescribed the time of death for everyone and only He knows when, where, or how a person is going to die. Islam encourages making the best use of all of God's gifts, including the precious gift of life in this world. At the time of death, there are specific rituals (bathing, wrapping the body in cloth, etc.) that must be done. Before moving and handling the body, it is preferable to contact someone from the person's mosque or Islamic Society to perform these rituals. | Permitted. However, there are some stipulations depending on the type of transplant/donation and its effect on the donor and recipient. It is advisable to contact the individual's mosque or the local Islamic Society for further consultation. | Humans are encouraged in the Qu'ran (Koran) to seek treatment. It is taught that only Allah cures. However, Muslims are taught not to refuse treatment in the belief that Allah will take care of them because even though He cures, He also chooses at times to work through the efforts of humans. |
| International Society for Krishna Consciousness (A Hindu movement in North America based on devotion to Lord Krishna) | Infant baptism is not performed. | The body should not be touched. The family may desire that a local temple be contacted so that representatives may visit and chant over the patient. It is believed that in chanting the names of God, one may gain insight and God consciousness. | There is no formal statement prohibiting this act. It is an individual decision. | Illness or injury is believed to represent sins committed in this or a previous life. They accept modern medical treatment. The body is seen as a temporary vehicle used to transport them through this life. The body belongs to God, and members are charged to care for it in the best way possible. |

(continued)

**Table 57–2**
**Religious Influences** *(continued)*

| Religious Sect | Birth | Death | Organ Donation/Transplantation | Beliefs regarding Medical Care |
|---|---|---|---|---|
| Jehovah's Witnesses | Infant baptism is not practiced. | There are no official rites that are performed before or after death, however, the faith community is often involved and supportive of the patient and family. | There is no official statement related to this issue. Organ donation isn't encouraged, but it is believed to be an individual decision. According to the legal corporation for the denomination, Watchtower, all donated organs and tissue must be drained of blood before transplantation. | Adherents are absolutely opposed to transfusions of whole blood, packed red blood cells, platelets, and fresh or frozen plasma. This includes banking of ones' own blood. Many accept use of albumin, globulin, factor replacement (hemophilia), vaccines, hemodilution, and cell salvage. There is no opposition to nonblood plasma expanders. |
| Judaism (Orthodox and Conservative) | Circumcision of male infants is performed on the 8th day if the infant is healthy. The mohel (ritual circumciser familiar with Jewish law and aseptic technique) performs the ritual. | It is important that the health care professional facilitate the family's need to comfort and be with the patient at the time of death. | Permitted and is considered a mitzvah (good deed). | Only emergency surgical procedures should be performed on the Sabbath, which extends from sundown Friday to sundown Saturday. Elective surgery should be scheduled for days other than the Sabbath. Pregnant women and the seriously ill are exempt from fasting. Serious illness may be grounds for violating dietary laws but only if it is medically necessary. |
| Lutheran | Infant baptism is practiced. If the infant's prognosis is poor, the family may request immediate baptism. | Family may desire visitation from clergy. Prayers for the dying, commendation of the dying, and prayers for the bereaved may be offered. | There is no formal statement regarding this issue. It is considered a matter of personal conscience. | Illness isn't seen as an act of God, rather, it is seen as a condition of mankind's fallen state. Prayers for the sick may be desired. |
| Methodist | Infant baptism is practiced but is usually done within the community of the church after counseling and guidance from clergy. However, in emergency situations, a request for baptism would not be seen as inappropriate. | In the case of perinatal death, there are prayers within the United Methodist Book of worship that could be said by anyone. Prayer, scripture, and singing are often seen as appropriate and desirable. | Organ donation/transplantation is supported and encouraged. It is considered a part of good stewardship. | In the Methodist tradition, it is believed that every person has the right to death with dignity and has the right to be involved in all medical decisions. Refusal of aggressive treatment is seen as an appropriate option. |

| | | | | |
|---|---|---|---|---|
| Pentecostal<br>Assembly of God, Church of God, Four Square, and many other faith groups are included under this general heading. Pentecostal is not a denomination, but a theological distinctive (pneumatology) | No rituals such as baptism are necessary. Many Pentecostals have a ceremony of "dedication," but it is done in the context of the community of faith/believers (church). Children belong to heaven and only become sinners after the age of accountability, which is not clearly defined. | The only way to transcend this life; is the door to heaven (or hell). Questions about "salvation of the soul" are very common and important. Resurrection is the hope of those who "were saved." Prayer is appropriate, so is singing and scripture reading. | Many Pentecostal denominations have no statement concerning this subject, but it is generally seen as positive and well received. Education concerning wholeness of the person and nonliteral aspects like "heart," "mind," etc., have to be explained. For example, a Pentecostal may have a problem with donating a heart to a "non-believer." | Pentecostals sometimes labeled as "in denial" due to their theology of healing. Their faith in God for literal healing is generally expressed as intentional unbelief in the prognostic statements. Many Pentecostals do not see sickness as the will of God, thus one must "stand firm" in faith and accept the unseen reality, which many times may mean healing. As difficult as this position may seem, it must be noted that, when death occurs, Pentecostals may leap from miracle expectations to joyful hope and theology of heaven and resurrection without facing issues of anger or frustration due to unfulfilled expectations. Prayer, scriptures, singing, and anointing of the sick (not a sacrament) are appropriate/expected pastoral interventions. |
| Presbyterian | Baptism is a sacrament of the church but is not considered necessary for salvation. However, it is seen as an event to take place, when possible, in the context of a worshipping community. | Family may desire visitation from clergy. Prayers for the dying, commendation of the dying, and prayers for the bereaved may be offered. | There is no formal statement regarding this issue. | Communion is a sacrament of the Church. It is generally celebrated with a patient in the presence of an ordained minister and elder. Presbyterians are free to make their own choices regarding the use of mechanical life-support measures. |
| Roman Catholic | Infant baptism is practiced. In medical facilities, baptism is usually performed by a priest or deacon, as ordinary members of the sacrament. However, under extraordinary circumstances, baptism may be administered by a layperson, provided that the intention is to do as the church does, using the formula, "I baptise you in the name of the Father, the Son, and the Holy Spirit." | Sacrament of the sick is the sacrament of healing and forgiveness. It is to be administered by a priest as early in the illness as possible. It is not a last rite to be administered at the point of death. The Roman Catholic Church makes provisions for prayers of commendation of the dying, which may be said by any priest, deacon sacramental minister, or layperson. | Catholics may donate or receive organ transplants. | The Sacrament of Holy Communion sustains Catholics in sickness as in health. When the patient's condition deteriorates, the sacrament is given as viaticum ("food for the journey"). Like Holy Communion, viaticum may be administered by a priest, deacon, or a sacramental minister. The church makes provisions for prayers for commendation of the dying that may be said by any of those listed above or by a layperson. |

*Source:* Adapted from Texas Children's Cancer Center–Texas Children's Hospital (2000), reference 10.

**Table 57–3**
**The Rights of the Newborn and Infant**

- I have the right to be listened to as a person with rights and am not the property of my parents, medical doctors, nurse practitioners, and society.
- I have the right to cry.
- I have the right to hope.
- I have the right of not being alone.
- I have the right to create fantasies.
- I have the right to interact with my siblings.
- I have the right to have my pain controlled.
- I have the right to have my needs taken care of.
- I have the right to be at home and not in the hospital if my parents choose to have me there.
- I have the right to receive help for my brothers and sisters in dealing with my illness.
- I have the right to comfort care.

*Source:* Adapted from Palliative Care Center and Hospice of the North Shore (1999).

---

**Table 57–4**
**Differences between Hospice Care for Newborns/Infants and Adults**

**Patient issues**
- Patient is not legally competent.
- Patient is in developmental process that affects understanding of life and death, sickness and health, God, etc.
- Patient has not achieved a "full and complete life."
- Patient lacks verbal skills to describe needs, feelings, etc.
- Patient is often in a highly technical medical environment.

**Family issues**
- Family needs to protect the child from information about his/her health.
- Family needs to do everything possible to save the child.
- Family may have difficulty dealing with siblings.
- Family feels stress on finances.
- Family fears that care at home is not as good as care at the hospital.
- Grandparents feel helpless in dealing with their children and grandchildren.
- Family needs relief from burden of care.

**Caregiver issues**
- Caregivers need to protect children, parents, and siblings.
- Caregivers feel a sense of failure in not saving the child.
- Caregivers feel a sense of "ownership" of children, even at the expense of parents.
- Caregivers have out-of-date ideas about pain in children, especially infants.
- Caregivers lack knowledge about children's disease processes.
- Influence of "unfinished business" on style of care.

**Institutional/agency issues**
- There is less reimbursement or none for children's hospice/home care.
- High staff-intensity caring is required for children at home.
- Ongoing staff support is necessary.
- Children's services have immediate appeal to public.
- Special competencies are needed in pediatric care.
- Assess how admission criteria may screen out children.
- Address unusual bereavement needs of family members.

*Source:* Adapted from Kuebler and Berry (2002), reference 25 (used with permission); and Children's Hospice International, reference 26 (prepared by Paul R. Brenner).

*in Ethical Decisions Treatment of Critically Ill Newborns*[20] and Rogers and colleagues[21] developed an educational program to address issues of moral distress in NICU nurses. The emphasis in this latter publication was to help nurses address the family needs during the dying process. It acknowledges the toll palliative care takes on the health professional.

Sometimes we underestimate what toll palliative and EOL care can take on us as caregivers. We often feel torn between spending quality time with a dying child and family and caring for our other patients. We are only human. We need to give ourselves permission to set priorities and to make the most of the time we do have with child and family. Sometimes a word, a gentle touch, a look across the room while providing care for another baby is enough for a parent to know we are there for them. Although it is not ideal to be multitasking while caring for a dying child, it is the reality of today's work environment. We also have to realize that sometimes we need to ask for help, to give someone else the opportunity to provide support when we cannot. Try to remember that for some parents this the first time they have lost a family member, let alone a child. They don't know what to expect or if that "ad" in the newspaper with funeral arrangements costs anything. We have to anticipate these questions, but we also have to realize that some days we deal better with these situations than others. For example, if you have just had a baby yourself, it may be very difficult to care for a newborn who is dying. That is okay. But make sure that someone knows this and, if possible, get reassigned. Communication is the key for others to know what you need—whether it is a new assignment, to have more time with the child and family, or to attend the funeral. You need to make it clear what you need. We practice asking families "Tell me what you need" but often neglect ourselves.

## New Trends

In the last 5 years the End-of-Life Nursing Education Consortium (ELNEC) has developed a neonatal/pediatric version. To date, 650 pediatric/neonatal nurses have received this education in the United States and abroad http://www.aacn.nche.edu/elnec. More institutions are interested in neonatal-specific content to start their own palliative care teams. Despite support from the American Academy of Pediatrics (AAP) and the World Health Organization (WHO) for the provision of palliative care, there are still many barriers. Kain[22] identified barriers to neonatal palliative care as formal educational needs on the part of staff, a feeling of failure (especially by the physicians), difficulty in communicating bad news to the parents, and ethical conflicts among the team members. These issues have not appreciably changed over the last decade. Yet, there is more evidence through the interest in ELNEC that nurses around the world wish to provide good palliative care as a standard part of neonatal care. For example, these authors presented an overview of ELNEC and precepts of palliative care to Children's Hospital #1 in

St. Petersburg, Russia. What is needed is more education and information as well as more evidence-based guidelines to support nursing and medical care interventions.

## Summary

Neonates who would benefit from excellent palliative care could die minutes, months, or years after birth with a life-threatening anomaly or illness. Because the prognosis is so difficult to predict, the professional is called upon to focus on providing care that is often changing and challenges existing health-care system structures. The period of life may be so unpredictable that the focus needs to be on excellent pain and symptom management, while promoting development of the child and family within their community. Families and professionals have the difficult task of helping the child live as fully as possible with complete dignity and comfort while preparing for and accepting that the child may not live a long time. This requires a committed interdisciplinary team with community linkages as appropriate.

Regardless of the length of life or the place where that life is lived, excellent palliative care includes optimum symptom relief for the neonate, honoring the parents' wishes, providing ongoing support to parents and family, planning for the death, and honoring the life by creating memories of the life. Even though the neonate cannot be cured, let it never be said that "there is nothing we can do." We always can.

## Appendix 57–1

### Neonatal End-of-Life Palliative Care Protocol*

*This protocol was published in Kenner C, Lott JW. Neonatal Nursing Handbook. St. Louis: Mosby, 2003:506–525. Adapted from Reference 10.

The purpose of this protocol of care is to educate professionals and enhance their preparation and support for a peaceful, pain-free, and family-centered death for dying newborns.

### Planning for a Palliative Care Environment

To begin a palliative care program, one must realize that some institutions find it difficult to confront the issue of a dying child. So to begin to create a palliative care environment, there must be staff education and buy-in. This education must address cultural issues that affect caregiving. Ethical issues must be addressed either by the group creating the environment or by consultants who specialize in ethics.

For the family, staff must treat the family as care partners and not visitors. They must recognize that someone needs to be available 24/7 to address issues such as advance directives and symptom and pain management both in the hospital and at home if discharge is possible. There must be a mechanism to prepare the community for the child's entrance home or to hospice. This preparation includes what is appropriate to say to friends, relatives, and visitors.

### Prenatal Discussion of Palliative Care

It is essential that fetal development and viability be discussed with all families as a part of prenatal care packages and classes and to all families receiving assisted reproductive therapies. As the course of prenatal care progresses, pregnant women should be made aware that newborns in the very early gestational periods of 22 to 24 weeks and birth weights of less than 500 grams may not be responsive to resuscitation or applied neonatal intensive care.

### Physician Considerations

The families need honest, straightforward language. They need to know their options and it is essential that they understand what to expect. Usually the physician delivers this information, but the nurse is generally the one that can help the parents sort through feelings and grasp what they were just told. If this incident is sudden, such as an unexpected premature or complicated birth, then the family's ability to comprehend and retain what is being said is limited. Reinforcement at a later time is advisable.

### Family Considerations

Peer support from families that have experienced a similar infant illness or death may help the family cope. If the family finds out that the pregnancy is not viable, then it is up the health-care team to help support their needs and to garner resources such as other family members, spiritual counselors, and friends. Helping the family to experience the normal parenting tasks such as naming the baby is very appropriate and helpful. This act helps the family gain some control and to be a parent first and build memories of that experience.

### Transport Issues

It is best that mothers not be separated from their newborn infants. Transport is considered both traumatic and expensive, and if the newborn's condition is incompatible with prolonged life, then arrangements to stay in the local hospital may generally be preferred. It is best to avoid transferring dying newborns to Level III NICUs if nothing more can be done there than at the local hospital. The local area is recognized as that location at which parents have their support system, rapport with their established health-care providers, a spiritual/religious community, and funeral availability.

The key to whatever decision is made, referral or not, requires good, clear communication with the family and between the two institutions. The family should not feel they are being sent away or given the wrong message by the nature of the transfer, or even return from a tertiary center once a referral is made if there is nothing to be done. The family needs a consistent message if trust is to be developed.

### Which Newborns Should Receive Palliative Care?

Although many aspects of palliative care should be integrated into the care of all newborns, there are infants born for whom parents and the health-care professionals believe that palliative care is the most appropriate form of care. The following list includes categories of newborns that have experienced the transition from life-extending technological support to palliative care. The individual context of applying palliative care will require that each case, in each family, within each health-care center, be explored individually. These categories of newborns are provided for educational purposes and may engender discussion at the local institutional level.

- Newborns at the threshold of viability.
- Newborns with complex or multiple congenital anomalies incompatible with prolonged life, where neonatal intensive care will not affect long-term outcome.
- Newborns not responding to intensive care intervention, who are deteriorating despite all appropriate efforts, or in combination with a life-threatening acute event.

### Introducing the Palliative Care Model to Parents

Speaking to parents about palliative care is difficult. There is heartache from the staff and heartfelt sympathy for the parents. The following points are offered to help physicians and nurse practitioners facilitate the process:

- Let the family know they will not be abandoned.
- Assist the family in obtaining all of the medical information that they want. Tell them that the entire medical team wishes the situation were different. Let them know you will support them every step of the way and that their infant is a valued and loved member of their family.
- Hold conversations in a quiet, private, and physically comfortable space.
- Give them your beeper number or telephone number to call you after they have digested the information and have more questions. Offer the ability to have a second opinion and/or an ethics consultation.
- Provide parents time to consult the local regional center that works with children with special needs or their area pediatrician, who can provide information on projected abilities and disabilities.
- Offer to introduce them to parents who have been in a similar situation.

- When possible, use lay-person language to clarify medical terms, and allow a great deal of time for parents to process the information.
- The terms "withdrawal of treatment," such as referring to the stopping of life support, or "withdrawal of care," referring to the stopping of feedings or other supportive interventions, should be avoided. The exact treatment or care that is to be terminated should be specifically explained so that the intention is clear.
- Use terms such as "change in care" or "change in treatment."
- Communicate and collaborate with parents at all times. Efforts should be made to clarify mutually derived goals of care for the infant. Give as many choices as possible about how palliative care should be implemented for their infant. Inform the parents of improved access to the infant for holding, cuddling, kangaroo care, and breastfeeding. Use of developmental care approaches such as these promotes the building of a relationship between the infant and parents.
- If the transition in care involves the removal of ventilatory support, explain that the use of ventilators is for the improvement of heart/lung conditions until cure, when cure is a likely outcome.
- Tell the parents that you cannot change the situation but you can support the infant's short life with comfort and dignity. Explain that discontinuing interventions that cause suffering is a brave and loving action to take for their infant.
- Validate the loss of the dreamed-for healthy infant, but point out the good/memorable features he/she has. Help parents look past any deformities and work to alleviate any blame they may express.
- Encourage parents to be a family as much as possible. Refer to the newborn by name. Assist them to plan what they would like to do while the infant is still alive.
- Encourage them to ask support persons to join them on the unit. Facilitate sibling visitation. Support siblings with child-life specialists on staff.
- In daily conversation, avoid terms that express improvement such as "good," "stable," "better" in reference to the dying patient so as not to confuse parents.
- Prepare the family for what may happen as the infant dies.
- Introduce families to the chaplain and social worker early in the process.

## Optimal Environment for Neonatal Death

When the decision is made that a newborn infant may be close to death, there are several components to optimizing the care. These include:

- Compassionate, nonjudgmental, consistent staff for each infant, including physicians knowledgeable in palliative care. If consistent staff is not an option in a particular unit, then agreement on the plan of care is essential, with proposed revisions to care discussed with the whole team.
- Nurses and other health-care staff educated in providing a meaningful experience for the family while caring for the family's psychosocial needs, including a period of time after the death.
- Parents who are educated in what to expect and who are encouraged to participate in, or even orchestrate, the dying process and environment of their infant in a manner they find meaningful.
- Flexibility of the facility and staff in responding to parental wishes, such as participation of siblings and other family members, and including wishes of parents and families who do not wish to be present.
- Institutional policies that allow staff flexibility to respond to parental wishes.
- Providing time to create memories, such as allowing parents to dress, diaper, and bathe their infant, feed him/her (if it is possible), take photos, and hold the infant in their arms. If they wish to take the infant outdoors to a peaceful and natural setting, that should be encouraged.
- Siblings should be made comfortable; they may wish to write letters or draw for the infant. Snacks should be available.
- Allowing the family to stay with the infant as long as they need to, including after death occurs.
- The process for treating the dying infant[12,17,19] is well-described in the literature and by the various bereavement programs.
- Parents should be assisted in making plans for a memorial service, burial, and so forth. Some parents might wish to carry or accompany the infant's body to the morgue, or take it to the funeral home themselves. Issues such as autopsy, cremation, burial, and who may transport the body should be discussed, especially if the parents are far from home and wish to take the body back to their home area for burial. In some states, hospitals may release a body to parents after notifying the county department of vital statistics. The family must sign a form for removal of the body. The quality assurance department should be notified. Further discussion of autopsy and organ/tissue donation issues is included.

Specific skills are needed by the staff to provide palliative care. These include:

- A physician leader of the team who is familiar with family-centered care and the tenets of palliative/hospice care
- A trained nursing staff, clinical social workers, and clergy supportive of this manner of care

- Agreement to cease all invasive care, including taking frequent vital signs, monitoring, medical machinery, and artificial feeding
- Removal of all medications other than those to provide comfort or to prevent or treat a troubling symptom, with continued IV access for pain medication and anxiolytics
- Maintenance of skin care, participation in discussion on the appropriateness of feeding, and prevention of air hunger
- Use of simple blow-by oxygen or suctioning if needed for comfort
- Continuous observation and gentle assessment by nursing staff as individualized by parent wishes
- Physicians' notes describing the need for ongoing physician observation and nursing staff interventions to provide the needed level of care
- Appropriate palliative care orders on the chart.

### Location for Provision of Palliative Care

Location is not as important as the "mindset" of persons involved in EOL care. The attitude of staff, their desire to care for dying newborns and their families, their training in observation, support, and symptom management, and their knowledge of how to apply a bereavement protocol are more important than the physical location of the patient. Many agree that an active NICU may not be the optimal place for a dying newborn. Whether the infant is moved to a room off of the unit (e.g., a family room), onto a general pediatrics ward, or kept on the postpartum floor, the best available physical space with privacy and comfort should be chosen.

The families need help to make the decision of how and where the infant is to be given care. If families take the infant home, coordination with the EMS personnel may be necessary to prevent undesired intervention. Parents need to be instructed not to call 911 because in some places emergency medical technicians (EMTs) are obligated to provide cardiopulmonary resuscitation (CPR). A letter describing the diagnosis, existence of in-hospital do-not-resuscitate (DNR) order, and hospice care plan for home with the full expectation that the patient will die should be provided to the parents, their primary physician, home-health agency/hospice, and perhaps the county EMS coordinator. Generally, hospice nurses are allowed to confirm a patient's death.

### Ventilator Removal, Pain and Symptom Management

At times, cessation of certain technological supports accompanies the provision of palliative care. The following information addresses (1) how to prepare the family, staff, and facility for discontinuation of ventilator support, and (2) the process of removing the ventilator in a manner that minimizes discomfort for the infant and the family. The latter includes who will be present at the time of extubation. A plan must be worked out with the family about what medications and support will be given to alleviate pain and suffering and

what they can expect the dying process to be like for their baby. Consideration of developmentally supportive care that is attuned to ambient light and noise as well as comfort measures are important. These should incorporate cultural considerations.

Mementos can be obtained by nurses, such as a lock of hair, hand or footprints in plaster, and photos and/or videotapes of the family together if this is culturally appropriate. If the infant has serious anomalies, photos of hands, ears, lips, feet can be provided. Ear prints and lip prints are possible. Some parents have indicated that mementos of a newborn who died are not acceptable in their culture.

### When Death Does Not Occur After Cessation of Aggressive Support

A private room somewhere in the hospital is recommended where nurses trained in palliative care are available. If the expected time for expiration passes and death does not take place, the infant could be discharged to home for ongoing palliative care services. The parents, NICU staff, and the hospice staff should meet to make plans for home care, including the investigation of what services are offered and what insurance will cover. Continued palliative care/hospice services with home nursing care is essential, including the possibility of ventilator removal at home.

If the infant is to go home, a procedure for dispensing outpatient medications should be in place. All needed drugs and directions for use should be sent along with the infant so that the parents do not have to go to a pharmacy to fill prescriptions. Identifying and communicating with a community health-care provider who will continue with the infant's home-care needs is essential.

Some families and health-care providers feel dying newborns should be fed, and if unable to suck, should be tube fed. Others feel that artificial feeding is inappropriate. However, withholding of feedings is an ethical dilemma for many health professionals and families and needs careful consideration.[23] Recent research indicates that feeding can be burdensome and that an overload of fluids can impede respirations.[24] In all cases, infants should receive care to keep their mouth and lips moist. Drops of sucrose water have been found to be a comfort agent if the infant can swallow, and they may be absorbed through the buccal membrane.

Parents who feel they cannot take the infant home should be assisted to find hospice care placement.

### Discussion of Organ and Tissue Procurement and Autopsy

At some point in the course of care, organ and tissue donation and autopsy will need to be discussed. Prior to discussion with families, the regional organ donation center should be contacted to see if a particular infant qualifies as a potential donor. In some areas, only corneas or heart valves are valuable in an infant under 10 pounds, but in different locations, other organs (e.g., heart) or tissues may be appropriate. It is important to know if a newborn has no potential donor use and to communicate this respectfully. Parents often desire the ability to give this gift and may be doubly hurt if they are hoping for the opportunity to help others and are turned down.

The person who discusses organ/tissue procurement must be specially trained. While the physician usually initiates this, a nurse, chaplain, or representative from donor services may conduct the conversation with tact and compassion. The provider should be aware of cultural, traditional, or religious values that would preclude organ donation for a specific family, as many cultures and religions would consider this desecration of the dead infant.

### Suggestions Concerning Autopsy

Requests for autopsies are not required in all states but may be considered appropriate in many instances of infant death. If the medical examiner or coroner is involved in the case, laws may require autopsy. Some providers feel that asking for an autopsy is important to potentially provide parents with some answers regarding their infant's illness and death. The placenta may also be used for testing to provide information. In the discussion, parents may wish to know all or some of the following:

- Autopsy does not cause any pain or suffering to the infant; it is done only after death.
- The body is handled with the ultimate respect.
- Some insurance companies pay for a physician-ordered autopsy.
- Final results are returned in approximately 6 to 8 weeks, at which time the primary physician can meet with the parents, conduct a telephone conference, or communicate by letter to discuss the results.

### Family Care: Cultural, Spiritual, and Practical Family Needs

The hospital social worker is an essential component of supportive palliative care. Families may immediately need financial assistance, access to transportation, and a place to stay.

*Practical Considerations.* Parents of multiples in which some lived and one died will need special attention to validate their bereavement as well as to support their love for their living child(ren).

Time should be permitted for the parents to contact the needed authority in their culture and to plan any necessary ceremony, some of which may require special permission; for example use of incense.

*Cultural Sensitivity.* These support needs should be anticipated and provided as much as possible.

- When using a translator, simple words and phrases should be used so that the translator can convey the message exactly as it is given. It is most appropriate to use hospital-trained and certified translators to ensure accuracy.
- Whenever possible, written materials should be given in the family's primary language, in an easy-to-read format, culturally and linguistically appropriate for the family.
- Culturally sensitive grief counseling and contact with a support group of other parents who have been through this is helpful.

### Family Follow-Up Care

Families who have experienced a neonatal death will likely leave the facility in a shocked state. Families can be best be served by:

- Establishing contact with a social worker, chaplain, or grief counselor prior to discharge.
- Receiving an information packet as described and a date for a follow-up discussion with the attending physician (which may be in conjunction with autopsy results).
- Notifying the family's obstetrician of the death no matter how long after delivery it occurred.
- A home visit by one of the staff or a public health nurse within a few days.
- Phone calls weekly, then monthly, then at 6-month intervals if parents agree. Also providing contact on significant days such Mother's Day, the infant's due date, or anniversary of death.
- Invite family to a group memorial service held by the hospital for those who have lost pregnancies or infants in the past year.
- Keep in mind that subsequent pregnancy may be difficult and offer support at that time; include genetic counseling if indicated.
- Keep snapshots and mementos on the unit if parents do not wish to take them at the time, as some parents may reconsider later.

### Ongoing Staff Support

The work of providing EOL care for newborns and their families is very intense. Staff needing support must not be limited to the nursing staff, and must include physicians and all health care and ancillary personnel who have interacted with the infant or family. Suggested support includes:

- Facilitated meetings of the multidisciplinary team during the process are needed, especially if some of the team members are reluctant to change to this mode of care.
- Debriefings after every infant's death and after any critical incident will be helpful for the staff.
- Meetings or counseling sessions should be part of regular work hours and not held on voluntary or unpaid time.
- Moral support for the nurses and physicians directly caring for the dying newborn is required from peers as well as the unit director, other neonatologists, chaplain, and nursing house supervisor.

- Nursing staff scheduling should be flexible and allow for overtime to continue with the family or to orient another nurse to take over.
- If they wish, the primary nurse and physician should be called if not present at the actual time of the infant's dying. With permission by the parents, they should be allowed to attend the funeral if desired and to take time off afterwards if needed.

☙❧

## Appendix Acknowledgments

Catlin and Carter wish to include the following acknowledgments for assistance in the development of this neonatal end-of-life palliative care protocol: We thank our reviewers Alex G. M. Campbell, MD, David Clark MD, Joel Frader, MD, John Lantos, MD and Bill Silverman, MD, and our Delphi methodology consultant, Dr. Carol Lindemann. The project was funded by the American Nurses Foundation Julia Hardy RN Scholar Award, with travel support from the Lambda Gamma Chapter of Sigma Theta Tau. We appreciate support from our institutions, Napa Valley College and Vanderbilt University College of Medicine, and from the IRB at Queen of the Valley Medical Center in Napa, California.

We sincerely thank our 101 participants for their time, wisdom, and commitment. Readers may contact us for participant names as space did not permit listing: acatlin@napanet.net; bcarter@ghsystem.com.

REFERENCES

1. Centers for Disease Control and Prevention (CDC). Fast Stats A-Z. Available at: http://www.cdc.gov/nchs/fastats/infmort. htm (accessed February 19, 2005).
2. Centers for Disease Control and Prevention (CDC). US Infant Mortality Rate Now Worse than 28 Other Countries. Available at: http://www.wsws.org/articles/2008/oct2008/mort-o18. shtml (accessed November 28, 2008).
3. Rip MR, Dosh, SA. The Neighborhood and Neonatal Intensive Care: A Population-Based Analysis of the Demand for Neonatal Intensive Care in Detroit, Michigan (1984–1988). Available at: http://www.uic.edu/sph/cade/mchepi/meetings/may2001/ nicu.ppt (accessed November 8, 2003).
4. Cassel CK, Foley KM. Principles of Care of Patients at the End of Life: An Emerging Consensus among the Specialties of Medicine. New York: Milbank Memorial Fund, 1999. Available at: http://www.milbank .org/reports/endoflife (accessed February 23, 2005).
5. Americans for Better Care of the Dying. Making Promises. Washington, DC: Americans for Better Care of the Dying, 2001. Available at: http://www.abcd-caring.org/tools/actionguides. pdf (accessed March 24, 2005).
6. Last Acts Partnership. Precepts of Palliative Care for Children, Adolescents and Their Families. National Association of Pediatric Nurse Practitioners, NAPNAP,

October 2003. Available at: http://www.napnap.org/index. cfm?page=54&sec=465 (accessed November 28, 2008).
7. Institute of Medicine. (IOM). To err is human: Building a safer health system., 1999. Available at: http://www.iom.edu/ CMS/8089/5575.aspx (accessed November 28, 2008).
8. Institute of Medicine. (IOM). Crossing the quality chasm: The IOM health care quality initiative, 2001. Available at: www. iom.edu/CMS/8089.aspx (accessed November 28, 2008).
9. Hockenberry MJ, Wilson D. Wong's Nursing Care of Infants and Children (8th ed). St. Louis, MO: Mosby, 2006.
10. Texas Children's Cancer Center–Texas Children's Hospital. End-of-Life Care for Children. Houston, TX: Texas Cancer Council, 2000.
11. Lundqvist A, Nilstun T, Dykes AK. Neonatal end-of-life care in Sweden. Nurs Crit Care 2003;8:197–202.
12. Oosterwal G. Caring for People from Different Cultures: Communicating across Cultural Boundaries. Portland, OR: Providence Health System, 2003.
13. Rebagliato M, Cuttini M, Broggin L, et al. Neonatal end-of-life decision making: Physcians' attitudes and relationship with self-reported practices in 10 European countries. JAMA 2000;284(19):2451–2459.
14. Shipman C, Gysels M, White P, et al. Improving generalist end of life care: National consultation with practitioners, commissioners, academics, and service user groups. BMJ 2008;337:a1720. Available at: http://www.bmj.com (accessed November 28, 2008).
15. Feudtner C, Feinstein JA, Stachell M, Zhao H, Kang TL. Shifting place of death among children with complex chronic conditions in the United States, 1989–2003. JAMA 2007;297(24):2725–2732.
16. Catlin A. Extremely long hospitalizations of newborns in the United States: Data, descriptions, dilemmas. J Perinatol 2006;26:742–748.
17. Catlin A, Carter B. Creation of a neonatal end-of-life palliative care protocol. J Perinatol 2002;22:184–195.
18. Anand KJS. Pharmacological approaches to the management of pain in the neonatal intensive care unit. J Perinatol 2007;27:S4–S11.
19. American Hospital Association (AHA). A Patient's Bill of Rights. Available at: http://www.injuredworker.org/Library/ Patient_Bill_of_Rights.htm (accessed March 28, 2005).
20. National Association of Neonatal Nurses (NANN). NANN Position Statement 3015: NICU Nurse Involvement in Ethical Decisions (Treatment of Crticially Ill Newborns). Adv Neonatal Care 2007;7(5):267–268.
21. Rogers S, Babgi A, Gomez C. Educational interventions in end-of-life care: Part I: An educational intervention responding to the moral distress of NICU nurses provided by an ethics consultation team. Adv Neonatal Care 2008;8(1):56–65.
22. Kain VJ. Palliative care delivery in the NICU: What barriers do neonatal nurses face? Neonatal Netw 2006;25(6):387–392.
23. McHaffie HE, Fowlie PW. Withdrawing and withholding treatment: Comments on new guidelines. Arch Dis Child 1998;79:1–2.
24. Craig F, Goldman A. Home management of the dying NICU patient. Semin Neonatol 2003;8:177–183.
25. Kuebler KK, Berry PH. End-of-life care. In: Kuebler KK, Berry PH, Heidrich DE, eds. End-of-Life Care: Clinical Practice Guidelines. Philadelphia: W.B. Saunders; 2002:25.
26. Children's Hospice International. Available at: http://www. chionline.org (accessed February 23, 2005).

# 58 ❧ Betty Davies, Rana Limbo, and Juhye Jin

# Grief and Bereavement in Pediatric Palliative Care

*Since Kristen died, we have tried to carry on as well as we can. Some days are better than others...we miss her so much—she's still with us in our minds when we sit at the table and see her empty high chair, or in the car when we think about where her car seat used to be. At first, I thought it was just me—that I think about those things more than my wife or the other kids— but one day, I said something about it, and I could tell that everyone's ears perked up...they knew what I was talking about. We all feel her absence, just in different ways. It's something that will always be with us—even with the younger kids...you don't ever really get over something like this.—Father, age 42 years, whose 18-month-old daughter died a year ago*

♦ **Key Points**
♦ *Bereavement care for all family members is an integral component of pediatric palliative care.*
♦ *Grieving after a death is a normal process; however, some grief reactions become complicated, and nurses must assess for factors that put family members at risk for such reactions.*
♦ *Grief assessment begins at the time of diagnosis of a child's life-limiting condition, applies to all family members, and continues into the bereavement period following the child's death.*
♦ *Nurses have a responsibility to create supportive environments in which family members feel free to express their grief.*
♦ *Caring for dying children requires nurses to attend to their own personal and professional responses to death, dying, and bereavement as a basis for providing optimal care to families.*

Effective and compassionate care for children with life-threatening conditions and their families is an integral and important part of care from diagnosis through death and bereavement.[1] This guiding principle, one of seven put forth by the Institute of Medicine report on the status of palliative and end-of-life care for children and their families, emphasizes that care continues for the family following the child's death. Though medical science has contributed significantly to the treatment of children with life-limiting illnesses or conditions, children still die from cancer, cardiac disease, respiratory conditions, genetic conditions, and more. Moreover, thousands of neonates die each year and thousands more children of all ages, particularly toddlers and adolescents, die as a result of trauma. Approximately 55,000 children die annually in the United States.[1] Regardless of the cause, the death of a child is a tragedy, an incomparable life event that has an impact on all family members, friends of the family, and the community in which the family lives. A child's death also affects the physicians, nurses, social workers, and other health-care personnel who provide care for the dying child. The purpose of this chapter is to define common words associated with grief; to describe factors that affect the grief of family members, the effects of grief upon them, and the nurse's role in helping grieving individuals and their families; and to discuss the needs of nurses who work in pediatric palliative care.

❧

## Grief as a Process

Death is a part of each individual life, something we all must face though we resist even the thought of our own mortality. The hoped-for pattern is that we experience deaths of others that are easier in earlier life, for us to build the skills to aid us with the more difficult deaths in later life. The death of one's child, though, sits outside of that hoped-for pattern.

The grief associated with a child's death begins even before the actual death event, as the child's parents and other family members anticipate the death and experience the child's dying, and their grief continues long past the child's death. Many parents feel they never "recover" from the death of their child. They may resume daily activities, adjust to life without their child's presence, and find new pleasures in life, but most parents feel they remain vulnerable and feel they are not the same people they were before the child's death.[2] The death of a child, or any beloved person, is not something one "gets over;" rather, over time, one learns to integrate the loss into one's life. Indeed, grief is a process that is not always orderly and predictable, and given that grief is the individual experience of each human being, it manifests in many diverse ways.

## Grief, Bereavement, and Mourning

The term *grief* is often used to refer to the emotional response to a loss.[3] But grief is much more than emotion—it is an overwhelming and acute sense of loss and despair; it is the personalized feeling and response that an individual makes to real, perceived, or anticipated death; it encompasses feelings, physical sensations, cognitions, and behaviors. Grief encompasses every domain of human life—physical, emotional, psychological, social, and spiritual. Sadness, anger, numbness, sleep and eating disturbances, inability to concentrate, fatigue, existential angst, and tension in interpersonal interactions are among the responses to a loved one's death.

Grief occurs when a loss is deemed as personally significant to the individual. For example, hearing the news about a child's death in a bicycle accident may produce sadness, but not necessarily a grief reaction. However, grief will ensue when it is learned that the child is your nephew. To a certain degree, who or what we consider to be personally significant is culturally defined. For example, in the contemporary United States, the death of one's child is expected to result in profound grief. In fact, a classic research study suggests that grief in response to a child's death is more intense than grief following the death of a spouse or parent.[4]

The term *bereavement* refers to the state of being bereaved or deprived of something. The word derives from an Old English word, "reave," which means to plunder, spoil, or rob.[5] This meaning implies that the loss object is a valued one, together with a suggestion of violence in the way in which the loss occurred. This definition is especially apt for bereaved parents, who often report feeling as if a part of them has been torn away. As the bereaved mother of a 22-month-old who died following a brain aneurysm sighed:

> When my son died, it was as if my heart had been stolen from my breast, and my arms that held him ripped from their sockets.

*Mourning* refers to the outward, social expression of grief, often through ritual and sometimes to the psychological process of adapting to loss.[6] How one expresses a loss may be dictated by cultural norms, customs, and practices, including rituals and traditions. Some cultures may be very emotional and verbal in their expression of loss, while others may appear stoic and businesslike. Religious and cultural beliefs may also dictate how long one mourns and how one behaves during the bereavement period. In addition, outward expression of loss may be influenced by the individual's personality and life experiences.[7]

## Types of Grief

It is important for nurses' understanding of grief and bereavement and for the implementation of appropriate interventions to be aware of several types, or variations, of grief that have been described in the thanatology literature, including anticipatory grief, disenfranchised grief, and pathological grief reactions or complicated grief. How these concepts apply to pediatric palliative care is particularly important.

### Anticipatory Grief

Anticipatory grief often occurs in advance of an expected loss. Rando[8] indicates that anticipatory grief entails grieving not just for future losses, but also for losses that have already occurred and for current losses. It may be associated with the losses of expectations for a "normal" life that are associated with a particular diagnosis, with acute and chronic illness, or with death. For example, parents may fear the potential loss of health in their child when a child is being tested for unusual symptoms. All family members may grieve the expected loss of a part of the child's body, mental function, or self-image; they may grieve the loss of the child's and their own independence, choice, and dreams. Anticipatory grief occurs while the ill child is still alive, and this allows for hope. This is a subtle difference that makes anticipatory grief unique, and helps account for what parents often describe as an "emotional roller coaster," particularly for parents of children with long-term chronic illness. Their experience of witnessing the child's physical deterioration and worsening of symptoms, interspersed with remissions, "good" days, and seeming progress toward health lays fertile ground for emotional ups and downs and hope for the child's recovery. Over time, however, the focus of hope changes, and nurses can play a critical role in facilitating the expression of that hope. Initially, parents of children with cancer, for example, focus their hope on the possibility of cure. Each exacerbation chips away at the hope for the child's full recovery, and family members hope for longer remissions. Eventually, they hope their child will be able to live until he reaches a particular milestone, such as graduation, a special birthday, or the next holiday. As the child's condition worsens, parents may hope that their wish to care for their child at home will be possible, and that their child will not suffer at the end. Hope is life-sustaining; health-care providers should support family members in their hope, refraining from crushing hope with overdoses of facts. In response to a mother's proclamation that her child will overcome a serious illness, the nurse can empathize, "I certainly do hope so." The death is anticipated, but it has not occurred, and in the parents' eyes, there is a chance, no matter how small, that it might not occur:

> *My son has been to the PICU three times. At his first transfer to the PICU, my sorrow was beyond description. At that time, I thought I would never see him again. But my son has fought against his cancer every time. Whenever he came back to the ward from the PICU...I remember recently that day was 3 days before his 13th birthday...it was so amazing and I prayed thanks to God for allowing me to hope for his life again.*

For more information on hope, see Chapter 26.

Though painful, anticipatory grieving does present an opportunity for families to begin to think about their future without the child. It can help family members begin to face the existential questions that arise when a child is dying. It can help families begin to the process of reorganizing their fractured lives. Anticipatory grieving can also take its toll, especially when the child's illness endures. Rando[9] interviewed parents whose child had died from cancer, and suggests there is an optimal length of anticipatory grief of 6 to 18 months. A shorter time did not give parents enough time to prepare for the loss, and a longer period had a debilitating effect on them.

Unacknowledged grief before the death may inhibit communication and preparation for death which, in turn, may contribute to strong feelings of subsequent guilt and regret.[1] However, anticipatory grief does not mean the grieving that occurs after the child's death is somehow easier or less painful for parents and other family members. Health-care providers cannot assume that family members whose child died following a long-term illness grieve "less" than those whose child dies suddenly and unexpectedly. In fact, every child's death is unexpected. Even when parents know their child will die, the actual moment of death is often unexpected, as reflected in parents' words: "*I knew the end was near, but I really thought he would make it until his brother got home from college.*" Or, as the 7-year-old sister wept following her brother's death a few days before her birthday: "*But, he was coming to my party.*"

### Disenfranchised Grief

Disenfranchised grief acknowledges the social context of grief. It refers to the grief that persons experience when they incur a loss that is not or cannot be openly acknowledged, publicly mourned, or socially supported.[10,11] Those at risk include, for example, classmates, teammates, teachers, coaches, school bus drivers, crossing guards, or past boyfriends/girlfriends of the child or adolescent who died—those whose relationship

with the now-deceased child/adolescent is not regarded as significant. Also feeling disenfranchised are those grieving a terminated pregnancy or a neonatal death where the significance of these losses may not even be acknowledged, or if it is, comments such as "You can try again" reflect insensitive misunderstanding of the parents' grief. Families of children with serious cognitive or physical limitations, from progressive neurodegenerative illnesses, for example, may experience disenfranchised grief when others perceive the child's death as a "blessing" rather than a loss for the family. Disenfranchised grief also occurs when bereaved persons are not recognized by society as capable of grief or needing to mourn. Young children, mentally-challenged children or adults, and abusing parents whose actions have caused the child's death are often disenfranchised in this way.

### Complicated or Troubled Grief

The processes of grief and mourning are normal and healthy aspects of human living. However, all human processes can go awry, especially in particularly difficult situations, and such grief is sometimes referred to as "complicated" grieving. However, as everyone who has experienced the loss of a loved one knows, all grief is complicated. It is just that sometimes, grief is more complicated than at other times. But common terminology differentiates complicated from uncomplicated grief, with the latter referring to the typical feelings, behaviors, and reactions to loss; complicated grief refers to a response to loss that is more intense and longer in duration than usual.[12] Worden[13] has outlined four basic types of complicated grief: (1) chronic grief is characterized by grief reactions that do not subside and continue over long periods of time; (2) delayed grief is characterized by grief reactions that are suppressed or postponed, and the family member consciously or unconsciously avoids the pain of the loss; (3) exaggerated grief occurs when the family member resorts to self-destructive behaviors such as suicide; and (4) masked grief occurs when the family member is not aware that behaviors that interfere with normal functioning are a result of the loss.

Those who are mourning the loss of a child are at risk for complicated grief. Other risk factors include: preexisting difficulties in the relationship with the deceased (such as between a parent and a delinquent daughter); the circumstances of the death (such as traumatic death through suicide or homicide); chronic illness; the survivor's own history of depressive illness; multiple losses or history of troubled grief reactions to previous deaths; difficulty with the dying process; when the death is socially negated; or a lack of social support system or faith system.

### Factors Affecting the Grief Process

Family responses to grief vary widely and depend on a multitude of factors. Some of these factors may be obvious, some less apparent, but all influence how individual family members cope with the pain of a child's death. Influencing factors fall into three broad categories. Individual variables have to do with attributes of the bereaved, including the relationship between the child who died and other family members; environmental factors have to do with the social, familial, and cultural environments; and situational factors pertain to the characteristics of the death. All factors interact with one another to provide the context of grief.

### Individual Factors

Individual, or personal, characteristics that affect the grief process may include history and relationship with the child, previous exposure to death, dying, grief and loss, developmental level, and temperament and coping styles.

### History and Relationship with the Child

Each parent, sibling, or grandparent has a unique history and relationship with the deceased child. Histories among siblings are closely intertwined because siblings often develop special bonds that are unlike any other. The closer two siblings are to one another before death, the more behavior problems the surviving sibling may have following the death.[14] Similarly, grandparents may be integrally involved in children's lives, whether they live geographically far apart or down the street; in other families, grandparents and children barely know one another. Some histories among the children and other family members will have been predominantly troubled (filled with tension and conflict) and others filled with laughter and harmony.

### Previous Experience with Death

Past experiences with death and the learned response to loss also affect how each family member will grieve a child's death. Other deaths of a similar nature may have occurred in the family, such as when more than one child suffers from the same life-limiting genetic disorder. How previous losses were handled in the family will influence the current situation.

In the R family, for example, when Grandfather R was 10 years old, his older brother was killed in a car accident. No one explained to the grieving child what had happened, he was not allowed to attend the funeral, and following the death, he regretted that he had not been the one to die because he felt his brother was so much smarter than he. As a young boy, he decided unconsciously that he would hide his pain behind a wall of silence; he seldom displayed or talked about emotions. When Mr. R's grandson died from cancer at age 11 years, Mr. R was flooded with memories and sadness. His previously-learned coping through silence and withdrawal resulted in his being unprepared for how to help his distraught son and himself with the current loss.

### Developmental Level

When we think of "developmental level," we often think only of children and adolescents. Variants of four subconcepts of death are commonly included in writings about children and death: irreversibility, nonfunctionality, universality, and inevitability.[15,16] But development is a lifelong process; therefore, the developmental level of each grieving individual must be considered. For example, magical thinking (i.e., the person will become alive again) is typically associated with children. Yet Joan Didion[17] entitled her recent book about her husband's sudden death

### The Year of Magical Thinking

She recounts numerous examples of her magical belief that he would return, such as deciding not to give away all of his shoes, since he would need them when he came home. Young parents who are facing the death of their child have not typically experienced many life crises; elderly grandparents may be struggling under the burden of having faced too many. A teenage mother, struggling to be independent from her parents, faces new challenges when she must rely on them for assistance because her baby becomes ill and dies. A midlife father, anxious about his family's financial future following his son's long-term illness, agonizes deeply over the expenses of his son's funeral and feels guilty about his feelings. A grandmother who overcame breast cancer at age 65 years laments over why her 20-year-old granddaughter was the one to die from cancer.

### Personality and Coping Style

Individuals of all ages vary in temperament and personality, and styles of interacting with the world are evident in even the youngest children. Some youngsters are naturally more extroverted; they talk easily with others and eagerly seek out resources and sources of support and comfort. Others are more introverted; they keep their thoughts and feelings to themselves and may prefer the solitude of reading or quiet play. Doka[10] describes styles of grieving among adults that occur along a continuum, with "instrumental" grieving at one end and "intuitive" grieving at the other. Most people fall in the middle, but describing the extremes of the continuum clarifies the differences and may be helpful in understanding how parents and other family members manifest their grief. Intuitive grievers fit the pattern of how we think individuals "should" grieve. They express strong affective reactions, their expression mirrors their inner feelings, and their adaptation involves expression and exploration of feelings. In contrast, the grief experience for instrumental grievers is primarily cognitive or physical, expressed cognitively or behaviorally, and adaptation generally involves thinking and doing. Gender, culture, temperament, and a variety of other factors influence grieving styles. Caution is advised against assuming that mothers are more intuitive in style and fathers more instrumental. Both parents must be assessed individually to determine where on the continuum their style rests. It is important, as well, to remember that these terms represent differences, not deficiencies, in grieving styles. Most parents in pediatric palliative care are young and likely inexperienced with illness, hospitals, technologies, dying, and death. Consequently, they typically have few skills for dealing with significant loss.

### Environmental Factors

Environmental factors include the role of the deceased child in the family and various aspects of the family itself.

### Role in the Family of the Child Who Died

Ordinal position often defines children's roles in the family. When a child dies, shifts occur among the other children. For example, Jose was the eldest of three sons. When he died, his father told Marco, the middle son, that he was now the "oldest." The three boys had shared very close relationships, and now they felt their father was "forgetting" Jose by no longer regarding him as the eldest son. Children also play particular social, spiritual, and physical roles in the family; the child's absence leaves their role unfilled and resultant adjustments can be difficult for remaining family members. Jose had been the "leader;" Marco did not want to assume his brother's leadership role. Also, how the child defined the other members of the family affects their grieving. Again, Jose particularly liked to joke about his "little" brother who was growing to be taller than Jose. Marco had enjoyed the teasing and did not want to displace his admired older brother. Tension grew between father and sons.

### Family Characteristics

Even before their child dies, families have characteristic ways of being in the world, of solving problems, of managing crises, of interacting with one another, and of relating to those outside the family. When a child is seriously ill and dies, families respond in the ways that are typical for how they manage other life events. These ways of coping are more or less functional. Earlier research with families of adult patients[18] and with pediatric patients[14,19] documented eight dimensions of family functioning: communicating openly, dealing with feelings, defining roles, solving problems, using resources, incorporating changes, considering others, and confronting beliefs. These dimensions occur along a continuum of functionality so that family interactions tend to vary along the continuum rather than being positive or negative, or good or bad.[14] In families where thoughts and opinions are expressed freely without fear of recrimination, where a wide range of feelings is expressed and differences tolerated, where roles are flexible, where problem solving instead of blaming is the pattern for dealing with challenges, where families are able to ask for and receive assistance from others, and where beliefs and values are confronted and examined, the children

and all family members are better able to manage their grief and support one another. The nurse's role is to assess each family's way of functioning, and to realize that some families are more difficult to assess and work with than others. For example, some families may not wish to share information in the presence of their children, others do not wish to discuss matters with any relatives in the room, while other families include everyone in most discussions. Thus, it is important for the nurse to gather information over time, and to talk with more than one family member to appreciate the varied perspectives. When families are less functional, practitioners may want to offer potential resources one at a time, with considerable attention paid to the possible disruption that would result from each suggestion. In more functional families, a list of possible options can be presented and considered all at once. The vast majority of families values the opportunity to tell their story, and thus listening becomes a central aspect of caring for all grieving families.

### Social/Cultural Characteristics

No one grieves in isolation from others. Individual responses are shaped by distinct social and cultural circumstances, and, in turn, each grieving person plays many roles in shaping family and community responses. Friends, extended family, and community support also influence how the family unit and individual family members function and come to terms with a child's death. A friend with a sensitive presence and listening ear can be of significant support to a grieving parent or sibling. Or, when grieving parents are challenged by the responsibilities of parenthood, a kind and supportive aunt or uncle can help to maintain a normal routine and a safe and understanding environment for the surviving siblings.

Individuals and families grieve within broader cultural contexts. Some turn to culture and tradition to find support and comfort in the answers, rituals, ceremonies, behavioral prescriptions, and spiritual practices they provide. Others do not strongly identify with the beliefs and mores of their cultures of origin, even when other members of their own family may do so. Too often culture is thought of in prescriptive ways, as if to say that we expect a member of a given community to express and process grief in the manner typical of that group. Surprisingly little attention has been paid to learning about the experiences of families from diverse cultural backgrounds when their child is seriously ill and dies. This seems a remarkable oversight, since it is broadly recognized that cultural values, beliefs, and practices play a central role in shaping how families raise and care for their children not only when they are healthy, but especially when they are seriously ill.[20] It is important to find out what each individual family member believes about the nature of death, the rituals that should surround it, and the expectations about afterlife. As well, we must remember that our modern health-care systems—hospitals in particular—have their own cultural mores, which may be in conflict with the cultural beliefs and practices of families in pediatric palliative care.

Watching a child fall sick and die is a crisis of meaning for families, and it is through their cultural understandings and practices that families struggle to explain and make sense of this experience.[21] In fact, though research is sparse on the topic, there are some universal themes across cultures. One is the use of ritual and ceremony, and the other is the struggle for meaning and the questions that come to all bereaved families, whether they are whispered or cried out loud: "Why did my child (my sister, my brother, my grandchild) have to die?" "Where is the child now?" and "Will I ever see her again?"[22] Spiritual or religious rituals may help families find meaning when their child dies. However, such rituals may interfere with the expression of grief if they prescribe, rather than foster creation of, meaning of the child's death for individual family members.

## Situational Factors

Situational factors refer to characteristics of the situation or the circumstances surrounding the child's death. These variables include, for example, characteristics of the child's illness, such as its duration, and of the death, such as the cause and place of death, and the extent of involvement in death-related events.

### Characteristics of the Child's Illness and Death

Where or when a child died, decision-making about the death, memories of sights and sounds, degree of medical intervention, and the cause of death are all subject matters that families discuss during bereavement while exploring their grief. Ideally, the location (home or hospital) of a child's death is based upon the family's specific needs and requests, but circumstances (insurance issues, nursing shortages, transportation issues) may preclude achieving this goal. Long-term outcomes for bereaved parents and siblings of home-care deaths suggest an early pattern of differential adjustment in favor of home-care deaths.[22,23]

Decisions at the end of life, such as withdrawal of life support, may have been made with parents feeling they had insufficient understanding of the situation. Lasting images or smells may be comforting or concerning to families depending upon their associations. In fact, pain or other distressing symptoms the child might have experienced provide powerful material for families to struggle with during their grief. A full code that ends with the child's death is very different than if a child slips into death from an unconscious state. Years of treatment followed by death is experienced very differently than one in which a child dies quickly.

### Involvement in the Illness and Death-related Events

Growing consensus supports informing children about their medical condition and involving them in discussions and decisions about their care, appropriate for their levels of cognitive and emotional maturity.[24–26] The same is true for involving siblings in the care of the ill child and in the events surrounding the death, such as the funeral, memorial service, and burial rituals. In one study, children who were more involved in such activities had fewer behavioral problems following the death.[14] At the same time, practitioners must consider not only the individual child's capacity for involvement, but also the family's values about discussions of death, medical care, and children's roles.

## Models and Theories of Grief

From Freud to the current day, several theories and models have been developed that offer conceptual frameworks for how grief manifests in human beings. It is not the purpose of this chapter to provide an in-depth description of these various theories and models, since that content is covered elsewhere within this text. But, since nursing practice is guided by such theories and models, it is important to outline the development of thinking about bereavement as a basis for implementing best practices. Theories and models of grief can be categorized into stages and phase models, medical models, and task models.

### Stage and Phase Models of Grief

Models of grief based on stages and phases work on the premise that there is a beginning and an end to the grief process, with some amount of sequential progression through grief. Among stage or phase theorists are Lindemann,[27] Bowlby,[28] Engel,[29] Kubler-Ross,[30] Parkes,[31] and Rando.[32] Common patterns among these theories are the sequential, although overlapping, nature they suggest and the emphasis of the physical, emotional, behavioral, social, and intellectual impact of grief.

### Medical Models of Grief

Some models of grief liken the process to that of healing secondary to disease, injury, or psychiatric illness. Lindemann,[27] Engel,[29] Parkes,[31] and Rando[32] are among those who discuss issues of symptoms, management, or need for clinical attention with complicated forms of grief. Beverly Raphael[33] urges that although pathological complications in grieving may be more readily equated with illness, the medical analogy is more difficult to sustain with uncomplicated grief. The overall process is articulated as a form of healing that might include issues such as helplessness, resistance to the reality of the death, preoccupation with the deceased, or identification with the deceased.

Stage, phase, and medical models have been subject to numerous criticisms in recent years. In particular, critics assert that the models do not capture the diversity of how we experience grief, either from an ethnocultural approach or from the perspective of the individual. Yet the phases may be *clinically useful* if used descriptively, rather than prescriptively, to help those who grieve—and their healthcare providers—anticipate, predict, and understand some of the nuances of their experience of loss. Recent support for the descriptive use of the stage or phase model is provided by Maciejewski and colleagues,[34] who used a revised stage model of grief to study widowed persons whose partner had died of natural causes. Their findings suggest that disbelief, yearning, anger, and depression overlap, yet peak at distinct time periods, all within the first six months after loss.

Critics of the stage, phase, and medical models assert that the three types of models erroneously suggest that we come to an end in our grieving as we complete uniform or predictable stages or at last recover or reach "acceptance." Yet Bowlby[35] describes his and Parkes' final phase of "reorganization" (p. 93) as the bereaved person's redefinition of self and situation, an idea compatible with reconstructed meanings.[36] Bowlby also notes that widowed persons, as part of reorganizing and redefining, "retain a strong sense of the continuing presence of their partner" (p. 96), evidence that connections and bonds continue after death as part of uncomplicated adjustment to significant loss. In truth, the questions of what happens after death or what is the meaning of life and relationship are never-ending existential mysteries for all of us. Clinicians are cautioned to avoid using these models to support the idea that grief is a passive response to loss, when, in fact, grief is hard, dynamic work that leads to maintaining, rather than ending, connections with the one who died.

Bowlby[35] specifically addresses grief in children, noting that they mourn much like adults, yearning, becoming angry, and keeping memories of the person who died close at hand. Bowlby asserts that—far from forgetting or detaching—when children establish new relationships after someone close to them dies (e.g., a parent), they do better when their attachments to the person who died are talked about and honored.

**Task Models of Grief**

Lindemann[27] was the first to coin the phrase "grief work," and he identified three tasks: relinquish attachment to the deceased, adjust to life without the deceased, and develop new relationships. Parkes and Weiss[37] and Worden[13] have also developed task models, with a central theme being the need to loosen ties to the deceased. Attig[38,39] describes the work of grieving as an active process of relearning the world, including physical surroundings, social surroundings, aspects of self, and the relationship with the deceased.

Attig's model of relearning the world may come the closest to describing how adults, as well as children and adolescents, relearn the world by summing the many smaller tasks that together make up the complex nature of living with grief. A bereaved parent may return to normal life functioning, but is never finished loving or remembering his or her child. Even if the characteristics of that grief modulate over time, there may well be some form of heartache when that child is present in parental thoughts decades after the death. In the words of a bereaved mother, "I buried my child in my heart. I will always be with him anytime and everywhere." Attig asserts that we relearn the world as whole beings, not all at once, but rather piecemeal in distinct and growth-filled encounters. Such a description aptly applies to bereaved children—they cannot take in the whole event at once, and only over time, with their whole beings, do they relearn their worlds.

A central question is how parents and other family members manage the relationship with the child who died. Given that the child is no longer physically present, what do parents, grandparents, aunts, uncles, siblings, or friends do with the bonds, feelings, thoughts, and past experiences with that child? Research studies document that grievers do, indeed, maintain lasting connections with the deceased.[14,38,40,41] In fact, nurses can do much to facilitate these ongoing connections by offering to assist the family to obtain a memento of their child, such as a lock of hair, a foot or handprint, a photograph taken in the hospital, a piece of artwork, or a poem written by the child.

## Impact of Grief and Bereavement on Family Members

### Dying Children

Children react to their own dying as they do to most of life's experiences—within their cognitive and emotional capabilities. They live and die as children, but often with much apparent wisdom, sometimes seeming to surpass that of their adult caregivers. One of the earliest studies of seriously ill children indicated that very ill children are, indeed, aware of death and are more anxious than children hospitalized for nonserious illnesses or nonhospitalized children.[42] Bluebond-Langner,[43] based on her ethnographic study of dying children, subsequently described a process of how they become aware of their own impending death (Table 58–1). The children may experience a wide range of feelings, including but not limited to anger, anxiety, sadness, loneliness and isolation, and fear. Behaviors may include avoiding deceased fellow friends' names or staying away from their belongings; reducing attention to non-disease-related chatter and play; being preoccupied with death and disease imagery, particularly in play; engaging in open talk about the death only with selected persons; feeling anxious about weakened body functions and doubts about going home; evading talk of the future; being concerned with things being done right away; regressing, such as refusing to cooperate with relatively easy, painless procedures; or having estranged relationships with others, demonstrated by anger or silence.

Of course, we need to recognize individual variations within the above patterns, but this work provides some

---

**Table 58–1**
**The Process of Children's Perceptions of Their Own Impending Death**

1. **I am ill.** For some children there is a clear beginning to their illness although there may be a gray period before their diagnosis. For others, with a progressive disease, the realization is likely to be more gradual but it is eventually reached.

2. **I have an illness that can kill people.** Some children reach this stage simply because they hear a word like leukemia and know perhaps rather vaguely that it is associated with death. Others are told by their parents, if for no other reason than to help explain why the treatment given is so awful. The understanding that comes at this stage is virtually academic and it is possible some children do not believe what they are told.

3. **I have an illness that can kill children.** When there are three boys with cystic fibrosis in a school one summer term and only two in the autumn, the remaining two have had the clearest possible lesson. We should always be on guard for the ripples that come to a hospital ward or the school class when a death occurs.

4. **I am never going to get better.** This may follow on quite quickly after Stage 3, or it may take some time. It is almost always associated with depression. This does not imply children know their death is imminent.

5. **I am going to die.** Some authors suggest that all children from 3 years and up are capable of reaching this stage. One must be open to the possibility that even very young children may have a full understanding not only of death, but of their own death.

*Source*: Goldman, A., & Lansdown, R. (1994), reference 2. Reproduced with permission of Oxford University Press (UK).

---

background for understanding terminally ill children, such as this 14-year-old boy whose death is imminent:

> My mother used to go to church to pray for me early every morning. I also prayed in my bed for my mother to stop her soundless sorrow. We were all sad and we pray separately in different places. Now, I am getting more worried about how sad she will be after my death, and she will feel lonely without me. How can I express my sorrow for her and thank her? She has lost so many things… money, time, and smiles, all because of me….

## Parents

Parent–child relationships are not contractual, but sacred. They are unique and complex. The connectedness between parent and child has its roots in the biological and emotional bonds and attachments that precede birth. It grows as the parent begins to know and care for the child. The child is a parent's link to the future.[44] Parental grief is all-consuming, affecting every aspect of parents' existence.

Parents often struggle with guilt following their child's death because of deep-rooted feelings of responsibility for their child's welfare. Because parents are responsible for protecting and sustaining their children, shielding them from all danger, many parents feel they should have protected their child from illness and death. When children die from an inherited disease such as cystic fibrosis or sickle cell anemia, parents know their child's condition results from their unknowingly passing on the genetic material. When the child dies, parents may still carry the burden of knowing they "gave" their child a terminal illness. Parents whose child died from an accident may also feel guilty for abdicating their protective role. Bereaved parents may cling to irrational guilt since it is often easier to accept blame, with its fantasy of control, than the total loss of control with which they must grapple. Or, they may blame someone else for their child's death. Sometimes this guilt is targeted toward a partner or spouse, another child or family member. Nurses need to be aware of these dynamics and help a family find an appropriate place for their anger and blame.[45]

Parents, as individuals, may have different styles of grieving as described earlier. Nurses can help by acknowledging the "normality" of a variety of grieving styles and encouraging parents to understand each other's ways of grieving. Differences in bereavement response also may lead to a strain on the couple's sexual intimacy. Sexual abstinence is frequently reported by bereaved couples due to a lack of sexual interest; others seek out comfort through sexual intimacy. Again, pointing out that such reactions can be expected may help couples realize the "normalcy" of their reactions. A long-standing myth is that divorce rates among bereaved parents are very high. In fact, it is not higher than the national divorce rate. And, when divorce follows a child's death, it is usually due to problems that existed before the child's illness or death.

Nurses must also be cognizant of the special needs of bereaved parents who cope with additional stressors in their everyday lives. Single parents or same-sex parents may not have as many options for support as married parents in a heterosexual relationship.

Moreover, nurses must pay attention to the indirect grief of parents who witness or coexperience the death of other terminally ill children in the same clinical setting as their child.[46]

## Grandparents

The grief of grandparents is twofold: they have to bear their own grief, as well as bear the agony of the grief of their own child, the parent of the deceased child. Grandparents can be a source of considerable strength for parents and siblings, or they can be an additional source of stress. Their advice may be sought but then ignored; often their practical help is accepted, but their own grief is barely acknowledged.[2] Grandparents may experience considerable helplessness and frustration; they question the meaning of life as they struggle with the "lack of order" of having the young one precede them in death.

## Siblings

Siblings have been called the "forgotten grievers." They have been typically ignored when a brother or sister dies, not for lack of parental concern, but because their parents are so overcome with grief, they have little energy to devote to the needs of their surviving children. The impact of a child's death on surviving siblings is manifested in four general responses, best characterized in the words of the children themselves[14]: "I hurt inside," "I don't understand," "I don't belong," and "I'm not enough." Not all children who have a brother or sister die experience all four responses, but most children through to adolescence demonstrate all responses to varying degrees.

### "I Hurt Inside"

The first response includes all the emotions typically associated with grief—sadness, anger, frustration, loneliness, fear, guilt, restlessness, and a host of other emotions that characterize bereavement. Unlike adults who are able to talk about their responses, children manifest their responses in various behaviors, such as withdrawing, seeking attention, acting out, arguing, fear of going to bed at night, overeating, or undereating. In response to children who are hurting inside, nurses need to allow, and even encourage, the expression of the hurt the children are feeling. They may endeavor to share their own thoughts and feelings with the children to let them know that they are not alone in this situation. If adults do not allow children to express their feelings, siblings learn there is something wrong with such feelings. When adults are impatient with children, or belittle their expression, siblings learn to stifle their feelings.

### "I Don't Understand"

Children's difficulty in understanding death is greatly influenced by their level of cognitive development. However, once children know about death, their cognitive worlds are forever altered. If they are not helped to understand what has happened in clear, simple, and age-appropriate ways, children make up their own explanations that usually involve taking responsibility for the death and their parents' distress. Without explanations, they become more frightened and insecure. Nurses must have a solid grasp of children's cognitive development, provide appropriate explanations for events that happen, and be open to questions from children.

### "I Don't Belong"

A death in the family tears apart the usual day-to-day activities and patterns of living. Parents are overwhelmed with their grief, with making arrangements, and with caring for their other children. Surviving children are overwhelmed with the flurry of activity and the depth of emotion surrounding them. They often feel as if they don't know what to do; they may want to help, but they don't know how, or, if they try, their efforts are not acknowledged. They begin to feel as if they are in the way, or as if they are not a part of what is happening. They feel different from their peers as well, and begin to feel as if they don't belong anymore. Nurses can play a critical role in including siblings in illness and death-related events, such as encouraging or teaching the child to participate in certain treatments (for example, by holding their sibling's hand or blowing bubbles together during painful procedures). After death, the nurse can help the parents by modeling what to say to the children.

### "I'm not Enough"

Assuming that they are somehow responsible for their parents' distress, siblings may feel as if they are not enough to make their parents happy ever again. They may feel that their deceased brother or sister was the favorite child, and they should have been the ones to die instead. Some siblings respond by striving to be as good as they can be, trying to prove that they are worthy. They must be made to feel special just for being themselves, and by not comparing them to their deceased brother or sister. Moreover, siblings may not want to burden their parents with their grief, knowing their parents are already overladen. Nurses can assist siblings to feel special by asking them questions about their lives and reassuring them of their value and unique characteristics or abilities.

## Adolescents

Teenagers who are dying, or who are the siblings or friends of another child, are often overlooked.[47] They face a particularly complicated situation when they encounter death and bereavement because adolescents are typically engrossed in achieving independence and in proving their invulnerability. Serious illness and grief catches them by surprise, as they seldom have developed the coping skills necessary to deal with their reactions. As well, many adults believe it is difficult to help adolescents cope with death because adolescents are reputed to turn away from adults and to talk only with other adolescents. This is not entirely true, as these young people often seek out and value the input and support of adults they respect, such as a teacher, a nurse, or a friend's parent. Moreover, when adolescents turn to their peers, if they do, they may often find that their peers have no significant resources to offer because they too are inexperienced with death.

Dying adolescents with a terminal disease struggle against physical pain, are sensitive to their parents' reactions, and have a strong desire to have relationships with their friends regardless of their illness status: "I couldn't say anything with my Mom. She pretends to smile to me, but I know how she feels so sad whenever looking at me. I want to come out and share my emotions with my friend at least. But, now there is nobody around me." In such cases, nurses are in a position to help an adolescent's family members to understand adolescent cognitive and psychosocial functioning. Self-help support groups for teens, either in person or via the Internet, often prove valuable to grieving adolescents. Adolescents are often open to writing, art, or music. Adults may come along on such journeys, or share the results, but they should take care to follow the adolescents' lead, respecting confidentiality and permitting them to interpret the significance of their work in their own way.

## Assessing Grief

Bereavement care is interdisciplinary in nature, focusing on assessment of the comprehensive pattern and character of the whole family, as well as of individuals within the family. Grief assessment focuses on the ill child, other family members, and their significant others. Grief assessment begins when the child is admitted to the hospital or at the time of diagnosis of acute, chronic, or terminal illness. It is ongoing throughout the course of the child's illness and comes to the forefront during the bereavement period after the death. As illustrated in Figure 58–1, an integrative model of bereavement care, as opposed to a series or parallel model, highlights the central role of bereavement support for a family from the moment they suspect their child is ill. Milstein[48] emphasizes the compatibility of goals for curing and palliation that include caregiver mindsets of relationship (being with) and intervention (doing to). Nurses, in particular, play a central role in a family's initial bereavement experience, holding in mind the family's sense of loss, while pursuing with other team members care that best addresses the child's well-being. Most children's deaths still occur in the hospital; nurses are most often present at the time of death. If not with the child at the moment of death, the nurse is usually the first one called to the child's bedside. The nurse's words and actions at that time leave indelible imprints upon parents. Even years after their child's death, parents recall vivid memories of the nurse's gentle approach in offering privacy, giving a hug, sharing the sadness, allowing families the amount of time they want with

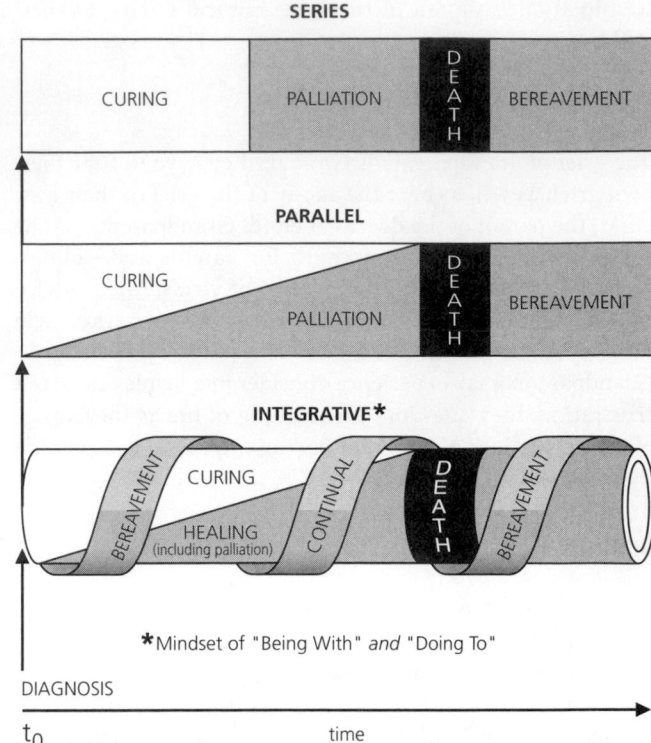

**Figure 58–1.** A Paradigm of Integrative Care: Heading with Caring Throughout Life.

their child before leaving the hospital. Unfortunately, other parents remember the nurse who spoke abruptly to them, or rushed them away because their child's room had to be made ready for the next patient. In even these brief interactions, nurses can do so much to prevent this devastating experience from being any worse than it already is for the family.

In assessing grief, clinicians should keep in mind the range of factors that impact upon the grief of family members, while noting those factors that put individuals and families at risk for disenfranchised or complicated grief. The passage of time is not a useful consideration in assessing grief responses; instead, we must assess the degree of intrusiveness into each individual's life and the extent to which family members can carry out their usual activities.

## Helping Bereaved Families

Grief assessment leads to a plan of care with the goal of facilitating and supporting the grieving process. Understanding grief as a normal, human process that is individually expressed enables practitioners to present an accepting, nonjudgmental attitude that helps create a respectful and trusting milieu. The approach to children or other family members experiencing anticipatory grief is the same as for family members whose child has died, but the focus of some interventions may differ. For example, prior to death, families should be offered information about the signs and symptoms of disease progression and the dying process; following death, the focus may be on listening to family members review the course of the child's dying.

## Grief Interventions

### For Families

Bereaved individuals need an opportunity to express their grief in a supportive environment. Nurses have a responsibility to create such an environment for parents and other family members following a child's death so that they feel it is okay for them to express whatever they are feeling. Such comments as "It must be very difficult for you right now" give permission for expression. The form of expression may vary among family members; some will verbalize, others will cry, some may leave the room. Still others may express anger, and others appreciation.

Nurses may fear "saying the wrong thing" to a family member, or may fear not knowing what to say, or feel they must have the "right thing to say." Attitudes are conveyed through words and more importantly, through actions. Thus, it is usually best to say very little, avoiding clichés and euphemisms that can be so distressing to grieving individuals. It is not appropriate to encourage anyone to "Keep a stiff upper lip" or to "Look on the bright side." It is disrespectful, and even cruel, to say "He is no longer suffering" or "You are young; you will have more children." These messages, whether given directly or indirectly, may compound the pain by making family members think the clinicians do not understand their loss. Instead, sit or stand quietly close to the family, let them know they can stay with their child for as long as they would like, comment on the child's special qualities and acknowledge your own sadness about the child's death. Offering to help in practical and concrete ways is also helpful. However, rather than asking if "there is anything I can help you with," offer to do specific things, such as making phone calls or getting them a glass of water. Most family members have a need to share their story, telling and retelling anecdotes about the child and the events of his living and dying. Listening to their stories is probably the most helpful action. For some families, reviewing what happened with their child with the care providers is critical. Follow-up phone calls or visits with the providers who cared for the child are much appreciated by families.

Many family members who are unaware of the normal manifestations of grief can find some comfort in knowing that their pain is normal. Providing information about the common facts of grief can be helpful; having written materials to send home with families is even better. Understanding that each person's grief experience is unique helps family members understand that there is "no right way to grieve." It also helps them to realize they are not "bad" or "crazy" if they express their grief differently from other family members; it also may prevent family member from telling other family members how they "should" grieve. Clinicians should identify any need for additional assistance and make referrals as needed. For example, a family member may have spiritual concerns that would be best addressed by the pastoral care person; a social worker may assist with funeral arrangements or financial concerns. In addition, the nurse should make referrals to bereavement specialists, psychologists, or physicians as needed.

### For Children

Since grief is a human response, children and adults alike feel denial, anger, sadness, guilt, longing in response to a loved one, and experience lack of sleep, lack of appetite, and difficulty concentrating and maintaining usual patterns of interaction with others. However, most children have limited ability to verbalize and describe their feelings; they also have very limited capacity to tolerate the emotional pain generated by open recognition of their loss.[49] Moreover, children's cognitive developmental level interferes with their ability to understand the irreversibility, universality, and inevitability of death, and to understand the reactions of their parents. They also deeply fear being different in any way from their peers, and so are often unable to find comfort, as adults do, in sharing their discomfort with their friends. As play is the work and the language of childhood, children are able to express their feelings through their play, as well as music and art. A summary of grief reactions in children, according to age level, and corresponding suggested interventions, is presented in Table 58–2.

### For Parents

Before the child's death, an important emphasis for clinicians is to facilitate connections between the parents and the ill child and their other children, as well as by helping them develop memories and keepsakes that they can hold and cherish long after the death. The earlier these can be collected, the better, so they reflect a longer period of time with the child and not simply the final days of life. Facilitating communication between family members and the caregiving staff, as well as among family members themselves, also creates positive memories and optimal coping. Informing parents about the dying process, and helping them with the concept of appropriate death consistent with patient, family, cultural, and spiritual goals is necessary. Assisting with planning funeral or memorial services also can be helpful, particularly for families who have limited support systems.

After the child's death, follow-up by the clinicians who cared for the child is much appreciated by families. Such follow-up also allows ongoing assessment (see Table 58–3 for questions to ask during an initial follow-up telephone call). Parents, overcome with their own grief, may need assistance in dealing with the needs of their other children; encourage parents to enlist the support of aunts, uncles, or good friends

**Table 58–2**
**Grief and Bereavement in Children**

| Characteristics of Age | View of Death and Response | What Helps |
|---|---|---|
| **Birth to six months** | | |
| Basic needs must be met, cries if needs aren't met. | Has no concept of death. | Progressively disengage child from primary care-giver if possible. |
| Needs emotional and physical closeness of a consistent caregiver. | Experiences death like any other separation—no sense of "finality." | Introduce a new primary caregiver. |
| Derives identity from caregiver. | Nonspecific expressions of distress (crying). | Nurture, comfort. |
| View of caregiver as source of comfort and all needs fulfillment. | Reacts to loss of caregiver. | Anticipate physical and emotional needs and provide them. |
| Developing trust. | Reacts to caregiver's distress. | Maintain routines. |
| **Six months to two years** | | |
| Begins to individuate. | May see death as reversible. | Needs continual support, comfort. |
| Remembers face of caregiver when absent. Demonstrates full range of emotions. | Experiences bona fide grief. | Avoid separation from significant others. |
| Identifies caregiver as source of good feelings and interactions. | Grief response only to death of significant person in child's life. | Close physical and emotional connections by significant others. |
| | Screams, panics, withdraws, becomes disinterested in food, toys, activities. | Maintain daily structure and schedule of routine activities. |
| | Reacts in concert with distress experienced by caregiver. | Support caregiver to reduce distress and maintain a stable environment. |
| | No control over feelings and responses; anticipate regressive behavior. | Acknowledge sadness that loved one will not return—offer comfort. |
| **Two years to five years** | | |
| Egocentric. | Sees death like sleep: reversible. | Remind that loved one will not return. |
| Cause-effect not understood. | Believes in magical causes. | Reassure child that he/she is not to blame. |
| Developing conscience. | Has sense of loss. | Give realistic information, answer questions. |
| Attributes life to objects. | Curiosity, questioning. | Involve in "farewell" ceremonies. |
| Feelings expressed mostly by behaviors. | Anticipate regression, clinging. | Encourage questions and expression of feelings. |
| Can recall events from past. | Aggressive behavior common. | Keep home environment stable, structured. |
| | Worries about who will care for them. | Help put words to feelings; reassure/comfort. |
| | | Reassure children about who will take care of them; provide ways to remember loved one. |
| **Five years to nine years** | | |
| Attributes life to things that move; may fear the dark. | Personifies death as ghosts, "boogeyman." | Give clear and realistic information. Include child in funeral ceremonies if they choose. |
| Begins to develop intellect. | Interest in biological aspects of life and death. | Give permission to express feelings and provide opportunities; reduce guilt by providing factual information. Maintain structured schedule, individual and family activities; needs strong parent. |
| Begins to relate cause and effect; understands consequences. | Begins to see death as irreversible. | |
| Literal, concrete. | May see death as punishment; may feel responsible. | |
| Decreasing fantasy life, increasing control of feelings. | Problems concentrating on tasks; may deny or hide feelings, vulnerability. | Notify school of what is occurring, gentle confirmation, reassurance. |
| **Pre-adolescent through teens** | | |
| Individuation outside home. | Views death as permanent. | Unambiguous information. |
| Identifies with peer group; needs family attachment. | Sense of own mortality; sense of future. | Provide opportunities to express self, feelings; encourage outside relationships with mentors. |
| Understands life processes; can verbalize feelings. | Strong emotional reaction; may regress, revert to fantasy. | Provide tangible means to remember loved one; encourage self-expression, verbal and non-verbal. |
| Physical maturation. | May somaticize, intellectualize, morbid pre-occupation. | Dispel fears about physical concerns; educate about maturation; provide outlets for energy and strong feelings (recreation, sports, etc.); needs mentoring and direction. |

*Source*: Fine, P. (Ed.) (1998), reference 50. Scottsdale, AZ: Vista Care Hospice, Inc. Reprinted with permission.

**Table 58–3**
**Questions for an Initial Follow-up Telephone Call to Parents Who Have Experienced the Loss of a Child of Perinatal Loss**

- "You might recall that you were told that someone from the hospital would call you in (number) weeks."
- "Is this a good time to talk?"
- "Are there any issues that you have been thinking about that perhaps I could follow-up on for you?"
- "Have you been back yet for a post partum check-up?"
- "Some parents have noticed a change in their sleeping or eating habits. Has this been a problem for you?"
- "How has (name of other parent) responded to your loss? Sometimes it is hard for both parents to talk about it. How has it been for you?"
- "Do you have other family members or friends that you have been able to talk to? What types of things have they been able to do for you?"
- "Do you have plans to work outside of your home? The first few days at work can be especially difficult. Have you thought about how it might be for you?"
- "Did you receive any information on support groups for parents?"
- "Are there any other materials you received in the hospital that you have questions about?"
- "Are there any other questions I can answer for you?"
- "During the call you stated that…"
- "I will call you again on (date)."

*Source*: Friedrichs, J., Daly, M.I., & Kavanaugh, K. (2000), reference 51. Reprinted with permission.

in this regard. For parents who are willing and interested in finding additional support, provide a listing of parental support groups and other parent bereavement resources in the community, such as Compassionate Friends, a self-help organization to help parents and siblings after the death of a child (www.compassionatefriends.org).

### Bereavement Programs

The development of pediatric palliative care programs, including bereavement programs, in health-care institutions has increased notably in the past decade despite budget and other resource concerns. Still, the dearth of consistency and excellence in both the training of professionals and the offering of services to families results in many gaps in the experiences of families. Such gaps must be addressed, especially for families of children who had a chronic illness that meant frequent trips to the hospital, sometimes over many years, and resulted in the development of close relationships with staff members. Such families worry that the staff will forget their deceased child; some families want to maintain an ongoing relationship with those who cared for their child. Thus, during the transition after the child's death, families and staff have to navigate the changing relationship.[52] A bereavement program within pediatric palliative care, or as part of an agency-wide program, can be of considerable service to both families and staff. These services typically include staff with specific training in bereavement care and a follow-up component. A bereavement program facilitates referral of families to grief therapists as needed; ensures that all families are made aware of the available services, such as support groups, memorial services, or grief workshops; and may facilitate

bereaved families connecting with one another as a source of support. The existence of a bereavement program gives a clear message that an institution and its staff are committed to the care of families. Perinatal palliative care guidelines are provided by Limbo, Toce, and Peck.[53]

### The Nurse: Death Anxiety, Cumulative Loss, and Grief

Professionals who help children and families with the serious illness and death of a child are witness to numerous heart-wrenching scenes, and are constantly reminded of the frailty and preciousness of life. Working with dying children can trigger nurses' awareness of their own personal losses and fears about their own death, the death of their own children, and mortality in general. Historically, nurses and other health-care professionals were taught to desensitize themselves to these experiences and to maintain an "emotional detachment." This approach, which still exists today in many situations, results in the nurses' use of defenses to allay their fears, including focusing only on physical-care needs, evading emotionally-sensitive conversations with children and families, and talking only superficially about topics that are comfortable for the nurse. These behaviors result in emotional distancing, avoidance, and withdrawal from dying children and their families at a time when children most need intensive interpersonal care and active involvement by the nurse. Death anxiety occurs when clinicians are confronted with fears about death and have few resources or support systems to explore and to express thoughts and emotions about dying

**Table 58–4**
**Coping with Professional Anxiety in Terminal Illness**

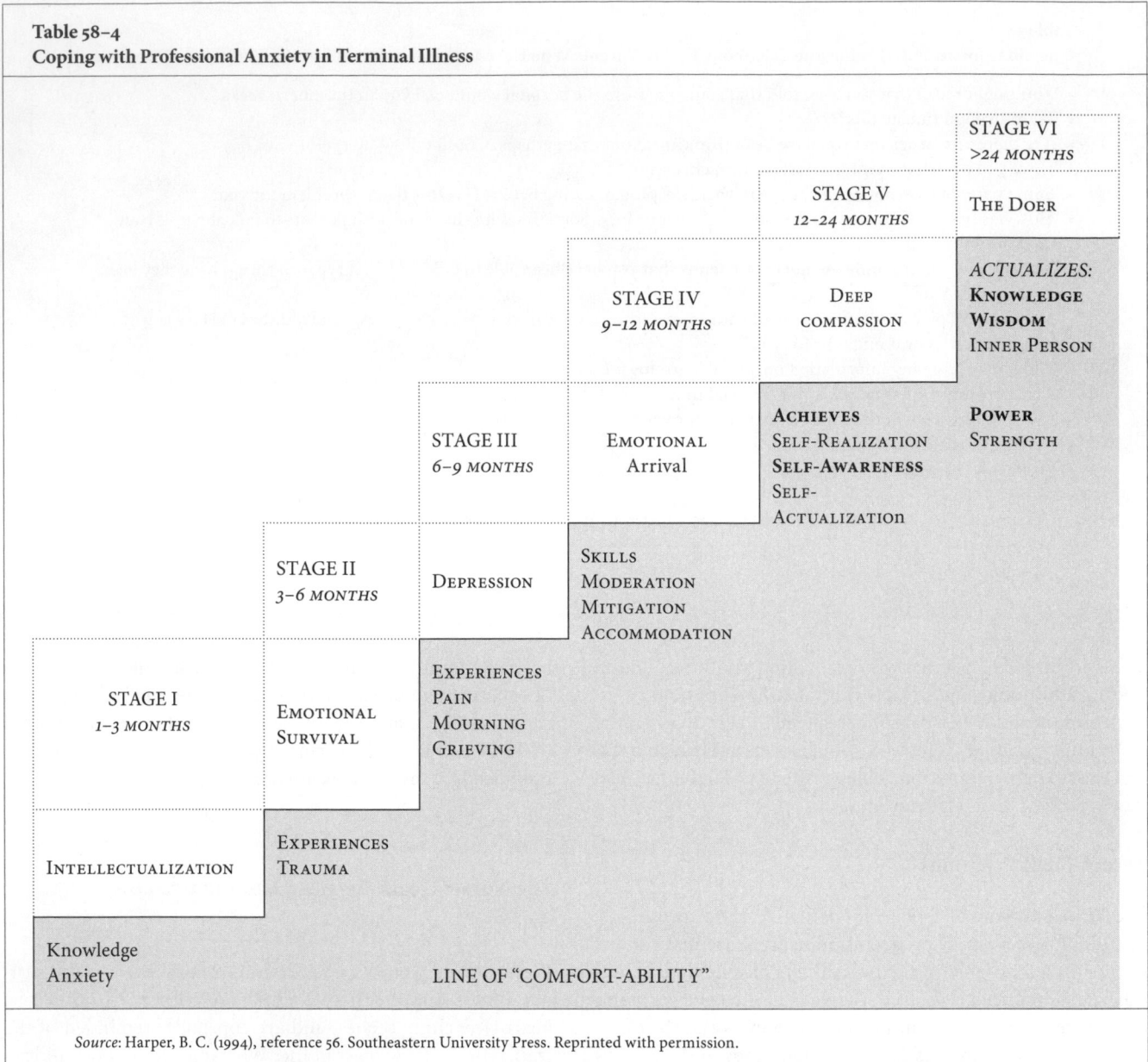

| | | | | | STAGE VI<br>*>24 MONTHS* |
| | | | | STAGE V<br>*12–24 MONTHS* | THE DOER |
| | | | STAGE IV<br>*9–12 MONTHS* | DEEP<br>COMPASSION | *ACTUALIZES:*<br>**KNOWLEDGE**<br>**WISDOM**<br>INNER PERSON |
| | | STAGE III<br>*6–9 MONTHS* | EMOTIONAL<br>Arrival | **ACHIEVES**<br>SELF-REALIZATION<br>**SELF-AWARENESS**<br>SELF-<br>ACTUALIZATION | **POWER**<br>STRENGTH |
| | STAGE II<br>*3–6 MONTHS* | DEPRESSION | SKILLS<br>MODERATION<br>MITIGATION<br>ACCOMMODATION | | |
| STAGE I<br>*1–3 MONTHS* | EMOTIONAL<br>SURVIVAL | EXPERIENCES<br>PAIN<br>MOURNING<br>GRIEVING | | | |
| INTELLECTUALIZATION | EXPERIENCES<br>TRAUMA | | | | |
| Knowledge<br>Anxiety | LINE OF "COMFORT-ABILITY" | | | | |

*Source*: Harper, B. C. (1994), reference 56. Southeastern University Press. Reprinted with permission.

and death.[54] Thus, rather than a "desensitization" of oneself, professionals are encouraged to sensitize to this powerful human material. Caring for dying children requires nurses to explore, experience, and express their personal feelings regarding death. Personal death-awareness activities and exercises, discussion of belief systems about death/afterlife with friends and colleagues, self-exploration, and reflection may promote an understanding and acceptance of death as part of life. The process is complicated by cumulative loss, a succession of losses experienced by nurses who work with patients with life-threatening illness and their families, often on a daily basis.[55] When nurses are exposed to death frequently, they seldom have time to grieve one child before another child dies.

Harper[56] has put forth a model of how professional caregivers learn over time to move through the pain of providing this kind of care. Her five-step model (Table 58–4) about caring for dying children starts with intellectualization of the experience, and is characterized by attainment of knowledge and anxiety about performance. She goes on to describe caregivers moving through emotional survival, depression, and emotional arrival. Finally, and only after working through the personal pain of grief work, caregivers arrive at a place of deep compassion for families, characterized by self-realization and self-actualization on the part of the caregiver. Self-awareness about one's own personal history of loss is necessary to know one's own set of beliefs about death, dying, and the afterlife. Without this awareness, our own beliefs and cultural/spiritual biases can interfere with the experience of the family. For caregivers, strong coping techniques, good self-care and ongoing education and support are necessary components to not only do the work, but also to avoid burnout.

Several factors influence nurses' adaptation to the inherent grief in pediatric palliative care. They include the nurses' professional training and other training in dealing with dying, death, and grief; nurses' personal and professional history of loss and possible unresolved issues of dealing with grief; personal and professional life changes; and the presence or absence of support systems.

In one study of nurses' experiences following the death of a child, participants described two types of distress. Moral distress resulted when the nurses knew the child's death was imminent and were required to carry out painful treatments they perceived as unnecessary. Grief distress occurred in response to the child's death. Both types of distress resulted from lack of open communication within the care team and lack of consideration of the nurses' viewpoints.[54] Thus, systems of support are critical to nurses' coping with the stress of working with seriously ill children and their families. In addition to helping bereaved families, as mentioned earlier, institutional bereavement programs also serve the needs of staff. Programs can be structured to offer help in debriefing after a death, validating staff feelings, offering support groups, and encouraging informal support through the one-one-one sharing of experiences with coworkers, peers, or pastoral care workers.[57,58] The presence of a supervisor, mentor, or instructor during the care of the dying, when a family member visits, or during the time of the child's death can greatly decrease anxiety and provide immense support to the nurse, particularly to novice nurses in pediatric palliative care.

Caregiver suffering is a contemporary term that includes moral distress and grief[56] and encompasses bearing witness to others' suffering.[59,60] Suffering is part of the human condition and provides opportunities for growth and transformation for both nurses and families.[61,62]

Education that enhances knowledge and skills in end-of-life care can promote competence and self-confidence and is associated with hopeful thinking.[63] Education helps make the experience both meaningful and bearable for families.[64] Education that describes families' experiences can be invaluable because it empowers clinicians to offer care that is more sensitive to the needs of families, more humanistic, and more family-centered and thus, more rewarding to staff. Nurses have responsibilities for acknowledging their own personal and professional limitations, seeking assistance, and engaging in self-care activities. Reflection is a key process for pediatric palliative care nurses in being with the child and family before, during, and after death.[65,66] Education specific to grief and bereavement in palliative care can be personally and professionally transformational when designed as relationship-based; inclusive of the caregiver's beliefs, values, and feelings and parents' stories; and focused on the caregiver as guide.[67–71] Davies et al.[72] identify the need for

more education to foster communication skills and increase overall comfort level of nurses and physicians who work in pediatric palliative care.

Pediatric palliative care is a challenging field, one that demands finding the balance between providing compassionate quality care and personal satisfaction as a professional nurse. In addition, working with dying children and their families provides meaning to life. Working with these children helps to develop a clear perspective of what is really valuable; it helps us grow as persons and professionals. From the children and their families, we learn that death is part of life, that human beings are remarkably resilient, and that hope is everlasting.

REFERENCES

1. Field MJ, Behrman RE, eds. Committee on Palliative and End-of-Life Care for Children and Their Families. When Children Die: Improving Palliative and End-of-Life Care for Children and their Families. Washington, DC: National Academy Press, 2003.
2. Goldman A. Care of the Dying Child. Oxford, England/New York, NY: Oxford University Press, 1994.
3. DeSpelder LA, Strickland AL. The Last Dance: Encountering Death and Dying. Mountain View, CA: Mayfield Pub, 1992.
4. Sanders CM. A comparison of adult bereavement in the death of a spouse, child, and parent. Omega 1979;10(4):303–322.
5. Murray JAH, Philological Society (Great Britain). The Compact Edition of the Oxford English Dictionary. Oxford: Oxford University Press, 1971.
6. Silverman PR. Never Too Young to Know: Death in Children's Lives. New York, NY: Oxford University Press, 2000.
7. Corless IB. Bereavement. In: Ferrell B, Coyle N, eds. Textbook of Palliative Nursing. New York, NY: Oxford University Press; 2001:35.
8. Rando TA. Clinical Dimensions of Anticipatory Mourning: Theory and Practice in Working with the Dying, Their Loved Ones, and Their Caregivers. Champaign, IL: Research Press, 2000.
9. Rando TA. Grief, Dying, and Death: Clinical Interventions for Caregivers. Champaign, IL: Research Press, 1984.
10. Doka KJ. Disenfranchised Grief: Recognizing Hidden Sorrow. Lexington, MA: Lexington Books, 1989.
11. Doka KJ. Disenfranchised Grief: New Directions, Challenges, and Strategies for Practice. Champaign, IL: Research Press, 2002.
12. Prigerson HG, Jacobs SC. Perspectives on care at the close of life. Caring for bereaved patients: "All the doctors just suddenly go." JAMA 2001;286(11):1369–1376.
13. Worden JW. Grief Counseling and Grief Therapy: A Handbook for the Mental Health Practitioner. New York, NY; London: Springer, 2008.
14. Davies B. Shadows in the Sun: The Experiences of Sibling Bereavement in Childhood. Philadelphia, PA: Brunner/Mazel, 1999.
15. Corr CA. Children's emerging awareness of death. In: Doka KJ, Tucci AS, eds. Living with Grief: Children and Adolescents. Washington, DC: Hospice Foundation of America; 2008:5–17.

16. Hunter SB, Smith DE. Predictors of children's understandings of death: Age, cognitive ability, death experience and maternal communicative competence. Omega (Westport) 2008;57(2):143–162.

17. Didion J. The Year of Magical Thinking. New York, NY: A.A. Knopf, 2005.

18. Davies B. Fading Away: The Experience of Transition in Families with Terminal Illness. Amityville, NY: Baywood Pub., 1995.

19. Davies B, Spinetta J, Martinson I, McClowry S, Kulenkamp E. Manifestations of levels of functioning and grieving families. J Fam Issues 1987;7(3):297–313.

20. Die Trill M, Kovalcik R. The child with cancer: Influence of culture on truth-telling and patient care. Ann N Y Acad Sci 1997;809:197–210.

21. McGrath BB. Illness as a problem of meaning: Moving culture from the classroom to the clinic. ANS Adv Nurs Sci 1998;21(2):17–29.

22. Lauer ME, Mulhern RK, Bohne JB, Camitta BM. Children's perceptions of their sibling's death at home or hospital: The precursors of differential adjustment. Cancer Nurs 1985; 8(1):21–27.

23. Mulhern RK, Lauer ME, Hoffmann RG. Death of a child at home or in the hospital: Subsequent psychological adjustment of the family. Pediatrics 1983;71(5):743–747.

24. Hilden JM, Emanuel EJ, Fairclough DL, et al. Attitudes and practices among pediatric oncologists regarding end-of-life care: Results of the 1998 American Society of Clinical Oncology survey. J Clin Oncol 2001;19(1):205.

25. Hinds PS, Oakes L, Furman W, et al. End-of-life decision making by adolescents, parents, and healthcare providers in pediatric oncology: Research to evidence-based practice guidelines. Cancer Nurs 2001;24(2):122–134.

26. Nitschke R, Meyer WH, Huszti HC. When the tumor is not the target, tell the children. J Clin Oncol 2001;19(2):595–596.

27. Lindemann E. Symptomatology and management of acute grief. Am J Psychiatry 1944;101(2):141–148.

28. Bowlby J. Attachment and Loss. New York, NY: Basic Books, 1969.

29. Engel GL. Grief and grieving. Am J Nurs 1964;64:93–98.

30. Kubler-Ross E. On Death and Dying. New York, NY: Macmillan, 1969.

31. Parkes CM. Bereavement: Studies of Grief in Adult Life. Philadelphia, PA: Routledge, 2001.

32. Rando TA. Parental Loss of a Child. Champaign, IL: Research Press, 1986.

33. Raphael B. The Anatomy of Bereavement. New York, NY: Basic Books, 1983.

34. Maciejewski PK, Zhang B, Block SD, Prigerson HG. An empirical examination of the stage theory of grief. JAMA 2007;297(7):716–723.

35. Bowlby J. Loss: Sadness and Depression. New York, NY: Basic Books, 1980.

36. Neimeyer RA, Baldwin SA, Gillies J. Continuing bonds and reconstructing meaning: Mitigating complications in bereavement. Death Stud 2006;30(8):715–738.

37. Parkes CM, Weiss RS. Recovery from Bereavement. New York, NY: Basic Books, 1983.

38. Attig T. How We Grieve: Relearning the World. New York, NY: Oxford University Press, 1996.

39. Attig T. The Heart of Grief: Death and the Search for Lasting Love. New York, NY: Oxford University Press, 2000.

40. Packman W, Horsley H, Davies B, Kramer R. Sibling bereavement and continuing bonds. Death Stud 2006;30(9):817–841.

41. Klass D, Silverman PR, Nickman SL. Continuing Bonds: New Understandings of Grief. Washington, DC: Taylor & Francis, 1996.

42. Waechter EH. Children's awareness of fatal illness. Am J Nurs 1971;7(6):1168–1172.

43. Bluebond-Langner M. How terminally ill children come to know themselves and their world. In: The Private Worlds of Dying Children. Princeton, NJ: Princeton University Press; 1978:166–197.

44. Arnold JH, Gemma PB. A Child Dies: A Portrait of Family Grief. Philadelphia, PA: Charles Press, 1994.

45. Worden JW, Monahan JR. Caring for bereaved parents. In: Armstrong-Dailey A, Zarbock SF, eds. Hospice Care for Children. New York, NY: Oxford University Press; 2001:137–156.

46. James L, Johnson B. The needs of parents of pediatric oncology patients during the palliative care phase. J Pediatr Oncol Nurs 1997;14(2):83–95.

47. Christ GH, Siegel K, Christ AE. Adolescent grief: "It never really hit me…until it actually happened." JAMA 2002;288(10):1269–1278.

48. Milstein J. A paradigm of integrative care: Healing with curing throughout life, "being with" and "doing to." J Perinatol 2005;25(9):563–568.

49. Webb NB. Helping Bereaved Children: A Handbook for Practitioners. New York, NY: Guilford Press, 2002.

50. Fine P, ed. Processes to Optimize Care During the Last Phase of Life. Scottsdale, AZ: Vista Care Hospice, 1998.

51. Friedrichs J, Daly MI, Kavanaugh K. Follow-up of parents who experience a perinatal loss: Facilitating grief and assessing for grief complicated by depression. Illness Crisis Loss 2000;8(3):302.

52. McKlindon D, Barnsteiner JH. Therapeutic relationships. Evolution of the Children's Hospital of Philadelphia model. MCN Am J Matern Child Nurs 1999;24(5):237–243.

53. Limbo R, Toce S, Peck T. Resolve Through Sharing (RTS) position paper on perinatal palliative care. Updated 2008. Available at: http://www.bereavementservices.org/documents/FINAL9.11.08.pdf (accessed December 3, 2008).

54. Davies B, Clarke D, Connaughty S, et al. Caring for dying children: Nurses' experiences. Pediatr Nurs 1996;22(6):500–507.

55. Vachon MLS. The nurse's role: The world of palliative care nursing. In: Ferrell B, Coyle N, eds. Textbook of Palliative Nursing. New York, NY: Oxford University Press; 2001:647–662.

56. Harper BC. Death: The Coping Mechanism of the Health Professional. Greenville, SC: Southeastern University Press, 1994.

57. Meadors P, Lamson A. Compassion fatigue and secondary traumatization: Provider self care on intensive care units for children. J Pediatr Health Care 2008;22(1):24–34.

58. Rushton CH, Reder E, Hall B, Comello K, Sellers DE, Hutton N. Interdisciplinary interventions to improve pediatric palliative care and reduce health care professional suffering. J Palliat Med 2006;9(4):922–933.

59. Ferrell BR, Coyle N. The nature of suffering and the goals of nursing. Oncol Nurs Forum 2008;35(2):241–247.

60. Lee KJ, Dupree CY. Staff experiences with end-of-life care in the pediatric intensive care unit. J Palliat Med 2008; 11(7):986–990.

61. Taubman-Ben-Ari O, Weintroub A. Meaning in life and personal growth among pediatric physicians and nurses. Death Stud 2008;32(7):621–645.

62. Hogan NS. Sibling loss: Issues for children and adolescents. In: Doka KJ, Tucci AS, eds. Living with Grief: Children and Adolescents. Washington, DC: Hospice Foundation of America; 2008:159–174.

63. Feudtner C, Santucci G, Feinstein JA, Snyder CR, Rourke MT, Kang TI. Hopeful thinking and level of comfort regarding providing pediatric palliative care: A survey of hospital nurses. Pediatrics 2007;119(1):e186–e192.

64. Churchill LR, Schenck D. One cheer for bioethics: Engaging the moral experiences of patients and practitioners beyond the big decisions. Camb Q Healthc Ethics 2005;14(4):389–403.

65. Rashotte J. Dwelling with stories that haunt us: Building a meaningful nursing practice. Nurs Inq 2005;12(1):34–42.

66. Rushton CH. A framework for integrated pediatric palliative care: Being with dying. J Pediatr Nurs 2005;20(5):311–325.

67. Browning D. To show our humanness—relational and communicative competence in pediatric palliative care. Bioethics Forum 2002;18(3–4):23–28.

68. Browning DM, Solomon MZ. Relational learning in pediatric palliative care: Transformative education and the culture of medicine. Child Adolesc Psychiatr Clin N Am 2006;15(3):795–815.

69. McNeilly P, Read S, Price J. The use of biographies and stories in paediatric palliative care education. Int J Palliat Nurs 2008;14(8):402–406.

70. Romanoff BD, Thompson BE. Meaning construction in palliative care: The use of narrative, ritual, and the expressive arts. Am J Hosp Palliat Care 2006;23(4):309–316.

71. Pridham K, Limbo R, Schroeder M, Krolikowski M, Henriques J. A continuing education program for hospital and public health nurses to guide families of very low birthweight infants in caregiving. J Contin Educ Nurs 2006; 37(2):74–85.

72. Davies B, Sehring SA, Partridge JC, et al. Barriers to palliative care for children: Perceptions of pediatric health care providers. Pediatrics 2008;121(2):282–288.

# 59

*Mary Layman Goldstein and Mayuko Sakae*

# Pediatric Pain: Knowing the Child Before You

*It's so painful and I'm embarrassed. I can't do anything about it. My brother and one of the nurses thinks it's funny. Nobody knows how much I hurt!—Alex , age 14 with sickle-cell disease, on being admitted with painful priapism*

♦ **Key Points**
♦ *Pain assessment depends on the child's age and cognitive developmental stage.*
♦ *Analgesic doses are initiated according to the child's chronological age and body weight (milligrams or micrograms per kilogram).*
♦ *Pain management plans are based on the child's past experiences, developmental level, present response, and physical, emotional, and cultural factors.*
♦ *The child and parent are the unit of care. Parental involvement is key to successful interventions. Parents/caregivers must be included in assessment and pain management plans.*

Pain, a source of suffering, is present in many children—those who are facing a potentially life-threatening illness and those who are not. Expert pain management is a necessary part of pediatric palliative care.[1] It is possible for very young children to feel and express pain. A child's ability to communicate pain is influenced by age and cognitive level.[2] Even a preverbal child can communicate pain. To effectively manage an individual child's pain, the nurse first must be aware of the possibility of pain, sensitively observe the child, and use developmentally-appropriate, objective assessments. Developmental factors (physical, emotional, and cognitive) play an important role in both pediatric pain assessment and pain management. Through knowledge of these factors and an awareness of how they affect an individual child, it is possible for nurses to effect better management of each child's pain (Table 59–1). Despite a significant increase in interest and in the study of pediatric pain and its control over the last 20 years, there often remains a gap between what is technically possible and what is clinically practiced.[3]

## Definitions of Pain and Other Relevant Terms

There are two very useful definitions of pain. The first states that pain is "an unpleasant emotional experience associated with actual or potential tissue damage or described in terms of such damage."[4] The second, which stresses the subjective nature of pain and was stated by Margo McCaffery, RN, in 1968, is that "pain is whatever the experiencing person says it is, experienced whenever they say they are experiencing it."[5]

Nociception is "the perception by the nerves of injurious influences or painful stimuli."[6] This term is frequently used in discussions of pain in the neonate because of the challenges in evaluating the newborn's ability to be conscious to the perception of pain. A neonate is a newborn baby who may be preterm or up to age 1 month.[7]

**Table 59–1**
**Questions to Answer When Evaluating a Child with Pain**

| Useful Questions | Clinical Implications of Answers |
|---|---|
| What is the chronological age of this child? | Age-related physiological development affects pharmacokinetic and pharmacodynamic effects of medications.<br>In the neonate, normal neuroanatomical and neurobiological developmental processes occur and allow for transmission of painful stimuli. |
| What is the developmental stage of this child?<br>• Neonate<br>• Infant<br>• Toddler<br>• Preschooler/young child<br>• School-age child<br>• Adolescent | Developmental age helps determine.<br>• How a child might express his or her pain.<br>• Which assessment tools may be useful.<br>• What cognitive-behavioral techniques might be considered. |
| What type of pain does this child have?<br>• Acute pain<br>• Chronic pain<br>• Procedural pain | The particular situation can guide the clinician to a developmentally appropriate assessment tool and a situation-specific pain management plan that includes both pharmacological and nonpharmacological interventions. |
| Does this child have a chronic illness? | Certain painful conditions have disease-specific, validated pain assessment tools. For example, the Douleur Enfant Gustave Roussy (DEGR) scale is available to assess prolonged pain in 2- to 6-year-olds with cancer.[*] |
| Is this child neurologically impaired? | Cognitively impaired children may process information and communicate distress differently from normally developed children.[†]<br>Besides knowing the science, and the individual child, it may help to know other children with similar conditions.[‡]<br>New pain assessment tools for children with intellectual disabilities are being validated to look at generic, procedural, and surgical pain. |
| Does this child and do the parents of this child speak the same language as the health care providers? | Find ways of obtaining translators.<br>Some pain assessment tools are available in translated versions.<br>It may be worth having pain assessment tools translated into languages common to certain practice settings. |
| What is the underlying cause of this pain? | If the underlying cause is treatable, the pain may be reduced or eliminated. |
| What is the weight in kilograms of this child? | Dosage of analgesics is expressed in milligrams or micrograms per kilogram.<br>For some medications, the starting dose depends on the child's being larger or smaller than a set weight. |
| Is the oral route of drug administration used whenever possible? | Besides being a cheaper and less invasive route (with less potential for pain and infection), the oral route in children provides more reliable absorption. |
| Are there any obvious, outstanding barriers that may be playing a role in this child's pain assessment and management? | Some barriers can be directly and quickly addressed with minimal effect and maximal positive impact. |
| Have nonpharmacological pain interventions been considered? | Nonpharmacological pain interventions based on the etiology of a child's pain can improve the comprehensiveness and effectiveness of a pain management plan. |

*Sources:* *Gauvain-Piquard et al. (1999), reference 119; †Van Dongen et al. (2002), reference 120; ‡Hunt et al. (1995), reference 121.

The concept of Patient Controlled Analgesia (PCA) is well-established. What is less understood is the term PCA by Proxy. The American Society for Pain Management Nursing (ASPMS) defines that term as the "activation of the analgesic infusion pump by anyone other than the patient (p. 6)."[8] They further define the term Authorized Agent Controlled Analgesia (AACA) as "a method of pain control in which a consistently available and competent individual is authorized by a prescriber and properly educated to activate the dosing button of an analgesic infusion pump when the patient is unable, in response to that patient's pain (p. 6)."[8]

The authorized agent may be the nurse who is responsible for a particular patient. In that case, AACA could be Nurse Controlled Analgesia (NCA). Or, the authorized agent could be a nonprofessional person such as a parent or significant other and the method could be referred to as Caregiver Controlled Analgesia (CCA).[8] The term "PCA by Proxy" is not encouraged as it implies that a potentially unsafe, uneducated, unauthorized individual is activating a child's PCA pump.[9]

One term that is frequently encountered in the subject of pediatric pain is procedural pain. Procedural pain is pain that is caused by procedures (e.g., needlesticks, heel punctures, lumbar punctures). All children who interact with the health-care system potentially experience procedural pain.

Conscious sedation has been defined by the American Academy of Pediatrics[10] as "a medically controlled state of depressed consciousness that (1) allows protective reflexes to be maintained; (2) retains the patient's ability to maintain a patent airway independently and continuously; and (3) permits appropriate response by the patient to physical stimulation or verbal command (p. 1110)."

## Prevalence of Pain in Children

Clinicians working with children in the general pediatric area will encounter pain in children who are undergoing immunizations and procedures and those who have pharyngitis, oral viral infections, otitis media, urinary tract infections, headache, or traumatic injuries. Pain continues to be present in child with cancer at the end of life.[11,12] Conditions such as meningitis and necrotizing colitis can cause pain in children. Children who experience chronic diseases such as cancer, human immunodeficiency virus (HIV) infection, sickle cell disease (SCD), hemophilia, juvenile chronic arthritis (JCA), and cystic fibrosis (CF) also will have pain.[6,13,14] Cassidy reported that chronic pain syndromes in pediatric rheumatology have increased during the last 25 years.[15] Chronic musculoskeletal pain is thought to range from 10% to 35 % in children who are not clinically ill.[16] Juvenile primary fibromyalgia syndrome (JPFS) occurs frequently.[16,17] Definitive studies focusing on the prevalence of pain in the pediatric population are lacking. At best, we have studies that look at the incidence of pain in various disease subpopulations. Children with certain conditions are prone to particular pain syndromes. Nurses working with children need knowledge of the pain syndromes they may commonly encounter in the populations they work with and need to feel comfortable assessing and managing those particular pain syndromes.

## Etiology of Pain in Children

### Neuropathic Pain

Neuropathic pain is less common in children than in adults. Many of the neuropathic pain syndromes seen in adults are not seen as frequently in children. Children may experience neuropathic pain from migraine headaches, scar neuromas after surgery, phantom limb pain after amputations for trauma, tumors, meningococcemia, and complex regional pain syndromes (reported in preteen and teenage girls).[18,19] Although diabetes is increasing in incidence in the pediatric population, it is rare to see a child who has diabetic neuropathy, a syndrome that takes years to develop. Brachial plexus avulsion, an injury that sometimes occurs to babies during childbirth, is thought by some to be less disabling and painful in babies than when it occurs (for other reasons) in adults. It is not clear whether this is due to inadequate assessment of infants or to the physical developmental functions of babies.[18]

### Burns

Burns, thermal injuries caused by hot liquids, flames, and electricity, are among the most common causes of injury to children and are associated with pain. This injury, which destroys the skin, can have significant morbidity and mortality depending on the extent of the burn. Intact skin is necessary for protection against bacterial infection, fluid and electrolyte balance, and thermoregulation. Treatment of severe burns is associated with significant pain. Undertreatment of this pain can make it difficult for the child to cooperate with burn treatment. It is postulated that use in children of an individualized pain management plan with high-quality pain control components, such as intravenous opioids, local block, or even general anesthesia, can avoid the development of a postburn hyperalgesia syndrome caused by continuous or repeated stimulation of nociceptive afferent fibers.[20] Researchers are also looking to see if aggressive pain management decreases the development of posttraumatic stress disorder, a long-term morbidity issue for some children who have been burned.[21]

### Cancer

As recently as 1998, the World Health Organization (WHO) stated that 70% of children with cancer will experience severe pain during their illness.[22] The types of pain in children with cancer, whether caused by procedures, by the disease or tumor, or by anticancer treatment, have been well-described for many years.[22–25] This pain can be acute or chronic. Children with chronic cancer-related pain frequently experience break through pain.[26] A study by Ljungman and colleagues[27] of children receiving treatment for cancer revealed that procedure- and treatment-related pain were significant problems initially and that procedure-related pain gradually decreased, but treatment-related pain remained constant. In addition, children with cancer may have pain for unrelated reasons, such as acute appendicitis.[23]

All children with cancer are at risk for procedural pain. Most procedure-related pain involves needle puncture. This procedure may be necessary for obtaining blood supplies, accessing implanted venous devices, administering intravenous chemotherapeutics, or giving intramuscular or subcutaneous medications. Lumbar punctures (using a spinal needle) or bone marrow aspiration (involving insertion of a large needle into the posterior superior iliac spine) are variations of needle puncture.[23] Some children develop prolonged postlumbar puncture headaches.[22] Despite significant efforts to avoid needlesticks in the pediatric population, sometimes a needle puncture is necessary and cannot be avoided. Removal of tunneled central venous catheters or implanted ports also causes procedural pain and must be addressed by clinicians caring for the children undergoing this procedure.[23]

For some children, it is the experience of tumor-related pain that leads their parents to seek medical attention and eventual diagnosis. This pain can be nociceptive or neuropathic. Nociceptive pain can be somatic, caused by tumor involvement with bone or soft tissue, or visceral, caused by tumor infiltration, compression, or distention of abdominal or thoracic viscera. Neuropathic pain can be caused by tumor involvement (i.e., compression or infiltration) with the peripheral or central nervous system.

Most children who receive a diagnosis of cancer, no matter what the stage, will receive some sort of anti-cancer treatment. Frequently this treatment causes some sort of pain, either acute or chronic. Surgery leads to acute, postoperative pain. Removal of limbs may lead to the development of phantom limb sensations and pain. This experience is thought to decrease over time in children.[23] Radiation therapy may lead to an acute dermatitis or pain. Children undergoing chemotherapy are at risk acutely for mucositis pain and gastritis from repeated vomiting (if nausea and vomiting are not successfully controlled)[24] and chronically for neuropathic pain from certain chemotherapies. Children who have been treated with high doses of steroids are at risk for development of avascular necrosis, a disabling condition that eventually causes the affected bone to collapse. Some chemotherapies, such as vincristine, asparaginase, and cyclophosphamide, can cause pain or painful conditions such as peripheral neuropathy, constipation, hemorrhagic cystitis, or pancreatitis. Complications of intravenous chemotherapy administration may lead to pain from irritation, infiltration, extravasation, tissue necrosis (if vesicants are used), or the development of thrombophlebitis. Children receiving intrathecal chemotherapy may develop arachnoiditis or meningeal irritation, also painful conditions. The child who is immunocompromised, whether from chemotherapy or from disease, is at risk for infection and infection-related pain. Skin, perioral, and perirectal infections are common. Children seem to be at less risk for acute herpes zoster and its related pain.[23] Bone marrow transplantation may lead acutely to severe mucositis and potentially to chronic graft-versus-host disease, which may manifest as severe abdominal pain if it effects the gastrointestinal system.[23]

Medications used to prevent or modify side effects of primary disease treatment can have painful effects. Use of corticosteroids in disease treatment may lead to bone changes that cause pain.[22] Colony-stimulating factors may lead to medullary bone pain shortly after administration and before the onset of neutrophil recovery.

Nurses caring for patients receiving new treatment protocols need to be alert to the development of pain syndromes associated with particular agents. For example, in recent years, the use of 3F8, an anti-ganglioside monoclonal antibody, in the treatment of advanced neuroblastoma has significantly improved survival but causes an acute episode of neuropathic pain affecting random body parts during infusion.[23] As more is known about the effects of new treatment agents, more effective preventive measures can be taken to improve the quality of life of children undergoing potentially life-sustaining or life-extending therapy.

As children live longer with cancer, they may live longer with pain. Pediatric tertiary care centers, such as Children's Hospital of Boston, have reported a variety of chronic pain problems, including causalgia of a lower extremity, chronic lower extremity pain caused by a mechanical problem with an internal prosthesis, and avascular necrosis of multiple joints in long-term survivors of childhood cancers.[23]

## Human Immunodeficiency Virus Infection

Children with HIV infection may experience pain for a variety of reasons, including disease, treatment, and procedures. Some factors are quite similar to those associated with cancer-related pain, and some are unique to HIV disease. For example, children with the acquired immunodeficiency syndrome (AIDS) may have abdominal cramping pain due to AIDS-associated diarrhea.[13]

## Sickle Cell Disease

One of the most common genetic diseases in the United States, commonly affecting individuals of African, Middle Eastern, Mediterranean, and Indian descent, is highly associated with a variety of painful conditions. Sickle cell disease (SCD) is characterized by a predominance of hemoglobin S (HbS), which becomes sickle shaped (as opposed to donut shaped) after deoxygenation. It is this stiff, sickle-shaped red blood cell that becomes trapped in small blood vessels, leading to vaso-occlusion, tissue ischemia, and even infarction.[28]

Some of the many painful states that are commonly associated with SCD include acute painful events, acute hand-foot syndrome, acute inflammation of joints, acute chest syndrome, splenic sequestration, intrahepatic sickling or hepatic sequestration, avascular necrosis of femur or humerus, and priapism. The reader is directed to the American Pain Society's *Guidelines for the Management of Acute and Chronic Pain in Sickle Cell Disease* (pp. 3–7)[29] for a review of the clinical signs and symptoms of these and other common SCD pain states, their underlying causes, and special features or considerations. These episodes can vary in frequency and severity among and within individuals with SCD. Although most would be considered to be frequently recurring acute pain episodes, some, such as those caused by vertebral collapse or avascular necrosis of the femoral or humeral heads, can lead to chronic, debilitating painful conditions. A child with SCD may require hospitalization for pain control. A multicenter study by Platt and associates[30] showed that 39% of patients with SCD had no pain episode that required hospitalization, whereas 1% had to be hospitalized for pain more than six times in a single year. For patients age 20 years and older, being hospitalized more than three times per year for pain is associated with an increased incidence of death.[29] Inconsistent pain management for individuals with SCD clearly leads to increased morbidity and mortality for affected children and adults[31] (Dumaplin).

## Cystic Fibrosis

Cystic fibrosis (CF), an eventually fatal genetic disease that is diagnosed in 1 of every 3,000 live births, has a different trajectory than other lethal childhood diseases. Throughout their lives, children with CF simultaneously receive preventive care to preclude future complications, therapeutic care to reverse the progress of current lung disease, and palliative care to relieve symptoms. Because of advances in medical science, individuals with CF are living longer and longer. Although they are most frequently cared by pediatric specialists, individuals with CF may live to be age 20, 30, or even 40 years. A study by Robinson and others[32] retrospectively reviewed the care received by 44 patients older than age 5 years with CF before their deaths from respiratory failure. Thirty-eight patients received opioids for chest pain or dyspnea or both. Although the pain present was not thoroughly described, the fact that it was noted is significant information for those who care for CF populations.

## Other Conditions Associated with Pain in Children

Other conditions children experience that may be associated with pain include muscular dystrophy and other degenerative neurological diseases and severe dermatological conditions.[33] A recent study of children with hemiplegic cerebral palsy identified from a population register revealed that 33% had mild pain and 18% had moderate-to-severe pain.[34] We continue to learn more about the prevalence, distribution, and description of pain syndromes in many life-threatening illnesses in children, but for many illnesses these facts have yet to be determined. This shortcoming may be a result of assessment difficulties in infants, preverbal children, and children with communication impairments. Or, it may be a consequence of the often single-minded focus on cure. As clinical interest broadens to also include increased attention to the comfort of these children, it is hoped that the pain and its treatment will be better defined and practiced.[13]

## Physiology and Pathophysiology of Pain in Children

Important factors relevant to the physiology and pathophysiology of pain are well covered in Chapter 7. Those working with children need to be aware of the normal neuroanatomical and neurobiological developmental processes that occur in neonates and allow for the development of transmission of painful stimuli (Table 59–2). It is possible to assess the severity of pain and the effects of analgesics in neonates. Neonates who do not cry, move, or show other behavioral response in response to painful stimuli may still be experiencing pain. It has been shown that increased neonatal morbidity may result from prolonged or severe pain. It has been shown that neonates who experience pain may respond differently to pain later on (e.g., pain from inoculation) than do those who have not experienced previous painful events.[7]

## Assessment of Pain in Children

The assessment of pain in children is a dialogue between the clinician, the child, and the parents. Through a series of questions, the nurse learns who the child in front of him or her is and how best to address this individual child's pain. To do this, nurses assessing pain in children, from preterm neonates through adolescents, need to be aware of barriers and other influencing factors that play a role in accurate, developmentally appropriate assessment.

Barriers to pain control in children are similar to those in adults. They primarily relate to (1) lack of assessment; (2) inadequate analgesics; (3) incorrect attitudes or misconceptions by patients, their families, or health-care providers about pain and its management; and (4) issues related to systems.[2,35] Table 59–3 reviews these barriers in detail.

To best assess and manage a child's pain, the nurse must ask a series of questions that lead him or her to better know who a particular child is. One of the first questions is, "What is the child's chronological age and what is his or her developmental stage?" Is this child a neonate, infant, toddler, preschooler/young child, school-age child, or adolescent? Nurses who work exclusively with children know that the answers to these questions have a huge impact on how a child is approached. Nurses who do not may find the review of developmental stages and factors relevant to pain useful (see Table 59–2). The following case study may also be helpful.

CASE STUDY
*Devon, 11 Months Old With Recurrent Otitis Media*

Devon is an 11-month-old with his fourth otitis media since birth. His mother reports that he had just finished his course of antibiotics 10 days ago but started having fever 2 days prior to presenting in Pediatric emergency room on Saturday night. She gave him Infant Tylenol every 4 hours, but it would only seem to relieve his pain for less than 2 hours, and he would start fussing, crying, tugging, and pulling at his right ear. He refused to eat and had only two wet diapers that day. He starts grimacing when a pediatrician approaches his right side with an otoscope, and upon otoscope insertion into the external ear canal, Devon starts screaming, kicking, and bashing his arms and legs about, shaking his head. His heart rate is 137 bpm. He has

**Table 59–2**
**Pain-Related Developmental Milestones**

| Age | Development | Assessment and Management Implications |
|-----|-------------|----------------------------------------|
| 7 wk gestation | Pain receptors present[*] | |
| 20 wk gestation | Full compliment of neurons in cerebral cortex[*]<br>Pain receptors spread to all cutaneous and mucosal surfaces[*] | |
| 26 wk gestation | Can respond to tissue injury as demonstrated by "specific behavioral, autonomic, hormonal, and metabolic signs of stress and distress" (p. 1094) due to sufficient development of peripheral, spinal, and supraspinal afferent pain transmission pathways[†] | |
| 30 wk gestation | Myelination usually complete[*]<br>Slower transmission of pain thought to be offset by decreased distance the impulse must travel[*] | |
| 40 wk gestation | Descending, inhibitory pathways, which alter and modulate pain perception, present[*] | |
| Neonate (preterm through 1 mo) | **Acute pain responses:**<br>• Physiological measures, such as increase in vital signs, are similar to those of older children and adults<br>• Behavioral indicators include vocalizations (crying, whimpering, groaning), facial expression changes (grimaces, furrowed brow, quivering chin, tightly closed eyes, squarish open mouth), body movement and posture (thrashing, limb withdrawn, fist clenched, flaccidity), and other behavior changes (sleep/wake cycle, feeding, activity, irritability or listlessness)[*]<br>• Chronic responses can include changes or disruptions in usual feeding, activity, and sleep/wake patterns | • Challenging to differentiate symptoms of pain (a stressful situation) from other life-threatening situations such as hypoxemia[‡]<br>• Validated composite measures include the Neonatal Infant Pain Scale, or NIPS[§]; the CRIES postoperative pain tool[§] (C = crying; R = requires increased oxygen administration; I = increased vital signs; E = expression; S = sleeplessness) and the Premature Infant Pain Profile, or PIPPS[¶]<br>• One-dimensional pain assessment measure: Neonatal Facial Coding System[#]<br>• Measures do not address neonates with chronic pain, those pharmacologically paralyzed for mechanical ventilation, or those with significant facial deformity[‡] |
| | **Physiological developmental issues[†]:**<br>• Increased water and volume of distribution for water-soluble medications<br>• Decreased fat and muscle<br>• Immature hepatic enzyme systems, leading to decreased metabolic clearances<br>• Decreased glomerular filtration rates, producing accumulation of renally excreted medications and active metabolites<br>• Many factors in respiratory function lead to increased risk of hypoventilation, atelectasis, or respiratory failure | • Need for increased dosing interval or decreased rates of infusion for many medications[†]<br>• Vulnerable to effects of decreased ventilatory reflexes[†] |
| Infants (older than 1 mo) | **Acute pain responses:**<br>• Behavioral changes, physiological responses, and facial responses of neonates exhibited[*]<br>• May cry loudly, thrash, arch, or exhibit body rigidity[*]<br>• Local reflex withdrawal of stimulated area in young infants[*]<br>• Deliberate withdrawal of affected area in older infants[*]<br>• Development of stranger anxiety after 7 mo[**] | • Examine infants older than 1 mo in parent's lap[**]<br>• Children's Hospital of Eastern Ontario Pain Scale (CHEOPS)[††] |
| | **Physiological developmental issues[†]:**<br>• Immature hepatic enzyme systems, leading to decreased metabolic clearances<br>• From birth to 7 mo, decreased glomerular filtration rates produce accumulation of renally excreted medications and active metabolites<br>• By 8 to 12 mo, renal blood flow, glomerular filtration, and tubular secretion increase to near adult values<br>• Many factors in respiratory function lead to increased risk of hypoventilation, atelectasis, or respiratory failure | • Need for increased dosing interval or decreased rates of infusion for many medications[†]<br>• Vulnerable to effects of decreased ventilatory reflexes in response to opioids or sedatives[†] |

*(continued)*

**Table 59–2**
**Pain-Related Developmental Milestones** (*continued*)

| Age | Development | Assessment and Management Implications |
|---|---|---|
| Toddlers | Behavioral changes (such as changes in eating, play/activity, and sleep/wake patterns) and physiological responses as described in neonates[*]<br>May also cry intensely, be verbally aggressive, or withdraw from play or social interaction[*,**]<br>May have words for pain by 18 mo[††]<br>Stranger anxiety persists[**]<br>From age 2 to 6 y, children have a larger liver mass per kilogram of body weight and this is thought to increase metabolic clearance of many medications | Give toddler time to get used to you and build trust[**]<br>Use play and minimized physical contact during physical assessment[**]<br>Language development varies and it is best to use words for pain that are most familiar to a particular child[**]<br>Often it is beneficial to have parents present during assessment and procedures[‡‡]<br>By age 2 y, dosing intervals may be decreased or infusion rates increased because of increased metabolic clearance[†] |
| Preschooler (young child, age 3–6 y) | Behavioral changes (such as changes in eating, play/activity, and sleep/wake patterns) and physiological responses as described in neonates[*]<br>Developmentally able to give meaningful, concrete information about location and severity of pain[‡,‡‡]<br>Able to anticipate painful events/procedures[*]<br>Behaviors may include clinging, lack of cooperation, attempts to push painful stimuli away before their application[*]<br>"Magical thinking" (mixes facts and fiction)[‡‡]<br>Pain may be viewed as a punishment or as a source of secondary gain[*]<br>From age 2 to 6 y, children have a larger liver mass per kilogram of body weight and this is thought to increase metabolic clearance of many medications | Physical and emotional support by adults present, especially parents, may be comforting<br>Consider building on "magical thinking" abilities when initiating nonpharmacological interventions[‡‡]<br>Offer realistic choices if possible, and provide positive reinforcement[**]<br>By age 2 y, dosing intervals may be decreased or infusion rates increased because of increased metabolic clearance[†] |
| School-age child | Behavioral changes (such as changes in eating, play/activity, and sleep/wake patterns) and physiological responses as described in neonates[*]<br>May exhibit rigid muscularity (gritted teeth, contracted limbs, stiff body, closed eyes, or wrinkled forehead)<br>May demonstrate more stalling behaviors to delay potentially painful experiences<br>Continued normal cognitive development influences ability to both report and learn information<br>May demonstrate influences of cultural group[*] | Child able to use more objective measures of pain, give more specific and detailed reports<br>Able to use more cognitive coping methods, including educational interventions<br>Cultural beliefs may influence child's pain experience[*] |
| Adolescent | Behavioral changes (such as changes in eating, play/activity, and sleep/wake patterns) and physiological responses as described in neonates[*]<br>May show more decreased motor activity in presence of pain<br>Continued normal cognitive development<br><br>Increased influence of peers and cultural group[*]<br>Increased needs for privacy and independence[**]<br>Adolescent not legally independent (except in special cases) but needs to have a larger emerging role in his or her care[**] | May deny pain in presence of peers<br>May be influenced by cultural factors regarding interpretations and expressions of pain[*,§§]<br>Parents remain advocate for child but teenagers, if they so desire, need to be involved in decision making[**] |

*Sources:* [*]Hockenberry et al. (2007), reference 6; [†]Berde and Sethna (2003), reference 48; [‡]American Academy of Pediatrics (2000), reference 7; [§]Lawrence et al. (1993), reference 122; [||]Krechel and Bildner (1995), reference 123; [¶]Stevens et al. (1996), reference 102; [#]Grunau and Craig (1990), reference 124; [**]Levetown (2000), reference 125; [††]Children's Hospital of Eastern Ontario Pain Scale, reference 126; [‡‡]Franck et al. (2000), reference 40; [§§]Hockenbery-Eaton et al. (1999), reference 81.

**Table 59–3**
**Pediatric-Specific Barriers to Pain Control**

| Issue | Barrier/Misconception |
|---|---|
| Inadequate assessment | *Misconception:* infants and children do not feel pain in the same way as adults do[*] |
| | *Misconception:* Children unable to provide useful, accurate information about the location and severity of their pain[†] |
| | Lack of knowledge about how to assess pediatric pain[†] |
| | Challenge of pain assessment in preverbal or noncommunicating children |
| | Choosing the correct population specific tool |
| Inadequate analgesics ordered or administered | Need for comprehensive assessment with pain etiology and contributing or modifying factors identified |
| | Need to select most appropriate medications, doses, dosing intervals, and route of administration for situation |
| | Nurses or parents may not administer the complete dose ordered or as frequently as ordered |
| | Prescriber's reluctance to send children home with the effective opioids that the child received while hospitalized[‡] |
| Incorrect attitudes or misconceptions by patients, families, or health care providers about pain and its management | Pain control in children too difficult or time-consuming[*] |
| | Lack of knowledge or incorrect knowledge of pharmacokinetics and pharmacodynamics of analgesics, especially opioids[†] |
| | Lack of knowledge of the consequences of unrelieved pain[†] |
| | *Misconception:* Children can tolerate pain better than adults can (this can lead to heightened pain and anxiety about pain control)[†] |
| | Fear of opioid-related side effects and lack of knowledge about how to manage them can also prevent appropriate use of opioids in children[†] |
| Systems-related issues | Need for systematic re-evaluation and reassessment of pain management plan's effectiveness[†] |
| | No systematic, evidenced-based approach to pain management despite rigorous approach to other aspects of a child's care, including disease diagnosis and treatment |
| | Lack of appropriate use of nondrug therapies to complement or supplement the pharmacological interventions[†] |
| | Lack of knowledge by health care professionals of simple and practical physical, cognitive, or behavioral strategies that can give children and their families more control and less anxiety about pain management |
| | Lack of clear delineation of who is responsible for a particular child's pain control, leading to gaps in management[†] |

*Sources:* [*]American Academy of Pediatrics (2001), reference 36; [†]McGrath and Brown (2004), reference 2; [‡]Field and Behrman (2003), reference 13.

sunken eyes and is crying without tears. He is admitted for IV hydration, antibiotics, maximum dose of Motrin q6h, and auralgan drops.

Other influencing factors that may make the assessment of pain challenging are language or cultural differences between the child or family and the health-care providers; the presence of chronic health conditions, developmental disabilities, cognitive, sensory, or motor impairments; and severe emotional disturbance.[36,37] Factors that can complicate the communication between a child and the health-care team increase the likelihood of suboptimal pain control.

In learning who an individual child is and what would work best in managing his/her pain, the nurse needs to talk with both the parents and the child. Although parents have varying abilities to recognize pain and its severity in their child, there is probably no one more sensitive to changes in their child's behavior or more motivated in looking out for the health and well-being of a child than his or her parents.[6] Researchers are beginning to explore maternal pain-related behavior in an effort to better understand chronic pediatric pain in the social context.[38] Hester and Barcus[39] developed a series of practical questions for both the child and the parents that reviews the pain experience of a particular child. With the child, the nurse explores what pain or hurt is to this particular child, whether he/she communicates the pain to others, what relieves the pain, what the child finds helpful, what the child wants to avoid from others when he or she is in pain, and anything unique to how the child acts when in pain. With the parents, the nurse explores the language a child uses and the behavior the parents observe when their child is in pain. The nurse reviews what painful experiences the child has had, how the child reacts, what tends to relieve a child's pain (including what the child does and what the parents do for the child), and any other special information about the child when he or she is in pain. By using this questionnaire, a nurse is better able to get a complete picture of the child in pain.

Choosing an appropriate tool that will be useful in particular clinical situations can be challenging at best. In choosing a tool, the developmental age of the child should be considered first, and then the type of pain or medical situation or illness that the child will be experiencing. Attempts at measurement of pain include physiological measures, behavioral observations, composite measures and self-report. Physiological measures may reflect the response to the stress of pain and not the pain itself. Although they are far from ideal, physiological measures are often used in situations in which the child is unable to report pain for himself or herself. Acute pain is often associated with increases of 10% to 20% in noninvasively measured blood pressure, heart rate, or respiratory rate. These changes may not be present in the child with chronic pain.

Observational pain assessment tools, also used when a child cannot self-report pain, are criticized for possibly measuring distress behavior instead of pain behavior.[40] Observational or behavioral scales are most often used in preverbal or cognitively-impaired children. The pain behaviors specific to certain conditions may be useful, such as the observation of guarding, bracing, and active rubbing in children with JCA.[41] The Pediatric Initiative on Methods, Measurement, and Pain Assessment in Clinical Trials (www.immpact.org) recently commissioned a review of observational scales of pain for children age 3 to 18 years with the purpose of identifying which scales might be used as an outcome measure in clinical trials. Although this review identified tools that were useful in specific acute pain situations, such as post-operative pain assessment in the hospital, it concluded that no single observational measure can be recommended for pain assessment across all contexts.[42]

Self-report measures, by far the most preferable, can be obtained in some children as young as age 3 years and generally by 6 years. Most pediatric self-report tools are not multidimensional and measure only pain intensity.[23] To adequately report detailed ratings of pain intensity, a child, usually of school age or older, must understand the concepts of order and numbering. To test this knowledge, a child could be given six different-sized pieces of paper and asked to place them in order from smallest to largest.[40] If a 0-to-10 scale is used, with 0 being no pain and 10 being the worst possible pain, older children and adolescents may be asked to rate their pain with an number and then asked, "Do you consider your pain to be none, slight, moderate, severe, or excruciating?" The comparison between the child's numeric pain rating and the categorical pain rating ideally will show some general agreement. Readers attempting to narrow their choices of pain assessment tools are referred to detailed reviews of pediatric pain assessment tools found in several references.[6,40,43,44]

The case study below demonstates a child who is able to self-report.

CASE STUDY
*Jimmie, A 9-Year-Old with Streptococcal Pharyngitis*

Jimmie is a 9-year-old with severe pharyngitis, able to quantify and describe his pain. He states that his throat became constantly hot and sore last night and today his pain is 8 out of 10; when trying to swallow even his own saliva, he experiences "sharp pain," and his pain level goes up to 10 out of 10. Upon exam, he has bilateral tonsillar erythema, enlargement, and exudates. Rapid Strep test in the office is positive. Because his mother thinks he cannot even swallow liquid amoxicillin, he is treated with a single dose of bicillin IM and discharged home.

In any one practice setting, it may be necessary to use several tools because of the broad range of child development and cognitive disabilities that may be present. In the ongoing stress of pain and illness, a child may regress cognitively and emotionally, which may necessitate the use of a simpler tool. This may also happen when a child is rendered cognitively impaired from medications administered. At present, there is a need for research that can make pain assessment tools more generalizable, with improvement of both specificity and sensitivity.[40,42]

Assessment for pain begins with screening for the possibility of pain. This can occur in a systematic way every time a child enters a health-care system through the use of documentation tools that ask about the presence of pain. In addition to the collection of this information in an initial nursing database, hospitalized children may be screened more than once a day for the new development of pain or for the presence of unsatisfactory pain control.[45] The so-called QUESTT approach to pediatric pain assessment is a self-explanatory one that summarizes the points stressed in this section and also leads to action and re-evaluation.[46] A slightly adapted version consists of the following:

Question the child and parent.
Use pain rating scales appropriate to developmental stage of the child and to the situation at hand.
Evaluate behavioral and physiological changes.
Secure parents' involvement.
Take the cause of pain into account.
Take action and evaluate results.

In every practice setting, a child with pain needs reassessment on a regular ongoing basis to improve or maintain the management of his or her pain.

## Management

No matter what the practice setting, one of the main principles in pediatric pain management is to anticipate and prevent pain whenever possible. If that is not possible, the next principle is to minimize the pain by treating the underlying disease (if possible), using pharmacological and nonpharmacological modalities as appropriate, and choosing the least painful necessary procedures.

## Pharmacological Management

Nurses working with children with pain must be aware of age-related physiological trends that are relevant to analgesic action and have an impact on dosage prescribed. Many pediatric analgesic studies in children are limited because they include a wide age range of children. The use of different age groups makes it challenging at best to distinguish between the effects of developmentally dependant physiological processes that play a role in analgegic effects.[47] The physiological processes that are involved include the body compartments, hepatic enzyme systems for medication metabolism, plasma protein binding, renal filtration and excretion of medications and their metabolites, and metabolic rate, oxygen consumption, and respiratory function.[48] Table 59–2 presents some of these developmental physiological changes and their clinical implications. Tables 59–4, 59–5, and 59–6 suggest starting doses for opioids and nonopioids that reflect these developmental aspects of pediatric pharmacology.

Although studies indicate that with proper age-related adjustments and dosing, children can safely receive pain medication, it is important to bear in mind that approximately 50% to 75% of medications used in pediatric medicine, including analgesics, have not been adequately studied to provide appropriate labeling information.[49] Clinicians who treat the pain of children have diligently tried to extrapolate data from experience with adults to determine what medications should be used and at what doses in children. This uncontrolled, undocumented, and unsystematic practice of off-label use, although well intended, is a systems problem that does not allow for medications used in children to be studied with sound scientific and ethical principles. It does not allow for the definition of age-dependent differences in pharmacokinetics and pharmacodynamics or for the establishment of which adverse events in children are similar to those in adults and which ones are unique to pediatric patients. This situation frequently occurs because of a result of lack of resources. The pediatric market is but a small segment of the total pharmaceutical market, and there is limited financial incentive to study medications in children.[50] Fortunately, the limited pharmacokinetic data that is available in children is steadily increasing and will assist clinicians in making appropriate medication choices for individual children.[51]

There are three main groups of medications used to treat pain in children: (1) nonopioids (acetaminophen, nonsteroidal antiinflammatory drugs [NSAIDs], and aspirin), (2) opioids, and (3) adjuvant analgesics. Use of these medications depends on the severity and cause of pain in an individual child. The nonopioids and opioids are most helpful in the treatment of nociceptive pain, and adjuvant analgesics work best for specific neuropathic pain. A general review of these medications and their use is presented in Chapter 6. What follows in this section are factors that are most relevant to the use of these drugs in children.

In 1998, the WHO published guidelines for cancer pain relief and palliative care in children.[22] They stressed four key concepts of analgesic use in children: "by the ladder, by the clock, by the appropriate route, and by the child" (p. 24). "By the ladder" refers to approaching a child's pain based on the presenting severity of pain, with steps clearly delineated for mild, moderate, and severe pain. For mild pain, nonopioids are indicated, with the addition of an adjuvant analgesic if a neuropathic contribution to the pain is suspected. If a child presents with or progresses to moderate pain, the nonopioid is continued (if not contraindicated), an appropriate adjuvant is continued if a neuropathic component is likely, and codeine, a "weak" opioid, is added to the child's analgesic

---

**Table 59–4**
**Nonopioid Drugs for Relief of Cancer Pain in Children**

| Drug | Dosage | Remarks |
|------|--------|---------|
| Paracetamol | 10–15 mg/kg orally, q4–6h | Has no gastrointestinal or hematological side effects, but lacks antiinflammatory activity. |
| Ibuprofen | 5–10 mg/kg orally, q6–8h | Antiinflammatory activity, but may have gastrointestinal and hematological side effects. |
| Naproxen | 5 mg/kg orally, q8–12h | Antiinflammatory activity, but may have gastrointestinal and hematological side effects. |

*Source:* World Health Organization (1998), reference 22.

**Table 59–5**
**Oral Dosage Guidelines for Commonly Used Nonopioid Analgesics**

| Drug | Dose Child <60 kg | Dose Child ≥60 kg | Interval | Maximum Daily Dose Child <60 kg | Maximum Daily Dose Child ≥60 kg |
|------|------|------|------|------|------|
| Acetaminophen | 10–15 mg/kg | 650–1000 mg | 4 h | 100 mg/kg[*] | 4000 mg |
| Ibuprofen | 6–10 mg/kg | 400–600 mg[†] | 6 h | 40 mg/kg[†,‡] | 2400 mg[†] |
| Naproxen | 5–6 mg/kg[†] | 250–375 mg[†] | 12 h | 24 mg/kg[†,‡] | 1000 mg[†] |
| Aspirin | 10–15 mg/kg[†,§] | 650–1000 mg[†] | 4 h | 80 mg/kg[†,‡,§] | 3600 mg[†] |

[*]The maximum daily doses of acetaminophen for infants and neonates are a subject of current controversy. Provisional recommendations are that daily dosing should not exceed 75 mg/kg for infants, 60 mg/kg for full-term neonates and preterm neonates of >32 wk postconceptional age. Fever, dehydration, hepatic disease, and lack of oral intake may all increase the risk of hepatotoxicity.

[†]Higher doses may be used in selected cases for treatment of rheumatological conditions in children.

[‡]Dosage guidelines for neonates have not been established.

[§]Aspirin carries a risk of provoking Reye's syndrome in infants and children. If other analgesics are available, aspirin should be restricted to indications for which an antiplatelet or antiinflammatory effect is required, rather than being used as a routine analgesic or antipyretic in neonates, infants, or children. Dosage guidelines for aspirin in neonates have not been established.

*Source:* Berde and Sethna (2003), reference 48, with permission.

regimen. If this proves ineffective, or if severe pain is present, the codeine is rotated to morphine or another opioid for moderate to severe pain and titrated to effect, with the rest of the regimen continued as appropriate.

"By the clock" reflects the concept that for pain that is almost continuous, a child will benefit most from nearly continuous analgesics administered on a regular schedule. This method promotes better pain control and decreases a child's anxiety regarding uncontrolled pain. "By the appropriate route" promotes the administration of analgesics by the simplest, most effective, least painful route. For most children this is the oral route, but for some situations other routes may be more effective. "By the child" indicates the need for individualization of each child's analgesic regimen. Starting doses listed on tables are just that—starting doses. Each child's dose must be titrated up or down based on his or her response. If uncontrolled pain is present, opioids should be titrated upward until analgesic relief is obtained or unmanageable side effects occur.

A prospective pediatric cancer pain management study that followed 240 hospitalized children with a median age of 9 years demonstated that safe, effective pain control can be achieved by closely following the WHO-guidelines.[52] Although the WHO guidelines were developed for the control of cancer pain, the four concepts can be applied to the use of analgesics in children in other chronic painful circumstances.

## Use of Nonopioids in Children

Nonopioids (acetaminophen, NSAIDs, and aspirin) have a ceiling effect and cannot be safely titrated beyond the dose per weight given at drug-specific intervals. Pediatric dosage guidelines for commonly used nonopioid analgesics can be found in Tables 55–4 and 55–5.

Aspirin is not routinely used as an analgesic in infants and children because of the risk of Reye's syndrome associated with its use in this population. The most widely-used mild analgesic for children is acetaminophen.[48] The recommended weight-based dosing of acetaminophen in children is based on the dose response for antipyretic effects, because the pediatric analgesic dose response is unavailable.[23] Currently there is no safety data on long-term acetaminophen use in children.[53] NSAIDs have been shown to be safe and effective analgesics for children. Children using NSAIDs have been shown to have greater weight-normalized clearance and volumes of distribution than adults but with similar drug half-lives. In order to decrease the change of dosage error and toxicitys, parents need to be educated regarding the proper use and administration of acetaminophen and NSAIDs.[54] Selective cyclooxygenase-2 inhibitors are not yet approved for use with children. Large-scale studies looking at the efficacy and risk-benefit and cost-benefit ratios of selective cyclooxygenase-2 inhibitors in children have yet to be done.[48,55]

## Use of Opioids in Children

There is growing evidence, beyond case studies, that supports the use of specific opioids in children and adolescents.[47,56–61] It takes until the age of 2 to 6 months for the weight-normalized clearance of many opioids to reach mature levels. Pharmacokinetic studies of morphine show an average serum half-life of 9 hours in preterm neonates, decreasing to 6.5 hours in full-term neonates and finally reaching 2 hours in the older infant. If not carefully monitored, neonates may be more likely to develop side effects from morphine due to decreased

**Table 59–6**
**Opioid Analgesic Dosage Guidelines for Opioid-Naïve Patients**[*]

| Opioid (Biological Half-life) | Equianalgesic Doses[†] | | Usual Intravenous or Subcutaneous Starting Dose[‡] | | Parenteral/ Oral Dose Ratio | Usual Oral Starting Dose[‡] | |
|---|---|---|---|---|---|---|---|
| | Parenteral | Oral | Child <50 kg | Child ≥50 kg | | Child <50 kg | Child ≥50 kg |
| **Short-half-life opioids** | | | | | | | |
| Codeine (2.5–3 h) | 130 mg | 200 mg | N/R | N/R | 1:1.5 | 0.5–1 mg/kg q3–4 h | 30 mg q3–4 h |
| Oxycodone (2–3 h) | N/A | 30 mg | N/A | N/A | N/A | 0.2 mg/kg q3–4 h | 5–10 mg q3–4 h |
| Pethidine[§] N/R (3 h) | 75 mg N/R | 300 mg N/R | 0.75 mg/kg q2–4 h N/R | 75–100 mg q2–4 h N/R | 1:4 | 1–1.5 mg/kg q3–4 h N/R | 50–75 mg q3–4 h N/R |
| Morphine (2.5–3 h) | 10 mg | 30 mg | *Bolus dose:* 0.05–0.1 mg/kg IV or SQ q2–4 h *Continuous infusion:* 0.03 mg/kg qh | *Bolus dose:* 5–10 mg IV or SQ q2–4 h *Continuous infusion:* 1 mg/h | 1:3 | 0.15–0.3 mg/kg q4 h | 5–10 mg q4 h |
| Hydromorphone (2–3 h) | 1.5 mg | 7.5 mg | 0.015 mg/kg q2–4 h | 1–1.5 mg/kg q2–4 h | 1:5 | 0.06 mg/kg q3–4 h | 2 mg q3–4 h |
| Oxymorphone (1.5 h) | 1 mg | N/A | 0.02 mg/kg q2–4 h | 1 mg q2–4 h | N/A | N/A | N/A |
| Fentanyl[‖] (3 h) | 100 mcg single dose | N/A | 0.5–2 mcg/kg qh as a continuous infusion | 25–75 mcg qh | N/A | N/A | N/A |
| **Long-half-life opioids** | | | | | | | |
| Controlled-release morphine | N/A | N/A | N/A | N/A | N/A | 0.6 mg/kg q8h or 0.9 mg/kg q12 h | 30–60 mg q12 h |
| Methadone[¶] (12–50 h) | 10 mg | 20 mg | 0.1 mg/kg IV or SQ q4–8 h | 5–10 mg IV or SQ q4–8 h | 1:2 | 0.2 mg/kg q4–8 h | 5–10 mg q4–8 h |

N/A, not applicable; N/R, not recommended.

[*]Important notes:

1. For all drugs for which a distinction is made between children <50 kg and those ≥50 kg, doses should be calculated in milligrams per kilogram for children <50 kg and the "usual adult dose" should be used for those ≥50 kg.

2. When a change is made to short-half-life opioids in an opioid-tolerant patient, the new drug should be given at 50% of the equianalgesic dose (because of incomplete cross-tolerance) and titrated to effect.

[†]Equianalgesic doses are based on single-dose studies in adults.

[‡]Usual starting dose is the commonly used standard dose and is not always based on equianalgesic principles (i.e., starting dose of hydromorphone may be 2 mg despite the parenteral ratio of 1:5). For infants <6 mo, starting doses should be ¼ to ⅓ of the suggested dose and titrated to effect.

[§]Pethidine is not recommended for chronic use because of its long half-life and the possibility of accumulation of a toxic metabolite.

[‖]Continuous infusion of fentanyl at 100 μg/h is approximately equianalgesic to a morphine infusion of 2.5 mg/h.

[¶]Methadone may cause irritation when administered SQ. Extreme care is needed when using methadone, both for initiation of therapy and when doses are increased, because of its extremely long biological half-life.

*Source:* World Health Organization (1998), reference 22, with permission.

renal clearance of metabolites. The respiratory reflex response to hypoxemia, hypercapnia, and airway obstruction does not reach full maturity until 2 to 3 months after birth in both full-term and preterm infants. This can lead the nonintubated neonate receiving opioids to be at higher risk for ventilatory depression.[48] Neonates receiving opioids or other agents that can compromise cardiorespiratory function must be continuously monitored in a setting that can quickly provide airway management. Those receiving prolonged opioid therapy may benefit from the use of continuous infusions to avoid the variation in plasma concentrations that occurs with bolus dosing. In neonates receiving synthetic opioids, the administration of infusions over several minutes or of small, frequent aliquots is recommended to avoid the adverse effects of glottic and chest wall rigidity that are associated with rapid bolus injection of medications such as fentanyl and sufentanil.[7]

When using opioids with infants, children, and adolescents, the goal is to control pain as quickly as possible. Repeated administration of small, ineffective doses that prolong the pain and worsen pain-related anxiety is to be discouraged. For moderate to severe pain, it is appropriate to use opioids such as morphine, fentanyl, and hydromorphone in optimal doses titrated to an individual child's response.[36] Initial pediatric opioid dose guidelines can be found in Table 59–6.

The following case illustrates how opioids can be given and adjusted for the benefit of an individual child.

CASE STUDY

*Andre, A 7-Year-Old with B-cell Lymphoma with Multiorgan Failure*

Andre is a 7-year-old with refractory B-cell lymphoma who failed third-line chemotherapy and first allogenic bone marrow transplant, and recently underwent a stem-cell transplant. He has mucositis, acute renal failure, pleural effusion, and chronic graft-versus-host-disease, is pancytopenic, confined to a negative pressure room in the Bone Marrow Transplant Unit. He has high fevers daily, severe diarrhea, excruciating attacks of abdominal pain, is on TPN, and requires oxygen most of the day. He initially received 0.05 mg/kg morphine IV PRN, but his pain level kept escalating requiring 0.15 mg/kg morphine Q2 hrs around the clock. He was started on morphine PCA and was titrated every 12 to 24 hours to comfort and started being able to rest without being awaken by sudden pain every hour. It also helped him with his air hunger. It also caused significant somnolence and his mother became very upset that he no longer had his normal attention span and alertness. He received dialysis daily and continued on multiple antibiotics and anti-fungal medications. Eventually he was on 75 mg/hr morphine and spent most of his day sleeping. His parents reported that after starting PCA, they felt comforted to see Andre no longer screamed in pain crisis and that he stopped having panic attacks in the middle of the night. Andre died peacefully in his sleep 2 months after his transplant in the bone marrow unit.

Any discussion of pain management in children with opioid analgesics would not be complete without a review of "PCA by Proxy" and AACA. PCA is well-established as a safe, effective method of pain control for children with moderate to severe pain in a variety of situations (including children in the last week of life). The risk of respiratoy depression is lessened because a child who is too sedated from his opioid pain medication would not be able to push the PCA dose button to give him or herself more.[62,63] When "PCA by Proxy" occurs, someone other than the patient pushes the dose button. The danger is that they may not be educated as to the appropriate use of a PCA pump and may overdose a patient who was not in need of the opioid medication. In 2004 the JCAHO issued a sentinel alert regarding this practice, and in 2005 the ISMP also issued a sentinel alert advising against this practice.

The challenge is that some children who are unable to push the dose button by thenselves would benefit from use of a PCA. Anghelescu[64] and colleagues identified four groups of patients who would benefit from AACA. They include those unable to control a PCA pump because of: *(1)* age (ususally <5 years) or cognitive ability; *(2)* neuromuscular impairment; *(3)* needing to undergo a painful procedure; and *(4)* being at the end of their life (p. 1625). These children are ususally opioid tolerant. The literature and the ASPMN advocate for AACM as a means of safe, effective pain control when a designated proxy is carefully chosen and educated about appropriate use of a PCA for an individual child.[8,9,64,65] Any organization or institution setting up AACM is referred to the recommendations of the ASOPMN along with Kenagy and Turner when writing their policies and procedures, when establishing criteria for proxy selection, patient monitoring, and education of proxy and health-care team members.

## Use of Adjuvant Analgesics in Children

Adjuvant analgesics are a heterogeneous group of medications that include psychostimulants, corticosteroids, anticonvulsants, antidepressants, radionuclides, and neuroleptics. Much of the evidence supporting their use in specific targeted pain syndromes comes from the adult literature. However, there has been some initial work looking at the use of adjuvants in children. The use of methylphenidate and dextroamphetamine in adolescents with cancer was reported to be safe, efficacious, and tolerable by Yee and Berde.[66] Intraarticular injection of corticosteroids is one of the mainstays of initial treatment of most children with JCA.[67] Although gabapentin has been studied as an anticonvulsant in children, it has yet to be investigated as an adjuvant analgesic in children despite widespread use as such.[2] A recent review article looking at the nonepileptic uses of antiepileptic drugs in children and adolescents concluded that although promising, there is insuffcient data (utilizing the Academy of Neurology's four-tiered classification scheme for a therapeutic article and translation to a recommendation rating) to recommend the use of antiepileptic medication for the treatment of pediatric neuopathic pain.[19] It is recommended that a child have baseline hematological and biochemical laboratory studies and an electrocardiogram performed to rule out Wolff-Parkinson-White syndrome and other cardiac conduction defects before initiation of tricyclic antidepressants and at periodic intervals if the child receives long-term therapy or exceeds standard dose/weight guidelines.[53] Ketamine, a phencyclidine derivative, has been established a useful medication to consider for procedural sedation and analgesia when used by individuals who are trained in pediatric analgesia in pediatric settings.[68,69] One case has been reported of the use of 131 iodine-meta-iodo-benzylguanidine to treat a boy's bone pain caused by neuroblastoma.[70] Future research in the use of adjuvant analgesics in the pediatric population is needed.

The following case is an example of the usefulness of adjuvant analgesics:

CASE STUDY

*Jonathan, 13-Year-Old with Spastic Quadriplegia Secondary to Near Drowning*

Jonathan is a 13-year-old male with static encephalopathy following a near drowning accident. Rescued after a 12-minute-long submersion, he was resuscitated with CPR by his father and EMS and woke up in PICU paralyzed 13 days later. Over the course of the following 2 years, he remained wheelchair-bound, and his arms and legs became progressively spastic. Unable to control the back and hip pain with worsening joint contractures, he was started on muscle relaxant and lortab elixir via PEG. The above medication combination made the general weakness worse and caused excessive sleepiness. After he had three episodes of aspiration pneumonia, he was referred to the Center for Pain Management at the local university hospital. He was placed on a baclofen pump and stopped missing school as frequently due to pain and discomfort as the time before the pump placement. He only needs to have the pump reloaded at an outpatient pain clinic and is able to stay home and continue his regular activities. After the baclofen pump placement, he has not been hospitalized for 16 months.

## Use of Local Anesthetics and Other Anesthetic Techniques

In the past, local anesthetics were not widely used in children because of concerns regarding cardiac depression and seizures. Today, they can be administered by a variety of routes and have acceptable safety as long as the maximum recommended doses are adhered to. For bupivacaine, with or without epinephrine, the maximum recommended dose is 2 mg/kg for neonates and 2.5 mg/kg for other children. The maximum recommended dose for lidocaine in neonates is 4 mg/kg without epinephrine or 5 mg/kg with epinephrine. For children, the maximum recommended dose of lidocaine with epinephrine is 5 to 7 mg/kg.[48]

Over the past 20 years, local anesthetics have been increasingly used to help prevent pain associated with needle puncture of skin.[71] Intradermal administration of lidocaine can be effectively used for skin anesthesia if painful punctures will occur. The lidocaine can be buffered with 1 part sodium bicarbonate to 10 parts 1% or 2% lidocaine to avoid the stinging effects of lidocaine administration.[6] Several preparations of local anesthetics can be obtained for topical or transdermal administration to control procedural pain. Of these, eutectic mixture of local anesthetics (EMLA) is available as a cream or anesthetic disc. One hour before puncture, the EMLA cream is placed over the potential site with an occlusive dressing applied to prevent or minimize puncture pain. Analgesic effectiveness is proportional to the amount of EMLA applied and the amount of time it is on prior to the needle stick.[71] Lidocaine/adrenaline/tetracaine (LAT) or tetracaine/phenylephrine may be applied to open wounds for suturing, providing skin anesthesia for approximately 15 minutes. LAT, because it contains adrenaline that causes vasoconstriction, must not be placed on distal arteries (located on tip of nose, earlobes, penis, fingers, and toes). "Numby Stuff" is a commercially available product that uses a novel delivery system, iontophoresis, to deliver 2% lidocaine and epinephrrine 1:100,000 approximately 10 mm into the skin. It takes approximately 10 minutes of use before dermal anesthesia is achieved. This device may be somewhat frightening to young children, who may not like feeling its mild current.[6] Recent advances in the technology of the noninvasive transdermal delievery systems has inproved the speed of analgesic onset to the benefit of children. Widespread clinical implimentaion will depend on several factors including cost, adverse effects/ events, and ease of use.[71]

The use of regional nerve blocks in anesthetized children to provide improved postoperative analgesia has expanded over the last 20 years and been shown to be both effective and safe.[48,72,73] This technique, which involves the injection of long-acting bupivacaine or ropivacaine into nerves that innervate a designated area, can also be used to provide local anesthesia for surgical procedures such as circumcision or reduction of fractures.[6,36]

Long-acting anesthetics (e.g., bupivacaine, ropivacaine) can be given intraspinally (epidurally or intrathecally) in children. Administration of epidural medications (opioids, local anesthetics, clonidine) can effectively control pain in children, including preterm neonates.[36,48] They are often given for postoperative pain control after specific procedures or in children with chronic pain who have not been helped by effective systemic therapy.[48] A case study of the use of an intraspinal infusion system in a 15-year-old girl dying of sarcoma demonstated its effectivness at the end of life in managing what had been intractable pain, minimizing side effects from systemic therapy, and symplifing a complex pain management plan. This allowed her to return home with her family to die in her country as they had desired.[74] The use of epidural analgesia in children requires special education and training on the part of the physicians and nurses. Careful calculation and administration of epidural medications and close postadministration observation with adequate nurse staffing are necessary to prevent serious complications. Nurses play a key role in setting the institutional standards for use of intraspinal analgesics in children.[2,7,48,75,76]

## Nonpharmacological Management

Nonpharmacological pain management interventions include psychological, physiatric, neurostimulatory, invasive, and integrative techniques. Components are frequently combined as part of a pediatric pain management plan; they are dependent on the comprehensive pain assessment of an individual child and are based on the presumed etiology of pain. In considering which nonpharmacological interventions might be beneficial, the nurse needs to look at several factors, including the child's and family's past experience with non-drug interventions. What has worked well and what has not? Are there religious or cultural issues or concerns that would make certain interventions inappropriate? Is the proposed intervention consistent with the developmental level of the child? What is the present cognitive status of the child? Has the stress and fatigue from a prolonged illness made it difficult for the child or family members to concentrate, follow directions, or learn new information? Also, the nurse should consider teaching potentially useful techniques before the skills are needed.[77]

Psychological interventions can include patient and family education, cognitive interventions, and behavioral techniques such as writing in a pain diary. Pain diaries may be especially useful in working with children who have recurrent or chronic pain, and their use has some value in pediatric pain research.[78] Children who enjoy writing may benefit from a private place to express themselves. Young children who have not mastered the written word may find drawing about their pain and pain experiences helpful.

The value of cognitive techniques such as distraction and relaxation is well established in children. A recent Cochrane review of the use of psychological nonpharmacological techniques found sufficient evidence to recommend using techniques such as coaching, distraction, and hypnosis to help children cope with procedural pain.[79] Across studies, distraction has been shown to reduce children's behavioral distress during procedural pain, although it has a variable effect on pain intensity. Various distractors have been used for children's pain management, including bubble-blowing, party blowers, puppetry, video games, and listening to music. The distractor is more likely to be effective if it is age-appropriate and complementary to the interests and preferences of the individual child.[80] Nurses working with infants and toddlers, to age 2 years, may distract them with mobiles, rocking, stroking, or patting. Children from 2 to 4 years of age may find blowing bubbles, breathing, puppet play, or storytelling useful distractions. Four- to six-year-olds like these activities and may also like television shows and talking about favorite places. School-age children can be distracted with these activities and may also be receptive to humor, counting, or thumb-squeezing. Progressive muscle relaxation exercise is used most effectively in older children and adolescents but can also be taught to children as young as age 5 years. Guided imagery, which ideally incorporates all of a child's senses, can help children "escape" to a safe favorite place unique to that child. Sometimes children like to imagine doing a favorite activity, such as swimming or skating.[81]

It is estimated that 30% to 84% of children use complimentary and alternative medicine such as acupuncture. Despite reports that acupuncture is offered in at least 30% of pediatric pain centers, there is little data regarding its use in children. It it postulated that this may be related to the possiblity of fear of needles that children may have.[82] More research is needed regarding the safety, efficacy and acceptability of the use of some complementary or integrative approaches (e.g., acupuncture) in children with pain in large, well-designed studies before these modalities can be routinely recommended. Such data can potentially establish other credible choices for assisting children with pain as well.[13,83–85]

Nurses caring for children with pain have both collaborative and independent functions when implementing nonpharmacological interventions. Psychological interventions that a nurse should feel comfortable initiating include patient-family education and cognitive techniques such as distraction, relaxation, positive self-statements, and pain diaries. An individual nurse might initiate the use of music as a relaxation or distraction technique. Independent physiatric interventions can include movement and positioning and swaddling of neonates. Collaborative efforts may involve massage, vibration, or use of superficial heat or cold. (Protecting the child's skin by placing the heat or cold source in commercially available animal wraps or using towels decorated with favorite characters may make the experience more enjoyable for young children.) The nurse needs to know which members of a child's primary team are knowledgeable in the use of nonpharmacological techniques and which special consultants are available to help if needed.[77] The American Massage Therapy Association (AMTA) is a resource in finding an accredited massage therapist.[86] Child-life specialists can be a resource for employing distraction and other psychological pain management techniques such as providing information/preparation, medical play, and positive reinforcement in children.[13,87] Promising cognitive techniques such as biofeedback and hypnosis, although potentially useful for children with chronic pain, require the use of trained instructors for initiation.[88] Also, more robust clinical studies of hypnosis and its effectiveness and acceptablity are needed prior to recommending it as part of a "best practice" guideline.[89,90]

The resources available to the nurse (including time available to initiate a particular intervention, education in a particular technique, availability of patient/family educational materials, and availability and affordability of particular devices) play a role in what techniques are initiated with an individual child.[81] The Institute of Medicine noted that the teaching of cognitive behavioral techniques, despite their demonstrated effectiveness, is not done in as rigorous or consistent a way as is observed for other clinical modalities.[13] A start has recently been made in teaching developmentally-appropriate, cognitive-behavioral strategies to nursing students. Results of a study that looked at the effects of this type of program revealed that program participants had an improved knowledge of these strategies and were bette able to implement them.[91] More detailed information regarding the use of nonpharmacological pain relief methods with children can be found in a variety of sources for those wishing to expand their practice.[5,6,88]

## Procedural Pain Management

Procedural pain is a widespread experience for most children interacting with the health-care system. Nurses who know how to successfully address procedural pain, using both pharmacological and nonpharmacological techniques, can help a very large number of children. Procedural pain is the one area in the pain literature that is much better developed for children than for adults, who may also experience this problem. The goals of successful procedural pain management include minimizing pain, maximizing patient cooperation, and minimizing risk to the patient.[92]

Anticipation is the key word. Having procedures performed by technically-competent individuals can reduce both risk of pain and risk of harm. The medical personnel involved must be knowledgeable in both pharmacological and nonpharmacological pain management appropriate to the child and the situation. Both children and parents need appropriate information regarding what will happen and how they can decrease stress.[36,93]

How pain is avoided or managed the first time a child undergoes a particular procedure influences how the child anticipates and copes with subsequent procedures. It is recommended that pain and anxiety be maximally treated the very first time a child undergoes a procedure.[94,95] Depending on the procedure and the individual child, this can be as simple as providing information and topical analgesics or vapocoolant immediately before needle punctures or as complex as administering conscious sedation with the combination of an opioid analgesic and a benzodiazepine. A recent review of the effectiveness of conscious sedation for anxiety, pain, and

procedural complications in young children suggests that its use should be considered and advocated if a child is experiencing a heightened stress reaction.[96] It is important to bear in mind that the use of anxiolytics or sedatives alone does not provide analgesia but does render a child unable to communicate distress.[36]

Conscious sedation/moderate sedation and analgesia are a part of the sedation continuum that is referred to as procedural sedation and analgesia (PSA). Procedural sedation and analgesia is a method of managing a child's pain and anxiety using pharmcologic agents by qualified practioners and should be tailored to each child's goal for a specific situation. Depending upon the child and situation, the goal could be for analgesia, anxiety relief, or both.[97,98] Many institutions are considering the additon of a Pediatric Sedation Team to promote safe and effective use of PSA.[99] A detailed review of PSA is beyond the scope of this chapter. Readers desiring practical information regarding safe and effective use of PSA for children in their practice setting are referred to articles listed in the reference section.[97–100]

It is useful to discuss coping strategies with the child and parents, if possible, long before the medical procedure. This enables them to mentally rehearse ways in which they can cope with the situation when it occurs.[80] Review of the literature by Christensen and Fatchett[101] revealed that distraction, relaxation, and imagery are effective for children in decreasing anxiety and pain associated with painful procedures. Therapeutic play and orientation to the room and equipment may help to promote patient cooperation. Risk can be minimized by having all equipment, supplies, and staff ready and available for both routine and emergency care.

Other things the nurse can do to facilitate comfort for children during stressful procedures include inviting the caregiver to be present and attending to environmental factors. This includes using a treatment room whenever possible; creating a pleasant environment; minimizing noxious noises, sounds, and sights; and maintaining a calm, positive manner. Attending to these details can not only increase the comfort of the parents and the child but also that of the health-care personnel involved.[102] Finally, during and after the procedure, the nurse needs to provide ongoing assessment of pain and anxiety and work to collaborate and modify the treatment plan if suboptimal control of either occurs.

## Where Improvement Is Needed

All children are vulnerable to inadequate pain assessment and management. Those most vulnerable include the preverbal child, the cognitively- or neurologically-impaired child, immigrant children, and children without homes or consistent caregivers. System issues that interact with the barriers discussed earlier also need to be addressed (see Table 59–3).[2] For example, children cared for in pediatric tertiary care centers may find that health-care professionals in their home environment lack up-to-date information about pain assessment and comprehensive pain control in children.[13]

Long-term follow-up and outcome expectations and monitoring are important in preventing, anticipating, and alleviating pain in the pediatric population. Implementing a successful pediatric pain management program is more complicated than just selecting a pain assessment tool and requires a commitment of resources.[40] To follow up in a systematic way and promote the timely and adequate use of appropriate medications and behavioral interventions for children, initiatives have been started that work to develop and implement evidence-based pediatric pain assessment and management protocols.[13,103,104] A recent study looking at opioid use in dying children during the last week of life in pediatric oncology units in 33 different children's hospitals in the United States revealed much variation in continuous prescription of opioids, even after controlling for the clinical characteristics of the patients. A study such as this is the beginning of the process to determine or establish quality indicators that could be used to assess quality of pediatric end-of-life care across practice settings.[105] Disease-specific guidelines have been developed for children with SCD[29] and JCA,[41] and a position paper has been published by the Association of Pediatric Oncology Nurses for pain management of the child with cancer at the end of life.[106] Groups are focusing on the analgesic needs of the neonatal population.[107,108] It is hoped that pain will receive this kind of attention in other pediatric populations.

Pediatric groups are striving to achieve organizational changes in pediatric pain management.[109,110] This can happen in many ways. In some settings it involves creating a formal pediatric pain or palliative care service. In othe settings it may involve basic qualitiy improvement programs.[111–114] To start to improve the process of pain management, it is necessary to collect information about the present process, to develop an awareness of all the various factors that may either promote or deter achievement of the desired outcome. The literature reveals several efforts to collect baseline information about pain management and areas for improvement.[115,116] One area to consider is that of pain medication errors. Sources of errors in pediatric medication administration include dilution errors, milligram-microgram errors, decimal point errors, and confusion between a total daily dose and a fractional dose.[48,117] Through application of the quality improvement process, nurses can play an important role in improving pain control for both the individual children they care for and other children that they may not be directly involved with.

## Summary

Despite the significant increase in knowledge about assessment and management of pain in infants and children, too many suffering children do not receive proper treatment. In today's age of "powerful, invasive medicine, we can save more lives, but any wrong choice turns medicine into torture, inflicting avoidable sufferings on patients" (p. 2).[118] To prevent suffering for children and their families, nurses and other health-care professionals must apply the most up-to-date techniques of pain assessment and management to all children they care for, especially from the time a child receives a diagnosis of a potentially life-threatening illness through his or her survival or death. By application of an integrated treatment plan that is based on the developmental level of the individual child, involves his or her family, and uses both pharmacological and nonpharmacological interventions, optimal pain control is possible.[2]

REFERENCES

1. Last Acts Palliative Care Task Force. Precepts of palliative care for children/adolescents and their families. 2003. Available at: http://pedsnurses.org/html/LastActsPrecepts03 (accessed March 29, 2005).
2. McGrath PA, Brown SC. Pain control. In: Doyle D, Hanks G, Cherny N, et al. Oxford Textbook of Palliative Medicine (3rd ed). New York, NY: Oxford University Press; 2004.
3. Walco GA, Cassidy RC, Schechter N. Sounding Board: Pain, hurt, and harm—the ethics of pain control in infants and children. N Engl J Med 1994;331:541–544.
4. Pain terms: A list with definitions and notes on usage. Recommended by the International Association for the Study of Pain Subcommittee on Taxonomy. Pain 1979;6:249–252.
5. McCaffery M, Pasero C. Pain: Clinical Manual (2nd ed). St. Louis, MO: Mosby, 1999.
6. Hockenberry M, Wilson D. Wong's Nursing Care of Infants and Children (8th ed). St. Louis, MO: Mosby Elsevier, 2007.
7. American Academy of Pediatrics, Canadian Pediatric Society. Prevention and management of pain and stress in the neonate. Pediatrics 2000;105:454–461.
8. Wuhrman E, Cooney M, Dunwoody C, Eksterowicz N, Merkel S, Oakes L. Authorized and unauthorized ("pca by proxy") dosing of analgesic infusion pumps: Position statement with clinical practice recommendations. Pain Manag Nurs 2007;8(1):4–11.
9. Kenagy A, Turner H. Pediatric Patient-controlled analgesia by proxy. AACN Adv Criti Care 2007;18(4):361–365.
10. American Academy of Pediatrics. Guidelines for monitoring and management of pediatric patients during and after sedation for diagnosis and therapeutic procedures. Pediatrics 1992;89:1110–1115.
11. Wolfe J, Hammel J, Edwards K, et al. Easing of suffering in children with cancer at the end of life: Is care changing? J Clin Oncol 2008;26(10):1717–1723.
12. Pritchard M, Burhen E, Srivastava D, et al. Cancer-related symptoms most concerning to parents during the last week and last day of their child's life. Pediatrics 2008;121(5):e1301–e1309.
13. Field MJ, Behrman R, eds. When Children Die: Improving Palliative and End-of-Life Care for Children and Their Families. Report of the Institute of Medicine Task Force. Washington, DC: National Academy Press, 2003.
14. Sherry D. Avoiding the impact of musculoskeletal pain on quality of life in children with hemophilia. Orthop Nurs 2008;27(2):103–108.

15. Cassidy JT. Progress in diagnosis and understanding of chronic pain syndromes in children and adolescents. Adolesc Med 1998;9:101–114,vi.

16. Connelly M, Schanberg L. Latest developments in the assessment and management of chronic musculoskeletal pain syndromes in children. Curr Opin Rheumatol 2006;18(5):496–502.

17. Anthony K, Schanberg L. Pediatric pain syndromes and management of pain in children and adolescents with rheumatic disease. Pediatr Clini N Am 2005;52:611–639.

18. Ingelmo PM, Locatelli BG, Carrara B. Neuropathic pain in children. Suffering Child 2003;2(February):1–15. Available at: http://www.thesufferingchild.net (accessed February 28, 2005).

19. Golden A, Haut S, Moshe S. Nonepileptic uses of antiepileptic drugs in children and adolescents. Pediatr Neurol 2006;34(6):421–432.

20. Busoni P, Bussolin L. Pain in acutely burned children. Suffering Child 2002;1(October):1–7. Available at: http://www.thesufferingchild.net (accessed February 28, 2005).

21. Gold J, Kant A, Kim S. The impact of unintentional pediatric trauma: A review of pain, acute stress, and psottraumatic stress. J Pediatr Nurs 2008;23(2):81–91.

22. World Health Organization. Cancer Pain Relief and Palliative Care in Children. Geneva, Switzerland: WHO, 1998.

23. Collins JJ, Berde CB. Management of cancer pain in children. In: Pizzo PA, Poplack DG, eds. Principles and Practice of Pediatric Oncology, 3rd ed. Philadelphia, PA: Lippincott-Raven Publishers; 1997:1183–1199.

24. Patterson KL. Pain in the pediatric oncology patient. J Pediatr Oncol Nurs 1992;9:119–130.

25. Bossert EA, Van Cleve L, Adlard K, Savedra M. Pain and leukemia: The stories of three children. J Pediatr Oncol Nurs 2002;19:2–11.

26. Friedrichsdorf S, Finney D, Stevens M, Collins J. Breakthrough pain in children with cancer. J Pain Symptom Manage 2007;34(2):209–216.

27. Ljungman G, Gordh T, Sorensen S, Kreuger A. Pain variations during cancer treatment in children: A descriptive survey. Pediatr Hemacol Oncol 2000;17:211–221.

28. Jakubik JD, Thompson M. Care of the child with sickle cell disease: Acute complications. Pediatr Nurs 2000;26:373–379.

29. American Pain Society. Guidelines for the Management of Acute and Chronic Pain in Sickle Cell Disease. Glenview, IL: APS, 1999.

30. Platt OS, Thorington BD, Brambilla DJ, et al. Pain in sickle-cell disease: Rates and risk factors. N Engl J Med 1991;325:11–16.

31. Dumaplin C. Avoiding admission for afebrile pediatric sickle cell pain: Pain management methods. J Pediatr Health Care 2006;20:115–122.

32. Robinson WM, Ravilly S, Berde C, Wohl ME. End-of-life care in cystic fibrosis. Pediatrics 1997;100:205–209.

33. Engel J, Kartin D, Jaffe K. Exploring chronic pain in yothe with duchenne muscular dystropy: A model for pediatric neuromuscular disease. Phys Med Rehabil Clin N Am 2005;16:1113–1124.

34. Russo R, Miller M, Haan E, Cameron I, Crotty M. Pain characteristics and their association with quality of life and self-concept in children with hemiplegic cerebral pasy identified from a population register. Clin J Pain 2008;24(4):335–342.

35. Nilofer S, Sunil S. Pain in neonates. Lancet 2000;355:932–933.

36. American Academy of Pediatrics. The assessment and management of acute pain in infants, children, and adolescents. Pediatrics 2001;108:793–797.

37. Jacob E, McCarthy K, Sambuco G, Hockenberry M. Intensity, location, and quality of pain in Spanish-speaking children with cancer. Pediatr Nurs 2008;34(1):45–52.

38. Hermann C, Zohsel K, Hobmeister J, Flor H. Dimensions of pain-related parent behavior: Development and psychometric evlauation of a new measure for children and their parents. Pain 2008;137(3):689–699.

39. Hester N, Barcus C. Assessment and management of pain in children. Pediatr Nurs Update 1986;1:3.

40. Franck LS, Greenberg CS, Stevens B. Pain assessment in infants and children. Pediatr Clin North Am 2000;47:487–512.

41. American Pain Society. Guideline for the Management of Pain in Osteoarthritis, Rheumatoid Arthritis, and Juvenile Chronic Arthritis (2nd ed). Glenview, IL: APS, 2002.

42. von Baeyer C, Spagrud L. Systematic review of observational (behavioral) measures of pain for children and adloescents aged 3 to 18 years. Pain 2007;127(1–2):140–150.

43. Ghai B, Kaur MakkarJ, Wig J. Postoperative pain assessment in preverbal children and children with cognitive impairmant. Paediatr Anaesth 2008;18:462–477.

44. Crellin D, Sullivan T, Babl F, O'Sullivan R, Hutchinson A. Analysis of the validation of existing behavioral pain and distress scales for us in the procedural setting. Paediatr Anaesth 2007;17(8):720–733.

45. Bookbinder M, Coyle N, Kiss M, et al. Implementing national standards for cancer pain management: Program model and evaluation. J Pain Symptom Manage 1996;12:334–347.

46. Baker C, Wong D. Q.U.E.S.T.: A process of pain assessment in children. Orthop Nurs 1987;6:11–21.

47. Duedahl T, Hansen E. A qualitative systematic review of morphine treatement in children with postoperative pain. Paediatr Anaesth 2007;17:756–774.

48. Berde CB, Sethna NF. Analgesics for the treatment of pain in children. N Engl J Med 2003;347:1094–1103.

49. Roberts R, Rodriquez W, Murphy D, Crescenzi T. Pediatric drug labeling: Improving the safety and efficacy of pediatric therapies. JAMA 2003;290:905–911.

50. Budetti PP. Ensuring safe and effective medications for children. JAMA 2003;290:950–951.

51. Stoddard F, Usher C, Abrams A. Psychopharmacology in pediatric critical care. Child Adolesc Psychiatric Clin N Am 2006;15:611–655.

52. Zernikow B, Smale H, Michel E, Hasan C, Jorch N, Andler W. Paediatric cancer pain management using the WHO analgesic ladder—results of a prospective analysis from 2265 treatment days during a quality improvement study. Eur J Pain 2006;10:587–595.

53. Collins JJ. Palliative care and the child with cancer. Hematol Oncol Clin North Am 2002;16:657–670.

54. Dlugosz C, Chater R, Engle J. Appropriate use of nonprescription analgesics in pediatric patients. J Pediatr Health Care 2006;20:316–325.

55. Hilario M, Terreri M, Len C. Nonsteroidal anti-inflammatroy drugs: Cyclooxygenase 2 inhibitors. J Pediatr (Rio J) 2006;82(5 Suppl):S206–S212.

56. Hain R, Miser A, Devins M, Wallace W. Strong opioids in pediatric palliative medicine. Pediatr Drugs 2005;7(1):1–9.

57. Zernikow B, Michel E, Anderson B. Transdermal fentanyl in childhood and adolescence: A comprehensive literature review. J Pain 2007;8(3):187–207.

58. Davies D, DeVlaming D, Haines C. Methadone analgesia for children with advanced cancer. Pediatr Blood Cancer 2008;51(3):393–397.

59. Lugo R, Satterfield K, Kern S. Pharmacokinetics of methadone. J Pain Palliat Care Pharmacother 2005;19(4):13–24.

60. Madadi P, Koren G. Pharmacogenetic insighs into codeine analgesia: Implication to pediatric codeine use. Pharmacogenomics 2008;9(9):1267–1284.

61. Ekemen S, Yelken B, Ilhan H, Tokar B. A comparison of analgesic efficacy of tramadol and pethidine for management of postoperatvie pain in children: A randomized, controlled study. Pediatr Surg Int 2008;24(6):695–698.

62. Lehmann K. Recent developments in patient-controlled analgesia. J Pain Symptom Manage 2005;29(5S):S72–S89.

63. Schiessl C, Gravou C, Zernikow B, Sittl R, Griessinger N. Use of patient-controlled analgesia for pain control in dying children. Support Care Cancer 2008;16:531–536.

64. Anghelescu D, Burgoyne L, Oakes L, Wallace D. The safety of patient-controlled analgesia by proxy in pediatric oncology patients. Anesth Analg 2005;101:1623–1627.

65. Czarnecki M, Ferrise A, Mano K, et al. Parent/nurse-controlled analgesia for children with developmental dely. Clin J Pain 2008;24(9):817–824.

66. Yee JD, Berde CB. Dextroamphetamine or methylphenidate as adjuvants to opioid analgesia for adolescents with cancer. J Pain Symptom Manage 1994;9:442.

67. Cron RQ, Sharma S, Sherry DD. Current treatment by United States and Canadian pediatric rheumatologist. J Rheumatol 1999; 26:2036–2038.

68. Morton N. Ketamine for procedural sedation and analgesia in pediatric emergency medicine: A UK perspective. Paediatr Anaesth 2008;18:25–29.

69. Dallimore D, Herd D, Short T, Anderson, B. Dosing ketamine for pediatric procedural sedation in the emergency room department. Pediatr Emerg Care 2008;24(8):529–533.

70. Westlin JE, Letocha H, Jakobson S, Strang P, Martinsson U, Nilsson S. Rapid, reproducible pain relief with [131]iodine-meta-iodobenzylguanidine in a boy with disseminated neuroblastoma. Pain 1995;60:111–114.

71. Houck C, Sethna N. Transdermal analgesia with local anaethetics in children: Review, update and future directions. Expert Rev Neurother 2005;5(5):625–634.

72. Dalens B. Periperhal blocks in children: Which techniques to begin with? Suffering Child 2002;1(October):1–24. Available at: http://www.thesufferingchild.net (accessed February 28, 2005).

73. Ecoffey C. Pediatric regional anesthesia—update. Curr Opin Anaesthesiol 2007;20:232–235.

74. Saroyan J, Schechter W, Tresgallo M, Granowetter L. Role of intraspinal analgesia in terminal pediatric malignancy. J Clin Oncol 2005;23(6):1318–1321.

75. Anghelescu D, Ross C, Oakes L, Burgoyne L. The safety of concurrent administration of opioids via epidural and intravenous routes for postoperative pain in pediatric oncology patients. J Pain Symptom Manage 2008;35(4):412–419.

76. Tsui B, Berde C. Caudal analgesia and anesthesia techniques in children. Curr Opin Anaesthesiol 2005;18:283–288.

77. Coyle N, Layman-Goldstein M. Pain assessment and management in palliative care. In: Matzo ML, Sherman DW, eds. Palliative Care Nursing: Quality Care to the End of Life. New York, NY: Springer; 2001:362–486.

78. Palermo TM, Valenzuela D. Use of pain diaries to assess recurrent and chronic pain in children. Suffering Child 2003;3:1–24. Available at: http://www.thesufferingchild.net (accessed February 28, 2005).

79. Uman L, Chambers C, McGrath P, Kisely S. Psychological interventions for needle-related procedural pain and distress in children and adolescents. Cochrane Database System Rev 2006;(4):1–77.

80. Piira T, Hayes B, Goodenough B. Distraction methods in the management of children's pain: An approach based on evidence of intuition? Suffering Child 2002;1(October):1–10. Available at: http://www.thesufferingchild.net (accessed February 28, 2005).

81. Hockenberry-Eaton M, Barrera P, Brown M, Bottomley SJ, O'Neil JB. Pain Management in Children with Cancer Handbook. Texas: Texas Cancer Council, 1999. Available at: http://www.childcancerpain.org/frameset_nogl.cfm?content=handbook.html (accessed February 28, 2005).

82. Kundu A, Berman B. Acupuncture for pediatric pain and symptom management. Pediatr Clin N Am 2007;54:885–899.

83. Evans S, Tsao J, Zeltzer L. Complementary and alternative medicine for acute procedural pain in children. Altern Ther Health Med 2008;14(5):52–56.

84. Rheingans J. A systematic review of nonpharmacologic adjunctive therapies for symptom management in children with cancer. J Pediatr Oncol Nurs 2007;24(2):81–94.

85. Libonate J, Evans S, Tsao J. Efficacy of acupuncture for health conditions in children: A review. Sci World J 2008;8:670–682.

86. Hughes D, Ladas E, Rooney D, Kelly K. Massage Therapy as a supportive care intervention for children with cancer. Oncol Nurs Forum 2008 35(3):431–442.

87. Bandstra N, Skinner L, LeBlanc C, et al. The role of child life in pediatric pain management: A survey of child life specialists. J Pain 2008;9(4):320–329.

88. Rusy LM, Weisman SJ. Complimentary therapies for acute pediatric pain management. Pediatr Clin North Am 2000; 47:589–599.

89. Wild M, Espie C. The efficacy of hypnosis in the reduction of procedural pain and distress in pediatric oncology: A systematic review. J Dev Behav Pediatr 2004;25(3):207–213.

90. Richardson J, Smith J, McCall G, Pilkington K. Hypnosis for procedure-related pain and distress in pediatric cancer patients: A systematic review of effectiveness and methodology related to hypnosis interventions. J Pain Symptom Manage 2006;31(1):70–84.

91. MacLaren J, Cohen L, Larkin K, Shelton E. Training nursing students in evidence-based techniques for cognitive-behavioral pediatric pain management. J Nurs Educ 2008;47(8):351–358.

92. Schecter N, Berde C, Yaster M. Pain in Infants, Children, and Adolescents (2nd ed). Philadelphia, PA: Lippincott, Williams & Wilkins, 2003.

93. Power N, Liossi C, Franck L. Helping parents to help their child with procedural and everyday pain: Practical, evidence-based advice. HSPN 2007;12(3):203–209.

94. American Academy of Pediatrics. Report of the subcommittee on the management of pain associated with procedures in children with cancer. Pediatrics 1990;86:827.

95. Young K. Pediatric procedural pain. Ann Emerg Med 2005;45(2):160–171.

96. Dresser S, Melnyk BM. The effectiveness of conscious sedation on anxiety, pain, and procedural complications in young children. Pediatr Nurs 2003;29:320–323.

97. Doyle L, Colletti J. Pediatric procedural sedation and analgesia. Pediatr Clin N Am 2006;53:279–292.

98. Bartolome S, Cid J, Freddi N. Analgesia and sedation in children: Practical approach for the most frequent situations. J Pediatr (Rio J) 2007;82(2 Suppl):S71–S82.

99. Davis C. Does your facility have a pediatric sedation team? If not, why not? Pediatr Nurs 2008;34(4):308–318.

100. Koh J, Palermo T. Conscious sedation: Reality or myth? Pediatr Rev 2007:28(7):243–248.

101. Christensen J, Fatchett D. Promoting parental use of distraction and relaxation in pediatric oncology patients during invasive procedures. J Pediatr Oncol Nurs 2002;19:127–132.

102. Stevens BJ, Johnson C, Petryshen P, Taddio A. Premature infant pain profile: Development and initial validation. Clin J Pain 1996;12:13–22.

103. Jacox A, Carr DB, Payne R, et al. Management of Cancer Pain. Clinical Practice Guideline No. 9. AHCPR publication No. 94–0592. Rockville, Md.: Agency for Health Care Policy and Research, U.S. Department of Health and Human Services, Public Health Service, 1994.

104. Agency for Health Care Policy and Research. Acute Pain Management in Infants, Children, and Adolescents: Operative and Medical Procedures. Quick Reference Guide for Clinicians. Rockville, Md.: U.S. Department of Health and Human Services, 1992.

105. Orsey A, Belasco J, Ellenberg J, Schmitz K, Feudtner C. Variation in receipt of opioids by pediatric oncology patients who died in children's hospitals. Pediatr Blood Cancer 2008;DOI 10.1002/pbc:1–6.

106. Hooke C, Hellstren MB, Stutzer C, Forte K. Pain management for the child with cancer in end-of-life care: APON position paper. J Pediatr Oncol Nurs 2002;19:43–47.

107. Kanwaljeet J, Anand J, Aranda J, et al. Summary proceedings from the neonatal pain-control group. Pediatrics 2006; 117:S9–S22.

108. Anand K, Aranda J, Berde C, et al. Analgesia and anesthesia for neonates: Study design. Clin Therap 2005;27(6):814–843.

109. Dowden S, McCathy M, Chalkiadis G. Achieving organizational change in pediatric pain management. Pain Res Manage 2008;13(4):321–326.

110. Oakes L, Anghelescu D, Windsor K, Barnhill P. An institutional quality improvement initiative for pain management for pediatric cancer patients. J Pain Symptom Manage 2008; 35(6):656–669.

111. Harper J, Hinds P, Baker J, Hicks J, Spunt S, Razzouk B. Creating a palliative and end-of-life program in a cure-oriented pediatric setting: The zig-zag method. J Pediatr Oncol Nurs 2007;24(5):246–254.

112. Meyer M. Integration of pain services into pediatric oncology. Int Anesthesiol Clin 2006:44(1):95–107.

113. Johnson D, Nagel K, Friedman D, Meza J, Hurwitz C, Friebert S. Availability and use of palliative care and end-of-life services for pediatric oncology patients. J Clin Oncol 2008;26(28):4646–4650.

114. Friedrichsdorf S, Remke S, Symalla B, Gibbon C, Chrastek J. Developing a pain and palliative care programme at a US children's hospital. Int J Palliat Nurs 2007;13(11):534–542.

115. Ellis JA, McCarthy P, Hershon L, Horlin R, Rattray M, Tierney S. Pain practices: A cross-Canada survey of pediatric oncology centers. J Pediatr Oncol Nurs 2003;20:26–35.

116. Ely B. Pediatric nurses' pain management practice: Barriers to change. Pediatr Nurs 2001;27:473–480.

117. Levine SR, Cohen MR, Blanchard NR, et al. Guidelines for preventing medication errors in pediatrics. J Pediatr Pharmacol Ther 2001;6:426–442.

118. Facco E, Giron G. The nature of pain and the approach to the suffering child. Suffering Child 2003;2(February):1–3. Available at: http://www.thesufferingchild.net (accessed February 28, 2005).

119. Gauvain-Piquard A, Rodary C, Rezvani A, Serbouti S. The development of the DEGR®: A scale to assess pain in young children with cancer. Eur J Pain 1999;2:165–176.

120. Van Dongen KAJ, Abu-Saad HH, Hammers JPF, Zwakhalen SMG. Pain assessment in the intellectually disabled child: The challenges of tool development. Suffering Child 2002; 1:1–18.

121. Hunt AM, Burne R. Medical and nursing problems of children with neurodegenerative disease. Palliat Med 1995; 9:19–26.

122. Lawrence J, Alcock D, McGrath P, Kay J, MacMurray SB, Dulberg C. The development of a tool to assess neonatal pain expression. Neonatal Netw 1993;12:59–66.

123. Krechel SW, Bildner J. CRIES: A new neonatal postoperative pain measurement tool. Initial testing of validity and reliability. Paediatr Anaesth 1995;5:53–61.

124. Grunau RVE, Craig KD. Facial activity as a measure of neonatal pain expression. In: Tyler EC, Krane EJ, eds. Advances in Pain Research Therapy: Pediatric Pain (Vol 15). New York, NY: Raven Press; 1990:147–155.

125. Levetown M, ed. Compendium of Pediatric Palliative Care. Alexandria, VA: National Hospice and Palliative Care Organization, 2000.

126. Children's Hospice of Eastern Ontario Pain Scale. Available at: http://www.cebp.nL/media/m333.pdf (accessed March 29, 2005).

# VIII

## Special Issues for the Nurse in End-of-Life Care

# 60

*Jay R. Horton and Rose Anne Indelicato*

# The Advanced Practice Nurse

*The advanced practice nurse brings a pivotal role and perspective to hospital palliative care teams, often embodying in a single person palliative nursing's focus on the whole person and the medical practitioner's ability to diagnose conditions, prescribe medications and order treatment interventions—while recouping salary costs through billing for consultations.[1]*

◆ **Key Points**
◆ *Palliative care relieves suffering and improves quality of life for patients with serious, debilitating, or life-threatening illness and their families by offering symptom management, care coordination, and psychosocial and spiritual support from the time of diagnosis and extending through the period of bereavement.*
◆ *Advanced practice nursing builds on the strong foundation of nursing practice by incorporating advanced knowledge and expertise in performing histories and physical examinations, ordering and interpreting diagnostic tests, and prescribing medications and other therapies appropriate for the management of particular symptoms or diseases.*
◆ *Advanced practice nursing in palliative care is recognized as a specialty with its own scope and standards of practice, education and training programs, and certification.*
◆ *Palliative care advanced practice nurses (APNs) practice in a broad range of treatment settings and bring their unique blend of compassionate, evidence-based care to patients of all ages.*
◆ *Palliative care APNs contribute to the financial viability of palliative care programs by providing cost-effective care and through billing and reimbursement.*

Numerous initiatives over the last two decades have identified the critical need for improved clinical care of patients with life-threatening illness and their families.[2–4] Palliative care aims to relieve suffering and improve quality of life for those patients with serious, debilitating illness and their families, whether or not they choose to be treated simultaneously with life-prolonging therapies.[5] It offers expert pain and symptom management, psychosocial support, and care coordination through an interdisciplinary team consisting of appropriately-trained physicians, nurses, and social workers with assistance and contributions from other professionals as required.[5] Palliative care provides support from the time of diagnosis, during active treatment, and throughout the period of bereavement.[5]

Within a changing health-care environment, advanced practice nurses (APNs) have demonstrated their ability to adapt to the new challenges they face as the population ages, their patients live longer with chronic, serious illness, and as patients and families struggle to navigate an increasingly complex and fragmented health-care system. Advanced practice nurses have also taken a leading role in the development and delivery of palliative care because they possess expert clinical, teaching, and advocacy skills and because the public trusts nurses to provide this kind of care.[6]

## History and Definition of Advanced Practice Nursing

In the early 20th century, nurses who had completed postgraduate coursework, or who had extensive expertise in a particular clinical area, were called specialists.[7] They were the predecessors of today's APNs. In 1954, the first clinical nurse specialist (CNS) program was created at Rutgers University in New Jersey, and in 1965 the first nurse practitioner (NP) program was established at the University of Colorado.[7,8] Initially, these roles were described as extending beyond the scope of nursing to include some practices and procedures from medicine and other disciplines. In the 1980s, however, the term "advanced practice" was adopted after growth within graduate nursing education allowed nurses to obtain advanced expertise within the field of nursing instead of looking only to other fields for advanced knowledge and skills.[7]

In addition to the clinical nurse specialist and NP roles mentioned above, there are two other distinct APN roles: the Certified Nurse Midwife (CNM) and the Certified Registered Nurse Anesthetist (CRNA). APNs have advanced knowledge and expertise in performing histories and physical examinations, ordering and interpreting diagnostic tests, and prescribing medications and other therapies appropriate for the management of particular symptoms or diseases.[9] APNs have varying degrees of prescriptive privileges in all 50 states. In the field of palliative care, the APN is most often educated and certified as either a clinical nurse specialist or an NP. Some authors have described a unique blended role for APNs whose education and practice is a combination of aspects traditionally considered to be in the domain of either the clinical nurse specialist or the NP.[10] These blended-role APNs may be particularly well-suited to the broad range of knowledge and skills required in the practice of palliative care.[11] In this chapter the term APN will be used to refer to the clinical nurse specialist, the NP, and the blended-role APN.

### The National Consensus Project and the National Quality Forum

Two significant developments within the past decade reflect a period of growth and standardization in palliative care. First, the National Consensus Project for Quality Palliative Care published the Clinical Practice Guidelines for Palliative Care (NCP Guidelines) in 2004.[5] The NCP is a partnership of five national palliative care organizations: The American Academy of Hospice and Palliative Medicine (AAHPM), the Center to Advance Palliative Care (CAPC), the Hospice and Palliative Nurses Association (HPNA), the Last Acts Partnership, and the National Hospice and Palliative Care Organization (NHPCO). The NCP Guidelines were intended to aid the development of palliative care programs, establish definitions of palliative care, set goals for access to quality palliative care, reduce variation, foster performance measurement and quality improvement, and promote continuity of palliative care across settings. The guidelines cover eight domains of palliative care: structure and process; physical aspects; psychological and psychiatric aspects; social aspects; spiritual, religious, and existential aspects; cultural aspects; imminently dying patients; and ethical and legal aspects.[5,12]

While publication of the NCP Guidelines helped establish the definition and scope of palliative care, the National Quality Forum's National Framework and Preferred Practices for Palliative and Hospice Care Quality (NQF Preferred Practices) was an essential next step in the acceptance and implementation of those guidelines by the larger health-care community.[13] The NQF is a nonprofit public-private partnership focused on improving the quality of health care through setting voluntary consensus standards. The NQF Preferred Practices are based on the NCP Guidelines and identify 38 preferred practices that will improve the quality of palliative and hospice care. It also recommends a framework for creating a quality measurement and reporting system that may be used to support improved reimbursement for palliative care services.[13] Taken together, the NCP Guidelines and the NQF Preferred Practices set the performance standards for new and existing palliative care programs.

Advanced practice nurses will find these two publications indispensible to their professional practice for at least four key reasons. The practice guidelines help clinicians identify and understand the standards of clinical care. For example, the NQF Preferred Practices advocate for screening and assessment of symptoms with standardized scales,[13] and the NCP Guidelines call for prompt response to psychological symptoms and regular documentation of response to treatment.[5]

Second, the NQF Preferred Practices address educational issues and assert that "all healthcare professionals, in the routine course of providing healthcare services, are expected to be adequately trained to provide basic elements of palliative care."[13] As will be discussed below in the section on education, APNs are ideally equipped as educators, both for their nursing colleagues as well as for other clinicians. To promote palliative care in all settings, the NCP Guidelines suggest that "educational experiences in the range of settings where patients receive care" must be provided to clinicians in training.[5] The consensus guidelines will help APN educators identify basic skills that should be integrated into curricula for all clinicians and insure that palliative care clinical training programs help advanced practice students develop specialist-level competency in all domains.

Advanced practice nurses are frequently involved in development projects for both new and existing palliative care programs. The NCP Guidelines and the NQF Preferred Practices will also help APNs identify the essential components of any such program and will serve as a yardstick by which they can measure their progress. For example, in determining the structure of the palliative care team, one could find guidance in the NCP Guidelines[5] and the NQF Preferred Practices[13] which state that the teams must be interdisciplinary and that patients and families must have access to palliative care expertise 24 hours per day, 7 days per week.

Finally, the NCP Guidelines and the NQF Preferred Practices serve as useful framing devices for research needs in palliative care. Any APN considering participation in research would be wise to study the recommendations made in these publications. For example, the NCP Guidelines call for new research methods to overcome the shortcomings of randomized controlled trials in palliative care, demonstration projects and multi-center research to test some of palliative care's central tenets, and more detailed studies analyzing reasons for late referrals to hospice.[5] The NQF Preferred Practices identifies gaps in palliative care's knowledge base and has extensive notes on directions for research in each of the domains and in cross-domain issues.[13]

## Competencies and Skills of the Advanced Practice Nurse in Palliative Care

The APN's expertise is built upon the strong foundation of skills possessed by the generalist registered nurse. Compared to the generalist, the APN has broader and deeper education and expertise in the areas of assessment, diagnosis, and treatment of disease as well as prevention, health maintenance, and provision of comfort. Additionally, the APN holds a graduate degree in nursing, is nationally certified at the advanced practice level, and has a practice focused on care of patients and families.[9] The APN is also expected to engage in more complex problem solving and typically has broader responsibility for patient care than the generalist nurse.

To address the developing role of hospice and palliative care nurses, including the growing importance of APNs in this field, HPNA has defined the breadth and depth of practice for both generalists and APNs via their publication, "Hospice and Palliative Nursing: Scope and Standards of Practice."[14] In the section on scope of practice, eight competencies are outlined for the generalist hospice and palliative nurse. Competencies are defined as the "quantifiable knowledge, attitudes, and skills" that the nurse demonstrates in the provision of palliative care.[15] For both the generalist and the APN, these include clinical judgment, advocacy and ethics, professionalism, collaboration, systems thinking, cultural competence, facilitation of learning, and communication.[14] In HPNA's companion publication for APNs, "Competencies for Advanced Practice Hospice and Palliative Care Nurses," the same eight competencies, plus a research competency, are defined and include details of additional criteria for the APN's expanded scope of practice.[15] To cite an example from within the clinical judgment competency, while both the generalist and the APN use "the nursing process to address the physical, psychosocial, and spiritual needs of patients and families,"[14] the APN further "assumes responsibility for the overall evaluating, documenting, and communicating of care to enhance continuity of palliative care across health care settings."[15]

The Hospice and Palliative Nurses Association has supplemented the scope of practice and competency statements by providing measurement criteria for each of 15 standards.[14] There are six standards of practice (assessment, diagnosis, outcomes identification, planning, implementation, and evaluation) and nine standards of professional performance (quality of practice, education, professional practice evaluation, collegiality, collaboration, ethics, research, resource utilization, and leadership).[14] In each case, generalist standards are described first, followed by additional practices for which the APN is responsible. For example, to meet the diagnosis standard, the generalist is responsible for deriving "the nursing diagnoses or issues based on assessment data, which includes actual or potential responses to alterations in health," while the APN "systematically compares and contrasts clinical findings with normal and abnormal variations and developmental events in formulating a differential diagnosis."[14]

## Palliative Care Education in Advanced Practice Nursing

The NCP Guidelines highlight improved education for all clinicians as a priority in palliative care. Advanced practice nurses will undoubtedly play a key role in fulfilling this mandate, but they first will need additional training themselves.[16] A decade ago, surveys confirmed that undergraduate and graduate nursing programs paid little attention to palliative care topics.[2,17,18] More recent data show that there is still a lack of adequate coverage.[19] A study that looked at 50 nursing textbooks used frequently in nursing curricula found that only 2% of all pages had any end-of-life content.[20] Increased palliative care content has been endorsed by HPNA[21] and the National Council of State Boards of Nursing (NCSBN).[22] Additionally, nurses should advocate for more palliative care content on other APN certification exams, such as the Adult Nurse Practitioner or Pediatric Nurse Practitioner exams. At the generalist level, palliative care content has already been successfully integrated into the National Council Licensure Exam for RNs (NCLEX-RN).[22]

Efforts to address these deficits have begun in several areas, including graduate coursework, clinical experiences, and continuing education. In the 1990s, the first graduate nursing programs specifically designed for training palliative care APNs were created. The first palliative care nursing master's program for clinical nurse specialists was established at Breen School of Nursing, Ursuline College in Pepper Pike, OH and for NPs at New York University College of Nursing.[23,24] Currently there are at least 13 programs in the United States that are designed to train APNs with a specialization in palliative care. For example New York University College of Nursing and Madonna University both offer integrated programs that prepare graduates eligible to sit for both the Adult Nurse Practitioner and the Advanced Certified Hospice and Palliative Nurse (ACHPN) certification exams. Other programs that offer a course of study in palliative care that can be pursued along with a different primary concentration include the Vanderbilt School of Nursing, the Columbia University School of Nursing, the Breen School of Nursing at Ursuline College, the University of Pennsylvania School of Nursing, and the University of California at San Francisco School of

Nursing. Some of the aforementioned programs also provide opportunities for APNs to receive post-master's certificates in palliative care. A current list of programs may be found on the HPNA website.[25] In 2004, the American Association of Colleges of Nursing (AACN) endorsed the Position Statement on the Practice Doctorate in Nursing[26] recommending that all advanced practice graduate nursing programs transition to Doctor of Nursing Practice (DNP) programs by 2015.[27] Many new DNP programs have begun enrolling students since then and others are currently in development. It remains to be seen what effect this initiative will have on advanced practice nursing in palliative care.

In addition to didactic coursework, palliative care APNs in training need clinical experiences. HPNA has published standards for the structure and content of three types of clinical practicums in palliative nursing: the observership, the preceptorship, and the fellowship.[28] Many hospital-based and other palliative care programs offer observerships (1–5 days) and preceptorships (2 weeks to 6 months). Although fellowships are a standard part of physician training, they are a relatively new educational opportunity for APNs. Currently there are at least four organizations offering palliative care fellowship training for APNs: the Beth Israel Medical Center offers the Nurse Fellowship in Pain Medicine and Palliative Care in New York City, Children's Hospital Boston and Dana-Farber Cancer Institute together offer the Pediatric Palliative Care Nursing Fellowship in Boston, Memorial Sloan-Kettering Cancer Center offers the Fellowship in Cancer Pain Management and Palliative Care for Nurse Practitioners in New York City, and the Department of Veterans Affairs (VA) offers Interprofessional Fellowships in Palliative Care at six VA facilities across the country. Both AAHPM and HPNA have also started formal mentorship programs that match APNs with peers who have expertise in clinical, educational, or research aspects of palliative care.[29,30]

Both palliative care and other APNs need continuing education in palliative care, which can be accomplished through self-study, clinical in-services, and professional conferences. It is important for APNs to become active members of national, regional, and local professional organizations so they will have access to continuing education opportunities, and so that those APNs with palliative care expertise can do the important work of providing education for the non-specialists. One self-study program developed for APNs in Michigan used nine self-teaching modules consisting of printed manuals, videos, slides, and test questions that were geared towards second-year graduate nursing students or post-graduate APNs.[31] In 1999, the AACN and the City of Hope National Medical Center formed the End-of-Life Nursing Education Consortium (ELNEC) to design a curriculum for teaching palliative care to nurses.[32] Over the course of 5 years, ELNEC presented the ELNEC-Graduate train-the-trainer curriculum with the goal of improving the coverage of palliative care content in graduate nursing curricula.[32] This National Cancer Institute (NCI)-funded program reached a total of 300 graduate

nursing program faculty members representing 63% of all graduate nursing programs in the United States.[32] Post-intervention follow-up indicated that trained faculty nearly tripled the average number of hours of palliative care content in their graduate curricula.[32] Although the NCI-funded ELNEC-Graduate training programs formally came to an end in 2006, the course continues to be offered through the AACN and some of the content has been integrated into the ELNEC-SuperCore program.[32] Programs such as these that use a train-the-trainer format can be particularly powerful because they have the potential to reach a much larger audience through the participants' efforts to replicate the training in other settings.

## Advanced Practice Nurse Certification in Palliative Care

Obtaining national certification of advanced-level nursing practice within a specialty has several benefits. Certification is a marker of professional competence and assures that care meets the established standards for quality and safety, and is necessary for APN billing and reimbursement.[9,33,34]

In response to the evolution of palliative and hospice care as an advanced practice specialty, the National Board of Certification of Hospice and Palliative Nurses (NBCHPN), together with the American Nurses Credentialing Center, created an advanced practice certification exam. The ACHPN exam, first offered in 2002, tests knowledge in five domains of practice (clinical judgment; advocacy, ethics, and systems thinking; professionalism and research; collaboration, facilitation of learning, and communication; and cultural and spiritual competence).[35,36] Advanced practice nurses who wish to sit for the exam must meet eligibility criteria including graduate-level education and a minimum of 500 hours of clinical practice in palliative care.[35] In 2005, the NBCHPN assumed sole responsibility for the examination process.[36] As of 2009, 520 APNs from 47 states and the District of Columbia were certified as ACHPNs.[37]

## State Law

Advanced practice nursing is governed by laws found in states' nurse practice acts and is regulated by the state board of nursing or, in some states, jointly via the board of nursing and the medical or pharmacy board.[8,33] There is considerable state-to-state legislative and regulatory variation regarding scope of practice; prescriptive authority; education, licensure, and certification requirements; and collaborative practice between APNs and physicians.[8,38] It is the APN's responsibility to be familiar with relevant state law and to maintain a practice that is guided by legal, ethical, and professional practice standards.

## Palliative Care APN Practice Settings

Advanced practice nurses provide palliative care in a wide range of care settings including home care programs, hospices, long-term care facilities, outpatient clinics, emergency rooms, acute care hospitals, and sub-acute rehabilitation units.[39] Numerous settings were highlighted in the publication "Advanced Practice Nursing: Pioneering Practices in Palliative Care."[40] Produced by Promoting Excellence in End-of-Life Care, a national program office of the Robert Wood Johnson Foundation, this publication described APN practice in diverse palliative care programs. Because APNs practice in such a variety of locations, they have the opportunity to reduce the fragmentation of care that can occur during transitions from one care setting to another.[6,41] Provision of expert symptom management by palliative care APNs early in the course of disease may improve quality of life and, in some cases, patient survival.[42] This early involvement also helps the patient and family develop a trusting therapeutic relationship with the APN over time.

## Billing and Reimbursement for the APN in Palliative Care

Employing APNs in palliative care programs may be cost-effective even without billing,[16] and it will be important to demonstrate this fact in a variety of practice settings. However, APN billing and reimbursement can be an essential part of a palliative care program's business model, and it is easier to demonstrate and to understand an APN's value to a program through documentation of revenue generated by reimbursement from third-party payers. In difficult economic times this may translate into the ability to keep a palliative care program afloat or to keep an APN on the team.[43] The following guidelines apply to reimbursement for APN services provided in inpatient hospital settings, outpatient clinics, skilled nursing facilities, and at home. Hospice will be covered separately at the end of the section. Medicare, the federally-administered health insurance available to those aged 65 years and older or who have end-stage renal disease or meet disability criteria, will be covered in some detail because it represents a large proportion of total reimbursement for hospital and office-based care, and because other third-party payers often follow Medicare's lead.[8] Billing and reimbursement guidelines will be described in greater detail for NPs than for clinical nurse specialists because these issues are more frequently addressed for NPs in the literature and in legislation.

Under the Omnibus Budget Reconciliation Acts of 1989 and 1990, APNs were first granted limited ability to bill Medicare in rural areas and in skilled nursing facilities.[44] Prior to this legislation, APNs could bill "incident to" physician services, but this applied only to patient encounters in which the physician provided direct personal supervision by being in the office suite at the time of the encounter, and APNs could not bill for new patients or new problems.[8,44] In the 1997 Balanced Budget Act, APN billing was expanded significantly. Advanced practice nurses in all geographic areas and practice sites were allowed to be reimbursed at 85% of the physician fee schedule under Medicare Part B.[8,44] "Incident to" billing continues to be an option, but applies to only a small number of encounters and is subject to numerous restrictions.[45]

To qualify for Medicare reimbursement, APNs must satisfy a variety of requirements. They must have a master's degree in nursing, advanced certification from a nationally recognized certification body, and a National Provider Identifier. The APN must satisfy all of the state's practice requirements, including state RN and APN licensure, and must document a collaborative arrangement with a physician even if the state does not have a collaborative practice law. The service being submitted for reimbursement must be a service for which a physician would be reimbursed, and the state must recognize the APN's legal authority to perform that service. In addition, the practice cannot be hospital-owned, and the APN's salary cannot be on the hospital nursing department's cost report because the hospital is reimbursed under Medicare Part A for those services.[46] The APN who satisfies the above requirements can bill Medicare Part B. These rules apply to both NPs and clinical nurse specialists, but clinical nurse specialists may have a more difficult time meeting the requirements either because of limits on their scope of practice or silence on the subject of scope of practice for clinical nurse specialists by the state.[8,44,46,47]

One potential difficulty currently facing palliative care APNs is the issue of state recognition of ACHPN certification. In 2007, the Centers for Medicare and Medicaid Services (CMS) added NBCHPN to the list of certifying bodies it recognizes, opening the way for ACHPN billing. The ACHPN specialty, granted by NBCHPN, is accredited by the American Board of Nursing Specialties (ABNS) and many states have formally recognized ACHPN certification. A current list may be found at the NBCHPN Web site.[48] However, because the NCSBN has not recognized palliative care as a specialty, those states that rely on NCSBN recognition may consider palliative care to be a subspecialty rather than a specialty and require those APNs with ACHPN certification to be certified in another recognized specialty in order to be reimbursed.[47]

To be eligible for Medicare reimbursement, a service must be defined as a "physician service" and assigned a Current Procedural Terminology (CPT) code to document the procedure done or the service provided.[8,44,49] The evaluation and management (E&M) CPT codes are the most frequently used in palliative care because rather than describe procedures (which make up a small part of palliative care practice), they describe cognitive services such as history-taking, conducting the physical exam, decision-making, and counseling.[43] There are different sets of CPT codes for different practice settings, and each set comprises a range of numbers reflecting distinct levels of service. The level of service may be determined on the basis of either complexity or time. If greater than 50% of a clinician's time is spent in coordination and counseling, then the clinician may bill based on time. This can be an effective way to document the intensity of work in palliative care, especially if the physical exam is limited.[43] For inpatients, the total time spent on the unit is what counts toward the E&M code and for outpatients, only face-to-face time counts.[49] For billing on the basis of complexity, the level of service is supported by documentation of the extent of the history, physical exam, decision-making, and counseling.[44,49]

A second set of codes for diagnoses is necessary to qualify a service for reimbursement. International Classification of Diseases, Ninth Revision, Clinical Modification (ICD-9-CM) codes are used to describe the disease or symptom that is treated.[49] Examples include acute respiratory failure, pain, and nausea. It is important to note that a payer will not reimburse more than one clinician per day for the same indication. For example, a palliative care APN who consults on a patient on a ventilator in an ICU, and who helps manage the patient's dyspnea should avoid submitting the ICD-9-M for acute respiratory failure because the critical care clinician or pulmonologist is likely to use that code. A better choice for the APN in such a case would be to use the ICD-9-CM code for dyspnea. If two clinicians submit bills listing the same ICD-9-CM code on the same day, only the clinician whose bill is processed first will be reimbursed. It is possible to bill for concurrent care, even if the clinicians are from the same specialty, as long as each clinician is providing a different service and can bill for a different diagnosis.[49]

In addition to Medicare reimbursement, APNs may be eligible for reimbursement from other third-party payers including Medicaid, commercial insurers, and managed care organizations (MCOs).[46] Although many of the billing and reimbursement guidelines for Medicare are applicable to these other payers, the Medicaid plans have considerable state-to-state variation, and each commercial insurer and MCO has its own policies.[46]

The 2003 Medicare Modernization Act specifies that NPs can directly bill Medicare Part B for services provided to hospice-enrolled patients, but only if they are the patient's attending, and only if they are not a paid or volunteer employee of the hospice. An NP who is a hospice employee, or who is consulting on a hospice-enrolled patient, can bill the hospice and then the hospice can bill Medicare Part A.[42] Currently, NPs cannot certify patients as hospice eligible and cannot serve as hospice medical directors.[46] The Medicare Modernization Act does not address hospice billing issues for clinical nurse specialists.

## Summary

The emergence of palliative care was spurred by the recognition that patients at all stages of serious, debilitating, or life-threatening illness had needs for symptom management, care coordination, and psychosocial and spiritual support that were not being met. The provision of high-quality palliative care to an aging population amid rising costs, an increasingly complex health-care system, and clinical workforce shortages poses serious challenges. Palliative care APNs have addressed these challenges by contributing to interdisciplinary patient care; providing education to patients, families, and colleagues; serving as consultants; conducting research; and taking on leadership roles. Reducing psychosocial and spiritual distress is a basic nursing role that palliative care APNs fulfill by addressing symptoms and responding to suffering through compassionate presence.[50] Through expert communication, the APN helps to improve continuity of care and alleviate feelings of abandonment. Palliative care APNs skillfully elicit patient and family care preferences and advocate for the construction of individualized, coordinated care plans that are aligned with those values and goals. Advanced practice nurses also contribute to the financial viability of palliative care programs and their institutions via cost reduction and through billing and reimbursement. The role of the palliative care APN will be strengthened in the future by pursuing improvements in education, conducting research to demonstrate the value of APN interventions, and advocating for legislation that supports APN practice and reimbursement.

CASE STUDY
### Palliative Care in Acute Myelogenous Leukemia

Patient RC was a 47-year-old man with acute myelogenous leukemia. He lived in another state, but had temporarily relocated so that he could receive a stem cell transplant at a large academic medical center. He was single, with no children, and worked as a teacher. He had close friends and family, but because of the great distance, they could visit only on weekends. RC was first brought to the attention of the palliative care team when the nurse manager from oncology spoke to the palliative care APN: "We have a patient who really needs your support." RC had already been in the hospital for one month and was experiencing severe graft versus host disease of his gastrointestinal tract resulting in diarrhea and abdominal pain. When the palliative care attending physician and physician fellow saw him for the initial consultation, he was also uncomfortable due to his bilateral lower extremity lymphedema, depressed, and in tears. Because a long hospitalization was anticipated, the interdisciplinary team decided that the APN would have primary responsibility for his ongoing, consultative follow-up to promote continuity. It was another 4 months before RC was discharged to acute rehabilitation, and he was seen over 60 times, mainly by two different APNs who billed for each encounter by submitting the appropriate CPT and ICD-9-CM codes. Both APNs were certified as ACHPNs. Each morning in a team meeting, the APN reviewed RC's progress with the palliative care interdisciplinary team and engaged the assistance of other team members as appropriate. In addition to the APNs and physicians, the palliative care chaplain, massage therapist, and social worker made important contributions to RC's care. Over the course of his hospitalization, RC suffered from a severe exacerbation of his abdominal pain which resolved after a cholecystectomy. He also had a left parietal stroke, an exacerbation of his depression, and numerous other complications that contributed to his suffering and delayed his discharge. With the occurrence of each setback or symptom the palliative care APN assessed RC and presented a treatment plan to the oncology team. Advanced pain assessment skills and knowledge of opioid pharmacology allowed the APNs to advocate for changes in RC's pain regimen that contributed to a dramatic improvement in his pain control. Training in the psychological impact of serious illness coupled with an understanding of psychopharmacology enabled the APNs to successfully advocate for the use of a psychostimulant which led to more rapid alleviation of RC's depression. There was often opportunity for cooperation and negotiation with the oncology team as they were concerned about the effects that some of the treatments, especially the opioids, might have on his gastrointestinal and mental function. With almost every visit, no matter how sick he was feeling, RC expressed his gratitude for the careful and patient-centered approach used by the palliative care APNs.

## CASE STUDY
### A Case Study with COPD

Mrs. B, a 78-year-old woman with chronic obstructive pulmonary disease (COPD) and hypertension, was hospitalized with shortness of breath and disorientation, and required a Bilevel Positive Airway Pressure (BiPAP) device to manage her respiratory failure. A right lower lobe pneumonia was identified and intravenous antibiotics were given. Recently, Mrs. B. had a number of hospitalizations related to her COPD, requiring intubation and mechanical ventilation from which she had been successfully weaned. A palliative care consultation was requested for support, symptom management, and clarification of the goals and plan of care. The palliative care APN met Mrs. B and her care aide. She was quite dyspneic despite use of BiPAP and was unable to engage in conversation. The patient's medical record was reviewed and a focused physical exam was performed. The APN recommended initiation of standing morphine, use of a bedside fan, consideration of an anxiolytic for management of dyspnea and anxiety, and use of a communication board to allow Mrs. B to make her needs known. Once the patient was more comfortable, further assessments and conversations could take place. Mrs. B's dyspnea responded well to the morphine, but she continued to experience oxygen desaturation, mostly due to retained secretions. The pulmonologist recommended a trial of intubation

with mechanical ventilation. The patient's four children were brought to the bedside for a conversation related to the plan of care. Although Mrs. B had a living will in which she declined aggressive therapy at the end of life, she agreed to intubation with reassessment of her respiratory status in a few days. She expressed her wish for full resuscitation attempts in the event of cardiac arrest. The patient was intubated and started on standing lorazepam in addition to morphine to help manage pain, dyspnea and anxiety.

Unfortunately, Mrs. B. was unable to be weaned from the ventilator and continued to retain secretions. The APN and palliative care team met with Mrs. B and her children. Her children discussed the possibility of palliative extubation, but Mrs. B stated she wanted to live and wished to go home if possible. She stated that she had the financial resources to enable her to go home, even if she required mechanical ventilation. However, when she was approached for consent to a tracheostomy tube for chronic ventilatory support Mrs. B declined to give a direct answer, asking team members, "What would you do?" The team agreed to revisit Mrs. B's wishes in a few days. At the next meeting with Mrs. B and her daughter, the attending physician and palliative care APN explained Mrs. B's options for care including a tracheostomy, a Percutaneous Endoscopic Gastrostomy (PEG), or palliative extubation. The APN assured both the patient and her daughter that no matter which decision was made, comfort would be maintained. The patient with her daughter agreed to the tracheostomy and PEG. Mrs. B. reported increased comfort, but still required around-the-clock morphine and lorazepam to manage dyspnea and anxiety. The APN recommended switching to a transdermal fentanyl patch to allow for a more consistent serum opioid concentration and better symptom control. Mrs. B. stabilized and conversations related to discharge planning were initiated. A meeting was held with Mrs. B, her children, her attending physician and the palliative care team. Mrs. B clearly stated her wish to go home, but concerns related to Mrs. B's capacity to make these decisions were voiced by some of the hospital staff, so a formal ethics consultation to establish the patient's decisional capacity was held. Numerous ethics committee members, including the palliative care APN, met at the patient's bedside with her daughter and aide. Discussion related to Mrs. B's understanding of her current medical condition and her wishes related to discharge. The committee members also offered Mrs. B the option to allow her family to decide for her if she was unable to make the decision for herself. The committee members agreed that Mrs. B. continued to retain decisional capacity and that she understood the possibility that she may die sooner if discharged home rather than to a skilled nursing facility. Mrs. B's children agreed to take her home with home care and mechanical ventilation. The patient died at home 10 days later. During bereavement follow up, Mrs. B's children were consoled by the knowledge that the patient was where she wanted to be during her last days.

REFERENCES

1. Meier DE, Beresford L. Advanced practice nurses in palliative care: A pivotal role and perspective. J Palliat Med 2006;9:624–627.

2. Field MJ, Cassel CK. Approaching Death: Improving Care at the End of Life. Washington, DC: National Academy Press, 1997.

3. Peaceful Death: Recommended Competencies and Curricular Guidelines for End-of-Life Nursing Care. Washington, DC: American Association of Colleges of Nursing, 1998. Available at: http://www.aacn.nche.edu/publications/deathfin.htm (accessed October 24, 2009).

4. The SUPPORT Principle Investigators. A controlled trial to improve care for seriously ill hospitalized patients: The study to understand prognoses and preferences for outcomes and risks of treatments (SUPPORT). JAMA 1995;274:1591–1598.

5. Clinical Practice Guidelines for Quality Palliative Care. Pittsburgh, PA: National Consensus Project for Quality Palliative Care, 2004. Available at: http://www.national consensusproject.org (accessed October 24, 2009).

6. Advanced Practice Nurses Role in Palliative Care: A Position Statement from American Nursing Leaders. Missoula, MT: Promoting Excellence in End-of-Life Care, 2002. Available at: http://www.dyingwell.org/downloads/apnpos.pdf (accessed October 24, 2009).

7. Keeling AW. A brief history of advanced practice nursing in the United States. In: Hamric AB, Spross JA, Hanson CM, eds. Advanced Practice Nursing: An Integrative Approach (4th ed). St. Louis, MO: Saunders; 2009:3–32.

8. Buppert C. Nurse Practitioner's Business Practice and Legal Guide (3rd ed). Sudbury, MA: Jones and Bartlett, 2008.

9. Hamric AB. A definition of advanced practice nursing. In: Hamric AB, Spross JA, Hanson CM, eds. Advanced Practice Nursing: An Integrative Approach (4th ed). St. Louis, MO: Saunders; 2009:75–94.

10. Hentz PM, Hamric AB. The blended role of the clinical nurse specialist and the nurse practitioner. In: Hamric AB, Spross JA, Hanson CM, eds. Advanced Practice Nursing: An Integrative Approach (4th ed). St. Louis, MO: Saunders; 2009:437–461.

11. Skalla KA. Blended role advanced practice nursing in palliative care of the oncology patient. J Hosp Palliat Nurs 2006;8:155–163.

12. Ferrell B, Connor SR, Cordes A, et al. The national agenda for quality palliative care: The National Consensus Project and the National Quality Forum. J Pain Symptom Manage 2007;33:737–744.

13. NQF. A national framework and preferred practices for palliative and hospice care quality. Washington, DC: NQF, 2006.

14. HPNA, American Nurses Association. Hospice and Palliative Nursing: Scope and Standards of Practice (4th ed). Silver Spring, MD: American Nurses Association, 2007.

15. HPNA. Competencies for Advanced Practice Hospice and Palliative Care Nurses. Dubuque, IA: Kendall/Hunt, 2002.

16. Coyne PJ. The evolution of the advanced practice nurse within palliative care. J Palliat Med 2003;6:769–770.

17. Ferrell BR, Grant M, Virani R. Strengthening nursing education to improve end-of-life care. Nurs Outlook 1999;47:252–256.

18. Hewitt M, Simone JV, eds. Ensuring Quality Cancer Care. Washington, DC: National Academy Press, 1999.

19. Paice JA, Ferrell BR, Virani R, et al. Graduate nursing education regarding end-of-life care. Nurs Outlook 2006;54:46–52.

20. Ferrell BR, Virani R, Grant M. Analysis of end-of-life content in nursing textbooks. Oncol Nurs Forum 1999;26:869–876.

21. HPNA. HPNA position statement: Value of advanced practice nurse in palliative care. Pittsburgh, PA: HPNA, 2006. Available at: http://www.hpna.org/PicView.aspx?ID=384 (accessed October 24, 2009).

22. Wendt A. End-of-life competencies and the NCLEX-RN examination. Nurs Outlook 2001;49:138–141.

23. Beach P. The evolution of hospice and palliative nursing. In: Perley MJ, Dahlin C, eds. Core Curriculum for the Advanced Practice Hospice and Palliative Nurse. Pittsburgh, PA: HPNA; 2007:3–11.

24. Sherman DW. Training advanced practice palliative care nurses. Generations 1999;23:87–90.

25. Hospice and Palliative Master's Education Programs. Pittsburgh, PA: HPNA, 2009. Available at: http://www.hpna.org/DisplayPage.aspx?Title=Degree%20Programs (accessed October 24, 2009).

26. AACN Position Statement on the Practice Doctorate in Nursing. Washington, DC: AACN, 2004. Available at: http://www.aacn.nche.edu/DNP/DNPPositionstatement.htm (accessed October 24, 2009).

27. DNP roadmap task force report. Washington, DC: American Association of Colleges of Nursing, 2006. Available at: http://www.aacn.nche.edu/DNP/pdf/DNProadmapreport.pdf (accessed October 24, 2009).

28. Standards for clinical practicum in palliative nursing for practicing professional nurses (CPPN). Pittsburgh, PA: HPNA, 2006. Available at: http://www.hpna.org/DisplayPage.aspx?Title=Standards%20for%20Clinical%20Practicum (accessed October 24, 2009).

29. Mentoring programs. Glenview, IL: AAHPM, 2008. Available at: http://www.aahpm.org/about/mentoring.html (accessed October 24, 2009).

30. Advanced practice mentoring program. Pittsburgh, PA: HPNA, 2009. Available at: http://www.hpna.org/DisplayPage.aspx?Title=Mentoring (accessed October 24, 2009).

31. Kuebler K, Moore C. The Michigan advanced practice nursing palliative care project. J Palliat Med 2002;5:753–754.

32. Malloy P, Paice J, Virani R, et al. End-of-life nursing education consortium: 5 years of educating graduate nursing faculty in excellent palliative care. J Prof Nurs 2008;24:352–357.

33. Hanson CM. Understanding regulatory, legal, and credentialing requirements. In: Hamric AB, Spross JA, Hanson CM, eds. Advanced Practice Nursing: An Integrative Approach (4th ed). St. Louis, MO: Saunders; 2009:605–626.

34. Lentz J, Sherman DW. Professional organizations and certifications in hospice and palliative care. In: Matzo ML, Sherman DW, eds. Palliative Care Nursing: Quality Care to the End of Life (2nd ed). New York, NY: Springer; 2006:117–132.

35. Candidate Handbook and Application. Pittsburg, PA: NBCHPN, 2009. Available at: http://www.nbchpn.org/DisplayPage.aspx?Title=Candidate%20Handbook%20and%20Application (accessed October 24, 2009).

36. Perley MJ, Dahlin C, eds. Core Curriculum for the Advanced Practice Hospice and Palliative Nurse. Pittsburgh, PA: HPNA, 2007.

37. Advanced practice registered nurse (APRN) map. Pittsburg,PA: HPNA, 2009. Available at: http://www.nbchpn.org/Certificants_ Map.aspx?Cert=APRN (accessed October 24, 2009).

38. Kuebler KK, Pace JC, Esper P. The advanced practice nurse in palliative care. In: Kuebler KK, Heidrich DE, Esper P, eds. Palliative and End-of-Life Care: Clinical Practice Guidelines (2nd ed). St. Louis, MO: Saunders; 2006:3–18.

39. Quaglietti S, Blum L, Ellis V. The role of the adult nurse practitioner in palliative care. J Hosp Palliat Nurs 2004;6:209–214.

40. Advanced practice nursing: Pioneering practices in palliative care. Missoula, MT: Promoting Excellence in End-of-Life Care, 2002. Available at: http://www.dyingwell.org/downloads/ apnrep.pdf (accessed October 24, 2009).

41. Kuebler KK. The palliative care advanced practice nurse. J Palliat Med 2003;6:707–714.

42. Whedon MB. Revisiting the road not taken: Integrating palliative care into oncology nursing. Clin J Oncol Nurs 2002;6:1–7.

43. Meier DE, Beresford L. Billing for palliative care: An essential cost of doing business. J Palliat Med 2006;9:250–257.

44. Frakes MA, Evans T. An overview of Medicare reimbursement regulations for advanced practice nurses. Nurs Econ 2006; 24:59–65.

45. Medicare reimbursement fact sheet. Washington, DC: American Academy of Nurse Practitioners, 2009. Available at: http:// www.aanp.org/NR/rdonlyres/D498CAF2–7BE6–4D89–A588– 9DBC9CBD901A/0/FactSheetMedicareReimbursement108. pdf (accessed October 24, 2009).

46. Buppert C. Billing Physician Services Provided by Nurse Practitioners. Annapolis, MD: Law office of Carolyn Buppert, 2006.

47. Campbell M, Dahlin C. Advanced Practice Palliative Nursing: A Guide to Practice and Business Issues. Pittsburgh, PA: HPNA, 2008.

48. State recognition of NBCHPN APN certification. Pittsburg, PA: National Board for Certification of Hospice and Palliative Nurses, 2008. Available at: http://www.nbchpn. org/DisplayPage.aspx?Title=State (accessed October 24, 2009).

49. Von Gunten CF, Ferris FD, Kirschner C, et al. Coding and reimbursement mechanisms for physician services in hospice and palliative care. J Palliat Med 2000;3:157–164.

50. Ferrell BR, Coyle N. The Nature of Suffering and the Goals of Nursing. New York, NY: Oxford, 2008.

## 61

*Mary L. S. Vachon and Jayne Huggard*

# The Experience of the Nurse in End-of-Life Care in the 21st Century: Mentoring the Next Generation

♦ **Key Points**

♦ *Hospice palliative care nursing can be both stressful and very rewarding.*

♦ *Hospice palliative care nursing is whole-person care in that the whole person of the patient and caregiver must be considered in the process of truly caring.*

♦ *To care for others effectively, we must care for ourselves.*

♦ *Spirituality, an important component of palliative care, is the amalgam of the positive emotions, including compassion, that bind us to other human beings—and to our experience of "God" as we may understand Her/Him.[2]*

♦ *Organizations have a responsibility to provide care for the caregivers.*

## Personal, Professional, and Organizational Responsibilities

Several events have led, albeit over a long time, to this research. First are the experiences my fellow student nurses and I had during our nursing training in the late 1960s when support for staff was noticeable by its absence. Informally debriefing ourselves in the Nurses' Home forged a strong bond which continues to this day; however, I believe the responsibility for our emotional safety should not have been left to us alone. A vivid and painful memory is finishing a night duty in a large medical ward after four people had died on my shift, and the shame I felt when the night supervisor "found" some of the "bodies," with her implying a lack of diligence on my behalf and presumably questioning my ability to be a good nurse. But I *was* a good nurse, and when I applied for a Charge Nurse position, it was because I wanted to make a difference. I wanted to challenge beliefs and attitudes. I knew the patients were getting the best care we could give them at the time, but I knew that the staff also needed more of that care themselves. My advocating for them caused a few requests for me to "see the matron and explain yourself." My passion for supporting staff has continued to this day. I strongly believe we have to put our staff first and, if we do, then the care our patients receive will be the very best we can give.[1]

The discipline of hospice palliative care nursing began more than 30 years ago. The first author has been involved in the field as a researcher, educator, and practicing clinician since before its early days and has written what might be seen as snapshots of stress and coping in hospice palliative care at various points over the past four decades.[3–7] In the Introduction to her Master's thesis the second author, living in New Zealand, wrote:

> *My father died of cancer in 1979, the same year Te Omanga Hospice in Lower Hutt (where we lived) was being established. He died alone in Wellington*

*Hospital; no one had told us he was dying. I wish he could have spent his last days in a hospice surrounded by his family and the grandchildren he loved. I knew back then that one day I would work in a hospice.*

Several years later, after increasingly feeling like I never had enough time as a nurse to really talk to patients and their families in order to get to the essence of what their issues and concerns were, I chose to do my counselor training. Again, I wanted to make a difference, and I wanted to continue to do work that was meaningful and would give me much satisfaction. I found this work as a grief counselor at Mercy Hospice Auckland, and started there the day before September 11th, 2001. When I saw how the hospice handled the subsequent shock, bewilderment and anger that staff, patients and families felt at the events that happened on the other side of the world, and how that grief was allowed expression and not seen as something that had to be hidden away, I knew I had found the place to be.

A couple of years later, and with my ongoing interest in staff support, I conducted two staff support audits at Mercy Hospice eighteen months apart; the second audit determined the effects of new staff support initiatives developed as a result of the first. These audits were carried out as partial fulfillment of postgraduate palliative care course requirements and with the encouragement and support of Mercy Hospice. The writings of Professor Mary Vachon in the area of occupational stress for health professionals working in palliative care became well known to me through reading the literature. Without her realizing, she had

become my unofficial mentor, so in 2004 I emailed her to see if I could visit her when I traveled to Canada the following year. Mary was amazingly generous to me with her time, her knowledge and her resources, and she is now my 'official' mentor!

This chapter focuses on the experience of hospice palliative care nursing primarily from 2006 to 2008. Elsewhere the first author has written of stress in the earlier years of the hospice palliative care nursing.[4,5]

## Method

The literature from 2006 to 2008 was reviewed. The first author, who is engaged in a full-time clinical practice, has included some of her reflections. The majority of new data in this chapter comes from Huggard's postal questionnaire[1] of 464 palliative care staff, representing 11 professional groups. The sample includes: nurses, managers, doctors, counselors, social workers, pastoral and spiritual care co-coordinators, physiotherapists, occupational and diversion therapists, administrators, fundraisers, hospice shop managers, volunteer co-coordinators and household staff from 30 hospices across New Zealand (see Table 61–1).[1] Volunteers were excluded as they would have increased the numbers several fold, and they had already been studied.[8] The purpose of the study was to gain a greater understanding of the support needs of interprofessional staff working

| Table 61–1 Sample[1] | |
|---|---|
| Occupation | Number |
| **Nursing staff** | |
| Registered nurses | 253 |
| Enrolled nurses (graduates of an 18-month training program, the equivalent of Licensed Practical Nurses, no longer being prepared) | 36 |
| Health-care assistants | 11 |
| **Physicians** | 39 |
| Senior doctors identifying as consultants or medical specialists and "other doctors" including house officer, senior medical officer, and medical officer special scale. | |
| **Administrators/coordinators—non-clinical responsibilities** | 52 |
| Principal nurses or directors of nursing, nurse managers, team leaders, charge nurses, clinical team or care coordinators. All but one, a social worker, are nurses. | |
| **Managers** | 18 |
| Chief Executive Officers, business managers, fundraising managers, accountants, human resource managers and quality managers. | |
| **Social workers** | 11 |
| **Counselors, psychotherapists, art therapists** | 19 |
| **Chaplains** | 13 |
| **Allied health professionals** | 5 |
| **Housekeeping staff** | 7 |
| Total | 464 |

*Source*: Reprinted with permission from Huggard, J. 2008.

in New Zealand hospices and to determine if staff had enough organizational, professional and personal support to do the job required of them. Over 1100 staff are employed in 37 New Zealand hospices. Forty-two percent of the sample population completed an anonymous postal questionnaire developed by the researcher. Questions were both quantitative and qualitative, and primarily questioned the amount and type of support available to staff, both within and outside the organization; how important they felt this support was; and how effectively it met their needs. For the purposes of this chapter, the data presented will focus primarily on the nursing staff studied.

## Frameworks for Viewing Hospice Palliative Care

In their powerful book, *Crossing Over: Narratives of Palliative Care*, which describes the experience of palliative care in two settings in the United States and Canada, Barnard and colleagues[9] stated, "Palliative care is whole-person care not only in the sense that the whole person of the patient (body, mind, spirit) is the object of care, but also in that the whole person of the caregiver is involved. Palliative care is, par excellence, care that is given through the medium of a human relationship" (p. 5). These authors documented the experiences of patients, families, and caregivers during some of their finest and not so fine moments. The reader comes to understand the humanity of all involved.

A more recent study of nurses in a European academic palliative care setting[10] ($n=14$) was undertaken to gain insight into the fact that many nurses were leaving feeling frustrated by the far-reaching medical orientation on the ward and unable to provide the care they wanted to give. These nurses were not neophytes. They were typically oncology nurses, age 35 to 55 years, who had been working on this unit from 6 months to more than years. They raised questions about the benefits and burdens of the medical treatment with which they collaborated. This study challenges whether the assumptions of Barnard[9] are completely generalizable at this point in time and may shed light on some of the conflicts hospice palliative care nurses are experiencing in the early years of the 21st century. Georges' group[10] observed that the concept of palliative care demands that relationships with dying patients and their family members must be grounded in a real encounter and shared mutual understanding, and not in self-conscious use of psychosocial skills and techniques. The concept of compassion to be discussed below will further elaborate on this concept.[2]

## Striving to Adopt a Well-Organized and Purposeful Approach versus Striving to Increase the Well-Being of the Patient

Georges and colleagues[10] found that on the unit they studied, which was having trouble retaining nurses, two methods of

practice described the nurses' actual activity. The first and more prominent method was "striving to adopt a well-organized and purposeful approach as a nurse on an academic ward" ($n=12$); the second was "striving to increase the well-being of the patient" ($n=2$). The categories in each method are:

### Striving to Adopt a Well-Organized and Purposeful Approach

- *Striving to Adopt a Well-Organized and Purposeful Approach in an Academic Setting*: Using a "scientific" classification system of nursing diagnosis, formulating nursing interventions in relation to the diagnosis, and working within the limits set by the policy of the ward and the hospital; "appropriate bed utilization"; making discharge arrangements at an early stage to avoid unnecessary occupation of beds. For these nurses, carrying out the nursing process in a professional manner was more important than investing in their relationships with patients.
- *Developing a Professional Attitude*: A "professional attitude" refers to the rational approach of nurses, which is principally directed to gaining information about patients' symptoms and gaining insight into their problems. The nurses had a more detached attitude, tended to focus on identified tasks and problems, and, when giving information to patients, paid much attention to clarity and completeness while failing to consider the emotional impact of the message.
- *Striving to Remain Objective*: Described patients' health problems in a formal language; avoided speaking about problems that could not be labeled well, because they were not sure members of the multidisciplinary team would understand them; argued that being objective was more in accordance with current professional developments in the field of nursing; used diagnostic instruments to establish their observations; felt this use of instruments allowed them to feel more comfortable speaking with physicians, to feel they were seen as more trustworthy, and hence involved in the decision-making process. These nurses consciously strived to avoid allowing their feelings to have an impact on the way they responded to situations.
- *Being Task Oriented*: Mostly committed to improving the situation of patients by solving or reducing their problems; found it important to see that their interventions actually did improve the situation; felt powerless and as if they had not been able to achieve something meaningful for their patients if it was not possible to find a solution for patients' problems (e.g., to achieve sufficient symptom control, especially pain).
- *Avoiding Emotional Stress*: Coping with the emotional aspects of palliative care was a leading theme; stress they experienced seemed to be related mainly to

their appraisal of, and approach to, palliative care; some said that the gravity of caring for dying patients would inevitably lead to burnout, so they did not plan to work too long in palliative care; tended to distance themselves from patients by focusing on tasks and the treatment of symptoms; some explained that their experience had taught them to remain more professional and detached while others decided consciously not to invest too much in their relationship with patients because it would be too demanding.

- *Embracing a Practitioner-Focused Perspective:* Working in accordance with rules, these nurses emphasized the need to respect important rules of the ward. By being mainly directed to using a rational and 'scientific' approach to their tasks, the nurses could fail to meet the real needs of patients and to pay sufficient attention to the development of a compassionate attitude. This perception is mainly characterized by a distant approach towards patients and a well-developed self-awareness to work on one's own development as a professional.[10]

## Striving to Increase the Well-Being of the Patient

- *Striving to Increase the Well-Being of the Patient:* These nurses felt that it was important to use their individual capabilities, such as being sensitive to patients' concerns, and they adapted their approach to individual patients. They found that when fully aware of the needs of patients, it was not difficult to explain them to other caregivers. Care appeared to be a central concern for these nurses and a main source of satisfaction. They were aware that thanks to their caring attitude, they could mean something to patients, even if only for a short time, and they felt this to be rewarding.
- *Adopting a Humble Attitude:* To act in accordance with the needs of patients, these nurses tried to put their own considerations aside and find a way to cope with their own emotions. They strove to adopt an unobtrusive approach and to show their availability to patients without forcing anything, even without expecting patients to answer their "invitation."
- *Giving Attention to Patients and Their Experience:.* Shaped by their sensitivity to the feelings of patients; awareness of patients. Awareness of patients' experiences is related to individual efforts to discover and understand what patients experience and why they react as they do. To be conscious of patients' experiences requires being really present. They were concerned that giving inadequate or incomplete information to patients could badly affect the direction of their decisions about further treatment. Through sensitivity to the experiences of patients, the

nurses became more connected with them and tried to really help them, even if they had to "break the rules."

- *Being Available:* Being truly present appeared to be a major virtue of nurses that allowed them to perceive the troubles and needs of a patient. They spoke about being sensitive to unspoken messages and about trusting their intuition. Being receptive to what is going on helped them see how they could contribute to the well-being of patients.
- *Valuing a Caring Attitude:* The meaning nurses assigned to their work was based mainly on their experience as nurses and their daily encounters with patient care; developed a caring attitude based on authentic relationships with patients.
- *Remaining Attentive and Thoughtful:* To find solutions to the problems they were confronted with, these nurses used self-reflection, striving to adopt a patient-centered attitude and improve their caring attitude. They were also attentive to the context of their work, particularly what should be changed so as to make it easier to express a caring perspective.
- *Trying to Accept and Cope with Emotional Strain:* Nurses recognized that by caring for patients whose lives were limited, they were exposed to painful moments. They tried to accept emotionally difficult situations as a part of their own reality, instead of attempting to avoid them. They strove to remain "authentic" and to stay close to patients even if they could not alleviate their problems.

These two nursing approaches can be compared with a recent study of 18 academic oncologists.[11] All participants viewed their role as including the provision of excellent biomedical care (e.g., treatment of cancer with appropriate therapies in hopes of cure or disease-free time). "Some oncologists viewed their role almost exclusively in these biomedical terms while other participants described providing excellent biomedical care and also described a clear psychosocial role; to help the patient and family to cope with and accept the dying process. These respondents identified the psychosocial role as a second core professional responsibility. The psychosocial role often included caring for both the patient and family through building relationships and communicating effectively" (p. 896).[11] In Notes from the Editor, von Gunten[12] refers to the physicians who perceive a clear psychosocial role as type I oncologists. Those who see their role as primarily biomedical are referred to as type II oncologists. He suggests that for the type I oncologist, specialist physician services may rarely be needed and any collaboration will need to acknowledge the professional satisfaction the oncologist derives from the practice. For the type II oncologist, a routine assumption of end-of-life care responsibilities without any shame is in order. It is possible that some academic palliative medicine programs may be more similar to the type II oncologist model. The anecdote below is a personal one reflecting a presumably, type II oncologist, as well as the tensions that can arise within a team when caregivers are operating from different perspectives. The stress for this woman and her husband is clear.

*My 34-year-old friend was married to a 65-year-old husband, with whom she had a 4-year-old child. I had first met her mother when we had babies and wanted to start a daycare program, many years ago. I had known my young friend from the time of her conception. As a 20-year-old she had been actively involved in the care of her mother, a nurse, who had died of pancreatic cancer. At 34 she was diagnosed with cervical cancer. She initially received curative radiotherapy and chemotherapy and relapsed within about 5 months of finishing treatment.*

*I spoke with a medical oncologist friend who specialized in gynecologic oncology. He said that if she were his patient, he would not treat her until she was symptomatic. There were no good treatments for her disease. She was not pleased with this response, and sought a variety of opinions, meanwhile engaging in a variety of alternative treatments, with considerable help from her husband and friends. She started treatment with one oncologist and her disease continued to progress. She switched to an oncologist closer to home in whom she and her husband had great confidence. The oncologist, living in a small community, said that if they were to go by his office late at night they would see his light on, trying to put together protocols to help his patients. He was initially very helpful. When, however, she relapsed, he stopped returning the phone calls she and her husband made to him. Her husband would call in frustration, begging the nurse to get the doctor to return their calls. The nurse would say in*

*frustration, "What do you want me to do, put the phone to his ear and force him to speak with you?"*

*When my friend died, under the care of a hospice program, her husband drove her body to the crematorium and sat beside her body as it was being cremated. While there he realized he was close to the oncology clinic. He wrote a letter to the oncologist telling him how distressed they both were at his failure to respond to their phone messages when things were not going well. He said that he was sitting beside the crematorium while he wrote the letter, and hoped that the oncologist would think of them with the next patient like his wife and respond differently. He then hand delivered the letter to the cancer clinic, showed it to the nurse, and asked if she agreed with his sentiments. She did. He received word a couple of weeks later that the oncologist left, giving only a few weeks notice. 'Can only think the poor guy was totally overwhelmed'.[13]*

### What Attracts Staff to Palliative Care?

In Huggard's study,[1] staff were asked what initially attracted them to work in palliative care. Thirteen themes were initially identified and then reduced to five. Table 61–2 shows these themes.

### Previous Death of a Close Family Member or Friend

*Having had a personal family experience which was an exceptional one, I thought how much I liked the*

---

**Table 61–2**
**Factors Attracting Staff to Work in Hospices (p. 92)[1]**

| Consolidated Themes | Initial Themes |
| --- | --- |
| Previous death of family member or friend | Interest developed following the death of family or friends/observed palliative care in action |
| Career development | Wanted change/saw job advertisement/was approached |
| | Natural progression/career decision |
| | Wanting more knowledge/educational opportunities |
| The work environment | Want to provide holistic care/nature of care/type of care |
| | Want to make a difference/job satisfaction/rewarding, meaningful, worthwhile |
| | Wanted to work with dying and bereaved/interest in loss and grief/good death/companion on the journey |
| | Time factor/have enough time to do job properly |
| | Being part of multidisciplinary team/team work |
| | Supportive place for staff to work/environment, people supportive |
| Values and philosophy | Values/belief in palliative care/mission/ethical care/hospice philosophy/personal values aligned with palliative |
| | Care ethos/acceptance of cultural considerations, respectfulness |
| | Personal, spiritual reasons/calling/God/service to others |
| Lifestyle factors | Hours/shifts/flexibility/close to home |

*environment and how extraordinary it would be to be part of something that gave such support at a time of such vulnerability.* —Manager

*Forty years ago seeing patients screaming in pain, and then 20 years ago seeing improvement with pain control but patients still suffering fear and apprehension. I wished to help* —Nurse

## Career Development

*I had been a district nurse, and always enjoyed the palliative care field. I decided to have a change.* —Community Nurse

*Progressed [from oncology] as wanted to gain more specialized skills.* —Nurse

## The Working Environment

*To be able to work holistically, always mindful of all aspects of care incorporating social, emotional, spiritual, and the physical.*—Nurse

*I was working in an [acute] ward with many end-of-life patients but in a busy hospital ward, and I was not able to give patients and family the 'time necessary' for palliative care.*—Nurse

*Being able to work as a nurse who can make independent decisions and whose contribution is valued by other members of the multi-disciplinary team.* —Community Nurse

## Values and Philosophies

*I feel that hospice / palliative care philosophy aligns with Maori values and beliefs; it is safe for staff and patients and their Whanau (extended Maori kinship system)...*—Nurse

*I believe dying with dignity is the greatest gift we can leave our families [nurse] For spiritual reasons...an opportunity for meaningful relationships with patients and families dealing with life and death.*—Nurse

## Lifestyle Factors

*In all honesty, the hours.*—Doctor

*Flexibility of work, no night shifts.*—Health Care Assistant

## Reflections and Reflective Practice

The work of Georges et al.[10] also stands in contrast with that of authors such as Harper,[14] Perry,[15–17] and Katz and Johnson.[18]

Dr. Harper[14] is a social worker whose initial work involved supervising other social workers at City of Hope Hospital in California. She states that health professionals must learn to cope with the anxieties which arise from such interpersonal experiences, coming to grips with their own feelings about mortality—both theirs and the patient's.[14] Her model proposes that "learning to be comfortable in working with the dying patient and his family must be preceded by a growth and developmental process or sequence including cycles of productive change, observable behavior, and feeling" (p. 124). She poses six stages of adaptation experienced by the nurse caring for dying patients: intellectualization, emotional survival, depression, emotional arrival, deep compassion, and the Doer.

A comparison of Harper's work[14] with that of Georges' group[10] shows that although Harper's model is very useful to describe the career path of some nurses in palliative care, there may be others who do not progress in the manner that Harper describes, perhaps because of a lack of suitable mentoring. From Harper's perspective, these nurses may never have evolved beyond the first stage of comfortability. They are still involved in an intellectual approach to their role and are defending against allowing emotions to intrude. However, the nurses in the category striving to increase the well-being of the patient could be seen to be in Harper's stage IV or higher, in which they have "the control to practice the art of one's science" (p. 71).

Perry[15–17] has used nursing narratives to explore exemplary nursing practice in palliative care and oncology nursing. She uses the themes of the dialogue of silence, mutual touch, and sharing the lighter side of life to illustrate aspects of exemplary nursing practice and identifies joint transcendence as the essence of exemplary nursing practice. Most recently[17] she did a phenomenological study of seven oncology nurses nominated by their colleagues as exemplary caregivers. Exemplary nurses were defined "as those nurses who did their work in a remarkable way and achieved outstanding outcomes for their patients and for themselves" (p. 87).[17] Three themes were identified: moments of connection, making moments matter, and energizing moments. Perry pursued the discusssion points rasied by the themes of attitude, the link between attitude and values, and strategies to promote a positive attitude. These issues will be explored below.

Perry's concept of joint transcendence,[15] which draws on the work of Watson,[19] captures some of what Harper[14] implies in her use of the term The Doer. "When both care providers and care receiver are co-participants in caring, the release can potentiate self-healing and harmony in both. The release can allow the one who is cared for to be the one who cares, through the reflection of the human condition that in turn nourishes the humanness of the care provider. In such connectedness they are both capable of transcending self, time, and space. Neither stands above the other."[15,19] Perry[16] speaks of the palliative care nursing experience as valuing each individual, experiencing the reciprocity of giving and receiving in relationships, a sense of interconnectedness and of mutual nurturing, being close to patients and sharing a part of one's self; the chance to make a difference in people's lives.

Katz[20] draws on the quantum physics concept that the whole is greater than the sum of its parts, similar to Kearney's *A Place of Healing: Working with Suffering in Living and Dying*,[21] Katz[20] speaks of the alchemical reaction which occurs when two individuals engage together at the most vulnerable time in human existence—the end of life. Alchemy is "that space" that takes its own place in the poignant relationship between helper and patient. Through the experience, both can be transformed.

During and following Dr. Veronique Benk's induction chemotherapy for treatment of her leukemia, a number of her friends and colleagues would spend the night at the hospital with her. I spent Tuesday nights.

*One Tuesday night Veronique awakened and said that she had a dream of two archangels, Gabriel and Raphael who told her they were Team 1.7. I suggested that maybe that meant they would be with her until her white blood count reached 1.7. On Thursday I received a call to say that Veronique had been transferred to the ICU with an acute respiratory syndrome which developed as her white blood count ascended to 1.7. She had been told that if she was ventilated there was only a 5% chance that she would survive.*

*I went to the ICU thinking that I would not be able to see Veronique, but maybe I could at least see her husband, Paul, for a couple of minutes. When I arrived Paul said that their daughter, Aude, then age 4 was in process of being admitted to the Hospital for Sick Children (HSC) with a ruptured appendix. I suggested that he go to HSC and I would stay with Veronique. She was afraid to go to sleep for fear that she would stop breathing. I told her to go to sleep and I would stay awake and pray all night.*

*In the morning when Veronique awoke she said that she was carried all night along the beach on a seat made by the crossed hands of her two angels, Team 1.7. She later said that night she had a near death experience and was asked whether she was ready to die, or still wanted to live. She chose to come back for the sake of her family. To this day, Aude insists that her mother was with her when she went for surgery that evening. On Friday when I went to my office I had my normal energy as though I had a full night's sleep (p. S50).[22]*

Today some nurses may be straddling the fence between a deep involvement in patient care and feeling challenged by bureaucratic issues; others may be carrying on their practice in the manner that Harper describes, whereas others may be practicing a type of nursing that might be more common to that seen in traditional medical settings. The preceding anecdote may seem normal to some palliative care nurses, and a bit "far out" to others. If the first author had seen such an anecdote several years ago, while working as a Consultant in Psychosocial

Oncology and Palliative Care in an academic cancer center, conducting research, writing and lecturing internationally, before getting cancer and having a spiritually transforming experience,[23] she too would have found it rather a far-fetched experience. We speak, however, of reflective practice. Schon[24] defines reflection as "knowing-in-action" "When the practitioner reflects-in-action in a case she perceives as unique, paying attention to phenomena and surfacing her intuitive understanding of them, her experimentation is at once exploratory, move testing, and hypothesis testing. The three functions are fulfilled by the very same actions. Situations do not present themselves as givens, but are constructed from events that are puzzling, troubling, and uncertain."[24]

Dr. Ira Byock speaks of trying to devise a palliative care system that is "cutting edge, medically crisp, but tender and loving."[25] What are some of the issues that keep this from happening? Meier and colleagues[26] described what might happen in physicians, and these comments hold true for nurses as well:

*Seriously ill persons are emotionally vulnerable during the typically protracted course of an illness. Physicians respond to such patients' needs and emotions with emotions of their own, which may reflect a need to rescue the patient, a sense of failure or frustration when the patient's illness progresses, feelings of powerlessness against illness and its associated losses, grief, fear of becoming ill oneself, or a desire to separate from and avoid patients to escape these feelings. These emotions can affect both the quality of medical care and the physician's own sense of well-being, since unexamined emotions may also lead to physician distress, disengagement, burnout, and poor judgment. (p. 3007)[26]*

These authors provided a model of reflective practice[26] for physicians to use to increase their awareness and improve their clinical practice.

This next section discusses the concepts of burnout and compassion fatigue as well as some of the stressors currently experienced in hospice palliative care and the ways in which stress may be expressed.

## Burnout and Compassion Fatigue

Burnout and compassion fatigue are two ways of understanding the stress that caregivers in palliative care may experience. Maslach and associates[27] reviewed the research on burnout over the past three decades. Burnout is a form of mental distress manifested in "normal" persons who did not suffer from prior psychopathology, who experience decreased work performance resulting from negative attitudes and behaviors.[28] The key dimensions of burnout include:

- Emotional exhaustion (EE), the basic *individual stress dimension* of burnout, refers to feelings of being overextended and depleted of one's emotional and physical resources. Exhaustion prompts action to distance oneself emotionally and cognitively from work, as a way to cope with work overload.[28]

- Feelings of **cynicism** and detachment from the job (**depersonalization** [DP]), the *interpersonal context* dimension of burnout, refers to a negative, callous, or excessively detached response to various aspects of the job. It is an attempt to put distance between oneself and various aspects of the job. Research shows a consistent strong relationship between exhaustion and cynicism from the presence of work overload and social conflict.[28]

- Sense of **ineffectiveness** and **lack of personal accomplishment** (PA), the self-evaluation dimension of burnout, refers to feelings of incompetence and a lack of achievement and productivity at work. PA arises more clearly from a lack of resources to get the work done (e.g., lack of critical information, lack of necessary tools, or insufficient time). It may be directly related to EE and DP, or be more independent.[29]

See Table 61–3 for the symptoms of burnout.

Six areas of work life encompass the major organizational antecedents of burnout. These include: workload, control,

---

**Table 61–3**
**Signs and Symptoms of Burnout**[36–38]

**Physical**
Fatigue
Physical and emotional exhaustion
Headaches
Gastrointestinal disturbances
Weight loss
Sleeplessness
Hypertension
Myocardial infarction

**Psychological**
Anxiety
Depression
Boredom
Frustration
Low morale
Irritability
May contribute to alcoholism and drug addiction

**Occupational**
Depersonalization in relationships with colleagues, patients, or both
Emotional exhaustion, cynicism, perceived ineffectiveness
Job turnover
Impaired job performance
Deterioration in the physician–patient relationship and a decrease in the quantity and quality of care

**Social**
Marital difficulties

---

reward, community, fairness and values.[27] Recent research in a university setting showed that fairness in the work environment may be the tipping point determining whether people develop job engagement or burnout.[28] Job engagement is conceptualized as being the opposite of burnout.[29] It involves energy, involvement, and efficacy. Engagement involves the individual's relationship with work. This includes a sustainable workload, feelings of choice and control, appropriate recognition and reward, a supportive work community, fairness, and justice and meaningful and valued work. Engagement is also characterized by high levels of activation and pleasure.[29] Engagement is defined as a persistent, positive-affective-motivational state of fulfillment in employees that is characterized by vigor, dedication, and absorption.[29]

Emotion-work variables (e.g., requirement to display or suppress emotions on the job, requirements to be emotionally empathic) account for additional variance in burnout scores over and above job stressors.[27] These stressors may be the same ones that in some situations could lead to compassion fatigue.[30,31]

Compassion fatigue is not as well researched as burnout,[7,32] but studies on compassion fatigue in palliative care are currently in process. Compassion fatigue symptomatology is closely related to that of Post Traumatic Stress Disorder, except that it applies to those emotionally affected by the trauma of another (usually a client or family member).[30] Numerous terms are used to describe the emotional component of work-related stress, including burnout, secondary traumatic stress disorder, vicarious traumatization, countertransference, traumatic countertransference, and emotional contagion. Although these terms are sometimes used interchangeably, the underlying constructs associated with each of these terms differ in their conceptual framework.[20,33–35] As a means of addressing these differences, and to capture the overall theme of emotionally-induced occupationally-related stress syndromes, the term traumatoid state has been suggested.[34] In contrast to one who has burned out, the caregiver with compassion fatigue can still care and be involved.[36] This ability to continue to be able to care and receive satisfaction from caring was described by Stamm as compassion satisfaction.[37]

---

### A Model for Understanding Occupational Stress

Recent research has focused on the degree of match or mismatch between the person and six domains of the job environment. The greater the gap or mismatch between the person and the environment, the greater the likelihood of burnout. The greater the match or fit, the greater the likelihood of engagement with work.[27] Mismatches arise when the process of establishing a psychological contract leaves critical issues unresolved or when the working relationship changes to something that the person finds unacceptable.

Mismatches lead to burnout. Six areas of work life come together in a framework that encompasses the major organizational antecedents of burnout; workload, control, reward, community, fairness, and values.[27]

Maslach and Leiter[28] describe the continuum between the negative experience of burnout and the positive experience of engagement. There are three interrelated dimensions to this continuum: exhaustion–energy, cynicism–involvement, and inefficacy–efficacy. Exhaustion and cynicism are the two primary measures of burnout. They "go together", both appearing strongly in people experiencing burnout, and they both fade away in people experiencing engagement with their work. A potential early warning sign of burnout is the appearance of one, but not the other of these signs. They suggest there is a push to move from an inconsistent pattern to a consistent one. A predictor of whether an inconsistent pattern will evolve towards burnout or engagement will be the presence of a negative incongruence between the person and the job. For someone who is experiencing one of the burnout dimensions, this level of incongruity can be the tipping point into burnout. In a university setting, the workplace incongruity (tipping point) that determined whether people changed was their perception of fairness in the workplace.[28]

The recent research on hospice palliative care nursing is now reviewed within this framework. Elsewhere, specific studies measuring burnout and stress in palliative care[5,38,39] and oncology[40] have been reviewed.

## Workload

Excessive workload exhausts the individual to the extent that recovery becomes impossible. Emotional work is especially draining when the job requires people to display emotions inconsistent with their feelings. Workload relates to the exhaustion component of burnout.[28] A recent review of the literature[5] showed that from the early 1970s there were perceived difficulties with workload, and insufficient staff to do the job at hand in both oncology and palliative care. From the 1970s through the ensuing decades to the 21st century, oncology staff in particular report being overwhelmed with the workload imposed by the increase in cancer and the chronic nature of the illness. Recent research[41] testing a new stress model in 403 fulltime undergraduate students found that the primary driver of perceived stress was neuroticism, rather than self-reported workload.

Hospice nurses initially prided themselves on having the time to spend with patients that was conducive to the best patient care. Current issues with managed care, the nursing shortage, and fiscal restraint have changed this situation in many settings. Payne[42] found that despite that fact that workload was a frequently reported stressor, it was not related to burnout, suggesting that some stress may be necessary for optimal functioning. In the New Zealand Study,[1] workload was not identified as being a stressor, nor was it identified as being related to a lack of organizational support.

## Control

The issue of control is related to inefficacy or reduced personal accomplishment. Mismatches often indicate that individuals have insufficient control over the resources necessary to do their work or insufficient authority to pursue the work in what they believe is the most effective manner.[28] From the 1970s to the present,[5] stress has resulted from a lack of knowledge in interpersonal skills and a lack of communication skills and/or management skills in both oncology and palliative care specialists.[43]

Research suggests that restructuring of high-demand, low-control jobs may enhance productivity and reduce disability costs.[44] Recent practices in hospice led by fiscal constraints have raised increasing concern. Nurses are sometimes expected to perform procedures in the community for which they have not been prepared and for which no supervision is provided. When people are expected to assume responsibility with inadequate training, they have difficulty functioning.[6]

Nurses report being in situations, both in the hospital and in the community, in which they feel responsible for alleviating the pain of a palliative care patient yet do not have a physician willing to order the medication they feel is sufficient to control pain.[6]

> I'm the admitting nurse. I have so many hours to get a patient on the service. I can't predict if the doctor will call back. He may not call back until the next day. It can happen that I am at X Hospital. The patient is going home. I call his doctor and tell him that the patient is short of breath and there isn't an order for Ativan. The doctor may not call back until tomorrow. We could use our hospice doctor, but I don't want to make the referring doctor angry.[6]

An American nurse said that when she reported that a dying patient was in severe pain and she felt that he needed to have his medication increased, the physician asked who he was treating—the patient or the nurse?[6]

Issues of control can also be related to physical safety. Nurses reported feeling unsafe when they were making visits to deserted country homes in the middle of snowstorms without access to cell phones or other ways of communicating if there is trouble; visiting in unsafe areas of the community, where the nurses do not feel safe during the day, and particularly at night; and visiting in homes where the family dynamics are such that nurses do not feel physically safe. If there are no organizational policies about how to handle these situations, staff can feel quite stressed.[6]

Nurses may also feel out of control if they begin to get emotionally involved with patients and families without sufficient supervision and support. Barnard and coworkers[9] noted the need to give full weight to both the promise and the fear of intimacy in palliative care and referred to palliative care as challenging caregivers to leap into the confrontation with the forces of chaos and disintegration (p. 26):

*We live in the tension between the promise of intimacy
and the fear of our own undoing. Surprised by
intimacy, we are exhilarated and lifted beyond
ourselves, as if we have not only made contact with
another person but also with another dimension of
living. At the same time we are brought face to face with
forces of chaos and destructiveness, internal as well as
external, and we fear that we ourselves shall be destroyed.*

These feelings can lead caregivers to feel out of control and
to experience significant role strain.

Nurses also feel out of control because of the timing of
patient referrals:

*Patients are referred later and sicker. They are more
acute. You don't have the time that you used to have.
Ten years ago we had patients for a couple of months
on average. Now it is just weeks. The doctors don't refer
until later because there is a fear of referring too soon
with reimbursement. There are more treatment
modalities. Patient's families want them to try more.
There is less time for me to do what I need to do, which
is (1) palliate symptoms, (2) prepare people for
impending death, (3) be a supportive presence so they
aren't so afraid, and (4) establish a trusting rapport.[6]*

## Rewards

Lack of reward may be financial when one doesn't receive a
salary or benefits commensurate with achievements, or lack
of social rewards when one's hard work is ignored and not
appreciated by others. The lack of intrinsic rewards (e.g.,
doing something of importance and doing it well) can also be
a critical part of this mismatch.[28] Funding issues have always
been an issue in palliative care[3] and continue to be.[45]

An American nurse noted some of the difficulties with the
financial reward of hospice palliative care nursing:

*The money isn't very good in a not-for-profit hospice,
but I can cope with the pay. I could make more, though,
in a for-profit hospice.[6]*

Huggard[1] stated that although not asked for, a small group
stated that it was not the monetary reward that kept them
working in this area.

## Community

Team communication problems have been a significant part
of hospice palliative care and, to a lesser extent, the field of
oncology since the early days of these specialties. The research
on this subject has been reviewed elsewhere.[3-7,38-40] Team
issues have been documented in numerous studies and across
many cultures.[38-40,45]

Lack of cooperation and discipline occurs when teams
have coordination without cooperation. If team members
are ordered about without consultation or participation, they
will not give their best effort and will fail.[6]

Studying hospice nurses in the United Kingdom, Payne[42]
found that dealing with death and dying, inadequate preparation, and workload were slightly more problematic than were
conflict with doctors, conflict with other nurses, lack of support, and uncertainty concerning treatment. However, in that
study conflict with staff contributed to both the emotional
exhaustion and depersonalization subscales of the Maslach
Burnout Inventory.[46] More recently palliative care specialist
registratrars in the UK were more likely than oncology registrars to report finding stress from low prestige of their specialty and from difficulties with nursing staff.[47]

Huggggard[1] found that of the support strategies she studied, "organizational support strategies appeared to be the
most important for hospice staff. The majority of participants
stated that they were well supported, especially by their line
managers and peers, and that they felt both supported and
valued by their organization" (p. 143).[1] Table 61-4 shows the
top five organizational initiatives most valued by registered
nurses. Participants were asked to rank the items on a scale
from 1 to 5, with 1 being "not effective" and 5 being "effective."
These include manageable rosters (shifts), informal support
from peers, orientation, management of staff conflict, and
feedback that acknowledges that you are doing a good job.

A large study of burnout in critical care nursing staff in
278 intensive care units ($n = 2,525$) in France[48] found that 33%
had severe Burnout symptoms on the French version of the
Maslach Burnout Inventory (MBI).[46] Four dimensions were
associated with severe burnout: *age* (younger and less experienced staff were more prone to burnout); *organizational
factors*, such as ability to choose days off or being able to participate in an ICU research group; *quality of work relations*,

---

**Table 61-4**
**Highest "Importance" Scores for Organizational Initiatives Professional Group: Registered Nurse**

| Q. No. | Organizational Initiative | Importance Mean | Available "Yes" (%) | Effective Mean |
|---|---|---|---|---|
| 14 | Manageable rosters | 4.66 | 90.0 | 4.03 |
| 7 | Informal support from peers | 4.65 | 98.3 | 4.38 |
| 11 | Orientation | 4.64 | 98.3 | 3.86 |
| 17 | Management of staff conflict | 4.49 | 87.3 | 3.26 |
| 21 | Feedback that acknowledges you are doing a good job | 4.48 | 87.8 | 3.61 |

such as conflicts with patients, relationship with head nurse or physicians; and *end-of-life* factors, such as caring for a dying patient and number of decisions to forego life-sustaining treatments in the last week.

Although teamwork has been seen as being the best and perhaps, only way of doing palliative care, and although teams will no doubt be the primary way in which palliative care will be delivered for the foreseeable future, particularly in academic palliative care units and hospices, a recent book by Peter Speck,[45] *Teamwork in Palliative Care: Fulfilling or Frustrating?*, questions some of the assumptions of palliative care teamwork.

Speck[49] writes: "Our personal identity is formed and shaped as a result of our interaction with other people as well as the expression of our basic genetic makeup. We, therefore, seek out and develop formal and informal social groups and networks in both our private and our working life which supplement the relationships we already have within our family unit..." (p. 7).[49] Social support from people with whom one shares praise, comfort, happiness, and humor affirms membership in a group with a shared sense of values (Ref. 29, p. 5).[27,29]

A random sample of 74 breast cancer teams[50] in the UK (548 members in six core disciplines, including nurses, used the 12-item GHQ that has been used in other studies and found the mental health of the breast cancer teams ("caseness"—15.7%) appeared to be significantly better than the mental health of other cancer clinicians in the National Health Service (NHS) ("caseness"—32%).[51] These teams were dealing with newly-diagnosed patients, which may have accounted for the decreased levels of mental health problems. The authors also suggested that the team shared responsibility for decision-making and team support, the better prognosis of breast cancer patients compared with those with other solid tumors and perhaps selection bias in those who returned their questionnaires could have contributed to this difference. They also noted that teams with shared leadership in clinical decision-making were most effective.

### Fairness

This mismatch arises when there is perceived unfairness in the workplace. Fairness communicates respect and confirms people's self-worth. Mutual respect between people is central to a shared sense of community. As already noted, fairness in the work environment may be the tipping point determining whether people develop job engagement or burnout.[28]

Rivalries between hospice and other settings of care and between different hospice programs have long been an issue.[3,6] Rivalries are encountered as programs try to determine with which agencies, if any, they will have preferred-partner arrangements. Other settings have developed palliative care programs in an apparent move to avoid referral to hospice and to gain access to funding that might be made available for dying persons.[6] In addition, there are financial barriers, including reimbursement systems that provide only for the options of cure or certain death.[52]

Whedon,[52] an oncology nurse whose practice changed to pain and symptom management, observed (p. 27): "Patients without a care provider; unwilling to forego beneficial palliative chemotherapy, radiation, or surgery; or with a prognosis that was not absolutely certain to be six months or less, were caught in the middle. This part of the path felt treacherous; we had no trail markers, no compass, and darkness was about to fall."

### Values

*When people come to work, they wish to engage with activities that are consistent with the values they hold. Values are what people believe to be right, wrong, good, desirable, moral etc. These values have developed in a variety of ways including: family life, education, belief system (religious and otherwise), peer group relationships and professional identity, and can affect how we function at work (pp. 3–4).[45]*

In Huggard's study[1] "values and philosophy" was one of the categories that explained caregivers' reasons for working in palliative care (Table 61–5). Stories about the mission, values and philosophy of palliative care featured again very strongly. Comments included the atmosphere, the environment, the beautiful surroundings that hospices are often set in, the positive way in which staff are treated, usually as well as the patients, the sense of purpose and the sacredness of the work. Repeated phrases include "making a difference", "loving the job", "passion for what I do", along with the "satisfaction" gained from working in this area and how "meaningful and rewarding" this type of work is. Issues of social justice, of caring for the poor and needy, of offering free care were also important, as were comments about helping society and services rendered to the community.

Some respondents talked of it being a "vocation," a "calling from God," or a "life's purpose." For most it was certainly not just a job.

Georges and coauthors[10] quoted James and Field,[53] who said that when the originating ethics of palliative care are marginalized, the heart and soul of care are endangered. "Expert" values based on medical technologies and psychosocial skills replace the compassionate help. Death is no longer a truth to confront but a process that must be managed as efficiently as possible. Nurses who participated in this study[10] were encouraged in this context to acquire knowledge and skills, whereas development of the moral qualities necessary to care for those who are dying was not addressed. Therefore, they became less sensitive to the moral values in situations. They responded less to problems because their moral values were endangered, mainly because they conflicted with their professional norms and established rules. In situations of pain and suffering, these nurses mainly tried to overcome their powerlessness through a medical approach, overlooking the possibilities of alleviating suffering by an authentic caring attitude based on really meeting with patients.

The findings of Georges and colleagues[10] illustrate the potential differences between applying palliative care in

**Table 61–5**
**Themes in Response to the Question "What Keeps You Working in Palliative Care?"**

| Initial Theme (16) | Consolidated Theme (7) |
| --- | --- |
| Supportive team/team work/being part of the multidisciplinary team | Team work and support |
| Support available/emotional safety/supervision/debriefs | |
| Type of care offered/hands on/primary care/quality care/excellent care/nature of work in palliative care | The nature and type of care |
| Importance of, and ability to give, holistic care | |
| Being able to care for families, importance of family needs/following families in their bereavement | |
| Time available to give proper care | |
| Variety of the work | |
| Challenges and complexity of the work | |
| Autonomous practice | |
| Ongoing learning/training, educational opportunities/developing more skills/mentoring | Professional and personal growth |
| Personal growth/life experiences/sense of vocation | |
| Working in the community/looking after patients at home/being part of larger community | Community |
| Life balance/hours/days/flexibility/close to home/need to work | Lifestyle |
| Making a difference to patient and family/satisfaction/rewarding/love my job/passionate about the work | Values and philosophy |
| Palliative care or hospice philosophy/social justice, mission /values/beautiful surroundings/ walk the talk | |
| Money | Money |

an academic hospital directed by a predominantly medical approach and applying it in the tradition of the hospice movement where care is at its most fundamental. Time will tell whether Byock's vision[25] of "cutting edge, medically crisp, but tender and loving care" can be realized.

## Emotion-Work Variables: Issues of Death and Dying

Although the literature has been somewhat divided as to whether or not the care of the dying is a major stressor in hospice palliative care,[3,4] recent research in the burnout area has focused explicitly on emotion-work variables (e.g., requirement to display or suppress emotions on the job, requirements to be emotionally empathic) and has found these emotional factors do account for additional variance in burnout scores over and above job stressors.[27]

The most problematic stressor reported by hospice nurses was "death and dying."[42] In contrast, Huggard's study[1] reporting results from all occupational groups working in hospices did not identify "death and dying" issues as a major contributor to creating a stressful work environment. Participants reported that these issues were manageable as long as there were sufficient and appropriate organizational support practices, such as acknowledgement of the deaths, the use of rituals, and the availability of debriefing, if required.

The difficulties associated with the care of dying persons may also be in part a result of the close connections palliative care nurses often develop with their patients. As has already

been noted, palliative care is, par excellence, care that is given through the medium of a human relationship.[9] Barnard and colleagues noted that education for palliative care involves the art of building and sustaining relationships and using the self as a primary instrument for diagnosis and treatment. This involves psychological risk-taking that may be unique in the health field.[9] As was clear from the work of Georges and associates,[10] not all nurses are prepared for this involvement, either personally or through their education, professional training, mentoring, and supervision.

Boston and coworkers[54] noted that dying persons experience disruption of the essence of day-to-day living and challenges to their perception of who they are. Through this process, they gain new wisdom and reshape their sense of meaning in life. A different way of knowing the world evolves, characterized by inner know-how and tacit knowledge that defines the self in relationship to others. Caregivers and others around them "are perceived to be in another place, or don't seem to be there at all" (p. 248). Patients and caregivers may feel that they just don't connect. Boston and coauthors[54] speak of palliative care as taking caregivers into emotional realms that are neither easy nor comfortable. The caregiver may be permanently changed through this encounter.

CASE STUDY
*A Story of Personal Growth*

While working on this article, the first author attended a lecture on Empathy and Spirituality and a workshop on Enhancing Empathy, given by nurse Margaret Baim at the conference on Spirituality & Healing in Medicine: The Resiliency Factor.[55] Baim spoke of the work of Edith Stein, author of On The Problem of Empathy,[56] asking if anyone knew the work of this woman, who had been executed in Auschwitz. She said Stein, a Jew, had been studying empathy and had become fascinated by the work of Saint Theresa of Avila and her empathy. Stein entered the Carmelites. I suddenly realized Stein was one of the modern-day saints, Saint Teresia Benedicta of the Cross, commemorated in the stained glass windows of the church I attend regularly. I had made a donation in honor of my clients for these windows, so [I] feel a connection to them. Bain then spoke of one of the miracles attributed to Stein. A young girl had been dying at Massachusetts General Hospital (my Alma Mater). The family was gathered, they had been prepared for her coming death. The young girl was unconscious. One of her aunts said she was named for St. Theresa, so maybe they should all pray to St. Theresa for a miracle. They did. The girl regained consciousness, and said she had a vision of Edith Stein.

Baum led the participants in the workshop through a Tonglen meditation on empathy.[57] She suggested we think of a time of joy in our life, and then think of someone in our life who was suffering and send the joy to that person.

I thought of a time a couple of years ago when my husband was very sick; his diagnosis and prognosis were at that point quite uncertain. I was trying to be supportive, while maintaining some of the structure of my normal life. On a beautiful spring May morning, I raced out to my car to go to the gym. Suddenly, between the garage door and the back gate, I was struck with a moment of internal joy, deep within my chest. I had this centered-feeling that no matter what happened all would be well.

I thought of a young, Jewish client who was dying at that point. We had conversations about whether there was something on the other side. She wasn't sure what to believe. Her mother believed there was something, but she didn't know, although she hoped that when she got there she would find there was something. I started to send her the joy I had felt, hoping it would help as she made her transition. I could feel myself "connect" with her, then suddenly it was as though she was sending me joy back. I started seeing colors, unlike any I had previously seen in a meditation. I thought to myself, "I wonder if she has died and is sending me the joy she is now experiencing." I spoke with my friend with whom I was staying, another author in this book, and shared the experience. When I returned home I found my client had died the day before I did the meditation. This experience will be one of the many that will stay with me and change me, particularly since part of the spiritual experience I had with my cancer diagnosis had to do with "connecting" with clients with whom I had worked who had died.[23]

## Multiple Losses

One does not have to work very long in palliative care before one begins to feel the accumulation of grief related to the experience of multiple losses. Early in the development of the field, Mount wrote of the concept of multiple losses within the context of oncology[58]; the concept became more recognized with the AIDS epidemic. Garfield[36] wrote of alternating between numbness and experiencing grief while caring for people dying of AIDS.

Papadatou[59] extended earlier work[3] to note that the losses nurses experience may extend beyond the deaths of their patients. These losses include:

- Loss of a close relationship with a particular patient
- Loss caused by the professional's identification with the pain of family members
- Loss of one's unmet goals and expectations
- Losses related to one's personal system of beliefs and assumptions about life
- Past unresolved losses or anticipated future losses
- The death of self.

## Satisfactions in Hospice Palliative Care

Although work in hospice palliative care can be stressful, it also has many rewards. Current research has focused on the experience of job engagement, which is conceptualized as being the opposite of burnout. It involves energy, involvement, and efficacy. Engagement involves the individual's relationship with work. As described by Maslach and colleagues,[27] it involves a sustainable workload, feelings of choice and control, appropriate recognition and reward, a supportive work community, fairness and justice, and meaningful and valued work. Engagement is also characterized by high levels of activation and pleasure. Clearly, for many caregivers, their work in hospice palliative care is very engaging, as was noted in the research reviewed in this section.

In Huggard's study,[1] caregivers gave the following reasons for continuing to work in hospice: teamwork and support, the nature and type of care, personal and professional growth, community, lifestyle, values and philosophy, and money.

### Team Work and Support

The supportive nature of the palliative care working environment was a major factor in retaining staff. Both the support from colleagues and being part of the wider team were mentioned frequently. Many spoke of the enjoyment of working in the team, they enjoyed the team dynamics, and the fact that everyone was working toward the goal of best practice for their patients. Also mentioned was the fact that each professional group had a voice in decision-making, something often not found elsewhere. Peer support was frequently cited as a key reason why staff chose to keep working in this field, and descriptive words used include: "amazing support," "fantastic colleagues," "understanding team mates," "warmth and friendship." The acknowledgement in some organizations of the commitment to making the team emotionally safe to do the work was also mentioned. This included the availability of debriefs, supervision, the ability to access Employee Assistance Programmes (EAP), counseling, and the level of training and supervision offered.

> *The supportive team and the support available, e.g. debriefs, trusted colleagues and regular monthly supervision with a committed group help me to be focused and safe.* —Nurse

> *The job enjoyment and the satisfaction is very fulfilling as an enrolled nurse. I enjoy the opportunity to work on an equal footing within the team. I know I would miss it too much if I ever left .*—Enrolled Nurse

## The Nature and Type of Care

As with the initial attraction for some staff, the opportunity to practice holistically in the field of dying and death and the nature of the therapeutic relationship were major factors for retaining staff. Others used the terms providing hands on care, or being able to offer quality care or excellent care. Comments such as the ability to provide "crisp symptom management" and relief of pain and other symptoms featured frequently in the stories. Caring for the family was again a source of satisfaction, both pre- and postdeath. Many spoke also of the variety of work within a working day and time featured strongly—time to do the care properly, time to spend sitting quietly with the dying patient, time to prepare family, time to educate and normalize what was happening. A sub-theme was the challenges and complexities of care that many found rewarding, and also the ability to practice autonomously.

> *In the 30 years I have been nursing, I knew there was something better than task nursing; it is a pity it has taken me so long to find holistic care...to me this is the epitome of nursing.* —Nurse

> *Definitely the patients...I am humbled and honoured to be sharing end of life experiences with them and their families.* —Nurse

> *Seeing [patients] relief at knowing someone understands, and cares, is priceless.*—Nurse

> *The challenge of working autonomously, liaising with GPs and other health professionals.* —Community Nurse

## Professional and Personal Growth

The privilege of working with patients, most of whom are at the end of their lives, and observing the resilience of families were key features of both the professional and the personal growth theme. Spiritual experiences, either new or constantly being reinforced, were well-documented. The degree of personal growth and awareness was described in a moving way. Working in hospice was called "life changing" and a perfect culmination of life's experiences. Professional growth was noted by many with ongoing learning, skill development, education, and mentoring opportunities cited. Learning something new every day was frequently recorded.

> *No matter how physically or emotionally drained you can feel at times there is a vitality about working with people who are dying. Also what other job is there where you are privileged to hear people's life stories.* —Nurse

> *Very contemplative work with lots of mystery.* —Nurse

> *I see this as the culmination of my life experience and professional skills.* —Community Nurse

> *No case is ever the same and I just keep learning and learning.* —Nurse

## Community

Three themes relating to community were identified: first, the satisfaction and the challenges of being able to work in the community, liaising with those in primary health-care service delivery, and how this differed from institutional care; second, the uniqueness and satisfaction of caring for patients in their own homes; and finally, for some, how important it was as a health professional to be part of the larger community, to give something back to their community or to have community involvement.

> *Sincere satisfaction with this field of nursing and responsibility to contribute to our wonderful community in ....* —Nurse

> *I enjoy the focus on the whole patient in the context of the patient in the community with their Whanau (extended family) .*—Nurse

## Lifestyle

Similar lifestyle factors to what initially attracted staff were found, such as proximity to work, shorter traveling distances, the availability of part time work and a good work/life balance.

Values and Philosophy (as discussed above):

> *Walking beside people in their last journey is a sacred task.* —Chaplain

*…and the meeting of Whanau from all over the motu [NZ], be they in support roles or as patients. Making the word palliative and hospice acceptable to Maori.* —Nurse

*The atmosphere of the place is such that I feel it is a privilege to work here.* —Nurse

*A welcome antidote to the insanities of public hospitals.* —Nurse

## Money

Although not asked for, a small group stated that it was not the monetary reward that kept them working in this area. The exclamation marks lend the researcher to assume this was in fact a reference to pay scales generally being lower in this field than in the public system, and the dissatisfaction of this, rather than the interpretation that money doesn't matter. It is known anecdotally that some staff choose not to apply to work in hospice because of the lower pay scales.

*Certainly not the money!* —Nurse

## Personality Variables and Palliative Care

In an earlier study of more than 600 caregivers from around the world,[3] the primary personal coping mechanism was a sense of commitment, control, and pleasure in one's work.[3] This characteristic is strongly linked with Antonovsky's sense of coherence,[60] with Kobasa's personality construct of hardiness,[61,62] with Hirshberg and Barasch's sense of congruence,[63] as well as with the concepts of job engagement[28] and compassion satisfaction.[37] A concept that is also reflected is resilience, which is recently gaining attention in palliative care.[64,65]

Resilience[7] is a "universal capacity which allows a person, group or community to prevent, minimize or overcome damaging effects of adversity." It is not just about reforming, but about the possibility of growth" (Ref. 65, p. 1).[65,66] "The promotion of resilience does not lie in an avoidance of stress, but rather in encountering stress at a time and in a way that allows self-confidence and social competence to increase through mastery and appropriate responsibility" (Ref. 64, p. 608).[64,67] Recent research shows that resilience can best be understood as the interplay between particular genes and the environment.[68] Researchers have discovered that a particular variation of a gene can help to promote resilience in the people who have it, acting as a buffer against the ruinous effects of adversity. In the absence of an adverse environment, the gene does not express itself this way, but drops out of the psychological picture. Caspi et al.[69] found the link between the gene *5-HTT* and childhood maltreatment in causing depression. *5-HTT* is critical for the regulation of serotonin to the brain. Proper regulation of serotonin helps promote well-being and protects against depression in response to trauma or stress.

In a study of 847 New Zealand adults[70] who had been either mistreated as children or experienced several "life stresses," there was an association between having at least one short allele on *5-HTT* and depression. Compared with children without the childhood trauma of being removed from their families because of physical abuse, sexual abuse, or neglect, the abused children with two short *5-HTT* alleles had a higher mean score for depression than those with two long alleles and the non-abused children, no matter what their alleles. Building on the research of other psychologists regarding contact with their most significant other, Kaufman[70] measured the quality of abused children's relationship with that person.[68,69] The mean depression scores for those children with two short alleles who rarely saw these people were "off the chart." If the children with two short alleles saw these people almost daily, their depression scores were close to those of children with two long protective alleles and within reach of those who had not been abused. The children with two protective alleles were far less affected by a lack of contact with the primary caregiver. The conclusion was that good social support ameliorated the effect of abuse and the high-risk genotype.[68,70]

Professional caregivers have been found to have a higher than normal level of deprivation in their childhoods.[71] Given the recent work on resilience, genetics, and social support, it is conceivable that some caregivers are more sensitive to the availability of social support within the work environment than are others. Current research on resilience is also looking at issues of attachment.[72,73] Recent research on hospice nursing staff has looked at attachment style.[73] Adult attachment style, stress, and coping were studied in 84 nurses recruited from five U.K. hospices. Attachment styles were characterized as follows:

- *Secure*—comfortable using others as a source of support when needed.
- *Preoccupied*—having a positive model of others, but a negative model of self, leading to becoming preoccupied with their attachment needs, actively attempting to get their needs for acceptance and approval met in close relationships.
- *Fearful*—having a negative model of self and a negative model of others.
- *Dismissing*—having a positive model of self but a negative model of others. Hospice nurses with a fearful or dismissing attachment style were found to be less likely to seek emotional social support as a means of coping with stress than hospice nurses with a secure or preoccupied attachment style.

The results of this study[73] were equivocal with regard to whether having an insecure attachment style predisposed nurses to a higher level of work-related stress. Although total scores on the Nursing Stress Scale and the General Health Questionnaire (GHQ) and episodes of absence from work were not significantly different in securely and insecurely attached nurses, the rate of high GHQ and days absent from work over the past 6 months were higher in the insecurely attached group. These findings may point to the need to have different types of support available for caregivers with different personality profiles.

## The Transformative Power of Positive Emotions

Vaillant,[2] who is known for his pioneering work in adult development has recently written of the transformative power of positive emotion. "Positive emotions—not only compassion, forgiveness, love and hope but also joy, faith/trust, awe, and gratitude—arise from our inborn mammalian capacity for unselfish parental love. They emanate from our feeling, limbic, mammalian brain and are thus grounded in our evolutionary heritage. All human beings are hardwired for positive emotions, and these positive emotions are a common denominator of all major faiths and of all human beings" (p. 3).[2]

He suggests that such positive emotions are essential to the survival of *Homo sapiens* as a species. This section will frame the concept of coping within a recognition of the importance of these positive emotions, for our survival in the field of palliative care.

Vaillant defines "spirituality as the amalgam of the positive emotions that bind us to other human beings—and to our experience of 'God' as we may understand Her/Him" (p. 5).[2] He discusses the spiritually important emotions of love, hope, joy, forgiveness, compassion, faith, awe and gratitude. He speaks of the difference between negative emotions, such as fear and anger, which are "all about me" and contrasts them with the positive emotions which have the power to free the self from the self. The emotions he chooses to discuss all involve human connection. Negative emotions are often crucial for survival, but in time present. Positive emotions "are more expansive and help us to build. They widen our tolerance, expand our moral compass, and enhance our creativity. They help us to survive in time future…while negative emotions narrow attention and miss the forest for the trees, positive emotions, especially joy, make thought patterns more flexible, creative, integrative and efficient…The effect of positive emotion on the automatic (visceral) nervous system has much in common with the relaxation response to meditation…In contrast to the metabolic and cardiac arousal that the fight-or-flight response of negative emotion induces in our *sympathetic* autonomic nervous system, positive emotion via our *parasympathetic* nervous system reduces basal metabolism, blood pressure, heart rate, respiratory rate, and muscle tension" (p. 5).[2]

## Resilience

Vaillant[2] notes that work from several investigators has confirmed the strong causal association between positive emotions and post-crisis resilience in events such as the World Trade Center bombings. The awareness of positive emotions after the crisis appeared to be a core ingredient in buffering students against depression by broadening their post-crisis resources. In a small study of resilience in palliative care

nurses, Ablett and Jones[64] compared the nurses' sense of purpose about their work and commitment with the two theoretical concepts of hardiness[61,62] and a sense of coherence.[60,74] Coherence sees one's life as being comprehensible, manageable and meaningful.[74] There was a divergence in the data about response to change, consistent with the main variance between a sense of coherence and a sense of hardiness. There is a need for stability inherent in a sense of coherence and change is seen as exciting opportunity for growth in hardiness. The authors suggest that a sense of coherence might explain resilience for some caregivers, while hardiness explains resilience for others. The key factor seems to be the individual's attitude towards change.

Monroe and Oliviere[65] feel the concept of resilience is important to the future delivery of end-of-life care and the significant challenges it faces. Resilient people are able to find positive meaning within stressors[75,76] "and have greater access to stored positive information that enables them to avoid being overwhelmed by the negative experiences and emotions that everyone goes through."[65]

In a cross-sectional national survey on predictors of career satisfaction, work–life balance, and burnout, mailed to 2,000 physicians (48% response rate)[77] factor analysis confirmed the presence of four domains: work–life balance, career satisfaction, personal accomplishment and emotional resilience. Measures of burnout strongly predicted career satisfaction. The strongest predictor of work–life balance was having some control over schedule. Both women and men reported moderate levels of emotional resilience (51% vs. 53%) and high levels of personal accomplishment (74%). The measures of burnout within personal accomplishment and emotional resilience (the opposite of emotional exhaustion) are both strong and significant predictors of career satisfaction, remaining strong predictors after adjusting for both work and demographic variables. Work–life balance, or having some control over schedule and hours worked, is the strongest work characteristic related to emotional resilience. Being older significantly predicted both Personal Accomplishment and emotional resilience.[77]

Possible neurochemical, neuropeptide and hormonal mediators of the psychological response to stress have been investigated.[78] The neural mechanisms of reward and motivation (hedonia, optimism, and learned helplessness), fear responsiveness (effective behaviors despite fear), and adaptive social behavior (altruism, bonding, and teamwork) were found to be relevant to the characteristic of resilience. A meta-analysis of 35 studies investigating mortality in initially healthy populations and 35 studies of disease populations[79] showed the protective effects of positive psychological well-being. Both positive affect (emotional well-being, positive mood, joy, happiness, vigor, energy) and positive trait-like dispositions (e.g., life satisfaction, hopefulness, optimism, sense of humor) were associated with reduced mortality in healthy population studies. Positive psychological well-being was significantly associated with reduced cardiovascular mortality in healthy populations, and with reduced death rates in patients with renal failure and with human immunodeficiency virus-infection.

## The Importance of Self-Care

Shanafelt et al.[80] found greater work satisfaction in oncologists who used wellness strategies in caring for themselves as they care for others. Vachon[81] has recently noted that as oncology nurses educate cancer patients about the importance of wellness strategies, they should take their own advice to heart and make wellness changes in their own lives. The reminder one receives when traveling on airplanes, "first, put on your own seat belt," applies to caregivers. First, make sure you are nurturing yourself.

Self-care has even been shown to be associated with mental wellbeing and increased empathy in internal medicine residents.[82] The importance of a number of personal wellness promotion strategies (aspects of self-care, relationships, work attitudes, religious/spiritual practice, personal philosophies, and strategies related to work–life balance) differed for residents with higher mental well-being on the SF-8. Higher mental well-being was associated with enhanced resident empathy in this cross-sectional survey.

Huggard[1] inquired into the personal coping mechanisms used by staff and found they fell into four categories: family/whanau, religion/spirituality, self-care and professional.

Considerable support was received from family members and friends. Religion and spirituality will be discussed below. Self-care practices included: relaxation practices, including massages and meditation; reading, gardening, and time spent with pets. Personal interests such as playing sports, running and jogging, or participating in hobbies were included as part of self-care and therefore were seen as supportive. Other forms of support of a professional nature included educational opportunities taken (courses or conferences), supervision, counseling, coaching or mentoring and opportunities for networking, all of these being paid for by the individual, and therefore seen as support received from outside the organization. Figure 61–1 shows the integration of the personal, professional and organizational responsibilities all placed within the palliative care community.

### Empathy, Compassion and Service

Vaillant[2] notes that the empathic response to pain, and accompanying emotion, compassion, does not have to be taught. We have evolved to be compassionate. "Compassion, like love, is a hallmark of all the world's great religions. But love and compassion are very different. Love is the desire to

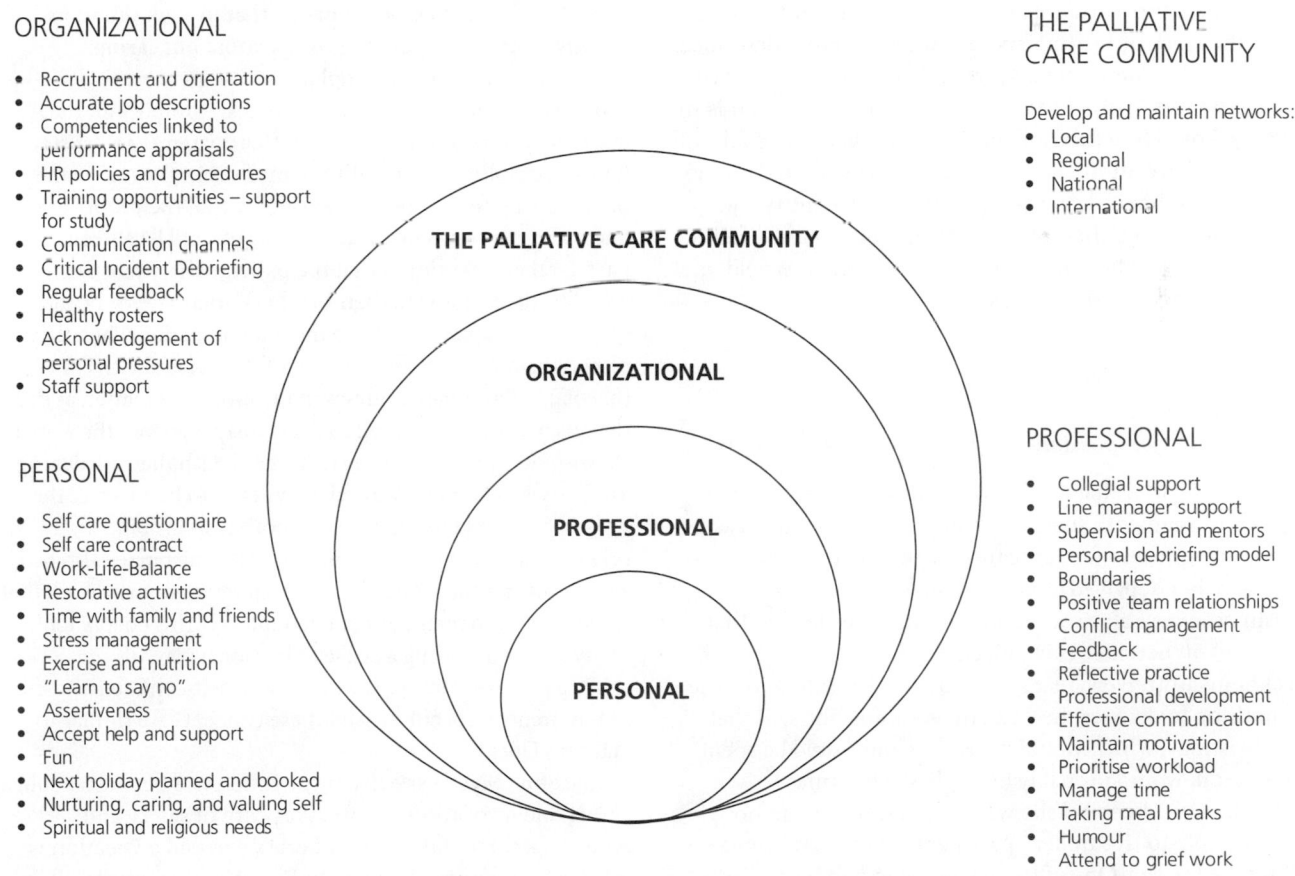

ORGANIZATIONAL

- Recruitment and orientation
- Accurate job descriptions
- Competencies linked to performance appraisals
- HR policies and procedures
- Training opportunities – support for study
- Communication channels
- Critical Incident Debriefing
- Regular feedback
- Healthy rosters
- Acknowledgement of personal pressures
- Staff support

PERSONAL

- Self care questionnaire
- Self care contract
- Work-Life-Balance
- Restorative activities
- Time with family and friends
- Stress management
- Exercise and nutrition
- "Learn to say no"
- Assertiveness
- Accept help and support
- Fun
- Next holiday planned and booked
- Nurturing, caring, and valuing self
- Spiritual and religious needs

THE PALLIATIVE CARE COMMUNITY

Develop and maintain networks:
- Local
- Regional
- National
- International

PROFESSIONAL

- Collegial support
- Line manager support
- Supervision and mentors
- Personal debriefing model
- Boundaries
- Positive team relationships
- Conflict management
- Feedback
- Reflective practice
- Professional development
- Effective communication
- Maintain motivation
- Prioritise workload
- Manage time
- Taking meal breaks
- Humour
- Attend to grief work

**Figure 61–1.** Personal, professional, and organizational responsibilities for health professionals working in palliative care. *Source:* © Jayne Huggard 2008. Reprinted with permission.

join with someone who is appealing; compassion is the desire to separate someone, even if unappealing, from his suffering. Few enjoy receiving the sympathy and pity that come from being loved as much as they do the empathy that comes from receiving compassion and that allows us to feel seen. If it is a blessing to be loved, it is also a blessing to be 'seen' a blessing that derives from the evolution of primate mirror neurons as much as from anywhere else" (p. 153).[2] Harper[14] says of stage VI in her model "The Doer" that to "some extent Doers have learned how to gather from the universe what they need to do their work. Their clients recognize something in them and feed back this information that can then be used to help others."

An image of compassion that illustrates Harper's concept of "gathering from the universe" and which has become central to the first author's professional work and life is The Man in Sapphire Blue, an illumination that was received by the 12th century mystic, Hildegard of Bingen. Mathew Fox[83] writes of this image and states that the color of the heart chakra is green. Hildegard built her entire theology on *viriditas* or "greening power." She felt that all creatures contained the greening power of the Holy Spirit, which makes all things creative and nourishing. In her picture of the Man in Sapphire Blue, the man's hands are outstretched in front of his chest. This gesture is an ancient metaphor for compassion, because compassion is about taking heart energy and putting it into one's hands—that is, putting it to work in the world. This is the work of healing and assisting. As Fox[83] described the image, "An energy field surrounds the man. Clearly this is a man whose 'body is in the soul' and not whose soul is in the body. Both Hildegard and later, Meister Eckhart, spoke of the body/soul relationship in this imagery of shared energy systems, with the soul energy being the greater entity" (p. 23). In the illumination, there is "an aperture at the man's head, so that this powerful healing energy can leave his own field and mix with others—and vice versa" (p. 23).

### CASE STUDY
#### *The Impact of Compassionate Presence*

While writing this chapter the first author was treating a divorced woman with metastatic lung cancer, who had two previous diagnoses of breast cancer. The woman began to speak of her deprived childhood, in which unhappy Christmases were a prime feature. As an adult she said that she turned off her answering machine on Christmas Eve, and hid at home until New Year's Day, so no one would know she had nothing to do over the Christmas season. She said that this Christmas, which would be her last and would be spent in a hospital, would probably be her best Christmas.

While in the hospital she was told that she would no longer be able to live in her apartment, which had been a real refuge for her. One of the nurses, who had been visiting her, mentioned the possibility of a hospice in her neighborhood, which was primarily for homeless people; she was now homeless. This hospice would have a homelike

atmosphere, so it would make giving up her apartment somewhat easier. She set her heart on it and two days before Christmas asked if there was anyway I could facilitate a transfer there. After a couple of phone calls and a little help from my colleagues, on January 2nd I found myself visiting her at Perram House Hospice. She sat in a large living room, surrounded by Christmas decorations and said that she couldn't believe her good fortune. She had begun to give away her possessions and said that it gave her great pleasure to know her precious objects would live on after her, giving pleasure to others. She was deriving great pleasure from giving her dining room set to an older couple, who had befriended her. They had never had a dining room set. The woman she gave it to had tears in her eyes as she said she never thought that she would ever be able to have a dining room set. The hospice nurse joined us and said they were looking forward to having help with their plants as the woman enjoyed gardening. We spoke of this chapter and the concept that it is in giving that we receive. This is compassion and empathy in action.

Dr. Christina Puchalski[84] notes that if one is practicing compassionate presence—being in the moment compassionately—burnout will be less and caregivers will not experience compassion fatigue. She feels that compassion fatigue comes from wanting to help the patient and being unable to so. Caregivers become less compassionate in order to protect themselves. She suggests that in such situations caregivers are not practicing compassion, but caring.

In her study of why exemplary oncology nurses avoid compassion fatigue, Perry[17] notes, "Simply put, the exemplary nurses connected with their patients and their families enabling them to put themselves in the role of the other. The nurses expressed repeatedly that their motivation and energy to continue to care at exceptional levels came, in part, by their realization that the patients they were caring for could be their mothers, their brothers, their sisters, or their neighbors. Respondents were moved into action when they placed themselves in the position of the person with cancer" (p. 89). In addition, the nurses made moments matter, as did the hospice nurse referered to previously who told the woman they would value having her help them with their gardening. The nurses in Perry's study felt privileged to be a part of the nurse-patient relationship, seeing both responsibilities and privileges as being inherent in their role. The nurses also had a zest-for-life attitude. They brought energy onto their work that spilled over into their patient encounters. "This energy took many forms, including a sense of humor, a playful spirit, a positive attitude, and a sense of self-confidence and self-awareness" (p. 90). Again, these concepts are similar to Harper's Doer.[14]

Caroline Myss[85] speaks of the difference between a job, a career and a vocation. A job takes care of safety and security, a career takes care of one's ego and a vocation is service to one's soul, similar to Puchalski's[84] "one's call," and Perry's[17] nursing as a privilege. Caregivers in hospice palliative care can see their roles as a job, a career, or a vocation. This perspective may further the understanding of different approaches caregivers take. As the first author was writing this article, an oncology nurse friend, with whom I have been in an oncology nurse support group for over 35 years, admitted an elderly friend of hers to a palliative care unit. She said things were going well, except for the fact that the night nurse, on her first night, showed no compassion.

For some, hospice palliative care is a job—simply a way to earn a living. For others, perhaps some of those nurses described by Georges and colleagues,[10] palliative care is a career, feeding their ego. This is not to say that the work they do is not good, but that in some ways the work is more about themselves and their own satisfaction than it is about entering into a deeply-caring relationship with patients. These nurses have been taught skills as opposed to reflecting on values. By mastering nursing diagnosis and being able to speak with physicians in a manner they believe is appropriate to an academic setting, these nurses can derive a great deal of satisfaction. However, some would say that something is missing from their care, which perhaps explains why so many staff were leaving the unit. For many caregivers in hospice and palliative care, their work is a vocation—service to their souls. In truly meeting the needs of others, they are meeting the needs of their own souls.

Dr. Rachel Naomi Remen[86] writes, "Basically service is about taking life personally, letting the lives that touch yours touch you" (p. 197). She contends that service is a relationship between equals. When you serve, the work itself keeps you from burnout. Unless you let the patients touch you, you will never last in this work.[86] Protecting ourselves from loss rather than grieving and healing our losses is one of the major causes of burnout[87]: "We burn out not because we don't care but because we don't grieve. We burn out because we have allowed our hearts to become so filled with loss that we have no room left to care" (p. 52).

Remen speaks of compassion, which, she says, "begins with the acceptance of what is most human in ourselves, what is most capable of suffering. In attending to our own capacity to suffer, we can uncover a simple and profound connection between our own vulnerability and the vulnerability in all others. Experiencing this allows us to find an instinctive kindness toward life which is the foundation of all compassion and genuine service."[86]

## Religion and Spirituality

Religion and spirituality have been found to be helpful to caregivers. In coping with work stress as well as perhaps being in a "better place" from which to meet the challenges of the work situation. Huggard's[1] respondents reported: *religious support* [including faith and prayer] was received from ministers, by attendance at church services and from the church community itself. *Spiritual support* was gained from spiritual directors, through prayer, belonging to a choir, or singing;

time spent communing with nature; and time away from home (e.g., weekends away or attending personal retreats); or reflective writing and journaling.

In a study at Memorial Sloan Kettering Cancer Center,[88] nurses were found to be more religious than other groups. Oncologists were more religious than fellows. Those who were "quite a bit" religious to "extremely" religious had significantly lower scores on diminished empathy or depersonalization and lower emotional exhaustion on the Maslach Burnout scale.[46] In a study of 155 members of the Israeli Oncology Society, spiritual well-being, extrinsic religiosity, and education demonstrated significant direct relationships in a path analysis toward attitudes toward spiritual care. Spiritual well-being of the nurse was the strongest predictor of Israeli oncology nurses' attitudes toward spiritual care.[89]

Vaillant[2] concludes his book by stating "…the human capacity for positive emotions is what makes us spiritual, and that to focus on the positive emotions is the best and safest route to spirituality that we are likely to find" (p. 186).[2] He quotes evolutionary biologist David Sloan Wilson[90] and evolutionary psychologist Mark Hauser[91] as suggesting that "maturity" and empathy have been positively selected for the evolution of *Homo sapiens*. "The biology of *Homo sapiens* has hardwired our brains to feel joy in communal efforts with strangers-but only under certain circumstances" (p. 186).[2] He contrasts spirituality with religion and says "spirituality refers to the psychological experiences of religiosity/spirituality that relates to an individual's sense of connection with something transcendent (be it a defined deity, truth, beauty, or anything else considered to be greater than self) and are manifested by the emotions of awe, gratitude, love, compassion, and forgiveness" (p. 187).[2] Where religion arises from cultures, spirituality arises from biology.

Sinclair et al.[92] studied spirituality in an interdisciplinary palliative care team and found that caregivers struggled to define spirituality. Respondents included concepts relating to integrity, wholeness, meaning, and personal journeying. For many, their spirituality was inherently relational, might involve transcendence, was wrapped up in caring, and often manifested in small daily acts of kindness and of love. For some participants, palliative care was a spiritual calling. A collective spirituality, stemming from common goals, values and belonging, surfaced.

The authors suggest that further research might explore spirituality on a collective level, including a more in-depth study of the relationship between spirituality and tacit skills such as empathy, "being present," and compassion employed by palliative care professionals in caring for the dying. The question arises whether the spiritual belief systems of those in palliative care might serve as a protection against burnout and compassion fatigue.

In Peter Huggard's study[32,93] of 230 New Zealand physicians, a positive and significant correlation was found between compassion satisfaction[37] and spirituality. This study examined the relationship between compassion fatigue, compassion satisfaction and burnout and resilience, spirituality, empathy, emotional competence, and social-support-seeking behaviors. Huggard found a positive correlation between religion and vicarious traumatization. High scores on the "relationship with a higher power" subscale were related to high scores on the compassion fatigue subscale. He also demonstrated a negative and significant correlation between spirituality and burnout.

Fricchione[72] spoke of spirituality specific resiliency factors including:

- Belief in a higher entity, the nature of which is love and beneficience, not retribution, on the health of the believer
- Elicitation of the relaxation response through prayer and meditation, with a proposed effect on the individual doing the praying and meditating
- Effects of pro-social behavior, based on the evolutionary mechanisms for empathy and compassion and forgiveness and love on the health of the organism
- Priming the human capacity for altruistic behavior and unlimited love through spirituality and true religious practice may uncover the malleability of the human being whose capacity for altruistic love may be epigenetically enhanced over and above genetic inheritance
- Benefits to health of increased positive expectation of the future
- Impact on health of acquiring or enhancing the role of meaning and purpose in one's life.

## Environmental Coping in Hospice Palliative Care

Despite the fact that the stressors of staff in hospice palliative care have been documented from the beginning of the field,[3–7] there is no substantial body of work documenting the impact of programs of intervention. A Cochrane Review assessed the prevention of occupational stress in health-care workers,[94] concluding there was limited evidence for the effectiveness of person- and work-directed interventions to reduce stress levels in health-care settings. Only two trials, one in oncology[95] were rated as being of high quality, based on receiving 75% on the internal validity subscales.

Figure 61–1 shows the model Huggard[1] developed to describe the personal, professional and organizational practices used by her respondents. Personal responsibilities for wellness were mentioned above. This section will discuss professional and organizational responsibilities.

## Professional and Organizational Responsibilities

Huggard notes that "at a personal support level, self-care strategies such as spiritual beliefs and reflective pastimes

were seen to be a necessary and integral component to the practice of palliative care professionals. However, what was identified was that organizational support strategies appear to be the most important for hospice staff" (p. 143).[1] "The five most *important* support practices reported—line managers/team leaders, orientation, rosters, peer support and feedback—were all of a managerial and organizational nature, and relate to organizational initiatives that value staff" (p. 121).[1]

Results of her study suggest that the overwhelming majority of participants felt well-supported by their peers (93%) with a majority also feeling well-supported by their managers and by their organizations (79%). This contrasts with Kulbe's[96] research which identified that 39% of nursing staff felt that support was inadequate. In general, staff in New Zealand hospices report being relatively well-supported[97] with one New Zealand hospice having an emotional safety policy that applies to all staff, both paid and volunteer.[5]

Huggard identified the following professional responsibilities for staff working in palliative care: collegial support, line manager support, supervision and mentors, personally debriefing model, being mindful of boundaries, positive team relationships, managing conflict, giving and receiving feedback, reflective practice, professional development, communicating effectively, maintaining motivation, prioritizing workload, managing time, taking meal breaks, humor, attending to grief work.

The organizational responsibilities included: appropriate recruitment and orientation, accurate job descriptions, competencies linked to performance appraisals, human resources policies and procedures, training opportunities and support for study, open communication channels, providing Critical Incident Debriefing, offering regular and timely feedback, healthy rosters, and acknowledgement of personal pressures, staff support.

In response to an inquiry, Barbara Monroe[98] from St Christopher's Hospice stated that organizational support was essential to support staff working in the hospice. They have moved away from offering "emotional support," concentrating instead on robust organizational procedures. St. Christopher's has appropriate recruitment, orientation and mentor programs. Individual or group supervision is available for all staff. Attention is paid to a performance review 6 months into working at the hospice, and annual appraisals are always held. Clinical reviews are held monthly, are well-attended and taken seriously. Specific training programs are held regularly, and include communication topics such as assertion and delegation skills. Staff can access occupational health for extra counseling and support and generous bereavement is offered as required. Critical incident stress management policies include debriefs. "The headlines are that we believe in good training opportunities. Clinical supervision for everyone. Clear competencies linked into the appraisal system and good organizational procedures and communication. We do not run staff support groups."

## Studies of Intervention

Puchalski[84] suggests that if health-care professionals are trained to be compassionate, if the practice is linked to spirituality, and if it is linked to one's call, the likelihood of burnout may be less. Caregivers need to be taught how to identify the emotions involved in caring for patients.[26] Puchalski and McSkimming[99] describe interventions to establish healing environments in hospitals. These included increasing awareness of the spirituality of the health-care professional through:

- Awareness of one's own spirituality
- Awareness of one's own mortality, woundedness, humanity
- Attention to spiritual life/having a spiritual practice.

Executive staff with decision-making capacity from a seven varied hospital sites met together to set goals related to improving patient care through recognition of the importance of the spiritual dimension in patients, families and caregivers. Interventions included the whole person—body, mind and spirit—and recognizing the body, mind and spirit of patients, families, and caregivers. The implementation strategies varied from hospital to hospital. Some of the approaches they took to meet their goals included:

- Brown bag lunches, workshops, grand rounds (didactic, experiential)
- Rituals, art work, posters (Catch the Spirit)
- Recognize excellence in spiritual care (beads, certificates)
- Institutionalized spiritual assessment
- Reminders of calling to profession (chimes, rituals, reinforcement from administration)
- Accountability measures for spiritual care
- Reported outcomes included:
- Cultural changes
- Improved patient satisfaction scores
- Increased staff satisfaction with work
- Waiting lists for staff from other units to work on the unit with the intervention
- Comments from other staff in hospital that "something different is happening on this unit"
- Frequency of patient call button ringing decreased.

## Meditation and Reflective Practice Interventions[7]

Recent interventions reflect approaches that build on concepts of job engagement and compassion satisfaction, enabling caregivers to learn approaches to sustain themselves, while acknowledging and indeed celebrating their engagement with their clients and in their work. Mindfulness meditation and narrative approaches have been used. These interventions have the potential to help caregivers enrich their personal lives, enhance their involvement with patients, and

avoid some of the team conflicts that have been noted earlier as having been a significant source of stress in palliative care in the past.

Based on the work of Kabat Zinn[100] Cohen-Katz et al.[101] conducted an 8-week Mindfulness-Based Stress Reduction (MBSR) program for nurses in a hospital system. Work had already been done to improve employee satisfaction and retention; a nursing advisory council had been set up; there was work to enhance the model of self-governance and increased opportunity for education and professional development.

Mindfulness is defined as being fully present to one's experience without judgment or resistance. Its emphasis on self-care, compassion, and healing makes it relevant as an intervention for helping nurses. The results of the study showed that the treatment group decreased scores on the Maslach Burnout Inventory and these changes lasted 3 months. Specifically, there was significantly decreased emotional exhaustion and depersonalization and a trend toward significance in personal accomplishment.

More recently, Fillion et al.[102] introduced a meaning-centered psycho-educational group intervention called Enhancing Meaning in Palliative Care Nursing, designed to support nurses providing palliative care. The intervention aims to increase job satisfaction and quality of life as well as preventing burnout. The work is based on Breitbart and his colleagues' earlier work with palliative patients.[103] The project has been piloted and is currently in process in a randomized, controlled clinical trial with 120 nurses. The intervention consists of four weekly meetings. The topics are (1) characteristics of meaning, (2) sources of meaning, (3) *creative values* explored in terms of personal historical perspective and a sense of accomplishment at work, (4) suffering as a source of *attitudinal change*, and (5) affective experiences and humor as *experiential avenues* to find meaning. Throughout the training, participants were also asked to participate in the creation of a collection of short essays related to meaningful experiences in their palliative care practice. The goal is to put together a small collection of texts that could eventually be used in training and therefore provide a sense of legacy for the participating nurses. The authors plan rigorous development and evaluation and then the program could eventually involve larger groups of palliative care nurses as well as other palliative care staff.

Wessel and colleagues[104,105] integrated reflective narratives into the practice of palliative care education for nurses. The narrative reflection allowed the nurses to document meaningful experiences in end-of-life care situations. In addition, on a local level, the process identified gaps in care and system issues enabling participant feedback. On a broader level, they affirm the nursing profession. Narratives can provide a helpful way for nurses to debrief and provide a means to find closure around emotionally charged experiences, especially when facilitated by an educated group of narrative experts.

Danieli,[106] a therapist, has adapted her group intervention developed over three decades of working with trauma, to use with caregivers dealing with counter-transference difficulties in end-of-life care. Although the intervention has been developed to be used with groups, it can also be used by individuals. Danieli's approach has two phases. In the first phase, the group or individual clinician enters into a state of deep relaxation, then connects with an end-of-life experience most meaningful to the individual, who then draws the image of this situation in as much detail as possible. There is then a word association with every word the image brings to one. The group or individual is then asked to reflect on the words written and check whether there is any affect or feeling that has not yet been included and to include those words and any others that come to mind. The individual is then asked to reflect in depth on when the *first* time he or she encountered this experience. The individual is then asked to reflect on choices and beliefs that may be based on this earlier experience, continuity and discontinuity of self, whether they have shared or kept secrets about this situation, and to reflect in a variety of ways about issues related to death.

In the second phase, which works best in a group, the caregivers share, explore, and comprehend the consequences of their experiences with dying and with death. The group experience serves to counteract their potential sense of isolation and alienation about working with the dying.

## Educational Interventions

A model for shifting established patterns is being conducted in the European Union with a goal of improving the interaction between mobile palliative care teams (PCMT) and the hospital staff with whom they interact.[107] In this model, recognizing the full range of convictions held by persons in a hospital setting, the concept of palliative care/terminal care has been bolstered by the concept of continuous care. Continuous care tends to articulate curative and palliative procedures focusing on the holistic care of patients and their family. "Promoting the integration of continuous care in the hospital' intends to identify the challenges in integrating continuous care through an inventory and analysis of the activity of palliative care mobile teams in several countries of Europe. Competencies for PCMTs have been derived and based on these, and a pilot three phase educational programme with PCMTs undertaken and evaluated" (p. 4).[107]

Mosenthal, Murphy, Barker, et al.[108] performed a structured palliative care intervention on consecutive trauma patients admitted to the Trauma Intensive Care Unit. The program included part 1, early (at admission) family bereavement support, assessment of prognosis, and patient preferences, and part II (within 72 hours) interdisciplinary team meeting. Data on goals of care discussions, do-not-resuscitate orders (DNRs), and withdrawal of life support (W/D) were collected from physician rounds, family meetings, and medical records. Eighty-three percent of patients received part I and 69% received part II intervention. Discussion of goals of care by physicians on rounds increased from 4% to 36% of patient-days. During intervention, rates of mortality (14%), DNR (43%), and W/D (24%) were unchanged, but DNR orders and W/D were instituted earlier in hospital course. ICU length of stay was decreased in patients who died. The authors concluded that "structured communication between physicians and families resulted in earlier consensus around goals of care for dying trauma patients. Integration of early palliative care alongside aggressive trauma care can be accomplished without change in mortality and has the ability to change the culture of care in the trauma ICU" (p. 1587).[108] This study built on earlier work by Mosenthal and Murphy,[109] a nurse, improving end-of-life care in the critically injured, an interdisciplinary model for palliative care, which was integrated into the trauma and surgical ICU (www.promotingex-cellence.org).

Meier, Back, and Morrison[26] have proposed an approach to physician awareness that involves identifying and working with emotions that may affect patient care. This involves looking at physician, situational, and patient risk factors that can lead to physician feelings and thus influence patient care.

More recently, Chochinov has proposed the A, B, C, and D of Dignity-Conserving Care.[110] Using empirical evidence, he shows that kindness, humanity, and respect, the core vales and behaviors of medical professionalism, often relegated to the "niceties" of care, embrace the true essence of medicine. These aspects of care—variably referred to as spiritual care, whole-person care, or Dignity-Conserving Care—involve *attitude, behavior, compassion, and dialogue.* Chochinov provides a core framework of Dignity-Conserving Care to guide health-care providers to incorporate this important facet of patient care. Hospice and palliative care specialists may feel that they have incorporated these values into their work, but there is still work to be done.

## Summary

Nurses work in palliative care for a variety of reasons. Some may regard the work as simply a job, perhaps to be done for only a few years so as not to become overly involved in the stress associated with caring for dying persons and their families. Others may see hospice palliative care nursing as a career. It may feed their ego to be able to get on top of symptoms, resolve psychosocial issues, communicate well with other disciplines, and perhaps even achieve recognition as an expert in their field. For others, hospice palliative care nursing is about service to their soul. As the Prayer of St. Francis, with which Vaillant[2] starts his book, says, "It is in giving that we receive."

This chapter explores the stressors in palliative care and draws heavily on new research in New Zealand about the professional and organization responsibilities involved in supporting caregivers in palliative care. It also draws on new research from evolutionary biology and psychology discussing the importance of the positive emotions, particularly compassion, discussing these concepts within the framework of resiliency and spirituality. Dealing with dying persons and their families can be difficult, but it can be extremely satisfying and rewarding as well. If done well, and with compassion, it enhances our own humanity.

## REFERENCES

1. Huggard J. A National Survey of the Support Needs of Interprofessional Hospice Staff in Aotearoa/New Zealand. Unpublished Master's Thesis. University of Auckland, Auckland, New Zealand, 2008.

2. Vaillant GE. Spiritual Evolution. New York: Broadway Books, 2008.

3. Vachon MLS. Occupational Stress in the Care of the Critically Ill, Dying and Bereaved. Washington, DC: Hemisphere, 1987.

4. Vachon MLS. Staff stress in hospice/palliative care: A review. Palliat Med 1995;9:91–122.

5. Vachon MLS, Sherwood C. Staff stress and burnout. In: Berger AM, Shuster JL, Von Roenn JH, eds. Principles and Practice of Palliative Care and Supportive Oncology. Philadelphia, PA: Lippincott, Williams & Wilkins; 2007:667–683.

6. Vachon MLS. The experience of the nurse in end-of-life care in the 21st century. In: Ferrell BR, Coyle N, eds. Textbook of Palliative Nursing (2nd ed). Oxford: Oxford University Press; 2006:1011–1029.

7. Vachon MLS, Müeller M. Burnout and Symptoms of Stress. In: Breitbart W, Chochinov HM, eds. Handbook of Psychiatry in Palliative Medicine, 2nd ed. New York: Oxford University Press; 2009:236–264.

8. Payne S. The role of volunteers in hospice bereavement support in New Zealand. Palliat Med 2001;15:107–115.

9. Barnard D, Towers A, Boston P, Lambrinidou Y. Crossing Over: Narratives of Palliative Care. New York: Oxford, 2000.

10. Georges JJ, Grypdonck M, De Casterle BD. Being a palliative care nurse in an academic hospital: A qualitative study about nurses' perceptions of palliative care nursing. J Clin Nurs 2002;11:785–793.

11. Jackson VA, Mack J, Matsuyama R, Lakoma MD, Sullivan AM, Arnold RM, Weeks JC, Block SD. A qualitative study of oncologists' approaches to end-of-life care. J Pall Med 2008;11:893–906.

12. von Gunten CF. Oncologists and End-of-Life Care. J Pall Med 2008;11:813.

13. Vachon MLS. Type II oncologists, letter to the editor. J Pall Med 2009;12:1:9.

14. Harper BC. Death: The Coping Mechanism of the Health Professional, rev. ed. Greenville, SC: Southeastern University Press, 1994.

15. Perry B. Beliefs of eight exemplary oncology nurses related to Watson's nursing theory. Can Oncol Nurs J 1998;8:97–101.

16. Perry B. Moments In Time: Images of Exemplary Nursing Care. Ottawa: Canadian Nurses Association, 1998.

17. Perry B. Why exemplary oncology nurses seem to avoid compassion fatigue. Can Oncol Nurs J 2008;18:87–92.

18. Katz RS, Johnson TA, eds. When Professionals Weep: Emotional and Countertransference Responses in End-of-Life Care. New York: Routledge, 2006.

19. Watson J. Human caring and suffering: A subjective model for health services. In: Watson J, Taylor R, eds. They Shall Not Hurt: Human Suffering and Human Caring. Boulder CO: Colorado Associated University, 1989.

20. Katz R. When our personal selves influence our professional work: An introduction to emotions and countertransference in end of life care. In: Katz RS, Johnson TA, eds. When Professionals Weep: Emotional and Countertransference Responses in End-of-Life Care. New York: Routledge; 2006:3–12.

21. Kearney M. A Place of Healing: Working with Suffering in Living and Dying. Oxford: Oxford University Press, 2000.

22. Vachon MLS. The soul's wisdom: Stories of living and dying. Curr Oncol 2008;15(Suppl 2):48–52.

23. Vachon MLS. The use of imagery, meditation, and spirituality in the care of people with cancer. In: Murray Edwards D, ed. Voice Massage: Scripts for Guided Imagery. Pittsburgh, PA: Oncology Nursing Society; 2002:21–41.

24. Schön D. The Reflective Practitioner. Basic Books: New York, 1983.

25. Byock I. Dying in America: Past, Present and Future. Paper presented at The Great Journey—Death, Dying and Bereavement, Tucson AZ, March 27, 2004.

26. Meier DE, Back AL, Morrison RS. The inner life of physicians and the care of the seriously ill. JAMA 2001;286:3007–3014.

27. Maslach C, Schaufeli WB, Leiter MP. Job burnout. Ann Rev Psychol 2001;52:397–422.

28. Maslach C, Leiter MP. Early predictors of job burnout and engagement. J Appl Psychol 2008;93:498–512.

29. Maslach C. Job burnout: New directions in research and intervention. Curr Dir Psychol Sci 2003;12:189–192.

30. Figley CR. Compassion Fatigue: Coping with Secondary Traumatic Stress Disorder in Those Who Treat the Traumatized. New York: Brunner/Mazel, 1995.

31. Figley CR. Treating Compassion Fatigue. New York: Brunner-Routledge, 2002.

32. Huggard, PK. Managing compassion fatigue: Implications for medical education. Unpublished Doctoral Thesis, University of Auckland, Auckland, New Zealand, 2008.

33. Pearlman LA, Saakvitne KW. Trauma and the Therapist. New York: W.W. Norton & Company, 1995.

34. Thomas RB, Wilson JP. Issues and controversies in the understanding and diagnosis of compassion fatigue, vicarious traumatization, and secondary traumatic stress disorder. Int J Emerge Mental Health 2004;6(2):81–92.

35. Sinclair HAH, Hamill C. Does vicarious traumatisation affect oncology nurses? A literature review. Eur J Onc Nurs 2007;11(4):348–356.

36. Garfield C, Spring C, Ober D. Sometimes My Heart Goes Numb: Love and Caring in a Time of AIDS. San Francisco: Jossey-Bass, 1995.

37. Stamm BH. Measuring compassion satisfaction as well as fatigue: Developmental history of the compassion satisfaction and fatigue test. In: Figley CR, ed. Treating Compassion Fatigue. New York, NY: Brunner-Routledge; 2002:107–119.

38. Vachon MLS. Staff stress and burnout in palliative care. In: Bruera E, Higginson IJ, Ripamonti C, von Gunten CF, eds. Textbook of Palliative Medicine. London: Hodder Arnold; 2006:1002–1010.

39. Vachon MLS. Stress and burnout in palliative medicine. In: Walsh D, Caraceni AE, Fainsinger R, et al., eds. Palliative Medicine. Philadelphia, PA: Elsevier; 2008:75–83.

40. Vachon MLS. Oncology staff stress and related interventions. In: Holland JC, Breitbart WS, et al. eds. Psycho-Oncology (2nd ed). New York: Oxford University Press, in press.

41. Conard MA, Matthews RA. Modeling the stress process: Personality eclipses dysfunctional cognitions and workload in predicting stress. Pers Indiv Diff 2008;44:171–181.

42. Payne N. Occupational stressors and coping as determinants of burnout in female hospice nurses. J Adv Nurs 2001;33:396–405.

43. Asai M, Morita T, Akechi T, et al. Burnout and psychiatric morbidity among physicians engaged in end-of-life care for cancer patients: A cross-sectional nationwide survey in Japan. Psycho-oncology 2007;16:421–428.

44. Yandrick RM. High demand low control. Behavioral Healthcare Tomorrow 1997;6(3):41–44.

45. Speck P. Teamwork in Palliative Care: Fulfilling or Frustrating? Oxford: Oxford University Press, 2006.

46. Maslach C, Jackson SE. The Maslach Burnout Inventory (manual) (2nd ed). Palo Alto, CA: Consulting Psychologists Press, 1986.

47. Berman R, Campbell M, Makin W, Todd C. Occupational stress in palliative medicine, medical oncology and clinical oncology specialist registrars. Clin Med 2007;7:235–242.

48. Poncet MC, Toullic P, Papazian L, et al. Burnout syndrome in critical care nursing staff. Resp Crit Care Med 2007; 175:698–704.

49. Speck P. Team or group-spot the difference. In: Speck P, ed. Teamwork in Palliative Care: Fulfilling or Frustrating? Oxford: Oxford University Press; 2006:7–24.

50. Haward R, Amir Z, Borrill C, Scully J, West M, Sainsbury R. Breast cancer teams: The impact of constitution, new cancer workload, and methods of operation on their effectiveness. Br J Ca 2003;89:15–22.

51. Taylor, C, Graham, J, Potts, HWW, Richards, MA, Ramirez, A. Changes in mental health of UK hospital consultants since the mid-1990's. Lancet 2005;366:742–744.

52. Whedon MB. Revisiting the road not taken: Integrating palliative care into oncology nursing. Clin J Oncol Nurs 2002;6:27–33.

53. James N, Field D. The routinization of hospice: Charisma and bureaucracy. Soc Sci Med 1992;34:1363–1375.

54. Boston P, Towers A, Barnard D. Embracing vulnerability: Risk and empathy in palliative care. J Palliat Care 2001;17:248–253.

55. Baim M. Empathy and spirituality, Presentation and Embracing empathy. Workshop presented at Spirituality & Healing in Medicine: The Resiliency Factor. Boston: Harvard Medical School and Massachusetts General Hospital, Benson-Henry Institute for Mind Body Medicine, December 13–14, 2008.

56. Stein E. On the Problem of Empathy (collected works of Edith Stein, Sister Benedicta of the Cross, Discalced Carmelite, vol. 3). The Netherlands: Kluwer Academic Press, 1989.

57. Varela FJ, Depraz N. Imagining: Embodiment, phenomenology and transformation. In: Wallace BA, ed. Buddhism and Science. New York: Columbia University Press; 2003:195–232.

58. Mount BM. Dealing with our losses. J Clin Oncol 1986; 4:1127–1134.

59. Papadatou D. A proposed model of health professionals' grieving process. Omega 2000;41:59–77.

60. Antonovsky A. Health, Stress and Coping. San Francisco: Jossey-Bass, 1979.

61. Kobasa SC. Stressful life events, personality and health: An inquiry into hardiness. J Pers Soc Psychol 1979;37:1–11.

62. Kobasa SC, Maddi SR, Kahn S. Hardiness and health: A prospective study. J Pers Soc Psychol 1982;42:172–177.

63. Hirshberg C, Barasch MI. Remarkable Recovery. New York: Riverhead Books, 1995.

64. Ablett JR, Jones RSP. Resilience and well-being in palliative care staff: A qualitative study of hospice nurses' experience of work. Psycho-Oncology 2007;16:733–740.

65. Monroe B, Oliviere D. Introduction: Unlocking resilience in palliative care. In: Monroe B, Oliviere D, eds. Resilience in Palliative Care: Achievement in Adversity. Oxford: Oxford University Press; 2007:1–7.

66. Newman T. What Works in Building Resilience? Ilford: Barnardo's, 2004.

67. Rutter M. Resilience in the face of adversity: Protective factors and resistance to psychiatric disorder. Br J Psychiatry 1985;147:598–611.

68. Bazelon E. A question of resilience. http://www.nytimes.com/2006/04/30/magazine/30abuse.html?ei=5070&en=2746fe42d76(accessed January 1, 2007.)

69. Caspi A, Sugden K, Moffitt TE, et al. Influence of life stress on depression: Moderation by a polymorphism in the 5-HTT gene. Science 2003;301:386–389.

70. Kaufman J. Stress and its consequences: An evolving story. Biol Psychiatry 2006;60:669–670.

71. Raphael B. The Anatomy of Bereavement. New York: Basic Books, 1983.

72. Fricchione G. Spirituality, and resiliency in health promotion. Presented at Spirituality & Healing in Medicine: The Resiliency Factor. Boston: Harvard Medical School and Massachusetts General Hospital, Benson-Henry Institute for Mind Body Medicine, December 13–14, 2008.

73. Hawkins AC, Howard RA, Oyebode JR. Stress and coping in hospice nursing staff. The impact of attachment styles. Psycho-oncology 2007;6:563–572.

74. Antonovsky A. Unravelling the Mystery of Health: How People Manage Stress and Stay Well. London: Jossey-Bass, 1987.

75. Fredrickson BI. The role of positive emotions in positive psychology: The broaden-and-build theory of positive emotions. Amer Psychol 2001;56:218–226.

76. Tugade MM, Fredrickson BI. Resilient individuals use positive emotions to bounce back from negative emotional experiences. J Pers Soc Psychol 2004;86:320–333.

77. Keeton K, Fenner DE, Johnson TRB, Hayward RA. Predictors of physician career satisfaction, work-life balance, and burnout. Obs Gyn 2007;109:949–955.

78. Charney DS. Psychobiological mechanisms of resilience and vulnerability: Implications for successful adaptation to extreme stress. Am J Psychiatry 2004;161:195–216.

79. Chida Y, Steptoe A. Positive psychological well-being and mortality: A quantitative review of prospective observational studies. Psychosom Med 2008;70:741–756.

80. Shanafelt TD, Novotny P, Johnson ME, et al. The well-being and personal wellness promotion strategies of medical oncologists in the North Central Cancer Treatment Group. Oncology 2005;68:23–32.

81. Vachon MLS. Meaning, spirituality and wellness in cancer survivors. In: Mayer DK, ed. Semin Oncol Nurs Issue Survivorship 2008;24:218–225.

82. Shanafelt TD, West C, Zhao X, et al. Relationship Between Increased Personal Well-Being and Enhanced Empathy Among Internal Medicine Residents. J Gen Intern Med 2005;20:559–564.

83. Fox M. Sins of the Spirit, Blessings of the Flesh: Lessons in Transforming Evil in Soul and Society. New York: Three Rivers Press, 1999.

84. Puchalski CM. Compassionate healthcare systems: Building resiliency and communities of support. Presented at Spirituality & Healing in Medicine: The Resiliency Factor. Boston: Harvard Medical School and Massachusetts General Hospital, Benson-Henry Institute for Mind Body Medicine, December 13–14, 2008.

85. Myss C. Advanced Energy Anatomy. Boulder, CO: Sounds True, 2001.

86. Remen RN. My Grandfather's Blessings. New York: Riverhead Books, 2000.

87. Remen RN. Kitchen Table Wisdom. New York: Riverhead Books, 1996.

88. Kash KM, Holland JC, Breitbart W, et al. Stress and burnout in oncology. Oncology 2000;14:1621–1637.

89. Musgrave CF, McFarlane EA. Israeli oncology nurses' religiosity, spiritual well-being, and attitudes toward spiritual care: A path analysis. Oncol Nurs Forum 2004;31:321–327.

90. Wilson DS. Darwin's Cathedral: Evolution, Religion and the Nature of Society. Chicago: University of Chicago Press, 2006.

91. Hauser M. Moral Minds: How Nature Designed Our Universal Sense of Right and Wrong. New York: HarperCollins, 2006.

92. Sinclair S, Raffin S, Pereira J, et al. Collective soul: The spirituality of an interdisciplinary palliative care team. Palliat Support Care 2006;4:13–24.

93. Huggard PK. Taking care of the health professional. Presentation at the Idaho Conference on Health Care, Health Care 2005: Emerging Issues, Pocatello, Idaho, October 27–28, 2005, personal communication.

94. Marine A, Ruotsalainen J, Serra C, Verbeek J. Preventing occupational stress in healthcare workers. Cochrane Database Syst Rev 2006;4:CD002892.

95. Delvaux N, Razavi D, Marchal S, Brédart A, Farvacques C, Slachmuylder J-L. Effects of a 105 hours psychological training program on attitudes, communication skills and occupational stress in oncology: A randomized study. B J Ca 2004;90:106–114.

96. Kulbe J. Stressors and coping measures of hospice nurses. Home Health Nurse 2001;19(11):707–711.

97. Huggard EJ. A Report of a Study of Staff Support Practices in UK and Canadian Palliative Care Units and Hospices. Wellington: Winston Churchill Memorial Trust, 2006.

98. Monroe B, personal communication, to Jayne Huggard, December 2, 2008.

99. Puchalski CM, McSkimming S. Creating healing environments. Health Progress 2006;May–June:30–35.

100. Kabat-Zinn J. Full Catastrophe Living: Using the Wisdom of Your Body and Mind to Face Stress, Pain, and Illness. New York: Delta, 1990.

101. Cohen-Katz J, Wiley SD, Capuano T, Baker D, Shapiro S. The effects of mindfulness-based stress reduction on nurse stress and burnout: A quantitative and qualitative study. Holist Nurs Pract 2004;18:302–308.

102. Fillion L, Dupuis R, Tremblay I, DeGrace G, Breitbart W. Enhancing meaning in palliative care practice: A meaning-centered intervention to promote satisfaction. Palliat Support Care 2006;4:333–344.

103. Breitbart W. Spirituality and meaning in palliative care: Spirituality and meaning-centered group psychotherapy interventions in advanced cancer. Support Care Cancer 2001;10:272–280.

104. Wessel EM, Garon M. Introducing reflective narratives into palliative care home care education. Home Health Nurse 2005;23:516–522.

105. Wessel EM, Rutledge DN. Home care and hospice nurses' attitudes towards death and caring for the dying: Effects of palliative care education. J Hosp Palliat Nurs 2005;7:2–8.

106. Danieli Y. A group intervention to process and examine countertransference near the end-of-life. In: Katz RS, Johnson TA, eds. When Professionals Weep: Emotional and Countertransference Responses in End-of-Life Care. New York: Routledge; 2006:255–265.

107. European Commission. Promoting the Development and Integration of Palliative Care Mobile Support Teams in the Hospital. Brussels: Directorate-General for Research Food Quality and Safety, 2004.

108. Mosenthal AC, Murphy PA, Barker LK, Lavery R, Retano A, Livingston DH. Changing the culture around end-of-life care in the Trauma Intensive Care Unit. Trauma 2008;64:1587–1593.

109. Mosenthal AC, Murphy PA. Interdisciplinary model for palliative care in the trauma/surgical ICU. Robert Wood Johnson Foundation demonstration project for improving palliative care in the ICU. Crit Care Med 2006;34:S399–S403.

110. Chochinov HM. Dignity and the essence of medicine: The A, B, C & D of dignity-conserving care. BMJ 2007;334:184–187.

# 62

*Maryjo Prince-Paul and Barbara J. Daly*

# Ethical Considerations in Palliative Care

*What a roller coaster of emotions making some of these decisions can be. I only want to do the best thing for mom. I feel so fortunate that we could talk about her wishes before she got really sick. It just puts my mind at ease to know what her thoughts are and how I can help in carrying them through her last days. Plus, it gives us time now to just be with each other.—A loved one's quote*

♦ **Key Points**

♦ *What constitutes "extraordinary care" will be almost entirely contingent upon the values and clinical situation of the patient.*

♦ *Enteral and parenteral nutrition and hydration are medical treatments that can be withheld or withdrawn under appropriate medical and ethical circumstances.*

♦ *Effective palliative care that rests on a sound ethical foundation requires on-going discussions about patient and family values and preferences.*

♦ *Decisions regarding ethical dilemmas and the choices that are necessary require thoughtful discussion and critical communication skills.*

## Ethics and Moral Reasoning

Ethics, broadly defined, is the branch of philosophy that is concerned with the study of human conduct, with the rational analysis of how human beings ought to behave and the methods by which we can identify good and evil, right and wrong.[1] In contrast, the term "morality" is conventionally used to refer to accepted and rational codes of conduct governing behavior, aimed to promote good and minimize evil.[2] As can be seen, these terms are closely related and are often used interchangeably.

Much of this text is concerned with the practical sense of nursing—that is, the application of natural and behavioral sciences in designing and implementing effective processes of care. This chapter will address what Bishop and Scudder refer to as the "primary sense of nursing practice," the moral sense.[3] The focus will be on the most common issues faced by nurses in palliative care. Our objective is to prepare the nurse for identifying, addressing, and resolving the complex questions that arise in caring for individuals and families facing life-limiting illnesses.

In confronting ethical questions, nurses may experience varying levels of moral quandaries. Given the complexity of the health-care system and individual patient situations, nurses often are uncertain about the right or most ethically sound action. Moral uncertainty can produce discomfort, but it is the hallmark of a morally sensitive agent. It signals doubt or confusion about values or rules, but can usually be resolved with careful analysis, as we will illustrate with case studies. Moral dilemmas are more troublesome and occur when the nurse finds her/himself in a situation with conflicting demands or one in which every possible action seems to involve violating an ethical duty. Dilemmas may be associated with significant stress and anxiety; resolution may require assistance of others to sort through the conflicts involved. Moral distress is the most damaging state and occurs when the nurse perceives a moral duty but is unable, often because of external constraints, to fulfill that duty. Persistent moral distress can lead to disillusionment, moral apathy, and eventual resignation.

Dealing with ethical questions before moral distress occurs requires knowledge and skill in ethical reasoning. While thorough exploration of ethical theories is beyond the scope of this chapter, a brief review of the major theories that are the basis for the commonly accepted principles of autonomy, beneficence, nonmaleficence, and justice will be helpful. Following this review, specific issues that the palliative care nurse is likely to face will be explored, with particular attention to analysis of the problems.

## Moral Reasoning

As mentioned, ethics as a discipline has its roots in philosophy. There are many ethical theories that have been developed over the years, each with its own justification. The best known of these are deontological theories and consequentialist theories. Consequentialist theories determine the justification for actions by examining consequences. The action that produces the best consequences for the greatest number is the preferred, or "right" action. Deontological theories, in contrast, argue that actions are right or wrong according to their adherence to duties and obligations, not by virtue of the consequences of the actions. Both types of theories generate principles, such as autonomy (the right of self-determination), beneficence (the duty to promote good), and nonmaleficence (the duty to do no harm). From principles, in turn, more specific moral rules can be derived. For example, the general duty to respect autonomy and the right of self-determination is the basis of the specific rule that we obtain informed consent before interventions.

Both deontological and consequentialist theories are forms of a principlist approach to ethics. Principlist approaches, although they may rest on differing theoretical premises, all use general and relatively universal principles as the central tool for ethical analysis. Universal principles play a key role in developing mature ethical agency, provide reliable rules of thumb for responding quickly in real life dilemmas, and reflect the considered wisdom of decades of philosophical analysis. Nevertheless, abstract and somewhat rigid principles can be insensitive to the nuances of specific clinical situations and conflict with deep intuitions of experienced clinicians. More recently, appreciation for the importance of context has grown.

Feminist ethics, an ethic of care, and narrative ethics are relatively new approaches to ethical analysis. The development of feminist ethics, an outgrowth of the feminist movement, was encouraged by the work of Carol Gilligan, who studied moral reasoning in children and found that boys relied on a rule-oriented, justice-based approach, while girls tended to analyze situations in terms of relationships and context,

seeking resolution in the details of the story or narrative.[4] Consistent with Gilligan's work, caring as a basis for ethics rests on the assumption that morality is rooted in human relationships and feelings. Nel Nodding, recognized as the originator of this theory, argues that morality must stem from the caring instinct and that the ethical ideal is located in the reciprocal caring relationship between and among persons.[5]

Narrative ethics uses the stories of patients and health professionals as the unit of analysis. In seeking understanding of ethical dilemmas from a narrative perspective, the elements of the situation are viewed as components of the story, and aspects such as the relation among participants, predominant voices, intentions of the actors, and consideration of whose voices are heard and not heard are central to developing understanding of the ethical dimensions.[6] As with the ethic of care and feminist ethics, understanding the relationships among all participants, the meaning of what is stated and unstated, and the motives of all involved is key to the evaluation of how best to respond in ethical dilemmas.

Sara Fry has argued that the traditional approach to medical ethics, which centers on application of objective principles and simply evaluating which principle takes priority, is no longer adequate as a foundation for nursing ethics.[7] She points out that caring, as an ideal, is a more comprehensive basis for the traditional values of autonomy and doing good for patients. Rather than relying on moral theory, Fry suggests that nursing ethics rests on a moral view of persons. Thus, in the discussion that follows, we will attempt to evaluate issues and illustrative cases with reference to the usual moral principles, but will also consider the moral obligations that may stem from the caring relationship that nurses have with their patients.

Regardless of the theoretical underpinnings of ethical analysis, the nurse who identifies ethical issues or questions will need to use a systematic process to examine the situation and reach a decision about what action to take. There are many suggested models for analyzing ethical dilemmas and any thoughtful, deliberative process can be helpful. One approach that is similar to the problem solving steps most nurses have learned is illustrated in Table 62–1. The process begins with identifying the issue or question; this step helps to focus the ethical issue, clarify what aspect of complex patient care situations is raising concerns, and differentiate the ethical dilemma from clinical problems. The second step, review facts and assumptions, directs the nurse to be clear about relevant data and to be sensitive to assumptions that may not be based on adequate data. The third step, list all options, is intended to prompt the nurse to think carefully about all possible actions, rather than fall into the temptation to dichotomize the possible answers (e.g., withdraw all treatment or continue all treatment, accept the patient's decision or do not accept it, etc.). The fourth step is the point at which the nurse must bring to bear considerations related to ethical principles, relevant professional norms, laws, policies, and personal values. In this step, each option is evaluated against these touchstones or criteria. Finally, having evaluated each

---

**Table 62–1**
**Steps of Ethical Problem-Solving**

1. Define the problem
   - Differentiate clinical problems, such as uncertainty or disagreement about prognosis, from ethical problems, such as determining how to balance duties to provide benefit and duties to respect autonomy; assure that everyone identifies the same issue.
2. Clarify facts and assumptions.
   - Differentiate known facts from assumptions about the situation, such as presumed motives of family members; assure that all parties have access to the same facts.
3. Develop list of all options.
   - Avoid collapsing options into "yes/no" absolutes, such as "continue all treatment" and "discontinue all treatment"; assure that all possible actions are evaluated, including intermediate steps such as continue all treatments and escalate as needed; continue all treatments but do not add anything further; discontinue ineffective interventions but continue non-invasive treatments; discontinue all interventions that do not promote comfort.
4. Evaluate all options.
   - Consider relevant laws, policies, and ethical principles; address rights, duties, and interests of all involved.
5. Choose the optimal option and implement.

---

option, the final decision is made as the fifth step. Most ethical dilemmas are multifaceted with conflicting demands. The case studies that follow in this chapter will demonstrate the complexity of these challenges, the need to address them in a methodical and logical process, and the essential caring role of the nurse in responding to such dilemmas.

## Common Ethical Dilemmas

### CASE STUDY 1

A 62-year-old man with a 12-year history of coronary artery disease, myocardial infarction, and heart failure enters the hospital with a left-sided CVA that has caused him to aspirate food of any consistency. His mental status is suspect and there is disagreement as to whether or not he has decisional capacity. He is able to answer "yes" and "no," although the responses are inconsistent. The attending physician is convinced that the patient lacks decision-making capacity while two family members (his wife and older brother) are equally convinced that he has decisional capacity. The patient does not have an Advance Directive. The patient's wife states that they have never held conversations about preferences for life-sustaining treatment. She believes he would not want to live in a condition that would not allow him to function as fully as he was prior to the CVA, but is ambivalent about the placement of a feeding tube. The patient's two daughters insist that a feeding tube should be placed because not doing so would be "killing him." The attending physician and the rest of the interdisciplinary health-care team are opposed to placing the feeding tube. In fact, several nurses who have cared for this patient during previous hospitalizations claim that the patient told them that

he would not want to be sustained by artificial means. The attending physician, as well as the neurological consultant, has verified that recovery is likely to be minimal due to dense damage to the cerebral cortex. They believe placing a feeding tube would be futile. The advanced practice nurse is not comfortable with claiming the feeding tube would be "futile" but is concerned about whether the patient would have wanted it and whether it will serve his best interests in the long term. She wonders how to get help in resolving the conflict.

## Goal-Setting and Advance Care Planning

Patients with advanced disease or near the end of life, their families, and health-care providers may encounter a variety of ethical dilemmas and subsequent choices. Although moral questions can arise about any aspect of nursing practice, including informed consent and duties to colleagues, the issues most frequently encountered in palliative care center around end-of-life decisions. These include withholding or withdrawing treatment (e.g. mechanical ventilation, hemodialysis, cardiopulmonary resuscitation, and cardiac assist devices), concerns about use of artificial nutrition and hydration, requests for hastened death (assisted suicide and euthanasia), and palliative sedation. For the most part, ethical analyses of these issues are grounded in patient choices, goals of care, preferences, prognosis, and communication. However, there are many important social, professional, and legal influences that have made these choices complicated. The explosion of technological advances and biomedical interventions over the past century has enabled the medical profession to prolong life through sophisticated interventions before adequate bioethical norms have been established. As a consequence, it is usually more helpful to focus on patient preferences for *outcomes* of treatments rather than preferences or choices for *specific treatments*.[8] Clearly this requires careful and repeated discussions with patients and their families. As can be seen in Case Study 1, it would have been much more helpful to know the patient's feelings and attitudes about what states or conditions would be acceptable to him rather than general statements about use of "artificial means."

The pace and demands of healthcare today add to the challenges of addressing ethical issues in the clinical setting and may lead to hasty and arbitrary decision-making. According to Levine-Ariff, "it is only with a thrust toward preventive ethics that decisions can be thoughtful and beneficial to patients and families" (p. 169).[9] "Preventive ethics" can be thought of as standards and norms that, when adhered to, can minimize the frequency with which difficult conflicts and dilemmas occur. The use of advanced care planning is an example of a "preventive ethics" intervention that nurses can implement.

Because of the many difficult decisions that will be faced by most people as they age and as they experience serious illnesses, assuring that thoughtful discussions take place before serious illness occurs can be quite helpful in preventing later uncertainties and dilemmas (see Case Study 1). Advance care planning is a process of communication and documentation to identify patients' preferences about goals of care and identify an authorized proxy who can provide competent, confident, and informed representation for choices when the patient is unable to express wishes. Advance directives are written instructions to health-care providers that are established before the need for medical intervention. Advance directives have three major purposes: provide a mechanism to enable providers to respect patient autonomy in situations in which the patient cannot express his wishes, provide guidance to health-care professionals and family members regarding how to proceed with decision-making about life-sustaining interventions, and provide immunity for professionals from civil and criminal liabilities when certain stated conditions are met.

A Living Will is one type of advance directive which is often accompanied by a durable power of attorney for health-care (DPAHC) or health-care proxy. Living Wills are used to declare wishes to refuse, limit, or withhold life-sustaining treatment under such circumstances that the individual is incapacitated or unable to communicate, while the DPAHC authorizes the agent or proxy to make all health-care decisions, presumably acting as the patient would have. A Living Will, as the patient's own treatment preference, takes precedence over the DPAHC if there are conflicts. However, in many states, the LW statute specifies that this document is only in effect when the patient is terminally ill, as determined by the physician, and thus it may not be helpful in situations such as major cardiovascular accident, persistent vegetative state, coma, or other serious illnesses that are not considered inevitably terminal.

Despite their shortcomings, advance directives are the best instruments we have to ensure that an individual's goals and preferences for care are met.[10] Unfortunately, because predicting and outlining all possible choices regarding health-care scenarios is difficult, advance directives are rarely defined as precisely as needed,[11] especially when a disease progresses and the context of the situation changes. Although it has been over a decade since the Patient Self Determination Act (PSDA) was made law in 1990,[12] empirical studies reporting effectiveness of advance directives have yielded disappointing results. Only 25% to 35% of patients have completed these, even among seriously ill populations such as persons with cancer,[13] and when present, they often do not direct care.[14,15] Nonetheless, advance care planning is an essential process that should begin to take place at the point of diagnosis and be revisited throughout the course of the disease trajectory to ensure that patients' preferences for care are preserved.

Other forms of advance directives include out-of-hospital do-not-attempt-resuscitation (DNAR) orders (discussed below), and the Five Wishes,[16] a detailed guide for discussions of preferences for end-of-life care. The Five Wishes document, now recognized in forty states, helps individuals who are seriously ill and unable to speak for themselves express how they want to be treated from a medical, personal, emotional, and spiritual perspective. In addition, this unique document helps patients discuss their wishes with family and the health-care team.

Health-care advance directives differ widely in format and content, making the already complex issues that palliative care nurses face even more difficult. Additional barriers exist when patients transfer from one care facility to another and the requirements change or the previously-existing document is not incorporated or honored.[17] In addition, some advance directives are not sufficient to direct care in some health-care institutions until a physician's order is written in the medical record. These barriers have led to an attempt to remedy these problems through the creation of other methods such as Physician Orders for Life-Sustaining Treatment (POLST)[18] and Medical Orders for Life-Sustaining Treatment (MOLST).[19] The overall aim of these newer forms of advance directives is to improve the communication of personal wishes about life-sustaining treatments, resulting in higher quality medical care that is consistent with patient choice.

The POLST program was originally developed in Oregon to improve end-of-life care by overcoming many of the shortcomings and pitfalls of advance directives.[20] The cornerstone of the program is a brightly colored standardized form that provides specific treatment orders for mechanical ventilation, antibiotics, cardiopulmonary resuscitation, and artificial nutrition and hydration. The POLST form is recommended for persons who have a life-limiting disease, who might die in the next year, or who want to further define their preferences for care and treatment. Other states have adopted similar programs with different names although all share the same core elements and with similar forms (POST in West Virginia; MOLST in New York). In 2006, the National Quality Forum[21] recommended that the POLST model be adopted nationwide because it more accurately reflects end of life preferences and produces higher medical adherence.[22,23] Unfortunately, many state statutes require modification before this goal can be reached.

Nursing responsibilities related to advance care planning include initiating conversations about patient overall goals and specific wishes related to hospitalization, use of cardio-pulmonary resuscitation, and other forms of advanced life support. These discussions will be most helpful if they focus on values rather than specific treatments. Patients and families should be asked about the existence of advance directives and education about both the formal documents and the process of advance care planning is a critical responsibility in palliative care. Patients and families also frequently need assistance in the actual completion of the documents, and nurses can be effective facilitators in providing access to the documents and showing patients how to complete them, as well as helping them think through their wishes.

## Do Not Attempt Resuscitation Orders

As noted, decisions about the level and type of interventions to be used must stem from consensus about the goals of care. For patients in acute care settings and those who have not yet elected to focus on comfort rather than cure, the specific issue of resuscitation status is a frequent source of distress for clinicians as well as patients and families. In addition to discomfort and inexperience with the topic, there continues to be widespread misunderstanding about the efficacy of cardiopulmonary resuscitation (CPR) efforts and the meaning of decisions to withhold CPR in the event of an arrest.

In acute care settings, cardiopulmonary resuscitation is successful in supporting survival to hospital discharge in only about 18% of instances of arrest.[24] This success rate has changed little in the 50 years since the technique of CPR was first developed. The relative ineffectiveness of CPR reflects the inappropriate widespread use of resuscitation efforts in situations in which multiple pre-existing chronic illnesses have led to an irreversible state and death is inevitable. Unfortunately, the public has little understanding of what actually occurs in CPR, the limited benefit except in situations of single-organ disease and immediate intervention, and the potential for cognitive impairment if circulation is restored.[25]

Clinicians, too, may inadvertently contribute to misunderstandings about this issue in several ways. In addition to the tendency to avoid discussions of goals of care, too often the topic of resuscitation status is raised in the form of a question to patients, or more commonly to families, as "What do you want us to do if his heart stops?" This approach reflects a well-intentioned but misguided attempt to identify patient/family preferences. It is misguided in that it places full responsibility for decision-making on the shoulders of family members and implies that it is possible to restore circulation through CPR.

As part of improving the standard of care in any institution, nurses can encourage providers to adopt the newer acronym, "DNAR." The American Heart Association, the recognized experts in emergency cardiac care, converted to the acronym "DNAR" (Do Not Attempt Resuscitation), rather then the former "DNR" in their 2005 standards,[26] signaling recognition that CPR, with its current wide application, more accurately is an *attempt* to restore cardiac function. This attempt is most often unsuccessful and this change in language will hopefully facilitate recognition that a DNAR order does not entail a decision to allow a preventable death to occur. Rather, a DNAR order indicates a decision to withhold a very invasive and aggressive intervention that has little chance in promoting survival to hospital discharge.

Clarification of resuscitation status is best done as part of overall care planning. All nurses can play a key role in raising this topic, encouraging sensitive but straightforward communication, and facilitating discussion. Because the intention to use CPR in the event of an arrest is the default in virtually all health-care settings today, resuscitation status must be addressed in every situation of life-limiting or serious illness. This is particularly important when patients change care settings or begin care with new providers, such as admission to a long-term care facility, home healthcare, or home hospice. In addition to discussion of overall goals and quality of life, the nurse can provide factual information about CPR and clarify the difference between a plan to withhold this ineffective intervention and the plan to use maximal efforts to prevent cardiac arrest.

Although use of DNAR orders is the standard method to indicate to health-care personnel that CPR is not to be used, these orders are only effective within the facility in which they are issued. The need to have portable orders and valid indicators of DNAR status for patients moving between facilities or patients being cared for at home has led to the creation of out-of-hospital forms and identifiers. Most states have passed legislation establishing a mechanism to reliably identify DNAR status for emergency response personnel.[27] In some cases this has been specific clauses in the Living Will and in others, a specific out-of-hospital standard order form has been developed. Unlike most advance directives, the out-of-hospital DNAR document is a valid physician order that takes effect as soon as it is signed; it is not limited by the patient's diagnosis or terminal status. When available, these forms should be initiated when the decision to forego CPR is first made so that patients can take them with them as they are discharged or transferred among facilities.

A frequent challenge nurses face is how to manage situations in which they perceive the patient's condition is deteriorating and no one has addressed the issue of resuscitation status with the patient or family. Common concerns are that initiating such a discussion is outside the boundaries of the nursing role, that physicians will be angry if the nurse raises the topic, that patients or families will be upset. Kirchhoff and colleagues[28] reported on the perceptions of obstacles and helpful behaviors that 199 critical care nurses discussed in providing end-of-life care to dying patients. The highest ranked "helpful" was "having all physicians agree about the direction of care." This ranking may reflect the degree of distress nurses feel when "stuck in the middle." It is important for nurses to recognize that it is within the professional role of nursing to identify the need to develop consensus around goals of care and treatment plans, and to facilitate discussions surrounding difficult decision-making.

## Proxy Decision-Making

Because patients with serious illness frequently lack cognitive capacity at some point during the illness, professionals must rely on family or friends to represent their wishes and participate in decision making. This creates a number of possible areas of conflict and uncertainty, including the need to make careful assessments of capacity, questions about the moral authority of family and friends to make decisions for patients, and, in some cases, the need to manage conflicts among and between families and the care team, as occurred in Case Study 1.

"Incompetency" refers to a status that is conferred by a court, establishing the inability of an individual to act as an autonomous and legally responsible person. Only the court can make a determination of *competence*; clinicians provide evidence to the court regarding the *capacity* of the individual, including data about diagnosis, cognitive and functional ability, and likelihood of recovery. An individual who has been deemed "incompetent" loses the right to make all decisions, including health-care decisions, and must have a guardian appointed by the court to manage all affairs.[29] Clinicians, therefore, cannot establish competency, but instead do have an on-going responsibility to assess capacity of the patient to participate in decision-making.

When patients are not able to express their wishes or make decisions and do not have a designated health-care agent, family members are asked to act as proxies. Although this is common practice, states vary in the extent to which this is authorized by law and the precise specification of which family members have priority in decision-making. The moral basis for allowing one adult to make decisions for another is the assumption that family members are committed to furthering the best interests of the patient and family members, who share background, experiences, religion, and culture with the patient, are well equipped to represent the preferences and values of the patient. These assumptions are usually quite valid, but there are situations in which nurses question the ability of the family member to act as a valid proxy for the patient. In these cases, establishing that the assumptions that are necessary to justify relying on the proxy are, in fact, not confirmed is important in making a plan to seek another representative for that patient. These situations are difficult and nurses must be prepared to seek guidance from the hospital ethics committee or hospital legal counsel, as well as collaborating with physicians and social workers on the care team.

Proxy decision-making, even under the best of circumstances, can be very burdensome to families already stressed by the realization of the seriousness of their loved one's illness. Several studies have demonstrated that family members are not able to consistently identify the preferences of their ill relative[30,31] even when an advance directive is in place. As mentioned earlier, this is related to reluctance to discuss end-of-life issues before a crisis and, when discussion does occur, the likelihood that the discussion was of a general nature and does not necessarily apply to the very specific decisions that have to be made in situations of prognostic uncertainty. An additional common occurrence is lack of consensus among family members about specific decisions, such as limiting treatment, DNAR status, or referrals to hospice.

There are several steps the nurse can take in an effort to prevent or minimize concerns related to proxy decision-making, particularly when initiating palliative care services. First, all patients who have a serious illness and do not have a DPAHC should be asked to identify a proxy to make decisions if they should become unable. This can be done on admission to the hospital or any other health-care delivery system in a nonthreatening manner, simply pointing out that sometimes patients become too ill or too sleepy due to medication. This will enable the team to know, if there are disagreements later, who has the strongest claim to the decision-maker role. Second, the time to obtain information about the patient's lifestyle, values, and preferences is before specific decisions about pursuing invasive diagnostic tests or procedures are needed. Talking with family members about what the patient was like, what he/she enjoyed, what was important, can be helpful in later discussions. Third, when it is necessary to ask a family proxy to provide input into the plan of care, it is essential to address the task as one of helping the clinicians to know what the patient would have wanted. This can be done by referring back to earlier discussions about what was most important to the patient. The goals here are twofold: to minimize the burden of responsibility the family member might feel and to remain focused on the ethical mandate to act according to the patient's wishes, not the family members' wishes. Table 62–2 provides some examples of ways to phrase questions that are not helpful and some ways that can be more useful in supporting family decision-making.

## Artificial Hydration and Nutrition

A fundamental care-giving task is to provide food and fluids. The provision of nutrition and hydration symbolizes the essence of care and compassion and eating serves as a symbol of health. In most societies, celebrations involve eating, and through these traditional social events we communicate sharing and well-being. Clearly, human life is represented as

**Table 62–2**
**Phrases to Avoid and Phrases That Can Be More Helpful**

| Do Not Say | Do Say |
|---|---|
| "What do you want us to do if your loved one's heart stops?" | "We need to talk about where we go from here if your loved one's condition continues to worsen." |
| "Would you want us to do CPR if your loved one's heart stops?" | "There are many things we can do, but it's very important that we talk together about what your loved one would want done in this situation. Have you and he/she ever known anyone who was this ill…did he/she say anything about what he/she would want in a situation like this?" |
| "We need your permission to do a (tracheostomy, PEG, angiogram, etc.)" | "Given what we've discussed about your loved one's situation and the most likely benefits and burdens of the procedure, we need your help to know if he/she would want us to proceed with the (tracheostomy, PEG, angiogram, etc.)" |
| "We'll do whatever you want us to…it's your decision…we'll support whatever you decide" | "We have to make some decisions about where to go from here. It's our job to give you information about the medical facts and our recommendations, and we need you to help us know what would be important to your loved one now. Then, we need to talk and come up with a plan together." |

social and communal through the provision of food.[32] When a loved one has an advanced illness, these opportunities wane and when one is dying, they are often lost. However, providing artificial nutrition and hydration is not synonymous with eating or feeding another person. In health, people eat in a socially acceptable form, with others, in a social setting. Medically provided nutrition and hydration do not share these social characteristics.

The technology of feeding tubes was developed to address specific temporary medical problems (e.g., postsurgical gastric motility issues, swallowing impairment following a stroke in a patient expected to recover). However, the use of feeding tubes and medically provided nutrition and hydration have become widely used in patients with very poor prognoses and for those with little likelihood of regaining functional abilities. Few decisions are more value-laden than those to withhold or withdraw a medical intervention that is thought to be able to prolong life. As with all decisions about the use of any medical device or treatment, this decision should be based on the patient's goals of care, the medical need, and the burdens and benefits of the treatment.

In general, patients (or their surrogates) have the right to withhold or withdraw artificial hydration and nutrition if they believe that the burden or risks outweigh the benefits. There is widespread agreement in ethics and law[33–35] that patients or their surrogates have a right to choose or refuse artificial nutrition and hydration. As with all decisions about medical interventions, decisions about nutrition and hydration should be made in light of patient's goals and outcomes of care. These goals of care may change during the course of the disease or as the disease progresses and the patient's cognitive and physical functioning decline. Consequently, nurses should create opportunities for discussion and negotiation of goals and priorities of care with the patient and family/surrogate on an ongoing basis.

Artificial nutrition and hydration (ANH) require the placement of a temporary or permanent feeding tube or the initiation of intravenous access. These interventions are associated with risks, including bleeding, tube displacement, and infection, as well as the potential need for repositioning and replacement.[36–39] In patients with impaired renal function, intravenous fluids may promote peripheral or pulmonary edema and increase the need for suctioning.[40] In addition, intravenous infusions can increase the risk of infections and phlebitis in a patient with an altered immune status simply related to an impaired functional status.[41] Tube feedings do not appear to prevent aspiration pneumonia and may increase the risk as compared to those patients who do not take anything by mouth.[42,43] Other potential side effects of tube feeding include diarrhea, nausea, vomiting, and aspiration of the feeding into the lung.[36] Many patients and family members have deep concerns about the issue of "hunger" and "starvation." Contrary to what many believe, a patient with a terminal disease, who is often anorexic from the effects of the disease, may not be bothered by hunger.[44] In fact, many patients in whom the disease is progressing tend to report a complete lack of hunger. Evidence suggests that natural physiological processes that accompany the cessation of food and fluid intake naturally suppress both hunger and thirst. In a study conducted with 32 terminally-ill patients during the final 6 months of their lives, 63% of the patients never experienced hunger, 34% expressed hunger states only transiently at the beginning of the study period, and 63% denied thirst.[45] Similarly, Sullivan[46] found that hunger and thirst issues in a similar population with terminal disease tended to cease after only a few days of decreased intake. Nursing interventions that can assist with the palliation of symptoms associated with dry mouth or thirst include small sips of oral intake, ice chips, meticulous mouth care, and lubrication of the lips.

Involving caregivers, family members, and loved ones in this activity may replace the family's desire and need to feed with another care-giving activity that can provide the family with the opportunity to provide physical comfort.

There have been several studies of the effect of withholding ANH on survival. A meta analysis conducted by Heyland and colleagues attempted to clarify whether total parenteral nutrition (TPN) affected morbidity and mortality in critically ill patients.[47] The overall conclusion of this study suggested that there was no benefit on mortality or major complication rates. A similar study validated these conclusions and went on to suggest that, given the potential increased costs and complications associated with the use of TPN and lack of effect on mortality or length of stay, further studies are needed before we assume who can benefit from this intervention.[48] Similarly, there is particularly strong evidence confirming the failure of percutaneous endoscopic gastrostomy tubes (PEGs) and tube-feeding to prolong survival in states of advanced dementia.[49-51]

Additionally, there may be both financial implication of these decisions and implications for discharge planning and home care. Some hospice programs cover the cost of ANH, based on the individual plan of care and the goals of care, but others do not. Some extended-care facilities (i.e., nursing homes) mandate medically-provided nutrition and hydration when a person stops eating and/or drinking, often related to misunderstanding and concern about state regulations or related to philosophy and religious missions. Consequently, discussions with families about decisions to use ANH, as in Case Study 1, should include consideration of these factors. In that case, the nurse would have several responsibilities, including clarifying the facts about the patient's previously stated wishes, educating all family members regarding the likely benefits and burdens of tube feedings, and focusing discussions with both physicians and family members on what was known about the patient's values and preferences.

Despite the lack of proven benefit in states of irreversible and advanced illness, artificial nutrition and hydration will remain an emotionally laden topic and one of the most difficult decisions. Nurses have a particularly important role in educating patients, families, and other members of the health-care team about the benefits and burdens of tube feedings. There is a persistent wide-spread belief, particularly among unlicensed assistive personnel and even among physicians,[52] that we have a duty to feed all patients and that the benefits of ANH always outweigh the burdens. This misunderstanding, in combination with concerns about causing suffering, is a significant barrier to careful ethical evaluation of the decision to use or withhold ANH. Assuring informed decision-making about this aspect of the care plan often must begin with addressing the concerns of the care team before developing a plan to make clear recommendations to families and providing family members with the necessary education about this issue.

CASE STUDY 2
*Withdrawal of Life Support in the Intensive Care Unit*

Ms. H was a 32-year-old caucasian woman. She was divorced from her husband and had custody of her son, age 6 years, and her daughter, age 3 years. Her parents and her fiancé were her significant others. Ms. H was diagnosed with a uterine leiomyosarcoma two years ago. She had undergone two regimens of chemotherapy following a hysterectomy, but the cancer had metastasized to her hip and her mediastinum. The thoracic lesion had grown to the point where it was compressing her bronchus and she was taken to the OR for stint placement as a palliative measure. This was not able to be done and she was then admitted to the ICU, intubated and on mechanical ventilation. Over the course of a week, several attempts were made to extubate her, but she was unable to maintain a patent airway without the positive pressure of the ventilator and the endotracheal tube. Each time the ventilator support was reduced, Ms. H became very anxious and short of breath, even with the use of increasing doses of lorazepam and morphine. She was awake and alert and able to write notes.

On rounds, the ICU attending physician mentioned to the team that it was time to think about doing a tracheostomy since it looked as if Ms. H was not able to be extubated. Ms. P, her nurse, was concerned that this would just subject Ms. H to another procedure and would not change the eventual outcome. She also was uncertain whether anyone had told Ms. H the details of her condition and the real possibility that she would never be able to leave the ICU. On the other hand, the fact that Ms. H was wide awake made it seem as if withdrawing life support (e.g., extubating her) might be cruel—how could this be done without causing suffering?

## Hastening Death

A central issue in decision-making in states of serious illness is the moral acceptability of actions that can be seen as hastening death. As has been noted throughout this chapter, it is well established in western bioethics that competent patients have an almost unlimited right to accept or refuse medical interventions, regardless of the established efficacy of the intervention or its necessity for survival. Supporting and advocating for this right is a critical function of the nurse and one which has been identified as a frequent source of ethical distress.[53]

The recognized right of the individual to elect to stop life-sustaining technology, such as mechanical ventilation or hemodialysis, has been used by some as the basis for arguing that there is no difference between this act and acts that intentionally hasten death, including both euthanasia and assisted suicide. Arguments that there is a difference usually rely on the distinction between allowing a death caused by disease, as occurs when removing unwanted or ineffective life-prolonging therapies such as mechanical ventilators and dialysis, and killing, which entails being the direct cause of death (see Case Studies 1 and 2). There is ongoing debate in the bioethics community about whether this is a morally relevant distinction and each nurse who cares for patients with life-limiting disease will have to carefully identify his/her own beliefs.

Euthanasia is defined as an intentional act performed for the purpose of causing the death of another for reasons of mercy, whereas assisted suicide is the provision of assistance in some form (e.g. supplying lethal medications or instructions) to an individual who then acts to take his/her own life. Euthanasia in all forms is illegal in the United States and is condoned by none of the professional associations (see Table 62–3). However, assisted suicide (also termed physician-aid-in-dying and physician-assisted suicide [PAS]) has been legalized in Oregon since 1997 and most recently approved by voters in Washington state.[54] At this time, professional nursing organizations do not condone nurses actively participating in assisted suicide (Table 62–3).

Nurses, as the health-care professionals who spend the greatest amount of time with patients and their families and who often have the most intimate relationships with them, are inevitably involved in situations involving the issue of hastening death. This may take the form of explicit requests from patients for some action that would precipitate death or shorten survival, patients and families may explicitly request information or counseling from the nurse regarding hastening death, or nurses may identify more subtle clues that the patient or family are considering hastening death. The desire for hastened death at some point in terminal illness has been found to occur with relative frequency. Emanuel, Fairclough, and Emanuel[55] reported an incidence of serious consideration for either euthanasia or PAS in 10.6% of 988 terminally ill patients. O'Mahoney, Goutlet, et al.[56] found that 34% of 131 patients admitted to a palliative care service had some level of desire for hastening death. In a large Dutch survey of nurses' involvement in end-of-life decisions in hospitals, nursing

---

**Table 62–3**
**Position Statements from Recognized Professional Organizations**

**Artificial hydration and nutrition**

- Hospice and Palliative Nurses Association (HPNA) Position Statement on Artificial Nutrition and Hydration in End-of-Life Care (http://www.hpma.org/DisplayPage.aspx?Title1=Position%20Statements)
- National Hospice and Palliative Care Organization (NHPCO)Commentary and Position Statement on Artificial Nutrition and Hydration (http://www.nhpco.org/files/public/ANH_Statement_Commentary.pdf)
- American Nurse's Association Position Statement(ANA): Foregoing Nutrition and Hydration (http://www.nursingworld.org/MainMenuCategories/HealthCareandPolicyIssues/ANAPositionStatements/)
- American Academy of Hospice and Palliative Medicine (AAHPM) Statement on Artificial Nutrition and Hydration Near the End of Life (http://www.aahpm.org/positions/nutrition.html)

**Physician assisted suicide**

- Hospice and Palliative Nurses Association (HPNA) Position Statement on Legalization of Assisted Suicide (http://www.hpna.org/DisplayPage.aspx?Title1=Position%20Statements)
- National Hospice and Palliative Care Organization (NHPCO) Commentary and Resolution on Physician Assisted Suicide (http://www.nhpco.org/files/public/PAS_Resolution_Commentary.pdf)
- American Nurse's Association Position Statement (ANA): Assisted Suicide (http://www.nursingworld.org/MainMenuCategories/HealthCareandPolicyIssues/ANAPositionStatements/)
- American Academy of Hospice and Palliative Medicine (AAHPM) Statement on Physician Assisted Death (http://www.aahpm.org/suicide.html)
- Oncology Nursing Society Nurse's Responsibility to the Patient Requesting Assistance in Hastening Death (http://www.ons.org/Publications/positions/AssistedSuicide.shtml)
- American Society for Pain Management Nursing Position Statement on Assisted Suicide (http://aspmn.org/pdfs/Assisted%20Suicide.pdf)

**Palliative sedation**

- Hospice and Palliative Nurses Association (HPNA) Position Statement on Palliative Sedation (http://www.hpma.org/DisplayPage.aspx?Title1=Position%20Statements)
- American Academy of Hospice and Palliative Medicine (AAHPM) Statement on Palliative Sedation (http://www.aahpm.org/positions/sedation.html)

homes, and home care, the nurse was the first person with whom the patient discussed a request for euthanasia or PAS in 45.1% of cases.[57] In a 1997 survey of New England Oncology Nursing Society members, 30% reported receiving requests for hastened death.[58] These situations require very careful attention from the nurse, awareness of legal and ethical considerations, and a well-developed and collaborative plan for responding.

The first, and perhaps most important, responsibility of the nurse is clarification and assessment. The expression of thoughts of hastening death may be an accurate report of a serious intention, it may be a relatively off-hand comment, it may be an expression of distress prompted by unrelieved symptoms, or it may be intended as a test of the nurse's views about hastening death. In addition to clarifying the meaning of the patient's statements, the desire for hastened death should always prompt a thorough evaluation of the adequacy of symptom management, particularly pain and depression. Ganzini found that, among 58 patients in Oregon who had sought PAS, 26% were assessed as depressed on psychiatric interview.[59]

There are a number of guidelines developed by professional associations and groups to assist the clinician in responding to requests for hastened death.[60–62] All of these emphasize both the right of professionals to withdraw from situations in which they are being requested to act in a way, such as participating in assisted suicide, which violates their moral principles. However, the duty to assure patients that they will not be abandoned, to work diligently to investigate and address correctable factors that may be leading to the request for hastened death, and the duty to refrain from withdrawing until an alternate source of care is in place are absolute.

## Special Questions: Cardiac Assist Devices, Palliative Sedation, Futility

There are three specific issues that present particularly challenging questions in palliative care. These are the acceptability and methods of withdrawing life-sustaining interventions that consist of cardiac assistive devices (pacemakers, automatic internal cardio-defibrillators [AICD]), concerns about requests for futile therapy, and terminal sedation.

### Cardiac Assistive Devices

One of the most concrete examples of the complexities created by advancing technologies is the situation of patients who have elected to forego continued use of cardio-assistive devices in order to allow a peaceful death. There are a number of implantable mechanical assistive devices intended to either support or replace normal cardiac electrical and mechanical function, including left ventricular assistive devices (LVADs), right ventricular assistive devices

(RVADs), total implantable hearts (TIH), internal automatic cardio-defibrillators (AICD), and pacemakers. Each of these raises unique issues.

Internal automatic cardio-defibrillators are very commonly used in the United States as treatment of recurrent ventricular fibrillation. Pacemakers have been a long-standing therapy for brady-arrhythmias and combined AICD-pacemakers are recommended for some forms of heart failure. In an international survey in 2005, 223,425 pacemakers and 119,121 AICDs were implanted in the United States.[63] It is therefore very likely that palliative care nurses will find themselves caring for patients with either or both of these devices. In most cases, both AICDs and pacemakers are on-demand therapy; that is, they are programmed to deliver therapy only on demand (when heart rate decreases or a lethal arrhythmia develops). Therefore, their function should be disabled when the plan of care is based on a goal of allowing a peaceful death with no further intervention. AICDs should be turned off so that they will not deliver a shock as the heart rate falls or ventricular arrhythmias occur. Demand pacemakers can have the rate and sensitivity decreased so they do not prolong the dying process. Cardiologists or cardiac technicians usually must be called and requested to make these changes using the device programming magnets.

When cardiac function is dependent on active device operation, as is the case with some pacemakers and most ventricular assist devices, there are more difficult challenges and unresolved questions. Some argue that discontinuing a cardiac assist device, with the expectation that death will follow, is no different, morally, than discontinuing mechanical ventilation for a patient who has elected (or whose family has elected) to have life-sustaining therapy discontinued. However, others believe that the fact that the device is implanted and has become, in a sense, part of the patient, makes discontinuation equivalent to an act of euthanasia and thus is impermissible.[64,65]

When caring for the patient with an implanted cardiac device, the nurse has several responsibilities. First, the exact status of the device's operation has to be determined. As with all components of the palliative care plan, the plan for adjusting the device should stem from a clear understanding of the patient's goals of care. If, for example, the goal is to make the most of whatever time is left and there is hope for more time, all cardiac devices should remain active and in place. On the other hand, if the patient is actively dying or has expressed a competent desire to remove any therapy that could interfere with the dying process (whenever that might occur), the devices should be inactivated (or turned to an inactive setting). Each of these decisions, of course, must be made in collaboration with the care team. If there is consensus about discontinuing a device on which cardiac function is entirely dependent, extra care must be taken to assure that the patient, family members, and the entire care team is in agreement. The timing of the discontinuation must be carefully considered and a plan to address likely symptoms put in place.

## Palliative Sedation

There are a very small number of situations at the end of life in which patient symptoms cannot be adequately relieved despite multiple pharmacologic regimens. In these cases the option of palliative sedation (also termed "terminal sedation") is sometimes raised. Palliative sedation refers to the use of medications to induce sedation, either intermittently or continuously, for the purpose of providing relief of intractable symptoms. The intention is not to cause death. Claessens, Menten, et al.[66] recently published the results of a comprehensive literature review on the subject of palliative sedation. They reported varying incidences among hospices and palliative care units of 1% to 50%. The most frequently used medication was midazolam, with or without other drugs such as haloperidol and barbiturates. The most common indication was refractory delirium, dyspnea, or pain, with some use for "existential suffering" (i.e., fear, emotional distress).

The wide variation in the reported use of palliative sedation and limited research evidence about best practice is likely a reflection of ambivalence and uncertainty about the ethical acceptability of the practice. Perhaps the most common objection to palliative sedation is the belief that deep sedation to the point of unconsciousness will directly hasten death. However, the review of published data by Claessens et al.[66] indicates that this is not the case. Nevertheless, use of deep sedation does require also addressing other interventions, such as the continuation of oral medications and the administration of food and fluids. In general, these other decisions should be made separately and before palliative sedation is begun. If there are adequate reasons to stop food, fluids, and other medications (i.e., if the patient is in the final stages of dying, has been refusing food and fluids, and other medications are not needed for promotion of comfort), there is no reason to insist they be used when palliative sedation begins. On the other hand, if nutrition and hydration were indicated before sedation, there may be good reason to continue their use or sedation should be stopped or lightened intermittently to offer food and fluid.

Case Study 2 is an example of a situation in which palliative sedation might be necessary. If Ms. H, who retained decisional capacity, chose to have ventilatory support withdrawn, it might be necessary to sedate her to the point of unconsciousness in order to prevent suffering. This act certainly would shorten her survival, compared to continuing mechanical ventilation. However, this act would be morally permissible and supported by the principle of double effect. This principle, well established in bioethics, asserts that acts that are intended to achieve a "good" effect (in this case, respecting autonomy and preventing suffering) are permissible even if the act also carries with it an unintended "bad' effect (hastened death). In addition to intending only the good effect, this principle requires that the good not be achieved by means of the bad (i.e., the relief of suffering is achieved by the sedation, not by causing death) and the weight of the good achieved must be greater than the bad effect.[32]

Although both the American Academy of Hospice and Palliative Medicine and the Hospice and Palliative Nurses Association (see Table 62–3) support the use of palliative sedation in carefully selected situations, both organizations emphasize the importance of clarity in the intended objective (relief of suffering) and the need for thorough discussion and informed consent from the patient. Davis and Ford[67] note that palliative sedation can be thought of as a kind of "social death" in that the patient loses the ability to interact and communicate. Given the importance of communication in the final stages of life, use of deep palliative sedation should be reserved for those few situations in which all other interventions have been ineffective and the patient finds continued consciousness to be intolerable.

## Futility

"Futility" is a term that refers to the inability of a specific intervention to lead to its intended outcome (e.g., prolonged survival, discharge from the hospital, shrinkage of tumor). This term has gained popularity in acute care over the past decade as clinicians have increasingly encountered situations in which patients and families request or demand therapies that the clinician believes have no meaningful chance of prolonging life or improving well being.[68-70] Over the years, there has been a growing consensus that the right of patients and families to accept or refuse therapies does not entail the right to demand therapies which the physician does not believe are medically justified.[71] The well-established right to accept or refuse therapy stems from the principle of autonomy. This principle establishes the duty to refrain from interfering in the life choices of competent persons; it is thus a "liberty right," not a right to demand access to any particular intervention.

The gradual move away from the paternalism of the past and a commitment to supporting patient autonomy has unfortunately led to a tendency to shift the responsibility for decision-making entirely to patients and families. This is sometimes seen in the reluctance of clinicians to advise or guide patients and families in decisions and, instead, to present options in a completely impartial fashion. Clinicians then may find themselves facing situations in which patients or families demand therapies that are thought to offer little benefit and significant probability of harm. Most often, this occurs with the question of resuscitation status or continued use of chemotherapy in advanced refractory cancer.[72,73] The frequency of futility dilemmas and the difficulty in resolving them has led professional organizations[74] and many other health-care organizations to develop policies for managing the conflict. At least one city, Houston, has developed a multi-institution, city-wide policy.[75] Although these policies are important in providing general guidelines for physicians and nurses, it is far more important to attempt to prevent futility conflicts from developing. As with most ethical dilemmas, effective communication and trusting relationships are key.

Specific steps that nurses can take in working to avoid the development of irreconcilable differences begin with talking early about goals of care, learning about the values and beliefs of the patient and his/her family, and establishing a collaborative model of decision-making. Not infrequently, families will express the wish to have "everything" done for their loved one. When this is said, the nurse or physician should respond by assuring the patient and family that they are heard and that their wish to receive all therapies that have any meaningful chance of maintaining or improving the patient's condition will be used. The use of shared decision-making should be emphasized from the start. As the condition of the patient deteriorates and it becomes apparent that continued interventions will not be helpful, it is best to set the stage for later decisions by affirming that the clinicians will provide honest and direct information and will identify when there are no further curative options, with assurances that the plan of care will always be discussed before changes are made. When the situation is such that CPR or other interventions are no longer indicated, this should be stated; patients or families should not be asked to give permission to withhold an ineffective intervention. If consensus appears to be unreachable, other resources, such as clergy or ethics consultants should be utilized.

In Case Study 2, the nurse, Ms. P, may have believed that performing a tracheostomy on Ms. H would indeed be futile. Although the procedure could be safely performed, it would not save the patient's life or even allow her to recover enough to leave the ICU—she would always require mechanical ventilation. To address this issue, Ms. P would need to first validate her assumption about the location of Ms. H's tumor and the ineffectiveness of a tracheostomy to relieve the obstruction. Next, a care conference with the entire multidisciplinary team would have to be arranged to develop consensus about the best approach. If the team reaches agreement about the lack of any effective treatment options for the cancer, a plan would have to be developed, including who would talk with Ms. H, what recommendation would be offered, what options would be acceptable, and how to manage her symptoms when she was ready to discontinue mechanical ventilation.

Although it is becoming increasingly recognized that clinicians have not only the right but the professional duty to refrain from interventions that are harmful, it is essential to be cautious in judging interventions as "futile." There are many treatments or therapies that offer neither cure nor improvement in patient condition, but which are effective in supporting survival, such as mechanical ventilation following anoxic brain injuries. The claim of futility should not be used to justify withholding therapies in situations in which the clinician believes that the proposed therapy would accomplish its intended purpose, but the resulting quality of life would be undesirable. Judgments such as this reflect the subjective opinions and values of clinicians and are not a valid basis for withholding therapy against the wishes of patients and families.

## Nursing Issues and Moral Distress

Decisions regarding ethical dilemmas and the choices that are necessary require thoughtful discussion and critical communication skills. Stemming from the priority of the principle of autonomy or self-determination, decisions about care should be made in accordance with patients' preferences for care, beliefs, and values. With increased medical technology, the advances in science, conflicting interests of patients and families, nurses stand in a pivotal position to lead the way in assuring patient access to quality palliative care. This charge does not come without the risk of the nurse feeling like he/she is "in the middle," trying to provide the best possible care to the patient, and supporting the family members, while bracketing personal values.[76]

Nurses and other members of the interdisciplinary healthcare team face ethical and legal issues in decision-making related to end of life care daily in clinical practice. These dilemmas have a strong potential to provoke conflict among those involved in patient care, sometimes between professionals and sometimes between patients, families, and professionals. The ANA Code of Ethics[77] states that nurses have the right to withdraw from providing care to patients when their own values conflict with that of patient, as so long as the patient's care can safely be transferred to another care provider. Caring for patients with advanced illness brings with it complex clinical situations and ethical challenges; nurses must find ways to support one another through talking and sharing experiences about moral uncertainty. Studies have demonstrated that nurses report having had to act against their conscience when confronted with ethical dilemmas[78] and describe emotional exhaustion related to the frequency of morally distressing situations.[79] In a large survey of nurses from a variety of health-care settings, including hospice, ICU, nursing facilities, and inpatient care, Ferrell[80] identified that nurses' greatest sources of moral distress originated from "aggressive care" and "aggressive care denying palliative care."

Ethics experts recognize that moral distress is often created in scenarios when nurses participate in activities that are perceived as medically futile. In fact, providing futile care undermines the core of the professional practice of nursing.[81] One of the most crucial elements in dealing with moral distress is knowing WHAT support is available and HOW to navigate the system in place. Ethics Committees are one source of support and serve to assist in resolving complicated ethical problems that affect the care and treatment of patients within health-care organizations. The Joint Commission on Accreditation of Healthcare Organizations requires hospitals and other health-care organizations to have a mechanism in place to address ethical issues in the provision of patient care.[82] Health-care organizations have different mechanisms by which to address ethical issues and it is therefore the responsibility of all nurses to know what resources are available in their organization and how to access them. Just as preventive ethics should be used before an ethical dilemma arises, so should they be used to guide nursing practice before a crisis occurs.

## Summary

There will always be new ethical dilemmas which require decision-making, and the answers to those dilemmas will not always be obvious or easily identified. It is often in states of uncertainty that serious wrongs occur. As partners in the care of patients and families with advanced illness who must make difficult decisions, nurses must be empowered to facilitate discussion and to be heard by all parties involved. The challenge for today is to ensure that all nurses acquire attributes of leadership, excellent communication skills, and self-reflection that enable them to fulfill the crucial role of nursing.

REFERENCES

1. Honderich T. The Oxford Guide to Philosophy. Oxford, UK: Oxford University Press, 2005.
2. Gert B. Morality: Its Nature and Justification. Oxford, UK: Oxford University Press, 2005.
3. Bishop AH, Scudder JR. The Practical, Moral, and Personal Sense of Nursing: A Phenomenological Philosophy of Practice. Albany, NY: State University of New York Press, 1990.
4. Sherwin S. Feminist and medical ethics: Two different approaches to contextual ethics. In Holmes HB, Purdy LM, eds. Feminist Perspectives in Medical Ethics. Indianapolis, IN: University Press; 1992:17–31.
5. Nodding N. Caring. Berkeley, CA: University of California Press, 1984.
6. Jones AH. Narrative based medicine: Narrative in medical ethics. BMJ 1999;318(7178):253–256.
7. Fry S. The role of caring in a theory of nursing ethics. In: Holmes HB, Purdy LM, eds. Feminist Perspectives in Medical Ethics. Indianapolis, IN: Indiana University Press; 1992:93–106.
8. Fried TR, Bradley EH, Towle VR, Allore H. Understanding the treatment preferences of seriously ill patients. N Engl J Med 2002;346(14):1061–1066.
9. Levine-Ariff J. Preventive ethics: The development of policies to guide decision-making. AACN Clin Issues Crit Care Nurs 1990;1(1):169–177.
10. Allen RS, DeLaine SR, Chaplin WF, et al. Advance care planning in nursing homes: Correlates of capacity and possession of advance directives. Gerontologist 2003;43(3):309–317.
11. Ditto PH, Danks JH, Houts RM, et al. Stability of older adults' preferences for life-sustaining medical treatment. Health Psychol 2003;22(6):605–615.
12. Greco PJ, Schulman KA, Lavizzo-Mourey R, Hansen-Flaschen J. The Patient Self-Determination Act and the future of advance directives. Ann Intern Med 1991;115(8):639–643.
13. Kish SK, Martin CG, Price KJ. Advance directives in critically ill cancer patients. Crit Care Nurs Clin North Am 2000;12(3):373–383.

14. Prendergast TJ. Advance care planning: Pitfalls, progress, promise. Crit Care Med 2001;29(2):N34.
15. Wallace SK, Martin CG, Shaw AD, Price KJ. Influence of an advance directive on the initiation of life support technology in critically ill cancer patients. Crit Care Med 2001;29(12):2294.
16. Five Wishes. http://www.agingwithdignity.org/5wishes.html (accessed November 15, 2008).
17. Meyers JL, Moore C, McGrory A, Sparr J, Ahern M. Physician orders for life-sustaining treatment form: Honoring end-of-life directives for nursing home residents. J Gerontol Nurs 2004;30(9):37–46.
18. Schmidt TA, Hickman SE, Tolle SW, Brooks HS. The physician orders for life-sustaining treatment program: Oregon emergency medical technicians' practical experiences and attitudes. J Am Geriatr Soc 2004;52(9):1430–1434.
19. Dunn PM, Tolle SW, Moss AH, Black JS. The POLST paradigm: Respecting the wishes of patients and families. Ann Long-Term Care 2007;15(9):33.
20. Hickman SE, Sabatino CP, Moss AH, Nester JW. The POLST (Physician Orders for Life-Sustaining Treatment) paradigm to improve end-of-life care: Potential state legal barriers to implementation. J Law Med Ethics 2008;36(1):119–140.
21. A National Framework and Preferred Practices for Palliative and Hospice Care Quality: A Consensus Report: National Quality Forum; 2007.
22. Hickman SE, Tolle SW, Brummel-Smith K, Carley MM. Use of the physician orders for life-sustaining treatment program in oregon nursing facilities: Beyond resuscitation status. J Am Geriatr Soc 2004;52(9):1424–1429.
23. Lee MA, Brummel-Smith K, Meyer J, Drew N, London MR. Physician Orders for Life-Sustaining Treatment(POLST): Outcomes in a PACE program. J Am Geriatr Soc 2000;48(10): 1219–1225.
24. Peberdy MA, Ornato JP, Larkin GL, et al. Survival From In-Hospital Cardiac Arrest During Nights and Weekends. JAMA 2008;299(7).785.
25. Jones GK, Brewer KL, Garrison HG. Public expectations of survival following cardiopulmonary resuscitation. Acad Emerg Med 2000;7(1):48–53.
26. American Heart Association. Guidelines for cardiopulmonary resuscitation and emergency cardiac care. Circulation 2005; 112(24):IV6–IV11.
27. Sabatino CP. Survey of state EMS-DNR laws and protocols. J Law Med Ethics 1999;27(4):297–315.
28. Kirchhoff KT, Spuhler V, Walker L, Hutton A, Cole BV, Clemmer T. Intensive care nurses' experiences with end-of-life care. Am J Crit Care 2000;9(1):36–42.
29. Post LF BJ, Dubler NN. Handbook for Health Care Ethics Committees. Baltimore, MD: Johns Hopkins University Press, 2007.
30. Zettel-Watson L. Actual and Perceived Gender Differences in the Accuracy of Surrogate Decisions About Life-Sustaining Medical Treatment Among Older Spouses. Death Stud 2008;32(3):273–290.
31. Shalowitz DI, Garrett-Mayer E, Wendler D. The accuracy of surrogate decision makers a systematic review. Arch Intern Med 2006;166(5):493–497.
32. Beauchamp TL, Childress JF. Principles of Biomedical Ethics. New York: Oxford University Press, 2001.
33. Cruzan et ux. v. Director, Missouri Department of Health, et al. (88–1503), 497 U.S. 261, 1990.

34. In the Matter of Karen Quinlan: The Complete Legal Briefs, Court Proceedings, and Decision in the Superior Court of New Jersey. Bethesda, MD: University Publications of America, 1975.

35. Michael Schiavo, as Guardian of the person of Theresa Marie Schiavo, Petitioner, v. Robert Schindler and Mary Shindler, No. 90-2908GD-003 (U.S. Dist., March 2004).

36. Finucane TE, Christmas C, Travis K. Tube Feeding in Patients with Advanced Dementia a Review of the Evidence. Am Med Assoc 1999:1365–1370.

37. Cogen R, Weinbryb J, Pomerantz C, Fenstemacher P. Complications of jejunostomy tube feeding in nursing facility patients. Am J Gastroenterol 1991;86(11):1610–1613.

38. Casarett D, Kapo J, Caplan A. Appropriate use of artificial nutrition and hydration-fundamental principles and recommendations. N Eng J Med 2005;353:2607–2612.

39. Ersek M. Artificial nutrition and hydration: Clinical issues. J Hospice Pall Nurs 2003;5(4):221.

40. Zerwekh JV, Rnc MA. The dehydration question. Nursing (Lond) 1983;13(1):47.

41. Ersek M, Wilson SA. The challenges and opportunities in providing end-of-life care in nursing homes. J Palliat Med 2003;6(1):45–57.

42. Finucane TE, Bynum JP. Use of tube feeding to prevent aspiration pneumonia. Lancet 1996;348(9039):1421–1424.

43. Kadakia SC, Sullivan HO, Starnes E. Percutaneous endoscopic gastrostoy or jejunostomy and the incidence of aspiration in 79 patients. Am J Surg 1992;164(2):114–118.

44. Moynihan T, Kelly DG, Fisch MJ. To feed or not to feed: Is that the right question? J Clin Oncol 2005;23(25):6256.

45. McCann RM, Hall WJ, Groth-Juncker A. Comfort care for terminally ill patients. The appropriate use of nutrition and hydration. JAMA 1994;272(16):1263–1266.

46. Sullivan RJ. Accepting death without artificial nutrition or hydration. J Gen Intern Med 1993;8(4):220–224.

47. Heyland DK, MacDonald S, Keefe L, Drover JW. Total parenteral nutrition in the critically ill patient a meta-analysis. Am Med Assoc 1998:2013–2019.

48. Heyland DK, Montalvo M, MacDonald S, Keefe L, Su XY, Drover JW. Total parenteral nutrition in the surgical patient: A meta-analysis. J Canad Chir 2001;44:102–111.

49. Murphy LM, Lipman TO. Percutaneous endoscopic gastrostomy does not prolong survival in patients with dementia. Am Med Assoc 2003:1351–1353.

50. Mitchell SL, Kiely DK, Lipsitz LA. Does artificial enteral nutrition prolong the survival of institutionalized elders with chewing and swallowing problems? J Gerontol Series A Biol Med Sci 1998;53(3):207–213.

51. Meier DE, Ahronheim JC, Morris J, Baskin-Lyons S, Morrison RS. High short-term mortality in hospitalized patients with advanced dementia lack of benefit of tube feeding. Am Med Assoc 2001;161:594–599.

52. Hanson LC, Garrett JM, Lewis C, Phifer N, Jackman A, Carey TS. Physicians' expectations of benefit from tube feeding. J Palliat Med 2008;11(8):1130–1134.

53. Austin W, Rankel M, Kagan L, Bergum V, Lemermeyer G. To stay or to go, to speak or stay silent, to act or not to act: Moral distress as experienced by psychologists. Ethics Behav 2005;15(3):197–212.

54. The Washington Death with Dignity Act. 2008. http://wei.secstate.wa/gov/osos/en/Documents/I1000-Text%20for%20web.pdf (accessed December 5, 2008).

55. Emanuel EJ, Fairclough DL, Emanuel LL. Attitudes and desires related to euthanasia and physician-assisted suicide among terminally ill patients and their caregivers. Am Med Assoc 2000:2460–2468.

56. O'Mahony S, Goulet J, Kornblith A, et al. Desire for hastened death, cancer pain and depression: Report of a longitudinal observational study. J Pain Symptom Manage 2005;29(5):446–457.

57. van Bruchem-van de Scheur GG, van der Arend AJG, Huijer Abu-Saad H, van Wijmen FCB, Spreeuwenberg C, ter Meulen RHJ. Euthanasia and assisted suicide in Dutch hospitals: The role of nurses. J Clin Nurs 2008;17(12):1618–1626.

58. Matzo ML, Emanual EJ. Oncology nurses' practices of assisted suicide and patient-requested euthanasia. Oncol Nurs Forum 1997;24(10):1725–1732.

59. Ganzini L, Goy ER, Dobscha SK. Prevalence of depression and anxiety in patients requesting physicians' aid in dying: Cross sectional survey. BMJ 2008;337:a1682.

60. Quill T, Arnold R. FAST FACT AND CONCEPT# 155: Evaluating Requests for Hastened Death.

61. Hudson PL, Schofield P, Kelly B, et al. Responding to desire to die statements from patients with advanced disease: Recommendations for health professionals. Palliat Med 2006;20(7):703.

62. Position Paper on the Death with Dignity Act. 1995. http://www.oregonrn.org/associations/3019/files/AssistedSuicide.pdf (accessed December 5, 2008).

63. Mond HG, Irwin M, Ector H, Proclemer A. The World Survey of Cardiac Pacingand Cardioverter-Defibrillators: Calendar Year 2005 An International Cardiac Pacing and Electrophysiology Society (ICPES) project. Pacing Clin Electrophysiol 2008;31(9):1202–1212.

64. Hansson SO. Implant ethics. J Med Ethics 2005;31:519–525.

65. Bramstedt KA, Nash PJ. When death is the outcome of informed refusal: Dilemma of rejecting ventricular assist device therapy. J Heart Lung Transplant 2005;24(2):229–230.

66. Claessens P, Menten J, Schotsmans P, Broeckaert B. Palliative sedation: A review of the research literature. J Pain Symptom Manage 2008;36(3):310–333.

67. Davis MP, Ford PA. Palliative sedation definitions, practices, outcomes and ethics. J Palliat Med. 2005;8(4):699–701.

68. Bernat JL. Medical futility. Neurocrit Care 2005;2(2):198–205.

69. Miles SH. Medical futility. J Law Med Ethics 1992;20(4):310–315.

70. Moseley KL, Silveira MJ, Goold SD. Futility in evolution. Clin Geriatric Med 2005;21(1):211–222.

71. Wicclair M. A conceptual and ethical analysis. In: Mappes TA, DeGrazia D, eds. Biomedical Ethics (6th ed). Boston: McGraw Hill; 2006.

72. von Gruenigen VE, Daly BJ. Futility: Clinical decisions at the end-of-life in women with ovarian cancer. Gynecol Oncol 2005;97(2):638–644.

73. Daly BJ. An indecent proposal: Withholding cardiopulmonary resuscitation. Am J Crit Care 2008;17(4):377–380.

74. Principles of Medical Ethics. 2008. http://www.ama-assn.org/ama/pub/category/2512.html (accessed December 5, 2008).

75. Halevy A, Brody BA. A multi-institution collaborative policy on medical futility. JAMA 1996;276(7):571–574.

76. Ferrell BR, Coyle N. The nature of suffering and the goals of nursing. Oxford: Oxford University Press, 2008.

77. Code of Ethics for Nurses. 2008. http://www.nursingworld.org/MainMenuCategories/ThePracticeofProfessionalNursing/

EthicsStandards/CodeofEthics.aspx (accessed November 12, 2008).

78. Puntillo KA, Benner P, Drought T, et al. End-of-life issues in intensive care units: A national random survey of nurses' knowledge and beliefs. Am J Crit Care 2001;10(4):216–229.

79. Meltzer LS, Huckabay LM. Critical care nurses' perceptions of futile care and its effect on burnout. Am J Crit Care 2004;13(3):202–208.

80. Ferrell BR. Understanding the moral distress of nurses witnessing medically futile care. Onc Nurs Soc 2006;33(5):922–930.

81. Daly BJ. Futility. AACN Clin Issues Crit Care Nurs 1994;5(1):77–85.

82. Organizations JCoAoH. Accreditation manual for hospitals. Oakbrook Terrace: Joint Commission on Accreditation of Healthcare Organizations, 2005.

# 63 Colleen Scanlon

# Public Policy and End-of-Life Care: The Nurse's Role

*Patients and families count on nurses to be their advocates as they receive healthcare. Additionally, the expectations of the public and of the nursing profession reflected in the Code for Nurses call for public policy advocacy by nurses to promote community, national and international efforts to meet health needs. As palliative care nurses, we bring a special trusted voice to public policy discussions based on our expertise, understanding and experience in caring for persons with life-threatening illness. We have an acute awareness of the physical, cultural, social, economic, and political barriers to excellent palliative care across the continuum and the resulting human suffering. With that awareness, comes a responsibility to use our individual and collective voices to inform our communities and our policymakers about palliative care excellence and measures that can eliminate or reduce current barriers. Advocacy goes hand in hand with the privilege of being called a nurse—a palliative care nurse—and new doors are now opening to be heard.—Karin Dufault, SP, PhD, RN Supportive Care Coalition: Pursuing Excellence in Palliative Care*

♦ **Key Points**
♦ *Public policy decisions have the potential to positively impact the quality and availability of palliative care services.*
♦ *There is a broad spectrum of public policies on state and national agendas that relate to end-of-life care.*
♦ *Public policy initiatives create a unique opportunity for nurses to influence present and future directions in palliative care.*

It has become clear that end-of-life care is not just the concern of health-care professionals, patients, and families. It is also a concern for the public at large and for governmental entities. There has been increasing interest and activity within the public policy arena at the state and federal levels of government that can create needed improvements in end-of-life care.[1] Institutions and individuals also have a responsibility to inform and influence pertinent public policy initiatives. Nurses, as the largest group of health professionals and with a rich history of concern and care for others, have a vital role in advocating for quality of life, particularly at life's end.[2]

Nurses and the nursing community have a unique opportunity to contribute to future directions in palliative care for individuals, communities and society. There are many important decisions impacting palliative care in the public policy arena that provide opportunities for professionals to influence care provided to the seriously ill.[3] It is important to build congruence between the illness experience of patients, families and caregivers and the development of public policy.[4] Public policy advocacy becomes another professional vehicle for nurses to improve palliative care.

## The Evolution of Palliative Care

The enormous strides in research, prevention, detection, and treatment of disease have been incredibly promising. Scientific and medical progress has created significant options and desired choices for those facing life-threatening illness, yet these possibilities have also created poignant questions and dilemmas for those at life's end, their families, and health-care providers. This reality has drawn the attention and activism of health-care professionals, the public, and policymakers.

Although significant changes in healthcare, including end-of-life care, have occurred, and although these have been mostly positive, it is recognized that a need for additional improvements persists. Intersecting trends have propelled palliative care to the forefront of American culture.

## Changing Nature of Death and Dying

Significant scientific and technological advances have created the possibility of extending life and delaying death. With the expansion of technology, there has been growing attention to the acceptability of limiting treatment interventions and focusing on the comprehensive, holistic needs of the person with life-threatening illness. Recent decades have witnessed the affirmation of the decisional authority of the individual, the dominance of self-determination, the acceptability of do-not-resuscitate (DNR) decisions, the use of advance directives, and the acceptance of withdrawal of life-sustaining therapies. Additionally, physician-assisted suicide (PAS) has become a more acceptable consideration.

## Judicial Decisions

End-of-life care has also been on the nation's judicial agendas. Judicial history is filled with cases, court decisions, and opinions that have influenced both directly and indirectly the course of end-of-life care. The courts and litigation process are often used to resolve conflicts that may more appropriately be made in other venues, including the legislature.[5] The adversarial nature of the judicial system magnifies the intensity and painfulness of very complex emotional dilemmas. Since the middle of the 1970s, starting with the Karen Ann Quinlan case,[6] the judicial system has dealt with complex issues in end-of-life care, including decisional authority, refusal of therapy, and physician-assisted suicide (PAS). Although each of these decisions dealt with discrete legal questions, these and other judicial cases drew notable attention to the broader questions and concerns in end-of-life care.

The recent case of Terry Schiavo, which attracted world-wide attention, drawing the intense interest of the media, public, and churches, was played out in the judicial system as well as the legislative and executive branches of government at the state and national levels. The case involved the right to refuse unwanted medical treatment, the role of surrogate decision-makers and the resolution of family disagreement.[7] Ultimately this case received direct intervention from President Bush and the United States Congress, leading to the passage and signing of a bill.[8] This tragic scenario reinforces the need for good end-of-life policy and public engagement in advance care planning.

## Research Data

The acquisition of quantitative and qualitative research data has influenced care at life's end and has the potential to shape public policy. Multiple clinical, attitudinal, experiential, and health professional studies have been generated in the last several decades. In addition, public opinion polls and surveys have drawn attention to the challenges in providing quality end-of-life care. Although these projects may generate important information, the ongoing challenge is to ensure that relevant data and knowledge garnered from research is integrated into care improvements that benefit individuals and communities. Research data on quality, cost, access, and utilization are necessary for public policy debate and action on needed reforms in end-of-life care.[9]

The Study to Understand Prognoses and Preferences for Outcomes and Risks of Treatment (SUPPORT) was the largest research project to examine end-of-life care and identify its inherent challenges and deficiencies.[10] SUPPORT was a 10-year project divided into two phases; the first phase focused on assessment of the experience of patients at the end of life, including decision-making and clinical outcomes, and the second phase involved testing of an intervention designed to improve communication and decision-making among patients, families, and physicians. Despite attempts to positively affect clinical outcomes, the conclusions of the study found the interventions to be ineffective in (1) ensuring that patient preferences were known and honored; (2) affecting the incidence and timing of DNR orders; (3) decreasing days in the intensive care unit or on a ventilator before death; (4) improving pain management; and (5) controlling the utilization of hospital resources.[10]

Since the SUPPORT study, numerous other investigational efforts have been initiated. A 2-year comprehensive study conducted by the Institute of Medicine (IOM) concluded that there were serious problems in end-of-life care and delineated steps to address this reality and improve care.[11] One of the committee's tasks was to propose steps that state and federal policymakers and others could take to improve the organization, delivery, financing, and quality of care for persons with terminal illness. An outcome of the study was six recommendations that could lead to significant improvements and provide a framework for public policy options (Table 63–1).

Also in the late 1990s, the Robert Wood Johnson Foundation, through the Last Acts project, promulgated a set of guiding principles, the "Precepts of Palliative Care," in an effort to explicate the nonnegotiables of palliative care for the professional community and the public.[12] The precepts have been endorsed by numerous national and local organizations and disseminated widely to the public. One precept states that "palliative care relies on the formulation of responsible policies and regulation by institutions and by state and federal governments."[12] The precepts also provide a starting point for needed reform in end-of-life care.

Several years later, Last Acts issued a report, *Transforming Death in America: A State of the Nation Report*, which outlined the current reality of dying in this country, the challenges, and the needed changes.[13] Last Acts' most recent study rated each of the 50 states and the District of Columbia on eight evaluative criteria on end-of-life care and was the

---

**Table 63–1**
**Institute of Medicine Recommendations for Improving End-of-Life Care**

- Create and facilitate patient and family expectations for reliable, skillful, and supportive care.
- Ask health-care professionals to commit themselves to improving care for dying patients and to using existing knowledge effectively to prevent and relieve pain and other symptoms.
- Address deficiencies in the health-care system through improved methods for measuring quality, tools for accountability by providers, revised financing systems to encourage better coordination of care, and reformed drug-prescribing laws.
- Develop medical education to ensure that practitioners have the relevant attitudes, knowledge, and skills to provide excellent care for dying patients.
- Make palliative care a defined area of expertise, education, and research.
- Pursue public discussion about the modern experience of dying patients and families and community obligations to those nearing death.

*Source*: Field and Cassel (1997), reference 11.

---

**Table 63–2**
**Approaching Just Access: Recommendations**

1. Health-care leaders, policymakers, and key stakeholder groups must come to consensus on the definition of palliative care and develop a framework for greater accountability in palliative care delivery in concert with financing mechanisms.
2. Public policy should expand the scope of hospice services.
3. Policymakers should act immediately to bring about policy reform of the absolute application of an individual's prognosis as a primary criterion for reimbursement of services.
4. Access and delivery of hospice care should be expanded to dying persons residing in long-term care facilities.
5. Leaders in the hospice community and in mainstream medicine must promote hospice–hospital partnerships to meet current and projected needs of the rapidly expanding volume of chronically and terminally ill patients.
6. Telemedicine should be developed to expand access to palliative care.
7. The business community should be engaged.
8. Educational programs should be developed to "reintroduce" hospice and palliative care to the public in light of their new capabilities, flexibility and accessibility.

*Source*: Jennings et al. (2003), reference 15.

---

first comprehensive measurement "report card"—a catalyst for dialogue and action.[14] Education of policymakers and regulators by individuals and communities is crucial to lay out a roadmap for improvement and action in various areas, including the enactment of needed legislation (Table 63–2).[13,15]

In 2007, U.S. Senator Ron Wyden (D-OR) requested that the Government Accoutability Office (GAO) examine end-of-life care in four states. The GAO report identified several integral elements of the states' end-of-life care programs: care management, support services, communication, and advance care planning.[16] Challenges were also identified. Information from the report can provide direction to government agencies addressing the care of persons at the end-of-life.

A recent report from the Center to Advance Palliative Care and National Palliaitive Care Research Center evaluated the availability of palliative care for patients in hospitals at the state level and the availability of palliative care programs at medical school teaching hospitals.[17] Although a general increase in the number of palliative care programs in the country is noted, there is significant state and regional variability. The report ends with recommendations including for elected officials and policymakers (Table 63–3).

## Legislation

Legislative initiatives have significantly influenced end-of-life care. From an historical perspective, one of the most significant pieces of legislation is the Patient Self-Determination Act (PSDA), which provides protection for the decisional authority of individuals.[18] The PSDA was the first federal act to require that all Medicare and Medicaid provider organizations recognize the legal rights of the recipients of care to make decisions about their healthcare. This monumental legislation provided

---

**Table 63–3**
**Recommendations for Elected Officials and Policymakers**

Palliative care has become the model for how high-quality, fiscally-responsible care can be provided to the sickest, most vulnerable patients and their families, and is emerging as a critical component of health reform. State governments and legislators need to be concerned about how their jurisdictions are performing—and should take action.

*If you are a state or federal policymaker, to ensure that your constituents facing serious illness have access to the highest-quality medical care, you should:*

- *Fund palliative care team training and technical assistance for all hospitals in your state.*
- *Include palliative care indicators in your state's quality programs for your state health plan and Medicaid programs.*
- *Ensure the development of palliative care programs in public and sole community provider hospitals, as these hospitals provide care to the underserved and most vulnerable patient populations.*
- *Promote and pass legislation requiring all hospitals to offer palliative care services as a condition of Medicare and Medicaid reimbursement.*
- *Promote and pass legislation requiring all state-supported medical schools to have affiliations with hospital palliative care programs.*
- *Create loan-forgiveness programs for nurses and physicians seeking postgraduate palliative care training.*
- *Create a statewide resource center for promotion of access to quality palliative care services (see New York Palliative Care Training Act—Public Health Law Article 28 at http://public.leginfo.state.ny.us/menuf.cgi).*
- *Support congressional initiatives that increase National Institutes of Health and Veteran's Health Administration funding for palliative care research.*
- For a state directory of hospital palliative care programs, visit *www.getpalliativecare.org.*

*Source*: America's Care of Serious Illness (2008), reference 17.

---

the impetus for legislative activity at the state level and the widespread acceptance of advance directives.

Simultaneous with legislative proposals related to protecting decision-making authority has been the initiation of legislation regarding DNR orders, financing mechanisms, pain management, surrogate decision-making, and PAS. These are explored further in later sections.

## Regulation

Once the legislative process is completed with the passage of a law, there is still the need to provide specificity through codified regulations and rules. Federal and state administrative agencies (e.g., Health and Human Services, Justice) assume responsibility for adding the needed details of the law so that it can be understood and implemented.[19] Public policy advocacy needs to include knowledge of relevant governmental agencies and access to them.

Generally, agencies release proposed regulations for public comment before the issuance of the final rule. The rulemaking process is a critical point of influence in the entire legislative process. Ensuring that regulations include relevant definitions, authority, eligibility, benefits, standards, and quality measures is essential to the delivery and financing of sustainable, efficient, and improved end-of-life care.[20,21] The significance of regulatory bodies and regulations should not be overlooked.

A recent example is the new Medicare Conditions of Participation (CoP) published by the Centers for Medicare and Medicaid (CMS) which includes a detailed list of patient rights related to end-of-life and hospice care.[22] It was the first

major overhaul of the regulations governing hospice care in several decades. Specifically, the rule states patients can choose hospice or palliative care over curative treatment, are entitled to participate in the treatment plan, to effective pain management, to refuse treatment and to choose his or her own physician.[22]

## Framework for the Development of Public Policy

An initial step in the process of developing relevant public policy proposals is to determine and clarify the particular issue or problem that needs to be addressed and to ascertain the perspectives of various stakeholders on the issue. Patients, providers, payers, and governmental entities may have very different goals and ends that they are seeking. The agendas and concerns of the multiple interested parties need to be considered, negotiated, and balanced. Ultimately, a priority issue focus needs to be crafted, messaged, and delivered to any and all audiences with the ability to advance the desired agenda.

## Spectrum of Issues Addressed in Palliative Care Public Policy Proposals at the State Level

In almost every state, public interest in improving end-of-life care and the momentum for legislative initiatives at the state level have been growing.[23,24] Decisions made at the state level can greatly impact the care provided to persons with serious illness.[3] There are town meetings, state commissions, community projects, grant allocations, seminars, active coalitions, and proposed legislation. Over recent years, statewide coalitions have had a significant role in end-of-life care policy reforms.[1,25] State governors, attorneys general, and the medical community have all begun to initiate activities related to end-of-life care. Although all of these interested parties may share a common goal, the focus can significantly vary from research, public dialogue, and grant projects to legislation.

Influence that develops through coalitions, multigroup partnerships or other collaborations can have a significant impact on future directions. A good example is the National Health Decisions Day of 2008. This effort brought together varied stakeholder groups that were interested in encouraging patients to express their wishes regarding healthcare, and for providers and families to respect their wishes.[26] Recognizing that most Americans have not engaged in advance care planning and formulated their preferences, this campaign, with its supporting organizations, launched a national effort with community involvement, media outreach and resources focused on this important issue. The effort was reinforced with concurrent resolutions, passed in the U.S. Senate and House of Representatives, encouraging everyone over age 18 years to prepare an advance directive.[27] The resolutions also called on all members of their respective Congressional bodies to execute an advance directive.

Some of the impetus for public and professional interest in state policy initiatives may be the presence of controversial issues such as PAS or just a growing awareness of the present deficiencies in end-of-life care. Many, if not most, Americans have directly experienced or heard of the plight of someone facing death.

The overwhelming majority of states have some legislative initiatives proposed within the domain of palliative care. The following are examples of issues that are being addressed at the state level with specific public policy initiatives.

### Advance Care Planning

Although all states have some type of advance directive legislation (e.g., living will, durable power of attorney for healthcare), there continues to be ongoing attention to the area of individual and surrogate decision-making through proposed acts or amendments to existing legislation.[23] The laws governing this area are in continual flux. Legislative proposals include general advance directive legislation, simplification of form and process, combining approaches into one document, awareness of advance care directives, role of surrogates in end-of-life decision-making, advance care registries and creating new approaches such as open-ended, situation-specific response forms. In addition, separate advance directives have been developed for mental health treatment and for long-term care.

Several states have begun to model legislation on Oregon's Physician Orders for Life Sustaining Treatment (POLST).[3]

The POLST document is not a typical advance directive, but is similar to out-of-facility DNRs or portable DNRs. They are designed to convey a person's end-of-life care wishes and become a set of physician's orders.

A growing trend within the states has been the establishment of some form of surrogate consent provision in legislative codes. Forty-four states and the District of Columbia have included some type of surrogate provision in their statutes.[28] Given the paucity of individuals who complete advance directives, this protection of appropriate decisional authority of others becomes increasingly important.[26] Although families have historically been considered the most natural decision-makers and their involvement in clinical decisions is generally normative in practice, in many states it is not always legally sanctioned. States have begun to rectify the problems created by this reality with specific legislation.

### Pain and Symptom Management

State laws, regulation and other governmental policy approaches are another avenue to address concerns about appropriate pain management, and the last decade has seen many positive developments in state pain policies.[29] The lack of meaningful federal pain policies has pushed this activity to the state level—whether to state legislatures, courts or executive committees.[30] Most efforts are attempting to address competing interests—one the untreated and undertreated pain, and the other the abuse and diversion of prescription-controlled substances.[29,31] There is a need to find balance between these two interests. Two significant policy improvements have occurred in recent years, in that state heath-care regulatory boards have policies encouraging pain management and state legislatures have changed ambiguous policy language, including problematic language in Intractable Pain Acts.[29]

The Federation of State Medical Boards updated its *Model Guidelines for the Use of Controlled Substances for the Treatment of Pain* to draw specific attention to the problem of the undertreatment of pain.[32] The revised *Model Guidelines* notes that the undertreatment of pain is inappropriate treatment and a departure from an acceptable standard of practice.[32]

Although limited, there have been some criminal prosecutions of physicians for providing end-of-life care, most commonly for prescribing opioid narcotic medications.[33] There is an ongoing need to mitigate the barriers to the appropriate role of physicians in prescribing controlled substances. Recently the National Association of Attorneys General (NAAG) hosted the Balance of Pain Policy Initiatives roundtable with a goal of establishing guidelines to assist law enforcement personnel with investigations related to physician alleged mishandling or diversion of controlled substances.[34] An outcome of the meeting will be the development of a document that will assist prosecutors at the local, state and federal level to achieve the goal of a balanced pain policy.[34]

States need to address legal, regulatory, and other policy barriers that may interfere with the effective management of pain, such as restrictive prescription monitoring laws (e.g., the requirement to use triplicate forms), dosage limitations, definitional language, and patient reporting.[31] If state pain policies are to continue to improve pain management, they will need to remove legislative and regulatory barriers (often focused on controlling substance abuse) that interfere with appropriate clinical care and medical decision-making.[29,31]

### Do-Not-Resuscitate (DNR) Orders

Periodically there are initiatives to expand and/or strengthen standard DNR laws that are used within inpatient settings, but the more significant activity concerns DNR orders in other settings, such as the home. Since the early 1990s, states have begun to address the needs of the seriously ill and dying in the community, and many changes have occured. Although previously EMS personnel were required to automatically institute cardiopulmonary resuscitation and other advanced lifesaving techniques in a crisis situation for the homebound, it has become more commonplace for states to have instituted nonhospital DNR orders to protect the wishes of individuals at home and to avoid interventions that are unwanted. States do continue to address some statutory improvements in DNR legislation.[24]

### Reimbursement

Financing and reimbursement options are also included in state legislative initiatives. These include expansion of hospice and home health benefits, changes in eligibility requirements, reimbursement rates, medication coverage, Medicaid waivers, long-term care and nursing home reform, and attention to the care of seriously ill children.[25] Except for hospice care, reimbursement for palliative care services is scattered among different payment sources. The different types of payment sources for palliative care services include Medicare, Medicaid, commercial insurance, out-of-pocket, and charity care and can vary according to setting and geographic area, making it difficult to understand the actual financing realities.[35]

### Physician-Assisted Suicide

There continues to be attention to legislation on PAS at the state level. The Oregon "Death with Dignity" bill, the first state legislative initiative to legalize PAS, passed in 1994 and was reaffirmed by public vote again in 1997.[36] Since the emergence of this issue at the state level, a wide spectrum of proposals and perspectives has been offered.[23] States have proposals to criminalize or to legalize PAS, and some have both pending simultaneously. The criminal laws of several states have been expanded to include harsher penalties, including civil actions and the revocation of medical licenses.

Although dialogue and legislative action within the states are present, Oregon remained the only state legally allowing PAS, despite ongoing challenges from the U.S. Justice Department until 2008. Each year, Oregon's Department of Human Services issues a report summarizing the number of requests, prescriptions issued, patients who took the prescribed medication and reasons offered. Oregon's most recent report shows there has been an increase in the number of patients taking lethal medication over the past several years, but that it is a relatively small number compared to total deaths in the state.[37]

On November 4, 2008, Washington state voters approved Initiative 1000, a ballot measure that legalizes physician-assisted suicide.[38] The measure is modeled after the Oregon Death with Dignity Act, which allows physicians to prescribe, but not administer, a lethal dose of prescription drugs to patients who have 6 months or less to live and who are able to make health-care decisions. Physicians, patients and others acting in good faith compliance would have criminal and civil immunity.[38]

As of December 5, 2008, Montana became the third state to allow physician-assisted suicide. A district court Judge ruled that Montana state constitution's protections for human dignity and individual privacy permit competent, terminally-ill Montana residents the right to die with dignity.[39] The Judicial decision concludes that a patient may use the assistance of his physician to obtain a prescription for a lethal dose of medications that the patient may take on his own, if and when he decides to terminate his life.[39] It is likely that this decision will be appealed to a higher court and possibly overturned.

### Federal Legislative Proposals

As is occurring at the state level, the federal government has been directing attention to issues of end-of-life care. Often, the attention occurs through the budgeting process when funds are allocated for Medicare and Medicaid services (e.g., hospice benefit) and through appropriations for health agencies (e.g., National Institutes of Health). Additionally, governmental entities have begun to address concerns about pain control, advance care planning, and PAS. Through the 1990s and 2000s, many federal legislative proposals were introduced; some had success in one or both congressional bodies (U.S. Senate and House of Representatives), but almost all failed to become law.[23] Examples of recent federal legislative proposals follow.

### Conquering Pain Act of 2005

This legislation was re-introduced in the Senate, but not the House after receiving very little attention as the Conquering Pain Act of 1999, 2001 and 2003. The bill was intended to address the public health crises of pain through the development of evidence-based practice guidelines, informational materials, quality improvement projects, rational models for improving pain and the elimination of reimbursement barriers for pain and palliative care services.[40]

## National Pain Care Policy Act of 2008

This legislation continues to be re-introduced in both the House and the Senate. It amends the Public Health Services Act to establish an office known as the Pain Consortium within the National Institutes of Health.[41,42] It is intended to set a national pain agenda to increase awareness, improve, and advance the quality, appropriateness, and effectiveness of pain management as well as address the barriers to appropriate pain care. This will be accomplished through research, grants, public campaigns, education, conferences and training programs. The House bill passed, but the Senate version received no further action after being introduced.

## Children's Compassionate Care Act of 2007

This legislation to improve palliative care for children was re-introduced only in the House of Representatives in 2007. The aim is to create pediatric palliative care demonstration projects and provide grants to expand services, training, and research.[43] Significant portions of the bill address the need to assess and improve the payment methadology for pediatric palliative care.

## Advance Directive Promotion Act of 2008

This House legislation amends the Social Security Act (Medicare and Medicaid) to increase awareness of the importance of end-of-life planning, improve policies related to the use and portability of advance directives and create a national information hotline for end-of-life decisionmaking and hospice care.[44] The bill received no further Congressional action after being referred to the House Subcommittee on Health.

## Life Sustaining Treatment Preferences Act of 2008

This legislation introduced into the House amends the Social Security Act, to extend Medicare coverage to consultations regarding an order for life-sustaining treatment for qualified individuals.[45] This bill is based on the Physician Orders for Life-Sustaining Treatment model (POLST), reinforcing the need for appropriate, informed conversation with clinicians, explaining treatment options to seriously ill patients and developing the necessary direction regarding life-sustaining treatment. The bill has not moved beyond the House Subcommittee.

## Life Span Respite Care Act of 2006

This bill was re-introduced in both chambers of Congress in 2006 and became law.[46,47] The law authorizes millions of dollars in grants and cooperative agreements to states and other qualifying entities to make respite care available to family caregivers.[47] The intent is to expand and enhance the quality and availability of respite care services to family caregivers, through improved dissemination and coordination of respite care with the goal of reducing family caregiver strain.

## Medicare Hospice Protection Act of 2008

This legislation was introduced into both the Senate and the House.[48,49] The sole intent of these bills is to eliminate the budget neutrality adjustment factor used to compute Medicare hospice reimbursement rates, which were issued by the Centers for Medicare and Medicaid (CMS). Without eliminating the adjustment factor, hospice payments would be reduced.

## Medicare Prescription Drug Improvement and Modernization Act of 2003

The Medicare Prescription Drug Improvement and Modernization Act of 2003 (the "Act") was signed into law (P.L. 108–173) on December 8, 2003.[50] The legislation has drawn attention primarily because of the new Medicare drug benefit, but there are many other significant provisions contained in the Act, including those that benefit the chronically ill and dying. There are several provisions to improve access to hospice care and to make services more available to patients and families earlier in their illnesses. The Act addresses hospice payments for beneficiaries and consultative education, expanded contracting opportunities, and rural hospice care.

The Act also recognizes nurse practitioners in the role of attending physicians to care for hospice patients. Under existing law, only an attending physician, medical director, or other physician at the hospice can certify a patient as terminally ill and determine the medical care to be delivered. The Act now expands the definition of attending physician in hospice to include nurse practitioners, although they are still not permitted to certify a patient as terminally ill for the purposes of receiving the hospice benefit.

## Medicare Improvements for Patients and Providers Act of 2008

The Medicare Improvements for Patients and Providers Act of 2008 was signed into law (P.L. 110–275) on July 15, 2008.[51] The legislation addresses many areas of the Medicare program, but does not have one specific section that addresses palliative care. In the preventive services section and requirements for the initial preventive examination for Medicare beneficiaries, end-of-life planning has been added. It specifies that verbal or written information should be obtained regarding the individual's ability to prepare an advance directive and whether or not the physician is willing to follow the individual's wishes as expressed in an advance directive.[51]

## Physician-Assisted Suicide Policy at the Federal Level

Similar to what has occurred at the state level, PAS has received escalating attention at the federal level of government throughout the last two decades. The highest court, the Supreme Court of the United States, addressed the issue of an individual's right to PAS. Although the court found there is no constitutionally protected right to PAS on behalf of terminally ill patients,[52] it did not prohibit states from legalizing such practices. The fact that this issue found its way to the nation's highest court and has been legalized in three states is a demonstration of the growing acceptability of PAS as a tenable choice.

Several pieces of federal legislation related to PAS have been introduced in Congress. Most recently, legislation to prohibit the use of controlled substances for the purpose of assisted suicide was introduced.[53] The bill received no congressional action beyond referral to a committee. There has not been federal effort to legislate the legalization of PAS.

The nursing community became actively engaged in the debate and activities surrounding the PAS issue. Major professional and specialty nursing organizations have struggled with the associated complex moral and professional issues. Nurses have invaluable experience and insight into care at the end of life, which informs the assisted-suicide debate and guides the profession's response. The development of position statements[54–56] and educational resources, involvement in professional collaborations and end-of-life coalitions, are important activities supported by and engaged in by the nursing profession. For more information on PAS, the reader is referred to Chapter 64.

## The Role of Nurses in Palliative Care Public Policy

Advocacy is generally considered a prominent component of professional nursing practice. Advocacy is most frequently understood by nurses in their clinical, patient-centered experiences; however, a broader perspective of advocacy is called for. Professional commitment must also express concern for the wider community, for society, and particularly for those who are most vulnerable. Nurses must advocate from the bedside through the provision of clinical care to public policy arena.[57,58] The skills that nurses use in their clinical, research, educational, and administrative roles can be extremely valuable and transferable into legislative and political arenas.[57]

Undoubtedly, public policy initiatives will continue to emerge at the state and federal levels, and nurses can assume an important role. Nurses are unequally positioned to influence the development of public policy that benefits patients, families and communities. Nurses need to remain in the forefront as advocates for improved end-of-life care, and they need to see public policy advocacy as yet another growing opportunity to demonstrate this commitment. To fully exercise this responsibility, nurses need to become aware of the issues, understand the legislative and regulatory practices, become politically skilled and get involved.[57,59] Advocacy requires motivation and the thoughtful design of sustainable efforts.

Nurses have most frequently been the professionals who have attempted to provide appropriate, competent, and compassionate care to individuals and families who confront the brevity of life. As the largest group of health professionals and those most connected to the comprehensive needs of the terminally ill and their families, nurses are obligated to provide leadership that advances improvements in end-of-life care.

Nurses, individually and collectively, must be interested in and become involved in the assessment of proposed end-of-life legislation and regulation. A proactive, responsible stance on the part of nurses can influence the creation and evaluation of needed end-of-life initiatives. Nurses bring an understanding of the present state of end-of-life care that helps in the analysis of appropriate public policy options and can craft future initiatives.

The Code for Nurses with Interpretive Statements (Code for Nurses), the profession's code of ethics, directs nurses "to engage in political action to bring about social change."[60] The Code for Nurses affirms the role of professional associations in acting on behalf of nurses to shape health-care policy. It affirms the emphasis on the citizenship responsibility of the nurse and the profession.[61] Ethical values that undergird professional responsibilities, such as respect for autonomy, justice, professional integrity, beneficence, and advocacy, interface with the goals of improving end-of-life care and provide a context for assessment of policy proposals.

Although nurses may individually engage in public policy initiatives, it is most often through their involvement in entities such as professional associations or coalitions that advocacy efforts are effectively advanced. The Oncology Nursing Society joined with the Oncology Social Workers to issue a joint statement on Palliative Care and End-of-Life Care, including a section on public policy.[62] Effective advocacy efforts rely on the mobilization and engagement of all feasible partners.

Unifying the voices of interested and invested constituencies can have a powerful impact on policymakers. Depending on the importance of a particular issue, the nursing community may assume different roles and levels of activism. At times, the nursing community may act as the leader, proactively advancing a particular public policy concern; at other times, it may choose to provide endorsement or support of an issue. Effective advocacy also includes halting the passage of policies that are viewed as detrimental to end-of-life care goals. The policy development and enactment process can be lengthy and calls for sustained engagement.

Nurses can and should become actively involved in the legislative and regulatory processes by gathering necessary

**Table 63-4**
**Dimensions of Advocacy Activities for Nurses**

**Agenda setting**

- Identify palliative care issues/legislation of greatest importance to the profession and the public (often these are not evident to policymakers).
- Define and prioritize those issues and decide where time and resources will be concentrated.
- Collect relevant data/information to validate the importance of particular health policy issues to the public, health-care providers, and legislative leaders.
- Evaluate policy proposals in light of professional goals and values.
- Develop consensus positions and form recommendations on issues of highest priority.
- Formulate new public policy proposals when needed.

**Coalition building**

- Identify other groups (e.g., health professionals, special-interest groups, consumers) with similar agendas with whom collaborative and coordinated efforts can be initiated.
- Seek opportunities for combining, allocating, and sharing advocacy work.
- Build grassroots networks within the profession through associations and coalitions such as the American Nurses Association, the Hospice and Palliative Nurses Association, and the Oncology Nursing Society.
- Recognize that, in coalition building, broad policy positions are more successful and compromise may be necessary to advance a proposal.
- Consider involving stakeholders who may not be typical partners in advocacy efforts, such as community members and employees.
- Educate others to the importance of particular palliative care policy proposals.

**Political activism**

- Become involved with associations and groups that influence palliative care policy.
- Develop strategic plans for advancing particular policy initiatives.
- Establish and maintain reliable relationships with key legislators and regulatory leaders.
- Mobilize and involve interested individuals in advocacy campaigns, including communicating (via letters, faxes, e-mails, phone calls) and visiting with key contacts.
- Invite policymakers and community leaders to environments where they can learn more about the experience of patients and families receiving palliative care services and the needs of providers.
- Engage the media in efforts through editorials, articles, and press conferences.
- Testify before public policy makers to put a human face on the issue.
- Monitor results of proposed public policy initiatives and communicate them to involved stakeholders.
- Follow up with policy makers, expressing either satisfaction and gratitude or disappointment with public policy outcomes.

*Source*: Scanlon (2001), reference 64.

information, providing the perspectives of not only professionals but also the recipients of care, evaluating policy proposals, communicating with policy leaders, and lobbying on specific bills.[3,57] Knowledge and skills are required for public policy success, as they are in other areas of professional competence. The more knowledgeable individuals are about the legislative process, the more effectively they can participate and influence outcomes. It is necessary to understand at least some of the dynamics that surround the policy and political environments.[57]

Health-care policy that is developed without the input of nurses lacks an important influence because of the unique and essential role that nurses have in the care of patients, families, and communities.[63] Involvement by nurses in public policy and political advocacy through various activities is yet another way to demonstrate professionalism and promote improvements in end-of-life care[64] (Table 63-4). Nurses can provide a critical and valuable voice in professional, public, and governmental discourse about end-of-life care.

## Conclusion

Public policy initiatives at state and federal levels of government can provide another avenue to advance improvements in end-of-life care. Nurses can inform and influence the process of developing, evaluating, and enacting palliative care public policy that benefits individual, family, and community end-of-life care. Involvement in public policy advocacy provides nurses an opportunity to assume their professional citizenship responsibilities and to positively affect the quality of end-of-life care provided throughout the United States.

REFERENCES

1. Schuster LJ Jr, Kabcenell A. Improving Care for the End of Life: A Source Book for Health Care Managers and Clinicians. New York, NY: Oxford University Press, 2000.

2. Hospice and Palliative Nurses Association. Value of the Professional Nurse in Palliative Care. Position Statement. Pittsburgh, PA: HPNA, 2008.

3. Meyer DE, Bereseford. Palliative care professionals contribute to state legislative and policy initiatives. J Pall Med 2008;11(8):1070–1073.

4. Lorenz KA, Schugarman LR, Lynn J. Health care policy issues in end-of-life care. J Pall Med 2006;9(3):731–748.

5. Miesel A. The role of litigation in end-of-life care: A reappraisal in improving end-of-life care: Why has it been so difficult? Hast Center Rep 2005;35(6):S47–S51.

6. In re Quinlan, 70 N. J. 10, 355 A.2d 647, 1976.

7. Kollas CD, Boyer-Kollas B. Closing the Schiavo case: An analysis of legal reasoning. J Pall Med 2006;9(5):1145–1163.

8. United States Senate. An Act for the Relief of the Parents of Theresa Marie Schiavo. 109th Congress (1st Session) Senate Bill 686. March 20, 2005.

9. Kyba FC. Legal and ethical issues in end-of-life care. Crit Care Nurs Clin North Am 2002;14:141–155.

10. SUPPORT Principal Investigators. A controlled trial to improve care for seriously ill hospitalized patients. JAMA 1995;274:1591–1598.

11. Field MJ, Cassel CK, eds. Approaching Death: Improving Care at the End of Life. Report of the Institute of Medicine Committee on Care at the End of Life. Washington, DC: National Academy Press, 1997.

12. Precepts of Palliative Care. Developed by the Task Force on Palliative Care, Last Acts Campaign, Robert Wood Johnson Foundation. J Palliat Care Med 1998;1(2):109–112.

13. Metzger M, Kaplan KD. Transforming Death in America: A State of the Nation Report. Washington, DC: Last Acts, 2001.

14. Last Acts. Means to a Better End: A Report on Dying in America Today. Washington, DC: November 2002.

15. Jennings B, Ryndes T, D'Onofrio C, Ball MA. Access to Hospice Care: Expanding Boundaries, Overcoming Barriers [Summary]. Hastings Cent Rep, March–April 2003.

16. U.S. Government Accountability Office. End-of-Life Care: Key Components Provided by Programs in Four States, GAO-08–66, December 2007. http://www.gao.gov (accessed October 13, 2009).

17. America's Care of Serious Illness: A State-by-State Report Card on Access to Palliative Care in our Nation's Hospitals. 2008. Center to Advance Palliative Care and National Palliative Care Research Center.

18. Omnibus Reconciliation Act of 1990. Publ. No. 101–508, Sect 4206, 4751.

19. Habgood CM, Welter CJ. Importance of the regulatory process and regulation. AORN J 2000;March:682–687.

20. Kapp MB. Legal anxieties and end-of-life care in nursing homes. Issues Law Med 2003;19:111–134.

21. Schuster JL, Myers D, Rogers SK, et al. Can we make the health system work? In: Morrison RS, Meier DE, Capello C, eds. Geriatric Palliative Care. New York, NY: Oxford University Press; 2003:345–356.

22. Centers for Medicare and Medicaid Services. CMS Outlines Rights of Medicare Hospice Patients: First Overall Since 1983 Aimed at Improving Quality of Care. Press Release. 2008. http://www.cms.hhs.gov (accessed January 5, 2009).

23. Miller KG, Health Policy Tracking Service—Issue Brief—Term Care and End-of-Life Care. September 29, 2008. Westlaw, Egan, Minnesota.

24. Health Care Decisions Statutes Enacted in 2008. American Bar Association. http://www.abanet.org (accessed January 1, 2009).

25. State Initiatives in End-of-Life Care. Focus: Community State Partnerships. Midwest Bioethics Center. Kansas City: Issue 19, June 2003.

26. Kottkamp N. Concept Paper for a National Healthcare Decisions Day 2008. http://www.nationalhealthcaredecisionsday. org (accessed December 30, 2008).

27. National Health Care Decisions Day 2008. 110th Congress, 2nd Session. S. Con. Res. 73, H.R. Con. Res. 323.

28. Surrogate Consent in the Absence of an Advance Directive. 2008. American Bar Association. http://www.abanet.org (accessed January 1, 2009).

29. Pain and Policy Studies Group. Achieving Balance in Federal and State Pain Policy: A Guide to Evaluation (5th ed). University of Wisconsin Paul P. Madison, WI: Carbone Comprehensive Cancer Research Center, 2008.

30. Imhof S, Kaskie B. How can we make the pain go away? Public policy to manage pain at the end of life. Gerontologist 2008;48(4):423–431.

31. Gilson AM, Joranson DE, Maurer MA. Improving state pain policies: Recent progress and continuing opportunities 2007. CA Cancer J Clinical 2007;57:341–353.

32. Federation of Sate Medical Boards of the United States. Model policy for the use of controlled substances for the treatment of pain. 2004.

33. Kollas CD, Boyer-Kollas B, Kollas JW. Criminal prosecutions of physicians providing palliative or end-of-life care. J Pall Med 2008;11(2):233–241.

34. National Association of Attorneys General. Balancing Law Enforcement and Pain Management: NAAG Holds Roundtable. September 2008. http://www.naag.org (accessed January 5, 2009).

35. von Guten CF, MD, PhD, FACP. Financing palliative care. Clin Ger Medicine 2004;20:767–781.

36. Oregon Death with Dignity Act. Ballot Measure 16. General Election, November 8, 1994.

37. Oregon Death with Dignity Act 2007 Annual Report. Oregon Department of Human Services, Division of Public Health. http://oregon.gov/DHS/ph/pas/index.shtml (accessed December 5, 2009).

38. The Washington Death with Dignity Act, Initiative Measure No. 1000, General Election, November 4, 2008.

39. Baxter v. Montana, ADV-2007–787, 1st Judicial Dist. Mont., January 6, 2009.

40. Conquering Pain Act of 2005, 109th Congress, 1st Sess. S. 999.

41. National Pain Care Policy Act of 2008. 110th Congress, 2nd Sess H.R. 2994.

42. National Pain Care Policy Act of 2008. 110th Congress, 2nd Session. S 3387.

43. Children's Compassionate Care Act of 2007. 110th Congress, 1st Sess H.R. 5192.

44. Advance Directive Promotion Act of 2008. 110th Congress 110th Congress, 2nd Session. H.R. 5702.

45. Life Sustaining Treatment Preferences Act of 2008. 110th Congress, 2nd Session. H.R. 5702.

46. Life Span Respite Care Act of 2006, 109th Congress, 2nd Sess, S. 1283, H.R. 3248.
47. Life Span Respite Care of 2006. P.L/ 109–442, December 21, 2006.
48. Hospice Protection Act of 2008. 110th Congress, 2nd Session. S. 3484.
49. Hospice Protection Act of 2008. 110th Congress, 2nd Session. H.R. 6873.
50. Medicare Prescription Drug, Improvement and Modernization Act of 2003, P.L. 108–173, December 18, 2003.
51. Medicare Improvements for Patients and Providers Act 2008. P.L. 110–275, July 15, 2008.
52. U.S. Supreme Court. (1997, June). No. 96–110, Washington et al., Petitioners v. Glucksberg et al. and No. 95–1858, Vacco et al. v. Quill et al.
53. The Assisted Suicide Prevention Act of 2006. 109th Congress, 2nd Session. S. 3788.
54. Hospice and Palliative Nurses Association. Position Statement on the Legalization of Assisted Suicide. Pittsburgh, PA: HPNA, 2006.
55. Oncology Nursing Society. Nurses' responsibility to patients requesting assistance in hastening death. Oncol Nurs Forum 2007;34(4):763–764.
56. American Nurses Association. Position Statements on the Nurses Role in End-of-Life Decisions. Washington, DC: American Nurses Association, 1996.
57. Scanlon, C. Advocacy: Central to the role of nurses, an interview with Colleen Scanlon Nurs Admin Quarter 2008;31(4):275–278.
58. Thacker KS. Nurses advocacy behaviors in end-of-life nursing care. Nursing Ethics 2008;15(2):174–185.
59. Aroskar MA. Three decades at the interface of nursing ethics and policy in health care settings. In: Pinch WJ, Haddad AM, eds. Nursing Health Care Ethics: A Legacy and Vision Silver Springs, MD: American Nurses Association Publishing; 2008:73–81.
60. American Nurses Association. Code for Nurses with Interpretive Statements. Washington, DC: American Nurses Association, 2001.
61. Fowler M. Provision 9 in Guide to the Code of Ethics for Nurses: Interpretation and Application. Silver Springs, MD: American Nurses Association; 2008:122–134.
62. Oncology Nursing Society and Association of Oncology Social Work Joint Position on Palliative and End-of-Life Care. Oncol Nurs Forum 2007;34(6):1097–1098.
63. Aroskar MA. Moldow DG, Good CM. Nurses' voices: Policy, practice and ethics. Nurs Ethics 2004;11(3):266–276.
64. Scanlon C. Public policy and end-of-life care. In: Ferrell B, Coyle N, eds. Textbook of Palliative Nursing. New York, NY: Oxford University Press; 2001:688.

# 64

## Palliative Care and Requests for Assistance in Dying

*Deborah L. Volker*

*I really hope or pray that this won't be a long, long drawn-out process of dying. I would prefer that it be a little faster.—Woman with end-stage colon cancer*

- *Key Points*
- *Palliative care nurses do encounter patient and family questions, concerns, and requests for assisted dying.*
- *Withholding and withdrawing life-sustaining measures and provision of pain relief are not acts of assisted dying.*
- *Individuals with life-limiting disease who may consider assisted dying include those experiencing unrelieved pain, depression, hopelessness, psychological distress, spiritual distress, poor social support, poor quality of life, or a perception of being a burden on others.*
- *Nurses should respond to requests for assisted dying in a manner that reflects professional guidelines and a sense of advocacy for patient rights for quality end-of-life care.*

The concept of palliative care, as described by the World Health Organization, is in direct conflict with the idea of deliberately hastening a person's death via the practice of assisted dying. Indeed, palliative care "intends neither to hasten nor postpone death."[1] Yet patients may be fearful of the extreme discomfort they anticipate, or they may simply want some certainty as to the timing or circumstances of death. Nurses who care for patients with life-limiting disease encounter patient and family questions, concerns, and requests for assisted dying. Receiving such a request can represent a morally troubling dilemma in which there is uncertainty about how best to respond. The purpose of this chapter is to review the ethical and legal status of assisted dying, summarize empirical findings regarding both professional and lay opinions and experiences with assisted dying, and offer guidelines for responding to requests for assisted dying.

### What Is Assisted Dying?

The term *assisted dying* is typically used to describe an action in which an individual's death is intentionally hastened by the administration of a drug or other lethal substance. This may take the form of either assisted suicide or active euthanasia. *Assisted suicide* is defined as "making a means of suicide available to a patient (e.g., providing pills, weapon) with knowledge of the patient's intention. The patient who is physically capable of suicide subsequently acts to end his or her own life."[2] *Active euthanasia* occurs when "someone other than the patient commits an action with the intent to end the patient's life."[3] Such an action can be voluntary (e.g., requested by a competent individual) or involuntary (administered without the individual's knowledge or consent).

It is important to distinguish between the concept of assisted dying and other actions designed to allow patients to die as comfortably as possible. Withholding and withdrawing life-sustaining measures are actions designed to not interfere with the natural trajectory of an illness. That is, life-sustaining measures such as artificial ventilation, renal dialysis, cardiopulmonary resuscitation, or artificial nutrition and hydration are withheld or stopped; the patient subsequently dies because of the effects of disease. In this instance, the intent of the action is to allow a natural death, and the cause of death is the underlying illness. In assisted dying, the intent of the action is to hasten death, and the cause of death is the lethal drug or other means administered to end life. Intent and causation are the key concepts that differentiate the two actions. Some practitioners worry that administration of sufficient doses of pain medication and other drugs designed to relieve suffering may hasten death and therefore may constitute assisted dying. However, this is *not* an action of assisted dying. It does not qualify as assisted dying because the intent is to relieve suffering, even though there may be a foreseen possibility that the medications could result in a hastened death. This is an example of the ethical principle of double effect, in which a good effect (relief of pain or other symptoms) is the goal despite the possibility of an unintended, harmful effect (a hastened death). The reader is referred to Chapters 7 and 62 for more information on the principles and ethics of proper pain management.

## What Are the Ethical and Legal Issues?

The ethical issues associated with assisted dying have been extensively described.[4-6] In essence, those who support the practice cite the patient's right to determine his/her own fate (autonomy), relieve untenable suffering, and maintain control over the end of life. Also relevant is the issue of equity, in that patients who are not dependent on life support do not have the same access to ending life as patients who can deliberately end life by discontinuing a ventilator, for example. Those who believe assisted dying is unethical worry that the practice will erode trust in health-care professionals, deny the sanctity of human life, discourage efforts to make palliative care available to all, and initiate a "slippery slope" in which vulnerable, underserved, or disenfranchised patients will feel pressured to take a quick way out with death. The health-care professions' ethical codes and position statements uniformly oppose the practice of assisted dying. Table 64–1 summarizes nursing organizations' relevant codes and statements.

Active euthanasia is illegal throughout the United States, whereas the Netherlands and Belgium have legalized both assisted suicide and active euthanasia under certain circumstances.[7] Australia briefly enacted a law that legalized both active euthanasia and assisted suicide; the statute was passed in 1996 and repealed a year later. Switzerland is unique in that it is the only country that allows assisted suicide to be performed by non-physicians and allows foreign citizens to engage in the practice within its borders.[8]

Worldwide, the Netherlands has had more experience with the practice of active euthanasia than any other country. Euthanasia was legally sanctioned via a series of court decisions in the Netherlands beginning in the 1970s; euthanasia and physician-assisted suicide were legalized in 2002 by the Dutch parliament.[9] Controversy exists as to whether increasing tolerance of these practices by physicians and the public has led to an increase in their use and a lesser emphasis on palliative and hospice care. Van der Heide and colleagues[10] studied end-of-life decision-making practices by physicians in the Netherlands after parlimentary approval. They concluded that the incidence of physician-assisted death had declined and the use of continuous deep sedation had increased since 2001. The practice of ending life without the request of the patient also declined from 0.8% of all deaths in 1990 to 0.4% in 2005. The researchers speculated that the decline in assisted deaths and increase in use of deep sedation may reflect consideration of high-quality end-of-life care as an alternative to deliberately hastening death. However, the study did not evaluate quality of end-of-life care and hospice use, nor did it obtain views of patients or family members. Ongoing study of assisted dying in the Netherlands is anticipated.

Assisted suicide was legalized in Oregon in 1997 with the passage of the Death with Dignity Act via two citizen referenda separated by 3 years. This Act allows a terminally ill person to obtain a prescription for a lethal dose of medication with the prescribing physician's understanding that the intent of the medication is to end life. Eligible patients must meet several criteria, including being at least 18 years of age, an Oregon resident, capable of making health-care decisions, and diagnosed with a terminal illness that will cause death within 6 months. The patient who requests a prescription must make two oral requests (separated by at least 15 days) to his/her physician and provide a written request that is signed in the presence of two witnesses. The prescribing physician and a consulting physician must confirm the diagnosis and prognosis and determine whether the patient is competent to make the decision. If either physician believes the patient's judgment is in question, the patient must be referred for a psychological examination. The prescribing physician must discuss alternatives to assisted suicide (comfort care, hospice care, and pain control) with the patient and must request (but not require) that the patient notify next-of-kin of his or her plans.[11] The Act was challenged in 2001 by the U.S. Attorney General, who asserted that physicians who prescribe lethal doses of drugs are violating federal laws regarding controlled substances. The U.S. Supreme Court ruled in 2006 that the Attorney General does not have the authority to determine what constitutes a legitimate medical practice and that individual states retain this responsibility.[12] Hence, the Oregon Act remains in place and physicians may continue to prescribe controlled substances for the purpose of hastening death.

**Table 64–1**
**Ethical Codes and Position Statements of Nursing Organizations Relevant to Patient Requests for Assisted Dying**

| Organization | Document | Guidelines |
|---|---|---|
| American Nurses Association | *Code of Ethics for Nurses with Interpretive Statements* | "Nurses may not act with the sole intent of ending a patient's life even though such action may be motivated by compassion, respect for patient autonomy and quality of life considerations" (p. 8). Nurses are charged with alleviating suffering and providing supportive care to the dying. |
| American Nurses Association | *Position Statement on Active Euthanasia* | "Moral opposition to actively taking a human life prohibits the nurse from participating in active euthanasia [but] does not negate the obligation of the nurse to provide proper and ethically justified end-of-life care which includes the promotion of comfort and the alleviation of suffering, adequate pain control, and at times forgoing life-sustaining treatments" (p. 2). |
| American Nurses Association | *Position Statement on Assisted Suicide* | "The nurse should not participate in assisted suicide" (p. 1). Responses should include a nonjudgmental approach; a search for understanding the meaning of the request and personal discomfort with the request; provision of counsel, support, and palliative care programs to manage chronic, severe bio-psycho-social and spiritual distress; collaboration with other health care team members; and a commitment to nonabandonment. |
| Oncology Nursing Society | *The Nurse's Responsibility to the Patient Requesting Assistance in Hastening Death* | "Nursing is charged with supporting the ethical mandates of the profession while simultaneously seeking to understand the meaning behind the request for hastening death" (p. 1). Responses should include "a thorough and nonjudgmental multidisciplinary assessment of the patient's unmet needs, and prompt and intensive intervention for previously unrecognized or unmet needs" (p. 1). |
| Oregon Nurses Association | *ONA Provides Guidance on Nurses' Dilemma* | Articulates the patient's right to self-determination and to have decisions regarding end of life be respected. Includes nurses' responsibility to share information about legal choices and right to refuse to be involved in the care of a patient who has chosen assisted suicide. Responses include providing care and comfort to the patient and family throughout the dying process and maintaining confidentiality of patient choice about end-of-life decisions. Allows nurses to be present during a patient's self-administration of a lethal dose of medication. Prohibits patient abandonment by a nurse who does not morally agree with assisted suicide but allows transfer of responsibility for patient's care to another provider. |
| International Council of Nurses | *The ICN Code of Ethics for Nurses* | Does not specifically address care of the dying. |
| International Council of Nurses | *Nurses' Role in Providing Care to Dying Patients and Their Families* | Emphasizes the nurse's role in providing skilled care at the end of life and the patient's right to choose or refuse treatment, and the right to a dignified death (p. 1). Does not address assisted suicide/active euthanasia. |

*Source:* Adapted from Volker (2003), reference 36, with permission.

In November 2008, voters in Washington state approved a Death with Dignity Act that is modeled after the Oregon law. If the law is enacted as scheduled in 2009, health-care providers in Washington will face the same challenges and opportunities that their Oregon colleagues encountered in their quest to improve end-of-life care.[13]

~☙~

## Who Wants Access to Assisted Dying and Why?

It is not unusual for terminally ill people to desire a hastened death. People who have life-limiting diseases such as cancer, degenerative neurological disorders, acquired immunodeficiency syndrome (AIDS), or end-stage cardio-vascular or renal disease have been identified as individuals who may be interested in access to assisted dying. Various studies have revealed characteristics of those who have expressed a desire for hastened death. Meier and coworkers[14] conducted a national survey of physicians who had received requests for assisted suicide to determine the demographic and illness characteristics of patients who had such requests denied or honored. Of the 1,902 physicians who responded, 63% described instances of receiving requests, and 80 requests were honored. Requesting patients were seriously ill, suffered from pain and other physical discomfort, and were near death. Physicians who honored requests were more likely to do so if the patient was in severe pain or discomfort, had a life expectancy of less than 1 month, and was not considered to be depressed.

Cancer is a major risk factor for an affected person's interest in suicide. In a case–control study of suicide risk in older Americans with medical illnesses, cancer was the only illness that was associated with a higher risk of sui-cide.[15] The study authors conjectured that contributing fac-tors may have included advanced disease and its treatment or social responses to progressive disease such as intracta-ble pain, poor prognosis, use of higher doses of analgesics, or social isolation. The study focused on analysis of actual suicides and did not capture desire for suicide that was not be enacted. Historically, risk for suicide in cancer patients has been associated with end-stage disease, depression, and hopelessness.[16] Indeed, in a study of attitudes of patients receiving palliative care for cancer, researchers found that 40% of respondents expressed an interest in requesting a physician-hastened death in the future.[17] However, Walker and colleagues surveyed approximately 3,000 outpatients with cancer to determine prevalence of suicidal thoughts.[18] About 8% reported suicidal thoughts; emotional distress, substantial pain, and older age were associated with this group of patients. This finding raises the concern that assess-ment for suicidal risk must go beyond that of cancer patients with terminal illness.

Patients with amyotrophic lateral sclerosis (ALS) are at higher risk for interest in hastening death via physician-assisted suicide or euthanasia. Typically, contributing variables include severe, advanced stage disease, treatment ineffective-ness, and increasing dependence on caregivers.[19] However, in a 40-year, case–controlled study of suicide in Sweden, people with ALS had a sixfold increased risk for suicide but that the risk was higher in earlier stages of the disease.[19] The study investigators hypothesized that severe emotional burden asso-ciated with a new diagnosis of ALS and physical inability to perform suicide at later stages of disease could have accounted for their findings.

Experience with legal assisted dying in Oregon reveals another picture. During the first 9 years of the Death with Dignity Act, 341 patients took lethal medications to end their lives, whereas 98,942 other Oregonians died from the same underlying illnesses.[20] The characteristics of Oregonians who died from assisted dying included older age (median: 69 years), non-Hispanic White race, and college-level education. Most had a diagnosis of either cancer or ALS and were enrolled in hospice care. The most common end-of-life concerns voiced included loss of autonomy, decreased ability to participate in enjoyable activities, and loss of dignity.[20]

Various studies of Oregon patients, families, and health-care providers' attitudes and experiences with assisted suicide have unfolded since the enactment of the Death with Dignity Act. In a longitudinal study of interest in physician-assisted suicide among Oregon advanced cancer patients, Ganzini and colleagues determined that most of the participants supported legalization of the practice.[21] Nine percent had a serious interest in obtaining a lethal prescription for assisted suicide; less than half of this group discussed their interest with their oncologists. Of the 161 patients in the study, two ultimately requested physician assisted suicide. Notably, the investigators found that patients who were dissatisfied with medical care were more likely to be interested in assisted suicide over time.

Despite access to legal assisted dying, or perhaps because of it, Oregon has become a national leader in improving plan-ning for end-of-life care. According to the Oregon Hospice Association, Oregon has the lowest rate of in-hospital deaths, highest rate of home deaths, and lowest cost of end-of-life care.[22] The Death with Dignity Act may be prompting more open communication between patients and health-care pro-viders about choices in end-of-life care, and improvements in delivery of expert palliative care.[9]

## How Do Nurses Respond to Requests for Assisted Dying?

Given their pivotal role in providing palliative care, nurses often may encounter patient requests for assisted dying. Survey studies have captured nurses' experiences with receiv-ing requests for assisted dying. For example, Matzo and Emanuel[23] surveyed 441 New England oncology nurses and discovered that 30% had received requests for assisted suicide, 1% had engaged in assisted suicide, and 4.5% had injected a drug to intentionally end a patient's life. In a national survey of more than 2,333 nurses,[21] 23% had received patient requests for assistance with obtaining a lethal prescription, and 22% had patients who requested that they be injected with a lethal dose of medication.

Qualitative studies have also been conducted to capture nurses' experiences with assisted dying. Volker[24] analyzed 48 anonymously-submitted stories of oncology nurses' experi-ences. Some of the nurses' stories reflected patient's, fam-ily's, or health-care provider's desires for control over an uncontrollable end-of-life experience. Many stories reflected nurses' moral conflicts over how to respond to patient or fam-ily requests for assisted dying; covert communication among nurses, physicians, and family members regarding agreement to intentionally hasten death; and a sense that the experience of receiving such a request had an enduring influence on future practice. Schwarz[25] interviewed 10 nurses from hospice, AIDS, critical care, and spinal cord injury practice settings to discern their experiences with being asked to help someone die. The nurses spoke both of unintentionally hastening death via clinically-appropriate symptom management (illustrative of the principle of double effect) and, on occasion, of knowingly intending death. Many expressed feelings of conflict, guilt, and moral distress. Notably, the context of a patient's request for assisted dying shaped the nurses' responses; neither codes of ethics nor professional position statements were used.

Coyle and Sculco[26] conducted a phenomenological study to investigate the meaning and uses of expressed desire for hastened death in seven patients living with advanced cancer. They concluded that expression of desire for hastened death constituted a communication tool used by the patients. Analysis of patient interviews revealed that meanings and uses of expression about desire for hastened death manifested in a variety of ways. Examples included expressions as a manifestation of the will to live, that the dying process itself was so difficult that an early death was preferred, and that the immediate patient situation was unendurable and required immediate action. The investigators observed that a request for hastened death may not be a literal expression of desire for suicide and may take on many meanings and uses for patients. Nurses should listen carefully to patient requests and associated stories to better understand what the patient is asking for.

The experience of Oregon nurses and social workers with hospice patients who requested physician-assisted suicide or voluntary refusal of food and fluids has also been examined. Harvath and colleagues interviewed 20 nurses and social workers regarding their experiences with patients who wished to hasten death.[27] The participants indicated that such requests presented opportunities to discuss patient concerns and fears about the dying process and to improve symptom-management strategies. But they also indicated that requests for aid in hastening death presented a dilemma between respect for patient autonomy versus honoring their commitment to uphold the goals of hospice care.

Given that euthanasia and assisted suicide are legal in the Netherlands, study of nurses' roles within this context is important. In a survey of 532 Dutch inpatient nurses, investigators examined the role of nurses in managing patient requests for euthanasia or assisted suicide, the decision-making process, and the administration of lethal drugs.[28] Findings revealed that patients often speak with their nurses first about their wishes for hastened death and that nurses respond by explaining legal requirements, hospital policies, and opportunities for palliative care. Most nurses reported discussing patient requests with physician colleagues. Notably, nurses administered a lethal drug with or without a physician present to 22 patients. Dutch law limits the administration of euthanatics to physicians only.

## How Should Nurses Respond to Requests for Assisted Dying?

Of the myriad communication skills expected of nurses, responding to requests for assisted dying can be the most difficult. Regardless of his or her personal feelings about the moral acceptability of assisted dying, the professional nurse has a responsibility to respond to a patient's request for assisted dying in a compassionate, sensitive way. The patient advocacy role of nursing is central to that response. Table 64-1 summarizes the guidelines that professional organizations offer to assist nurses in formulating responses to requests for assisted dying. In particular, the Oncology Nursing Society[29] has emphasized that "a request for hastening death prompts a frank discussion of the rationale for the request, a thorough and nonjudgmental multidisciplinary assessment of the patient's unmet needs, and prompt and intensive intervention for previously unrecognized or unmet needs" (p. 2). Table 64–2 outlines the American Academy of Hospice and Palliative Medicine's guidelines for exploring a request for assisted dying.[30] For nurses who practice in Oregon, the Oregon Nurses Association[31] has published detailed guidelines for nurses who choose to be involved in an assisted suicide, as well as guidelines for those who choose *not* to be involved but transfer the patient's care to another colleague. In either case, nurses may *not* inject or administer medication intended to end life; subject the patient, family, or other health care team members to judgmental comments or actions; or refuse to provide comfort and safety measures to the patient.

## Are There Alternatives to Assisted Dying?

The wish for a peaceful, comfortable death is not unreasonable. Given that assisted dying is not a viable moral or legal option for many individuals, what are the alternatives that could fulfill a desire to control the circumstances of the dying process? The obvious answer is universal access to expert palliative care. Indeed, there is strong moral consensus among health care providers that untreated suffering must never be a justification for assisted dying. However, there are legally and ethically sanctioned options other than assisted dying that may be palatable for some individuals. Refusal of medical treatment is a widely respected means for allowing the dying process to unfold unimpeded by treatments that will not fulfill the patient's personal goals for the end-of-life experience. Refusal may be in the form of withholding or withdrawing a life-sustaining treatment.

The individual who is not dependent on medical interventions to sustain life and wishes to control the timing of his or her death is faced with a more perplexing challenge. Voluntary refusal of food and fluids has been identified as a possible option. Although such action requires no direct

**Table 64–2**
**Approaches to Exploring a Request for Physician-Assisted Death: Guidelines from the American Academy of Hospice and Palliative Medicine**

- **Determine the nature of the request**

  Is the patient seeking assistance right now? Is he seriously exploring the clinician's openness to the possibility of a hastened death in the future? Is he simply airing vague thoughts about ending life?

- **Clarify the cause(s) of Intractable suffering**

  Is there severe pain or another unrelieved physical symptom? Is the distress mainly emotional or spiritual? Does the patient feel he is a burden? Has he grown tired of a prolonged dying?

- **Evaluate the patient's decision-making capacity**

  Does the patient have cognitive impairment that would affect his judgment? Does the patient's request seem rational and proportionate to the clinical situation? Is his request consistent with his past values?

- **Explore emotional factors**

  Do feelings of depression, worthlessness, excessive guilt, or fear substantially Interfere with the patient's judgment?

  Initial responses to requests for hastened death:

  - Respond empathically to the patient's emotions.
  - Intensify treatment of pain and other physical symptoms.
  - Identify and treat depression, anxiety, and/or spiritual suffering when present.
  - Consult with specialists in palliative care and/or hospice.
  - Consult with experts in spiritual or psychological suffering, or other specialty areas depending on the patient's circumstances.
  - Utilize a caring and understanding approach to encourage dialogue and trust and to assure the best chance of relieving distress.
  - Commit to the patient to work toward a mutually acceptable solution for his suffering.

  When unacceptable suffering persists, despite thorough evaluation, exploration, and provision of standard palliative care interventions as outlined above, a search for common ground is essential. In these situations, the benefits and burdens of the following alternatives should be considered:

  - Discontinuation of potentially life-prolonging treatments, including corticosteroids, insulin, dialysis, oxygen, or artificial hydration or nutrition.
  - Voluntary cessation of eating and drinking as an acceptable strategy for the patient, family, and treating practitioners.
  - Palliative sedation, even potentially to unconsciousness, if suffering is intractable and of sufficient severity. (AAHPM *Statement on Palliative Sedation:* www.aahpm.org/positions/sedation.html).

*Source:* American Academy of Hospice and Palliative Medicine (2007), reference 30, with permission.

participation by the health-care team, nurses can support patients who choose this option by ensuring optimal comfort measures and family support. Depending on the patient's underlying condition, death usually occurs within one to three weeks.[32] Concern has been voiced regarding discomforts that could accompany this action. To evaluate this possibility, Ganzini and associates[33] surveyed hospice nurses who had cared for terminally ill patients who deliberately hastened death by cessation of eating and drinking. Thirty-three percent of their 307 respondents reported that they had cared for such patients. The most common reasons given by patients for this choice were readiness for death, poor quality of life or fear of poor quality of life, belief that continued existence was pointless, and desire to die at home. Most of the patients had either cancer or a neurological disease; 85% of the patients died within 15 days after ceasing intake of food and fluids. The nurses were asked to rate the quality of these patients' deaths on a scale from 0 (a very bad death) to 9 (a very good death); the median score for this sample was 8. The authors concluded that, from the perspective of the nurse participants, most of the patients died a good or peaceful death. Notably, no family or patient perspectives were obtained in this study. Future research should focus on evaluating these perspectives.

The practice of palliative sedation represents another alternative to assisted dying. Palliative sedation refers to the use of sedative medications to reduce a patient's awareness of symptoms that have not been sufficiently controlled by other therapies.[34] According to the American Academy of Hospice and Palliative Medicine, sedation to the point of unconsciousness should only be used for "the most severe, intractable suffering at the very end of life" (p. 1).[34] The goal of palliative sedation is to relieve suffering, not to cause death. A detailed discussion of this practice is provided in Chapter 26. Palliative sedation may be ethically troubling for both family and professional caregivers because some do not differentiate between this practice and active euthanasia. Palliative care experts can provide guidance to assist patients, families, and professionals with appropriate use of sedation and to distinguish palliative sedation from hastened death. In addition, some patients may not find this choice acceptable because they view induction of unconsciousness until the time of death as undignified and as prohibiting communication with loved ones in those final days or hours.

CASE STUDY
*When Pain Is Intolerable at End of Life*

In the following scenario, a hospice nurse described a patient's plan to hasten death in the event she developed intolerable pain.[35]

"After a few weeks of visiting Beverly, a 55-year-old woman in the terminal stages of metastatic breast cancer, Beverly and her son confided that Beverly was a member of the Hemlock Society. Beverly planned with the support of her family to use certain drugs as described in the book, *Final Exit*, when she could no longer tolerate the pain of her disease. She wanted to know my feelings on her decision and plans. While maintaining a calm exterior, my heart beat accelerated. Somehow I knew that Beverly and her son were testing me, testing our relationship. I am not an advocate of assisted dying or suicide, but I am a strong believer in being non-judgmental of the beliefs of others. I decided to explore the reasons for Beverly's plan and in doing so found an area where we could work together to achieve her goal and possibily eliminate the need to take her life."

"Beverly admitted that it was the pain that concerned her the most. We made an informal contract that day that I would work closely with her physician to provide pain and symptom management so that she, hopefully, would not reach the point of needing to take her own life. When I contacted the physician and explained Beverly's tentative plan, he admitted that he was aware of her intentions. He agreed to the plan for aggressive pain and symptom management. For the next several months, her family, physician, and I worked diligently in adjusting medications to control her pain, anxiety, and depression. Beverly died at home of natural causes surrounded by her family."

This case illustrates the disturbing consequences of untreated suffering that can occur at the end of life. The patient's discussion of her plans and the Hemlock society, a lay organization focused on supporting patient access to legal assisted dying, were the prompts for assessment and interventions to address her needs. The nurse upheld professional standards by exploring the patient's concerns in a nonjudgmental manner and immediately initiating actions in consultation with the physician.

## Conclusion

Although many requests for assisted dying can be resolved by the application of expert palliative care, a small subset of individuals may seek assisted dying despite such care. Nurses are responsible for responding to patient requests in a manner that reflects professional guidelines and a sense of advocacy for patient rights for quality end-of-life care. Regardless of personal values or discomfort with a request for assisted

dying, nurses must apply open communication techniques that allow exploration of patients' needs and fears about the final phase of life.

REFERENCES

1. World Health Organization. WHO definition of palliative care. Available at: http://www.who.int/cancer/palliative/definition/en/ (accessed December 15, 2008).

2. American Nurses Association. Position Statement on Assisted Suicide. Washington, D.C.: American Nurses Association, 1994.

3. American Nurses Association. Position Statement on Active Euthanasia. Washington, D.C.: American Nurses Association, 1994.

4. Dieterle JM. Physician assisted suicide: A new look at the arguments. Bioethics 2007;21:127–139.

5. Darr K. Physician-assisted suicide: Legal and ethical considerations. J Health Law 2007;40:29–63.

6. Hurst SA, Mauron A. The ethics of palliative care and euthanasia: Exploring common values. Palliat Med 2006;20:107–112.

7. Bosshard G, Broackaert B, Clark D, Materstvedt LJ, Gordijn B, Müller-Busch HC. A role for doctors in assisted dying? An analysis of legal regulations and medical professional positions in six European countries. J Med Ethics 2008;34:28–32.

8. Pereira J, Laurent P, Cantin B, Petremand D, Currat T. The response of a Swiss University hospital's palliative care consult team to assisted suicide within the institution. Palliat Med 2008;22:659–667.

9. Quill T. Legal regulation of physician-assisted death—the latest report cards. N Engl J Med 2007;356:1911–1913.

10. Van der Heide A, Onwuteaka-Philipsen B, Rurup M, et al. End-of-life practices in the Netherlands under the Euthanasia Act. N Engl J Med 2007;356:1957–1965.

11. Oregon Public Health Division. Death with Dignity Act Requirements. 2006. Available at: http://www.oregon.gov/DHS/ph/pas/docs/Requirements.pdf (accessed December 15, 2008).

12. Tucker, KL. In the laboratory of the states: The progress of *Glucksberg*'s invitation to states to address end-of-life choices. Mich Law Rev 2008;106:1593–1611.

13. Steinbrook, R. Physician-assisted death—from Oregon to Washington State. N Engl J Med 2008;359:2513–2515.

14. Meier DE, Emmons C, Litke A, Wallenstein S, Morrison S. Characteristics of patients requesting and receiving physician-assisted death. Arch Intern Med 2003;163:1537–1542.

15. Miller M, Mogun H, Azael D, Hempstead K, Solomon D. Cancer and the risk of suicide in older Americans. J Clin Oncol 2008;26:4720–4724.

16. Quill T. Suicidal thoughts and actions in cancer patients: The time for exploration is NOW. J Clin Oncol 2008;26:4705–4707.

17. Wilson KG, Chochinov HM, McPherson CJ, et al. Desire for euthanasia or physician-assisted suicide in palliative cancer care. Health Psychol 2007;26:314–323.

18. Walker J, Waters R, Murray G, et al. Better off dead: Suicidal thoughts in cancer patients. J Clin Oncol 2008;26:4725–4730.

19. Fang F, Valdimarsdóttir U, Fürst CJ, Hultman C, Fall K, Sparén P, Ye W. Suicide among patients with amyotrophic lateral sclerosis. Brain 2008;131:2729–2733.

20. Oregon Public Health Division. Record and reports data on the Act. 2007. Available at: http://www.oregon.gov/DHS/ph/pas/ (accessed December 15, 2008).

21. Ganzini L, Beer TM, Brouns M, Mori M, Hsieh Y. Interest in physician-assisted suicide among Oregon cancer patients. J Clin Ethics 2006;17:27–38.

22. Oregon Hospice Association. Hospice in Oregon 2008: A historical perspective. 2008. Available at: http://www.oregonhospice.org/data_research_law.htm (accessed December 15, 2008).

23. Matzo M, Emanuel E. Oncology nurses' practices of assisted suicide and patient-requested euthanasia. Oncol Nurs Forum 1997;24:1725–1732.

24. Volker DL. Oncology nurses' experiences with receiving requests for assisted dying from terminally ill patients with cancer. Oncol Nurs Forum 2001;28:39–49.

25. Schwarz JK. Understanding and responding to patients' requests for assistance in dying. J Nurs Scholarsh 2003; 35:377–384.

26. Coyle N, Sculco L. Expressed desire for hastened death in seven patients living with advanced cancer: A phenomenological inquiry. Oncol Nurs Forum 2004;31:699–709.

27. Harvath TA, Miller LL, Smith KA, Clark LD, Jackson A, Ganzini L. Dilemmas encountered by hospice workers when patients wish to hasten death. J Hosp Palliat Nurs 2006;8:200–209.

28. Van Bruchem-van de Scheur GG, van der Arend A, Abu-Saad H, van Wijmen F, Spreeuwenberg C, ter Meulen R. Euthanasia and assisted suicide in Dutch hospitals: The role of nurses. J Clin Nurs 2008;17:1618–1626.

29. Oncology Nursing Society. Oncology Nursing Society position on the nurse's responsibility to the patient requesting assistance in hastening death. 2007. Available at: http://www.ons.org/Publications/positions/AssistedSuicide.shtml (accessed December 15, 2008).

30. American Academy of Hospice and Palliative Medicine. Position statement: Physician-assisted death. 2007. Available at: http://www.aahpm.org/positions/suicide.html (accessed December 15, 2008).

31. Oregon Nurses Association. Assisted suicide: ONA provides guidance on nurses' dilemma. 1998. Available at: http://www.oregonrn.org/associations/3019/files/AssistedSuicide.pdf (accessed December 15, 2008).

32. Quill T, Lee B, Nunn S. Palliative treatments of last resort: Choosing the least harmful alternative. Ann Intern Med 2000;132:488–493.

33. Ganzini L, Goy E, Miller L, Harvath T, Jackson A, Delorit M. Nurses' experiences with hospice patients who refuse food and fluids to hasten death. N Engl J Med 2003;349:359–365.

34. American Academy of Hospice and Palliative Medicine. Statement on palliative sedation. 2006. Available at: http://www.aahpm.org/positions/sedation.html (accessed December 15, 2008).

35. Volker DL. Oncology nurses' experiences with requests for assisted dying from terminally ill cancer patients. Doctoral dissertation, The University of Texas at Austin, 1999. Dissertation Abstracts International, 61(01), 199B.

36. Volker DL. Assisted dying and end-of-life symptom management. Cancer Nurs 2003;26:392–399.

# 65

*Denice K. Sheehan and Pam Malloy*

# Nursing Education

*It is very sad that palliative care is not more mainstream in everyone's care of the patient. Too few of us have "walked the walk" with a patient in pain, or with nausea, or shortness of breath for a significant period of time. To me, the real bottom line teacher is the experience.—Janice Mecklenburg, BSN student, the Breen School of Nursing*

♦ **Key Points**
♦ *There is a need for palliative care nursing education.*
♦ *Knowledge deficits exist among nurses regarding palliative care.*
♦ *Model academic programs are available for education in palliative care nursing.*

One of the earliest responsibilities of the professional nurse was care of the dying. Florence Nightingale and other nurses provided care to soldiers dying on battlefields as well as to civilians dying as a result of epidemics. A major shift in patterns of disease and treatment began in the 20th century as more effective treatment modalities became available. Today, student nurses are exposed primarily to curative-oriented care and are less likely to encounter comfort-oriented care. Although many health-care providers work with people at the end of their lives, nurses spend the most time with the dying and their families. Most nurses will provide palliative care to patients and their families no matter where they practice. Therefore, education in palliative care should begin in the nursing schools and extend through clinical inservices, continuing education courses, and professional conferences.

## The Need for Improved Palliative Care Nursing Education

It is imperative that nurses learn through both didactic and clinical experiences. Working with a palliative care or hospice team provides the best experience for learning about the interdisciplinary approach to patient care as the team members model excellence in care for the student. Many studies of end-of-life knowledge, attitudes, and skills of nurses provide evidence of the need to improve the education of nursing students, practicing snurses, and nursing faculty.[1–7] This chapter focuses on the role of nursing education in palliative care. An overview of the need to improve palliative care nursing education includes a brief history of nursing care of the dying, knowledge deficits, and the current focus on these deficits. Issues and challenges in palliative care education are discussed. Several models of nursing education programs are presented.

Many people, especially nurses and physicians, have been instrumental in developing a framework for care of the dying and their families. Dame Cicely Saunders is credited as the founder of the modern hospice movement. She was educated first as a nurse, then as a social worker, and later as a physician in London. Her interest in pain management led her to care for the dying. With support from the community and the national government, she founded St. Christopher's Hospice in Sydenham on the outskirts of London in 1967.[8] At about the same time, Dr. Elizabeth Kubler-Ross, a psychiatrist, began interviewing dying patients in hospitals. She found it difficult to find these patients because doctors and nurses repeatedly told her that there were no dying patients in their hospitals. She later proposed a model that described the five stages of dying.[9]

Jeanne Quint's landmark study in 1967 revealed little emphasis throughout the nursing curriculum on teaching nursing students to care for dying patients.[10] Teaching and support were particularly lacking in the clinical setting. Nursing instructors were inadequately prepared to teach or support the students in care of the dying and were not comfortable with nursing problems associated with dying patients. She recommended that faculty standardize death education curricula so that they could be offered consistently throughout schools of nursing and continuing education.

## Recognizing Deficits in Pain Education in the 1980s and 1990s

Many research studies have documented the lack of knowledge about pain management among student nurses, practicing nurses, and nursing faculty.[11-13] Studies have documented serious misconceptions in the assessment and treatment of pain and knowledge deficits in basic areas such as opioid pharmacology, use of adjuvant medications, and treatment of side effects. A recent national report documented poor pain management among nursing home residents and deficits in state pain policies.[3] These studies have been instrumental in encouraging greater emphasis on pain management in nursing education programs and the significant need to provide pain education to practicing nurses.

The awareness of educational deficits in the specific area of pain education extended in the late 1990s to the broader area of end-of-life content in nursing education. Many studies have documented the inadequate preparation of nurses to care for patients and their families at the end of life.[14-20] Several research studies have described important nursing behaviors in the care of the dying.[21,22] Inadequate professional education is often cited as a major barrier to appropriate end-of-life care. In Webster's 1981 study,[22] more than 30% of the student nurses reported that they were not always told which of their patients were expected to die. Additionally, 60% were not told whether the patients knew they were dying. Care of the dying patient was not routinely incorporated into their curriculum. The type and amount of knowledge and support were dependent on the instructor. Although the students may have learned these skills by working with more experienced nurses, observations revealed that 25% of the students worked alone with the dying, and the remaining 75% had only intermittent supervision.

Rittman and colleagues[23] identified five themes that were common among expert oncology staff nurses. They included knowing the patient and the stage of the disease, preserving hope, easing the struggle, providing for privacy, and responding to the spiritual aspects of living and dying. The nurses were able to maintain a high standard of practice by incorporating these themes into their clinical practice to provide for a peaceful death for their patients. They found that nurses who were able to deal with their own mortality became more comfortable with death.

Several studies have analyzed end-of-life content in nursing textbooks.[24,25] Kirchhoff and colleagues[24] analyzed 14 critical care nursing textbooks using the American Association of Colleges of Nursing (AACN) end-of-life competencies for undergraduate nursing education as their framework. Four additional end-of-life content areas were identified during the analysis. None of the textbooks contained all of the content areas. Although there was extensive information on ethical and legal issues, organ donation, and brain death in six or seven of the textbooks, the remaining textbooks contained no information on these topics. Pharmacological information was either mentioned briefly or absent. Approximately half of the textbooks had some information on patient/family communication.

Ferrell and colleagues[25] completed an analysis of nine areas of end-of-life content in nursing textbooks. Their review of 50 nursing textbooks revealed that only 2% of overall content was related to end-of-life care, and much of the information was inaccurate (Table 65–1). Deficiencies were found in all areas. Palliative care was usually discussed in terms of the hospice model of care rather than the broader concept of palliative care. There was little information on quality of life, which was surprising in view of the recent explosion of research in this area. Pain was often included in the textbooks, but usually in the context of acute rather than chronic pain. Pain management during the end of life was virtually absent. Major gaps were found in symptom assessment and management. Information about communicating with patients and families at the end of life was also lacking. There was little information about the roles and needs of family caregivers or about issues of policy, ethics, and law. A paucity of information was found about death awareness, anxiety, imminent death, and preparing families for the death. The stages and process of grief were described, but there was little information about nursing interventions or the nurse's personal grief.

Another component of this project was the collaboration with the National Council of State Boards of Nursing. (NCSBN).[26] The goal of this project was to improve end-of-life content in the national nursing licensure examination for registered nurses (NCLEX-RN). End-of-life content was

**Table 65–1**
**Analysis of End-of-Life (EOL) Content in Nursing Textbooks**

| Category of Nursing Text | No. of Texts Reviewed | % of Texts | No. of Pages | No. of EOL-Related Pages | No. of Chapters | No. of Chapters Devoted to EOL Content |
|---|---|---|---|---|---|---|
| **AIDS/HIV** | 1 | 2 | 526 | 20 | 16 | 0 |
| Assessment/diagnosis | 3 | 6 | 1783 | 15.3 | 80 | 0 |
| Communication | 2 | 4 | 767 | 38 | 35 | 0 |
| Community/home health | 4 | 8 | 3108 | 21.3 | 116 | 0 |
| Critical care | 4 | 8 | 4116 | 80.8 | 181 | 2 |
| Emergency | 4 | 8 | 1006 | 14.5 | 69 | 1 |
| Ethics/legal issues | 5 | 10 | 2018 | 143 | 88 | 4 |
| Fundamentals | 3 | 6 | 4353 | 114.9 | 140 | 3 |
| Gerontology | 3 | 6 | 2515 | 84.8 | 72 | 2 |
| Medical-surgical | 5 | 10 | 9969 | 146.3 | 298 | 2 |
| Oncology | 2 | 4 | 3264 | 107.5 | 149 | 7 |
| Patient education | 2 | 4 | 636 | 8.0 | 26 | 0 |
| Pediatrics | 3 | 6 | 2599 | 33.5 | 70.0 | 2 |
| Pharmacology | 4 | 8 | 3476 | 22.0 | 236 | 0 |
| Psychiatric | 3 | 6 | 2886 | 35.3 | 127 | 1 |
| Nursing review | 4 | 8 | 2661 | 17.0 | 47 | 0 |
| **Total** | **50** | **100** | **45,683** | **901.9 (2%)** | **1,750** | **24 (1.4%)** |

*Source:* Ferrell (1999), reference 25. Reprinted with permission.

increased in the NCLEX beginning with the April 2001 examination by incorporating the 15 competencies set forth by the AACN in the *Peaceful Death* document.[27] This was a significant force in increasing end-of-life content in the nursing curriculum.

Each of these studies has consistently echoed the strong message that improved patient care is contingent on adequate preparation of nurses. The deficits cited in these studies provide direction for needed areas of education.

## The Issues and Challenges in Palliative Care Education

The World Health Organization (WHO) has recognized the need for the development of national policies and programs for palliative care and has issued several recommendations regarding the education and training of health-care professionals. In addition, WHO has suggested that palliative care programs be incorporated into the existing health-care system.[28]

Another key document, the Institute of Medicine's 1997 report on improving end-of-life care,[4] made several recommendations specific to improving professional knowledge. Three of these related specifically to education:

*Recommendation 2:* Physicians, nurses, social workers, and other health-care professionals must commit themselves to improving care for dying patients and to using existing knowledge effectively to prevent and relieve pain and other symptoms.

*Recommendation 4:* Educators and other health professionals should initiate changes in undergraduate, graduate, and continuing education to ensure that practitioners have relevant attitudes, knowledge, and skills to care well for dying patients.

*Recommendation 5:* Palliative care should become, if not a medical specialty, at least a defined area of expertise, education, and research. Palliative care experts should provide expert consultation; serve as role models for colleagues and students; supply leadership for undergraduate, graduate, and continuing education; and organize and conduct research.

The Institute of Medicine report cited major deficiencies in professional education for end-of-life care. These included the relative absence of death in the curriculum, a lack of educational materials pertaining to the end stages of most diseases and neglect of palliative strategies, and the lack of clinical experiences with dying patients and those close to them. The report[3] suggested that educators could improve care by doing the following:

1. Conferring a basic level of competence in care of the dying patient for all practitioners
2. Developing an expected level of palliative and humanistic skills considerably beyond this basic level
3. Establishing a cadre of superlative professionals to develop and provide exemplary care for those approaching death, to guide others in the delivery of such care, and to generate new knowledge to improve care of the dying.[4]

A 2002 national report card on dying in America encouraged the development of hospice or palliative care service rotations in nursing education and requirements for continuing nursing education in end-of-life care.[3] Other groups have recently supported the recommendation for continuing education in hospice and palliative care for all health-care professionals.[29,30]

Educational programs for nurses in palliative care vary widely throughout the world. There are established courses and programs in palliative care at universities as well as seminars, workshops, and conferences in the Americas, Australia, the United Kingdom, and elsewhere in northern Europe. In other parts of the world, education in palliative care is woven into other courses. Palliative care concepts are taught within oncology courses in Japan and Thailand. Since 1990, the Nairobi Hospice in Kenya has provided palliative care courses for health-care professionals and has extended this program to nursing schools throughout Kenya. They are working to incorporate palliative care into the nursing curriculum. An increase in the availability of charitable sources has resulted in support for the development of palliative care in Russia and the Czech republic.[31]

There are many challenges in improving palliative care education. All educators struggle with how best to integrate more content into an already packed curriculum. Nurse educators have described undergraduate programs designed to incorporate end-of-life content into the curriculum through didactic and practicum courses.[32,33] Other academicians have described the process of developing interdisciplinary courses at the graduate level.[34] There also is tremendous need to increase the knowledge of faculty in palliative care so that they can lead the change in curriculum. Faculty also require current teaching guides such as audiovisual materials, case studies, and other resources to present this challenging content.

Teaching palliative care is not only a matter of didactic content. Preparing nurses to care for the terminally ill necessitates attention to the student's values, beliefs, personal experiences, and culture. It is essential that palliative care education not only incorporate knowledge and skills but also strive to identify methods to best enhance compassion, empathy, and the existential aspect or "art" of palliative nursing.[35–39]

## The Nursing Profession's Response to the Need for Change

In recent years, major professional nursing organizations have recognized the importance of nursing response to the mandate for improved end-of-life care. In 1997, the International Council of Nurses mandated that nurses have a unique and primary responsibility for ensuring that individuals at the end of life experience a peaceful death.[38,40] In the same year, the AACN convened a roundtable of expert nurses and other health care professionals to address this topic. The report from that meeting was titled *Peaceful Death*.[27] This document outlined 15 competencies necessary for nurses to provide high-quality care to patients and families during the transition at the end of life. These competencies should be attained before graduation from undergraduate programs of nursing. The group also made recommendations concerning the curriculum content areas in which these competencies could be addressed (Table 65–2).

At about the same time, the Nurses Section of the National Hospice Organization, under the direction of Cindy Yocum Scott and Nancy English, developed the *Guidelines for Curriculum Development on End of Life and Palliative Care in Nursing Education*.[41] Separate guidelines were prepared for undergraduate and graduate nursing programs. They included the biological, psychosocial, and spiritual responses to dying. Theory, assessment, interventions, and clinical placement were addressed within this conceptual framework (Table 65–3). National groups have recently developed clinical practice guidelines for palliative care.[29,30] They are especially useful for curriculum development.

Dr. Cynda Hylton Rushton, faculty of the School of Nursing of Johns Hopkins University, and colleagues at the Institute for Johns Hopkins Nursing convened a meeting of 23 nursing specialty groups in 1999 to design an agenda for the nursing profession on palliative and end-of-life care.[42] The group, the Nursing Leadership Consortium on End-of-Life Care, consisted of nursing organizations with administration, research, practice, and policy responsibilities and created a priority map for the nursing profession. The Nursing Leadership Academy for Palliative and End-of-Life Care continued the work of the Consortium.[43,44] In 2000, leaders from 22 nursing organizations met for 5 days to develop action plans to address key issues in end-of-life care in their organizations. This effort was repeated with another cohort in 2002, raising the number of participating organizations to 44. The project was funded by Project on Death in America.

In 2001, Dr. Ira Byock convened a group of palliative care advanced practice nurses (APNs) with expertise in clinical practice, education, and research to discuss the state of advanced practice nursing in palliative care in the United States and to make recommendations for the future development of this emerging nursing specialty. They recommended that nurse educators become more familiar with palliative

**Table 65-2**
**Competencies Necessary for Nurses to Provide High-Quality Care to Patients and Families During the Transition at the End of Life**

1. Recognize dynamic changes in population demographics, health-care economics, and service delivery that necessitate improved professional preparation for end-of-life care.
2. Promote the provision of comfort care to the dying as an active, desirable, and important skill and an integral component of nursing care.
3. Communicate effectively and compassionately with the patient, family, and health-care team members about end-of-life issues.
4. Recognize one's own attitudes, feelings, values, and expectations about death and the individual, cultural, and spiritual diversity existing in these beliefs and customs.
5. Demonstrate respect for the patient's views and wishes during end-of-life care.
6. Collaborate with interdisciplinary team members while implementing the nursing role in end-of-life care.
7. Use scientifically-based standardized tools to assess symptoms (e.g., pain, dyspnea [breathlessness], constipation, anxiety, fatigue, nausea/vomiting, and altered cognition) experienced by patients at the end of life.
8. Use data from symptom assessment to plan and intervene in symptom management using state-of-the-art traditional and complementary approaches.
9. Evaluate the impact of traditional, complementary, and technological therapies on patient-centered outcomes.
10. Assess and treat multiple dimensions, including physical, psychological, social, and spiritual needs, to improve quality at the end of life.
11. Assist the patient, family, colleagues, and one's self to cope with suffering, grief, loss, and bereavement in end-of-life care.
12. Apply legal and ethical principles in the analysis of complex issues in end-of-life care, recognizing the influence of personal values, professional codes, and patient preferences.
13. Identify barriers and facilitators to patients' and caregivers' effective use of resources.
14. Demonstrate skill at implementing a plan for improved end-of-life care within a dynamic and complex health-care delivery system.
15. Apply knowledge gained from palliative care research to end-of-life education and care.

*Source:* American Association of Colleges of Nursing. (1997), reference 27.

care, develop continuing education to prepare current APNs in palliative care competencies, integrate the competencies into the education of all APNs, and develop clinical tracks for APN students who intend to specialize in palliative care. The Robert Wood Johnson Foundation funded this project through the Promoting Excellence in End-of-Life Care national program.[45,46]

Another group reviewed certification examinations administered by nursing specialty organizations to encourage end-of-life content. The quantity and quality of end-of-life content in certification examination blueprints, specialty nursing scope and standards of practice documents, and specialty nursing core curriculum textbooks were analyzed and found to be lacking. This project, coordinated by the Oncology Nursing Certification Corporation, was designed to promote changes in nursing practice by introducing changes in continuing education materials focused on preparing candidates for the certification examinations and by promoting increasing content on end-of-life care in the examinations.[47]

Involvement of the certification corporations is a vital force in promoting palliative nursing care. In addition to integrating end-of-life content across multiple specialty organizations, the Hospice and Palliative Nurses Association (HPNA) has provided leadership to this evolving discipline. HPNA is the leading nursing organization supporting the development of palliative nursing. This organization provides numerous educational programs, publishes extensive educational materials, and also has a certification arm, the National Board for Certification of Hospice and Palliative Nurses (NBCHPN), that administers the specialty certification in Hospice and Palliative Nursing for registered nurses (Certified Hospice and Palliative Nurse, CHPN), for Advanced Practice Nurses (Advanced Certified Hospice and Palliative Nurse, ACHPN), for licensed practical/vocational nurses (Certified Hospice and Palliative Licensed Nurse, CHPLN) and for nursing assistants (Certified Hospice and Palliative Nursing Assistant, CHPNA). The Center for Medicare and Medicaid Services (CMS) recognizes the NBCHPN as a national certifying body for nurse practitioners and clinical nurse specialists at the advanced practice level. The APN application requires practice verification forms and official academic transcripts demonstrating completion of courses in advanced health assessment, advanced pathophysiology and advanced pharmacology as outlined in the Consensus Model for APN Regulation.[48] Table 65-4 summarizes the content for the Hospice and Palliative Advance Practice Nurse Certification Examination. Table 65-5 outlines the content for the Hospice and Palliative Nurse Certification Examination. The reader is directed to the National Board for Certification of Hospice and Palliative Nurses website (http://www.nbchpn.org) for additional information on certification tests.

**Table 65–3**
**The Human Response to Dying (Approaching Death)**

Level I (entry-level nursing students):
Theory and clinical practice to be integrated within the two years of a generic nursing education curriculum.

| Biological Response | Psychosocial Response | Spiritual Response |
|---|---|---|
| **Theory** | | |
| Physiology of dying (physical decline) | Family dynamics in crisis | Death as a final stage of growth |
| Adaptive responses to approaching death | Loss-grief continuum | Meaning of death from a philosophical view |
| Palliative nursing care | Exploration of attitudes regarding death and dying | Meaning of the human spirit |
| | Legal issues: | Meaning of suffering |
| | • Advance directives | Fears surrounding dying: Loneliness and abandonment |
| | • Proxy decision maker | Role of hospice interdisciplinary team |
| | Ethics—Dying | |
| | Community health nursing aging caregivers | |
| | Belief systems and cultural customs (rural/urban, minority, etc.) | |
| **Nursing theory** | | |
| | | Carative model of nursing practice |
| | | Role of hospice-caring and comfort |
| | | The carative role of the nurse |
| | | Palliative nursing |
| **Assessment/nursing diagnosis** | | |
| Nutritional needs | Coping strategies in response to loss: | Patient/family assessment of needs |
| Fluid volume needs and processes | • Anticipatory grieving | Assess the process: |
| Elimination needs | • Powerlessness | • Spiritual distress |
| Skin and tissue integrity | Age-related responses to loss | • Fear |
| Delirium | | • Anxiety |
| Pain: acute, chronic, terminal | | • Ineffective coping, individual/family |
| Confusion | | |
| Cycles sleep–rest | | |
| Cardiovascular processes | | |
| Respiratory processes: | | |
| • Agitation | | |
| • Anoxia | | |
| **Interventions** | | |
| Palliative care (symptom management to provide comfort and alleviate suffering) | Communication: | |
| Emphasis on comfort measures | • Therapeutic vs. nontherapeutic use of reflection storytelling | |
| Complementary therapies | • Empathetic listening | |
| Pain management guidelines | | |
| **Complementary therapies as a focus of interventions** | | |
| | | Touch with intent |
| | | Therapeutic Touch |
| | | Massage |
| | | Music therapy |
| | | Prayer |
| | | Imagery |
| **Clinical placement** | | |
| Nursing care centers (nursing homes) | Same as those listed under biological responses | Same as those listed under biological responses |
| Assisted-living centers | Psychosocial competencies identified | |
| Inpatient hospice centers | | |
| Senior-level optional community health nursing | | |
| Hospice in the home | | |

*(continued)*

**Table 65–3**
**The Human Response to Dying (Approaching Death)** *(continued)*

Level II (Registered Nurses with 6 months to 1 year of experience in clinical nursing):
Time required to complete Level II: three semesters (or four quarters) in a university setting, including at least 12 weeks in a palliative care hospice setting.

| Biological Response | Psychosocial Response | Spiritual Response |
|---|---|---|
| **Theory** | Palliative nursing care role | Philosophical and historical role of healers |
| Palliative care: | Nursing role in hospice: | The spiritual process and spiritual distress: |
| • History and present day | • In-home vs. residential care | • Religiosity vs. spirituality |
| • Application in health care | • Teaching: families, caregivers, | Meaning of suffering |
| Pathophysiology (end-stage disease | and nursing assistants | Consciousness and dying |
| processes): | • Liaison with community health | Transpersonal meaning of existence |
| • Malignancies | organizations/resources | Theories of Jung-Cassel |
| • Immune deficiency disease | Recognition of personal needs and | Nursing theory |
| • Dementia | attitudes regarding death/pain/loss | Carative model |
| • Chronic illness | Interdisciplinary team | Addressing the intuitive process within the |
| Neurophysiological mechanisms of | Family dynamics—pathological | nurse: |
| acute/chronic/terminal pain | families: | • Centering |
| Principle of pain management Physiology | • Abuse and neglect | • Journaling |
| of symptoms: | • Closed systems | |
| • Anoxia | • Addictive/manipulative | |
| • Dyspnea | • Enmeshed | |
| • Fluid volume changes | Cultural differences: | |
| • Changes in antidiuretic hormone | • Rituals | |
| and kidney function | • Customs | |
| • Nutritional changes—nausea, | • Values | |
| constipation | • Funeral preparations | |
| • Restlessness | • Religious influence | |
| Agitation | Symbolic communication | |
| Delirium | Communication/interaction: | |
| | • Interviewing techniques | |
| | • Reflection | |
| | • Empathetic listening | |
| | • Silence | |
| **Assessment/nursing diagnosis** | | |
| Emphasis on physical assessment, | Human response to loss of | Suffering |
| symptoms and behaviors in end-stage | individual/family | Spiritual distress |
| processes | Coping strategies: | Hopelessness |
| Pain assessment—types and analogies of | • Denial/anger/bargaining/ | Powerlessness |
| measurement | depression/acceptance | Anxiety |
| Age-related pain behaviors: | • Grief and grieving | Fear |
| • Infants | • Anticipatory grief | |
| • Children | Bereavement meaning and | |
| • Preadolescents | importance in hospice: | |
| • Adolescents | • High-risk families | |
| • Middle adulthood | Social isolation | |
| • Aging | | |

*(continued)*

**Table 65–3**
**The Human Response to Dying (Approaching Death)** *(continued)*

**Level II (Registered Nurses with 6 months to 1 year of experience in clinical nursing):**
**Time required to complete Level II: three semesters (or four quarters) in a university setting, including at least 12 weeks in a palliative care hospice setting.**

| Biological Response | Psychosocial Response | Spiritual Response |
|---|---|---|
| **Interventions** | | |
| Palliative nursing role | Therapeutic communication: | Establishing criteria for the efficacy of |
| Advanced practice role | • Patient/family | complementary therapies |
| Common approaches to symptom | • Hospice team | Scientific and historical evidence in support of |
| management: | Crisis intervention | complementary therapies |
| • Pharmacological | Teaching: | • Therapeutic Touch |
| • Nonpharmacological | • Patient/family | • Massage |
| Complementary therapies | • Staff | • Acupressure |
| Pain management: | • Community | • Aroma therapy |
| • Cancer pain | Conflict resolution: | • Music therapy |
| • Acute pain | • Patient/family | • Guided imagery |
| • Chronic pain | • Staff | • Visualization |
| Terminal pain | • Hospice team | • Prayer |
| | Complicated bereavement | • Relaxation techniques |
| | | • Breathing |
| | | • Homeopathy |
| **Clinical experience** | | |
| Inpatient hospice | | |
| Assisted living | | |
| In-home hospice or residential setting | | |
| Correctional institutional (hospice center) | | |
| **Management role of the nurse** | | |
| Strategies for reimbursement | Supportive intervention for staff | |
| Health maintenance organization | Facilitate communication with | |
| Medicare/Medicaid | team members | |
| Regulatory agencies | For profit vs. nonprofit hospice | |
| • Federal | Regulations interval | |
| • State | • Policy | |
| Standards/Accreditation | • Procedural guidelines | |
| • Joint Commission on Accreditation of | Education/training | |
| Healthcare Organizations (JCAHO) | • Inservice/staff | |
| • National Hospice and Palliative Care | • Community | |
| Organization (NHPCO) | • Management/leadership training | |
| • National Consensus Project (NCP) | Support and interface with | |
| Guidelines[52] | community | |
| Liaison with specialized agencies | | |
| Quality assurance standards | | |

*Source:* National Council of Hospice Professionals (1997), reference 41.

## Model Nursing Programs

### Undergraduate and Graduate Education

The co-author of this chapter (Sheehan) has identified many important strategies in teaching palliative care to nursing students. It is important to include both didactic and clinical components in both undergraduate and graduate curriculums.

An example of an undergraduate model includes content on loss, grief, and bereavement, as well as pharmacological interventions for symptom management, at the sophomore level. Content on the physiology of dying, psychosocial and spiritual issues, and the hospice model of care is presented at the junior level, with a minimum of 12 hours with nursing faculty at an inpatient hospice facility and a freestanding home for the dying. At the senior level, content on the dying child is covered in the Developing Families rotation.

**Table 65–4**
**Hospice and Palliative Advance Practice Nurse Certification Examination: Detailed Content Outline**

I. Clinical Judgment 54%
  a. Assessment
  b. Order and Interpret Common Diagnostic Tests and Procedures
  c. Differential Diagnoses
  d. Planning
  e. Interventions
  f. Evaluation and Revision of the Care Plan
  g. Special Populations

II. Advocacy and Ethics and Systems Thinking 13%
  a. Ethical Principles
  b. Ethical Issues / Conflicts Related to Progressive Illness, Dying and Death
  c. Advance Care Planning
  d. Vulnerability of the Population
  e. Resource Access and Utilization
  f. Settings for Care
  g. Quality Improvement
  h. Financing

III. Professionalism and Research 10%
  a. Palliative and Hospice Care (History, Philosophy, Precepts)
  b. Standards and Guidelines Relevant to Hospice and Palliative Care
  c. Roles of Advanced Practice Nurse
  d. Evidence-Based Practice
  e. Self-Care and Collegial Support
  f. Public Policy Involvement
  g. Professional Boundaries
  h. Leadership and Self-Development
  i. Process
  j. Human Subject Considerations

IV. Collaboration, Facilitation of Learning and Communication 17%
  a. Care Team Models
  b. Scope of Advanced Practice Nursing
  c. Principles of Adult Learning and Teaching. Methodologies
  d. Patient / Family Education
  e Community and Health Professional Education
  f. Theory and Principles
  g. Processes Related to Therapeutic Communication

V. Cultural and Spiritual Competence 7%
  a. Influence of Personal Values and Biases on Practice
  b. Responses to Illness within Cultural, Spiritual, Racial, Ethnic, Age and Gender Groups
  c. Responses to Loss, Grief, Bereavement
  d. Communication
  e. Assessment
  f. Interventions

**Table 65–5**
**Hospice and Palliative Nurse Certification Examination: Detailed Content Outline**

I. Patient Care: Life-Limiting Conditions in Adult Patients 14%
  a. Identify and respond to indicators of imminent death
  b. Identify specific patterns of progression, complications, and treatment

II. Patient Care: Pain Management 25%
  a. Assessment
  b. Pharmacologic Interventions
  c. Nonpharmacologic and Complementary Interventions
  d. Evaluation

III. Patient Care: Symptom Management 27%
  a. Neurological
  b. Cardiovascular
  c. Respiratory
  d. Gastrointestinal
  e. Genitourinary
  f. Musculoskeletal
  g. Skin and Mucous Membrane
  h. Psychosocial, Emotional, and Spiritual
  i. Nutritional and Metabolic
  j. Immune/Lymphatic System
  k. Mental Status Changes

IV. Care of Patient and Family 11%
  a. Resource Management
  b. Psychosocial, Spiritual, and Cultural
  c. Grief and Loss

V. Education and Advocacy 9%
  a. Caregiver Support
  b. Education
  c. Advocacy

VI. Interdisciplinary/Collaborative Practice 8%
  a. Coordination and Supervision
  b. Collaboration

VII. Professional Issues 6%
  a. Practice Issues
  b. Professional Development

Students tend to learn best during teachable moments. These include real events with real people. For student nurses, this usually means the clinical setting. During day 1 of the hospice clinical rotation, the students work with experienced hospice nurses and a clinical nursing instructor. The students work with the nursing instructor to provide care for residents of Malachi House, a home for the dying, during the second clinical day.

Two models have been implemented at the inpatient hospice facility. In the first model, students attend the morning report and choose one or two patients with the guidance of the hospice nurse. The nursing instructor asks questions of the student and hospice nurse to facilitate learning. The instructor also meets with the students as a group early in the day to clarify the assignments for the day and to check on how the students are feeling in this environment. In a second model, two students are assigned to do morning care for one patient. Patients who are actively dying or identified by the staff as good storytellers are chosen to be the "teachers." In both models, the nursing instructor brings the students together as specific learning opportunities arise, such as the death of a patient, unusual dressing changes, or pharmacological interventions.

Students experience a nonmedical approach to care at Malachi House. They are encouraged to interact with the residents to know them as people, rather than patients. The students quickly realize that they can do a physical assessment without their stethoscopes. They "see" the person differntly based on their nursing education and clinical experiences.

The use of reflection is a powerful tool to assist students and faculty to learn about themselves and about their practice from situations they encounter in the clinical setting and to integrate personal and professional learning experiences. For this reason, the students write a reflection on practice for each hospice clinical day. Students are prepared for the hospice experience during a group meeting with the nursing instructor early in the day. The following is an example of a 2-day hospice clinical rotation in a junior-level course:

**Day 1, Hospice House**

1. Students' experiences with end-of-life care
2. Hospice history and philosophy
3. Brief overview of symptom management and spirituality
4. Clinical expectations
   a. Clinical assessments, nursing interventions, evidence-based practice
   b. Clinical assignment
5. Tour Hospice House
6. Clinical assignments
7. Debriefing and reflection throughout the day

**Day 2, Malachi House**

1. Tour Malachi House
2. Clinical assignments
3. Debriefing and reflection throughout the day

**Undergraduate Clinical Preparation**

1. You may feel exhausted by the end of the day even if you have done very little physical work. You may be emotionally drained.
2. Take time to discuss your fears and experiences with death with your clinical instructor, the hospice nurse, or your peers.
3. You may leave the unit (or classroom) at any time. Please let your instructor know how you are feeling.
4. You may be given the opportunity to see someone who has just died to discuss physical changes in the body and the feeling in the room.
5. Take time to reflect on your practice.
6. Be open to learning from a variety of people, including patients, families, interdisciplinary team members, peers, and yourself.

**Undergraduate Clinical Assignments**

1. Listen to the full report on your unit. (Model I)
2. Review Patient/Family Guidelines for Signs and Symptoms of Approaching Death.
3. Make rounds with the hospice nurse to see all of his or her patients. (Model I)
4. Choose one or two patients with guidance from the hospice nurse. (Model I)
5. Review patient/family information with the hospice nurse.
6. Assess one specific physical symptom that is most important to the patient. Use the literature to link the diagnosis with the pathophysiology. List the appropriate nursing interventions and expected outcomes. This information will be presented during the clinical conference.
7. Listen to the patient's story throughout the day.
8. Reflection on practice: What happened today that made a difference in the way you will practice nursing?

**Undergraduate Hospice Clinical Written Assignment**

1. Assess at least one physical or psychosocial symptom. Use the literature to link the symptom with the pathophysiology. List appropriate nursing interventions and expected outcomes.
2. Assess spirituality in one patient/resident. Use the literature to describe spirituality, appropriate nursing interventions and expected outcomes.
3. Describe the physical, psychosocial, and/or spiritual manifestations of approaching death in at least one person. Use the literature to link the symptom with the pathophysiology. List appropriate nursing interventions and expected outcomes.
4. Talk with at least one patient at Hospice House and one resident at Malachi House. Ask them what advice they would you give to you as a nursing student working with people near the end of their lives.
5. Describe experiences you have had at Hospice House and Malachi House that you have not had in previous clinical settings. How will these experiences inform your clinical practice?

**Undergraduate Hospice Clinical Written Assignment (Makeup)**

(This assignment is given when the student misses one of the two hospice clinical days)

1. Discuss hospice admission criteria and the hospice philosophy of care.
2. Discuss hospice Medicare reimbursement.
3. Describe the signs and symptoms of dyspnea in someone with COPD at the end of life. Use the literature to link dyspnea with the pathophysiology. List appropriate nursing interventions and expected outcomes.
4. Describe signs and symptoms of spiritual distress at the end of life, appropriate nursing interventions and expected outcomes.
5. Describe the signs and symptoms of imminent death. Use the literature to link the symptom with the pathophysiology. List appropriate nursing interventions and expected outcomes.

Madonna University in Livonia, Michigan, was the first institution in the United States to offer interdisciplinary hospice education programs under the direction of Sister Mary Cecilia Eagan. The hospice education department, under the direction of Kelly Rhoades, PhD, offers associate's, bachelor's, and master's degrees in hospice education. Students in the Master of Science in Hospice (MSH) program complete 30 semester hours of coursework and select one of five cognate specialties in bereavement, pastoral ministry, business, education, or nursing. Students may enroll in certificate programs at both the graduate and undergraduate levels in hospice education or bereavement. Madonna University College of Nursing and Health offers the following graduate programs in nursing: Adult Acute and Palliative Care Nurse Practitioner Dual Track, Adult Primary and Palliative Care Nurse Practitioner Dual Track, and Adult Advanced Practice Palliative Care post master's certificate.

The Breen School of Nursing at Ursuline College in Pepper Pike, Ohio, was the first graduate program in the United States to prepare APNs in palliative care. The Master of Science in Nursing program officially began in August 1998, under the direction of Dr. Denice Sheehan, although the first course was offered during the 1998 spring semester. The program builds on the college's mission to provide an education based on values. Contemplation and reflection on practice are hallmarks of this program. The core curriculum of the master's program concentrates on theory, informatics, research, critical thinking, evidence-based practice, and leadership. The APN courses include pathophysiology, pharmacology, and health assessment. Students in the palliative care program also take one specialized palliative care course including 600 hours in the palliative care practicum. Table 65–6 lists the required courses. A post-master's certificate is offered to nurses with a Master of Science in Nursing (MSN) degree. These students complete 500 practicum hours.

Introduction to Palliative Care and Hospice is an interdisciplinary web-based course. It is the first course offered in the post-master's certificate program. The content is taught in the core courses in the MSN program. This introduction course provides an overview of palliative care with respect to history, philosophy, the interdisciplinary team model, and reimbursement mechanisms. Students have opportunities to explore personal beliefs, attitudes, and reactions to progressive illness, dying, and death. They discuss ways in which these attitudes can influence the care of people with life-threatening illnesses and their families. Ethical issues are explored in relation to treatment decisions and quality of life. Spirituality is explored within a framework of individual values and beliefs. The essence of the self as the physical being deteriorates at the end of life is analyzed. Religious and cultural beliefs, traditions, and rituals are discussed as they pertain to end-of-life issues. Loss, grief, and bereavement are also explored as they relate to the terminally-ill person and the family. Communication and counseling techniques are woven throughout this course. Research, case studies, and personal and professional experiences are used to emphasize key concepts. Classical literature is woven throughout this course in the form of case studies. Most of the students in the post-master's certificate program have extensive hospice or palliative care experience and clinical expertise. They live and work in urban and rural areas across the United States. This combination of expertise, diversity, and openness to new ideas creates complex discussions and innovative approaches to care.

In Palliative Care I, students have an opportunity to analyze personal attitudes toward progressive illness, dying, and death and compare their current analysis to that developed in earlier courses. They also continue the discussion about how these attitudes can influence the care of patients with life-threatening illnesses and their families. Ethical issues are explored in relation to treatment decisions and quality of life. This course integrates pathophysiology, pharmacology, psychosocial issues, and spirituality in the assessment and management of symptoms. Current research in palliative care is analyzed and applied in the clinical setting.

The practicum is incorporated into the Palliative I course.

During the Palliative Care Practicum, students have opportunities in the clinical area for direct contact with expert palliative care practitioners. This includes direct patient–family contact during home visits, team conferences, and clinical forums with the clinical group and the instructor. The students work with the dying and their families in the home, hospice, and palliative care inpatient facilities, hospitals, and extended-care facilities. Students meet with an assigned faculty member to tailor the practicum to meet the learning needs of the student. The students work with patients and their families through the dying process and participate in grief support groups. They keep a clinical journal, including learning objectives, personal/professional strengths identified during the practicum, and reflections on their thoughts and feelings during the clinical experience. They also participate

**Table 65–6**
**Ursuline College's Master of Science in Nursing Program and Post Master's Certificate in Palliative Care**

Master of Science in Nursing
  I.  Core Courses: 30 credits
     Concepts and Theories
     Advanced Research Concepts I
     Advanced Research Concepts II
     Health Care Informatics
     Advanced Physiology/Pathology
     Advanced Health Assessment
     Advanced Pharmacology
     Health Care Organization and Finance
     Health Promotion, Maintenance and Restoration
     Health Policies, Roles and Issues
  II.  Adult Nurse Practitioner Track: 9 credits
     APN: Adult
     APN: Women's Health
     APN: Adult Nurse Practitioner Practicum
  III.  Family Nurse Practitioner Track: 12 credits
     APN: Adult
     APN: Women's Health
     APN: Pediatric
     APN: Family Nurse Practitioner Practicum
  IV.  Palliative Care Concentration: 4 credits
     Palliative Care I (includes Practicum)

Post Master's Certification: 21 credits
Introduction to Palliative Care
Palliative Care I
Palliative Care II
Palliative Care Practicum
Advanced Physiology/Pathology
Advanced Health Assessment
Advanced Pharmacology

in team meetings, research, and educational presentations to staff, patients and their families, and the community.

Another model nursing program is located at New York University (NYU) in New York City. NYU was the first institution in the United States to offer a Palliative Care Nurse Practitioner program under the direction of Dr. Deborah Witt Sherman. The joint Adult Primary/Palliative Care program has replaced the the Palliative Care NP Program. The new program builds on the core curriculum of the master's program, focusing on theory, research, evidence-based practice, critical thinking, human development, cultural competence, community health-care systems, and leadership. In addition to advanced science courses in pathophysiology, pharmacotherapeutics, and advanced health assessment, students take primary care and three specialized palliative care courses, along with 500 hours each of palliative care and primary practicum. A post-master's certificate is an option for those individuals who already have a master's in nursing. Table 65–7 includes a summary of the curriculum.

Schools of nursing are incorporating palliative care into existing graduate curricula as a subspecialty or focus. Vanderbilt University School of Nursing in Nashville, Tennessee, offers two opportunities at the graduate level to prepare nurses to care for people with life-threatening illnesses and their families across the palliative care trajectory. The first is an adult nurse practitioner program (ANP) with a palliative-care focus under the direction of Professor James C. Pace, DSN, MDiv, RN, ANP-CS, FAANP. Graduate nursing students complete 39 semester hours of coursework and 700 practicum hours in a variety of outpatient clinics, long-term care facilities, palliative care programs, and hospice settings. At the conclusion of the program, students are eligible for ANP certification and with additional hours post-graduation in a palliative-care setting, certification in advanced-practice palliative care. The second option includes joint degree initiatives leading to either the MSN/MDiv or MSN/MTS dual degrees offered in cooperation by the Schools of Nursing and Divinity at Vanderbilt University. Students complete individually designed programs of study in both nursing and divinity and course credit can be shared between schools. Students can fulfill the 700-hour practicum requirement in the school of nursing and satisfy part of the field education requirements of the divinity school. The ANP Program with a palliative care focus can also be taken as a post-masters option.

The reader is directed to the HPNA website (www.hpna.org) for additional information on graduate education programs in palliative care.

## Continuing Education

Although palliative care education in undergraduate and graduate programs provides an important foundation for the nursing profession, continuing education is also needed to reach nurses already in practice. Continuing education is needed to reach nurses in all settings involved in end-of-life care. A wide range of methods, including conferences, self-study courses, computer- and web-based approaches, and simulated clinical experiences, are needed.

In 1999, the AACN and the City of Hope National Medical Center initiated collaboration to develop a national education program on end-of-life care for registered nurses.[49] This national project, the End-of-Life Nursing Education Consortium (ELNEC), followed the efforts by the medical profession to address end-of-life care through the Education for Physicians in End-of-Life-Care (EPEC) program. The ELNEC project was funded by The Robert Wood Johnson Foundation (RWJF).[50] The nine components of the ELNEC curriculum included Nursing Care at the End of Life, Pain Management, Symptom Management, Ethical/Legal Issues, Cultural Considerations, Communication, Grief/Loss/Bereavement, Achieving Quality Care, and Care at the Time of Death. The ELNEC project was developed as a 3-day training program

---

**Table 65–7**
**New York University's Master of Science in Nursing Program in Adult Primary/Palliative Care**

I. Nursing Core: 15 credits
Introductory Statistics for the Health Professions
Research in Nursing
Nursing Issues and Trends within the Healthcare Delivery System
Theories of Nursing and Social Science: Implications for Advanced Professional Practice
Population Focused Care

II. Advanced Practice Core: 15 credits
Advanced Pathophysiology I
Advanced Pathophysiology II
Clinical Pharmacotherapeutics
Advanced Comprehensive Health and Physical Assessment
Contemporary Clinical Practice: Advanced Practice Roles

III. Specialty Component: 27 credits
APN: Nursing Strategies: Adult and Aged
APN: Common Health Problems Across the Lifespan (with Palliative Care Breakout Sessions)
APN: Pain and Palliative Care: Advanced Nursing Care to Address the Multidimensional Nature of Pain and Suffering
APN: Adult Primary Care II
APN: Adult Primary Care Practicum II
APN: Adult Primary Care III
APN: Adult Primary Care Practicum III
APN: Advanced Palliative Care Theory: Assessment and Management of Advanced Progressive Illness and Related Symptoms
APN: Adult Palliative Care Practicum: Nursing Leadership and Management of Complex Patient/Family Issues in Palliative Care

Post Master's Advanced Certificate Program: 27 credits for non-NPs; 12 credits for NPs interested in palliative care specialization

I. Advanced Practice Core: 15 credits
Advanced Pathophysiology I
Advanced Pathophysiology II
Clinical Pharmacotherapeutics
Advanced Comprehensive Health and Physical Assessment
Contemporary Clinical Practice: Advanced Practice Roles

II. Specialty Component: 12 credits
Common Health Problems Across the Lifespan (with Palliative Care Breakout Sessions)
Advanced Palliative Care Theory: Assessment and Management of Advanced Progressive Illness and Related Symptoms
Adult Palliative Care Practicum: Nursing Leadership and Management of Complex Patient/Family Issues in Palliative Care

---

that included many educational modalities such as lectures, role-plays, small-group work, case discussion, and other experiences. The "Train-the-Trainers" model was used: individuals attending the ELNEC course were expected to gain knowledge of the content as well as skills in teaching the content. A very extensive application process was designed to ensure that ELNEC participants had established goals for their dissemination of the curriculum before attending the course and had the support of the Dean or administrators to ensure success in their implementation. The RWJF funding provided eight initial courses targeted for 100 participants per course. These courses included five focused on faculty teaching in undergraduate nursing programs and three targeted for continuing education providers. The five training programs were held in 2001 and 2002 and addressed continuing education providers and nurse educators from hospices, palliative care programs, and community agencies. Table 65–8 lists the components of the ELNEC program.

The ELNEC project subsequently received funding from the National Cancer Institute to reach educators in graduate nursing programs for an APN version of the curriculum. By 2009 total of 367 graduate nursing faculty, representing every state in the United States and 285 out of 438 (65%) graduate nursing programs have attended ELNEC-Graduate. In 2003 the project received funding to initiate a curriculum specific for oncology nurses. The oncology project was conducted in collaboration with the Oncology Nursing Society (ONS). In attendance were 264 oncology nurses, representing 141 of 222 (64%) ONS chapters. From 2001 to 2003, the ELNEC investigators developed and tested a pediatric version of ELNEC, with the first national training program held in August 2003. Over 650 pediatric nurses, including those working in perinatal nursing and neonatal intensive care units (NICU) have attended an ELNEC-Pediatric Palliative Care train-the-trainer program. The ELNEC Project Team worked with national nursing leaders to incorporate more parinatal and

**Table 65–8**
**End-of-Life Nursing Education (ELNEC) Consortium**

| Module | Description of Content |
|---|---|
| 1. Nursing care at the end of life | Goals of care; cost issues in palliative care; use of aggressive interventions, personal death awareness, board review of end-of-life care, to encompass all age groups and across various disease trajectories or acute illness |
| 2. Pain management | Assessment; pharmacological, nonpharmacological, and complementary therapies |
| 3. Symptom management | Assessment; pharmacological, nonpharmacological, and complementary therapies |
| 4. Cultural considerations in end-of-life care | Cultural assessment; beliefs regarding death and dying, after life, and bereavement |
| 5. Ethical/legal issues | Assisted suicide, euthanasia, advance directives, decision-making, advanced care planning |
| 6. Communication | Breaking bad news; communicating with other disciplines; interdisciplinary collaboration |
| 7. Grief, loss, bereavement | Assessment; interventions; nurses' experiences with cumulative loss and grief |
| 8. Preparation and care for the time of death | Nursing care at the time of death, including physical care, support of family members, saying good-bye |
| 9. Achieving quality of life at the end of life | Physical, psychological, social, and spiritual well-being; needs of special populations |

neonatal material throughout the ELNEC- Pediatric Care (ELNEC_PC) curriculum. The revised curriculum became available in 2009. The critical care version of ELNEC was also launched in 2006. By 2009, a total of over 550 intensive care, coronary care, emergency room nurses and other critical care professionals had attended a national ELNEC-Critical Care train-the-trainer program. ELNEC-Geriatric was first presented in 2007, with a total of 370 nurses attending one of these national courses.[51] Geriatric nurses who work in long-term care, skilled nursing facilities, acute care facilities, and Schools of Nursing have attended these courses. in excellent palliative care. Table 65–9 illustrates examples of implementing/disseminating ELNEC in schools of nursing.

In 2006 and 2007, the Open Society Institute (OSI) provided funding for an ELNEC International training conference in Salzburg, Austria. At the 2007 course, each participant from Eastern Europe received the ELNEC curriculum in the Russian language. An additional OSI-supported ELNEC train-the-trainer course was provided in Tajikistan in the fall of 2008. In 2007, the Oncology Nursing Foundation provided funds for four ELNEC faculty to offer ELNEC training in Tanzania. By having the ELNEC curricula translated into 3 languages—Russian, Spanish, and Japanese—ELNEC has an increased international presence. In the first 8 years of providing national ELNEC courses, over 10,000 nurses have received training in national and international courses. Those 10,000 nurses have returned to their institutions and have trained thousands of other members of the interdisciplinary team. Many publications have described the ELNEC project and its curriculum.[46–48,52–56] The reader is directed to the ELNEC website (www.aacn.nche.edu/ELNEC) for additional information.

In December 2008, the ELNEC Project announced a new relationship with the Hospice Education Network (HEN), a comprehensive, innovative service that offers staff orientation programs, annual in-services, volunteer training and specialized learning modules addressing the educational needs of hospice programs and end-of-life care professionals. HEN and ELNEC offer the hospice industry, and other interested individuals or groups, online subscription access to eight ELNEC modules presented by national ELNEC faculty. The programs being offered are part of the ELNEC core trainings that are provided across the country by individuals who have completed the ELNEC train-the-trainer program. ELNEC will continue to offer the national train-the-trainer courses, in addition to the online courses with HEN. To obtain more information about accessing these modules, go to www.hospiceonline.com.

Continuing education opportunities are offered by specialty nursing organizations. All of these organizations hold annual conferences and publish palliative care articles in their journals, many with continuing education credit. In addition, the HPNA offers teleconferences online for nurses and nursing assistants. The ONS hosts an annual Institute of Learning and a biennial Cancer Nursing Research Conference. Virtual Sessions uses streaming video to showcase instructional sessions from the ONS Congress and Institutes of Learning. Sigma Theta Tau International offers online sessions in end-of-life care. The American Association of Crtical Care Nurses has a website dedicated to palliative care in critical care settings www.aacn.org.

ELNEC trainers use many different models to deliver the content on end of life care. Delaware's ELNEC project is one model. The Delaware End of Life Coalition (DEOLC), led by Dr. Madeline Lambrecht, provided the ELNEC Super-Core Curriculum in distance learning format. The video lectures were recorded, replicated on DVDs and given to the

**Table 65–9**
**Examples of Implementing/Disseminating ELNEC in Schools of Nursing**

**Classroom setting**

Included ELNEC modules into Professional Nursing Issues Course

Developed elective theory and practicum courses on palliative care

Provided case studies for pharmacology class to practice using the 3-level World Health Organization (WHO) ladder and equianalgesic charts

Included ELNEC information into nursing skills lab, including signs and symptoms of impending death, preparing for autopsy and organ donation, administering cultural sensitive post-mortem care, preparing the body for cremation and funeral ceremonies

Provided role plays to practice "breaking bad news" or "picking-up the pieces after being told bad news"

Partnered with physician colleagues who are "Education on Palliative and End-of-Life Care" (EPEC) trained to provide interdisciplinary education for MD and RN students

Worked with students to complete living wills so they can learn about decisions that must be made regarding end-of-life issues

Developed a one-hour elective that focused on clinical, spiritual, and ethical issues, using ELNEC content entitled "From Cure to Care: Dealing with End of Life Issues"

Chaired doctoral dissertation committees with students interested in palliative care

Designed a Master's track in palliative care

Integrated ELNEC curriculum in various general nursing courses (i.e. ethics, culture, pharmacology, research, etc.)

Provided a course where graduate students "practiced" having a family meeting and obtaining an advanced directive

Collaborated with other disciplines in various professional schools within the university (i.e. medicine, dentistry, pharmacy, religious studies, social work, psychology, etc.) to develop an interdisciplinary graduate course

Developed on-line undergraduate and graduate nursing courses using the ELNEC curriculum (powerpoint slides, case studies, supplemental teaching materials)

Received government and private grants to develop palliative care track in graduate nursing education

Designed an Advanced Practice Palliative Care Certificate Program

Provided content mapping of palliative care in current nursing curriculum

Developed an end of life course for students that covered the life span by partnering with ELNEC-Pediatric Palliative Care trainer and an ELNEC-Geriatric trainer to develop this as an elective

**Clinical settings**

Forged clinical contracts with local hospices (both in-patient and homecare)

Arranged for senior nursing students to have an opportunity to visit patients in the community through hospice programs associated with the Visiting Nurses Association (VNA)

Worked with clinical partners in providing ELNEC training to staff nurses and other members of the interdisciplinary team

---

nurses to view according to their individual schedules. The nurses were also given the ELNEC syllabus, CD and other resources to teach the materials. The initiative was expanded to long term care facilities in 2009. This group received the ELNEC Super Core curriculum and the ELNEC Geriatric curriculum.

## Future Directions

Clearly, there is much work to be done to advance nursing education in palliative care. Improving the care of patients will be accomplished only when nursing education within undergraduate, graduate, and continuing education is improved and supported by research. Progress over the next decade will require collaboration internationally and a close commitment by nursing education, research, and practice. Collectively, these efforts can advance the profession of palliative nursing and dramatically improve care at the end of life.

## Evaluation of Palliative Care Education

Evaluation of education is a challenge in any program and for any content, but it is a special challenge in palliative care education. As the core content of this education evolves, so will the methods of evaluation. There is a need for standard knowledge assessment measures, as well as means for evaluating clinical skills, decision-making, and a broad range of physical, psychosocial, and spiritual care skills necessary in palliative care.[57-59] New technologies, such as web-based teaching and evaluation tools, will be important resources for educators.

REFERENCES

1. Meraviglia MG, McGuire C, Chesley DA. Nurses' needs for education on cancer and end-of-life care. J Cont Educ Nurs 2003;34(3):122–127.

2. Durkin A. Incorporating concepts of end-of-life care into a psychiatric nursing course. Nurs Educ Perspect 2003;24(4):184–185.

3. Last Acts. Means to a Better End: A Report on Dying in America Today. Washington, DC: Last Acts, 2002.

4. Field MJ, Cassel CK, eds. Approaching Death: Improving Care at the End of Life. Report of the Institute of Medicine Task Force on End of Life Care. Washington, DC: National Academy of Sciences, 1997.

5. Proctor M, Grealish L, Coates M, Sears P. Nurses' knowledge of palliative care in the Australian Capital Territory. Int J Palliat Nurs 2000;6:421–428.

6. Bowden V. End-of-life care: A priority issue for pediatric nurses. J Pediatr Nurs 2002;17:456–459.

7. Institute of Medicine. Priority Areas for National Action: Transforming Healthcare Quality. Washington DC: National Academy Press, 2003.

8. Bennahum DA. The historical development of hospice and palliative care. In: Forman WB, Kitzes JA, Anderson RP, Sheehan DK, eds. Hospice and Palliative Care: Concepts and Practice (2nd ed). Boston, MA: Jones and Bartlett; 2003:1–11.

9. Kubler-Ross E. On Death and Dying. New York, NY: Macmillan, 1969.

10. Quint JC. The Nurse and the Dying Patient. New York, NY: Macmillan, 1967.

11. Hollen CJ, Hollen CW, Stolte K. Hospice and hospital oncology unit nurses: A comparative survey of knowledge and attitudes about cancer pain. Oncol Nurs Forum 2000;27:1593–1599.

12. Grant MM, Rivera LM. Pain education for nurses, patients, and families. In: McGuire DB, Yarbro CH, Ferrell BR, eds. Cancer Pain Management. Boston, MA: Jones and Bartlett; 1995:289–319.

13. Glajchen M, Bookbinder M. Knowledge and perceived competence of home care nurses in pain management: A national survey. J Pain Symptom Manage 2001;21:307–316.

14. Arber A. Student nurses' knowledge of palliative care: Evaluating an education module. Int J Palliat Nurs 2001;7:597–598, 600–603.

15. Field D, Kitson C. Formal teaching about death and dying in UK nursing schools. Nurse Educ Today 1986;6:270–276.

16. Pickett M, Cooley ME, Gordon DB. Palliative care: Past, present, and future perspectives. Semin Oncol Nurs 1998;14(2):86–94.

17. Samaroo B. Assessing palliative care educational needs of physicians and nurses: Results of a survey. Greater Victoria Hospital Society Palliative Care Committee. J Palliat Care 1996;12:20–22.

18. Sellick SM, Charles K, Dagsvik J, Kelley ML. Palliative care providers' perspectives on service and education needs. J Palliat Care 1996;12:34–38.

19. Webber J. New directions in palliative care education. Support Care Cancer 1994;2:16–20.

20. Degner LF, Gow CM, Thompson LA. Critical nursing behaviors in care of the dying. Cancer Nurs 1991;(14)5:246–253.

21. McClement SE, Degner LF. Expert nursing behaviors in care of the dying adult in the intensive care unit. Heart Lung 1995;24:408–419.

22. Webster NE. Communicating with dying patients. Nursing Times 1981;June 4:999–1002.

23. Rittman M, Paige P, Rivera J, Sutphin L, Godown I. Phenomenological study of nurses caring for dying patients. Cancer Nurs 1997;(20)2:115–119.

24. Kirshhoff KT, Beckstand RL, Anumandla P. Analysis of end-of-life content in critical care nursing textbooks. J Prof Nurs 2003;19:372–381.

25. Ferrell BR, Virani R, Grant M. Analysis of end of life content in nursing textbooks. Oncol Nurs Forum 1999;26:869–876.

26. Wendt A. End-of-life competencies and the NCLEX-RN examination. Nurs Outlook 2001;3:138–141.

27. American Association of Colleges of Nursing. A Peaceful Death. Report from the Robert Wood Johnson End-of-Life Care Roundtable. Washington, DC: November 1997.

28. World Health Organization. Cancer Pain Relief and Palliative Care. WHO Technical Report Series 804. Geneva: WHO, 1990.

29. National Quality Forum. A National Framework and Preferred Practices for Palliative and Hospice Care Quality, 2007. Available at: http://www.qualityforum.org/publications/reports/palliative.asp (accessed December 23, 2008).

30. National Consensus Project. Clinical Practice Guidelines for Quality Palliative Care, 2004. Available at: http://www.nationalconsensusproject.org/Guidelines_Download.asp (accessed December 23, 2008).

31. Jodrell N. Nurse education. In: Doyle D, Hanks G, MacDonald N, eds. Oxford Textbook of Palliative Medicine (2nd ed). Oxford: Oxford University Press; 1998:1202–1208.

32. Birkholz G, Clements PT, Cox R, Gaume A. Students' self-identified learning needs: A case study of baccalaureate students designing their own death and dying course curriculum. J Nurs Educ 2004;43:36–39.

33. Pimple C, Schmidt L, Tidwell S. Achieving excellence in end-of-life care. Nurs Educ 2003;28:40–43.

34. Gelfand DE, Baker L, Cooney G. Developing end-of-life interdisciplinary programs in universitywide settings. Am J Hosp Palliat Care 2003;20:201–204.

35. Scanlon C. Unraveling ethical issues in palliative care. Semin Oncol Nurs 1998;14:137–144.

36. Redman S, White K, Ryan E, Hennrikus D. Professional needs of palliative care nurses in New South Wales. Palliat Med 1995;9:36–44.

37. Sheldon F, Smith P. The life so short, the craft so hard to learn: A model for post-basic education in palliative care. Palliat Med 1996;10:99–104.

38. Vachon ML. Caring for the caregiver in oncology and palliative care. Semin Oncol Nurs 1998;14:152–157.

39. Yates P, Hart G, Clinton M, McGrath P, Gartry D. Exploring empathy as a variable in the evaluation of professional development programs for palliative care nurses. Cancer Nurs 1998;21:402–410.

40. International Council of Nurses. Basic Principles of Nursing Care. Washington, DC: American Nurses Publishing, 1997.

41. National Council of Hospice Professionals. Guidelines for Curriculum Development on End-of-Life and Palliative Care in Nursing Education. Arlington, VA: National Hospice Organization, 1997.

42. Rushton C, Scanlon C, Ferrell B. Designing an Agenda for the Nursing Profession on End of Life Care. Report of the Nursing Leadership Consortium on End of Life Care. Aliso Viejo, CA: Association of Critical Care Nurses; 1999:1–14.

43. Rushton CH, Spencer KL, Johanson W. Bringing end-of-life care out of the shadows. Nurs Manage 2004;35:34–40.

44. Rushton C, Sabatier K, Gaines J. Uniting to improve end-of-life care. Nurs Manage 2003;34:30–33.

45. Advanced Practice Nurses' Role in Palliative Care: A position statement from American Nursing Leaders, July 2002. Available at: http://www.dyingwell.com/downloads/apnpos.pdf (accessed December 15, 2008).

46. Advanced Practice Nursing. Pioneering practiced in palliative care. Promoting Excellence in End-of-Life Care, July 2002. Available at: http://www.promotingexcellence.org/i4a/pages/Index.cfm?pageID=3775 (accessed December 15, 2008).

47. Esper P, Lockhart JS, Murphy CM. Strengthening end-of-life care through specialty nursing certification. J Prof Nurs 2002;18:130–139.

48. Consensus Model for APN regulation: Licensure, accreditation, certification and education, July 2007. Available at: http://www.nursingworld.org/DocumentVault/APRNs/ConsensusModelforAPRNRegulation.aspx (accessed December 17, 2008).

49. Ferrell BR, Dahlin C, Campbell ML, Paice JA, Malloy P, Virani R. End-of-Life Nursing Education Consortium (ELNEC) Training Program: Improving palliative care in critical care. Crit Care Nurs Q 2007;30:206–212.

50. Malloy P, Paice J, Virani R, Ferrell BR, Bednash G. End-of-Life Nursing Education Consortium: 5 years of educating graduate nursing faculty in excellent palliative care. Prof Nurs 2008;24:352–357.

51. Kelly K, Ersek M, Virani R, Malloy P, Ferrell B. End-of-Life Nursing Education Consortium Geriatric Training Program: Improving palliative care in community geriatric care settings. J Gerontol Nurs 2008;34:28–35.

52. Paice JA, Ferrell BR, Virani R, Grant M, Malloy P, Rhome A. Graduate nursing education regarding end-of-life care. Nurs Outlook 2006;54:46–52.

53. Malloy P, Ferrell B ,Virani R, Wilson K, Uman G. Palliative care education for pediatric nurses. Pediatr Nurs 2006;32:555–561.

54. Paice J, Ferrell BR, Virani R, Grant M, Malloy P, Rhone A. Appraisal of the graduate end-of-life nursing education consortium training program. Palliat Med 2006;9:353–360.

55. Paice JA, Ferrell BR, Coyle N, Coyne P, Callaway, M. Global efforts to improve palliative care: The International End-of-Life Nursing Education Consortium Training Programme. J Adv Nurs 2007;61:173–180.

56. Malloy P, Sumner E, Virani R, Ferrell B. End-of-Life Nursing Education Consortium for pediatric palliative care (ELNEC-PCC). Am J Matern Child Nurs 2007;32:298–302.

57. MacLeod RD. Education in palliative medicine: A review. J Cancer Educ 1993;8:309–312.

58. Sowell R, Seals G, Wilson B, Robinson C. Evaluation of an HIV/AIDS continuing education program. J Cont Educ Nurs 1998;29:85–93.

59. The SUPPORT Principal Investigators. A controlled trial to improve care for seriously ill hospitalized patients: The Study to Understand Prognoses and Preferences for Outcomes and Risks of Treatments (SUPPORT). JAMA 1995;274:1591–1598.

# 66

*Betty R. Ferrell, Marcia Grant, and Virginia Sun*

# Nursing Research

*Nurses are expected to deliver the highest possible quality of care in a compassionate manner...In today's world, nurses must become lifelong learners, capable of reflecting on, evaluating, and modifying their clinical practice based on new knowledge. And, nurses are increasingly expected to become producers of new knowledge through nursing research.—Polit and Beck (2004).[1]*

♦ **Key Points**
♦ *The goal of nursing research is to improve care for patients and caregivers.*
♦ *Nurses have been instrumental in the field of palliative care research.*
♦ *Palliative nursing research includes many sensitive topics such as pain, quality of life, and fatigue.*
♦ *Nurse researchers face many obstacles in conducting research, such as obtaining informed consent, dealing with high subject attrition, and openly discussing end of life issues with patients and families.*
♦ *Palliative nursing research should utilize an interdisciplinary model that includes all supportive care disciplines.*
♦ *Caregivers and patients' families should be included in palliative nursing research.*

A major component of palliative care research is nursing research.[2] The patient experience of dying is an ideal healthcare concern appropriate for nursing inquiry.[3] Because nurses are concerned with patient responses to illness, the physical, psychological, social, and spiritual responses of the terminally ill and their families are prime areas for nursing research.

The ultimate goal of nursing research, and indeed of nursing knowledge, is to improve care for patient care. Palliative care offers a rich opportunity for research to directly influence patient care in areas such as symptom management, psychological responses to a terminal illness, and the family caregiver experience of terminal illness.[4-7]

Some of the earliest contributions to palliative care research were made by nurses.[8] Pioneering work by Jeanne Quint Benoliel and others raised awareness of deficiencies in care of the dying.[9,10] Early descriptive studies documented the influence of nursing attitudes and beliefs about death on the care provided to patients.

From the earliest studies in the 1960s to the "awakening" of attention to palliative care in the late 1990s, research in palliative care has been limited. Nurse investigators have addressed aspects of end-of-life care such as pain management, bereavement, settings of care, and care of special populations such as patients with the acquired immunodeficiency syndrome (AIDS). However, there has been a lack of cohesive commitment to palliative care nursing research.

In 1997, the National Institute of Nursing Research (NINR) led an initiative regarding end-of-life care research across several institutes of the National Institutes of Health (NIH). Specific recommendations of an NINR-sponsored conference on end-of-life care are described later in this chapter.[11] NINR has been designated as the lead institute at the NIH in the area of end-of-life care. It is appropriate and commendable that the NINR is providing leadership at the NIH in this research agenda.

As has been true in other areas of healthcare, the research agenda has lagged behind the demands of clinical practice and education. Hospice programs and palliative care settings face increased demands for improved end-of-life care with little scientific knowledge to guide clinical decisions.[12] Nursing schools have begun to develop undergraduate and graduate courses in palliative care, and some have launched degree or certificate programs in palliative care, again with limited research as a scientific foundation of their programs. Obviously, development of a solid research agenda and support of nursing science in palliative care are overdue.[13]

## Goals of Palliative Care Research

The goals of palliative care nursing research are similar to goals of other areas of nursing inquiry. Nursing research serves multiple functions, including quantification of information, discovery, description of phenomena, quality improvement, and problemsolving.[1] Quantification is accomplished through descriptive studies or through epidemiologic approaches. For example, there is a need to quantify the symptoms present in terminal illness, as well as their severity and impact. The field of palliative nursing care is relatively unexplored, and therefore, there is great opportunity for discovery. What are the greatest needs of terminally ill patients and their family caregivers? What is the unique role of nursing within the interdisciplinary team?

The subjective nature of terminal illness and the existential experience of dying require research methods that describe phenomena. Death, as a subject that has been avoided in society, is still a relatively unknown aspect of life. On a more specific level, palliative care is also a field that would benefit tremendously from research linked to quality improvement. Numerous reports have identified serious deficits in end-of-life care, and efforts to improve the quality of end-of-life care will undoubtedly benefit from research.[14,15] Finally, a major goal of palliative care research should be basic problemsolving. What drugs are most beneficial for dyspnea or agitation? What is the best treatment for pressure ulcers in a dying patient? What education best prepares family caregivers for signs and symptoms of approaching death?

## Ethical and Methodological Considerations in Palliative Care Research

There are many unique aspects of research in palliative care. The multidimensional nature of care at the end of life and the vulnerability of the population are but two examples of factors that pose special challenges to this area of research.

The challenges of nursing research in palliative care should be prefaced by a discussion of the benefits. Although even the mention of conducting research with dying patients and their burdened families immediately creates concerns, there are in fact many benefits to participants. Participating in research, even at this most vulnerable and sensitive time of life, provides the opportunity for research subjects to contribute to others. Research participation often provides an opportunity to derive meaning from illness and to feel that one's suffering will provide benefit to others.[3,13,16]

In the authors' research at the City of Hope, involving numerous studies in sensitive areas such as pain, quality of life, and fatigue, positive feedback has consistently been received from research subjects. Patients and family caregivers often have thanked the researchers for studying these topics, which they perceive to be of great importance. Subjects have also frequently related that completing written instruments or participating in interviews provided a mechanism for communicating needs that had not previously been voiced.

However, research in palliative care is very challenging and includes many obstacles. Nurses are often conflicted in balancing the role of clinician with that of researcher. For example, in conducting research related to pain in terminally ill cancer patients, the authors have often had to carefully balance these roles. Identifying a patient with severe pain has often meant that the patient's participation in a study must be ended in order to seek treatment for the pain. Researchers must always respect the more important ethical consideration of protecting the patient's well-being.[16]

Seeking informed consent in rapidly declining, weak patients is a challenge, as is the need to constantly protect patient and family autonomy. Subjects in palliative care research may feel obligated to participate, particularly if they have been the recipients of good care. Although all patients in palliative care are considered vulnerable, certain subgroups, such as the cognitively impaired, the poor, and the elderly, are of special concern.[17–20]

The sensitive nature of palliative care research provides inherent challenges. The areas of concern at the end of life are highly emotional and may invoke heightened distress. Exploring areas such as grief, fears, spiritual concerns, family conflict, and other common dimensions of terminal illness is highly challenging. Participation in research can bring to the forefront previously undisclosed problems. The authors have found, in their research experience, that palliative care research necessitates a highly skilled research staff. Collecting data from palliative care subjects is very different from research in healthy or chronically ill subjects. Research nurses in palliative care studies must be clinically competent, highly skilled nurses equipped to balance the rigor of research with extreme sensitivity.[12,21]

Palliative care research, perhaps more than any other field of inquiry, must carefully weigh subject burden. The time required of research subjects in palliative care, a precious commodity for those with terminal disease, must be carefully protected. Special consideration must be given to the selection of research instruments and procedures to minimize subject burden.[22–27]

A useful resource for nurse-researchers in palliative care is a "Tool Kit" project, supported by a grant from the Robert

Wood Johnson Foundation of researchers at the University of Rhode Island. This project reviewed and compiled a list of research instruments recommended for use in palliative care. The tool kit is available online at http://www.chcr.brown.edu/web-pubs.htm#top.

Subject attrition is another common problem area in palliative care research.[28] Higher attrition has serious implications when determining sample sizes and also has budget implications. This problem area becomes an even greater concern in longitudinal studies, which are a definite need in palliative care.[20] New approaches to handling data are needed to improve data analysis.[29]

Palliative care research also necessitates diversity in research methods. The authors' experience has been that a combination of qualitative and quantitative approaches is needed.[23] Appendix 66–1 includes examples of two palliative nursing studies (one quantitative, one qualitative) that serve as models for application of these methods for palliative care research. Quantitative approaches are essential when studying symptoms and QOL, their frequency and nature, and response to treatment. Qualitative approaches are especially important in descriptive studies, and are a useful approach in describing "the lived experience" of terminally ill patients using their own narratives.

The authors also have found that nursing research in palliative care is greatly enhanced by interdisciplinary collaboration. The problems studied are multidimensional and are best defined from the viewpoints of various members of the health-care team. Participation from colleagues in psychology, theology, social work, and other disciplines has enhanced our work considerably.

A final special consideration in palliative care research is the importance of including family caregivers.[30] Terminal illness is a shared experience, and including family caregivers as subjects enriches the benefits to be derived from the research.[30]

Table 66–1 summarizes some of the key challenges of conducting palliative care research. Advancement of the nursing profession in palliative care will require attention to overcome these obstacles.

## A Research Agenda in Palliative Nursing

The Institute of Medicine (IOM), the health arm of the National Academy of Sciences of the United States, identified priority areas for end-of-life care research, including pain, cachexia-anorexia-asthenia, dyspnea, cognitive, and emotional symptoms. Also addressed was the need for social, behavioral, and health services research. Nursing as a profession has much to contribute to each of these identified priorities.[3]

There is a tremendous need to bring together nurse researchers and nurse clinicians in palliative care. Historically, few nurse researchers have focused on palliative care; likewise, few expert clinicians in palliative care have had opportunities or expertise in research.

Although an exhaustive review of research methods or grant writing is not possible in this chapter, a few comments are worthy of attention. Palliative care clinicians are encouraged to seek collaboration with nurse researchers to initiate clinically relevant and scientifically sound studies.[31] Another key issue of advice is to begin small. Conducting small pilot studies is an essential foundation to launching larger-scale studies. Potential sources for funding are found in Table 66–2.

Table 66–3 includes an example of criteria used in evaluating small-scale research projects. These criteria, adapted from the Oncology Nursing Foundation, depict the essential elements of a research proposal. Many professional organizations

---

**Table 66–1**
**Barriers to Nursing Research in Palliative Care**

- Overall limitations in funding for nursing research and in the limited number of nurse researchers.
- Research establishment and associated funding that has been focused on rehabilitation or cure.
- Lack of political or consumer advocates to promote a research agenda in end-of-life care.
- Limited focus on palliative care in graduate nursing education to promote end-of-life research within master's or doctoral nursing education.
- Few established relationships between nurse researchers and clinical settings of palliative care.
- Ethical considerations of conducting research with vulnerable populations, including issues related to ability to provide consent.
- Rapidly declining status, which limits subject accrual and opportunity for longitudinal measures.
- Lack of conceptual frameworks appropriate for palliative care research.
- Interference with demands of patient care caused by participation in research.
- Late referrals to hospice or palliative care programs, which severely restricts opportunities for accrual to studies.
- Lack of research instruments and methods appropriate for this population.
- Challenge of conducting research in a sensitive area.
- Need to balance demands of rigorous research, such as the need for randomization, with awareness of patient needs.

*Source:* Adapted from Field and Cassel (1997), reference 44, and Doyle et al. (2004), reference 45.

**Table 66-2**
**Funding Sources for Pilot Studies**

Hospital Continuous Quality Improvement programs
Oncology Nursing Foundation
Sigma Theta Tau
American Nursing Foundation
American Society of Pain Management Nurses
Local community foundations
Pharmaceutical companies
Hospice and Palliative Nursing Association

provide small grant support to novice investigators. Table 66–4 includes some general tips for preparing a research proposal. Steele and colleagues published a two-part series on their pilot study on transitioning families into pediatric hospice care. The first part of the series described the planning phase of their pilot study. The investigators described their rationale in conducting the study and provided a detailed description of the study site, recruitment of subjects, study procedures, data collection plan, and data analysis plan, as well as the challenges of conducting the study.[32] In the second part of the series, the investigators reported their findings.[33] The authors

**Table 66-3**
**Research Proposal Evaluation Criteria**

**Abstract**
• Abstract accurately reflects the proposal.
• Abstract includes problem statement and purpose.
• Abstract summarizes key variables, sample, and methods.

**Study aims, hypotheses, or study questions**
• Clearly stated
• Hypotheses or study questions are consistent with the study aim.
• All proposed study procedures and data to be collected are encompassed.

**Significance of the study**
• The research contributes to the science of palliative nursing care.
• The research has the potential to lead to further investigation.
• The research offers a unique contribution to the literature.
• The research is clinically relevant to end-of-life care.

**Literature review**
• Relevant and current literature is reviewed.
• Literature primarily includes research rather than opinion.
• Literature is critiqued, synthesized, and analyzed.

**Conceptual/theoretical framework**
• Framework identified is appropriate to the study and consistent with study questions and methods.
• Framework is consistent with the philosophy of palliative care.

**Procedures**
• The procedures are feasible.
• Procedures include methods for training and supervision of personnel.
• Procedures provide sufficient description of precisely what will be required of subjects.

**Data analysis**
• Specific statistical procedures are identified.
• Analysis is appropriate for the type of data and study design and answers the study questions.
• Computer facilities and consultation are described.
• Investigator has sought consultation if necessary in preparing the proposal.

**Human subjects considerations**
• Institutional Review Board approval is given or documentation of pending review is given.
• The investigator is clearly aware of the impact of participation in the study on the subject.
• The investigator addresses concerns regarding length, intrusiveness, and energy expenditure required.
• The investigator has acknowledged special considerations of terminal illness.

**Investigators and research team**
• Consultation is available for the less experienced researcher.
• The role of co-investigators or consultants is established.

**Overall**
• The proposal strictly adheres to format restrictions and page limitations

*Source:* Adapted from reference 46.

**Table 66–4**
**General Tips for Preparing Research Proposals**

- Grant writing is not a solo activity—seek consultation and collaboration from others. Seek opportunities to involve clinical palliative care settings, such as hospices, in nursing research.
- Have your proposal reviewed by peers before submitting it for funding. A proposal submitted for funding is generally the product of numerous revisions.
- Follow the directions in detail, including margins, page limits, and the use of references and appendices. Communicate directly with the funding source to clarify any directions you are unsure of.
- State ideas clearly and succinctly. Word economy is essential to a fine-tuned proposal.
- Use high-quality printing and use a good-quality copier. Give attention to spelling and grammar.
- Plan ahead and develop a time frame for completing your grant. Avoid the last-minute rush that will compromise the quality of your proposal. It is better to target a future deadline for submission than to compromise your score due to a lack of time for preparation.
- Use appendices to include study instruments, procedures, or other supporting materials. Adhere to funding agency criteria, but maximize the opportunity for a complete proposal.
- Include support letters from individuals who are important to the success of your study. This includes medical staff, nursing administration, consultants, and co-investigators.
- Do not hesitate to contact experts in your subject area to seek their input. They are often able to review your work and direct you toward related instruments or literature.
- Start small. Successful completion of a pilot project is the best foundation for a larger study. Efficient use of small grant funding is influential when seeking larger-scale funding for major proposals.
- Be realistic. Design research projects that can be realistically accomplished within the scope of your other responsibilities and the limitations of your work setting.
- Keep focused on the patient. Design and implement research that is relevant to patient care and improves quality of life at the end of life for patients and families.

*Source:* Ferrell et al. (1989), reference 47.

---

concluded that study findings will help with the development of a nursing intervention to aid families with transitioning to pediatric hospices. Palliative care research that also publishes the study development process is helpful in assisting novice palliative care researchers to understand the challenges, limitations, as well as rewards in designing quality palliative care studies.

Another useful guide for nurses initiating research proposals is included in Table 66–5. This includes the review considerations used by grant reviewers at the NIH. The five criteria of significance, approach, innovation, investigation, and environment can serve as a useful guide in designing research proposals.[11]

Several initiatives have begun to establish an agenda for palliative care research. Topics frequently identified as priority topics for palliative care research include pain, symptom management, epidemiological studies of terminal illness, family caregiver needs, bereavement, cultural considerations, spiritual needs, and health systems considerations such as costs of care.[34,35] Examples of palliative care research topics by nurse researchers include understanding the meaning of QOL domains such as social and spiritual well-being,[36,37] the experience of palliative care in the urban poor,[38] providing palliative and end-of-life care for nursing-home residents,[39] and evaluating innovative end-of-life programs in nursing homes.[40]

At the City of Hope, we have developed a framework of nine areas of palliative nursing care that is used in our nursing education efforts (see Chapter 64). Table 66–6 includes a summary of these nine topic areas, with examples of potential research that is needed.[41]

Another excellent resource for identifying future areas of palliative care research comes from the conference convened by the NINR described previously.[11] An excerpt of the Executive Summary from this NIH research workshop, which focused on symptom management in terminal illness, is included as Appendix 66–2, together with the specific recommendations from that conference, which identified research needs regarding the symptoms of pain, dyspnea, cognitive disturbances, and cachexia.[11]

## Summary

Advances in the care of patients and families facing terminal illness are contingent on advances in palliative nursing research. Control of symptoms, comfort for families, and attention to psychosocial and spiritual needs will improve when nurse clinicians have a stronger scientific foundation for practice.[15,42] Research will require collaboration with other disciplines and unity of nurse clinicians and researchers.

| Table 66–5 |
| --- |
| **Review Considerations for Research Sponsored by the National Institutes of Health** |
| **Significance**<br>Does this study address an important problem? If the aims of the application are achieved, how will scientific knowledge be advanced? What will be the effect of these studies on the concepts or methods that drive this field? |
| **Approach**<br>Are the conceptual framework, design, methods, and analyses adequately developed, well integrated, and appropriate to the aims of the project? Does the applicant acknowledge potential problem areas and consider alternative tactics? |
| **Innovation**<br>Does the project employ novel concepts, approaches, or methods? Are the aims original and innovative? Does the project challenge existing paradigms or develop new methodologies or technologies? |
| **Investigator**<br>Is the investigator appropriately trained and well suited to carry out this work? Is the work proposed appropriate to the experience level of the principal investigator and other researchers (if any)? |
| **Environment**<br>Does the scientific environment in which the work will be done contribute to the probability of success? Do the proposed experiments take advantage of unique features of the scientific environment or employ useful collaborative arrangements? Is there evidence of institutional support? |
| **Additional considerations**<br>In addition, the adequacy of plans to include both genders and minorities and their subgroups as appropriate for the scientific goals of the research are reviewed. Plans for the recruitment and retention of subjects is also evaluated. |
| *Source*: Adapted from reference 46. |

APPENDIX 66–1

## Two Examples of Palliative Nursing Studies

### Symptom Concerns and Quality of Life in Hepatobiliary Cancers

*Virginia Sun, RN, MSN, ANP*
City of Hope

The purpose of this study was to describe the symptoms concern of hepatocellular carcinoma (HCC) and pancreatic cancer patients and explore the impact of symptoms on overall QOL.

Hepatobiliary cancers are often diagnosed at advanced stages with poor prognosis. This poor prognosis is coupled with multiple symptom occurrences that result in a rapid decline in patient function and QOL. Only a modest number of studies in the literature have addressed symptoms and QOL in this understudied cancer population. Study framework is based upon the City of Hope QOL model and on the Functional Assessment of Chronic Illness Therapy (FACIT) model. This framework demonstrates that disease and treatment-related symptoms may influence QOL across the physical, social, emotional, functional, and spiritual domains. Intervening variables include patient and disease characteristics, treatment, and comorbidities. A prospective, longitudinal design was used to complete study aims. Participants were recruited from ambulatory clinics of one comprehensive cancer center. Eligibility criteria included a diagnosis of

HCC or pancreatic cancer, at least age 18 years, and ability to understand English. Forty-five HCC and pancreatic cancer patients were accrued and followed for 3 months, and outcome measures were administered monthly. Descriptive analysis of demographic, treatment, and symptom data was conducted, followed by two-way repeated measures Analysis of Variance (ANOVA) of QOL scores by diagnosis. Overall, symptoms concerns were high for weight loss, appetite, fatigue, ability to perform usual activities, and abdominal pain. There was a trend of worsening of these symptoms over time. Overall QOL scores were low in both the HCC and pancreatic cancer groups, and continued to decrease over time. At baseline, QOL subscale scores were highest for social well-being ($X = 22.6$, SD = 4.3). Conversely, scores were lowest for functional well-being ($X = 13.7$, SD = 5.9). At 3 months evaluation, social well-being remained highest ($X = 22.9$, SD = 5.3), whereas physical well-being was lowest ($X = 10.8$, SD = 7.1). Spiritual well-being in the pancreatic cancer group was significantly higher than the HCC group at three month evaluation. Pearson's correlations suggest that symptoms were highly correlated with physical well-being, functional well-being, emotional well-being, and overall QOL scores. Findings will be discussed in light of the Vulnerable Populations Model, where the relationship between resource availability, risk factors, and health status will be explored in this sample population. Hepatobiliary cancers are associated with high symptom burden and declining QOL, which continues through treatment and disease progression. Further understanding through research of the symptoms experience

**Table 66-6**
**Potential Areas for Research in End-of-Life (EOL) Care**

| Critical Areas of End-of-Life Care | Examples of Area Content | Examples of Potential Areas of Inquiry |
|---|---|---|
| 1. The Concept of Palliative Care | A. Importance of palliative care for nurses<br>B. Definitions of palliative care<br>C. Important goals/characteristics of palliative care:<br>   1. Dignity/Respect<br>   2. Relief of symptoms<br>   3. Peaceful death<br>   4. Ethical issues<br>   5. Patient control/choices<br>D. Importance of interdisciplinary collaboration<br>E. Recognition of nurses' own discomfort/anxiety | • Refinement of definitions/criteria for palliative care<br>• Descriptive studies of interdisciplinary involvement and related outcomes<br>• Evaluation of methods to provide staff support in palliative care |
| 2. Quality of Life (QOL) at the EOL | A. Recognition of multiple dimensions of QOL at the EOL<br>   1. Physical well-being<br>   2. Psychological well-being<br>   3. Social well-being<br>   4. Spiritual well-being | • Development/testing of QOL instruments for use in palliative care<br>• Refinement of research methods to decrease patient burden in QOL assessment<br>• Development/testing of QOL instruments for family caregivers |
| 3. Pain Management at EOL | A. Definition of pain<br>B. Assessment of pain<br>C. Assessment of meaning of pain<br>D. Pharmacological management of pain at EOL<br>E. Use of invasive techniques<br>F. Principles of addiction, tolerance, and dependence<br>G. Nonpharmacological management of pain<br>H. Physical pain vs. suffering<br>I. Side effects of opioids<br>J. Barriers to pain management<br>K. Fear of opioids hastening death<br>L. Equianalgesic dosing<br>M. Recognition of nurses' own burden in pain management at EOL | • Methods of assessing pain in the nonverbal or confused patient<br>• Refine methods for pain assessment to decrease patient burden<br>• Development of pain measures that incorporate all dimensions of pain at EOL (e.g., spiritual pain)<br>• Intervention studies to treat common pain syndromes at EOL<br>• Testing of protocols to treat pain at EOL, including changing routes of analgesia<br>• Development/evaluation of teaching programs for patients/families to decrease fears regarding pain management<br>• Development/evaluation of programs to educate/support nurses in managing pain |
| 4. Other Symptom Management at EOL | A. Assessment and management of common EOL symptoms<br>   1. Dyspnea/cough<br>   2. Nausea/vomiting<br>   3. Dehydration/nutrition<br>   4. Altered mental status/delirium/terminal restlessness<br>   5. Anxiety/depression<br>   6. Weakness/fatigue<br>   7. Dysphagia<br>   8. Incontinence<br>   9. Skin integrity<br>   10. Constipation/bowel obstruction<br>   11. Agitation/myoclonus | • Descriptive studies to better understand<br>• Symptom prevalence and patterns at EOL<br>• Evaluation of pharmacologic treatments for each symptom<br>• Development of patient/family caregiver education for symptom management, including pharmacological and nonpharmacological treatments<br>• Evaluation of protocols/algorithms to<br>• Enhance nurses' effectiveness in symptom<br>• Assessment and management |

*(continued)*

**Table 66–6**
**Potential Areas for Research in End-of-Life (EOL) Care** *(continued)*

| Critical Areas of End-of-Life Care | Examples of Area Content | Examples of Potential Areas of Inquiry |
|---|---|---|
| 5. Communication with Dying Patients and Families | A. Definition/goals of communication<br>B. Importance of listening<br>C. Barriers to communication<br>D. Delivering bad news/truth-telling<br>E. Recognizing family dynamics in communication<br>F. Sensitivity to culture, ethnicity, values, and religion<br>G. Discussion of options/decisions with patients/family<br>H. Communication among interdisciplinary team members/collaboration<br>I. Responding to requests for assisted suicide | • Descriptive studies to better determine common areas of concern regarding communication at EOL<br>• Studies that describe the role of nursing in communication<br>• Evaluation of protocols for delivering/ reinforcing bad news<br>• Studies that explore cultural issues influencing communication<br>• Evaluation of methods that support communication (e.g., written materials, family conferences)<br>• Exploration of decision making by patients and family caregivers<br>• Exploration of causes of requests for assisted suicide and preparation of nurses to respond to requests |
| 6. Role/Needs of Family Caregivers in EOL Care | A. The importance of recognizing family and caregivers needs at EOL<br>B. Assessment of family needs<br>C. Family dynamics<br>D. Recognizing ethical/cultural influences<br>E. Coping strategies and support systems | • Descriptive studies to enhance under-standing of the family caregiver perspective of terminal illness<br>• Studies that explore family dynamics and the family as a unit rather than focus only on single caregivers<br>• Exploratory studies to enhance understanding of cultural influences |
| 7. Care at the Time of Death | A. The nurse's personal death awareness<br>B. Death as natural process<br>C. Recognizing signs/symptoms of impending death<br>D. Patient/family's fears associated with death<br>E. Preparing for the death event<br>   1. Health care providers<br>   2. Patient<br>   3. Family caregivers<br>F. Physical care at the time of death<br>G. Spiritual care at the time of death | • Evaluation of educational/support approaches to enhance personal death awareness<br>• Evaluation of teaching approaches to prepare families for impending death<br>• Development and evaluation of protocols for care at the time of death—i.e., physical and spiritual care |
| 8. Issues of Policy, Ethics, and Law | A. Patient preferences/advance directives<br>B. Assisted suicide<br>C. Euthanasia<br>D. Withdrawing food/fluids<br>E. Discontinuing life support<br>F. Legal issues at the EOL<br>G. Need for changes in health policy<br>H. Confidentiality | • Evaluation of approaches to enhance use of advance directives<br>• Testing of educational methods to enhance nurses' ability to respond to requests for assisted suicide/ euthanasia<br>• Development and evaluation of protocols that promote patient comfort while discontinuing food/ fluids and life support<br>• Identification of legal and regulatory barriers to optimal EOL care |
| 9. Bereavement | A. Stages/process of grief<br>B. Assessment of grief<br>C. Interventions/resources<br>D. Recognition of staff grief | • Descriptive studies of grief by patients, families, and staff with attention to cultural considerations<br>• Refinement of efficient methods of grief assessment<br>• Testing of approaches to facilitate staff grieving |

## Meanings and Uses of an Expressed Desire for Hastened Death in People Living with Advanced Cancer

*Nessa Coyle, PhD, APRN, FAAN*
Memorial Sloan-Kettering Cancer Center

An exploratory qualitative study, using an interpretive phenomenological approach, explored the impact of advanced cancer on seven individuals living with the disease. These individuals had received the majority of their care at an urban research cancer center and had expressed, at least once, a desire for hastened death.[31] The hypothesis was that by providing an individual the space to talk about his or her lived experience through a series of in-depth, semistructured interviews, the grounds for the expression of desire for hastened death for that individual would be uncovered. A total of 25 interviews were held.

Through an interpretive analysis of the narratives of the seven individuals, four themes and two overarching themes were identified. The four themes were "Listen to Me," in which the participants described their relationships to the healthcare system; "Who Am I Now and Where Do I Belong?," in which the participants dealt with changes in themselves and their place in the world; "Up Against the Wall—There Is No Way to Live with Such Pain," in which the participants described their experiences with excruciating or chronically uncontrolled pain; and "The Existential Slap," the moment of realization by the participants that death was imminent. The two overarching themes were "The Hard Work of Living in the Face of Death" and the "Existential Paradox"—that is, that although the participants had expressed at least once a desire for death, what they were seeking was life.

The overarching themes appeared to capture the paradox of an expressed desire for hastened death and informed the interpretive analysis of the narratives—that an expressed desire for hastened death in these participants was a tool of communication reflecting:

1. A manifestation of the will to live
2. That the dying process itself was so difficult that an early death was preferred
3. That the immediate situation was untenable and required immediate action
4. That a hastened death was an option to extract oneself from an unendurable situation
5. A manifestation of the last control the dying can exert
6. A way of drawing attention to "me as a unique individual"
7. A gesture of altruism
8. Manipulation of the family in order to avoid abandonment
9. A despairing cry depicting the misery of the current situation

The overall interpretation was that an expressed desire for hastened death in these individuals was not a literal request for death but a tool of communication to get needs met.[43]

APPENDIX 66-2

## NIH Research Workshop on Symptoms in Terminal Illness—Executive Summary

Patients at the end of life experience many of the same symptoms and syndromes, regardless of their underlying medical condition. Pain is the most obvious example, but others are difficult breathing (dyspnea), transient episodes of confusion and loss of concentration (cognitive disturbances and delirium), and loss of appetite and muscle wasting (cachexia), as well as nausea, fatigue, and depression. Taken together, these and other symptoms add significantly to the suffering of patients and their families, and to the costs and burden of their medical care. Yet in many cases the symptoms could be treated or prevented.

Pain, for example, is a multibillion-dollar public health problem in the United States. More than half of all cancer patients experience pain related to their disease or its treatment. Similarly, half of all cancer patients and 70% of all hospice patients experience shortness of breath in the last weeks of life. Yet dyspnea remains underdiagnosed and undertreated. Forty percent of all patients experience cognitive disturbances during the final days of life, and high numbers of terminally ill patients experience cachexia regardless of their primary disease. Significantly, these symptoms occur not in isolation but in clusters, with most patients experiencing combinations of symptoms that vary greatly in their prevalence and severity, as well as in the suffering they cause.

Basic research has improved understanding of the underlying mechanisms of symptoms that are commonly experienced at the end of life, particularly with respect to pain. Clinical research has in some cases translated this knowledge into new drugs and other interventions that can effectively relieve or prevent these symptoms, even if the underlying disease cannot be cured. However, there remain a number of important gaps in knowledge.

Clinical care would benefit from an integrative, multidisciplinary research initiative that brings basic and clinical researchers together to address the constellation of symptoms at the end of life. The following areas should receive priority:

- Epidemiology—There is a need for better data on the incidence and combinations of symptoms that are experienced at the end of life in specific populations. Epidemiological data will demonstrate the magnitude and costs of the problem and suggest specific topics for basic and clinical research.
- Basic research—Additional research is needed on the mechanisms and interactions of these symptoms,

including biochemical, neuronal, endocrine, and immune approaches. The possibility of common factors, mechanisms, and pathways across different symptoms should be examined. There is also a need for research on the mechanism of action of successful therapies, with particular attention to the role of opioid receptors. This research could lead to therapies that are better targeted and more selective in their action, and thus produce fewer side effects.

- Clinical research—Because these symptoms have multiple determinants, and occur in clusters, successful interventions will also be multifactorial, including behavioral as well as pharmacological approaches. Combination therapies and off-label drugs should be explored. Researchers should be alert to differences in outcome based on age, gender, and underlying disease. Interventions to mobilize psychosocial and spiritual resources may be of help in mediating the perception and interpretation of symptoms. The goal of research should be to test a wide range of interventions that could be successfully implemented in the home or hospice, as well as in the hospital.
- Methodology—Researchers need better tests for diagnosing and assessing the level of severity of these symptoms, as well as for monitoring the effectiveness of interventions. Standardized terminology and definitions of symptoms should be established. Particular attention should be paid to validating subjective and nonverbal measures. Better data and tools are also needed for evaluating outcomes, in order to determine costs and strengthen accountability for the quality of care at the end of life. It is important to develop and use measures that reflect the subjective experience of the effects of symptoms on quality of life.

Research is also needed on the ethical issues that may be barriers to research at the end of life, including the needs and protection of vulnerable populations, especially the role of privacy during this important phase of life. Attention must be paid to community and individual preferences about the relative value of symptom management at different points in the dying trajectory, and to the development of comprehensive strategies for early detection and treatment of the full range of symptoms at the end of life—an approach that will reduce costs as well as burdens, while preserving the patient's dignity and quality of life.

## Recommendations for Research on Specific Symptoms

The following preamble for the recommendations reflected the consensus of the entire workshop:

> To adequately address symptom control in the terminally ill, an important first step is to invest resources in the development of new methodologies for assessing symptoms and evaluating treatments. These tools will allow us to elucidate the extent of

the problem and to set national priorities to improve quality of life for those facing life-limiting illness.

### Pain

1. Epidemiology—There is still a great need for epidemiological data on the incidence and types of pain at the end of life. Research in this area will provide direction for researchers regarding what specific topics should be tackled next.
2. Treatment—There is a clear need to discover new drugs for the treatment of pain, including analgesic combinations. Neuropathic pain, because of its incidence and burden, should be a particular priority. There should also be studies of the relationship between disease, pain, and suffering at the end of life, which would also include psychosocial mediators. Clinical Trials Groups should be developed to study promising interventions.
3. Measurement—Methods should be developed for collecting valid data on pain in the home, in nursing homes, and so on, possibly using telephones or computer technology. Measurement of other outcomes of subjective experience, such as the suffering caused by pain, should also be developed and utilized.

### Dyspnea

1. Epidemiology—What are the incidence and impact of dyspnea in different populations? There is some information about dyspnea in patients with cancer or chronic obstructive pulmonary disease (COPD), but almost none about patients with cardiac disease or other terminal conditions.
2. Mechanisms—Relatively little is known about the various determinants of dyspnea, including respiratory muscle strength, exercise capacity, respiratory controller, gas exchange, and psychosocial factors. Neurobiological models, like those developed for pain, will be useful, but the overall approach must be integrative. The determinants are almost certainly multifactorial, necessitating multidisciplinary strategies.
3. Measurement—Research is needed to refine available instruments and develop new ones for measuring both the causes of symptoms and the effects of treatments. There is at present no standardized approach for assessing the degree of dyspnea in a given disease (e.g., chronic vs. acute, COPD vs. cancer). The goal would be to formulate guidelines for optimal assessment, which would point to optimal treatment.
4. Treatment—Numerous potential treatments are available, but there is little information on their relative effectiveness. Particular attention should be given to the choice and timing of anxiolytics, phenothiazines, oxygen, opiates, and exercise. Attention should also be given to the timing and

management of terminal weaning (removal of ventilation), including the role of families.

The collaborative and integrative nature of this research is well suited to sponsorship and funding by NIH. It would be useful, for example, for the various NIH Institutes to sponsor a series of joint workshops that would characterize the clinical experience and impact of therapies on dyspnea in diseases other than lung cancer.

## Cognitive Disturbances

There is a considerable amount of epidemiological data on delirium already, and although it might be useful to gather additional information on specific patient populations, this symptom is known to be under recognized and under treated. Consequently, the research priorities in this symptom area are as follows:

1. Measurement—Research is needed to enhance the recognition of delirium in different treatment settings (homes, hospices, hospitals), including common diagnostic criteria and terminology. Also needed are better instruments to describe and rate the severity and course of episodes of delirium. This research will lead to a better understanding of the phenomenology of delirium—its signs, patterns, and subtypes—which in turn should produce benefits in terms of newer, more sensitive, and more effective treatments.
2. Treatment—Two aspects of treatment research deserve simultaneous attention. First, there should be randomized, placebo-controlled trials to systematically assess the efficacy of currently available therapies as well as emerging approaches, including both pharmacological and nonpharmacological strategies. Second, there should be research on the relation between the mechanism of action of these therapies and the underlying pathophysiology of delirium. In both cases, studies should include both random populations and populations with delirium of homogeneous etiology.
3. Epidemiology—Finally, there is a need for additional research on the interactions between delirium and other symptoms at the end of life.
4. A concurrent policy issue that must also receive priority attention is the need for guidelines for research in patients who are incapable of giving informed consent because of serious medical illness.

## *Cachexia*

1. Epidemiology—High priority should go to epidemiological studies of anorexia-cachexia, to establish the magnitude of the problem, its impact on the patient and family, and its costs to society. However, it is important that cachexia not be studied in isolation from other symptoms. If the ultimate goal of cachexia research is prevention and early intervention, then it would be useful to conduct studies that examine the epidemiology of several related symptoms (e.g., pain, dyspnea, delirium) at an earlier stage in their development.
2. Mechanisms—Basic and clinical research on cachexia should be done in parallel. Basic research should emphasize the interactions among multiple underlying pathophysiological mechanisms, both central and peripheral, including biochemical, neuronal, metabolic, endocrine, and immunological. Research is also needed on the varying clinical manifestations of these mechanisms, both neuropsychiatric and gastrointestinal. This calls for a multidisciplinary approach.
3. Treatment—Similarly, because it is unlikely that any single therapeutic intervention will be successful, clinical research should emphasize multiple combination therapies that include nutritional, pharmacological, and nonpharmacological components. Combination therapies should be evaluated for their effects on other symptoms such as pain, dyspnea, and delirium. Particular attention should also be paid to differences in outcome based on age, gender, and underlying disease. In considering drug trials, NIH should concentrate on studies that would not otherwise be funded by drug companies.

Given the wide range of mechanisms and therapeutic strategies in cachexia, it would be useful to convene a preliminary, integrative workshop that would include both basic and clinical researchers

## *Cross-Cutting Recommendations*

Methods issues that need to be addressed in all four symptom areas include the following:

1. Statistical handling of missing data.
2. Proxy reporting for subjective symptoms.
3. Outcome measures that indicate quality care.
4. Ethics issues are also important. What are the barriers to research at the end of life, including the needs and expectations of vulnerable populations? What are community and individual preferences with respect to symptom management of dying persons?
5. Economics questions include the direct and indirect costs and burdens of symptoms.

REFERENCES

1. Polit D, Beck C. Nursing Research: Principles and Methods. Philadelphia, PA: Lippincott Williams & Wilkins, 2004.
2. Payne SA, Turner JM. Research methodologies in palliative care: A bibliometric analysis. Palliat Med 2008;22(4):336–342.
3. Kristjanson LJ, Coyle N. Qualitative research. In: Doyle D, Hanks G, Cherny N, Calman K, eds. Oxford Textbook of

Palliative Medicine (3rd ed). Oxford: Oxford University Press; 2004:138–144.

4. King CR, Hinds PS, eds. Quality of Life from Nursing and Patient Perspectives (2nd ed). Sudbury, MA: Jones and Bartlett, 2003.

5. Dawson S, Kristjanson LJ. Mapping the journey: Family carers' perceptions of issues related to end-stage care of individuals with muscular dystrophy or motor neurone disease. J Palliat Care 2003;19:36–42.

6. Patterson LB, Dorfman LT. Family support for hospice caregivers. Am J Hospice Palliat Care 2002;139(5 Pt 2):410–415.

7. Brazil K, Bedard M, Willison K, Hode M. Caregiving and its impact on families of the terminally ill. Aging Ment Health 2003;7:376–382.

8. Bailey C, Froggatt K, Field D, Krishnasamy M. The nursing contribution to qualitative research in palliative care 1990–1999: A critical evaluation. J Adv Nurs 2002;40(1):48–60.

9. Benoliel JQ. Death influence in clinical practice: A course for graduate students. In: Benoliel JQ, ed. Death Education for the Health Professional. Washington, DC: Hemisphere Publishing, 1982:31–50.

10. Benoliel JQ. Health-care providers and dying patients: Critical issues in terminal care. Omega 1987;18:341–363.

11. National Institutes of Health. Symptoms in Terminal Illness: A Research Workshop. September 22–23, 1997. Available at: http://www .nih.gov/ninr/end-of-life.htm (accessed December 8, 2008).

12. Prince-Paul M, Daly BJ. Moving beyond the anecdotal. Identifying the need for evidence-based research in hospice and palliative care. Home Healthc Nurse 2008;26(4):214–219; quiz 20–21.

13. Kuebler KK, Lynn J, Von Rohen J. Perspectives in palliative care. Semin Oncol Nurs 2005;21(1):2–10.

14. Flemming K, Adamson J, Atkin K. Improving the effectiveness of interventions in palliative care: The potential role of qualitative research in enhancing evidence from randomized controlled trials. Palliat Med 2008;22(2):123–131.

15. Kaasa S, Hjermstad MJ, Loge JH. Methodological and structural challenges in palliative care research: How have we fared in the last decades? Palliat Med 2006;20(8):727–734.

16. Casarett D, Ferrell B, Kirschling J, et al. NHCPO tast force statement on the ethics of hospice participation in research. J Palliat Med 2001;4:441–449.

17. Cohen SR, Mount BM. Quality of life in terminal illness: Defining and measuring subjective well being in the dying. J Palliat Care 1992;8:40–45.

18. American Geriatric Society Panel on Chronic Pain in Older Persons. AGS Clinical Guidelines: Management of Persistent Pain in Older Persons. 2002. Available at: http://www. americangeriatrics.org/education/executive_summ.shtml (accessed March 22, 2005).

19. Calman K, MacDonald N, Downie R, et al. Ethical issues. In: Doyle D, Hanks G, Cherny N, Calman K, eds. Oxford Textbook of Palliative Medicine. Oxford: Oxford University Press; 2004:55–97.

20. Boult L, Dentler B, Volicer L, Mead S, Evans JM; Ethics Committee of the American Medical Directors Association. Position statement: Ethics and research in longterm care. J Am Med Dir Assoc 2003;4:171–174.

21. Meier DE, Beresford L. Advanced practice nurses in palliative care: A pivotal role and perspective. J Palliat Med 2006;9(3):624–627.

22. Cheung YB, Goh C, Thumboo J, Khoo KS, Wee J. Variability and sample size requirements of quality-of-life measures: A randomized study of three major questionnaires. J Clin Oncol 2005;23(22):4936–4944.

23. Ferrans CE. Differences in what quality-of-life instruments measure. J Natl Cancer Inst 2007;(37):22–26.

24. Granda-Cameron C, Viola SR, Lynch MP, Polomano RC. Measuring patient-oriented outcomes in palliative care: Functionality and quality of life. Clin J Oncol Nurs 2008;12(1):65–77.

25. Jordhoy MS, Inger Ringdal G, Helbostad JL, Oldervoll L, Loge JH, Kaasa S. Assessing physical functioning: A systematic review of quality of life measures developed for use in palliative care. Palliat Med 2007;21(8):673–682.

26. Kaasa S, Loge JH. Quality of life in palliative care: Principles and practice. Palliat Med 2003;17(1):11–20.

27. Kelly B, McClement S, Chochinov HM. Measurement of psychological distress in palliative care. Palliat Med 2006;20(8):779–789.

28. Steinhauser KE, Clipp EC, Hays JC, et al. Identifying, recruiting, and retaining seriously ill patients and their caregivers in longitudinal research. Palliat Med 2006;20(8):745–754.

29. Hopkinson JB, Wright DN, Corner JL. Seeking new methodology for palliative care research: Challenging assumptions about studying people who are approaching the end of life. Palliat Med 2005;19(7):532–537.

30. McClement SE, Woodgate RL. Research with families in palliative care: Conceptual and methodological challenges. Eur J Cancer Care 1998;7(4):247–254.

31. Gelfman LP, Morrison RS. Research funding for palliative medicine. J Palliat Med 2008;11(1):36–43.

32. Steele R, Derman S, Cadell S, Davies B, Siden H, Straatman L. Families' transition to a Canadian pediatric hospice. Part one: Planning a pilot study. Int J Palliat Nurs 2008;14(5):248–256.

33. Steele R, Derman S, Cadell S, Davies B, Siden H, Straatman L. Families' transition to a Canadian paediatric hospice. Part two: Results of a pilot study. Int J Palliat Nurs 2008;14(6):287–295.

34. Smith TJ, Coyne P, Cassel B, Penberthy L, Lopson A, Hager MA. A high-volume specialist palliative care unit and team may reduce in-hospital end-of-life care costs. J Palliat Med 2003;6:699–705.

35. Lynn J, Nolan K, Kabcenell A, Wessman D, Milne C, Berwick DM; End-of-Life Care Consensus Panel. Reforming care for persons near the end of life: The promise of quality improvement. Ann Intern Med 2002;137:117–122.

36. Prince-Paul M. Understanding the meaning of social well-being at the end of life. Oncol Nurs Forum 2008;35(3):365–371.

37. Prince-Paul M. Relationships among communicative acts, social well-being, and spiritual well-being on the quality of life at the end of life in patients with cancer enrolled in hospice. J Palliat Med 2008;11(1):20–25.

38. Hughes A, Gudmundsdottir M, Davies B. Everyday struggling to survive: Experience of the urban poor living with advanced cancer. Oncol Nurs Forum 2007;34(6):1113–1118.

39. Ersek M, Wilson SA. The challenges and opportunities in providing end-of-life care in nursing homes. J Palliat Med 2003;6(1):45–57.

40. Ersek M, Grant MM, Kraybill BM. Enhancing end-of-life care in nursing homes: Palliative Care Educational Resource Team (PERT) program. J Palliat Med 2005;8(3):556–566.

41. Ferrell BR, Virani R, Grant M. Analysis of end of life content in nursing textbooks. Oncol Nurs Forum 1999;26:869–876.

42. Fainsinger RL. Global warming in the palliative care research environment: Adapting to change. Palliat Med 2008; 22(4):328–335.

43. Coyle N. Expressed desire for hastened death in a select group of patients living with advanced cancer: A phenomenological inquiry. Dissertation Abstracts International 2004;63–11B:5156.

44. Field M, Cassel C. Approaching death: Improving care at the end of life. Committee on Care at the End of Life. Washington, DC: Institutes of Medicine, National Academy Press, 1997.

45. Doyle D, Hanks G, Cherny N, Calman K, eds. Oxford Textbook of Palliative Medicine (3rd ed). Oxford: Oxford University Press, 2004.

46. NIH announces updated criteria for evaluating research grant applications. Notice Number: NOT-OD-05-002. October 12, 2004. Available at: http://grants.nih.gov/ grants/guide/notice-files/ NOT-OD-05-002.html (accessed November 24, 2008).

47. Ferrell BR, Nail IM, Mooney K, et al. Applying for oncology nursing society and oncology nursing foundation grants. Oncol Nurs Forum 1989;16:728–730.

# 67

### Shirley Otis-Green and Iris Cohen Fineberg

# Enhancing Team Effectiveness

*By the third day that he was in the ICU I felt as confused as he was and nearly as frightened. Everyone came in and seemed to be telling us different things, but I had no idea what any of it really meant. It wasn't until the family meeting that I finally got a better idea of what we really faced. It was so helpful to have someone give us the big picture and explain what all those tests meant and to know who we could turn to for what!—A 57-year-old spouse of patient in critical care unit*

♦ **Key Points**

♦ *Palliative care is by definition team care. A team approach is necessary to best address the complex multidimensional bio-psychosocial-spiritual concerns of patients and their families.*

♦ *The National Consensus Guidelines for Quality Palliative Care, the National Quality Forum, and the Institute of Medicine recommend a team approach as the optimal delivery system for patient/family-focused care.*

♦ *Health-care professionals are socialized in their own unique disciplines yet are expected to work in a team environment. This makes it imperative that health-care professionals seek opportunities to enhance team skills necessary for effective communication, shared leadership, conflict resolution, role clarification, and addressing boundary issues.*

♦ *Further research is needed to better evaluate the effectiveness of team composition, leadership style, and interventions for different patient populations and settings, as well as a determination of core team competencies needed by differing staff members and how best to prepare participants for effective family meetings.*

The 2009 National Consensus Project (NCP) Guidelines for Quality Palliative Care, the 2006 National Quality Forum (NQF), and the 2008 Institute of Medicine Report all recommend a team approach as the optimal way to provide patient/family-focused care, yet our current socialization of professionals remains discipline-specific. This chapter will provide readers an opportunity to consider various strategies useful in increasing team effectiveness. The use of family meetings is highlighted as an important palliative care team intervention.

#### Professional Socialization and Models of Teamwork

A palliative care team has a collective identity and shared goals of care, recognizing that the patient and family are the "ultimate authority" whose perspective must be integrated in all assessment, implementation, and evaluation plans.[1] Palliative care teams typically include physicians, nurses, social workers, spiritual care professionals, and others with the shared goal of providing whole-person, patient/family-focused care. A team perspective means that individuals have consciously come together with a shared identity to address a common goal.[2] This shared identity differentiates them from a mob (a loose grouping of people with no shared purpose); an ad hoc group (that comes together for a specified need and has typically a reactionary focus); or a single-discipline work group.

Teams exist along a continuum from a multidisciplinary team (typically a consultation-based model, with information shared passively through the medical record); an interdisciplinary team (a more collaborative model but most frequently physician or nurse led) or transdisciplinary/interprofessional team (with intense collaboration and interaction, shared decision-making, and the recognition that there will be significant role overlap).[3]

This transdisciplinary (the term used more commonly in the United States) or interprofessional model, (the more frequently used European or Canadian word), invites professionals to share responsibility for team outcomes, teach and learn from each other, collaborate closely together to meet patient-identified goals and replaces hierarchal decision making with consensus-based decisions that are reflective of the needs of the individual patient/family.[4,5] Transdisciplinary teams seek to exploit discipline diversity as a strategy to best address the complex bio-psychosocial-spiritual needs of patients and their families.[6,7] This trans-disciplinary approach to care evolved from the hospice philosophy and has anthropologic and educational roots and was adopted first in healthcare by pediatric and geriatric care providers.[8-10] Bruder[11] describes this approach in more detail:

> "A transdisciplinary approach requires the team members to share roles and systematically cross discipline boundaries. The primary purpose of this approach is to pool and integrate the expertise of team members so that more efficient and comprehensive assessment and intervention services may be provided. The communication style in this type of team involves continuous give-and-take between all members...on a regular, planned basis. Professionals from different disciplines teach, learn, and work together to accomplish a common set of intervention goals...The role differentiation between disciplines is defined by the needs of the situation rather than by discipline-specific characteristics. Assessment, intervention, and evaluation are carried out jointly by designated members of the team." (p. 61)

As chronic illnesses increase and the bio-psychosocial-spiritual model evolves, health-care systems are challenged to adapt to changing contexts and diversity of expectations. Flexible boundaries and blended roles are expected and accepted based upon a recognition of clinical self-awareness regarding limitations of one's skills and scope of practice.[12] Palliative care teams are evolving now in settings where systems were designed and clinicians were trained to work in the traditional medical model that focused on acute situations. This creates opportunities for new models of care delivery to be evaluated for effectiveness in different environments.

Depending on the setting, team membership might include physicians, nurses, social workers, spiritual care professionals, a variety of integrative therapists (including a range of professionals skilled in the expressive arts), dieticians, occupational therapists, pharmacists, physiotherapists, psychologists, volunteers and the patients and families themselves. Each of these professionals was socialized within their discipline and area of specialization which results in boundary and turf issues that need to be addressed if the team is to be maximally effective. Professionals working together in teams come to that experience with training in their own disciplines with their own vocabulary and theoretical perspective.[13,14] Each discipline has its own ethics, history, and culture.[15] Health-care professionals typically have little formal education in team function and collaboration and may be unaware of normal team processes.[16-21] Each profession conveys to its students and members the norms, expectations, and skills of that profession.[22-24]

This process of socialization, often subtle and unnoticed, teaches people about how to behave as a member of a profession.[25] Although some of the teaching is formal and explicit, much of it is conveyed by less obvious mediums such as our observations in our personal experiences and in the media, modeling of behaviors by senior colleagues, and informal discussions.[26] As a result of our professional education being separate and specific to each discipline within healthcare, most of us know relatively little about how our colleagues on the team were trained and socialized, both generally and specifically in relation to teamwork and collaboration.[27,28] And, we know even less about the unofficial yet powerful socialization that our colleagues have received in clinical settings outside of the formal classroom.[29]

Yet, understanding that each profession socializes its members differently is critical to realizing that the behaviors we see in other team members and behaviors that they see in us, may be a reflection of deeply embedded professional norms in addition to individual views.[28] At the same time, we must be careful to avoid stereotyping a colleague based on their professional group. It is natural to make assumptions about why people behave as they do, but making such assumptions leads us then to react in particular ways. For example, we may assume that a team member's dominating approach to the team results from a lack a respect for colleagues' contributions when it may be a result of professional socialization that equates leadership and quick decision-making with a demonstration of responsibility. If we refrain from making assumptions about why someone behaves as they do, we can use the opportunity to learn more from them about what is behind their behavior or viewpoint. Occasions where differences among team members come to light can serve as opportunities to engage the entire team in a discussion about the norms and teachings of their professions.[30] Thus, differences may transform to strengthening opportunities for the team, especially as the team builds shared views centered on the needs of patients. Learning about the professional socialization of our team members can provide important insights into why people behave as they do, what unspoken assumptions might influence team behavior, and what areas of teamwork might be helpful to explore for the team to optimize its functioning.

Teamwork brings together a group of professionals, each from a different professional culture. If we were bringing together a group of people from different countries to work together, we would recognize the need for dedicated learning about each other's backgrounds, norms, and cultures. This awareness encourages us to be especially open-minded when faced with a conflict, and perhaps less likely to make assumptions about people or their motivations. Taking a similar approach to colleagues and recognizing that team members bring a variety of professional cultures to the team enhances the process and outcomes of teamwork.[14]

## Systems Perspective/Team Evolution

Viewing the team as a system can help us both to understand it and influence it. A systems perspective reminds us that in a system, when any part of the system is changed or affected, there is an impact on the rest of the system. This is true for both positive and negative influences. Using the systems perspective helps us to keep in mind that in a team, no one works in isolation (even if there are people who work as if they are in isolation). What we do influences those around us, and because of this, we have an opportunity to influence our team toward positive change and greater effectiveness.

Teams are noted to evolve over time in typical patterns. Tuckman[31] developed a framework that postulates that teams begin with a period he characterized as "forming" in which the focus of activity is in team development. During the "storming" period that follows, the various members of the team are coming to terms with the idiosyncrasies of their talents. The "norming" phase is noted as the period during which the team develops standard operating procedures. The "performing" period is the most productive time in the life of the team as members are free to concentrate on the tasks that brought the group together. Work tends to be at its most harmonious during this period. Unfortunately, for many health-care teams in teaching hospitals, this period is transitory, as new team members are periodically rotated through the team, resulting in frequent disequilibrium as the team adjusts to each person's coming and going.

## Support for a Team Approach in Palliative Care

A consensus of leading organizations and experts recommend a coordinated interdisciplinary team approach as the best way of delivering patient and family-centered palliative care. The NCP[32] developed evidence-based guidelines that validate the team focus as an ideal strategy to best meet the eight domains identified as necessary for quality palliative care. The eight domains are:

- Structure and processes of care
- Physical aspects of care
- Psychological and psychiatric aspects of care
- Social aspects of care
- Spiritual, religious, and existential aspects of care
- Cultural aspects of care
- Care of the imminently dying patient
- Ethical and legal aspects of care

These domains were adopted in their entirety by the NQF[33] and have been integrated into their 38 preferred practices for the provision of palliative care. The NQF outlines ongoing training and credentialing recommendations for the various members of the team and identifies the benefits of a team approach in developing comprehensive patient-driven care plans. And in 2008, the Institute of Medicine Report: Cancer Care for the Whole Patient: Meeting Psychosocial Health Needs[34] again recommended an integrated team approach as the most effective way to meet patient and families' complex, multidimensional concerns.

## Common Challenges to Optimal Team Functioning

Despite this growing support for a team approach to the delivery of care, there are many challenges to effective team functioning in clinic practice. Prior to instituting actions to foster team effectiveness, it is important to recognize the unique history of each individual health-care team and the institutional context within which it exists.[35] Each setting brings unique demands, whether critical care, an emergency department, an outpatient clinic, a specialized inpatient setting, a long-term care community, a home health agency, or a hospice program.[36]

Attention to improving the functioning of the team calls on members of the team to think about the team as a whole and to dedicate time and group energy to the process of team functioning and team dynamics. Rather than focusing solely on individual professional roles, members of the team collectively determine the shared vision of the team: vision for the role of the team, vision for the organization of the team, and vision for how the team will function and act. Questions to consider when forging a shared vision may include examples such as: How do you want non-team colleagues to view the team? What kind of care do you want this team to provide and to be known for? What does this team see as standards for high-quality functioning for itself? What would team members like from each other? Although the process of exploring and agreeing on a shared vision may take some time and require re-evaluation over time, it is recommended as a worthwhile investment of team effort.

When evaluating an existing team, consider its history of decision-making and its leadership style, its internal communication patterns and how well it collaborates with others outside the team. Are members of the team considered experts within the institution? It is not uncommon for palliative care consult teams to be perceived by others as adopting an attitude of superiority that impedes collaboration. This unintended perspective may not be easily recognized by the existing team, but determining how others view the team provides important insights into its overall effectiveness. For those teams that require referrals to its services, establishing a baseline measurement of where referrals come from and what types of referrals are missing also provides data for later evaluation of areas of needed growth.

The leadership style of a team has tremendous impact on how the team functions.[37,38] Although different leadership models may work better for different teams, a model that has been noted to foster team effectiveness is one of shared vision and shared accountability.[39] This differs dramatically from the model of hierarchical leadership in which one person "at the top" dictates the actions of the group; this "quarterback" model has been historically common in medicine but is no longer viewed as productive in the arena of palliative care.[40] Team meeting facilitators encourage positive support and pay attention to those who feel they have less power or status, building in time to regularly debrief and celebrate personal events and the professional accomplishments of one another.

The tendency for most health-care systems is to default into personal "fiefdoms"[41] with competing and parallel tracks of care versus an integrated delivery of services. Teams constantly struggle with how to share expertise within settings filled with blurred boundaries. Most practitioners have had the experience of working with a professional who behaves like he/she "owns" a patient and may determine all aspects of care that the patient receives. This can be a challenging dynamic as the remaining team members may feel they are not recognized for their expertise and professional contribution.

Although numerous professionals are caring for a patient, this does not automatically mean that people are functioning as a team.[42] How these care providers relate to each other can differ dramatically. We often see people working in their professional "silo,"[43] a situation where they practice their profession in isolation, not accounting for the holistic view of the patient or what other providers are doing for the patient. Such "silo" work leads to professionals providing parallel but disconnected care that may be redundant or competitive, neither of which is beneficial to the patient. The focus of the professionals' actions is on their particular tasks and roles regarding a patient, rather than the patient himself. While the patient might be getting "good care" from each professional, the focus remains on the clinicians rather than on the patient. The difficulties that arise when professionals' roles overlap and competition develops may be addressed by emphasizing care of the patient as the point of focus.

Teamwork grows from recognizing that differing members of the team will each have strengths and weaknesses, and unique areas of expertise, but that these characteristics do not exclude the place for other team members to offer patients assistance in an area of need to which they can contribute. Thus, while spiritual care might be the special expertise of the chaplain on the team, it may be beneficial for a particular patient to receive care from other team members that allows room for discussion of spiritual issues and concerns. The key to the success of the collaboration is to maintain the focus of the team on the shared goal of the well-being of the patient/family being served.

It must be remembered that systems are exquisitely designed to achieve the results they routinely get and that change will be resisted by those who are entrenched in and rewarded by the status quo. Implicit challenges to hierarchical decision-making require mutual adaptation, create confusion and ambivalence and challenge the comfort of conformity. Sharing leadership responsibilities increases professional visibility. Less "powerful" team members may paradoxically resist efforts to increase the transparent accountability that is inherent in more transdisciplinary decision-making team models. This tendency of normal resistance makes change efforts suspect and motives for change can be frequently misinterpreted.[44]

Healthcare is only recently integrating business and psychology models of change into its institutional change efforts. Gladwell's "Tipping Point"[45] and Hackman's "Leading Teams"[46] use successful business models to illustrate change strategies that have applicability within healthcare. Identifying areas of expected resistance will assist one in leveraging change-efforts to achieve maximum team effectiveness.

Poorly functioning teams may suffer from a culture of rivalry, subsystems, scapegoating, and mutual mistrust. In this setting, role confusion and ambiguity can lead to demoralization.[36,47] If divergent views are not tolerated, then members may remain silent and at risk of becoming a "moral accomplice" to unethical behavior when the loyalty to the team replaces loyalty to patient and family.[48] Another danger in teamwork is that one's work becomes exposed creating the potential for personal vulnerability by critical teammates.[49] Fears may develop on a number of levels: concern that others will demonstrate that they can do "your" job as much or better than you can, the sense that working closely with people will show them the areas where you feel less confident and able as a professional, the overall sense of vulnerability that accompanies inviting others into your world of practice, and the difficulty of asking others to trust you and having to trust them in return.

Recognizing one's sense of vulnerability is essential for differentiating between the treatment by others and fears of one's own. Equally essential for assuring that a sense of vulnerability does not translate to defensive or self-defeating behavior in the team is a strong understanding of one's role as a professional and the ability to convey that role to others. Confidence in one's role and value should be strengthened by the knowledge that each profession on the team needs the information and expertise of others' on the team to practice successfully.[50]

## Strategies to Enhance Team Effectiveness

Communication in teams is a critical factor to the functioning of the team.[39,43] As in any relationship, team communication has a tremendous impact on how team members perceive and understand each other, how coordinated the actions of the team are, how responsive the team can be, and how the team is perceived by people outside the team. Most critically, team communication has an impact on the quality and experience of patient care.[51] Poor communication is a tremendous barrier to team behavior, making the goal of excellent communication a crucial one for any team. Communication may be enhanced using numerous approaches:

- Scheduling regular team meetings[52]
- Finding an uninterrupted space for the team to meet
- Creating a structured approach to the team meeting
- Building in dedicated time during team meetings for discussion of team issues
- Creating ground rules for communication within the team, such as agreeing to disagree respectfully and ensuring that all members of the team have an opportunity to speak
- Giving specific attention to improving team listening skills

Negotiation is another ongoing and central activity in teamwork.[53] The term negotiation should be understood as an iterative process where multiple parties each try to have their needs met. It is not inherently adversarial though some people perceive it as such. The most effective negotiation keeps in focus an agreed-upon goal, such as the best interests of the patient. With such a focus, although team members may have different approaches to the ultimate goal, discussion has the opportunity to lead to a productive outcome.

Together with the ability to effectively communicate and negotiate, several additional qualities are associated with productive teams. These attributes include:

- Clear goals and mission[54]
- Sufficient resources including people, time, and money
- Individual expertise and a commitment to reflective practice[55,56]
- Open communication and a commitment to mutual cooperation and collaboration[57-60]
- Commitment to both process and outcome
- Continuous evaluation of roles, norms, values, and performance
- Trust and support
- Strong leadership through empowerment of all[61]
- Organizational support
- Systems thinking and synergy[62,63]

By contrast, vicarious traumatization from chronic caregiving puts palliative care teams at special risk for members to suffer from compassion fatigue. Attrition occurs when team members feel that their talents and contributions are underappreciated and poorly rewarded. Teams with a tendency to "default" to the side of mistrust, with members' jumping to assumptions and assuming the worst about their colleagues suffer from higher rates of burn-out and become decreasingly effective. Being a part of a poorly functioning team invites a downward spiral of less investment in team outcomes and poorer performance and lessrisk taking. Conversely, more effective teams have a willingness to "roll up one's sleeves and do what needs to be done" to achieve identified goals.

This high degree of functional nimbleness is associated with role flexibility and a conscious playing to team members' strengths while supporting other members' weaknesses (without focus on fault finding or blaming). Developing a shared network of support with like-minded individuals who you trust and respect provides an anecdote to compassion fatigue by increasing members' self-esteem and sense of self-efficacy.

Just as we recognize that building a trust relationship with patients and their families is critical to effective care, so we can understand that building trust with the team will have a major influence on the team's capacity to function well.[50] Trust and mutual respect need to be thoughtfully built and nurtured. It involves taking the time to become familiar with team colleagues as people, taking an interest in their work and their perspectives. It involves building shared experiences that enable team members to support each other and share the challenges of providing high-quality palliative care. Trust also involves being able to appreciate differences and knowing that those differences among colleagues will be handled with respect.[37]

Authenticity is important if teams are to be robust and long-lived. Members do best when they feel good about their skills and that there is a good "fit" with what they have to give and what the team values. This authentic use of team member's individual gifts and talents comes when there is a match between team goals and a member's personal vision.

Conflicts among team members will naturally occur and require a commitment to constructive conflict resolution[2] if they are not to impede team functioning:

- Identify symptoms, degree, and sources of conflict: competing organizational priorities, interpersonal differences, differing agendas and time constraints, differing conceptual approaches to problem-solving, differing commitments, fear of change, etc.
- Explore root causes rather than having an over-focus on symptoms (identify process barriers and systems challenges)
- Explore range of possible outcomes then identify a preferred outcome and clarify who should be involved in process
- Consider who is the community of practice (both intrinsic and extrinsic members)[36,47,62,63]

Teams operate best when members have a shared vision of "success." If the purpose of a palliative care team is to improve patient quality of life and enhance functioning, then team success should be measured accordingly. Analysis of how effectively members communicate with others (both within the team and outside of it) becomes an important indicator for team success. Establishing shared accountability for such successes requires consensual goals. Developing a perspective of "we're all in this together" (with shared credit and shared responsibility) creates an atmosphere of trust. A quick measurement of the degree that members have a team perspective occurs when compliments or complaints are given by others regarding a team interaction. If members respond with "thanks, our team did a great job" to what could have been a personal compliment, then a team culture is in place. Similarly, if members accept accusations of blame to an individual instead of reframing the situation as an opportunity for the team to learn from its mistakes and do better next time, then the culture of the team is in need of improvement.

One of the most effective strategies for team building occurs through shared learning that supports professional development of individual and team.[64] This can occur through numerous ways, such as:

- Regularly scheduled team trainings, such as rotating monthly "lunch and learn" sessions or annually scheduled team "retreats," offer ongoing opportunities to share responsibility to develop the training schedule, and identify topics and provide curriculum and content. These regularly occurring trainings or round-robin facilitated lectures can be focused upon the internal educational needs of the team, or can be an outreach effort (in the form of in-services or grand rounds) by the team toward the larger institution. In either case, increasing an understanding by constituents of what services the team offers and how the team can best be used enhances team effectiveness. The goal becomes to expand common core of knowledge while increasing individual expertise.[63]

- Mutual mentorship encourages the transmission of expertise across disciplines and provides concrete opportunities for more junior staff to benefit from the wisdom of senior staff. Adopting a universal mentorship model demonstrates the team's commitment to support life-long learning and institutionalizes the value of peer-to-peer training. In recognition that every team member has an area of expertise valuable to the team at large, all members are expected to develop mentorships, whether with students or colleagues. Mentorship can enhance member skills in regard to clinical care, research, patient and professional education, and advocacy skills.

- Journal clubs are a frequently used method to enhance team learning. These lend themselves to transdisciplinary education sessions where representatives from the differing disciplines share the responsibility to identify topics of interest and select evidence-based articles to share with the wider team. Rotating these responsibilities increases the relevancy of the materials to the greater whole.

- Inviting guests from differing disciplines to team in-services allows team members opportunities to learn from established leaders in fields outside their own. For those teams without honoraria funds, creativity may be called for in identifying speakers. Teams have successfully established networks of shared educational efforts with other community organizations to exchange presenters. Others

have coordinated presentations with established organizationally funded continuing educational offerings to fold-in an extra engagement at lessened or no additional expense. This strategy can allow a team the opportunity to have small-group interaction with big-name speakers for little additional team expense.

- A schedule of rotating leadership of patient-rounds or team meetings ensures that all members of a team have an opportunity to hone their leadership skills. Although initially awkward for some, developing a policy of shared leadership responsibilities demonstrates a team's commitment to honor the expertise of each team member in a concrete and tangible way. Importantly, this provides supervisors with an opportunity to identify leadership skills-training needs of supervisees that otherwise might be difficult to directly ascertain.

- Rotation of responsibilities for continuous quality improvement activities demonstrates the team's commitment to developing an evidence base to improve the delivery of care by each team member. Too often, the collection of data becomes optional for certain team members. Developing a broad definition of what constitutes "research" and integrating its responsibilities to the team as a whole ensures that concepts such as "continuous quality improvement" are not just the personal responsibility of a few, but a genuine priority of the team as a whole.

- Encouraging professional development through the attendance of courses and conferences outside of the institution or agency with an expectation that members return to the team and present "lessons learned" from the experience. This expectation that each member will contribute to the education of others through regular presentations within and beyond the team codifies the team's commitment to life-long learning and recognizes that the best learning tool is the expectation that one will teach the skill being learned.

Teams, like other organic systems, benefit from periodic re-assessments. Setting aside time to re-examine the balance of power within the team assures that more timely adjustments can be made. Consideration of how vertical or lateral leadership and group decision-making has become is important to recalibrate to maintain team integrity. Developing a consensus regarding what aspects of care are the shared responsibility of all team members will require frequent revisiting. Patient advocacy, cultural sensitivity, education, anticipatory guidance, and pain/symptom distress are examples of concepts that may be recognized as shared responsibilities of all members of the team. Decisions about what is the patient's role in the team's collaborative dynamic will require frequent re-assessment due to the myriad of factors that influence this (including culture, age, access to needed resources, etc.). This is important because, for many patients, the team is invisible and must be consciously brought into the patient and family's awareness.

## Family Meetings as a Team Intervention

Family meetings, (also called family conferences), serve as one of the most powerful communication tools available to palliative care teams.[65-68] Such meetings often involve the patient (if he or she is able to participate), multiple family members, and the care team. Family meetings are recommended as an optimal palliative care team intervention, especially useful with decision-making and in identifying goals of care. Altilio, Otis-Green, and Dahlin[69] provide concrete examples of how family meetings can be used to create a plan of care that meets the social aspects of care domain of the 2004 NCP Guidelines. Family meetings are typically held at times of transition, such as when there are changes in treatment or changes in prognosis.[70] Those with complicated care needs, such as those with multiple co-morbidities, those for whom English is not their primary language, or those who are facing end of life are especially good candidates to benefit from a family meeting.

Family meetings offer a tremendous opportunity for coordination both within the team and between the team with other care providers and the patient and family.[71] Meetings usually have a particular purpose or goal, although the vision of the agenda may differ among team members and between team members, the patient, and the family.

The most effective communication from the professionals in a family meeting occurs when the team members have come together prior to the meeting to discuss their shared goals for the meeting, potential concerns, and anticipated roles of different team members at the meeting.[72] A coordinated approach from the team is important to the family meeting in a number of ways. It creates a sense of cohesion and confidence in the team that may be reassuring to patients and families. It demonstrates a holistic approach to the care of the patient and family, recognizing the complexity of people and their experiences. Furthermore, it helps to build the basis for a shared understanding in the family meeting. Perhaps most significant about a coordinated team approach to the family meeting is what it prevents. It minimizes the likelihood that team members will argue with each other or present conflicting information in such a way that burdens stressed patients and families with team "issues." In the family meeting, the results of positive collaborative teamwork can be profound and invigorating to all who participate.

Because family meetings so often focus on difficult decision-making and education regarding complex medical options, it can be useful to structure the meeting to allow differing team members an opportunity to address each of the various issues that need to be covered. Attention to the medical indications and treatment options; identification of patient preferences; clarification regarding the social situation and family context

and attention to the quality-of-life issues important for this particular patient and family at this particular moment in time can be helpful formatting devises[73] to ensure that the family meeting ends with an action plan that is meaningful and timely.

## Potential Directions for Research

Although there is a growing evidence base for the effectiveness of team interventions in healthcare, more research is needed[74,75]:

- How do we measure the "quality" of teamwork provided? How do we evaluative the effectiveness of team interventions?[76,77]
- What is the role of team research?[78]
- Is patient satisfaction with the team an adequate proxy for evaluating quality care?[54,79]
- What team composition is most effective (including considerations of cost)?[80]
- What is the best way to prepare participants (including professionals, patients and families) for their roles in family meetings?
- What core competencies are necessary for each discipline to maximize team effectiveness? How should these be taught and evaluated?[81-83]
- What patient populations or settings are most helped by a team approach to care?[84]

## Summary

Effective palliative care teams require fluid boundaries and a blending of areas of expertise. Clinicians must assess and intervene from their own individual expertise with a cross-pollination of ideas, perspectives, and knowledge. The goal is for the patient family system to experience an enhanced relationship with the team rather than increased numbers of relationships with various team members. Ideally, leadership decisions vary based on knowledge and experience rather than functions or titles and depend on the needs of the individual patient care plan. Successful team meetings alternate with a focus on patient care and with meetings focused in team development, team dynamics, process, and goals.

*Patient Narrative 1*
*The complexity of Interdisciplinary Team Work*

Ms. H is a 55-year-old Latina woman with advanced metastatic breast cancer. She has had difficulty coping with her illness in recent weeks as the severity of her illness has increased. Her partner of 20 years, Ms. K, has been extremely supportive of her, helping her with physical care and providing positive emotional support. Although

Ms. H and her partner have been together for two decades, they do not have any legal documentation between them that provides Ms. K with legal rights to make decisions for Ms. H in the event that Ms. H is unable to do so for herself. Ms. H has had a challenging relationship with her family of origin, including her parents, who are intermittently involved in her life. They have never recognized the relationship between Ms. H and Ms. K and do not acknowledge their partnership.

The palliative care team has attempted to engage Ms. H in a discussion of her wishes and priorities for end of life, but she has adamantly refused to discuss the subject of her declining health. Ms. K is aware that the team has been attempting to approach the topic of end of life with Ms. H and would be willing to be present for such a discussion, but Ms. K does not want to distress Ms. H any more than she already is at this time. The palliative care team is finding itself divided in terms of how they think the situation should be handled. The physician is eager to have clear indication from Ms. H regarding whether she would or would not want certain measures in place, such as antibiotics in the event of a severe infection or a DNR order on her chart. Other members of the team are also concerned to whom they would turn in the family in the event that Ms. H is unable to speak for herself. They do not have contact information for Ms. H's family of origin, but her partner, Ms. K, does not have written indication of being Ms. H's proxy.

The team is concerned that Ms. H is demonstrating signs of clinical depression, although it has been difficult to differentiate this because of the medications she is taking and the recent timing of the change in her condition. During the week's palliative care team meeting, team members find themselves disagreeing on how to proceed with Ms. H's care regarding discussions of future care. Team members disagree about how strongly to push the topic of discussing end-of-life care with the patient and how to handle a situation of proxy decision making if it arises. The team also disagree about how to proceed regarding care for her symptoms of depression. The meeting ends with no resolution regarding how to proceed, although team members eventually agree that no member of the team will take immediate or singular action on these topics. The team agrees to meet again about Ms. H in 2 days.

Two days later, the team meets hurriedly for an *ad hoc* meeting regarding Ms. H. No major changes have occurred in the situation, although Ms. H's symptoms are becoming more severe and her resolve not to discuss end of life remains strong, as she continues to state that she has faith that "God will send a miracle." The social worker on the team suggests that the team try a different approach to their discussion, in which they make a brief list of their concerns and goals of care for Ms. H. Each team member does so and then shares their ideas with the team, and the social worker takes notes on the exchange. The brief exercise allows the team to see where members overlapped on concerns and priorities. This provides several points of focus

on which the team can proceed on topics they all agreed were priority. The team continues by taking each point in turn and listing several potential actions they can take, enabling all team members to contribute equally to the discussion and provide input. Although there are clearly varied perspectives, discussion is productive and remains focused on the identified goals.

In the end, the team comes to agreement on several actions. Although not all members are equally happy about all conclusions, all members feel that the process for reaching them was sound. It is decided that a family meeting will be scheduled between the palliative care team, Ms. H, Ms. K, and other people whom Ms. H might wish to have involved. The team agrees that the agenda of the meeting will focus on concern for the family situation and the role of Ms. K in Ms. H's life, without emphasizing (at least initially) the topic of end-of-life decisions. The team agrees that the chaplain will be the team leader for the meeting given their positive relationship and the patient's strong faith. Ms. H's symptoms of depression will be monitored for a few more days to help evaluate whether they were situational or clinical in nature, but the team then agrees that a plan of offering Ms. H antidepressant medication along with directed psychotherapeutic intervention will be implemented. The team agrees to re-evaluate the results in a few days at their weekly team meeting.

---

*Patient Narrative 2*
*The Central Role of the Nurse in Interdisciplinary Team work*

Mr. G was a 72-year-old Iranian man being cared for by the palliative care team at his community hospital. He had been hospitalized twice before and was now familiar to the team from his previous visits. Mr. G's daughter, his primary source of support and designated proxy in the event that he loses the ability to make decisions, mentioned to Mr. G's palliative care nurse concerns about Mr. G's recent levels of pain. After further discussion with Mr. G's daughter, the nurse recognized that the daughter's concerns were beyond Mr. G's immediate experience of pain. His daughter, though concerned about the current pain, was clearly concerned about pain treatment options and their implications as Mr. G's condition worsened in the future.

At the meeting of the palliative care team later that week, the palliative care nurse brought this issue to the attention of the team. The nurse detailed her conversation with Mr. G's daughter and identified a number of issues she considered significant in the daughter's expression of her concerns. Other members of the team asked questions of the nurse for further clarification, acknowledging her key role in identifying and highlighting the situation. The team then proceeded to discuss a cohesive plan to address the situation. Several suggestions arose from the team members, and each was considered thoughtfully for its advantages and disadvantages. Finally, the team determined that a family meeting would be beneficial for creating an open forum for discussion among Mr. G, his daughter, and all members of the team. The team further discussed strategies that specific members of the team would discuss in the family meeting, drawing upon the diverse approaches of the different disciplines to the subject of pain, pain treatment, and the psychosocial concerns that accompany both. Throughout the meeting, the team maintained the focus of the discussion on the needs and well-being of the patient.

## REFERENCES

1. Loscalzo MJ, Von Gunten C. Interdisciplinary team work in palliative care. In: Chochinov H, Breitbart W, eds. Handbook of Psychiatry in Palliative Medicine (2nd ed). New York, NY: Oxford University Press; 2009:172–185.
2. Rees F. How to Lead Work Teams: Facilitation Skills (2nd ed). San Francisco, CA: Jossey-Bass Publishers, 2001.
3. Simpson D. From interdisciplinary to transdisciplinary: Strengthening the hospice team. Hosp Palliat Care Insights 2003;4:8–15.
4. D'Amour DE, Ferrada-Videla M, Rodriquez LSM, Beaulieu MD. The conceptual basis for the interprofessional collaboration: Core concepts and theoretical frameworks. J Interprof Care 2005;19(Suppl 1):116–131.
5. McDaniel A, Champion V, Kroenke K. A transdisciplinary training program for behavioral oncology and cancer control scientists. Nurs Outlook 2008;56:123–131.
6. Grey M, Connolly C. "Coming together, keeping together, working together": Interdisciplinary to transdisciplinary research and nursing. Nurs Outlook 2008;56:102–107.
7. Otis-Green S, Ferrell B, Spolum M, et al. An overview of the ACE Project—advocating for clinical excellence: Transdisciplinary palliative care education. J Cancer Educ 2009;24(2):120–126.
8. Takamura J. Introduction: Health teams. In: Campbell LJ, Vivell S, eds. Interdisciplinary Team Training for Primary Care in Geriatrics: An Educational Model for Program Development and Evaluation. Washington, DC: Government Printing Office; 1985:II:64–II:67.
9. Zeiss AM, Steffen AM. Interdisciplinary healthcare teams: The basic unit of geriatric care. In: Carstensen LL, Edelstein BA, Dornbrand L, eds. The Practical Handbook of Clinical Gerontology. Thousand Oaks, CA: Sage Publications; 1996:423–450.
10. Zeiss AM, Steffen AM. Interdisciplinary health-care teams in geriatrics: An international model. In: Bellack AS, Hersen M, eds. Comprehensive Clinical Psychology: Clinical Geropsychology. New York, NY: Elsevier Science; 1998:551–570.
11. Bruder MB. Working with members of other disciplines: Collaboration for success. In: Wolery M, Wilbers JS, eds. Including Children with Special Needs in Early Childhood Programs. Washington, DC: National Association for the Education of Young Children; 1994:45–70.
12. Skalla KA. Blended role advanced practice nursing in palliative care of the oncology patient. J Hosp Palliat Nurs 2006;8:155–163.
13. Hall P, Weaver L. Interdisciplinary education and teamwork: A long and winding road. Med Educ 2001;35(9):867–875.
14. Hall P. Interprofessional teamwork: Professional cultures as barriers. J Interprof Care 2005;19(Suppl 1):188–196.
15. Fineberg IC. Preparing professionals for family conferences in palliative care: Evaluation results of an interdisciplinary approach. J Palliat Med 2005;8:857–866.
16. Cadell S, Bosma H, Johnston M, et al. Practicing interprofessional teamwork for the first day of class: A model for an interprofessional palliative care course. J Palliat Care 2007;23:273–279.
17. Interprofessional education & core competencies: Literature review. Vancouver, Canada: Canadian Interprofessional Health Collaborative, College of Health Disparities, University of British Columbia, 2007. Available at: http://www.cihc.ca/resources-files/CIHC_IPE-LitReview_May07.pdf (accessed October 28, 2008).
18. Knowledge translation in interprofessional education: A review of literature and resources. Vancouver, Canada: Canadian Interprofessional Health Collaborative, University of British Columbia, 2007. Available at: http://www.cihc.ca/resources-files/CIHC-KT%20Review%20of%20KT%20and%20IPE%20Literature%20-%20May%202007.pdf (accessed October 28, 2008).
19. Interprofessional mentorship, preceptorship, leadership, & coaching (IMPCL) super toolkit. Toronto, Canada: University of Toronto, 2007. Available at: http://ipe.utoronto.ca/docs/IMPLC_SUPER_TOOLKIT.pdf (accessed October 28, 2008).
20. Christie C, Smith A, Bednarzyk M. Transdisciplinary assignments in graduate health education as a model for future collaboration. J Allied Health 2007;36:67–71.
21. Lawrie I, Lloyd-Williams M. Training in the interdisciplinary environment. In: Speck P, ed. Teamwork in Palliative Care: Fulfilling or Frustrating? New York, NY: Oxford University Press; 2006:153–165.
22. Wear D. On white coats and professional development: The formal and the hidden curricula. Ann Intern Med 1998;129(9):734.
23. Oandasan I, Reeves S. Key elements of interprofessional educations: Part 1—the learner, the educator, and the learning context. J Interprof Care 2005;Suppl 1:21–38.
24. Oandasan I, Reeves S. Key elements of interprofessional educations: Part 2—factors, processes, and outcomes. J Interprof Care 2005;Suppl 1:39–48.
25. Lockhart-Wood K. Specialist nursing. Collaboration between nurses and doctors in clinical practice. BJN 2000;9(5):276–280.
26. Horsburgh M, Perkins R, Coyle B, Degeling P. The professional subcultures of students entering medicine, nursing and pharmacy programmes. J Interprof Care 2006;20(4):425–431.
27. Rudland JR, Mires GJ. Characteristics of doctors and nurses as perceived by students entering medical school: Implications for shared teaching. Med Educ 2005;39(5):448–455.
28. Whitehead C. The doctor dilemma in interprofessional education and care: How and why will physicians collaborate? Med Educ 2007;41(10):1010–1016.
29. Heinemann GD, Zeiss AM. A model of team performance. In: Heinemann GD, Zeiss AM, eds. Team Performance in Healthcare: Assessment and Development. New York, NY: Kluwer Academic/Plenum Publishers; 2002:29–42.

30. Ekedahl M, Wengstrom Y. Coping processes in a multidisciplinary healthcare team—a comparison of nurses in cancer care and hospital chaplains. Eur J Cancer Care 2008;17:42–48.

31. Tuckman BW. Developmental sequence in small groups. Psychologic Bull 1965;63(6):384–399.

32. National Consensus Project for Quality Palliative Care. Clinical practice guidelines for quality palliative care, 2009. Available at: http://www.nationalconsensusproject.org (accessed on January 2, 2009).

33. National Quality Forum. A National Framework and Preferred Practices for Hospice and Palliative Care: A Consensus Report, 2006. Available at: http://www.qualityforum.org/pdf/reports/palliative/txPHreportPUBLIC01-29-07.pdf (accessed January 2, 2009).

34. Institute of Medicine. Cancer Care for the Whole Patient: Meeting Psychosocial Health Needs. Washington, DC: The National Academies Press, 2008.

35. Drinka T, Clark PG. Health-care Teamwork: Interdisciplinary Practice and Teaching. Westport, CT: Auburn House, 2000.

36. Lickiss JN, Turner KS, Pollack ML. The interdisciplinary team. In: Doyle D, Hanks G, Cherny N, Calman K, eds. Oxford Textbook of Palliative Medicine. Oxford, UK: Oxford University Press; 2004:42–46.

37. Xyrichis A, Lowton K. What fosters or prevents interprofessional teamworking in primary and community care? A literature review. Int J Nurs Stud 2008;45(1):140–153.

38. Costa L, Poe SS. Nurse-led interdisciplinary teams: Challenges and rewards. J Nurs Care Qual 2008;23:292–295.

39. McCallin A. Interdisciplinary practice—a matter of teamwork: An integrated literature review. J Clin Nurs 2001;10(4):419–428.

40. Rock W. Interdisciplinary teamwork in palliative care and hospice settings. Am J Hosp Palliat Care 2003;20(5):331–333.

41. Herbold RJ. The Fiefdom Syndrome: The Turf Battles That Undermine Careers and Companies—and How to Overcome Them. New York, NY: Doubleday Business, 2004.

42. Gearon CJ, Fields H. Medicine's turf wars. US News World Rep 2005;138:57–60.

43. Curtis JR. Caring for patients with critical illness and their families: The value of the integrated clinical team. Respir Care 2008;53(4):480–487.

44. Otis-Green S. The Transitions Program: Existential care in action. J Cancer Educ 2006;21:23–25.

45. Gladwell M. The Tipping Point: How Little Things Can Make a Big Difference. New York, NY: Little Brown & Company, 2000.

46. Hackman JR. Leading Teams: Setting the Stage for Great Performances. Boston, MA: Harvard Business Press, 2002.

47. Speck P. Teamwork in Palliative Care Fulfilling or Frustrating. New York, NY: Oxford University Press, 2006.

48. Pellegrino ED. The ethics of collective judgment in medicine and healthcare. J Med Philos 1982;7:3–10.

49. McCallin A, Bamford A. Interdisciplinary teamwork: Is the influence of emotional intelligence fully appreciated? J Nurs Manag 2007;15(4):386–391.

50. Lindeke LL, Sieckert AM. Nurse-physician workplace collaboration. Online J Issues Nurs 2005;5:43–46.

51. Barclay J, Blackhall L, Tulsky J. Communication strategies and cultural issues in the delivery of bad news. J Palliat Med 2007;10:958–977.

52. Rutherford J, McArthur M. A qualitative account of the factors affecting team-learning in primary care. Educ Prim Care 2004;15(3):352–360.

53. Ellingson LL. Communicating in the Clinic: Negotiating Frontstage and Backstage Teamwork. Cresskill, NJ: Hamptom Press, 2005.

54. Weaver TE. Enhancing multiple disciplinary teamwork. Nurs Outlook 2008;56:108–114.

55. Hermsen MA, Ten Have H. Palliative care teams: Effective through moral reflection. J Interprof Care 2005;19:561–568.

56. Teno JM. Palliative care teams: Self-reflection–past, present, and future. J Pain Symptom Manage 2002;23:94–95.

57. Bronstein LR. A model for interdisciplinary collaboration. Social Work 2003;48:297–306.

58. Broome ME. Collaboration: The devil's in the detail. Nurs Outlook 2007;55:1–2.

59. Junger S, Pestinger M, Elsner F, Krumm N, Radbruch L. Criteria for successful multiprofessional cooperation in palliative care teams. Palliat Med 2007;21:347–354.

60. Karnstrom S. Difficulties in collaboration: A critical incident study of interprofessional healthcare teamwork. J Interprof Care 2008;22:191–203.

61. Wilson NL, Gleason M. Team roles and leadership. In: Long DM, Wilson NL, eds. Houston Geriatric Interdisciplinary Team Training Curriculum. Houston, TX: Baylor College of Medicine's Huffington Center on Aging; 2001:1–32.

62. Briggs MH. Team talk: Communication skills for early intervention teams. J Childhood Commun Disord 1993;15:33–40.

63. Briggs MH. Building Early Intervention Teams: Working Together for Children and Families. Gaithersburg, MD: Aspen Publishers, 1997.

64. Shaver JL. Interdisciplinary education and practice: Moving from reformation to transformation. Nurs Outlook 2005;53:57–58.

65. Hudson P, Quinn K, O'Hanlon B, Aranda S. Family meetings in palliative care: Multidisciplinary clinical practice guidelines. BMC Palliat Care 2008;7:12.

66. Miller RD, Krech R, Walsh TD. The role of a palliative care service family conference in the management of the patient with advanced cancer. Palliat Med 1991;5:34–39.

67. Powazki RD, Walsh D, Davis MP, Bauer A. The Family Conference: How we do it. J Palliat Care 2006;22(3):240.

68. Azoulay E. The end-of-life family conference: Communication empowers. Am J Respir Crit Care Med 2005;171:803–804.

69. Altilio T, Otis-Green S, Dahlin C. Applying the national quality forum preferred practices for palliative and hospice care: A social work perspective. J Soc Work End Life Palliat Care 2008;4:3–16.

70. Deja K. Social workers breaking bad news: The essential role of an interdisciplinary team when communicating prognosis. J Palliat Med 2006;9:807–809.

71. Kristjanson LJ, Aoun S. Palliative care for families: Remembering the hidden patients. Can J Psychiatry 2004;49(6):359–365.

72. Lautrette A, Ciroldi M, Ksibi H, Azoulay E. End-of-life family conferences: Rooted in the evidence. Crit Care Med 2006;34(Suppl 11):364–372.

73. The Decision Making Tool for Comprehensive Care Planning. Seattle, WA: Pediatric Palliative Care Consulting Service, 2003. Available at: http://www.seattlechildrens.org/our_services/pdf/Decision%20Making%20Tool.pdf (accessed January 2, 2008).

74. Fernandez R, Vozenilek JA, Hegarty CB, et al. Developing expert medical teams: Toward an evidence-based approach. Acad Emerg Med 2008;15:1025–1036.

75. Salas E, Cooke NJ, Rosen MA. On teams, teamwork, and team performance: Discoveries and developments. Hum Factors 2008;50:540–547.

76. Schofield RF, Amodeo, M. Interdisciplinary teams in health-care and human services settings: Are they effective? Health Soc Work 1999;24:210–219.

77. Delva D, Jamieson M, Lemieux M. Team effectiveness in academic primary health-care teams. J Interprof Care 2008;22:598–611.

78. McCallin AM. Interdisciplinary researching: Exploring the opportunities and risks of working together. Nurs Health Sci 2006;8:88–94.

79. Sargeant J, Loney E, Murphy G. Effective interprofessional teams: "Contact is not enough" to build a team. J Contin Educ Health Prof 2008;28:228–234.

80. Batorowicz B, Shepherd TA. Measuring the quality of transdisciplinary teams. J Interprof Care 2008;22:610–620.

81. McNair RP. The case for educating health-care students in professionalism as the core content of interprofessional education. Med Educ 2005;39:456–464.

82. Hallin K, Kiessling A, Waldner A, Henriksson P. Active interprofessional education in a patient based setting increases perceived collaborative and professional competence. Med Teach 2009;31:151–157.

83. Salas E, DiazGranados D, Weaver SJ, King H. Does team training work? Principles for healthcare. Acad Emerg Med 2008;15:1002–1009.

84. Higginson IJ, Finlay I, Goodwin DM, et al. Do hospital-based palliative care teams improve care for patients or families at end of life? J Pain Symptom Manage 2002;23:96–106.

# IX

# International Models of
# Palliative Care

# 68 🙰 *Nessa Coyle*

# International Palliative Care Initiatives

An aging population, a growing incidence and prevalence of cancer, and a growing HIV/AIDS epidemic has brought increased attention to palliative care as a public health issue and a human right.[1] Each year worldwide, 10 million people are diagnosed with cancer and 6 million die from the disease. According to the UNAIDS 2006 report, the number of people worldwide living with HIV ranges from 33.4 million to 46.0 million. During 2005, an estimated 4.1 million became newly infected with HIV worldwide, and an estimated 2.8 million lost their lives to AIDS. In predicting the future need for palliative care, HIV/AIDS projections for 53 of the most affected countries in Africa indicate that excess mortality due to HIV will increase by a factor of 5 by 2050, from 53 million excess deaths in the current decade to 278 million by 2050. Global cancer rates will increase by 50% from 10 million in 2002 to 15 million new cases in 2020.[1]

Fifty percent of the world's new cancer cases are now occurring in developing countries, and 80% of these individuals are already incurable at the time of diagnosis.[2] Many of these individuals die without adequate pain or symptom control and most lack access to assessment and management of psychological, social, and spiritual concerns. As a result, widespread and needless suffering is a common global phenomenon for those with life-threatening illnesses.[2]

These figures are daunting, and yet with the increasing awareness of palliative care as a public health issue and human right, national and international government healthcare policies are beginning to identify palliative care as an essential component of care.[3-5] This includes support for children with life-threatening illness, the elderly, and people with cancer, HIV/AIDS, neurodegenerative disorders, as well as other life-limiting conditions. The WHO Cancer, Aids, and Aging Units as well as UN-AIDS have conceptualized palliative care as a fully integrated component of a care system that provides concurrent disease treatment with an emphasis on the patients quality of life by ensuring symptom control and supportive therapy combined, when possible, with disease-specific treatment.[2] The Council of Europe has also issued recommendations that provide a framework for member states to define the role and scope of palliative care in a regional, national, and international context.[2]

The challenge remains to integrate palliative care into all health-care systems worldwide. Barriers are numerous, especially in resource-poor countries where disease burden and poverty are high and man-power limited. Many of these countries do not have established hospice-palliative care services. Despite these many challenges, country-specific innovations shine through with the ultimate goal of improving quality of life for those facing life-threatening illnesses. The countries highlighted in this international section illustrate a growing number of countries, albeit still in the minority, with model strategies that have been developed for integrating palliative care into national health programs, delivery systems, and professional and public education. Both resource-rich and resource-poor countries are represented. Particular emphasis has been placed on access and availability of essential drugs for pain relief and symptom management as well as professional education. The International Narcotics Control Board, that monitors opioid consumption globally, supports palliative care initiatives and has advocated for a balanced opioid drug policy to ensure adequate availability of opioid drugs for medical purposes. The Council of Europe has also issued recommendations that provide a framework for member states to define the role and scope of palliative care in a regional, national, and international context.[2]

The following nine chapters explore the evolution and various levels of development of palliative care in both developed and developing countries. Nurses from Africa, Australia and New Zealand, Canada, Europe, Japan, Israel and Palestine, South Korea, South America and the United Kingdom describe the challenges in their particular countries and describe strategies for the future. A wide range of models is seen. In some countries, palliative care is recognized as a specialty or sub-specialty, whereas other countries have developed an extensive community home-based system. Always there is advocacy for the poor. The nurses' role in patient advocacy and in moving palliative care forward is evident. Because nurses are often closest of all the professions to patients and their families, and typically spend the most time with them, they are uniquely placed to serve as clinicians, advocates, and educators. They provide care across the lifespan, throughout the disease trajectory, and in virtually every health-care setting, including inpatient, outpatient, home care, and many others. As a result, they have the greatest potential to change the way care is provided to those with life-threatening illness and to support families. Unfortunately, many nurses in developing and marginalized countries still have little access to palliative care education. This is changing. Examples of educational programs for nurses in hospice-palliative care are reflected in the countries detailed in the following chapters. Growing collaboration between nurses in resource-rich countries and nurses in resource-poor countries has benefited both. As war and conflict remain a reality in today's world, one chapter has been included that specifically addresses the challenge of providing palliative care in areas of conflict. The author's observations are based on his experience in working with Palestinian and Israeli patients in a Jewish hospital in Jerusalem.

## REFERENCES

1. Callaway M, Ferris FD. Foreword—advancing palliative care: The public health perspective. J Pain Symptom Manage 2007;33:483.
2. De Lima L. Palliative care: Global situation and initiatives. In: Bruera E, Higginson I, Ripamonti C, von Gunten C, eds. Palliative Medicine. United Kingdom: Arnold Publishers, 2006:117–126.
3. Stjernsward J, Gomez-Batiste X. Palliative medicine—the global perspective: Closing the know-do gap. In: Caraceni AT, Fainsinger R, Foley K, et al., eds. Palliative Medicine. Philadelphia, PA: Saunders; 2009:2–8.
4. Stjernsward J, Foley KM, Ferris FD. The public health strategy for palliative care. J Pain Symptom Manage 2007;33:486–493.
5. Brennan F. Palliative care as an international human right. J Pain Symptom Manage 2007;33:494–499.

# 69

*Dennie Hycha and Lynn Whitten*

# Palliative Care in Canada

◆ **Key Points**
◆ *The development and service delivery of hospice palliative care in Canada has further developed in the past 5 years because of initiatives at federal, provincial, and local levels.*
◆ *Some of the current factors impacting hospice palliative service delivery include the status of the nursing workforce, technology, the shift from hospital to community based services, the concept of advance care planning, and rural and remote-area service delivery.*
◆ *Hospice palliative care nursing in Canada has evolved to a recognized nursing specialty that enables nursing to provide leadership in integrated models of interdisciplinary service delivery.*

Canadians highly value their publicly funded health-care system and believe that quality end-of-life care is imperative. Indeed, quality and available end-of-life care is consistent with the very values that resulted in the creation of a national health-care system.[1] Access to end-of-life care is influenced by the diseases from which Canadians die, whether they live in a city or rural or remote areas, the province in which they reside, the nature of their private health insurance plans, and their personal wealth.[2] Federal reports are calling for federal action to ensure that palliative care services are included in community based services, particularly in the home.[1] Increased attention on end-of-life care and acknowledgment that services are inequitable across our country challenge those responsible for health services delivery to develop initiatives and to address models of care for palliative care delivery.

This chapter discusses palliative and end-of-life care from national, provincial, and local perspectives, describes population and health-care trends contributing to the development of palliative care and provides examples of models of service delivery and best-practice program development which influence palliative care programs in the country. As the delivery of services continues to evolve and develop, so does the terminology. For the purposes of this chapter, end-of-life care will be identified as the terminal stage of the continuum of hospice palliative care.

To provide a context within Canada, an overview of the Canadian health-care system, the responsibilities of the federal and provincial governments and local health authorities are described, as these three levels of government are accountable for health-care delivery. Additionally, the impact of the national not-for-profit advocacy association, the Canadian Hospice Palliative Care Association (CHPCA), is discussed.

## Health Care in Canada

Health care in Canada is publicly funded and universally accessible. The Canada Health Act is federal legislation that facilitates reasonable access to health services without financial or other barriers through the five key principles of public administration, comprehensiveness, universality, portability, and accessibility.[3] Although the Constitution Act of Canada (1982) defines health care as a provincial rather than federal responsibility, in practice, responsibility for health care is shared between the federal and provincial governments. The federal government can influence health care through legislation and control of financial resources. The federal government can also impact areas of health care through regulations, commissions, and activities of its various departments. For example, Health & Welfare Canada has initiated several key reports and meetings that have increased national discussion about health care and end-of-life care issues.

## Foundational National Activities

In June of 1995, a special Senate Committee on Euthanasia and Assisted Suicide was developed and chaired by Senator Sharon Carstairs. This Senate Committee developed suggestions that would improve access, services, and standards of care, and increase knowledge and skill and the need for palliative and end-of-life care education for health professionals. In June 2000, a subcommittee was formed from the Senate Committee on Social Affairs, Science and Technology which tabled a report *Quality End-of-Life Care: The Right of Every Canadian.*[4] This report identified that federal leadership and the development of a national strategy were required to improve care. They made reference to support for family caregivers; access to home care and pharmaceuticals; training and education of health professionals; and the need for research and monitoring of indicators/outcomes.[4]

In December 2000, a blueprint for action was developed by the Quality End-of-Life Care Coalition. This was comprised of 24 national stakeholders under the umbrella of the CHPCA. This blueprint identified five key priorities from the Subcommittee report. These included:

1. Availability and access
2. Professional education
3. Research and data collection, including surveillance
4. Family and caregiver support
5. Public education and awareness

In February 2001, the Canadian Strategy for Cancer Control—Palliative Care Working Group[5] affirmed that palliative care was a fundamental component of cancer care and recommended improving the integration of palliative care delivery within existing cancer care centers and in health-care delivery systems across the country. In March 2001, the Prime Minister of Canada appointed Senator Sharon Carstairs as Minister with Special Responsibility for Palliative Care and as an advisor to the Minister of Health on palliative and end-of-life care.

In June 2001, the Secretariat on Palliative and End-of-Life Care was established. This was the first step in Health Canada's work to develop a coordinated national strategy promoting collaboration within and with federal and provincial governments and with key stakeholders in palliative and end-of-life care provision. This initiative worked toward creating greater awareness of the need for quality care at the end of life.[6] The strategy developed would reflect a holistic approach and include accepted core principles in palliative and end-of-life care. In March 2002, a National Action Planning Workshop was sponsored by the Secretariat where 150 national, provincial, and regional clinicians, researchers, and administrators were brought together to recommend action. The workshop focused on the priorities and action plans already determined by the work done previously in the country. The strategy served as a focus for hospice palliative care from 2002 to 2007 with the following key achievements:

- Development of accreditation standards and a core set of measures for hospice palliative care
- Development of pediatric hospice palliative care guiding principles and norms of practice
- Identification of core and intra-professional competencies as well as collaborating with the nursing, physician, and social work national professional associations to further develop discipline specific competencies
- Development of a palliative and end-of-life care medical curriculum through creation of the Educating Future Physicians in Palliative and End-of-Life Care (EFPPEC)
- Creation of a forum to share knowledge through creation of an Education Commons accessed at www.chpca.net
- Increase in understanding of advance care planning through development of a glossary of terms entitled *Advance Care Planning: the Glossary project*
- Creation of a hospice palliative care research network

In October 2002, the Senate Standing Committee on Social Affairs, Science and Technology Final Report: *The Health of Canadians—The Federal Role* released the Kirby report. This report identified five key areas for further development and to date some of the recommendations were implemented. These included a 6-week compassionate care leave for Canadians choosing to care for their family members; expansion of tax measures for families caring for the dying; and all provinces and territories have a standard process for assessing hospice palliative care needs and criteria for palliative home care.

In November 2002, a Commission on the Future of Health Care in Canada was established and the Romanow report was developed. This was the largest Canadian consultation process that had ever occurred on health care. From this consultative process, conclusions to expand the Canada Health Act for medically necessary home-care services, one of which included palliative and end-of-life care, and to develop supports for informal caregivers through Human Resources Canada were reached. The second recommendation provided further support to the findings from the Kirby Report. The most notable actions following these reports resulted from the 2004 First Ministers Health Accord. The Accord identified as one of several priorities access to home-care services that included end-of-life care for case management, nursing, palliative-specific pharmaceuticals, and personal care at the end of life.[7]

## Canadian Hospice Palliative Care Association

The Canadian Hospice Palliative Care Association (CHPCA) is the voice for hospice palliative care in Canada. It is a national charitable nonprofit association whose mission is to provide leadership and an advocacy role in hospice palliative care in the country. The organization strives to achieve this mission by supporting research, promoting education and training, improving public awareness of hospice palliative care, and by advocating for increased programs and services. CHPCA works in close partnership with other national organizations and continues to move forward with the goal of ensuring that all Canadians, regardless of where they may live, have equal access to quality hospice palliative care for themselves and their family.[8]

Historically, the terms "hospice" and "palliative care" were used in Canada in a variety of ways. The term hospice may have indicated a philosophy of care, a free-standing building, a unit in a long-term care facility, or a home-based program. New terminology in Canada was proposed in 2002. The words *hospice* and *palliative care* were combined to recognize the convergence of hospice and palliative care into one movement. The national organization for palliative care adjusted their name to include the term "hospice palliative care."[9] Their updated definition is: "Hospice palliative care is aimed at relief of suffering and improving the quality of life for persons who are living with or dying from advanced illness or are bereaved." It is appropriate for any person and family living with a life-threatening illness resulting from any diagnosis, regardless of age and prognosis.[9] This definition calls for hospice palliative care intervention earlier in the disease trajectory for all diagnoses. The CHPCA is also currently in the process of identifying a definition of end of life to reflect the broader population that may benefit form hospice palliative care.

A priority of the CHPCA has been the development of national standards to guide the development of palliative and hospice care service delivery across the country. Following 10 years of extensive consensus building and collaboration across Canada, a model to guide hospice palliative care was

published in 2002.[10] The model is comprised of the values, principles, and foundational concepts that underlie all aspects of hospice palliative care; a conceptual framework for the delivery of care called the "Square of Care"; and a conceptual framework to guide organizational development and function called the "Square of Organization".

The CHPCA has also been an active partner in the establishment of palliative care as a specialty within the Canadian Nursing Association (CNA). The CHPCA Nursing Interest Group provided the venue through which nurses across Canada collaborated to establish the Hospice Palliative Care Nursing Standards of Practice, which were developed in 2002.[11] These standards and the CHPCA Model of Care provided the foundation for the development of palliative care nursing certification. The first sitting of the certification occurred in April 2004. Now more than 1100 nurses are registered.[12]

## Palliative Care Service Delivery in Canada

Several key events have occurred since 1992 in Canada that have strongly influenced what exists today in the provision of hospice palliative care.[1–4,13–17] It is generally agreed that service delivery models for palliative and hospice care need to include essential components such as pain and symptom management, interdisciplinary teams, consultation services, psychosocial/counseling care, spiritual care, and volunteer and bereavement programs.[18] Services to support care in the community include home care, outpatient clinics, daycare, respite care, hospice (home support, freestanding, and integrated into long-term care facilities), and community consultation teams.

In 1992, the Palliative Care 2000 for Cancer[17] provided recommendations for priorities and coordination of cancer care, which has traditionally been the focus of care within the palliative care context. Over two decades ago, this palliative care expert panel identified the need for an integrated and coordinated palliative care service delivery. This seminal report was the first report to identify a system of care that spanned the health-care continuum as well as identify primary-to-tertiary palliative services. This report provided recommendations on priorities and coordination for cancer care to national cancer agencies. It strongly recommended support of development-based services in local or regional planning.[17] The report contained essential components such as home-based care, acute care, chronic palliative care beds, consultation services, and a tertiary, regional unit that would act as a learning and research center.[17] The development of secondary and tertiary levels of care were noted as necessary for the collaborative management of complex cases and for the much-needed education and research development in this field.

In Canada, hospice palliative care is provided in a variety of settings and by a range of providers. With the shift of health-care services to primary care, the predominant amount of end-of-life care occurs in the community with health care provided by family physicians and community based services such as home care. These health-care providers have various levels of expertise as well as variable access to consultation or advice from palliative consultants. Secondary level services are provided by designated interdisciplinary teams of hospice palliative care experts who can provide support to primary care providers in all care settings. These services may be advisory or consultative, providing expert assessments for pain and symptom management, psychosocial and/or spiritual and, as a liaison to other services or through focused education. Access to such services 24 hours per day 7 days a week is critical. This level of expertise often contributes to the development of local standards and is key to implementing best practices in hospice palliative care.

Highly specialized services provided by academically prepared health professionals and with a palliative care clinical specialty are often provided in specialized palliative care units in tertiary health-care facilities. Experts at the tertiary level of palliative care often provide education to secondary and tertiary level experts, conduct research and are affiliated with academic institutes.

During the past decade, numerous strategies have been developed that are applied across the country, such as national hospice palliative care standards and accreditation standards, which are discussed later in further detail. Clinically, a core set of clinical assessment tools has been adopted as a standard of palliative care in all service levels and throughout Canada. These tools include the Edmonton Symptom Assessment Score (ESAS), the Palliative Performance Scale (PPS), the CAGE, and the Mini Mental State Exam (MMSE). Various comprehensive pain assessment tools are also used for specific patient populations.

## Factors Influencing Palliative Care Health Care

Multiple factors are influencing the delivery of palliative services in terms of care providers, settings of care, and services. This undoubtedly impacts the delivery of hospice palliative care services as well. Although not exclusive, the factors that currently are having considerable impact on palliative care in Canada include: our changing culture, end-of-life care in the aboriginal culture, hospice palliative care in a changing health-care system, the changing role of nursing, the use of technology, the emergence of advance care planning, and providing service to rural and remote areas. Each of these aspects will be further discussed.

### Impact of Culture on Models of Care

Canada is a rich tapestry of cultures from around the world. Canada's population in 2005 was approximately 32,107,000, reflecting a growth of 300,000 people from the previous year with two-thirds a result of a migratory increase.[19] Canada has

experienced the most rapid rate of growth of all G8 countries, with about 240,000 newcomers annually since 2001.[19] Although there has been a decrease since 2002, 57% to 62% of Canada's immigrants are persons migrating from Asia.

The four main cultural groupings include the Aboriginal peoples, British and French "founders" of Canada, and more recently, immigrants from Asia, Africa, and other non-European nations.[20] The larger urban centers in Canada, where the "third wave" of immigrants from Asia and Africa as well as an increasing number of Aboriginal people tend to settle, are challenged to respond to the linguistic and cultural diversity.[21]

Palliative care practitioners are particularly challenged by this diversity on several fronts. In regard to access, research has suggested that ethnic minorities are underrepresented in palliative care programs.[22] Access is further compromised because of the lack of translated materials and clinical assessment tools.[23] The foundations of the modern palliative care/hospice movement are based on Christian tradition and teachings and a growing recognition of the futility and indignity of continuing expensive and intrusive treatments for people who are clearly dying. Guiding palliative care principles are based on the western ethics of "truth telling" and patient autonomy.[24] These principles are often in direct conflict with the beliefs and values of many of the persons that we care for, resulting in culturally insensitive decision-making and health policies.[20] In Canada, there has been greater emphasis on addressing this culture diversity through the various reports, formation of cultural specific practices such as addressing aboriginal needs, as well as translation of clinical tools such as the ESAS in multiple languages. However, palliative care programs in Canada need to continue to focus on developing cultural competence by reflecting values, behaviors, attitudes, knowledge, and skills that are respectful and inclusive of diverse cultural backgrounds.[23]

### Aboriginal Health

In Canada, the aboriginal population is defined by the Constitution Act of 1982 to include North American Indian, Inuit, and Métis.[25-27] Canada's Aboriginal people total just over 3% of Canada's total population.[28] The North American Indian makes up 62% of the aboriginal population with 30% Métis and 5% Inuit. The Aboriginal population has the highest population growth rate with half of the aboriginal population under 25 years contrasted with half of the non-Aboriginal population under 38 years of age. Quality-of-life indicators indicate that more Aboriginal people live in overcrowded housing conditions, experience higher unemployment, and have not completed high school.[25]

The unique cultural, end-of-life care needs of the Aboriginal population and the continued interest in aboriginal hospice palliative care have been identified through several federal government, national organizations, and Aboriginal forums and papers.[29] In the report, Cross-Cultural Considerations in Promoting Advance Care Planning in Canada,

Con (2008 #27) identifies guidelines for caregiving in the aboriginal community to include: (1) respect of individuals; (2) practice conscious communication; (3) use of interpreters; (4) involvement of family, including extended family; (5) recognition of alternatives to truth telling; (6) practice of noninterference; and (7) allowing the practice of traditional medicine.[27] In addition to the areas of growth that have occurred in the past decade with regards to aboriginal hospice palliative care, Hanson identifies significant gaps that need to be addressed.[29] These gaps include: the acquisition of knowledge and evidence to inform program and policy development and service delivery; jurisdiction and policy clarity around service provision on and off reserve, limitations of Aboriginal issues in health-care education curriculum; cultural competence; practical aspects of health service delivery on and off reserve settings and with vulnerable populations; fragmentation and effective funding and reporting models; aboriginal grief and bereavement models and services; and basic housing, food, and clothing needs that impact daily Aboriginal living and dying.[2,29]

## Incorporating Hospice Palliative Care in Canada's Changing Health-Care System

Palliative care was formally recognized in Canada through the development of palliative care units at St. Boniface Hospital in Winnipeg, Manitoba, in 1974 and at the Royal Victoria Hospital in Montreal, Quebec, in 1975. In accordance with the health-care delivery models of the time, services for individuals who were dying were located primarily in the acute care model of health-care delivery. Since then, the services have evolved and shifted to include community, hospice, and long-term care models of service delivery.

As with multiple health service areas, the evolution of our approach to service delivery for end-of-life care continues to be influenced by several other changes in our broader health-care system. Although not exhaustive, these factors include:

- A need to increase the capacity of primary care givers to enhance palliative and end-of-life care delivery;
- Expanded scope of hospice palliative care to include end-of-life care for broader disease and illness populations beyond the traditional cancer diagnoses, thus greatly expanding the volume and increased knowledge required for end-stage chronic diseases;
- Increased understanding of the need for care to be integrated across care settings;
- Workforce issues requiring care providers across the continuum to enhance palliative care knowledge and skills as well as requiring how this specialized care can be delivered for larger populations;
- A need to examine critical areas in hospice palliative care to determine the most effective and efficient way systems deliver quality and safe care; and
- Increased upsurge of information and technology and the application across settings as well as in rural and remote areas that are challenged with access to specialized hospice palliative care expertise.

Additionally, consumers have become more engaged in and knowledgeable of their options while ensuring the need for quality and safe care. It is expected the baby-boomer generation will have a major impact on health care because of their high expectations, demand for choice, and involvement in decision-making. These factors impact how practitioners communicate and support individuals and families requiring hospice palliative care.

## The Changing Role of Nursing

The changing demographics, longer life expectancies, healthier lifestyles of some segments of the population, new populations, technology, and emerging challenges reflective of lifestyle patterns, all have accelerated the need for a health-care system that can respond quickly. The previously established health-care system centered around single point of entry through medical and hospital based care performed well in the past, but is no longer meeting the current need. This realization has seen the move from the traditional acute-care illness treatment model to one focused on wellness and community-based service delivery.[30]

In planning for the future, the Canadian Nurses Association report, *Toward 2020 Visions for Nursing*, calls for nurses to provide leadership in this change by "setting an agenda to create a health-care system that truly serves and reflects the priorities of Canadians. But no one will appoint them to the task."[30] This provides incredible opportunities and challenges for nursing staff as well as for those who specialize in hospice palliative care. This report also identifies several scenarios for a preferred future that can be applied to hospice palliative care nursing such as:

- Providing leadership in education of nursing, interdisciplinary team and the public as well as leading and/or participating in research regarding the impact of individual and family coping and decision-making;
- Increasing the knowledge, skill, and research to be able to respond to changing disease patterns;
- Identifying and supporting effective coping mechanisms as well as identifying at risk individuals and families in order to contribute to the wellness trend with an expectation of increased education and engagement in personal health;
- Promoting advanced practice hospice palliative care nurses such as clinical nurse specialists and nurse practitioners (NPs) who are well placed to provide increased integration of a holistic health movement into mainstream medicine; and
- Identifying global environmental issues that already contribute to major health changes and would benefit from palliative and end-of-life care.

Additionally, the future will consist of various health system trends that continue to see a shift to community-based services, use of technology, increased focus on long-term and end-of-life care, expectations and support for increased family involvements and funding ratio changes. It is clear, however, that if new delivery models are not developed, the current shortage of health-care professionals will impact health care adversely. There is an urgent need to work differently.[23] This provides incredible opportunity for hospice palliative care nurses to engage in community development and enhancing communities' capacities to provide compassionate and effective hospice palliative care services in the most appropriate settings of care.

The scopes of practice for health-care providers are front and center in the evolution of health-care practices. Licensed Practical Nurses (LPNs) have assumed several pre-existing functions of the registered nurse (RN). Registered nurses, clinical nurse specialists and NPs have assumed functions that were within the scope of general practitioners less than two decades ago. Hospice Palliative Care nurses in Canada need to find ways to have discussions and debates, yet speak with one voice and to identify strategies to transform nursing practice to better meet the needs of the individuals who are dying and their families and community needs in a changing national and global environment. Identification of hospice palliative care as a national nursing specialty as well as development of a national list server registry housed at the CHPCA website are beginning steps that are facilitating cohesion and dialogue.

## Technology

There is a great need for patient information and utilization data to flow between various health-care providers, care settings, and across provincial settings and beyond. It is vital to look for solutions that will strengthen the coordination of care through innovation and creativity and facilitate seamless patient movement regardless of the location of care delivery.[31] As the Canadian Institute for Health Information identified, we need to implement new models of end-of-life care, and by doing so we need to make an investment in standards, information systems, access to technology, and the education of nurses in how to use technology in their work with colleagues, patients, and families.[32] The vision statement of the Canadian Society for Telehealth works towards achieving "optimal health for all."[33]

One of the barriers to use of technology is the comfort level of nurses in using computer technology.[34] As a result of these trends, some innovative solutions have been developed in the country, which will be highlighted later in the chapter. Critical is the need for common data bases to enable comparison across the country and the need to develop a surveillance system to clearly identify the scope of the palliative care population to develop appropriate services and determine the impact of these services.

Several recent Web-based innovations in Canada will help to address some of the challenges experienced in the provision of rural and remote areas in palliative care. In 2001, Health Canada announced funding to support the development of the Canadian Virtual Hospice (CVH).[35] Canadian Virtual Hospice goals are to facilitate, via a Web-based forum, equitable distribution of mutual support, the exchange of information, communication and collaboration between and among health-care professionals, researchers, the terminally ill, and their families. Another example is the rural palliative telehealth project funded by Alberta Health and Wellness in 2007. This project determined that telehealth technology offers an e-health solution to the challenges faced with a widely dispersed rural population.[36] This project demonstrated that there was improved access to secondary-level palliative care consultation, improved home support, reduced emergency visits and hospitalizations, reduced need for travel, and improved symptom management for rural and home-bound patients.

## Advanced Care Planning

Advanced care planning was identified as a priority at a National Action Planning Workshop for End-of-Life Care held in 2002. This workshop brought provincial and territorial governments, regional health authorities, and stakeholder organizations together. The outcomes of the workshop included the need to develop an inventory of tools for Canadians, standards for health-care settings, and information for health professionals around advanced care planning.[37] Identification and clarification of advance care planning concepts and terms understood by professionals and consumers is provided in the Health Canada The Glossary Project report.[38]

The development of a national guide for planning and implementation of advanced care planning initiatives was informed by the work and progress made by the Calgary Health Region and Fraser Health Authority. With support from Health Canada, a guide was developed that proposes a four-part model that is patient and family centered. The four tenets include: engagement; organizational and community education; system infrastructure; and continuous quality improvement. These four basic building blocks are linked to provincial/national policy, regulatory bodies such as accreditation and to the environment in which it functions.[39] The CHPCA is taking a leadership role to advance this work and has established an Advanced Care Planning Task Group.

## Rural and Remote Areas

There is a need to support Canadians who live in rural and remote regions with palliative and end-of-life care needs. Rural or remote nursing is a practice that varies in roles and responsibilities according to the health needs of the population and the services available within that specific community.[40] A key challenge is that communities are often complex, linked to a broad range of economic, geographic, and environmental factors. Romanow identified that geography is actually a determinant of health.[2] Nurses practicing in rural and remote areas must practice proficiently in multiple areas of health. Factors contributing to the complexity are low service volumes, lack of health service, human resources, and physical access. The literature repeatedly identifies the needs for rural and remote nurses to be able to crosstrain and be flexible in their knowledge and skills.[11] Health services are often designed for urban environments and do not necessarily meet the needs of rural/remote populations. One of the challenges for persons living in rural/remote areas is that people have to travel outside of their communities for health services, which in turn creates emotional and financial stress. Most patients and families identify the desire to be cared for in their home communities by their primary health-care team.[41] In the Romanow report, a recommendation to establish a Rural and Remote Access Fund to support new initiatives for delivering health care for populations living in rural/remote areas was made.[2]

One of the key strategies in addressing the challenges in rural/remote communities is the use of telehealth. The Canadian Nurses Association recognizes telehealth as being within the scope of nursing practice.[42] It has created the ability for the exchange of knowledge regardless of geography or environmental barriers. It has been shown to be a time-efficient and cost-reducing form of health-care access.[43] Research has continually demonstrated the effectiveness of the use of telehealth in health-care provision. It is used to access nursing and other health services, skills training, and development of assessment techniques and to allow nurse's access to specialized consultants in palliative and end-of-life care issues when required. The body of evidence continues to grow, demonstrating that telehealth visits are as effective as face-to-face consultations.[43]

## Major National Hospice Palliative and End-of-Life Care Initiatives

Ongoing initiatives and activities are continually being developed and implemented at national and local service delivery levels. First to be discussed, are initiatives developed at the national level that impact local service organization and provision.

### Quality End-of-Life Coalition

In 2000, the Quality End-of-Life Coalition of Canada (QELCC) was established to serve as an advocate for quality end-of-life care of all Canadians. The Coalition network includes representatives from thirty national professional and family caregivers, volunteers, health-care professionals, those with terminal illness, families, and others interested in quality end-of-life care.[44] Governed by an Executive Committee,

the Coalition operates through five working groups with the CHPCA as the secretariat providing administrative support. Achievements have included providing a status report on end-of-life care, *Dying for Care* (2004), advocating for changes to the Compassionate Care Benefits resulting in eligibility in 2006.In May 2008, the QELCC released a progress report on the status of hospice palliative home care in Canada. Twelve provinces and one territory were part of the QELCC survey. Their determinations were that:

- All jurisdictions have a standard process to assess clients care needs and have developed eligibility criteria for hospice palliative home care;
- All patients/families have access to advice from pharmacists;
- Twelve/thirteen report some medical supplies and equipment have costs covered or an equipment lending service;
- Eleven/thirteen report some coverage for pharmaceuticals receiving end-of-life care at home;
- Eleven/thirteen have a team-based approach and interprofessional education on hospice and palliative care is provided.

### Canadian Home Care Association (CHCA)

This organization is a national forum and "promotes excellence in home care through leadership, awareness, and knowledge to shape strategic directions."[45] Literature supports that Canadians prefer to be at home when faced with a terminal or end-stage illness.[32,46] In 2004, a 10-year *Plan to Strengthen Health Care* was developed where levels of government recognized that there was a need for coverage for hospice palliative care in the home. In this plan, federal, provincial, and local leaders made a commitment to provide coverage by 2006 for some home care services, which included case management, nursing, palliative-specific pharmaceuticals, and personal care at the end of life.[47]

A progress report on this 10-year plan, prepared by the QELCC, noted that there was significant progress in access to a range of services.[44] However, timely access to comprehensive home care services was limited by workforce issues, geography, and lack of training. The progress report indicated that improvement is required for access of other settings of care such as long-term care and hospices as well as with marginalized populations. Case management, personal care services 24/7, research activities, and the strategies to collect data for wait times to access to palliative home-care services were less clearly defined.

### Educating Future Physicians in Palliative and End-of-Life Care (EFPPEC)

This initiative resulted from a 2001 survey of Faculties of Medicine in Canada indicating concerns with inadequate training in end-of-life care. The surveyors recommended increased clinical exposure, curriculum development, student assessment, and evaluation in the curriculum of medical students. They also emphasized the need for faculty development and improved infrastructure to support the required needs for education. In 2002, 14 of 16 Faculties of Medicine representatives met with a group of palliative care experts to begin to develop ways to address these inadequacies. EFPPEC emerged from these discussions with the development of a joint project by the Association of Faculties of Medicine of Canada and the CHPCA with funding support from Health Canada.

Following the 3-year period of funding, participants strongly supported continuation to build upon the strengths gained through this process. Common themes were identified by the participants, which included:

- Education needed to be truly inter-professional to reflect the real work environment;
- Continuing to create linkages between licensing/accrediting bodies, the schools/faculties, and practicing professionals;
- Development of accreditation standards for palliative and end-of-life care were a necessity;
- Continued strengthening of provincial networks of palliative care by aligning with shared resources, which is already established.[48]

EFPPEC participants agreed to continue to influence and shape interprofessional palliative and end-of-life care education in the ways identified at the final conference.

### Accreditation Canada

Accreditation Canada has been conducting health services reviews for 50 years. Their goal is to "ensure that safe, efficient and reliable care is being delivered within the health systems."[49] Accreditation Canada released their 2008 Canadian Health Accreditation Report stating that there were 977 service organizations that were surveyed in 2007.[49]

To influence organization and health-system changes it was crucial to develop nationally accredited standards for palliative and end-of-life care. Accreditation Canada began to develop hospice palliative and end-of-life care standards in 2003. It identified its guiding principles as sustainability, timeliness, relevance, efficiency, rigor, specificity, client/family focus, flexibility, and adaptability. This project was funded through Health Canada's Secretariat on Palliative and End-of-Life Care and included the provision of a national set of standards, an accreditation program for hospice organizations, and a core set of performance measures or indicators.[50,51] These standards were released in May 2006. The standards focus on:

- Investing in hospice palliative and end-of-life services;
- Engaging prepared and proactive staff;
- Providing safe and appropriate services;
- Enhancing quality of life;

- Maintaining accessible and efficient clinical information systems; and
- Measuring quality and achieving positive outcomes.[52]

Although not inclusive, five initial core indicators that were developed include: availability of hospice palliative care 24/7; continuity of care; identification of the degree and management of distress (measured using ESAS); family/caregiver satisfaction with end-of-life care; and documentation of client and family service goals.[52]

### Research

Another important need identified by the national forums is the importance of palliative and end-of-life care research. Health providers in palliative care continue to identify the need to develop a body of evidence. There are many challenges in researching this population. The Canadian Institute of Health Research (CIHR) developed a strategic initiative in 2003 to encourage and stimulate either new investigators or investigators currently working and who have an interest in palliative and end-of-life care. The identified outcomes were to: promote innovative pilot or feasibility studies; develop evidence necessary to determine viability of new research avenues; and build research capacity.[53]

As well, the CIHR of Cancer Research determined in 2003 that palliative and end-of-life care is one of their most important strategic directions for research. There were three components to the initiative:

- One-year pilot projects to target and assess innovative approaches;
- Five-year New Emerging Team grants to build capacity and to promote new research teams or increase existing teams; and
- One-year career transition awards to attract new researchers into this area of specialty.

Networks are being formed through Canada to conduct research to better understand the scope and care needs of palliative and end-of-life populations and their families. Examples of these networks include the Victoria Palliative Research Network (Victoria, British Columbia), the Division of Palliative Medicine (Edmonton, Alberta), and Network for End of Life Studies in Nova Scotia. Examples of research initiatives include:

- Network for End of Life Studies in Nova Scotia has identified its beginning steps for developing a surveillance strategy for its palliative population identified in The End of Life Care in Nova Scotia Surveillance Report (2008) NELS ICE.[54]
- Research on Family Care-giving in Palliative and End-of-Life Care—initiated through Canadian Institute of Health Research funding in 2004, this group is focused on studying family caregiving.[55]
- A research collaboration between four western provinces is reported in Health Care Use at the End

of Life in Western Canada. Identified in this report is the use of hospital and pharmacy services specifically analyzing the location of death, hospital use in the last year of life and use of community-dispersed drugs and supplies.[21]

- Prognostication studies conducted through collaborative research projects with University of Victoria and University of Alberta.[56]

Since the majority of Canadians die from nonmalignant causes, the Institute of Circulatory and Respiratory Health (ICRH) is also a key stakeholder in conducting research in this vital area as well.[57]

## Provincial Programs That Support Palliative Care at Home

### Palliative Drug Benefits Programs

Provinces have jurisdiction over the delivery of hospice palliative care services resulting in various initiatives, support, and service models. Manitoba and British Columbia, acknowledge palliative care as a core health-care service. Quebec has committed support through its palliative end-of-life care and strategic planning policy documents.[58,59] Others, such as Saskatchewan and Alberta, have developed provincial guidelines for services.[60] British Columbia has developed a provincial strategy for end-of-life care.[61] Quebec has begun to integrate palliative care into its existing local community centers known as CLSC, supporting home care with a dedicated phone line and on-call physicians, nurses, and pharmacists.[62] In 2005, the Ontario Ministry of Health and Long-Term Care committed $115.5 million to an end-of-life strategy over 3 years. The goals of the strategy were to shift care to the community, to enhance interdisciplinary approaches to care delivery, and to improve access, coordination, and consistency of services and supports. Though the strategy reflected progress, gaps in service delivery were also highlighted.[63]

Barriers to accessing medications in the home are being addressed by some provinces. For example, several provinces will now cover the cost of palliative medications such as opioids and laxatives for persons who are designated as palliative by their physicians. Alberta and British Columbia also provides coverage of equipment such as hospital beds and supplies. In 2008, Prince Edward Island announced the implementation of their provincial palliative care drug program.[64]

Canadian physicians have adequate access to a wide variety of analgesics for pain management and do not have to contend with the daunting regulatory impediments faced by care providers in many other countries.[24]

### Primary Care Models

There is increasing recognition of the need for adequate reimbursement for family physicians to provide home visits, spend the necessary time with patient and family, work with team members, and provide 24-hour coverage.[65–67] One example of a response to the need for resources was the development of a primary care initiative (PCI), established in Alberta in 2003 in collaboration with Alberta Health and Wellness, the Alberta Medical Association and Alberta's Regional Health Authorities. This was established to improve access to family physicians and other front-line health-care providers in Alberta. The purpose of the PCI is to develop Primary Care Networks (PCNs) and support them in meeting the objectives of the program.[68] One PCN developed a project charter, which focused on resource enhancement specifically for palliative patients and their families. The intent is to enable palliative patients to remain in their respective communities through use of flexible funding, provide opportunity for building capacity, and remove barriers for primary care physician involvement as well as to enhance linkages with palliative care specialists.[68]

### British Columbia Telenursing

Leaders in the Fraser Health regions of British Columbia identified the need to improve access for palliative and end-of-life care. There was a need to provide 24/7 access to nurses who are generalists and deal with a broad range of health problems, and to address questions related specifically to hospice palliative care. The exploration of how information and communications technology could be used to achieve this kind of support for home based palliative patients and their families began.[69] This was a collaboration between the Fraser Health Hospice Palliative care program and B.C. Nurse Line.

A pilot project was conducted where hospice palliative care content was incorporated into the provincial call system for after hours call. At any one time, 750 home-based hospice palliative care clients had access to after-hours telephone lines. "Healthwise Knowledge base triage protocols" include specialized content specific to palliative care were added to enhance the existing tools.[69] The results of the project demonstrated that 80% of calls met the needs of the patients and/or families. With this support, 91% of the patients were able to stay home throughout the night.[70] Only six home visits have been made in the 2 years since implementation of this after-hours service.

The nurses involved in the project were able to leverage their experience and develop training tools, a resource manual for using the HPC protocols, and templates to enable other health authorities to develop these types of programs.

## Technology Projects that Support Hospice Palliative Care

### InterRAI

The interRAI assessment tools are at various implementation stages for select provinces. British Columbia, Alberta, and

Ontario are planning to or have implemented the InterRAI MDS Home Care and/or MDS 2.0 for continuing care assessment tools to improve quality of care and access to services. Alberta is using the tool to determine the most appropriate service, to monitor current trends and outcomes, as well as to assist in forecasting future needs and projections.[71] Critical to the Albertan experience is the linkage in the use of the interRAI tools with standard and policy development. The continuing care standards in Alberta include palliative care and related components such as goal setting, pain, and symptom management. Strategies to identify key triggers within the tools that identify the need for consultation to palliative care services are in their preliminary phases of development.

The interRAI palliative care assessment tool has been used primarily for research purposes in Canada. In research, Brink and Frise Smith[72] have used the tool to identify the determinants of home death among individuals receiving home-care services. Results from this study reinforce that the presence of a supportive family and consideration for the individual and family as a unit of care is significant in the ability to allow a home death.[72]

### Electronic Health Record

There was a desire in Alberta's former Chinook Health Region to look at some form of integrated electronic health information platform. The ideal solution would ensure a common platform for all health services. In 2004, a decision was made to pull rural health services into a shared forum called Regional Shared Health Information Program (RSHIP) to develop a common database that would be used by various departments such as finance, pharmacy, and for clinical care documentation. This would also create the capability to complete documentation at the point of care and allow for data to be compared with the areas involved in the project.

A collaboration which involved the former seven non-metro Regional Health Authorities in Alberta including: Chinook, Palliser, David Thompson, East Central, Aspen, Peace Country, and Northern Lights was formed. Their vision was "to develop a Center of Excellence for the delivery of a full suite of integrated clinical and financial applications and the creation of a shared Enterprise Medical Record."[73] The creation of the Patient Care System, which was a clinical documentation system in Meditec software, occurred. The intent was to design documentation to assist multiple disciplines working in a variety of health-care settings. The goals of the project were to:

- Reduce duplication of entry and minimize narrative charting on progress notes;
- Meet legal and professional requirements;
- Facilitate provincial and national reporting requirements;
- Utilize evidence-based practices and standards;
- Incorporate provincially recommended systems (ACORN, MORE, STROKE, etc.);

- Standardize assessment tools, protocols, abbreviations, and create common content;
- Select consistent taxonomy from universally accepted classification tables (e.g., ICD-10); and
- Ensure the system is patient-focused with workload and acuity measurements for utilization data needs.

This initiative, implemented in June 2008, has allowed patient information to be accessed from any point in the health-care system within these participating former seven regional health authorities. As yet, measurable outcomes have not been reported but anecdotal reporting from health professionals indicates good uptake and staff are pleased with the ability to access patient information in a timely manner. This also resulted in incorporation of the common palliative care assessment tools such as the Palliative Performance Scale and the Edmonton System Assessment Tool into the electronic health record. This has assisted health professionals to use identified measures to help shape the clinical picture for palliative patients across the continuum of care.[73]

### Palliative Care Nursing in Canada

#### Hospice Palliative Care Nursing Standards

Recognition of hospice palliative care nursing in Canada began in 1993, in Winnipeg, where nurses met to form a special interest group.[74] The intent was to develop a formal network that would meet at national and international palliative care conferences held in Canada. The goal of the network was to establish a national voice to advance hospice palliative nursing care in policy development, education, and research.

This network was recognized by CHPCA through the formation of the Nurses Interest Group. With the use of technology, the network moved beyond conference discussions to development of a national list serve that continues to serve as a mechanism for networking and information exchange.

In 2002, the first Standards for Hospice Palliative Care Nursing were developed. These standards, based on the Supportive Care Model, identified six dimensions that reflected hospice palliative nursing at that time and included valuing, connecting, empowering, doing for, finding meaning, and preserving integrity.[75] Following the endorsement of these standards and competencies by hospice palliative care nurses in Canada, the Canadian Nurses Association (CNA), in conjunction with the CHPCA Nurses Interest Group, initiated the process of specialty certification for hospice palliative care nursing. CNA certification "requires adherence to rigorous practice standards, a commitment to continuous learning."[69] Review and revision of the hospice palliative care nursing standards is currently underway to recognize the changing role of the hospice palliative care nurse within the interdisciplinary team and projected future roles.

## Hospice Palliative Care Nursing Certification in Canada

Since its inception as a Canadian Nurses Certification specialty in 2003, the number of nurses certified in hospice palliative care in 2008 alone was 20.4%. This is an increase from 916 to 1,247 nurses compared to a 3% increase of all of the 17 certification specialties combined.[76] In spite of this significant growth, the continued development and need for succession planning for hospice palliative care nurses in Canada is essential. The CNA report, *Towards 2020*, indicates that is it critical to is critical to look through a different lens for nursing to provide leadership to create a health-care future that meets the needs of the population. Hospice palliative care nurses in Canada have an opportunity to engage in this discussion through the current revision of the CHPCA Hospice Palliative Care Nursing Standards.

## Hospice Palliative Care Nursing Education

The Canadian Association of Schools of Nursing (CASN) recognized that though research indicates that nursing students have concerns for caring for individuals who are dying, they lack the necessary preparation.[77] In 2004, a CASN Task Force was established to address this gap in palliative care nursing education. Sponsored by Health Canada, a survey was distributed, through purposive sampling, to education administrators, CASN members and hospice palliative care practitioners.

The results of the survey indicated that although hospice palliative care education is being addressed in most programs that participated in the survey, there is a need to further develop palliative and end-of-life curriculum. Challenges to do so include adding additional content to full curriculum; the tension to balance generalist and specialist competencies in undergraduate education; and faculty and organizational approval and practicum placement sites.[77]

## Summary

There has been tremendous change in palliative and end-of-life care in Canada over the past 5 years. Numerous influences, national and provincial developments, and best practice models have emerged to continually enhance care provision for Canadians. The establishment of the Health Canada Secretariat on Palliative and End-of-Life Care provided a mechanism for the palliative care community to collectively initiate key strategies to further enhance hospice palliative care nationally.

There are areas identified by colleagues and the literature for future growth. One of the major areas is the use of technology in health care and the many opportunities that have yet to occur. The CNA position statement on nursing information and knowledge management encompasses several aspects of technology in the provision of nursing care. It cites that information management and communication technology are vital to nursing practice.[78]

The enhanced support for community based services and family caregivers are significant in continuing to broaden the scope of palliative care services. Further development of palliative and end-of-life care standards, measurable outcomes, and indicators to create common methods to be able to compare and measure various programs and services across the country are needed.[79] The need to define the scope of the palliative and end-of-life care population through the establishment of a nationwide surveillance process is critical.

Several challenges continue to exist today with inconsistency among programs and services; access to pharmaceuticals, equipment, and supplies; and lack of access to palliative and end-of-life care by patients and families. Advocacy for improvement of these factors will continue to be required in moving hospice palliative care forward in the country.[80]

Recommendations identify the need for inter-professional education in palliative and end-of-life care. To accomplish this there would need to be collaboration and linkages with licensing/accrediting bodies, schools/faculties, and practicing professionals. The interprofessional approach to education reflects how care is provided in health-care settings. There is also a strong recommendation for hospice palliative care curriculum development needing to be incorporated into universities education for health professionals.[81]

There is also a need to ensure accessible, comprehensive palliative and end-of-life education is available for those health professionals currently practicing in health care to build their knowledge base and skill. It is vital to ensure that these education programs are flexible, meet adult learning needs, and can be adapted to a variety of work settings and within the workforce constraints that exist.

With courage to vision beyond traditional approaches of care delivery and to collectively develop the hospice palliative nursing voice within collaborative and intraprofessional models, hospice palliative care nurses are well-positioned to provide leadership in the provision of exceptional integrated and intraprofessional care, education, and research to further enhance and ensure quality palliative and end-of-life care to all Canadians.

## Acknowledgments

Sandy McKinnon was an original author of the 2000 chapter on Canada. Sandy died in 2000, yet her ongoing influence on this chapter is acknowledged.

The authors would like to thank Carleen Brenneis, Pam Brown, and Pat Selmser for editing the chapter, and to thank our many colleagues across the country who shared information and continue to champion hospice palliative and end-of-life care in Canada.

## REFERENCES

1. Commission on the Future of Health Care in Canada. Building on values. The future of health care in Canada. Final Report. November, 2002. Available at: http://www.healthcarecommission.ca (accessed March 20, 2005).

2. End-of-life care coalition. Brief to Roy Romanow, Commissioner. Future of Health Care in Canada. April 30, 2002.

3. Canada Health Act, 1984, C.6, s.1, 1–12. Canadian Centre for Analysis of Regionalization & Health. What is regionalization? Available at: www.regionalizaton.org/Regionalization/Regionalization.html (accessed April 25, 2005).

4. Standing Senate Committee on Social Affairs, Science and Technology. The Health of Canadians—the Federal Role, Vol. 6, Recommendations for Reform 2002. Available at: http://www.parl .gc.ca/37/2/parlbus/commbus/senate/com-e/soci-e/rep-e/repfin nov03-e.htm (accessed October 2008).

5. Canadian Strategy for Cancer Control—Palliative Care Working Group. Available at: www.phac-aspc.gc.ca/publicat/prcc-relcc/chp_6-eng.php (accessed December 2009).

6. Health Canada. Canadian Strategy on Palliative and End-of-Life Care: Final Report. 2007. Available at: http://www.hc-sc-gc.ca/hcs-sss/pubs/palliat/2007-soin_fin-end?life/evolution-eng.php (accessed December 2, 2008).

7. Health Canada. First Minister's Meeting on the Future of Health Care 2004. A 10-year plan to strengthen health care. Available at: http://www.hc-sc.gc.ca/hcs-sss/delivery-prestation/fptcollab/2004-fmm-rpm/index-eng.php (accessed March 2, 2009).

8. Canadian Hospice Palliative Care Association. Strategic Plan and Progress Report. 2006–2009. Available at: http://www.chpca.net/about_us/CHPCA_Strategic_Plan_2006_2009.pdf (accessed December 2008).

9. Canadian Hospice Palliative Care Association. Available at: http://www.chpca.net/menu_items/faqs.htm#faz_whatis (accessed October 2008).

10. Ferris FD, Balfour HM, Bowen K, et al. A Model to Guide Hospice Palliative Care. Ottawa: Canadian Hospice Palliative Care Association, 2002.

11. Sevean P, Dampier S, Spadoni M, Strickland S, Pilatzke. Bridging the distance: Educating nurses for telehealth practice. J Contin Educ Nurs 2008;39:413–418.

12. Canadian Nurses Association, Department of Regulatory Policy. Number of RN's with Valid CNA certification by Year and Specialty, 2003–2007.

13. Subcommittee to update "of Life and Death" of the Standing Senate Committee on Social Affairs Science and Technology. Quality End-of-Life Care: The Right of Every Canadian. Ottawa: Government of Canada, 2001.

14. Hospice palliative care nursing standards of practice. CHPCA Nursing Standards Committee. February 2002. Available at: http://www.chpca.net/interest_groups/nurses/Hospice_Palliative_Care_Nursing_Standards_of_Practice.pdf (accessed November 2008).

15. Chochinov HM, Kristjanson L. Dying to pay: The cost of end-of-life care. J Palliat Care 1998;14:5–15.

16. National Consensus Project Guidelines. Available at: http://www.nationalconsensusproject.org/Guidelines_Download.asp (accessed October 28, 2008).

17. Report to Cancer 2000 Task Force. The Expert Panel on Palliative Care, 1991.

18. Salisbury C, Bosanquet N, Bilkinson EK, et al. The impact of different models of specialist palliative care on patients' quality of life: A systematic literature review. Palliat Med 1999;13:3–17.

19. Statistics Canada, Portrait of the Canadian Population in 2006: National portrait Available at: http://www12.statcan.ca/english/census06/analysis/popdwell/NatlPortrait1.cfm (accessed December 2008).

20. Hall P, Stone G, Fiset VJ. Palliative care: How can we meet the needs of our multicultural communities? Palliat Care 1998;14:46–49.

21. Mackay B. Changing face of Canada is changing the face of medicine. CMAJ 2001;168:599.

22. Eve A, Smith AM, Tebbit P. Hospice and palliative care in the UK 1994–95, including a summary of trends 1990–95. Palliat Med 1997;11:31–43.

23. Bon Bernard C, Feser L. Enhancing cultural competence in palliative care; perspective of an elderly Chinese community in Calgary. J Palliat Care 2003;19:133–139.

24. Maddock I. Is hospice a western concept? In: Clark D, Hockly J, Ahmedsa S, eds. New Themes in Palliative Care. Buckingham: Open University Press; 1997:195–238.

25. Statistics Canada, 2007, Overview 2007—aboriginal peoples. Available at: http://www41.statcan.ca/2007/10000/ceb10000_000_e.htm (accessed November 16, 2008).

26. Aboriginal self-government in the Northwest Territories: Our government today. 1999. Available at: http://www.gov.nt.ca/publications/asg/pdfs/ourg.pdf (accessed December 2008).

27. Con A. Cross-cultural consideration in promoting advance care planning, Prepared for Health Canada, CIHR Cross-Cultural Palliative NET, p. 6, 2008. Available at: http://www.bccancer.bc.ca/NR/rdonlyres/39C930BB-1AAA-4700-98BB-9004835F3BD/28582/COLOUR030408_Con.pdf (accessed December 2008).

28. Statistics Canada, Aboriginal Peoples in Canada in 2006: Inuit, Metis and First Nations, 2006 Census. Available at: http://www12.statcan.ca/english/census06/analysis/aboriginal/surpass.cfm (accessed December 23, 2008).

29. Canadian Hospice Palliative Care Association. A discussion document on aboriginal hospice palliative care in Canada, Health Canada, Prepared for Canadian Hospice Palliative Care Association by Hanson and Associates, 2007.

30. Canadian Nurses Association. Toward 2020 Visions for Nursing, Principal Investigators M. Villeneuve & J. MacDonald. 2006. Available at: www.cna-aiic.ca/CNA/documents/pdf/publications/Toward-2020-e.pdf (accessed December 2008).

31. Calgary Health Region. Available at: www.albertahealthservices.ca (accessed December 2008).

32. Canadian Institute for Health Information, 2007. Health Care Use at the End of Life in Western Canada.

33. Canadian Society for Telehealth, 2006. Vision Statement. Available at: http//:www.sct.org (accessed January 2, 2009).

34. Lupoli J, Rizzo V. The impact of technology on the "older" nurse. Home Healthc Nurse 2003;21(10):691–692.

35. Health Canada. Canadian virtual hospice: Knowledge development and support in palliative care. November 2001. Available at: http://www.hc-sc.gc.ca/english/media/releases/2001/2001_121ebk1.htm (accessed November 2008).

36. Rural Palliative Telehealth Project, final project report, October, 2007.

37. Advanced care planning: An implementation guide for health authorities in Canada, March 2008.

38. Health Canada. Advance Care Planning the Glossary Project—Final Report, 2006. Available at: http://www.hc-sc.gc.ca/hcs-sss/pubs/palliat/2006-proj-glos/index-eng.php#Toc144091361 (accessed March 2, 2009).

39. ACP, An implementation guide for health authorities in Canada, March 2008; Health Canada 2006. Executive Summary, Advanced Care Planning, the Glossary Project: Final Report.

40. Macleod ML, Misener RM, I'm a different kind of nurse: Advice from nurses in rural and remote Canada. Nurs Leadersh (Tor Ont) 2008;21(3):40–53.

41. Rural Palliative Telehealth Project, Alberta Health and Wellness, Clinical Grant Fund, October 15, 2007.

42. Position Statement: Nursing Information and Knowledge Management Canadian Nurses Association 2008. Available at: www.cna-nurses.ca (accessed November 28).

43. Sevean PS, Dampier S, Spadoni M, Strickland S, Pilatze S. Patients and families experiences with video telehealth in rural/remote communities in Northern Canada. J Clin Nurs 2008;10:1365–2702.

44. CHPCA, Quality End-of-Life Care Coalition of Canada, History and Background of the Coalition. Available at: http://www.chpca.net/qelccc/information_and_resources/3_History_and_Mandate-nov2007.pdf (accessed December 2008).

45. Canadian Home Care Association, Available at: www.cdn.homecare.ca (accessed November 2006).

46. CHCA, Nov 2006; Pan-Canadian Gold Standard for Palliative Home Care, December 2006; Hospice Palliative Home care in Canada: A Progress Report, May 2008; 2007 Canadian Institute for Health Information, Health Care Use at the End of Life in Western Canada.

47. 10-year plan to strengthen health care, Government of Canada, 2004. Available at: www.hc-sc.gc.ca/hcs-sss/delivery-presentation/fptcollab/2004-fmm-rpm/index_ehtml (accessed December 2008).

48. Educating Future Physicians in Palliative and End of Life Care, Symposium, November 2007—Making Change Happen.

49. Accreditation Canada, 2007. 2008 Canadian Health Accreditation Report. Available at: http://www.accreditation-canada.ca (accessed January 29, 2009).

50. Accreditation Canada: Hospice palliative and end-of-life care. Available at: http://www.accreditation-canada.ca/default.aspx?page=58 (accessed December 2008).

51. Accreditation Canada: Strategy. Available at: http://www.accreditation-canada.ca/default.aspx?page=47&cat=34 (accessed December 5, 2008).

52. Accreditation Canada, Qmentum Program 2009, Hospice, Palliative, and End-of-Life Services Available at: http://www.accreditation-canada.ca (accessed December 2, 2008).

53. Canadian Institute of Health Research. Available at: www.cihr-irsc.gc.ca/e/15919 (accessed December 2008).

54. End of Life Care in Nova Scotia Surveillance Report. Network for End of Life Studies (NELS) Interdisciplinary Capacity Enhancement (ICE), Dalhousie University, Halifax, Nova Scotia. Available at: http://nels.schoolofhealthservicesadministration.dal.ca/ (accessed February 2, 2009).

55. Family Caregiving in Palliative and End-of-Life Care. Available at: http://www.coag.uvic.ca/eolcare/ (accessed February 2, 2009).

56. Victoria Hospice, Palliative Care Research. Available at: http://www.victoriahospice.org/health-care-professionals/palliative-care-research/palliative-care-research-projects (accessed February 2, 2009).

57. Canadian Institute of Health Research. Available at: www.cihr-irsc.gc.ca/e/12874 (accessed December 2008).

58. Canadian Hospice Palliative Care Association, Quebec End-of-Life Care Policy, Available at: http://www.chpca.net/public_policy_advocacy/Quebec_policy.pdf (accessed December 2008).

59. Canadian Hospice Palliative Care Association Provincial Association. Available at: http://www.reseaupalliatif.org/ (accessed December 2009).

60. Palliative Care: A Policy Framework. Alberta Health, December 1993.

61. Minister of Health Services, British Columbia. Discussion paper on a provincial strategy for end-of-life care in British Columbia. October 2002. Available at: http://www.healthservices.gov.bc.ca/hcc/pdf/elcpaper.pdf (accessed October 2002).

62. Rachlis M. Prescription for Excellence. Toronto, Canada: HarperCollins Publishers, 2004.

63. Seow H, King S, Vaitonis V. The impact of Ontario's end-of-life care strategy on end-of-life care in the community. Healthc Q 2008;11(1):56–62.

64. CHPCA annual conference, 2008 (this was from an announcement at the CHPCA 2007 conference by the premier of PEI on October 27, 2008).

65. Burge F, McIntyre P, Twohig P, Cummings I, Kaufman D, Frager G. Palliative care by family physicians in the 1990's. Can Fam Physician 2001;47:1989–1995.

66. Brenneis C, Bruera E. The interaction between family physicians and palliative care consultants in the delivery of palliative care: Clinical and educational issues. J Palliat Care 1998;14:58–61.

67. MacKenzie MR. The interface of palliative care, oncology and family practice: A view from a family practitioner. CMAJ 1998;158:1705–1707.

68. Primary Care Network, Calgary Rural. Primary Care Service—Project Charter. Available at: www.albertapci.ca (accessed September 24, 2008).

69. Canadian Nurse, Telenursing in Hospice Palliative Care, May 2007.

70. Roberts D, Tayler C, MacCormack D, Barwich D. Canadian Nurse, Telenursing in Hospice Palliative Care, May 2007.

71. Lai V, Laing G. Making the quality connection between RAI processes and continuing care policy/standards, 2008 Canadian RAI Conference Making the Quality Connection, Edmonton, May 2008. Available at: www.capitalhealth.ca/NR/rdonlyres/eqn3a60rb4jz7lewfctpvdg3bicenpbtl7huxh6pf7wyet5dwr75ssn7dflcukvahochjqojy7hqdhj6jmqwxpsh5uc/RAI-C1-Handout_LaiLaing.pdf (accessed December 2008).

72. Brink P, Frise Smith T. Determinants of home death in palliative home care: Using the interRAI palliative care to assess end-of-life care. Am J Hosp Palliat Care 2008;25(4):263–270.

73. E-Doc for Palliative Care, Chinook Health, PowerPoint, June 20, 2008.

74. Hospice palliative care nursing standards of practice. CHPCA Nursing Standards Committee. February 2002. Available at: http://www.chpca.net/interest_groups/nurses/Hospice_Palliative_Care_Nursing_Standards_of_Practice.pdf (accessed November 2008).

75. Davies B, Oberle K. Dimensions of the supportive role of the nurse in palliative care. Oncol Nurs Forum 1990;17(1):87–94.

76. Canadian Nurses Association, Department of Regulatory Policy. Number of RN's with Valid CNA certification by Year and Specialty, 2003–2007.

77. Canadian Association of Schools of Nursing, 2008, Certification Bulletin, 5, April 2008. Available at: http://www.cna-nurses.ca/cna/documents/pdf/publications/Cert_bulletin_5_April_08_e.pdf (accessed December 2008).

78. CNA, Nursing Information and knowledge management. 2008. Available at: www.cna-nurses.ca/CNA/issues/position/practice/default_e.aspx (accessed December 2, 2008).

79. CHPCA, Strategic Plan and Progress Report. 2006–2009.

80. CHCPA, annual report 2006–2007; Quality End-of-Life Care Coalition of Canada, Hospice Palliative Home Care in Canada: A Progress Report, May 2008.

81. The Pan-Canadian Gold Standard for Palliative Home Care; Toward Equitable Access to High Quality Hospice Palliative and End-of-Life care at Home; December 2006.

# 70    *Margaret O'Connor and Peter L. Hudson*

# Palliative Care in Australia and New Zealand

- **Key Points**
- *There are commonalities and differences between models of palliative care in Australia and New Zealand, based on aspects like geography, historical models, culture, and community involvement.*
- *Palliative care nurses in both countries are increasingly taking on advance practice leadership roles in research, education, and policy.*

Palliative care nursing in Australia and New Zealand shares many features of palliative care nursing as practiced elsewhere in the world. The similarities between Australasian palliative care nursing and palliative care nursing in other countries is evident in the Australasian contribution to journals such as the International Journal of Palliative Nursing and in the adoption of *texts written or co-edited by Australians and accepted by international publishers.*[1,2] The purpose of this chapter is to both profile palliative care in Australia and New Zealand and to provide insights into some of the key innovations in care where nurses are providing a leading role.

In developing this chapter, we acknowledge the work of our colleagues (and friends) Sanchia Aranda and Linda Kristjanson who contributed to the former chapters and allowed us to include and build on their foundational content. We have retained and updated those sections of the chapter that provide an overview of palliative care in Australia and New Zealand. The survey, utilized to gain information from practicing nurses in Australia and New Zealand for the first edition, has been repeated for this edition (see Acknowledgements). We have also maintained the specific focus on particular issues from the second edition, but included new content on education and training, research, policy and international links, and advanced practice roles. The chapter concludes with some reflections on future directions.

## Some Essential Differences between Australia and New Zealand

Australia and New Zealand are often considered together—consistently labeled as "down under" and far away in world consciousness. Despite being close geographically and sharing a predominantly British heritage, these countries have significantly different personalities that are important to understand before exploring palliative care developments of the two countries.

New Zealand is a small country consisting of two large islands and one smaller, sparsely populated island. The total population is 4.1 million, according to the 2006 census.[3] The population is unevenly spread between the two main islands, with almost 75% living in the North Island. European/Pakeha (white) make up almost 80% of the population; with 13.6% Maori and 6.4% Pacific Islanders.[3] The population is very young with the total average age being 33.1 years. Industry is predominantly agricultural.

Specialist health services are likely to be confined to large cities in each of the two main islands, but most general health services are available locally. However, New Zealand's population density, 16 people per cubic square kilometer compared to 234.5 per km[3] in Britain, has some effect on access to health services, with those in less densely populated areas having less access to specialized services, including palliative care.[4]

In contrast, Australia is the smallest continent, but one of the largest countries in the world, being a large island and one very small island state of Tasmania, and ordered into six regional states and two territories. The population is about 20,600 million (www.abs.gov.au) with a population density of 2.7 people per square kilometer. However, about 90% of the population lives in about 3% of the land area, making city living very dense. According to the 2006 census (www.abs.gov.au), Indigenous Australians make up only 2.6% of the population, although the total number of 517,000 individuals has increased over the last 10 years. Australia has undergone significantly more migration than New Zealand, with 25% of the population born overseas at the 2006 census. Overseas-born Australians are predominantly from the United Kingdom (24%), New Zealand (9%), Italy (5%), and China and Vietnam (4%; www.abs.gov.au). The most recent new immigrant groups come from the Sudan, Afghanistan, and Iraq. This makes for a very diverse population with one dominant cultural group and many minorities.

Because of the size of its land mass, Australia's rural and remote populations may be very isolated, with the nearest neighbor a day's drive away; this has implications for models of health service. Despite the Aboriginal population constituting only a small percentage of the total population, they make up 30% of the population of central Australia, and in some communities are the main clients of health services.

It is clear, then, that Australia and New Zealand have similarities and differences. Both countries feature a predominance of people from Anglo-Celtic origins and were populated by these settlers at a similar time, although under different circumstances—Australia was established as a penal colony and New Zealand with free settlers. Both were colonialist settlements featuring disenfranchisement of the existing population—in Australia the native Aboriginal people, and in New Zealand the Maori. Since that time, New Zealand has remained largely bicultural despite limited migration from other parts of the world, while Australia is considered a diverse multicultural society. Despite many languages being spoken in Australia, English is the only official language. In contrast, both English and Maori are recognized national languages in New Zealand, and significant effort has been made to maintain Maori cultural identity and influence at a national level. Resurgence in Maori nationalism over recent years has been more effective in influencing national policy than has similar Indigenous nationalism in Australia.

## Australian and New Zealand Models of Health and Palliative Care

Both countries have a long history of universal health insurance systems that provide basic healthcare to all people, supplemented by a limited system of private healthcare, which is more extensive in Australia. There is a consistent valuing of universal access to adequate healthcare within the two populations despite increasing trends toward user payment for some services.

Both countries feature a trend toward privatization of public facilities that affects health-care services, perhaps most noticeable in residential aged care. Privatization of residential aged care facilities has resulted in fewer not-for-profit providers and an increased need to profit from care of the elderly, with considerable potential impact on access to palliative care services when combined with the shift toward user payments. Despite this, healthcare remains at a high standard, with access to a range of generalist and specialist services at a level consistent with that of the United States and Europe. Spending on health is 8% to 9% in Australia and 6.2% in New Zealand of Gross Domestic Product. In both countries, most generalist services are available to rural communities, but specialist services, such as radiotherapy, usually require travel to a large city. In remote areas of Australia, access to healthcare may be limited to a regular monthly clinic by the Royal Flying Doctor Service and limited access to outreach telephone services. In some remote settings, nursing care may be provided through remote nursing stations where nurses are expected to serve as advanced generalists attending to a range of health-care concerns within the community.

## Structure and Delivery of Palliative Care

Hospice and palliative care developments in Australia and New Zealand are well advanced, with services required to meet established standards of service delivery.[5,6] Models of palliative care delivery in both these countries feature inpatient, home care, and hospital support teams, with New Zealand evidencing more use of daycare services than Australia. Urban cities tend to feature all service elements, with home-care provision showing the most variation. In larger rural cities, small specialist services provide support and consultancy services to generalist nurses and local doctors. Palliative care developments in both countries are notable for their lack of homogeneity, with models of care dependent on historical factors, financial support, population density, and the local community environment.

The first hospice service in New Zealand opened in 1979,[4] with services now operating in the main cities across the country (www.hospice.org.nz). Palliative care in New Zealand features the development of small community inpatient hospices that link strongly with local community nursing services in the provision of home care, and highly dependent on local fundraising. The system is well-organized through a national association that facilitates communication between members, including a bi-annual national conference. A national election and change of government at the end of 2008 promised an increase in government funding support for hospice and palliative care services throughout the country.

The first Australian hospices predate the opening of St. Christopher's in London (1969) by 79 years—the establishment by the Irish Sisters of Charity of hospices in Sydney (1890) and Melbourne (1938). These traditional large bed-based facilities followed the Irish model and philosophy of caring for dying people in a facility linked to, but separate from, an acute hospital. Over time, the skills and expertise in caring for dying people were seen to be concentrated in the hospice, resulting in a separation of this knowledge from other healthcare settings.[7] Following the global spread of modern hospice, Australia's response during the 1980s and 1990s occurred largely through the development of community based palliative care services with a particular emphasis on care in the home. However, significant change has taken place in service delivery, with increased emphasis in both state and federal government health policy to improve access to palliative care by equitable service distribution across the community and health-care systems. To this end, Palliative Care Australia promotes a needs-based model of care, necessitating the significant involvement of primary care providers, which ensures people receive the right level of care commensurate with their stage of illness, symptom burden, and other needs.[8,9] New inpatient developments are increasingly linked to acute services to assist in the availability of appropriate beds for people in acute settings. There is increasing recognition of the need for the expertise of palliative care being available across hospital systems and of the applicability of palliative care principles for people dying of any illness. Hospital-based palliative care consultancy teams, often nurse-led, have become increasingly utilized in acute hospitals.[10,11]

Palliative care services in both countries uphold the principle of supporting a person's decision to be cared for and to die where they choose. Australian government policy directions clearly support the care of people in their own homes.[12] This emphasis includes specific attention to respite care and 24-hour access to supportive advice.

## Cultural Issues

A key feature of New Zealand healthcare is its responsiveness to Maori nationalism, which calls for greater control over their own health and services compatible to cultural beliefs. Cultural safety is a feature of Maori demands for appropriate health service development, and is a concept that moves beyond cultural sensitivity, featuring both acknowledgment and respect for difference, toward implementation of strategies to promote and nurture the cultural identity of the person who is ill.[13] In New Zealand, nurses have taken the lead on cultural issues in health with the production of guidelines in 1992,[13] which were updated in 2002.[14] These guidelines define cultural safety as "an outcome of nursing and midwifery education that enables safe service to be defined by those who receive the service" (p. 5). Ultimately, this means that people of one culture feel able to utilize a health service provided by another culture without feeling at risk. The New Zealand Palliative Care Strategy, released in February 2001,[15] specifically detailed expectations for Maori and Pacific people, including development of linkages with Maori organizations, local service plans, and the employment of care coordinators in conjunction with local Maori providers.

In contrast, the Australian indigenous people remain a marginalized group with a health status significantly below that of other Australians, despite strong government programs to address their health issues. A long history of neglect and suffering as a result of earlier ethnocentric government policy has left a legacy of difficulties for indigenous peoples. And chronic illnesses like diabetes and kidney failure are endemic.

In 2004, Australia's peak health research body, the National Health and Medical Research Council (NHMRC) released ethical guidelines for conducting research with Aboriginal and Torres Strait Islanders, a move highly significant in raising the importance of respecting different values and ethics.[16] And under the National Palliative Care strategy[17] there was a need identified, for services "...to cater sensitively and flexibly for the needs of Aboriginal and Torres Strait Islanders" (p. 6). Under this program, a project addressing culturally appropriate palliative care has developed a resource kit to assist work with these population groups (www.health.gov.au). Building on a needs study, practice principles and educational resources were developed to support mainstream healthcare workers to provide culturally appropriate palliative care. The key goals of this project were to ensure communication and other systems were in place to increase health worker awareness of the needs of Aboriginal and Torres Strait Islander peoples, as well as Aboriginal and Torres Strait Islander awareness of the services that mainstream palliative care services can provide.

Working with indigenous people, culturally responsive models of palliative care delivery are starting to be developed, to ensure that traditional practices that surround care of dying people and death are understood, respected, and incorporated into care. For example, an in-patient facility constructed in Darwin incorporated the ability to move a bed outside the room, so that a patient could be cared for and die in the open air. The facility also has the ability to undertake the traditional smoking ceremony, conducted in the facility after a person has died, to drive their spirit away.[18]

Importantly, Kanitsaki's research[19] has challenged a dominant palliative care nursing belief in open discussion about death and dying. Participants in her studies of Italian, Chinese, and Greek Australians often perceived nurses "who attempted to discuss with them death and dying" as "negative, insensitive, and transmitted to them a sense of hopelessness" (p. 39). In addition, nurses who were accepting of death and told them they were dying were interpreted as giving up on them, producing fears that they would stop caring.

Of particular relevance in both Australia and New Zealand, are the expectations of people from Asian cultures living in both countries. In a multicultural country like Australia, the barriers of culture and language have been the basis for examining communication patterns and styles between health providers and patients, and a lack of effective communication may mean less than satisfactory exchanges between health providers, patients, and their families.[20,21] In particular, ways of breaking bad news, decision-making processes, and other forms of communication differ between cultures as to what is acceptable.[22] During the past decade, several projects have developed culturally appropriate information on palliative care services for the particular cultural community, aimed at improving service provision and access,[23] but because information is most often introduced through service providers, it is limited to those who access such services. Systematic attention to cultural safety should move beyond access to interpreters, multilingual information, and liaison with ethnic community organizations and religious groups.

### Rural and Remote Communities

Nurses working in rural areas believe there is significant work needed to provide for the palliative care needs of rural communities.[24] Rural and remote communities in both Australia and New Zealand are not homogeneous; they offer various challenges to health delivery based on demographics, local culture, physical environment, and distance from health services. Rural nurses, providing palliative care as one aspect of a broader health role in the community, suffer significant professional isolation. In some settings, particularly in remote areas, the nurse may be the sole health practitioner in a community, receiving telephone support from a doctor located some distance away. The challenge is to develop sustainable models of palliative care provision in many of these communities.

One successful primary health-care program has been the Program of Experience in the Palliative Approach (PEPA; http://www.pepaeducation.com). Supported by the Australian Government under the National Palliative Care Program, the program aims to improve access and quality of services across Australia, through the up-skilling of mainly primary health-care providers. The program has three components to develop the knowledge and skills of participants: funded clinical workforce placements; integration of learning into the workplace, and networks of support. Travel, accommodation, and backfill are also provided to facilitate the participation of clinicians, especially those in rural areas.

### Models of After Hours Service Provision

Consistent with the standards of Palliative Care Australia, is the requirement to plan coordinated care among service providers, so that a patient and their caregivers are well-supported, particularly in the home environment.[6] In many places this will include provision of 24-hour access to support. The nature of this support differs across services and between rural and metropolitan areas and maintaining the after-hours service can place significant strain on small services in terms of small numbers of nurses sharing after-hours responsibilities. Two models of metropolitan after-hours provision have developed that address this strain. The first consists of a triage model where a related inpatient service receives calls from patients or family members at home regarding their needs. In an evaluation of this model,[25] the triage nurse was able to manage 30% (192 calls) of calls alone. The remaining 70% (437 calls) were transferred to the specialist community palliative care nurse on call. Of these, a further 43% (186 calls) were managed by the specialist nurse with telephone support. The remaining 57% (251 calls) required a home visit. Importantly, the identity of the triage nurse was significantly related to whether the call could be managed alone, suggesting improvements in training and support for the triage nurse could increase the number of calls managed in this way and further reduce burden on the specialist community palliative care nurse.

The second model consists of sharing after-hours responsibilities between specialist palliative care services and generalist community nursing services. Across Australian metropolitan areas generalist community nursing services already offer after-hours care and are already available to visit patients at home requiring palliative care. All of these nurses are provided with basic palliative care knowledge and skills and have access to updated information about the specific palliative patients seeking after-hours support on a daily basis. In some settings this service is supplemented by telephone support after hours by a specialist palliative care nurse, increasing the capacity of the general community nurse to meet the patients' needs.

Night respite can be another means of improving after-hours support. An Australian study undertaken by Kristjanson and colleagues,[26] described the benefits of night respite for patients receiving a home palliative care service and their families. The investigators developed and tested a brief assessment tool to determine those patients and families most in need of night respite. Care aides were then specifically trained to provide night respite support and 53 patients received this support over an 11-month period. Results indicated that the assessment tool was reliable and feasible for use in practice. Findings from this study revealed that the types of patients most in need of night respite support were confused, agitated, or incontinent. As well, families with high levels of caregiver fatigue were particularly in need of this type of respite. Patients and family caregivers reported high levels of satisfaction with the night-respite service and 70% of patients who died during the study were able to die at home. Cost estimates indicated that the home-care and night-respite service was delivered for approximately one third the cost for an equivalent period of inpatient palliative care.

## Palliative Care in Aged Care Settings

During the last two decades, research has indicated that the proportion of people dying in Australian residential aged care facilities has steadily increased. The increased number of residents dying in residential aged care facilities has focused attention on the need for a palliative approach that may enhance the care already provided to both residents and the families. A palliative approach[27] aims to improve the quality of life for individuals facing the end stage of their life, by reducing their suffering, treating pain, and assessing other physical, cultural, psychological, social, and spiritual needs. The palliative approach should be able to be provided by all health professionals in all settings of care, with referral to specialist palliative care services where patient needs require this.

In response to the developing recognition of the needs of people dying in residential aged care, in 2002 the Australian Government Department of Health and Ageing commissioned the Australian Palliative Residential Aged Care (APRAC) Project Team to develop palliative care guidelines for the residential aged care setting (www.aprac.org). The interdisciplinary team was led by nurses in palliative care and aged care and included individuals with special expertise in guideline development, dementia, and cultural issues.

The guidelines provide all levels of staff working in these facilities with evidence-based criteria against which their services can be monitored. The guidelines will also assist in the identification of local strengths and weaknesses in the provision of a palliative approach in residential aged care facilities, providing a mechanism by which changes in service delivery may be evaluated over time. More recently, this work has been extended, to produce Guidelines for a Palliative Approach for Aged Care in the Community, to incorporate the care provided by medical practitioners, nurses, and other health professionals, as well as volunteers, in the community setting. A related project has also commenced to engage medical practitioners in their work in residential aged care environments (www.palliativecare.org.au).

In early 2008, the Australian Government introduced a new Aged Care Funding Instrument (ACFI) to allocate an additional subsidy for residents with additional care needs like those requiring palliative care. The ACFI is based on an assessment of a resident's care needs and is intended to better match funding to the increasing complex care needs of residents as they approach their end of life. Residents in aged care facilities with palliative care needs are eligible for the maximum funding assessment rating under ACFI's Complex Health Care Supplement, where ratings on medications and complex health-care questions are used to determine a resident's suitability for the supplement.

## Research

Increasingly, palliative care research in Australia is led from a multidisciplinary team of investigators with nurses commonly taking lead roles. The National Health and Medical Research Council, Australia's peak research body, has acknowledged the importance of palliative care and allocated specific funding in a way that targets improvements in research outputs and building research capacity.

Several states in Australia have active multidisciplinary academic palliative care centers. There is an increasing trend towards formalized research collaborations to maximize research outcomes and palliative care research in Australia is no exception. The Centre for Palliative Care Education and Research (St Vincent's and The University of Melbourne) is currently undertaking a large project to discern optimal ways of promoting research collaboration in order to avoid duplication, and promote capacity building. As part of this project, 95% of respondents to a statewide survey ($n = 76$), many of whom were nurses, reported a desire for a structured research collaboration. The top two responses in other key areas related to palliative care research are noted in Table 70–1.

The Palliative Care Clinical Studies Collaborative (PaCCSC) is a research collaboration of a number of universities that aims to improve quality of care for patients through access, awareness, and quality use of palliative care medicines in the community through clinical studies (www.caresearch.com.au).

The Psycho-Oncology Co-operative Research Group (PoCoG) is again, a national collaboration which aims to improve the outcomes of patients experiencing a diagnosis of cancer, their families, and caregivers through evaluation and implementation of psycho-social and supportive care interventions for patients, caregivers, health professionals, and the health-care system. Although its focus is not specifically palliative care research, some activities are related, and therefore, worth highlighting in this review (www.pocog.org.au).

The International Palliative Care Family Carer Research Collaboration (IPCFRC) under the auspices of the European

| Table 70-1 |
| --- |
| **Research Priorities, Enablers and Barriers in Victoria, Australia** |
| **Research priorities** |
| 1. Symptom management |
| 2. Rural settings |
| **Enablers to undertaking palliative care research** |
| 1. Funded research positions |
| 2. Ability to combine clinical work with research |
| **Barriers to undertaking palliative care research** |
| 1. Funding |
| 2. Lack of research experience/expertise |
| **Enablers to dissemination of research findings** |
| 1. Funding to attend palliative care conferences |
| 2. Palliative care peer review journals |
| **Barriers to dissemination of research findings** |
| 1. Time |
| 2. Lack of knowledge regarding the process surrounding publishing research findings |
| **Enablers to translation of research results to clinical care** |
| 1. Close partnerships between researchers and service care providers. |
| 2. Organizational culture |
| **Barriers to translation of research results to clinical care** |
| 1. Lack of time to keep up to date with literature |
| 2. Lack of organizational support |

Association of Palliative Care but operating out of Australia, was established by two nurses.[28] This group aims to develop a strategic approach to palliative care research planning related to family caregivers of people requiring palliative care by establishing international partnerships and promoting information exchange (www.ipcfrc.unimelb.edu.au). The collaboration operates a major initiative to assist with the transfer of knowledge to practice is CareSearch (www.caresearch.com.au). It is an electronic evidence-based on-line resource of palliative care literature not typically available in existing anthologies, which was developed for palliative care practitioners, educators, and researchers.[29] Indexed and reviewed literature includes unpublished abstracts, government- and organization-sponsored documents, theses from Australian universities, and international published palliative care literature missing from standard electronic databases.

Given the global environment in which nursing and healthcare is informed, several Australian and New Zealand nurses are actively participating in international palliative care initiatives. Typical organizations in which nurses are involved on Boards incorporate: International Association of Hospice and Palliative Care, Asia Pacific Palliative Care Network, IPCFRC, and Worldwide Palliative Care Alliance. In addition, palliative care nurses in Australian and New Zealand are regularly presenting work at international palliative care congresses.

## Policy

As indicated in various sections of this chapter, Australia has enjoyed a period of healthy development of service-related palliative care policy. The National Palliative Care Strategy has enabled the development of many national, state, and local palliative care projects and nurses are involved in all key areas. There are four main areas that have been addressed in the Strategy: support for patients, families, and caregivers in the community; increased access to palliative care medicines in the community; education, training, and support for the workforce; and research and quality improvement for palliative care services. All these areas have translated into policy in order to influence practice. A summary of this work can be found at www.health.gov.au/palliativecare.

Palliative care nurses in New Zealand have been actively involved in Ministry of Health policy work in both cancer and palliative care. Of particular note is the recently released National Cancer Control and Action Strategy Plan (http://www.moh.govt.nz/moh.nsf/indexmh/cancercontrol-strategyandactionplan), providing direction in this area of health for the country for the next 5 years. In response to this plan, District Health Boards, which include membership of nurses, have provided their regional implementation responses.

As part of developing the New Zealand nursing workforce, the National Professional Development Framework for Palliative Care Nursing in Aotearoa New Zealand (www.moh.govt.nz), aims to develop palliative care nursing in order to improve end-of-life care for patients. A set of competency indicators, together with resource materials to help nurses acquire these competencies, have been developed.

Of particular note in the last few years has been the development of national palliative care special interest groups for nurses in both countries. This has provided a vehicle for the voice of nursing to be heard in this discipline and an opportunity to promote nursing work in policy development, education, and research, through nursing-specific conferences. The Australian government has utilized this group to seek advice on particular issues.

## Education, Training, and Advanced Practice

Although almost all nurses are exposed to end-of-life and palliative care issues, undergraduate nursing education in palliative care is inconsistent in both countries. From the survey undertaken for this chapter (see Acknowledgments), nurses in both countries said that despite being able to undertake clinical placements in palliative care, there remains significant work to routinely include palliative care in the core undergraduate curriculum. Reflecting these sentiments, a survey of the deans of 41 Australian universities showed that only a few had established dedicated course time for palliative care.[30]

To help address this issue, both Australia and New Zealand have National Palliative Care Strategies,[15,17] which specifically include the fostering of education of palliative care professionals. One example, is the Palliative Care Curriculum for Undergraduates program (PCC4U) to promote the inclusion of palliative care in undergraduate curricula and the ongoing education of all health professionals (http://www.caresearch.com.au/).

It is still apparent however, that most palliative care education occurs at post-graduate level and as such, is optional and self directed.[31] The nurses surveyed for this chapter described many and varied opportunities available at this level of education in both countries. Of note are the on-line and distance courses, that have developed, probably as a response to the isolation of many rural work environments in both countries. There are a variety of continuing education (short course) and postgraduate (University auspiced) courses available in Australia (http://www.caresearch.com.au/caresearch/Education). There has also been a recent focus on establishing specialist multidisciplinary education initiatives, which have demonstrated effectiveness.[32] Such initiatives have been used as the basis for developing a University accredited specialist training program that seeks to become the minimum requirement for health professionals to work in the specialist palliative care setting (http://www.mccp.unimelb.edu.au/courses/award-courses/specialist-certificate/palliative-care).

In New Zealand, palliative care nursing has seen an increased focus on multidisciplinary teamwork, shared care in the community, and nurse specialists in hospital consultancy and plans to recognize nurse practitioners with limited prescribing rights. Nursing competencies were incorporated into several of the main tertiary courses for hospice nurses by 2002.[31]

Regarding scope of practice, numerous senior role titles were described by the nurses in the survey. Clinical nurse consultants, clinical nurse specialists, and nurse practitioners undertake consultative roles in a variety of settings like acute hospitals, specialist palliative care units, aged care, and the community. Constraints on practice discussed were the workloads, a lack of available time for the number of patients, resistance from medical colleagues, limited prescribing rights, and fear of litigation. Despite these difficulties, advance practice roles continue to develop and interest seems to be increasing. The minimal education requirement for endorsement is a completed Masters of Nurse Practitioner (MNP). Part of this course includes a therapeutic medication module(s) and a clinical internship. Further information about endorsement can be found via www.nbv.org.au/web/guest/endorsements-nurse-practitioner. National competency standards for practitioners in Australia are available from www.anmc.org.au/docs/Publications/Competency%20Standards%20for%20the%20Nurse%20Practitioner.pdf.

## Current Issues and Looking to the Future

The current issues described by the nurses surveyed, fell into a number of categories. In relation to workforce, there were many comments about the ageing and retirement of nurses with expertise in palliative care, leaving inexperienced staff to carry more and more caseloads. This has implications for planning models of healthcare, including palliative care, into the future.

A number of comments noted in the survey were made about the lack of support from medical staff and how poorly informed they are, probably reflective of insufficient education in palliative care. In looking to the future, the nurses saw a growing divide between palliative medicine and palliative care generally.

Funding, together with increased workloads, was a frequently noted concern; for example, one nurse specifically bemoaning the removal of two vehicles from a large rural service with no commensurate reduction in the travel expectations. With more care being planned to be delivered in people's homes, the nurses suggested that funding models will need to maintain community-focused priorities, to enable people not only to die in their place of choice but also, to save unnecessary hospital admissions.

In relation to the performance of their own role, the nurses wished they had more clinical supervision. They saw that the community-based and consultative aspects of their role would continue to develop into the future, in line with developing health policy. All these issues will impact on the way palliative care develops in the future.

## Conclusion

Palliative care nursing in Australia and New Zealand continues to develop and grow. Nurses now perform significant leadership roles in both countries and evident in clinical practice, education, and research. The continued development of academic positions in palliative nursing is becoming increasingly successful in attracting research funding competitive research funding bodies. These academic positions have continued to be established with close relationships with clinical facilities, maintaining a research agenda that is clinically relevant.

Looking to the future, the surveyed nurses suggest that workforce issues will continue to impact on the shape of palliative care. Issues like the ageing of the health workforce and the need to continually upskill generalist staff by making education readily available were regarded as key. Continuing to work closely with both Government and peak body policy will influence the further development of palliative care and particularly the work in primary health-care environments that makes palliative care equitably available across regions, settings, and populations. Improvements in community awareness and understandings of palliative care are regarded as essential in future planning.

This chapter demonstrates that nurses are at the forefront of developing service systems able to meet the needs of people requiring palliative care in our communities and are committed to sustainable models of palliative care delivery. Mainstreaming and primary health-care models, together with the important integration of policy, research, and practice, will allow palliative care nurses in Australasia to continue their leadership roles in advancing palliative care practice and ensuring its place in healthcare.

## Acknowledgments

This chapter is informed by the responses of twenty nurses from Australian and New Zealand, who responded to an online survey repeating the questions asked in the first edition of this chapter. The questions were placed on a website (survey monkey) for one month from mid-October 2008. Nurses were accessed through Palliative Care Nurses Australia and the National Palliative Care Conference, held in Palmerston North New Zealand in October 2008. The questions were:

- To what extent is palliative care included in the undergraduate curricula in your country?
- What opportunities exist for education of specialist palliative care nurses in your setting/country?
- What is the scope of practice of nurses working in palliative care in your context? What other roles exist? What constraints are there on practice?
- What are the current issues facing nurses in the delivery of palliative care in your setting?
- What impact are the changing directions in nursing likely to have on palliative care nursing in the near future?
- What are the future directions in palliative care that will have an impact on nursing in palliative care?

REFERENCES

1. O'Connor M, Aranda S, eds. Palliative Care Nursing: A Guide to Practice (2nd ed). Oxford: Radcliffe Medical Press Ltd, 2003.
2. Hudson PL, Payne S, eds. Family Care and Palliative Care: A Guide for Health and Social Care Professionals. Oxford: Oxford University Press, 2008.
3. New Zealand Population Census. 2006. Available at: www.stats.gov.nz/statsweb.nsf (accessed December 2, 2008).
4. Payne S. To supplant, supplement or support? Organizational issues for hospices. Soc Sci Med 1998;46:1495–1504.
5. Standards for the Provision of Hospice/Palliative Care. Hospice New Zealand, Wellington, 1998.
6. Standards for Palliative Care Provision (4th ed.). Canberra: Palliative Care Australia, 2005.
7. O'Connor Margaret. The veils of death: Understanding dying in residential aged care. A discourse analysis of policy. Unpublished thesis, La Trobe University Victoria, Australia: 2002.
8. Palliative Care Australia, A Guide to Palliative Care Service Development—a population-based approach. Canberra: Palliative Care Australia, 2005.
9. Palliative Care Service Provision in Australia: A planning guide (2nd ed). Canberra: Palliative Care Australia, 2003.
10. O'Connor M, Chapman Y. The palliative care clinical nurse consultant: An essential link. Collegian 2008;15:151–157.
11. O'Connor M, Peter L, Walsh K. Palliative care nurse consultants in Melbourne, Australia: A "snap shot" of their clinical role. Int J Palliat Nurs 2008;14/7:350–356.
12. Department of Health and Ageing. Community attitudes to palliative care issue. Canberra: Department of Health and Ageing, 2003.
13. Ramsden I. Kawa Whakaruruhau: Guidelines for nursing and midwifery education. Wellington: Nursing Council of New Zealand, 1992.
14. Guidelines for Cultural Safety, the Treaty of Waitangi, & Maori Health in Nursing and Midwifery Education and Practice. Wellington: Nursing Council of New Zealand, 2002.
15. The New Zealand Palliative Care Strategy. Wellington: New Zealand Ministry of Health, 2001.
16. National Health and Medical Research Council. Values and ethics: Guidelines for ethical conduct in aboriginal and Torres Strait Islander health research. Canberra: National Health and Medical Research Council, 2003.
17. National Palliative Care Strategy: A Framework for Palliative Care Service Development. Commonwealth of Australia, 2000.
18. McGrath P, Phillips E. Insights on end of life ceremonial practices of Australian Aboriginal peoples. Collegian 2008;15:125–133.
19. Kanitsaki O. Palliative care and cultural diversity. In: Parker J, Aranda S, eds. Palliative Care: Explorations and Challenges. Sydney: MacLennan & Petty; 1998:32–45.
20. Shanmugasundaram S, Chapman Y, O'Connor M. Development of palliative care in India: An overview. Int J Nurs Prac 2006;12:241–246.
21. Chiung-Hin Hsu, O'Connor M, Lee S. Issues affecting access to palliative care services for older Chinese people in Australia. ACCNS J Community Nurses 2005;10(3):9–11.
22. Fallowfield LJ, Jenkins VA, Beveridge HA. Truth may hurt but deceit hurts more: Communication in palliative care. Palliat Med 2002;16:297–330.
23. Payne S, Chapman A, Holloway M, Seymour JE, Chau R. Chinese community views: Promoting culture competence in palliative care. J Palliat Care 2005;21(2):111–116.
24. McCarthy A, Hegney D. Rural nursing in the Australian context. In: Aranda S, O'Connor M, eds. Palliative Care Nursing: A Guide to Practice. Melbourne: Ausmed Publications; 1999:83–101.
25. Aranda S, Hayman-White K, Devilee L, O'Connor M, Bence G. Inpatient hospice triage of 'after hours' calls to a community palliative care service. Int J Palliat Nurs 2001;7(5):214–220.
26. Kristjanson L, Cousins K, White K, et al. Evaluation of a night respite community palliative care service. Int J Palliat Nurs 2004;10(2):84–90.

27. Finlay IG, Jones JVH. Definitions in palliative care. BMJ 1995;311:754.
28. Hudson PL, Payne S. Collaboration on research into family careers moves a step forward. Eur J Palliat Care 2007;14(5):218.
29. Tieman J. Multiple sources: Mapping the literature of palliative care. Palliat Med 2009;23:425–431.
30. Yates P, Nash R, Parker D, et al. Scoping undergraduate palliative care education in the health profession. Implications for the future. 3rd Annual Research Conference, Centre for Palliative Care Research and Education, Brisbane, Australia, 2004.
31. Spruyt O, Macleod R, Hudson P. Australia and New Zealand In: Wee B, Hughes N, eds. Palliative Care Education: Building a Culture of Learning. Oxford: Oxford University Press; 2007:59–67.
32. Quinn K, Hudson AM, Thomas K. "Palliative care the essentials": Evaluation of a multidisciplinary education program. J Palliat Med 2008;11(8):1122–1129.

# 71

*Penny Hansford*

# Palliative Care in the United Kingdom

~~~

## The Historical Context

The birthplace of the modern hospice movement, St Christopher's Hospice in South East London, is now over 40 years old. Founded by Dame Cicely Saunders in 1967 as a 62-bed inpatient unit, the home care service was developed some 2 years later. The bereavement and daycare services were established in 1970.

The founding of St Christopher's was Dame Cicely's impassioned response to the deep-seated shortcomings in the care of the dying. Dame Cicely's philosophy was greatly influenced by Professor John Hinton's seminal book *Dying*. According to Hinton, these failings reflected on society as a whole: "We emerge deserving of little credit: we who are capable of ignoring the conditions that make muted people suffer. The dissatisfied dead cannot noise abroad the negligence they have experienced."[1] Those with a terminal illness were often sent away with the words "there is nothing more we can do," and given little or no honest information about their medical condition. Symptoms were inadequately managed, strained relationships between professionals, patients, and families led to isolation and fear. Psychological, social, and spiritual needs were largely ignored. It was this realization and the belief in the possibility of change that together with her firm Christian beliefs, motivated Dame Cicely. She envisioned hospices as a model of care that would permeate mainstream healthcare services. Writing in the 1970's, she said "A few Hospices will be needed for...intractable problems, research and teaching...but most patients will continue to die in hospitals, cancer centres, or their own homes. The staff they will find there should be learning how to meet their needs."[2]

However, years of planning would be needed to achieve the revolution in care required by this new model. Cicely herself qualified in three different professional fields, first as a nurse, then as a medical social worker, and finally, at age 39 years, as a doctor. In 1958, just after completing her medical

| | Adult Inpatient Units | | | | | | Children's Inpatient Units | |
|---|---|---|---|---|---|---|---|---|
| | Total Units | NHS Units | Vol Units | Total Beds | NHS Beds | Vol Beds | Units | Beds |
| London | 16 | 6 | 10 | 359 | 86 | 273 | 4 | 30 |
| Midlands and East of England | 45 | 15 | 30 | 646 | 182 | 464 | 11 | 87 |
| North | 60 | 8 | 52 | 851 | 79 | 772 | 12 | 81 |
| South | 52 | 11 | 41 | 773 | 143 | 630 | 9 | 71 |
| **England** | **173** | **40** | **133** | **2,629** | **490** | **2,139** | **36** | **269** |
| Scotland | 24 | 10 | 14 | 355 | 96 | 259 | 2 | 17 |
| Wales | 15 | 9 | 6 | 143 | 65 | 78 | 2 | 15 |
| N Ireland | 5 | 1 | 4 | 67 | 4 | 63 | 1 | 10 |
| Channel Islands | 2 | 0 | 2 | 11 | 0 | 11 | 0 | 0 |
| Isle of Man | 1 | 0 | 1 | 12 | 0 | 12 | 1 | 4 |
| **TOTAL** | **220** | **60** | **160** | **3,217** | **655** | **2,562** | **42** | **315** |

The voluntary adult units include nine Marie Curie hospices with 228 beds and six Sue Ryder hospices with 107 beds.
The remainder are independent local charities including two services exclusively for HIV patients with 18 beds.
The children's units include the two Zoe's Place baby hospices, which care for infants up to the age of five. Between them they have 12 beds.

**Figure 71–1.** Hospice and palliative care inpatient units. *Source*: Help the Hospices.

training, she observed, "It appears to me that many patients feel deserted by their doctors at the end. Ideally the doctor should remain at the centre of a team who work together to relieve where they cannot heal, to keep the patient's own struggle within his compass, and to bring hope and consolation to the end."[3]

Dame Cicely recognized that dying was a social experience, and that patients needed individualized, holistic care. Her model of care was to take account of the many facets of a patient's life and illness: the emotional burden of dying, practical concerns such as financial worries, careful symptom control, and support for family and friends during the illness and into bereavement. This approach encompassed both the science and the art of nursing and medicine: "You matter because you are you and you matter to the last moment of your life."[4]

From the beginning, the identity of St Christopher's was more than just the building or inpatient wards; the aim was that care should be capable of being adapted to different settings. At the basis of Dame Cicely's philosophy was a trilogy of care, education, and research, "St Christopher's will try to fill the gap that exists in both research and teaching concerning the patients dying of cancer, and those needing skilled relief in other long term illnesses and their relatives."[5] Indeed, the early studies conducted at St Christopher's in the use and effectiveness of morphine to control malignant pain were to change the face of medicine.[6]

The speed at which this approach has spread and influenced service provision is remarkable. Day-care centers mushroomed in the 1980s and children's hospices were established

from 1982 onward. The first hospital palliative care service was set up at St Thomas's Hospital, London, in 1976. Today, there are palliative care support teams in acute hospitals all over the United Kingdom.

In the United Kingdom, the Hospice Information Service, a partnership between "Help the Hospices" and St Christopher's,[7] collates information on service provision both in the United Kingdom and worldwide. Figure 71–1 shows the number of beds and inpatient units in the United Kingdom. Figure 71–2 shows community and hospital palliative care provision. The National Council for Specialist Palliative Care collects UK-wide activity data through the "minimum data set."[8]

Two of the leading national charities that promote good end-of-life care are Marie Curie Cancer Care Foundation and Macmillan. Marie Curie has 10 inpatient units often known as Marie Curie centers. Two hundred and thirty-two beds are available in these units. They also have a nationwide nursing service that supplements and enhances care at home, and works alongside the statutory nursing service (district nursing), thus enabling many people to die at home. Macmillan (formerly known as Macmillan Cancer Relief) traditionally pump-primed clinical nurse specialist posts in the community. At the end of a 3-year period the primary care trust was expected to continue the funding. This initiative lead to a phenomenal growth in community service provision, resulting in over 400 home care teams in the United Kingdom today.

The spread of palliative care services worldwide has also been significant; services are now established in 115 countries.

| | Home Care Teams* | Hospice at Home Services | Day Care Centres* | Hospital Support Nurse Services | Hospital Support Teams |
|---|---|---|---|---|---|
| London | 26 | 11 | 15 | 0 | 39 |
| Midlands and East of England | 60 | 36 | 70 | 12 | 60 |
| North | 72 | 22 | 76 | 9 | 74 |
| South | 68 | 26 | 64 | 4 | 55 |
| **England** | **226** | **95** | **225** | **25** | **228** |
| Scotland | 47 | 1 | 25 | 15 | 39 |
| Wales | 26 | 7 | 22 | 1 | 23 |
| N Ireland | 9 | 2 | 7 | 0 | 14 |
| Channel Islands | 1 | 1 | 2 | 0 | 2 |
| Isle of Man | 1 | 1 | 1 | 0 | 1 |
| **TOTAL** | **310** | **107** | **282** | **41** | **307** |

\* A single service may provide more than one home care team/day centre

**Figure 71–2.** Community and hospital support services—2008. *Source*: Help the Hospices.

## Political Development

In 1987, palliative medicine became a recognized speciality for doctors in the United Kingdom and a 4-year training program was introduced. Shortly after this, palliative nursing degrees and diplomas were developed, building on the shorter English National Board courses in "care of the dying." Palliative care had become an acceptable career path for doctors and nurses.

The Department of Health produced its first major report on cancer services in 1985, the Calman Hine Report,[9] and this began to change the balance of cancer care from the acute sector to the community. The report made reference to the importance of palliative care but provided no suggestions or recommendations as to how to organize or achieve good quality care.

With the launch of the National Cancer Plan[10] in 2000, Cancer Networks came into being throughout the United Kingdom. Isolated hospices and specialist palliative care services had the opportunity to join mainstream health-care services, to identify gaps in service provision and think creatively about how these could be filled. In the United Kingdom, 75% of specialist inpatient palliative care and 65% of specialist community care is provided by the voluntary sector; and the government is increasingly pushing for statutory services to recognize and work with voluntary organizations. A 2008 Department of Health report[11] set out a vision of having a "set of new voluntary agreements between the government, private, and third-sector organizations on actions to improve health outcomes."

In 2003, the National Institute for Clinical Excellence (NICE) published its report on palliative and supportive care with recommendations on how palliative care services should

be structured and what they should provide.[12] However, without adequate funding these comprehensive palliative care services will not be realized. In 2007, on average, 31% of hospice funding came from statutory sources. The 2006 Department of Health publication "Our Health, Our Care Our Say: A New Direction for Community Services,"[13] recognized the need for investment in palliative care services, particularly in the community, where most patients would prefer to be cared for. Over the years, government pledges to fund 50% of hospice running costs have not materialized, and recent initiatives to develop a common tariff have stalled. Although attempts have been made to redistribute income from acute hospitals to community services, they have been unsuccessful.

Nevertheless, palliative care (now often termed "end-of-life care") is rising up the political agenda. Since 2005, numerous disease or patient group-specific National Service Frameworks have been produced by the Department of Health. These refer, for example, to older people[14] or to diseases such as renal failure[15] and dementia,[16] and each has a section on end-of-life care, thus recognizing that the same principles as those developed by Dame Cicely for a cancer population should be extended to other diseases and patient groups.

The first ever UK National End of Life Care Strategy was published in July 2008.[17] This is an important milestone in the development of the care of the dying; it emphasises that good end-of-life care should be available for any disease in any setting. But this goal is still a distant one. Most deaths in England occur in hospital (58%), with 18% of people dying at home, 17% in care homes and only 4% in hospices. Several large-scale surveys have been undertaken in recent years to ascertain preferences for place of care and place of death,[18,19] and some research has also been carried out on the subject.[20] Although people's preferences and priorities change over time,[21] the findings indicate that most people would prefer to be cared for and to die at home. They generally do not wish to die in an acute hospital setting, which is where most people die today. The same surveys unsurprisingly reveal that patients want to receive high quality, well coordinated care and to be able to discuss their personal needs and preferences with health-care professionals. Dying people wish to be treated with dignity and respect and for those close to them to receive support. Those at home want rapid response services and access to advice and support 24 hours a day and 7 days a week.

The Strategy acknowledges the pioneering work of Dame Cicely and the importance of paying close attention to the physical, psychological, social, and spiritual needs of patients and their families. Generalist health-care providers are urged to undertake education and training so that the "gold standard" of hospice care reaches all people who are dying of life-limiting illnesses, wherever they are. This is entirely consistent with Dame Cicely's original vision at St Christopher's.

The strategy outlines the ways in which this can be achieved and recommends the introduction of three specific tools.

## The Gold Standards Framework (GSF)

The GSF provides a framework for a planned system of care in consultation with the patient and family. It promotes better coordination and collaboration between health professionals, helps to optimise out-of-hours care, and aims to prevent crises and inappropriate hospital admissions. The tool was developed by Dr Keri Thomas, a GP with a special interest in palliative care, and was initially planned for use in primary care. It has now been introduced to over one-third of GP practices in the United Kingdom. In 2004, it was modified for use in care homes.

The three key processes of GSF are:

1. Identification of a patient in need of palliative care. In primary care, discussions take place between the GP and nursing staff who decide, with the help of specially produced prognostic indicators,[22] which patients might be expected to live for less than a year. These patients are entered onto a supportive care register, which is used to plan, record, and monitor patient care at regular health-care team meetings in the GP practice, or care home. In the care home setting, all residents are assessed using a "traffic light" coding system based on expected prognosis:

   - A (blue) = years
   - B (green) = months
   - C (yellow) = weeks
   - D (red) = days

2. Assessment of need, symptoms, and any preferences and considerations that are important to the patient and family.

3. Planning ahead, particularly for the "out-of-hours" situation. Ensuring that handover forms have been sent to ambulance services and that medications that might be needed are available in the home or care home.

A GSF co-coordinator is appointed within the practice or care home and is responsible for implementing and maintaining the framework. The whole program is overseen by the National Gold Standards Framework team,[23] which provides training for the GSF coordinators. Implementing GSF in care homes has been an important lever for changing practice because the focus of care has traditionally been rehabilitation with little emphasis on good end-of-life care, despite the fact that the average length of stay in homes with nursing care is 18 months. The GSF care home program therefore needs competent external facilitators to guide care homes so that they can implement the tool and achieve the quality mark of accreditation. The program is currently being implemented in 400 care homes in the United Kingdom.[23]

## The Liverpool Care Pathway

The strategy recommends the adoption of this pathway, or something similar, for patients in their last days of life. The tool aims to standardize the care delivered during this period. It details the steps that should be taken to bring about and maximize good quality support for dying patients. The documentation can also be used to audit practice.

The pathway was developed in 1997 for use in hospitals by Dr John Ellershaw,[24,25] but it has now also been adopted by many hospices and more recently care homes. A patient commences on the Liverpool Care Pathway (LCP) after a multiprofessional team decision that the patient is dying and meets certain criteria. After this, medical and nursing staff are required to carry out and document assessments aimed at promoting comfort, such as reducing the number of unnecessary medications, and ensuring that all interventions for symptom control are planned in advance. This might mean anticipatory prescribing of common medications needed at the end of life for pain, restlessness, and excess secretions. Other goals include prompting staff to ascertain whether family members (including those not present at the initial assessment) are aware that their relative is dying, and identifying the needs of any children in the family.

The LCP can only be used once the dying process has been acknowledged, yet many clinicians still have difficulty making that judgement. In acute hospitals, the culture of care remains oriented toward cure. Invasive procedures may be pursued at the expense of patient comfort.[25] One London Trust that had been using the LCP for over 5 years carried out an audit in the elderly care unit.[26] The findings indicated that patients were on the LCP in only 25% of deaths. Another 25% of deaths were patients who had died suddenly but there were a further 50% of deaths that could have been anticipated but the patients were not started on the pathway. A review of relevant patient notes suggested that that patients could have benefited from a systematic approach to end-of-life care. In many cases, active medical management obscured the patient's actual physical, psychological, social, and spiritual needs.

Information elicited from completed documentation does not of course measure the quality of the death. The LCP is a tool designed to trigger care processes and needs to be supported by educational programs.

Sustainability of both GSF and LCP remain a concern. Used well, both tools can radically improve quality of care offered to dying people, but they depend on adequate facilitation and training in the implementation phase, followed by a maintenance phase with external facilitation. In addition, "insider" champions are needed for both tools in the relevant care settings.[27]

## Advance Care Planning

The third recommended tool in the End of Life Strategy is the Preferred Priorities of Care (PPC) document,[28] developed by Les Storey in 2001. Again, the strategy is not prescriptive about using this tool but emphasizes the importance of professionals having open discussions with the patient and family members about treatment and place of care. This process has become known as advance care planning (ACP) and the PPC tool is an example of this. With the patient's consent, decisions are noted on the patient-held record, regularly reviewed, and communicated to key professionals involved in the patient's care. An ACP discussion might include what the patient and family understands about the patient's illness and prognosis, as well as their preferences for types of care and treatment. Also included are their important values or personal goals for care and any individual or family concerns. The document provides an opportunity for health-care professionals to engage in what can be difficult and painful discussions with patients and their families about subjects that might not otherwise be broached. Having these difficult conversations can significantly contribute to achieving the care that patients and families want. The recent Mental Capacity Act[29] strengthens the right for people to make decisions for themselves and makes provision in the best interests of those who do not have capacity.

With the advent of the End-of-Life Care Strategy all primary care trusts are expected to complete a needs assessment of their population and to develop a local strategy. Although the government has made a commitment to double their investment in palliative care, there is insufficient information to cost the care accurately. Alongside the strategy, a set of national quality standards are being produced. It is understood that these will consist of a set of structure and process measures rather than outcome measures.

Another recently published document on end-of-life care has been produced by the National Audit Office.[30] Their report illustrates the variations and inequalities in service provision around the United Kingdom. The researchers studied the records of 200 patients who had died in hospital in the city of Sheffield, UK, during October 2007. They found that 40% had no medical needs at the point of admission and that they could therefore have been cared for elsewhere. These patients had used 1,500 bed-days. Assuming the cost of an inpatient day in an acute hospital to be £250, the total cost of patients dying unnecessarily in hospital was £375,000. An extrapolation of these figures suggests that if such admissions could be avoided, up to £4.5 million over a year might be made available for end-of-life care in the community in Sheffield. The figures are even more startling if one considers the picture nationwide: if reductions of admissions to the acute sector were reduced by 10%, £104 million could be made available for redistribution.

The National Audit Office Report[30] also provides insight into local health-care priorities and highlights the need to develop partnerships between providers and to use existing funding creatively to meet local needs. It supports the messages in the End-of-Life Care Strategy and makes the case for its implementation.

## The Future of Hospices and Specialist Palliative Care Services

There is no doubt that hospices and specialist palliative care services are seen as exemplars of good practice and that they have highlighted and championed the importance of good palliative care. However, the allegation made by Douglas eighteen years ago that palliative care provides "deluxe dying for the privileged few," remains a challenge today.[31] Hospices overall continue to deliver care predominantly to a cancer population. Less than 5% of non-cancer patients in the United Kingdom access specialist palliative care, with only 0.2% receiving inpatient hospice care.[32] Hospices and specialist palliative care services do not provide equal access to black and minority ethnic groups [33] and other vulnerable populations; e.g., refugees and asylum seekers, prisoners, the homeless and travellers, those with learning disabilities. The public image of hospices is "white, middle-class, and Christian" The End-of-Life Care Strategy, predicated on the belief that "the care of all dying people must improve to the level of the best,"[17] challenges hospices to consider how they can contribute to the vision it describes. Many hospices, although delivering excellent care to the few, have been preoccupied with funding issues and have remained separate from the challenges faced by mainstream health care. But now the gauntlet has been thrown; hospices need urgently to develop a collective voice. They "must move beyond the dichotomy between hospices working in splendidly isolated independence, delivering a 'lot to a few,' and the bureaucratically controlled state vanilla version delivering 'a little to a lot.' With sensible integration it must be possible to deliver 'rather more to rather more.' "[33]

## How Can Specialist and Palliative Care Services Become More Relevant?

### Community and Hospital Support Teams

The majority of palliative care is delivered by nurses. Some of the earliest specialist roles for nurses were in palliative care community and hospital teams. Specialist nursing posts have generally been called "clinical nurse specialists." The expansion of this role was driven through the Calman-Hine report,[9] which saw the reorganization of cancer services and the development of specialist nurses for each tumor group. The absence of an educational pathway and the failure to regulate the title of clinical nurse specialist has led to varying levels of skills and competencies among these practitioners. The clinical nurse specialist has traditionally been responsible for five distinct areas of work: clinical work, consultation with others, teaching, leadership, and research.[34] In the past, community and hospital support teams have not been planned strategically and little attention has been given to integrating them into the right organizational structure or to providing clinical leadership. It is not surprising, therefore, that an evaluation of the role revealed ambiguity and role conflict.[35] Coupled with this is a failure to demonstrate the benefits of having clinical nurse specialists. Finding a reliable measure for outcomes in palliative care is a complex task and no research to date has conclusively demonstrated the value of the role. Thankfully, regulation of the specialist nurse title is now being addressed by the UK Nursing and Midwifery Council (NMC), who provide a helpful definition of the role, now termed "advanced practice nurse." Advanced practice nurses "are highly experienced, knowledgeable, and educated members of the care team who are able to diagnose and treat your health-care needs or refer you to an appropriate specialist when needed." They can:

- Carry out physical examinations
- Use expert knowledge and clinical judgement to decide whether to refer patients for investigations and make diagnoses
- Decide on and carry out treatment, including the prescribing of medicines
- Use their extensive practice experience to plan and provide skilled and competent care to meet patients health and social needs, involving other members of the health-care team as appropriate
- Ensure the provision of continuity of care including follow-up visits
- Assess and evaluate, with patients, the effectiveness of the treatment and care provided and make changes where needed
- Work independently, although often as part of a health-care team that they will lead
- As a leader of a team, make sure that each patient's treatment and care is based on best practice.[36]

It is expected that only when nurses have achieved the competencies set out by the NMC will they be able officially to join the advanced practice register and use the title. It is also probable that they will need to be qualified to Master's degree level. However, the timescale for setting up this register remains unclear.

Another significant development in nursing, and palliative care nursing in particular, is the advent of nurse prescribing which commenced in 1998 in district nursing. To begin with, the prescribing role was limited to medications that could be bought in a pharmacy and medications that could be applied topically. In 2002, the "Nurse Prescriber's Extended Formulary" was introduced and then expanded in 2003 and 2005.[37,38] From May 2006, regulations changed to enable the extended formulary independent prescribers (now called nurse independent prescribers) to prescribe any licensed medicine for any medical condition within their competency.[39] The Department of Health identified palliative care as one of the first areas where nurses could take on this independent role. Nonetheless, nurse prescribing in the United Kingdom remains controversial. The process of setting up the service has been described as hastily implemented for reasons of political expediency.[40] However, the facility for clinical nurse specialists to prescribe in the home during a consultation, rather than make recommendations to the patient's General Practitioner, undoubtedly makes for better and more efficient symptom control and reduces the need for the family to collect prescription scripts.[41] Although Department of Health funded evaluations have acclaimed nurse prescribing as a success,[42,43] an editorial in the British Medical Journal[44] has pointed out that evaluations do not permit us to draw conclusions as to the safety and appropriateness of extended nurse prescribing. A postal survey conducted in 2007 explored the views of 2252 palliative care clinical nurse specialists on extended nurse prescribing. Of the 70% who responded, only 11% were trained as independent nurse prescribers[45] and only half of these[45] were using their newly acquired skills in prescribing. This group reported training deficits and also that courses were too short and general to meet the needs of those working in palliative care. It also highlighted a lack of medical mentorship. The survey revealed little enthusiasm among cancer and palliative care nurses for undertaking prescribing training.[45] Clearly, for the majority of palliative care nurses the structure and content of the courses need to be reviewed and an organizational commitment required to achieve implementation.

In a cash-strapped National Health Service, there is considerable cynicism about the role of clinical nurse specialist. Their traditional role of "advising and supporting" their health-care colleagues is disappearing. To remain relevant to the changing health-care scene, they must develop into advanced practitioners and become interventionist as well as advisory. Skills in prescribing and clinical assessment will help demonstrate their worth.

A few studies show the effectiveness of the hospital palliative care team. A Scottish study in 2004 demonstrated clinically significant improvements in all aspects of pain, mood, and sleeping in the group of patients who had experienced the involvement of the hospital palliative care team. These patients were more satisfied than the control group with the information provided about their illness, medication, and treatment. They were also more likely to be involved in discharge planning and were less likely to be readmitted in the months following discharge.[46]

A systematic review undertaken by Hearn and Higginson[47] examined palliative care interventions and found that there were significant improvements in outcomes for those cared for by a specialist palliative care team compared to those receiving standard care. They reviewed 18 studies including five randomized controlled trials and found that specialists were effective in improving satisfaction and identifying and dealing with a wider range of patient and family needs. The improved outcomes for patients included: more time spent at home, better symptom control, greater satisfaction for both patients and caregivers, and a greater likelihood of patients dying where they wished.

However, the key challenge for specialist teams remains whether they succeed in empowering and improving practice in their generalist colleagues or whether they simply take over, so deskilling them. Further research in this area is vital.

Another development in nursing that has the potential to impact upon palliative nursing is the new role of Nurse Consultant. The posts were a political initiative aimed at encouraging senior skilled nursing staff to remain in clinical practice rather than move to a managerial or purely educational role. Guidance issued by the Department of Health in 1999[48] stated that each post should be structured around four core functions:

- Expert practice function
- Professional leadership and consultancy function
- Education training and development function
- Practice and service development, research, and evaluation.

It was expected that the time allocated to discharge the tasks and responsibilities associated with each function would vary from post to post, however, 50% of the post holder's time was to be spent in clinical practice, working directly with patients, clients, or communities. There was initially an attempt to protect the title "Nurse Consultant." All proposals for posts had to be submitted to the Department of Health and were scrutinized by a panel. Without the regulation of the role by the Nursing and Midwifery Council, this proved to be an impossible task. Furthermore, the role was initially open only to employees from the National Health Service (NHS) and not to those from the voluntary sector, despite the fact that the voluntary sector provides most of the services to patients and

their families in specialist palliative care. However, in 2003, the Department of Health backtracked on the need for proposals to be submitted for agreement and left it to the Strategic Health Authorities to oversee the creation of new posts. The posts were also opened up to the voluntary sector with the first non-NHS palliative nurse consultant being appointed at St Christopher's Hospice in London in 2005.

To the detriment of nursing, there remains no agreed level of education, training, or function required for nurse consultants. However, in palliative care, the roles, tasks, and relationships between nurses and doctors are being restructured. Nurse-led services are common in community settings, and in some inpatient settings patients are beginning to be admitted by nurses. This is testing for both professional groups who must respond to the need to deliver cost effective palliative care to all. Services have had to find ways of complying with the 2000 NICE guidance.[12] The emphasis on providing specialist advice and support 24 hours a day, 7 days a week in both hospital and community services, with access to specialist inpatient units on the same basis, has been a considerable challenge.

## Daycare

Specialist daycare has grown in popularity over the last 20 years and the involvement of artists and complementary therapists has also flourished. Many of these resources are centered on daycare services, further perpetuating inequitable distribution of scarce resources. Patients report high levels of satisfaction with daycare services but recent research reports have been critical of the benefits and appropriateness of such services.[49] Patients who require day care often need a complex mix of care and support. It is likely that these people will have social needs which will need to be addressed, such as isolation because of difficult family dynamics or the absence of informal care arrangements.[50]

The challenge for day care is to meet patient needs and be cost-effective. This may mean, for example, disaggregating the arts and complementary therapists from the day-care setting and making them available wherever the need (e.g., in care homes). Group work and models of care that bring people together can help patients to find new interests and strengths at a critical time in their lives.[50]

## Inpatient Hospices

Hospice beds remain a tiny subset of the health-care system. However, they provide important opportunities to demonstrate the outcomes of good nursing care and effective multiprofessional teamwork. As indicated earlier, many hospices are dogged by funding issues that threaten to paralyze them and prevent them from delivering a creative response to the challenges of health care in the early 21st century. It remains unclear whether hospices are going to succeed in negotiating an appropriate and standardized funding mechanism with the NHS. Nonetheless, they remain beacons of good practice. Hospices have always managed to attract large number of volunteers and in the United Kingdom it is estimated that they benefit from the services of 100,000 volunteers with an economic value of £110m per annum. They not only operate as trustees (charitable hospices are required by UK charity law to have a board of trustees to oversee their strategic direction and these trustees must be volunteers), but also support individual patients and carry out a wide range of other tasks, such as raising funds. In addition, they fulfil an important role in integrating the hospice into the local community. In fact, volunteers can help to influence public attitudes to death and dying.

## Care Homes

The most neglected setting for the care of the dying is the care home. In the United Kingdom, "care home" is the term used for all types of community institutional settings, including care homes with nursing, residential care homes, sheltered housing, and extra-care housing. In March 2007, there were 18,557 registered adult care homes in England offering a total of 441,958 places. Approximately 4,048 of these care homes were care homes with nursing and 14,515 care homes providing personal care. Around 80,000 people die there each year, representing 16% of all deaths. Specialist palliative care teams have historically had little involvement in the care-home sector, partly because most people in care homes do not have a cancer diagnosis. Nonetheless, care homes could be said to be the hospices of tomorrow. Over the past 10 years, most long-stay facilities in hospitals for the frail elderly have been closed and these patients now live in care homes with nursing. Here, they have considerably less access to nursing and medical expertise, even though they are living longer with multiple pathologies, including dementia.

Despite the number of deaths they see, support of dying has been found to be peripheral to the culture of care homes.[27] These homes are mostly privately owned businesses and retention and recruitment of staff is problematic.[51] Most staff are untrained and many do not come from the same cultural backgrounds as the residents and may have different attitudes to death and dying. In addition, the homes are often poorly served by family doctors or visiting medical officers. As a result, old and frail residents are often admitted inappropriately to hospital for their last days of life. The fact that care homes have not benefited from the developments in palliative care or the collaboration with specialist nurses, and the limited involvement of doctors raises concerns over the quality of care in these settings. Fortunately, early results from the implementation of the Gold Standards Framework in Care Homes are encouraging.[52]

## Death and Dying in Society

Despite the rapid growth of the hospice movement, death remains a taboo subject in UK society. In a large-scale survey conducted by the BBC in 2005, only 34% of the general public reported that they had discussed their wishes about how they would like to die.[53] Even for those over age 65 years, the figure was only 51%. Patients being admitted to hospitals and their relatives often hope that cure is possible. It might even be said that older people do not seem to have the right to die of natural causes. Of course all of us will die, but the increasing medicalization of care, the availability of tests, and trial treatments, can make it harder for patients and families to come to terms with dying. The offer of "active treatment" also pervades hospices, making transfer to a hospital setting for consultations and treatment or investigations more common.

Therefore, there needs to be a sustained effort to develop a public health and community-based approach to death, dying, and loss. There will never be enough professional resources to meet all needs and people and communities have to learn to respond sensitively and appropriately to the needs of the dying and those caring for them. In Australia, promising work has been performed to promote healthier attitudes to death and dying,[54] and at St Christopher's a school's project,[17] commended in the End of Life Care Strategy, has sought to do something similar with children, and is being extended to other parts of the United Kingdom.[55]

Key challenges for the future delivery of effective end-of-life care include:

- Ensuring a competent specialist palliative care workforce
- Creating effective mentoring and training partnerships to ensure the competence of the generalist workforce
- Offering a needs led service that demonstrates equitable delivery for all disease groups
- Improving service access for black and minority ethnic populations and others
- A determined focus to meet the needs of older people
- Ensuring access to services 24/7 in all settings including the home
- Focussing on the development and implementation of measures of cost effectiveness. These are vital if funding is to improve.

## REFERENCES

1. Hinton J. Dying. London: Penguin Books, 1967.
2. Saunders CM. The philosophy of terminal care. In: Saunders CM, ed. The Management of Terminal Disease. London: Edward Arnold; 1978:195.
3. Clarke C. Cicely Saunders Founder of the Modern Hospice Movement. Selected letters 1959–1999. Oxford: Oxford University Press, 2002.

4. Saunders CM. Care of the dying the problems with euthanasia. Nursing Times 1976;72(26):1003–1005.

5. Saunders CM. St Christopher's Hospice. Br Hosp J 1967;77: 2217–2130.

6. Twycross R. Relief of pain. In: Saunders CM, ed. The Management of Terminal Disease. London: Edward Arnold; 1978:65–92.

7. Help the Hospices. The Annual Hospice and Palliative Care Directory. http://www.helpthehospices.org.uk/our-services/information-service/uk-hospice-and-palliative-care-services/?locale=en (accessed October 16, 2009).

8. National Council for Palliative Care. Minimum Data Set. http://www.ncpc.org.uk/publications/freedownloads.html (accessed October 16, 2009).

9. Department of Health. A Policy Framework for commissioning cancer services. A report by the expert advisory group on cancer to the Chief Medical Officer of England and Wales. London, Department of Health, 1985.

10. Department of Health. The NHS Cancer Plan: A Plan for Investment, a Plan for Reform. London: Department of Health, 2000.

11. Department of Health. Next Stage Review. London: Department of Health, 2008.

12. National Institute for Clinical Excellence (NICE). Improving supportive and palliative care for adults with Cancer. London: National Institute for Clinical Excellence, 2004.

13. Department of Health. Our Health, Our Scare, Our Say: A New Direction for Community. London: Department of Health, 2006.

14. Department of Health. National Service Framework for Older People. London: Department of Health, 2001.

15. Department of Health. National Service Framework for Renal Services. London: Department of Health, 2005.

16. Department of Health. National Dementia Strategy. London: Department of Health, 2009.

17. Department of Health. End of Life Strategy: Promoting High Quality for all at the end of life. London: Department of Health, 2008.

18. Higginson IJ. Priorities and preferences for end of life care in England, Scotland and Wales. London National Council for Specialist Palliative Care Services, 2002.

19. Addicot R, Dewar S. Improving Choice at the end of life. A descriptive analysis of the impact and costs of the Marie Curie Delivering Choice Programme in Lincolnshire London: The King's Fund, 2008.

20. Higginson IJ, Sen Gupta GJA. Place of Care in advanced cancer: A qualitative systematic literature review of patient preferences. J Palliat Med 2000;3(3):287–300.

21. Hinton J. Can Home Care maintain an acceptable quality of life for patients with terminal cancer and their relatives? Palliat Med 1994;8(3):183–196.

22. Gold Standards Framework. Prognostic indicator guidance. http://www.goldstandardsframework.nhs.uk/Resources/Gold%20Standards%20Framework/PIG_Paper_Final_revised_v5_Sept08.pdf (accessed October 16, 2009).

23. Gold Standards Framework. About GSF. http://www.goldstandardsframework.nhs.uk/About_GSF/ (accessed October 16, 2009).

24. Improving end of life care. Liverpool Care Pathway. http://www.endoflifecare.nhs.uk/eolc/lcp.htm (accessed October 16, 2009).

25. Ellershaw J, Wilkinson S. Care of the Dying. A Pathway to Excellence. Oxford, England: Oxford University Press, 2003.

26. Edmonds P, Preston M. Audit of the use of the Liverpool Care Pathway. (Unpublished). London: King's College Hospital, 2004.

27. Hockley J. Developing High Quality End of Life Care in Nursing Homes: An action research study. Un published thesis, University of Edinburgh, 2006.

28. National Health Service. End of life Care Programme. Preferred Priorities of Care. http://www.endoflifecareforadults.nhs.uk/eolc/ppc.htm (accessed October 25, 2009).

29. National Council for Palliative Care. Good Decision Making—The Mental Capacity Act and End of Life Care. Summary Evidence. London: National Council for Palliative Care, 2009.

30. National Audit Office. End of life Care. London: Stationary Office, 2008. http://www.nao.org.uk/publications/0708/end_of_life_care.aspx (accessed October 25, 2009).

31. Douglas J. For all the saints. BMJ 1991;304:579.

32. Guneratnum Y. Ethnicity and Older People, Palliative Care. London: National Council for Palliative Care, 2006.

33. Monroe B, Hansford P, Payne M, Sykes N. St Christopher's and the future. Omega 2007;56(1):63–75.

34. Clarke D, Seymour J, Douglas HR, et al. Clinical Nurse Specialists in palliative care. Part 2. Explaining diversity in the organization and costs of Macmillan Nursing Services. Palliat Med 2002;16(5):375–385.

35. Seymour J, Clarke D, Hughes P, et al. Clinical nurse specialists in palliative care part 3. Issues for the Macmillan nurse role. Palliat Med 2002;16(5):386–94.

36. National Midwifery Council. Framework for the Establishment of Advanced Nurse Practitioners and Midwife Practitioner posts. London: National Council for the Professional Development of Nursing and Midwifery, 2001.

37. Department of Health. Extending Independent Prescribing within the NHS in England. A Guide for Implementation. London: Department of Health, 2002.

38. Department of Health. Nurse and Pharmacist Prescribing Powers Extended. London: Department of Health, 2005.

39. Department of Health. Nurse Prescribers Extended Formulary: Additional Controlled Drugs. London: Department of Health, 2006.

40. Horton R. Nurse prescribing in the UK: Right but also wrong. Lancet 2002;359(9321):1875–1876.

41. Kinley J, Hancock D, Casterton J. Nurse prescribing in palliative care: Putting training into practice. Nurse Prescr 2004;2(2):60–64.

42. Luker K, Fergusson B, Austin L. Evaluation of Nurse Prescribing: Final Report. London: Department of Health, 1997.

43. Latter S, Maben J, Myall M, et al. An Evaluation of Extended Formulary Independent Nurse Prescribing. Final Report. Southampton: University of Southampton, 2004.

44. Avery A, Pringle M. Extended Prescribing by UK nurses and pharmacists. BMJ 2005;331(7526):1154–1155.

45. Ryan-Woolley B, McHugh G, Luker K. Prescribing by specialist nurses in cancer and palliative care: Results of a national survey. Palliat Med 2007;21(4):273–277.

46. Scottish Executive Health Department Chief Scientist Office. 2004. An Evaluation of a Multidisciplinary Hospital based Palliative Care Team (HPCT). http://www.sehd.scot.nhs.uk/cso/Publications/ExecSumms/OctNov04/farrer.pdf (accessed October 26, 2009).

47. Hearn J, Higginson IJ. Do specialist palliative care teams improve outcomes for cancer patients? A systematic review. J Palliat Med 1998;12(5):317–332.

48. Department of Health. Health Service Circular 29th September 1999. HSC 1999/217 Nurse Midwife and Health Visitor consultants: Establishing posts and making appointments. London: Department of Health, 1999. http://www.dh.gov.uk/en/Publicationsandstatistics/Lettersandcirculars/Healthservicecirculars/DH_4003972 (accessed February 13, 2009).

49. Higginson IJ, Hearne J, Myres K, et al. Palliative day care: What do services do? J Palliat Med 2000;14(4):277–286.

50. Hartley N, Payne M, eds. The Creative Arts in Palliative Care. The palliative care community—using the arts in different settings. Hartley N 40–51.

51. O'Kell S. Care staff recruitment and retention: What is happening in the independent care sector? Hous Care Supp 2002;5(2):21–24.

52. Gold Standards Framework. Evaluation of GSFCH Programme. http://www.goldstandardsframework.nhs.uk/GSFCareHomes/Evaluation_GSFCH_Programme.htm (accessed October 25, 2009).

53. ICM RESEARCH. How to Have a Good Death—General Public Survey. London: ICM Research, 2006.

54. Kellehear A. Compassionate Cities. Public Health and End of Life Care. Milton: Park Routledge, 2005.

55. Hartley N, Kraus F. The St Christopher's Schools Project. London: St Christopher's Hospice, 2008.

# 72 Palliative Care in Europe

*Marianne Jensen Hjermstad and Stein Kaasa*

Palliative care begins from the understanding that every patient has his or her own story, relationship, and culture and is worthy of respect as an individual. This implies that palliative care should be patient-oriented, guided by the needs of the patient, taking into account his or her values and preferences, and that ethical issues are considered with cultural variation in needs and values.

In 2002, the World Health Organization (WHO) definition stated that palliative care is "an approach that improves the quality of life of patients and their families facing the problems associated with life-threatening illness, through the prevention and relief of suffering by means of early identification and impeccable assessment and treatment of pain and other problems, physical, psycho-social, and spiritual."[1] These aspects are specifically emphasized in the specific document on palliative care from the Council of Europe, Committee of Ministers: "Recommendation REC (2003) 24 of the Committee of Ministers to Member States on the Organization of Palliative Care."[2]

Palliative care should be offered at all levels in the health-care system and could be regarded as an integral part of all medical services. However, based on the above, it becomes evident that palliative care has its own special characteristics that are not entirely covered by the mainstream health-care system. Thus, the emergence of palliative care as a medical and nursing specialty is rapidly progressing, and palliative medicine and nursing increasingly being acknowledged in many countries as a medical specialty beyond the basic level.[3,4]

In the Nordic countries for example, a 2-year specialist training program for physicians working in palliative medicine was started in 2003, and attracted huge interest. The course is offered every other year, has a duration of 21 months, and is composed of six 1-week slots of teaching with working assignments in the intervals. All participants conduct a small research project and many write a paper for publication, preferably for international journals. More than 80 participants will have completed the course in the spring of 2009.[5]

The cancer incidence rate is steadily increasing by 1% to 2% every year in most European countries. The cancer mortality rates have remained relatively stable or slightly decreased in the western world, and the scientific advances in cancer therapy have not led to a dramatic reduction in cancer incidence. This means that more patients are living longer with metastatic disease. A recent EUROCARE 4 analyses[6] showed slight increases in survival and decreases in geographic differences over time compared with the figures from the previous EUROCARE study for all cancer studied. This was interpreted as a result of improvements in health-care services in countries with poor survival and taken as an indication of better cancer care.

Because palliative care goes far beyond opioid availability and pain treatment and encompasses all the key elements of the holistic nursing approach—the care needs, the suffering, and the dignity and the quality of life of patients and relatives toward the last stages of life—it seems inappropriate to draw artificial lines between disease-modifying therapy and palliative care. This becomes even more evident when we know that many cancer patients are not cured from their disease, and that palliative care should be offered early in the stage of disease to provide the essential part of this care to all patients. Thus, the development and improvement of palliative care is an important, growing, and large public health issue across nations and cultures.

The purpose of this chapter is to present some of the European experiences with respect to the development, organization, and delivery of palliative care, educational issues, and research.

### The Situation in Europe

Because of increasing life expectancy and declining birth rates, the age distribution in many European nations is skewed toward a larger proportion of older people. Because the overall cancer incidence rises with advanced age, more people with cancer are expected in the near future. Predictions for causes of death in Europe for the next 15 years also show a changing pattern (Table 72–1), with more people living with and dying from chronic diseases.[1,7]

Palliative care is often associated with cancer, but the principles and definitions of palliative care are universal for several diseases.[1] Although different diseases present with various symptoms along the illness trajectory, epidemiological studies show that many symptoms and problems in the last year of life are similar.[8] This represents a challenge to the health-care systems in the delivery of effective and adequate end-of-life care to an increasing number of people.

Europe has gone through great political changes in the last decade, economically and culturally. From 2004, twelve new countries, primarily the former eastern European states, have become members of the European Union (EU), now counting 27 membership states. Despite an economic growth in Europe in general, there is still great diversity related to industrial, economic, cultural, and health policy aspects, as well as

| Table 72–1 |
|---|
| **Predicted Causes of Death in Europe for 2020 Compared with the 1990 Figures** |

| Disorder | Predicted Ranking 2020 | Previous Ranking 1990 |
|---|---|---|
| Ischemic heart disease | 1 | 1 |
| Cerebrovascular disease (including stroke) | 2 | 2 |
| Chronic obstructive pulmonary disease | 3 | 6 |
| Lower respiratory infections | 4 | 3 |
| Lung, trachea, and bronchial cancer | 5 | 10 |

*Sources:* Davies (2004), reference 1; Murray (1997), reference 7.

significant differences in population size, from 4.7 million in Norway to 83 million people in Germany. These diversities represent a challenge for the development of palliative care across Europe. Nevertheless, the gradually increasing medical and scientific collaboration across borders has led to the development of various models for palliative care. Some European centers are influenced by the Canadian model in Edmonton, Alberta,[9] the Beth Israel Medical Center program in New York City, New York,[10] or by the WHO project on palliative care implementation that influenced the development of palliative medicine throughout Spain.[11,12] However, directly adopting a model from another nation with a different health-care system is not always feasible. An example of this is the integration of the departments of pain service and palliative medicine into one, as has been successfully done at Beth Israel in New York. The pain programs in Europe are most often closely linked to anesthesiology, and, as such, not only are caring for palliative care patients but also taking care of patients with postoperative pain, chronic nonmalignant pain, chronic back pain, and so forth. Although pain treatment is an essential part of palliative care, the linkage between departments in Europe is more often based on cooperation and consultation services and, to some extent, translational research. Several services in Europe have begun either from pain/anesthesiology and/or oncology teams. It seems that the most successful programs have been able to combine the skills and knowledge across specialties.

A recently published report "The EAPC Review of Palliative Care in Europe"[4] gives a good overview of the development of palliative care in Europe. This is based on (1) a systematic review of the palliative care scientific literature in the decade from 1995 to 2005; (2) a summary of the findings, supplemented by bibliographic reports; and (3) an outline of the methodology and additional references. This gives information about the national palliative care activities with respect to implementation of palliative programs, finances and funding, delivery of care through palliative care units/hospices/home care, as well as education, specialist training, and research. There has been a gradual growth in this medical field during the last three decades, with significant innovations in the last 10 years. The first national palliative care units (PCUs) were opened in Great Britain in 1967, in Cyprus in 1974, and in Norway in 1993. Germany, France, Poland, and Finland followed before 1999. After this, Romania, the Netherlands, Belgium, Hungary, Portugal, Austria, Switzerland, Slovakia, Denmark, and Luxembourg all established their units before the change of the millennium. However, the survey revealed major international as well as intranational variations with respect to most of the issues that were evaluated.

To place palliative care on the health policy agenda, strategic interventions based on evidence-based knowledge and consensus among international experts in the field are mandatory to gain the necessary influence. This can be achieved through the establishment of professional organizations, such as the European Association for Palliative Care (EAPC), www.eapcnet.org.[13] The EAPC was established in 1988 with 42 members, on the initiative of Professor Ventafridda and the Floriani Foundation in Italy. The aim of the EAPC is to promote palliative care in Europe at the scientific, clinical, and social levels. In 1998, the EAPC was awarded the status of Non-Governmental Organization (NGO) of the Council of Europe and was transformed to "Onlus" (nonprofit organization with social utility). The EAPC has participated in two Expressions of Interest presented to the European community for the EU 6th and 7th Framework Research Programs. As a result of this work, research programs related to palliative care and advanced cancer have been brought to the forefront of the agenda for advanced research. Thanks to the development in palliative care research during the last decade, several projects have received funding from the European Union during these framework programs.[14]

The first of these, the European Palliative Care Research Collaborative (EPCRC) translational research collaborative with members from eight European countries and collaborators from Canada and Australia, aims to develop novel genetic methods for the prediction of opioid responses and individual variation in cachexia, in addition to developing consensus and evidence-based methodology for assessment and classification of pain, cachexia, and depression.[15] The development of European evidence based guidelines for treatment and assessment will be based on the results from research. The European Commission's Executive Agency for the Public Health Program (PHEA) received funding for the development of mechanisms for reporting and analyses of health issues and producing public health reports, focusing on best practices and models in palliative care—that is, the provision of specialist versus basic palliative care as dependent and integrated approaches. Two other initiatives, the PRISMA (reflecting the positive diversities of European priorities for research and measurement in end of life care) and a European Collaboration to optimize research for the care of cancer patients in the last days of life (OPCARE9) were also recently funded by the European Union.[16]

## Criteria for Excellence

At present, there is no uniform European consensus regarding the minimum set of indicators that constitutes a center of excellence in palliative care. Although this is a universal problem that exists outside Europe as well, a major challenge is related to the agreement on a definition of these criteria. Furthermore, the conceptual definitions of home care and hospice for example differ. The latter has negative connotations in Southern European cultures.[4] The national models for delivery of palliative care are not identical, and they are not equally prioritized in each country, either economically or politically. In Norway, the health authorities recently launched a National palliative care program with clinical guidelines.[17] The Norwegian Association for Palliative Care (NFPM) has developed a Standard for Palliation,[18] which describes the organization of palliative care services and defines the standard for palliative care in Norway for the years to come. An English version of the document can be downloaded from the NFPM website (www.nfpm.no).

Because of the relatively large economic, political, and cultural diversities across Europe, it might not be feasible to aim for the implementation of one particular model of excellence everywhere. However, there are certain key criteria that can be used in all models of palliative care to ensure the sufficient comprehensive provision and quality of care. These criteria include the following.

### Delivery and Content of Care

- Inpatient professional palliative care services in PCUs or hospices.
- Outpatient palliative care services or home care, organized by the PCU or through the established health-care services.
- Size of the unit and patient case mix.
- Multidisciplinary approach.
- Consultation services.
- A systematic approach to symptom assessment and classification, and common indicators for the quality of care.

### Education and Advanced Training

- Basic levels, medical/nursing schools.
- Continuing medical/nursing education.
- Palliative medicine specialists, palliative care nurse specialists.
- University chairs of palliative medicine.
- Systematic training of clinicians and clinical scientists in palliative care research.
- Opportunities for part-time work assignments, 50/50 clinical work and research.

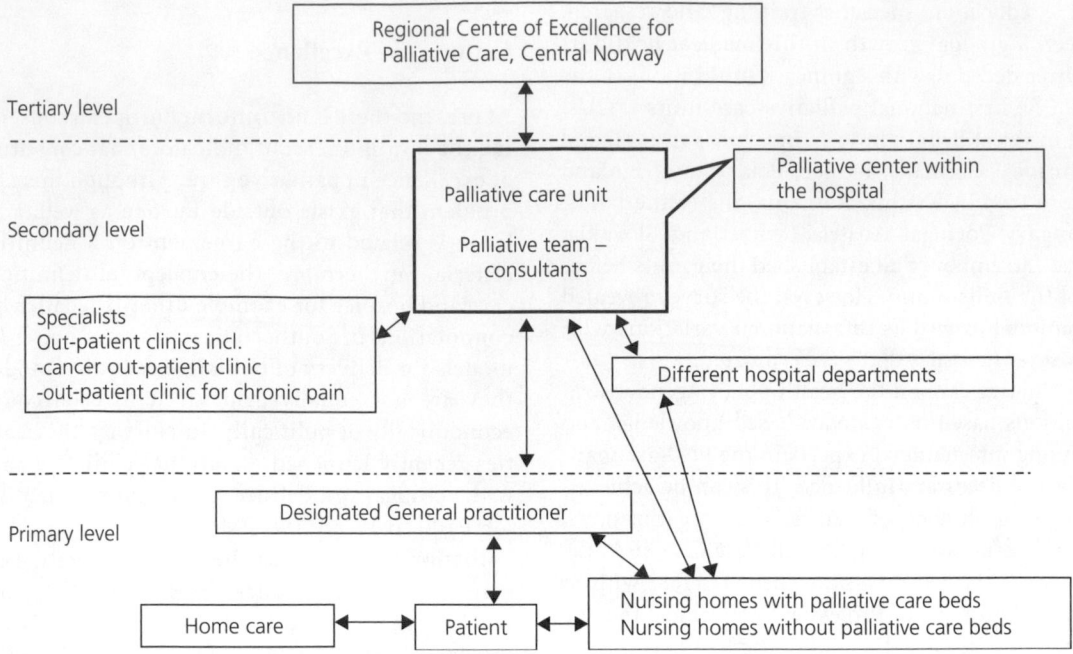

**Figure 72–1.** The Trondheim organizational model for palliative care.

## Research

- Continuous evaluation of the quality of palliative care services (structure, process, delivery).
- Consensus of indicators for the classification and assessment of subjective patient reported outcomes.
- Evidence-based knowledge to provide guidelines for treatment.
- National and international multicenter studies, and the development of formal research collaboratives.
- Translational research to close the gap between basic sciences and clinical practice.
- National and international networking, such as the EAPC Research Network and other formal structures.

## Integration of Palliative Medicine and Care in Public Healthcare

- Policy, advocacy, lobbying.
- Earmarked funding to palliative care research on a national level, possibly similiar to the British or Canadian models, preferable with incentives for national and international collaboration.

At the University Hospital in Trondheim, a fully integrated model has been developed during the last decade (Figure 72–1). The program started with the development of a 12-bed inpatient unit (acute palliative care) and an outpatient program, including a consultation service at the various wards and departments at the University Hospital. The staff composition is interdisciplinary with highly trained nurses and doctors. A close collaboration with the municipality of Trondheim has been organized as an integrated part of the palliative care program. This has resulted in establishment of designated palliative care units or beds in several nursing homes, combined with specialist palliative care service in patients' homes in collaboration with the general practitioners (GPs) and home-care nursing services in the community. The outpatient clinics, both for cancer patients and for chronic nonmalignant pain, and the palliative medicine unit have succeeded in joining forces regarding their clinical, educational, and research-related activities.

## The EAPC Activities: An Example of International Networking

### EAPC Initiatives

The EAPC serves as a catalyst for international collaboration and networking, with respect to distribution and delivery of care, clinical collaborative work, and research. There is a steadily growing number of activities, task forces, and individual and collective members (Figure 72–2).

One of the top priorities of the EAPC is the development of high-quality palliative care in Eastern Europe. The EAPC coordination center at Stockholm's Sjukhem Foundation in Stockholm, Sweden, was established in 2002. The major aims of the EAPC East project, which was established as a task force in 2001, were to support and improve the development of palliative care and to coordinate the activities and initiatives in Eastern Europe. In most of these countries, the care is

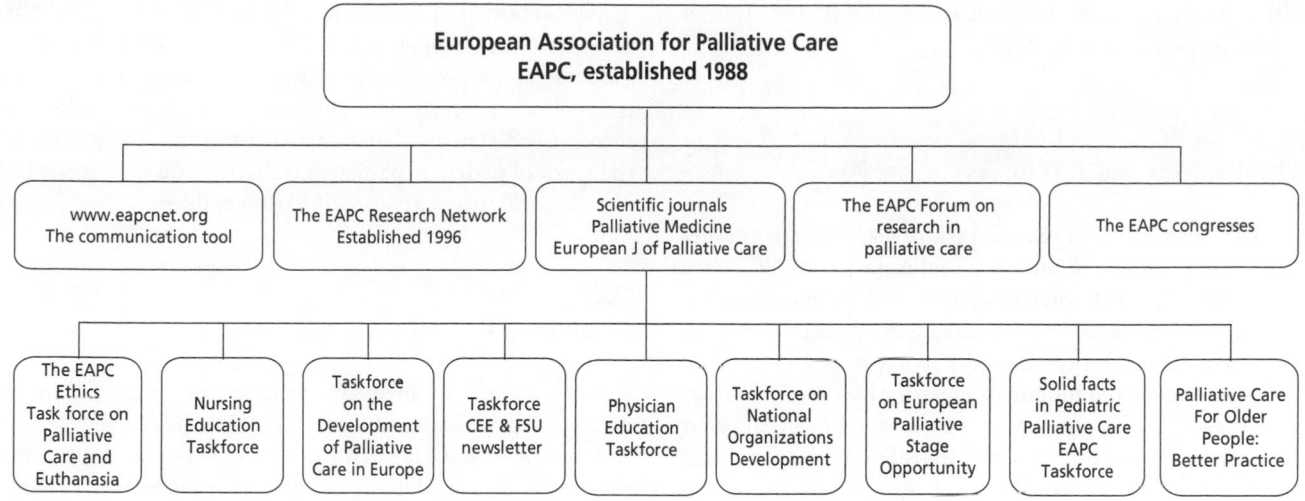

**Figure 72–2.** Overview of EAPC activities and task forces.

unevenly distributed and poorly developed, and drugs such as opioids are not readily accessible everywhere.[19] For example, recent reports show huge variation of access to medication depending on geographical area in Albania[20] and a lack of certain formulas in Romania.[21] Some national laws and regulations prohibit the prescription of opioids for use outside of the hospitals,[22] and only allow treatment for a few days.[20,21,23] Through international networks and collaboration with people and organizations interested in and working with palliative care in Eastern Europe, palliative care is put on the health policy agenda, a prerequisite for funding and change of practice. The first peak in this work was in the fall of 2004. Media campaigns, seminars, and discussions occured in order to disseminate the recommendations from the Council of Europe documents, that "legislation should make opioids and other drugs accessible in a range of formulations and dosages for medical use,"[2] as well as the recommendations from EAPC and national organizations.

The development of educational, training, and twinning projects between EAPC member institutions and Eastern European health-care professionals constitutes a major part of the work. Also important are the identification of national and international donors for hospice and palliative care development. The current aims of the project include the work on common minimal standards for palliative care services. Both the eastern and western part of Europe are engaged in this work. Education and training on a pedagogic level, quality assurance programs, and the realization of centers with minimal standards demonstrated by audit were other important activities. The EAPC coordination center for Eastern Europe was the launch pad of the CEE & FSU Newsletter Task Force (www.eapcnet.org/CeeFsuNlt/index.html).

The official website, www.eapcnet.org,[13] has become an important communication tool, for members and nonmembers, providing continuously updated information on activities, conferences, publications, and reports.

The EAPC Research Network was founded in 1996, based on the fact that research is a key issue for palliative care. This collaborative effort has organized eleven expert working groups on topical issues in palliaitive care for which a common European position or recommendation is needed, for example, on pain measurement tools[24] regarding prognostic factors in advanced cancer[25] or on fatigue.[26]

In addition, cross-sectional surveys on pain and pain treatments[27] and patient demographics and Center descriptions respectively in European palliative care units have been undertaken.[28] Two research projects have been initiated: the European Pharmacogentic study (EPOS) and the PAT-C project, the precursor of the EPCRC project.[15] Papers from these and other activities are published and downloadable from the EAPC website (www.eapcnet.org/publications/research.asp).

Recently, the Junior International Forum (JIF)[29] was established adjacent to the EAPC Research Network, with the intention of fostering international collaboration and providing a meeting place for PhD and postdoctoral students and other young scientists in the field of palliative care. The first meeting was held during the 5th EAPC Research Forum in Norway, 2008.

The two journals of the EAPC, the European Journal of Palliative Care and the peer-reviewed Palliative Medicine, with a steadily increasing impact factor (1.7 in 2007), have gained wide attention among a variety of researchers, clinicians, and other health professionals working in palliative care.

Two major activities by the EAPC are the The EAPC Forum on Research in Palliative Care and the EAPC congresses. These are each held every other year and hosted by different European countries. The 5th Research Forum was organized in Trondheim, Norway, in 2008. There were 1085 participants and 446 abstracts were presented, compared with 342 participants in the first Forum in Berlin in 2000. The last EAPC congress in Budapest had more than 2000 registrered participants, with an increasing distribution of participating countries.

## EAPC Projects and Taskforces

The EAPC has initiated several taskforces. Some also function as expert groups or advising bodies to the EAPC board of Directors. The Taskforce on Ethics and Euthanasia is an example and represents the official EAPC position on these issues. The major aim of this Task Force was to revise the EAPC's statement and judgment of palliative care and euthanasia. These issues created much debate; the original paper with comments[30] is found on the website www.eapcnet.org/projects/ethics.asp. The guidelines have been translated from English into French, Italian, Hungarian, German, Greek and Finnish, (downloadable from the EAPC website). The EU-funded research project PALLIUM is also concerned with the elucidation of ethical principles within European palliative care services and has finalized specific country reports from a survey undertaken in 1999.[31]

Education and research are imperative for palliative care to become acknowledged as a medical and nursing specialty. The EAPC task forces on nursing and medical education are in the process of developing recommendations for the curricula on basic educational levels, advanced and specialty levels. A downloadable file, www.eapcnet.org/ projects/nursingeducation.htm; "A Guide for the Development of Palliative Nurse Education in Europe," is available in English, French, and Dutch. From the EAPC Task Force on Medical Education, a recommendation in the form of a "Report of the Curriculum in Palliative Care for Undergraduate Medical Education" is also accessible on the website http://www.eapcnet.org/projects/TF-EducForPhys.html.

The delivery and development aspects of palliative care are addressed by the EAPC Task Force on the Development of Palliative Care in Europe. The aim is to explore, assess and summarize the care activity and development of palliative care in Europe. The recent overview[4] and the EAPC Atlas in printed and electronic versions[32] is the result of the work of the Task Force.

To foster networking and improve the communication between Central and Eastern Europe (CEE) and the former Soviet Union (FSU) states, and bridge the gap in communication between east and west, a Hungarian initiative was taken to establish the CEE and FSU Newsletter Taskforce.

Currently, a survey is underway by the taskforce on National Association Organizations Developments. The survey addresses organizational development, identification of problems, and functionality of the national associations.

The Task Force on European Palliative Stage Opportunity was initiated by the Dutch palliative care network and the Nursing education group. The aim is to prepare a Web-based catalog for people who would like to perform clinical work in a foreign country. This initiative is also aimed at increasing collaboration.

A new task force that was established in 2007 on Palliative Care for Older people, Better Practice, builds on two WHO guides[1,33] and aims to improve care practice for the increasing proportion of elderly. This corresponds with the EAPC taskforce in Pediatric palliative care that facilitates and supports the work of pediatric palliative medicine and provides a link between palliative care for adults and children.

## Delivery of Palliative Care Models

As pointed out earlier in this chapter, the organization and delivery of palliative care services in Europe is unevenly distributed. A recent German survey for example, showed that the quality and availability of palliative care beds have developed rapidly, but that only a minority of the units surveyed had a ratio of nursing staff to inpatient beds of 1.4:1 or more as recommended by the German Association for Palliative Medicine.[34] The Spanish region of Catalonia has about 46% of the nation's palliative care programs but only 15% of the entire Spanish population.[35]

Palliative care is delivered through various channels, and the degree to which it is integrated, co-existing, or separated from the formal health-care system varies considerably. In many countries, health professionals, as well as volunteers, private, charitable, and religious organizations, in primary care and through general hospitals, carry out much palliative care. In Spain, for example, private organizations are providing home-based palliative care to a substantial number of people, and likewise through volunteers in countries such as Hungary, Italy, and France. However, there is little tradition for volunteer work as a separate work-force in the Nordic countries. With the increasing knowledge and recognition of the complexity in the symptomatology of incurable diseases, a common model of providing care in Europe has been to concentrate expertise in multi-professional teams. These teams work in hospitals, inpatient units, hospices, or in the community in direct patient care or acting as consultants. To fully integrate palliative care into the general health-care system, political guidelines from the health-care authorities are necessary. In 2001, the Italian National Health Service passed a law saying that palliative care programs should be provided free to patients and families. This built on a previous law on hospice development that was followed by a budget allocation to the regional administrations. Several other European countries, for example, the United Kingdom, France, Norway, and Spain, also have health policy directives on palliative care implementations.

An all-inclusive and comprehensive overview of all European centers is not possible to present. Because the statistical and reporting guidelines vary so much, it is difficult to obtain sufficient documentation for valid comparisons across countries. In addition, the field is rapidly developing—perhaps a quality criteria in itself! Table 72–2 presents the activities of 15 centers in Europe according to the previously mentioned criteria.

**Table 72–2**
**Overview of Some European Palliative Care (PC) Centers**

| Country | Name | Palliative Care Unit (PCU), Size, Team Composition[a] | Outpatient Unit | Home Care[b] | Patients | Education/Training Consultation Services | Research | Specific Activities |
|---|---|---|---|---|---|---|---|---|
| Denmark, Copenhagen | Department of Palliative Medicine Bispebjerg Hospital | Acute PCU, 12 beds. Multidisciplinary team: doctors, nurses, social worker, physical and occupational therapists, psychologists, chaplains | Yes | Yes | All cancer patients | Collaborating with the medical and nursing schools and the university. Postgraduate/specialist training for nurses and doctors. Consultants in other units and home care | Clinical intervention research and psychosocial research. Multidisciplinary, PhD students | Continuous quality monitoring. In charge of establishing a national palliative care quality and research database |
| France, Lyon | Centre de Soins Palliatif, Hospices Civils de Lyon | Acute PCU, 12 beds. Multidisciplinary team: doctors, nurses, psychologist, art-therapy, esthetic therapy, social worker, chaplains, volunteers | Yes, pain clinic | In progress with another organization | 99% cancer patients | Collaborating with the medical and nursing schools and the university. Postgraduate training for nurses, hospital doctors and general practitioners. Specialist training for physicians | Clinical research on pain assessment, phase 2 and phase 4 pain studies, PhD students | Active in consensus meetings of the national palliative care development |
| Germany, Achen | Department of Palliative Medicine, University Hospital of Aachen | Acute PCU, 9 beds. Multidisciplinary team: doctors, nurses, psychologist + physical therapist, social worker, chaplain from hospital | Yes | PC team serves as consultants in close collaboration with home care | 98% cancer patients | Collaborating with the medical and nursing schools and universities. Undergraduate education with lectures and seminars, (20 hours are mandatory), post graduate 40 hours course, advanced PC course. Involved in development of PC curriculum in Germany. Consultation services for other units and home care, other professionals | Clinical drug trials, epidemiological studies, qualitative research, case reports, research on outcome and quality assurance. Multidisciplinary | Active in political activities to advance PC, through ie. media to inform patients, relatives, and medical staff |
| Hungary, Budapest | Budapest Hospice House | Acute PCU (Sept. 2004), 10 beds. Multi-disciplinary team: doctors, nurses, physical therapist, social worker, psychologist, psychiatrist, bereavement counsellor | Yes, pain clinic and psycho-oncology and bereavement services | Yes | Primarily cancer patients | Continuous PC training of staff, and several courses for other professionals and the public. Accredited 1-week training for nurses. Organizing international courses with other former eastern European states | New psycho-oncology research program (2003), focusing on anxiety/depression and distress, first Hungarian protocol on these issues | |

*(continued)*

**Table 72–2**
**Overview of Some European Palliative Care (PC) Centers** (*continued*)

| Country | Nam | Palliative Care Unit (PCU), size, team Composition[a] | Outpatient Unit | Home Care[b] | Patients | Education/Training Consultation Services | Research | Specific Activities |
|---|---|---|---|---|---|---|---|---|
| Italy, Milan | Cure Palliative, Istituto Tumori | Acute PCU, 10 beds, day-hospital (9 beds). Multidisciplinary team: doctors, nurses, social worker, physical therapists, volunteers | Yes | Yes | All cancer patients | Collaborating with Postgraduate education for doctors (master courses, specialty schools). Pain and PC consulting service for other units. | Assessment and treatment strategies for difficult cancer pain: neuropathic, chronic iatrogenic, breakthrough, bone pain, management of end-of-life care. Multidisciplinary, PhD students | EAPC coordinating office located here |
| Lancaster, UK | St Johns Hospice and Lancaster University | Hospital and community teams, full multidisciplinary membership | Yes | Yes | Majority cancer patients (85%), but increasing number of other diagnoses | Regular undergraduate teaching and post-graduate training for specialist doctors, regional teaching programme for clinical nurse specialists and general practitioners. | Clinical studies on pain, end of life care decisions. Lead unit for regional network of research active hospices | |
| London, UK | Cicely Saunders Institute of Palliative Care, Palliative care teams at Guy's and St Thomas' Hospitals, Palliative care team at King's College Hospital | Cicely Saunders Institute of Palliative Care, Palliative care teams at Guy's and St Thomas' Hospitals, Palliative care team at King's College Hospital | Yes | Yes | 70% cancer around 30% non-cancer, special heart failure, renal, and neurological interests | Large undergraduate medical school—over 450 medical students per year. Nursing school. Multi-professional research based MSc program to train those needing advanced skills in palliative care. Around 40% of those attending are from outside of UK, mostly from Europe. Local education for staff in the hospitals and community. | Active program of multiprofessional applied, clinical and health-care research, joint with rehabilitation. Approx 40 publications in peer review journals per year. PhD students and training, some visitors and placements accepted. Extended facilities including video conference links for lectures at Cicely Saunders Institute once this opens in 2009. See www.kcl.ac.uk/palliative | Leading EU PRISMA collaborative on end of life care measurement. Specific interests in evaluating new treatments and models of care, non-cancer, palliative care in Africa, place of death, home care, breathlessness, needs assessment, outcome measurement. Validated POS and STAS tools. Designated as a WHO Collaborating Centre for Palliative Care and Older People |
| Netherlands, Amsterdam | VUmc | Acute PCU (sept. 2004), 4 beds in close collaboration with hospice, 10 beds for terminally ill. Multidisciplinary | Yes. Multidisciplinary Anesthesiology/ pain clinic and palliative oncology clinic | PC team serves as consultants in close collaboration with home care | 90% cancer patients | Education program for medical students, regular PC pain management courses for physicians/ nurses. Consultation services and regional courses for professionals | Government funded research program in PC, public health and extra—mural medicine, symptom management. PhD students | Partner in Network Palliative Care Amsterdam. Organized a regional Helpdesk with PC help team for professionals |

| Location | Centre | Clinical service | PC team/clinics | Consultants | Patient population | Education | Research | Links |
|---|---|---|---|---|---|---|---|---|
| Netherlands, Nijmegen | UMC St Radboud | PCU in dept. of oncology, 5 beds. Multidisciplinary team: doctors, nurses, supported by specialist nurses, psychologist | Yes. Multidisciplinary through the PC team | PC team serves as consultants in close collaboration with home care | Majority cancer patients | Continuous PC education/ courses for staff. Consultation services for other units and home care, other professionals | Symptom management, improvement of PC, ethics. Multidisciplinary. PhD students | Partner in Network Palliative Care Rotterdam. A multidisciplinary regional PC team is coordinated for phone consultations |
| Netherlands, Rotterdam | Erasmus MC | Acute PCU, 11 beds. Multidisciplinary team: doctors (neuro-oncologist, anesthesiologist), specialist nurses, social worker, home care technology expert, psychiatrist, dieticians, chaplain | Yes | Yes | All cancer patients | Continuous PC education/training for oncologists, nurses and general practitioners. Educational programme for nursing home physicians. Post-graduate courses for medical students, oncology nurses, others. Specific focus on development and implementation of intervention programs | Clinical and epidemiological research: symptom prevalence, development of clinical interventions, end-of-life decision-making, organisational aspects of PC. Multidisciplinary, PhD students | |
| Norway, Oslo | Avdeling lindrende behandling | Acute PCU, 8 beds + out-patient clinic. Multidisciplinary team: doctors, nurses, social worker, physical therapists, dieticians | Yes | No | 99% cancer patients | Continuous PC education and training for medical students, physicians and nurses in collaboration with the University. Consultants in other units | Link to the University through the Regional Center for Excellence in Palliative Medicine which holds a chair in palliative medicine. PhD/master students | |
| Norway, Trondheim | Seksjon lindrende behandling (SLB) | Acute PCU, 12 beds + 12 beds in a designated nursing home. Multidisciplinary team: doctors, nurses, social workers, physical therapists, dieticians, chaplains | Yes | Yes | 99% cancer patients | Continuous PC education and training for medical students, physicians and nurses in collaboration with the University. Regular internal education, courses and training on basic/ specialist levels. Consultants in other units, home care and the nursing homes | Close link to the University, chair in palliative medicine. Specific research seminars, high degree of translational research, substantial number of scientific publications on PC every year. Multidisciplinary, several | |
| Scotland, UK | Edinburgh Cancer Centre. Edinburgh Cancer Research Centre | No PCU but access to Oncology Beds. Multidisciplinary team of consultants, nurses, social worker, with access to physiotherapy, occupational therapy and chaplaincy | Yes. General, Research and Complex Pain Clinics | No. Provided by local hospices | 90% cancer and 10% non-malignant patients | Formal program of education for Palliative Medicine. Postgraduate MSc in Palliative Care | University Chair of Palliative Medicine. Co-ordinator of National Research Program, including multicenter RCTs. Several MD and PhD students. | Local links with Oncology and Hospices. National links through NCRI. EU links through EAPC. |

*(continued)*

**Table 72–2**

**Overview of Some European Palliative Care (PC) Centers** *(continued)*

| Country | Name | Palliative Care Unit (PCU), Size, Team Composition[a] | Outpatient Unit | Home Care[b] | Patient | Education/Training Consultation Services | Research | Specific Activities |
|---|---|---|---|---|---|---|---|---|
| Spain, Barcelona | Institut Català d'Oncologia | Acute PCU, 16 beds. Multidisciplinary team: doctors, nurses, social workers, psychologist, psychiatrist, physical therapist | Yes | Yes | All cancer patients | University hospital support team to serve other units. Individually based continuous education and training for staff. Master of PC located on site, doctors/nurses | Active research department, center based and multicenter studies. Multidisciplinary research | CATPAL (Catalan multicenter cooperative group), 1998, design of studies and trials Grupo de Cuidados Paliativos en el seno de la Red Temática de Investigación Cooperativa en Cáncer (RTICC) OMS COLLABORATIVE CENTRE |
| Sweden, Stockholm | Stockholms Sjukhem (SSH) | Acute PCU, 38 beds (19 × 2). Multidisciplinary team: specialist doctors in oncology, geriatrics, algology, neurology, internal medicine, nurses, social workers, physical therapists, occupational, therapists, chaplains | Yes | Yes | The vast majority are cancer patients | Continuous PC education and training for medical students, physicians, nurses in collaboration with the Karolinska Intitutet, University Hospital. One medical training position. Educational unit. Continuous education and courses for team members at the unit and other health-care professionals | Collaborating with the University, chair in palliative medicine and nursing. Specific research seminars. Substantial no. of scientific publications on PC every year. Multidisciplinary research, several PhD students. Translational research and development projects. International collaboration. A web-based multicenter research network including the research tool "PANIS" | The Swedish Palliative Network (SPN), a web-based information service developed and based here Executive office for the Swedish National Council for Palliative Care, NRPV |

[a]No differentiation between part-time and full-time employment.
[b]Defined as PC services provided out of hospital by the PC team.

## Comprehensive Care

Most studies on delivery of care uncover the importance that patients and families place on receiving a well-organized package of care.[36] Quite often these professional teams take care of the most advanced patients with complex symptomatology and rapidly changing needs. Despite this, there is evidence that such specialized teams are effective in relieving distressing symptoms and can improve the quality of life of the patients and families toward the end of life.[36,37] Research studies concerning patient preferences in relation to end-of-life care show that many respondents (43%–75%) would prefer to die at home.[38,39] However, preferences may change as the disease progresses.[39] Scandinavian trials on different ways of coordinating palliative care services across the different settings of hospital, home, and community have found that a higher proportion of people can be helped to remain and to die at home as they wish to, and to spend less time in nursing homes.[40]

Most European palliative care units have a limited number of inpatient beds, normally around 10, as shown in Table 72–2. This is in line with the numbers in Figure 72–3, still demonstrating an insufficient coverage of PCU and hospice beds on national levels in some Western European countries. The range is from 10 to a maximum of 75 per 1 million inhabitants.[32] Nevertheless, this represents a positive development compared with the 2003 figures, when the maximum number of beds was 50 per 1 million inhabitants. The ratio of Palliative care beds to population in the former Eastern European states ranges from less than five to a maximum of 50 per 1 million inhabitants, with the majority of countries reporting from 15 to 25.[32]

Palliative care models encompass the provision of comprehensive care, and most centers presented in Table 72–2 also have outpatient/daycare facilities and home-care services. However, there is no universal way of delivering palliative care, because the national health services are organized and reimbursed for this work in different ways. In many PCUs, the hospital palliative care teams provide direct patient care after discharge (see Table 72–2). In certain parts of Spain, private organizations have a car service to take palliative experts from the hospital to the patients' homes. In Norway, there was no tradition for physicians to leave the hospital to take care of the patients at home. The financial system was prohibitive of such activities, with no reimbursement for extramural activities. Through intense and evidence-based lobbying, however, local politicians were convinced that the hospitals, not the individual physicians, should be reimbursed for this work. Thus, the Trondheim model was implemented in one region, enabling more people to stay in their homes.[40] In the Netherlands, on the other hand, the home care services are generally well-functioning, and the hospital palliative care teams basically serve as a facilitator and consultant to ease the transition between the PCU and the home. A Dutch evaluation showed that the team served the needs of the professional caregivers in a variety of settings, and that most consultations concerned physical and pharmacological problems.[41]

Some of the PCUs shown in Table 72–2 are closely collaborating with nursing homes, for example, in the Netherlands and Norway, as recommended by Norwegian governmental committees.[42] Extending intensive services to sites of more traditional care represents a challenge on the political, personal, organizational, economical, and educational levels. Hospitals and nursing homes often have different budgets,

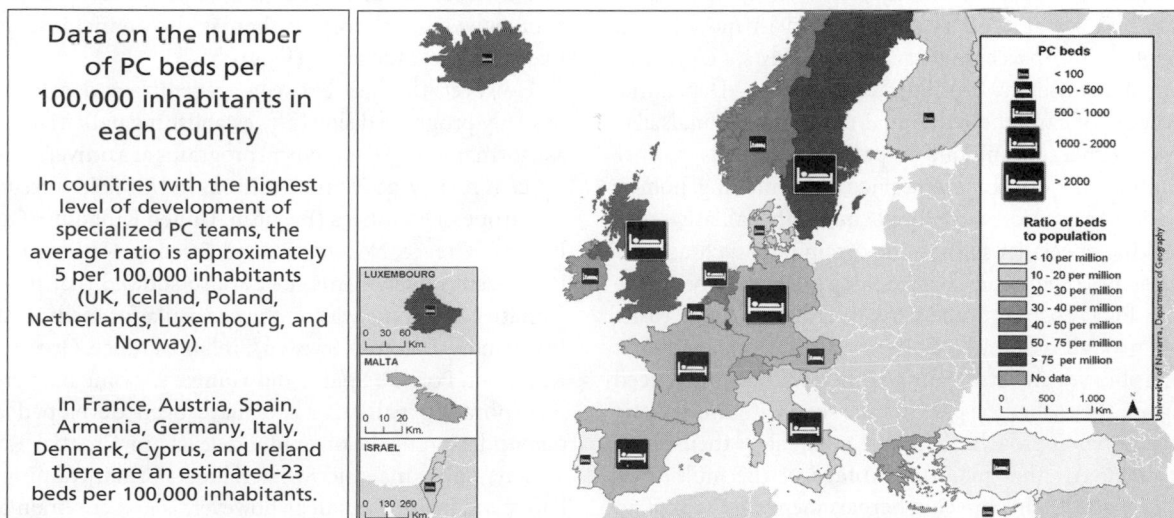

**Figure 72–3.** PC beds per 100,000 inhabitants in the Western European countries. *Source*: Adapted from EAPC Atlas of Palliative Care, reference 32.

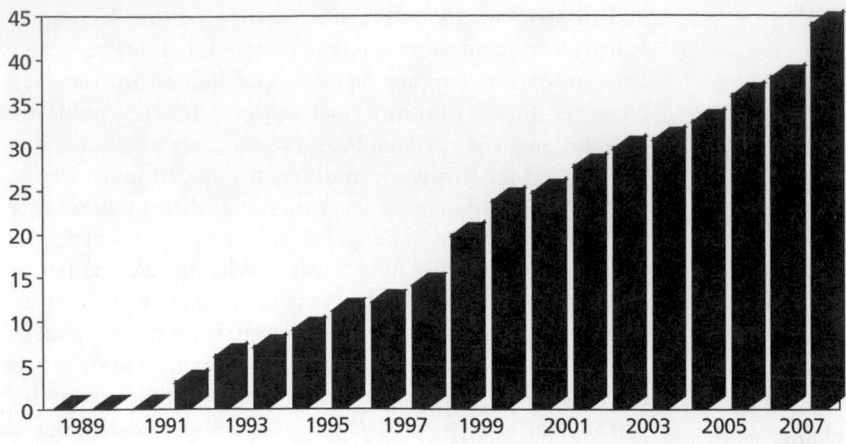

**Figure 72–4.** Overview of the development of collective member associations in the EAPC, 1989 to 2008. *Source*: Adapted from EAPC Review of Palliative Care in Europe, 2008, p. 218.[4]

and cost containment might be difficult when expensive drugs, fluids, and transfusions become part of daily care. This also increases the workload for the PCU care teams with respect to direct out-of-hospital patient care, extended consultation services, and specifically designed educational programs at basic and advanced levels.

## Multidisciplinary Approach and Consultation Services

The increasing complexity of the tasks involved in palliative care makes it clear that multidisciplinary teams are necessary for the identification and interventions needed to meet the rapidly changing needs of patients and families. Professionals in specialist palliative care settings may form relatively permanent teams, as is the case in most of the European centers presented in Table 72–2. Physicians, nurses, physical therapists, and social workers are included in most teams, supplemented by psychologists, psychiatrists, dietitians, bereavement counselors, chaplains, and others. Depending on the context of care, the individual team professionals also may serve as expert consultants for palliative patients in other hospital units, the home-care service, and nursing homes. The situation may also be the opposite, with palliative care teams seeking specialist services in disciplines such as neurology, anesthesiology, and pharmacology. Continuity of care across the PCU/hospice/home-care interface is more easily achieved through a multidisciplinary team composition if the responsibilities and strategies for the care plan are agreed upon. Again, the earlier the patients are seen with this holistic interprofessional approach, the more adequately their needs might be met. Another major advantage of the multidisciplinary teamwork is the aspect of bereavement care of staff, in cases with bereavement overload, an area traditionally better managed by professions other than physicians. The increasing numbers of professions involved in palliative care is directly

reflected in the membership of palliative care organizations. The German Association for Palliative Medicine was founded by 17 physicians in 1994. There were 50% physicians and 40% nurses among the 1100 members in 2003. At the EAPC 2009 Congress in Vienna, Austria, there were more than 2700 participants from 77 countries. Around 50% of the 1047 submitted abstracts were from physicians and 10% from nurses. Altogether, the abstract submittors represented 24 professions in contrast to almost 100% physicians at the first Research Forum in 2000 (www.eapcnet.org).[13]

## Education and Advanced Training

Rapid progress in the growth of professionals interested in palliative care began from 1995/96 and onward. This is evidenced by the steadily increasing number of members in the EAPC, from around 8300 in 1996 to more than 50,000 in 2008 (www.eapcnet.org).[13] There is also an increase in collective member association (Figure 72–4).

However, the link between academics and palliative care has only progressed slowly by establishing palliative medicine as a formal part of the medical programs at a university level. In a recent review, academic positions in this field were found in 10 European countries (Belgium, United Kingdom, Germany, Finland, Greece, Norway, Poland, Sweden, Netherlands, Italy) in a recent review.[3] This review also showed that teaching in palliative medicine was on the curricula for medical students in Germany, Norway, Sweden, Finland, France, Greece, United Kingdom, Poland, Spain, and Hungary.[3] Some new programs incorporating palliative care have been developed at various under-graduate or graduate levels in Croatia, Romania, Turkey, Lithuania, and Switzerland.[4] Formal training as palliative medicine specialists however, is less common and can be found in United Kingdom, Romania, Poland, Germany, Norway, Sweden, Denmark, Iceland, and Finland.[3] Specialized palliative textbooks in indigenous language are available in 12 countries. The situation is basically the same for the nursing curricula, with few countries having palliative care as formal parts of the graduate or postgraduate levels or as an accredited specialization. The United Kingdom has been in the forefront regarding palliative care nursing, all basic nurse education (advanced diploma level) includes teaching about core palliative care knowledge and skills. At a postbasic qualification level, there are approximately 10 university-based courses offering master's level courses in palliative care and psychosocial palliative care. These courses are usually taught in a multidisciplinary context. According to Larkin,[43] the United Kingdom remains a beacon of palliative care learning, offering not only theoretical but clinical learning. These opportunities are less readily available in many European countries and which are essential to the translation of theory to practice.

The recent extension of the EU has led to a more flexible employment market, with less restriction on crossing borders for work. A priority of the EU to facilitate this flexibility is the process toward more universal educational programs. Revising the different medical school curricula and the postgraduate specialist education programs to make them more standardized is an example of this.

## Palliative Care Research

Palliative care had its origin in the hospice movement emerging in the United Kingdom in the late 1960s. For quite some time, it was erroneously believed that research had no priority in this context. The development of palliative care in most countries in the 1960s and 1970s took place outside of the mainstream health-care system and outside academic institutions. It was primarily directed towards developing different clinical programs in hospitals, hospices, and consultant team activities.[14] However, many of the European stakeholders in palliative care at the time, Vittorio Ventafridda (Italy), Cicely Saunders, Geoffrey Hanks, and Robert Twycross (UK), as well as Kathey Fowley in the US were conducting high quality palliatiave care research. This research makes it clear that palliative care ideology is based not "only on compassion but equally on skills preferably founded on scientific evidence."[44,45]

## The Need for Research

Research is indispensable for the further development and improvement of palliative medicine and nursing.[46,47] We have witnessed an increased interest and development in interdisciplinary palliative care research during the last decade. For example, within the United Kingdom there is recognition of the importance of palliative care nursing research and involvement of nurses in multidisciplinary research teams. In addition, there is evidence of the growth in scholarship and publication of research from a bibliometric analysis[48] although there remain concerns about the number of small-scale studies. Although nursing in general makes a very small contribution to UK National Health Service (NHS) research in comparsion to the number of nurses involved in delivering care, palliative care represents one area of research that nurses have readily engaged with.[49] The steadily increasing number of international collaborative efforts in clinial and translational research in palliative care and advanced cancer are promising, yet there are many challenges ahead.[50,51]

Research is poorly embedded in the clinical work with patients in advanced stages of disease. This may partly result from to the traditional focus on compassion and the perceptions of the health-care providers that patients should not be bothered with interventions or self-report questionnaires for assessment of symptoms. This is also called "gate-keeping." Routine symptom assessment as a step toward better pain and symptom management has continued to have low priority in routine clinical activity. There remains a lack of evidence-based medicine and nursing in nursing homes and hospices.

There is an increasing demand for documentation on quality and costs of care, through scientifically based evaluation of outcomes. Furthermore, inadequate symptom management has been identified as the single most important barrier to adequate symptom relief.[52] Additionally, the use of standardized questionnaires providing immediate results, has been demonstrated to positively influence the doctor–patient communication,[53] and is endorsed by patients.[54]

However, there are many obstacles to the prioritization of research in palliative care: both methodologically clinically, and attitudinal as well as ethical, these problems can be overcome. Based on experience, most patients are willing to participate in various topics of palliative care research, including randomized trials on the impact of palliative care services,[55,56] evaluation of pain programs,[57] palliative radiotherapy,[58] and an intervention study on physical training.[59]

Funding still remains a major obstacle for research. Despite the fact that about 50% of cancer patients eventually die from their disease, less than 0.05% of funding goes to research in palliative care.[33] In the best-case scenario, only 0.18% of the oncology research budget is invested in palliative care, relative to 0.9% in the United States.[60] Nevertheless, Canadian and British national programs have funded the establishment of long-lasting, multidisciplinary groups covering a broad spectrum of palliative care research[61] (Table 72–3). Because a sound body of scientific research increases the chances of receiving funding for research projects, it is important that national and international research collaboratives are able to rely on predictable and sustainable funding over time.

Despite the difficulties involved in palliative care research, there is general consensus that the benefits of conducting research outweigh the many clinical and ethical challenges. The future looks bright, however, as evidenced in a recent EAPC European survey, displaying great enthusiasm for research in the palliative care community across Europe.[28]

Table 72–3
Examples of Basic and Clinical Research Topics for Multidisciplinary Research

| Areas | Content—Some Examples |
| --- | --- |
| Biomedical—Basic | Pain, cachexia, anorexia, fatigue |
| Biomedical—Basic and clinical | Mechanisms of drug actions: Inter-individual variability—adverse effects |
| | Pharmacokinetics—the elderly |
| Biomedical—Clinical | Controlled clinical trials |
| | Symptom control/medical interventions |
| Psychological—Clinical | Classification and assessment of pain |
| | Prognostication of pain relief |
| | Classification and assessment of cachexia |
| | Classification and assessment of anxiety/depression |
| | Cognitive function (in palliative care) |
| Sociological | Family |
| | Bereavement |
| | Areas for delivery of care |
| Health-care provision | Standards for palliative care |
| | Consensus on a minimum set of indicators present in a center of excellence in palliative care |
| | Quality assurance |
| Philosophical | Euthanasia/patient assisted suicide |

## Evidence-Based Medicine (EBM) and Palliative Care

A definition of EBM states that it is the conscientious, explicit, judged use of the best available evidence in order to offer the patient the most optimal individual care.[62] Thus, retrieving and applying the best available evidence is important to every clinician in the diagnostic workup and treatment of patients.[63] There are no contradictions between the philosophy of palliative care and EBM, although this debate has been going on for decades.

Many of the decisions made in palliative care are based on inferior quality studies, clinical experience, or extrapolation from studies performed in other populations, as seen, for example, in pain management. The need for EBM in palliative care is evident. Treatment of patients with a complex pathophysiology depends on research that focuses on the specific patient population and their problems.

There are at present two major areas in palliative care research and attention. The first is to work toward achieving consensus on how to assess and classify the most prevalent symptoms experienced by patients in advanced stages of cancer.[14,51] Recent reviews have shown that more than 80 different assessment tools were used to measure pain[64] and that the development of new tools is a continuously ongoing process without a defined rationale for doing so.[65] Furthermore, agreed upon definitions are of the utmost importance for making comparisons across studies, providing a valid basis for drawing conclusions about selection of medication or other treatment options. It is a major problem in clinical palliative care trials that study populations vary considerably in several characteristics associated with the symptom being studied.[66] Stringent definitions of patient characteristics and observations are required to identify to which class or subclass the patient belongs. Agreement on a minimum set of characteristics for a palliative care population is necessary to increase the evidence base of research.[67]

Other areas that need more in-depth studies are related to cancer and noncancer pain and symptoms, barriers to accessing care, and differences in the social, psychological, cultural, and spiritual aspects of palliative care from the point of patients, relatives, and caregivers (Table 72–3). One example is related to the fact that most patients in palliative care are elderly. This is in contrast to most studies in mainstream oncology, internal medicine, and even in pain treatment, where the upper age limit often is 70 to 75 years. The validity of extrapolating data from these age groups into older populations is questionable, and the need for appropriate research programs in the elderly is warranted.[33]

## Research Collaboration

In palliative care research, national or international multicenter collaborative studies are usually prerequisites for obtaining sufficiently large samples. The EAPC research network has established collaborations in the area of clinical and basic scientific studies, including the combining of clinical data with pharmacology (phenotyping) and genetic mapping (genotyping).[68] Eleven expert working groups have been working on various topics aiming for European consensus. Results from this work include the EAPC recommendations on morphine and alternative opioids in cancer pain,[69] and the previously mentioned recommendations on prognostication[25] and fatigue.[26]

Important information for palliative care providers as well as for policymakers can be gained by exploring already existing data on palliative care. This includes evaluation of different models of palliative care and the huge variation in costs of care. Other data to explore include the spending on palliative care versus other healthcare, and the number of people who die in hospices versus in home care. This might be facilitated through networks such as the EAPC, channels for communication and education such as telemedicine for educational and consulting purposes in Norway, or through new national European databases such as the OICP (Italian Observatory of Palliative Care) and PANIS (Palliative Assessment Network in Sweden). The OICP's website (www.oicp.org) and has two main contents: a directory of all Italian palliative services and a research center with annual exclusively online surveys on palliative care issues. The PANIS network (www.panis.se) conducts semiannual nationwide e-mail surveys on prevalent symptoms, with rapid online feedback to attending physicians.[70]

Several well-funded palliative care research initiatives have been established in Canada, United States, Australia, and Europe during the last 5 to 6 years.[14,48] Financial support from 7th Framework program of the European Union to the PRISMA and OPCARE9 program[16] and to the EPCRC through the 6th Framework program before that,[15] are important steps in the right direction to foster international collaboration. To succeed in achieving consensus with respect to assessment and classification of symptoms and on how to define a palliative care population, a systematic, stepwise approach in a multiprofessional and international collaborative composed of clinicians, researchers, and basic scientists is necessary. An example of this is the stepwise systematic work of the EPCRC toward a better method for symptom assessment, as shown in Figure 72–5.[51] In relation to pain, the goal is to develop a computer-based assessment tool that is both for and by the patient and the clinician, with a software content that is based on international consensus and is applicable for clinical work and research with a high degree of user-friendliness.

Computers used interactively have the potential to process, report, and communicate results reliably, efficiently, and cost-effectively between people. By applying Computer Adaptive Testing (CAT) new measurement systems can be developed. Item response theory (IRT) is being investigated by many groups as a potential methodology for CAT.[71,72] By taking advantage of modern computer technology, symptom assessment may be facilitated, questions may be tailored to the individual patient and skip sessions for irrelevant questions incorporated.

To develop the appropriate and user-friendly software, the EPCRC has placed great emphasis on design, input, and review by patients and clinicians during the development process meetings, steps 1 and 5 (Figure 72–5), and during the data collection process, steps 2 and 7. The EPCRC project recently embarked on the step 7 (Figure 72–5), the international data collection study, in 12 European, 4 Australian,

| Step 1. | Definition of content and selection of items based upon systematic literature review |
|---|---|
| | • Determine the content of the measure based upon the literature, the content of widely used forms, the clinical expert experience and advice from an expert panel |
| | • Generate an item pool for pain assessment, primarily based on existing pain assessment tools and reflecting the recommended dimensions. |
| Step 2. | Data collection number 1 |
| Step 3. | Analyses of data and functional specification of a computerized pain assessment tool |
| Step 4. | International expert evaluation II |
| Step 5. | Patient involvement, qualitative interview, and focus groups to document qualitative evidence of content and face validity |
| Step 6. | Development of a computerized analyses model (software based upon collected data) |
| Step 7. | International data collection number 2 |
| Step 8. | Data analysis |
| Step 9. | Programming of first version of the computer based pain assessment tool |

**Figure 72–5.** The EPCRC stepwise approach. *Source*: Adapted from Kaasa et al., JCO 2008, p. 3870.[51]

and 2 Canadian palliative care and oncology centers. The entire study is performed by touch-screen computers. The majority of questions are related to pain assessment and classification, primarily in the domains previously identified as most important;[64,65] intensity, temporal pattern, localization, exacerbating/relieving factors, and interference. Additional questions on depression, physical function, and cachexia are also included, as well as the Edmonton Classification System for Cancer Pain (ECS-CP)[73] and the Alberta Breakthrough pain questionnaire.[74] The upcoming data analyses will focus on user-friendliness, feasibility issues and validity, reliability, and psychometrics. This analysis will be used to develop the next and improved version of the computerized tool.

## The European Way to Promote Research

To further develop and improve the assessment and classification of cancer pain in general, the initiatives taken within the European and international palliative care community should be continued.[14,47,50] Many of the European centers presented in Table 72–2 were engaged in research activities on various levels. To successfully integrate multidisciplinary research in a palliative care program, certain criteria have to be accomplished:

- Professional leadership.
- Agreement on and promotion of a clear strategy and research agenda.
- Parallel development of clinic and research.
- An infrastructure that ensures interaction with scientists not working in the palliative field.
- Translational research.
- Multicenter national and international cooperation.

- Research programs at all levels: undergraduate, PhD students, postdoctoral, and researchers.
- Continuous application for funding at all levels.
- Dissemination of results.
- Leading journals.
- Conferences.
- Involvement of the public.

The pain and palliation research group in Trondheim, Norway, is an example of a multiprofessional group that is active in international collaboration (see Figure 72–1). Main areas are pharmacogenetics, genetic variability related to pain control, pain management, subjective symptom assessment, development and use of computer technology for symptom reporting, physical function, ethical issues, communication, and symptom palliation. Several PhD students are pursuing their dissertations in this group, and 183 scientific papers have been published during the last 5 years. The Instituto Tumori in Milan, the Dutch university hospitals, and King's College in the UK (Table 72–2) are other examples of successful collaboration between research and clinical palliative work.

An ultimate goal is to ensure that palliative care is represented at all local and national research forums. For Europe as a whole, the promotion and financing of palliative care research within the EU framework represents a major step forward.

## The Challenges

Although palliative care in Europe has undergone a remarkable development from its start in the 1960s and into the first decade of a new millennium, there are still several challenges ahead. As we have demonstrated in this chapter, there are still major differences within Europe, on the social, political, financial, and developmental levels, all which impact on the distribution, delivery, and access to palliative care. One problem relevant to the collection of survey data on palliative care is that there is no clear definition of the minimum number or set of indicators characterizing a palliative care program, a hospice, or a palliative care unit in a nursing home. To be able to describe and compare programs across countries, it is urgent to agree on minimum criteria for developing a palliative care program at various levels of the health-care system.

The EAPC is in the progress of establishing a new task force on "Centres of Excellence" in palliative care. The aim is to create a network of European countries at the university hospital level to establish common criteria of success and failure for developing a standard at all levels.

The challenges appear to be universal. The first is related to the total integration of palliative care into the general health-care system both in the inpatient and outpatient sector and the policy implications of such an integration. This would include education and specialist training at basic and advanced levels through universities and medical associations and a multi-disciplinary approach. In addition, special national and EU research programs in palliative care have started on the road of evidence-based palliatiave medicine. Striving for these goals is evidence-based practice with compassion—the cornerstone in the professional encounter with patients.

## Acknowledgments

The following persons have contributed to the writing of this chapter:

CJ Fürst, Stockholm, Sweden;
K Muszbek, Budapest, Hungary;
M Nabal, Barcelona, Spain;
M Filbet, Lyon, France;
M Groenvold, Copenhagen, Denmark;
A Rhebergen, Amsterdam, Netherlands;
A Caraceni, Milan, Italy;
L Radbruch, Aachen, Germany;
MI Bennett, Lancaster, UK;
H Blumhuber, Milan, Italy;
IJ Higginson, London, UK;
S Payne, Lancaster UK;
M Fallon, Edinburgh, UK.

### REFERENCES

1. Davies E, Higginson IJ, eds. Palliative Care. The Solid Facts. WHO Regional Office for Europe, Copenhagen 2004. Available at: http://www.euro.who.int/document/e82931.pdf (accessed December 20, 2008).
2. Council of Europe website. Available at: http://www.coe.int/T/E/Social_Cohesion/Health/Recommendations/Rec(2003)24.asp# (accessed December 20, 2008).
3. Kaasa S, Hjermstad MJ, Loge JH. Methodological and structural challenges in palliative care research: How have we fared in the last decades? Palliat Med 2006;20:727–734.
4. Rocafort J, Centeno C. EAPC review of palliative care in Europe. European Association for Palliative Care. EAPC Head Office, Milan, Italy, 2008.
5. Nordic Specialist Course in Palliative Medicine. Available at: www.nscpm.org (accessed December 20, 2008).
6. Berrino F, De Angelis R, Sant M, et al. Survival for eight major cancers and all cancers combined for European adults diagnosed in 1995–99: Results of the EUROCARE-4 study. Lancet Oncol 2007;8(9):773–783.
7. Murray CJL, Lopez AD. Alternative projections of mortality and disability by cause 1990–2020: Global burden of disease study. Lancet 1997;349:1498–1504.
8. Edmonds P, Karlsen S, Khan S, Addington-Hall J. A comparison of the palliative care needs of patients dying from chronic respiratory diseases and lung cancer. Palliat Med 2001;15:287–295.
9. Bruera E, Sweeney C. Palliative care models: International perspective. J Palliative Med 2002;5:319–327.

10. Portenoy R, Heller KS. Developing an integrated department of pain and palliative medicine. J Palliat Med 2002; 5:623–633.

11. Stjernswärd J, Colleau SM, Ventafridda V. The World Health Organization cancer pain and palliative care program. Past, present and future. J Pain Symptom Manage 1996;12:65–72.

12. Gòmez-Batiste X, Porta J, Tuca A, et al. Spain: The WHO Demonstration project of palliative care implementation in Catalonia: Results at 10 years (1991–2001). J Pain Symptom Manage 2002;24:239–244.

13. European Association for Palliative Care. Available at: www.eapcnet.org (accessed December 20, 2008).

14. Kaasa S, Radbruch L. Palliative care research—priorities and the way forward. Eur J Cancer 2008;44:1175–1179.

15. European Palliative Care Research Collaborative (EPCRC). Available at: http://www.epcrc.org (accessed December 20, 2008).

16. European Commission's Directorate-General for Research, Seventh Framework Programme (FP7). Available at: http://cordis.europa.eu/fp7/projects_en.html (accessed December 20, 2008).

17. Norwegian Directorate of Health [Nasjonalt handlingsprogram for Palliasjon, Norwegian version] National palliative care program with clinical guidelines. IS-1529 Oslo, SHDir, 2007.

18. Norwegian Association for Palliative Medicine. [Standard for Palliation, Norwegian]. Available at: http://www.palliativmed.org/?id=76086 (accessed December 20, 2008).

19. Clark D, Wright M. Transitions in End of Life Care. London: Open University Press, 2003.

20. Newton M. The development of terminal care in Albania. Eur J Palliat Care 2001;8 (6):246–249.

21. Mosoui D, Andrews CC, Perrols G. Palliative care in Romania. Palliat Med 2000;14 (1):65–67.

22. Costello J, Gorchakova A. Palliative care for children in the Republic of Belarus. Int J Palliat Nurs 2004;10 (4):197–200.

23. Salmon I. A British nurse's view of palliative care in Russia. J Palliat Nurs 2001;7(1):37–43.

24. Caraceni A, Cherny N, Fainsinger R, et al. Pain measurement tools and methods in clinical research in palliative care: Recommendations of an Expert Working Group of the European Association of Palliative Care. J Pain Symptom Manage 2002;23:239–255.

25. Maltoni M, Caraceni C, Brunelli C, et al. Prognostic factors in advanced cancer patients: Evidence-based clinical recommendations—a study by the steering committee of the European association for palliative care. J Clin Oncol 2005; 23:6240–6248.

26. Radbruch L, Strasser F, Elsner F, et al. Fatigue in palliative care patients—an EAPC approach. Palliat Med 2008;22:13–32.

27. Klepstad P, Kaasa S, Cherny N, Hanks G, De Conno F, the Research Steering Committee of the EAPC. Pain and pain treatments in European palliative care units. A cross sectional survey from the European Association for Palliative Care Research Network. Palliat Med 2005;19:477–484.

28. Kaasa S, Torvik K, Cherny N, Hanks G, de Conno F. Patient demographics and centre description in European palliative care units. Palliat Med 2007;21(1):15–22.

29. Gretton SK, Droney J, Branford R, Stene GB, Knudsen AK, Kaasa S. EAPC Research Network: The Junior Forum. Eur J Palliat Care 2009;16:232–235.

30. Materstvedt LJ, Clark D, Ellershaw J, et al. Euthanasia and physician-assisted suicide: A view from an EAPC Ethics Task Force. Palliat Med 2003;17:97–101.

31. Clark D, ten Have H, Janssens R. Common threads? Palliative care service development in seven European countries. Palliat Med 2000;14:479–490.

32. Centeno C, Clark D, Lynch T, et al. EAPC Atlas of Palliative Care in Europe. Valladolid: European Association for Palliative Care, 2007.

33. Davies E, Higginson IJ, eds. Better palliative care for older people. WHO Regional Office for Europe, Copenhagen, 2004. Available at: http://www.euro.who.int/document/ E82933.pdf (accessed December 20, 2008).

34. Radbruch L, Nauck F, Fuchs M, Neuwohner K, Schulenberg D, Lindena G. What is palliative care in Germany? Results from a representative survey. J Pain Symptom Manage 2002;23(6):471–483.

35. Centeno C, Hernansanz S, Flores LA, Rubiales AS, Lopez-Lara F. Spain: Palliative care programs in Spain, 2000: A national survey. J Pain Symptom Manage 2002;24:245–251.

36. Higginson IJ, Finlay I, Goodwin DM, et al. Do hospital-based palliative teams improve care for patient and families at the end of life? J Pain Symptom Manage 2002;23:96–106.

37. Higginson IJ, Finlay IG, Goodwin DM, et al. Is there evidence that palliative care teams alter end-of-life experiences of patients and their caregivers? J Pain Symptom Manage 2003;25:150–168.

38. Beccaro M, Costantini M, Giorgi Rossi P, et al. Actual and preferred place of death of cancer patients. Results from the Italian survey of the dying of cancer (ISDOC). J Epidemiol Community Health 2006;60(5):412–416.

39. Agar M, Currow DC, Shelby-James TM, Plummer J, Sanderson C, Abernethy AP. Preference for place of care and place of death in palliative care: Are these different questions? Palliat Med 2008;22(7):787–95.

40. Jordhøy MS, Fayers P, Saltnes T, Ahlner-Elmqvist M, Jannert M, Kaasa S. A palliative care intervention and death at home: A cluster randomised trial. Lancet 2000;356:888–893.

41. Schrijinemaekers V, Courtens A, van den Beuken M, Oyen P. The first 2 years of a palliative care consultation team in the Netherlands. Int J Palliat Nurs 2003;9:252–257.

42. Kaasa S, Breivik H, Jordhoy M. Norway: Development of palliative care. J Pain Symptom Manage 2002;24:211–214.

43. Larkin P. Education and scholarship in palliative care. In: Payne S, Seymour J, Ingleton C, eds. Palliative Care Nursing: Principles and Evidence for Practice (2nd ed). Maidenhead: McGraw-Hill Press; 2008:591–607.

44. Saunders C. Watch with me. Nurs Times 1965;61:1615–1617.

45. Saunders C. A personal therapeutic journey. BMJ 1996; 313:1599–1601.

46. Kaasa S, Dale O. Pain and Palliative Research Group. Building up research in palliative care: An historical perspective and a case for the future. Clin Geriatr Med 2005;21:81–92.

47. Kaasa S. Palliative care research: Time to intensify international collaboration. Palliat Med 2008;22:301–302.

48. Payne S, Turner M. Research methodologies in palliative care: A bibliometric analysis. Palliat Med 2008;22(4):336–342.

49. Rafferty AM, Traynor M. Assessing research quality. J Adv Nurs 2006;56(1):2–4.

50. Fainsinger RL. Global warming in the palliative care research environment: Adapting to change. Palliat Med 2008;22:328–335.

51. Kaasa S, Loge JH, Fayers P, et al. Symptom assessment in palliative care: A need for international collaboration. J Clin Oncol 2008;26:3867–3873.

52. Von Roenn JH, Cleeland CS, Gonin RR, et al. Physician attitudes and practice in cancer pain management. A survey from the Eastern Cooperative Oncology Group. Ann Intern Med 1993;119:121–126.

53. Velikova G, Booth L, Smith AB, et al. Measuring quality of life in routine oncology practice improves communication and patient well-being: A randomized controlled trial. J Clin Oncol 2004;22:714–724.

54. Brundage M, Leis A, Bezjak A, et al. Cancer patients' preferences for communicating clinical trial quality of life information: A qualitative study. Qual Life Res 2003;12:395–404.

55. Jordhøy MS, Kaasa S, Fayers P, Ovreness T, Underland G, Ahlner-Elmqvist M. Challenges in palliative care research; recruitment, attrition and compliance: Experience from a randomised controlled trial. Palliat Med 1999;13:299–310.

56. Jordhøy MS, Fayers P, Loge JH, Ahlner-Elmqvist M, Kaasa S. Quality of life in palliative cancer care: Results from a cluster randomised trial. J Clin Oncol 2001;19:3884–3894.

57. Hanks G, Robbins M, Sharp D, et al. The imPaCT study: A randomised controlled trial to evaluate a hospital palliative care team. BMJ 2002;87:733–739.

58. Sundstrøm S, Bremnes R, Aasebø U, et al. The effect of hypofractionated palliative radiotherapy (17Gy/2 fractions) in advanced non-small cell lung carcinoma (NSCLC) is comparable to standard fractionation for symptom control and survival. Results from a national phase II trial. J Clin Oncol 2004;22:801–810.

59. Oldervoll LM, Loge JH, Paltiel H, et al. The effect of a physical exercise program in palliative care; a phase II study. J Pain Symptom Manage 2006;31(5):421–430.

60. Higginson IJ. End-of-life care. Lessons from other nations. J Palliat Med 2005;8(Suppl 11):S161–S173.

61. Payne S, Addington-Hall J, Sharpe M. Supportive and palliative care research collaboratives in the United Kingdom: An unnatural experiment. Prog Palliat Care 2007; 21:663–665.

62. Sackett D, Richardson WS, Rosenberg W, Haynes B. Evidence Based Medicine. London: Churchill Livingstone, 1996.

63. McQuay HJ, Moore A, Wiffen P. Research in palliative medicine. The principles of evidence-based medicine. In: Doyle D, Hanks G, Cherny N, Calman K, eds. Oxford Textbook of Palliative Medicine (3rd ed). Oxford, England: Oxford University Press; 2003:119–128.

64. Holen JC, Hjermstad MJ, Loge JH, et al. Pain assessment tools: Is the content appropriate for use in palliative care? J Pain Symptom Manage 2006;32:567–580.

65. Hjermstad MJ, Gibbins J, Haugen DF, Caraceni A, Loge JH, Kaasa S. On behalf of the EPCRC, European Palliative Care Research Collaborative Pain Assessment Tools in Palliative Care; an urgent need for consensus. Palliat Med 2008;22:895–903.

66. Borgsteede SD, Deliens L, Francke AL, et al. Defining the patient population: One of the problems for palliative care research. Palliat Med 2006;20:63–68.

67. Currow DC, Wheeler JL, Glare PA, et al. A framework for generalizability in palliative care. J Pain Symptom Manage 2008;37:373–386.

68. Klepstad P, Cherny N, Hanks G, et al. Protocol: European Pharmacogenetic Opioid Study. EPOS, 2004.

69. Hanks GW, de Conno F, Cherny N, et al. On behalf of the Research Network of the European Association for Palliative Care. Morphine and alternative opioids in cancer pain: The EAPC recommendation. BMJ 2001;84:587–593.

70. Lundstrom S, Strang P. Establishing and testing a palliative care network in Sweden. Palliat Med 2004;18:139.

71. National Institutes of Health (NIH): PROMIS: Patient Reported Outcomes Measurement Information System, 2007. Available at: http://www.nihpromis.org (accessed December 20, 2008).

72. European Organisation for Research and Treatment of Cancer (EORTC), 2007. Available at: www.eortc.be (accessed December 20, 2008).

73. Fainsinger RL, Nekolaichuk CL. A "TNM" classification system for cancer pain: The Edmonton Classification System for Cancer Pain (ECS-CP). Support Care Cancer 2008; 16:547–555.

74. Hagen NA, Stiles C, Nekolaichuk C, et al. The Alberta Breakthrough Pain Assessment Tool for cancer patients: A validation study using a delphi process and patient think-aloud interviews. J Pain Symptom Manage 2008;35:136–152.

# 73

*Nathan I. Cherny and Ora Rosengarten*

# Palliative Care in Situations of Conflict

*If I don't look after my interests, then who will; but, if I look after my interests only, then what am I?—Rabbi Hillel (30 BC–9 AD)*

Situations of political conflict are characterized by enmity and potential for, or actual, violence. Conflict of this ilk may be manifested as outright war, a cycle of terror and reprisals, or a grumbling enmity between religious, national, ethnic, or cultural groups.

Incurable, life-threatening illness is endemic and it often occurs in places of conflict. In these circumstances, care delivery is often compromised or complicated. Situations of conflict occur in many places in the world and, at any time, a substantial proportion of the world population is involved in conflict of one sort or other. Conflicts, such as war or terror, traumatize the involved populations.[1–3] The nature of conflict has changed particularly with regard to the likelihood of civilian casualty, which accounted for around 5% at the beginning of the century and which is as high as high as 90% in some ongoing conflicts.[4] In this situation, bereavement, fear, anxiety, and depression become commonplace. Persistent conflicts may generate feelings of hopelessness and helplessness.

These observations are derived from my experience in working with Palestinian and Israeli patients in a Jewish hospital in Jerusalem over the past 15 years.

## Our Context

Jerusalem is a city that has existed in a situation of conflict over the past 100 years. Historically this has been the ancient capital of the Jewish people and currently it is the capital of the modern state of Israel. Jerusalem, however, is also claimed by the Palestinian Arab population as their capital. Indeed, Palestinians and Jews have in conflict over the destiny of this small strip of land between the Mediterranean and the Jordan River since the inception of the plan to re-establish a Jewish state in the area.

Attempts to achieve some form of rapprochement between the Jewish and Palestinian peoples have been intensified over the past 15 years. The breakdown of negotiations in 2000 has been accompanied a violent Palestinian uprising characterized by a wave of terror against Israeli citizens with subsequent restrictions on Palestinian movements and reprisals against terror organizations and their supporters. Thousands of peoples have been killed on both.[5]

In the midst of this, The Cancer Pain and Palliative Medicine Service, in the Department of Oncology at Shaare Zedek Medical Center has provided palliative care for both Israeli and Jewish patients. Shaare Zedek Medical Center is a Jewish general hospital that serves the entire population of Jerusalem. Reflecting the demographics of the city, 20% of the population are Palestinian Arabs, most of whom are Moslems.

The Cancer Pain and Palliative Medicine service is an integral part of the oncology service and it is based in the Oncology day hospital. The service consists of two physicians, a palliative care nurse coordinator and education and research coordinator, three social workers (Hebrew, Arabic, and Russian), a chaplain and liaison psychiatrist and psychologist. The service provides ambulatory and inpatient care. Community care is provided in cooperation with a number of home hospice services. Although most of the clinicians are Jewish, both the Arabic-speaking social worker and thoracic surgeon (who works very closely with the service) are Palestinian.

## Uniting and Dividing Experiences

Peoples on different sides of a political conflict of this ilk share a common traumatized existence.[2,3,6,7] Both sides suffer from risk of violent death or injury; both sides are vexed by injustices wrought by the other. Two peoples with different readings of history, different cultures and yet a common home, a common homeland often common cities, neighborhoods, and health-care services.[8]

Conflict breeds bias, and this is often manifest both among patients and health-care providers.

Illness is a unifying experience. The experiences of physical and psychological distress, fear of deterioration or death are universal. Similarly, the desire to care for the ill and to alleviate suffering is, fundamentally, universal. Indeed, even in the situation of very awful conflict, healthcare can provide opportunities to bridge between communities and peoples.

Nurses have a very special role to play in this situation. Given the greater opportunity for intimate contact and often, greater time for dialogue and compassionate care, their role is critical. This is true both regarding care delivery and also for the critical role of developing bonds of trust. Communication is critical to the success of this endeavor and this will often require the use of a translator to ensure that the patient is understood and that they understand the care provider.

## Barriers to Care in Situations of Conflict

*Infrastructural:* Conflicts commonly disrupt the flow of persons (patients and health care providers), the availability of care and the delivery of healthcare. Often patients are unable to get to the needed healthcare and health-care providers may be hampered in their ability to get to their patients. Physical resources may be limited by diversion of resources for other purposes, lack of free movement of goods or utilization of limited health-care resources by the combatants or victims. In times of war or conflicts, medications, sterile dressings, hospital beds and health-care providers may be in short supply. Often, the cost of medications may be inflated because of the collapse of health insurance arrangements or shortage.

*Bias and Access:* Both patients and health-care providers may be affected by bias against persons on the other side of the conflict barrier. This bias may be generated by resentment, fear, cultural misunderstanding or demonization. Bias may hinder patients from seeking healthcare that may involve contact with health-care providers or other patients from the other side of the conflict divide. Similarly bias may influence health-care providers in their attitudes or in delivery of care to persons on the other side of the divide. This can be as mild as personal distaste or as severe as overt hostile neglect or sabotage of treatment.

*Distrust and Enmity:* Neither patients or heath-care providers are protected from the political and social environment. Both parties may carry and project distrust and/or enmity that may be manifest in the carer/patient interaction. Distrust or enmity can interfere with all aspects of care delivery. Distrust and/or enmity may also affect other relationships: patients sharing the same waiting-room or adjacent hospital beds, health care providers form different sides of the conflict or patient's family members' relationships with the health-care providers.

*Safety:* Death or injury to health-care providers is, sadly, common in war and conflict. Beneficently minded health care providers often feel naively protected by the nature of the humanitarian work that they undertake. The enmity of conflict is often such that it is stronger than any compunction about the killing of carers.[9] Similarly, patients seeking medical assistance may be endangered en route to care; they may be confused for combatants, suspected of malice, or may simply be traversing a conflict zone.[10,11]

### Narrative: "I almost killed a patient today"

Monday night; 11 p.m. I almost killed a patient with methadone today. She was (and thankfully still is) a 68-year-old lady who came to see me from Natanya. She has a huge inoperable cancer deep in her abdomen, and even with high doses of morphine, her pain hadn't been adequately relieved.

Under close supervision I gave her two doses of methadone. Over the next 2 hours her pain subsided. She was able to get up and walk about. She seemed to have good relief without excessive drowsiness, confusion, or sleepiness.

Methadone is not widely available, and in Jerusalem, there is only one pharmacy that carries it. At 3:15 this afternoon, I wrote out a prescription and sent this lady and her husband to buy the methadone before they headed back to Natanya. To avoid parking problems, they went to the pharmacy by cab.

The pharmacy is in the middle of town… on Jaffa road near Zion Square. Half an hour later I was called to the emergency room. A terrorist had shot some 30 people in the center of town…exactly outside the pharmacy. I was quietly panicked. They didn't arrive in our emergency room. I checked with the emergency coordination center. They weren't on any of the emergency room lists. That meant that they were both alive and well or, possibly, dead but unidentified.

It was a very long hour until they returned to hospital to ask where else they could possibly get the methadone. The shooting had broken out as they approached the area and their cab driver was diverted.

Few things scare physicians, and particularly physicians relieving pain with opioids, than almost killing a patient with a medication intended to help. I am an expert in the side effects of methadone, but this would have been a new side effect for me. These are strange and evil times.

*Abuse*: In some instances health-care resources are seconded or abused to facilitate violence.[12] The harboring of combatants or weapons in hospitals or clinics and the ferrying of arms or combatants in ambulances or disguised as doctors, medics or nurses undermines the assumption of benevolence.[13] To be respected, it is essential that the credibility of the beneficence of health-care providers must be maintained. Without the assumption of benevolence, ambulances, health-care providers or even patients may be submitted to justifiable suspicion, which may cause delays in genuine care delivery as a result of security concerns and suspicion of potentially hostile intentions.[14]

## Why Provide Care in Conflict

Medicine is a fusion of humanity, science, and compassion. Humanity and compassion dictate that the suffering of illness must be addressed, and, when possible relieved. This holds true for all who suffer, be they friends or foes. One need not love a foe, but their suffering can be acknowledged and should be relieved when possible. Through this process, new opportunities for understanding and for mitigating enmity can be developed. Geneva Convention clearly recognizes the special status of the wounded or sick, be they civilians or combatants, an emphasizing the separation of medical care from the military conflict.[15]

Depersonalization and dehumanization of the enemy are common processes in conflict.[16] Often members of the "enemy" are demonized such that they are perceived as fundamentally hostile, evil, unworthy or even, worthy of harm (such as abuse, torture and punishment without due process).[16] These processes of depersonalization, dehumanization and demonization are re-enforced by lack of intimate contact between peoples. Social contacts are limited by perceived or real issues of fear, risk of harm, distrust, and enmity. All of these processes make the possibility of cooperation or conflict resolution more difficult.

Medicine has the potential to be a positive agent of change. Provision of care across lines of enmity creates the potential to reverse some of these processes.[17] Given that suffering at the end of life is universal, there is a very special opportunity for palliative care clinicians working is regions of conflict. Where end-of-life care is so often ignored or neglected, palliative care emphasizes humanity and respect for human dignity in a very special way. This focus on humanity stands in stark conflict to the disregard for the value of human life that is so much part of war and terror. Through the delivery of care, there is a potential to break barriers of suspicion and hatred and to reverse the processes of depersonalization, dehumanization, and demonization.[18]

### CASE STUDY 1
*You Are Now My Brother*

Mr. A was a 40-year-old husband of a young Palestinian woman with metastatic colon cancer. Together they had 4 children and they lived in East Jerusalem. In September 2000, he had been at the site of a violent clash between Palestinian protesters and the Israeli armed services. The young man who stood beside him was shot and killed and he carried the body away from the battle scene.

When he initially came with his wife to an Israeli hospital he was full of anger at Israelis and Jews and he had little reservation about hiding his hostility. The treating oncologist was an orthodox Jewish Israeli, Dr. S. They communicated with the help of a Palestinian social worker.

Over 2 years, Dr. S cared for this young family. Mrs. A underwent several lines of chemotherapy; some successful, others less so. When she developed a bowel obstruction, Dr. S arranged for a diverting colostomy and supported the family through the ordeal. The treating nurses would hold her hands, stroke her hair and extended the same care and support that they would to any other patient.

Slowly, enmity faded and Mr. A, his wife, and family became a part of the routine in the oncology day hospital. As her illness progressed she became increasingly dependant on help from the palliative care nurse. Because they lived in an Area that had became increasingly unsafe for Israelis, and in the absence of a Palestinian home care program, we had to make do with telephone support and hospital based ambulatory care.

Mrs. A ultimately developed a severe pain problem with lumbosacral plexopathy. She was admitted for pain stabilization. She did not achieve adequate relief with PCA morphine and she was switched to methadone which provided reasonable relief. It became clear however that she would not be able to return home and she died in the oncology/palliative care ward, surrounded by her family and friends and her mainly Israeli doctors and nurses.

A week after her death her husband returned with his four children with gifts and thanks for the staff. To Dr. S he said, "You are now my brother"

୭ଈ୯

୭ଈ୯

## Facilitating Care Delivery Across Lines of Enmity

*Advertise Availability and Neutrality*: Unless it is known that care is available irrespective of conflict and irrespective of "sex, race, nationality, religion, political opinion or other similar criteria,"[15] many potential patients may not seek help. Advertisement can be in the form of letters to doctors, commercial advertisements, or the print or video media.[19]

*Demilitarize Hospitals and Clinics*: It is absolutely unacceptable for hospitals to be militarized by any party in the conflict; they must be respected neutral territory. Then this principle is not adhered to, those in need of help may be too afraid to seek care. The abuse of hospitals either as bases for attack or as asylum for health combatants undermines impartiality and potentially invites incursion or conflict. As stated in the Geneva Convention I: Art. 2. *No persons residing, in whatever capacity, in a hospital zone shall perform any work, either within or without the zone, directly connected with military operations or the production of war material.*[15] This is further highlighted in the Convention for the Amelioration of the Condition of the Wounded in Armies in the Field, which states *Ambulances and military hospitals shall be recognized as neutral, and as such, protected and respected by the belligerents as long as they accommodate wounded and sick.*[20]

*Finances and Payment*: Health-care provision costs money and, unless supported by charity, costs must be covered to ensure ongoing ability to provide care. Emergency care should be available to all whom presenting need irrespective of ability to pay. For patients without insurance or financial resources, providing ongoing care can present logistic challenges. Several options are possible: provision of care at cost, arranging for care to be provided by health care services across the divide of conflict, or providing subsidized or charitable care. Arranging care, at lesser expense to the patient, across the lines of conflict requires the development and maintenance of lines of communications with health care practitioners on the other side of the conflict. In our experience, even in the setting of political animosity and differences, this sort of humanitarian cooperation has been possible and positive.

*Physical Access*: Patients, their caregivers, and family members may need specific permits to enable them to reach health-care facilities across lines of enmity. Members of the health-care team are often able to liaise directly with the civic or military authorities to facilitate the granting of permits. In doing so, there is an element of responsibility insofar as that the clinicians need to be adequately convinced that these permits will not be abused to ferry either arms or combatants. Because the authorities at check posts may, sometimes, be hostile to the patients or their families, it is helpful to provide them with written testimony to the fact that they are seeking health care with a specific contact name and telephone number for verification purposes. This is often a challenging situation since medical practitioners may be doubtful about exposing themselves to the risks of misuse of this kind of request.

*Cost Containment*: To protect the interests of the patient and the health-care provider, the clinician has a duty of care to try to contain costs of care provision as far as possible. This concern reflects itself in clinical decision making both regarding diagnostic investigations and therapeutics. One needs to be aware of the cost of medications and the most effective formulations to provide ongoing care. Commonly available formulations of controlled release opioids may be prohibitively expensive and cheaper options such as immediate release morphine or methadone may be preferred.

*Physician Liaison and Cooperation*: Physicians caring for individuals on both sides can initiate dialogue between the factions. Often patients can get adequate care without enduring all of the logistic barriers involved in crossing lines of enmity. It is often useful to liaise with physicians across the lines of enmity, to evaluate the availability of care and the limits of care resources. In suggesting to a patient that they not cross lines of enmity and that they seek care locally, one must first be sure that there is a real possibility of receiving adequate care. In so doing, it is appropriate to invite open lines of communication to address any medical issues that may arise. This approach requires effort in creating and maintaining an efficient medical network, based on reciprocal respect of a common ethical framework as and commitment to quality of care. Telemedicine and phone consultations are often useful to maintain clinical follow-up despite movement restrictions.

*Address the Needs of Children*: War and conflict inflicts a very severe price on the psychological and physical well being of children.[3,17,21–24] Building on the axiom that children need to be protected from the effects of war, physicians can work together in promoting child health. This can take the form of collaborative research, shared patient management, and joint conferences focusing on child welfare.[17]

*Create a Bank of Returned Medications*: Returned and unused medications are usually discarded or destroyed. When there are potential patients who do not have the resources to pay for medication, this is wasteful and inappropriate. Returned medications should be stored appropriately and may be used in the care of patients who do not have resources to pay for them. In our setting, we have successfully done this with cytotoxics, analgesics and antiemetcs and other potentially expensive medications.

*Creative Improvisation*: Often, normal care structures, such as home hospice services or day clinic availability will be unavailable or inaccessible. In such cases the available care resources need to be evaluated to explore the possibility of some form of improvisation, which may be suboptimal, but at least fills a modicum of care needs. This may involve a compromise on care plan; for example when a PCA could not be maintained at home because home care staff could not safely visit, we switched the patient to methadone suppositories which were both cheap and effective. Often family members, or sometime friends and neighbors will need to be trained to provide for care needs or even to do simple procedures such as tube feeding, suction, and wound care.

CASE STUDY 2

*Meeting the Needs of a Dying Patient When Cross Border Conflict Restricted Access*

Mrs. FW was a 60-year-old Palestinian woman from a small village just outside Jerusalem who presented to an Israeli hospital with metastatic breast cancer with liver and bone metastases. She received palliative antitumor therapies in two Israeli hospitals. She was regularly reviewed in the day hospital by the palliative care service who managed her pain with transdermal fentanyl and oral morphine.

Her condition deteriorated just as the conflict in Jerusalem worsened. Because of excessive personal risk, home hospice services were unable to attend her. The danger was understood by the patient and her family who not only accepted this with sorry resolve but who actively discouraged staff from placing themselves at risk.

Contact was made with a local doctor and nurse; with the support and instruction of the palliative care service they undertook a program of home care. When she was unable to take oral medication, a PCA pump was provided and serviced by the local medical team with daily telephone support form the palliative care service. This arrangement was successfully maintained until the patient's death at home.

## International Organizations

Several international organizations have created special infrastructures to assist in the provision of care in situations of conflict. It is very helpful to know and to develop relationships with those services and agencies active locally.

*The World Health Organization (WHO):* Sponsored by the United Nations, this international organization has widely accepted and acknowledged credibility that usually crosses all lines of conflict. Indeed, the WHO is mandated by its Constitution (article 2) to "furnish appropriate technical assistance and, in emergencies, the necessary aid upon the request or acceptance of Governments." In such situations, national authorities have the prime responsibility to respond to the needs of the affected population but in protracted conflict situations the situation can often deteriorate to a degree

that undermines the capacity of the local authorities to meet the urgent public health needs. Through its presence in all countries, its regional structure, its technical units and programmes at headquarters, its use of the existing health partnerships (such as the well-established polio network) and its system of collaborating centres, WHO is well-structured to deliver its technical advisory support to national and local authorities, sister agencies, the donor community and international NGOs and local self-help groups.

*Médecins Sans Frontières (also known as Doctors Without Borders or MSF):*[25] Doctors Without Borders (DWB) is a private, nonprofit organization that is at the forefront of emergency healthcare as well as care for populations suffering from endemic diseases and neglect. Health-care professionals working for DWB deliver emergency aid to victims of armed conflict, epidemics, and natural and man-made disasters, and to others who lack healthcare because of social or geographical isolation. They provide primary healthcare, performs surgery, rehabilitates hospitals and clinics, runs nutrition and sanitation programs, trains local medical personnel, and provides mental healthcare.

*Physicians for Human Rights:*[26] Physicians for Human Rights is less involved with providing actual care but can contribute to health-care provision in the work in protecting human rights.[27] When the ability to provide care has been hampered by bias, malice or draconian rule, they have been helpful as an international advocate. They provide teams of experts to investigate and expose violations of human rights.

*International Medical Corps:*[28] Similarly to Doctors without Borders, the International Medical Corps (IMC) is a global nonprofit organization dedicated to providing care in places of distress and conflict through health care training and relief and development programs. By offering training and healthcare to local populations and medical assistance to people at highest risk, and with the flexibility to respond rapidly to emergency situations, IMC rehabilitates devastated healthcare systems and helps bring them back to self-reliance.

## Narrative: Me and Muhammad

Dr Muhammad Natshe is dying. A father of five, a devout Moslem, a sweet man of peace who has lived almost all of his life through the tumult of Middle East Conflict. Tonight, as I write these words, he lies in a three-bedroom in Internal Medicine A at Shaare Zedek Medical Center (an Orthodox Jewish Hospital in West Jerusalem). He is weak and tired. Three of his sons were at his bedside when I bid him farewell tonight. As I left, I saw his eldest son prostrate and barefoot on his prayer mat, face to Mecca, deep in prayer.

Formerly a handsome man with a strong resemblance to the late King Hussein of Jordan, Dr Natshe is now withered and prematurely aged. The whites of his eyes are yellow tinged with an early jaundice from his now failing liver. His abdomen is distended with fluid; his legs are bloated by edema. His eyes are bright and his broad loving smile breaks through the misery, sadness and fear of his current circumstances. Like many Palestinian men, he has smoked most of his adult life. Now the lung cancer, that presented 9 months ago, has erupted through the brief response to chemotherapy and threatens the function of his vital organs.

Today, I am Mohammed's doctor; his oncologist and palliative medicine physician. That was not always the case. I first encountered him as a colleague. He was a highly respected general practitioner in East Jerusalem. There, close to the spectacular hubbub of the Damascus Gate of the Old City of Jerusalem, he tended to a large practice. Patients he referred were among the first Palestinians that I treated when first I arrived in Jerusalem some 7 years ago. He was a caring and involved family doctor. I was impressed and touched by his devotion: be it visiting his patents when they were admitted to our hospital, or caring, alongside the Home Hospice Service, for his patients who were approaching their deaths.

Dr Natshe was a general practitioner by default. He had initially wanted to be a surgeon and had, indeed, started a surgical residency at Hadassah Hospital in early 1973. Shortly after it began, his residency was interrupted by the surprise attack of the Yom Kippur War. The Jewish world was shocked, and outraged at the surprise attack. Most Palestinians supported the Egyptian/Syrian alliance. Dr Natshe took leave from Hadassah during the war and, in the aftermath, he felt too embarrassed to return to his residency in surgery. After 3 years of general practice, he applied and was accepted back to Hadassah as a radiology resident. The medical world of Israel, The West Bank and Jordan is small, and word of Dr Natshe's appointment quickly reached Amman. The Jordanian Medical Association dispatched a strongly worded letter of reprimand, intimating that it would be treasonous to work in an Israeli hospital. Thus, Mohammed returned to his general practice, where he worked until the toll of the lung cancer and the adverse effects of its treatment made it impossible to continue.

Faith and pragmatism: Dr Natshe's eyes twinkle with enthusiasm as he explains his love of Islam and the word of The Prophet. He is a deeply religious man and, in the encroaching shadow of death, his faith in God's ultimate beneficence underscores his inner strength and courageous coping. His sons are dapper, deferential and attentive to their frail father. Even in his ill-fitting hospital pajamas, I can see his tired chest rise with pride at the sight of them. He tells me that he insisted that each of them learn a trade before entering tertiary education. He has successfully assured them of short and long term economic opportunity. His eldest son, a part time hairdresser, studies computer engineering at an Israeli Technical School; the second, a part time truck driver, studies industrial chemistry at the Hebrew University. The boys speak to me in Hebrew and English. He tells them that they will need to look after their mother, as he will soon be gone.

Tomorrow, I plan to discharge Dr Natshe back to his home in East Jerusalem. After three days in hospital, his pain and vomiting are now controlled. He is very weak. In a week, I anticipate I will need to again drain his abdomen of the reaccumulating fluids that painfully distend his abdomen and compress his viscera. By then, he will probably be too weak to return to the hospital, so I will attend to him at home.

Dr Mohamed Natshe, Palestinian physician, man of Islam, man of God, father and husband.. is my colleague, my patient and my friend. I will care for him and his family with all of the skill and devotion that I can muster. I have promised him my commitment and my service as long as it is needed. Sadly, that won't be long.

That I am a Jew, that I am Israeli, that our peoples are in conflict in an awful time of violence and hatred, are irrelevant to the humanity that binds us. I will miss him when he's gone.

Behind the headlines, behind the shocking and awful images of violence, death, cruelty and humiliation small acts of caring, cooperation and love play themselves out…daily. This is another reality of the Intifada. Gladly, this is part of my reality; my source of hope and strength.

## Summary

War and conflict are among the major challenges to man's humanity. The provision of palliative care in times and places of conflict is fraught with personal and infrastructural difficulty. In meeting these challenges, medicine and health-care providers have the potential to be positive agents of change. The challenges are great but the potential rewards, even greater.

REFERENCES

1. Shalev AY, Freedman S. PTSD following terrorist attacks: A prospective evaluation. Am J Psychiatr 2005;(6):1188–1191.
2. Lavi T, Solomon Z. Palestinian youth of the Intifada: PTSD and future orientation. J Am Acad Child Adolescent Psychiatr 2005;44(11):1176–1183.
3. Solomon Z, Lavi T. Israeli youth in the Second Intifada: PTSD and future orientation. J Am Acad Child Adolescent Psychiatr 2005;44(11):1167–1175.
4. Downes AB. Targeting Civilians in War. Itheca, NY: Cornell University Press, 2008.
5. B'Tselem. Statistics, Fatalities 29.9.2000–30.11.2008, 2008.
6. Shuter J. Emotional problems in Palestinian children living in a war zone. Lancet 2002;360(9339):1098.
7. Khamis V. Post-traumatic stress and psychiatric disorders in Palestinian adolescents following intifada-related injuries. Social Sci Med 2008;67(8):1199–1207.
8. Minear L, Weiss TG, eds. Humanitarian Action in Times of War—A Handbook for Practitioners. Boulder: Lynne Rienner, 1993.
9. Siegel-Itzkovich J. David Applebaum. BMJ 2003;327(7416):684.
10. Giacaman R, Husseini A, Gordon NH, Awartani F. Imprints on the consciousness: The impact on Palestinian civilians of the Israeli Army invasion of West Bank towns. Eur J Pub Health 2004;14(3):286–290.

11. Miranda JJ. Ambulances and curfews: Delivering health care in Palestine. Lancet 2004;363:176.

12. Pearl MA. Ambulances and curfews: Delivering health care in Palestine. Lancet 2004;363(9412):895;author reply, 896.

13. Cohn JR, Romirowsky A, Marcus JM. Abuse of health-care workers' neutral status. Lancet 2004;363(9419):1473.

14. Viskin S. Shooting at ambulances in Israel: A cardiologist's viewpoint. Lancet 2003;361(9367):1470–1471.

15. Geneva Conventions. Geneva Convention (I) for the Amelioration of the Condition of the Wounded and Sick in Armed Forces in the Field. Geneva, Switzerland: Geneva Conventions, 1949.

16. Vetter S. Understanding human behavior in times of war. Military Med 2007;172(12 Suppl):7–10.

17. Wexler ID, Branski D, Kerem E. War and children. JAMA 2006;296(5):579–581.

18. Ashkenazi T, Berman M, Ben Ami S, Fadila A, Aravot D. A bridge between hearts: Mutual organ donation by Arabs and Jews in Israel. Transplantation 2004;77(1):151–155;discussion, 6–7.

19. Rees M. Amid the killing, E.R. is an oasis. Time 2003; 161(25):36–38.

20. Geneva conventions. Convention for the Amelioration of the Condition of the Wounded in Armies in the Field, Article 1. 1864.

21. Qouta S, Punamaki RL, Montgomery E, El Sarraj E. Predictors of psychological distress and positive resources among Palestinian adolescents: Trauma, child, and mothering characteristics. Child Abuse Neglect. 2007;31(7):699–717.

22. Elbedour S, Onwuegbuzie AJ, Ghannam J, Whitcome JA, Abu Hein F. Post-traumatic stress disorder, depression, and anxiety among Gaza Strip adolescents in the wake of the second Uprising (Intifada). Child Abuse Neglect 2007; 31(7):719–729.

23. Berger R, Pat-Horenczyk R, Gelkopf M. School-based intervention for prevention and treatment of elementary-students' terror-related distress in Israel: A quasi-randomized controlled trial. J Trauma Stress 2007;20(4):541–551.

24. Abdeen Z, Greenough PG, Chandran A, Qasrawi R. Assessment of the nutritional status of preschool-age children during the second Intifada in Palestine. Food Nutrition Bull 2007;28(3):274–282.

25. Doctors Without Borders. http://www.doctorswithoutborders. org (accessed December 2008).

26. Physician for human rights. http://www.phrusa.org (accessed December 2008).

27. Shauer A, Ziv H. Conflict and public health: Report from physicians for human rights—Israel. Lancet 2003;361(9364): 1221.

28. International Medical Corps. http://www.imc-la.com (accessed December 2008).

# 74 ❧ Marta H. Junin

# Palliative Care in South America

*In life we cope, we get by with what we have.\*—Family member of dying patient with few resources (\*En la vida hay que arreglarse con lo que se tiene, no con lo que falta)*

South America occupies a territorial area of 18,678,047 square kilometers and is populated by 357 million inhabitants[1] distributed in 12 countries: Argentina, Bolivia, Brazil, Chile, Colombia, Ecuador, Guyana, Paraguay, Peru, Suriname, Uruguay, and Venezuela (Figure 74–1). There are different geographical regions with distinctive characteristics: the ocean coasts, the tallest mountain chain of the Andes, the long rivers, such as the Amazon, large forests, wild jungles, prairies, lakes, deserts, such as the Puna of Atacama, and islands, each with its own cultural characteristics.

South America offers one of the more complex demographic realities from the point of view of ethnic composition, history of conquests, colonialism, and immigration. The indigenous populations over many generations have accumulated their own scientific knowledge, traditions, and holistic approaches to their lands, natural resources, and the environment. These populations are extremely vulnerable in today's society.[2]

The early indigenous populations were largely replaced at the end of the 14th and 15th centuries by Spanish and Portuguese colonization and, to a lesser extent, by the French, English, and Dutch. African slaves populated parts of the coastal regions at a later date. At the end of the 19th century to the middle of the 20th century, there was increasing European migration to South America by Spaniards, Italians, Poles, and Germans, as well as Arabian and Japanese.

The official language in the majority of South American countries is Spanish, with Portuguese spoken primarily in Brazil. Indigenous groups also have their own languages, for example, Mapuche, Quechua, Aymara, Guaraní, and Yámana. These are considered a secondary language in some countries. The South American population is mainly a mixture of races, descendants of European conquerors and American aborigines. There is a constant migration of people from areas of extreme poverty to more developed urban regions. This has resulted in problematic, uncontrolled urban growth. The large cities contain 50% of the total population. At the same time,

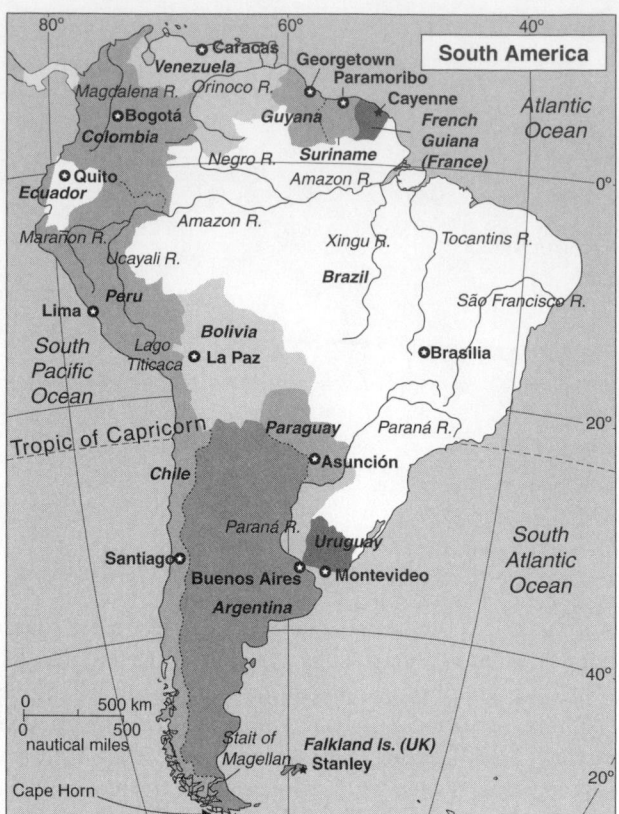

**Figure 74–1.** Countries of South America. *Source*: http://www.infoplease.com/atlas/southamerica.html. Copyright MAGELLAN Geographix.

however, there has been a large population emigration, mainly to the United States and Spain.[2]

## Political and Social-Economic Situation

The government systems, after long periods of authoritarian regimes, military dictatorships, and political instability, are mainly democratic, with constitutional republics and presidents. The establishment of democratic regimes and greater societal participation in the political arena are considered important achievements in the last two decades. However, the return to democracy hasn't yet been sufficient to reduce the social and economic inequities that threaten a country's stability, social integration, and ability for sound government. Ways to strengthen democratic principles and practices present ongoing challenges. This is especially true in situations of economic poverty, uncertainty, and struggles between peace and violence. All of these issues affect a population's health.

The conditions and levels of social and economic development in South America are generally heterogeneous. However, these factors significantly mould the health and welfare of the population. The economic and social transformations

experienced by South American countries in the 20th century have been characterized by governmental efforts to reduce inflation, increase investment, and privatize companies, all in response to recommendations of the International Monetary System.

State reform, with its emphasis on efficacy and modernization, underscores the important role of government and civil society in economic and social development. A population's health is defined by its economic situation.[2] A country's social and economic crisis presents an opportunity to promote programs with quality, efficacy, and equal access. Palliative care programs are one example.

## The Health Systems

South America is a region with large income differences. At the beginning of the 21st century, large variations in life conditions were noted between countries and within countries. Differences in educational levels, technical knowledge, income, health resources and organization, health service accessibility, and other social characteristics that determined a population's state of health were also noted.

In South America, there are different health systems. These are organized around three main providers that cover different percentages of the population in each country:

- The public system, with national, provincial and municipal-communal jurisdiction, supplies free clinical care through primary health centers in the community and general-specialist public hospitals for inpatients and outpatients. In some countries, the national health system provides assistance to the whole population without distinctions of race, economic situation, or religion.
- The insurance social system for working people is administered by trade unions. Employers and employees each pay a fixed fee. The cost of medical care and medicines in varying proportions are covered. Differences between the fixed fee and the actual treatment fee are paid by the patient.
- The private sector is for individuals with a good income. In this system, patients meet the total cost of their care. In some countries, all nonworking people are referred to this sector, with the risk that some will not be able to access healthcare because of lack of income. In general this health system assists a small percentage of the population.[2]

All South American countries are considered "in development" by the World Health Organization (WHO). In addition, the population is aging, with an average life expectancy of 70 years. The elderly face special problems. They have a high prevalence of chronic disease, and this occurs in the setting of poverty, insufficient health-care access and the absence of efficient social and political support. These issues are further compounded by the progressive deterioration of family ties and responsibilities.[2]

All age groups, including those who are especially vulnerable (children, people with low incomes, and those suffering from life-threatening illnesses such as cancer, HIV/AIDS, congestive heart failure, cerebrovascular disease, neurodegenerative disorders, and chronic respiratory diseases), have brought increased attention to palliative care as a public health issue. Palliative care is an integral part of comprehensive care for adults and children with life-limiting illnesses. The lack of good health-care policies can lead to unnecessary suffering and costs for these patients, families, and society. Yet the challenge remains to integrate palliative care into health-care systems worldwide and especially in resource-poor countries.

## Overview of the Health Context and World Health Organization Palliative Care Programs

The WHO estimates that 7.6 million people died of cancer in 2005 and 84 million people will die in the next 10 years if action is not taken. More than 70% of all cancer deaths occur in low and middle income countries where resources available for prevention, diagnosis and treatment of cancer are limited or nonexistent. Some of the most common cancers are curable if detected early and treated. Even with late cancer, the suffering of a patient can be relieved with good palliative care. The principles guiding the development of palliative care within a cancer control program are very similar to those needed to improve palliative care for people with other chronic disease.[3]

The neoplastic diseases are the second leading cause of death in all countries of the region.

In response to these statistics, WHO and the Pan American Health Organization (PAHO) designated palliative care as a priority in the Cancer Relief Program. They adopted measures for the development of palliative care programs in South America that were responsive to regional needs and specific problems. Attention was paid to the different income levels, disease presentations, technical expertise, resources allocated to health organizations, and access to health services in each country.

The WHO has pioneered a Public Health Strategy for integrating palliative care into existing health-care systems. This offers the best approach for translating new knowledge and skills into evidence-based, cost-effective interventions that can reach everyone in the population. It includes advice and guidelines to governments on health-care priorities and how to implement both national palliative care programs and national cancer control programs. In these programs, palliative care is one of the four key pillars of comprehensive cancer control. For public health strategies to be effective, they must be incorporated into all levels of the health-care system and be "owned" by the community. In other words, this strategy will be most effective if it has societal "buy in" within the

context of the culture, disease demographics, socioeconomics, and health-care system of the country. For each component of the public health strategy for integrating palliative care into existing health-care systems, there are short, intermediate, and long-term outcomes that must be measured.[4]

The WHO public health model for effective national palliative care programs consists of the following four parts:

1. National palliative care-appropriate policies and guidelines that incorporate palliative care into the public health system.
2. Laws and regulations that make readily and responsibly available opioid analgesics and other essential palliative care drugs.
3. Education in palliative care for health-care providers, policymakers, the public, and patients and caregivers.
4. Implementation of palliative care programs at all levels of society.

Good policies lay the groundwork for an effective health-care system. To ensure the best possible implementation of palliative care in a country, it must be incorporated into the National Health Plan and related policies and regulations. Goals include that affordable medications become widely available and palliative care education and services are integrated into the health-care system and society at all levels.

The WHO has included palliative care in a series of manuals on Integrated Management of Adolescent and Adult Illness. These manuals provide guidance for combining primary, preventive, and palliative care with disease-modifying treatment for HIV/AIDS at community levels in poor settings. National and local governments are encouraged to provide these services as a package. Several innovative programs have begun integrating community-based palliative and disease-modifying therapy for poor patients with HIV/AIDS or cancer.[5-7]

In summary, the WHO has based its approach to improving palliative care in the region on the following three components: government policies, opioid availability, and education. It describes the need for an additional measure of "implementation" to serve as an umbrella for the well-recognized WHO triangle.

## Government Policy

Three quarters of cancer patients worldwide are incurable when diagnosed. Because the size of the problem and the suffering associated with cancer are enormous, development of a national cancer control policy is an effective point of entry to begin integrating palliative care into a country's health-care system. Ideally, palliative care is incorporated as a priority within all aspects of each country's national health plan, so that all patients living with or dying from any chronic disease may have their suffering relieved. This includes both children and the elderly.[8]

The WHO identified palliative care as a priority for national cancer programs. The WHO has requested that governments revise their policies as to how they allocate resources in cancer treatment. In South America's developing countries, most patients with cancer are incurable at the time of diagnosis and need palliative care. Nonetheless, many developing countries assign a large proportion of their cancer resources to sophisticated treatments that have a low impact on the majority of the population. WHO recommendations are that more than half of these health-care resources be directed towards palliative care, which will benefit a much greater proportion of the population. In addition, WHO suggests using the information in the program to open up discussions with regulators and institutions interested in establishing or extending palliative care services. Although palliative care professionals are aware that this approach to care offers the most holistic treatment for both patients and their families, some health authorities still think that palliative care is "second-rate" medicine, and they prefer to invest their money in newer and more expensive technology. People involved in palliative care have some responsibility for this because they have not demonstrated to the health authorities the benefit and cost-effectiveness of this work.

Despite the strong endorsement and encouragement from WHO that all countries examine their system of national cancer control programs (and if one does not exist, develop one), many countries in South America do not have such programs. As stated by WHO, "A national cancer control program is a public health program designed to reduce cancer incidence and mortality and improve quality of life of cancer patients, through the systematic and equitable implementation of evidence-based strategies for prevention, early detection, diagnosis, treatment and palliation, and making the best use of available resources."[3]

Pain relief and palliative care can improve the quality of life of patients and their families. With careful planning, implementation, monitoring, and evaluation, the establishment of national cancer control programs offers the most rational means of achieving a substantial degree of cancer control, even where resources are severely limited. The establishment of a national cancer control program is recommended wherever the burden of the disease is significant. There is a rising trend of cancer risk factors, and there is a need to make the most efficient use of limited resources.

At this time, palliative care in South America still reaches only a tiny proportion of those who could benefit from it. The challenge for palliative care in the 21st century is to develop models and coverage appropriate to those in need, whatever their diagnosis, income, or setting without losing the original principles of the hospice movement.[9] Although cancer has been the disease focus for the majority of national policies in palliative care, there is an enormous need to incorporate palliative care policies into national health strategies for HIV/AIDS, the elderly, and pediatric populations.

National policies are the cornerstone for facilitating the implementation of palliative care programs that will provide care for all people in need of these services. These policies can be empowering and can ensure equitable access to affordable medications and therapies, or can be restrictive and lead to unnecessary suffering by patients, families, and the society.[8]

## Availability of and Access to Opioid Analgesics and Other Essential Palliative Care Drugs

In palliative care, one of the basic principles is the relief of pain with the use of the WHO Analgesic Ladder and the use of opioids. All the South American countries have adopted the WHO Guidelines. However, changes in legislation and regulations are urgently needed to allow adequate access to opioids.[10]

There are still some difficulties with the treatment of cancer pain in this region. The health policy does not endorse opioid analgesics. As a result, many cancer patients still die with their pain uncontrolled. Additionally, many patients and their families retain taboos and fears related to the use of opioids, necessitating that palliative care teams spend much time educating the family about the importance of opioids such as morphine to control pain and dyspnea.

In addition to the numerous myths regarding palliative care and morphine, many health-care professionals do not know how to adequately assess and treat pain. The misplaced fear of respiratory depression or hastening death through the use of opioids remains common. Opiophobia among regulators is illustrated through their concern that making opioids available for therapeutic use would increase the illicit drug market.

Although opioids can be easily found in the capital cities, prescriptions for controlled substances require many copies. Ready availability of opioids is not a reality for the inner-country people. These people must come to the capital city to get opioid medications for pain relief.

The most frequently used opioid for pain is morphine (ampules, syrup, pills) because of its availability, effectiveness, and cost. Morphine is available in all South American countries but laws and regulations make it difficult to prescribe adequate amounts of opioids to control pain. Morphine consumption by terminally ill patients remains low in many South American countries. The underlying cause continues to be fear surrounding morphine use, both on the part of health professionals and the general population. This underscores the need for governments to support teaching about palliative care, including the safe and effective use of morphine to control pain, in public education programs.[11]

In many situations, opioids are available but their high cost limits such availability to those who can pay. The cost of opioids in developing countries is higher than the cost of opioids in developed nations. In some South American countries such as Argentina, the high cost of opioid therapy can be more than 200% of the average monthly income. This problem reflects politics where expensive and sophisticated opioid preparations such as ampules and controlled-release oral morphine are available, whereas cheaper preparations such as immediate-release oral morphine tablets or elixir are not available.

Many countries, in their eagerness to prevent opioid misuse, have adopted laws and regulations that have resulted in restrictions affecting the medical use of opioids. For example, imposing limits on opioid doses and days of treatment allowed per patient. This is contrary to good palliative care and pain control practices where the maximum monthly quantity of medication allowed in each prescription is guided by patient need and not restricted through an arbitrary cut-off number. Only allowing a small number of pills per prescription can impose hardship on families who may have to travel long distances to acquire each prescription.[8]

Established in 1996 at the University of Wisconsin Comprehensive Cancer Center (now the Paul P. Carbone Comprehensive Cancer Center in the University of Wisconsin School of Medicine and Public Health), Pain & Policy Studies Group (PPSG) has been developing methods to evaluate and improve national policies that govern availability and access to the medicines that are essential for relieving severe pain throughout the world. The PPSG was recently redesignated as a World Health Organization Collaborating Center (WHOCC) until 2010.[12]

For many years, the Pain and Policy Studies Group have given advice and technical support to Pan American Health Organization and South American countries to find a solution to the problem of guaranteeing the availability of opioid analgesics for the whole population. Their guidelines are intended to help governments and health workers identify barriers in laws and regulations that make access to the tools of palliative care (e.g., opioids) impossible or difficult to obtain.

In summary, South America uses less than 1% of the world's morphine consumed for medical purposes.[13] Some of the reasons are: restrictions or excessive bureaucracy in the importation process of drugs, which increase the final cost of the product; legislation and restrictive control that impose maximum limits in the daily doses; delivery systems that are insufficient to make availability of these drugs uncomplicated in the rural area; health staff that are uneducated in the use of opioids for the relief of pain; concerns about addiction; and reticence to prescribe or store opioid drugs because of concern about legal liability if the drugs are stolen. Compounding the problem is a lack of authorized pharmacists for the preparation and delivery of generic formulations of opioid drugs.

An additional factor is that governments are underfunded to finance health-system infrastructure, assistance centers, infectious disease control, prenatal assistance, and malnutrition, etc. But these same health systems continue to pay for life-prolonging, and sometimes futile, interventions, rather than providing quality palliative care.

Because improving access to opioids is an international effort, we are all affected to some degree by the decisions and actions taken by others. We need to become aware that opioid availability is not just a local issue, but, rather, one without borders. All stakeholders in this process, including patients, professionals, multilateral organizations, the pharmaceutical industry, policymakers, and health-care professionals, must be included in the development of strategies to improve this situation.

In response to a request from WHO, the International Association for Hospice and Palliative Care (IAHPC) developed a List of Essential Medicines for Palliative Care. This list was based on the consensus of palliative care workers from around the world, using two criteria: efficacy and safety. The IAHPC List of Essential Medicines for Palliative Care includes 33 medications, which can be applied in all countries and are especially valuable in resource-poor settings. The esential drug list was created to increase access to treatment for patients who have uncontrolled symptoms. The goal is that Governments, policymakers, and health-care providers will take the necessary steps to ensure that all patients in need have access to these medications.[14,15]

## Education

In order to implement palliative care effectively across the South America countries, there are many different target audiences who require palliative care education. Typically these include the media and public; medical, nursing, social work, psychology, and pharmacy health-care professionals; policymakers, and regulators; and spiritual leaders, patients, and families. An example of one way to approach this would be to develop educational interventions and advocacy tools to engage the media, and heighten public and policymakers' awareness of the need for and benefits of palliative care for patients and their families. Some initiatives have started in relation to the community offering general information about palliative care and volunteers training.

A goal is that all health-care workers (doctors, nurses, social workers, psychologists, pharmacists, etc.) become knowledgeable and skilled in the core competencies of palliative care. This could be accomplished through policies that encourage or mandate palliative care education in the curricula and examinations of undergraduate and postgraduate health-care students; in continuing education programs for practicing health-care professionals; and for health-care professionals requesting or renewing licenses.[8]

This education in palliative care is intended to change the experience of illness for patients and families. In some South American countries, there are regional and local initiatives to promote graduate education programs for health professionals. However, standards in palliative care education are lacking. Training is generally sought out by the individual professional on her/his own initiative, and it is mainly theoretical, with few opportunities for clinical practice. However, a fundamental change is occurring in palliative care education opportunities. A variety of training systems have been implemented, including university or non-university courses, single discipline or interdisciplinary methodology, long-distance learning, and educational activities with a strong clinical emphasis. These activities include, workshops, advanced seminars, classroom-bedside teaching, and distance-learning courses. Some training programs have collaborated with foreign universities (e.g., Oxford, UK, and Calgary, Canada).[16,17] It is also recognized that communication skills training is important and can have a beneficial effect on behavior change in professionals working with cancer patients.[18]

Pain treatment, palliative care, and grief and bereavement are topics that are included at the undergraduate level in medicine, social work, psychology, and nursing. In some university hospitals, access to the palliative care training is possible for health-care students. In these institutions, there are either obligatory or optional lectures or modules on palliative care available to students in the last year of their training. This surely is one important way to improve patients' access to palliative care in the future. At a postgraduate level, activities are carried out at the main educational centers. The current focus on palliative care in the educational system gives hope for real change in the future.

One of the main obstacles to palliative care team members' training is the high cost of medical and nursing education. Nevertheless, in recent years, several Latin American programs have generated free education resources for professional training in symptom control and palliative care. This includes access to an international bibliography and medical and nursing scholarships. Financial support is given mainly by NGOs to individuals who are willing to travel abroad for training in palliative care and for leaders to attend major scientific conferences.

In some countries, for example Argentina, an interdisciplinary palliative care residency is available in public hospitals of Buenos Aires (two years, 40 hours per week). The residency program was started in 2005 and includes training in interactive multi-professional team work. There is also palliative medicine certification for physicians. In 2006, the Medical College of one Province, recognized palliative care as a discipline.[16]

## The Historical Perspective and Current Status of Palliative Care

During the early 1980s, because of the influence of the Hospice Movement and WHO's Cancer Pain Program, modern palliative care concepts began to spread in an organized manner across South America. The development was unlike that in Europe or North America, because social, cultural, and economic characteristics made it difficult to follow those models exactly.

The historical context of palliative care was similar in many South American countries, with a lack of support from governments and health authorities. The palliative care movement began with small, motivated groups of health professionals working with terminally ill patients in public and private institutions. This movement coincided in some countries with the beginning of democracy and ending of dictatorships and years of violence. Progress was slow, largely resulting from lack of financial support. However, once links were established with European and North American centers or universities, physicians and nurse leaders gained an opportunity to receive palliative care experience in more developed services and programs outside of South America.

Eventually, palliative care units were established in public hospitals, with programs that provide hospital-based care to terminally ill patients. In some cases, close and collaborative relationships were built between the oncology departments and palliative care services. During these early stages, support from the international palliative care community and NGOs was invaluable. Advice on educational, philosophical, and organizational skills was sought from experienced palliative care practitioners in the United Kingdom and the United States.

Overall, palliative care in South America was not the result of a strategic plan for the region. National programs are reported to exist only in Chile and Colombia.[19] The experience of Chile in the 1990s shows what can be achieved with support from national health administrators. It began with the development of several interdisciplinary palliative care teams organized as "local programs" in their respective health centers. Later, each one of these teams was consolidated as a "motor team"—the driving force of the future national program. The aim was to create awareness in the health sector about palliative care. Up until this time, there was little awareness. These pioneer groups became the National Committee. The committee reviewed the international literature and similar programs in other countries and organized standards. A high level of interest and financial support from the Health Ministry regarding "Pain Relief and Palliative Care National Programs" was officially recognized for cancer patients. Primary health services and public hospitals introduced a consulting team for inpatients and for patients cared for in the ambulatory setting. Today these centers cover 70% of the Chilean territory.

Despite the progress made in South America in the past 20 years, there is evidence that in general, quality of life during the dying process remains poor. Fragmented assistance and poor communication among professionals, patients, and families results in uncontrolled suffering and a great burden on family caregivers. Most of the regional health systems still fail to provide appropriate care for dying patients. The failures are clinical, educational, organizational, and ethical.[20] In some countries, there are national laws that guarantee access to palliative care throughout the health system, but these regulations have little real impact on practice and are frequently ignored.

In 1990, the First Palliative Care Latin American Meeting took place in Argentina. The participants recommended that a National Association of Palliative Care be created to promote national standards in palliative care education and practice, and to protect the interests of their members. Today, most South

American countries have their own scientific Palliative Care Association. The Latin American Palliative Care Association (ALCP) was created in 2002. The aims were: to promote the development of palliative care in the region; to coordinate actions by international funding agencies to ensure the access to essential medications and appropriate palliative care; to promote changes in the health legislation and regulations to establish apprioriate policies; to develop an international network to cooperate with others in the region; and to coordinated the Latin American Palliative Care Congress.[21] The last Congress took place in Lima, Perú, in March 2008 with professional participation from all Latin American countries.

## Proposals to Implementation of Palliative Care Programs in South America

Palliative care has been developing in South America since the mid-1980s, but there is a paucity of information on hospice and palliative care provision and only a weak evidence base upon which to develop policy and practice. It is necessary to create a committee to assess the current state of palliative care across the continent, This would provide an evidence base regarding what provisions for palliative care currently exist in the countries of South America and what barriers impede its development. Such information would set the stage for an informed debate on how to engage intergovernmental and governmental organizations and policymakers in addressing the problems facing individuals at end-of-life care in the region.[22] The goals for those already involved in palliative care in the region are to: map the existence of services in each country; draft national quality standards and clinical audit; design and develop research strategies; advocate for ongoing funding; and achieve "palliative care for all."

## Categorizing Development of Countries

The International Observatory on End of Life Care (IOELC)[23] Institute for Health Research, established in 2003 at Lancaster University, United Kingdom, have shown it is possible to map and measure the levels of palliative care development, country by country, throughout the world. Its aims are to provide clear and accessible research-based information about hospice and palliative care provision in the international context, especially in resource-poor regions. The information could be grouped into four categories as "Categorizing Development of Countries": (1) no known hospice or palliative care activity; (2) capacity-building activity is underway to promote hospice and palliative care delivery; (3) localized provision of hospice and palliative care is in place, often heavily supported by external donors; and (4) countries where hospice and palliative care services are approaching integration with the wider public health system and policy recognition.[24]

Using the IOELC typology, South America and each country were allocated to one of the four categories with the following results: (1) All South American countries had some hospice or palliative care activity; (2) Bolivia, Paraguay, and Suriname had capacity-building activities underway; (3) Brazil, Colombia, Ecuador, Guyana, Perú, Uruguay, and Venezuela had localized provisions for hospice or palliative care in place; and (4) Argentina and Chile had hospice or palliative care approaching integration with the wider public health system.

Using the IOELC typology, country reports were used to categorize current palliative care services, including how these are funded and reimbursed, estimates of the workforce capacity and coverage, and details of educational programs. Information was also provided on opioid availability, the public health context in which it was provided, the population, epidemiology, health-care system, the economy, and significant ethical issues in the delivery of hospice and palliative care. The level of development is depicted in a series of regional maps. To further assist those engaged in policy and service development in South America, further work is needed in constructing a broader evidence base for informed decision-making, and to form a globally appropriate system of service identification.[25]

## National Quality Standards and Clinical Audit

It is recommended that the Ministries of Health form an advisory committee consisting of experts from health institutions to draft national quality standards for palliative care and to create a national-regional network. The goal is to promote the growth and development of clinical programs that encompass the highest quality practices to guide the work of palliative care professionals. In addition, it is important to create a set of voluntary clinical practice guidelines to guide the growth and expansion of palliative care in South American countries. Guidelines on policies and strategies for the establishment of public health programs for the effective implementation and development of palliative care are also extremely important.[26–29]

It is recognized that the provision of quality palliative care requires the commitment and cooperation of a multiplicity of health-care service providers, community organizations, professionals, and volunteers. The overall objective of such collaboration is to ensure efficient, high-quality palliative care across the continuum of care.

The need is also recognized for evaluating the effectiveness and implementation of common assessment tools.[30] Use of validated tools is considered an essential cornerstone to maintaining standards of symptom control, evaluating outcomes, and developing an evidence base for symptom management guidelines.[31] Communication and integration of palliative care service across organizations and every sector of the health-care system is a goal to be strived for.[32]

In summary, implementation of quality palliative care starts with careful strategic planning followed by a systematic development of guidelines, outcome measures, indicators, standards, and a performance-improvement process through an inclusive consensus-building process. The process is must always be customized to the situation that exists within the community/country.

If there is to be consistent high-quality palliative care, every individual in the organization will need to know, accept, and agree to work with all elements of the quality strategy that are pertinent to his/her day-to-day activities.[33]

## Clinical Audit

A central goal of palliative care is to ensure the best possible quality of life until the end of life is reached. A clinical audit, understood as the systematic assessment of the quality of care delivered, is recognized as the means to measure this. Unfortunately, clinical audit in palliative care is not a common practice in many parts of the world. That is the case in South American countries, where there is a lack of adequate validated tools to assess palliative care outcomes. One initiative underway is the cross-cultural adaptation and validation of the Palliative Outcome Scale (POS) into a Spanish (Argentina) language and cultural context. The POS has undergone similar adaptation and development in diverse languages and cultural settings. It has been demonstrated to have good construct validity and internal consistency, sensitivity to change, and acceptability among multiprofessional teams.[34]

## Research Strategies

The lack of palliative care outcome measures developed and validated in South America is a fundamental challenge to establishing evidence-based practice for the continent.[35] There is, however, a growing interest in establishing an evidence base to underpin palliative care service provision in South America. This is part of a wider impetus to advance a global palliative care research agenda, as embodied in the "Venice Declaration."[36]

The Declaration calls to develop and promote a global palliative care research initiative, with special focus on developing countries specific to their geographical, socioeconomic, and cultural contexts.[37,38]

There is a general consensus that rigorous palliative care research must be undertaken if we are to ensure evidence-based health practice.[39,40]

## Funding for Programs

The funding necessary to cover essential palliative care services exceeds the financial means of many South America

countries. In addition, governments may not have the political will to implement palliative care policies. Services may have to be complemented by nongovernmental organizations (NGOs). These organizations are often dependent on fundraising and voluntary donations from a variety of sources.

Coordinated action by international funding agencies is needed to ensure that the poorest people have access to essential medications and appropriate palliative care. To this end, international networking in the palliative care field is vital. There are now numerous collaborative networks that have made a significant contribution to the development and sustainability of hospice and palliative care across many resource-poor regions of the world.

Palliative care programs and initiatives in South America need to identify sources and activities capable of generating funding streams. Long-term financial survival is the key to solving critical economic and human resource issues that interfere with the development of palliative care activity.[41]

## "Palliative Care for All"

This principle must underpin National Palliative Care Programs in South American countries. Although palliative care services may start in one or more health-care organizations that will become centers of palliative care excellence, it is always important to keep in mind the vision of striving to integrate palliative care into all levels of the society. It will be impossible to develop a palliative care system that is separate from the existing health-care system and social support network—there is simply not the capacity to do this. It will be critical for all palliative care experts to spend 40% to 50% of their time educating and supporting other health-care professionals and community support systems, in addition to providing consultation and direct patient/family care.[4]

The Neighborhood Network in Palliative Care Initiative (NNPC, a WHO Demonstration Project) in Kerala, India, demonstrates how to achieve meaningful palliative care coverage for everyone when citizens themselves take responsibility and ownership for community members with advanced illnesses and the dying. By creating a movement within the community that has embraced the existing community support and health-care systems, the community has integrated "palliative care for all" through a system that came "from the people, for the people, by the people."[42] Some of the features of this program might be applicable to some South American countries.

## The Palliative Care Teams

There are unknown numbers of palliative care teams and programs in South America, and there is no information on how many are successful in their development or their service delivery. What is known is that they vary among countries, cities, and also each other. These teams operate differently, depending on their level of development, and are located in the community or in hospitals. Some teams work exclusively in home care or inpatient facilities, other teams work in both settings. Most patients followed, have a diagnosis of cancer.[16]

The teams are multidisciplinary consisting of doctors from different specialties, registered and practical nurses, pharmacists, psychologists, social workers (as part- or full-time staff), spiritual/religious representatives, and volunteers. The coordinator is generally a doctor. The number of team members varies according to availability of resources. The teams work in a similar way to other palliative care teams throughout the world, but in many cases there are limited resources and no specific government or institutions facilities. The team's areas of activities include symptom control, psychosocial support to the patient and the family, counseling services, bereavement support, education and training, and clinical research. The team members in general are available via a 24-hour telephone-contact service.

Different program and team models have been developed, including palliative care units in general hospitals with designated beds, mobile consulting teams without designated beds for inpatients and patients in the ambulatory setting, and day care. In some areas of home care services run by hospitals, hospices or volunteer networks are available. Home visits are limited by lack of government funding. There is, however, a movement to provide such care with the support from NGOs. Some palliative care services have only informal support from the national health system. Contributing to this lack of support is that palliative care is not recognized as a medical or nursing specialty and is still considered to be unimportant.

Lack of government support for palliative care services has resulted in different approaches to obtain funding and or to provide care to patients in need. Examples are obtaining resources from charititable organizations, working for free on a volunteer basis, and care paid by the patient when this is feasable. Professional volunteer services are usually time limited. Volunteers frequently join the team because they are both interested in this new discipline and also wish to learn its practice. Eventually most withdraw from the team activity unless they can be reimbursed. This results is teams with cyclic staffing which impacts on team effectiveness.

Plans for future palliative care development include improvement of home care public programs specific to palliative care. Some teams that provide private care already exist, but there are few health institutions similar to hospice. In some places, there are charitable, nongovernment associations designed to provide clinical care to hospital inpatients and outpatients. Some countries, with large urban institutions in main cities provide such care, but in general, palliative care teams do not exist in rural communities. There is a great need in South America for palliative care services to be available in all settings where patients receive their care both in the community and in acute and long-term care facilities.

Despite the presence of functioning palliative care teams in some countries, in many hospitals in South America, the concept of teamwork is not evident. Professionals work more as individuals within a group, each with his/her own tasks and objectives. One influencing factor is that some doctors fear losing their patients for a variety of reasons both finacial and others. Consequently there may be an element of competition for patients among colleagues. The atmosphere among nurses, however, tends to be more passive. The doctors' competition and the nurses' passivity contribute to poor, interprofessional communication, which affects patient care. The concept of interdisciplinary teamwork is poorly developed in most centers, influenced in part by the different status of nurses and doctors. Nurses are seen as having a lower status than their medical colleagues. Encouraging communication between the two groups and the development of interdisciplinary palliative care training programs is important to enhance the understanding of the role of the other.

## The Nurse's Role in Palliative Care Teams

Although well-trained and financially supported palliative care teams are still absent in many regions, the number of interdisciplinary teams working in palliative care is expanding in South America. Nursing interventions in inpatient hospital settings, day care, outpatient and home care, are increasing day by day, and nurses have independent roles in this area. There are specific characteristics and substantial differences between the role of palliative care nursing and those in other medical specialties.

In all care settings, registered nurses training and working in palliative care assume key roles in the following areas: patient and family assessment; provision of direct care such as bathing comfort, wound dressings, and other treatment; management of distressing symptoms; administration and monitoring of the medication's therapeutic effects and any side effects; liaison with related services, particularly local doctors; referral to and coordination of volunteers; informing patients and families about available resources; professional and community education; and provision of counselling and bereavement support. One of the most important nursing tasks is family support, education, and training on various aspects of symptom management. Without appropriate education, care of the terminally ill patient by the family at home becomes impossible. The nurse supervises home care through visits and telephone support. In addition to these responsibilities, the nurse participates in multidisciplinary patient consultations, takes an active part in the assessment, diagnosis, treatment, and decision-making processes with the patient and family and actively participates in the palliative care team meetings.

## Barriers to Palliative Care Nursing

Despite these expectations of palliative care nursing there are many barriers for the nurse. In many South American countries, working conditions are difficult. Hospital wards are overcrowded and understaffed, often with many patients per nurse. This situation causes a high level of nursing stress. The nurse's status is relatively low, and consequently nursing is not a profession that many people enthusiastically pursue. There are few nurses working full-time in palliative care, and many working part-time. In addition, as discussed earlier, interprofessional communication is not on an equal level. Multidisciplinary–interdisciplinary workshops have been encouraged, and palliative care is one of the first disciplines in medicine-nursing to be taught in such a collaborative fashion. Nurses now have a voice in medical meetings, and they are beginning to be recognized as an independent profession with a significant contribution to offer. Another innovation in nursing is the use of interactive teaching sessions rather than the traditional didactic methods common in unidisciplinary nursing and medical teaching.

Nurses working in rural areas believe there is significant work to be done to help them provide for the palliative needs of the community. Rural and remote communities are not homogeneous; they offer various challenges to health-care delivery based on demographics, local culture, physical environment, and distance from health services. Rural nurses providing palliative care in the community suffer significant professional isolation. But interestingly, people living in these regions do not have the profound negative beliefs and thoughts about death and dying as seen in large cities. In some settings, particularly in remote areas, the nurse may be the sole health practitioner in a community, receiving telephone support from a doctor located some distance away. The challenge is to find sustainable models of palliative care provision in many of these communities which lack specialist services and technological advances.

It is important to understand the different levels of nurse training that exist in South American countries: those with a doctoral or master's degree in nursing, those with a college or university degree, licensed nurses, and auxiliaries. There is a lack of consistent inclusion of palliative care in undergraduate curricula across the countries. In general, a discrete module in the form of an elective is offered to a small group of students. This situation is changing, and there are more nursing colleges and universities, including palliative care content in their curriculum.

The demand for ongoing palliative care education has increased. There are education programs available to prepare nurses for their role in some government institutions. These courses range from one day seminars to 50- to 100-hour programs on different aspects of palliative care. Nurses with experience and knowledge set up palliative nursing inservice programs for their unit and for nurses from surrounding hospitals.

One of the issues that is very important to development in nursing training is how to manage the patient in pain. The inadequate treatment of pain remains a pervasive clinical problem in hospitalized patients. This results in significant physiological, psychological, and financial consequences for the patient and family. Barriers that lead to the undertreatment of pain continue to be lack of knowledge, inappropriate attitudes, and lack of pain management skills in those healthcare professionals who provide the treatment. Well-trained nurses can play a crucial role in reversing this process. Nurses often act as mediators between the doctor and the patient and serve as the main observer of pain and discomfort in the patient. However, they frequently lack the necessary pain management knowledge for this role.[43]

Therefore, in some public hospitals a pain education program has been implemented for nurses who act as "first-line" in assessing and managing pain. The program consists of two components: a theoretical component and clinical demonstration of the implementation of daily pain assessment and treatment. After implementation of the pain education program, nurses demonstrated a significant increase in their pain knowledge, skills, assessment and attitudes.[44]

Access to postgraduate palliative care education largely depends on geographic location, with more educational opportunities in large urban centers than elsewhere. Because of this, there is increasing emphasis on the provision of specialist courses via distance education. In some cases, this is supported by information technology such as teleconferencing and internet delivery. These approaches overcome some of the access issues. Importantly, the Nursing Committee of the Latin American Association of Palliative Care has developed a Post Graduate Nursing Curricullum to address the needs for palliative care education for Latin American nurses.[45]

One recommendation is that postgraduate continuing education should be structured in such a way as to ensure the development of nurses prepared for clinical nursing roles in specialist areas. Also recommended is that links with higher-education institutions be developed to accredit such courses for nurses and that all courses be subjected to a joint professional and academic validation and accreditation. Currently there are no postgraduate diplomas or master's degree nursing programs in South American countries.

Health-care research in South America is primarily carried out by medical doctors, with minimal participation by nurses. The overall number of nurses involved in research is very low. The reasons for this are many, including: inadequate training at an undergraduate level on the principles of clinical research; lack of time as many nurses hold two or three jobs because of low salaries; and the limited number of grants available for nursing research. However, some institutions have generated initiatives for nursing participation in research, including participation in presenting work guidelines, explaining patient informed consent, gathering information personally or by phone, entering statistical data for future analysis, and presenting and discussing results in quantitative and qualitative research.

Despite the emotional and interpersonal challenges that palliative care nursing staff face in providing care to patients near the end of life, there is currently no survey that has been designed specifically to evaluate the work environment that is provided to the staff.

Surveys of team attitudes and relationships need to be developed in areas such as: individual work rewards, teamwork, management support, organizational support, workload issues, and job satisfaction. There is substantial evidence to suggest that job satisfaction is related to the quality of care that patients receive.[46,47]

## Sociocultural, Religious, and Spiritual Issues Influencing Palliative Care

In spite of South America's cultural diversity, the predominant religion is Catholicism. Most people have a deep faith and the spiritual aspect of care is very important to terminally ill patients. A patient who realizes that he/she is dying may lean heavily on religion, as does the family. As a result, most patients prefer to spend their last days at home, surrounded by relatives. In addition, the presence of a spiritual assistant at the hour of death and confession to a Catholic priest may be very important at this time. In South American cultural groups, many patients think that illness is a punishment by God and that only God can grant salvation, relief, and healing.

Nurses have a difficult but humanistic role to carry out in accordance with Catholic principles. They are usually the first and the last contact when the patient consults at a health institution, and they frequently hear and are exposed to family problems, worries, anxieties, emotions, and grief. Nurses recognize the need for palliative care training to learn how to respond appropriately to the patient's religious and spiritual needs. Some people in rural areas adopt a stoic attitude in the face of painful experiences. In villages far away from large cities there is also a strong influence of folk medicine, quackery, healers, and popular herbal alternative treatments not prescribed or sanctioned by medical doctors. These beliefs and practices may hinder a dying person from seeking and or accepting medical treatments for the effective relief of pain and other symptoms.

In South America's multicultural environment, the lower social status of most patients in relation to doctors makes it difficult for them to communicate their fears, needs, and queries. As a result, it is almost impossible for them to understand the implications of treatment. In most settings, nurses act in an advocacy-and-treatment translator role. Direct and honest communication between patients and doctors is rare. Constraints on the doctor's time make meaningful explanations difficult. In addition, the relatives may see the doctor first and tell the doctor not to tell the patient about a diagnosis and prognosis. A "siege of silence" isolates the patient early on, denying him/her the opportunity to attend to "unfinished business," and imprisons the person in a lonely world of silence and secrecy. The traditional strong family support network in South America is currently under threat.

It still exists, but the culture is changing. More women go out to work as opposed to working at home, and more families are becoming isolated from the larger family unit. The move away from the village to the cities continues as people search for work. There are reports of patients with advanced cancer being abandoned by their families because financial resources are so drained or because family members cannot cope with their own terrible suffering and feeling of impotence at the sight of someone they love in uncontrollable pain. In the community, numerous voluntary groups and religious communities have developed networks to help in the care of patients at home or in hospital through visiting regularly and providing food, medicines, and/or money.

Sometimes families are not involved in the care of their terminally ill relatives because patients are frequently sent to hospitals far away from their homes. This also means that family doctors are infrequently involved in this type of care. The main responsibility for end-of-life care therefore lies in the hands of the hospital doctors and nurses. Although these doctors and nurses are improving their knowledge and skills in palliative care, the challenges remain great. Most patients and families do not participate in the decision-making process.

However, when the hospital the patient is admitted to is near to the patient's home, in keeping with the family structure and South American traditions, a relative is required to stay at the health center when the patient is admitted. The relatives are involved in a training program for inpatient care during this period. The training given is as follows: importance of cleanliness and patient hygiene and comfort; wound care and dressings; how to feed the patient; pain treatment including the use of morphine and other medications as well as the patient's medication timetable at home. In addition, the family is expected to keep the patient entertained, occupied, and supported. The team staff are acutely aware of the patient's needs and transmit this to the family.

Traditionally in South American countries people died at home, but the situation is changing. Because most of the patients who come to a palliative care service arrive from the rural areas of the country or from surrounding towns, they prefer to stay in the hospital. Acute care beds are used for palliative care, where some patients feel safer because of staff presence. They have added spiritual and psychological support from the palliative care team. Most of these patients do not have a home care service to ensure that they will be cared for properly in their homes.

There are regional differences in availability of home support. In some South American countries, palliative care can be provided in the home through national, provincial, and municipal programs. But providing community-based palliative care programs for the whole population remains a challenge for most countries. Although many patients would prefer to die at home, there are multiple reasons to explain why the majority now die in hospitals.[48] These include: lack of socioeconomic resources, low educational level, fears harbored by relatives about the development of the disease and end of life, past bad experiences with a death, lack of relatives, and difficulty in symptom control. Educational family programs are important helping families become aware of their importance and role in the care of a dying patient at home. Minimizing patient and caregiver distress is a central principle of palliative care delivery. Being the caregiver of someone dying at home without adequate support can be a confronting and daunting experience. Feelings of isolation and overwhelming responsibility can be compounded when health-care providers are not accessible, particularly after-hours. Unfortunately, access to this level of service is variable and particularly limited in rural and remote communities.

Although often not a reality in the region, 24-hour access for patients and families receiving palliative care is accepted as a gold standard for palliative care service delivery, particularly in regional and rural settings. In this way, palliative care teams keep in touch with relatives by phone to offer help in case of unexpected home events. The role of telephone support for patients and their caregivers after-hours, especially at the end of life provides information and reassurance not only in alleviating distress of patients and caregivers but also in avoiding hospitalization and emergency department presentations.[49–51] The availability and accessibility of comprehensive and coordinated home care services is critical in making death at home a rewarding and realistic option.

Inpatient hospices are not yet the chosen place to die for most patients. Two reasons contributing to this are the lack of such hospices and the stigma and fear sometimes associated with this type of institution in South American.

The disproportionate suffering of the South America's poor from cancer, AIDS, and other advanced life-threatening illnesses has generated efforts to promote palliative care as a more achievable and affordable alternative to expensive disease-modifying therapies. These well-intentioned efforts stem from a wish to respond to the suffering of the poor as quickly and widely as possible, and from the view that only inexpensive interventions are feasible in poor settings. Although palliative interventions to relieve the disproportionate physical, psychological, and social suffering of the poor are essential, they should be integrated with preventive and disease-modifying interventions. By calling attention to the injustice of massive and unnecessary poverty-related suffering and death, and by calling for an effective response, proponents of palliative care are promoting social justice too.[52,53] If palliative care is truly "just," it must respond to suffering with whatever it takes to relieve it, within the limits of what is available, but without losing sight of and advocating actively for what is possible.[54]

## Ethical Issues Influencing End-of-Life Care

Because of cultural barriers existing in South American countries, most doctors have difficulty in communicating with patients regarding their cancer disease diagnosis and terminal prognosis. The doctor usually informs the family, but the relatives often want to protect the patient from knowing the truth resulting in a "siege of silence." The patient progressively loses his/her autonomy, and the family makes decisions without the patient's explicit consent. Freedom of choice is compromised for patients because of:

- A patriarchal, protective presence of family members in medical decision-making
- A paternalistic attitude toward patient care by the physicians
- The strong influence exerted by the Catholic church on public debate
- A lack of communication skills among health-care professionals.

In recent years, increasing attention has been given to patient self-determination and autonomy, especially in decisions surrounding the end of life. The challenge of addressing public and professional attitudes to truth-telling within a multicultural society is experienced by some countries. "Truth telling with compassion," with the patients determining how much they wish to know and who should have access to their information, is the goal of communication. Ideally, making decisions regarding end of life care includes discussions about the use of hydration, antibiotics, and artificial feeding, as well as the potential use of cardiopulmonary resuscitation. Palliative care has initiated a change from the long-established practice of not telling a patient his or her diagnosis, to one that respects the patient's right to know and facilitates open communication. The concept of patient autonomy is just starting to emerge in some South American countries.

In large cities, one of the problems confronting palliative care teams is the high expectations of both professionals and the public regarding the preservation of life at all costs. This is most prominent when the dying person is in the intensive care unit (ICU). Some patients with advanced cancer are die alone in ICUs, wired up to machines without a nurse in constant attendance. Outside the ward, the patient's family may be denied access to the bedside, and wait in the waiting room for the inevitable to happen. Both family and patient therefore suffer the final stage of separation alone, at a time when they most need to be united.

In South America countries, discussions about resuscitation or the benefit-versus-burden of admitting a dying patient to an ICU if chances for improvement are held infrequently. Most patients and families have difficulty addressing these issues, and few palliative care teams approach them. The use of living wills and other advance directives are still uncommon, and do not carry much legal weight. Some palliative care teams, however, appear to be making inroads in addressing these issues.

Communicating diagnosis and prognosis to the patient and recognition of the ethical responsibility of obtaining informed consent from the patient regarding treatment and other important decisions is occurring more frequently and with less discomfort for some palliative care teams. The need for ongoing discussion of ethical issues and for continuing education in palliative care and ethical dilemmas is esential for physicians in training and nurses who provide end-of-life care. Some nurses express feelings of guilt when they asked by a doctor to sedate a patient feeling that they are being asked to practice euthanasia by following the medical orders.

Overall, in South American countries, there is a growing consensus that end-of-life issues must be debated more fully, including the country's position and laws regarding euthanasia and physician-assisted suicide.

Ethicals issues need to be handled sensitively in palliative care settings, within the framework of the traditions and culture of the society. Ethics committees if available can be very helpful in thinking through these ethical concerns.[55]

The relief of suffering of the sick is a medical and moral imperative. Palliative care pursues its goal through relief of pain and other distressing symptoms and psychosocial support for patients and their families. The importance of these tasks has prompted assertions that palliative care is a fundamental human right. Yet, palliative care, like HIV/AIDS and cancer treatment, is unavailable to most in the developing South America countries.[56]

There have been several requests and publications calling for palliative care and pain treatment to be recognized as human rights but not an international declaration joining palliative care, pain, cancer, AIDS and other related organizations for this same purpose. The International Association for Hospice and Palliative Care (IAHPC) and the Worldwide Palliative Care Alliance (WPCA) joined efforts and worked together to develop a "Joint Declaration and Statement of Commitment," which unites all organizations working in this field in the Declaration: "Palliative Care and Pain Treatment as Human Rights."[57]

A summary of the strengths, weaknesses and challenges for palliative care in South American countries can be found in Appendix 74–1.

### The Nurse's Role in the Palliative Care Team in South American Countries—What is Needed

- Achieve standards of training in palliative care and relief of pain for all nursing levels.
- Include palliative care in schools' and universities' nursing curriculum.
- Create awareness of the nurse's role in the interdisciplinary palliative care team and as agent of change in the society.
- Increase the nurse's participation in clinical updates and research with colleagues and other members of the team.

### Sociocultural, Religious, and Spiritual Issues

- Adapt international models to the South American multicultural/sociopolitical environment, reality, and resources, and define each country's own palliative care model.
- Respect cultural values in different ethnic groups and be aware of the need for cross-cultural palliative care

teams appropriated for aboriginal culture of South America.
- Establish volunteers and social networks to provide resources.
- Make communities aware of their rights to increase requests for palliative care's efficient services.
- Develop palliative care in all places with own resources, even in poor countries and among marginalized communities.
- Emphasize the important role of the family in providing care in places with few palliative care human resources.

### Ethical Issues Influencing End-of-Life Care

- Provide widespread information to the population about end-of-life decision-making in relation to incurable diseases.
- Ensure greater participation of palliative care professionals in the discussion about euthanasia.
- Collaborate with authorities and legislators to advance knowledge about palliative care's objectives and scopes to guarantee the right to die with dignity.
- Ensure that health professionals within institutions provide ethical and quality palliative care for dying patients.
- Empower the public to demand respect for human rights and ethical basic principles from health professionals, including autonomy, beneficence, nonmaleficence, and justice.

### Summary

Palliative care as a medical and nursing discipline began to grow throughout South America in the mid-1980s thanks to the pioneer initiatives of multiprofessional health teams, working with a holistic approach to promote the care of dying people. These first initiatives were supported by the enthusiasm of their leaders and were able to prosper with few available resources, both inside and outside of the hospital setting. At that time, institutional recognition was either partial or nonexistent. The teams were small and the job was hard; however, they have grown a lot and been an instrument of change in improving citizens' quality of life. Many difficulties still remain, and the need to provide skilled and compassionate care for seriously ill and dying patients is now being recognized as a major challenge in most South American countries.

In recent years, WHO has proposed providing more palliative care at the time of diagnosis for patients in developing countries. The reasoning behind this was that by the time many patients get to their doctor, it is either too late in the course of their disease for curative therapy, or the country/institution is unable to offer curative therapy, or the patient is unable to access curative options for economic or other reasons. Consequently, the need for palliative care is recognizes as being huge. Allocation of health-care resources in developing countries should reflect this situation and health-care resources should be balanced accordingly. The developing countries need technological and financial support to develop palliative care programs that cover the patients with advanced and progressive disease and family needs. International and nongovernmental organizations play an important role in this process continue to offer assistance. The WHO and PAHO have been important to the continued growth and development of new programs and in the consolidation of the existing ones.

In South America, there is evidence of growth in palliative care initiatives to improve availability of opioid analgesics for the treatment of cancer pain, as well as more educational opportunities for physicians, nurses, social workers, psychologists, and community level volunteers.

There is still a great need to develop national health policies that promote and implement palliative care. The social and economic crises of South American countries is an opportunity to encourage these programs which can have such a significant medical and social impact. These programs have been demonstrated to be cost-effective. Today, the majority of people in South American cities die in hospitals, and care must be provided in this setting. But it is also important not forget the Latin American tradition that identifies relatives as the main caregivers. This means active participation of families in care, even in the hospitals. In providing palliative care, it is essential to recognize the diverse needs of a multicultural society.

The aim of palliative care has been a model of care based on the concept of an interdisciplinary, multiprofessional team including nurses, physicians, social workers, psychologists, religious care providers, pharmacists, physio/occupational therapists, and volunteers. In South American countries, palliative care strongly highlights the nurses' role, and their importance as a members of the team. However, the role of doctors has been traditionally hierarchical, with a paternalistic relationship to other team members. Such attitudinal tradition can be slow to change but change is occuring in South American countries.

South American nurses remain in the front line fighting against the difficulties in providing palliative care for those in need.

## REFERENCES

1. United Nations. Population and Vital Statistics Report. Available at: http://unstats.un.org/unsd/seriesa/introduction.asp (accessed January 2009).
2. Pan American Health Organization. Health in the Americas, Vol I & II. Scientific and Technical Publication. Washington, DC: PAHO, 2007.
3. World Health Organization. Cancer Control. Knowledge into Action. WHO Guide for Effective Programmes. Palliative Care, Module 5. WHO 2007; Geneva. Available at: http://www.who.int/cancer/modules (accessed January 2009).
4. Stjernswärd J, Foley K, Ferris F. The public health strategy for palliative care. J Pain Symptom Manage 2007;33(5):486–493.
5. Gilks CF, Crowley S, Ekpini R, et al. The WHO public-health approach to antiretroviral treatment against HIV in resource-limited settings. Lancet 2006;368:505–510.
6. Defilippi KM, Cameron S. Promoting the integration of quality palliative care—the South African mentorship program. J Pain Symptom Manage 2007;33(5):552–557.
7. Clark D, Wright M, Hunt J, Lynch T. Hospice and palliative care development in Africa: A multi-method review of services and experiences. J Pain Symptom Manage 2007;33(5):698–710.
8. Stjernswärd J, Foley K, Ferris F. Integrating palliative care into national policies. J Pain Symptom Manage 2007;33(5):514–520.
9. Graham F, Clark D. The changing model of palliative care. Medicine 2008;36(2):64–66.
10. Foley KM, Wagner JL, Joranson DE, Gelband H. Pain control for people with cancer and AIDS. In: Jamison DT, Breman JG, Measham AR, et al., eds. Disease control Priorities in Developing Countries (2nd ed). New York, NY: Oxford University Press; 2006:981–994.
11. Wiffen PJ, Mc Quay HJ. Oral morphine for cancer pain. Cochrane Review. In The Cochrane Library Plus, Issue 3, 2008.
12. Joranson D, Ryan K. Ensuring opioid availability: Methods and resources. J Pain Symptom Manage 2007;33(5):527–532.
13. Pain and Policy Studies Group. Global, regional, and national consumption statistics for 2006. Madison, WI: PPSG; 2008. Available at: http://www.painpolicy.wisc.edu/news/international.htm (accessed January 2009).
14. WHO Model List of Essential Medicines (15th ed). Geneva, WHO 2007. Available at: http://www.who.int/medicines/services/essmedicines_def/en/index.html (accessed January 2009).
15. De Lima L, Krakauer E, Lorenz K, Praill D, Mac Donald N, Doyle D. Ensuring palliative medicine availability: The development of the IAHPC list of essential medicines for palliative care. J Pain Symptom Manage 2007;33(5):521–526.
16. Wenk R, Bertolino M. Palliative care development in South America: A focus on Argentina. J Pain Symptom Manage 2007;33(5):645–650.
17. Bugge E, Higginson I. Palliative care and the need for eduaction. Do we know what makes a difference? A limited systematic review. Health Educ J 2006;65(2):101–125.
18. Fellowes D, Wilkinson S, Moore P. Communication skills training for health-care professionals working with cancer patients, their families and/or carers. Cochrane Review. In: The Cochrane Library, Issue 4, 2008.
19. Torres Vigil I, Aday LA, De Lima L, Cleeland CHS. What predicts the quality of advanced cancer care in Latin America? A look at five countries: Argentina, Brazil, Cuba, Mexico, and Peru. J Pain Symptom Manage 2007;34(3):315–327.
20. Wenk R. The development of palliative medicine in Latin America. In: Bruera E, Higginson I, Ripamonti C, Von Gunten Ch., eds. Textbook of Palliative Medicine. Great Britain: Hodder Arnold; 2006:37–41.
21. De Lima L. Palliative care in Latin America. Medicina Paliativa 2006;13(1):1–3.

22. Clemens KE, Kumar S, Bruera E, et al. Palliative care in developing countries: What are the important issues? Palliat Med 2007;21:173–175.

23. The International Observatory on End of Life Care (IOELC). Institute for Health Research, Lancaster University, Lancaster, United Kingdom. Available at: http://www.eolc-observatory.net/global_analysis/regions_main.htm (accessed January 2009).

24. Clark D, Wright M. The international observatory on end of life care: A global view of palliative care development. J Pain Symptom Manage 2007;33(5):542–546.

25. Wright M, Wood J, Lynch T, Clark D. Study mapping levels of palliative care development: A global view. J Pain Symptom Manage 2008;35(5):469–485.

26. Ferrell B, Connor S, Cordes A, et al. The National Consensus Project for Quality Palliative Care Task Force Members. The National Agenda for Quality Palliative Care: The National Consensus Project and the National Quality Forum. J Pain Symptom Manage 2007;33(6):737–744.

27. National Consensus Project. Available at: http://www. nationalconsensusproject.org (accessed January 2009).

28. National Quality Forum. Available at: http://www.qualityforum.org (accessed January 2009).

29. Center to Advance Palliative Care. Available at: http://www.capc.org (accessed January 2009).

30. Higginson I, Hart S, Koffman J, Selman L, Harding R. Needs assessments in palliative care: An appraisal of definitions and approaches used. J Pain Symptom Manage 2007;33(5):500–505.

31. Doyle D, Woodruff R. The IAHPC Manual of Palliative Care (2nd ed). Published by IAHPC Press, 2008. Available at: http://www.hospicecare.com/iahpc-manual/IAHPCmanual.htm (accessed January 2009).

32. Dudgeon D, Knott Ch, Eichholz M, et al. Palliative Care Integration Project (PCIP) quality improvement strategy evaluation. J Pain Symptom Manage 2008;35(6):573–582.

33. Ferris F, Gómez-Batiste X, Furst C, Connor S. Implementing quality palliative care. J Pain Symptom Manage 2007;33(5):533–541.

34. Eisenchlas J, Harding R, Daud M, Perez M, De Simone G, Higginson I. Use of the Palliative Outcome Scale in Argentina: A cross-cultural adaptation and validation study. J Pain Symptom Manage 2008;35(2):188–202.

35. Bakitas MA, Lyons KD, Dixon J, Ahles TA. Palliative care program effectiveness research: Developing rigor in sampling design, conduct, and reporting. J Pain Symptom Manage 2006;31:270–284.

36. Declaration of Venice. Available at: http://www.hospicecare.com/dv (accessed January 2009) or http://www.eapcnet.org/latestnews/VeniceDeclaration.html (accessed January 2009).

37. Adoption of a declaration to develop a global palliative care research initiative. Prog Palliat Care 2006;14(5):215–217.

38. Kaasa S, Jensen M, Loge H. A 25 year perspective on the development of palliative care research in Europe. Venice, Italy, May 25–27, 2006. Palliat Med 2006;20(3):231.

39. Harding R, Powell R, Downing J, et al. Generating an African palliative care evidence base: The context, need, challenges, and strategies. J Pain Symptom Manage 2008; 36(3):304–309.

40. Webster R, Lacey J, Quine S. Palliative care: A public health priority in developing countries. J Pub Health Policy 2007;28(1):28–39.

41. Callaway M, Foley K, De Lima L, et al. Funding for palliative care programs in developing countries. J Pain Symptom Manage 2007;33(5):509–513.

42. Kumar S. Kerala, India: A regional community based Palliative Care Model. J Pain Symptom Manage 2007;33(5):623–627.

43. Zhang CH, Hsu L, Zou BR, Zhu XP. A survey of pain management in clinical nurses. Chinese J Nurs Sci 2006;21(10):6–9.

44. Zhang CH, Hsu L, Zou BR, et al. Effects of a pain education program on nurses' pain knowledge, attitudes and pain assessment practices in China. J Pain Symptom Manage 2008;36(6):616–627.

45. Latin American Association of Palliative Care. Nursing Curriculo for a Palliative Care Posgrade Program. Published by IAHPC Press, 2008. Available at: http://cuidadospaliativos.org/archives/curriculo-de-enfermería-alcp.pdf (accessed January 2009).

46. Qaseem B, Shea J, Connor S, Casarett D. How well are we supporting hospice staff? Initial results of the survey of team attitudes and relationships (STAR) Validation Study. J Pain Symptom Manage 2007;(4):350–358.

47. Castle NG. An instrument to measure job satisfaction of nursing home administrators. BMC Med Res Methodol 2006;6:47–58.

48. Beccaro M, Costantini M, Rossi PG, et al. Actual and preferred place of death of cancer patients. Results from the Italian Survey of the Dying Of Cancer (ISDOC). J Epidemiol Commun Health 2006;60:412–416.

49. 49.. Phillips J, Davidson P, Newton P, Di Giacomo M. Supporting patients and their caregivers after-hours at the end of life: The role of telephone support. J Pain Symptom Manage 2008;36(1):11–21.

50. Worth A, Boyd K, Kendall M, et al. Out-of-hours palliative care: A qualitative study of cancer patients, caregivers and professionals. Br J Gen Pract 2006;56(522):6–13.

51. Kerr C, Hawker S, Payne S, Lloyd-Williams M, Seamark D. Out-of-hours medical cover in community hospitals: Implications for palliative care. Int J Palliat Nurs 2006;12(2):75–80.

52. Krakauer E. Just palliative care: Responding responsibly to the suffering of the poor. J Pain Symptom Manage 2008;36(5):505–512.

53. Harding R. Palliative care in resource-poor settings: Fallacies and misapprehensions. J Pain Symptom Manage 2008;36(5):515–517.

54. Selwyn P. Palliative care and social justice. J Pain Symptom Manage 2008;36(5):513–515.

55. Chaturvedi SK. Ethical dilemmas in palliative care in traditional developing societies, with special reference to the indian setting. J Med Ethics 2008;34:611–615.

56. Brennan F. Palliative care as an international human right. J Pain Symptom Manage 2007;33:494–499.

57. International Association Hospice and Palliative Care and Worldwide Palliative Care Alliance. Palliative Care and Pain Treatment as Human Rights. IAHPC and WPCA, 2007. Available at: http://www.hospicecare.com/resources/pain_pallcare_hr (accessed January 2009).

APPENDIX 74-1
## Palliative Care in South America: Strengths, Weaknesses, and Challenges

### Strengths

*Government Policy:*
- Some countries beginning to develop of palliative care national or regional programs and policies.
- Integration of the different health professions and scientific societies creating government approved organization, rules, and standards,

*Availability of and Access to Opioid Analgesics:*
- Availability of analgesic opioids but still limited access for the whole population.
- Opioid consumption increased over the last few years.

*Education:*
- Some educational activities for health professionals before and after graduation although still not systematic training.
- Some palliative care training opportunities for professionals together with experienced palliative care teams locally and abroad.
- Nongovernmental organizations' support of palliative care advanced-education programs.
- Human resources of healthcare with specific training in palliative care beginning to be available.

*The Palliative Care Team:*
- An increase in palliative care teams with active assistance programs for adults and children, most of them in public hospitals.
- Support of the initiatives and programs by international organizations, with the agreement of leaders.
- Exchange of experiences and resources with other regional groups or countries.
- Possibility to work in an interdisciplinary way in some cities and regions.
- An increasing use of rules and symptom-control protocols and standards.
- Associations of palliative care that coordinate scientific activities in most South American countries.

*The Nurse's Role in the Palliative Care Team:*
- Historical hierarchical position of the nurse in the interdisciplinary palliative care team.
- More closeness to the patient than most health professionals.
- Sensitivity to family's needs and feelings.
- Ability to communicate with people of different social and cultural status.
- Ability to creatively adapt to lack of resources.

*Sociocultural, Religious, and Spiritual Issues:*
- Beginning change in attitudes relating to palliative care in people and professionals: "cure" attitude vs. "care" approach.
- Family inclusion in care of the patient at home and in the hospital setting.
- Increased family, friends', or neighbors' role in providing care to ease the process of adaptation.
- Patient's and families' satisfaction with the palliative care team's assistance at home.
- Volunteers and social community networks for providing resources locally.
- Acceptance and approval of palliative care by different religions, with official recognition, especially by the Catholic church.

*Ethical Issues Influencing End-of-Life Care:*
- More hospital ethics committees collaborating with palliative care teams regarding the difficulties in end-of-life decision-making.

### Weaknesses

*Government Policy:*
- Lack of recognition of palliative care needs in the national and regional health programs.
- Difficulties in all the health sectors: public, private, and social-security, with insufficient fulfillment of palliative care requests.
- Lack of institutional financial support because palliative care programs are not a priority.
- Failure to uphold the WHO recommendations in practice regarding cancer relief and palliative care.

*Availability of and Access to Opioid Analgesics:*
- Lack of suitable legislation; state bureaucracy; passivity and inequality regarding the Prescription, availability and allocation of opioids.
- Excessive cost, inefficiency in the management and administration of analgesic drug supplies.
- Prevalent popular and professionals' negative attitudes regarding morphine prescriptions, and myths and fears about addiction.
- Economic difficulties of the poor population to pay for medications and other treatments, and lack of government analgesic provision.

*Education:*
- Absence of informative and educative programs about palliative care benefits for the community.
- No systematic training activities for the health professionals before and after graduation.
- Little and expensive palliative care advance education.
- No master, specialized degree, or diploma levels in palliative care education.
- Misconceptions about the use of morphine and other strong opioids by health professionals.

- Difficulty accessing palliative care education for health professionals in rural areas.
- Lack of professional training about how to listen and how to communicate bad news.
- Limited academic connection among palliative care professionals.

### The Palliative Care Team:

- Absence of palliative care standards, professional certification, and systematic service accreditation.
- Lack of an operational network of palliative care providers among different cities, regions, and countries.
- Unequal interprofessional communication.
- Lack of professionals trained in palliative care.
- Insufficient financial support of palliative care teams.
- Low salaries, and sometimes none, for palliative care professionals.
- Difficulties in guaranteeing volunteer work and charitable funding.
- Few researcher opportunities because of a low priority given to research in the culture, and a lack of time, and rigor in scientific methodology, resources, and industry support.

### The Nurse's Role in the Palliative Care Team:

- Medical community unaware of the importance of the nurse's role in the interdisciplinary palliative care team and as agent of change in the society.
- Widespread acceptance in the medical community of the paternalistic attitude of the physicians.
- Palliative care training needs not considered essential in order to achieve safe practices.
- Many dying patients, and yet few nurses with training in palliative care.
- Low nurse status in relation to other health professionals.
- Lack of participation in clinical updates and research with colleagues and other members of the team.

### Sociocultural, Religious, and Spiritual Issues:

- High level of distressing, unbearable pain and low expectations of relief in cancer patients.
- Difficulty of communication between rural population and palliative care centers in big cities because of large distances.
- Barriers to access of palliative care teams because of economic problems in poor populations.
- Family feelings of isolation, distress and overwhelming responsibility in taking care of the patient at home.
- Rural population's beliefs about traditional folkloric medicine with traditional alternative therapies in symptom control used more frequently than Western medicine.

- Religious and family obstacles about end-of-life decision-making.
- Difficulties in addressing the spiritual suffering associated with chronic, advanced, and progressive disease by health professionals.

### Ethical Issues Influencing End-of-Life Care:

- Difficulties in end-of-life decision-making: terminal sedation vs. euthanasia; truth telling and communicating bad news; "siege of silence"; diagnosis and prognosis disclosure.
- Inequality in the distribution of health resources.
- Indiscriminate use of health-care high technology and medical futility in the end-of-life ICUs in many hospitals.
- Failure to address or resolve issues surrounding death and dying.
- Lack of palliative care quality-of-life standards.

## Challenges for Palliative Care in South America

### Government Policy:

- Integrate palliative care programs into national, provincial, municipal, and regionals health systems.
- Implement palliative care teams, services, or designated beds in all countries according to individual needs.
- Establish rules, standards, handbooks, and team directories, by professional team leaders, according to international guidelines, with regional and cultural adaptations.
- Ensure governmental and nongovernmental institutions work together to identify communities' palliative care needs and, by integrating resources, determine the most effective care delivery.
- Improve distribution and access of health resources.
- Detect and resolve obstacles blocking implementation of palliative care programs.
- Develop regional strategies and communication among South American countries, and request for international founding and support.

### Availability of and Access to Opioid Analgesics:

- Develop a list of essential palliative care medicines as a national formulary to be included in the medicine policy.
- Include universal availability and allocation of recommended opioid analgesic and other essential palliative care drugs with free access for the whole population.
- Design laws that assure coverage of treatment for palliative care patients.
- Decrease the cost of opioids.

*Education:*
- Distribute information about palliative care throughout the population.
- Identify attitudes and myths regarding morphine prescription and myths and address through public education.
- Assure systematic palliative care training activities for health professionals both before and after graduation, with inclusion in the curriculum.
- Provide masters, specialized degree, and diploma levels in palliative care professionals' education.
- Provide exchange of professionals with training in palliative care for education programs in developing countries.

*The Palliative Care Team:*
- Develop communication between government and health institutions' administrators to implement and consolidate palliative care programs, using community resources.

- Design own palliative care standards, professional certification, and systematic services accreditation.
- Include palliative care in the early stages of disease[21] to improve care management and to provide complementary services with other medical specialities.[22]
- Eliminate interprofessional communication barriers in the team.
- Include psychotherapists with training in palliative care team support to decrease staff burn-out.
- Develop a supportive group that includes volunteers.
- Create an operational network of palliative care providers among different cities, regions, and countries.
- Design and develop research strategies and increase opportunities for researchers of different teams to work together.
- Create palliative care associations throughout South America.
- Organize multidisciplinary committees of special interest groups.

# 75

*Faith N. Mwangi-Powell, Henry Ddungu, Julia Downing,*
*Fatia Kiyange, Richard A. Powell, and Abby Baguma*

# Palliative Care in Africa

*My mother spent the last days of her life in terrible pain, treated only with panadol. We reached*
*a point where we all wished she would die rather than continue in her pain.—25-year-old*
*Kenyan male*

◆ ***Key Points***

◆ *Palliative care in Africa originated over 25 years ago. Today,*
*provision of palliative care on the continent is inconsistent,*
*often provided from isolated centers of excellence rather than*
*integrated into the mainstream health-care system.*

◆ *The primary mode of palliative care service delivery is home-*
*based care. Predominantly dependent upon volunteers, this*
*has implications for staff recruitment and retention, and the*
*maintenance of an acceptable standard of patient care.*

◆ *Pain in Africa is disturbingly under-treated among adults*
*and children, with opioid analgesic consumption remaining*
*extremely low in relation to medical need. There is an emerging*
*trend to alter existing legal provisions to enable other specially*
*trained cadres (e.g., nurses) to prescribe opioids for patients in*
*moderate-to-severe pain.*

◆ *Whilst some governments are adopting Basic Care Packages*
*(BCP), comprised of interventions that address the major causes*
*of a country's disease burden, in most African countries, BCP*
*excludes palliative care, as it is equally absent from the vast*
*majority of national health policies.*

◆ *Nurses have a pivotal role in palliative care provision on the*
*continent given they are present at all levels of the health-care*
*system, from the facility to the community.*

◆ *Traditionally children have been relatively neglected by palliative*
*care service development on the continent.*

The second largest continent, stretching across five time
zones, Africa covers an area of 30.2 million square kilometers (11.7 million square miles), including its adjacent islands,
approximately 20% of the global land area. Its estimated 967
million inhabitants, amounting to 14.4% of the world's total
population,[1] are distributed across five regions and 53 independent nations: Eastern Africa (17 nations); Central Africa
(9); Northern Africa (6); Southern Africa (5); Western Africa
(16) (Figure 75–1).

In general terms, the vast expanse of the Sahara desert
acts as a natural geographic separator between the predominantly Arabic coastal north and the African south. However,
there is a rich heterogeneity of ethnic groups (including non-
African ones) that currently populate the continent. This
extensive diversity is partly revealed by the estimated 1,000
to 2,000 indigenous languages, based around four major linguistic families: the Afro-Asiatic languages; Nilo-Saharan
languages; the Niger-Congo languages; and the click conso-
nants-based Khoisan languages. Post-colonial governmental
attempts to forge national unity from such linguistic variation have meant that, in many countries, English and French
are used for official public discourse.

## Political and Socioeconomic Situation

Following increasing commercial and missionary interest in
the "Dark Continent" among mid-19th century explorers, a territorial "scramble for Africa" occurred in the late 19th century
among European powers. With the exception of Liberia and
Ethiopia, between 1880 and 1912 colonial nation states were
established across the continent. For many nations, this
caused artificial delineation of national boundaries, exerting
a socially destabilizing effect. In those countries with numerically significant colonizing populations, however, the effects

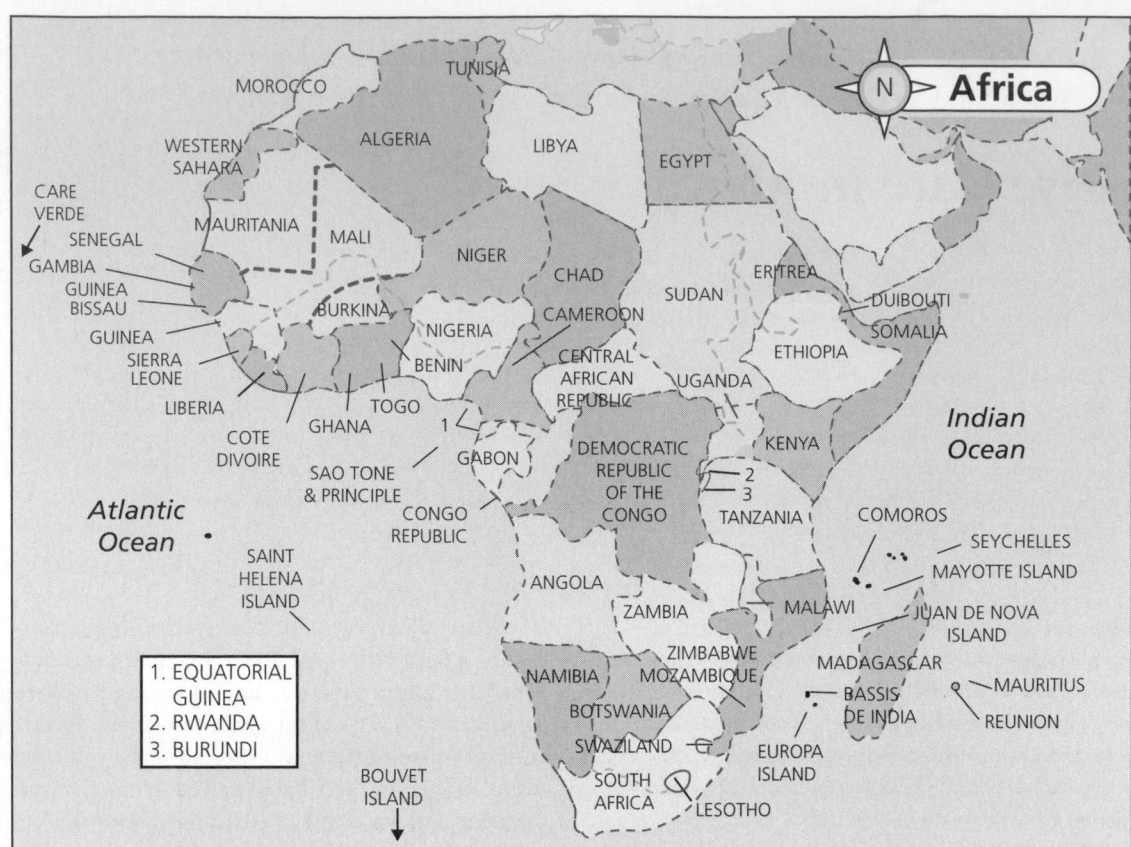

**Figure 75–1.** Countries of Africa. *Source*: http://www.infoplease.com/atlas/africa.html. Copyright MAGELLAN Geographix.

of the "scramble" were more significant: systems were established that ensured disproportionate political influence to Europeans over indigenous Africans.

Confronted by rising nationalism, in the 1950s and 1960s European powers granted independence to most territories. In the post-colonial 1970s and 1980s, however, many African states were characterized by episodes of sociopolitical instability, corruption, violence, and authoritarian rule. African nations failed to deliver democratic regimes underpinned by principles of good governance. In the late 1980s and early 1990s, some states attempted to initiate democratic reforms. However, this ongoing democratic transition has proven problematic, and the political and social narrative continues to stereotype the continent. Political instability and civil strife have continued to stain some countries; for example, nearly 1 million people were killed in the Rwandan genocide of 1994.

Economically, despite extensive natural resources (e.g., oil, gold, diamonds), Africa remains an overwhelmingly underdeveloped continent, with the vast majority of its predominantly rural population engaged in cash crop production. Indeed, the bottom 27 ranked countries (from 151st to 177th) reported in the 2007 *United Nations' Human Development Report* were all African.[2]

## Health Systems in Africa

Following independence, many African countries sought to address the social inequities of colonization. As such, improving people's well-being by overcoming the discriminatory restrictions that had underpinned colonial social policy and advancing social development were prioritised.[3] Consequently, up to the end of the 1970s many African health systems, as well as the education sectors, expanded as a result of centralized funding, with an increase in trained health professionals. Despite this expansion, inequitable access to health services persisted, as did unmet need for health services given various capacity limitations. Additionally, during this period there was recognition of the qualitative difference in service provision in urban and rural health settings, with the former receiving greater resources. As a result, the primary health-care system was introduced in many nations to address this health care imbalance, an agenda embodied in the Declaration of Alma-Ata in 1978.[4]

By the 1980s, economic crises across Africa resulted in inequities in health systems re-entering public discourse. In response, governmental austerity measures, and externally driven structural adjustment programs entailed commitments to cost recovery and user charges, as well as the introduction of marketization as the principle determining policy and practice. The diminution of the public sector, compounded by reductions in real income occasioned by repeated currency devaluations, meant that health cadre relocated from the public health sector to more financially rewarding employment, while reduced public funding resulted in deterioration of the physical infrastructure and equipment of public health facilities.

Today, and in general terms, there are three different types of health systems: the *public system,* which is based around specialist, regional, district and home-based care (HBC) providers, with services provided free to inpatients and outpatients; an *insurance-based system,* which is either based around individual, private contributions or around an employer-related health scheme; and the *private-sector system,* which is for a relatively small percentage of the population with sufficient financial resources.

In most African countries, however, health inequalities and differential service access continue to pose a considerable challenge, with impoverished households excluded from accessing affordable quality health-care services resorting to self-medicating (sometimes with fake medicines), home-based health-seeking behaviors as a consequence.[3] Health systems across the continent remain weak, with an estimated more than 20% of total health expenditure in 48% of the 46 countries in the WHO African Region provided by external sources.[5] This weakness in part arises from poverty; the overwhelming communicable and noncommunicable disease burden; inadequate institutional capacity (e.g., for cancer treatment); inefficient use of potential national expertise; weak coordination of health development partners; frequent and often inconsistent changes in government policies; inadequate legislation; weak accountability and lack of transparency; nonmaximization of international agreements and regulations; and a crisis in human health resources.

## The Historical Perspective and Current Status of Palliative Care

The disease burden in sub-Saharan Africa is significant. By 2008, an estimated 22 million people in the region were living with the human immunodeficiency virus/acquired immune deficiency syndrome (HIV/AIDS)—67% of the global disease burden—with 1.9 million new infections reported in that year alone.[6] Moreover, there were over 700,000 new cancer cases and nearly 600,000 cancer-related deaths in Africa in 2007,[7] whereas cancer rates on the continent are expected to grow by 400% over the next 50 years.[8] Furthermore, there is a growing concern that, as people's lifestyle, nutritional preferences, and non-sedentary work patterns on the continent change, Africa may experience an increase in the incidence of chronic, life-limiting diseases.[9]

The development of palliative care in Africa originated over 25 years ago, when Island Hospice was founded in Harare, Zimbabwe, in May 1979.[10] Many of its pioneer services were advanced by highly motivated, charismatic individuals with minimal financial resources. Today, however, provision of palliative care on the continent is, inconsistent, often provided from isolated centers of excellence rather than integrated into the mainstream health-care system. Indeed, for the overwhelming majority of Africans who currently endure progressive, life-limiting illnesses, access to culturally appropriate, holistic palliative care (that includes effective pain and symptom management) is at best limited, and at worst nonexistent.[11] Indeed, a survey of hospice and palliative care services on the continent found not only that 44.7% (21 of 47) of African countries had no identified hospice or palliative care activity but that only 8.5% (*n* = 4) could be classified as having services approaching some measure of integration with mainstream service providers.[12]

Despite the reported need among care providers, the evidence base that underpins much of current palliative care service provision on the continent is inadequate.[13] Indeed, although donor demands (primarily led by the President's Emergency Plan for AIDS Relief [PEPFAR]) for the proven impact of funded projects have impelled monitoring and evaluation onto the African palliative care agenda, palliative care research remains embryonic.[14]

However, there are positive palliative care developments occurring on the continent. For example, in November 2002, nearly 30 African palliative care trainers met in South Africa and produced the "Cape Town Declaration," which advanced that palliative care (and pain and symptom control) is the right of every adult and child with life-limiting illness, and as such should be incorporated into national health-care strategies, making it accessible and affordable for all in sub-Saharan Africa.[15]

The meeting also served as the impetus for the development in Arusha, Tanzania, in 2004, of the African Palliative Care Association (APCA), with a regional remit to promote palliative care for all in need on the continent. One of its leading achievements has been a series of subregional advocacy meetings oriented toward improving access to opioid pain management. In September 2007, APCA held its 2nd regional conference, attracting nearly 500 delegates from across the continent and beyond to discuss palliative care issues.

## The Public Health Approach to Palliative Care in Africa

Based on earlier guidance to national governments, the World Health Organization (WHO) recently revealed an enhanced model of palliative care provision. For the public heath approach—which is population and risk-factor oriented rather than symptom- or disease-oriented—to work, it must be founded upon appropriate government policies, adequate drug availability, the education of health professionals, implementation of palliative care at all levels (see Figure 75–2),[16] and be integrated into national health-care systems.[17]

## Government Policy

The adoption and promotion by government of appropriate health policies is the cornerstone of an effective health-care system. These include a national health policy, an essential medicines policy, and education policies.

## National Health Policy

The failure of the Declaration of Alma-Ata (1978), which formally adopted primary healthcare as *the* means for bringing comprehensive, universal, equitable, and affordable health-care services closer to people, and the Bamako Initiative (1987), among others, to improve access and quality of healthcare in Africa, was ultimately replaced by the **United Nations' Millennium Development Declaration** and its eight Millennium Development Goals (MDGs) to be realized by 2015: (1) eradicate extreme poverty and hunger; (2) achieve universal primary education; (3) promote gender equality and empower women; (4) reduce child mortality; (5) improve maternal health; (6) combat HIV/AIDS, malaria and other diseases; (7) ensure environmental sustainability; and (8) develop a global partnership for development. This declaration has been underpinned by a plethora of funding initiatives—not least being the Global Fund against AIDS, TB and Malaria, the U.S. President's Malaria Initiative, and PEPFAR—resulting in new rounds of national health policies

and strategic plans in the health sector or revision of existing ones.[18] To date, however, the region is struggling to meet the health-related MDGs.

Additionally, although some governments are adopting BCP, comprised of interventions that address the major causes of a country's disease burden and serve as the primary means of public fund allocation in the health sector, for the vast majority of African countries, BCP excludes palliative care, and it is equally absent from the vast majority of national health policies. Consequently, rather than being provided nationally, palliative care is primarily limited to nongovernmental organizations, faith- and community-based organizations, and hospices that are unable to reach all those in need. However, some of these organizations are excellent demonstration sites for national palliative care scale-up.

## Essential Medicines Policy

African governments are urged by the WHO to institute a policy on essential medicines for adults and children that includes palliative care medicines (including opioids, such as oral morphine, for effective pain management as part of the WHO analgesic ladder) and is supported by a policy on their importation to ensure that all can access medications that are affordable and effective.

In most parts of Africa, however, current legislation restricts the prescribing of opioids to doctors. Given the poor physician:patient ratios in most African health systems, and the predominantly non-facility-based care received by rural populations, there is an emerging trend to alter existing legal provisions to enable other specially trained cadres

Policy
- Palliative care part of national health plan, policies, related regulations
- Funding/service delivery models support palliative care delivery
- Essential medicines
(Policy makers, regulators, WHO, NGOs)

Drug Availability
- Opioids, essential medicines
- Importation quota
- Cost
- Prescribing
- Distribution
- Dispensing
- Administration

(Pharmacists, drug regulators, law enforcement agents)

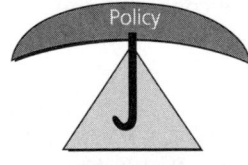

Policy

Implementation
- Opinion leaders
- Trained manpower
- Strategic & business plans – resources, infrastructure
- Standards, guidelines measures

(Community & clinical leaders, administrators)

Education
- Media & public advocacy
- Curricula, courses – professionals, trainees
- Expert training
- Family caregiver training & support

(Media & public, healthcare providers & trainees, palliative care experts, family caregivers)

**Figure 75–2.** Enhanced WHO public health model. *Source*: Reprinted with permission from Journal of Pain and Symptom Management, Sternsward J, Foley K, Ferris F. The public health strategy for palliative care,[33] 486–493, 2007, with permission from Elsevier.

(e.g., nurses) to prescribe opioids for patients in moderate-to-severe pain.

## Education Policies

In 2004, the WHO recommended that governments develop policies that include palliative care in training curricula for health workers at all levels, equipping them with the discipline's knowledge and core competencies. Currently, however, integration of palliative care into the institutes of higher learning is not widespread in Africa but APCA is currently (2009) working in Botswana and Kenya to support its integration into the core curricula of nurses and doctors.

## Drug Availability

Access to palliative care medicines is crucial to ensure effective pain and symptom management. Notwithstanding the development of an essential medicines list, many medications remain unavailable. As such, and despite its prevalence among cancer and HIV/AIDS patients, pain in Africa is disturbingly undertreated among adults and children. Opioids, such as morphine, are critical to the effective relief of moderate-to-severe pain. In many African countries, however, opioid analgesic consumption remains extremely low in relation to medical need (see Figure 75–3).[19]

Barriers to the opioid analgesics supply on the continent include, among others, *Supply* (e.g., central stores not stocking adequately, overly restrictive control, unreliable stocks, and insufficient numbers of dispensers); *Legislation* (e.g., punitive and prohibitive regulations, lack of national policies on opioid use, and bureaucratic processes); *Education* (e.g., existing clinicians unaware of how to assess and treat pain, the fear of addiction—that is, "opiophobia"—poor patient compliance, palliative care stressing its specialty to the point of exclusion, and doctors lacking interest in terminally ill patients); and *Practical issues* (e.g., storage requirements, not enough prescribers, unqualified staff in HBC, poor infrastructure to follow discharged patients home, and the short shelf-life of morphine in the absence of sufficient demand).[20]

The United Nations' Economic and Social Council has called upon Member States to remove such barriers to the medical use of analgesics, and the International Narcotics Control Board has requested governments promote the rational use of opioid analgesia for pain management. Given that such appeals require supplementary advocacy with national policymakers, APCA has recently undertaken policy-influencing work across eastern, southern, and western Africa to promote the availability and accessibility of pain-relieving medicines, especially opioids. Consequently, 18 participating countries have formed national teams to advocate to this end with their respective governments.

Additionally, and as mentioned, the relative lack of doctors on the continent means that there is a growing acceptance of " 'task-shifting," enabling other appropriately trained specialist health cadre (e.g., nurses) to prescribe opioids. However, task-shifting does not negate the imperative to educate doctors in the need for effective pain management, and address the "opiophobia" that perceives such medicines as addictive and health workers vulnerable to legal prosecution. Moreover, there is a need for African governments to use cheaper, but still effective, generic opioids (including reconstituted morphine sulphate powder) that governments can afford without fear of stock outs.

## Education

Palliative care education should target diverse audiences (e.g., policymakers, health-care workers, and the general public) to increase their awareness, skills, and knowledge of, and change their attitudes to, the discipline. One critically important group, however, is those national leaders (both clinical and academic experts) who are responsible for education, and it is vital that palliative care professionals work collaboratively with them to change existing, and develop new, palliative care educational curricula.

There are numerous educational initiatives in Africa that seek to address the holistic needs of patients and their families, with an emphasis on pain and symptom management, psychosocial, cultural, and spiritual needs. These programs range from short certificate courses, to diploma, undergraduate, and masters-level degrees. In South Africa, for example, there is a masters course for doctors conducted at the University of Cape Town that from 2009 was made available to other disciplines.

In some African countries, such as South Africa, Zimbabwe, and Uganda, palliative care is incorporated into medical and nursing curricula and is examinable at both undergraduate and postgraduate levels. In other African countries, educational programs to build the capacity of tutors and lecturers of health-teaching institutions to teach palliative care are being implemented.

## Implementation

Without effective implementation, the three additional components of the enhanced WHO public health model are redundant. Consequently, most African governments need to ensure there are sufficient funding and appropriate service delivery models in place to support the expansion of palliative care in their respective countries.

The primary mode of palliative care service delivery is HBC, which is predominantly dependent on volunteers. In addition to addressing the issues of staff recruitment and retention, it is imperative that African palliative care providers ensure that the HBC services provide an acceptable standard of patient care. Of particular importance in this respect is the development and adherence to national quality care standards, work that is presently (2009) being developed by APCA. Moreover, to ensure widespread implementation, it is important that palliative care is integrated into all levels of the health-care system, including the specialist, regional, and district (as well as HBC) facilities.

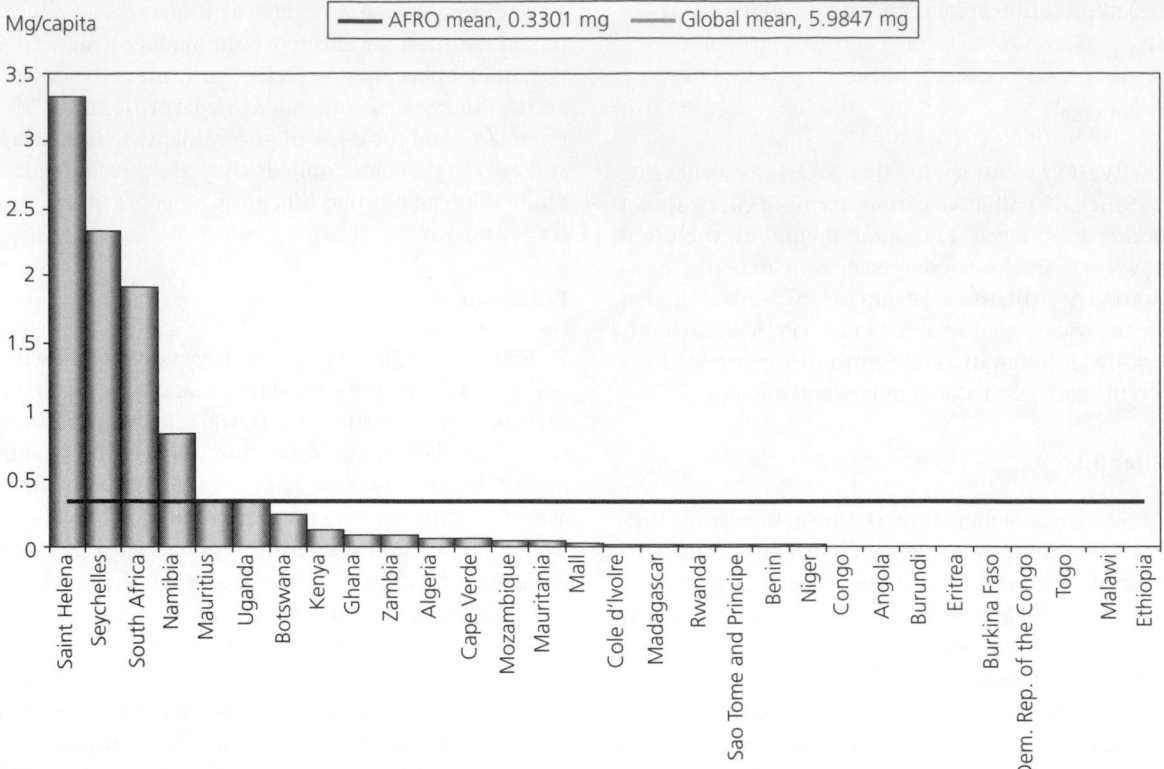

**Figure 75–3.** Consumption of morphine, Africa, 2006 mg/capita. *Source*: Copyright Pain and Policy Studies Group, University of Wisconsin/WHO Collaborating Centre (2008). Reprinted with permission from Pain and Policy Studies Group, University of Wisconsin, USA, AFRO Region 2006 consumption, www.painpolicy.wisc.edu/internat/AFRO/index.htm.

### CASE STUDY—UGANDA

One of the palliative care success stories on the continent is found in Uganda. Established in 1993, Hospice Africa Uganda (HAU) (with its subsequent affiliates, Mobile Hospice Mbarara and Little Hospice Hoima), working with other in-country palliative care providers, has not only persuaded the national government to make palliative care for people with AIDS and cancer a priority in its National Health Plan—where it is classified as "essential clinical care"—but, and importantly for a country where the doctor:patient ratio is so low, succeeded in changing legislation to authorize palliative care nurses and clinical officers to prescribe morphine.

### The Multi-Disciplinary Team and Palliative Care

In Africa, where there are limited numbers of health professionals, the multidisciplinary team should include whoever is considered most appropriate (e.g., nurses, doctors, social workers, counselors, and allied health professionals, working alongside others such as traditional, religious and community leaders, teachers and community health workers).

Despite the theoretical ideal, the reality in rural Africa is that the team may be comprised of only one or two members (e.g., a nurse and community volunteer working alongside family members). The precise nature of the team will vary according to the care model provided, be that a specialist palliative care unit, a hospital, a road-side clinic, or HBC service. Few hospitals (e.g., Mulago Hospital in Uganda, Kenyatta Hospital in Kenya, and several hospitals in South Africa) have access to dedicated palliative care teams. Consequently, it is important that these teams network effectively with other services to ensure that the patient is able to receive care in a home and facility setting.

For the vast majority of services, no distinct palliative care team exists, with health-care providers working with different people at different times. Despite the challenges such working arrangements pose, multidisciplinary teamwork is slowly being developed across the region, often with nurses leading such teams.

### The Nurse's Role in Palliative Care in Africa

Nurses have a pivotal role in palliative care provision on the continent given they are present at all levels of the health-care system, from the facility to the community. The merits of the holistic focus and broad skills base of the nursing profession is supplemented by the fact that for the vast majority of African patients—especially in rural areas—nurses are the only health-care professionals available (as indicated earlier). For example, in Tanzania, there are two physicians per 100,000 people and 37 nurses; in Mozambique, there are three physicians per 100,000 people and 21 nurses; and in Cote d'Ivoire, there are 12 physicians per 100,000 and 60 nurses.[21]

Nurses' roles within palliative care in Africa are varied, including vital roles in the development of teamwork, assessment, communication, and counseling, treatment and prescribing as appropriate, training and supervision, advocacy, and health promotion.[22]

As outlined above, to ensure accessibility to palliative care services (particularly in the rural areas) some countries are changing existing legislation so that palliative care-trained nurses are enabled to prescribe medications such as oral morphine. Following Uganda's work in this area, other countries (e.g., South Africa, Malawi, Zimbabwe, and Namibia) are attempting to emulate their success.

Education and mentorship, both for the patient, family, community health workers and other nurses, is another vital part of the nurses' role in palliative care in Africa. Training family members to care for their loved ones and providing them with support and mentorship to accomplish this, is an important part of enabling HBC delivery. Additionally, the significant workforce role played by community-based volunteers means that nurses also have a pivotal role to play in equipping the former with the necessary skills and supporting them through supervision.

The important role of research in African palliative care development is now recognized, with nurses increasingly trained to develop and implement research programs. This is an important advance not only in the development of palliative care in the region, but in the valuation of the nurses' role. However, despite this positive development, the inadequate incorporation of palliative care into preservice (undergraduate) training for nurses, the lack of clear career pathways for nurses interested in specializing in palliative care, and the lack of recognition of palliative care qualifications by local Ministries of Health and Education, continue to be a challenge.

## Sociocultural, Religious, and Spiritual Issues Influencing Palliative Care

Africa has a rich diversity of cultures that provide people with a framework with which to understand their experiences and influence the way in which palliative care is delivered to patients and their families. Common social, cultural, religious and spiritual needs of the patient and their family include: overwhelming social needs; communication around issues of death, grief, and bereavement; and perceptions and beliefs and practices surrounding illness and death among others.

Deprivation for many in Africa means that social needs are central to palliative care provision, with patients concerned for the welfare of their children (including their school fees, care arrangements when death comes, and their inability to afford their basic needs).

Patients and their families experience the common phases of grief, including denial, anger, depression, bargaining, and acceptance. They additionally experience understandable fear and anxieties, and sometimes self-blame for contributing to the disease's cause, especially HIV/AIDS. Many African patients who are in denial do not prioritize their medical treatment, but instead resort to traditional healing in the belief that their ancestors could be angry with them. Moreover, the taboo that surrounds death in most African countries means that communication regarding this important topic is problematic, a fact that is compounded by the overwhelming number of patients presenting at health facilities that render meaningful discussion of sociocultural, religious, and spiritual issues impossible.

Although variation exists for the preferred location of death (i.e., home or facility-based), for many patients, a domiciliary death is the desired choice, provided appropriate care is accessible.[23] Although there is a need to sensitize communities and health-care workers to respect such dying patients' priorities, there is also recognition that the facility-based alternative to a domiciliary death is unaffordable for the majority of patients. Consequently, training programs for family caregivers and community volunteers are widely implemented to ensure the provision of basic HBC, supplemented with support and supervision from professional teams.

Africa is characterized by multiple religious denominations, with most following Christianity (45%) or Islam (40.6%), the adherents of which can also simultaneously practice traditional African religions.[24] These religious and spiritual beliefs and practices can prove very important to the terminally ill as they influence their attitude and insight toward illness and death.

Many Africans believe there are four main categories of diseases: African disease; foreign disease; chronic disease; and plague.[25] Consequently, some diseases are primarily addressed using indigenous African medicines and traditional healers (which are extensively used on the continent), whereas others are treated using modern scientific medicine and medical professionals. However, given that many pharmaceutical products currently remain largely unaffordable and inaccessible to the majority of Africans, many patients interact with their local traditional healers, whose dispensed herbal medicines can interact negatively with medically prescribed treatments. Consequently, some African countries have established collaborative medical programs (e.g., for HIV/AIDS) between traditional and modern health practitioners to nurture an environment of joint learning and care provision.[26] Moreover, given the lack of health-care providers trained in assessing patients' psychosocial, religious, and spiritual needs, some palliative care organizations recruit social and spiritual care professionals to support clinical teams with complex cases, and train their team members.

## Special Populations

For some patients, palliative care service provision can be problematic because of multiple factors (e.g., stigma, especially for HIV/AIDS, and various financial, social, or legal barriers). This is especially the case in Africa for internally displaced persons (IDPs), prisoners, and the armed forces, among others.[27]

### Internally Displaced Persons

Defined as "someone who has been forced to flee his or her home, but who has not reached a neighboring country and therefore, unlike a refugee, is not protected by international law and is not eligible to receive many types of aid,"[28] there is in excess of an estimated 4.5 million refugees/IDPs across Africa who have fallen through the safety net provided to many ordinary citizens who are not receiving palliative care.

### Prisoners

Millions of people are imprisoned across Africa, in conditions that are commonly and extremely basic, often characterized by deficient sanitation, poor nutrition, limited access to medical services, and heightened risk of infection (e.g., in 1998 the HIV prevalence in Ugandan prisons was 20%, higher than the general population).[29] For released prisoners, poor discharge planning and follow-up, compounded by the stigmas of illness and being an ex-convict, mean that accessing care can remain problematic.

### Armed Forces

The armed forces (i.e., army, navy, air force, presidential guard, police, etc.) are another unique subpopulation for African palliative care services. Often members are forced to live apart from their families for considerable durations of time (often exposing them to risky health behaviors; e.g., unprotected sex with commercial sex workers), whereas the suspicion that a diagnosis of ill health will impact adversely on their career prospects and living situation means that they can often present in the advanced stages of life-threatening illnesses. It is important that armed forces recognize and integrate palliative care within their military health system. This approach has been followed in Uganda, where members of the Ugandan People's Defence Force have established their own branch of the country's national palliative care association, and work to identify and treat soldiers and their families.

Key to the provision of palliative care among such subpopulations is the establishment of trust, adapting services to ensure that those who feel marginalized, stigmatized and are distrustful of society can receive the benefits of its healthcare system.

## Children's Palliative Care

In 2007, an estimated 1.8 million children under the age 15 years in sub-Saharan Africa were living with HIV/AIDS, with about 240,000 dying in that year alone.[7] Additionally, despite the deficiencies of existing systems to enumerate its incidence and prevalence, it is reasonable to assume that a considerable percentage of the estimated 7.6 million new cancer cases and 6 million cancer-related deaths in Africa in 2007 were children.

The palliative care needs of children differ from those of adults. For example, children's differential development stages will affect their understanding of their illness; they are not legally competent to consent to medical treatment; they may have deficient skills to verbalize their needs, or express their pain and discomfort; and they may protect their parents or loved ones at their own expense.

Traditionally, children have been relatively neglected by palliative care service development on the continent, despite the fact that they may well have already experienced parental and sibling deaths and now face their own mortality. This neglect is exacerbated by the limitations of existing community and health service physical and human resources, including: restricted access to pediatric medical formulations; lack of understanding of the disease process in children; limited access to affordable and accessible chemotherapy and antiretroviral therapy services, which are often centered around urban areas; societal myths concerning whether children can neurologically feel pain; and familial financial destitution that forces parents to make exacting decisions on who among their needy should receive their finite resources (i.e., the dying child or their caregiver).

However, the growing awareness of the positive impact that it can exert upon children has resulted in an increasing demand that children's palliative care should no longer be the "orphan" of its adult equivalent. This demand recently manifested itself in the International Children's Palliative Care Network's charter of rights for children with life-limited and life-threatening illnesses, which promises to be an important advocacy tool for the development of children's palliative care on the continent.

There is also a recognition that, given it is often the same nurse (particularly in rural areas, in the absence of specialist children's hospitals and palliative care services) who has responsibility for delivering care to adults and children, the distinct differences that characterize children mean it is imperative that pediatric palliative care is integrated into all palliative care trainings, whereas a small number of health professionals can receive specialist children's palliative care training to enable them to provide support and mentorship to others. This should be supplemented by effective networking and collaboration between organizations involved in pediatric palliative care (e.g., general home-based programs, children's daycare programs, inpatient programs, and hospital-based programs).

## Ethical and Legal Issues

In most African countries, legal and ethical frameworks for palliative care are in their infancy or indeed nonexistent. As stated above, the Cape Town Declaration advanced palliative care and pain and symptom control as a human right. For the vast majority of countries in the region, however, this remains an ideal; restricted health-care budgets and multiple competing demands mean that populations cannot access even basic public health requirements, such as clean water, sanitization, or rudimentary healthcare. Consequently, for many palliative care professionals in the region, advocating for palliative care as a right of every adult and child is tempered by the need to advocate for other more basic human rights that will also improve the quality of life of those with life-limiting illnesses.

Generic palliative care ethical issues include truthtelling, informed consent, patient autonomy, and doing no harm to patients. However, specific ethical challenges exist in Africa resulting from its varied cultures, and the high prevalence of HIV/AIDS, which compounds usual ethical considerations with stigma, disclosure, and blame. Additionally, many African health professionals believe that human life must be preserved at all costs, resulting in terminally ill patients being transported back to their local hospital for medical procedures they neither need nor can afford.

Within the African context, there is widespread disparity in gender power relations that can affect women not only in sexual issues but also in terms of adequate access to information regarding their illness, their economic dependency, loss of inheritance property following their spouse's death, and lack of control over end-of-life treatment preferences. In palliative care, respect for patient autonomy entails the individual making their own decisions, something that is premised on adequate information regarding potential treatment and care options. However, this premise is undermined in those parts of Africa where sociocultural norms dictate that the needs of the family and community supersede those of the individual. For example, in some cultures any decisions regarding treatment will be made by the senior familial male member, sometimes at the patient's expense. This situation can be compounded by the paternalistic nature of heath-care systems, where women and girls may be discouraged from asking questions and health-care workers may be reluctant to discuss illness, death, and dying.[30]

Although advance directives and living wills are gradually being introduced and discussed in the region (mainly in southern Africa), they remain in many areas embryonic concepts and philosophical discussion points. Euthanasia is also a topic of philosophical discussion by some in the region.

## Challenges to Palliative Care in Africa

- *Delayed health-seeking behavior:* Palliative care has traditionally been viewed as an "end-stage" intervention, signaled by the conclusion of the need for curative treatment, despite clinical evidence that patients need pain, symptom management, and psychosocial care throughout the disease trajectory.[31] With the advent of highly active antiretroviral therapy (HAART), this perception is further misplaced. However, the fact remains that large numbers of people infected by HIV/AIDS and cancer delay seeking medical assistance (e.g., because of the stigma associated with HIV/AIDS as well as the cost of treatment).

- *Lack of trained palliative care professionals:* Not only is there a worldwide health workforce crisis, as noted at the first Global Forum on Human Resources for Health in 2008, that is characterized by widespread global shortages, maldistribution of personnel within and between countries, migration of local health workers, and poor working conditions,[32] but there is a significant deficit in skilled palliative care professionals (with limited opportunities for health workers to acquire palliative care training), while the preponderant reliance on HBC volunteers raises questions regarding the quality and sustainability of services significantly dependent upon their contribution.[33]

- *Unfavorable drug environments:* As stated earlier, despite the overwhelming medical need, access to even the simplest pain-relieving medication—notwithstanding the strong painkillers (i.e., opioids)[34]—and antibiotics to treat opportunistic infections in many African countries is provided within very restrictive policy and operational environments (e.g., limited legitimate prescribers).

- *Logistical challenges to service provision:* The geographical and topographical challenges facing effective palliative care provision cannot be understated. Given the relatively low level of urbanization in many African countries (e.g., 2.2 people per km$^2$ in Namibia), services sometimes have to be provided to low-density populations across vast rural areas. Additionally, the preference of many health professionals to work in urban locations means that rural health-care provision is primarily left to community- and home-based volunteers, offering care that is often no more than supportive in nature.

- *Limitations of existing service models in an era of HAART:* Although HAART is pivotal to effective HIV/AIDS management, the extent to which current African HBC models are able to integrate it into their existing services is a challenge. Many current models are, to varying degrees, largely non-medicalized. However, efforts to address this challenge have shown that HAART can be provided as part of a palliative care service by community-based indigenous health-care workers as long as training and resource needs are adequately addressed.[35]

- *Other challenges include*: lack of rigorous research evidence indicating the benefits of palliative care; poor public awareness and understanding of the discipline; uncommitted national governments; lack of funding; entrenched attitudes within the medical profession; cultural taboos surrounding death and the disclosure of diagnosis; and the absence of a consensus that regards palliative care as a basic human right.

## Summary

The discipline of palliative care started relatively late in Africa, advanced over the preceding three decades by highly committed individuals with access to limited resources to meet an overwhelming need. The agenda for the coming years is significant, encompassing the need to overcome government indifference and effect high-level policy change, training for its primarily volunteer cadre as well as orthodox pre- and in-service health workers (to include recruitment, training, and retention issues), improving societal and medical understanding and use of opioids for effective pain management, building effective linkages between relevant stakeholders (e.g., academics, oncologists, pediatricians, those working with the aged, etc.), and developing and utilizing a methodologically rigorous research base to inform service development and, ultimately, maximize the quality of patients' lives.

REFERENCES

1. Population Reference Bureau. 2008 World Population Data Sheet. New York, NY: Population Reference Bureau, 2008.
2. United Nations Development Programme. Human Development Report—Fighting Climate Change: Human Solidarity in a Divided World. New York, NY: United Nations Development Programme, 2007.
3. Council for the Development of Social Science Research in Africa. 2005. Access and Equity in African Health Systems. www.codesria.org/Archives/Training_grants/health/health05.htm (accessed on January 20, 2009).
4. World Health Organization. Alma-Ata 1978: Primary Health Care, HFA Sr. No. 1. Geneva: World Health Organization, 1978.
5. Kirigia JM, Diarra-Nama AJ. Can countries of the WHO African Region wean themselves off donor funding for health? Bull World Health Org 2008;86:889–892.
6. Joint United Nations Programme on HIV/AIDS. Report on the Global AIDS Epidemic. Geneva: UNAIDS, 2008.
7. Garcia M, Jemal A, Ward EM, et al. Global Cancer: Facts and figures 2007. Atlanta, GA: American Cancer Society, 2007.
8. Morris K. Cancer? In Africa? Lanc Oncol 2003;4:5.
9. World Health Organization The African Regional Health Report: The health of the people. Geneva: World Health Organization, 2006.
10. Wright M, Clark D. Hospice and palliative care in Africa: A review of developments and challenges. Oxford, England: Oxford University Press, 2006.
11. Harding R, Higginson IJ. Palliative care in sub-Saharan Africa: An appraisal. Lancet 2005;365(9475):1909–1911.
12. Clark D, Wright M, Hunt J, Lynch T. Hospice and palliative care development in Africa: A multi-method review of services and experiences. J Pain Symptom Manage 2007;33(6): 698–710.
13. Harding R, Powell RA, Downing J, et al. Generating an African palliative care evidence base: The context, need, challenges and strategies. J Pain Symptom Manage 2008;36(3):304–309.
14. Powell RA, Downing J, Radbruch L, Mwangi-Powell FN, Harding R. Advancing palliative care research in Africa: From Venice to Nairobi. Palliat Med 2008;22(8):885–887.
15. Sebuyira LM, Mwangi-Powell F, Pereira J, Spence C. The Cape Town palliative care declaration: Home-grown solutions for Sub-Saharan Africa. J Palliat Med 2003;6(3):341–343.
16. Sternsward J, Foley K, Ferris F. The public health strategy for palliative care. J Pain Symptom Manage 2007;33:486–493.
17. World Health Organization. Cancer Pain Relief and Palliative Care. Technical Report Series 804. Geneva: World Health Organization, 1990.
18. Oluwole D. Health policy development in Sub-Saharan Africa: National and international perspectives. Washington DC: World Press, 2008. www. worldpress.org/Africa/3251.cfm (accessed January 20,2009).
19. International Narcotics Control Board. Narcotic drugs: Estimated world requirements for 2008—Statistics for 2006. New York, NY: United Nations, 2008. Pain & Policy Studies Group, University of Wisconsin/WHO Collaborating Center, 2008.
20. Harding R, Powell RA, Kiyange F, Downing J, Mwangi-Powell F. Pain-relieving drugs in 12 African PEPFAR countries: Mapping current providers, identifying current challenges, and enabling expansion of pain control provision in the management of HIV/AIDS. Kampala, Uganda: African Palliative Care Association, 2007.
21. World Health Organization. World Health Report. Geneva: World Health Organization, 2006.
22. Downing J, Finch L, Garanganga E, et al. Role of the nurse in resource-limited settings,. In: Gwyther L, Merriman A, Mpanga Sebuyira L, Schietinger H, eds. A Clinical Guide to Supportive and Palliative Care for HIV/AIDS in Sub-Saharan Africa. Kampala, Uganda: African Palliative Care Association; 2006:345–56.
23. World Health Organization. A community health approach to palliative care for HIV/AIDS and cancer patients in sub-Saharan Africa. Geneva: World Health Organization, 2004.
24. McLaughlin A. In Africa, Islam and Christianity are growing—and blending. The Christian Science Monitor, January 26, 2006. www.csmonitor.com/2006/0126/p01s04-woaf.html (accessed on January 20, 2009).
25. Waliggo JM, Gwyther L, Mguli E, Mini C, Nieuwmeyer SM, Salie NM. Spiritual and cultural care. In: Gwyther L, Merriman A, Mpanga Sebuyira L, Schietinger H, eds. A Clinical Guide to Supportive and Palliative Care for HIV/AIDS in Sub-Saharan Africa. Kampala, Uganda: African Palliative Care Association, 2006:233–248.
26. Hills SY, Finch L, Garanganga E. Traditional medicine, In: Gwyther L, Merriman A, Mpanga Sebuyira L, Schietinger H, eds. A Clinical Guide to Supportive and Palliative Care for HIV/AIDS in Sub-Saharan Africa. Kampala, Uganda: African Palliative Care Association, 2006:219–232.

27. Downing J. Special populations, In: Gwyther L, Merriman A, Mpanga Sebuyira L, Schietinger H, eds. A Clinical Guide to Supportive and Palliative Care for HIV/AIDS in Sub-Saharan Africa. Kampala, Uganda: African Palliative Care Association; 2006:323–334.

28. United Nations High Commission on Refugees. Refugees by Numbers. Geneva: United Nations High Commission on Refugees, 2004.

29. Kaddu M, Nabatanzi F. Palliative care in the Uganda Prisons Service. PCAU J Pall Care 2004;17:25–27.

30. Sebuyira LM, Gwyther L. Ethical and human rights issues. In: Gwyther L, Merriman A, Mpanga Sebuyira L, Schietinger H, eds. A Clinical Guide to Supportive and Palliative Care for HIV/AIDS in Sub-Saharan Africa. Kampala, Uganda: African Palliative Care Association; 2006:309–322.

31. Breitbart W, McDonald MV, Rosenfeld B, et al. Pain experience in ambulatory AIDS patients—I: Pain characteristics and medical correlates. Pain 1996;68:315–321.

32. World Health Organization. The global shortage of health workers and its impact. Fact Sheet No 302. 2006.

33. Powell RA, Mwangi-Powell FN. Improving palliative care in Africa: Selection, training, and retention of community-based volunteers is a priority. Br Med J 2008;337:1123–1124.

34. Harding R, Higginson IJ. Palliative care in sub-Saharan Africa: An appraisal. London: The Diana, Princess of Wales Memorial Fund, 2004.

35. Campbell C, Nair Y, Maimane S, Sibiya Z. Home-based carers: A vital resource for effective ARV roll-out in rural communities? AIDS Bull 2005;14:22–27.

# 76

*Sayaka Takenouchi and Keiko Tamura*

# Palliative Care in Japan

## Transition of Palliative Care in Japan

### Establishment of Hospice

The modern hospice movement began with the establishment of St. Christopher's Hospice in the suburbs of London, United Kingdom, in 1967. Thereafter, the hospice movement spread from the United Kingdom to the United States and around the world. The hospice concept was introduced in Japan in the 1970's and the discussion of the need for hospice programs was started. In 1981, the first in-hospital independent hospice unit was founded within Seirei Mikatahara General Hospital of Shizuoka prefecture. This was followed in 1984 by the creation of an in-hospital hospice floor at Yodogawa Christian Hospital. Since their establishment, not only medical professionals, but the general public has shown a high interest in death and dying topics. This has led to a growing implementation of hospice care services within medical facilities in Japan.[1] Table 76–1 outlines the history of palliative care in Japan from 1973 to 2008.

### Governmental Approach

In an effort to improve end-of-life care and palliative care services in Japan, the Ministry of Health and Welfare released a report in June of 1989 from the "Investigative Committee for the Role of Terminal Care." This report was followed in April of 1990 by the introduction of the "Palliative Care Unit Admission Fee."[1] This new system provided a fixed amount of money to cover medical services provided in palliative care wards as long as the stipulated facility and staff criteria were met. This resulted in an increased number of facilities providing hospice or palliative care services in Japan. However, the "Palliative Care Unit Admission Fee" applied only to end-of-life care provided to limited illnesses such as cancer and AIDS. In addition, it only applied to medical care

**Table 76–1**
**The History of Hospice/Palliative Care in Japan**

| | |
|---|---|
| 1973 | Activities by the Organized Care of Dying Patients (OCDP) started at Yodogawa Christian Hospital. |
| 1977 | The activities by St. Christopher's Hospice in the UK were introduced in the newspaper. |
| | The first meeting of the Japanese Association for Clinical Research on Death and Dying was held. |
| 1981 | The first Japanese hospice was opened at Seirei Mikatahara General Hospital. |
| 1984 | A hospice was opened at Yodogawa Christian Hospital. |
| 1989 | Ministry of Health, Labor, and Welfare announced a report by the "Investigative Committee for the Role of Terminal Care." |
| 1990 | Ministry of Health, Labor, and Welfare introduced the "Palliative Care Unit Admission Fee" as the remuneration for medical services under health insurance. |
| 1991 | Japan Hospice Palliative Care Foundation (presently, a nonprofit organization "Hospice Palliative Care Japan") was founded. |
| 1996 | The first meeting of Japanese Society of Palliative Medicine was held. |
| | Japanese Nursing Association launched accreditation of Oncology Certified Nurse Specialist. |
| 1997 | Japanese Nursing Association launched accreditation of Certified Nurse Specialist for hospice care, cancer pain care, etc. |
| 2002 | "Additional Charge for Palliative Care" was started as remuneration for medical services under health insurance. |
| 2006 | Cancer Control Act enacted. |
| 2007 | Cancer Control Act enforced. |
| 2008 | The number of Palliative Care ward reaches: 182 facilities, 3534 beds (as of April). |

*Source*: Adapted from reference 2.

**Table 76–2**
**Facility Criteria for Palliative Care Unit Admission Fee**

2008 Ministry of Health, Labor, and Welfare Notification No. 62: Facility Criteria, etc., for Basic Medical Service Fee
Excerpt from "Facility Criteria for Palliative Care Unit Admission Fee"[3]

1. Patients with malignant tumors or acquired immune deficiency syndrome shall be admitted to the palliative care unit, and palliative care should be provided in the ward as a unit.
2. Within this ward, care must be always provided by a minimum of no less than 1 RN for every 7 patients. However, if the number of RN is higher than the specified number above, the number of RN on night shift shall be two or more.
3. Sufficient equipment and structure must be prepared to provide the adequate treatment.
4. Sufficient building and facility must be prepared to provide the adequate treatment.
5. Structure to determine the hospitalization/discharge of patients must be in place.
6. The ratio of hospital rooms must be appropriate for providing special treatment environment as optional medical treatment, as stipulated in subparagraph 4 of paragraph 2 of Article 63 of the Health Insurance Law and subparagraph 4 of paragraph 2 of Article 64 of the Act for the Assurance of Medical Care for the Elderly.
7. The facility must be evaluated by Japan Council for Quality Health Care.
8. Training must be provided to physicians and nurses of related medical institutions.

provided within the ward that fulfilled the stipulated criteria.[2] The result was that many patients in need did not have the opportunity to benefit from palliative care.

To correct this, the "Remuneration for Medical Services" was revised in 2002 to include an "Additional Medical Fee for Palliative Care." This was a new step in the development of hospice and palliative care in Japan. In addition to the in-hospital medical services within the hospice and palliative care wards, the fee revision provided additional medical service fees for palliative care provided in general wards by a full-time team of staff that engaged in alleviation of symptoms. This provided a catalyst to expand hospice and palliative care consultation services to the general wards as well as home-based services including out-patient care and home visits. Table 76–2 shows the criteria for facilities that can provide in-patient hospice/palliative care within the current Japanese health coverage.

Facilities offering hospice/palliative care are increasing year by year, as can be seen in Figure 76–1, with 182 hospice/palliative care wards (3534 beds) country-wide as of April 2008.[4]

However, of the patients who die from cancer every year, only 4% (as of 2002) spend the last days of their lives receiving hospice or palliative care. The numbers show that there are still an inadequate number of facilities. The government added requirements for palliative care facilities to be authorized in 2002. One of those requirements was the need to be approved by the Japan Council for Quality Health Care

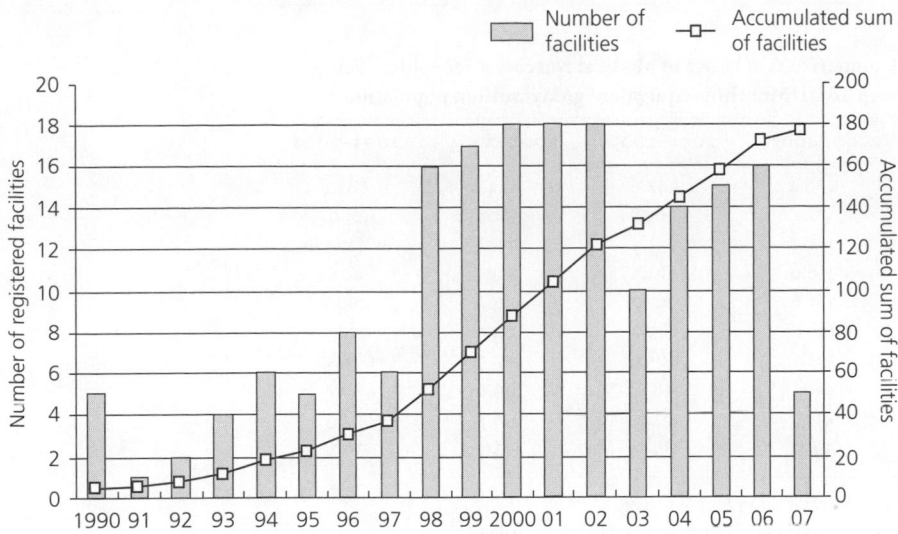

**Figure 76–1.** Changes in number of registered/approved facilities for palliative care unit admission fee and number of beds in each year (as of April 1, 2008). *Source*: Hospice Palliative Care Japan (2008), reference 4.

(JCQHC). Some organization failed to qualify by the JCQHC standard and could not register their new palliative care facilities. This led to a decline in facilities in 2003 (Figure 76–1). A further decline of facilities in 2007 is considered to be due to the "Remuneration for Medical Services," which was revised in 2006. Each facility has struggled to ensure a nurse-to-patient ratio of a minimum of one RN for every seven patients in general medical or post-surgical care units. This nurse-to-patient ratio is required in order to obtain the increase in revenues as outlines in the revision. This has resulted in a delay of plans to open new palliative care facilities.

**Cancer Control Act**

In response to the unmet needs of cancer patients, the "Cancer Control Act" was approved in June 2006 and implemented in April of 2007. The aim was to create a nationwide structure for receiving specialized medical treatment for cancer. Patients having to "roam" around many medical facilities in order to receive comprehensive cancer care led to the term "Cancer Refugee" being used. This was recognized as a social problem. Demands from the patients and citizens to improve this situation resulted in the Cancer Control Act.

The "Cancer Control Act" focused on three areas: *(1)* Prevention and early detection of cancer; *(2)* Equalization of cancer medical services; and *(3)* Research. The second area—Equalization of cancer medical services—stipulated that palliative care be promoted in order to maintain and improve the quality of life of cancer patients under medical treatment.

In addition, in June of 2007, based on the Cancer Control Act, the Japanese government formulated the "Basic Plan to Promote Cancer Control Programs." Feedback from the Cancer Control Promotion Council, which included cancer patients and their families as its members, was taken into account. The "Basic Plan to Promote Cancer Control Programs" placed "initiation of palliative care at an early stage of treatment" as a priority.[5,6] The Act stipulated that

alleviation of physical symptoms and support for psychological problems be provided, not only in the terminal phase of the disease, but from the early stages of treatment. The goal was for cancer patients and their families to maintain as high a quality of life as possible. Thus, the foundation to seamlessly provide palliative care to patients and their families in various situations of life-threatening illness was laid.

**Modes of Hospice Care/Palliative Care**

In Japan, hospice care and palliative care are provided in many forms: In-hospital Independent type, In-hospital Floor type, In-hospital Segmented type, Home Care, and Free Standing type.[1]

In-hospital Floor type uses one of the wards of a general hospital as a hospice or palliative care ward, while In-hospital Segmented type has no independent building or ward but has a consultation palliative care team to provide palliative care at the request of the staff or patient. The Home Care type, has no inpatient facility (or has only a short-term inpatient facility) and practices mainly home-based hospice/palliative care. Finally, the Free Standing type is independent from any general hospital, in terms of relationship and location. There are only a few such facilities offering hospice/palliative care in Japan. An example is the Life Planning Center Foundation Peace House Hospice.[7]

**Training of Medical Professionals with Specialized Knowledge Regarding Palliative Care**

Opioid consumption in Japan for medical use remains approximately one tenth of that of the developed Western

**Table 76–3**
**International Comparisons of Usage of Medical Narcotics Morphine, Fentanyl, and Oxycodone in Total (Morphine equivalent g/day/million population).**

|           | 2000–2002 | 2001–2003 | 2002–2004 | 2004–2006 |
|-----------|-----------|-----------|-----------|-----------|
| Austria   | 469.2     | 542.8     | 624.0     | 882.1     |
| Canada    | 371.2     | 461.8     | 580.6     | 1,090.3   |
| Australia | 220.1     | 235.9     | 250.5     | 427.3     |
| USA       | 458.0     | 574.2     | 700.5     | 1,403.4   |
| France    | 271.6     | 301.7     | 326.1     | 460.1     |
| UK        | 147.6     | 143.0     | 171.0     | 298.5     |
| Germany   | 338.5     | 405.6     | 551.3     | 1,088.7   |
| Japan     | 25.9      | 38.6      | 49.0      | 69.1      |
| Italy     | 46.4      | 72.2      | 94.5      | 140.3     |
| Korea     | 19.4      | 19.3      | 17.0      | 36.7      |

Note: (1) No data for oxycodone in 2003 or earlier.
(2) Data before 2000 cannot be compared because of changes in method.
*Source*: International Narcotic Control Board, reference 8.

countries (Table 76–3). This reflects a lack of appreciation of the critical importance of opioid availability and use in the relief of suffering and the control of pain and dyspnea, especially at the end of life.[8]

When the "Basic Plan to Promote Cancer Control Programs" was approved by the cabinet on June 15th 2007, a goal was set that "within 10 years, all doctors engaging in cancer treatment would acquire basic knowledge about palliative care through training." The Prime Minister announced that he would work to realize the goal "within 5 years" so as to be ahead of schedule for the "within 10 years" plan. The Japanese government is strongly encouraging doctors working with cancer patients to complete their palliative care training as quickly as possible to meet the goal of "completing within 5 years."[6]

In this way, in addition to preparing a structure to provide comprehensive palliative care to patients and their families, specialized education and training in this field are being promoted. The goal is to increase the number of doctors with specialized knowledge and skills in palliative care at the same time as establishing a number of medical institutions that offer cancer treatment through palliative care teams.[6]

## Nurse Specialists in Palliative Care

A certification system for Oncology Certified Nurse Specialist was introduced in Japan in 1996. In 1999, a certification process was introduced by the Japanese Nursing Association for hospice care nurses and cancer pain management nurses. Following the revision of the Medical Service Fee in 2002, the number of nurse specialists working in general wards increased. With support and encouragement from their own Departments, many of these nurses signed up for training on "how to set up a palliative care team."[9]

Certified Nurses are nurse specialists whose proficient skills and knowledge have been certified for the purpose of raising the quality of nursing care in clinical practice. Currently there are 19 certification fields in Japan. Certification fields especially relevant to palliative care are "Hospice Care" and "Cancer Pain Management". The Certified Nursing Specialist Curriculum, approved by the Japanese Nursing Association, is a 6-month program that includes practical training. Nurse specialists with 5 years or more of clinical practice experience may enter the program, and, after completion, are eligible to take the certification examination. The roles of the Certified Nurse Specialists include hands-on practice, teaching, and consultation. The sites of practice include general wards, home care, and as a member of a palliative care team.[10]

Apart from the educational structure, to train specialists in particular fields[11] there is a wide variance in palliative care education within basic nursing training programs and for new staff or generalists working on hospice/palliative care units. There was recognition that this was an important issue for nurses to be addressed[12] and palliative care training within basic nursing education/continuing nursing education was re-evaluated. The need to train instructors that provide the palliative care education was identified [13]. To this end, in 2007, the educational program End-of-Life Nursing Education Consortium (ELNEC) developed by the American Association of Colleges of Nursing (AACN) and the City of Hope National Medical Center in the United States, was translated into Japanese and adapted to fit the present situation in Japan. This resulted in the "ELNEC Japan Train-the-Trainer Program." The expectation was that with this training, nurse educators would improve the quality of palliative nursing care and end-of-life care for practicing nurses as well as nursing students in Japan. Three ELNEC courses have been held, and over 150 nurses from throughout the country have been trained.

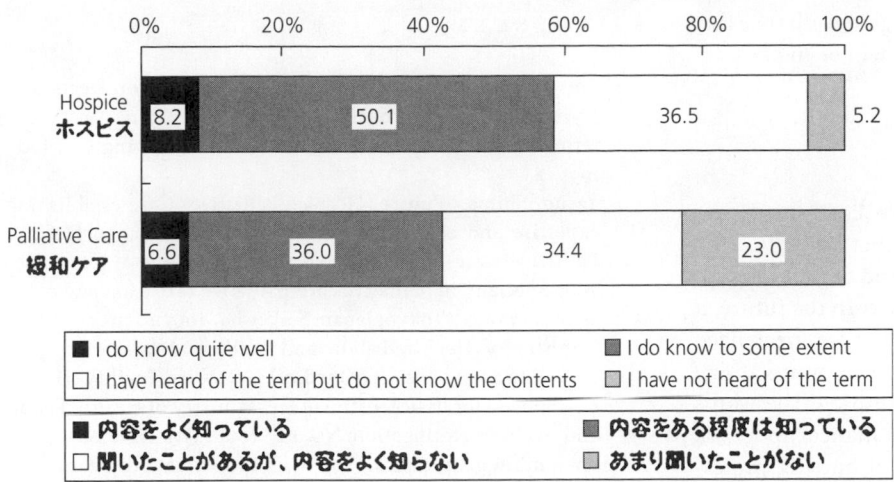

**Figure 76–2.** Level of awareness of hospice/palliative care. *Source*: Adapted from reference 15.

## Dissemination and Awareness of Palliative Care to the General Public

With governmental and professional activities in place to strengthen the overall quality of palliative care, the next step was to disseminate this information to patients and their families so that such care could be accessed if needed. However, the concept of palliative care as part of comprehensive medical and nursing care is still not widely known or accepted by the Japanese general public. The belief that palliative care is medical care for patients that have "given up and simply await their death" or that opioids, even when medically indicated, are "dangerous" are still fairly common attitudes.[14]

Since 2007, a project for dissemination and awareness of palliative care has been in effect. The goal is to increase public awareness and understanding of palliative care and what it has to offer. The Japan Hospice and Palliative Care Foundation conducted a survey in February of 2008 to assess the general publics' knowledge of hospice and palliative care. Of the 1010 people who participated in the survey (age range from 20 years to 89 years), in response to the question "Are you familiar with what a hospice is?," 50.1% responded "I do know to some extent," while 8.2% answered "I do know quite well." To the question "Are you familiar with palliative care?," 42.6% answered "yes," whereas 6.6% answered "I do know quite well," and 36.0% answered "I do know to some extent" (Figure 76–2).[15] The term "Palliative Care" is still quite new to the general public in Japan, and many people are still unfamiliar with the concept.

To increase public awareness of, and accurate information about palliative care, the Ministry of Health, Labor, and Welfare, in April 2007, developed plans for the "Dissemination and Awareness Project." The project called "The Orange Balloon Project" was entrusted to the Japanese Society for Palliative Medicine.[16] There are high hopes that this project will result in increased awareness of palliative care among the general public and requests for such care.

## Challenges for Palliative Care in Japan

### Challenges Connected to the Sociocultural Background

There is a social trend to avoid conversations about death and facing death or dealing with death related situations within the sociocultural background of Japan.[1] This barrier creates delays in introducing palliative care to the patients and their families early on in the disease process based on need not prognosis.

### Educational Challenges

Although the previously described activities to educate medical and nursing professionals who engage in palliative care are well under way, many patients and their families continue to report experiencing feelings of hurt or abandonment when the focus of their care shifts from cancer treatment to palliative care. There is an urgent need to include "communication skills" as an essential skill to be taught to all medical and nursing professionals, but especially those involved in palliative care and end-of-life care.

### Enhancement of Home Care

The "Basic Plan to Promote Cancer Control Programs" includes as one of the objectives "accommodating the wishes of patients, by increasing the number of patients that can choose to receive treatment in the comfort of their home or region with which they are familiar."[6] This objective requires preparation for a structure and environment to provide palliative care, not only in hospitals but also in the homes of patients. Coordination and cooperation between sites of care, depending on the changing needs of the patient, will be necessary to achieve this objective. In addition, it is important that each region take into consideration characteristics of their particular area so that a systematic approach to initiating home medical treatment and to constructing a regional alliance that can support the patients and their families will be in place.

## Expansion of the Role of Hospice/Palliative Care Wards

At this time in Japan, hospice/palliative care wards are expected to provide control of symptoms that are difficult to handle within general wards or at home, and to provide support for home treatment and end-of-life care. In the future, it is envisioned that the wards will be able to offer specialized care to alleviate the patients' pain and other symptoms at various steps of disease and treatment. In addition, the wards would function as a base for the regional alliance, and work towards providing training to medical and nursing professionals in palliative care. In this way the quality of palliative care would be enhanced throughout the entire region.

## Summary

Since 1990, the Japan Ministry of Health, Labor, and Welfare has actively advocated for and facilitated palliative care by designating palliative care as eligible for national health insurance. Because of the significant suffering experienced by cancer patients and using that as an impetus—the Ministry of Health, Labor, and Welfare has launched multiple nationwide projects to facilitate the dissemination of palliative care. In 2007, one of these actions of great significance was to change the criteria of palliative care admissions to include all cancer patients with a considerable level of suffering irrespective of stage of the disease. The Ministry also mandated that all 353 regional cancer centers throughout Japan establish palliative care teams, and approved palliative care teams as eligible for national health coverage.[17] These are all big steps, which are applicable to other chronic and debilitating life threatening illness. With the implementation of these measures, palliative care provided to patients and their families in Japan is expected to steadily improve.

Notably, the field of medicine and general culture in Japan differ from other nations. The palliative care approach to patients and families also differs from the approach to care provided by other departments. For example, in palliative care, appreciation of the family and culture that surround the patient play a significant role in planning their care.

There is a need to establish Japan's unique approach to palliative care and palliative care education that will fit with the medical background and culture of the nation. Even if palliative care at home becomes well developed, there will always be patients who will choose to spend the last days of their lives in the general hospital. It is therefore essential for any medical facility that provides care to patients facing life threatening illness and terminal disease to have available high quality palliative care for those in need.

REFERENCES

1. The Japanese Association for Clinical Research on Death and Dying. Clinical Approaches on Death and Dying IV. Future terminal care. Tokyo, Japan: Chuo Seihan Printing Co., Ltd., 1995:12.

2. Yasuo Shima. Future Hospice/Palliative Care-establishing expertise and community dissemination. In: Japan Hospice Palliative Care Foundation. Hospice/Palliative White Paper 2007 Specialty in palliative care-palliative care team and palliative care ward. Tokyo, Japan: Seikaisha, 2007:10–16.

3. Ministry of Health, Labor, and Welfare. Notification, etc., regarding 2008 revision of medical service fee. Facility criteria, etc., applied for basic treatment fee. Ministry of Health, Labor, and Welfare Notification No. 62, 2008. Available at: http://www.mhlw.go.jp/topics/2008/03/dl/tp0305–1at.pdf (accessed December 18, 2008).

4. Hospice Palliative Care Japan. Available at: http://www.hpcj.org/what (accessed December 18, 2008).

5. Ministry of Health, Labor, and Welfare. Health Service Bureau General Affairs Division Cancer Control Promotion Office. The first conference of dissemination and awareness regarding cancer. Data: Cancer-related statistics, 2007.

6. Masashi Kato. Yasuhisa Takeda. The Structure of Japan's Medical Services and Palliative Care Movements in Japan's Cancer Control and The Future Directions for Palliative Care—Based on the Plans of the "Basic Plan to Promote Cancer Control Programs." In Japan Hospice Palliative Care Foundation. Hospice/Palliative White Paper 2008 Structure of Medical Services and Regional Networks for Palliative Care. Tokyo, Japan: Seikaisha; 2008:6–13.

7. Tetsuo Kashiwagi. Sadamoto Hospice/Palliative Care. Tokyo, Japan: Seikaisya; 2006:140–148.

8. Center for Cancer Control and Information Services of National Cancer Center. Cancer statistics 2008 Data section, Consumption of narcotic for medical use, 2008; 99.

9. Toshiko Matsumoto. The Present Situation and Foresight into Postgraduate Training of Nurses for Palliative Care Certified Nurses. In Japan Hospice Palliative Care Foundation. Hospice/Palliative White Paper 2006 Education and Human Resource Development for Palliative Care. Tokyo, Japan: Seikaisha; 2006:17–19.

10. Japanese Nursing Association. What is a Qualification Certifying System? Available at: http://www.nurse.or.jp/nursing/qualification/howto/index.html (accessed December 17, 2008).

11. Megumi Umeda. Expertise of Nurses and Palliative Care. In Japan Hospice Palliative Care Foundation. Hospice/Palliative White Paper 2007. Expertise in Palliative Care, Palliative Care Team, and Palliative Care Ward. Tokyo, Japan: Seikaisha; 2007:47–50.

12. Noriko Futami. Present situation and issues of nursing education in palliative treatment for cancer. Palliat Med 2006;8:27–33.

13. Sayaka Sakamoto, Atsushi Asai, Shinji Kosugi. Evaluation of ethical teaching method in terminal care using the education program of End-of-Life Nursing Education Consortium (ELNEC) by Japanese nurse-practitioners engaging in end-of-life phase treatments. Kumamoto University Press. Adv Ethics Res 2007;2:54–65.

14. Minister's Secretariat, Public Relations Office. Survey on Cancer Control. Summary of Results. Cancer Information 2007. Available at: http://www8.cao.go.jp/survey/h19/h19-gantaisaku/2-3.html (accessed December 17, 2008).

15. Japan Hospice Palliative Care Foundation. Survey on Hospice/Palliative Care: Report Summary of Questions to 1000 Male/Female Participants—If the remainder of your life was limited, what kind of medical services would you like to receive; how would you like to spend the last days of your life; and the ratio of people that know the terms "Hospice" and "Palliative Care." Available at: http://www.hospat.org/research2-04.html (accessed December 17, 2008).

16. Japanese Society for Palliative Medicine. Orange Balloon Project. Entrusted Survey on Palliative Care in Cancer Treatment in 2007. Available at: http://www.kanwacare.net/ (accessed December 19, 2008).

17. Morita T, Miyashita M, Tsuneto S, et al. Palliative care in Japan: Shifting from the stage of disease to the intensity of suffering. J Pain Symptom Manage 2008;6:e6–e7.

# 77

*Hyun Sook Kim and Boon Han Kim*

# Palliative Care in South Korea

Located at the crossroads of Northeast Asia, Korea lies between Japan, the Russian Far East, and China. After World War II, a republic government was set up in the southern half of the Korean Peninsula while a communist-style government occupied the northern half of the Korean Peninsula. The Korean Demilitarized Zone serves as the buffer between North Korea and South Korea. South Korea rose out of absolute poverty but became one of the most economically successful countries among developing countries since the Korean War (1950–1953).

As of the end of 2008, South Korea's total population was estimated at 48.6 million with a density of about 500 people per square kilometer (Korea National Statistical Office, 2009a; http://www.korea.net). Although the population grew by about 3% annually during the 1960s, the rate decreased to below 1% over the decades that followed due to aggressive government-driven family planning. The rate was 0.21% in 2005 and is expected to be 0.02% by the year 2020. In the 1960s, the population distribution of Korea was pyramidal with a high birth rate and relatively short life expectancy. Today the age-group distribution is more bell shaped due to the low birth rate and extended life expectancy. People who are 15 and younger will make up a decreasing portion of the total, while those 65 and older will account for 15.7% of the total by the year 2020 (http://www.korea.net). As of 2007, life expectancy at birth was 76.1 years for males and 82.7 years for females, which is 20 years longer than the life expectancy in 1960 (Korea National Statistical Office, 2009a; http://www.korea.net).

## Attitudes Toward Death

In 2008, there were 246,113 deaths (672 per day on average). The primary causes of mortality and morbidity have shifted from acute, infectious disease to chronic disease over the last half century. By 2008, the top five causes of death in Korea were cancer, cerebral vascular accident (CVA), cardiovascular diseases, suicide, and diabetes mellitus (Korea National Statistical Office, 2009b). Every year, approximately 110,000 people are diagnosed with cancer in Korea (National Cancer Control Program, http://www.ncc.re.kr) and 68,912 die from the disease (Korea National Statistical Office, 2009b; National Cancer Control). Cancer became the first leading cause of death in Korea in 1983. Cancer mortality has been steadily increasing over the last two decades and cancer deaths accounted for 28% or over one-quarter of all deaths in 2008. Leukemia is the leading cause of death for those under 20, stomach cancer for people in their 30s, liver cancer for ages 40–50, and lung cancer for those over 60. Cancer in the circulatory system is a main cause of death for Koreans 40 and under, while cerebral vascular accident (CVA) is responsible for deaths in people 50 and over. About 20 % of these deaths are acute and sudden while the rest are chronic.

A national study conducted in 2004 showed that over half of Koreans (54.8%) chose their home as the preferred place of death.[1] Despite their preference, Koreans who died in their home decreased substantially from 72.9% in 1992 to 45.1% in 2003,[2] while those who died in hospitals increased from 16.6% in 1992 to 39.9% in 2001.

That same 2004 national study also showed that 82.3% of Koreans would prefer to withdraw from medically futile life-sustaining treatment.[1] The most important criteria for dying with dignity was (1) removing burdens for other people (27.8%), and (2) being with family and significant others (26.8%).[1] In reality, however, many Koreans still receive futile treatment even after their conditions are diagnosed as terminal. Furthermore, Korean law does not allow doctors to remove life-sustaining treatment regardless of the patient's condition or desires, or those of family members. The limited hospice/palliative care that is offered often demand a high degree of family responsibility; the caregivers of terminal patients are usually immediate family members or private caregivers hired by the family. For these reasons, Korean family members of terminally ill patients experience heavy physical, emotional, and social stresses much more so than families in the West.[3] Depression is common among family caregivers of the cancer patients.[4]

Recently, the Supreme Court granted the right to die to a 77-year-old patient, identified by her surname Kim, who had been in a coma for 456 days. The decision was that all medical treatment to prolong her life would be stopped and the respirator was taken off line on 6/24/2009. Kim first visited the hospital for a bronchial endoscopy in February 2008 for suspected lung cancer. During the biopsy, Kim suffered unexpected profuse bleeding and lapsed into a coma. Kim's family sued for permission to let her die in peace on the grounds that living on a respirator would not be her wishes. The core question was how to confirm that this was Kim's opinion while she was in coma. The Supreme Court said Kim's case satisfied four conditions to die with dignity:

that the patient must be examined by a third medical party to prove that he or she has no chance of recovery; that the patient should have expressed a strong desire to halt life-sustaining treatment; that the only means of death is to remove life-sustaining treatment; and that only medical doctors have the right to stop treatment.

This is the first recognized case in Korea of a person's right to die with dignity, and the case has led to heated debate. A discussion is ongoing within the medical society to reach consensus and to establish guidelines on the withdrawal of life-sustaining treatment. With this ruling, the number of similar cases of terminally ill patients is expected to grow. The importance of hospice/palliative care has now been brought to the public's attention.

⁓⁓

## History of Hospice Palliative Care

Hospice care in Korea began in 1965 at the Calvary Hospice in Gangneung City by the Sisters of the Little Company of Mary. The societal chaos and turmoil in a post-Korean War environment made it almost impossible to build new facilities for terminal patient care. Even during these trying times, the Calvary Hospice and the Australian Sisters of the Little Company of Mary persisted in providing care for terminally ill patients by following the mission provided by founder Mary Potter: "Tomorrow will be too late. Let us pray for those dying today."

The concept of hospice care was introduced to Korea in the 1970s, as the entire nation strived to work toward a better future. Hospice care expanded in the 1980s through the revolutionary care provided for the terminally ill by the Catholic University of Korea at Seoul St. Mary's Hospital. The first physician to introduce hospice care in South Korea was Gyung-Sik Lee, a hematology/oncology specialist who was an assistant professor in internal medicine at the Catholic University School of Medicine in 1981. Most of the academic focus in the early 1980s was on prolonging the lifespan of patients, and thus hospice care was not a widely discussed topic. However, Dr. Lee's experiences showed him that some patients would become terminally ill and pass away regardless of technological advances. Dr. Lee believed that the process of dying was as important as the process of living and surviving in many of his cancer patients.[5] Student hospice care began in September 1981 under the supervision of Catholic University medical and nursing students, and the concept of hospice care was further advanced and implemented through an oncology conference in June 1982 at St. Mary's Hospital. A department dedicated to hospice care centered on the nursing staff was established at St. Mary's Hospital, and began operation in March 1987. The first hospice units (10 total) were established at St. Mary's Hospital in October 1988. A program for home hospice care was also initiated in the oncology department of Severance Hospital in 1988, while another project on home hospice care began that same year in the nursing department of Ewha Women's University under the supervision of a resident nurse. Saint Columban Hospital opened its doors in 1989 by providing house calls that eventually evolved into family hospice care. Thereafter, hospice programs blossomed around the nation: the three hospice programs available in 1965–1980 grew to 17 in 1980–1990; 73 in 1990–2000; 125 in 2000–2004; and 130 in 2007.[6] Yun et al. reported the present condition of 64 different programs in 2002.[7]

The increase of hospice facilities led to the establishment of the Korean Hospice Association in 1991 and the Korean Catholic Hospice Association in 1992. These two associations have greatly influenced the expansion of hospice care in Korea, despite the religious undertones that were inextricably linked to their missions.

In 1995, So Woo Lee, a professor of the Seoul National University College of Nursing conducted a study, "The National Hospice Care Service Development in Korea,"[3] (outsourced by the Ministry for Health and Welfare), reporting on the status of terminal patients and their family caregivers. So Woo Lee then developed the Internet-based hospice information service system.[8] That same year (1995), The Catholic University of Korea's nursing school was selected as WHO's Collaborating Center for Hospice and Palliative Care, and the school began medical training for structured hospice and palliative care, focusing on nursing (http://hospice.catholic.ac.kr).

The researchers who participated in The National Hospice Care Service Development in Korea realized the need for establishing an academic society. Some of the researchers and the medical cadre of the Catholic University of Korea who were operating the hospice inpatient unit at the time joined forces to form an eight-member steering committee (Chair, Gyeong-Sik Lee and three nurses included). After three months of preparation, the Korean Society for Hospice and Palliative Care (KSHPC) was established in 1998 (www.hospicecare.co.kr). The purpose for the establishment of the KSHPC was to advance academics pertaining to hospice and palliative care in Korea; to increase the quality of life for terminal cancer patientsl to factor in the public health policies and medical regulations which would help them to lead a comfortable life; to interact with the international hospice and palliative care academic societies and associations; and to exchange information. Professor So Woo Lee, a nurse and one of the committee members, served as the second president of this academic society. In 1998, hospice and palliative care were unfamiliar to many doctors. In fact, there were many who held negative views about hospice. Thus, it is not surprising that nursing is the leading occupation among members of the KSHPC.

KSHPC hosted the hearing session on the hospice systemization in 1999 along with the Korean Catholic Hospice Association and Korea Hospice Association at the National Assembly Member Center. In 2002, it published "Guidance for the cancer patient pain management"' jointly with the Korean Cancer Study Group. In 2003, it organized a symposium on the "Korean Hospice and Palliative Care Systemization" jointly with the National Cancer Center, and submitted a draft hospice law to the Ministry for Health,

Welfare, and Family Affairs. The Korean society is trying hard to systemize hospice care. On March 2005, it supervised the Asia Pacific Hospice Conference (APHC) that is held every two years. Likewise, it is involved heavily in the interchange with foreign nations. Moreover, KSHPC published *The Korean Journal of Hospice and Palliative Care s* first edition, Volume 1 on December 1998—the year when the academic society was established. Until 2001, it had published the journal at least once a year, twice a year from 2002 to 2006, and quarterly since 2007, contributing to the academic development of the hospice and palliative care scholars, including the nurses.

However, nurses were very passionate about the organizations that define their inherent roles and that can help them increase their knowledge. Thus, the Korean Hospice Palliative Nurses Association (KHPNA) was established on August 29, 2003. Professor So Woo Lee of the Seoul National University, who was the Chair of the steering committee for the launch of the society, served as the first president of KHPNA. Presently, Professor Boon Han Kim of the Hanyang University is serving as the president. Due to the effort made by the KHPNA, nurses in the area of hospice and palliative care are now recognized as specialized nurses. In March 2004, graduate level training for nurses (APN) specializing in hospice and palliative care began. As of 2009, numerous nurses are active as the members of the KSHPC and KHPNA.

The establishment of academic organizations has served as a turning point in increasing interaction between Korean experts on hospice and palliative care with overseas institutions. APHC agreed to develop a hospice and palliative care model that is appropriate for our culture along with the people of the Asia Pacific region. The medium used is the academic conference that is hosted every two to three years in the Asia Pacific region. The sixth conference was held in 2005 in Seoul, Korea with the theme of Changing Society and Human Life with Hospice and Palliative Care. The sixth academic conference promoted the advancement of the hospice and palliative care system in Korea, and stimulated related academic researches. Moreover, it publicized the need to increase attention to terminal cancer patients' quality of life. This international trend will advance hospice and palliative care. In 2001, Asia Pacific Hospice Palliative Care Network (APHN) was established as an academic forum for the hospice and palliative care professionals of the Asia Pacific region and Hong Kong, Japan, Taiwan, Singapore, Indonesia, India, Thailand, Malaysia, Vietnam, Myanmar, Nepal, Pakistan, Sri Lanka, Australia, New Zealand, and Korea of the Asia Pacific region subscribed as member nations. After the establishment of the APHN, the network was in charge of the APHC. Professor Young Sun Hong was the figure who represented Korea ever since the academic society was established, and he eventually moved into the vice chair position. In 2007, Professor Young-Seon Hong was appointed as the President in Manila, and is serving for two years. In 2009, Hyun Sook Kim, a nurse, was recommended as a council member to represent Korea in the APHN council, which is made up primarily of medical doctors.

Systemization is continuing slowly compared to the academic advancement of hospice and palliative care. Several studies were done and evidence provided to support Korean standardization of a Hospice palliative care service by National Cancer Center.[9,10] Systemization at the government level involves creating and submitting guidelines on the standards and regulations pertaining to hospice and palliative care.

In March 2006, representatives of hospice-related organizations in the nation gathered to declare a day of global palliative care and presented a declaration on this occasion. The Korea declaration calls for the expansion of the government's support on the policy level, drafted based on the "Barcelona declaration on the hospice and palliative care" which was published in the Worldwide Global Summit for National Association of Hospice Palliative Care on December 9, 1995. It is used as a symbolic sign to encourage medical service targeting the terminal cancer patients from different parts of the world.[5]

Thanks to the constant effort of the academic society and National Cancer Center since 2003, the central government selects the institutions offering hospice service to the cancer patients who are at the final stage. Since 2009, support is provided to 34 sites. Moreover, the Ministry for Health, Welfare and Family Affairs (www.mw.go.kr) is recently recruiting institutions for a pilot to be conducted in eight hospice units starting in November 2009.

## Hospice Palliative Care Nursing Education

### Master Program; Advanced Practice Nurse(APN) in Hospice Palliative Care

The Ministry of Education and Human Resources Development is the government body responsible for the formation and implementation of educational policies. The government provides guidance on basic policy matters as well as financial assistance. The Ministry of Health, Welfare and Family affairs regulates the number of students to admit heath related fields (medicine, nursing, physical therapy, etc) in Korea. The Korean Accreditation Board of Nursing, founded in 2004, is the body responsible for the nursing education accreditation, APN education institution appointment and evaluation, national certification examination for APN, and the national licensing examination for nurses (www.Kabon.or.kr).

The name of specialized nurse was changed to advanced practice nurse (APN) by revised medical law on January, 2000. The recognized specialized areas are geriatric and home care nursing by 2003. The areas of APN have expanded from 4 areas to 10 areas in 2003 and to 13 areas in 2006. The APN program became the master program, and APN in hospice palliative/palliative care program started in March 2004.

As of 2008, 11 graduate nursing schools have been appointed as the APN in hospice/palliative care. Seventy-five students per each year are admitted to become APN's in hospice/palliative care. As of 2008, 176 out of 3,032 APN are specialized in hospice palliative care in Korea .

As for the curriculum for APN in hospice palliative care, they must complete at least 13 credits in the basic core curriculum, 10 credits in the classes in their major that address theories, and 10 credits in Practicum classes. All in all, they must complete at least 33 credits to be eligible to take the nationally administered board examination for APN. At least 220 hours of the basic core classes, at least 160 hours of the classes essential for their major, and at least 300 hours of the practical training in their major must be taken in order to be eligible to take the certification exam. And master thesis is not a requirement. Thus, this is handled by the individual schools. Detailed curriculum is shown in Table 77–1. The APN certification examination is operated by the Ministry for Health, Welfare and Family Affairs in a way that the Korean Nurses Association (KNA) can act as a proxy. National certification is granted to those who passed the first test (written test) and the second test (practical test).

As for the roles for APN in hospice palliative care, they are specified into nine duties and 46 tasks, and the classes on the theories and on the practical training and test on the practical training are formed according to the analysis of these roles. The role of APN in Korea is very similar to APN in USA except Korean APN doesn't have prescription privileges yet.

### Certified Program for Hospice Palliative Care Nurses

The Catholic University of Korea College of Nursing was authorized as Collaborating Centre for Hospice and Palliative Care from WHO on September 28, 1995. The following year, the "Research Institute for Hospice Palliative Care" was established within The Catholic University of Korea College of Nursing that is in charge of the hospice and where research and training are conducted, to plan for and to implement structured work. This research institute operates over 300 hours of education program for hospice and palliative care nurses since 1996. There are 588 graduates of this education program as of 2008 (http://hospice.catholic.ac.kr). Besides these institutions, short-term and ad hoc training programs (which range from one to six months) take place at nursing schools or hospice institutions.

Moreover, the need to supply specialists was raised in the academic community prior to the systemization of the hospice and palliative care. At The Korean National Cancer Center, a minimum of 60 hours training was suggested[9] in order for the nurses to work in the hospice and palliative care institutions. Based on this criterion, a pilot program for the hospice of terminal cancer patients was conducted during 2004 and 2005. As for the details on this pilot program, basic training program was developed for the MDs, nurses, social workers, clergies and volunteers who are working in hospice palliative care, and training was conducted touring the nation for two years. Moreover, the demands of the nurses who participated in this training were factored in to suggest 78-hour long training curriculum for nurses.[11]

**Table 77–1**
**Curriculum for APN in Hospice Palliative Care**

| Classification | Subject | Credit | Hour | Remarks |
|---|---|---|---|---|
| Core curriculum for APN in all areas | Nursing theory | 2 | 32 | |
| | Advanced nursing role | 2 | 32 | |
| | Pharmacology | 2 | 32 | |
| | Advanced physical examination & practice | 3 | 64 | |
| | Thesis research | 2 | 32 | |
| | Pathophysiology | 2 | 32 | |
| | **Subtotal** | **13** | **224** | |
| Theory education for APN in hospice palliative care only | Introduction to hospice palliative nursing | 2 | 32 | |
| | Pain & symptom management | 2 | 32 | |
| | Psychosocial spiritual nursing care | 2 | 32 | |
| | Bereavement, family care and counseling | 2 | 32 | |
| | Hospice management | 2 | 32 | |
| | **Subtotal** | **10** | **160** | |
| Practical training | Hospice palliative nursing practicum I-1 | 1 | 32 | Home hospice |
| | Hospice palliative nursing practicum II-1 | 1 | 32 | Bereaved family |
| | Hospice palliative nursing practicum III | 2 | 64 | Community health center |
| | Hospice palliative nursing practicum IV | 2 | 64 | Hospice unit |
| | Hospice palliative nursing practicum I-2 | 2 | 64 | Hospice unit |
| | Hospice palliative nursing practicum II-2 | 2 | 64 | Hospice unit |
| | **Subtotal** | **10** | **320** | |
| **Total** | | **33** | **704** | |

*Source:* Graduate School of Information in Clinical Nursing, Hanyang University Bulletin (2009). Hanyang University Press.

**Table 77–2**
**Professional Development Aims in Hospice Palliative Care from Government's Second Term 10-Yr Plan for Cancer Control**

| | Year 2006 | Year 2010 | Year 2015 |
|---|---|---|---|
| Train-the-trainer | 20 (2007) | 120 | 200 |
| Physician | Develop course | 130 | 260 |
| • Palliative medicine diploma certification | | | |
| Nurse | Develop course | 900 | 1,800 |
| • APN in hospice palliative care (100/year) | | | |
| Social worker | Develop course | 65 | 130 |
| Clergy | Develop course | 65 | 130 |
| Volunteer | Develop course | 10,000 | 20,000 |

*Source:* The Ministry for Health, Welfare and Family Affairs (2005). National Cancer Control.

While conducting these diverse educational programs, it was necessary to train the trainers who were to be responsible for the development of standard training program that use standardized training materials and who will be responsible for training in individual regions. To this end, the National Cancer Center with the backing of the government selected eight nurses, doctors and social workers to attend the Education on Palliative and End-of-life-care (EPEC) training (http://www.epec.net/EPEC/webpages/index.cfm) in 2007. They then developed a 60-hour long basic training program for all interdisciplinary team in hospice palliative care based on the EPEC project.[6]

The National Cancer Center has a further plan for development of an advanced level curriculum for each interdisciplinary team, and the first work is for the nurses (Table 77–2). In March 2009, a task force team (TFT) for developing curriculum

**Table 77–3**

**Frequency of Nursing Interventions for Hospice Clients According to the NIC System—Home Care Hospice, Hospice Unit, Home-Based Cancer Patient Hospice Through Public Health Center**

| Domain | Interventions (Frequency) | Home Care Hospice (%) | | Hospice Unit (%) | | Home-Based Cancer Patient Hospice Through Public Health Center | |
|---|---|---|---|---|---|---|---|
| Physiological basic | Activity & exercise | 0.13 | | 0 | | 5.65 | |
| | Elimination management | 4.79 | | 9.65 | | 1.51 | |
| | Immobility management | 0.76 | 12.23 | 2.97 | 41.02 | 0 | 15.33 |
| | Nutrition support | 1.56 | | 7.75 | | 3.64 | |
| | Physical comfort promotion | 2.82 | | 6.79 | | 0 | |
| | Self-care facilitation | 2.19 | | 13.86 | | 4.53 | |
| Physiological Complex | Electrolyte & acid–base management | 0.84 | | 0.95 | | 4.8 | |
| | Drug management | 11.8 | | 12.09 | | 7.22 | |
| | Neurological management | 5.92 | 40.13 | 2.23 | 37.24 | 0 | 18.27 |
| | Respiratory management | 1.47 | | 5.10 | | 4.93 | |
| | Skin/wound management | 5.84 | | 5.10 | | 1.32 | |
| | Tissue perfusion management | 14.2 | | 11.77 | | 0 | |
| Behavioral | Coping assistance | 5.55 | 11.13 | 0.96 | 6.39 | 0 | 14.27 |
| | Patient education | 5.57 | | 5.43 | | 14.27 | |
| Safety | Risk management | 28.4 | 28.40 | 3.21 | 3.21 | 0 | 0 |
| Family | Lifespan care | 2.94 | 2.94 | 1.62 | 1.62 | 0.68 | 0.68 |
| Health system | Health system mediation | 0.42 | | 2.23 | | 23.75 | |
| | Health system management | 1.09 | 4.62 | 4.46 | 10.52 | 2.96 | 44.45 |
| | Information management | 3.20 | | 3.83 | | 17.74 | |
| Spiritual care | | | | | | 6.66 | |
| Dying patient care | | | | | | 0.34 | |
| Total | | 100 | | 100 | | 100 | |

*Source*: Ro et al., reference 12; Yong, et al., reference 13; Kim, reference 14.

for certified generalist hospice palliative care nurses was established and is working to develop the curriculum collaborating with KHPNA. KHPNA is the body to develop guidelines for certified generalist hospice palliative care nurses (Table 77–3). The education and training subcommittee of National Cancer Center, Cancer Control Institute is the body to develop the curriculum. TFT has agreed that the hours of education for the certified generalist hospice palliative care nurses will be over 130 hours (98 hours in theory and 32 hours in practice): palliative nursing care (6 hours), understanding life and death (4 hours), pain and symptom management (23 hours), psychosocial care (7 hours), spiritual care (6 hours), complementary intervention (8 hours), communication (8 hours), final hours and bereavement (9 hours), hospice management (11 hours), end of life care for special population (10 hours), and practicum (32 hours). The developing direction of this curriculum is to provide web based training. The materials of End-of-Life Nursing Education Consortium (ELNEC) international training program (http://www.aacn.nche.edu/elnec/) will be used and adopted to develop the contents of this curriculum with permission by ELNEC project. By the end of this year, the content of this curriculum will be developed, and the pilot course

will be operated in 2010, and the certified hospice palliative nurse education program will be operated in 2011.

### The End-of-Life Nursing Education Consortium (ELNEC) Core Train-the-Trainer Program

An ELNEC core train-the trainer program was held from August 20th to 21st in Seoul by City of Hope National Medical Center (COH), the American Association of Colleges of Nursing (AACN) and ELNEC Project-Korea collaborating with KHPNA. The ELNEC Project is a national end-of–life education program administered by COH and AACN designed to enhance palliative care in nursing. The ELNEC Project-Korea team consists of four nurses who were trained as ELNEC trainer in USA and two nurses who are key board members of KHPNA. The faculties of the courses were ELNEC principal investigator Dr. Betty Ferrell, ELNEC consultant Dr. Judith Paice, and four Korean nurses who were trained in the USA. One hundred seventy-eight nurses and other interdisciplinary team members attended the course, and 145 nurses, who represented all provinces of South Korea, were certified as ELNEC trainers.

## Hospice/Palliative Care Setting

As of 2007, there were 113 hospice palliative care institutions in Korea including 21 home hospice institutions, 19 hospice units, 19 mixed types, 12 free standing hospice institutions and 42 other type institutions. Hospice team members include MDs, nurses, social workers, clergies, volunteers, pharmacists, nutritionists, physical therapists, art therapists, music therapists and speech therapists. There were 43 hospice institutions with beds for hospitalization. In Korea, the institutions that provide hospice palliative care can be divided into three major groups: home hospice palliative care, inpatient hospice palliative care of hospitals or free standing hospice institutions, and home-based cancer patient hospice through regional public health centers.

## Systematization of Hospice Palliative Care

### The Policy Development of Hospice Palliative Care

Compared to the advancement in education and research, systemization is progressing slowly in Korea. Systemization of the Korean government's hospice palliative care has been conducted only for the patients suffering from cancer, considered the number one cause of death, and their family members. In response to the growing cancer burden at the government level, the Cancer Control Division was built within the Bureau of Health Promotion, the Ministry of Health & Welfare in 2000. Also, the National Cancer Center was founded in March 2000 as a government-funded institution devoted to research, patient care, education & training in cancer. The Cancer Control Act, another important legal framework for controlling cancer in Korea, was legislated in 2003. This law authorizes the Health & Welfare Minister to formulate and implement cancer control programs including supportive palliative care and promote international collaboration as well. In early 2006, the comprehensive second-term cancer control plan for the next ten years (2006–2015) was forged to strengthen the cancer control efforts at the government level. According to the government's second term 10 year-long plan to conquer cancer, it plans to secure 2,500 beds until 2015—thereby providing hospice palliative care to 40,000 terminal cancer patients (about 50% of the target population).

## Future of Hospice Care

Since the concept of hospice was introduced to Korea 40 years ago, it has not yet consolidated its position firmly within Korean society. Obstacles include non-standardization of hospice palliative care, lack of structured training for palliative care, operation of this system by religious organizations as not-for-profit initiatives, non-vitalization of the home hospice, non-structured operation of the hospice palliative care provided mostly by hospitals and from the respect of voluntarism based on religious principle, lack of experts, lack of awareness and negative perception of the hospice by the general public, and lack of financial support and medical subsidy.[15]

A system of financial support should be established and systemized as a first measure. Medical charges for hospice from health insurance will be implemented in the form of a pilot starting from November 2009 and should be set at an appropriate level. This medical charge should be applied not only to patients who are in palliative care while hospitalized, but also to the home hospice. Second, it is necessary to vitalize the home hospice, and it is necessary to turn around the current focus on the palliative care based on hospitalization to a home hospice-centered policy. Moreover, a service delivery system needs to be developed so that hospice and palliative care while hospitalized and home hospice can be offered as a continuum. In Korea, people prefer to benefit from hospice palliative care while at home, which in turn increases satisfaction level. People prefer to spend their final hours at home due to strong feelings of affinity with family members. Third, standardization of training and operation of advanced training program are required not only for nurses but for people from all types of professions who participate in the interdisciplinary team. According to the Government Cancer control action plan, standardization will take place under the supervision of the National Cancer Center. However, the National Cancer Center needs to develop their curriculum by conferring with the academic organizations of each specialized field as the nurses confer with the KHPNA. Fourth, hospice and palliative care that is currently targeting only the terminal cancer patients and their family members needs to be rolled out to the non cancer terminal patients as well. Moreover, it is necessary to provide service to special groups such as pediatric or geriatric palliative care. Fifth, hospice and palliative care should be provided under special circumstances such as for patients dying in the emergency room due to acute illness or accident or at the intensive care unit, as well as their family members.

Because death is an unavoidable part of life, it is necessary to provide hospice palliative care to anyone in need, from any place.

REFERENCES

1. Yun YH, Rhee YS, Nam SY, et al. Public attitudes toward dying with dignity and hospice palliative care. Korean J Hosp Palliat Care 2004;7(1):17–28.
2. Yun YH. Issues and current status of the hospice palliative institutionalization. Paper presented at the 2005 National Cancer Center Symposium on the direction of policymaking for hospice palliative care in Korea, 2005.
3. Lee SW, Lee EO, Ahn HS, et al. The national hospice care service development in Korea. Korean Nurse 1997;36(3):49–69.

4. Rhee YS, Yun YH, Park S, et al. Depression in family caregivers of cancer patients: The feeling of burden as a predictor of depression. J Clin Oncol 2008;26(36):5890–5895.

5. Korean Society for Hospice & Palliative Care. History of Korean Society of Hospice & Palliative Care for 10 Years. Seoul: Korean Society for Hospice & Palliative Care, 2008.

6. National Cancer Center. Basic Level Standard Curriculum for the Hospice Palliative Interdisciplinary Team. Ilsan: National Cancer Center, 2009.

7. Yun YH, Choi ES, Lee IJ, et al. Survey on quality of hospice palliative care programs in Korea. Korean J Hosp Palliat Care 2002;5(1):31–42.

8. Lee SW, Lee EO, Park HA, et al. Development of internet based hospice information service system. J Korean Soc Med Inform 1999;5(1):109–118.

9. National Cancer Center. Korean Hospice Palliative Care Standards and Regulations. Ilsan: National Cancer Center, 2003.

10. Kim SY, Yun YH, Park SM, et al. Development of the Service Model for Hospice Palliative Care in Terminal Cancer Care. Policy research study of cancer control, the Ministry of Health, Welfare & Family affair, 2004.

11. Choi ES, Yoo YS, Kim HS, Lee SW. Curriculum development for hospice and palliative care nurses. Korean J Hosp Palliat Care 2006;9(2):77–85.

12. Ro YJ, Han SS, Yonh JS, Sonh MS, Hong JU. A Comparison of Nursing I interventions with Terminal Cancer Patients in a Hospice Unit and General Units. J Korean Acad Soc Adult Nurs 2002;14(2):543–553.

13. Yong JS, Ro YJ, Han SS, Kim MJ. A comparison between home care nursing interventions for hospice and general patients. Korean Acad Nurs J 2002;31(5):897–911.

14. Kim BH. 2009'Evaluation Report of Home Hospice Palliative Service in Seongnam City Hospice Palliative Center (first half), 2009. Unpublished.

15. Hong YS, Yeum CH, Lee KS. The past & present of hospice palliative in korea. Korean J Hosp Palliat Care 2000;3(2): 185–189.

# X
# Conclusion

# 78

## A Good Death

*Betty R. Ferrell*

The chapters of this textbook span the broad scope of the practice of nurses in providing palliative care across populations and settings. Palliative nursing care is simple in its mission to provide comfort while also a complex and masterful practice of deliberate intention. Palliative care nurses recognize the very limited opportunity to orchestrate meaningful and sacred days in the last chapter of a life. Ultimately, all of the preceding pages of this book, diverse in their content, speak to the ultimate goal of palliative care nurses of *insuring a good death.*

### A Good Death Honors the Life of the Person Facing Serious Illness and Death

John Rolling was an 89-year-old man who had spent a lifetime avoiding the healthcare system. As a child of "dirt farmers" in Texas born in 1916, his childhood came to an abrupt end when at age 7 he and his 9-year-old brother became the breadwinners for their mother and five sisters on the death of his father from what he described as a "lung infection." His farm labor continued until he was drafted in World War II and served 4 years in the Army. He returned home, where he began a simple life as a construction worker, husband, and father. As a man with only a second grade education, his life was rich in wisdom and dedication to his family. His basic life values were best manifested when, after 55 years of marriage, he became caregiver to his wife, who was dying of lung cancer. For 7 months, his days were spent with the most detailed and deliberate care of feeding, lifting, toileting, and bathing his wife in a way that would put an experienced nurse to shame. All of this was done, without ever a complaint, because "it's what a man does."

John sought medical care only three times in his life—for a medical exam on entering the Army, a broken bone from a construction injury, and a "dizzy spell" at age 70 when his family panicked and took him to the local hospital. Seven years after his wife's death, his own death came not from an abrupt diagnosis of cancer, acute stroke, or heart failure but in a subtle trajectory perhaps parallel to his own gentle life, a calm slope that finally lead to his life's end.

Over a matter of days, a mild respiratory infection lead to functional decline and just enough fever, dehydration, and insult to an aged man. This stable, elderly person became a seriously ill patient with onset of severe infection, sepsis, and the cascade of medical events to follow that are not easily reversed. Soon, this man who avoided anything technological or heroic became a hospitalized patient with the usual barrage of scans, tubes, consultants, antibiotics, and a medical solution to the evolving multitude of symptoms. Over 2 weeks the man whose idea of a good day was watching "Gunsmoke" reruns and spending time in the rose garden with his dog became the victim of a healthcare machine determined to avoid death, ready with a solution to every bodily failure.

A family meeting was convened, and the lure of medicines, an attractive offer of long-term parenteral antibiotics, enteral nutrition, and transfer to a skilled care facility were instead overruled by a decision to stop the medical machine and return home with hospice care for this man's last days of life with care that would honor the 89 years he had lived.

### A Good Death Is Made Possible Through Expert Attention to Symptoms and Ultimate Care of the Physical Body

Although gradual in one sense, in yet another it is alarming how an independent adult can transcend to total bodily dependence. Upon return to home hospice, the man who only 2 weeks earlier had dutifully cared for himself became dependent on every aspect of care. The transformation to adult diapers, blue pads, spoon-feeding, and turning quickly transformed a man who had cared for others since age 7 years to total dependence. A good death through palliative care shifts the goals of care to allow that transcendence in all its physical and emotional meaning to a sacred time of family care.

A good death is not a perfect, problem-free existence but, rather, death that often includes a physical decline and cessation of bodily function fraught with a multitude of symptoms. John's life of dignity and health became a daily evolution complete with both predictable and unexpected problems, including delirium, agitation, diarrhea, and pain. It was the expert knowledge of a palliative care nurse, Judy, who intervened with skillful assessment to suggest medications that resolved the delirium and myoclonus, and in so doing she helped him avoid a death that could have left memories of agitated jerking in favor of a peaceful, dignified death. Beyond the pharmacological expertise, she offered

compassionate presence to an exhausted daughter at a time when these uncontrolled symptoms were the fatal blow to this ultimate loss. Palliative care nurses respond to physical needs and suffering and support family caregivers in what is often the most difficult work of their lives.

### A Good Death Is Achieved When Palliative Care Responds to the Depths of Emotional Suffering

Serious illness steals away the physical attributes of life and also the elements of a meaningful life and psychological integrity. While tending to the physical body and relief of symptoms, palliative care nurses also respond to the emotions associated with declining health and approaching death.

John was a man of few words but experienced a life long in physical labor. His life from childhood to adulthood meant doing—from farming to construction work to taking on household tasks as his wife's health declined, his being as a protector and provider was in action. But his actions were unlike many in the hectic world where getting things done as quickly as possible is the aim. His "doing" was full of his "being," infused with care and limitless commitment. A prime example occurred when in the last weeks of his wife's life his daughter, 40 years his junior, became exhausted by the physical care whereas he became energized by the opportunity to provide the physical care that might relieve his wife's suffering.

When his daughter's attempts at feeding her mother with "store-bought" pudding and applesauce failed to entice her rapidly declining appetite in end-stage lung cancer, John responded by preparing a roast complete with vegetables, slow-cooked to perfection. Although far from being an expert chef (his culinary skills were more inclined to a can of Campbell's soup), on this day he prepared with the attention of a gourmet chef this roast dinner and then proceeded to blenderize to perfection the just right combination of juice, meat, and vegetables to create the finest puree ever witnessed! In this act, both were nourished by the rare gifts of genuinely serving another and receiving a gift of love.

Now, as the roles reversed and John was the recipient of hospice care, an apparent challenge was to honor a life of purpose and "doing" rather than succumb to the threats of serious illness that often prohibit meaningful days. Palliative care is not passive waiting for death amidst depression, fear, or suffering. It is active care that preserves meaningful life, although this often requires a significant reevaluation of what constitutes purposeful life.

Upon his return home for hospice care, John's daughter awoke on his first morning home and cut a bouquet of roses and took them to his room as proof that they indeed had escaped from the hospital and were at home. John, while in a markedly altered cognitive state induced by his failing body and medications, responded initially with a broad simile, but then a look of panic as he realized that he was no longer able to tend the roses. The look of panic was short-lived, followed by a contemplative look and soon after by a look of absolute peace. His gentle voice then explained the emotions as he explained that he felt so bad that he could no longer do "his jobs," but he was thinking that because all he could do was sit in a chair, his "job" would be to "pray for everyone."

*Palliative Care Has as its Goal a Good Death, Made Possible When Final Days Are Not Filled With Failure, Abandonment, and Desperation, but, Rather, Are a Time of Meaning, Service, Purpose, and the Legacy of a Life Well-Lived*

*A good death* is a sacred act. Regardless of the presence or absence of religious affiliation, patients and families facing death have the opportunity to experience the essence of life. When patients and families are supported and symptoms are relieved, when a sense of calm and control are restored, final days may become the most meaningful days of even a full and long life.

On admission to hospice, John's nurse assessed his needs—not only as a patient, but as a person, acknowledging his life history and values and not only his problems, but the strengths that had sustained him through life. A few days later, a hospice chaplain called, and although the daughter's immediate thought was that this must be an offer of formal ritual or prayer, instead the enthusiastic voice of the chaplain said "Your father's nurse tells me he was a Southern Baptist—I was thinking maybe I could come visit with my guitar and play some old hymns and gospel songs. Would that be OK?"

Hours later, the chaplain arrived. He accompanied the daughter upstairs where John sat propped up with pillows but in an ever-advancing stage of weakness, confusion, and limited communication. The chaplain braced his guitar and began to play selections clearly influenced by his intimate understanding of the man before him, a man he just met.

The daughter sat on the floor next to her father, intending to insure he was able to sit upright and listen, to do yet another task of caregiving. Within moments, the room was transposed from sick room to sacred space.

The chaplain strummed "Amazing Grace" and both daughter and father recalled the momentous times of life when these words were sung. They heard together "His Eyes Are on the Sparrow" and sensed peace and then "The Old Rugged Cross" as the daughter witnessed her father's physical being infused with a state of grace that was almost incomprehensible. Most of all, it was in this moment that patient and caregiver were moved to a place of being father and daughter—a place where the trauma of the previous weeks of hospitalization was replaced by a comforting "coming home" and recognition of the circle of life and the naturalness of a life ending. It was the kind of healing that hospice provides, removed from the concept of curing often seen as the only goal of care. These are the moments hard to explain to a congressional hearing arguing details of hospice reimbursement, yet known by any family who has received such care as priceless and essential in any society that claims to provide humane care.

*Palliative Care Nurses Work Closely With Their Interdisciplinary Colleagues So That the Gifts of Nursing, Medicine, Social Work, Nursing Assistant, and Chaplain Woven Together Provide a Quilt of Comfort*

Although the legacy of 21st century healthcare is a population that equates death with pain, isolation, critical care units, and failure, the work of palliative care is now creating a legacy where fathers' and daughters' stories encompass comfort, dignity, meaning, and the sacredness of dying.

This *Oxford Textbook of Palliative Nursing* is both a blueprint of the technical expertise of our field and a vision of the art of our profession. The story of John—my father—is the story of *a good death*.

APPENDIX  *Rose Virani and Licet Garcia*

# Palliative Care Resource List

## Bibliographies/References/Texts

American Journal of Nursing, Palliative Nursing Series
   http://www.AJNonline.com
City of Hope Pain/Palliative Care Resource Center
   http://prc.coh.org
End-of-Life Nursing Education Consortium (ELNEC)
   http://www.aacn.nche.edu/ELNEC/ELNECSeries.htm
Journal of the American College of Surgeons, Palliative Care
   in Surgery Series
   http://www.facs.org/cqi/jacsarticles.html
Mary Ann Liebert, Inc.—Unipac Series
   http://www.liebertpub.com/publication.aspx?pub_id=119
   - *UNIPAC One:* The Hospice/Palliative Medicine Approach to
     End-of-Life Care
   - *UNIPAC Two:* Alleviating Psychological and Spiritual Pain
     in the Terminally Ill
   - *UNIPAC Three:* Assessment and Treatment of Pain in the
     Terminally Ill
   - *UNIPAC Four:* Management of Selected Non-pain
     Symptoms in the Terminally Ill
   - *UNIPAC Five:* Caring for the Terminally Ill-Communication
     and the Physician's Role on the Interdisciplinary Team
   - *UNIPAC Six:* Ethical and Legal Decision Making When
     Caring for the Terminally Ill
   - *UNIPAC Seven:* The Hospice/Palliative Medicine Approach
     to Caring for Patients with HIV/AIDS
   - *UNIPAC Eight:* The Hospice/Palliative Medicine Approach
     to Caring for Pediatric Patients
Oxford University Press
   http://www.oup-usa.com
Shaare Zedek Cancer Pain and Palliative Care Reference Database
   http://www.chernydatabase.org

## Guidelines

Agency for Healthcare Research and Quality (AHRQ) Pain
   Guidelines (formerly Agency for Health Care Policy and
   Research [AHCPR])
   http://www.ahrq.gov/clinic/cpgsix.htm

National Comprehensive Cancer Network (NCCN)—palliative
   care clinical practice guidelines
   http://www.nccn.org/professionals/physician_gls/PDF/
   palliative.pdf
National Consensus Project for Quality Palliative Care
   http://www.nationalconsensusproject.org
World Health Organization (WHO)
   http://www.who.int/medicines/areas/quality_safety/Scoping_
   WHOGuide_malignant_pain_adults.pdf

## Journals/Newsletters

American Journal of Hospice & Palliative Care
   http://www.pnpco.com
Americans for Better Care of the Dying Exchange Newsletter
   http://www.abcd-caring.org/newslettermain.htm
Cancer Care News Newsletter
   http://www.cancercare.org
The European Journal of Palliative Care
   http://www.ejpc.eu.com
International Association for Hospice and Palliative Care
   http://www.hospicecare.com
International Journal of Palliative Nursing
   http://www.markallengroup.com/healthcare
Journal of Hospice and Palliative Nursing
   http://www.jhpn.com
Journal of Pain and Palliative Care Pharmacotherapy
   http://www.haworthpress.com
Journal of Pain and Symptom Management
   http://www.elsevier.com
Journal of Palliative Care
   http://www.ircm.qc.ca/bioethique/english
Journal of Palliative Medicine
   http://www.liebertpub.com
Journal of Psychosocial Oncology
   http://www.haworthpress.com
Journal of Supportive Oncology
   http://www.supportiveoncology.net
National Comprehensive Cancer Network (NCCN)
   http://www.nccn.org

National Hospice and Palliative Care Organization (NHPCO)
Newsline
http://www.nhpco.org

National Quality Forum (NQF) Framework and Preferred
Practices for Palliative and Hospice Care:
http://www.qualityforum.org/publications/reports/
palliative.asp

Oncology Nursing Form (ONF)
http://www.ons.org

Pain: Clinical Updates International Association for the Study
of Pain
http://www.iasp-pain.org

Palliative & Supportive Care
http://journals.cambridge.org

Palliative Medicine
http://pmj.sagepub.com/

Psycho-Oncology
http://www.wiley.com

Progress in Palliative Care
http://www.leeds.ac.uk/lmi

Southern California Cancer Pain Initiative (SCCPI) Newsletter
http://sccpi.coh.org

Supportive Care in Cancer
http://www.springerlink.com

## Organizations and Websites (Patient, Professional, and State Pain Initiatives)

AARP (American Association of Retired Persons)
http://www.aarp.org/life/endoflife

Aging With Dignity
http://www.agingwithdignity.org

Alliance of State Pain Initiatives
http://aspi.wisc.edu/

American Academy of Hospice and Palliative Medicine (AAHPM)
http://www.aahpm.org

American Academy of Pain Medicine (AAPM)
http://www.painmed.org

American Academy of Pediatrics (AAP)
http://www.aap.org

American Association for Therapeutic Humor
http://www.aath.org

American Board of Hospice & Palliative Medicine
http://www.abhpm.org

American Cancer Society (ACS)
http://www.cancer.org

American Geriatrics Society (AGS)
http://www.americangeriatrics.org

American Holistic Nurses Association
http://www.ahna.org

American Hospice Foundation
http://www.americanhospice.org

American Medical Association (AMA)
http://www.ama-assn.org

American Nurses Association (ANA)
http://nursingworld.org

American Pain Foundation
http://www.painfoundation.org

American Pain Society (APS)
http://www.ampainsoc.org

American Society for Bioethics and Humanities
http://www.asbh.org

American Society of Clinical Oncology (ASCO)
http://www.asco.org

American Society of Law, Medicine and Ethics
http://www.aslme.org

American Society for Pain Management Nursing (ASPMN)
http://www.aspmn.org

Americans for Better Care of the Dying (ABCD)
http://www.abcd-caring.org

Approaching Death: Improving Care at the End of Life
http://www.nap.edu/catalog.php?record_id=5801

Association for Death Education and Counseling (ADEC)
http://www.adec.org

Association of Oncology Social Work (AOSW)
http://www.aosw.org

Association of Pediatric Oncology Nurses (APON)
http://www.apon.org

Before I Die: Medical Care and Personal Choices
http://www.thirteen.org/bid

Beth Israel Medical Center, Department of Pain Medicine and
Palliative Care
http://stoppain.org

Candlelighters Childhood Cancer Foundation
http://www.candlelighters.org

Caregiver Network
http://www.ltcplanningnetwork.com

Caregiver Regional Resources
http://www.caregiver911.com

Catholic Health Association of the United States
http://www.chausa.org

Center to Advance Palliative Care
http://www.capc.org

Center for Applied Ethics and Professional Practice (CAEPP)
http://caepp.edc.org

Center for Palliative Care (Harvard Medical School)
http://www.hms.harvard.edu/cdi/pallcare

Center for Palliative Care Studies (formally known as Center to
Improve Care of the Dying)
http://medicaring.org

Center for Practical Bioethics
http://www.midbio.org

Children's Hospice International (CHI)
http://www.chionline.org

Children's Project on Palliative/Hospice Services (CHIPPS)
http://www.nhpco.org

City of Hope Pain/Palliative Care Resource Center (COHPPRC)
http://prc.coh.org

Compassion in Dying Federation
http://www.compassionandchoices.org

The Compassionate Friends, Inc. (TCF)
http://www.compassionatefriends.org

Department of Health and Human Services, Healthfinder
http://www.healthfinder.gov

Dying Well: Defining Wellness Through the End of Life
(Missoula Demonstration Project)
http://www.dyingwell.org

Edmonton Regional Palliative Care Program
http://www.palliative.org

Education for Physicians on End-of-Life Care Project (EPEC)
http://epec.net/EPEC/webpages/index.cfm

The End of Life: Exploring Death in America
    http://www.npr.org/programs/death
End-of-Life Care for Children
    http://www.childendoflifecare.org
End-of-Life Nursing Education Consortium (ELNEC)
    http://www.aacn.nche.edu/ELNEC
End-of-Life Physician Education Resource Center (EPERC)
    http://www.eperc.mcw.edu
European Association for Palliative Care (EAPC)
    http://www.eapcnet.org
FACCT: Foundation for Accountability Family Caregiver Alliance
    (Markle Foundation)
    http://www.markle.org/resources/facct/index.php
Family Caregiver Alliance
    http://www.caregiver.org
Grief.Net
    http://www.griefnet.org
Growth House, Inc.
    http://www.growthhouse.org
GROWW: Grief Recovery Online for All Bereaved
    http://www.groww.org
Gundersen Lutheran
    http://www.respectingchoices.org
Hospice Association of America
    http://www.nahc.org/haa/
Hospice Foundation of America
    http://www.hospicefoundation.org
Hospice Net
    http://hospicenet.org
Hospice and Palliative Nurses Association (HPNA)
    http://www.hpna.org
Hospice Resources.Net
    http://www.hospiceresources.net
International Association for the Study of Pain (IASP)
    http://www.iasp-pain.org/
The International Work Group on Death, Dying and Bereavement
    http://www.iwgddb.org
Life's End Institute (Missoula Demonstration Project)
    http://www.missoulademonstration.org
Mayday Pain Project
    http://www.painandhealth.org
Medical College of Wisconsin, Center for the Study of Bioethics
    http://www.mcw.edu/bioethics
Medical College of Wisconsin Palliative Care Center
    http://www.mcw.edu/pallmed
National Association for Home Care (NAHC)
    http://www.nahc.org
National Cancer Institute (NCI)
    http://www.cancer.gov
National Consensus Project (NCP)
    http://www.nationalconsensusproject.org
National Hospice and Palliative Care Organization (NHPCO)
    http://www.nhpco.org
The National Institute of Aging
    http://www.nia.nih.gov
National Institute of Health
    http://www.nih.gov
National Prison Hospice Association
    http://www.npha.org
National Public Radio (NPR)
    http://www.npr.org

Not Dead Yet
    http://www.notdeadyet.org
On Our Own Terms
    http://www.pbs.org/wnet/onourownterms
Oncology Nursing Society (ONS)
    http://www.ons.org
Open Society Institute
    http://www.soros.org
Oregon Health Sciences University, Center for Ethics in
    Health Care
    http://www.ohsu.edu/ethics
Patient Education Institute
    http://www.patient-education.com
Pediatric Pain
    http://pediatricpain.ca
Promoting Excellence in End-of-Life Care
    http://www.promotingexcellence.org
The Robert Wood Johnson Foundation (RWJF)
    http://www.rwjf.org
Southern California Cancer Pain Initiative (SCCPI)
    http://sccpi.coh.org/
Supportive Care of the Dying
    http://www.supportivecarecoalition.org
University of Wisconsin Pain and Policy Studies Group
    http://www.painpolicy.wisc.edu
Wisconsin Cancer Pain Initiative
    http://aspi.wisc.edu/wpi

## Position Statements

American Nurses Association (ANA)
    http://nursingworld.org
    • Active Euthanasia
    • Assisted Suicide
    • Foregoing Nutrition and Hydration
    • Nursing and the Patient Self-Determination Acts
    • Nursing Care and Do-Not-Resuscitate (DNR) Decisions
    • Pain Management and Control of Distressing Symptoms in
      Dying Patients
American Nursing Leaders
    http://www.dyingwell.com/downloads/apnpos.pdf
    • Advanced Practice Nurses Role in Palliative Care
American Society of Pain Management Nurses (ASPMN)
    http://www.aspmn.org
    • Assisted Suicide
    • Pain Management at the End of Life
    • Authorized and Unauthorized ("PCA by Proxy") Dosing of
      Analgesic Infusion Pumps
    • Pain Assesment in the Non-verbal Patient
    • Balancing Pain Relief and Abuse
    • Pain Management in Patients with Addictive Disease
    • Use of Placebos in Pain Management
    • Joint Statement:The Use of As Needed Range Orders for
      Opioid Analgesics in the Management of Acute Pain
    • Promoting Pain Relief and Preventing Abuse of Pain
      Medications: A Critical Balancing Act
Hospice and Palliative Nurses Association (HPNA):
    http://www.hpna.org
    • Complementary Therapies in Palliative Care Nursing
      Practice

- Evidence-Based Practice
- Legalization of Assisted Suicide
- Pain Management
- Palliative Sedation
- Role of Palliative Care Nursing in Organ and Tissue Donation
- Shortage of Registered Nurses
- Spiritual Care
- The Ethics of Opiate Use within Palliative Care
- Value of Advanced Practice Nurse in Palliative Care
- Value of licensed Practical/Vocational Nurse in Palliative Care
- Value of the Nursing Assistant in End-of-Life Care
- Value of Nursing Certification
- Value of the Professional Nurse in End-of-Life Care
- Withholding and/or Withdrawing Life Sustaining Therapies

Oncology Nursing Society (ONS):
http://www.ons.org
- Cancer Pain Management
- End of Life Care
- The Impact of the National Nursing Shortage on Quality Cancer Care
- The Nurse's Responsibility to the Patient Requesting Assisted Suicide
- ONS and Association of Oncology Social Work Joint Position on End-of-Life Care
- Use of Complementary and Alternative Therapies in Cancer Care

## Reports

Center for Palliative Care Studies
- Living Well at the End of Life: Adapting Health Care to Serious Chronic Illness in Old Age—http://medicaring.org/whitepaper

Institute of Medicine
- Approaching Death: Improving Care at the End of Life— http://www.iom.edu/report.asp?id=12687
- Improving Palliative Care for Cancer—http://www.iom.edu/?id=12684&redirect=0
- When Children Die: Improving Palliative and End-of-Life for Children and their Families—http://www .iom.edu/report.asp?id=4483

National Hospice and Palliative Care Organization (Children's International Project on Palliative/Hospice Services-ChIPPS)
- A Call for Change: Recommendations to Improve the Care of Children Living with Life-Threatening Illness— http://www.nhpco.org/files/public/ChIPPSCallforChange.pdf

Promoting Excellence in End-of-Life Care
- Advanced Practice Nursing: Pioneering Practices in Palliative Care— http://www.promotingexcellence.org/apn

Robert Wood Johnson Foundation Funded Reports
- Disparities at the End of Life— http://www.rwjf.org/pr/product.jsp?id=20792

- Means to a Better End— http://www.rwjf.org/files/publications/other/meansbetterend.pdf
- Precepts of Palliative Care— http://www.sgna.org/resources/statements/statement10b.html
- Precepts of Palliative Care for Children, Adolescents and Their Families— http://www.apon.org/files/public/last_acts_precepts.pdf

## Research Instruments

Brown University Center Toolkit of Instruments To Measure End-of-Life Care (TIME)
http://www.chcr.brown.edu/pcoc/toolkit.htm
Center to Improve Care of the Dying/Toolkit of Instruments to Measure End of Life
http://www.gwu.edu/~cicd/toolkit/toolkit.htm
City of Hope Pain/Palliative Care Resource Center
http://prc.coh.org (refer to Research Instruments section)
Edmonton Assessment Tools
http://www.palliative.org/PC/ClinicalInfo/AssessmentTools/AssessmentToolsIDX.html
Patient-Reported Outcome and Quality-of-Life Instruments Database
http://www.proqolid.org
Promoting Excellence in End-of-Life Care
http://www.promotingexcellence.org/i4a/pages/index.cfm?pageid=3276
State of the Art Review of Tools for Assessment of Pain in Nonverbal Older Adults
http://prc.coh.org (refer to Pain in the Elderly section)
Supportive Care of the Dying
http://www.careofdying.org

## Videos

Applied Vision
http://www.appliedv.com/catalog.htm
Aquarius Productions, Inc.
http://www.aquariusproductions.com
City of Hope Pain/Palliative Care Resource Center
http://prc.coh.org (refer to End-of-Life/Palliative Care section for extensive video listings)
Fanlight Productions
http://www.fanlight.com
Initiative for Pediatric Palliative Care (IPPC)
http://www.ippcweb.org/video.asp
PBS Home Video
http://www.pbs.org
Lippincott Williams & Wilkins Electronic Media Division
http://www.lww.com/browsemediaspec/Video/0,0,0,00.html
University of Michigan (Evan Mayday)
http://www.med.umich.edu/nursing/EndOfLife/mayday.htm

# Index